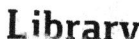
MEDICAL
SCIENCES

Dedication

I would like to dedicate this book to all medical students, past and future, and to all future doctors. You have to know the science in order to understand the practice of medicine.

Jeannette Naish

Commissioning Editor: **Ellen Green, Pauline Graham**
Development Editor: **Hannah Kenner, Carole McMurray**
Project Manager: **Christine Johnston**
Designer: **Sarah Russell, Stewart Larking**
Illustration Manager: **Bruce Hogarth**
Illustrators: **Robert Britton, Antbits**

MEDICAL SCIENCES

EDITED BY

JEANNETTE NAISH
MBBS MSC FRCGP

Clinical Senior Lecturer, Institute of Health Science Education, Barts and The London School of Medicine and Dentistry, London, UK; Wolfson Institute for Preventive Medicine, London, UK

PATRICIA REVEST
BA PHD

Non-clinical Senior Lecturer, Institute of Health Science Education, Barts and The London School of Medicine and Dentistry, London, UK

DENISE SYNDERCOMBE COURT
C BIOL MIBIOL CSCI FIBMS DMEDT PHD

Non-clinical Senior Lecturer, Institute of Cell and Molecular Science, Barts and The London School of Medicine and Dentistry, London, UK

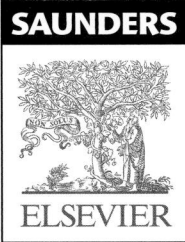

SAUNDERS
ELSEVIER

Edinburgh London New York Oxford Philadelphia St Louis Sydney Toronto 2009

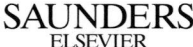

SAUNDERS
ELSEVIER

Main edition ISBN: 978 0 702 026 799
  Reprinted 2009, 2011
International edition ISBN: 978 0 702 026 805

British Library Cataloguing in Publication Data
A catalogue record for this book is available from the British Library

Library of Congress Cataloging in Publication Data
A catalog record for this book is available from the Library of Congress

Notice
Knowledge and best practice in this field are constantly changing. As new research and experience broaden our knowledge, changes in practice, treatment and drug therapy may become necessary or appropriate. Readers are advised to check the most current information provided (i) on procedures featured or (ii) by the manufacturer of each product to be administered, to verify the recommended dose or formula, the method and duration of administration, and contraindications. It is the responsibility of the practitioner, relying on their own experience and knowledge of the patient, to make diagnoses, to determine dosages and the best treatment for each individual patient, and to take all appropriate safety precautions. To the fullest extent of the law, neither the Publisher nor the Authors assume any liability for any injury and/or damage to persons or property arising out or related to any use of the material contained in this book.

The Publisher

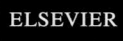
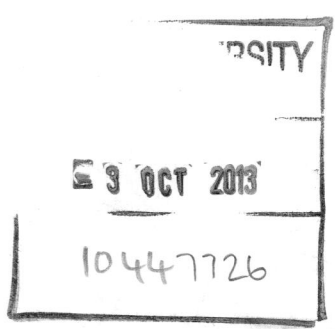

Contents

Contributors

Alison Chambers BSc
Department of Human Nutrition, Barts and The London School of Medicine and Dentistry

Paola Domizio BSc MBBS FRCPath
Professor of Pathology Education, Institute of Cell and Molecular Science, Barts and the London School of Medicine and Dentistry; Department of Cellular Pathology, Royal London Hospital

Gavin Donaldson BSc PhD
Senior Lecturer, Academic Unit of Respiratory Medicine, University College Medical School, London, UK

Mark Holness BSc PhD
Reader in Diabetes and Metabolism, Institute of Cell and Molecular Science, Barts and The London School of Medicine and Dentistry

David P Kelsell BSc PhD
Professor of Human Molecular Genetics, Institute of Cell and Molecular Science, Barts and The London School of Medicine and Dentistry

Alan Longstaff BSc PhD BSc FRAS
Associate Lecturer in Earth Sciences, Open University, Milton Keynes, UK; formerly Senior Lecturer in Physiology and Pharmacology, University of Hertfordshire, Hatfield, UK

Adrian C Newland BA MB BCh MA FRCP(UK) FRCPath
Professor of Haematology, Institute of Cell and Molecular Science, Barts and the London School of Medicine and Dentistry; Department of Haematology, Royal London Hospital

Jeremy Powell-Tuck MD FRCP
Professor of Clinical Nutrition, Institute of Cell and Molecular Science, Barts and the London School of Medicine and Dentistry

Drew Provan BSc MBChB MD FRCP FRCPath
Clinical Senior Lecturer, Institute of Cell and Molecular Science, Barts and the London School of Medicine and Dentistry; Department of Haematology, Royal London Hospital

Lesley Robson BSc PhD
Senior Lecturer, Institute of Cell and Molecular Science, Barts and the London School of Medicine and Dentistry

Malcolm Segal BSc PhD MPS
Senior Lecturer, Emeritus Reader in Physiology, Centre for Neuroscience Research, GKT School of Biomedical Sciences, King's College London, UK

Mary Sugden MA DPhil (Oxon) DSc (Lond)
Professor of Cellular Biochemistry, Institute of Cell and Molecular Science, Barts and The London School of Medicine and Dentistry

Walter Wieczorek MIBiol PhD
Lecturer, Institute of Dentistry, Barts and The London School of Medicine and Dentistry

John Wilkinson BSc (Hons) PhD
Academic Manager (Retired), School of Life Sciences, University of Hertfordshire, Hatfield, UK

Nigel Yeatman MBBS BSc MRCP DCH DRCOG
Senior Lecturer, Institute of Health Science Education, Barts and The London School of Medicine and Dentistry; Department of Clinical Immunology, Royal London Hospital

Preface

Towards the end of the twentieth century, massive progress was made in the basic medical sciences, and this is continuing, particularly in the understanding of cellular mechanisms and genomics. The discovery and mapping of the human genome, together with the rapid advances in clinical medicine, has meant that the amount of scientific knowledge required for the effective practice of medicine can become overwhelming for the undergraduate. A competent doctor, whether a specialist or generalist, has, however, always needed to be able to use scientific knowledge for understanding and solving their patients' clinical problems. Worldwide, the vast, and ever increasing, amount of scientific information has led to the development of undergraduate curricula aimed at enabling students to integrate the understanding of basic sciences with clinical medicine.

Clinical teachers have sometimes found that medical students are unable to recall important, basic scientific facts that are relevant to diagnosing and treating medical conditions. Despite the large amount of cellular biology, anatomy, physiology, biochemistry and pharmacology that they have been taught, students often appear to have difficulty with the synthesis and application of factual knowledge to solving clinical problems. In *Medical Sciences*, we have tried to explain clinical phenomena in the context of the science that underpins diagnostic and therapeutic decisions. As well as the traditional basic sciences, we have included epidemiology and public health as a basic science for practicing the art of medicine, where the epidemiological approach provides the scientific framework for how health problems occur, how diseases behave and whether interventions are effective. We have also included nutrition, because of the role of malnutrition, including both over- and unbalanced-nutrition, in so many of the diseases of the twenty-first century.

We have tried to be scientifically comprehensive, but limiting the amount of core information to focus on the facts that are relevant and important to clinical medicine. There is also benefit from integrating information from separate basic science disciplines, such as cellular biology, anatomy, biochemistry and physiology, to support the understanding of health and disease. We have used clinical examples to illustrate how disordered function leads to pathology, and to set the wealth of scientific knowledge in a clinical context. We have also included some aspects of recent research to alert the reader to potential areas of future development in medicine. Because *Medical Sciences* is not a textbook of clinical medicine, our greatest challenge has been to find the appropriate level of scientific detail and the right balance between the scientific and clinical information needed by undergraduates, from the recent school leaver to the finalist. The trend in the UK, and internationally, to widen participation in higher education to more non-traditional groups of students increases the variability in the prior knowledge that students bring to institutions for medical education. This book tries to support students who do not have a traditional science background.

Modern medical curricula that integrate the teaching of basic sciences with clinical medicine have often meant that students have to refer to a range of basic science textbooks to seek out the relevant materials. One of our aims was to integrate information from the diverse branches of medical science in a book based on all the systems of the human body in health. This is a new approach for a medical textbook. Collaboration between the basic science contributors and clinicians has contributed to the end result. We hope that *Medical Sciences* will engage students' interest, and inspire deep lifelong learning.

Jeanette Naish
Patricia Revest
Denise Syndercombe Court

Acknowledgements

Medical Sciences has had a long gestation. We thank everyone who has supported and helped us through this time. Ellen Green had the original idea of a book about the science for medicine that covered all the systems of the human body. Alison Whitehouse, from whom we learned so much, expertly helped with editing early versions of the chapters. Pauline Graham, Carole McMurray and Christine Johnston saw us through the later stages of production. Lotika Singha did the copy-editing, Ceinwen Sinclair, Carrie Walker and Barbara McAviney ensured that the proofs were properly read and Lynda Swindells created the index. Warm thanks are also due to the design and illustration team.

Special thanks are due to the following people who gave their time to read and make invaluable comments on the various chapters: Professor Robert Cohen, Professor of Medicine at the London Hospital Medical College (retired) (Ch. 3); Dr Barbara Boucher, Research Physician at the Royal London Hospital (retired) (Chs 3 and 10); Professor Ben Sacks, Professor of Neuropsychiatry at Imperial College School of Medicine (retired) (Chs 3 and 4); Dr Mark Carroll, Associate Dean (Education Quality) (Ch. 3); Dr John Patterson, Associate Dean (Undergraduate Medical Studies) (Ch. 13); Professor Athol Johnston and Dr Sabih Huq of the William Harvey Institute (Ch. 4); Dr. Richard Coleman of the Aberdeen Royal Infirmary (Ch. 8); Mrs Enid Hennessy, Senior Lecturer at the Wolfson Institute of Preventive Medicine (Ch. 7); Dr Jeremy Sayer, Consultant Cardiologist at Princess Alexandra Hospital, Harlow (Ch. 11); Professor Peter Schneider, University of Cologne (Ch. 6) and Dr Emma Dunne (Ch. 5).

A very special thank you to Rosemary Hall who was meticulous when helping to read proofs.

1 Introduction

Patricia Revest

PHYSIOLOGICAL CONTROL MECHANISMS AND HOMEOSTASIS

The French scientist Claude Bernard (1813–78) first described the 'mileau interieur', and observed that this 'internal environment' remains remarkably constant despite changing conditions in external conditions. Shortly afterwards, the American physiologist Walter Cannon (1871–1945) first used the word **homeostasis** to describe this constancy.

Homeostasis is the physiological process by which the internal systems of the body are maintained at equilibrium despite variations in the external conditions. It comes from the word homeo-, which means the sameness, and stasis, that is, standing still. However, equilibrium is not an unchanging state, so this is not strictly true – it is a dynamic state of equilibrium causing a dynamic constancy of the internal environment. It arises from the variation in response to changes in the external environment.

Homeostasis is responsible for maintaining physiological systems and there are many examples which can be used to describe the way in which systems work together. Two of the most well known and understood are the control of acidity of the body fluids, better know as acid–base balance, and the control of the fluid volumes of the body, fluid balance.

TYPES OF CONTROL SYSTEM

All control systems have a common basic structure. In control system theory the factor that is being controlled is called the **variable**. In order to control the value of a variable all control systems need at least three components:

- A **sensor** – which monitors the current value of the variable

- A **control centre** – which stores the desired value of the variable and can compare this to the current value as provided by the sensor
- An **effector** – which changes the value of the variable in a way that is determined by the control centre.

NEGATIVE FEEDBACK MECHANISMS

The most common type of control system is **negative feedback** (Fig. 1.1). A negative feedback system causes the variable to change in the opposite direction to the initial change, returning it to its set point. An everyday example of a negative feedback system is a central heating system. The sensor is the temperature sensor on the wall that monitors the room temperature. The control centre is the thermostat that compares the measured temperature to the temperature set on the thermostat; if it is too low, the heating is turned on. In most domestic systems this control system can only function to increase the temperature when it gets too cold but in more sophisticated systems, if the temperature becomes too high, the thermostat could then turn on the air conditioning. In these circumstances the temperature is constantly maintained at the set temperature.

Control of body temperature

A good example of a physiological homeostatic negative feedback system is the control of body temperature. Human beings live in a wide range of environments where the temperature may range from –50 to +50 °C. But body temperature is normally controlled between 36° and 38 °C. Biochemical processes in the body will not function if the temperature becomes too low or too high. At very high temperatures enzymes lose their activity and at low temperatures there is insufficient energy to maintain metabolic processes. Hyperthermia occurs when the core temperature rises above 40 °C and hypothermia occurs below 35 °C.

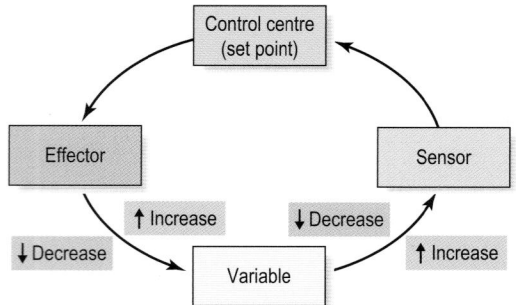

Fig. 1.1 Negative feedback loop. An increase in the variable produces an effector response to decrease it and vice versa.

Thermoneutral zones

The metabolic rate is at a minimum when heat gain or heat loss mechanisms are at a minimum. In naked humans who are resting, this **thermoneutral zone** occurs around 27 °C. At ambient temperatures above and below this, energy must be expended to control the body temperature. Body temperature also rises during activity, as the series of chemical reactions that cause muscular contraction do not convert all the energy to mechanical energy. The efficiency is low and as much as 75% is lost as heat. Other mammals have a thermoneutral zone that is much colder. Arctic foxes can live comfortably at temperatures below −50 °C, protected by their thick coats.

Heat loss mechanisms

An increase in body temperature is detected by sensors in the skin, which measure **peripheral temperatures**, and in the hypothalamus, which measure **core temperature** (Fig. 1.2). One of the effectors that enables the body to lose heat is the rings of smooth muscles in the walls of blood vessels in the skin, which can change the rate of blood flow in the region just under the skin surface. By relaxing the smooth muscle, the diameter of the blood vessels increases and the resistance to flow falls. By increasing the amount of blood flow, heat can be lost by radiation, reducing both the local temperature and the core temperature by returning cooler blood to the central blood volume. This can be clearly seen on pale-skinned people on a hot day when they become very red. If they have been exercising this redness can be widespread, but if the increase in heat is more localised, such as on bare arms in the sun, then the redness may be very local and show up as distinct lines.

Another effector that is particularly effective in hot, dry climates is the sweat glands in the skin. An increase in the rate of sweat produced causes more water to be evaporated from the surface of the body. As the latent heat of evaporation of water is high, large amounts of heat can be lost by this mechanism. However, in hot, wet climates, this mechanism is ineffective as evaporation requires a gradient of humidity between the skin and the air. In tropical climates the humidity may be 100% so evaporation does not occur. The other problem with this method of heat loss is that it requires large amounts of body water. If this is not replaced then dehydration can occur.

Heat gain mechanisms

If there is a fall in body temperature the responses are more varied. The same effectors – the vascular smooth muscle and

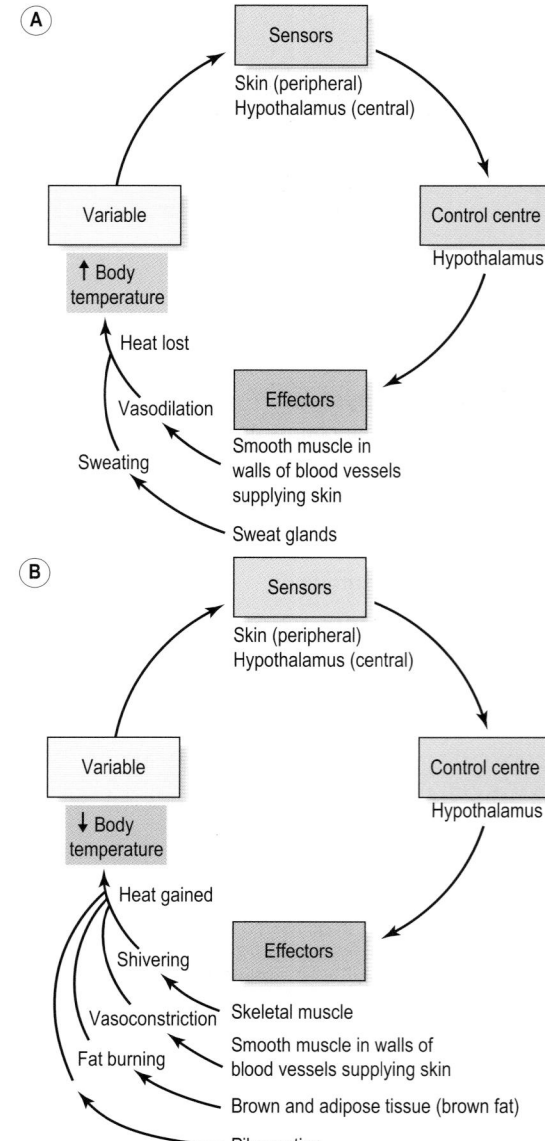

Fig. 1.2 Control of body temperature by negative feedback. (A) Responses to an increase in body temperature; (B) responses to a decrease in body temperature.

the sweat glands – that can reduce body temperature can work in reverse to increase the temperature. Constriction of vascular smooth muscle in the skin can reduce the blood flow in the upper layers of the skin to almost nothing. This prevents heat loss and gives the pale, slightly blue tinge to the skin surface. The pallor is due to the very small amounts of blood in the skin and the blue tinge is due to the fact that the rate of blood flow is so slow that most of the haemoglobin is deoxygenated and so appears bluish.

Two other mechanisms are also brought into play. In adult humans, a fall in core temperature can induce an increase in muscular activity. Voluntary activity includes stamping the feet, tapping the hands and generally increased fidgeting. Involuntary movements also occur as shivering; the rapid contraction and relaxation of skeletal muscle that is controlled by the autonomic nervous system. This can range from an increase in muscle tone to vigorous shaking.

In the cold, humans also show piloerection, when the body hairs stand up. In mammals with thick fur this can significantly decrease heat loss by trapping more air close to the skin, where it is warmed and forms an insulating layer. However, most humans are not hairy enough for piloerection to affect their heat balance and the behavioural practice of wearing clothes produces the same effect much more efficiently. Humans who fall into cold water survive longer if clothed than if naked, as a similar blanket effect is produced by water trapped inside the clothes. Because of this, thrashing about, which disrupts this warm layer, causes the heat to be lost faster.

Long-term temperature control

Long-term mechanisms to control body temperature include changes in metabolic rate, changes in feeding, and behavioural mechanisms such as seeking shade in the heat or shelter in the cold. The wearing, and discarding, of clothes has reduced the need for much temperature regulation. However, babies become overheated quite easily if clothed too much, as they cannot discard clothes at will.

Fever

The set point for temperature control is not always fixed. In infection, toxins released from bacteria and chemicals produced by cells of the immune system change the set point upwards (see Ch. 6). The normal mechanisms to generate heat, such as shivering, are triggered leading to an increase in body temperature known as fever or **pyrexia**. The cause for this fever is thought to be a mechanism to help kill off bacteria. The higher rate of metabolism will also produce a faster rate of healing and more rapid induction of defence mechanisms. However, if the temperature becomes too high, the proteins inside the cells are damaged.

POSITIVE FEEDBACK MECHANISMS

Whilst many physiological control systems compensate for change, to produce constancy of the internal environment, there are a few cases where the opposite occurs. That is, the change triggers a control system that further amplifies the change. This is called **positive feedback** (Fig. 1.3). The change becomes self-perpetuating, and in the process, small changes are also amplified into something much larger. These types of event are often called cascades, when there are obviously no set points to defend as the system triggers a runaway change in the variable.

Using the analogy of central heating, imagine a system where the rise in temperature causes the heating to switch

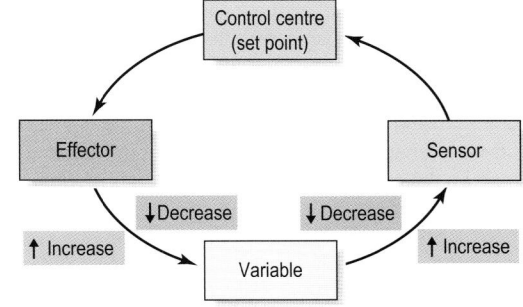

Fig. 1.3 **Positive feedback loop.** An increase in the variable produces an effector response to increase it, and vice versa, until the loop is terminated.

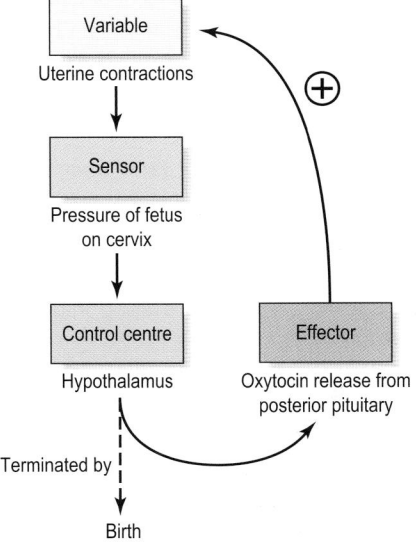

Fig. 1.4 **Control of childbirth by a positive feedback mechanism.**

ON, which increases the temperature still further. The most dramatic example of a positive feedback system is the atomic bomb. The injection of neutrons into the fissile material causes more neutrons to be released, which trigger the release of still more neutrons, until the entire system explodes.

A positive feedback system, once triggered, could continue forever. To prevent this becoming a runaway event, there has to be a way of terminating it. One way is when there is a single critical event that must occur, a self-limiting mechanism.

Positive feedback during childbirth

A good example of a positive feedback system with a self-limiting mechanism is the control of the contractions of the uterus during childbirth (Fig. 1.4). The actual trigger for birth is a complex series of events that are thought to be, in part, regulated by signals from the fetus. However, the key event that triggers the positive feedback loop is the pressure of the fetus on the cervix, which is the lowest part of the uterus.

Nerve impulses from the cervix are transmitted to the brain where they stimulate the hypothalamus. This causes the release of a chemical, the hormone oxytocin, from the posterior pituitary gland at the base of the brain into the bloodstream. Oxytocin acts on the smooth muscle of the uterus to increase the force and rate of contractions, pushing the fetus harder against the cervix, which produces more oxytocin causing further contractions. This continues until the uterus manages to expel the baby, thus relieving the pressure on the cervix, so oxytocin secretion is stopped and the uterine contractions cease. In this case, the positive feedback loop is terminated by the birth of the baby, a significant self-limiting event.

FEEDFORWARD CONTROL MECHANISMS

In many circumstances, it is beneficial to anticipate a change and compensate before the variable has changed too much. This ensures the variables do not vary too much and reduces, and sometimes eliminates, the amount of time during which the change occurs. It is like looking out of the window on a cold day. You observe that the weather outside the house looks cold so you put on extra clothes before you leave the house, rather than getting cold first and then putting on a coat.

An example of this type of **feedforward mechanism** occurs during exercise. The increased demand for oxygen that is needed by muscles during exercise, has to be provided by two main mechanisms. Firstly, the rate and depth of breathing must increase in order to draw more oxygen into the lungs. Secondly, the blood passing through the lungs must be propelled more quickly to the tissues in order to supply the oxygen. This means that the heart rate, and also the amount of blood pumped at each beat, must increase.

The motor nerves in the brain that trigger the muscle movements have branches that go to the areas that control breathing and the heart. At the start of exercise, even before exercise has altered blood levels of oxygen and carbon dioxide, the breathing rate, heart rate and strength of contraction are all increased. Other feedback mechanisms also contribute – sensors in muscles and joints send signals to the brain to produce changes that ensure adequate oxygenation.

HOMEOSTATIC IMBALANCES CAUSE DISEASE

When the mechanisms of homeostasis fail or are overwhelmed, then the normal biochemical and physiological balance in the body is lost. Most disease is a result of **homeostatic imbalance**.

A disease is a recognisable set of **signs** and **symptoms**. Symptoms are states that are not obviously observable, which are reported by the patients, such as feeling tired. Signs are changes that can be observed and measured by a doctor, such as increases in blood pressure. The diagnosis of disease is made by considering information provided by the patient – their symptoms, medical history and personal circumstances – and information gathered from physical examination and laboratory tests.

ACID–BASE BALANCE

One of the most important homeostatic mechanisms in the human body is the precise regulation of the concentration of hydrogen ions in the body fluids, known as **acid–base balance**.

HYDROGEN ION CONCENTRATIONS

The free hydrogen ion concentration is the concentration of hydrogen ions in solution that are not bound to other molecules and therefore free to react. Hydrogen ion concentrations are described using the **pH scale.**

$$pH = -\log_{10}[H^+] \qquad \text{(Eq. 1.1)}$$

where $[H^+]$ is the hydrogen ion concentration.

This is a logarithmic scale where each pH unit represents a 10-fold change in hydrogen concentration. On this scale a concentration of 10^{-9} molar equals pH 9 (Table 1.1). The logarithmic scale can easily represent a very large range of concentrations.

On the pH scale neutral pH is 7 because the hydrogen ion concentration of pure water contains 10^{-7} moles/L of free hydrogen ions. Solutions that contain more hydrogen ions have a lower pH and are **acidic**. Those with fewer hydrogen ions have a higher pH and are **alkaline**, also known as more basic. The range of possible hydrogen ion concentrations is very wide (Table 1.2). However, in body fluids it is normally maintained within very strict limits.

Physiological pH ranges

There is a very narrow range of pH that is compatible with life. The normal pH of blood is around 7.4 with blood in the arteries being slightly less acidic at pH 7.45 than the venous blood (pH 7.35). This is a very low concentration of H^+; at pH 7.4 this corresponds to a $[H^+]$ of only 40 nmoles/L. If the pH falls below 7.35 this is called **acidosis** and above 7.45 is **alkalosis**. If the pH of blood falls below 6.8 or rises above 8 for a significant period of time then death occurs. This represents a very small change in the concentration of H^+ as the difference between pH 6.8 and 8 is only 148 nmoles/L (1.48 $\times 10^{-7}$ moles/L).

Body fluids other than blood have a different pH. The fluid bathing the brain, the cerebrospinal fluid, is usually about pH 7.3. Intracellular fluids have a lower pH that varies with

Table 1.1	The pH scale of hydrogen ion concentrations			
[H+]/moles/L	10^{-9}	10^{-8}	10^{-7}	10^{-6}
pH	9	8	7	6

Table 1.2	pH values for some different fluids
Solution	**pH**
Hydrochloric acid (0.1 moles/L)	1.0
Gastric juice	1.0–2.5
Lemon juice	2.1
Tomato juice	4.1
Urine (average)	6.0
Saliva	6.8
Milk	6.9
Pure water (25 °C)	7.0
Blood (average)	7.4
Sea water	7.9–8.3
Ammonia (NH_3, 0.1 moles/L)	11.1

metabolic activity. In resting muscle cells, the pH is between 6.8 and 7, but with increased activity this falls as low as 6.4. Some intracellular compartments such as lysosomes have even lower pH (i.e. they are more acidic).

pH sensitivity

Many physiological processes within the body are pH sensitive. Many of the chemical reactions that occur inside cells are sensitive to the hydrogen ion concentration. Most of the chemical processes have an **optimal pH** at which they occur faster. If the pH is higher or lower than this then the reactions may proceed at a slower rate or not at all. In most cases the optimal pH is ~7.4, but this varies according to the normal pH of the compartment where the reaction occurs. In the case of lysosomes, the chemical reactions that occur within them require the low pH and so the biomolecules within the compartments are adapted to this environment and are not damaged (see Ch. 2).

Changes in pH have profound effects on the excitability of nerves and muscles. A reduction in pH (acidosis) causes a reduction in excitability, especially in the brain, which can cause confusion and, in extreme cases, coma and death. Conversely, an increase in pH (alkalosis) will produce unwanted nervous activity in the peripheral and central nervous system. Nerves become hypersensitive and transmit signals even in the absence of normal stimuli. This can produce symptoms such as tingling in the fingers, caused by overactivity of sensory nerves. Overactivity in the nerves that excite the muscles can cause muscle spasms, which can paralyse the muscles required for breathing. Overactivity in the central nervous system can cause convulsions.

One of the potentially most serious effects of a fall in pH is the effect on cardiac muscle. A compensatory response to an increase in H^+ is an increased secretion of H^+ from the kidney (see below), which leads to an increase in the levels of potassium (K^+) in the blood – hyperkalaemia (see Ch. 14). This can produce alterations in the rate and rhythm of the heart (cardiac arrhythmia or dysrhythmia) and if severe can lead to a heart attack.

Biological sources of acid and alkali

Acids are continually produced within the body as part of the chemical reactions that break down food to provide energy for metabolic processes. A major byproduct of energy generation is carbon dioxide (CO_2), which reacts with water to form acid (see below). Other acids are produced specifically from the proteins and fats we consume as food. More acid is produced during exercise, particularly lactic acid, which is generated when the exercise level exceeds the oxygen intake – anaerobic exercise. It is the lactic acid produced during heavy exercise that produces the pain, the 'burn' of lactic acid.

Bases are not generated in the body but vegetables are a major source of alkali. On balance, people consuming a Western meat-containing diet generate excess acid in their bodies, but the acid load of vegetarians is less. However, despite the average daily increase in acid load, there are mechanisms within the body that, under normal conditions, are perfectly able to cope with the excess acid. There are two ways in which balance is maintained:

- In the short-term, chemicals called **buffers** act as storage for H^+, in order to prevent the free concentration from changing too much.
- In the long-term, there is excretion of excess CO_2 and H^+ by the lungs and the kidneys.

BUFFERS

A **buffer system** is a solution that can minimise changes in free $[H^+]$. It does not eliminate the H^+ but transiently removes it from free solution. An acid in solution can dissociate to give a hydrogen ion whereas a base is a hydrogen ion acceptor. Together, an acid and a base make a **conjugate pair**.

$$\text{acid} \rightleftharpoons H^+ + \text{base} \qquad \text{(Eq. 1.2)}$$

A **strong acid** completely dissociates in solution. An example of this is hydrochloric acid (HCl), which completely dissociates into protons (H^+) and chloride ions (Cl^-). **Weak acids**, such as carbonic acid (H_2CO_3), only partly dissociate and do not yield as many hydrogen ions. Bases can bind free H^+. Strong bases, such as NH_3, bind H^+ more readily than weak bases, such as HCO_3^-. The terms acid and base are relative. A molecule can be an acid in one system and a base in another. An example of this is bicarbonate (HCO_3^-), which can act as a base in a conjugate pair with carbonic acid but as an acid with carbonate (Table 1.3). The reaction of a buffer pair is reversible and is dictated by the law of mass action. This means that the reaction depends on the concentration of the chemicals involved. In the buffer systems described above this means that if you add H^+, then more acid is formed. If you add more acid then more H^+ plus base is formed.

The degree to which a particular acid will dissociate is a constant for each acid. This **dissociation constant** (K) is the proportion of the acid that is dissociated and is expressed as:

$$K = [H^+][\text{base}]/[\text{acid}] \qquad \text{(Eq. 1.3)}$$

where [base] and [acid] are the concentrations of the base and acid, respectively. Using a notation that is similar to that used for $[H^+]$, the constant is usually quoted as **pK** where pK $= -\log_{10} K$. When a buffer solution has a pH that is the same

---

Clinical box 1.1   Hyperventilation

Rapid, deep breathing, or overbreathing (for example during a panic attack) could lead to the excessive breathing out of CO_2 and low levels of CO_2 in the blood. This can give rise to an increase in pH (alkalosis) due to a loss of the buffering activity of CO_2 in the blood (see below). The symptoms of numbness and tingling (paraesthesia) in the hands and around the mouth (perioral numbness) are due to unprovoked nervous activity caused by alkalosis. Alkalosis can further alter the electrolyte balance in the blood, where hypocalcaemia (low calcium) causes muscle spasms, particularly in the hands and feet (carpopedal spasm) – **hyperventilation tetany**.

Table 1.3	Examples of conjugate pairs	
	Acid	**Base**
	HCl	Cl^-
	H_2CO_3	HCO_3^-
	HCO_3^-	CO_3^{2-}
	NH_4^+	NH_3
	H_2O	OH^-

as the pK, half of the buffer is acid and half is base; that is, it is 50% dissociated. A buffer is therefore most effective at buffering changes in H⁺ if its pK is near the desired pH.

BIOLOGICAL BUFFER SYSTEMS

Biological buffer systems use weak acids to prevent large changes in [H⁺]. They consist of buffer pairs which, at pH levels found in the body, are only partially dissociated so both acid and base are present. If hydrogen ions are added to the system, they can bind to the base and form acid. This prevents a fall in pH. If hydrogen ions are removed, then more acid dissociates to form H⁺ and base and, again, the pH does not change. The amount of change that can be prevented depends on the quantity of the buffer pair present. Three major buffer systems are involved in maintaining a relatively constant pH in body fluids. These are:

- Bicarbonate/carbon dioxide
- Proteins, particularly haemoglobin
- Phosphate.

Each buffer system is able to buffer a certain amount of H⁺, called the **buffer capacity** (Table 1.4). Changes in H⁺ that are less than the available buffer capacity are not seen as changes in pH. Changes in pH are only seen when the available buffer capacity is exceeded.

The blood contains all of the main buffer systems: bicarbonate, proteins (especially haemoglobin) and phosphate. However, in the extracellular fluid outside the blood vessels there is very little protein and all buffering is done by the bicarbonate and phosphate buffer systems. Inside the cells there are large amounts of protein and phosphate as well as bicarbonate, although the bicarbonate concentration is lower than that of extracellular fluid (see Ch. 2, Table 2.15).

The bicarbonate/carbon dioxide buffer system

Carbon dioxide and **bicarbonate** are both involved in the most important buffer system in the blood. It is the primary buffer system in the extracellular fluid that can buffer hydrogen ions produced by mechanisms that do not involve either bicarbonate or carbon dioxide themselves. For example, it can buffer hydrogen ion changes produced normally, during exercise, by the production of lactic acid or in disease states, such as diabetes, where excess acid is produced due to changes in the fuels used in metabolism.

This system uses a set of linked reactions, with carbon dioxide and water on one side and bicarbonate and hydrogen ions on the other.

$$CO_2 + H_2O \rightleftharpoons H_2CO_3 \rightleftharpoons H^+ + HCO_3^- \qquad \text{(Eq. 1.4)}$$

In water, carbon dioxide first forms a solution. About 5% of the CO_2 transported in blood does so in solution (Fig. 1.5). Some of this dissolved CO_2 reacts slowly with water to produce **carbonic acid**, but inside red blood cells the reaction is accelerated by the enzyme **carbonic anhydrase**. The carbonic acid then dissociates into a hydrogen ion and a bicarbonate ion (the base). Although this is a two-stage process, as opposed to the simple buffer pairs described above, it is still possible to work out a dissociation constant for the overall reaction.

The effective pK of the carbon dioxide/bicarbonate system is 6.1. This is quite acidic compared with the normal pH inside red blood cells, but it is a very effective buffer because of the high concentration of bicarbonate in blood, at almost 24 mmoles/L. The reason that this buffer system cannot buffer changes in pH due to production of carbon dioxide or bicarbonate is that these ions are a part of the buffer system itself. If there is an increase in CO_2, for example due to an increase in metabolism during exercise, then the law of mass action will push the equilibrium of equation 1.4 to the right, generating more H⁺. The only way of removing this H⁺ is either by adding more bicarbonate, which is relatively slow, or by buffering the H⁺ using a different buffer pair.

Buffering by proteins

The extracellular fluid surrounding cells contains few proteins but, inside cells, proteins are plentiful and the acidic and basic side chains that are attached to them can accept or donate H⁺ in order to limit changes in pH. The carboxyl and amino groups found at the ends of each protein chain can also buffer H⁺. In the blood plasma, proteins such as albumin can also buffer significant amounts of H⁺, including that derived from carbonic acid.

The haemoglobin buffer system

The protein **haemoglobin**, which is present in large amounts inside red blood cells, is the most important buffer of any H⁺ derived from carbonic acid. It is involved in the transport of carbon dioxide from the tissues, where the gas is produced as a waste product of metabolism, to the lungs where it is exhaled. This prevents the generation of large quantities of acid in the venous blood; in fact venous blood is only slightly more acidic than that in the arteries.

In the tissues, CO_2 diffuses into the blood. Here it forms H_2CO_3, which dissociates into HCO_3^- and H⁺. The HCO_3^-

Table 1.4	Buffer capacity of the main buffer systems in the blood	
Buffer system	**Capacity (mmoles H⁺/L)**
Bicarbonate/carbon dioxide	18
Protein	1.7
Haemoglobin	8
Phosphate	0.3
Total	28

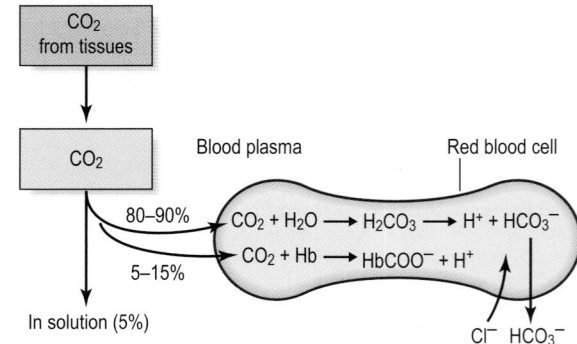

Fig. 1.5 Carriage of CO₂ in the blood. Most of the CO_2 is converted to HCO_3^-, the remainder is either in solution (5%) or combined with haemoglobin (5–15%).

diffuses out of the red blood cell and is carried to the lungs in the plasma. Most (80–90%) of the CO_2 transport from the tissues to the lungs is in the form of bicarbonate. In the red blood cell, the H^+ then combines with haemoglobin, aided by the fact that **deoxyhaemoglobin** has a higher capacity for H^+ binding than **oxyhaemoglobin** (HbO_2). As O_2 is released from HbO_2 in the tissues, the binding of haemoglobin to H^+ increases and more H^+ is bound to Hb (HHb).

$$H^+ + Hb \rightleftharpoons HHb \qquad \text{(Eq. 1.5)}$$

On reaching the lungs, as O_2 binds to haemoglobin, H^+ is released. The H^+ combines with HCO_3^- giving H_2CO_3, which dissociates into CO_2 and H_2O. The CO_2 is then exhaled. However, if the ability of the lungs to remove CO_2 is impaired, this system fails (see below).

Haemoglobin also carries some CO_2 as **carbamino-haemoglobin**. This reaction combines four molecules of CO_2 with each haemoglobin molecule releasing four H^+. However, this does not increase the pH, as the effect of CO_2 in hae-moglobin is more complex. Binding of CO_2 to haemoglobin causes the affinity of O_2 for haemoglobin to be reduced. This encourages unloading of O_2 in the tissues where CO_2 levels are high. This is known as the Bohr effect (see Ch. 12). As described above, deoxyhaemoglobin binds more H^+, so any H^+ produced by the reaction of haemoglobin with CO_2 is more than made up for by the increased binding capacity of haemoglobin. About 5–15% of the CO_2 carried in the blood is in combination with haemoglobin.

The phosphate buffer system

Although extracellular fluid does not contain much **phosphate**, this, along with proteins, is an important buffer inside cells. It is also an important buffer in urine. Humans normally excrete phosphate which, along with ammonia, can buffer H^+ secreted into the urine in the kidneys. This is important as it allows larger amounts of H^+ to be secreted than would be possible without buffering. The secretion of H^+ is necessary as buffers do not remove excess H^+ from the body, they only prevent it affecting body systems. Any excess H^+ must eventually be removed otherwise the buffering capacity of the body would become completely saturated and unable to buffer any further H^+.

The phosphate buffer system consists of the acid, dihydrogen phosphate, which can give up H^+ to form hydrogen phosphate.

$$H_2PO_4^- \rightleftharpoons HPO_4^{2-} + H^+ \qquad \text{(Eq. 1.6)}$$

HENDERSON–HASSELBALCH EQUATION

This equation expresses the relationship between $[H^+]$ and the concentrations of the buffer pair.

For a given buffer pair the **Henderson–Hasselbalch equation** is given as:

$$pH = pK + \log_{10}[\text{base}]/[\text{acid}] \qquad \text{(Eq. 1.7)}$$

For the bicarbonate/carbon dioxide buffer system it can be expressed as:

$$pH = pK + \log_{10}[HCO_3^-]/[H_2CO_3] \qquad \text{(Eq. 1.8)}$$

Because most of the CO_2 is converted to H_2CO_3, the $[H_2CO_3]$ is a direct reflection of the $[CO_2]$ so equation 1.8 can be rewritten as:

$$pH = pK + \log_{10}[HCO_3^-]/[CO_2] \qquad \text{(Eq. 1.9)}$$

This equation can be used to predict the pH at any given levels of CO_2 and HCO_3^- and as the pK is constant for any acid, this means that changes in the ratio of CO_2 and HCO_3^- will change the pH. The normal ratio of $HCO_3^-:CO_2$ is 20:1 in the extracellular fluid. Substituting these values in equation 1.9 gives:

$$pH = 6.1 + \log_{10}(20/1) = 7.4 \qquad \text{(Eq. 1.10)}$$

where $[HCO_3^-]$ = 24 mmoles/L and $[CO_2]$ = 1.2 mmoles/L.

CONTROL OF PH

As the bicarbonate/carbon dioxide system is the buffer system with the highest buffer capacity then changes in either CO_2 or HCO_3^- will largely determine the pH.

Respiratory control of pH

As described above, CO_2, which is generated by tissue metabolism, is removed from the body by the lungs. This prevents the generation of large amounts of H^+, so it is not surprising that part of the control of breathing is regulated by pH (see Ch. 12). This is a negative feedback system, where the variable being controlled is the pH: the sensor is in the brain, where cells in the medulla respond to the pH of the cerebrospinal fluid, and the effectors are the nerve cells, which stimulate the increased rate of respiration.

Under normal conditions, if there is a decrease in the pH of the blood there is a proportional rise in respiration, by an increase in the rate and/or depth of breathing. Similarly, an increase in pH causes a fall in respiration. However, as the driving force for the increase in respiration is pH, which is determined by the $[CO_2]$, as the levels of CO_2 return to normal, the driving force is reduced. This means that respiratory compensation is not completed. For this, it requires the action of the kidneys.

Renal control of pH

The kidneys can control pH by controlling the amounts of both H^+ and HCO_3^- excreted in the urine. Small molecules, such as H^+ and HCO_3^-, can enter the urine by two ways:

- Passive filtration in the first part of the kidney, the Bowman's capsule. This fluid, the primary filtrate, is subsequently modified to form urine.
- Addition to the urine by transport mechanisms in the kidney tubules.

H^+ secretion

Almost all of the H^+ found in the urine is actively secreted by the kidney; this is because the $[H^+]$ of plasma is very low (40 nmoles/L at pH 7.4). CO_2, derived either from H^+ and HCO_3^- in the plasma or directly from plasma CO_2, diffuses into the kidney tubule cells (Fig. 1.6). Carbonic anhydrase converts CO_2 and H_2O to H_2CO_3, which dissociates into H^+ and HCO_3^-. The H^+ is transported out of the cells into the urine, while the HCO_3^- is returned to the blood. The H^+ in the urine is then buffered by one of two mechanisms:

- H^+ combines with phosphate (HPO_4^{2-}) and sodium ions (Na^+) to form NaH_2PO_4, which is excreted.
- If there is insufficient phosphate available, ammonia (NH_3), synthesised from glutamine in the tubule cells, is

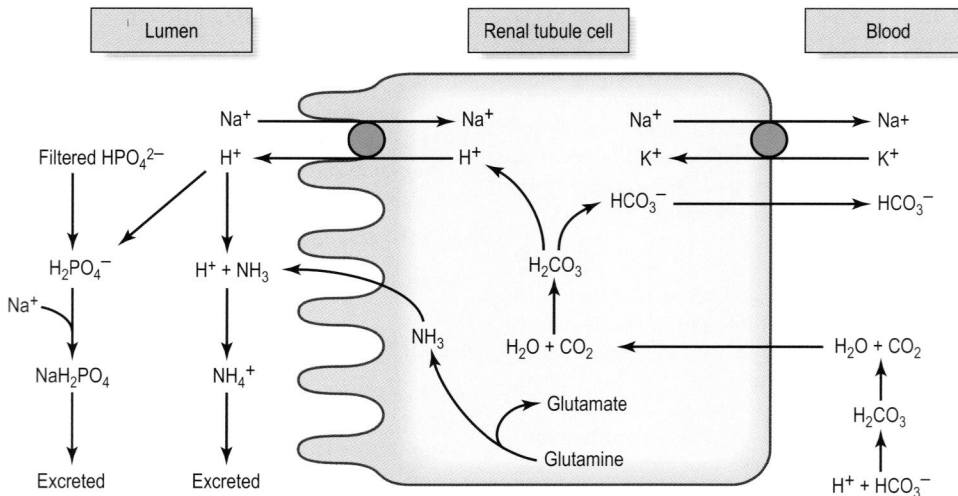

Fig. 1.6 Renal excretion of H⁺. H⁺ combines with phosphate or ammonia before being excreted.

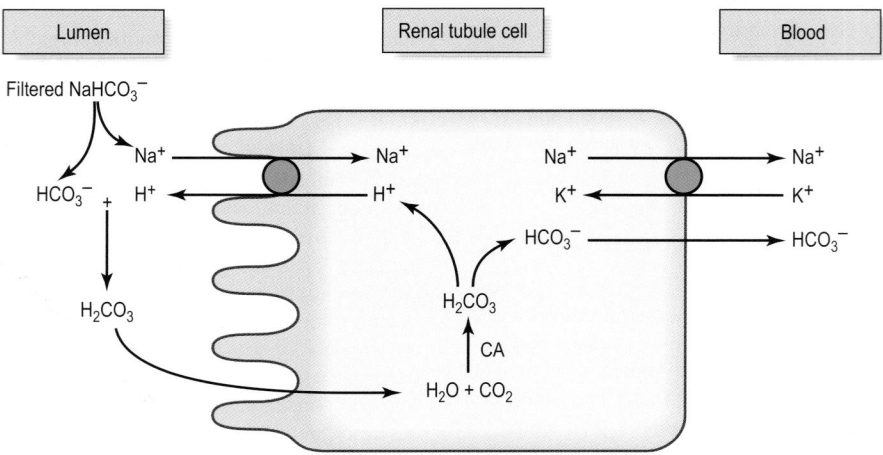

Fig. 1.7 Renal reabsorption of HCO₃⁻. The net result is the transfer of a molecule of HCO_3^- from lumen to blood. CA, carbonic anhydrase.

secreted into the urine where it combines with the H⁺ to form ammonium ions (NH_4^+) which are then excreted.

This ensures that the pH of the urine does not fall below the limiting level of 4.5 and H⁺ does not diffuse back into the body.

Bicarbonate reabsorption

As well as the HCO_3^- that is added to blood by the secretion of H⁺, bicarbonate can also be reabsorbed from urine. Bicarbonate is freely filtered from blood, but the cells lining the renal tubules are impermeable to HCO_3^- so it must be reabsorbed indirectly. The HCO_3^- reacts with secreted H⁺ to form H_2CO_3 (Fig. 1.7). On the surface of the tubule cells, carbonic anhydrase converts H_2CO_3 to H_2O and CO_2. The CO_2 diffuses freely into the tubule cells where intracellular carbonic anhydrase catalyses the reverse reaction to produce H_2CO_3. This then dissociates into HCO_3^- and H⁺. The H⁺ is secreted into the urine and the HCO_3^- diffuses into the blood. The net result is the transfer of a molecule of HCO_3^- from the urine to the blood.

Table 1.5	Changes in the HCO₃⁻:CO₂ ratio in acid–base disorders	
Disorder	**HCO₃⁻:CO₂ ratio**	**Change**
Respiratory acidosis	<20:1	Increase [CO₂]
Respiratory alkalosis	>20:1	Decrease [CO₂]
Metabolic acidosis	<20:1	Fall in [HCO₃⁻]
Metabolic alkalosis	>20:1	Rise in [HCO₃⁻]

ACID–BASE DISTURBANCES

Acid–base disturbances occur when there is a change in the HCO_3^-:CO_2 ratio. Respiratory acid–base disorders cause changes in the arterial pCO_2, the partial pressure of CO_2 in arterial blood, whereas metabolic acid–base disorders lead to changes in either [H⁺] or [HCO_3^-] (Table 1.5) (see also Chs 12, 13 and 15). Changes in acid–base balance caused by changes in respiration can only be corrected by non-respiratory mechanisms. However, changes in pH caused by metabolic disturbances, except those due to renal causes, can be corrected by both respiratory and renal mechanisms.

Clinical box 1.2   Example of an acid–base disturbance

An elderly man who has chronic emphysema (a respiratory disorder) has the following results:

- pH = 7.30
- pCO_2 = 50 mmHg
- Standard $[HCO_3^-]$ = 32 mM

Using Table 1.6:

- The pH is below 7.35 so he has acidosis
- The pCO_2 is greater than 45 mmHg so the primary cause of the acidosis is respiratory
- The standard $[HCO_3^-]$ is greater than 28 mM so he has respiratory acidosis with renal compensation.

A diagram has been constructed using data from patients with different respiratory and metabolic acid–base disorders to show the range of changes in H^+, HCO_3^- and pH (Fig. 1.8). This diagram can be used to help identify the particular disorder, but can also be used to plot the progress and effectiveness of treatment as sequential measurements can be plotted and changes towards (or away from) the normal range can be observed.

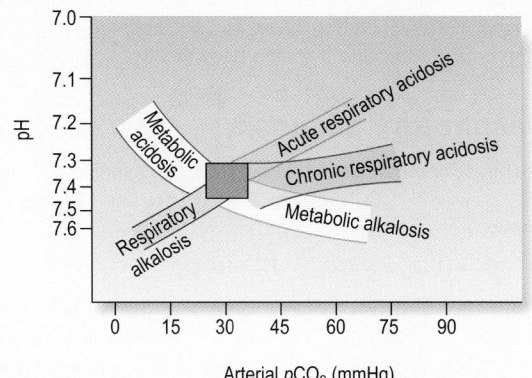

Fig. 1.8 **Acid–base diagram, showing ranges of H^+ and pCO_2 for acid–base disturbances.** Normal range = *red shaded area*.

Table 1.6   Acid–base disturbances

1. Determine blood pH (normal values 7.35–7.45)

If less than 7.35: acidosis		If more than 7.45: alkalosis	
Determine arterial pCO_2 and $[HCO_3^-]$ (standard bicarbonate) normal values pCO_2 35–45 mmHg (4.8–6.1 kPa) $[HCO_3^-]$ 22–28 mM			
If pCO_2 > 45 mmHg (6.1 kPa) there is: **Respiratory acidosis**	If $[HCO_3^-]$ < 22 mM there is: **Metabolic acidosis**	if pCO_2 < 35 mmHg (4.8 kPa) there is: **Respiratory alkalosis**	If $[HCO_3^-]$ > 28 mM there is: **Metabolic alkalosis**
Then		**Then**	
If $[HCO_3^-]$ > 28 mM there is:	if pCO_2 < 35 mmHg (4.8 kPa) there is:	If $[HCO_3^-]$ < 22 mM there is:	if pCO_2 > 45 mmHg (6.1 kPa) there is:
Respiratory acidosis with renal compensation	**Metabolic acidosis with respiratory compensation**	**Respiratory alkalosis with renal compensation**	**Metabolic acidosis with respiratory compensation**

Information box 1.2   Determining the type of acid–base disorder

In order to determine the type of acid–base disorder, as well as noting signs and symptoms and taking a patient history, it is necessary to measure three things:

- pH
- pCO_2
- Standard bicarbonate concentration.*

Arterial blood samples are taken anaerobically in a tube containing the minimum necessary of an anticoagulant such as heparin. Although heparin is itself acidic, a dilute solution does not affect samples too much. The anticoagulant citrate should not be used as that will significantly change the pH. Samples should exclude air bubbles and be capped to exclude any gas exchange with air which has a lower CO_2 content. The samples should be processed immediately or stored in ice, as white blood cell metabolism will increase levels of CO_2 and reduce O_2.

*As the concentration of HCO_3^- in a sample will vary with the concentration of CO_2, this is always measured in a sample at body temperature which has been fully oxygenated and equilibrated at a normal CO_2 (40 mmHg).

Initially changes in H^+ will be buffered, so there will be alterations in either CO_2 or HCO_3^-, but if the condition lasts long enough for compensatory mechanisms such as those described above to occur, then changes in both CO_2 and HCO_3^- will be seen (Table 1.6).

Respiratory acidosis

Respiratory acidosis occurs when there is hypoventilation and a reduction in the excretion of CO_2 by the lungs. Driving the reaction:

$$CO_2 + H_2O \rightleftharpoons H_2CO_3 \rightleftharpoons H^+ + HCO_3^-$$

to the right will cause the $[H^+]$ to rise and the pH will fall. Although in this reaction HCO_3^- is produced in the same Quantities as H^+, the rise in $[HCO_3^-]$ is insignificant. So, if the pH falls to 7.0, for example, this is a rise in $[H^+]$ of 60 nmoles/L, which added to the normal 40 nmoles/L gives a total of 100 nmoles/L. Also, 60 nmoles/L of HCO_3^- are produced but this is added to an existing $[HCO_3^-]$ of about 24 mmoles/L. This increases the $[HCO_3^-]$ by less than 0.00003%, which is essentially an insignificant change. Common causes of respiratory acidosis are lung diseases that reduce ventilation, such as bronchitis and emphysema, and drugs which inhibit ventilation, such as barbiturates and opioids (for example morphine).

As the primary cause of the acidosis is hypoventilation, this cannot be compensated for by an increase in ventilation. However, there can be renal compensation by a number of mechanisms which can help to limit the change in pH:

- All filtered HCO_3^- is reabsorbed (see Fig. 1.7)
- H^+ is secreted, which also adds new HCO_3^- to blood (see Fig. 1.6).

If the hypoventilation causes a doubling of the pCO_2 then the ratio of $HCO_3^-:CO_2$ would be 20:2 in the extracellular fluid, which would give pH = 6.1 + $\log_{10}$ (20/2) = 7.1 (see equation 1.10). In order to compensate for this acidosis the plasma [HCO_3^-] would have to be doubled (to about 48 mmoles/L) to bring the ratio back to 20:1.

Respiratory alkalosis

Respiratory alkalosis is caused by excess ventilation which will 'blow off' CO_2 causing the pH to rise. Driving the reaction:

$$CO_2 + H_2O \rightleftharpoons H_2CO_3 \rightleftharpoons H^+ + HCO_3^-$$

to the left will cause the [H^+] to fall and the pH will rise. A decrease in the pCO_2 by half will change the ratio of $HCO_3^-:CO_2$ to 20:0.5 or 40:1, which would give a pH of 6.1 + $\log_{10}$ (40/1) = 7.7. This occurs with a reduced oxygen level (hypoxaemia) at high altitude or with normal O_2 levels in conditions such as pneumonia and pulmonary oedema. Again, this cannot be compensated by a decrease in respiration, but the kidneys will conserve H^+ and excrete HCO_3^-.

Metabolic acidosis

Metabolic acidosis can be caused by a variety of conditions. One type increases [H^+] by changes in metabolism that produce abnormally high levels of H^+. An example of this is during starvation where a lack of adequate calories leads to the body consuming its fat and protein reserves, which produces large quantities of non-carbonic acids. These are then buffered by plasma HCO_3^- so the production of these acids results in a reduction in plasma HCO_3^-. Another cause of this type of metabolic acidosis occurs during cardiogenic shock. This occurs most commonly following a heart attack. Damage to the heart reduces its ability to pump effectively, so tissues do not receive adequate oxygen. Instead of normal aerobic respiration, which uses oxygen and generates CO_2, they then start to respire anaerobically, which generates lactic acid. In other conditions, a decrease in pH can be caused by losses of HCO_3^-. An example of this is severe diarrhoea such as occurs in cholera, where a rapid loss of the intestinal and pancreatic secretions, which are rich in HCO_3^-, prevents the reabsorption of HCO_3^- in the intestinal tract.

A compensatory response to metabolic acidosis is rapid breathing – which is the respiratory system exhaling more CO_2 in an effort to increase the pH. This may serve to buffer some of the increase in H^+ but, as mentioned above, once the pH returns towards normal, the drive to increase ventilation is reduced. The excess H^+ (or reduced HCO_3^-) must eventually be restored to normal values by the kidneys. If the cause of the metabolic acidosis is renal disease then this is extremely dangerous as the kidney loses the ability to secrete H^+ and ammonia.

Metabolic alkalosis

Metabolic alkalosis is rare, as the kidneys are usually very good at excreting excess HCO_3^-. However, it can be produced by acute losses of [H^+] or an increase in [HCO_3^-]. A loss of H^+ can be caused by vomiting of stomach contents, which are highly acidic (see Table 1.2) and lead to a loss of H^+ that has to be replaced from the blood. A common cause of an excess of HCO_3^- is overuse of either soluble analgesic preparations or antacid tablets, both of which contain large quantities of alkali. An increase in HCO_3^- can also be caused

by severe constipation, which leads to excess HCO_3^- being reabsorbed from the intestine. Both conditions will lead to a respiratory response of reduced ventilation. However, because of other factors that drive respiration, this response is limited and most of the compensation must occur by renal mechanisms.

FLUID BALANCE

The example of homeostasis and homeostatic imbalances shown by acid–base balance is only one of very many homeostatic systems that act throughout the body to maintain a constant internal environment. A large number of other examples can be used to show how important this balance is and the consequences of its failure, but one of the most critical is the maintenance of the correct fluid balance.

The human body contains large quantities of water in a number of different compartments, and the maintenance of the correct amounts of fluid, of the correct composition, in the different compartments is essential. Water is essential for all chemical reactions. Virtually all biochemistry happens in solution. Chemicals moving around and through the body either diffuse through water for short distances or, for longer distances, in bulk flow, in the blood.

BODY FLUIDS AND FLUID COMPARTMENTS

The **total body water** (TBW) of a 70 kg person is about 60%. This percentage varies with age and weight. Babies, at birth, are about 80% water, while an elderly person may only have about 50% water. As the amount of adipose tissue increases, the proportion of body water decreases. An average 70 kg person has about 20% fat and 60% water whereas a 100 kg person with 40% fat will only have 44% water.

The TBW is divided into two main compartments (Fig. 1.9) which have different ionic compositions (see Ch. 2, Table 2.15).

- **Intracellular fluid** (ICF), which is contained inside all cells, is about two-thirds of the TBW (or 40% body weight).

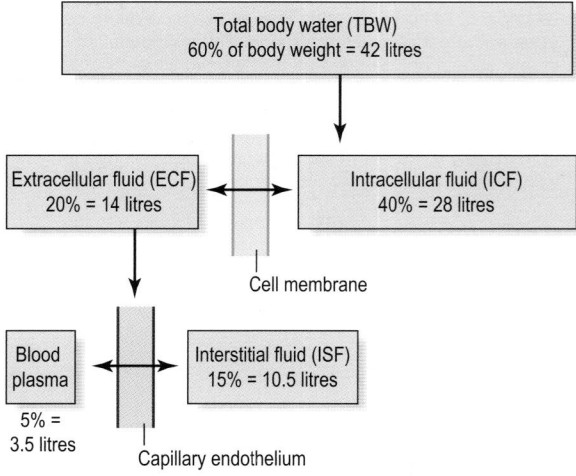

Fig. 1.9 Fluid compartments of the body. These are approximate values for a 70 kg person (per cent of total body water (TBW)).

High blood viscosity is dangerous

Blood plasma alone is slightly more viscous than water (1.2 times) but at a haematocrit of 0.45 the viscosity of blood is more than twice that of water (actually 2.4 times). This means that blood is thicker and harder to move round the body than pure water.

Anything which either increases the number of red cells, or decreases the plasma volume will increase the viscosity of the blood. If the haematocrit rises to 0.70, then the viscosity more than doubles. The blood becomes stickier and harder to move and there is a danger of blood clots, strokes and heart failure.

An increase in the number of red cells in the blood (a condition called **polycythaemia**) also increases the oxygen-carrying capacity. Athletes who cheat by injecting erythropoietin (EPO; a synthetic version of the hormone which stimulates red cell production) are at risk, especially during a long race in which they may also become dehydrated, which would increase the blood viscosity still further.

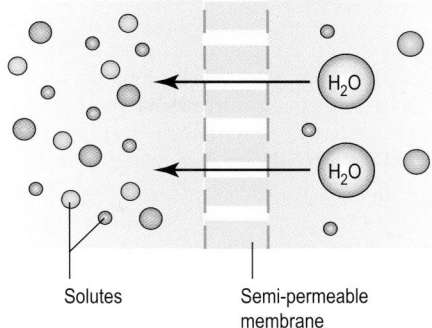

Solutes   Semi-permeable membrane

Fig. 1.10 Osmotic movement of water. Water flows across a semi-permeable membrane driven by osmotic pressure. The membrane is permeable to water but not to solutes.

- **Extracellular fluid** (ECF), which surrounds all cells, is about one-third of the TBW (or 20% body weight). The ECF itself is divided into two main compartments:
  - **Interstitial fluid** (ISF). This is about three-quarters of the ECF (or about 15% TBW). The ISF surrounds the cells but is outside the blood vessels. Unlike the blood plasma, it contains very little protein and few cells in suspension.
  - **Blood plasma**. This is one-quarter of the ECF (or about 5% TBW). It is the fluid inside the blood vessels and carries the other components of blood, such as red and white blood cells and plasma proteins, in suspension around the body.

Fig. 1.9 shows the volume in various compartments in an adult weighing 70 kg. As well as the fluid in the spaces between cells in the body tissues, the interstitial fluid includes extracellular fluids in particular areas such as the cerebrospinal fluid, which bathes the brain, the fluid inside the eye, fluid inside joints and fluid secreted into the intestines.

The total blood volume is about 5.5 L for a 70 kg person. Only 3.5 L of this is blood plasma, the remainder is mainly red blood cells. The ratio of the volume of red blood cells to the volume of whole blood is the **haematocrit** and is usually between 0.36 and 0.53 (men 0.42–0.53, women 0.36–0.45).

Separation of fluid compartments

The different fluid compartments are separated by **semi-permeable barriers** with different characteristics. In tissues, the cells are surrounded by membranes which allow water movement in and out of cells, but restrict the movement of the main extracellular ion, sodium. The ISF is separated from the blood plasma by a layer of cells, the endothelium. Gaps between the cells allow free movement of water and ions, but under normal conditions restrict the blood cells and proteins to the vascular compartment. This means that water can move freely between the compartments but that sodium does not move into cells, and proteins and blood cells are restricted to blood.

Fluid movements

The movement of water between the compartments is determined by the differences in hydrostatic and osmotic pressure in the different compartments. **Hydrostatic pressure** is produced by the pumping action of the heart, and **osmotic pressure** by the concentration of solute particles. Water moves osmotically from dilute to concentrated solutions, moving from a high concentration of water to a low one (Fig. 1.10). The more solute particles there are in a solution the greater the 'pull' on the water molecules. Osmolarity is determined by the number of osmotically active particles per litre and the normal osmolarity of body fluids is 290 mOsm/L.

Tonicity

The **tonicity** of a solution is the actual effect of a solution on a living cell. A solution bathing a cell that does not cause the cell to osmotically take up or lose water is said to be isotonic. A **hypertonic** solution, which contains more osmotically active particles than the cell, would cause cells to lose water and shrink. More dangerous for the cell are **hypotonic** solutions. These contain fewer osmotically active particles. In a hypotonic solution, the cell takes up water until it bursts (lysis).

The tonicity of a solution not only depends on the solute concentration but on the nature of the solute. For example, a solution of sodium chloride that has an osmolarity of 290 mOsm/L has no effect on the cells, so it is isotonic. However, a solution of urea of 290 mOsm/L causes cell lysis; it is hypotonic. This is because the cells are impermeant to sodium, which does not move into the cells, but urea can cross the cell membrane. So it moves into the cell, increasing the number of osmotically active particles inside the cell, then water follows and the cell swells and bursts. This shows that it is not only the volume of water surrounding the cells that is important but the solutes as well. In situations where body fluids are lost, such as in bleeding (haemorrhage) or burns, the types of fluids given as replacement will determine which fluid compartments they replace.

Under normal conditions, while there are large exchanges of fluid between the different fluid compartments over time there are no net changes in the volumes in each compartment. This is because the different compartments have the same tonicity. However, if there was a change in either the water content or solute concentration in a compartment then net changes would occur.

Solute contents

The three major fluid compartments have different solutes within them. The major **extracellular ions** are sodium (Na^+) and chloride (Cl^-). The major **intracellular ions** are potassium (K^+) and large anions such as protein and phosphate. The distribution of Na^+ and K^+ are determined by the action of specific transporters, the Na^+/K^+-ATPases (see Ch. 2), which simultaneously move K^+ into cells and Na^+ out of cells. The cell membranes are permeable to K^+ but not to Na^+, so K^+ can diffuse out of cells but the Na^+ cannot move in.

The ISF is also different from blood plasma in that blood contains large amounts of protein that cannot diffuse out of the blood because of the endothelium. This means that while the ionic content of the plasma and ISF is the same, the added protein in the plasma has an osmotic pull (called the **colloid osmotic pressure**) that opposes the hydrostatic pressure of the blood, which would tend to push fluid out of the blood into the ISF. This means that the volume of the blood compartment remains constant.

DAILY FLUID BALANCE

Fluid balance means balancing water intake with water losses and maintaining the appropriate water and solute content of the fluid compartments. The amount of sodium in extracellular fluid is controlled by processes occurring in the kidney, detailed in Ch. 14. Overall fluid balance is controlled by both behavioural and hormonal mechanisms.

Fluid intake and output

The amount of water that needs to be ingested every day varies according to climate and activity, but for adults in temperate climates it is an average of about 2.5 L/day (Fig. 1.11). Most of the water intake is via ingested fluids, either as drinks or in food, but about 10% is produced by metabolic processes within the body.

Water output occurs mainly by the production of urine in the kidney, but there are other losses in faeces and sweat as well as loss by evaporation from the lungs and skin. The amount of water lost in these different ways will vary enormously depending on levels of activity. The amount and concentration of urine can vary enormously. On a low-protein and low-salt diet, a minimum of 300 mL of urine per day needs to be produced in order to eliminate accumulated solutes, particularly nitrogenous waste, from blood. Higher

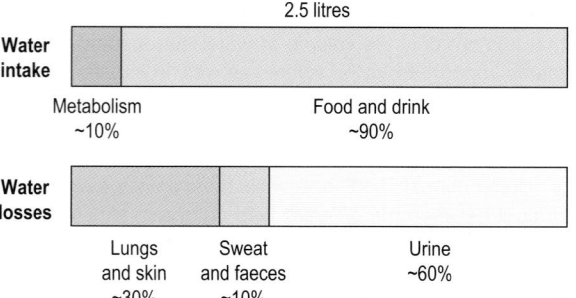

Fig. 1.11 **Approximate daily water intake and water losses for an average adult in a temperate climate.**

protein diets require higher minimum urine production. However, much more is produced, as water intake normally exceeds the minimum necessary.

Thirst

One of the ways in which the fluid intake is controlled is by the sensation of **thirst**. Thirst is stimulated either by an increase in the osmolarity of blood, which is sensed by receptors in the hypothalamus of the brain, or a fall in the total blood volume. Immediately on drinking and before water is absorbed in the intestine, the sensation of thirst is quenched, preventing excessive consumption. This tends to encourage multiple small drinks until fluid balance is restored. Very salty foods stimulate thirst, e.g. salty crisps and peanuts sold in bars to go with beer.

Regulation of water loss in the kidneys

The kidneys filter the plasma to form urine. This filtration is driven by hydrostatic pressure of the blood. The volume of filtrate produced is partly determined by the blood pressure and partly by the blood flow to the kidneys. If blood volume is low, then the blood flow to the kidneys is reduced so less filtrate is produced. If blood volume is high, then blood flow to the kidneys is high and more filtrate is generated.

Large volumes of filtrate are produced daily. This is necessary in order to filter the waste solutes from blood. On average 120 mL/min of filtrate are produced, which would amount to 170 L/day. So obviously most of the water filtered in the kidney must be recovered. After being filtered, the primary filtrate passes through the tubules of the kidney where its composition is modified by transport processes. The urine then passes into the collecting ducts before being passed into the bladder.

Vasopressin

The main mechanism for controlling the volume of the urine depends on the production of a hormone that controls water losses in the urine. **Vasopressin**, also known as anti-diuretic hormone (ADH), is released into the blood from the posterior pituitary gland, situated at the base of the brain. This release is stimulated by osmoreceptors in the hypothalamus in response to an increase in osmolarity of the blood. Vasopressin is also secreted in response to a fall in blood pressure, sensed by pressure receptors found in the heart and large blood vessels.

Much of the water in the primary filtrate (75%) is recovered by osmotic processes in the early part of the kidney tubules (the proximal tubule). Here, movements of sodium from the filtrate to the blood produce an osmotic gradient that reabsorbs much of the filtered water. The final concentration of the urine, however, is determined in the latter part of the tubules. When the urine needs to be concentrated, vasopressin is released and acts on cells in the distal tubule and collecting ducts to increase their permeability to water. The tissue surrounding the collecting ducts is hyperosmotic compared with the dilute urine, so water then passes back into the tissues and hence into blood. If blood pressure is high or the blood is hypo-osmotic (too dilute) then no vasopressin is produced and dilute urine passes into the bladder, allowing water loss. The amount of urine produced can vary enormously from 0.5–20 L/day and in osmolarity from 50–1200 mOsm/L. However, there are many conditions where either too much or too little urine is produced, or it does not have the correct concentration.

Other hormones control the excretion of sodium (and potassium) in the urine and this has a large effect on water movements. A high concentration of sodium chloride in the urine will tend to draw water into the urine and vice versa. However, up to certain limits it is possible for the sodium and water losses to be controlled independently (Ch. 14).

FAILURES OF FLUID BALANCE

If too much urine is produced then the body fluids become depleted and **dehydration** occurs. If too little urine is produced then the body becomes overloaded with water.

Dehydration

If water intake is insufficient to cover water losses over a period of time, then eventually water is lost, not just from the plasma but also from the ISF. Water then moves out of cells and cells shrink. Early symptoms are dry mouth, thirst, dry skin and a low volume of urine. This can lead to weight loss, fever and confusion. Concentration of the blood can increase the work load of the heart and may cause blood clots (see Clinical box 1.3).

Excess urine production occurs in both forms of diabetes. In the more common diabetes mellitus, excess sugar in the urine increases the osmolarity of the urine and prevents water reabsorption. In diabetes insipidus up to 40 L/day of dilute urine is produced due to either failure of vasopressin secretion or a failure of the kidney to respond to vasopressin. Both types of diabetes are characterised by the production of large volumes of dilute urine accompanied by thirst and frequent drinking. In diabetes mellitus the urine contains lots of sugar, hence the name mellitus or honey, whereas in diabetes insipidus the urine has very little taste, hence insipidus or tasteless.

Both the very young and the elderly are prone to dehydration. Newborn infants do not have fully developed kidneys and cannot concentrate urine up to the age of 2 months. Because of this, infants produce a lot of urine and in hot weather must take in large amounts of fluid to compensate for these losses. Infants with diarrhoea lose large quantities of fluid and so proportionally must take in more fluid than adults. Kidney function declines with age, with tissue atrophy and loss of function. By aged 70 about half of kidney function is lost. Combined with a reduction in the size of the bladder, this means that many elderly people have to get up in the night to urinate (nocturia). Recently, the death of elderly people in care homes during hot weather, particularly in France, has been ascribed to dehydration as they were unable to obtain sufficient fluids.

Water intoxication

When too much water is drunk too fast or there is a complete blockage of urine production, there is a dilution of body fluids. The sodium concentration of the ECF is reduced causing an osmotic shift of water into cells and cell swelling. This is particularly dangerous in the brain, where swelling can cause convulsions, coma and death.

Oedema

Swelling of the tissues due to the accumulation of fluid is called **oedema**. It has many different causes, several of which have little to do with overall fluid balance. As mentioned earlier, there are large quantities of fluid exchanged between different compartments. Over 4000 L/day of fluid leaves the smallest blood vessels, the capillaries, due to a very slight excess of hydrostatic pressure over the colloid osmotic pressure. However, under normal circumstances, all of this fluid returns to the circulation. If only a very small proportion of this fluid is retained by the tissues then oedema can occur (Ch. 11).

A modest example of this occurs every day when a pair of shoes which seem perfectly comfortable in the morning are tight by the evening. This is because during the day some of the fluid leaving the capillaries in the legs accumulates in the feet due to gravity, making the feet swell. During the night, the fluid is redistributed returning the feet to their previous size.

FAILURES OF HOMEOSTASIS

The two examples of homeostasis described in detail here illustrate how multiple body systems are involved in maintaining homeostatic balance for a single variable. Acid–base balance requires the effort of both the respiratory (Ch. 13) and renal systems (Ch. 14), coordinated by the nervous system (Ch. 8), in order to keep [H$^+$] within suitable limits. Fluid balance is achieved by the coordinated actions of the renal (Ch. 14), cardiovascular (Ch. 11), endocrine (Ch. 10) and nervous systems (Ch. 8).

Throughout this book you will come across many other examples of both how homeostasis is achieved and the consequences of its failure. There are some diseases that are currently on the increase and seem to be a consequence of modern living. Humans evolved to survive in a very different type of environment from that in which we now live, and there are occasions where adaptations for that environment are no longer adaptive to the current situation. Some diseases seem to be made worse by homeostatic compensations that have not evolved to deal with modern circumstances.

DIABETES AND OBESITY

A serious failure of homeostasis that is becoming more common in affluent societies is the failure of blood sugar regulation known as type 2 (or late-onset) **diabetes mellitus**. Diabetes currently affects more than 30 million people and the current rate of increase is so rapid that the World Health Organization (WHO) estimates that by 2025, more than 300 million people worldwide will have diabetes. Although diabetes can be treated with drugs, including insulin, even those people with diabetes who have reasonable control of their blood sugar levels have a reduced life expectancy and have a higher incidence of strokes, heart attacks (myocardial infarction) and vascular diseases. Diabetes damages many organs in the body, especially the eye, the kidney and the nervous system; damage to the nerve sheaths in the nervous system causes subsequent damage to the underlying nerve fibres all around the body.

This type of diabetes is often associated with excessive food intake and lack of exercise, which lead to **obesity**. More than 18% of the world's population are either overweight or obese (ironically a similar number are underfed). Modern humans, at least in Westernised societies, are exposed to an abundance of high-calorie foods and also cars, which allow us to avoid physical activity in almost all situations. While many of the infectious diseases which plagued human societies for millennia are now curable or preventable, leading to increased life expectancy, new ones such as HIV/AIDS are now reversing that trend, and changes in our lifestyles are presenting new problems. In the distant past, humans rarely had access to the types of high-calorie food freely available today at every shop and supermarket. We are adapted to store food efficiently for times of need and now, for a significant part of the world's population, the lean times never come.

HIGH BLOOD PRESSURE

Another way in which our own biology seems to works against us is in the case of high blood pressure. **Hypertension** is a serious cardiovascular problem for increasing numbers of people (Ch. 11). Using the World Health Organization (WHO) criteria to define hypertension, as many as 36% of males in the USA between 18 and 74 have hypertension. Hypertension is often a silent killer, as it has few symptoms of its own, but leads to a much higher risk of heart disease and strokes. The first time many people are aware of the problem is when they have a heart attack or stroke, or, if they are lucky, when they have their blood pressure checked at a routine medical check-up.

There are a number of theories about why the blood pressure is raised initially, but it is clear that once the higher blood pressure is established then homeostatic mechanisms work to maintain the blood pressure at the elevated value. That is, the set point is altered to the higher value. One of the adaptations in hypertension is the thickening of the rings of smooth muscle which control blood flow into the tissues, the arterioles. Under normal conditions when the blood pressure is raised, for example during exercise, the arterioles contract to reduce the lumen size in order to prevent the high pressure being transmitted into the smallest blood vessels, the capillaries, which could be damaged by these higher pressures. However, during exercise the rise in blood pressure is transient and the arterioles can relax immediately afterwards.

In hypertension the increase in blood pressure is sustained, and, just as muscles trained by weightlifters increase in size in response to increased work, the arterioles which are being constantly stressed respond by thickening. This thickening decreases the size of the lumen, through which blood flows and, as the ease with which blood flows through the arterioles is related to their diameter (just as water flows more easily through big pipes than small ones), this reduces the blood flowing into the tissues. In order to compensate for this the heart has to work harder to push the blood through the narrowed arterioles. This increases the blood pressure still further, setting up a positive feedback loop. A reduction in the blood flow to the kidneys will reduce urine production, which leads to increased blood volume. This raises the blood pressure further. Although there are effective drugs to treat hypertension, the underlying causes are complex and epidemiological evidence suggests that for many patients lifestyle factors play a role in the development of the disease.

Knowledge of the normal physiological mechanisms that underpin homeostatic control can help in understanding how these go wrong and produce disease, and how helping the body's own systems to regain control can reduce or eliminate the problems.

2

Biochemistry and cell biology

Patricia Revest

INTRODUCTION

The human body is mainly water plus a wide variety of biologically active chemicals which subserve all the functions of the body. **Biochemistry** describes how these molecules are made and the interactions between them at molecular level. **Cell biology** then goes on to describe how the biochemicals are organised into cells and cellular components, which then form the tissues of the body. Normal processes within the body are called **physiological**, whereas processes that cause disease are called **pathological**.

Metabolism

All the processes of replication, growth, repair and so on that are vital to the survival of a cell require energy. Much of the economy of any cell is taken over by the chemistry required, firstly, to generate that energy, and, secondly, to harness it to drive crucial processes or to build molecules needed by the cell to maintain itself. All this chemistry is termed **metabolism**. We can think of cells as being extremely complex chemical machines. At any time a cell may have many thousands of individual chemical reactions going on simultaneously, each a part of a **metabolic pathway** that may result in the breakdown of larger molecules, or the assembly of large molecules from smaller ones, or simply the conversion of one molecule into another. All of these pathways need to be controlled so that molecules are produced in the right place in the right amounts.

Catabolism and anabolism

In general, metabolism that involves degrading complex molecules to simpler ones, called **catabolism**, is the route by which chemical energy is generated. By contrast, the metabolism that results in the synthesis of more complex molecules from simpler components, **anabolism**, has a net requirement for chemical energy. It is these synthetic metabolic pathways that produce the components needed for cell growth, repair and replication.

Cells

The **cell** is the basic unit of living organisms. All living things consist of cells and although there are many organisms which exist as single cells, such as bacteria and amoeba, the largest living organisms on Earth, such as the great blue whale, also consist of aggregates of the same basic cellular units, although in rather large numbers. An adult human has somewhere in the region of 10^{15} cells.

All living organisms are made up of one of two types of cell: **prokaryotes** and **eukaryotes**.

Table 2.1	Eukaryotic kingdoms	
Kingdom	**Examples**	**Examples of pathogens**
Protists	Protozoans, algae, slime moulds	*Plasmodium* spp. (malaria)
Fungi	Yeasts, moulds, mushrooms	*Candida albicans* (candidiasis or thrush)
Plants	Mosses, ferns, conifers, flowering plants	None, although many plants are poisonous to humans
Animals	Sponges, corals, arthropods, amphibians, reptiles, birds, mammals	*Taenia solium* (tapeworm)

Table 2.2	Chemical elements of the human body	
	Element (atomic symbol)	**Abundance (% wet weight)**
Major elements	Oxygen (O)	65.0
	Carbon (C)	18.5
	Hydrogen (H)	9.5
	Nitrogen (N)	3.3
	Total	96.3
Minor elements (in order of abundance)	Calcium (Ca), phosphorus (P), potassium (K), sulphur (S), sodium (Na), chlorine (Cl), magnesium (Mg)	
	Total	3.7
Trace elements (in alphabetical order)	Aluminium (Al), boron (B), chromium (Cr), cobalt (Co), copper (Cu), fluorine (F), iron (Fe), manganese (Mn), molybdenum (Mo), selenium (Se), silicon (Si), tin (Sn), vanadium (V), zinc (Zn)	

Prokaryotes

Two of the major kingdoms into which organisms are classified are the Eubacteria and the Archaebacteria. These are all prokaryotes. Prokaryotic cells lack a nucleus and other internal structures. All prokaryotic organisms are single celled; they are extremely numerous and can be found in almost all environments, including some which seem too hostile to support living things. The earliest organisms on Earth were prokaryotes, and they were the only living things for more than 2 billion years. From the point of view of medicine, the bacteria are important in that they cause many of the infectious diseases.

Many chemicals and chemical processes which occur in the human body are similar to those found in many other organisms, including prokaryotes. However, there are also significant differences and sometimes these can be exploited, for example in the use of antibiotics that can kill bacterial cells that have invaded the body, without killing the host, by exploiting differences in their biochemistry.

Eukaryotes

The other four kingdoms are made up of organisms with **eukaryotic** cells (Table 2.1). These cells have a nucleus and other internal structures which allow compartmentation of chemical processes within a single cell. The Protista contains both unicellular and multicellular organisms and it is thought that the organisms in the other three kingdoms evolved from ancient protists.

Viruses

Although **viruses** are not cells and as such are not strictly living organisms, they are dependent on the host's cells to reproduce, i.e. they are parasites. The effects of this parasitism are the symptoms of many viral infections. However, as with bacteria, differences in chemical processes used by viruses can be exploited to produce antiviral drugs.

Cells and viruses exist on different scales. Viruses are very small (60–80 nm), which is smaller than some of the intracellular components of eukaryotic cells. Most bacteria are between 1 μm and 10 μm and many eukaryotic cells are 10–100 mm.

BASIC CHEMISTRY

Chemical composition of the human body

The chemicals which make up the human body are mainly compounds consisting of combinations of carbon, hydrogen and oxygen atoms (Table 2.2) with small quantities of other elements. These are known as **organic** compounds because they contain carbon. Together with nitrogen, carbon, hydrogen and oxygen make up 96.3% of the body weight. The remaining 3.7% is made up of seven **minor elements**. As well as these major and minor elements there are a number of **trace elements** which are required in very small amounts (less than 0.01%). Many of these are needed as special components of proteins called enzymes and are required for their activation (see Regulation of enzyme activity).

CHEMICAL BONDS

In order for atoms to combine to form molecules, chemical bonds must be formed between the individual atoms (Fig. 2.1). There are three main types of chemical bonds:

- Ionic
- Covalent
- Hydrogen.

The strength of the different types of bond varies enormously (Table 2.3). Stronger bonds are more stable but, often, large numbers of weaker bonds stabilise molecular interactions.

Atomic structure

In order to understand how chemical bonds are formed it is necessary to know something about the structure of atoms. All atoms of a particular element have a nucleus of **protons**

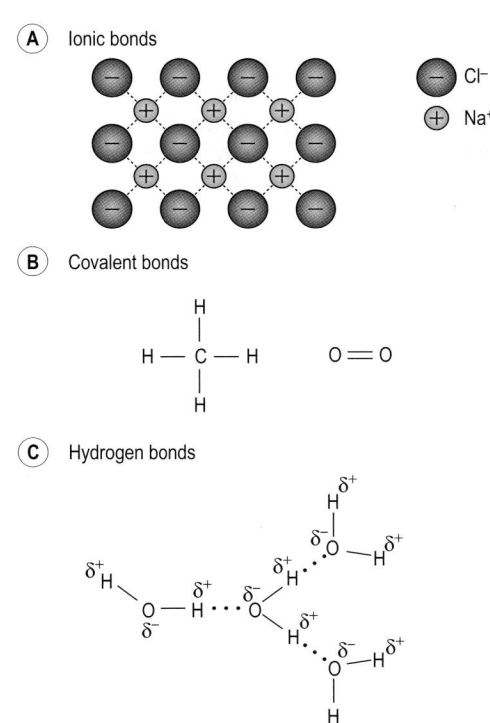

Fig. 2.1 **Different types of chemical bond.**

Table 2.3	Energy of some typical chemical bonds in biological systems	
Type of bond		**Energy (kJ/mol)**
Ionic		12.6–29.3
Covalent (single)		210–460
Covalent (double)		500–710
Covalent (triple)		815
Hydrogen		4.2–8.4
Van der Waals interaction		4.2

and **neutrons** (except ordinary hydrogen which has a single proton as a nucleus) surrounded by a cloud of electrons. The total number of protons in an element gives its **atomic number**, and the total of protons and neutrons (which may vary between different forms or **isotopes** of an element) gives the **atomic mass**. Carbon has six protons and an atomic number of 6, but it can have six, seven or eight neutrons. Its atomic mass is thus the average of the mass of the different isotopes: 12.01. This reflects the much greater abundance of carbon-12 (where 12 is the atomic mass) than the other isotopes, carbon-13 and carbon-14.

Atomic shells

The electrons which surround the nucleus are found in fixed energy levels called shells and there are strict rules about how many electrons can occupy each shell:

- The innermost shell can contain a maximum of two electrons
- The next shell can contain eight electrons
- The third shell can hold up to 18.

Atoms are at their most stable when their outermost shell is either full or contains eight electrons. The most stable

elements which exist are the noble gases such as helium or neon, which, with two and 10 electrons, respectively, have full outer shells. These atoms are chemically inert, their full outer shells rendering them non-reactive, and they rarely form compounds with other atoms. Atoms with unfilled outer shells are more reactive.

Ionic bonds

When dissolved in water many atoms are able to form charged particles called **ions** by either losing or gaining electrons from their outer shell:

- Atoms which gain an electron become negatively charged **anions**.
- Atoms which lose an electron become positively charged **cations**.

These ions will be attracted to each other by the opposite electrical charges, resulting in the formation of **ionic bonds**. The tendency of an atom to lose or gain electrons depends on the number of electrons already present.

Sodium chloride: an example of an ionic bond

Common salt, or sodium chloride, is a compound formed by the combination of sodium and chlorine atoms. Sodium has 11 electrons: both its inner two shells are full and it has a single electron in its outer shell. Chlorine has 17 electrons, again with full inner shells but with seven electrons in its outer shell. In water, sodium (Na) atoms lose a single electron to become sodium (Na^+) cations with a single positive charge. Chlorine (Cl) atoms gain the electron lost by the sodium to become chloride (Cl^-) anions with a single negative charge. When sodium chloride solution is dehydrated, then the ions form a lattice of interlocking anions and cations held together by the ionic bonds between the ions to give white salt crystals (Fig. 2.1A). The resulting sodium chloride has completely different properties from its component parts. Sodium is a highly reactive metal and chlorine is a poisonous green gas, but sodium chloride is the main ionic constituent of seawater, where life was thought to have evolved, and forms the major ions in the extracellular fluid which bathe all the cells in the body.

Ionic bonds are frequently formed between molecules such as potassium (K) or calcium (Ca), which have either one or two electrons in their outer shell – forming K^+ and Ca^{2+}, respectively – and fluorine or iodine, which like chlorine require only one electron to fill their outer shell.

Hydrogen ions

Hydrogen ions are formed by losing its single electron to form a cation (H^+). This ion is stable because its nucleus with its lone proton has an empty electron shell. However, hydrogen can also form an anion (H^-) with more reactive metals, called a hydride, with two electrons in its single shell. Water forms a small number of ions when it dissociates into H^+ and OH^- (hydroxyl) ions. This is depicted as $H_2O \rightleftharpoons H^+ + OH^-$ and is reversible, as indicated by the double arrows. These ions are important in many chemical reactions.

Covalent bonds

It is not necessary for an atom to completely lose or gain an electron in order to participate in chemical bonding. Atoms can share their electrons with other atoms to fill their outer electron shells part of the time. Up to three pairs of electrons can be shared, producing increasingly strong links known as **covalent bonds**. These bonds can form between atoms of the same element, as in the formation of O_2, where two oxygen atoms, each with six electrons in the second shell, share two pairs of electrons forming a double bond (O=O). Two hydrogen atoms form molecules of H_2 by sharing their electrons with a single bond (H–H). When a single atom of oxygen shares electrons with two atoms of hydrogen the result is the most abundant biological molecule of them all, water or H_2O.

Carbon bonds

Carbon can form a wide variety of covalent bonds with other atoms by sharing four of its electrons to form pairs (Fig. 2.1B). When a single carbon atom combines with four hydrogen atoms the simplest organic molecule, methane (CH_4), is formed. However, carbon can form long chains of atoms both with other carbon atoms and with other atoms to form complex biochemicals.

Stereoisomers

The four covalent bonds around a carbon atom are arranged in a tetrahedral pattern. When the four chemical groups are different this means that the molecule can exist as two mirror images, which cannot be superimposed. The asymmetric carbon atom is said to be **chiral** and the two molecules are called **stereoisomers**. Stereoisomers rotate polarised light in either a clockwise, or dextrorotatory (+), direction or in an anticlockwise, or levorotatory (–), direction.

Stereoisomers can only be converted, one to the other, by breaking and re-forming the covalent bonds. A molecule with one chiral centre has two stereoisomers, and one with n chiral centres has 2^n possible stereoisomers. This means that many organic molecules with identical formulae and chemical groups can exist in different forms depending on the number of asymmetrical carbon atoms. This is particularly important in the structures of macromolecules such as proteins and carbohydrates, in which the building blocks consist of specific stereoisomers.

Carbon–carbon double bonds

Carbon atoms can also share two pairs of electrons to form carbon–carbon double bonds. These bonds are planar and rigid and do not rotate. When they occur in carbon chains they produce either *cis* or *trans* **isomers** depending on whether the next carbon atoms are:

- On the same side of the double bond (*cis*)
- On opposite sides (*trans*).

This isomerism is important in the structures of fatty acids, which are components of many lipids. Most important dietary fatty acids are in the *cis* form but commercially processed fats in foods such as some margarines and peanut butter contain *trans* forms, which are known to raise blood cholesterol. Recent nutritional guidelines recommend that consumption of these types of fatty acids be limited.

Polar and non-polar covalent bonds

In covalent bonds between atoms, the electrons are not always equally shared between the atoms. When the electrons are more attracted to one of the atomic nuclei, then the bond has two poles of charge called a **dipole** and the bond is called a **polar** covalent bond. This occurs in H_2O, where the electrons are closer to the oxygen atom than the hydrogen atoms. The oxygen then has a partial negative charge (δ^-) and the hydrogen atoms partial positive charges ($\delta+$). These partial charges affect the way these molecules react, and are particularly important in the way water molecules interact. In compounds such as methane, where the electrons are shared equally, the bonds are called **non-polar** covalent bonds.

Hydrogen bonds

The partial positive charges caused by the unequal sharing of electrons by hydrogen atoms are attracted to the partial negative charges on atoms such as oxygen and nitrogen. This forms a weak bond called a **hydrogen bond**. Although this type of bond is only about 1/20 as strong as a covalent bond, the presence of a large number of hydrogen bonds can produce a significant cohesive force. Many large molecules contain numerous hydrogen bonds between different parts of the molecule and these help to maintain the structure.

Hydrogen bonds can be disrupted easily, by heat and by excess acidity, causing a molecule to lose its shape and possibly its function. This is shown clearly in the formation of ice crystals where the regular lattice of the frozen water molecules is held together by the hydrogen bonds between the molecules (see Fig. 2.1c). When ice is heated, the hydrogen bonds are disrupted and ice becomes liquid water.

Other molecular interactions

Two types of interaction between non-polar molecules produce attractive forces between molecules:

- Van der Waals interactions
- Hydrophobic interactions.

Van der Waals interactions happen when transient dipoles occur in the electron clouds of uncharged molecules in close proximity. The resultant force depends on the distance between the molecules, as these interactions can only occur when the atoms are 0.3–0.4 nm apart.

Van der Waals interactions are weaker than hydrogen bonding and are very dependent on the precise molecular shapes of the interacting molecules. However, two interlocking molecules can form very many of these contacts and, because of this, van der Waals interactions are particularly important in specific interactions between biological molecules, such as enzymes and their substrates.

Hydrophobic interactions take place between non-polar molecules, which do not contain either ions or dipoles and so do not interact with water molecules and are almost completely insoluble in aqueous solution. These molecules will aggregate together to exclude water. Such hydrophobic interactions are due to the fact that the insertion of a non-polar molecule into water requires energy because it involves distorting the interactions between the polar water molecules. Thus the most stable conformation of non-polar molecules is to exclude water and to form structures that have the least possible surface area exposed to water.

This exclusion of water by hydrophobic forces is the basis of cell membrane structure. Cell membranes are largely made up of molecules that are polar at one end, where they interact with water, attached to long, non-polar carbon and hydrogen chains which aggregate together and do not react with water.

BASIC CHEMICAL REACTIONS

In order for molecules to be formed, chemical bonds must be made or broken between the constituent atoms. There are three basic types of chemical reaction:

- **Synthetic** or **combination** reactions in which bonds form between two molecules or atoms to form a larger molecule, e.g. $X + Y \rightarrow XY$.
- **Decomposition** reactions where a molecule is broken down into smaller parts, e.g. $XY \rightarrow X + Y$.
- **Exchange** reactions where atoms are exchanged between molecules, e.g. $XY + AB \rightarrow XA + YB$.

Some reactions are thermodynamically irreversible; that is they will only proceed in a single direction. However, many reactions can be reversed, although sometimes this may require special conditions.

Oxidation–reduction (redox) reactions

A commonly occurring biochemical reaction is the **oxidation–reduction** or **redox** reaction. In this reaction one molecule loses electron(s) in a process called oxidation, with the lost electron(s) being transferred to another molecule in a process called reduction. The name 'redox' derives from the fact that, in biological systems, the molecule which often receives the transferred electron is oxygen.

Many redox reactions also involve the loss of two hydrogen atoms in the form of a hydrogen ion (H^+) and a hydride ion (H^-). Oxidation–reduction reactions allow energy, in the form of chemical bonds, to be transferred from the molecule that is oxidised to the molecule that is reduced. The process is best thought of as two tightly linked processes in which there is a reduction in the potential energy of the oxidised molecule, whereas the potential energy of the reduced molecule is increased.

For example, one of the basic reactions used to provide energy to cells by the metabolism of glucose is summarised as:

$$C_6H_{12}O_6 + 6O_2 \rightarrow 6CO_2 + 6H_2O$$

glucose + oxygen $\rightarrow$ carbon dioxide + water

This is an oxidation–reduction reaction: glucose is oxidised to carbon dioxide, losing hydrogen, and oxygen accepts the hydrogen and is reduced to water. However, in cellular metabolism it does not occur in a single step. In a series of linked reactions, the energy liberated in the oxidation of the glucose is transferred to other molecules which can then be used to drive other reactions.

Energy in chemical reactions

The breaking of chemical bonds requires energy input, whereas the formation of new bonds releases energy.

Thus chemical reactions produce:

- Either a net release of energy (**exergonic** reactions)
- Or a net absorption of energy (**endergonic** reactions).

In exergonic reactions the energy required to break existent bonds is less than that released by the newly formed bonds. The products have a lower potential energy than the reactants. The reverse occurs in endergonic reactions, where the products have a higher potential energy than the reactants. Many biochemical reactions (e.g. the redox reactions) couple exergonic and endergonic reactions to transfer energy between molecules.

Activation energy

The energy initially required to break the chemical bonds in the reactants is the **activation energy**. In order to react, molecules and atoms must collide with sufficient kinetic energy to overcome the repulsive force between their electron clouds, and this kinetic energy can be increased by raising the temperature. Increasing the concentration of the reactants also increases the chance of favourable collisions. Some reactions also require energy input to alter certain properties of the covalent bonds and others may require the excitation of electrons from inner electron shells into the outermost shell before the reaction can occur.

Catalysts

Special transport systems and mechanisms of compartmentation within cells can help to increase the effective concentration of a compound. However, large increases in temperature are undesirable in biological systems and many biochemical reactions would not occur without the presence of a **catalyst**. Reactions between molecules occur more readily if the reactants collide in the correct orientation. Catalysts act to lower the activation energy of the reaction by helping the reactant molecules to collide in a more favourable direction. The catalysts themselves are unchanged by the process so they can be used again and again. Biological catalysts called enzymes allow a large number of chemical reactions to occur at an appropriate rate and under normal physiological conditions, such as at normal body temperature. (see Enzymes, below)

INORGANIC MOLECULES AND IONS

We tend to think of life as being carbon-based. However, as well as the large number of carbon-containing organic molecules, there are large numbers of molecules which do not contain carbon but are also essential for life. These include water and many salts, acids and bases.

Water

Water makes up about 60% of the human body by weight. The large amount of water which is present in and around the cells has a number of functions. The most important of these is as a **solvent** for all the molecules, the **solutes**, which need to be in **solution** in order to participate in chemical reactions. Water is also an important **substrate** in many of these reactions. Many chemicals are transported around the body in solution and, without water, the gases oxygen and carbon dioxide could not be moved between the lungs and the blood.

A 70 kg human has approximately 42 L of total body water divided into two main compartments:

- **Intracellular fluid** contained within cells: about 28 L (approximately 40% of body weight).
- **Extracellular fluid**: about 14 L (approximately 20% of body weight), divided between the interstitial fluid of about 10.5 L and the blood plasma volume of about 3.5 L.

Water acts as a **lubricant**, preventing solid structures rubbing against one another and causing damage. It also cushions the brain within the solid skull, reducing the pressure applied by the brain's own weight to the base of the brain. This cushioning prevents some of the damage which could occur due to sudden movements of the head banging the brain against the inside of the skull (see Ch. 8).

The high thermal capacity of water also allows it to be used to dissipate heat easily from areas of high temperature, preventing cell and tissue damage, and the large amount of heat required to evaporate water released as sweat is a very efficient cooling mechanism.

Acids, bases and salts

Acids, bases and salts are organic or inorganic compounds which, when dissociated in water, form ions:

- Acids form hydrogen ions (H^+) and anions
- Bases form hydroxyl ions (OH^-) and cations
- Salts form anions and cations.

Acids and bases are crucially important in the control of the acidity (pH) of the body, which is maintained within very strict limits close to the neutral pH of 7 (see Ch. 1).

The salts sodium chloride (NaCl) and potassium chloride (KCl) are the main ionic constituents of the fluids outside and inside cells, respectively. Sodium and potassium ions are essential for the transmission of nerve impulses, and calcium is required for muscle contraction. However, the commonest salts present in the body are the calcium phosphates which make up the bones and teeth (see Ch. 9).

BIOLOGICAL COMPOUNDS

SIMPLE ORGANIC COMPOUNDS

The simplest types of organic molecules are the **hydrocarbons**, which are composed of carbon and hydrogen. They are divided into two groups:

- Those that do not contain double bonds and are called **saturated**
- Those containing double bonds and are called **unsaturated**.

Hydrocarbons are **non-polar** and **hydrophobic**. Long hydrocarbon chains form the fats that make up cell membranes and form dense energy stores. Another distinctive type of hydrocarbon is produced when carbon atoms form a ring structure with six carbon and six hydrogen atoms, known as benzene. These ring structures, called aromatic rings, may also contain nitrogen.

Common chemical groups

Apart from hydrocarbons, all of the other biochemicals in the body consist of molecules in which hydrogen has been replaced by other atoms or groups of atoms. Potentially, although there is a huge range of possible groupings of atoms that can be formed, there are a limited number of distinctive functional groups found on biological molecules (Table 2.4). The reactivity of these groups determines the roles played by the molecules that contain them and determine their interactions with other molecules.

Table 2.4	Common functional groups and classes of compounds (R represents the rest of the molecule)	
Group	**Formula**	**Class**
Hydroxyl	R—OH	Alcohols
Aldehyde	R—COH	Aldehydes
Carbonyl	R—CO—R′	Ketones
Carboxylate	R—COOH	Carboxylic acids
Ester	R—COO—R′	Esters
Amino	R—NH_2	Amines
Imino	R—NH	Imines
Amide	R—$CONH_2$	Amides
Phosphate	R—PO_4	Organic phosphates
Sulphydryl	R—SH	Thiols

Table 2.5	Macromolecules	
Macromolecule	**Monomer**	**Major functions**
Proteins (15%)*	Amino acids	Structural material, biological catalysts
Carbohydrates (2%)*	Sugars	Energy source, cell surface markers
Nucleic acids	Nucleotides	Genetic information (DNA and RNA)
Lipids (20%)*	(Many lipids are triacylglycerols)	Energy storage, cell membranes

*Note the percentages quoted are very variable due to the difference in fat and protein content in different individuals. The values shown here are a guide to their relative abundance.

MACROMOLECULES

Although a large number of small molecules are involved in biochemical processes, it is only in the formation of large molecules that the complexity of life becomes evident. There are three major groups of **macromolecules** present in the body. Each of these groups is formed from a number of related small molecules, **monomers**, which can be linked together by covalent bonds into polymers. The three groups of macromolecules are:

- Proteins
- Carbohydrates
- Nucleic acids.

A fourth group of molecules, which are not macromolecules in the same sense, are the **lipids**. These form macromolecular complexes by hydrophobic bonding.

Together, these four groups of molecules make up most of the remaining 40% of the human body, after water (Table 2.5). Although each of these groups has a particular type of building block, they often contain other molecules in varying amounts. For example, proteins often have carbohydrates covalently linked to them.

PROTEINS

Proteins have an enormous diversity of roles in the body and have the most complex structures of all of the macromolecules. Although all proteins are made in a similar manner and formed from similar building blocks, they have a wide variety of structures and functions, some examples of which are described below.

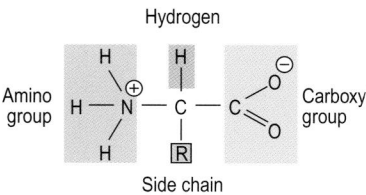

Hydrogen

Amino group

Carboxyl group

Side chain

Fig. 2.2 Generalised amino acid with ionised NH₃⁺ and COO⁻ groups in its two stereoisomers. The two molecules are mirror images of each other and cannot be superimposed.

Amino acids

Amino acids are the building blocks from which proteins are made. They also have other roles as neurotransmitters, as a source of energy, and as key intermediates in the maintenance of nitrogen balance.

Amino acid structure

Amino acids are a group of molecules with a common structure, which consists of a central carbon atom, attached to which are four different groups:

- A hydrogen atom (—H)
- An **amino** group (—NH₂)
- A **carboxyl** group (—COOH)
- A **side chain** (—R), which varies between the different amino acids.

At the normal pH of body fluids the amino and carboxyl groups of amino acids are ionised to NH₃⁺ and COO⁻, respectively (Fig. 2.2). This produces a molecule with positive and negative charges at opposite ends called a **zwitterion**. However, when amino acids bond together to form proteins, these charged groups combine. Thus it is only the side chains (and the terminal groups) that remain charged in proteins.

A wide range of amino acids are found in living things, but only 20 of these are made into human proteins (Table 2.6). The side chains vary in size and complexity, from a single hydrogen atom in glycine to the large side chains of tryptophan and arginine (Fig. 2.3). Each amino acid has a three-letter and a single-letter abbreviation.

Essential amino acids

There is a continual turnover of proteins in the body. This varies from minutes, in the case of some enzymes involved in metabolic control, to months, in the case of the main structural protein, collagen. Although some of the amino acids are reused many are metabolised, which means that even adults (who are not growing) require a daily dietary intake of protein. Eight of the 20 amino acids found in human proteins are called **essential amino acids** and must be included as components of the diet because they cannot be manufactured from metabolic intermediates (see Ch. 16). Dietary protein must be broken down in the gut to its constituent amino acids, which are then absorbed into the blood.

Table 2.6	Amino acids found in human proteins		
Classification	**Amino acid**	**Abbreviations**	
Non-polar aliphatic	Glycine	Gly	G
	Alanine	Ala	A
	Valine	Val	V
	Leucine	Leu	L
	Isoleucine	Ile	I
	Proline	Pro	P
Non-polar aromatic	Phenylalanine	Phe	F
	Tyrosine	Tyr	Y
	Tryptophan	Trp	W
Polar uncharged	Serine	Ser	S
	Threonine	Thr	T
	Asparagine	Asn	N
	Glutamine	Gln	Q
Polar negatively charged	Glutamic acid	Glu	E
	Aspartic acid	Asp	D
Polar positively charged	Lysine	Lys	K
	Arginine	Arg	R
	Histidine	His	H
Sulphur-containing	Cysteine	Cys	C
	Methionine	Met	M

Enantiomers

The central carbon atom is called the α-**carbon**. In all the amino acids except glycine, the presence of four different groups around the α-carbon means that each amino acid can exist in two **stereoisomers**. These pairs of amino acids are called **enantiomers** and are named D– (**dextro** = right) and L– (**laevo** – left). With very few exceptions, only L-amino acids are incorporated into proteins. However, D-amino acids are important constituents of the cell walls of bacteria, and as such are targets for antibiotics such as penicillin. One of the 20 amino acids, proline, is not actually an α-amino acid but an α-imino acid with an —NH— group instead of the amino (—NH₂) group. This has important structural consequences for proteins that contain this particular amino acid (see below).

Classification of amino acids

Amino acids are classified into groups according to the chemical properties of their side chains, R. For example, amino acids with polar side chains, and particularly charged ones, will form hydrogen bonds with water and will thus tend to be found on the parts of the protein exposed to the aqueous environment. Non-polar amino acids will be **hydrophobic** and will be found in parts of the protein not exposed to water. Amino acids are classified as follows:

- **Non-polar aliphatic**: these have side chains which consist of carbon and hydrogen atoms with no double bonds. These saturated hydrocarbons are hydrophobic.
- **Non-polar aromatic**: these side chains all contain aromatic rings. They are generally hydrophobic except for tyrosine, which has a hydroxyl group that can be found on the hydrophilic part of proteins.
- **Polar uncharged**: these neutral amino acids have polar hydroxyl or amide groups. The hydroxyl groups on serine and threonine, like tyrosine, are often on the hydrophilic surface of proteins where they are often modified to change the activity of the protein by phosphorylation.
- **Polar negatively charged**: these acidic amino acids have carboxyl groups that are negatively charged at pH 7.

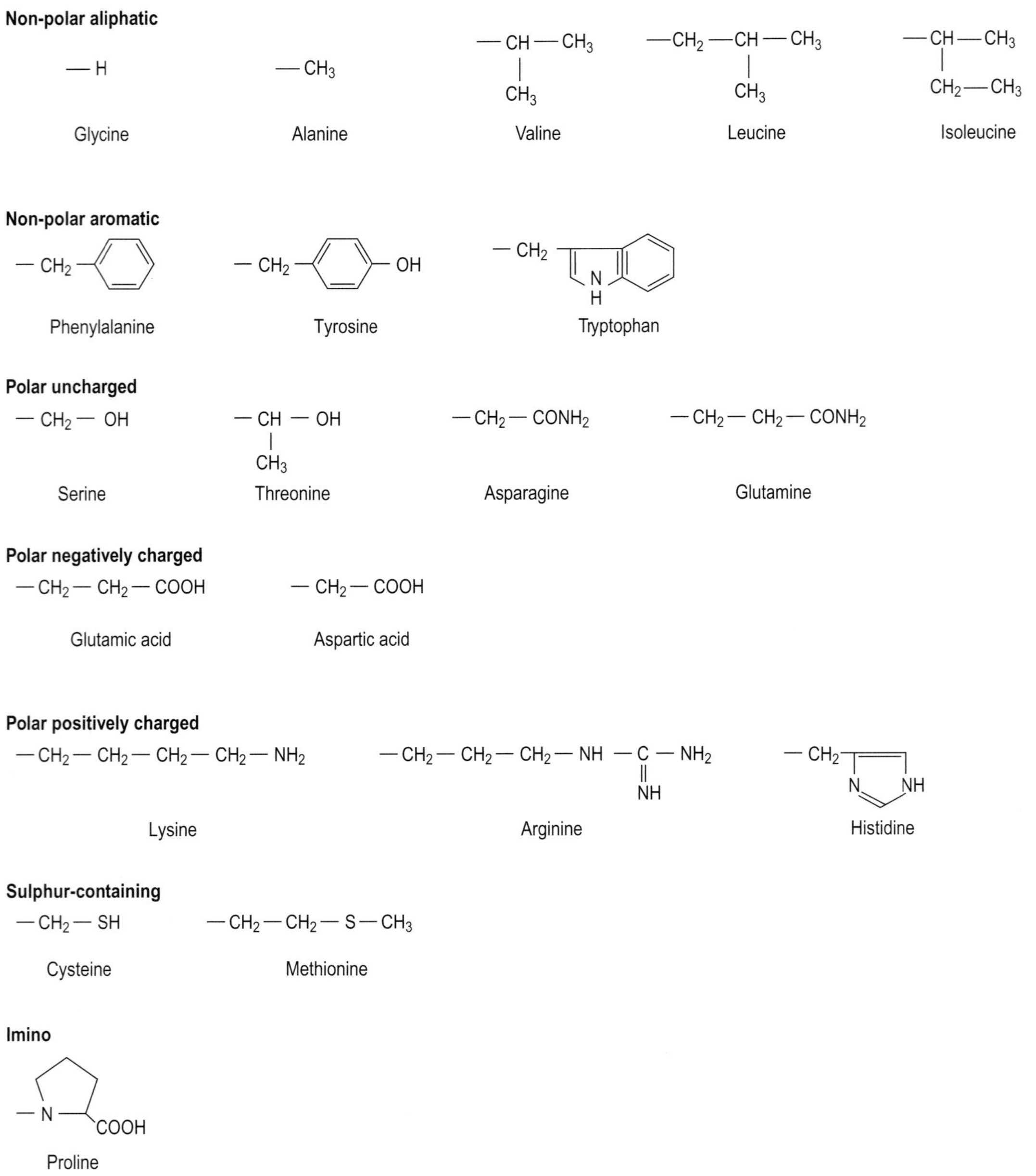

Non-polar aliphatic

— H	— CH₃	—CH—CH₃ | CH₃	—CH₂—CH—CH₃ | CH₃	—CH—CH₃ | CH₂—CH₃
Glycine	Alanine	Valine	Leucine	Isoleucine

Non-polar aromatic

Phenylalanine   Tyrosine   Tryptophan

Polar uncharged

— CH₂ — OH	— CH — OH | CH₃	—CH₂— CONH₂	—CH₂— CH₂— CONH₂
Serine	Threonine	Asparagine	Glutamine

Polar negatively charged

—CH₂— CH₂— COOH	— CH₂— COOH
Glutamic acid	Aspartic acid

Polar positively charged

—CH₂— CH₂— CH₂— CH₂— NH₂	—CH₂— CH₂— CH₂— NH —C— NH₂ || NH	—CH₂ ... N ... NH
Lysine	Arginine	Histidine

Sulphur-containing

—CH₂— SH	—CH₂—CH₂— S—CH₃
Cysteine	Methionine

Imino

Proline

Fig. 2.3 Structures of the 20 common amino acids. This diagram shows only the R group of each amino acid.

- **Polar positively charged**: lysine and arginine are both positively charged at pH 7. However, the side chain of histidine is mainly charged at a pH of 6.8 and mainly uncharged at a pH of 7.8. Variations in pH can therefore influence whether histidine residues are charged or not.
- **Sulphur-containing**: adjacent cysteine residues on protein chains can form bonds between their sulphur atoms called disulphide bonds. These are important in maintaining the structure of the protein and in forming links between separate protein chains.

Peptide bonds

Amino acids are linked together to make proteins by the formation of bonds between the carboxyl group of one amino acid and the amino group of the other, with the elimination of a water molecule. The reaction leaves an amide bond called a **peptide bond**.

$$^{+}H_3N\text{—}CHR\text{—}COO^{-} + {}^{+}H_3N\text{—}CHR\text{—}COO^{-} \rightarrow$$
$$^{+}H_3N\text{—}CHR\text{—}COHN\text{—}CHR\text{—}COO^{-} + H_2O$$

This reaction can be repeated, adding more amino acids to form a chain of amino acid residues with a carboxyl group at one end, the C-terminal, and an amino group at the other end, the N-terminal. Molecules containing two amino acid residues are called **dipeptides**, those with three, **tripeptides**. Usually peptides with more than 50 residues are called **proteins**, or **polypeptides**, and they can be made up of thousands of amino acids. Amino acid residues in a protein are numbered from the N-terminal end, which is the end from which protein synthesis starts.

The single covalent peptide bond has some of the rigidity of a double bond because electrons are unevenly shared between the COHN atoms (Fig. 2.4). This means that rotation around the C—N linkage is limited. However, rotation can still occur around the α-carbon atom and this rotation affects the way that the chains can fold.

Fig. 2.4 The peptide bond. The peptide bond is relatively rigid but rotation can occur around the α-carbon.

Protein structure

Although proteins can be thought of as a linear sequence of amino acids, this does not convey the fact that, in order to function properly, each protein chain must be formed into the appropriate three-dimensional shape. There are four levels of structure that are used to describe proteins.

1. **Primary**: the amino acid sequence of the protein linked by peptide bonds.
2. **Secondary**: regular structures determined by hydrogen bonding between the atoms of the backbone.
3. **Tertiary**: precise folding patterns of the polypeptide chain stabilised by a wide range of bonds between the amino acid side chains.
4. **Quaternary**: in multimeric proteins, the number and arrangement of the subunits.

Primary structure

The primary structure of a protein is the sequence of amino acids that makes up the protein chain. A chain with a large number of hydrophobic residues will have completely different properties from one with many polar, charged side chains. Likewise, the characteristics of a particular region of a protein will depend on the average properties of the amino acids in that region. Proline residues produce a very rigid molecule with kinks in the protein chain, and glycine residues have only a single hydrogen as their side chain and so take up only a small space. Glycine and proline residues are, therefore, often found in the regions of a protein where it loops back on itself.

Secondary structure

The primary structure of a protein determines the overall folding pattern of the polypeptide chain. However, there are a number of regular patterns of folding which occur, stabilised by hydrogen bonding between the atoms of the backbone of the peptide chain. These secondary structures are not dependent on the nature of the side chains as the hydrogen bonds form between the carbonyl group (C=O) of one peptide bond and the hydrogen atom of another.

There are two common types of secondary structure (Fig. 2.5), one forms a helical structure known as an **α-helix** and another forms ribbons which can interact with one another to form extensive **β-sheets**. A third important structural motif is the **U-turn**, which allows protein chains to rapidly change direction.

The α-helix

An α-helix is formed when the polypeptide chain is twisted into a rod, with the carbonyl group of each peptide bond hydrogen bonded to the hydrogen of the amide, which is four residues further down the chain (Fig. 2.5A). This coiling is

---

ⓘ Information box 2.1 Sickle cell anaemia

Changes in a single amino acid in a protein chain can have extreme consequences in the function of that protein. In sickle cell anaemia, the haemoglobin protein of red blood cells has a single change in one of the 146 amino acids which make up the β-globin chain. This is due to a mutation in the DNA which changes a single base from A to T, resulting in a glutamate (glutamic acid) residue at position 6 in the normal protein being replaced by a valine. This substitution of a negatively charged side chain by a non-polar hydrophobic one allows the proteins to form rigid rods under low oxygen conditions, changing the shape of the cells and making them inflexible and unable to travel through small blood vessels as readily. These rigid cells are phagocytosed more readily than normal cells, producing the characteristic anaemia.

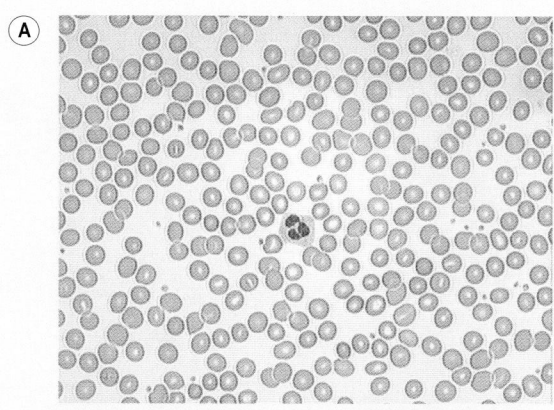

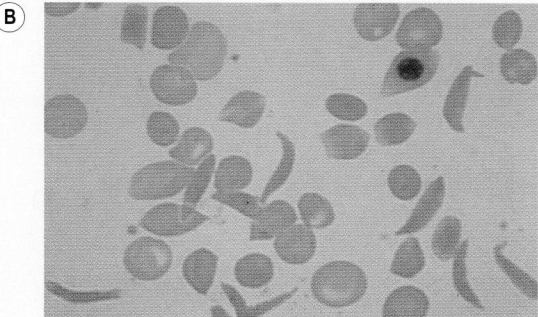

Blood films: (A) normal; (B) with sickle cells.

---

always right-handed (clockwise) and has a pitch of 3.6 residues per turn. Each amino acid adds 0.15 nm to the length of the helix. The structure is rigid and all the side chains face outwards. This means that the overall hydrophobicity of these α-helical regions of the protein are determined by the side chains and not by the backbone. Proline residues are rarely found in α-helices because their rigid structure would not allow them to twist at the appropriate angle.

β-Sheets

β-sheets occur where hydrogen bonds form between peptide chains that lie alongside each other (Fig. 2.5B). Because the four bonds around the α-carbon atom are arranged in tetrahedral fashion, the chains cannot lie completely flat and the β-sheet has a pleated appearance with the side chains protruding above and below the plane of the sheet. Some proteins are formed from multiple layers of β-sheets stacked on

i   **Information box 2.2**   α-Helical structures can cross cell membranes

The α-helix is commonly found in proteins that cross the cell membrane. These proteins have regions in which there are sequences of hydrophobic amino acid side chains that are about 25 residues long. An α-helix formed in these regions gives a rod with a hydrophobic exterior about 3.75 nm long, i.e. the length required to span the hydrophobic interior of the cell membrane.

Some of the helices have hydrophobic residues on one side of the helix and charged, hydrophilic residues on the other side. These are called amphipathic helices and they are found in proteins which form pores or channels in the cell membrane.

top of each other. An example of this is silk: its flexibility results from β-sheets sliding over one another, while its strength is due to the axis of the protein backbone lying parallel to the silk fibres.

U-turns

A third type of secondary structure formed due to hydrogen bonding is the **U-turn**. A U-turn consists of three to four residues, commonly glycine and proline, which form a short loop often found on the surface of proteins. The absence of a large side chain in glycine and the kink produced by proline allow the polypeptide chain to fold tightly back in the protein, facilitating a compact tertiary structure.

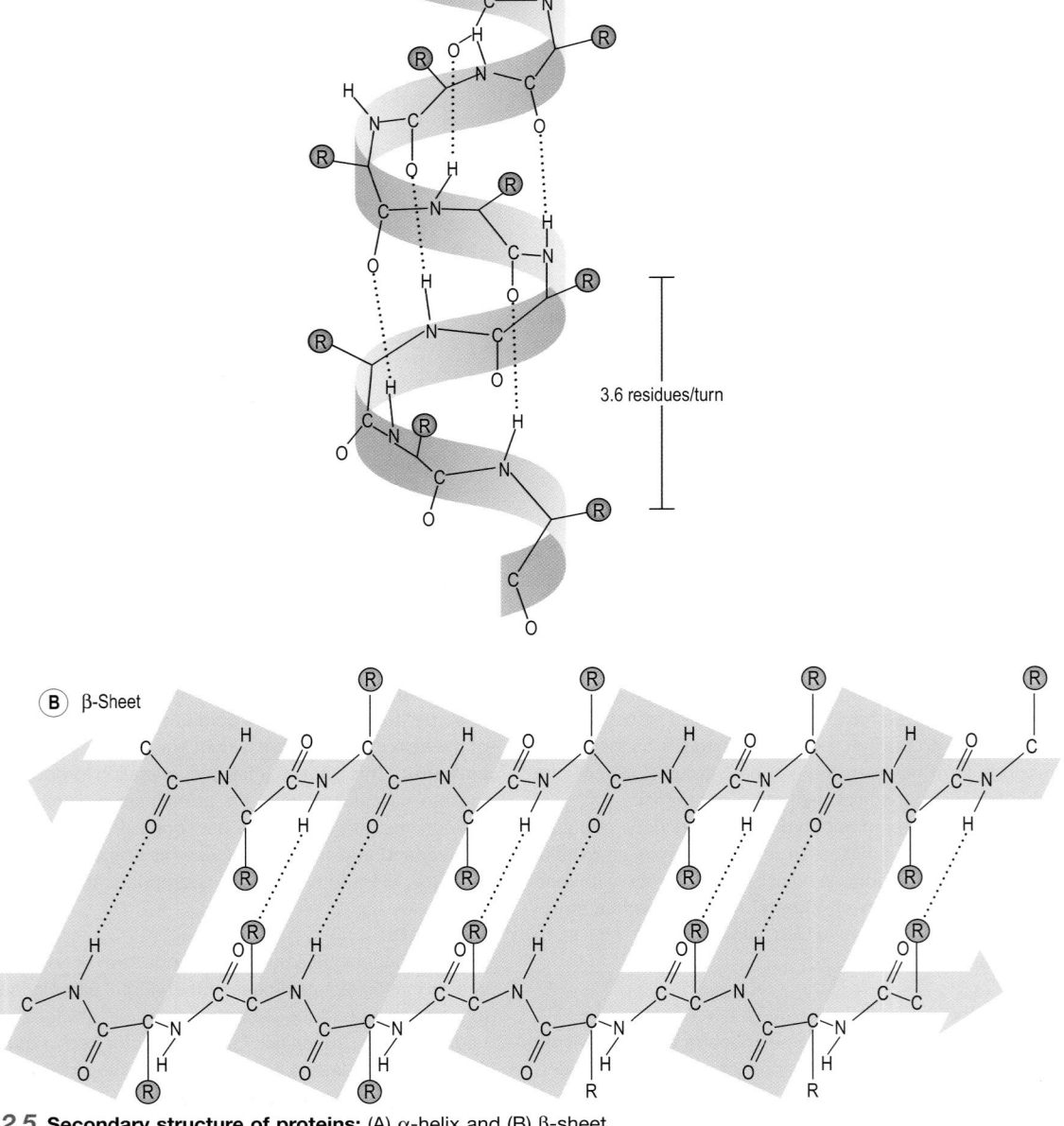

Fig. 2.5 **Secondary structure of proteins:** (A) α-helix and (B) β-sheet.

Tertiary structure

The next level of three-dimensional organisation of the polypeptide chain, the tertiary structure, results from a variety of interactions between the amino acid side chains. These interactions may include all the types of bonding already described. Tertiary structure specifies exactly how the entire protein is folded.

The type of interactions include:

- **Disulphide bonds**, between cysteine residues on the polypeptide chains
- **Hydrogen bonding** between side chains that have partial positive (δ^+) and negative (δ^-) charges, e.g. hydrogen bonding between serine and asparagine side chains
- **Ionic bonds** between oppositely charged side chains, e.g. between lysine and glutamate, sometimes called salt bridges
- **Hydrophobic interactions** in regions of the protein where there are large numbers of non-polar, aliphatic and aromatic side chains, which are excluded from the aqueous surroundings.

Denaturation

The tertiary structure of many proteins can be disrupted by heating, treatment with high concentrations of substances such as urea, or reducing agents which can break disulphide bonds. This is called **denaturation** and it leads to a loss of both tertiary and secondary structure, abolishing the protein's biological activity (which itself is often used as an assay of the degree of denaturation). The fact that some proteins can recover their activity when the denaturing agent is removed shows that the tertiary structure of these proteins is entirely determined by the primary structure. Examples of such proteins are lysozyme (an enzyme found in tears and saliva) and RNase (an enzyme which breaks down RNA).

Molecular chaperones

Not all denatured proteins can recover their structure and activity. The recent discovery of proteins called **molecular chaperones** or **chaperonins**, which aid the folding of the protein chain, has shown that at least some proteins require other factors to achieve the correct tertiary structure. These chaperonins may also be involved in increasing the rate at which naturally folding proteins can fold. Although many proteins are able to fold correctly in vitro this is a slow process and in vivo the chaperones make this process much more efficient.

ℹ Information box 2.3 | **Hair is made up of many α-helices**

Hair is made up largely of a protein called keratin. Single hairs are made up of hundreds of microfibrils embedded in a protein matrix. Each microfibril is formed from a number of α-helices that are wound around each other in a superhelix. Hairs can be stretched by elongating the α-helices, which breaks the hydrogen bonds in the helices. When the hair is released it reverts to its previous length because the covalent disulphide bonds between cysteine residues in the α-helix and the protein matrix remain intact. Hair can be permanently curled or straightened by applying chemicals which first break these disulphide bonds and then re-form them in the new conformation.

Quaternary structure

Although some proteins consist of a single chain, there are many **multimeric proteins**. These consist of multiple proteins held together by non-covalent bonds. These proteins have an additional level of **quaternary** structure which specifies how many of each type of subunit is included (stoichiometry) and how they are arranged.

An example of this is the most common type of antibody molecule, immunoglobulin G (IgG) (see Ch. 6). This type of immunoglobulin is composed of four protein chains, called heavy and light chains. The Y-shaped structure consists of two heavy and two light chains, joined by disulphide bonds and hydrogen bonds. Breaking the disulphide bonds between the chains destroys the quaternary structure, and separately the proteins chains have no biological activity.

Protein modification

Almost all proteins are modified in some way after they have been synthesised. Some of these modifications are permanent while others are reversible. Some involve chemical modification of either the terminal carboxyl or amino groups and/or modification of the side chains. Other changes involve removal of regions of the protein after it has been assembled.

Acetylation

The most common modification involves the addition of an acetyl (CH_3CO) group to the N-terminal. The effect of this covalent change is to reduce the rate at which these proteins are degraded, thus increasing their lifespan.

Glycosylation

Another common modification is the addition of carbohydrate molecules to the surface of the protein, a process called glycosylation. These **glycoproteins** and **proteoglycans** have many diverse roles including cell-to-cell recognition and as components of the extracellular matrix.

Glycoproteins

Only serine, threonine or asparagine side chains can be directly glycosylated. Serine and threonine are linked to carbohydrates via their hydroxyl groups (O-glycosylation) and asparagine via the amide group (N-glycosylation) of the asparagine side chain. Another amino acid, lysine, can have carbohydrates added to it after it has been modified to hydroxylysine.

The carbohydrates found on glycoproteins are often complex, branched molecules. Many of these glycoproteins are components of the plasma membrane and have their carbohydrate residues facing outwards and are thought to be involved in cell-to-cell recognition processes.

Proteoglycans

The other types of protein which have carbohydrates linked to them are called proteoglycans. They are protein chains where the core protein is linked to large, linear carbohydrates with a repeating unit.

Lipid modifications of proteins

Some proteins have fatty acids attached, which, through their hydrophobic interactions can then be inserted into the lipid bilayer of the cell membrane. These proteins are thus concentrated at the inner face of the cell membrane where they can interact more easily with other membrane proteins.

Phosphorylation

The activity of many proteins can be reversibly modified by **phosphorylation**. Enzymes called **kinases** add phosphate groups to the hydroxyl groups of serine, threonine and tyrosine residues found on many proteins. This change can have the effect of increasing or decreasing the activity of the protein. Other enzymes, **phosphatases**, can remove these phosphate groups. These changes in structure can act as a molecular switch that regulates the protein's activity.

Protein cleavage

Many proteins are formed from a precursor, which is then modified to make the mature protein. An example of this is the hormone, insulin, which is originally formed from a single peptide chain with 84 amino acids (pro-insulin). After the protein has been folded and disulphide bonds formed between two parts of the chain, part of the central part of the chain, called the C-peptide, is removed, leaving the two ends of the polypeptide, called the A and B chains, connected by the disulphide linkages. If the protein is denatured, for example by using mercaptoethanol which disrupts disulphide bonds, the A and B chains are separated. When the mercaptoethanol is removed the two chains do not reassociate, presumably because the most stable state for the separate chains is different from that of the original single, pro-insulin chain.

Enzymes

Almost all the biochemical reactions that take place in the body require the presence of protein catalysts called **enzymes**. Possibly as many as half of all proteins are enzymes, each with their own unique structure. They are globular proteins with irregular structures. They may contain short stretches of α-helices and β-sheets, but their overall forms vary enormously. Some enzymes fundamental to general metabolism are found in all cells, whereas others may only be found in specialised tissues. Enzymes act in the same way as inorganic catalysts in that they lower the activation energy of the reaction so that it can proceed under physiological conditions, i.e. at temperatures and pressures found in the human body. They can speed up the rate of reaction between 10^6- and 10^{12}-fold. Enzyme activity may be increased in some diseases and reduced, or absent, in others. Enzyme analysis can be an aid to the diagnosis of many conditions.

The general mechanism of enzymic action is as follows:

1. The reactants called **substrates** bind to the enzyme to form an enzyme–substrate complex.
2. The binding of the substrate causes changes in shape to occur within the enzyme–substrate complex. These internal rearrangements produce changes to bonds that favour the formation of the **product**.
3. The product is released from the enzyme, which reverts to its former shape. It can then go on to bind another substrate molecule.

Specificity

The substrates bind to the enzyme at the active site by a combination of ionic and hydrophobic interactions. The

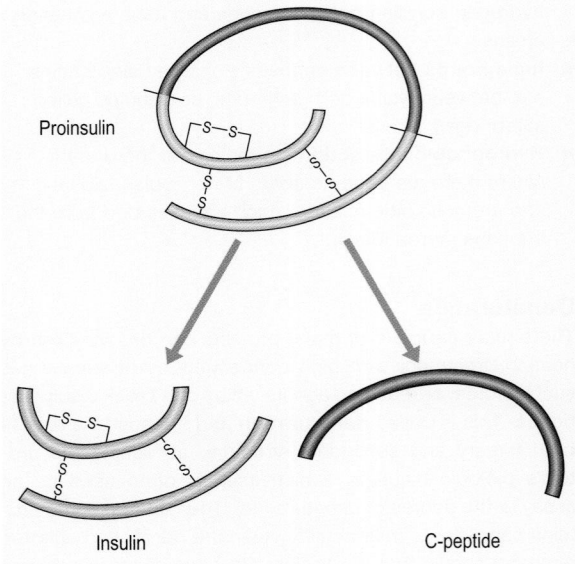
active site of each enzyme has a specific size and structure that allows the substrate to fit into it exactly, a characteristic that is often called a **lock and key mechanism**.

Some enzymes are very specific in their substrates, only catalysing the reaction of a single substrate, whereas others may accept a range of related substrates. Protease enzymes break down proteins by breaking peptide bonds, and different proteases act on different proteins. For example, trypsin is a proteolytic enzyme that will only hydrolyse those peptide bonds to which arginine or lysine contribute the carboxyl group. Pepsin, another gastric protease, is less specific in its substrates and will hydrolyse a wider range of peptide bonds.

Enzymes are very specific in the reaction they catalyse. The same substrate can be converted to a number of different products by the action of different reaction-specific enzymes. For example, pyruvate can be converted to lactate, alanine, oxaloacetate or acetyl CoA by different enzymes.

Enzyme nomenclature

Enzymes have specific names, depending on the reaction catalysed, the substrates and the products. They are classified into six classes, depending on the type of reaction catalysed (Table 2.7). However, many enzymes have a less formal 'common' name, which, for general use, describes their action and often their substrate.

Table 2.7	Classes of enzymes		
Class	**Type**	**Action**	**Examples of common names**
I	Oxidoreductases	Oxidation–reduction reactions, often with coenzymes, such as NAD$^+$	Dehydrogenase, oxidase, peroxidase, reductase
II	Transferases	Transfer of amino, carboxyl, acyl, carbonyl, methyl, phosphate groups from one molecule to another	Transaminase, transcarboxylase
III	Hydrolases	Cleave bonds between carbon and another atom by inserting water	Esterase, peptidase, amylase, phosphatase, pepsin, trypsin
IV	Lyases	Break carbon–carbon, carbon–sulphur and carbon–nitrogen (but not peptide) bonds	Decarboxylase, aldolase
V	Isomerases	Racemisation of optical or geometric isomers	Epimerase, mutase
VI	Ligases	Formation of bonds between carbon and oxygen, sulphur, nitrogen, etc, often hydrolysing ATP (adenosine triphosphate) to provide the required energy	Synthetase, carboxylase

Factors affecting enzyme activity

Enzyme activity (the rate of the enzyme-catalysed reaction) is affected by a number of factors:

■ Temperature
■ pH
■ Substrate concentration.

Temperature

Although normal body temperature is 37°C, a large number of enzymes increase their activity as the temperature is increased. This is because of the increased kinetic energy of the molecules and the increased likelihood the electrons will be excited. If the temperature falls the rate of reaction falls and sometimes the reaction will cease entirely. However, if the temperature returns to normal, the enzyme activity is regained.

If the temperature is increased above a certain level, the protein 'melting' point, the thermal excitation will be great enough to break essential weak bonding forces and the enzyme will become permanently disabled. At very high temperatures proteins become insoluble, as shown by the precipitation of egg white proteins during cooking.

Even though they catalyse the same reaction, some enzymes isolated from different tissues have different temperature resistance. For example, the differing denaturation temperatures of lactate dehydrogenase (LDH) have been used to distinguish heart and liver disease in assays where LDH of cardiac origin appears more heat stabile than that from the liver. The difference is due to LDH being present in different forms.

Optimal pH

All enzymes have an **optimal pH** at which they function at their fastest. Below or above this the enzyme's activity is reduced. For many enzymes the optimal pH is close to pH 7. However, there are some enzymes which have their optimal pH at very different acidities, reflecting the environment in which they work. For example, the enzyme pepsin, which digests proteins in the stomach has an optimal pH of about 2 which is the pH of the gastric juice in the stomach (see Ch. 15). Control of pH can also be a way of regulating enzyme activity. Enzymes which are inactive under normal conditions can become active when specific conditions change the pH.

Substrate concentration

The other major factor which determines the rate of reaction of an enzyme is the concentration of the substrate which is written as [S], where the square brackets represent the concentration. As the **substrate concentration** [S] is increased, the rate of the reaction increases: at first the increase is linear, then at higher [S] the rate of increase slows until the rate reaches a plateau, where any further increase in [S] does not produce any increase in the **reaction rate**.

This occurs because at low [S] the rate of reaction is limited by the limited number of substrate molecules which are bound to the active site. The initial increase in the rate is due to the increase in the binding of the substrate to the enzyme as the amount of substrate increases. As [S] increases further, more and more of the substrate binding sites are occupied until, at high [S] the enzyme is **saturated** with substrate, i.e. all the binding sites are occupied by substrate. At this point, even though there are more substrate molecules available, there are no binding sites available. The rate of the reaction is now limited by the rate at which the enzyme can catalyse the reaction and the rate at which the products leave the active site, making it available to more substrate. The maximum rate of the reaction is called the V_{max}. V_{max} is dependent on the quantity of enzyme present and the conditions such as temperature and pH, which affect the rate of catalysis.

Enzyme kinetics

If the initial rate of the reaction (v) at different [S] is plotted, the resulting curve is a **rectangular hyperbola**, described by the Michaelis–Menten equation. This is derived from the rate equation:

$$E + S \rightarrow ES \rightarrow E + P$$

where E is the enzyme, S is the substrate and P is the product.

$$v = (V_{max} \times [S])/(K_m + [S])$$

V_{max}, the maximum reaction rate, can be estimated from the plateau of the curve in Figure 2.6 where the rate of reaction is plotted against concentration. The other constant of the Michaelis–Menten equation is K_m. This is defined as the substrate concentration at which the rate is half V_{max}. The constant K_m is informative, as it describes the ease with which the substrate binds to the enzyme, or its **affinity**. K_m is inversely proportional to the affinity, with a low value of K_m indicating a high affinity. In other words, only a low concentration of substrate is required to saturate the enzyme and vice versa. The two constants, V_{max} and K_m, are characteristic for the enzyme–substrate combination under the conditions under which they are measured.

Curve fitting and linear transformations

Without using statistical curve-fitting programs it is very difficult to get accurate estimates of V_{max} and K_m from the Michaelis–Menten curve, especially as it is often difficult to see where the plateau stops rising, which occurs at very high levels of substrate. This leads to inaccurate estimates of V_{max} and because estimates of K_m use this inaccurate value, they themselves are inaccurate. This can be solved by using one of two possible rearrangements of the Michaelis–Menten equation that produce straight lines when plotted, where the kinetic constants can be easily identified from the slopes and the intercepts. These plots are called **Lineweaver–Burk** and **Eadie–Hofstee** plots (Fig. 2.7 and Table 2.8). Both of these linear transformations have some drawbacks because the use of reciprocals tends to underestimate errors in the data at different parts of the range. However, in the absence of curve-fitting programs, they are much better than the standard plot for estimating the kinetic constants.

The same mathematical models can be used to describe:

- **Membrane transport** (where J_{max} is the maximum rate of transport and K_m the affinity of the transport system for the substrate Carrier mediated transport)
- **Receptor binding** (where the constants are called B_{max} and K_d, see Ch. 3).

They can also be used to model drug interactions with a variety of targets.

The Michaelis–Menten equation applies only to a simple reaction with a single substrate. Reactions that involve multiple substrates can have different shaped curves, depending on the mechanism by which the substrates bind. In particular, reactions arising from cooperative interactions between substrate molecules, such as the binding of oxygen to haemoglobin, have sigmoidal curves,

Enzyme inhibition

Many enzymes involved in metabolic pathways are inhibited by the end-products or intermediates of those pathways. This is an important mechanism for controlling the production of metabolites in appropriate amounts. Many drugs used therapeutically act by inhibiting enzymes in order to reduce the amount of a particular reaction product. Inhibition can be reversible or irreversible.

Reversible inhibition

There are two types of reversible inhibition:

- Competitive inhibition
- Non-competitive inhibition.

They can be distinguished easily by looking at the effect of the inhibitor on the kinetic parameters of the reaction.

Competitive inhibition
Competitive inhibition occurs because the inhibitor binds reversibly to the same site on the enzyme as the substrate.

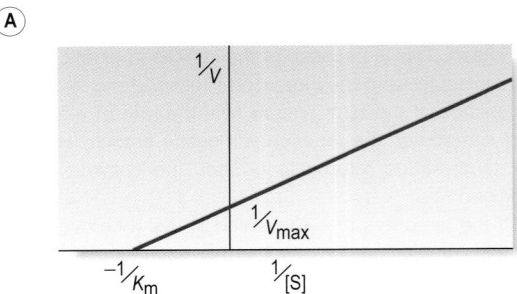

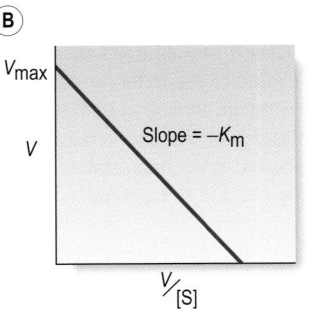

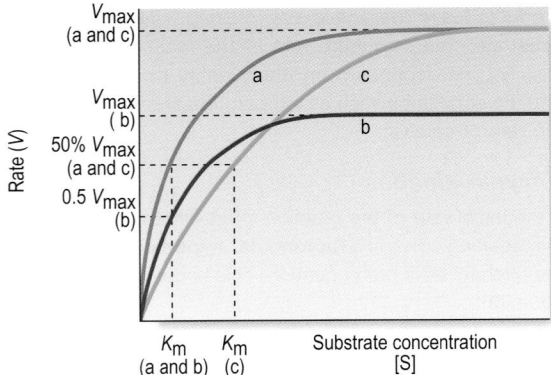

Fig. 2.6 **Michaelis–Menten curves.** Curves *a* and *c* have the same V_{max}, whereas curves *a* and *b* have the same K_m.

Fig. 2.7 **(A) Lineweaver–Burk plot:** x-intercept = $-1/K_m$, y-intercept = $1/V_{max}$. **(B) Eadie–Hofstee plot:** y-intercept = V_{max}, slope = $-K_m$.

Table 2.8	Kinetic constants from different plots				
Type of plot		**X-axis**	**Y-axis**	**V_{max}**	**K_m**
Michaelis–Menten		[S]	v	Plateau of curve	[S] at $\frac{1}{2} V_{max}$
Lineweaver–Burk		1/[S]	1/v	1/y-intercept	-1/x-intercept
Eadie–Hofstee		v/[S]	v	Y-intercept	$-$slope

Competitive inhibition of alcohol dehydrogenase can be used to treat poisoning by methanol and ethylene glycol

Methanol is poisonous to humans and can cause blindness. It can be formed accidentally in the production of homemade spirits, or can be ingested intentionally as 'meths' by alcoholics. The metabolism of both methanol and ethanol (and the antifreeze, ethylene glycol) involves the enzyme, alcohol dehydrogenase. Part of the treatment of poisoning by both methanol and ethylene glycol is the administration of ethanol in order to block their breakdown, as it is the breakdown products of methanol and ethylene glycol that are toxic. Ethanol has a higher affinity (lower K_m) for the active site of alcohol dehydrogenase than either methanol or ethylene glycol and so blocks their binding to the enzyme, and therefore their subsequent breakdown. They can then be removed from the blood by dialysis.

At low concentrations of substrate the enzyme activity is reduced, but as [S] rises the inhibitor is displaced and at very high [S] the enzyme activity returns to normal. This can be seen by an increase in the K_m of the enzyme; more of the original substrate is now required to saturate the enzyme than before, with V_{max} unchanged. Competitive inhibition often occurs between alternative substrates for the same enzyme. The substrate with the lowest K_m will be preferentially metabolised.

Non-competitive inhibition

Non-competitive inhibition occurs when the inhibitor binds to a site on the enzyme other than the active site and by doing so reduces the rate at which products are formed. The binding of the substrate is unaltered so the K_m remains the same. However, at all [S] the rate of reaction is reduced, so V_{max} is reduced. Several chemotherapeutic drugs act in this way.

Irreversible inhibition

Irreversible inhibition occurs when the inhibitor is so tightly bound to the enzyme that it cannot be removed and the only way that the effect can be reversed is by the removal of the enzyme and its replacement by newly synthesised enzyme. For example, penicillin covalently inactivates a key enzyme in bacterial cell wall synthesis.

Regulation of enzyme activity

Enzyme activity is regulated in several ways:

- **Feedback inhibition** by the product of the pathway. Many enzymes are inhibited by the products of their metabolic pathways. The product of the pathway can bind to a site on the enzyme and reduce the rate of reaction.
- **Allosteric regulation**: this is regulation by other small molecules which can either activate or inhibit the enzyme. The binding of the allosteric regulator to a site other than the active site causes a change in the tertiary structure of the protein, which alters the enzyme activity.
- **Gene expression**: the amount of an enzyme is altered by increased production of the enzyme in response to a metabolic signal.

- **Phosphorylation**: as described earlier, the activity of many proteins, including enzymes, can be reversibly altered by the addition (with kinases) or removal (with phosphatases) of phosphate groups.
- **Proteolysis**: enzymes can be irreversibly activated or inactivated by being broken down by other, proteolytic, enzymes. The lifespan of enzymes can be changed by altering their rate of proteolytic degradation in the cell.

Cooperativity between multiple subunits

In multimeric proteins **cooperativity** can occur between multiple subunits. This happens when the binding of a molecule, which can be a substrate or a regulator, to one subunit induces a change in the quaternary structure of the protein, which changes the affinity of the substrate-binding sites. This means that small changes in the concentration of the molecule cause a large change in the rate of catalysis.

For example, the oxygen-carrying protein, haemoglobin, can bind four oxygen molecules. The binding of a single oxygen molecule to one of the substrate-binding sites of deoxyhaemoglobin (the deoxygenated form of haemoglobin) causes a conformational change in the other subunits that increases their affinity for oxygen so that the second oxygen molecule binds more easily. This, in turn, increases the affinity of the other binding sites and so on, until all four sites are filled. The reverse also occurs in that if one oxygen molecule is unbound then the other molecules are lost more easily. This cooperativity enables haemoglobin to become fully oxygenated in the lungs and to lose this oxygen readily in the tissues (see Ch. 13).

Isoenzymes

Many enzymes exist in different tissues in slightly different forms, called **isoenzymes**. They may differ in their primary structure or their subunit composition. Isoenzymes catalyse the same reaction but may have different properties. For example, they may have different affinities for their substrates. They may also show different patterns of inhibition that help to regulate their function in different tissues.

Lactate dehydrogenase isoenzymes can be used to diagnose heart disease

Five different types of LDH are found in different human tissues. Each type consists of a combination of four subunits of two possible types called A and B. Type 1 consists of four B subunits, type 5 of four A subunits with types 2–4 being combinations of A and B subunits. The different subunits determine how the enzyme is inhibited by its substrate, pyruvic acid, and because of this, the degree to which the particular tissue can undergo anaerobic respiration (i.e. without oxygen). Heart muscle contains virtually only type 1, whereas skeletal muscle and liver have mainly type 5. When someone has a myocardial infarction (MI) and their heart muscle is starved of oxygen, then muscle cells in the heart die and release their contents into the blood. Analysis of the LDH isoenzymes in the blood can confirm an MI as there would be more LDH-1 in the blood than normal. In contrast, in someone with liver disease, you would tend to see increased levels of LDH-5 in the plasma.

Coenzymes

Many enzymes require the presence of an additional component in order to function. These are called **coenzymes**, or **cofactors**. They may consist of metal ions such as copper or iron, or they may be more complex organic molecules. Some enzyme cofactors are derived from vitamins. **Vitamins** are organic molecules that are required in small amounts in the diet and without which deficiency diseases, such as scurvy (vitamin C deficiency) or beriberi (vitamin B_1 deficiency), can occur. Coenzymes are often involved in oxidation–reduction reactions, where they act as either electron donors or acceptors. For example, the coenzymes, flavine adenine dinucleotide (FAD) and nicotinamide adenine dinucleotide (NAD), which are derived from vitamin B_2 (riboflavin) and niacin, respectively, have a central role on the transduction of energy in the electron transport chain of mitochondria.

Structural proteins

Many of the proteins that form the structural elements of the body are fibrous proteins made up of long repeating units, arranged in bundles, which give strength and stability. These make up the muscles, bones, skin and connective tissues. They often have a simple repeated secondary structure of α-helices and β-sheets, but because they are often multimeric they may also have a quaternary structure.

The three major groups of structural proteins are:

- Collagens
- Muscle proteins
- Cytoskeletal proteins.

Collagens

The most abundant types of fibrous protein, which make up about 25% of the total protein of the body, are the **collagens**. They form the major component of the **extracellular matrix** (ECM) which is the material that surrounds the cells. There are a large number of different types of collagen (at least 20 have been described to date); they vary according to their protein chains but they all have a similar quaternary structure.

Collagen is made up of three polypeptide chains each of which can be up to 3000 amino acids in length. Each chain forms a left-handed helix that is tighter than the standard α-helix, with just three amino acids per turn. This tight helix can be achieved because every third amino acid is a glycine, which, with its single hydrogen, can fit into the core of the molecule. The other amino acids are very often proline and its derivative, hydroxyproline. The three helices are then wound round each other into a right-handed triple superhelix, which is stabilised by hydrogen bonding. The commonest form of collagen (type I) can be found in a variety of tissues and forms fibrils, with its molecules packed side by side that confer great strength. Other types of collagen, such as type IV, form sheets in which the molecules produce large flexible networks. The basement membrane underlying epithelial cells is partly made up of type IV collagen.

Muscle proteins

The main proteins that make up the contractile elements of muscle cells are **myosin** and **actin**. They form the thick and thin filaments of skeletal muscle, which interact to produce muscle movement (see Ch. 9, Fig. 9.16). The two types of filaments are formed in very different ways. Myosin is made up of six polypeptide chains, two heavy chains and four light

Table 2.9	Cytoskeletal proteins	
Filament types	**Main protein constituent**	**Major role**
Microfilaments	Actin	Cell movement Form core of microvilli
Intermediate filaments (IFs)	Keratins*	Mechanical strength
Microtubules	Tubulins	Chromosome separation Intracellular transport

*The proteins making up IFs vary between cell types. They are made up of keratins in many cells, but there are six different classes of IFs. For example, nerve cells have IFs made from neurofilament proteins.

chains. The two heavy chains form α-helices, which then coil around each other. At their N-terminals they form two globular head regions, with the four light chains. These globular heads contain binding sites which interact with the actin and adenosine triphosphate (ATP) to power muscle movement. The strands of myosin aggregate into thick filaments made up of 300–400 myosin molecules.

The other filaments are composed of actin. Actin filaments are made by the polymerisation of molecules of globular actin (G-actin) into long fibrous strands of F-actin. These strands can be continuously extended and shortened by the addition and removal of G-actin.

Cytoskeletal proteins

All cells contain cytoskeletal proteins that make up three different types of filament, each made up of fibrous proteins (Table 2.9). Each has a different role.

Other structural proteins

Elastin is a flexible protein, associated with collagen in tissues which need to be elastic. It is found mostly in ligaments and blood vessel walls, and is also found in skin, tendons and connective tissues in much smaller amounts. Many globular elastin molecules are cross-linked covalently between lysine residues. When the tissue is stretched the globular proteins can extend, but when the tension is released they shorten back to their globular form. A mixture of collagen and elastin allows a certain degree of stretch, the degree of which is controlled by the amount of collagen.

Two other groups of glycoproteins, important in forming the basement membrane, the layer of material which lies under sheets of cells, are laminin and fibronectin. These both form part of the basal lamina, the part of the basement membrane closest to the cell surface membrane. These molecules can bind to proteins on the cell surface, as well as to collagen and other ECM proteins.

Signalling proteins and receptors

Hormones and neurotransmitters

Some, but not all, of the signalling molecules which travel from cell to cell, are proteins. These can be either **hormones**, which are released into the bloodstream or **neurotransmitters** which are released from nerve endings.

An example of a protein hormone is insulin, which regulates blood glucose levels. Insulin is secreted from cells in the pancreas into the bloodstream when blood glucose levels are high and acts on other tissues to promote the uptake and storage of the glucose. Hormonal responses are relatively slow because hormones are often released at an area distant from the site of action.

In contrast, when a rapid signal is needed, nervous impulses can produce a rapid action through the release of neurotransmitters (see Ch. 8) at the nerve terminals very close to the site of action. In fact, many nerves secrete more than one neurotransmitter. In response to low levels of stimulation, they secrete one of a number of small molecules, such as acetylcholine or noradrenaline (norepinephrine). However, in response to higher levels of stimulation, many nerves also secrete a peptide neurotransmitter. An example of a peptide neurotransmitter is the natural painkiller β-endorphin. This acts on opioid receptors, so called because they are also activated by the opiate drugs, such as morphine.

Proteins are also involved in the signalling pathways inside cells. For example, **transcription factors** are small proteins which, when activated, bind to the genetic material, DNA, to alter the type and amount of protein being produced in the cell.

Receptors

Signalling molecules produce an effect on target cells by interacting with proteins called **receptors**. The ability of a cell to respond to any chemical signal (or **ligand**) depends on the presence of receptors for that molecule. If the receptor is not present then the cell cannot respond.

Cell surface receptors

For many ligands their receptors are embedded in the cell membrane, with the binding site on the cell surface. Binding of the ligand causes a conformational change in the receptor that produces some effect inside the cell. This is called **signal transduction**.

Intracellular receptors

Some signalling molecules, such as the sex hormones, testosterone and oestrogen, can enter the cell and act on receptors present inside the cell. Some of these are present in the cytoplasm, and others are located in the nucleus. The intracytoplasmic receptors have two binding sites, one for the hormone and one for DNA. When the hormone is bound, the receptor moves to the nucleus, binding with acidic proteins of the DNA. The ligand-bound receptors, bound to the DNA, produce changes in protein production, thus effecting cell growth and metabolism.

Immune system proteins

Immunoglobulins

The body defends itself from attack by foreign bodies such as bacteria and viruses with its immune system (see Ch. 6).

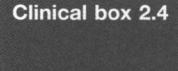

Clinical box 2.4 | **The absence of testosterone receptors produces babies that look like girls who should have been boys**

Androgen insensitivity syndrome is a condition in which the male fetus lacks the receptors for the male sex hormone, testosterone. Genetically they are XY males, but a mutation causes them to lack testosterone receptors. Despite producing testosterone, these individuals cannot respond to it and do not develop male genitalia because proteins necessary for the appropriate cell growth and metabolism are not transcribed. They do, however, produce normal amounts of other hormones, which means that they develop external female features such as breasts. Unfortunately, they do not develop internal female organs, so cannot function as normal females.

One of the key elements of the immune system is the production of vast numbers of different proteins called **immunoglobulins** or **antibodies** which can bind to the invading organism or antigen, enabling the latter to be removed and destroyed.

Antibodies have a common basic structure but include a variable region which produces the binding site. These proteins are produced with an enormous variety of variable regions to cope with the large number of possible exogenous (i.e. of foreign origin) antigens. Problems can occur, however, when the body produces antibodies that recognise its own, endogenous, molecules as antigens. This failure to recognise self results in autoimmune conditions, where the body's own cells are destroyed. A well-known example of this problem is rheumatoid arthritis (RA).

Cytokines

Another group of proteins involved in both the immune response and in the body's response to inflammation are the **cytokines**. More cytokines continue to be reported as new research techniques are developed. Cytokines mainly act locally, but some have been identified that have wide-ranging effects on metabolism. One of the better-known groups of cytokines are the **interferons**, which have actions against viruses and cancer cells. One of them, interferon beta, is currently being tested as a possible treatment for some forms of multiple sclerosis.

Transport proteins

Many substances have to be transported around the body in the extracellular fluids, and then subsequently into and out of cells.

Transport in blood

Many proteins travel around the body in the fluid phase of the blood: the plasma. **Albumin** is the major protein found in blood plasma at a concentration of 35–45 g/L, making up 50% of the total plasma protein. It has two major functions:

- To increase the osmotic pressure of the blood, thereby ensuring the correct distribution of fluid between the vascular and interstitial compartments (see Ch. 11)
- To act as a non-specific transport protein for many substances in the plasma.

Table 2.10	Some of the binding proteins in plasma
Protein	**Ligand/s**
Albumin	Metal cations, free fatty acids, steroids, bilirubin, haem
Transferrin	Iron
Thyroid-binding globulin	Thyroxine (T_4), triiodothyronine (T_3)
Cortisol-binding globulin	Cortisol
Sex-hormone-binding globulin	Androgens and oestrogens

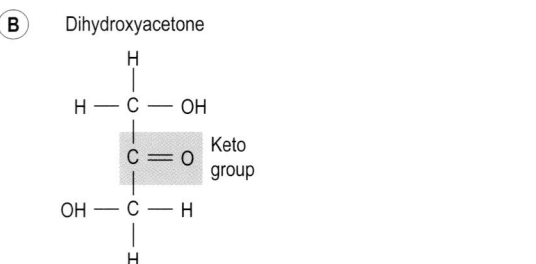

Fig. 2.8 Triose sugars: (A) aldoses and (B) ketoses.

Albumin has an overall negative charge at physiological pH, which means that it can easily bind metal cations such as copper and iron. Many molecules, some of which are extremely hydrophobic, can be transported in the aqueous environment of the plasma, bound to albumin. This increases the length of time they remain in the blood, due to reduced degradation and elimination (see Ch. 2).

Other plasma proteins are specific binding proteins for signalling molecules, such as sex steroids (Table 2.10).

Transport into cells

Hydrophobic substances can move into cells by simple diffusion but many substances, including glucose, cannot move into cells without the presence of specific proteins called **transporters**. These transporters are proteins embedded in the cell membranes that bind the transported molecule on one side of the membrane and move it through to the other side. Inside cells, substances can be moved into separate compartments by the action of other specific transport proteins.

CARBOHYDRATES

Carbohydrates form about 2% of body mass. They consist of carbon, oxygen and hydrogen, with a ratio of hydrogen to oxygen of about 2:1, hence the name 'hydrated carbon'. The most common organic compound on the planet is a carbohydrate, **cellulose**, which forms the principal component of plant cell walls. Unfortunately, humans cannot digest significant amounts of cellulose, although it is important to digestion as a bulk element of food. Of more importance is the carbohydrate, **glucose**, which is one of the central molecules in energy metabolism and forms the backbone for the synthesis of many other compounds. The simplest forms of carbohydrates are called **sugars**. These are either **monosaccharides**, which are single units or **disaccharides**, formed from two monosaccharides. Larger carbohydrates, called **polysaccharides** are polymers, formed from many monosaccharides.

Sugars

Monosaccharides

The basic units of all carbohydrates are called **monosaccharides**, or simple sugars. These can be obtained directly from the diet or derived from the breakdown in the gut of more complex carbohydrates. They can also be manufactured from non-carbohydrate sources when carbohydrate sources have been used up. Although food is the main source of sugars there is no dietary requirement for carbohydrates as such.

Triose sugars

Sugars have the general formula $(CH_2O)_n$ where n is the number of carbons in the sugar. The simplest of these are the three-carbon trioses. Two types of **triose sugars** contain either an aldehyde group, aldoses, or a ketone group, ketoses (Fig. 2.8). In **aldose sugars**, the carbon atom of the terminal aldehyde group is numbered carbon-1. In **ketose sugars**, carbon-1 is the end carbon next to the carbonyl group. The central carbon of glyceraldehyde, the simplest of the aldose sugars, is chiral, and therefore it can exist as two stereoisomers, D- and L-glyceraldehyde.

D and L sugars

All sugars larger than trioses have two or more chiral groups, and so exist as a number of stereoisomers. By convention they are divided into D- and L-series, depending on the arrangement of atoms around the asymmetrical carbon furthest from the carbon-1 end. The sugar is a D-sugar if the arrangement around this carbon is the same as D-glyceraldehyde, and an L-sugar if it is like L-glyceraldehyde. Virtually all sugars found in biological systems are **D-isomers**.

Different forms of glucose

D-Glucose, also known as **dextrose**, is found in all cells and in blood plasma, where its concentration is strictly controlled. Glucose is a six-carbon sugar, or **hexose**, and has the formula, $C_6H_{12}O_6$. It can exist in four different forms, all of which are freely convertible in aqueous solution (Fig. 2.9). The straight chain form (which exists as less than 1%) has an aldehyde group at one end (where the carbon is always called carbon-1). This reacts with the hydroxyl group on carbon-5 to give a six-member ring form called a **pyranose ring**. Depending on the arrangement of the —H and —OH on carbon-1, the glucose molecule forms either α- or β-glucose (also known as α-D-glucopyranose and β-D-glucopyranose). These different forms are known as **anomers**. While the cyclic form of D-glucose is usually a pyranose ring, rarely it can also form a five-member **furanose ring**, D-glucofuranose.

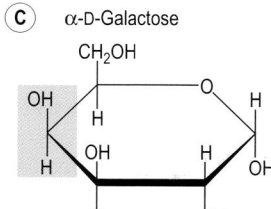

Fig. 2.9 Different forms of glucose. Each of these molecules has an identical chemical composition. A reaction between the hydroxyl group on C5 and the aldehyde on C1 produces the pyranose ring structure (B, C). If the hydroxyl group is on C4 then the furanose ring is produced (D).

Due to the tetrahedral arrangement of bonds around the carbon atoms, the pyranose and furanose rings are not planar molecules. They form two different arrangements, known as the **chair and boat conformations**. Both of these conformations are important for the packing of the molecules, although the chair conformation is the more stable.

Common hexose sugars

Other common hexoses are mannose, galactose and fructose (also known as fruit sugar) (Fig. 2.10). **Mannose** and **galactose** are both aldoses and tend to form pyranose rings. They are only different from glucose in the configuration of the other carbons, and are called **epimers**. Mannose is identical to glucose, except for the arrangement around the carbon-2. Similarly, galactose only differs from glucose by the arrangement around carbon-4. **Fructose** is a ketose sugar and forms both furanose and pyranose rings.

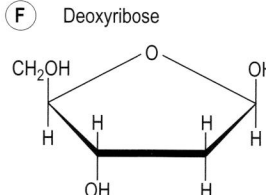

Fig. 2.10 Structures of some common sugars. In (B) and (C) the part of the molecule which differs from glucose is highlighted.

Pentose sugars

Two important **pentose** sugars are **ribose** and **deoxyribose**, which are found as components of the nucleic acids, DNA and RNA. These are both aldoses and form cyclic furanose rings.

Table 2.11	Principal disaccharides				
Disaccharide	**Carbon-1 sugar**	**Other sugar**	**Linkage**	**Digestive enzyme**	
Sucrose	α-Glucose	β-Fructose	1→2	Sucrase-isomaltase	
Lactose	β-Galactose	β-Glucose	1→4	Lactase	
Maltose	α-Glucose	β-Glucose	1→4	Maltase	
Isomaltose	α-Glucose	β-Glucose	1→6	Sucrase-isomaltase	

Other simple sugars

Other carbohydrates can be derived from basic carbohydrates by the inclusion of other elements. **Glucosamine** and **galactosamine** are derived from glucose and galactose, both having amino groups replacing the hydroxyl groups on carbon-2. These two sugars are major components of the proteoglycans, which make up the ECM.

Among other possible substitutions are:

- Phosphates – widespread in energy metabolism
- Sulphates and carboxylates: commonly found in proteoglycans.

Disaccharides

Monosaccharides can be linked together by **glycosidic linkages** to form disaccharides. These links are formed by a dehydration reaction between the hydrogen on carbon-1 atom of one sugar and the hydroxyl group of another, with the loss of a water molecule. This reaction is reversible. These are either α or β linkages, depending on the orientation around carbon-1 atom. This means that there are a large number of different possible bonds that could occur between two sugars, each of which gives a different product (Table 2.11). For example, glucose has five different —OH groups (on carbons 1, 2, 3, 4 and 6), so could potentially form dimers in 10 different conformations. If two different sugars are combined the second sugar could be either an α-sugar or a β-sugar, increasing still further the possible combinations. However, enzymes are able to distinguish between the different conformations ensuring that the required linkage is either made or broken in order to produce the required product.

Dietary sugars

The compound known as ordinary sweet-tasting sugar is actually a **disaccharide, sucrose**, which is made up of α-glucose and β-fructose in an α (1→2) linkage. Two other important dietary disaccharides are **maltose**, which is a dimer of two glucose molecules, and **lactose** (called milk sugar, because milk is its only significant source), which is made from galactose and glucose. Dietary disaccharides are hydrolysed by specific enzymes found in the intestine. The resulting monosaccharides are then absorbed by specific transport mechanisms (see Ch. 15).

Polysaccharides

Polysaccharides are polymers of monosaccharides and may contain thousands of units. They allow large amounts of glucose to be stored in a highly concentrated form, without the osmotic problems that would be associated with high aqueous concentrations of separate glucose molecules.

Starches

These are a group of polysaccharides which are used as sugar storage in plants. They consist of polymers of glucose

Clinical box 2.5	In certain populations adults cannot digest lactose

The enzyme, lactase, which breaks down lactose into galactose and glucose, is usually present only in children and only persists in adults of northern European descent. Lactase deficiency is common in Mediterranean countries, parts of Africa and Asia. In the absence of lactase, consuming milk products containing lactose produces watery diarrhoea, flatulence and abdominal pain. This is because the unabsorbed lactose is fermented by bacteria in the small intestine, producing gas and large numbers of metabolites that draw water into the intestine by osmosis, producing diarrhoea. This can be avoided to some extent by fermenting the milk, to produce yoghurt, for example, because the lactose is converted to lactic acid during fermentation.

linked in two different ways. The simplest starch, **amylose**, consists of long linear chains of glucose molecules, linked via α 1→4 bonds. **Amylopectin**, which makes up about 80% of the starch in foods, also has 1→4 linked glucose chains, but additionally every thirtieth glucose molecule is also linked via a 1→6 bond, producing a branched molecule. The starches found in grains, such as wheat or rice and potatoes, are the major source of dietary carbohydrates. They can be broken down to glucose in the human gut by **amylases** secreted by the pancreas and the salivary glands. These enzymes break starches into glucose, maltose and isomaltose (from the 1→6 linkages in amylopectin).

Non-starch polysaccharides

Cellulose is an unbranched glucose polymer with β 1→4 linkages. Humans have no enzymes capable of hydrolysing these linkages, although a small amount of cellulose is broken down by bacteria in the colon. However, cellulose, along with other non-metabolised polysaccharides, are the major component of dietary fibre. They produce bulk in the intestine which aids defecation.

Glycogen

Glycogen is the storage form of glucose in animals, including humans. Like the starches, it is a large glucose polymer. It is similar in structure to amylopectin, except that the branch points occur every tenth glucose molecule. The high level of branching of the molecule means that it has a large number of free ends to allow glucose molecules to be added or removed rapidly. Glycogen stores are not very large in humans, with about 75 g in the liver and about 250 g in skeletal muscle. Each gram can produce 16.7 kJ (4 kcal), so glycogen stores can provide sufficient glucose for 12–18 hours in the absence of other sources of glucose. Dieting rapidly depletes glycogen, with an apparent rapid weight loss. However, this loss is mainly due to the loss of water molecules that are associated with glycogen.

Table 2.12	Major glycosaminoglycans (GAGs)
GAG	**Main source**
Hyaluronic acid	Joints
Chondroitin sulphate	Cartilage
Keratan sulphate	Cornea
Dermatan sulphate	Skin
Heparan sulphate	Basement membranes
Heparin	Mast cells

Functions of carbohydrates

Glucose, as mentioned above, is a major metabolic fuel, and it is the only fuel used by the brain under normal circumstances. Red blood cells are completely reliant on glucose for energy because they lack the ability to metabolise fats. Also, at the beginning of exercise, muscle preferentially uses glucose rather than other fuels. Glucose is oxidised by cells in a process called glycolysis, which liberates 16.7 kJ (4 kcal) per gram of glucose. The intermediates of glycolysis can also provide precursors for many amino acids, nucleotides and lipids.

Other functions of carbohydrates include forming structural elements surrounding cells and playing a part in the mechanisms by which cells recognise each other.

Structural carbohydrates

The proteoglycans, which form the gel part of the ECM, typically contain 95% carbohydrate. They are formed from two components: a linear polypeptide chain, to which are attached large, linear polysaccharide chains called **glycosaminoglycans** (GAGs) or **mucopolysaccharides** (Table 2.12). These GAGs consist of repeating disaccharide units. Many of these are negatively charged and thus attract cations and large amounts of water, drawn into the gel by osmosis. This results in a gel-like structure around the collagen fibres of the ECM, imparting a degree of flexibility to the tissue and acting as a shock absorber. In contrast, the GAG, heparin, although having a similar structure to the other GAGs, has a very different function. It is released from mast cells and acts as an anticoagulant (see Ch. 12).

Cell recognition by cell surface glycosylation

The carbohydrates found in glycoproteins are of two types. One type, which consists of one or two simple mono- or disaccharides, are linked to serine and threonine residues by **O-glycosylation**. The linkage is between the hydroxyl group of the amino acid side chain and the carbon-1 of N-acetylgalactosamine.

The other way that sugars are linked to proteins is via **N-glycosylation** to asparagine. This always occurs at specific amino acid sequences in the protein, either asparagine-X-serine or asparagine-X-threonine, where the linkage is between the amide group of asparagine and the carbon-1 of N-acetylglucosamine. Monosaccharide units are then added, in a specific pattern, to give highly branched carbohydrates. Many of these carbohydrates contain the sugar N-acetylneuraminic acid (sialic acid). This sugar is negatively charged, giving many cell surfaces a net negative charge. Lipids in the cell membrane are also glycosylated.

These distinctive patterns of glycosylation are particularly important in cell-to-cell recognition and how the immune system recognises self. An example of this specificity can be seen on red blood cells.

Blood groups

The surface of the red cell is covered with patterns of carbohydrates attached to protein and lipids, making the many different **antigens** that determine different **blood groups**. The most studied of these is the **ABO blood group system**. The O antigen is a small polysaccharide, present on all red cells of all blood groups. The A and B antigens are produced by the addition of N-acetylgalactosamine or galactose sugar, respectively, to this O antigen. These are added by specific transferase enzymes; individuals with the AB blood group have both enzymes and their erythrocytes have both A and B antigens (see Ch. 12).

LIPIDS

In adults who are not overweight or underweight, lipids make up about 20% of body mass, usually more in women. Unlike proteins, carbohydrates and nucleic acids, lipids are not large covalently bonded molecules. However, because of the interactions that occur between lipid molecules, they form large structures of repeating molecules. Lipids have a number of crucial roles:

- They form the membranes surrounding every cell and the compartments within the cells.
- They are also the major form of energy storage.
- They have important roles in cell signalling.

Abnormalities in lipid transport are associated with the development of atherosclerosis, where arteries are clogged with fatty deposits, and excess storage of lipids results in obesity. Diseases such as diabetes mellitus and pancreatitis have associated lipid abnormalities, and there are also rare inherited lipid storage diseases.

Triacylglycerols

The simplest type of lipids, the **triacylglycerols**, also called triglycerides or neutral fats, are formed from two components, **fatty acids** and **glycerol** (Fig. 2.11). Triacylglycerols have three ester bonds, formed by dehydration reactions between the carboxylate group of three fatty acids and each of the three hydroxyl groups of glycerol (Fig. 2.11D).

Fatty acids

Fatty acids are chains of carbon and hydrogen (Fig. 2.11A, B), with a carboxylate (COOH) group at one end (the α-carbon) and a methyl group (CH_3) at the other (the ω-carbon):

- If all the carbon atoms in the chain are single bonded then the fatty acid is **saturated**.
- If there is a single double bond it is **monounsaturated**.
- If there is more than one it is **polyunsaturated**.

Most of the double bonds in biological molecules are in the *cis*-configuration, which puts a rigid kink in the hydrocarbon chains. Many of the fatty acids found in cells have 16, 18 or 20 carbon atoms and up to three double bonds.

Glycerol

Glycerol is a sugar alcohol, a modified triose sugar formed by the reduction of the aldehyde group to hydroxyl (Fig. 2.11C).

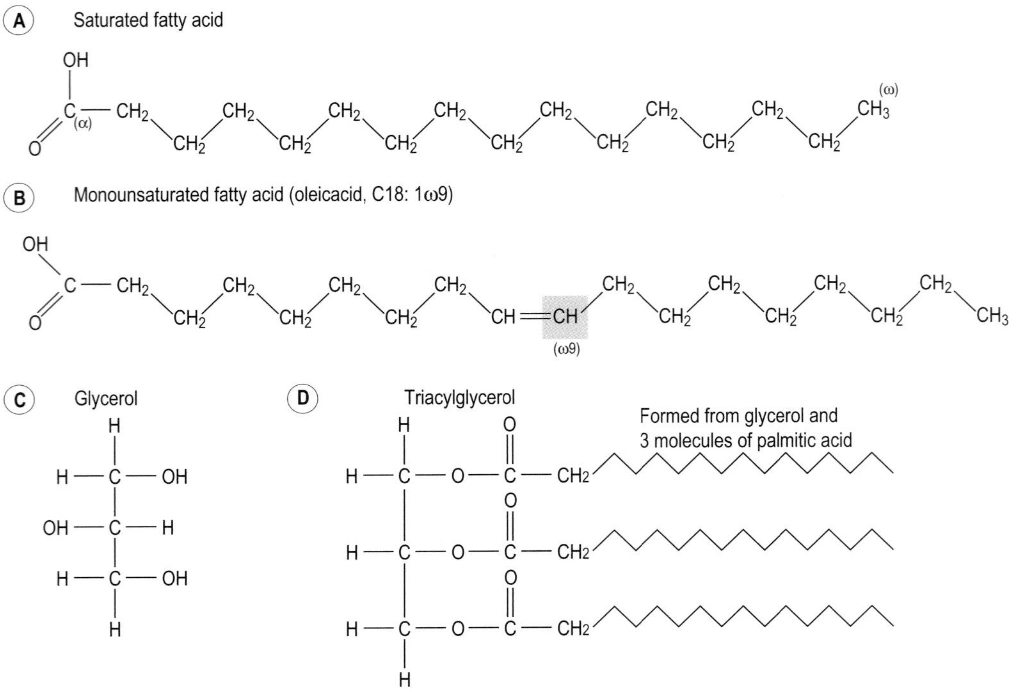

Fig. 2.11 **Components of triacylglycerols.**

> ℹ️ **Information box 2.5** **Fatty acids can be named in several ways**
>
> Many of the different fatty acids have common names which reflect their original source, but all fatty acids can be described according to the number of carbon atoms in the chain and the number and position of the double bond/s.
>
> A shorthand notation that is widely used gives the number of carbon atoms, the number of double bonds and the position of the first double bond, counting from the ω-carbon. For example, the saturated fatty acid found in palm oil is called palmitic acid. The formula for palmitic acid is $CH_3(CH_2)_{14}COOH$, its chemical name is n-hexadecanoic acid and the shorthand notation is C16:0, indicating that it has 16 carbon atoms and no double bonds.
>
> Another fatty acid, arachidonic acid, is called *cis*-5,8,11,14-eicosatetraenoic acid, which is shortened to C20:4 ω-6. Another type of shorthand indicates the positions of all of the double bonds: C20:4 All *cis*-$\Delta^5, \Delta^8, \Delta^{11}, \Delta^{14}$ (see Fig. 2.14).

Dietary fats

Dietary fats, both solid and liquid (oils), are mainly composed of triacylglycerols. The fatty acids which make up the triacylglycerol molecules in each type of fat determine the physical properties of the fat. If the triacylglycerol has fatty acid chains that are predominantly short, or contains unsaturated fatty acids, it will be liquid at room temperature. Examples of these are the oils such as olive oil (which contains oleic acid) and sunflower oil, which contain polyunsaturated fatty acids. If there are more saturated fats and longer fatty acid chains then the resulting fat will be solid at room temperature, for example, butter and the fats found in meat.

Adipose tissue

Triacylglycerols tend to aggregate with the formation of hydrophobic bonds between them which exclude water. This can be seen clearly when oils are added to water. They do not mix and form droplets. Instead they form a thin layer over the surface. In the body, triacylglycerols form the major energy store. They are stored in white adipose tissue. This is found mainly under the skin, and also surrounding the abdominal organs and on the hips. Adipocytes, specialised mesenchymal cells, each consist almost entirely of a single droplet of triacylglycerols. The molecular aggregation of the lipid molecules means that the lipids do not have an osmotic effect; i.e. despite the presence of large numbers of molecules, they do not act like individual particles. Obesity is characterised by increased size and number of these cells.

Fats yield 37.7 kJ (9 kcal) per gram and the amount of fat stored in the adipose tissue in a lean average human would be enough to survive for more than two months without food. There is no specialised storage site for proteins or amino acids. In severe starvation the body will break down tissue and plasma proteins in order to produce fatty acids. Glycogen also has no specialised storage cell; it is simply accumulated in the cytoplasm, particularly in liver and muscle.

Membrane lipids

The lipids which form cell membranes are of three types:

- Phospholipids
- Sphingolipids
- Cholesterol.

Two of these have broadly similar structures. These are the **glycerolipids**, which are mainly **phospholipids**, and the **sphingolipids**.

(A) Phosphatidylserine

Phosphate

COO⁻
|
CH — CH₂ — O — P — O — CH₂
| || |
NH₃⁺   **Serine**   O   CH — O — O — [R]
                     |
                     O⁻   O
                                                   ||
Hydrophilic   **Hydrophobic**

R = Fatty acid hydrocarbon chains   CH — O — C — [R]
                                    Glycerol

(B) Sphingomyelin

```
        CH₃    Phosphocholine    O              H    H                    Hydrophobic
        |                        ||             |    |
CH₃ — N⁺ — CH₂ — CH₂ — O — P — O — CH₂ — C — C — CH = CH — (CH₂)₁₂ — CH₃
        |                        |                  |
        CH₃                      O⁻   Sphingosine   OH

                                          NH — C — [R]
                                               ||
        Hydrophilic                            O

R = Fatty acid hydrocarbon chains
```

Fig. 2.12 Two membrane lipids.

Types of membrane lipids

Phospholipids

Phospholipids (Fig. 2.12A) consist of glycerol, with fatty acids attached to two adjacent OH groups via ester linkages to give two acyl groups, and with a third group attached, which is a phosphate group. The phosphate is itself linked to one of a number of possible molecules, including serine, ethanolamine (a derivative of serine), choline and inositol. The resulting molecular structure looks somewhat like a tuning fork, with hydrophobic prongs and a hydrophilic handle.

Sphingolipids

Sphingolipids (Fig. 2.12B) have a similar structure to phospholipids, but the hydrophobic portion is formed from **sphingosine**. Sphingosine contains a long hydrocarbon chain and as part of a sphingolipid it is linked to a fatty acid, giving the sphingolipid two long hydrocarbon chains. This in then linked to either a phosphate-containing group, phosphocholine, or a group of sugar residues to produce a glycolipid.

Cholesterol

A third component of cell membranes is **cholesterol**. This has a structure completely different from the other membrane lipids (Fig. 2.13), as it is formed from a four-ringed hydrocarbon called a **steroid**. Although cholesterol is almost entirely hydrocarbon, it has a hydroxyl group attached to the first ring, which can interact with water. The ring structure is quite rigid and has important effects on the fluidity of membranes.

Arrangement of membrane lipids

All the membrane lipids are **amphipathic**; that is they have a hydrophilic head group and a hydrophobic tail. They aggre-

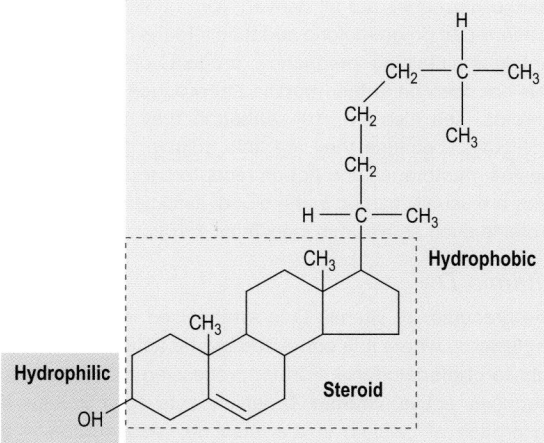

Fig. 2.13 **Structure of cholesterol.** The figure inside the dotted blue lines is the basic steroid structure.

gate with their head groups facing the aqueous medium and their tails excluding water. It is this arrangement which underlies the formation of all cell membranes (see Fig. 2.28). Many, although not all, of the head groups are negatively charged, giving the surface of the aggregated lipids an overall negative charge.

Different membranes vary in their relative composition. For example, the myelin sheath around nerves has a very high concentration of sphingolipids, whereas phospholipids are more prevalent in the red cell membrane.

An alternative arrangement of amphipathic lipids in aqueous solution leads to the formation of spherical micelles (see Ch. 15), structures generated, for example, by bile salts during the digestion of dietary fat.

Cholesterol and other steroids

Cholesterol is the major **sterol** (a steroid alcohol) in the human body, having both structural and transport functions. It can be synthesised in the liver or absorbed in the diet.

Studies have shown a relationship between raised plasma cholesterol (in the form of low-density lipoprotein (LDL)-cholesterol; see Ch. 16) and increased mortality from heart disease. It is therefore thought to be beneficial to reduce plasma cholesterol levels. However, reducing dietary cholesterol has less of an effect on plasma cholesterol levels than reducing the intake of saturated fats. Diets that are rich in polyunsaturated fats can also reduce serum cholesterol.

As well as forming an important part of membranes, cholesterol is the precursor of many important molecules that are formed by modifications of the basic **steroid** structure (see Fig. 2.13). These are:

- Bile salts
- Steroid hormones
- Vitamin D.

Bile salts

Bile salts act as detergents, helping to break up fats, so aiding their digestion and absorption. They are produced in the liver and are secreted from the gall bladder into the intestine (see Ch. 15).

Steroid hormones

Steroid hormones are all derived from cholesterol, which is converted to pregnenolone and then into the hormone important in maintaining pregnancy, progesterone (Table 2.13). This can then be further modified to produce all of the other steroids (see also Ch. 10). Although they are quite large molecules, because they are lipid soluble, they can cross plasma membranes and act on receptors found inside cells. They are usually carried in the blood, associated with binding proteins such as albumin (see Table 2.10).

Vitamin D

The precursor of vitamin D is synthesised in the skin from cholesterol, where it is converted by the action of ultraviolet light to **cholecalciferol**. Further processing of this molecule produces active **vitamin D** which acts to influence the absorption of calcium in the intestine, reabsorption in the kidney and bone resorption and calcification. When skin exposure to light levels are low, such as might occur in countries outside the tropics in combination with a cultural tradition of not exposing the skin, then dietary sources of vitamin D are important (see Ch. 16).

Essential fatty acids

While most of the fatty acids used in the body are supplied in the diet (Fig. 2.14), there is almost no requirement for any fat in the diet. Saturated fatty acids can be synthesised from the breakdown products of carbohydrates and proteins in a process called lipogenesis (see Ch. 3). The requirement for mono- and polyunsaturated fatty acids is met by enzymes that convert saturated fatty acids to unsaturated fatty acids.

However, some fats **are** required:

- To aid the absorption in the gut of fat-soluble vitamins
- As precursors to the eicosanoids.

These **essential fatty acids** are **linoleic acid** and **linolenic acid**, both of which were originally identified in linseed oil. They cannot be manufactured in the body as none of the enzymes which convert fatty acids can include double bonds beyond carbon-10, and an important group of lipids, the **eicosanoids** are all made from 20 carbon fatty acids with between three and five double bonds. **Arachidonic acid**, the precursor for a large number of different eicosanoids, is synthesised from linoleic acid (see below).

Eicosanoids

These are a large group of locally acting hormones derived from fatty acids (Fig. 2.14). They are extremely potent

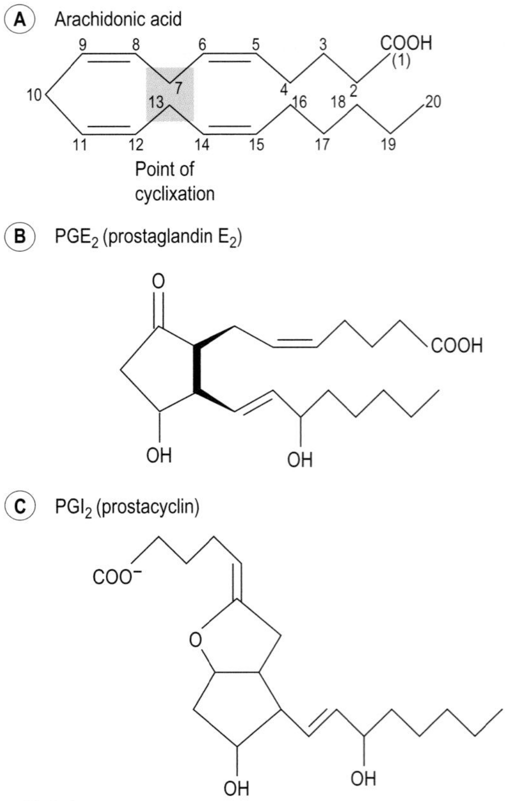

Fig. 2.14 **Arachidonic acid. All cis, 5, 8, 11, 14 eicosatetraenoicacid (or alternatively C20: $4\omega6$ C-20 Δ^5, Δ^8, Δ^{11}, Δ^{14}) and two of the many eicosanoids derived from it (PGE$_2$ and PGI$_2$ (prostacyclin)).**

Table 2.13	Important steroid hormones	
Group	**Example**	**Major actions**
Glucocorticoids	Cortisol	Formation of glucose, breakdown of proteins and lipids
Mineralocorticoids	Aldosterone	Sodium and potassium homeostasis
Progestogens	Progesterone	Pregnancy and ovarian cycles
Androgens	Testosterone	Male sexual development and characteristics
Oestrogens	Oestradiol	Female sexual development and characteristics

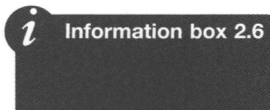

Prostanoids facilitate normal blood flow through vessels and aspirin acts by inhibiting the synthesis of prostaglandin

Blood is protected from clotting in blood vessels, under normal conditions, due to the release of a compound, prostacyclin, from the vessel wall. Prostacyclin acts as a vasodilator, thus encouraging flow, and inhibits the sticking together of blood platelets, which form the basis of clot formation. If the vessel wall is broached substances are released that stimulate platelets to release another prostaglandin, thromboxane A_2. In contrast to prostacyclin, thromboxane A_2 acts as a vasoconstrictor, thus reducing blood loss through the leaking vessel wall, and stimulates platelets to aggregate, plugging the hole in the vessel.

The enzyme which acts on arachidonic acid in the first step of the production of the prostanoids is cyclo-oxygenase (COX). Aspirin (acetylsalicylic acid) is one of a group of drugs called non-steroidal anti-inflammatory drugs (NSAIDs) which inhibit COX and reduce inflammation and pain. Aspirin is also used to inhibit blood clotting by daily consumption of a low-dose, since, in the absence of COX, thromboxane A_2 cannot be produced. Because of the enzyme inhibition by NSAIDs, gastric bleeding is seen as a common side effect. COX is seen in two isoforms, COX-1 and COX-2. While COX-1 is continuously produced, the other isoform, COX-2, is only induced in response to inflammatory mediators. Although current NSAIDs inhibit both COX-1 and COX-2, it is thought that if specific COX-2 inhibitors were developed, they might be able to reduce inflammation without the side effects of current NSAIDs.

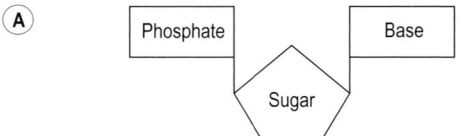

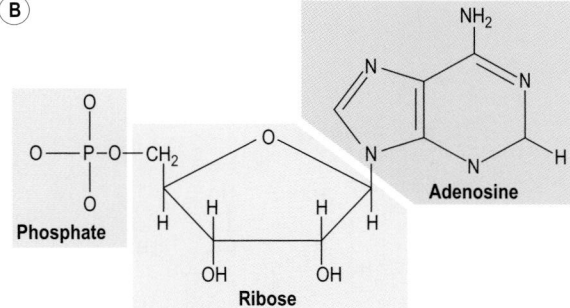

Fig. 2.15 Nucleotide structure: (A) components of a nucleotide; (B) structure of ribo-adenosine monophosphate (rAMP), usually referred to more simply as adenosine monophosphate.

substances and are all broken down quickly after being released, so they act only over short distances. They have important roles in responses to inflammation and in the control of physiological processes, showing a wide range of functions. For example, some stimulate smooth muscle cell contraction, producing vasoconstriction, while others act as vasodilators.

The different groups of eicosanoids are:

- Prostaglandins
- Thromboxanes (together these are called the prostanoids)
- Leukotrienes.

Arachidonic acid, or **eicosatetraenoic** acid, is one of the fatty acids incorporated into membrane phospholipids. It can be released from the membrane by the action of the enzyme phospholipase A_2 (PLA_2) on phosphatidylcholine, one of the most common membrane phospholipids. PLA_2 is stimulated by a range of different signals in different tissues, including general cell damage.

Another fatty acid, **eicosapentaenoic** acid, is the precursor to a group of prostaglandins with three double bonds. One of the double bonds is at carbon-17, which is three carbons from the ω-carbon, hence the name of this type of fatty acid which is ω-3 fatty acids. It is thought to be beneficial to include this polyunsaturated fatty acid, which is found in fish oils, in the diet.

NUCLEIC ACIDS

Deoxyribonucleic acid (DNA) and the **ribonucleic acids** (RNAs) contain and transmit the genetic information in all biological organisms. Nevertheless, they are not very complex, in the sense that they are regularly arranged

molecules made from a limited number of monomers. Nucleic acids, like proteins, are unbranched chains of units that are all linked with a similar type of bond. However, instead of the 20 possible different subunits which can make up proteins, each of the nucleic acids has only four different subunits. In this way they would seem to be much simpler molecules than proteins, but the way in which the nucleic acid chains are used to store and transmit the genetic information of every cell indicates that the information contained within these macromolecules is complex (see below).

In addition to their genetic role, some of the subunits of nucleic acids also have important roles in energy transfer and as cell signalling molecules.

Nucleotides

Nucleotides form the basic units from which the larger nucleic acids are made. Nucleotides have three components (Fig. 2.15):

- A sugar
- A phosphate
- A base.

Nucleotide sugars and phosphates

Two different sugars are found in nucleotides, **deoxyribose** and **ribose**. These pentose sugars are both aldoses with a furanose ring (see Fig. 2.10E,F).

Attached to the hydroxyl on carbon-5 of these sugars by an ester bond is one of three possible phosphate-containing groups. These phosphate-containing groups can have either one, two or three phosphates attached to each other via phosphoanhydride (pyrophosphate) bonds between the phosphates.

Nucleotide purines and pyrimidines

There are two types of **bases** found in nucleotides: the **purines** and the **pyrimidines** (Fig. 2.16). Purines have two fused rings, while pyrimidines have only one. The rings contain both carbon and nitrogen atoms and form planar

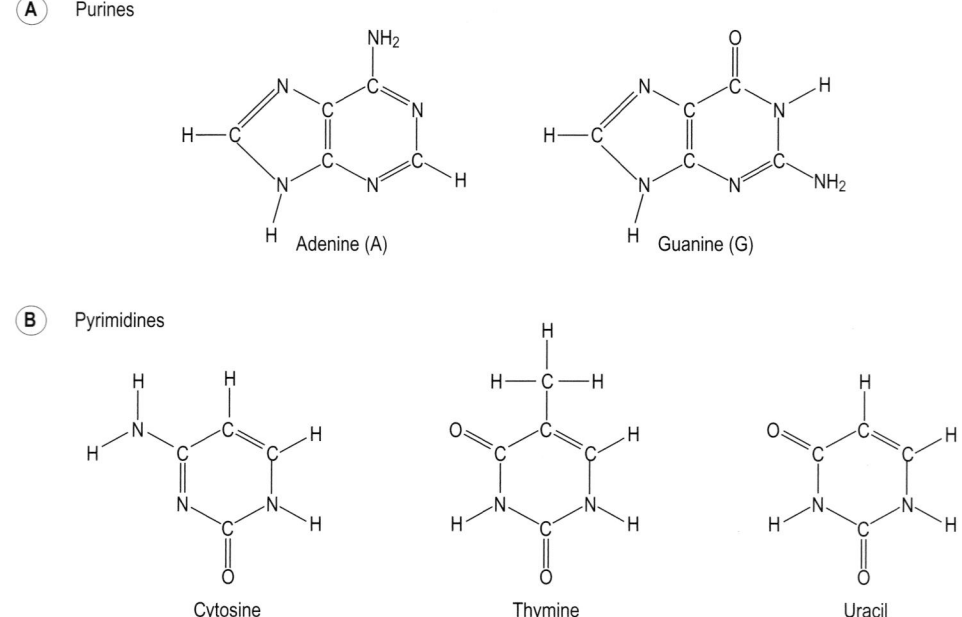

Fig. 2.16 Structure of purine and pyrimidine bases.

Table 2.14	Nucleoside phosphates*				
Base	Nucleoside	Nucleoside monophosphates	Nucleoside diphosphates	Nucleoside triphosphates	Cyclic nucleotides
Adenine	Adenosine	AMP	ADP	ATP	cAMP
Guanine	Guanosine	GMP	GDP	GTP	cGMP
Cytosine	Cytidine	CMP	CDP	CTP	
Uracil	Uridine	UMP	UDP	UTP	
Thymine	Thymidine	TMP	TDP	TTP	

*The nucleosides A, G, C and U can contain ribose or deoxyribose, but AMP infers the ribose form, which strictly is called rAMP, the deoxyribose form being called dAMP. The thymidine nucleotides are only produced as deoxynucleotides and are usually written without the d (e.g. TTP).

molecules. The nitrogen atoms are uncharged at neutral pH, which means that the bases are non-polar and hydrophobic. The major purines are adenine and guanine and the major pyrimidines are cytosine, thymine and uracil. The coenzyme NAD (nicotinamide adenine dinucleotide) contains a pyridine base, nicotinamide.

Nomenclature of nucleotides

There are two different ways of naming nucleotides, which can cause confusion. **Nucleosides** are nucleotides without the phosphate; that is, they have a pentose sugar and a base. Nucleotides with one phosphate can be called mononucleotides or nucleoside monophosphates and so on. Many of the different nucleoside phosphates can be found in cells and have a variety of functions (Table 2.14).

Nucleoside phosphates

Adenosine triphosphate

The most important of the nucleoside phosphates is **adenosine triphosphate** or ATP (Fig. 2.17). The covalent phosphoanhydride bonds which attach the second (β) and third phosphate (γ) groups to the mononucleotide, **adenosine monophosphate** (AMP), can be broken to release energy for other reactions, about 7.3 kcal/mol each. This is under standard laboratory conditions, although in the conditions

within the cell, energy released may be as high as 50 kJ (12 kcal). These bonds are usually shown as ~ indicating, that they are high-energy bonds. They can be formed in two ways, either by the transfer of a phosphate group from another phosphorylated compound, called **substrate-level phosphorylation**, or by a process called **oxidative phosphorylation**, where electrons are transferred between a number of intermediates in order to power the enzyme ATP synthase.

Using these mechanisms, the metabolism of a single molecule of glucose can generate 36–38 molecules of ATP (from ADP). This is an energy transfer of about 1130 KJ (270 kcal/mol) of glucose. This energy can then be used to power other cellular processes.

Other nucleoside phosphates

Many of the nucleoside phosphates have been identified as signalling molecules, both outside and inside cells. ATP has been identified as a neurotransmitter at nerve terminals of the autonomic nervous system (see Chapters 4 and 8), as have ADP and AMP. Intracellular ATP can bind to a number of enzymes and receptors to regulate their action.

The cyclic nucleotides, cyclic AMP (**cAMP**) and cyclic guanosine monophosphate (**cGMP**), are important intracellular messengers called **second messengers**, involved in signal transduction between membrane receptors and intra-

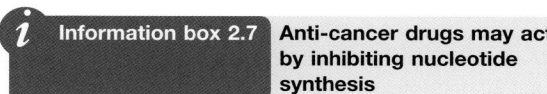

Fig. 2.17 **Structure of adenosine triphosphate (ATP).** The symbol ~ denotes the so-called high-energy bonds.

> ### ⓘ Information box 2.7 | Anti-cancer drugs may act by inhibiting nucleotide synthesis
>
> One of the ways in which cancer is treated is to prevent the rapid proliferation of the cancer cells by blocking cell division. As the majority of normal cells will not be dividing they will not be affected by drugs which block cell division. Many of the side effects of anti-cancer drugs can be accounted for by their effect on cells that are normally rapidly dividing, such as hair and intestinal cells.
>
> A commonly used anti-cancer drug methotrexate, acts by inhibiting an enzyme involved in the production of thymidine nucleotides. It is an analogue of dihydrofolate, which acts as a competitive inhibitor of the enzyme DHFR (dihydrofolate reductase). Other cytotoxic agents act by inhibiting other points in the production of nucleic acids.
>
> See also Chapter 4.

cellular proteins. The coenzymes **NAD**, nicotinamide adenine dinucleotide phosphate (**NADP**), flavin adenine dinucleotide (**FAD**) and **coenzyme A** are all derived from nucleotides.

Sources of nucleotides

The nucleotides required to make DNA and RNA can be synthesised de novo by all cells. The first step involves the synthesis of ribose, as ribose 5-phosphate, which is then converted to a precursor for all the nucleosides, PRPP (5-phosphoribosyl pyrophosphate). This precursor is then used to produce either rUMP (see Table 2.14) from which the other pyrimidines are produced or rIMP (inosine monophosphate), which is the precursor for the purines. The nucleoside monophosphates are then phosphorylated by nucleoside kinases to generate the bi- and triphosphates.

Ribonucleotides are required continually by all cells but dividing cells also require deoxyribonucleotides in order to make new DNA. These are produced from the corresponding ribonucleoside diphosphates. The deoxyribonucleotide TMP is produced from dUMP by a series of reactions requiring the vitamin folic acid.

Recycling of nucleotides

The synthesis of nucleotides de novo requires a large input of energy and there are mechanisms by which free bases, either salvaged from endogenous sources or from nucleotides present in the diet, can be combined with PRPP to produce new nucleotides. This recycling is important in some cells, particularly in T lymphocytes. Also many obligate parasites, such as viruses, do not have the enzymes required to manufacture nucleotides and are completely dependent on their hosts for a supply of nucleotides.

Deoxyribonucleic acid and ribonucleic acids

Deoxyribonucleic acid

Only a single type of nucleic acid is made from the deoxyribonucleotides, **deoxyribonucleic acid**, or **DNA**, and this is found in all cells capable of dividing.

Most of the DNA within a cell is found in the nucleus, from which derives the name nucleic acids. It is absent from red blood cells, which do not have a nucleus. It is also found in the cytoplasm of prokaryotic cells (bacteria) and some viruses (DNA viruses). A small amount of DNA is also found inside intracellular structures called mitochondria. DNA occurs as a double-stranded molecule, which has a characteristic double-helical structure. This structure was first proposed by James Watson and Francis Crick in 1953, after seeing the X-ray crystallography data obtained by Rosalind Franklin and Maurice Wilkins.

Ribonucleic acids

Nucleic acids made from **ribonucleotides** are more diverse. Three types of **ribonucleic acid** (RNA) are found in eukaryotic cells. These are:

- **Messenger RNA** (mRNA): which is copied from DNA and used as the template for the synthesis of proteins
- **Transfer RNA** (tRNA): small molecules which transfer amino acids to the site of protein synthesis, the ribosome
- **Ribosomal RNA** (rRNA): ribosomes consist of a combination of RNA and protein in two subunits. They are involved in binding mRNA and tRNA during protein synthesis.

Details of how these molecules are involved in the manufacture of proteins are covered below. RNAs are found in all cells (except red blood cells), including prokaryotes, and in some viruses (RNA viruses). All viruses have either DNA or RNA as their genetic material.

Clinical box 2.6 Excess purines can cause disease

In humans, excess purines are broken down to uric acid. If large amounts of uric acid are produced and not removed by the kidneys, uric acid crystals are deposited in joints and soft tissues, resulting in gout. One treatment of gout blocks the enzyme, xanthine oxidase, which catalyses the last steps in the production of uric acid. The intermediate breakdown products are more water soluble than uric acid and can be excreted.

Deficiencies in one of the enzymes involved in the recycling pathways leads to increased purine synthesis and a concomitant increase in uric acid, leading to a condition known as Lesch–Nyhan syndrome. One of the features of Lesch–Nyhan syndrome is gout. Patients may also go on to develop arthritis and severe mental disorders.

Constituent bases of DNA and RNA

Each nucleic acid contains two purines and two pyrimidines. The purines adenine (A) and guanine (G) are found in both DNA and RNA. However, DNA and RNA differ in one of their pyrimidines. DNA contains the pyrimidines cytosine (C) and thymine (T), but in RNA thymine is replaced by uracil (U).

Nucleotide bonds

The nucleic acid chains are formed by the sequential linkage of nucleoside triphosphates by phosphodiester bonds between the sugar and phosphate groups (Fig. 2.18), a reaction catalysed by the enzymes DNA polymerase and RNA polymerase. The free hydroxyl group of carbon-3 of the sugar is linked to the triphosphate on the carbon-5 on the next nucleotide, with the loss of a pyrophosphate (PPi). The chain grows in the direction 5′→3′. This forms a sugar-phosphate chain with bases attached to the other side of each sugar (carbon-1). At physiological pH the phosphate groups are anions, so the nucleic acids have a negative charge.

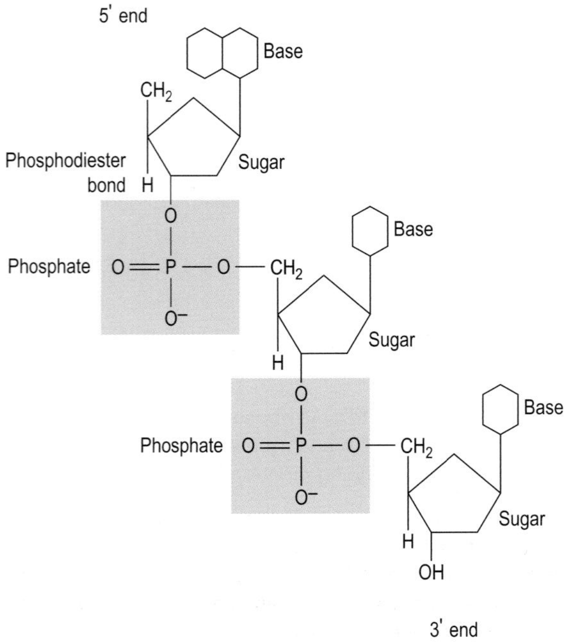

Fig. 2.18 **Nucleotide bond formation.**

Nucleic acid structure

While the subunits which make up DNA and RNA are fairly similar, there are great structural differences between the macromolecules themselves.

Primary structure

The primary structure of DNA and RNA consists of chains of nucleotides held together by nucleotide bonds. DNA molecules are very large. The genetic material in eukaryotes is organised in units called chromosomes, each of which contains a single DNA molecule. In humans, the largest of these is nearly 10 cm long when fully extended and has $2–3 \times 10^8$ nucleotides in each of its two strands.

RNA molecules vary enormously in size. Each mRNA molecule is used to code for a protein. Therefore the length of the mRNA is related to the size of the protein. Due to the way in which the coding occurs, the mRNA for a protein has at least three times more nucleotides than the number of amino acids in the protein and may have many more. Their sizes range from 500 to 6000 nucleotides. About 50 different tRNA molecules are produced in animal cells, each between 70 and 90 nucleotides long.

Secondary structure of DNA

The secondary structure of DNA is relatively simple, but it nevertheless gives clear indications of how the molecule can function as a source of information and also how it can be duplicated. It is dependent on interactions called **base pairing** between the bases that project from the sides of the sugar–phosphate backbone of each of the two strands. The two strands of the DNA molecule run in opposite directions from one another; they are anti-parallel, with one 3′→5′ chain and one 5′→3′ chain.

Base pairing

Hydrogen bonds form between pairs of bases projecting from each strand, each **base pair** consisting of a purine and a pyrimidine. The bases can only form specific pairs, depending on the number of hydrogen bonds formed between them (Fig. 2.19). Pairs consisting of **adenine** and **thymine** can form two hydrogen bonds, and pairs between **cytosine** and **guanine** have three hydrogen bonds. The two types of pairs are the same width, which means the double strands are held at the same distance apart throughout their length, with the two carbons from the sugar–phosphate backbone being 1.08 nm apart.

The planar base pairs are thus stacked one on top of another along the core of the DNA, where hydrophobic interactions occur between the non-polar base pairs. The negatively charged phosphate groups and the sugar backbone are on the outside.

The entire DNA molecule is extremely stable because of the large number of hydrogen bonds between the bases and the hydrophobic interactions between the base pairs.

Helical structure of DNA

The double-stranded DNA molecule forms a regular helical structure with 10 base pairs (bp) for each turn, advancing 3.4 nm (0.34 nm per base pair). The geometry of the backbone favours a right-handed helix, which is the normal structure. This type of DNA is called the B form. The two helical grooves along the outside of the molecule have different widths, called the major and minor grooves. The DNA mol-

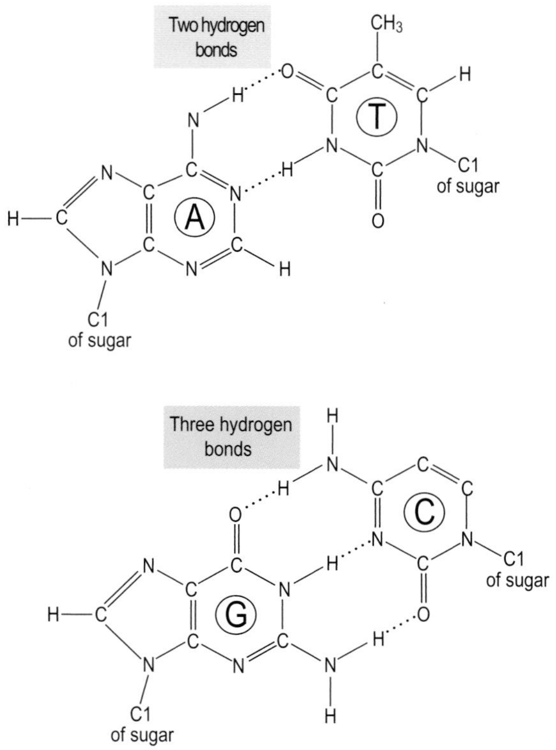

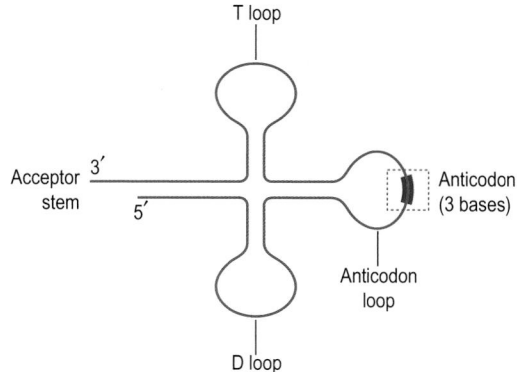

Fig. 2.19 **Base pairing between A-T (or U) and C-G.**

ecule is stable as well as being quite flexible as there are no hydrogen bonds between nucleotides above or below which would make the double helix more rigid. While most DNA exists in the B form, other forms of DNA are known to exist which may be involved in interactions between DNA and proteins or different regions of DNA.

Complementary strands of DNA

The two strands of the DNA are **complementary**. Because of the constraints of base pairing (A with T and G with C) a particular sequence on one strand must be reflected by a specific sequence on the other. For example the sequence TGCT in one strand would be reflected by the sequence ACGA in the other. In this complementarity lies the key to the way in which the sequence of bases can act as a template for the production of identical copies.

Secondary structure of RNA

RNA molecules are single-stranded and many have a well-defined secondary structure. Stem-loops are loops of RNA that have a base-paired sequence at the beginning and end, or hairpins (which are shorter loops that are almost all paired). These can form between regions of the single-stranded RNA by base pairing between complementary regions.

The small tRNAs all have a similar structure (Fig. 2.20). They form a cloverleaf pattern with four stem-loops, each of which forms a short double helix. rRNA forms a complex secondary structure containing many stem-loops. This pattern seems to be common among a wide variety of organisms, suggesting a common evolutionary origin.

Tertiary structure of RNA

Only some RNAs have a unique folding pattern and, as previously described for proteins, the primary structure is all that is required to reassemble the molecule if it is denatured. The

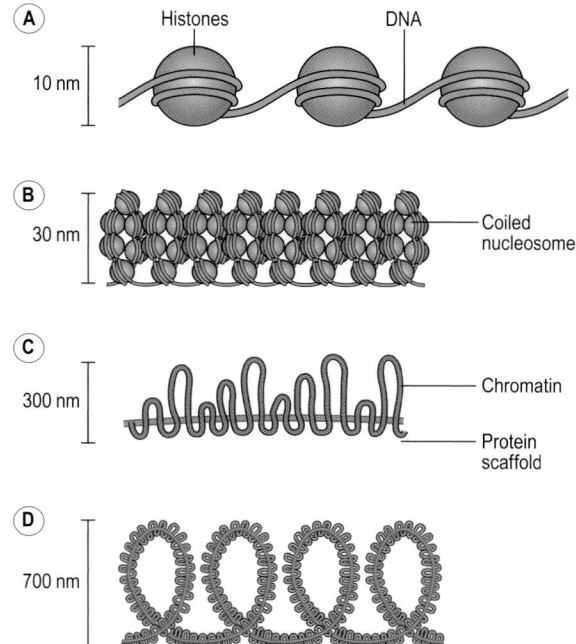

Fig. 2.20 **Generalised structure of tRNA.**

Fig. 2.21 **Tertiary structure of DNA.**

tertiary structure of tRNAs involves hydrogen bonding, which holds two of the loops parallel to the rest of the molecule in an L-shaped molecule, with a site for binding to mRNA at one end and a site at the other end where the amino acid can be attached.

Tertiary structure of DNA

In a human cell there are about 3×10^9 base pairs of DNA that must be packed into the nucleus. The largest **chromosome** has over 200 million base pairs, which, if extended completely, would give a DNA molecule that would be much larger than the cell. In addition, the packing must allow this DNA to be easily accessible by uncoiling, in order to copy segments.

Chromatin and nucleosomes

In the chromosome, DNA is combined with some RNA and about the same mass of protein, producing a structure called **chromatin**. Chromatin consists of a series of units called **nucleosomes** (Fig. 2.21). Each nucleosome is composed of globular proteins called histones, around which are wrapped two loops of DNA 140 bp long, with a piece of linker DNA between each nucleosome about 80 bp long (Fig. 2.21A).

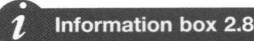

The Human Genome Project has sequenced the entire human genome

A project to map and sequence the entire human genome of approximately 3 billion base pairs was started in 1990 and the first stage, described as a 'working draft', was declared complete on 26 June 2000, by two groups, the Human Genome Project led by Francis Collins, and Celera Genomics led by Craig Venter. The groups used different techniques to produce the draft, which was fully completed by 2003. Surprisingly the total number of genes in the human genome turned out to be much lower than expected (20000–40000) although many genes produce more than one gene product through alternative splicing. Much effort is now concerned with identifying the role of these genes and it is expected that this will lead to further advances in medicine.

This produces a 10 nm width fibre which is then coiled into a fibre 30 nm wide with 6 nucleosomes per turn (Fig. 2.21B). The coils are then formed into a supercoiled structure 300 nm in diameter (Fig. 2.21C). This multiple folding reduces the length of the DNA molecule by about 8000-fold. When cells are about to divide the chromatin is concentrated still further and the DNA molecules become visible under a light microscope as chromosomes (Fig. 2.21D). How DNA uncoils in order to be copied is an obvious topological problem.

Human cells have 23 pairs of chromosomes, each with a specific size and shape.

Mitochondrial DNA

The tertiary structure of mitochondrial DNA is very different from nuclear DNA. It is a circular molecule, which is similar to the DNA in bacteria. This is used as evidence that mitochondria originated as free-living bacteria, before forming a symbiotic relationship with what later became eukaryotic cells.

BASIC CELL STRUCTURE

The defining difference between prokaryotic and eukaryotic cells is the presence, in all eukaryotic cells, of a nucleus and other intracellular structures. In the same way that macromolecules contained within cells have similarities across a wide range of organisms, so there are common structures found in cells of different types. However, the specific structure of a particular cell varies enormously, both between cells of different organisms and between cells within a multicellular organism. While there are many multicellular organisms, such as sponges, which consist of aggregates of largely similar cells, most multicellular organisms have cells with different specialised functions. Furthermore, animals and plants have significant differences in their organelles and cell membranes.

HISTOLOGY

Cellular structures can be identified using either light microscopy or electron microscopy (EM). The study of tissue structure by microscopy is termed **histology**. Naturally, the thin layers of cells or tissues on a slide are transparent and featureless, so both types of microscopy require that the cell or components within the cell are made opaque in some way, which usually kills the tissue. Specialised forms of light microscopy, such as phase contrast, can be used to observe living specimens, although their resolution is fairly poor. The light microscope can resolve objects which are about 0.2 μm apart with magnification up to about 1000 times.

Histochemistry

Cells can be treated by a wide range of methods so that they become visible under the light microscope. These methods rely on specific chemical reactions between the chemicals being applied and the molecules making up or contained within the cellular organelles. One of the most useful stains is a combination called haematoxylin and eosin (H and E). Haematoxylin is a basic dye that stains acidic components in the cell blue. Eosin is an acidic dye that stains basic components pink. In most cells, H and E stains the nucleus, containing the acidic DNA and RNA, blue, and the cytoplasm, most of whose proteins are basic, pink.

Other staining methods have been developed in order to label specific tissues; for example enzyme histochemistry can identify cells or parts of cells containing a particular enzyme. The recent development of methods using immunological markers, a technique referred to as immunohistochemistry, enables identification of specific proteins or other macromolecules within cells.

Electron microscopy

The detailed ultrastructure of cells can be revealed only by **electron microscopy**, where the image is formed by bombarding the specimen with electrons. This can resolve objects which are 1 nm apart, with a maximum magnification of about 100000-fold. There are two types of EM:

- Scanning EM – used to image the surface of objects.
- Transmission EM – which uses thin sections of tissue treated with heavy metals that bind to cell components in varying amounts and reflect electrons. Those components with a large amount of bound metal reflect many electrons, are electron dense, and look dark in EM, and vice versa.

All EM images are black and white only, although false colour processing can be used to highlight differences in grey scale.

Artefacts

Care must be taken in interpreting images from both types of microscopy. Artefacts can be introduced during the many steps involved in the preparation of a specimen, and interpreting two-dimensional images as three-dimensional (3D) objects takes a lot of thought. However, computer software nowadays assists in reconstructing 3D structures from sequential sections.

ORGANELLES, STRUCTURE AND FUNCTION

Organelles are distinctive structures found within cells. Many are enclosed by one or more membranes, but there are a few structures which are not (called non-membranous organelles) (Fig. 2.22). Organelles enable cells to compartmentalise biochemical processes into different regions of the cell. Enzymes needed to carry out a particular reaction can

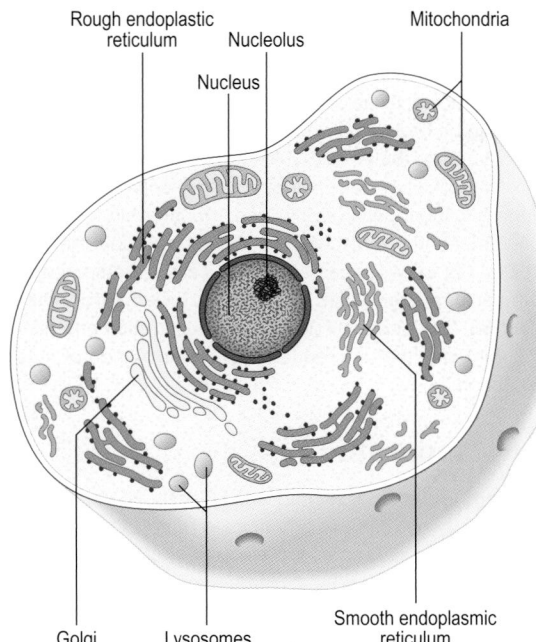

Rough endoplasmic reticulum
Nucleolus
Nucleus
Mitochondria
Golgi
Lysosomes
Smooth endoplasmic reticulum

Fig. 2.22 **An idealised eukaryotic cell showing the major organelles.** Not all organelles are present in all cells.

> **ⓘ** **Information box 2.9** **Gram staining of bacterial cell walls**

Gram staining was invented by Hans Christian Gram in 1884 and is used to identify different types of bacteria. The method consists of soaking the sample of the bacterial culture firstly in a violet dye (Gentian violet), followed by treatment with iodine. The slide is then washed with alcohol and counter-stained with a red dye, safranine.

Gram-positive bacteria are coloured blue-black and Gram-negative bacteria are stained red. The different colours obtained are due to the different amounts and accessibility of the peptidoglycan in the cell walls of bacteria. Gram-positive bacteria have a thick layer of peptidoglycan surrounding their plasma membranes. This takes up the violet dye and appears blue to purple.

Gram-negative bacteria have less peptidoglycan, which is surrounded by a second outer cell membrane.

Mycobacteria, such as those causing tuberculosis, have cell walls that have a very different composition and are not stained by the Gram stain.

be put in the same compartment as the substrates for the reaction, and the products can be passed onto the next enzyme in the chain by placing it in the same compartment. Conditions can be maintained within the restricted volume of organelles that would be harmful to the cell overall.

Cell membranes

All cells, both prokaryotic and eukaryotic, are surrounded by a **plasma membrane**, also called the **cell membrane**. It maintains the integrity of the cell and separates the fluids inside the cell from those on the outside and is typically about 9 nm thick. Under the electron microscope it is seen to consist of two outer dark layers, with a clearer inner layer. The plasma membrane regulates the movement of molecules in and out of the cell. The major component of all membranes is lipid, which on its own would make the cell impermeable to all hydrophilic molecules. However, it also contains proteins that allow the movement of hydrophilic molecules through the membrane. The outside of the plasma membrane is also studded with carbohydrates, attached to the proteins and the lipids, which have roles in cell-to-cell interactions and cell recognition. The membranes which surround the membrane-bound organelles also have a banded, double-layered appearance in electron micrographs but are thinner (about 6 nm).

Plant and bacterial cell walls

Plant cells have a rigid cell wall outside their plasma membrane, which gives the plant cell strength. Plant cell walls contain cellulose and sometimes lignin and suberin, which form wood and cork, respectively. Most bacteria also have cell walls. They often contain peptidoglycan, a polymer of amino sugars cross-linked with short peptide chains. The presence and concentration of this macromolecule is used as a way to categorise bacteria. Peptidoglycan is not found in eukaryotic cells and many antibiotics, including the penicillins, inhibit bacterial cell growth by inhibiting its synthesis.

Cytoplasm

Between the plasma membrane and the nucleus is the **cytoplasm**, which contains all the other cellular elements suspended in the **cytosol**. This is a viscous aqueous solution that contains salts, proteins, sugars and the countless other molecules that are involved in the metabolic pathways. It is criss-crossed by the fibrous cytoskeleton. It has been estimated that there are about 300 mg/mL of protein and RNA in the cytosol, which makes it very crowded indeed.

Nucleus

The most prominent organelle in most eukaryotic cells is the **nucleus**, which is often at the centre of the cell, although some cells, such as skeletal muscle cells, have their nuclei displaced to one side. Some cells have more than one nucleus, whereas mammalian red blood cells lose their nucleus as they mature (see Ch. 12). The nucleus is the only organelle that can be seen under the light microscope without staining.

The nucleus contains the chromosomes in the form of chromatin, which is not normally visible as an organised structure. Actively transcribed chromatin, called **euchromatin**, is diffuse. This is where mRNA and tRNA are being transcribed. More condensed chromatin, called **heterochromatin**, is inactive.

Inside the nucleus are one or more dark-staining spherical areas called **nucleoli**. These are areas of the nucleus where ribosomes are assembled. These areas contain large amounts of RNA and proteins, and in cells which are actively secreting large amounts of protein they can be very large. Surrounding the chromatin and the nucleoli is a gel-like suspension called the **nucleoplasm**.

The nucleus is surrounded by a double layer of membrane, the **nuclear envelope**. The inner membrane is smooth, whereas the outer membrane may be continuous with the

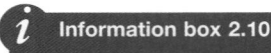

endoplasmic reticulum and the outer face may be covered with ribosomes. The nuclear envelope is studded with pores. These are about 9 nm in diameter and are surrounded by an octet of protein complexes in each membrane, forming a channel through which molecules of protein and RNA can move.

Endoplasmic reticulum

Extending from the nucleus and into the cytoplasm are a series of interconnected flattened tubules and sacs called the **endoplasmic reticulum** (ER). This network of membranes extending into the cytoplasm, which is continuous with the outer nuclear membrane, encloses cavities called cisternae. There are two types of ER within the cell, one called rough ER, whose membranes are covered with dense granules, and smooth ER, which does not have these granules.

Ribosomes and rough ER

The granules which are studded all over the rough ER are called **ribosomes**. They are made from two subunits, each made up of a combination of RNA and protein which is assembled in the nucleolus. The large subunit contains a large RNA molecule of 4800 nucleotides with two smaller RNAs of 160 and 120 nucleotides, all associated with about 50 proteins. The small subunit has a single RNA of 1900 nucleotides and about 33 proteins.

Ribosomes are involved in the synthesis of proteins, which may be destined for insertion into membranes, used in lysosomes, or exported from the cell. Rough ER is very extensive in cells that have high levels of protein secretion. Many of these proteins are then processed by enzymes within the ER, which can add sugars and proteins to them. Small vesicles bud off from the ER and are seen to combine with the Golgi apparatus (see below).

Ribosomes are also found in the cytoplasm, unattached to the ER. These free ribosomes are involved in the manufacture of cytoplasmic and nuclear proteins. Mitochondria also contain ribosomes, whose rRNA is coded for by mitochondrial DNA.

Smooth ER

Smooth ER is continuous with rough ER, but is generally more tubular in nature. Smooth ER manufactures membrane phospholipids and also makes cholesterol and steroid hormones. Cells, such as those in the adrenal cortex, the testes and the ovaries, which secrete large amounts of steroid hormones, have very extensive smooth ER. In the liver, cells called hepatocytes have rough ER, which is involved in the production of plasma proteins, such as albumin. However, a large proportion of the ER in these cells consists of smooth ER. This smooth ER is associated with granules of glycogen, which can be broken down to maintain blood glucose levels. The enzymes in the smooth ER in the liver are involved in the detoxification of a wide range of lipid-soluble molecules, including carcinogens and drugs, transforming them into polar metabolites that can then be excreted by the kidney (see Ch. 14). In two types of muscle cells, cardiac and skeletal muscle, a specialised smooth ER, called **sarcoplasmic reticulum**, has a critical role in the sequestration and release of calcium ions that are required for the activation of muscle contraction.

Golgi apparatus

The **Golgi apparatus**, named after Camillo Golgi, who first described it in 1898, appears as a number of flattened membrane-bound sacs called **cisternae**, stacked on top of each other and surrounded by large numbers of small spherical membrane-bound organelles called **vesicles**. It is involved in the concentration, modification (mainly glycosylation and phosphorylation) and packaging of proteins produced in the rough ER. The Golgi apparatus has a definite polarity. Small vesicles, called transport vesicles, derived from the ER and containing proteins and lipids, fuse onto the *cis* Golgi. After processing through the *medial* Golgi, where they are glycosylated, vesicles containing protein bud off from the *trans* Golgi, where they are sorted for a number of different destinations including secretory vesicles and lysosomes. The proteins move through the Golgi stack by being shuttled in small transport vesicles from cisterna to cisterna.

Secretory vesicles

Proteins destined to be exported from the cell are contained in vesicles derived from the *trans* Golgi. Mature vesicles are called **secretory granules**, and in some cells (for example, in the exocrine pancreas) these are some of the most prominent structures, filling a large proportion of the cytoplasm. During maturation the contents of the vesicles are concentrated and the proteins can be modified; for example modification of the insulin molecule, which removes the C-peptide, occurs in the secretory granules (see Clinical Box 2.1).

Secretion

Proteins are released into the extracellular space by a process called **exocytosis**, which involves the fusion of the vesicle's membrane with the plasma membrane. Release of the proteins may be continuous, or vesicles may be stored. Continuous secretion, called **constitutive secretion**, occurs in some immune cells called plasma cells, which continually secrete immunoglobulins.

Most secretion occurs in response to a signal, often a rise in intracellular calcium levels, and this **regulated secretion** releases stored secretory granules. Many neurons release more than one type of chemical and it is possible to identify different populations of vesicles in nerve terminals. The different chemicals, which often consist of a small non-protein and a protein, are released under different patterns of stimulation (see Ch. 8).

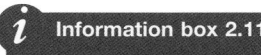

Enzyme histochemistry can be used to identify lysosomes

Despite their variable and relatively unremarkable structure, lysosomes can be easily identified using a staining technique called enzyme histochemistry, as they contain acid phosphatases. The cells are incubated with a substrate for the acid phosphatase. The reaction between enzyme and substrate releases phosphate ions. These ions react with lead ions to form the insoluble product lead phosphate, which is deposited at the location of the acid phosphatase. This is then treated with ammonium sulphide to give a black precipitate of lead sulphide, clearly visible with a light or electron microscope.

Clinical box 2.7 **Tay–Sach's disease is one of a number of lysosomal storage diseases**

The absence of a particular enzyme in the breakdown pathways inside lysosomes leads to the accumulation of the substrate for that enzyme. In Tay–Sach's disease, the absence of the enzyme, hexosaminidase leads to the accumulation of a membrane glycolipid, G_{M2}, which is particularly common in nerve cells. The disease, which is inherited, causes mental retardation and central nervous system disorders, with death occurring by about the age of 5.

Lysosomes and proteasomes

One of the destinations for vesicles derived from the Golgi are the **lysosomes**. These are spherical or oval organelles with a variety of sizes up to 400 nm diameter. They contain about 40 different acid hydrolase enzymes which can digest most biological molecules. As well as vesicles from *trans* Golgi, other membrane-bound structures fuse with lysosomes, where their contents can be digested. These include particles such as bacteria and viruses that have been retrieved from the extracellular medium by two processes called endocytosis and phagocytosis. The lysosome is also used to destroy aged cell organelles that are first engulfed by the ER, forming a vesicle that is passed to lysosomes for destruction.

Acid hydrolases

The fluid inside lysosomes is much more acidic, at about pH 4.8, than the normal pH of about 7.0–7.3. This is the optimal pH for the activity of the **acid hydrolase** enzymes present in the lysosomes. The low pH denatures many macromolecules, which aids their degradation. However, fortunately, the acid hydrolase enzymes are relatively inactive at the pH of the cytoplasm, so if a single lysosome is ruptured little digestion of cytoplasmic contents occurs. Hydrogen ions will tend to leak out of the lysosome so the pH gradient between the cytoplasm and the interior of the lysosome is maintained by special protein pumps in the lysosomal membrane that pump hydrogen ions into the lysosome. Other pumps transport the products of the lysosomal digestion, such as amino acids and sugars, into the cytoplasm where they can be recycled.

The lysosomal membrane has an important role in compartmentalising the degradative enzymes because, if many lysosomes were ruptured, the cell could self-digest. This process is known as **autolysis** and can occur physiologically, such as, for example, during the breakdown of the uterine lining during menstruation.

Proteasomes

While membrane components and aged organelles are degraded in lysosomes, another pathway exists to degrade cytosolic proteins. **Proteasomes** are large complexes of proteins arranged in four rings around a central core. Proteins destined for destruction are first tagged with multiple copies of a protein called **ubiquitin** by specific enzymes. This acts as a signal to direct the protein into the core of the proteasome where it is broken into small peptides. These are then further digested in the cytoplasm by peptidases. Only proteins tagged with ubiquitin are able to enter the proteasomes, ensuring that normal cytosolic proteins are protected.

Many proteins are continually being turned over and each protein has its own rate of degradation. Some enzymes are replaced rapidly but others such as collagen have an almost imperceptible turnover rate. In starvation, proteins, particularly skeletal muscle proteins, are broken down to provide precursors for glucose synthesis.

Peroxisomes

Peroxisomes are small vesicles, also called **microbodies**, which superficially resemble lysosomes, but contain completely different enzymes that are transported into the peroxisome from the cytosol. Some of these enzymes are oxidases and catalases:

■ The oxidases break down a variety of substrates, such as fatty acids, with the production of hydrogen peroxide (H_2O_2). Although potentially highly toxic to cells, H_2O_2 is produced inside some cells of the immune system in order to kill bacteria.
■ The catalase enzymes use H_2O_2 to oxidise other potentially toxic compounds, or break down H_2O_2 to water.

Other peroxidase enzymes are also involved in the biosynthesis of cholesterol and other membrane components. Peroxisomes are particularly abundant in the hepatocytes of the liver.

Mitochondria

All the organelles described so far are involved in the production, processing, targeting and degradation of the proteins and other molecules made within the cell. However, most of these processes require **energy** in the form of ATP. **Mitochondria** are the organelles where ATP is generated, and so they are particularly plentiful in cells which consume large amounts of energy.

Structure of mitochondria

Mitochondria vary in size and shape but are generally sausage-shaped and about 1 μm wide and 7 μm long. They have a complex internal structure with two layers of membranes. The outer membrane is smooth and the same thickness as in other organelles. It is highly permeable to small molecules, due to the presence of a pore-forming protein called **porin**. The intermembrane space between the outer and inner membrane is usually narrow. The inner membrane is studded with many proteins that are involved in oxidative phosphorylation, and the subsequent generation of ATP. This membrane is thinner and has multiple folds projecting inwards, called **cristae**, producing a very large surface area for ATP production. The innermost region is called the **matrix**. It is here that pyruvate, derived from the metabolism of glucose in the cytosol, and fatty acids are metabolised to provide the substrates for oxidative phosphorylation.

Mitochondrial DNA

The mitochondria are unique among the organelles in that they contain their own DNA and the mechanism to make proteins. The matrix contains **mitochondrial DNA** (mtDNA), which codes for some of the molecules needed by the mitochondrion, including its own rRNA and tRNA. However, many of the proteins required by mitochondria are manufactured in the cytoplasm and have to be imported into the mitochondrial matrix. Receptors on the surface of mitochondria act to transfer these proteins required in the matrix through the outer and inner membranes.

Evolutionary origin of mitochondria

Bacterial cells do not contain mitochondria but mitochondria themselves have many similarities with a group of bacteria called purple bacteria. This has led to the hypothesis called the **endosymbiotic theory**: that mitochondria and other intracellular organelles of eukaryotes could have arisen when one type of bacteria was engulfed by another, without digesting it. The two bacteria could have become dependent on one another until they could no longer exist separately. Another piece of evidence for the bacterial origin of mitochondria is that the genetic code which translates the bases of the mitochondrial DNA molecule into amino acids is slightly different from that used by the rest of the cell, and can vary both between different mammals and other organisms.

Inheritance of mitochondrial DNA

Mitochondria are passed from parent to child during reproduction, but because the volume of the cytoplasm contributed by the sperm is very small compared to that of the ovum, virtually all the mitochondria (estimated at 99.99%) are inherited from the mother. mtDNA is therefore passed, virtually unchanged, down the maternal line and geneticists interested in the evolution of humans have utilised mtDNA lineages to examine population movements.

Plant 'mitochondria'

In plants, the equivalent organelle is the chloroplast, which generates glucose from light, water and CO_2 by photosyn-

thesis. This reaction not only provides all the food we eat, but also produces oxygen as a 'waste product', without which we could not live.

Non-membranous organelles

Non-membranous organelles are cellular structures not bound by membranes. These include ribosomes and lipid droplets, which are composed of triacylglycerols, seen in fat-storing cells called adipocytes. In liver hepatocytes, large numbers of glycogen granules can be seen in the cytoplasm either as single particles or as aggregates called rosettes.

Cytoskeleton

All cells have an internal skeleton of protein fibres called the **cytoskeleton** (Table 2.9). These are made up of:

- Microfilaments
- Intermediate filaments
- Microtubules.

Microfilaments

Microfilaments are composed of twisted double strands of actin (Fig. 2.23A) and are the thinnest of the cytoskeletal fibres at 7 nm in diameter. They enable cells to move in an amoeboid fashion and change their shape. They form a mesh of fibres below the plasma membrane attached to proteins embedded in the membrane, which themselves connect with

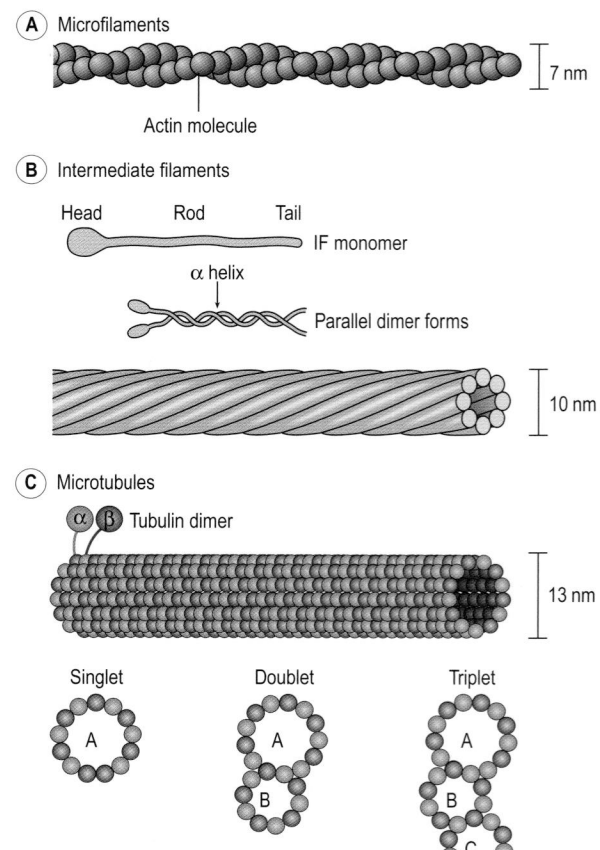

(A) Microfilaments

Actin molecule

7 nm

(B) Intermediate filaments

Head   Rod   Tail

IF monomer

α helix

Parallel dimer forms

10 nm

(C) Microtubules

α β Tubulin dimer

13 nm

Singlet   Doublet   Triplet

A   A   A
       B   B
              C

Fig. 2.23 **Structure of cytoskeletal elements.** IF, intermediate filament.

> ℹ **Information box 2.12** **Mutations in mitochondrial DNA are inherited maternally**
>
> Any mutations that occur in mtDNA are passed from a mother to all her children. Because many of these mutations occur in the enzymes responsible for energy metabolism and impair ATP production they often result in an increase in anaerobic metabolism, with the production of lactic acid. This may cause cell death in tissues such as skeletal and cardiac muscle which are heavily dependent on ATP, causing myopathies.

molecules of the ECM. This enables a cell to fix its shape with respect to the external environment and, if necessary, move around in it. Cells move by extending either thin finger-like structures, called **filopodia**, or thin sheets, called **lamellipodia**, which contain large amounts of F-actin that is continuously added to in the direction of movement. The fibres are thought to be moved forward by the movement of myosin pushing the actin fibres against the plasma membrane. They are attached to long actin fibres, called stress fibres, which extend backwards. Microfilaments also form the core of the specialised plasma membrane structures, microvilli and stereocilium.

Intermediate filaments

Intermediate filaments (IFs) are made from a variety of proteins. However, they all form filaments 10 nm wide which are extremely stable. They all form α-helical dimers, which twist around one another forming rope-like structures (Fig. 2.23B), which give mechanical support to structures such as the nucleus and the plasma membrane. IFs do not change dynamically like microfilaments and microtubules, and so they form the most stable element of the cytoskeleton.

There are five classes of IFs, which are characteristic of each cell type. In epithelial cells, IFs made from keratin are anchored to structures called desmosomes, which link cells together, and hemidesmosomes, which link cells to the ECM. In nerve cells, neurofilaments form the core of axons which can stretch for long distances.

Microtubules

Microtubules are made up of two globular proteins, α- and β-tubulin, which form a dimer. These proteins are polymerised into a protofilament of alternating α- and β-tubulin. These are then arranged to form a tube from 13 protofilaments, which is 25 nm wide, called a singlet (Fig. 2.23C). Other arrangements involve adding extra protofilaments around the singlet to form doublets and triplets. The microtubule can be extended by the addition of further dimers to the '+' end of each protofilament, the end furthest away from the nucleus. Microtubules can be shortened from both ends by disassembly, which, using electron microscopy, looks as if the tube is being frayed. The growth of microtubules requires GTP, which is hydrolysed to GDP when the dimer of tubulin is incorporated into the growing protofilaments.

A number of different proteins are attached to microtubules, called **microtubule-associated proteins** (MAPs). One type of MAP cross-links microtubules in the cytoplasm, or binds to IFs. One of the MAPs found in nerve cells is called **tau**. A model of Alzheimer's disease suggests that accumulation and cross-linking of tau proteins can lead to the formation of the neurofibrillary tangles which are found in the brains of many people with Alzheimer's.

Transport along microtubules

Inside the cell, organelles and proteins are moved to specific locations. Microtubules are used as tracks along which organelles can be moved. For example, in nerve cells, the distance between the nucleus and the synapse, the point at the end of the axon where chemicals are released, can be several metres. The synapse does not contain the ribosomes required for protein synthesis, and in any case the DNA is in the distant nucleus. Proteins and membrane components required in the synapse are manufactured in and near the nucleus in the cell body and must be transported along microtubules to the synapse. This process is called **fast axonal transport**.

Transport occurs in both directions along the same microtubule and is rapid (1–2 μm/s):

- **Anterograde transport** carries new material from the cell body to the synapse.
- **Retrograde transport** carries unwanted materials back to the cell body for destruction by lysosomes.

Anterograde transport

The anterograde transport, from the − end to the + end of each microtubule, is carried out by proteins called **kinesins**. These consist of four peptide chains: two heavy chains that bind to tubulin at their head end, and which are then coiled in an α-helix until they reach the tail end, where there are two light chains which bind to the transported substance. The force required to move material is provided by the heavy chains which, like the muscle protein myosin, change their shape on the hydrolysis of ATP.

Retrograde transport

Another type of motor protein, **dynein**, is responsible for retrograde transport. Dyneins have a different structure from kinesins but they are similar in that a globular head region binds to the microtubules and moves with the consumption of ATP. In nerve cells, microtubules do not extend all the way to the synapse; they stop at the end of the axon, where they are replaced by microfilaments. Materials transported along the microtubules are taken the rest of the way along these microfilaments, the movement being powered by a type of myosin and ATP. Other, slower transport may involve IFs.

Microtubule structures

Three distinct structures are formed from microtubules:

- Centrosomes
- Cilia
- Flagella.

Centrosomes

Most cells contain a **centrosome** which is found near the nucleus. This is the organising centre for microtubules, which radiate from here to the plasma membrane. The centrosome contains two **centrioles**, each of which is composed of a cylinder made up of nine microtubule triplets. This arrangement is called a 9 + 0 array. Centrioles are essential to the movement of the chromosomes to the opposite ends of a cell during cell division.

Cilia and flagella

Cilia and **flagella** (singular: cilium and flagellum) are mobile projections from the plasma membrane that are also composed of microtubules. The arrangement is slightly different from that found in centrioles, as the **core** or **axoneme** is formed from nine microtubule doublets, arranged around a doublet running down the central axis, in what is called a 9 + 2 array. Just underneath the plasma membrane, cilia and flagella are anchored to the **basal body**, which is identical in structure to the centrioles. The doublets of the cilia and flagella merge into the triplets of the basal body. The entire structure is covered in extensions of the plasma membrane. Inner and outer arms attached to the nine doublets are dyneins, which move the cilia and flagella using energy derived from ATP.

Cilia are hair-like projections up to 10 μm long, whereas flagella are much longer and occur individually or in pairs. Many cells are covered with cilia, which serve to move fluids or particles across their surface. There may be up to 300 cilia on each cell and they move in a coordinated manner. In the lungs, the cells which cover the larger airways are covered in cilia, which move mucus and particulates out of the lungs – the **mucociliary escalator**.

In single-celled organisms, cilia and flagella are the means by which the organism propels itself through the medium in which it lives. The only human cells that have flagella are sperm. Each sperm moves by beating the flagellum that forms its tail. Many bacteria also have flagella but these are completely different in structure, consisting of a protein strand that is rotated in its basal body, using energy derived from proton gradients.

INTRACELLULAR AND EXTRACELLULAR FLUIDS

All cells contain fluid and are bathed in fluid, but the composition of the intracellular and extracellular fluids is very different (Table 2.15). The **extracellular fluid** resembles a dilute version of seawater, possibly reflecting our evolutionary origins as single-celled marine organisms. It is rich in sodium and chloride ions, with quite high levels of calcium but very little protein compared with intracellular fluids. The **intracellular fluid** has a high concentration of potassium and a large number of intracellular anions such as phosphates and protein side chains, which balance the positively charged potassium ions. It also has a relatively high concentration of

protein. Free calcium levels inside cells are very low, reflecting its role as an intracellular messenger.

Ion gradients

While a pure lipid bilayer is virtually impermeable to ions, there are a number of transport processes acting across cell membranes which not only allow the dissipation of the ion gradient but also use the energy contained within it. The concentration gradients of Na^+ and K^+ across the plasma membrane are maintained by the activity of a special transport protein called the Na^+/K^+–ATPase, which transports sodium ions out of the cell and potassium into it. Without the activity of this pump the ion gradients would disappear and many cellular processes would cease to function.

Resting membrane potential

The differential distribution of sodium and potassium cations, and the fact that cells are more permeable (at rest) to potassium than sodium, leads to the establishment of an electrical potential. This is called the **resting membrane potential** which acts across the cell membrane. In most cells it is of the order of −60 mV (inside negative), but is higher in **excitable cells**, such as neurons and muscle (see Ch. 8). Variations in this electrical potential underlie the electrical signalling carried out by excitable cells, which is entirely dependent on the ion gradients of sodium and potassium. The resting membrane potential is very sensitive to the external potassium concentration, which must always be closely controlled otherwise the electrical signalling will be disrupted (Clinical box 2.9).

Osmotic pressure

Osmolarity

Osmosis is the movement of water by diffusion through a semi-permeable membrane from a region of high water concentration to a lower concentration. If two solutions of differing solute concentration are separated by a semi-permeable membrane water will tend to move from the lower solute concentration to the higher one until the solutions have equal concentrations of both water and solute. The solution with the higher solute concentration is said to have a higher **osmotic potential**.

Water is a polar molecule and pure phospholipid bilayers, which are non-polar, only allow limited water movement across them. However, in many cells, particularly in erythrocytes and water-absorbing cells of the collecting ducts of the kidney, there are large numbers of specific water channels, formed by proteins called **aquaporins**. Using these channels

Table 2.15	Composition of intracellular and extracellular fluids	
Ion	Extracellular concentration (mM)	Intracellular concentration (mM)
Na^+	145	12
K^+	4	139
Cl^-	116	4
Bicarbonate, HCO_3^-	29	12
Phosphates	2	13
Protein anions	9	138
Ca^{2+}	1.8	<0.0002
Mg^{2+}	1.5	0.8

water moves freely across these plasma membranes. Therefore the internal and external media must have the same osmotic potential (they must be **isotonic**), otherwise cells would shrink or swell and burst. If cells, for example erythrocytes, are put in a dilute solution which has a lower osmotic potential (it is hypotonic) than normal plasma, then water will move into the cells and they will swell and eventually break open (lysis). Equally, if they are put into a more concentrated hypertonic solution then water would move out of the cells and they would shrink. The osmotic pressure of the intracellular and extracellular fluids is normally the same at about 285 milliosmoles per litre (mOsm/L (see Ch. 14)).

Vascular compartment

The **intravascular** compartment, which contains the blood, is separated from the **extracellular** fluid surrounding most tissues by a barrier, which in the smallest blood vessels, the capillaries, consists of endothelial cells. Although in some tissues, such as the liver, this barrier is very permeable to both water and solutes, in most tissues there is a significant difference between the intravascular and extracellular fluid composition. Although they both contain sodium as their predominant cation, the blood also contains significant amounts of protein, mainly in the form of albumin. This means that blood has a higher osmotic potential than extracellular fluid, which tends to draw water out of the interstitial spaces between the cells. This does not mean that all the fluid around cells moves into the blood. The blood has a significant hydrostatic pressure and this tends to push water out of the blood and into the interstitium. While this varies around the body, the net effect is that the movement of water into and out of the vasculature is balanced (see Clinical box 2.11 and Ch. 11).

PROTEIN SYNTHESIS AND PROCESSING

The central dogma of molecular biology is that, briefly stated, 'DNA makes RNA makes protein' and not the other way round. That is, you cannot make protein from protein or DNA from RNA. This holds true for all cellular organisms. Only in some viruses, which are obligate parasites, is this rule broken (see Information box 2.14).

The synthesis of proteins involves two processes which convert the base sequence of the appropriate DNA into a polypeptide chain.

1. Transcription: the conversion of a specific section of DNA into a complementary strand of mRNA. This transcription occurs in the nucleus after which the mRNA is processed and translocated to the cytoplasm where it is attached to a ribosome.
2. Translation: the strand of mRNA is used as a template to assemble the sequence of amino acids which make up the protein. This involves converting the code within the bases of the mRNA into amino acid residues and each of the 20 possible amino acids is coded for by three bases in what is called the genetic code. Both tRNA and rRNA are involved in this process.

GENES AND THE GENOME

The entire complement of double-stranded DNA within a cell is called the **genome**, but only about 10% of the DNA in mammals is thought to carry information in the form of sequences that are expressed. The sequences of bases within the long DNA molecules are of two different types:

- Those which only occur in single or a few copies, which are the **genes**
- Regions of repeated sequences, which may be repeated millions of times within the genome.

Some of these repeated sequences code for proteins which are needed in large amounts, such as histones. But the function of much of this DNA is unknown, hence the term **'junk' DNA**. Some of this DNA may be 'old' genes which have undergone mutations and are no longer transcribed. However, it has also been suggested that this DNA may act as a reservoir for the evolution of new genes.

Genome size

The size of the genome varies enormously between organisms; the well-studied bacterium *Escherichia coli* has about 5 million base pairs, compared to the 3 trillion base pairs of the human genome. In humans there are estimated to be about 30 000 genes, each of which contains the information for a gene product. Most gene products are proteins; the only other gene products are the RNA molecules that form rRNA and tRNA.

Table 2.16 The genetic code (RNA to amino acids)

First position	Second position				Third position
	U	**C**	**A**	**G**	
U	Phe	Ser	Tyr	Cys	U
	Phe	Ser	Tyr	Cys	C
	Leu	Ser	Stop	Stop	A
	Leu	Ser	Stop	Trp	G
C	Leu	Pro	His	Arg	U
	Leu	Pro	His	Arg	C
	Leu	Pro	Gln	Arg	A
	Leu	Pro	Gln	Arg	G
A	Ile	Thr	Asn	Ser	U
	Ile	Thr	Asn	Ser	C
	Ile	Thr	Lys	Arg	A
	Met (start)	Thr	Lys	Arg	G
G	Val	Ala	Asp	Gly	U
	Val	Ala	Asp	Gly	C
	Val	Ala	Glu	Gly	A
	Val (start)	Ala	Glu	Gly	G

The code given here translates mRNA codons into amino acids; the original sequence of DNA would be complementary to the mRNA and would contain thymine (T) instead of uracil (U).

THE GENETIC CODE

DNA is only made up of a sequence of four different nucleotides (A, G, C and T) which are used to code for 20 amino acids. Obviously this could not be achieved by one-to-one coding as, with only four different nucleotides, it would only be possible to specify four different amino acids. If each amino acid were coded by two nucleotides, there would still only be 16 (4^2) different possible combinations. The way in which DNA codes for different amino acids uses sets of three nucleotides to code for each amino acid giving 64 (4^3) possible combinations. Each group of three nucleotides is called a **codon**. The genetic code is usually shown as a table showing the sequence of three nucleotides in the mRNA codons and the corresponding amino acid (Table 2.16). It can be seen from the table that not all of the codons represent an amino acid. There are three codons that cause the protein chain to terminate, called **stop codons**, and one codon (AUG) that codes for methionine but also acts as a **start codon** to initiate the protein synthesis. The codon GUG usually codes for valine, but occasionally also acts as a start codon.

All 64 possible codons are used, many amino acids being coded for by more than one possible codon, but this is not evenly spread. Some amino acids are represented by six different codons, whereas others only have a single one. The code is said to be 'degenerate'. The code is virtually the same in all organisms and this universality is used as an argument that life on Earth evolved once only. However, there are minor differences in the genetic code in mitochondria, in some protozoans and in single-celled plants. These minor changes are thought to be later mutations.

Reading frame

In most cases the code has to be read, in threes, starting at the AUG codon, to one of the stop codons. This is known as the **reading frame**, and most mRNAs are read within a single frame, although in some cases it has been found that by starting at a different AUG codon the same mRNA can produce a different protein. Also some unusual RNAs contain sites where either four or two bases are read and then the remaining RNA is read with a **frame shift**.

Information box 2.13 Deletion of a single base from DNA will frame shift the protein

If a single nucleotide is removed from a gene then the resulting protein will be very different. The protein chain will be normal up to the point of the deletion. After this all the resulting codons will be read out of phase. This results in different amino acids being substituted and the frame shift will continue adding the wrong amino acids until one of the 'new' codons corresponds to a stop codon. If the deletion is near the end of the coding sequence, then the protein may be nearly normal, but if it is close to the beginning then changes can be catastrophic. Normal haemoglobin is composed of two polypeptide chains, α- and β-globin, folded to hold the haem molecule. β-thalassaemia is an inherited anaemia characterised by a point mutation in the β-globin chain. The resulting frame shift produces a protein that contains a series of unexpected amino acids, rendering the chain unstable and the molecule unbalanced. Precipitation of the globin chains results in red cells that are vulnerable to haemolysis, producing a severe anaemia in those individuals who have inherited the abnormality from both parents.

TRANSCRIPTION

Transcription is started by the binding of the enzyme **RNA polymerase** (RP) to the appropriate section of the appropriate strand of the DNA (Fig. 2.24). RNA polymerases can start a new RNA strand (initiation) and extend it (elongation). In mammals, there are three types of RNA polymerase (RPI, RPII, RPIII), which make pre-rRNA, pre-mRNA and pre-tRNA, respectively.

As stated previously, the two strands of DNA are anti-parallel and complementary. Starting at the same end of each strand would yield two different sequences of bases, so the RP must bind to the correct strand. The strand serving as a template is called the **antisense** strand. The other strand, the coding strand, is not usually transcribed and is called the **sense** strand.

The sequence of bases represented by the sequence of the mRNA is the same as the original coding strand of the

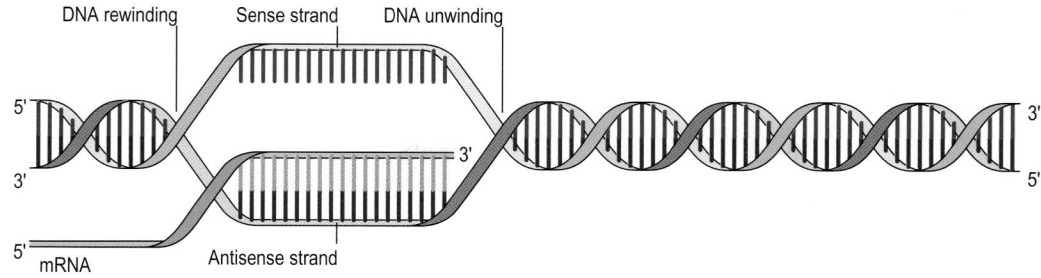

Fig. 2.24 **Transcription of DNA into RNA.**

Table 2.17	**Complementary DNA and mRNA sequences**	
Sequence	**Direction**	**Codons or amino acids**
DNA coding strand (sense)	5′→ 3′	ATG AGA CTA TTC AGC TAA
Complementary DNA (antisense)	3′→ 5′	TAC TCT GAT AAG TCG ATT
mRNA	5′→ 3′	AUG AGA CUA UUC AGC UAA
Amino acids	N → C	Met Arg Leu Phe Ser (start)

Spaces are shown between the codons for clarity.

DNA, except that mRNA contains uracil instead of thymine. This is because a complementary copy of a complementary copy produces the original sequence. This can be followed through step by step as shown in Table 2.17. It used to be thought that only the antisense strand was used; however, in very limited sections of DNA, there are proteins encoded on both strands.

Starting transcription

The antisense strand is read from its 3′ end to the 5′ end, and the RNA chain grows from the 5′ end to the 3′ end. Each gene has a region called the initiation site, where the RP must bind to start transcription. In many genes, upstream (25–35 bp) from the transcriptional start site is a sequence called the **TATA box**, which contains the sequence TATA(A or T)A, that binds transcription factors that initiate transcription. Other regions contain areas called **promoters**, which are sequences that control the rate at which the gene will be transcribed. They are located both upstream and downstream from the gene to be transcribed and bind molecules called **trans-acting factors**, which can either enhance gene transcription or silence it. Many slow-acting hormones, such as the steroid hormones and thyroid hormones, change the rate of gene expression, causing changes in the rate of transcription of specific mRNAs by forming a ligand–receptor complex that binds to promoter regions of DNA.

Binding of RNA polymerase

The binding of RP produces separation of the two strands of DNA in the region of the gene. This separation occurs more easily between T-A pairs than G-C pairs, because T-A pairs are joined by two hydrogen bonds whereas G-C pairs have three. The weaker links of the TATA box may help the DNA to unwind more easily. The first exposed base then binds the complementary free nucleotide from the cytoplasm. The first nucleotide of the RNA chain at the 5′ end is different from all

the others because, being at the beginning of the chain, it remains a triphosphate. The second base of the DNA then binds the corresponding free nucleotide, which is then linked to the first by the RP enzyme. As each nucleotide is added to the chain, a pyrophosphate is lost, leaving only the single α-phosphate in the backbone of the growing chain. Travelling along the DNA in the 3′ to 5′ direction the RP adds each successive complementary base to the growing RNA chain. As the RP proceeds, the DNA unwinds, while areas that have already transcribed will rewind.

Transcription can proceed quite rapidly at about 40 bases/s. At this rate a very large gene can take many hours to transcribe. The gene which codes for dystrophin, the protein that is absent in Duchenne muscular dystrophy, is more than 2×10^6 bp and would take more than 13 hours to transcribe. However, most gene transcripts are considerably smaller. The error rate in copying RNA is about 1 error every 10^4–10^5 nucleotides. This is high compared to the error rate in DNA replication but, because RNA is a short-lived molecule and is not repeatedly copied, this rate of error is not significant.

Termination of transcription

After the gene has been transcribed, elongation terminates and the RP is dislodged from the DNA strand. How this occurs in eukaryotes is not yet understood, although it may involve the formation of hairpin-like secondary structures in the mRNA that destabilise the RP. Termination often occurs up to 2000 bp past the end of the last exon (see below) of the gene. The excess mRNA will be ignored, because nothing after the stop codon is translated. The mRNA has a number of nuclear proteins associated with it, which are necessary for the transport out of the nucleus.

Post-transcriptional processing

All eukaryotic mRNAs are modified after they have been transcribed and before they are translated into protein in the cytosol. While the rest of the gene is being transcribed, and after only about 35 nucleotides have been added, the **primary transcript** of mRNA is capped at the 5′ end by the addition of 7-methylguanosine to the 5′ triphosphate group via an unusual 5′-5′ linkage. The two 5′ end nucleotides may also be 2′-methylated. This capping is thought to have a number of functions that aid further processing and protect the mRNA from destruction by nuclease enzymes.

Poly-A tails

Next, the 3′ end is cleaved at a region called the poly-A site at the sequence AAUAAA (or rarely AUUAAA). This 3′ end of the mRNA then has a sequence of up to 300 adenosine (A) nucleotides added, hence the term poly-A tail. These adenosine nucleotides bind proteins to help prevent degradation of the mRNA. This polyadenylation does not occur in all RNAs; for example it is absent in histones. However, the poly-A tails make it easier to isolate mRNAs for experimental use by 'fishing' for them with molecular probes that consist of poly-T nucleotides.

RNA splicing: introns and exons

Most eukaryotic genes are much longer than would be predicted by the number of amino acids in the resulting protein. This is because these genes contain regions, called **exons** (short for expressed sequences), which code for the protein, interspersed with non-coding regions, called **introns**. Many genes have multiple introns, which are removed from the initial primary transcript of mRNA to produce the mature mRNA.

The final modification to the pre-mRNA involves the removal of the **introns** by a process called **splicing**. This is done by a protein–RNA complex called a **spliceosome**. The positions of the sections to be removed are indicated by special sequences in the introns which allow the correct positioning of the different proteins involved in removing the intron.

Splicing of the same pre-mRNA does not always yield the same mature mRNA. Exons may also be removed. This **alternative splicing** can produce mRNAs with different exons, which will give different proteins. This can be controlled in a tissue-specific manner. For example, the extracellular protein fibronectin, which is secreted by different cell types, has two exons that code for parts of the protein which interact strongly with cell surface receptors. These are included in the mRNA produced in fibroblasts but are removed in the mRNA from hepatocytes. This change results in a functional difference such that that the hepatocyte fibronectin does not attach to cells very readily and circulates easily in the plasma.

RNA editing

This is a recently discovered process, which changes the sequence of an mRNA. This process is widespread among protozoans and plants, particularly in the chloroplast. In mammals, a few examples have been shown. For example, in a particular protein, by changing a single base in a specific position from A to G this changes the codon from CAG to CGG. This changes the amino acid inserted at that position from glutamine to arginine, with a subsequent change in the behaviour of the protein.

Processing rRNA and tRNA

The other gene products, rRNA and tRNA, are also processed before they leave the nucleus. In their mature form, tRNA molecules contain a number of modified bases. These modifications are important in determining the secondary structure of the tRNAs and the way in which they recognise the enzymes involved in protein synthesis. Ribose sugars are also modified by methylation, which makes them more stable.

Assembly of ribosomes

Ribosomal subunits are assembled in the nucleolus, where the rRNA is produced. Proteins are imported from the cytoplasm to be combined with the rRNA to make the small and large ribosomal subunits. The pre-rRNA is split into two subunits from a single original transcript. This is a way of ensuring that the separate subunits are produced, as needed, in equal amounts.

TRANSLATION

After the mRNA has been transcribed and modified in the nucleus it is transported to the cytoplasm where the production of the proteins occurs by translation of the mRNA transcript.

Transport from the nucleus

It has been estimated that more than one million molecules pass in or out of the nucleus every minute through approximately 4000 pores. These include the mRNAs, as well as other molecules exported from the nucleus such as ribosomal subunits and tRNAs. Moving in the opposite direction are nuclear and ribosomal proteins.

Nuclear pores

After it has been processed in the nucleus, the mature mRNA is transported to the cytoplasm through one of the **nuclear pores**. The normal diameter of the pores is 9 nm, but they can open to a maximum of 25 nm. It is thought that mRNAs that are ready for export include a sequence designating them for transport to the cytoplasm. Additionally, nuclear proteins are associated with their 5′ end, and these possibly act as a signal sequence to guide the RNA. The 5′ end leaves the nucleus first, then the nuclear proteins are removed and returned to the nucleus for reuse.

tRNAs

The function of tRNA is to link a particular amino acid onto the acceptor stem (see Fig. 2.20) and to bind to mRNA, through base pairing of three complementary base pairs, the **anticodon**, which corresponds to the linked amino acid on the opposite loop, called the anticodon loop. Because of the way that tRNA is folded into a clover leaf, the acceptor stem contains both the 3′ and 5′ ends of the molecule. The amino acid is attached to the 5′ end of the tRNA in a sequence of reactions involving the enzyme, aminoacyl-tRNA synthetase. Using ATP, the enzyme forms an AMP-amino acid, which is then transferred to the tRNA, releasing AMP. This reaction is referred to as **charging**, because the energy from the ATP bond is passed to the tRNA bond, and is later used to form the peptide bond, when the amino acid is incorporated into the protein chain. There are different synthetase enzymes for each of the amino acids; this ensures that each specific amino acid is charged with the correct tRNA.

Codon wobble

While there are 61 different codons that code for amino acids – remember that three of the 64 codons are stop codons – there are only about 50 different types of tRNA found in animal cells. This is also more than the number that would be required if only one tRNA was used for each amino acid. The reason for this anomaly lies in the fact that each tRNA is able to recognise more than one codon, a phenomenon called **wobble** (Table 2.18). This happens because the first base in the anticodon can recognise different bases in the third position on the mRNA. These non-standard base pairings are particularly common between G-U bases, which

Table 2.18	Codon/anticodon base pairings
Third base of the codon	**First base of the anticodon**
Normal base pairing	
A	U
G	C
U	A (rare)
C	G
Unusual base pairing	
G	U
U	G
A or C or U	I
I, inosine.	

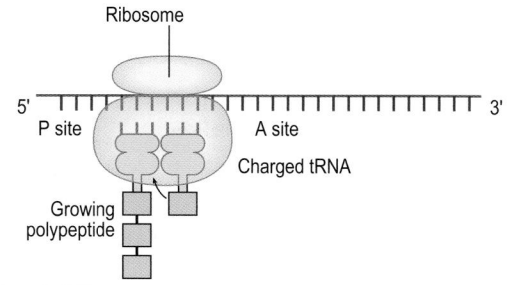

Fig. 2.25 Translation of mRNA.

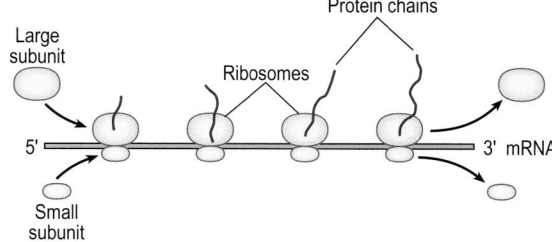

Fig. 2.26 Polysomes produce multiple copies of a protein from a single mRNA.

are formed almost as easily as the normal G-C pairing. Thus the mRNA codons for phenylalanine, UUU and UUC, are both recognised by the tRNA anticodon GAA.

Ribosomes and protein synthesis

Ribosomes direct protein synthesis in the cytoplasm in a cycle that consists of three phases:

1. The **initiation phase**, when the ribosomal subunits combine with the mRNA and move to the start codon.
2. The **elongation phase**, when the mRNA is translated into protein.
3. The **termination phase**, when the protein is released and the ribosome dissociates.

Initiation phase

The first part of the **initiation phase** is when the small ribosomal subunit binds to the cap at the 5′ end of the mRNA. It then travels along the mRNA until it reaches the start codon, AUG. This then binds Met-tRNA and the large ribosomal subunit then binds to form the complete ribosome.

There are two tRNA binding sites on the ribosome, A and P (Fig. 2.25). The A site receives the tRNA carrying the next amino acid to be added to the chain. The P site holds the tRNA attached to the growing peptide chain.

Elongation phase

Elongation starts with the Met-tRNA bound to the P site and the ribosome assembled. The next codon of the mRNA is in the A site of the ribosome and is then base paired with the appropriate tRNA. A peptide bond is formed between the carboxyl group of the first amino acid, which becomes the N-terminal amino acid, and the amino group of the second. The ribosome moves one codon down the mRNA and the first tRNA is released to be recharged in the cytoplasm. The second tRNA is shifted to the P site of the ribosome and a new tRNA occupies the A site. The energy required to form the peptide bond comes from the tRNA-amino acid bond, but the movement of the ribosome and the movement of the tRNA from the A site to the P site requires the hydrolysis of GTP to GDP.

Termination phase

The process of elongation continues, with each step adding another amino acid to the peptide. When the A site is occupied by a stop codon the elongation ceases. The last step, which also requires GTP, removes the peptide chain from its attachment to the last tRNA and dissociates the ribosome into its subunits.

Polysomes

A given mRNA can be translated simultaneously by more than one ribosome. Once the first ribosome has moved far enough down the mRNA, the initiation site can be occupied by another ribosome. This gives rise to a structure called a **polysome**, which consists of a single mRNA molecule with many ribosomes attached to it, each with a lengthening peptide chain attached (Fig. 2.26).

Lifetime of mRNAs

A given mRNA can be translated many times until it is degraded. Enzymes in the cytoplasm gradually remove the A residues from the poly-A tail. When this becomes too short then the 5′ cap is also removed. The mRNA is then degraded by exonucleases, which remove nucleotides from each end of the mRNA. Most mRNAs last a few hours, but some only last a few minutes and others last a few days. Many of the short-lived mRNAs code for proteins that are involved in the control of gene transcription. The half-life of these mRNAs – the time required for the concentration to halve – is determined partly by sequences in their genetic code, which allow them to be targeted for degradation, and partly by regulation depending on cellular requirements. An example of this is the mRNA coding for the milk protein, casein. In the presence of the hormone prolactin, which stimulates milk production, the rate of transcription of the casein gene rises about threefold. However, the amount of casein mRNA is increased 100-fold. This is due to a large increase in the stability of the mRNA, which in some cases is due to the binding of specific proteins to sequences in the 3′ region after the stop codon.

Rate of protein synthesis

Protein synthesis is a major activity of cells; it is estimated that, in an average mammalian cell, about one million amino acids are being added to growing polypeptide chains each second. A single polypeptide grows at the rate of three to five amino acids per second. This implies that at any given time a cell is busy making some 200 000 proteins. Clearly,

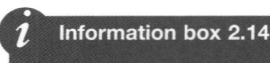

Information box 2.14 Some viruses break the rules

In some viruses, the rule observed in cellular organisms, 'DNA makes RNA makes protein' is not followed. Viruses can have either DNA or RNA as their genetic material and they rely on the synthetic machinery of the host cell to make more copies. In many of the RNA viruses, DNA is not generally involved in that process as the virus directs the manufacture of more RNA particles, which also make the proteins necessary to make more viruses. There are, however, a group of RNA viruses, called retroviruses, which use a specific viral enzyme, reverse transcriptase, which is packaged in the virus along with the RNA, to make a DNA copy of the viral RNA. This DNA is then incorporated into the host cell genome, from where it can make more copies of the viral RNA and proteins.

The most well-known retrovirus is the human immunodeficiency virus (HIV). One of the consequences of this packaging of DNA is that the virus can 'hide' in the genome and remain undetected for years until activated and new virus particles are produced.

Knowledge of reverse transcriptase enzymes has revolutionised the study of molecular biology, enabling researchers to reverse engineer DNA from mRNAs, which are more easily accessible, allowing the identification of products.

See also Chapter 5.

small proteins of 100 to 200 amino acids can be made in less than a minute. However, many proteins are larger. The largest protein known, titin, which is found in muscles, has about 30 000 amino acids and, at the rate of five amino acids per second, it would take over 1.5 hours to synthesise each molecule.

PROCESSING PATHWAYS FOR PROTEINS

As described previously, almost all proteins are modified after they are translated. Many modifications are not permanent but serve to help the targeting of proteins to the appropriate destinations. As they are produced, proteins are folded into their final shapes. This is partly determined by their primary structure and partly by the presence of molecular chaperones, which aid folding.

Protein can be produced in three different sites:

1. Some proteins are synthesised entirely on 'free' ribosomes within the cytosol. These are the proteins that are either destined to remain in the cytosol or those which are used in the nucleus, mitochondria or peroxisomes.
2. Proteins destined for the other organelles (ER, Golgi, lysosomes), insertion into membranes (organelle or plasma), or for secretion, are synthesised on ribosomes on the rough ER.
3. Some mitochondrial proteins are synthesised on ribosomes within mitochondria themselves using mitochondrial DNA.

Regardless of their final destination, all proteins start their synthesis on cytoplasmic ribosomes. Their subsequent fate is determined by the presence (or not) of a signal sequence of 16–30 amino acids at the N-terminal end of the protein.

PROTEIN PRODUCTION IN THE CYTOSOL

Proteins for use in the nucleus are transported through the nuclear pores. These pores are large enough for the protein to be transported without being unfolded. Nuclear localisation sequences, often rich in positively charged lysine and arginine residues, interact with the nuclear pores to facilitate uptake.

Those mitochondrial proteins not made in mitochondria are manufactured on cytosolic ribosomes. The proteins are targeted by N-terminal signal sequences, which not only determine that the protein will be transported into the mitochondria but also specify whether it will end up in the outer or inner membrane, or in the matrix or intermembrane space. Mitochondrial proteins have to be transported through the membrane unfolded. They are unfolded by molecular chaperones, transported through the membrane/s, and then refolded using other chaperones inside the mitochondria.

The enzymes within peroxisomes are made in the cytosol and imported into the organelles. They are thought to bind to receptors on the surface of the peroxisomes before entering through a transport protein. Rare disorders such as Zellweger's syndrome, which is characterised by central nervous system, liver and renal abnormalities, seems to involve a defect in protein import into peroxisomes.

Protein production in the ER

For proteins destined for insertion into the rough ER, as the signal sequence emerges from the free ribosome it is bound to a complex of protein and RNA, called a **signal recognition particle** (SRP). This inhibits further elongation of the protein until the ribosome reaches the ER. The cytoplasmic surface of the ER has receptors that bind the SRP and stimulate the formation of a transmembrane channel, through which the signal sequence can pass. The SRP then dissociates and is free to bind another signal sequence. The peptide continues to grow, but with the N-terminal end being extruded into the lumen of the ER. The signal sequence is then cleaved by an enzyme in the ER and degraded. As the protein grows, it is modified by the addition of carbohydrate and other residues, folded using chaperones, and when the C-terminal is reached it is released into the lumen of the ER. The ribosome is released from the rough ER and dissociates, as does the transmembrane channel. Many of the varying signal sequences contain a series of hydrophobic amino acids, particularly leucine, which help the signal sequence to cross the membrane. When these are cleaved, the resulting protein is more hydrophilic and will be retained within the ER.

Transmembrane proteins

Proteins that are destined to be part of a membrane are inserted into the membrane as it is being made. For a simple protein with only one transmembrane segment (one end of the protein inside the cell and one end outside, with the middle section spanning the membrane), this is achieved due to the presence of a second signal sequence. The first part of the protein, the N-terminal end, is made in the same way as secreted proteins. This will eventually become the external part of the protein, and it has the signal sequence removed and is glycosylated as normal. However, when this part reaches its appropriate size, there is a second signal sequence that consists of about 22 hydrophobic amino

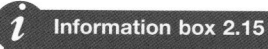

Information box 2.15   **One type of cystic fibrosis is due to a protein not being processed correctly**

The most common form of cystic fibrosis is caused by a deletion of a single amino acid (a phenylalanine at position 508) in the gene that codes for the membrane protein, CFTR (cystic fibrosis transmembrane regulator). This results in the ER being unable to export the CFTR protein which is needed to produce the proper ion channels needed for cAMP-regulated chloride transport across the plasma membrane. At normal body temperature, there is an error in folding of the protein which prevents its export from the ER. However, curiously, it was found that at lower temperatures (25°C) the proteins fold normally.

These channels are found particularly in the specialised linings of the bowel and lung. Defective ion transport results in salt imbalance, drawing water from the airways and producing the thick lung secretions typical of this disease. Defective ion transport explains the high concentration of salt ions in sweat secretions in patients with CF (the 'sweat' test).

See also Chapter 14.

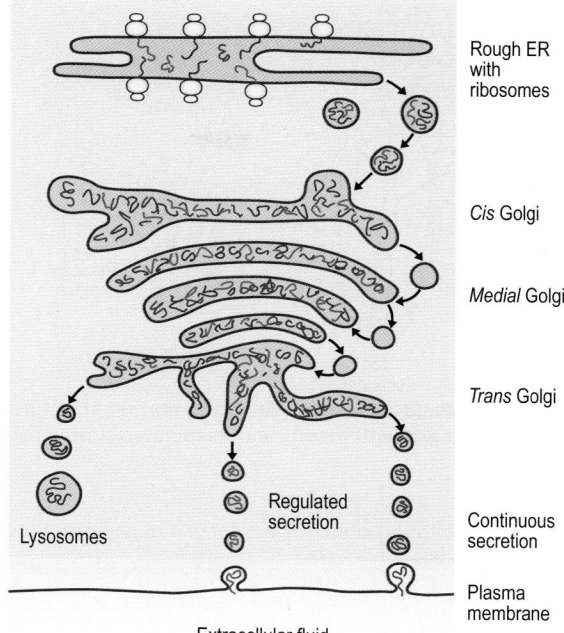

Fig. 2.27 **Destinations of proteins.**

acids. This forms an α-helix, which spans the membrane and is anchored in it. This signal is called the stop-transfer membrane-anchor sequence. The transmembrane channel is disassembled leaving the ribosome to finish the C-terminal end of the protein on the cytosolic side of the ER.

Protein processing in the ER

In the ER, a number of important steps take place:

- Multimeric proteins are formed into oligomers.
- Mutated proteins which misfold are identified and retained.
- Unwanted excess protein subunits are degraded.
- Asparagine residues undergo *N*-linked glycosylation.
- Precursors of the lysosomal enzymes, prohydrolases, are glycosylated.

Processing in the Golgi

Proteins move from the ER to the Golgi (Fig. 2.27) where they are processed further. In the Golgi, as in the ER, there is a wide range of modifications which occur before proteins can be sent to their final destinations.

Glycosylation

Many of the *N*-linked sugars that are added in the ER are modified, and other sugars are added by *O*-linked glycosylation to serine and threonine residues, and then further modified. Many proteins, especially peptide hormones, are converted from pro-hormones to their active forms by cleavage of peptides by proteolytic enzymes. Sphingolipids are manufactured in the Golgi and glycosylated.

Phosphorylation

The phosphorylation of glycosylated lysosomal pro-hydrolase enzymes generates terminal mannose-6-phosphate groups, which are then used to target them to **lysosomes**. These mannose-6-phosphate groups bind to receptors on the internal face of the *trans*-Golgi. These are clustered into an area of membrane that is coated on the cytoplasmic side by the protein, clathrin. The areas of

membrane coated with clathrin bud off from the Golgi, after which the clathrin is removed. After a number of complicated steps, involving other vesicles called **late endosomes**, a vesicle containing the dephosphorylated enzyme fuses with the lysosome, and another vesicle containing the empty mannose receptors returns to the Golgi.

Secretory proteins

Proteins in the Golgi that are destined for secretion do not have mannose-6-phosphate and are not targeted to lysosomes. However, they are separated according to whether or not they are continuously secreted, or their secretion is regulated (Fig. 2.27). Regulated secretion requires that vesicles are stored in the cytoplasm and attached to the cytoskeleton before they are secreted. A large number of proteins have been identified that carry out the necessary docking, priming and fusion. Research carried out in the secretion of neurotransmitters has helped determine these mechanisms (see Ch. 8).

MEMBRANE STRUCTURE AND FUNCTIONS

FLUID MOSAIC MODEL OF MEMBRANES

A typical cell membrane has hundreds of different types of protein, which may be pictured as floating in the phospholipid sea. This model of proteins embedded in a lipid bilayer, some of them free to diffuse and some fixed, was originally proposed by Singer and Nicholson in 1972 and is called the **fluid mosaic model** (Fig. 2.28).

It is largely the proteins in a cell membrane which determine its biological function. So, for example, a given cell responds to a particular chemical signal because its plasma membrane contains a specific protein. Any cell lacking the particular protein in its membrane would be completely

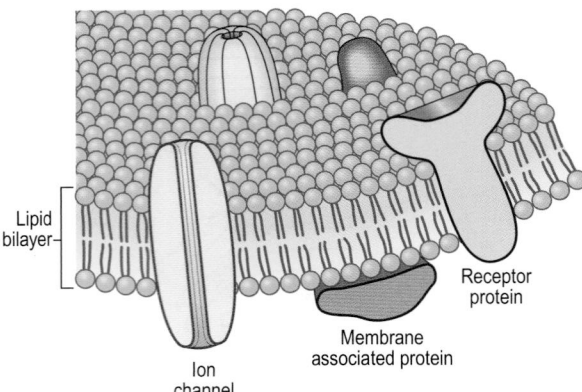

Fig. 2.28 **Fluid mosaic model of membrane structure, showing integral and membrane-associated proteins.**

unresponsive to the signal. The functions of cell membrane proteins include:

- Enzymes
- Transporters
- Transmembrane channels
- Receptors
- Cell markers
- Linking the cytoskeleton and the ECM.

Lipid bilayer

All cell membranes, including the plasma membrane, consist in part of a **bilayer** of phospholipids, sphingolipids and cholesterol. Phospholipids are all **amphipathic** molecules because they have two acyl groups that are hydrophobic, and a substituted phosphate, which is hydrophilic because it is polar. Similarly, sphingolipids and cholesterol both have hydrophobic and hydrophilic regions. Because of this property, in an aqueous environment phospholipids aggregate so that the acyl tails are as far away from the water as possible. One configuration that permits this is a bilayer.

Movement of lipids in the bilayer

Of itself, a phospholipid bilayer is remarkably dynamic. Individual phospholipid molecules are free to rotate rapidly around their long axis and migrate rapidly within their side of the bilayer. However, transfer of a phospholipid between the sides of the bilayer (flipping) is very rare. Overall, a phospholipid bilayer has the fluidity of olive oil, and it is a highly impenetrable barrier to most materials. It will, however, allow the passage of small molecules, such as water, oxygen and carbon dioxide, and anything that is fat soluble, but it will exclude almost all polar molecules or charged solutes.

Differential distribution of lipids in the bilayer

Different membranes have different lipid compositions, including the two leaflets of the same bilayer. An example of this is the red cell plasma membrane, which has sphingomyelin and phosphatidylcholine as the major components of the outer face of the membrane (called the **exoplasmic leaflet**), and phosphatidylethanolamine and phosphatidylserine as the main lipids in the inner side (the **cytoplasmic leaflet**). The difficulty with which lipids flip between the two leaflets helps to maintain this differential distribution. Phospholipids can be moved between organelles by exchange proteins. Proteins called **flippases** are found in some membranes,

particularly in the ER and in erythrocytes. These can move phospholipids from one side of the bilayer to the other.

Cholesterol in membranes

At normal human body temperature the presence of cholesterol reduces the fluidity of the membrane. It inserts itself between the phospholipids with its hydrophilic hydroxyl group facing outwards where the planar structure of cholesterol reduces the movement of phospholipids. The plasma membrane of cells has more cholesterol than the intracellular membranes, which makes it more rigid, less permeable to small molecules and thicker than intracellular membranes. Some intracellular membranes such as the ER contain very little cholesterol.

Membrane proteins

The second major component of membranes is protein. Membrane proteins are of two main types:

- Integral (intrinsic)
- Peripheral (extrinsic).

Integral membrane proteins can be removed only by disrupting the membrane structure. Many of these proteins span the bilayer and have hydrophobic amino acid residues on the part of the protein in contact with the membrane, while the parts inside and outside the cell are hydrophilic and may also carry charged groups. These charged groups are often glycosylations in the extracellular face, and phosphate groups on the intracellular face.

Peripheral membrane proteins, in contrast, may be removed without disrupting the membrane. They may be associated with the cytoskeleton, or involved in signal transduction across the membrane, or they may be attached to the ECM.

Protein composition of different membranes

The amount of protein varies enormously between different membranes. The erythrocyte plasma membrane is about half lipid and half protein with about 8% carbohydrate. In contrast, the myelin membrane, which surrounds nerve cell axons and acts as an insulator, is almost 80% lipid. The inner mitochondrial membrane, which contains all the enzymes associated with metabolism, is over 75% protein, with no carbohydrate.

SPECIALISED PLASMA MEMBRANE STRUCTURES

Many cells, particularly those that make up the solid tissues of the body, are polarised. That is, different functions are observed in different parts of the cell. Given the fluidity of the plasma membrane, and the ability of membrane lipids and proteins to move laterally within the membrane, in order for cells to have polarity there needs to be a way of separating the different areas of membrane. Cells adhere to one another through interactions of cell adhesion molecules (see below), but cells that form sheets, separating different body compartments, must have structures which link them together with sufficient strength to maintain the integrity of the layer.

Sheets of epithelial cells

Epithelial cells form layers covering most body surfaces. A typical polarised epithelial cell has an apical surface in contact with the lumen (e.g. the intestinal lumen). This may have one of a number of membrane specialisations (Table 2.19). The basolateral surface is in contact with the basement membrane, which consists of the basal lamina and the reticular lamina. The proteins in the plasma membrane are restricted to the apical and basolateral domains by junctions between the cells (Fig. 2.29).

Junctions between cells

There are a number of different types of junctions between cells, and between cells and the ECM (Fig. 2.29). Many sheets of cells sit on a fibrous network of collagens, proteoglycans, laminin and fibronectin called the basal lamina.

These junctions can be classified as:

- **Tight junctions** – ones that prevent movement of substances
- **Adhering junctions** – ones that maintain cellular positions
- **Gap junctions** – ones that allow movement of substances.

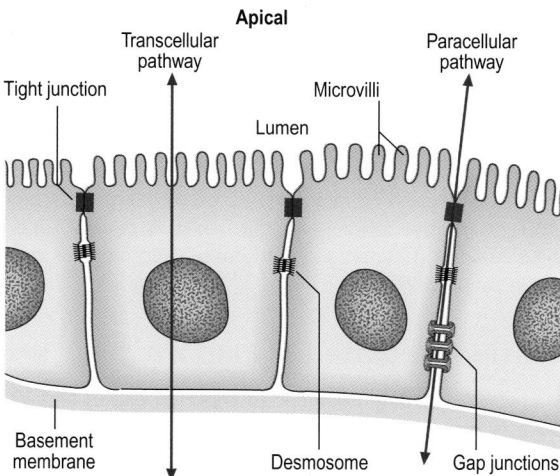

Fig. 2.29 **A sheet of epithelial cells.**

Tight junctions

Tight junctions, also known as **occluding junctions**, form a belt around the cell attached to the neighbouring cells known as the zonula occludens. The zonula occludens is formed from a complex of proteins (ZO1-3, AF-6 and occludin) that connect the two membranes tightly together in a series of studs appearing as interconnected ridges with no visible extracellular space. Tight junctions are not connected to the cytoskeleton and prevent the movement of membrane components between the separated regions of the cell. This mechanism allows each part to have its own set of proteins and lipids. Tight junctions also prevent the passage of molecules across the sheet of cells through the route passing between the cells, the paracellular pathway. This barrier is produced by a family of proteins called claudins.

Adhering junctions

Three types of **adhering junctions**, also known as **anchoring junctions**, are all different types of **desmosomes**. These are formed from plaques just below the plasma membrane, bound to cytoskeletal elements. The plaque is attached to the plaque of another cell, or to the ECM, by proteins which span the intercellular space (Table 2.20). Zonula adherens form a belt around the cell, whereas the macula adherens only contact the other cell at spots around the cell.

Gap junctions

Gap junctions, also known as **communicating junctions**, are formed from integral membrane proteins called **connexins**. A pore in the membrane, called a **connexon**, is formed from six connexins, and this is aligned with a connexon in the opposing cell. This forms a channel between the cells which allows the free passage between the cytoplasms of the cells of water, small molecules (up to 1.2 nm diameter), including some signalling molecules, and ions. It is this electrical coupling of cells via gap junctions that allows the movement of excitation across sheets of muscle. This is particularly important in smooth muscle and cardiac cells. The connexons tend to cluster in patches on the membrane. The pore is closed by high concentrations of calcium, which may be important during apoptosis.

Microvilli and stereocilia

In cells that are required to absorb substances from the extracellular medium, such as those found in the intestine and kidney, the surface area for absorption can be increased up to 30-fold by the presence of **microvilli**. There may be up to 3000 microvilli per cell, forming what is known as the **brush border**. Microvilli are small (<1 μm) projections of the plasma membrane, with a core formed of actin microfilaments. They are attached to the terminal web, a network of actin filaments running under the apical surface of the cell. **Stereocilia** are longer and branched, with a similar actin core

Table 2.19	Specialisations of the apical membrane	
Specialisation	**Function**	**Example**
Cilia	Movement across surface	Bronchial epithelium
Microvilli	Increased area for absorption	Intestinal epithelium
Stereocilium	Sperm maturation	Epididymal epithelium

Table 2.20	Different types of adhering junctions		
Adhering junction	**Alternative name**	**Interaction**	**Linker**
Belt desmosome	Zonula adherens	Actin–actin	Cadherins
Spot desmosome	Macula adherens	IFs–IFs	Cadherins
Hemidesmosome	–	IFs–basal lamina	Integrin and laminin
IF, intermediate filament.			

to microvilli. They are rare, mainly being found in the epididymis.

CELLULAR TRANSPORT PROCESSES

In order for chemical reactions to occur, the reagents must be placed appropriately along with their enzyme catalysts. The products and reaction waste products may need to be moved elsewhere. All cells have a plasma membrane, which is a barrier to the movement of substances that are not membrane soluble. The movement of compounds across this and other intracellular membranes depends on the chemistry of the molecule and often requires specialised transport mechanisms.

Passive diffusion

Small molecules such as water, oxygen, carbon dioxide, and fat-soluble molecules are able to move through cell membranes readily by **simple** or **passive diffusion**. Net diffusion occurs from high concentration to low concentration, that is, down the concentration gradient. The shorter the distance a molecule has to diffuse, the quicker the journey will be. Electron microscopy shows that cell membranes are only some 9 nm across, so the diffusion distance is extremely short.

    This is important for respiration in the lungs, in which oxygen and carbon dioxide must diffuse through five cell membranes. To enter the red blood cell, oxygen in the lung must cross the alveolar cell lining the lungs (two cell membranes), the endothelial cell lining the capillary through which blood flows (two cell membranes) and must then diffuse across the red cell membrane; carbon dioxide takes the reverse journey. The total diffusion distance is about 1 μm and only 3 s is required for this **gas exchange** to be completed.

Fick's first law of diffusion

Passive diffusion occurs through a series of random steps, which result in the molecule being equilibrated between the compartments. Molecules can move randomly in all directions but the net movement occurs down the concentration gradient, and the relationship between the rate of transport and the concentration gradient is linear (Fig. 2.30). Diffusion across a plasma membrane can be described by Fick's first law of diffusion:

$$J = -DA\,\Delta c/\Delta x$$

where J is the net rate of diffusion; D is the diffusion coefficient; A is the membrane area; Δc is the concentration difference across the membrane and Δx is the thickness of the membrane.

    The diffusion coefficient (D) is defined as:

$$D = kT/(6\pi r\eta)$$

where k is Boltzmann's constant; T is the absolute temperature; r is the molecular radius of the diffusing compound and η is the viscosity of the medium.

Diffusion coefficient

From the equation above it can be seen that the diffusion coefficient (D) is dependent on the viscosity of the diffusing medium and the molecular radius of the diffusing compound. The larger the compound and the thicker the medium, the

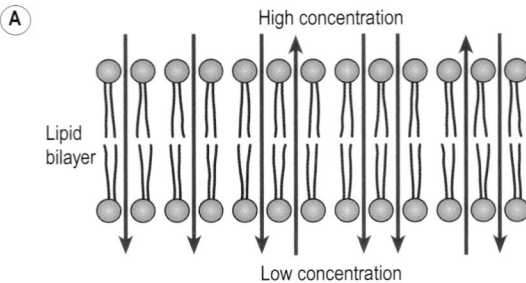

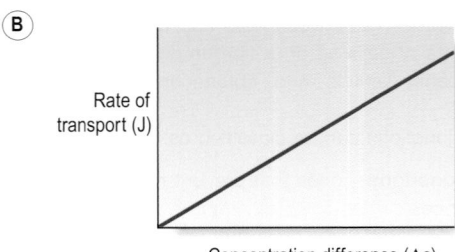

Fig. 2.30 Passive diffusion: (A) transport and (B) relationship between rate and concentration difference.

slower the rate of diffusion. An 'average' small water-soluble molecule, with a diffusion coefficient of 1×10^{-5} cm/s, will only take 0.5 ms to diffuse 1 μm (the thickness of a capillary wall), but it will take 5 s to move 100 μm (the length of many cells), and 14 hours to diffuse 1 cm.

    In prokaryotic cells there are no membrane-bound structures within the cytoplasm, so all compounds can diffuse within the cell to their target. However, over large distances, this type of transport is very slow, which is possibly one of the size-limiting factors for both prokaryotic organisms and within single cells.

Carrier-mediated transport

Many materials that cells need to import or export are either polar or charged, and so will not diffuse through cell membranes. These charged molecules go via special proteins within the membrane, called **transporters**. Any transport of materials that requires transporters is said to be **carrier-mediated transport**. Transporters are specific, in the same way that enzymes are specific; they have preferred substrates and the kinetics of transport show the same characteristics as enzymes. Transporters are both specific and saturable, so the maximum rate of transport and the affinity of the transporter for the substrate can be described using the Michaelis–Menten equation.

    There are three types of carrier-mediated transport:

- Facilitated diffusion
- Active transport
- Secondary active transport.

Facilitated diffusion

In **facilitated diffusion** the substrate diffuses from high to low concentration – just as in passive diffusion – except that a transporter is essential for diffusion to occur (Fig. 2.31). These transporters are protein channels – pores, also called **permeases** – that span the entire width of the membrane. It is the size and chemistry of the channel lining that allows specific substrates to pass through it.

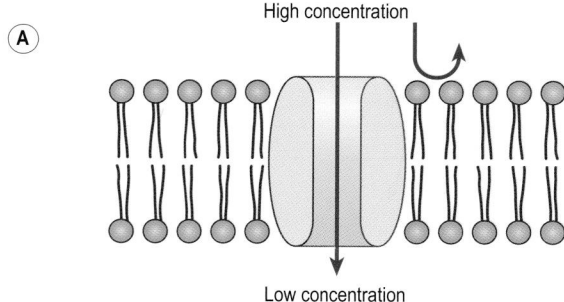

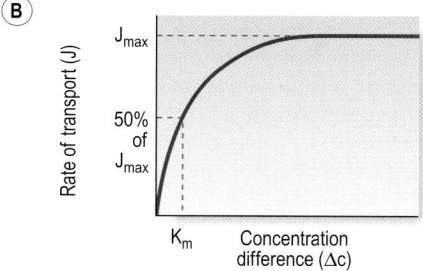

Fig. 2.31 Facilitated transport via an ion channel: (A) transport and (B) relationship between rate and concentration difference.

Transport of glucose into red blood cells is one of many possible examples of facilitated diffusion. Glucose permease is a transporter found in red blood cells that allows the facilitated diffusion of glucose. Once inside the cell the glucose is phosphorylated to glucose-6-phosphate by the enzyme hexokinase. The transporter does not recognise glucose-6-phosphate, and so it remains trapped inside the erythrocyte. Many of these transporters allow transport in both directions where the transport is dependent only on the concentration gradient. Without the action of the hexokinase glucose would accumulate inside the cell and when the gradient was reversed could diffuse out through the same permease.

This permease is one of a number of glucose permeases called GLUT1–5 that are found throughout the body. Transporters like this, which bind a single substrate, are called **uniporters**. The erythrocyte transporter, GLUT1, can transport a number of sugars, but each sugar has a different K_m. The K_m for D-glucose is about 1.5 mM, whereas the K_m for D-galactose is about 30 mM. In the presence of both sugars, the amount of each sugar transported will depend to some extent on their relative concentrations, but glucose will bind more readily to the transporter and so will be preferentially transported.

Ion channels

Another important example of facilitated diffusion involves the movement of ions. Although charged ions cannot cross a pure phospholipid bilayer they can diffuse across plasma membranes – under some circumstances – via protein pores called **ion channels** (see Ch. 4). These channels are selective for specific ions, so it is possible to talk of sodium channels, potassium channels and calcium channels. About 40 different types of ion channel have been discovered so far. Many channels are normally closed. Some are opened in response to chemical signals, either directly **(ligand-gated ion channels)** or indirectly **(receptor-operated channels)**.

Other ion channels are opened by small changes in the electrical potential that exists across the membrane, and hence are termed **voltage-dependent ion channels**.

Binding of substrate

The mechanism of transport across the membrane using transporters is thought to involve the binding of the substrate to a specific site on the extracellular face of the transporter. This stimulates a conformational change in the transporter that moves the transported molecule through the protein until it is exposed on the intracellular face, from which it then dissociates. Many of these transporters are able to work in reverse if the concentration gradient is inverted.

Rates of transport

Maximal rates of transport through permeases are in the order of 10^2–10^4 molecules per second. Ion channels allow a faster rate of transfer than do transporters: 10^7–10^8 ions per second. When the pore is open, more than one ion or water molecule at a time can enter the channel. This means that more than one molecule can move through the membrane simultaneously.

Active transport

Sodium and potassium ions are differentially distributed across the plasma membrane, with higher concentrations of sodium outside the cell and higher concentrations of potassium inside (see Table 2.15). A number of processes, including diffusion through ion channels, can allow these concentration gradients to dissipate.

If the only form of transport available was diffusion, both passive and facilitated, then very quickly all the cellular compartments would be at equilibrium, with all molecules at the same concentration throughout the body, and transport would cease. A second type of carrier-mediated transport uses the energy contained in ATP to power transport against the concentration gradient, i.e. to concentrate a compound. The process is called **active transport**, and the enzymes that carry this out are called **ATPases**, a number of which are critical for cell function. They use the energy stored in the high-energy phosphoanhydride bonds of ATP to transport molecules against their concentration gradients. The ATP is converted to ADP and the energy released moves the molecule.

Na$^+$/K$^+$-ATPases

One of the most important of these ATPases is a cation pump which moves the cations, sodium and potassium, across the plasma membrane. This is achieved by a transporter called the **Na$^+$/K$^+$-ATPase**. This membrane protein takes Na$^+$ from inside the cell and pumps it out. In exchange, and simultaneously, the protein pumps K$^+$ from outside the cell into the cytoplasm. Any transport process that uses metabolic energy directly, in the manner of the cation pump, is called active transport, sometimes referred to as direct active transport because the ATP is used directly by the pump.

The Na$^+$/K$^+$-ATPase consists of four protein subunits, $\alpha2\beta2$, all of which span the membrane and have multiple transmembrane helices. There are binding sites for ATP on the internal sides of the α subunits, and a site on the outer surface of the α subunits which can bind a number of drugs, including digoxin (see Information box 2.16). In the most common type of Na$^+$/K$^+$-ATPase, in each cycle three Na$^+$ are removed from the cell, and two K$^+$ are added to the internal

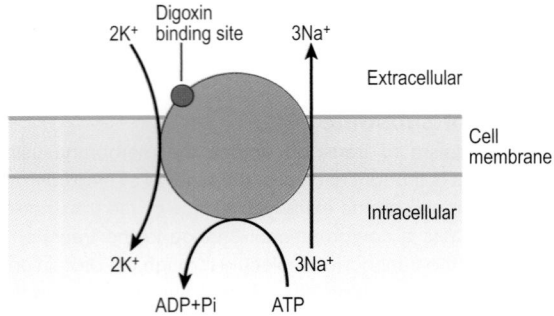

Fig. 2.32 Na$^+$/K$^+$-ATPase activity. Pi, phosphate.

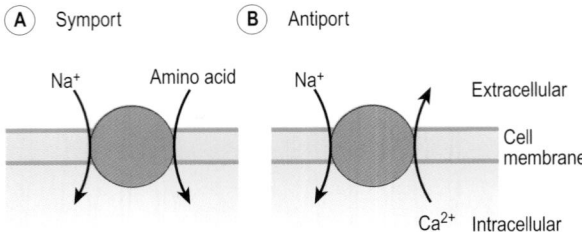

Fig. 2.33 Secondary active transport.

medium (Fig. 2.32). However, there are Na$^+$/K$^+$-ATPase molecules with other stoichiometries.

The Na$^+$/K$^+$-ATPase cycle is as follows:

1. Pump open to intracellular fluid binds ATP
2. Three Na$^+$ bind to pump
3. ATP phosphorylates α subunits
4. Conformational changes and three Na$^+$ released into extracellular fluid
5. Two K$^+$ bind from extracellular fluid
6. Dephosphorylation of the α subunits
7. Pump reverts to previous conformation
8. Two K$^+$ released into cell.

Virtually all cells have cation pumps in their plasma membranes. It is estimated that as much as 30% of all ATP generated is used to power cation pumps, a reflection of just how important they are.

Other ATPases

Another example of active transport is the H$^+$-ATPase found in the membranes surrounding lysosomes. This transports H$^+$ into the lysosome, reducing the pH to about 5.5, the optimal pH for the activity of the acid hydrolases. Ca^{2+}-ATPases are active in removing calcium from the cytoplasm, either by pumping it into organelles or across the plasma membrane.

In mitochondria, an H$^+$-ATPase with two subunits F$_0$ and F$_1$, also known as **ATP synthase**, runs in reverse, using the energy of the H$^+$ gradient to produce ATP.

P-glycoprotein

A relatively recently discovered active transport mechanism explains why some drugs do not cross the blood–brain barrier into the brain, despite being theoretically able to cross the plasma membranes of the capillary endothelial cells. The transporters, called **P-glycoprotein** or **MDR1** (multidrug resistance) and **MDR2**, are present on the endothelial cells and are able to transport a wide variety of hydrophobic compounds out of the endothelial cell cytoplasm into the blood and thereby prevent them entering the brain. This protects the brain from toxins by preventing hydrophobic compounds entering the brain by passive diffusion, and any toxic polar molecules cannot cross the endothelial cells without a specific transport mechanism.

However, unfortunately, a number of drugs which can be used to treat cancer, such as vincristine and vinblastine, are substrates for P-glycoprotein and, because of the activity of P-glycoprotein, do not enter the brain readily. In many cases,

where tumours become resistant to chemotherapy, this is because they express a large number of these P-glycoprotein transporters on their membranes, a process selected for by continued treatment.

Secondary active transport

A major role of the cation pump is to maintain a large difference in the concentration of Na$^+$ ions across the cell membrane. This gradient stores energy in the form of potential energy. A large group of transporters work by allowing Na$^+$ ions to diffuse from outside to inside the cell, providing the energy to pump other materials up their concentration gradients. A good example of this type of transport, called **secondary active transport**, is the movement of many amino acids into cells. Some amino acids are in low concentration in the blood, but in higher concentration inside cells. To import these amino acids into cells requires energy. This is provided by a co-transport mechanism, which couples the diffusion of Na$^+$ to the import of amino acids. Many transport processes harness the energy of Na$^+$ diffusion in this way, which is also described as **indirect active transport**. In this example, transport is active because energy is required to import the amino acid. Ultimately, the energy is supplied by ATP, but in indirect active transport the protein transporter does not, itself, require ATP; the energy comes from sodium diffusing down its concentration gradient.

Symport and antiport

There are two types of secondary active transporter (Fig. 2.33). In the example above, the amino acid and the sodium move in the same direction; this is called **symport**. In **antiport**, the sodium moves one way across the membrane and the other solute moves up its concentration gradient in the other direction. An example of this is the Na$^+$/Ca^{2+} antiport found in heart muscle (see Information box 2.16 and Ch. 4).

Coordinated action of transporters

The movement of substances through layers of cells usually requires the coordinated activity of a number of transport systems working together (Table 2.21). A good example of this is the movement of glucose from the lumen of the intestine into the blood (Fig. 2.34). This entails crossing both membranes of the epithelial cells which line the lumen. This requires the activity of three different types of transport:

- Secondary active transport by a sodium-linked glucose transporter
- Facilitated diffusion by a glucose permease
- Active transport by the Na$^+$/K$^+$-ATPase.

Table 2.21	Summary of transport processes		
Type of transport	**Transporter/s**	**Energy source**	**Rate (molecules/s)**
Passive diffusion	None	Concentration gradient of substrate	Depends on substrate and medium
Facilitated diffusion	Uniporter	Concentration gradient of substrate	10^2–10^4
	Ion channel	Concentration gradient of substrate	10^7–10^8
Active transport	ATPase	Direct ATP $\rightarrow$ ADP	Up to 10^3
Secondary (indirect) active transport	Symporter	Indirect ATP $\rightarrow$ ADP	10^2–10^4
	Antiporter	Indirect ATP $\rightarrow$ ADP	10^2–10^4

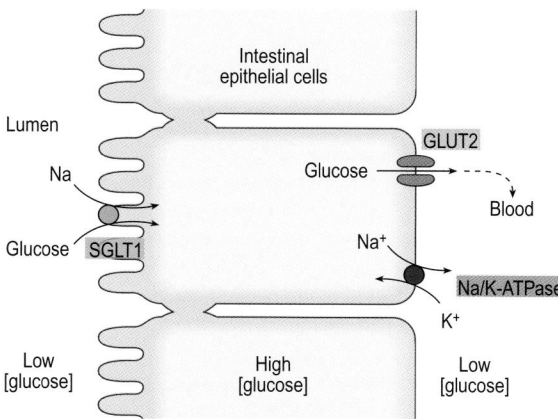

Fig. 2.34 **Transport of sugars across the intestinal lumen.**

Sodium-linked glucose transport

The transport of glucose across the luminal brush border of the intestinal epithelial cells (enterocytes) is carried out by secondary active transport via a sodium-dependent cotransporter called **SGLT1** (Sodium/Glucose Linked Transport). This is an example of a cotransporter where both the sodium and the glucose travel in the same direction, a symport. Sodium moves down its concentration gradient into the cell and glucose moves from the low concentration in the lumen to the higher concentration in the cell.

Glucose permease

Glucose then exits the cell into the extracellular space through the glucose permease, GLUT2, on the basolateral membrane. This **uniporter** moves the glucose by facilitated diffusion down its concentration gradient. It then diffuses from the extracellular space between the endothelial cells into the blood.

Na$^+$/K$^+$-ATPase

The sodium, which would otherwise accumulate in the cell and inhibit further transport, is removed from the cell by active transport using the Na$^+$/K$^+$-ATPase. This is situated on the basolateral membrane and ensures that sodium is also absorbed by this process and is not lost into the gut lumen. A number of similar transport systems also exist for the absorption of amino acids, both in enterocytes and in the epithelial cells lining the renal tubules.

Endocytosis and exocytosis

Transport using transporter proteins is usually very specific. Except in the case of P-glycoprotein, there is a limited range of substrates that can bind to a given transporter. In some cases only a single molecular species will be transported. Very large compounds cannot be moved into the cell by this method, as the energy required to move them through the membrane is too large. However, molecules and particles in the extracellular fluid can be internalised by a process called **endocytosis**. This involves the enclosure of these external substances by the plasma membrane, which is pinched off inside the cell (Fig. 2.35).

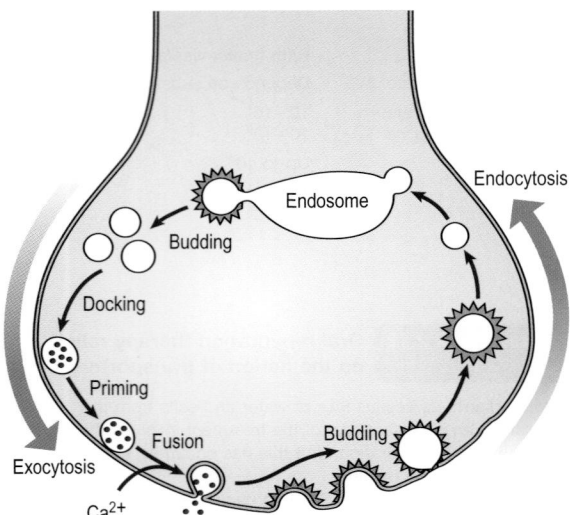

Fig. 2.35 Endocytosis and exocytosis.

Endocytosis

There are three major categories of endocytosis:

- Phagocytosis
- Pinocytosis
- Receptor-mediated endocytosis.

Phagocytosis

Phagocytosis (cell eating) involves the uptake of large particles into large vesicles called **phagosomes**. This is mainly carried out by phagocytic cells of the immune system – macrophages and neutrophils – where it is a part of the body's defence against pathogens. Phagocytosis involves the recognition of the bacteria, or other particles, by the phagocyte, perhaps through antibodies bound to the invading organism (see Ch. 6). This triggers a rearrangement of the actin cytoskeleton of the phagocytes so that the plasma membrane is extended around the particle, forming an intracellular membrane-bound organelle called a phagosome. Once the particle is engulfed, the phagosome is moved using motor proteins to the lysosomes, where the acid hydrolases can break down the particle into its component parts. These can then be utilised by the cell. Anything that cannot be degraded remains in the lysosome as a residual body. In long-term smokers, for example, lung tissue is blackened by the accumulation of macrophages in the septa of the alveoli that contain black substances derived from inhaled smoke.

Pinocytosis

Pinocytosis (cell drinking) is carried out by small vesicles (**pinocytes**) that take up external fluid and solutes. Cells can also ingest large amounts of bulk fluid and solutes by **macropinocytosis**, where an extension of the plasma membrane spreads around an area of extracellular fluid that can be large, up to 100 nm. For example, cells in the thyroid gland use this method to take up thyroglobulin.

Receptor-mediated endocytosis

Many compounds present in the extracellular fluid, especially those that are too large to be taken up by transporter proteins, can be specifically transported by **receptor-me diated endocytosis**. This is a mechanism for concentrating and internalising substrates, often proteins, glycoproteins or carbohydrates. It is also referred to as **clathrin-dependent endocytosis**, as it involves the formation of vesicles in specific areas of cell membrane that are coated with an intracellular lattice of a protein called clathrin. The substrate binds to cell surface receptors, which are clustered on the area of membrane marked by the clathrin. The binding of the ligand causes the membrane to fold inward, forming a **coated pit**. The edges of the pit fuse together and an intracellular vesicle coated with clathrin is formed. The clathrin then dissociates from the vesicle, now called an **early endosome**. This fuses with another endosome, which has a low internal pH (about 5), becoming a **late endosome**, or CURL. The low pH is due to the active transport of H$^+$ into the enzyme by a H$^+$-ATPase. Due to the low pH the ligands then dissociate from their receptors. The membrane, with its inserted membranes, is returned to the cell surface and the ligand is delivered to a lysosome, where it is either broken down into the required components or transported into the cytoplasm.

Two substances taken up by most cells using receptor-mediated endocytosis are **low-density lipoproteins** (LDLs), which carry about 75% of the plasma cholesterol around the body, and **transferrin**, which carries iron into the cell.

LDL particles are spheres, about 20 nm in diameter, composed of a single phospholipid layer plus some cholesterol, surrounding a core of cholesterol esters (cholesterol plus a fatty acid). Embedded in the phospholipid monolayer is a single protein, called apoB, which binds to LDL receptors on the cell surface. Once bound to LDL receptors, the LDL particle is ingested in a clathrin-coated vesicle. The LDL receptor is eventually recycled to the cell surface and the LDL particle is degraded into cholesterol, fatty acids and amino acids (from the apoB protein). Cells balance their requirement for cholesterol by regulating both the synthesis of cholesterol and the number of LDL receptors in their surface.

Another example of receptor-mediated endocytosis, followed by sorting in endosomes, is the transport of transferrin. Transferrin receptors bind **ferrotransferrin**, a combination of the iron-binding protein, **transferrin**, found in plasma, along with bound iron. Ferrotransferrin is endocytosed in clathrin-coated vesicles. However, after the fusion with a late endosome, the transferrin is not dissociated from the receptor, but iron is dissociated from the transferrin. This allows the iron-free **apotransferrin** to be recycled to the plasma when the transferrin receptors are returned to the plasma membrane.

Exocytosis

The process by which the receptors are returned, along with their membrane, is the inverse of endocytosis, a process called **exocytosis**. This involves the fusion of intracellular vesicles with the plasma membrane, releasing their contents into the extracellular fluid. Exocytosis is not only the mechanism by which endocytotic receptors are returned to the cell surface but it is the main mechanism by which hormones and neurotransmitters are secreted from cells (see Ch. 8).

Transcytosis

Some molecules are moved across a sheet of cells, such as the intestinal epithelia, by a combination of endocytosis and exocytosis, called **transcytosis**. The molecules are moved by receptor-mediated endocytosis into endosomes, which travel across the cell and fuse with the opposite plasma

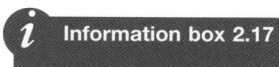

Information box 2.17 | **High levels of plasma cholesterol can be caused by a defect in LDL receptors**

A relatively common genetic disorder known as familial hypercholesterolaemia, causes a raised level of cholesterol in the blood. This defect occurs in about 1 in 500 of the normal population and is associated with a family history of early heart disease.

There are a number of genetic mutations responsible for causing the disease, but the common theme is a reduction in the clearance of LDL particles via the LDL receptors. In some cases the receptor numbers are reduced. In others it is the receptor which is defective.

Another form of familial hypercholesterolaemia that is relatively common is caused by a defect in the apoB protein which prevents binding of the LDL particles to the receptor.

While many heterozygotes (who only carry one copy of the defective gene) have mild symptoms, children who have inherited the disorder from both parents are severely affected, most dying from heart disease before adulthood if untreated. Even in those treated individuals about 50% will die by the age of 60.

See also Chapter 3.

membrane, where the molecules are released. The cycle is completed by the endocytosis of the vesicle membrane containing the receptors and its exocytosis on the other side, returning the receptors to their original place. An example of transcytosis is the movement of immunoglobulins across the intestine of the newborn from the mother's milk. Interestingly, the receptors will bind the immunoglobulins at the slightly acid pH (pH = 6) of the intestinal lumen, but release them at the neutral pH of the interstitial fluid. These ingested immunoglobulins confer significant levels of immunity to the newborn while its own immune system is developing.

Bulk flow in the blood

Diffusion and membrane transport processes are sufficient for moving substances short distances, but for large distances the time required would be impossible. The fastest way for substances to move around the human body is in the blood. Propelled by the contraction of the heart, the **bulk flow** of blood, with its suspension of cells, lipid particles and proteins, allows the movement of large quantities around the body at high speed. In humans, this bulk flow can move oxygen from the lungs to the furthest blood vessels in the limbs in 30 s, from where it can diffuse the 10 μm or so into the tissues (see Ch. 11).

CELL-TO-CELL COMMUNICATION

The human body is a large structure that needs to behave in a coordinated fashion. This can be achieved through signalling mechanisms, which transfer information about biochemical events between cells. Signalling requires two interacting elements:

- A signalling molecule
- A receptor molecule so the signal can be recognised and acted upon.

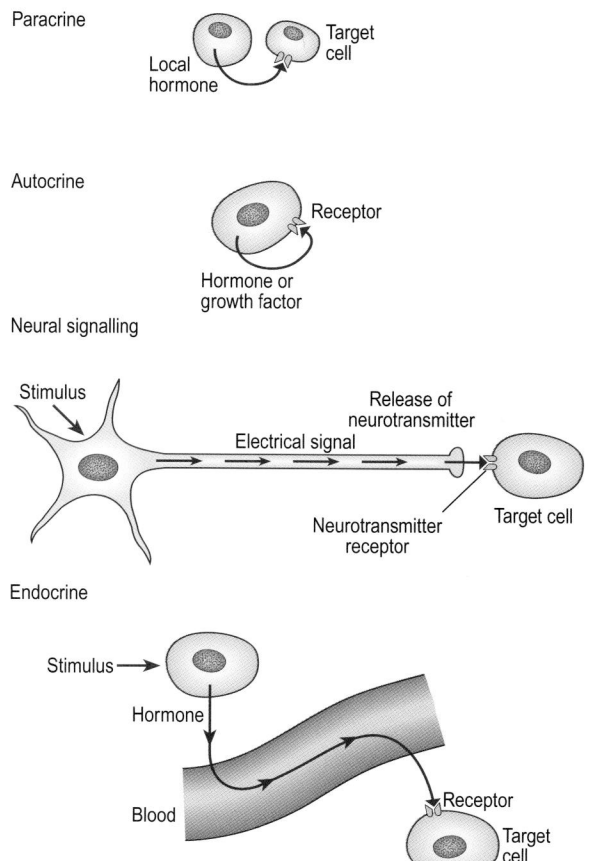

Fig. 2.36 **Different types of cell signalling.**

The signal molecule, or **ligand**, binds to the receptor at a specific binding site, causing a change in the receptor, which can produce an effect in the target cell, the **effector**. This process is called **signal transduction**.

TYPES OF SIGNALLING

There are four main forms of signalling (Fig. 2.36):

- **Paracrine**: this is where molecules called local hormones are released into the local environment of the cell producing the signal. These act on cells in the immediate environment.
- **Autocrine**: these molecules act on the cell releasing the signal. This is the mode of action of many growth hormones. Unregulated release of growth hormones can lead to the formation of tumours.
- **Neural signalling**: this is a particular type of signalling that can be both paracrine and autocrine. A signal generated in a nerve cell travels along nerve fibres to the effector. These signals travel electrically down these fibres until the target is reached, where a chemical called a **neurotransmitter** is released locally (see ch. 8). This signal can act either on the releasing nerve cell (autocrine), or on the nearby target (paracrine), which may be an effector, such as a muscle or gland, or another nerve.
- **Endocrine**: the signal is called a **hormone** and is released into the blood where it can circulate to the whole body. However, it will only affect cells and tissues that have receptors for the hormone (see Ch. 10).

Another type of local signalling occurs when proteins in the cell membrane are attached to receptors on adjacent cells. These are involved in cell-to-cell recognition and cell adhesion.

While paracrine and autocrine signalling rely on the passive diffusion of the signalling molecule and so are only active over a small distance, both neural and endocrine signalling allow information to be transmitted over large distances in a short time. Hormones released into the bloodstream can travel throughout the body within seconds, and although neurotransmitters themselves only have to diffuse very short distances, the electrical signals which trigger their release can travel for many metres. The longest nerves in the human body connect the lower spinal cord to the toes; the same nerves in a giraffe are many metres long.

LIGANDS AND RECEPTORS

The **ligands** involved in cell signalling are extremely varied. Some are small molecules derived from amino acids, such as noradrenaline, which is synthesised from tyrosine, while others are proteins, like insulin. An unusual ligand only recently discovered is **nitric oxide** (NO). Known previously only as a poisonous gas, this is now known to be released from endothelial cells (and some neurons) where it acts locally. It also has a role in the immune response, where it combines with superoxide anions to produce a compound poisonous to bacteria and parasites.

Many molecules can act as ligands for more than one type of signalling (Table 2.22). For example, noradrenaline acts as both a hormone and a neurotransmitter. It is released from many nerve terminals in the autonomic nervous system (see Ch. 4) but it can also be released into the blood from the adrenal medulla.

Receptors, like enzymes and transporters, show specificity in their binding and the kinetics of binding can be

Clinical box 2.13 | Nitric oxide relieves the pain of angina

In 1867 the pharmacologist Lauder Brunton observed that amyl nitrite inhalation relieved the pain of angina, but the mechanism of this effect was unknown. Amyl nitrite has since been superseded by nitroglycerin (glyceryl trinitrate), which acts by being degraded in the blood, releasing nitric oxide. This acts to relax smooth muscle cells found in blood vessel walls, thus increasing the diameter of the vessel and increasing blood flow. The pain of angina is due to the heart muscle not receiving enough oxygen delivered in the blood; increasing the blood supply through vasodilation thus reduces the pain.

described in a similar way to transport kinetics using the Michaelis–Menten equation. Specific receptors also mediate a specific response.

Receptors fall into two main categories depending on their ligands:

- **Cell surface receptors**: these are integral membrane proteins with an extracellular binding site for the ligand. The ligands for these receptors are either hydrophilic molecules, which cannot diffuse across the cell membrane, or are molecules which are too large to be easily transported across the membrane.
- **Intracellular receptors**: these bind to their ligands either in the cytosol or in the nucleus. The cytosolic receptors then translocate to the nucleus. Many of the ligands for these receptors are the steroid hormones, which are derivatives of cholesterol, and can diffuse across the cell membrane. Others include thyroid hormone, which is transported into the cell as an inactive prohormone (T_4) and is subsequently converted into the active form (T_3), which binds to nuclear receptors, and the retinoids which include vitamin A.

Cell surface receptors

The cell surface receptors fall into three main groups

- G-protein-coupled receptors
- Ligand-gated ion channels
- Receptor kinases.

G-protein-coupled receptors

The most abundant type of cell surface receptors are called either **G-protein-coupled receptors** (GPCR) or **7TM receptors**. Both of these names derive from the fact that they all share a similar transduction mechanism, changing intracellular biochemistry via a group of proteins called **G proteins**, which bind guanine nucleotides (GTP and GDP). The receptors also share a similar structure, in that they consist of an integral membrane protein with seven transmembrane segments, with an extracellular binding site for the ligand and an intracellular region that interacts with the G protein. They are also called **metabotropic receptors** because of their actions on intracellular metabolism. Many of these receptors exist in multiple isoforms. For example, the receptors which respond to smells are GPCRs; in humans there are thought to be over 500 different genes which code for GPCRs (compared to over 1000 in mice).

Table 2.22	**Some cell signalling molecules**	
Type of signalling	**Example**	**Example of effect***
Paracrine	Glucagon	Increases insulin release
	Nitric oxide	Local vasodilator released from endothelial cells
Autocrine	Prostaglandins	Inflammatory mediator
	Noradrenaline	Regulation of noradrenaline release via autoreceptors
Neural	Glutamate	Excitation of nerves in the central nervous system
	Acetylcholine	Excitation of skeletal muscle
	Noradrenaline	Vasoconstricts blood vessels
Endocrine	Adrenaline/noradrenaline	Increases heart rate
	Glucagon	Increases blood glucose
	Testosterone	Male sex hormone

*Many of the compounds listed have multiple effects, only a single example is given here.

Table 2.23	**Some G proteins and their associated enzymes and second messenger systems**			
G protein family*	**Enzyme affected**	**Second messenger (or effect) produced**	**Other effects**	
G_s	Adenylate cyclase	Increased cAMP	Opens Ca^{2+} channels and closes Na^+ channels	
G_i	Adenylate cyclase	Decreased cAMP	Closes Ca^{2+} channels and opens K^+ channels	
G_q	Phospholipase C	IP_3, DAG	IP_3 releases intracellular Ca^{2+} from stores which acts as another second messenger	
G_o	Phospholipase C	IP_3, DAG	IP_3 releases intracellular Ca^{2+} from stores, closes Ca^{2+} channels	
G_t	cGMP phosphodiesterase	cGMP		

*Strictly, these are the names of the α-subunit family of the G protein.
cAMP, cyclic adenosine monophosphate; IP_3, inositol trisphosphate; DAG, diacylglycerol; cGMP, cyclic guanosine monophosphate.

G proteins

The G proteins are activated by the receptors and in turn activate other intracellular signalling processes, often involving the production of intracellular signalling molecules called **second messengers**. Despite the very wide range of different GPCRs, the number of different second messengers produced seems to be limited. Some of the best known are cAMP, cGMP, calcium, inositol trisphosphate (IP_3) and diacylglycerol (DAG).

The G proteins in their inactive form are trimers consisting of α, β and γ subunits. When they are activated by the receptors, the α subunit separates from the β and γ subunits (which remain together). The α subunit then interacts with an effector, which is often an enzyme, but may also be a membrane ion channel. The effect of the G protein is to a large extent determined by the identity of the α subunit. There are known to be at least 16 different genes coding for α subunits, which fall into five or six groups (depending on the system used) according to their actions and locations (Table 2.23). This means that many different receptors must activate the same G protein. The different G proteins affect only a small number of intracellular enzymes. These enzymes produce the second messenger molecules, which themselves activate protein kinases and phosphatases to influence cell biochemistry.

Light receptors are GPCRs

As well as being responsible for the sense of smell, GPCRs also mediate vision where the ligand is a photon of light (see Ch. 8). In humans there are four types of light-sensitive GPCR in the eye. One of these, **rhodopsin**, absorbs a wide range of photons at low intensity and is responsible for black and white vision in cells called **rods**. Colour vision is mediated by three types of **coneopsin**, which preferentially absorb either red, green or blue light. These are found in **cone cells**, and in the brain the signals from these three kinds of receptor are processed in a way that identifies the 16 million different colours which it has been estimated that humans can distinguish.

Ligand-gated ion channels

Another major group of cell surface receptors are the **ligand-gated ion channels**. These are multimeric integral membrane proteins that have an extracellular binding site for the ligand. Binding of the ligand causes a conformational change in the protein which opens up a pore that crosses the membrane, through which ions can move. Each type of ligand-gated receptor allows a specific ion to move through it, and this is determined by the amino acid sequence of the amphipathic helices which line the pore. An example of this type of receptor is the **acetylcholine receptor** found on all skeletal muscle. When this is activated by acetylcholine, a pore opens, which allows Na^+ to flow into the muscle cell and depolarise it, a process which initiates muscle contraction (see Ch. 9).

Receptor kinases

Other cell surface receptors activate intracellular tyrosine or serine/threonine **kinases**. These kinases may either be an integral part of the receptor, as in the case of the insulin receptor, or in the case of the cytokine receptors the receptor may activate cytosolic tyrosine kinases. Other receptors, such as the receptor for atrial natriuretic peptide, activate a different membrane-integral enzyme, guanylate cyclase, to produce cGMP. Guanylate cyclases are also the target for nitric oxide, although these ones are cytosolic. Nitric oxide activates them to increase cGMP levels, which in turn leads to smooth muscle relaxation. Other receptors for growth factors and cytokines activate pathways that influence gene activity via transcription factors.

Intracellular receptors

The **intracellular receptors** for the steroid and other intracellular ligands are very different from the cell-surface receptors. When activated they all affect gene transcription because the receptors bind directly to DNA. These receptors consist of large monomeric proteins with a hormone-binding site and a region of about 60 residues, called the **DNA-binding domain**, which has a similar structure in all of the different receptors. It contains two loops of about 15 residues, called zinc fingers, which contain four cysteine residues surrounding a zinc atom. It is these fingers that are thought to bind to the DNA. Binding of the ligand to the receptor causes the protein to form dimers, which then bind to a specific sequence on the DNA, found about 200 base pairs from the start of the appropriate gene, the hormone-response element. The binding of the receptor–ligand complex causes an increase in transcription of the gene.

Nuclear and cytoplasmic receptors

Thyroid hormone receptors are found in the nucleus, permanently bound to DNA, but the steroid receptors are found, initially, in the cytoplasm. When they have bound their ligand they move to the nucleus and bind to DNA.

CELL RECOGNITION

In multicellular organisms, cells must have a way of interacting with the surrounding cells and the extracellular components. This is particularly important during development, where cells are forming tissues and there are considerable movements of cells from place to place. However, even in the adult, cells need to divide and grow in order to replace themselves and respond to changes in demands. In order for cells to grow in a controlled manner they need to be aware of their surroundings. They do this by means of a small variety of **cell adhesion molecules**. Many of the cell–cell interactions are relatively permanent, as in muscle, which must bind to other muscle cells and to tendons, and in skin, where cells must adhere to each other and the underlying matrix. Other interactions are much less permanent, such as that between capillary endothelial cells and white blood cells (see below).

CELL ADHESION MOLECULES

Four main types of molecules allow cells to make connections between each other and the ECM. Firstly, the two types of calcium-dependent molecules, the **cadherins** and the **selectins**, and secondly, the calcium-independent molecules, the **integrins** and the immunoglobulin superfamily of cell adhesion molecules known as **CAMs**. They are all transmembrane proteins with intracellular and extracellular domains.

Homophilic binding occurs when both ligand and receptor are the same molecule. Heterophilic binding joins two different molecules, although which is referred to as the receptor and which as the ligand is not important. As well as these major types there are a number of other adhesion molecules that do not fall into these four groups.

Cadherins

There are more than 80 different types of **cadherins** so far identified. The intracellular domain interacts with actin via proteins called catenins, and the extracellular section consists of a protein dimer with four calcium-binding sites. The dimer then binds to cadherin dimers on the opposing cell. E-cadherins are found on most epithelial cells, while N-cadherins and P-cadherins are found on neural (plus some muscle) and placental cells, respectively. The removal of calcium reduces cell adhesiveness, a factor taken into account when preparing tissue extracts for cell culture.

Selectins

Selectins belong to a group of molecules called **lectins**, which are proteins that bind to carbohydrates. They bind to the carbohydrate portion of glycoproteins, especially on the surface of white blood cells (leucocytes), helping them to target sites of inflammation. One of the selectins, P-selectin, is usually found in vesicles inside endothelial cells lining the blood vessels. When the endothelial cell is stimulated by factors released during inflammation, these selectins are inserted into the cell surface membrane, where they can interact with circulating leucocytes. The leucocytes can then move across the endothelial cells to reach the required tissue.

Integrins

The **integrins** are mainly used in interactions between the cell and the ECM, binding to adhesion proteins in the ECM

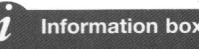

called **laminin** and **fibronectin**. These, in turn, bind to the proteoglycans of the ECM, ensuring that the cells and the ECM are bound together. Inside the cell the integrins bind to cytoskeletal proteins. Many tumour cells do not have fibronectin on their surface, aiding their migration through the ECM. This is a critical factor in their ability to spread to other parts of the body (metastasis).

CAMs

The cell adhesion molecules known as **CAMs** have a similar structure to the G-type immunoglobulins (IgG). They can bind homophilically or heterophilically to other CAMs. N-CAMs are found on neural cells where they mediate adhesion, while intercellular (I)-CAMs and vascular (V)-CAMs are involved in the interactions with leucocytes.

CELL DIVISION AND DNA REPLICATION

Proteins are continually being replaced inside cells and, at the same time, cells themselves are continually dying and in many cases being replaced. Cells have many different forms and mature cells are said to be **differentiated**. The replacement of cells is carried out by one of two processes:

- An undifferentiated precursor cell, a **stem cell**, is stimulated to develop into the required cell type.
- A fully differentiated parent cell divides into two by a process called **mitosis**, producing two smaller daughter cells which then grow into two parent cells.

Another type of cell division, called **meiosis**, is required to produce the **gametes**, e.g. the eggs and sperm of mammals. Both mitosis and meiosis require **DNA replication**.

STEM CELLS

Some cells do not undergo mitosis. Once formed, mature erythrocytes and nerve cells cannot divide – they are post mitotic. Other cells will undergo mitosis, although the rate at which this occurs varies enormously. At the other end of the spectrum, **stem cells** divide continually and can be stimulated to differentiate into mature cells. Some stem cells can produce all of the different cell types in a tissue – they are **pluripotent**. Others are **multipotent**, that is, they can produce some but not all of the cells in a tissue.

In different adult tissues there are stem cells that can be induced to form the different cells of which that tissue is

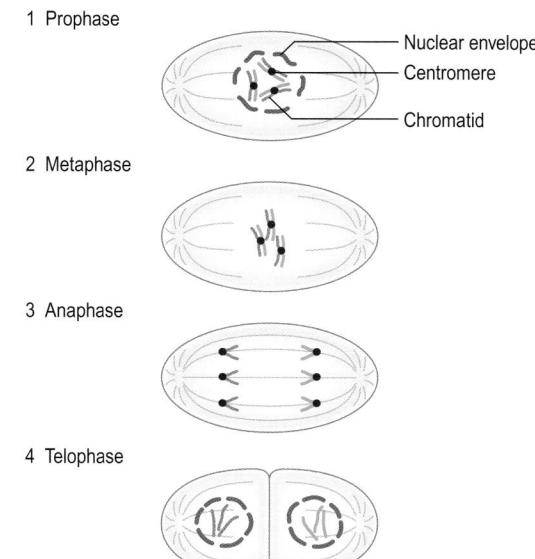

Fig. 2.38 **Phases in mitosis (for clarity only three chromosomes are shown).**

While adult stem cells from different tissues may be used to produce replacement cells of that tissue type, there is a great deal of interest in the use of embryonic stem cells, which produce all the different tissues of the embryo (except the placenta). One line of current research aims to treat a type of diabetes (juvenile onset type 1), where the insulin-producing β-cells of the pancreas are destroyed, by replacing them with β-cells derived from stem cells. Other studies are looking at replacing damaged heart muscle using stem cells. However, the advantage of using adult stem cells from the patients themselves ensures that there are no problems with rejection and therefore no need for immunosuppressive drugs.

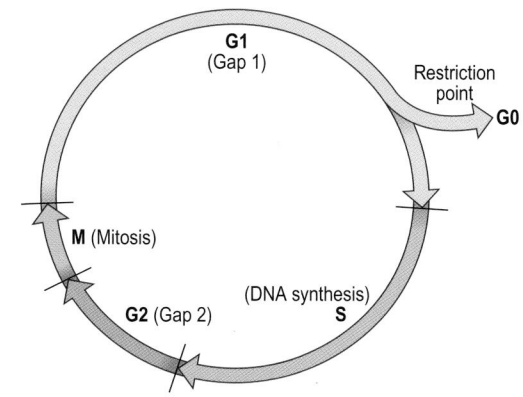

Fig. 2.37 **The cell cycle.**

made. For example, in the bone marrow, pluripotent stem cells can divide and form the red blood cells, platelets and the full variety of white blood cells (leucocytes) that are found in the blood. Bone marrow transplants from donors, which contain these stem cells, require matching of the major cell surface antigens in order to avoid donor–versus–host reactions. Some tissues only have very few stem cells, although there is some evidence that the numbers may increase following stress.

PHASES OF THE CELL CYCLE

The term **cell cycle** describes the life cycle of a cell from the time at which it is produced to when it divides into two daughter cells. The cycle consists of two major parts: **mitosis** and **interphase** (Fig. 2.37). During mitosis, also called the M phase, the cell divides rapidly. In a cell which is dividing every 24 hours, the M phase lasts about 1 hour. Interphase is divided into three phases, G1, S and G2.

In the absence of specific growth factors there is a point in late G1, called the **restriction point**, when the cell enters a quiescent phase called G0. However, if the appropriate growth factors are produced, the cell continues through G1 until it reaches the S phase where the DNA of the cell is replicated. This produces a cell containing two copies of the DNA, one for each of the daughter cells. This process takes about 8 hours. The cell then remains in G2 until it divides. There are a very few cell types which can remain in G2, but

most cells, once they pass the restriction point are committed to dividing.

The human karyotype

The number and type of chromosomes in a particular species or individual is called the **karyotype**. Humans normally have 46 chromosomes: 22 pairs of autosomal chromosomes, which are the same in males and females, and a pair of sex chromosomes. Normal males have one Y chromosome and one X chromosome, whereas normal females have two X chromosomes. The cells are said to be **diploid** because they have $2n$ chromosomes, where n is the number of chromosome pairs. So in humans n is 23.

In mitosis, a single cell that has already duplicated its DNA, so that it contains twice the normal amount ($4n$), divides into two virtually identical daughter cells. Each of the daughter cells is diploid: it has its own nucleus, which contains the normal amount of DNA ($2n$), and half the cytoplasm and cytoplasmic organelles of the parent cell.

In meiosis, the starting point is the same: a cell with $4n$ chromosomes. However, this is followed by two cycles of cell division, so that the resulting cells are **haploid** ($1n$). Sexual reproduction requires the fusion of two gametes, one from each parent. When female and male gametes (an egg and a sperm) combine they each contribute $1n$ chromosomes to produce a diploid ($2n$) fertilised ovum or **zygote**.

MITOSIS

Mitosis is the division of the single nucleus into two identical daughter nuclei and is divided into four periods (Fig. 2.38):

1. **Prophase.** This begins when the replicated DNA condenses into visible chromosomes. This condensation involves each chromosome becoming more and more coiled until it is dense enough to be observed under a light microscope. The nucleoli disappear and the nuclear envelope breaks down. Each pair of replicated chromosomes, called sister **chromatids**, are joined at a

characteristic point where the chromosome appears to be constricted, called a **centromere**. The **centrioles**, which are also duplicated during interphase, move apart in pairs, towards opposite ends, or poles, of the cell to form a **centrosome**, or microtubule-organising centre, with a radiating array of microtubules that is visible between the two centrosomes forming the **mitotic spindle**.

2. **Metaphase**. In the region of each centromere develops a **kinetochore**, which attaches the chromosome to the microtubules. The chromosomes align themselves on the microtubules at the centre of the cell, the **equatorial** or **metaphase plate**. These kinetochore microtubules are used to pull the chromosomes – one from each pair – towards opposite poles of the cell.

3. **Anaphase**. This occurs when the centromeres of each chromosome pair split and the kinetochore microtubules shorten, pulling each chromosome to opposite ends of the mitotic spindle. This is balanced by other microtubules (**radiating microtubules**) that anchor the centrosome to the plasma membrane. Once the chromosomes have reached the centrosomes, the poles separate further by elongation of the polar microtubules.

4. **Telophase**. This is marked by the uncoiling of the chromosomes and the re-formation of a nuclear envelope around each group of chromosomes. Around the equator of the cell an indentation forms where a contractile ring, formed from actin and myosin, pinches the cell until it cleaves into two daughter cells.

Strictly speaking, mitosis is the division of the nucleus only. **Cytokinesis** is the name given to the division of all of the cell except for the nucleus. Mitochondria, ribosomes and other organelles need not be distributed equally, just as long as each cell has some of them, and there is no mechanism which ensures their equal distribution. Usually the cytoplasm is divided equally between the two daughter cells, but this is not always the case.

The replication of mitochondria occurs throughout interphase. As mitochondria grow in size, other mitochondria are pinched off in a similar way to the division of some bacteria.

Daughter cells may not be completely identical to each other. This may be because they have different mitochondria, which do not all have identical DNA but also because DNA replication may not be perfect and one of the daughter cells may carry a mutation. Furthermore, if the chromosomes are not divided correctly between the two daughter cells, then the resulting cells will have an abnormal number of chromosomes, which is called **aneuploidy**.

As only a small proportion of cells in a population are dividing at any one time, it is difficult to observe the chromosomes. However, cells can be blocked at metaphase by the alkaloid colchicine, which prevents the chromosomes dividing. Cells then accumulate in metaphase and the chances of observing the chromosomes are much higher.

MEIOSIS

While mitosis produces virtually identical daughter cells with a full complement of chromosomes, during meiosis (Fig. 2.39) two processes occur.

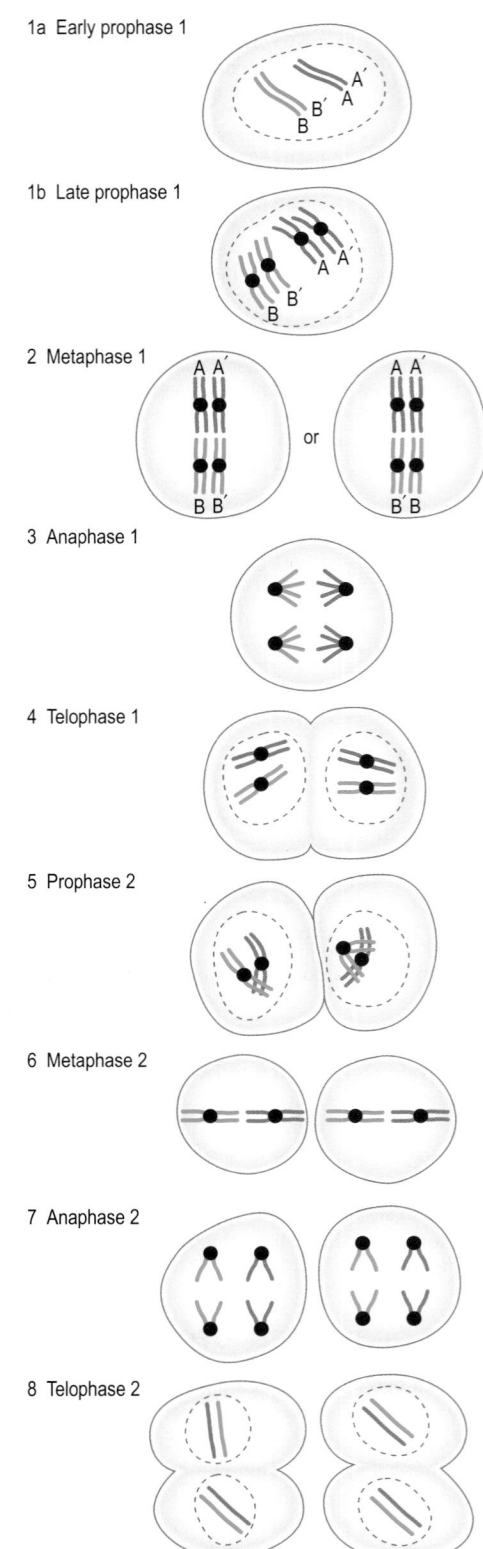

1a Early prophase 1

1b Late prophase 1

2 Metaphase 1   or

3 Anaphase 1

4 Telophase 1

5 Prophase 2

6 Metaphase 2

7 Anaphase 2

8 Telophase 2

Fig. 2.39 **Phases in meiosis.**

Prior to meiosis, during interphase, the DNA is replicated (just like mitosis), which increases the number of chromosomes to $4n$, four of each type. But, unlike mitosis, this is followed by **two** cycles of cell division. These are called meiosis I and II and each consists of the same four phases as in mitosis. This produces cells with half the number of

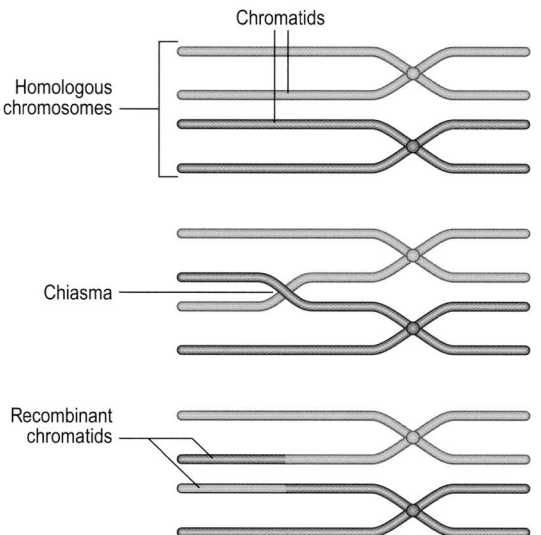

Fig. 2.40 Recombination during prophase 1 of meiosis.

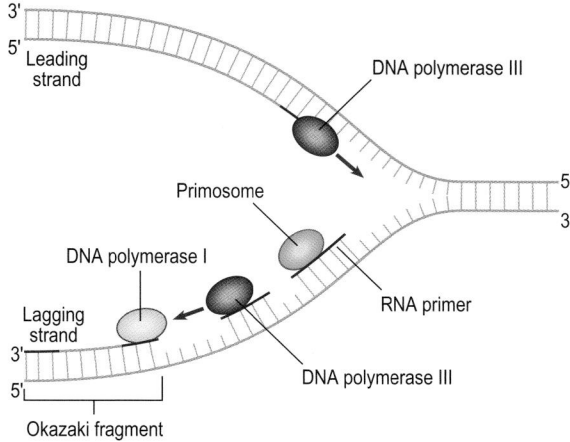

Fig. 2.41 DNA replication.

chromosomes (1*n*), one of each of the 22 autosomal pairs and either an X or Y chromosome.

During meiosis, genetic material is exchanged between chromosomes in a process called **recombination**, or **crossing over**, so that each resulting gamete has a different combination of genes. This is what produces the genetic diversity between individuals, as each person, while inheriting their parents' genes, gets them in a unique combination.

The phases of meiosis

1. **Prophase 1**. Firstly, the chromosomes condense, with each chromosome consisting of two chromatids joined by a centromere. The homologous pairs of chromatids form pairs along their whole lengths, a process called **synapsis**. During this time, recombination exchanges parts of chromatids. This can be seen by the formation of structures called **chiasmata** between pairs of chromosomes (Fig. 2.40). This recombination allows for novel combinations of genes to occur in the chromosomes. In late prophase 1, the nuclear envelope breaks down.
2. **Metaphase 1**. The pairs of chromosomes line up on the equator of the cell and attach to the microtubules via the kinetochores.
3. **Anaphase 1**. The chromosomes separate, with one pair of chromatids going to each pole.
4. **Telophase 1**. The chromosomes form into nuclei and the nuclear envelope starts to reform. The cell then divides into two.
5. **Prophase 2**. After a very brief interphase, when the DNA does not replicate, the chromosomes condense again.
6. **Metaphase 2**. The chromosomes line up on the equators of the new cells.
7. **Anaphase 2**. The chromatids separate, one going to each pole.
8. **Telophase 2**. The chromosomes gather into nuclei and the cells divide again.

The whole process of meiosis gives rise to four haploid gametes, each with a different assortment of chromosomes and, due to recombination, a different combination of genes

from the chromosomes of the parent. When combined with a haploid gamete from the other parent they will form part of a unique individual, who inherits 50% of their genes from each parent.

DNA REPLICATION

During interphase, which precedes both mitosis and meiosis, the entire DNA of each cell is copied. This process is a **semi-conservative** one in which a new complementary strand is formed against each of the two parent strands. The replicated strands will contain one parent strand and one daughter strand, so only half of the replicated DNA is new at each cycle of DNA synthesis.

In order to be copied, the double-stranded DNA is unwound by the action of a number of enzymes, including helicases, which separate the strands at a position called the **origin of replication**. In eukaryotes there are many of these replication sites. In order to prevent the strand reassembling during replication, single-stranded binding proteins bind to each of the separate strands. Replication can proceed in both directions, producing two **replication forks** that travel away from the origin as DNA is unwound and replicated (Fig. 2.41) . An enzyme called **RNA primase**, which, with other proteins, forms the **primosome**, makes a short strand of complementary RNA that acts as a primer for the manufacture of DNA.

The enzyme responsible for the manufacture of new strands is **DNA polymerase III** and, like RNA polymerase, it reads the parent strand only in the 3′ to 5′ direction, so new nucleotides are only added to the 3′ end of the new strand. This means that only one of the parent strands, the 3′-5′ strand, called the leading strand, can be made in one continuous stretch, starting at the 5′ end. The other strand, the lagging strand, is made by the synthesis of multiple short stretches of about 100–200 base pairs long, called **Okazaki fragments**. The enzyme DNA polymerase I then replaces the RNA primer with DNA, and the fragments are then joined together by DNA ligase at the points where they meet.

DNA checking and repair

DNA polymerase III also controls the accuracy of replication by checking that the base pair on the original strand and the new strand are complementary. If they are not, then the incorrect nucleotide is excised and replaced. This leads to a very low error rate in replication (Clinical box 2.14). It is estimated that the error rate before this proofreading is about 1 in 10000, but with the replacement of wrong nucleotides this falls to 1 in 10^8–10^{12}. However, this still means that many genes will contain errors that could be deleterious to the daughter cell.

Damage to DNA

The DNA of a cell not only contains copying errors but is continuously being subjected to damage by high-energy radiation, mutagenic chemicals (particularly reactive oxygen intermediates) and spontaneous chemical reactions. These different processes have been estimated to produce up to 60000 modifications per day. Many of these modifications may produce no discernible effect, possibly because they occur in non-essential DNA or do not change the activity of the gene product. However, some may cause the death of the individual cell. In multicellular organisms with their many other cells, this can be relatively unimportant. However, more damagingly, mutations in gametes can lead to damage in future offspring. This occurs particularly in ova because the ova are all formed in the early embryo and can therefore accumulate damage throughout their life from before birth until the menopause. Mutations in somatic cells can lead to cancers, with the uncontrolled proliferation of cells.

DNA repair

Two major mechanisms repair DNA continually. They have been studied extensively in bacteria, but similar mechanisms are thought to exist in eukaryotes:

- Small lesions are repaired by **DNA glycosylase** enzymes that check the DNA for mispaired bases, chemically modified bases, or strands with excess bases. These are then excised and replaced.
- Larger lesions are repaired by removing the section of DNA containing the damage using **DNA helicase**, and then replacing it with a new section made by DNA polymerase, with the new fragment being attached by **DNA ligase**.

CELLULAR AGEING AND CELL DEATH

At the same time that new cells are being created, old cells die. Under normal conditions the adult organism remains a constant size because cell birth and cell death are balanced.

Hayflick limit

When cells are removed from the body and placed in tissue culture, they will grow and divide until they cover the surface of a dish, forming a monolayer. They then cease dividing and become quiescent. If the cells are removed from the dish and re-plated at a lower density, they will start dividing again until they form a new monolayer. However, normal cells do not continue in this way indefinitely. Depending on their age when they were removed from the body, cells continue to divide about 50 times. This is called the **Hayflick limit**. Cells derived from an adult have already divided a number of times, so they will not divide as many times as those removed from an embryo. For this reason, cell cultures are usually prepared from either fetal or young material. Once they reach their limit, the cells then become senescent and die.

Telomeres

A key element in determining when a cell dies depends on both the existence of regions of DNA sequences called **telomeres** and the activity of the enzyme **telomerase**, which consists of a combination of protein and RNA. Found at the end of each chromosome, telomeres are regions of single-stranded DNA composed of repeated nucleotide sequences. In human telomeres the sequence TTAGGG can be repeated up to 100 times. The telomeres prevent enzymes that normally join broken ends of DNA from linking the chromosomes together and allow the chromosome to be copied all the way to the end. Without the telomeres, the lagging strand would not be copied to the end, because DNA polymerase cannot copy the strand underneath the last RNA primer.

Somatic cells do not usually have telomerase activity, so at each mitotic cell division the telomeres are shortened due to the failure of DNA polymerase to copy the chromosomal ends. When the telomeres become too short the chromosomes tend to fuse together and the cell dies. In contrast, in germ cells, and in some stem cells, the enzyme **telomerase** extends the 3′ end of DNA, by a form of reverse transcription: the RNA template of the enzyme is copied into DNA which is added to the end of the chromosome, thus maintaining its length.

The action of telomerase in maintaining cell viability is shown by cancer cells which are often immortal; that is they continue to divide beyond the Hayflick limit, seemingly indefinitely. These cells have regained active telomerase activity, maintaining the telomere length. Interestingly, in individuals with premature ageing diseases, the telomeres are often found to be unusually short.

Mechanisms of cell death

Cells can die in two ways:

- Necrosis
- Apoptosis.

These two mechanisms occur under different conditions and have very different consequences.

Oxygen toxicity

While oxygen is essential for life on earth, because of its reactivity, it can also damage cells. Oxygen can react with a wide range of metabolites via reactions with **superoxide anions**. First, molecular oxygen is reduced to the superoxide anion:

$$O_2 \rightarrow O^{\cdot}_{2}{}^{-}$$

This is a type of **free radical** (denoted by the dot on the right) as it has an unpaired electron in its outer shell, making it highly reactive. Oxygen radicals can react with almost any biological molecule. They react with lipids to form peroxides, a process called **peroxidation**. Most damagingly they react with DNA, which can produce mutations that may be deleterious. They can also damage proteins and carbohydrates and they are particularly important in the development of the arterial disease, atherosclerosis. This is due to the fact that oxidised LDLs cannot be taken up in the liver, but are scavenged by macrophages, which go on to form the foam cells that are central to the formation of atherosclerotic plaques (see Ch. 11).

Occasionally, free radical generation can be beneficial when macrophages use the production of oxygen free radicals to kill invading bacteria. NADPH (nicotinamide adenosine dinucleotide phosphate (reduced form)) is used to convert oxygen to superoxide anions. These are then converted to hydrogen peroxide (H_2O_2) by the enzyme superoxide dismutase and also, with the addition of chloride, to hypochlorous acid (HOCl). These compounds are released by the macrophage in order to degrade bacterial cells. The consumption of oxygen required to produce these molecules results in a respiratory burst that is associated with phagocytosis (see Ch. 6).

Antioxidants

Damage caused by free radicals can be prevented by the action of a number of protective compounds, called **antioxidants**. Many of these compounds, such as vitamin E, form stable radicals which do not react. An important antioxidant is glutathione, which is especially important in red blood cells. Because they carry large amounts of oxygen, red cells are particularly prone to damage. This is shown by the appearance of methaemoglobin, an inactive oxidised form of haemoglobin, which cannot transport oxygen. Glutathione maintains the proteins and enzymes in a reduced state, particularly the sulphydryl groups, and is also important in reconverting peroxylipids and proteins, using the enzyme glutathione reductase. A cofactor for this enzyme is selenium, which is required in trace amounts in the diet. Other antioxidants include vitamin C and β-carotene, present in fruit and vegetables (see Ch. 16).

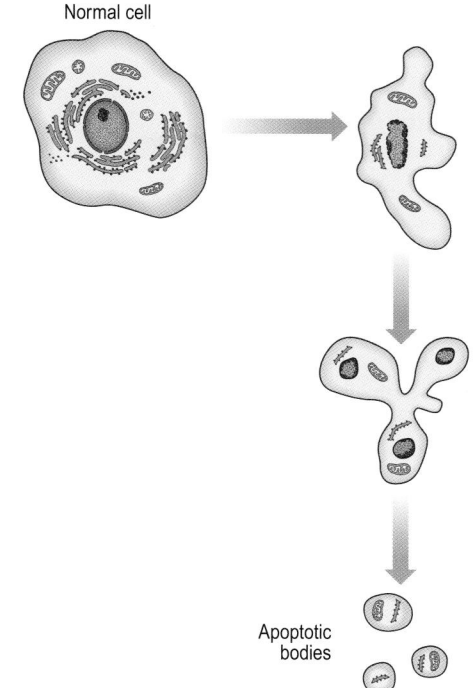

Normal cell

Apoptotic bodies

Fig. 2.42 Apoptotic cell death.

Necrosis

When cells are damaged by an acute injury, such as when they are starved of oxygen by blockage of a blood vessel, as in a stroke, or poisoned by toxic substances, they die by **necrosis**, or accidental cell death. The cells swell and burst, releasing their cytoplasmic and nuclear contents into the extracellular space, triggering an inflammatory response. While this response is a necessary defence mechanism its effects can also be life-threatening (see Ch. 6).

Apoptosis

Apoptosis, also called programmed cell death (Fig. 2.42), is the type of cell death that occurs during the normal turnover of cells in the adult and also under a number of other circumstances in apparently healthy cells:

- Elimination of excess neurons during the development of the nervous system
- During development of organs, such as loss of webbing between the fingers in the human embryo
- Death after a fixed time, such as in the epithelial lining of the gastrointestinal tract, or in the skin keratinocytes
- Shedding of the endometrium during the menstrual cycle
- Death of lymphocytes during their maturation in the thymus in order to prevent autoimmune reactions (see Ch. 6).

Apoptosis also occurs when cells are damaged by chronic injury through viruses, toxins and genetic mutations, but unlike necrotic cell death, this does not produce a potentially harmful inflammation.

Cells undergoing apoptosis first lose contact with their neighbours and shrink. The nuclear chromatin condenses against the nuclear membrane. The cell then breaks up into several membrane-bound fragments called apoptotic bodies, which are phagocytosed by macrophages or shed from epithelial surfaces. Importantly, the cell contents are not released and there is no inflammatory response.

Triggers for apoptosis

Two main interrelated pathways trigger apoptosis in cells:

- the **Fas pathway**: this involves the expression of cell surface receptors, called **death receptors**, which bind a ligand called Fas. This may be a paracrine or an autocrine signal. This activates an enzyme, **caspase-8**, which in turn activates other caspases (a family of intracellular proteases) that induce the breakdown of chromatin.
- the **Bax pathway**: this also involves caspase-8, which activates the channel protein, Bax. Bax is inserted into the mitochondrial membrane, allowing cytochrome c to be released. ATP synthesis in the mitochondria is thus prevented and cytochrome c also activates other protease enzymes, which then break down the intracellular structures.

KEY METABOLIC PATHWAYS

Chemical reactions in the body consist of **catabolic reactions**, which break down large precursor molecules and release energy, and **anabolic reactions**, which use energy in order to build up large molecules. ATP acts as a form of energy storage, to be consumed to fuel **exergonic** or energy-requiring reactions. The metabolic pathways are a highly integrated network of chemical reactions occurring within cells. They rely on the energy supplied by the breakdown of large molecules that may be stored in the body, mainly as fats or carbohydrates, but which ultimately are derived from ingested nutrients.

> **ℹ Information box 2.20**   **Cancer cells do not undergo apoptosis**
>
> The protein **p53** is expressed by cells in response to damage to DNA. If the damage is slight, p53 induces the cells to delay entry to the S phase of the cell cycle, until the DNA has been repaired. However, if the damage is too great, then p53 can trigger apoptosis.
>
> A link to cancer is the observation that cancer cells do not respond to the normal signals that induce apoptosis, and it has been shown that about 50% of all human cancers have non-functional p53 genes, hence another name for p53, the **tumour-suppressor gene**. p53 also controls the expression of the Fas and Bax genes. The lack of p53 expression in cancer cells that have been exposed to ionising radiation during radiotherapy results in the survival of these cells, which can then continue to proliferate.

As well as ATP, which transfers phosphate groups from one molecule to another, a number of other **coenzymes** are involved in metabolism and also transfer groups between molecules. Some of these are given in Table 2.24.

In summary:

1. Carbohydrates and fats are broken down and converted into glucose and fatty acids, respectively.
2. These are used as substrates in the production of ATP through a series of pathways that converge on a common intermediate, **acetyl coenzyme A (acetyl CoA)** (Fig. 2.43).
3. Acetyl CoA is further metabolised by a common pathway called the **tricarboxylic acid cycle** (TCA), also known as the **citric acid cycle**, or **Krebs cycle**, after Sir Hans Krebs who first described it in 1937. Under conditions of decreased carbohydrate and fat intake, proteins can be broken down into amino acids, and these can also be metabolised by the same reactions.
4. The reduced coenzymes produced by the TCA cycle are then used in the conversion of ADP to ATP in a series of reactions called the **electron transport chain**. These chain reactions are all driven by the final step, where oxygen is required to oxidise cytochrome a.
5. The electron transport chain produces a gradient of protons across the mitochondrial inner membrane. This proton gradient is finally dissipated in the conversion of ADP to ATP by the enzyme ATP synthase in a process called **oxidative phosphorylation**.

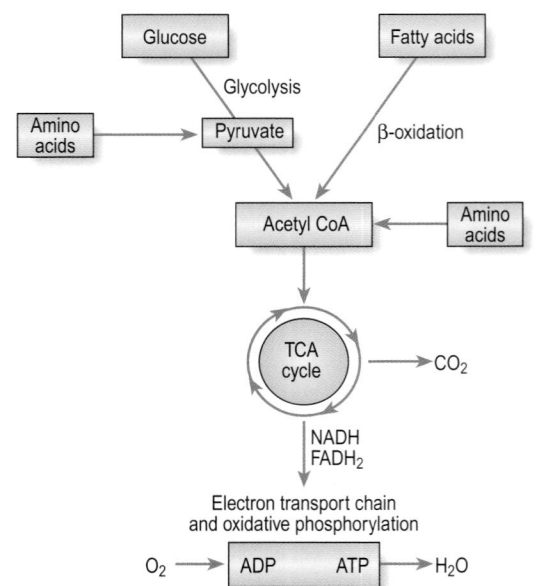

Fig. 2.43 **Metabolic pathways to produce acetyl CoA.**

Table 2.24	Some coenzymes involved in metabolism		
Coenzyme	**Group transferred**	**Oxidised**	**Reduced**
Nicotinamide adenine dinucleotide (NAD)	2H	NAD^+	$NADH + H^+$
Nicotinamide adenine dinucleotide phosphate (NADP)	2H	$NADP^+$	$NADPH + H^+$
Flavin adenine dinucleotide (FAD)	2H	FAD^+	$FADH + H^+$
Coenzyme A (CoA)	Acyl groups ($CH_3(CH_2)_nCO$), for example, the acetyl group (CH_3CO, where $n=0$)	CoA	Acetyl CoA

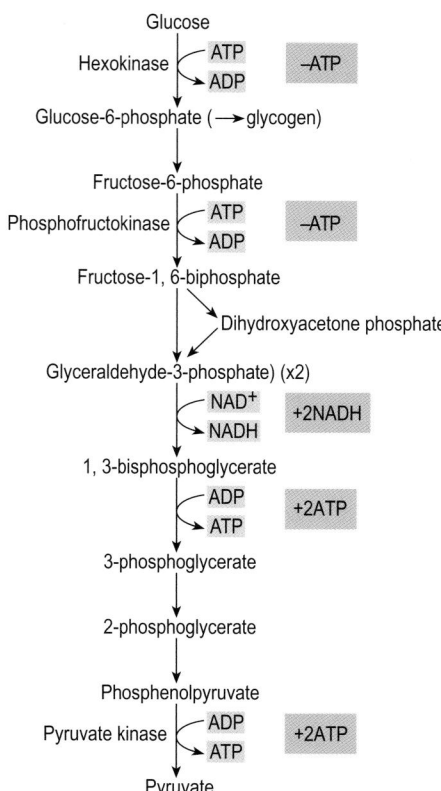

Fig. 2.44 **Steps in glycolysis.**

GLYCOLYSIS

Glycolysis occurs in the cytosol of cells and, via a series of enzyme-linked reactions, converts the 6-carbon **glucose** molecule into two molecules of the 3-carbon **pyruvate** (Fig. 2.44). Some of these reactions use ATP (which is converted to ADP) and others convert ADP to ATP. During glycolysis there is a net gain of two molecules of ATP for each molecule of glucose; however, two molecules of NAD are also reduced, producing two molecules of NADH. None of these reactions require the presence of oxygen and therefore they can operate under anaerobic conditions. However, unless the NADH can be regenerated, the reactions will stop. NADH regeneration normally occurs by the transfer of the NADH to the mitochondria where it can be reoxidised.

In strenuous exercise, the rate of this reoxidation is insufficient and, in order to continue the breakdown of glucose, NADH is oxidised by the reduction of pyruvate to lactate. This is exported to the liver, where it can be used to resynthesise glucose (see Ch. 3). Many of the intermediate molecules of glycolysis can also be used in the synthesis of other biomolecules.

Hexokinase and glucokinase

The first step in glycolysis is the phosphorylation of glucose to **glucose-6-phosphate**, either by the enzyme **hexokinase**, present in all tissues, or **glucokinase**, which only occurs in the liver or in the insulin-secreting pancreatic β-cells. This important reaction traps the glucose within the cell as glucose-6-phosphate, which is not a substrate for the glucose transporters in the cell membrane. Glucokinase has a lower affinity for glucose than hexokinase and, unlike hexokinase, is not inhibited by glucose-6-phosphate. This produces two effects:

- The liver can take up large amounts of glucose from the glucose-rich blood arriving via the hepatic portal vein from the intestine after a carbohydrate-rich meal.
- In pancreatic β-cells, because the enzyme does not saturate at normal levels of blood glucose, the concentration of glucose inside the cells continues to rise even after the ingestion of large amounts of glucose. As the secretion of insulin is linked to the amount of glucose-6-phophate inside the cells, this ensures that, after a large meal, sufficient insulin is released.

In some types of diabetes there are mutations of the glucokinase gene, which may prevent glucose being trapped inside the pancreatic β-cells. This then prevents glucose-6-phosphate levels rising sufficiently inside the cells, and patients secrete lower amounts of insulin than normal. Red blood cells lack mitochondria, which contain the enzymes necessary for further metabolism of pyruvate, so they obtain all their energy from anaerobic glycolysis.

Control of glycolysis

The rate of glycolysis in red blood cells is regulated by controlling the activity of three enzymes in the glycolytic pathway. These are:

- Hexokinase
- **Phosphofructokinase** (PFK-1), which converts fructose-6-phosphate to fructose-1,6-bisphosphate
- **Pyruvate kinase**, which catalyses the last step in glycolysis, which produces pyruvate.

All these three enzymes catalyse irreversible reactions (although some reactions can be reversed by other enzymes) which, because of their low activity levels (low V_{max}) relative to other glycolytic enzymes, are rate limiting steps.

Hexokinase
Hexokinase is inhibited by its product, glucose-6-phosphate, and has the lowest activity of all the glycolytic enzymes.

PFK-1
The dominant role in the control of glycolysis is the allosteric regulation of PFK-1. Binding of ATP to the enzyme lowers its affinity for the substrate (i.e. it increases K_m). This enzyme is also stimulated by ADP and AMP, so its overall activity depends on the ratio between ATP and (ADP + AMP) concentrations.

Pyruvate kinase
The third enzyme, pyruvate kinase, is activated by the product of the PFK-1 reaction, fructose-1,6-bisphosphate. This type of regulation, known as **feed-forward activation**, ensures that intermediates of glycolysis do not accumulate. Glycolysis is inhibited by other metabolites such as pyruvate and citrate (which is an intermediate in the TCA cycle; see below).

Control mechanisms in other cells

The control mechanisms described above occur in red blood cells, which seem to have relatively simple requirements, and their metabolism remains fairly constant. In other tissues such muscle and liver, however, where energy requirements fluctuate more, the control of these key enzymes is more complicated, involving other allosteric modulators and covalent modification, such as phosphorylation.

Link reaction

Pyruvate produced by glycolysis is transported into the mitochondria where the rest of energy metabolism takes place. The oxidation of pyruvate to acetyl CoA occurs via a **link reaction** catalysed by the enzyme complex **pyruvate dehydrogenase**, which requires the coenzyme thiamine pyrophosphate (derived from vitamin B_1) as well as other coenzymes. During this reaction, for each molecule of pyruvate a single carbon is lost as CO_2 and a molecule of NADH produced (Fig. 2.45). As well as being converted to acetyl CoA and lactate, pyruvate can also be converted to alanine, which can be used in protein synthesis, or to **oxaloacetate**, to be used by the liver to synthesise glucose.

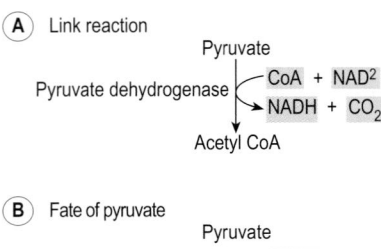

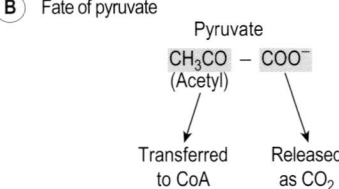

Fig. 2.45 Link reaction between glycolysis and the TCA cycle.

Clinical box 2.16 **Vitamin B_1 deficiency impairs glucose metabolism**

Vitamin B_1 is the source of an essential coenzyme involved in carbohydrate metabolism. The body stores very little vitamin B_1 (thiamine) and so it has to be ingested at regular intervals. Thiamine is present in the husks of rice, in wheat germ and in seeds. Thiamine is phosphorylated in the tissues to produce both the coenzyme, thiamine pyrophosphate (also known as thiamine diphosphate), and thiamine triphosphate, which has a role in nerve conduction. In thiamine deficiency there are raised levels of pyruvate, which will inhibit glycolysis. This can lead to the accumulation of glucose in the blood. The accumulation of both pyruvic acid and lactic acid causes acidosis which, in severe cases, can lead to coma and death.

The commonest form of thiamine deficiency, beriberi, occurs in populations dependent on rice diets where, if the rice is polished, thiamine is removed. Alcohol inhibits the absorption of thiamine in the intestines, so deficiency conditions are relatively common in alcoholics. Wernicke–Korsakoff's syndrome is the result of thiamine deficiency associated with the combination of chronic misuse of alcohol and malnutrition.

See also Chapter 16.

THE METABOLISM OF FATTY ACIDS

All tissues except the brain and red blood cells take up free fatty acids from the blood and use them in the production of **acetyl CoA** (see Ch. 3). Fats are energy-rich foods as they produce more ATP per mole when oxidised than glucose, owing to the large number of H atoms in the fat molecules.

The carnitine shuttle

The first step involves the conversion of fatty acids to a CoA derivative (**acyl CoA**) as they enter the cell, which prevents the fatty acids dissolving cell membranes. While small acyl CoA molecules derived from fatty acids with fewer than about 12 carbons can passively diffuse into mitochondria, larger acyl CoA molecules are transported across the mitochondrial membranes by a shuttle mechanism. This involves their conversion to acylcarnitine, with the replacement of the CoA by carnitine, leaving CoA in the cytoplasm. The resulting acylcarnitine is transported across both the outer and inner membranes, before being converted back to acyl CoA and carnitine in the matrix. The carnitine is then returned to the cytosol where it can pick up another acyl CoA. As the transporters on both membranes use antiport mechanisms, the ability to transport fatty acids into the mitochondrial matrix is regulated by the level of free CoA in the matrix. If fatty acid levels are high then most of the CoA will be acylated and no further transport can occur.

β-Oxidation

The catabolism of acyl CoA molecules is carried out in the mitochondrial matrix by a process called **β-oxidation** (Fig. 2.46). This occurs via the stepwise removal of two carbon units to produce acetyl CoA. This process not only produces large amounts of acetyl CoA, but each step produces one **NADH** and one **FADH$_2$**. For each fatty acid of n carbon atoms, there are $n/2$ molecules of acetyl CoA produced and $(n/2 - 1)$ of each of NADH and FADH$_2$.

Each cycle is a series of four steps:

1. An oxidation reaction of the β-carbon (hence the name β-oxidation) to form a double bond (Fig. 2.46 step 1), yielding one FADH$_2$.
2. This double bond is then hydrated to produce a hydroxyl group (Step 2).
3. The hydroxyl group is then oxidised (Step 3), yielding one NADH.
4. This is then cleaved by a thiolase enzyme to give a molecule of acyl CoA that is shorter by two carbon atoms and a molecule of acetyl CoA (Step 4).

The enzymes which carry out these four steps are thought to be closely associated in the membrane so that the product of each reaction is passed directly to the next enzyme. As a consequence none of the intermediates can be detected in the mitochondrial matrix.

There are three different **acyl CoA dehydrogenase enzymes** which catalyse step 1, each with specificity for either short, medium or long chain acyl CoA. Very-long-chain fatty acids (>20 carbons) are shortened in peroxisomes to enable their uptake by mitochondria. Peroxisomes can also carry out β-oxidation of fatty acids with the production of hydrogen peroxide (H_2O_2), instead of FADH$_2$.

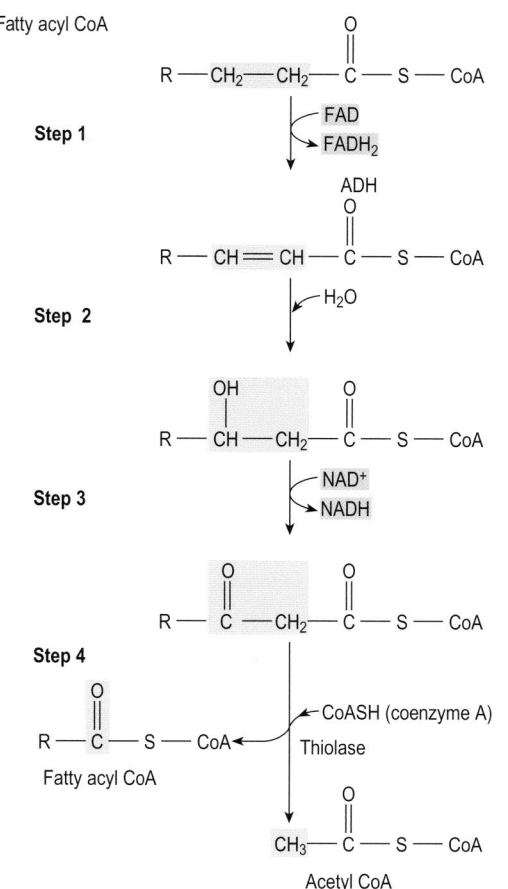

Fig. 2.46 **β-Oxidation of fatty acids.** R = CH₃—(CH₂)ₙ

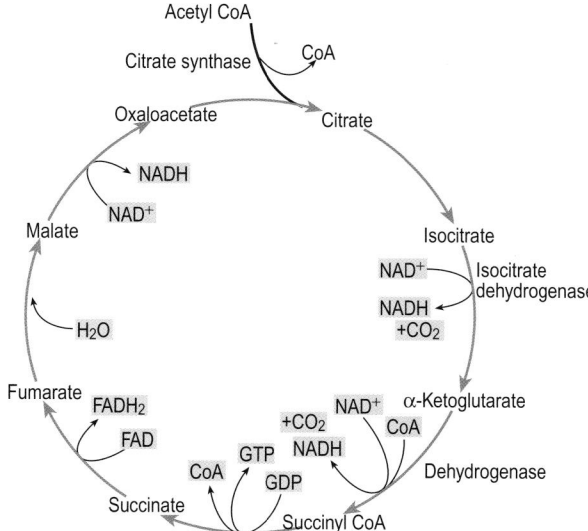

Fig. 2.47 The TCA cycle.

Fatty acids that are unsaturated or have uneven numbers of carbons can also be converted to acetyl CoA, but there are additional steps involved.

- In the case of unsaturated fatty acids, enzymes alter the position and shape of the double bonds.
- With odd numbers of carbons the last reaction produces propionyl CoA (which contains an extra CH_2 group), which is converted to the TCA cycle intermediate, succinyl CoA.

Ketones

In the liver any surplus acetyl CoA produced from fatty acid breakdown can be converted to **ketones bodies or ketones**, which can be exported to other organs. Ketone bodies consist of acetoacetate, β-hydroxy butyrate and acetone, which are water soluble. This type of metabolism is important for many tissues (except the liver) in fasting, starvation and in diabetes mellitus. However, high levels of acetoacetate and β-hydroxy butyrate can cause an increase in the acidity of the blood, a type of **metabolic acidosis** (see Ch. 1). During starvation, brain tissue may acquire 50% of its energy from ketone bodies. This reduces the demand for glucose and also thereby reduces the need for glucose production from other sources (see Ch. 3), particularly from the breakdown of body protein – a potentially survival-enhancing metabolic switch.

TCA CYCLE

The **TCA cycle** starts with the formation of citrate from a condensation reaction between acetyl CoA and the four-carbon oxaloacetate. This releases the CoA, which can then react with a further molecule of pyruvate. This series of reactions is called a cycle rather than a pathway because it eventually produces oxaloacetate which can react with another molecule of acetyl CoA. However, during these reactions, for each molecule of acetyl CoA, three molecules of NADH, one of FADH₂ and one molecule of GTP are produced (Fig. 2.47).

Control of the TCA cycle

The TCA cycle is regulated by three enzymes. **Citrate synthase**, which catalyses the condensation reaction between acetyl CoA and oxaloacetate, is sensitive to the availability of its substrates, particularly oxaloacetate. This enzyme is also inhibited by ATP and allosterically activated by ADP. In this way it is sensitive to the energy state of the cell. The other key regulatory enzymes, **isocitrate dehydrogenase** and **α-ketoglutarate dehydrogenase**, are both regulated by the levels of NAD⁺ and NADH. In this way the cycle can respond to the cell's need for energy.

Uses for TCA cycle intermediates

As well as providing reduced coenzymes for the electron transport chain, many of the intermediates of the TCA cycle can be used as substrates for other anabolic pathways (Fig. 2.48).

Examples are:

- Citrate – can be used as a substrate for fatty acid synthesis
- Oxaloacetate – can be converted to aspartate from which it can be used in many ways, including the manufacture of amino acids, nucleic acids and in the urea cycle, or as the starting point for the synthesis of glucose (gluconeogenesis)
- succinyl CoA – can be used as the starting point for the synthesis of haem.

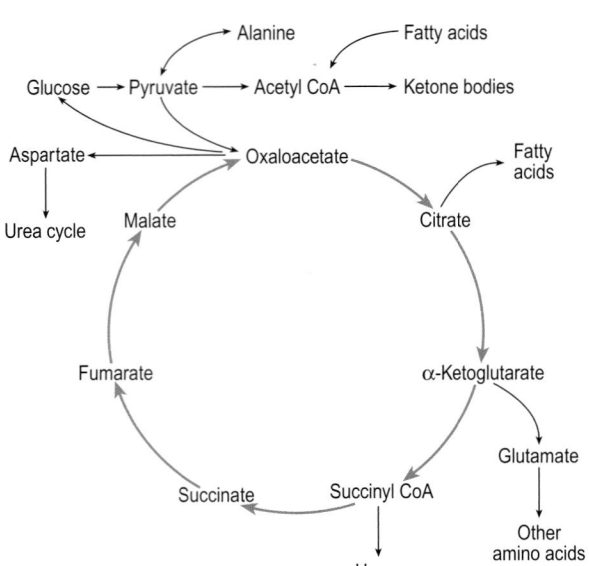

Fig. 2.48 TCA cycle intermediates are substrates for many other reactions.

Table 2.25	Glucogenic and ketogenic amino acids
Type	**Amino acids**
Glucogenic only	Alanine, arginine, asparagine, aspartate, cysteine, glutamate, glutamine, glycine, histidine, methionine, proline, serine, valine
Ketogenic only	Leucine, lysine
Both glucogenic and ketogenic	Isoleucine, phenylalanine, threonine, tryptophan, tyrosine

AMINO ACID METABOLISM

Proteins are broken down into amino acids (see also Ch. 3). Many of these are used directly in the production of other proteins and a number of important metabolites, including the purines and pyrimidines used in nucleic acid synthesis, some neurotransmitters, and the haem portion of haemoglobin. Amino acids can also be used to provide energy, particularly during fasting.

Deamination and transamination

Before amino acids can be used as fuel their amino groups must be removed, leaving the corresponding **α-keto acid**. This occurs either by **deamination**, which directly oxidises the amino acid to its keto acid with the removal of ammonia, or **transamination**, in which the amino group is transferred to an acceptor, another keto acid, which is thus converted to an amino acid. For example, the removal of the amino group from alanine ($CH_3CH(NH_2)COOH$) produces pyruvate ($CH_3COCOOH$). Similarly, the removal of the amino group from glutamate converts it to α-ketoglutarate, one of the TCA cycle intermediates. In this way amino acid derivatives can be integrated directly into energy metabolism.

Urea cycle

Ammonia is highly toxic, so it is immediately converted to **glutamine** or **alanine**. These are eventually removed, mainly by conversion into urea, carried out by the **urea cycle** in the liver. The urea is subsequently excreted in the urine.

Glucogenic and ketogenic amino acids

When the carbon skeletons derived from amino acids are catabolised, depending on metabolic requirements, they can be converted into glucose or ketone bodies. Different amino acids yield different products, so they are called **glucogenic**, or **ketogenic**, or both (Table 2.25). Ketogenic amino acids can yield either acetyl CoA or acetoacetyl CoA, while gluco-

genic amino acids give rise to pyruvate or a number of TCA cycle intermediates.

Essential amino acids

While many of the 20 amino acids used to manufacture proteins can be synthesised in the body there are a number that cannot. Adults require adequate dietary amounts of eight amino acids:

- Isoleucine
- Leucine
- Lysine
- Methionine
- Phenylalanine
- Threonine
- Tryptophan
- Valine.

Infants also require histidine and arginine as well because the amounts they can synthesise may not be enough to support their growth rate (see Ch. 16). Cysteine and tyrosine can only be made from the essential amino acids methionine and phenylalanine, respectively, so if they are not present in the diet, more methionine and phenylalanine must be ingested.

ELECTRON TRANSPORT CHAIN AND OXIDATIVE PHOSPHORYLATION

The final part of the transformation of glucose and other energy supplies into a source of energy usable by metabolic reactions occurs on the inner membrane of the mitochondrion. The enzymes responsible are mostly integral to the inner membrane and are arranged as a sequence of protein complexes called the **electron transport chain**.

Electron transport chain

Starting with the reduced coenzymes, electrons are passed from complex to complex, with the complexes acting as proton pumps (Fig. 2.49). The energy required to pump protons, against their concentration gradient, into the space between the inner and outer mitochondrial membranes is obtained from the free energy released as the electrons move from complex to complex, down a gradient of **redox potentials**. The final electron acceptor in the chain is oxygen, which combines with hydrogen to give water.

The overall reaction is therefore: glucose plus oxygen gives carbon dioxide and water.

$$C_6H_{12}O_6 + 6O_2 \rightarrow 6CO_2 + 6H_2O \text{ plus 38 ADP molecules converted to ATP}$$

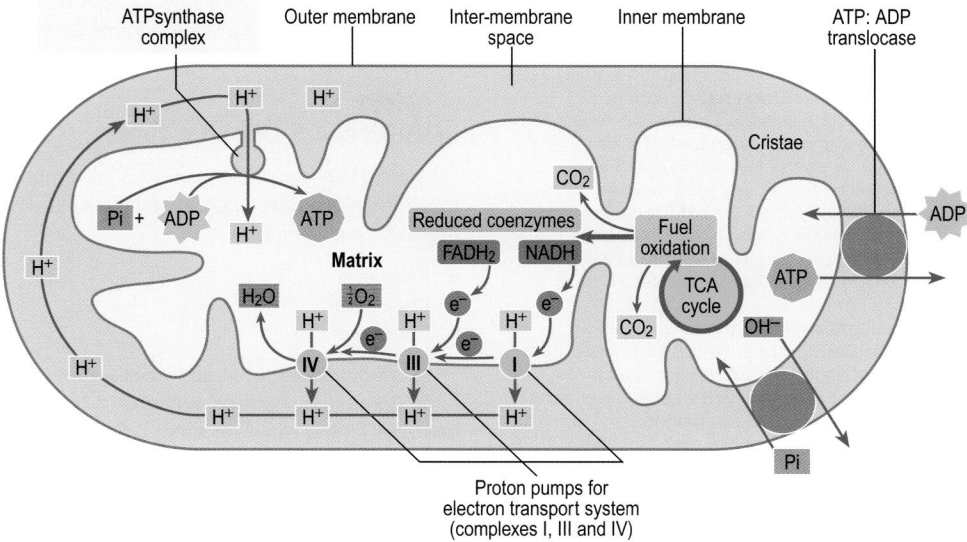

Fig. 2.49 Energy transfer in the mitochondrion. Adapted with permission from Baynes J, Dominiczak M 2005 Medical biochemistry, 2nd edn. Elsevier Mosby, Edinburgh.

Electrons from NADH can combine with **complex I**, while those from FADH$_2$ are transferred via **complex II**. These pathways converge at ubiquinone (coenzyme Q10). The electrons are subsequently passed to **complex III** and then via cytochrome c to **complex IV**, from where the electrons are finally accepted by oxygen. Each of complexes I, III and IV acts as a proton pump, increasing the concentration of H$^+$ ions in the intermembrane space.

Redox potentials drive metabolic reactions

The redox potential is the force that transfers electrons from one compound to another in oxidation–reduction (or redox) reactions. The gain of electrons is a **reduction**, and the loss an **oxidation**. When a reducing agent loses electrons, energy is transferred to the reduced product. Each molecule in the electron transport chain has a lower potential energy (a lower redox potential) than its predecessor, resulting in progressive release of energy. This energy is transferred to the gradient of hydrogen ions across the inner mitochondrial membrane. Because hydrogen is concentrated in the intermembrane space and not at equilibrium, the energy released by the redox reactions is stored as the potential energy of the pH gradient.

Chemiosmotic theory of oxidative phosphorylation

The **chemiosmotic theory** was devised to explain how the proton gradient is used to produce ATP. Inserted into the inner mitochondrial membrane, the multimeric protein **ATP synthase**, also known as **complex V**, consists of two major components, known as **F$_0$** and **F$_1$**. Hydrogen ions flow down their electrochemical gradient through F$_0$, which is a transmembrane protein with a central channel.

Attached to F$_0$ via a stalk region is the F$_1$ protein which converts ADP to ATP in a process called **oxidative phosphorylation**. Each pair of electrons passing along the electron transport chain reduces one atom of oxygen (½ O$_2$), and each of the three proton pumps moves enough H$^+$ to power the production of 1 molecule of ATP.

Table 2.26	Summary of ATP generated during the complete oxidation of glucose	
Stage	**Net change in coenzymes (per mole glucose entering glycolysis)**	**ATP equivalents***
Glycolysis	2 ATP	2
	2 NADH	6
Link reaction	2 NADH	6
TCA cycle	2 GTP	2
	6 NADH	18
	2 FADH	4
		Total 38

*During aerobic metabolism 1 NAD = 3 ATP and 1 FAD = 2 ATP.

Thus, when it is fully oxidised, each molecule of NADH will produce three molecules of ATP, while FADH$_2$ (which enters via complex II, bypassing the proton pump of complex I) only produces two. It is therefore possible to calculate the number of moles of ATP that can be produced by the metabolism of a mole of glucose (Table 2.26). The exact ratio between proton pumping and ATP synthesis varies, however, so 38 moles of ATP per mole glucose is an approximation.

A comparative calculation for the 16-carbon fatty acid, palmitic acid, gives a total of 129 moles of ATP per mole. This increases by 17 moles of ATP for each subsequent 2-carbon increase in fatty acid length. So stearic acid (C18) metabolism yields 146 moles of ATP per mole, which shows why fats provide so much more energy than carbohydrates.

Coupling of the electron transport chain and oxidative phosphorylation

The electron transport chain and oxidative phosphorylation are tightly coupled. This can be shown in vitro by measuring oxygen utilisation (a measure of the end point of the electron transport chain) while controlling ATP synthesis. If ADP is not added to the reaction then oxygen utilisation stops. When ADP is included, oxygen use increases until it is all converted to ATP. Blocking the proton channel of F$_0$ with oligomycin in

Information box 2.21 **Cyanide and other poisons**

Studies of the effect of a number of compounds, including cyanide, on in vitro preparations of mitochondria (usually from rat liver) have helped to elucidate the sequence of steps involved in the electron transport chain and oxidative phosphorylation. At the same time, because of their mode of action, they can also act as potent poisons in vivo.

In the presence of inhibitors of complex I, such as the insecticide **rotenone**, NADH cannot be oxidised but FADH can. The addition of succinate, which is metabolised in the TCA cycle to yield FADH, can stimulate the production of ATP while malate, whose metabolism yields NADH, does not.

A compound called **antimycin A** inhibits complex III. However, while the oxidation of both NADH and FADH are blocked, the addition of ascorbate (which can directly reduce cytochrome c, and which normally passes electrons from complex III to IV) restores ATP production.

Cyanide and **carbon monoxide** both inhibit complex IV, as well as binding to haemoglobin. As electrons can no longer be passed from complex IV to oxygen, the movement of all electrons stops, and hence both proton pumping and ATP production cease. In the absence of aerobic respiration, anaerobic lactate metabolism is switched on, resulting in a lactic acidosis, which can lead to death. One antidote is **methylene blue**, which removes the inhibition by accepting electrons from complex III; another is **thiosulphate**, which converts cyanide to thiocyanate.

the presence of ADP stops oxygen use, showing that it is the dissipation of the proton gradient that determines the rate of the electron transport chain. This is because the electron transport chain can only generate a gradient equivalent to two pH units. If the gradient exceeds this, then the proton pumps cannot generate sufficient energy to continue.

Uncoupling of the electron transport chain

Compounds called **uncouplers**, such as **2,4-dinitrophenol (DNP)**, do not affect the electron transport chain but act in a way that allows the proton gradient to dissipate, without the production of ATP. In the presence of DNP, oxygen utilisation increases in an attempt to restore the proton gradient. Uncoupling of the proton gradient allows the energy stored in the gradient to be dissipated as heat.

This mechanism is very important in newborn babies as a source of heat. Neonates do not shiver when they get cold, possibly because their nervous systems are not sufficiently developed to coordinate the muscular activity required. So, in specialised areas of adipose tissue called **brown fat** (so called because of the high number of mitochondria), an uncoupling protein called **thermogenin** allows the electron transport chain to be used under controlled conditions to generate heat rather than ATP.

TISSUES AND ORGANS

Although a 'typical cell' can be described and the function of its organelles explained, almost all the cells in the body show some specialisation, and most cells are organised into tissues and organs. Tissues are defined as a collection of cells that are adapted to perform a specific function. Organs are where more than one tissue forms a structural unit with a particular function.

ORIGINS OF CELLS

During the very early development of the embryo, by 16 days, the embryo has developed three layers of cells, called (from the surface inwards):

- Ectoderm
- Mesoderm
- Endoderm.

It is from these three germ cell layers that all cell types form. Some cells, such as epithelial cells, form from all three germ cell layers. However, other cells are derived from single layers. For example, nervous tissue is derived from ectoderm, muscle and connective tissue mainly from mesoderm, and most mucosae from endoderm.

In the adult only some cell types remain highly mitotic, such as epithelial and blood-forming cells. Others, such as nervous tissue, rarely divide. Some cells are produced by division of mature differentiated cells, but many new cells are derived from relatively undifferentiated stem cells. Stem cells have now been found in many different tissues. Of great interest is the possibility of using stem cells from easily accessible sources, such as the blood, to produce replacement cells in organs such as the brain where stem cells are rarer (see Information box 2.22).

BASIC TISSUE TYPES

There are four primary tissue types in the body. These are:

- Epithelial tissues
- Connective tissues (including blood)
- Muscle tissues
- Nervous tissues.

Epithelial tissues

Epithelial tissues, also called **epithelium**, are sheets of cells which cover or line body surfaces and form secretory glands. They are derived from all three of the germ cell layers found in the early embryo and have a variety of functions, which include secretion, absorption, protection and transport. They are characterised by a high cell density (a high cellularity). Epithelial tissues have a well-defined polarity with the basal end of the cell, which sits on a **basement membrane**, and a luminal end, which normally faces the surface, such as the intestinal lumen or the bloodstream. They are joined in sheets by intercellular junctions. The basement membrane provides mechanical support and attachment for the epithelial cell. In the kidney, the basal lamina also provides a barrier for the filtration of blood components during the formation of urine (see Ch. 14). Many epithelial cells have specialisations of their apical surfaces, such as **microvilli** and **cilia**.

Classification of epithelial cells

Epithelial tissues, which form linings, are usually classified according to three criteria (Table 2.27 and Fig. 2.50):

- **How the sheets are made up**. Epithelial sheets may be made up of either a single layer of cells, a simple

Table 2.27   Types of lining epithelium

Type	Cell shape	Examples	Function
Simple			
Simple squamous	Flattened	Pulmonary alveoli; loop of Henle; parietal layer of Bowman's capsule; endothelium of blood vessels and lymphatic vessels; mesothelium of pleural and peritoneal cavities	Limiting membrane; fluid transport; gaseous exchange; lubrication; reducing friction; lining membrane
Simple cuboidal	Cuboidal	Ducts of many glands; covering of ovary; kidney tubules	Secretion; absorption; protection
Simple columnar	Columnar	Oviducts; uterus; small bronchi; much of digestive tract; gall bladder; large ducts of some glands	Transportation; absorption; secretion; protection
Pseudostratified columnar	While all cells are in contact with the basement membrane they do not all reach the luminal surface. Those that do are columnar	Respiratory epithelium; most of trachea; primary bronchi; epididymis; vas deferens; large secretory ducts	Secretion; absorption; lubrication; protection; transportation
Stratified			
Stratified squamous (non-keratinised)	Flattened (with nuclei)	Mouth; oesophagus; vagina	Protection; secretion
Stratified squamous (keratinised)	Flattened (without nuclei)	Epidermis of skin	Protection
Stratified cuboidal	Cuboidal	Ducts of sweat glands	Absorption; secretion
Stratified columnar	Columnar	Conjunctiva of eye; some large secretory ducts; portions of male urethra	Secretion; absorption; protection
Transitional	Dome-shaped (relaxed) flattened (distended)	'urothelium' urinary tract from renal calyces to urethra	Protection; distension

epithelium, or from several layers, called stratified epithelium.

- **The cell shape**. The cells may have different shapes: cuboidal, squamous (flattened), columnar, or transitional (where the cells vary in shape across the different layers of the stratified epithelial sheet).
- **The type of surface specialisation**, for example cilia or keratin.

Glandular epithelial cells

Glandular epithelial cells store and secrete many compounds such as hormones and enzymes. The most simple type of glandular epithelium are the unicellular goblet cells, which secrete mucus into the intestinal lumen. Epithelial cells are also organised into glands. Glandular epithelia form either **exocrine glands**, which are continuous with the body surfaces and secrete either to the outside of the body or into luminal spaces via an excretory duct, or **endocrine glands**, which are ductless and where the secretions pass directly into the bloodstream. For example, the sweat glands are continuous with the skin surfaces. In contrast, endocrine glands, such as the adrenal gland, surround blood vessels and secrete hormones into the blood.

Exocrine secretion

Exocrine glands have a secretory portion, where the secretory product is released into the lumen of the gland, and an excretory portion consisting of a duct, by which the secretory product is transported to the outside. Exocrine glands are classified as either **simple** (such as the sweat glands), where the duct is unbranched, or **compound** where the secretory duct is branched and the gland is divided into units called lobes, which themselves are further subdivided into lobules.

A compound gland, such as the salivary gland, contains many different types of epithelial cells in different parts of the gland.

There are three types of secretion:

- **Merocrine**, where the release is by exocytosis
- **Apocrine**, where part of the apical surface is pinched off with the secretions inside it
- **Holocrine**, where the entire cell disintegrates to release the stored product.

In the mammary glands, milk proteins are secreted by merocrine secretion (exocytosis) and milk lipids are secreted by apocrine secretion. An example of holocrine secretion occurs in the sebaceous glands where sebum stored in the cytoplasm is released when the entire cell disintegrates.

Connective and supporting tissues

There are four types of connective and supporting tissues, all of which are derived from mesenchymal multipotent stem cells in the mesoderm. Between them they provide the structural, metabolic and defensive support within all tissues and organs. These are:

- Fibrocollagenous tissues
- Cartilage, bone and teeth
- Adipose tissue
- Blood.

ECM

Characteristically, **connective tissue** contains two components, the **ECM** and the **cells**, which are relatively sparse when compared to epithelial tissues. The ECM contains **ground substance**, made up of three main elements:

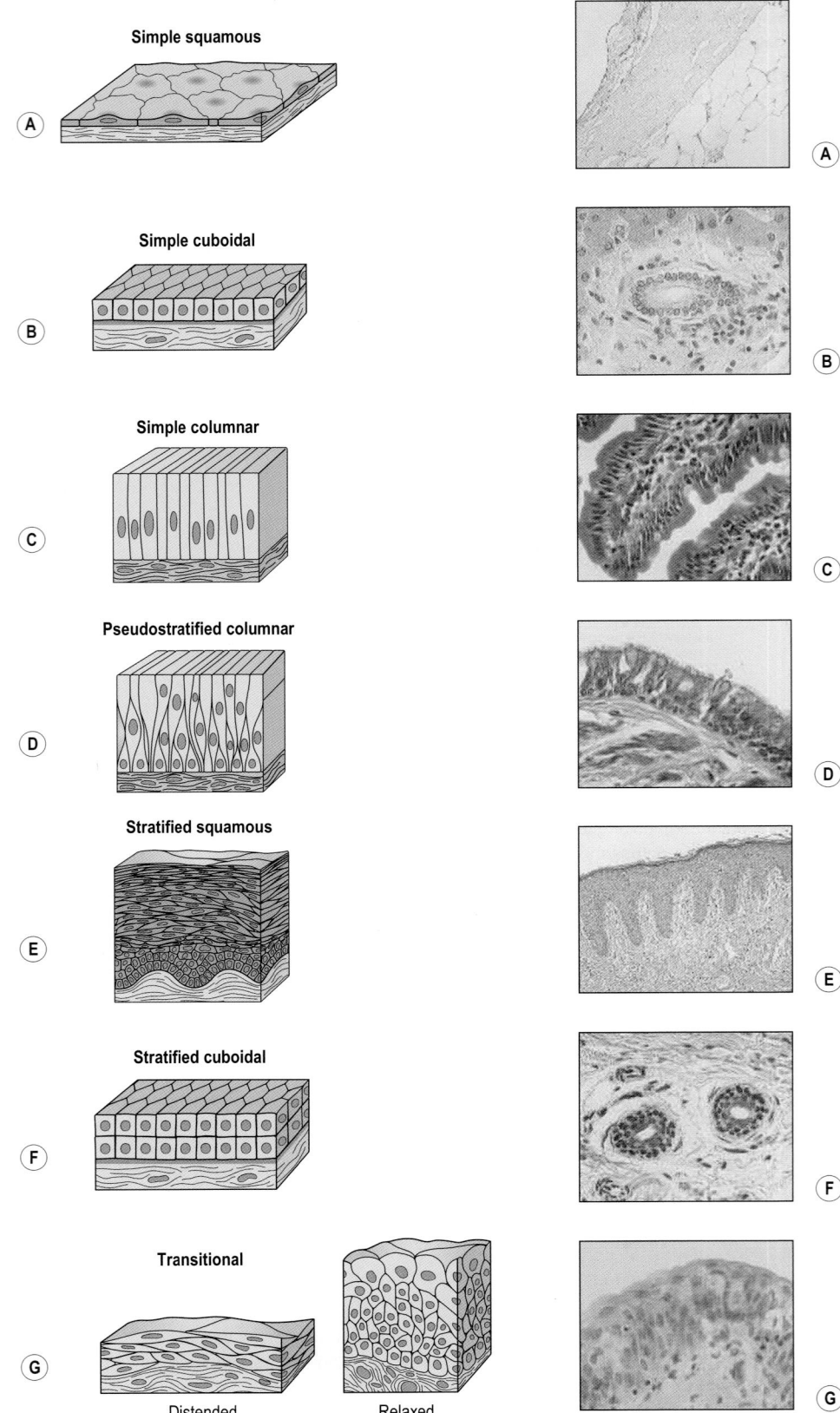

Simple squamous

(A)

Simple cuboidal

(B)

Simple columnar

(C)

Pseudostratified columnar

(D)

Stratified squamous

(E)

Stratified cuboidal

(F)

Transitional

(G)

Distended   Relaxed

(A)

(B)

(C)

(D)

(E)

(F)

(G)

Fig. 2.50 **Epithelial cell types.**

Loose or areolar connective tissue
Submucosa of large intestine

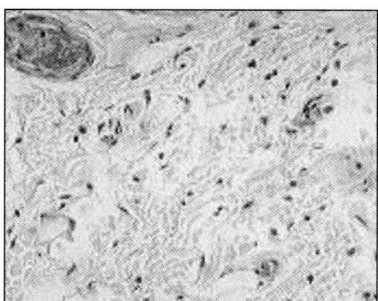

Dense connective tissues
Dermis of the skin

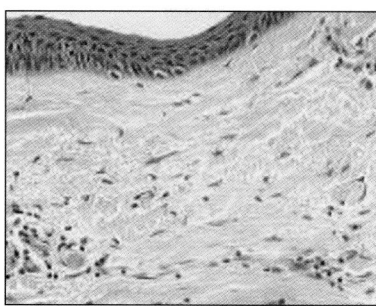

Tendon

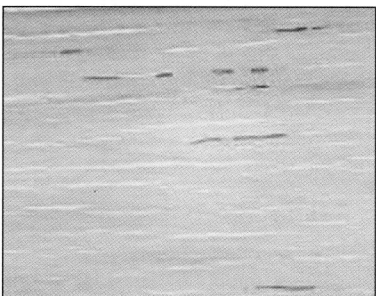

D

Reticular tissue
Liver

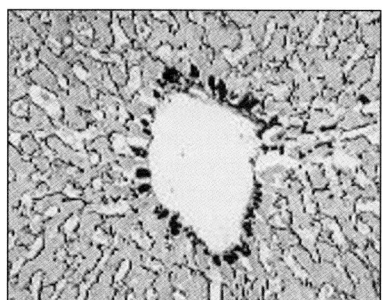

Fig. 2.51 **Types of fibrocollagenous tissue.**

- Structural carbohydrates, the **glycosaminoglycans (GAGs)** which form large proteoglycan complexes
- Structural proteins such as **laminin** and **fibronectin**
- Fibres, which are either **collagen** or **elastin**; collagen provides strength while elastin provides elasticity and support.

Fibrocollagenous tissues

Fibrocollagenous tissues can be divided into three main types (Fig. 2.51):

- Areolar or loose connective tissue, with abundant ground substance, which gives it a gel-like consistency, some collagen and elastic fibres, as well as many cell types.
- Dense connective tissue, which has little ground substance and abundant collagen and a few cells. These tissues provide mechanical support and tensile strength. Two types of dense connective tissue are defined according to the organisation of the collagen fibres:
    - **Irregular** – which is found in the dermis of the skin and the submucosa of the digestive tract
    - **Regular** – which is found in tendons and ligaments. This type of tissue is the most dense, with the least blood supply.
- Reticular connective tissue, which only occurs in organs with a high cellularity, such as the liver, where reticulin fibres (type III collagen) form a fine network around the many epithelial cells.

Fibroblasts

A number of different cells are found in fibrocollagenous connective tissue. **Fibroblasts** are spindle-shaped cells with an oval nucleus. They have a well-developed ER and a Golgi apparatus, which is indicative of their role in the secretion of ECM components. They produce the mature proteoglycans of the ECM as well as the precursors of the collagens (**tropocollagen**) and the elastins (**tropoelastin**). Fibroblasts are very active in wound healing, producing new connective tissue to bridge the wound. Fibroblasts which can contract, myofibroblasts, are involved in the shrinkage of the scar tissue.

Other cells in connective tissue

Also present in fibrocollagenous tissue are **blood vessels**, small numbers of **adipocytes** which store fat, **stem cells** (mesenchymal cells which can differentiate into a variety of cell types to replace, repair or grow existing tissues) and a wide variety of cells of the immune system (see Ch. 6). These include:

- macrophages – cells of the immune system which can engulf (phagocytose) and digest bacteria, cell debris and other unwanted material.
- mast cells – cells of the immune system that contain granules. Some of these contain histamine and other mediators of inflammation, which are released following exposure to environmental allergens.
- plasma cells – these are antibody-secreting mature B cells of the immune system.

Cartilage

Cartilage is denser than dense connective tissue, but less dense than bone. It is solid but flexible and resists compression while allowing diffusion of water through the matrix. It lacks blood vessels, so all metabolites must be exchanged by diffusion. The ground substance of cartilage has large amounts of the GAGs **chondroitin sulphate** and **hyaluronic acid**, bound to a lattice of **type II collagen**. Growing cartilage contains **chondroblasts**, metabolically active cells which secrete proteins and contain energy reserves in the form of lipids and glycogen. In adult cartilage the much less active mature **chondrocytes** are found in cavities, called lacunae, in the ECM.

The three types of cartilage reflect the varying amounts and types of fibres:

- **Hyaline cartilage** – contains type II collagen only, forms most of the embryonic skeleton, and in the adult forms the sternal part of the ribs and also the cartilage found in the nose, trachea and larynx. It also covers the ends of the long bones where it can absorb some of the compressional stresses.
- **Elastic cartilage** – this has more elastic fibres than hyaline cartilage. It supports the pinna of the external part of the ear and forms the epiglottis.
- **Fibrocartilage** – has less matrix than hyaline cartilage and also contains type I collagen. It is more compressible than hyaline cartilage and is found in areas where there are high pressures, such as the intervertebral discs and the knee joint.

Both hyaline and elastic cartilage are surrounded by a layer called the **perichondrium**, which consists of a fibrous layer that is continuous with the periosteal bone and the surface of surrounding connective tissue.

Bone

Bone is similar in some ways to cartilage, except that the ECM has more collagen fibres (type I) and the matrix has become mineralised. This produces a very rigid tissue that forms the skeleton (see Ch. 9). The ground substance contains glycoproteins, which specifically bind calcium, called **osteocalcin**. Bone is initially formed by **osteoblasts**, which produce the matrix called **osteoid**; this is followed by the deposition of **calcium phosphate**. Crystals of **calcium hydroxyapatite** are formed by the addition of hydroxide and bicarbonate ions to the amorphous calcium phosphate. This accumulates around the osteoblast, which becomes an **osteocyte**.

Woven and lamellar bone

There are two major types of bone:

1. **Woven bone** is an immature form, which is relatively weak and has randomly organised collagen fibres. Woven bone is produced when osteoid is being formed rapidly, as in the embryo or during the early repair of a fracture.
2. Woven bone is then remodelled into **lamellar bone**, where the collagen is highly organised into layers, or lamellae. Lamellar bone has a highly organised structure, which is highly vascularised.

Mature bone is continually being remodelled due to the activity of **osteoclasts**, which break down bone, and osteoblasts, which replace it.

Clinical box 2.17 **Osteoporosis is caused by an increased reabsorption of bone**

In post-menopausal women one of the effects of the lack of the sex steroid hormone, oestrogen, is a reduction in bone density. This makes the bones fragile and more likely to fracture. This is due to an increase in the numbers of osteoclasts leading to an increased bone reabsorption. This can be reversed in post-menopausal women by hormone replacement therapy (HRT), plus dietary calcium supplements and vitamin D if necessary.

Teeth

Teeth are made up of three layers. The external surface, or crown, of the tooth is covered by **enamel**, the hardest substance in the body. It is principally made up of calcium phosphate. The middle layer consists of a mineralised matrix, called **dentine**, similar to bone although it does not contain cells. Inside the dentine is the **pulp cavity**, which contains the cells which produce the dentine, the odontoblasts, as well as the nerves and blood vessels supplying the tooth. These enter the tooth through the **root canal**, a narrow channel at the root of the tooth. The part of the tooth which is embedded in the jaw bone is covered by a thin layer of a calcified tissue called cementum, which serves both to anchor the tooth and protect it.

Adipose tissue

While small numbers of adipocytes are found either isolated or in clumps throughout all loose supporting tissues, in **adipose tissue** they form the major cell type. There are two types of adipose tissue: **white** and **brown**. These are both derived from a common precursor cell, the **preadipocyte**, which itself is derived from the mesenchymal stem cell.

White adipose tissue

White adipose tissue contains **adipocytes** whose entire cytoplasm is taken up by a single large droplet of fat. The nucleus is flattened and pushed to one side and the cytoplasm, which contains mainly mitochondria, exists only as a ring around the fat droplet. Adipose tissue not only provides a large energy store, containing about 80% triacylglycerol, but also acts as a shock absorber and insulator. It is found throughout the body, particularly under the skin and around abdominal organs. The amount of adipose tissue varies with age and gender, typically increasing with age and being higher in women.

Brown adipose tissue

Brown adipose tissue is only extensive in newborn mammals and some hibernating animals. It is highly vascularised and contains multiple droplets of fat that surround a large central nucleus. The cells contain large numbers of mitochondria that metabolise the fat without the production of ATP. This uncoupling produces heat when the cells are stimulated by the sympathetic autonomic nervous system. The name **brown fat** derives from the colour of the large amount of cytochromes (electron transport chain molecules) present in the mitochondria. In adults, brown fat may have a role in burning off excess fat and preventing obesity.

Blood

Although blood does not provide mechanical support or connections between tissues, it is classified as a connective

Understanding the control of adipose tissue is of interest in the fight against obesity

People who are above average weight have a higher mortality than those who weigh less. The most commonly used measure of obesity is the body mass index (BMI), which is calculated from the weight (w) in kg and height (h) in m, where $BMI = w/h^2$. The longest life expectancy is associated with a BMI between 20 and 25, with higher mortality for those underweight (BMI <20) and overweight (BMI >25). Those individuals with a BMI >30 are classified as obese. However, although BMI is widely used, the amount of body fat is a more important predictor of mortality and morbidity. Levels of body fat are controlled by many different factors, but one which has been of great interest recently is a peptide released by adipocytes, called **leptin**, which acts on receptors in the hypothalamus. Genetically obese mice that lack leptin lose weight when given synthetic leptin. This discovery was hailed as a cure for obesity, but unfortunately there are very few obese people who have this type of genetic mutation. It has now been suggested that obese people, because they have more fat and secrete more leptin, have a problem with the sensitivity of their leptin receptors.

See also Chapter 16.

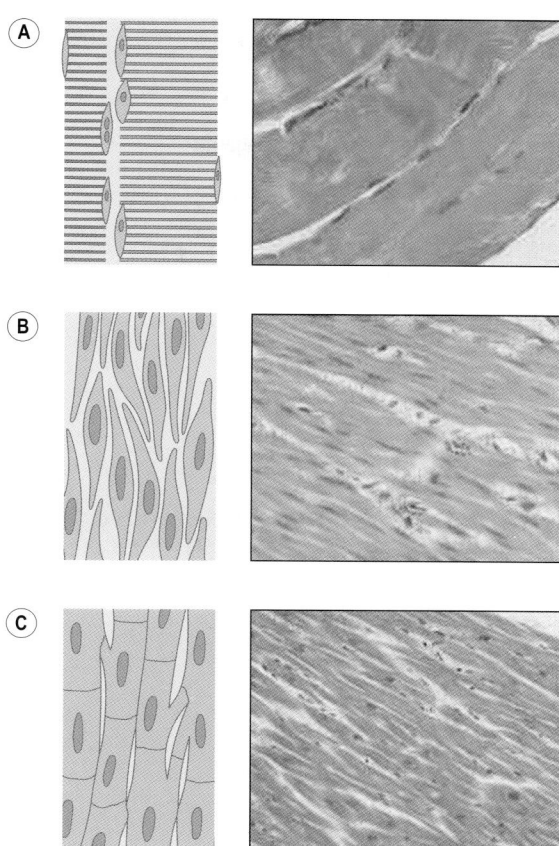

Fig. 2.52 Muscle types: (A) skeletal muscle; (B) smooth muscle; (C) cardiac muscle.

tissue because it is derived from the same germ layer as the other connective tissues, the mesoderm, and because it also consists of cells – **red blood cells**, **white blood cells** and **platelets** – in a matrix, the blood plasma. Blood contains the soluble protein **fibrinogen**, which is converted into insoluble fibrin fibres during blood clotting. The different elements of blood provide metabolic support by carrying nutrients and waste products and immune protection, by transporting white blood cells and antibodies around the body. **Platelets** are crucial in the control of bleeding, by plugging small holes in blood vessels and by their involvement in the clotting cascade (see Ch. 12).

Muscle

Muscle tissue is made up of **contractile cells**. While there are some cells in the body that do not form muscle tissues but are contractile, such as **pericytes** which surround blood vessels, most muscle cells (Fig. 2.52) form one of three types of muscle:

■ Skeletal muscle
■ Smooth muscle
■ Cardiac muscle.

All muscle cells contain the contractile proteins, **actin** and **myosin**, although their arrangement differs between muscle types. Some classifications separate muscle into:

■ **Voluntary muscles** (in that they are under conscious control, such as the muscles that move elements of the skeleton)
■ **Involuntary muscles** (which are controlled by the autonomic nervous system and circulating hormones).

In this classification skeletal muscle is classed as voluntary, and smooth muscle as involuntary (Table 2.28).

Skeletal muscle

This is made up of long, multinucleated cells, called **muscle fibres**, which are formed from the fusion of many single cells during development. Between 10 μm and 100 μm in diameter

and sometimes extending the whole length of the muscle (i.e. many centimetres), they have a distinct banded appearance. This is due to the regular arrangement of the myosin and actin filaments into repeating units called **sarcomeres**. The banded appearance gives rise to the name **striated muscle**. The **myofilaments** which make up the sarcomeres are arranged in cylindrical **myofibrils**, which are themselves grouped together to form the muscle fibres.

The shortening of muscle during contraction occurs due to overlap between the thin actin and thick myosin filaments, a process that is stimulated by the release of calcium from intracellular stores. The stores are called **sarcoplasmic reticulum** and form a network of flattened sacs surrounding the sarcomeres and connected via **T-tubules** to the surface of the fibre (see Ch. 9). The contraction of all skeletal muscle is controlled by the central nervous system via specialised nerve junctions known as **neuromuscular junctions**.

Muscle fibres are studded with muscle precursor cells called **satellite cells**. These quiescent cells can resume proliferation when the muscle is either damaged or stressed in order to replace or increase the muscle mass. This activity is particularly obvious in weight lifters and body builders, who can remodel their muscles by increasingly stressing them.

Smooth muscle

Smooth muscle is made up of elongated spindle-shaped cells that taper at the ends. They usually have a single nucleus and are much shorter than skeletal muscle cells. They are often joined together in sheets and the cells are electrically coupled through gap junctions between adjacent

Table 2.28	Comparing the different types of muscle		
	Skeletal	**Smooth**	**Cardiac**
Morphology	Multinucleated, long, thin	Single nucleus, spindle-shaped	Single or double nuclei, cylindrical, branched, prominent intercalated discs
Appearance	Striated appearance due to overlapping bands of actin and myosin	No obvious striations	Striated appearance, but less organised than skeletal muscle
Unit of excitation	Groups of fibres called motor units	Linked by gap junctions	Linked by gap junctions
Source of calcium	Calcium stores in extensive SR	Variable, calcium release can be induced from rudimentary calcium stores in SR, calcium can also enter from extracellular fluid	Calcium enters from extracellular fluid and releases more calcium from less extensive SR (calcium-induced calcium release)
Role of calcium	Calcium removes inhibition	Calcium increases phosphorylation of contractile proteins	Calcium removes inhibition
Contraction	Discontinuous	Usually continuous (resting tone), often rhythmic (wavelike), can maintain very high forces	Continuous, rhythmic
Regenerative ability	Can undergo limited regeneration (from satellite cells)	Can regenerate	No regeneration
Activation	Only contracts on nervous activation by motor nerves	Myogenic but also under autonomic and hormonal control	Myogenic but also under autonomic and hormonal control
Receptor/s	Nicotinic cholinergic	Various but include α- and β-adrenergic	β-adrenergic, muscarinic cholinergic
Neurotransmitter	Acetylcholine	Adrenaline, noradrenaline plus others	Adrenaline, noradrenaline, acetylcholine

SR, sarcoplasmic reticulum.

cells to form a functional **syncytium**. This enables cells to contract in a coordinated manner with quite diffuse inputs. Smooth muscle is specialised in producing relatively slow, low force contractions with a low energy requirement. However, it can also produce very forceful contractions under certain circumstances; for example, the contractions of the uterus during labour.

Muscle contraction is often spontaneous and may be affected by input from the autonomic nervous system, hormones and local factors, such as stretching. In this sense it is not thought to be under conscious control, hence the term involuntary muscle, although some smooth muscle can be controlled consciously.

Smooth muscle cells retain their ability to divide and **hypertrophy** in response to increased stress. This is a problem in high blood pressure, **hypertension**, where the response of many blood vessels to the increase in blood pressure is to increase the thickness of the smooth muscle layer. This reduces the diameter of the lumen, which in turn increases the resistance to blood flow and thus further increases the arterial blood pressure (see Ch. 11).

Cardiac muscle

Cardiac muscle makes up the walls of the heart and is in some ways intermediate in type between skeletal and smooth muscle. In appearance, cardiac muscle contains myofibrils and the muscle appears striated, although the muscle cells are much shorter than in skeletal muscle. Cardiac muscle fibres (and myofibrils) are branched and the cells connected by **intercalated discs**. These have large numbers of **gap junctions**, allowing electrical communication between cells, and **adhering junctions**, which bind the cells together to form a network of electrically and mechanically interconnected cells. Due to their high metabolic demands they have

large numbers of mitochondria and have a rich blood supply.

Specialised regions of heart muscle are electrically unstable and form **pacemaker** areas that trigger rhythmic muscular contraction in the absence of nervous input. These electrical signals, and their subsequent contractions, are then transmitted throughout the heart via low resistance pathways that ensure the coordinated contraction of the different areas of the heart, in order to ensure the pumping of blood. This **intrinsic rhythm** is modified by both nervous and hormonal inputs (see Ch. 11).

There are no stem cells in cardiac muscle, so that, when heart muscle is damaged, it cannot regenerate and healing replaces dead muscle with fibrous scar tissue. Heart muscle can also hypertrophy due to an increase in the size of individual cells and the addition of myofibrils. Current research is investigating whether stem cells from other parts of the body can be injected into heart muscle and be induced to replace damaged cardiac muscle.

Nervous tissue

The nervous tissue of the body is divided into:

- The **central nervous system (CNS)**, which consists of the brain and spinal cord
- The **peripheral nervous system (PNS)**, which consists of all nervous tissue found outside the brain and spinal cord.

Both the central and peripheral nervous systems are principally made up of two types of cells: **neurons** and **glia** (see also Ch. 8). There are a few other minor types of cells also present in the brain: **ependymal cells** (epithelial cells, which line the cavities of the brain, or ventricles) and **choroid**

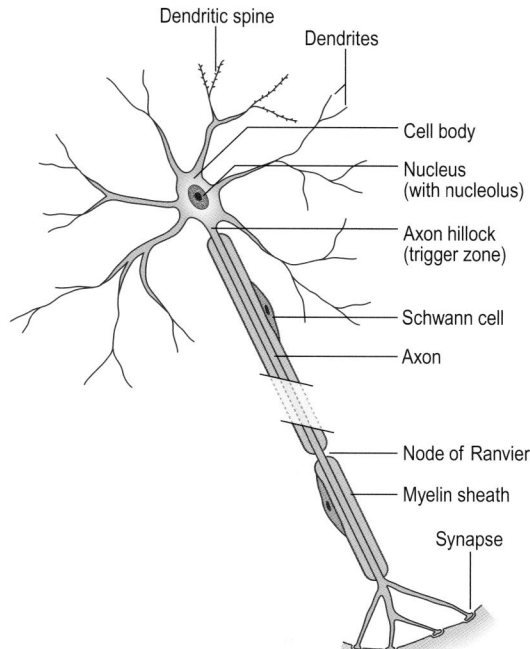

Fig. 2.53 **A typical multi-polar neuron.**

Labels: Dendritic spine; Dendrites; Cell body; Nucleus (with nucleolus); Axon hillock (trigger zone); Schwann cell; Axon; Node of Ranvier; Myelin sheath; Synapse

 Information box 2.22 | **Neural stem cells**

During the development of the nervous system, cells in the neural tube become **multipotent stem cells** that can divide into all the different cells of the brain. Other types of stem cells in other tissues produce other cells; for example **haematopoietic stem cells** in the bone marrow can produce all the blood cells. While these blood stem cells remain active throughout life, continually replacing cells, until recently it was thought that stem cells were not present in the nervous system after the initial phase of brain development. However, neural stem cells have now been isolated from both fetal and adult brains. These cells do not normally divide in adults, but current research is trying to identify the exact conditions under which these cells can be stimulated to divide and grow into mature functioning brain cells.

epithelial cells (which are involved in the secretion of the cerebrospinal fluid which bathes the brain).

Neurons

Neurons are the cells of the brain that receive signals, process them and transmit the appropriate response either to another neuron or to an effector, such as a secretory cell or a muscle. Neurons come in many different shapes and sizes but in their most basic form consist of three elements (Fig. 2.53):

1. A central **cell body** that contains the cell nucleus and other intracellular organelles concerned particularly with protein synthesis and secretory processes. The large numbers of ribosomes, particularly those associated with the rough ER or present as polyribosomes, appear as darkly staining **Nissl bodies**.
2. Highly branched processes extending from the cell body called **dendrites**, which may be covered with small **spines**, are the sites of the inputs from other cells. Dendrites form the main receiving portion of the neuron.
3. A single **axon** extending from the cell body to the target cell. Axons may extend just a few millimetres to a nearby cell or, as in the case of the motor neurons supplying muscles distant from the spinal cord, they may extend for metres. At the start of the axon is an area called the **axon hillock** or **trigger zone** where electrical signals, known as action potentials, can be generated. These are then propagated along the axon.

Most neurons can be classified into one of three major types, depending largely on the position and number of dendrites and the position of the trigger zone. They are:

- Multi-polar neurons
- Bipolar neurons
- Pseudo-unipolar neurons.

Due to their very active nature, neurons in general have a very high metabolic rate, which means that they need a continuous secure supply of oxygen and glucose. Because of this, interruption in the supply is critical, since deprived neurons will start to die very rapidly. This is particularly problematical as under most conditions mature neurons do not divide. During development epithelial cells lining the neural tube give rise to **neuroblasts**. These cells divide mitotically to produce amitotic neurons, which then migrate to their final positions in the brain. As this occurs during fetal development and is completed in early childhood, the mature brain does not contain neurons which can divide (however, see Information box 2.22). Thus neurons that die cannot usually be replaced. One result of this is that brain tumours derived from neurons are very rare and occur almost exclusively as **neuroblastomas** in children.

Glial cells

The other main category of cell in the nervous system are **glial cells**. They make up about half the brain mass and outnumber neurons about 10-fold. These cells have a number of functions, including structural and metabolic support, immune functions and electrical insulation of axons. There are three types of glial cells:

- Astrocytes
- Microglia
- Oligodendrocytes and Schwann cells.

Astrocytes

In the CNS the most common type of glial cells are **astrocytes**. They can be distinguished from neurons by the presence of a specific protein, **glial fibrillary acidic protein (GFAP)**. **Fibrous astrocytes** contain large numbers of filaments and are found in the nerve bundles of the white matter of the brain. **Protoplasmic astrocytes** have fewer filaments and are found mainly in the grey matter. They have a number of fine processes that surround neurons, capillaries and the ependymal cells lining the ventricles. These **astrocytic endfeet** do not touch the capillaries but release factors that induce blood–brain barrier characteristics in the capillary endothelial cells (see Ch. 8). As well as this role, astrocytes are important in regulating K⁺ levels around neurons and providing a store of glycogen that can be supplied to neurons, in the form of lactate, when required.

Astrocytes surrounding neurons have an important role in controlling the distribution of neurotransmitter chemicals released by the neurons. They do this in two ways, firstly by restricting the diffusion, and secondly by transporting neurotransmitters into the astrocyte, where they can be metabolised or recycled. The precursors of astrocytes are **radial glial cells** which, during early development, span the cerebral cortex forming a scaffolding for the migration of new nerve cells to their destinations.

Microglia

Microglial cells are small cells of the CNS with long spiny processes. During development, in addition to releasing growth factors, they act as macrophages, removing debris produced by the programmed cell death which occurs at this time. In the adult they are normally relatively inactive; however in the presence of almost any type of injury or insult to the nervous system, they revert to the role of phagocytotic macrophages, when they are said to be **reactive**.

Oligodendrocytes and Schwann cells

Oligodendrocytes and **Schwann cells** are both involved in electrically insulating axons in the CNS and PNS, respectively. They are large cells with few processes that wrap around the axons forming multiple lipid bilayers with their plasma membranes, called a **myelin sheath**. These membranes have a high lipid to protein ratio which makes them excellent insulators. Oligodendrocytes can myelinate more than one axon and the cell body lies between them. Schwann cells only myelinate a single axon and the cell body is closely apposed to the myelin sheath.

Schwann cells have a role in the regeneration of peripheral axons following injury. In order for a peripheral nerve to re-grow, the tip of the axon must make contact with a Schwann cell. This stimulates mitosis in the Schwann cell, which then extends processes towards the **growth cone** of the axon. The axon re-grows at between 2 mm and 5 mm per day along the Schwann cells, which then re-myelinate the new axon.

Damaged neurons in the CNS do not seem to regenerate successfully because CNS glial cells release factors that specifically inhibit axon growth, although current research into the supply of neuronal growth factors is encouraging. The implantation of fetal cells as in the experimental treatment of Parkinson's disease may prove useful, and other strategies involving the use of neural stem cells are ongoing.

Not all axons are myelinated, and this can be seen in the brain and spinal cord as **grey matter**, which consists of cell bodies and unmyelinated axons, as opposed to **white matter**, which consists of axons, most of which are myelinated. Dendrites are never myelinated.

ORGANS AND SYSTEMS

Organs are made up of at least two tissues, although many organs contain many more. Organs form distinct structural units with a particular function/s. Examples of specific organs are:

- Liver
- Kidney
- Lung
- Heart.

Many functions of the body require more than one organ. For example, the **cardiovascular system** requires that both the heart and blood vessels work together in a coordinated fashion. Some of these divisions may seem somewhat artificial; for example the **endocrine system**, which consists of all the organs which secrete hormones, is stimulated by feedback from almost all the other organs of the body, and has effects on the entire organism.

Coordinated activity of many organ systems

At the next level up the whole organism requires the action of all the organ systems acting together to perform many functions. For example, the relatively simple activity of running:

- The respiratory system needs to increase its activity to increase the oxygenation of the blood to meet the increased oxygen demand.
- The cardiovascular system needs to pump more blood and redirect blood to the appropriate muscles, without compromising the supply to the brain and the heart.
- The nervous system has to initiate and coordinate the muscular activity, which depends on the locomotor system for its execution.
- The metabolic activities of the liver and other tissues need to be changed in order to supply the energy required for the muscle to continue to contract.
- When the person stops running, the alimentary system will absorb the necessary nutrients to replace those used and the urinary system will excrete waste products and regulate fluid and acid–base balance.
- The immune system will clear away any damaged cells, and repair mechanisms will rebuild damaged tissues.

3

Energy metabolism

Mark Holness, Mary Sugden and Jeannette Naish

INTRODUCTION TO METABOLISM

The human organism needs a constant supply of energy:

- For survival (e.g. for the chemical reactions that take place in the processes of transport and storage, and in the biosynthesis of new molecules for tissue repair)
- To maintain body temperature
- To perform work (see Ch. 16).

Clinical box 3.1	Diabetes mellitus – a disorder of fuel metabolism

Importance of diabetes mellitus
- A common condition in which the normal pathways for fuel metabolism are disrupted by defective insulin secretion and/or action.
- Characterised by persistently high concentrations of blood glucose (hyperglycaemia) leading to life-threatening complications and long-term organ damage.
- Although no 'diabetic gene' has been identified, the patterns of family history and a higher incidence in some racial groups suggest genetic susceptibility, particularly for type 1 diabetes (see below).

There are **two main types** of diabetes mellitus:
- Type 1 diabetes – onset predominantly in children and young adults, but can occur at any time in adult life.
- Type 2 diabetes – usually of late onset, but is increasingly being seen in younger people, adolescents and even children.

Other forms of diabetes mellitus include:
- Gestational diabetes (during pregnancy)
- Maturity-onset diabetes of the young (MODY).

Fuel for producing energy is taken in as food, which is processed through digestion and absorption (see Ch. 15) into the circulation, and energy is produced from the breakdown – metabolism – of metabolic fuels. Glucose and fatty acids are the main energy substrates (metabolic fuels), with amino acids being used during fasting, illness and injury.

ENERGY IS RELEASED BY CATABOLISM AND CONSUMED BY ANABOLISM

The main metabolic fuels – carbohydrates, fats and proteins – are ultimately metabolised to yield energy, carbon dioxide (CO_2) and water (H_2O), and in the case of amino acids derived from proteins, urea. The two types of metabolic pathway in fuel metabolism are:

- Catabolism, when biochemical reactions break down large molecules of fuel substrate to release energy
- Anabolism, when chemical reactions consume energy in the synthesis of new molecules (see Ch. 2).

Energy is mainly trapped and stored in adenosine triphosphate (ATP), to be released and used in energy-requiring reactions. Energy is used to synthesise:

- Glycogen (the storage form of glucose)
- Lipids for storage
- Proteins for tissue regeneration and cell growth (Fig. 3.1).

Carbohydrates, amino acids and lipids are metabolised in separate pathways, but there are intricate adaptive processes for integrating fuel metabolism (Information box 3.1). Acetyl-coenzyme A (acetyl-CoA) is a major common metabolite. These acetyl residues are further metabolised in a

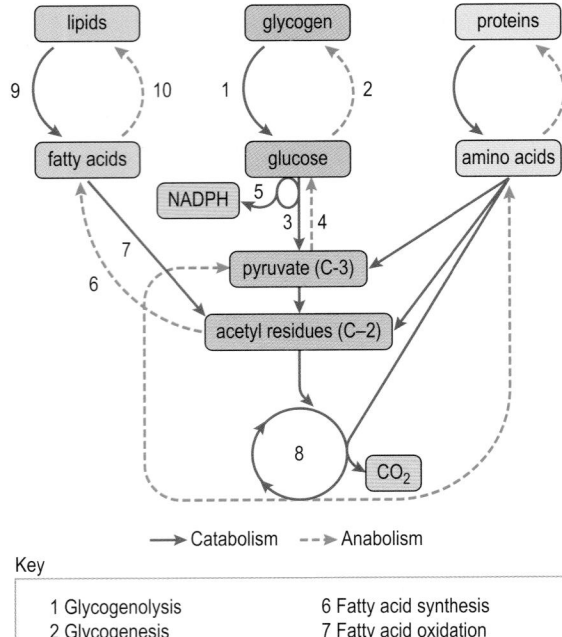

Key

1 Glycogenolysis	6 Fatty acid synthesis
2 Glycogenesis	7 Fatty acid oxidation
3 Glycolysis	8 Tricarboxylic acid cycle
4 Gluconeogenesis	9 Lipolysis
5 Pentose phosphate pathway	10 Triacylglyerol synthesis (esterification)

Fig. 3.1 **General layout of fuel metabolism.**

ⓘ Information box 3.1 Metabolic pathways are dynamic, interrelated networks

- Some of the products of metabolic pathways – intermediary metabolites – are activators or inhibitors of enzymes in the pathway, or in the pathway of another substrate.
- Catabolic and anabolic pathways are at least partially reversible in response to the availability of fuel substrates and to the changing energy requirements of the body.
- The pathways intersect; for example, variation in the plasma concentration of glucose can activate or inhibit pathways in lipid metabolism, and vice versa.
- Metabolic intermediates from one substrate can enter the pathway of another; for example, intermediates from glucose breakdown serve as substrates for amino acid and fatty acid synthesis.

---

common pathway, the tricarboxylic acid cycle (TCA cycle), also known as the citric acid cycle or Krebs' cycle (see Fig. 3.1 and Ch. 1).

TRICARBOXYLIC ACID CYCLE

The tricarboxylic acid (TCA) cycle is the metabolic 'engine' in the mitochondria, where acetyl-CoA is oxidised to produce CO_2 and reduced nucleotides (conversion of NAD^+ to NADH) (see Ch. 2). Reduced nucleotides are substrates for mitochondrial oxidative phosphorylation, which provides energy for ATP synthesis. Among other major functions, the TCA cycle contributes to the following processes:

- Glucose synthesis from amino acids and lactate
- Conversion of carbohydrate to fat for storage
- Synthesis of non-essential amino acids
- Formation of haem for haemoglobin.

REGULATION OF FUEL METABOLISM

Generally, metabolism takes place in cells, within the cytoplasm and in cellular organelles (see Ch. 2). The processes of human metabolism are tightly regulated to maintain internal functionality, but have to be flexible at the same time to respond to changes in the external environment of the cells.

The overall rate of reaction in a complex metabolic pathway is limited by its slowest process: the 'rate-limiting' (also known as flux-generating) step. The key enzyme in the 'rate-limiting' step regulates the metabolic pathway. Methods for controlling metabolism include:

- Binding of small molecules (allosteric effectors) to sites on an enzyme to increase or inhibit its affinity for substrates
- Reversible activation/deactivation of enzymes by covalent modification
- Regulation of gene expression and transcription in response to changing metabolic demands (see Ch. 5)
- The action of hormones.

Binding of allosteric effectors to an enzyme to alter its affinity for substrate

The binding of allosteric effectors to a site on an enzyme that is separate from the substrate binding site can alter the enzyme affinity for the substrate. For example, when the demand for energy is low, e.g. while resting after a meal, cellular ATP and NADH accumulate to allosterically inhibit isocitrate dehydrogenase (a major regulatory enzyme in the TCA cycle). Whereas when energy demand is high, e.g. during exercise, ADP and NAD^+ accumulate to allosterically stimulate isocitrate dehydrogenase (see Ch. 2).

Reversible activation and deactivation by covalent modification

Phosphorylation (by protein kinases) or dephosphorylation (by protein phosphatases) is a commonly used mechanism in the regulation of enzyme activity.

Regulation of gene expression and transcription in response to changing metabolic demands

Changes in metabolic demands can alter gene expression and transcription. For example, iron is necessary to produce haemoglobin for oxygen transport and is stored as ferritin. When iron concentrations are low, a repressor protein binds to ferritin mRNA so that no more ferritin is made. When iron is plentiful, iron binds to the repressor protein, so altering its shape, which releases the mRNA, again allowing ferritin to be produced (see Ch. 12). There are many other examples in carbohydrate and vitamin metabolism.

Action of hormones

Hormones (see Ch. 10) inhibit or activate essential enzymes in response to the body's internal environment (e.g. arising from a high-fat or a weight-reducing diet, or in response to stress and disease). This regulation may take effect rapidly, over days or gradually over weeks.

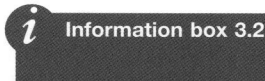

Maintenance of normal blood glucose concentration is the starting point in regulating fuel metabolism

Maintenance of a normal blood glucose concentration within a narrow range of 3.5–8.0 mmol/L is essential for life (see Ch. 2), and abnormal variation in this level triggers alternative metabolic pathways:

- Hypoglycaemia occurs when plasma glucose falls below 2.1 mmol/L, which can lead to acute neurological complications because glucose is an essential requirement for brain function in the short term. Although hypoglycaemia may occasionally occur in healthy people after fasting, exercise or alcohol consumption, it is most commonly seen as a complication of the treatment of diabetes mellitus by insulin.
- Consistently elevated fasting blood glucose concentrations above 7 mmol/L (hyperglycemia) are a consequence of failed regulation of glucose metabolism by insulin, as in untreated diabetes mellitus, and can lead to both acute complications, due to increased production of ketone bodies (ketones, diabetic ketoacidosis), and long-term potentially life-threatening complications of micro- and macrovascular disease (i.e. hypertension, coronary artery disease, diabetic glomerulosclerosis leading to renal failure, neuropathy, and retinopathy that can lead to blindness).

The hormones insulin, glucagon, adrenaline (epinephrine), cortisol and growth hormone are involved in the regulation of all metabolic fuels – carbohydrates, lipids and proteins – and can exert short-term effects on the direction of fluxes in metabolic pathways.

Both the catabolic and anabolic pathways of carbohydrate and lipid metabolism have to be partially reversible to adapt to environmental changes because we alternately eat food (feed) and fast between meals. The fasting state can begin just a few hours from the last meal. The processes of fuel metabolism are reversible within this feed–fast cycle.

When nutrients are plentiful

When nutrients are plentiful (the fed or absorptive state), the active pathways are fuel breakdown and storage of excess metabolic fuel through glycogen and lipid synthesis, and also protein synthesis for regenerating tissues (anabolism).

Glucose uptake into cells, the storage of carbohydrates and lipids, and protein synthesis are promoted by insulin, an anabolic hormone. For example, insulin stimulates lipoprotein lipase to break down dietary triacylglycerols to glycerol and fatty acids. Fatty acids are then transported into adipose tissue for storage (Information box 3.2).

Metabolic adaptation to changes in energy requirement

During the fasting state, the direction of the metabolic pathways is reversed to break down stored fuels (catabolism) – glycogen, lipid stores, proteins – to produce energy, while biosynthesis slows down.

The complex interactions between the biochemical pathways also have to adapt to changes in energy requirements, as in increased physical activity – the difference between a 100 m sprint versus a marathon – and some extreme changes from changing diets, fasting and starvation (see Ch. 16).

The action of insulin is opposed by glucagon, growth hormone, adrenaline and cortisol, which promote endogenous glucose production.

FURTHER CONSIDERATIONS IN FUEL METABOLISM

The processes by which different tissues metabolise different energy substrates, store and transport fuel are integrated and adapted for varying functions.

Different tissues metabolise different energy substrates

Red blood cells, the main carrier and transporter of oxygen (O_2), do not have mitochondria and rely on breaking down glucose through anaerobic glycolysis. This process does not consume O_2, thus maximising red cell capacity for carrying and delivering O_2.

Under normal circumstances, the brain uses only glucose as metabolic fuel, but under starvation conditions, it can use ketone bodies.

How fuel is stored and transported between tissues

The liver and skeletal muscle are both involved in the storage of fuel as glycogen, but:

- The liver is able to release glucose into the bloodstream to prevent hypoglycaemia in other tissues
- Muscle cannot release glucose into the circulation because it lacks glucose-6-phosphatase (see below). The glucose produced by muscle glycogenolysis is used within the muscle to produce energy for contraction.

CARBOHYDRATE METABOLISM

Carbohydrates are present in high concentration in plants, making up most of the dry tissue weight. For the body to make use of the many ingested carbohydrates, they must first be broken down by digestive enzymes into monomer sugars (e.g. glucose, fructose) and disaccharides (e.g. maltose, lactose). Disaccharide sugars can be converted to glucose, the major carbohydrate fuel for all tissues.

Even more importantly, some tissues (including the brain and red blood cells (RBCs), see above) have an obligatory requirement for glucose as a metabolic fuel. Blood glucose concentration (glycaemia) is governed by the balance between:

- Glucose absorption from the intestine
- Glucose production by the liver and kidneys
- Glucose uptake and metabolism by all tissues of the body.

REGULATION OF BLOOD GLUCOSE (GLYCAEMIA)

Glucose is the only metabolic fuel used by red cells, and under normal fed conditions, glucose is the only fuel that brain can use. Glucose is also the preferred fuel for skeletal muscle during short bursts of exercise. A continuous supply of glucose is therefore needed to ensure that there is adequate energy for the vital functions performed by these and other tissues. Fuel metabolism is highly regulated to ensure adequate energy for cellular function.

SOURCES OF BLOOD GLUCOSE

Metabolic fuels are stored for use in times of fuel shortage.

- Carbohydrates are stored as glycogen, the liver being the main glycogen source for maintaining blood glucose concentrations. However, liver glycogen stores are sufficient to last no more than a 16-hour fast.
- Dietary fat that is surplus to requirement is stored in adipose tissue (fat), and its glycerol moiety can be converted to glucose via gluconeogenesis (see below) to generate energy. The fatty acid moiety cannot be converted to glucose.
- Protein from muscle breakdown can also be converted to glucose via gluconeogenesis in the liver.
- Carbohydrates can also be converted to fats for storage.

FOUR KEY PATHWAYS MAINTAIN AND UTILISE BLOOD GLUCOSE

Maintenance of blood glucose levels and glucose utilisation are governed by four key interacting metabolic processes (Fig. 3.2):

- Glycolysis – the process by which glucose is broken down to form pyruvate and energy in the form of ATP
- Glycogenesis – the process by which glucose is converted to glycogen
- Glycogenolysis – the process by which glycogen is broken down
- Gluconeogenesis – the process by which glucose can be produced when glycogen stores are depleted.

GLUCOSE TRANSPORT

Before glucose can be metabolised, it must be transported into the cell. Molecules such as sugars cannot move through membranes by simple diffusion. Instead this is achieved via special transmembrane proteins by facilitated diffusion. Glucose transporters (GLUTs) are uniporters, moving only one type of molecule in one direction. They are specific for glucose (or, in certain cases, fructose), and generally facilitate the movement of glucose down a concentration gradient and do not require energy (see Ch. 2).

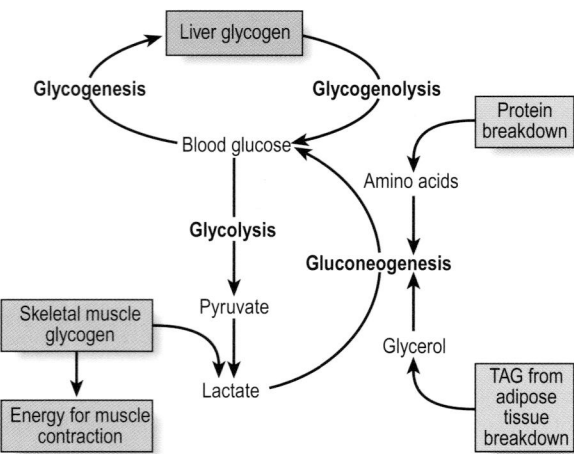

***Fig. 3.2* Pathways involved in the maintenance and utilisation of blood glucose.** TAG, triacylglycerol.

Originally, five members of the GLUT family were identified, GLUT1–5, which have been well characterised. However, a further eight have been identified through cloning of the human genome. GLUT1–4 are primarily glucose transporters with distinct tissue distribution and kinetic characteristics (Table 3.1). GLUT5 is a fructose transporter.

GLUT1

GLUT1 molecules do not require the stimulus of insulin and transport glucose under most conditions, including fasting (glucose concentration ≤5 mmol/L). They also work with GLUT3 (which does not have to be activated by insulin) to allow glucose to cross the blood–brain barrier, enter neurons and the placenta.

GLUT2

GLUT2 only transports glucose into pancreatic β cells and liver cells when blood glucose concentration is high, such as after a high carbohydrate meal, allowing glucose entry. It acts as a metabolic trigger to coordinate insulin secretion with high blood glucose concentration.

- In the pancreas: GLUT2 mediates the uptake of glucose into pancreatic islet cells. The increase in intracellular glucose stimulates the β cell to secrete insulin. GLUT2 thus acts as a 'glucose sensor' in the β cells.
- In the liver: GLUT2 activity facilitates glucose transport into hepatocytes from the blood for glycogenesis (temporary glucose storage), and from the liver into the blood after glycogenolysis (see Fig. 3.2).

GLUT4

GLUT4 is present in intracellular vesicles in insulin-sensitive tissues (liver, muscle, fat). When blood glucose concentration is high (e.g. fed state), insulin is released from the β cells, which binds to insulin receptors in the cell membrane, activating the insulin signal pathway; GLUT4 translocates to the cell membrane, allowing glucose transport into the cell. This process is reversed when blood glucose concentration falls, with a concomitant fall in insulin concentration. GLUT4 is recycled back to intracellular vesicles so that it can no longer transport glucose into the cell.

GLYCOLYSIS – THE ANAEROBIC CATABOLISM OF GLUCOSE

Glycolysis is the first step in the production of energy from glucose. It is a metabolic pathway that breaks down

Table 3.1	Tissue location of glucose transporters	
Transport protein	Tissue location	Characteristics
GLUT1	Most, including red cells	Low K_m*
GLUT2	Liver and pancreatic β cells	High K_m
GLUT3	Mainly brain	
GLUT4	Liver, muscle and adipose tissue	Insulin sensitive
GLUT5	Mainly intestinal tissue, kidney and spermatozoa	Fructose transporter

*K_m is a property of enzymes, defined as the concentration of the substrate that allows 50% of the *maximal* rate of enzyme reaction at normal body temperature and pH (see Ch. 2).

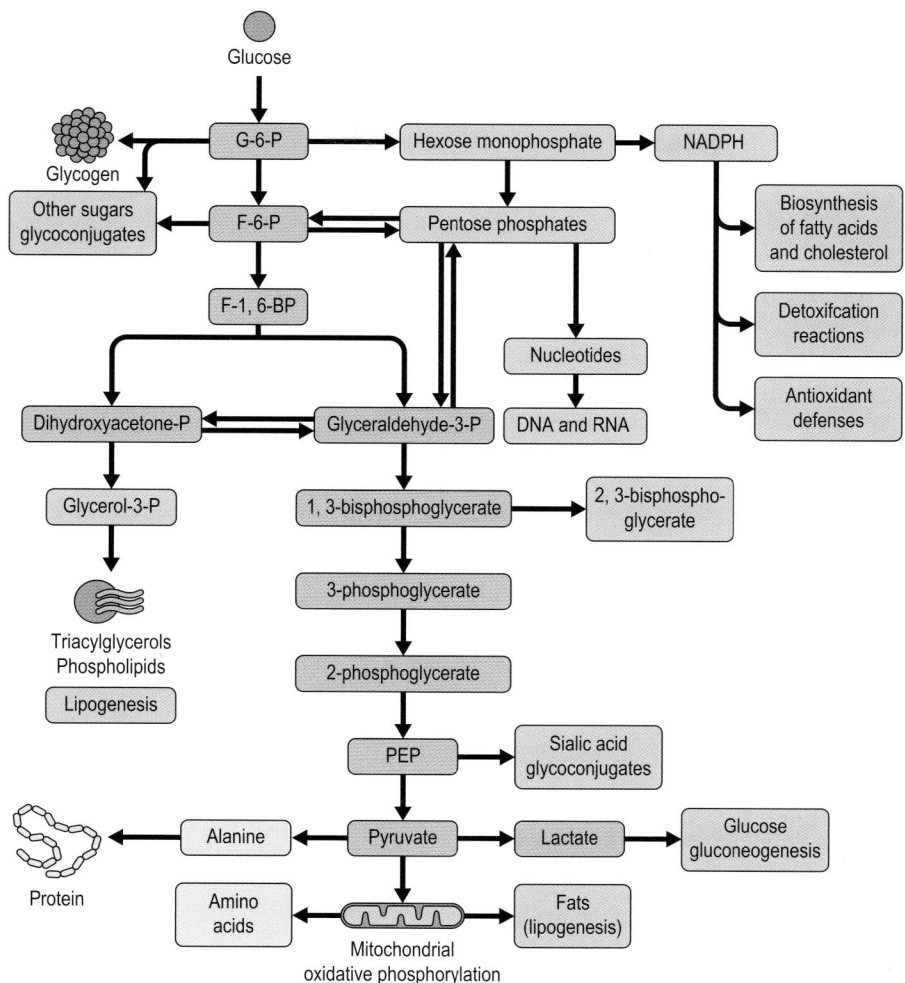

Fig. 3.3 Glycolysis and associated metabolic pathways. Adapted with permission from Baynes J, Dominiczak M 2005 Medical biochemistry, 2nd edn. Elsevier Mosby, Edinburgh. F, fructose; G, glucose; P, phosphate; PEP, phosphoenolpyruvate.

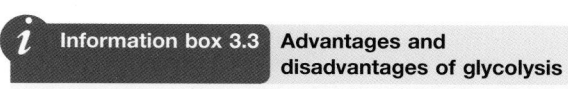

> ### *i* Information box 3.3 — Advantages and disadvantages of glycolysis
>
> **Advantages**
> - Ability to provide ATP without using oxygen for RBCs and when a tissue loses its oxygen supply.
> - Provides many intermediates, which interlink with the metabolic pathways of proteins and fats (see Fig. 3.3).
>
> **Disadvantages**
> - A relatively inefficient pathway for producing energy – the first part uses energy (two molecules of ATP for each molecule of glucose), though it continues with the release of four molecules of ATP – therefore it recovers only about 5% (two molecules) of the 36–38 ATP molecules that can be produced by the complete oxidative metabolism of glucose, which occurs in any cell containing mitochondria, provided that there is a sufficient supply of oxygen.

(catabolises) glucose to lactate without using oxygen (anaerobic). Insulin stimulates glycolysis in skeletal muscle and adipose tissue.

Glycolysis is also the main final pathway for the metabolism of other important dietary components, including fructose (found in sugar (sucrose)) and galactose (found in milk (lactose)). It also produces several intermediate metabolites

that are the starting points for the synthesis of amino acids, proteins, lipids, DNA, RNA and nucleotides (Fig. 3.3).

Importance of the anaerobic nature of glycolysis

The crucial biomedical significance of glycolysis is in its ability to provide ATP in the absence of oxygen (anaerobic metabolism).

For red blood cells

Mature RBCs have no mitochondria, and so cannot carry out oxidative metabolism nor oxidise fats for energy purposes (see later). RBCs rely entirely on glucose as fuel, but do not consume oxygen during metabolism, thus fulfilling their primary role of oxygen transport and delivery.

When a tissue's oxygen supply is cut off

When the oxygen supply to a tissue is cut off (anoxia), ATP levels can still be maintained by glycolysis for a short period of time. The capacity for glycolysis is particularly important in the brain, skeletal muscle during exercise, in ischaemic heart muscle, and during birth. The brain is most sensitive to oxygen lack – irreversible damage may occur after only three minutes of anoxia.

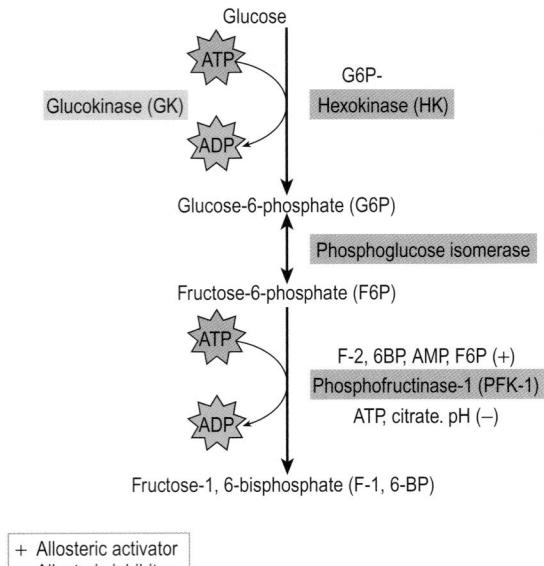

+ Allosteric activator
− Allosteric inhibitor

Fig. 3.4 **Energy-utilising steps in glycolysis.**

Energy-using reactions in glycolysis – glucose phosphorylation

Glycolysis proceeds through the formation of a series of phosphorylated intermediate metabolites, which are eventually metabolised to pyruvate and lactate with the production of ATP. In the first part of the pathway, two molecules of ATP are used up per molecule of glucose metabolised (Fig. 3.4), but this deficit is more than made up in the remainder of the pathway.

Glycolysis is initiated by the formation of the phosphorylated intermediate glucose-6-phosphate (G6P) from glucose. Glucose is phosphorylated to G6P in β cells and liver, catalysed in an irreversible process by hexokinase at normal blood glucose concentrations and by glucokinase at higher blood glucose concentrations (e.g. after a meal).

Synthesis of G6P is energy dependent, using one molecule of ATP as a phosphate donor, per molecule of G6P. However, ATP expenditure at this stage is a long-term investment because it enables the production of ATP later as G6P is broken down.

Phosphate esters are charged and water soluble, rather than lipid soluble, so do not readily penetrate lipid-rich cell membranes (see also Chs 1, 2 and 4). Because there are no transport systems for sugar phosphates in the plasma membranes of mammalian cells, the phosphorylated product, G6P, is trapped within cells, and glucose is thus committed to intracellular metabolism.

Hexokinase

The enzyme hexokinase (HK) is found in most tissues, including red blood cells and muscle. It has a low K_m (0.1 mM) for its substrate, glucose, relative to blood glucose concentration (approximately 5 mM). HK is normally saturated with both ATP and glucose. By phosphorylating all the glucose that enters the cell (because of the low K_m), HK maintains a large glucose concentration gradient between the blood and the intracellular environment, ensuring a continued intracellular supply of glucose, even at low blood glucose concentrations.

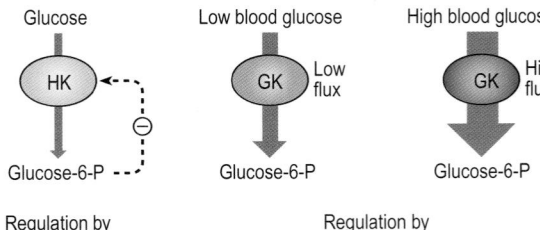

Regulation by feedback inhibition

Regulation by substrate concentration

Fig. 3.5 **Regulation of glucokinase (GK) and hexokinase (HK).** Hexokinase has a low K_m for glucose and is inhibited allosterically by its product, glucose-6-phosphate. In contrast, glucokinase has a higher K_m for glucose and is not inhibited by glucose-6-phosphate. Glucokinase phosphorylates glucose only when blood glucose levels are high.

HK is inhibited, allosterically, by its product G6P (i.e. feedback control, Information box 3.4). This is an important regulatory feature because it prevents HK from sequestering all the inorganic phosphate (Pi) of the cell in the form of phosphorylated glucose, which would make Pi unavailable for other biochemical reactions (Fig. 3.5). As well as acting on glucose, HK can also catalyse the phosphorylation of other hexoses (e.g. fructose), but at a much slower rate.

Glucokinase

Glucokinase (GK) is an isoenzyme of HK with strikingly different kinetic properties from other hexokinases. It is specific for glucose and found only in liver parenchymal cells and pancreatic β cells where GK assumes a more primary role than hexokinase. In contrast with HK:

- GK has a much higher K_m for glucose than HK, and operates optimally at blood glucose concentrations above 5 mM.
- GK is not inhibited by G6P, so neither the liver nor the pancreatic β cell is subject to any feedback inhibition as the result of G6P accumulation.
- GK activity in liver cells (not the pancreas) is inhibited by a GK regulating protein (GKRP), that competes with glucose for binding to GK.

This means that, when glucose concentrations are high, GK is the only enzyme responding to increases in glucose concentration. Its high concentration in the liver and pancreas provides for the synthesis of glycogen, the storage form of glucose. Because the K_m of GK for glucose (approximately 10 mM) is considerably greater than normal blood glucose concentrations (approximately 5 mM), any increase in glucose concentration leads to a proportional increase in the rate of glucose phosphorylation by GK and vice versa (see Fig. 3.5) – this is called substrate concentration regulation. Therefore:

- GK is the rate-limiting enzyme for glucose uptake in liver cells. The liver uses glucose at a significant rate only when blood glucose levels are greatly elevated. Mice with liver-specific knockout of GK have a mild hyperglycaemia and cannot synthesise liver glycogen.
- In the pancreatic β cell, glucose utilisation and oxidation closely track the release of insulin as glucose concentrations increase. GK in the pancreatic β cell has been termed the glucose sensor (glucostat) for insulin secretion (Information box 3.4).

One of the intermediate metabolites of glycolysis is G6P and at this point the pentose phosphate pathway branches off

Pentose is a sugar containing five carbons. The pentose phosphate pathway (or hexose monophosphate shunt) is present in all cells, branching from the glycolysis pathway at the G6P stage (see Fig. 3.3). The pathway is sited in the cytosol. It is the main pathway for the formation of pentose phosphates, necessary for the synthesis of DNA, RNA and nucleotides. It is also important as a generator of reduced nicotinamide adenine dinucleotide phosphate (NADPH) in the cytosol.

G6P enters into an irreversible redox stage to synthesise NADPH and pentose phosphates (see Fig. 3.3). There is also a reversible interconversion stage where excess pentose phosphates are recycled back into glycolysis.

Red cells have no nuclei and so have little need for DNA and RNA synthesis, and G6P is rerouted back into the next stage of glycolysis. About 90% of red cell glucose is metabolised to pyruvate, but the rest is diverted through the pentose phosphate shunt to provide NADPH, which is particularly important to red cells (Clinical box 3.2). NADPH is also needed in the redox reactions used for the biosynthesis of fatty acids, steroid hormones, cholesterol and bile acids. The first part of the conversion of G6P into NADPH is dependent on oxidation by the enzyme glucose-6-phosphate dehydrogenase (G6PD).

Phosphofructokinase-1 (PFK-1)

The second stage in glycolysis is the conversion of G6P into fructose 6-phosphate (F6P) by the enzyme phosphoglucose isomerase (see Fig. 3.4). This process is freely reversible and not subject to regulation. The product, F6P, may then be phosphorylated at a specific carbon, C-1, by another enzyme termed phosphofructokinase-1 (PFK-1) to yield the product fructose-1, 6-bisphosphate (F-1,6-BP). This is the second-energy requiring stage of glycolysis, consuming one molecule of ATP for each molecule of F-1,6-BP produced.

PFK-1 catalyses a reaction that is biochemically reversible, but physiologically irreversible. Like HK, PFK-1 is a key regulatory enzyme in glycolysis that accepts a phosphate group from ATP to form a more phosphorylated product. PFK-1 has the dominant role in the regulation of the overall rate at which glycolysis operates. By controlling the flux of F6P through glycolysis, PFK-1 indirectly controls the level of G6P and therefore the activity of HK.

PFK-1 activity is highly sensitive to the energy status of the cell

ATP serves both as a substrate and allosteric regulator of PFK-1. As an allosteric regulator, ATP can bind at a second site within the enzyme structure that is quite distinct from the

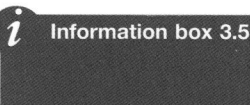

Information box 3.4 Glucokinase affects insulin release into the systemic circulation

There is evidence to suggest that glucokinase (GK) participates in the mechanism by which the pancreatic β cell monitors an increase in blood glucose concentration and delivers an appropriate quantity of insulin into the systemic circulation:

- Genetic mutations of GK can inactivate the enzyme, leading to diabetes, or activate it to cause hypoglycaemia.
- Mutations in the GK gene are associated with one form of maturity-onset diabetes of the young (MODY).
- In sustained hyperglycaemia, and when there are high levels of insulin (e.g. in people with insulin resistance leading to increased risk of type 2 diabetes), GK gene expression is enhanced, leading to increases in GK enzyme protein and activity that takes place over several hours. In this way the liver also contributes to the lowering of blood glucose levels.
- In hypoglycaemia (as a result of starvation or as a complication of the treatment of diabetes mellitus), GK gene and protein expression is decreased. This change both influences hepatic glucose handling, with a sustained switch to increase net glucose output, and impairs blood glucose 'buffering'. Insulin release by the pancreas is also impaired.

Clinical box 3.2 G6PD deficiency is a cause of haemolytic anaemia

G6PD deficiency is a common genetic defect that results in an inability to synthesise NADPH. NADPH is used to maintain reduced glutathione, which protects the cell from the toxic effects of oxidation (i.e. provides antioxidant protection). Red cells are particularly vulnerable to G6PD deficiency because they have no nucleus and so cannot make proteins for repair. As a result of oxidation, haemoglobin is oxidised to methaemoglobin and cannot deliver O_2 to the tissues; the red cell membrane becomes rigid and breaks up.

Acute, life-threatening intravascular haemolysis may be precipitated in G6PD deficiency by:

- Drugs (e.g. aspirin, some antimalarials and antibiotics) undergo redox reactions in red cells to produce oxidants (e.g. superoxide, hydrogen peroxide) that set off a toxic chain reaction, which disrupts the cells (see Ch. 16).
- Ingestion of fava beans
- Infections.

The prevalence of G6PD deficiency is highest in certain African, Mediterranean, Middle Eastern and South East Asian populations.

Information box 3.5 Life or death can depend on intense muscle activity and there must be a large supply of energy available at all times

One mechanism for providing this energy is to increase production through glycolysis, and glycolysis is therefore amplified:

- During exercise (when ATP is used for muscle contraction)
- During hypoxia and in anaerobic muscle (which limits ATP production by oxidative ATP-generating electron transport pathways within mitochondria).

Mechanism for increasing ATP production through glycolysis
- In muscle, ATP is used up during bursts of activity, with the accumulation of ADP.
- ADP is then converted to AMP + ATP by adenylate kinase (also referred to as myokinase).
- As a result, when ATP is used up there is a large increase in AMP concentration. (This is because sum of ATP + ADP + AMP remains nearly constant and the intracellular ATP concentration is much greater than that of AMP at equilibrium (approximately 50 times); relatively small fractional changes in ATP concentration therefore lead to relatively large fractional changes in the concentration of AMP.)
- AMP, the positive allosteric effector of PFK-1, acts as a metabolic amplifier – PFK-1 is therefore activated, increasing glycolysis.

substrate site (involved in the enzyme reaction) and inhibit PFK-1. PFK-1 is inhibited by high intracellular levels of ATP. Adenosine monophosphate (AMP) and adenosine diphosphate (ADP) relieve the inhibition of PFK-1 by ATP. Therefore, the rate of glycolysis depends on the ratio of (AMP + ADP) to ATP (Information box 3.5).

Regulation of PFK-1

PFK-1 is pivotal in regulating the rate and direction of glycolysis, being highly sensitive to the energy requirements of the cell. The enzyme is regulated by several molecules (see Fig. 3.4):

- Protein kinase (AMPK)
- Fructose-2,6-bisphosphate (F-2,6-BP)
- Citrate and pH
- ATP
- AMP

Protein kinase

In muscle, a change in AMP concentration coordinates glycolytic flux with glucose uptake via glycolysis. This involves the activation of a specific regulatory enzyme, a protein kinase (PK). PKs add phosphate groups by covalent mechanisms (phosphorylation) to specific amino acid residues in enzymes and proteins. This often results in altered catalytic activity in enzymes.

One particular PK, AMP-activated protein kinase (AMPK), is sensitive to cellular energy status because its activity is acutely increased when AMP levels rise. Activation of AMPK by AMP is achieved directly by an allosteric mechanism, as well as by phosphorylation induced by other kinases that phosphorylate AMPK itself. This constitutes a phosphorylation cascade, which regulates the rate of glycolysis.

Activation of AMPK, like insulin, leads to recruitment of GLUT4 protein to the plasma membrane. This allows increased glucose entry into the cell for ATP production, and is of particular importance for fast-twitch skeletal muscle during anaerobic exercise.

Fructose-2,6-bisphosphate

PFK-1 has a second potent allosteric effector, F-2,6-BP, which is not an intermediate of glycolysis, but a key regulator. F-2,6-BP activates PFK-1 and counters the inhibition by ATP of PFK-1.

F-2,6-BP is formed by phosphorylation of F6P through the regulatory enzyme phosphofructokinase-2 (PFK-2), which is also responsible for F-2,6-BP breakdown to F6P. PFK-2 is therefore a bifunctional enzyme that also has F-2,6-bisphosphatase (F-2,6-BPase) activity, exhibiting kinase activity when dephosphorylated and phosphatase activity when phosphorylated.

In the liver

In the liver, PFK-2 is under the allosteric control of F6P. High concentrations of F6P (due to an abundance of glucose) stimulate the kinase activity and inhibit the phosphatase activity, thereby stimulating glycolysis. This is an important mechanism for determining whether the predominant direction of hepatic glucose flux is towards glycolysis or towards glycogen synthesis.

During starvation, the hormone glucagon is released (by pancreatic α cells) in response to low blood glucose concentration. The hepatic priority then becomes glucose synthesis (gluconeogenesis) for export to extrahepatic tissues. Con-

sumption of the newly synthesised glucose by hepatic glycolysis would be wasteful. Under the influence of glucagon, PFK-2 exhibits F-2,6-BPase activity, bringing about a fall in cellular F-2,6-BP levels, simultaneously:

- Inhibiting glycolysis (PFK-1)
- Reducing the inhibition on gluconeogenesis.

In muscle

Muscle contains a different form of the bifunctional enzyme PFK-2, both in its amino acid sequence and its response to phosphorylation by protein kinase. Muscle PFK-2 is an isoenzyme, catalysing the same reaction, but it has different regulatory properties. Unlike the liver, muscle has no glucagon receptors. Instead, as part of the 'flight-or-fight' mechanism, a rise in the catecholamine stress hormone adrenaline (epinephrine) stimulates glycolysis in the heart muscle. This is part of a mechanism to meet the increased demand for ATP caused by an adrenaline-induced increase in workload (increased cardiac output).

Citrate and pH

PFK-1 is inhibited by citrate (from TCA cycle) and hydrogen ions (low pH) (see Fig. 3.4).

In oxidative tissues such as the heart during increased exercise, a rise in cytosolic citrate concentration signals the availability of fuels that are alternatives to glucose, namely fatty acids and ketone bodies. This occurs in starvation, when it is necessary to conserve available glucose for tissues that contain few mitochondria (where anaerobic glycolysis predominates) or that have a poor oxygen supply.

Crossover analysis (Information box 3.6) has demonstrated that inhibition of PFK-1 by citrate is important in suppressing cardiac glycolysis when the heart is oxidising fat during starvation. This decreases glucose utilisation and conserves glucose for tissues such as RBC and the central nervous system.

Hydrogen ions shut off glycolysis through inhibition of PFK-1. Unless lactic acid and the H⁺ ions formed by glycolysis are transported out of the cell, the intracellular pH will drop, decreasing PFK-1 activity so that further lactic acid

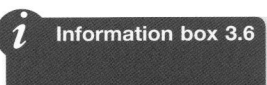

Information box 3.6   **Crossover analysis is used in experiments to determine the likely regulatory enzymes in a metabolic pathway**

For a hypothetical pathway with the intermediates A, B, C, D (A → B → C → D), the crossover theorem proposes that in the conversion of C to D:

- If a regulatory enzyme is inhibited the amount of substrate C will build up and the concentration of D will decrease. This is described as a crossover in the metabolic profile between C and D. (In the absence of an inhibitor the substrate C will decrease in concentration as D production increases under control of the enzyme.)
- Inhibiting a non-regulatory enzyme will cause little change in the intermediates concerned, unless the enzyme is completely inhibited.
- When steady-state concentrations of intermediates in the presence or absence of an inhibitor are compared, the intermediates before the site of inhibition (i.e. C) accumulate in response to the inhibitor, whereas the intermediates after the site (i.e. D) are depleted.

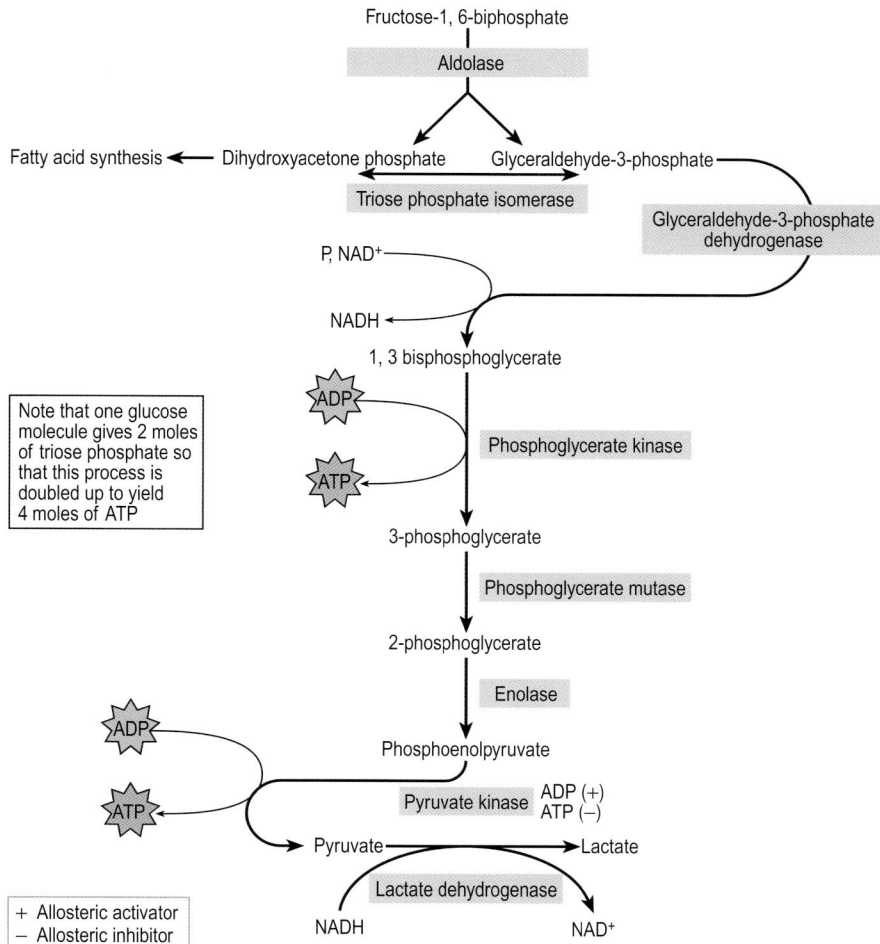

Fig. 3.6 **Energy-producing stage of glycolysis.**

production by glycolysis is stopped. This helps to prevent intracellular pH falling to a level where the cell is rendered non-viable. An accumulation of lactate in muscle results in the severe muscle cramp experienced by athletes during prolonged exercise.

Energy-producing stage of glycolysis – production of pyruvate and lactate

In the energy-producing stage of glycolysis, four molecules of ATP are produced.

Once F-1,6-BP is formed, the molecule is split into two 3-carbon phosphorylated intermediates (triose phosphates: dihydroxyacetone phosphate (DHAP) and glyceraldehyde 3-phosphate). These two compounds are interconvertible, but only glyceraldehyde 3-phosphate enters the later stages of glycolysis (Fig. 3.6). DHAP enters a pathway for fatty acid synthesis (see later). Each triose phosphate can provide one phosphate, which is subsequently transferred to ATP.

Two additional phosphate molecules are recruited in the next stage (one for each triose phosphate) as glyceraldehyde 3-phosphate traps soluble phosphate in the form of an acyl phosphate. This reaction is catalysed by glyceraldehyde 3-phosphate dehydrogenase (G3PDH) to form 1,3 bisphosphate glycerate (1,3-BPG), with the simultaneous reduction of NAD$^+$ to NADH.

Reactions yielding ATP

During the next stage of glycolysis, ATP is produced by substrate-level phosphorylation in which a 'high-energy' phosphate intermediate of the pathway (a pathway substrate) transfers its phosphate to ADP to form ATP. The two reactions that yield ATP and pyruvate are catalysed by the enzymes phosphoglycerate kinase and pyruvate kinase, which together yield 2 moles of ATP per mole of triose phosphate, a total of 4 moles of ATP per mole of glucose. The energy-producing stage of glycolysis also generates reduced nicotinamide adenine dinucleotide (NADH) from the coenzyme NAD$^+$ in the reaction catalysed by G3PDH.

After adjustment for the ATP invested in the phosphorylations catalysed by the HK and PFK-1 reactions, the conversion of glucose to pyruvate yields a net gain of two molecules of ATP, together with two molecules of NADH. Pyruvate now enters oxidative phosphorylation, the process by which energy is released in the form of ATP as pyruvate is broken down into CO_2 and water.

Pyruvate kinase

Pyruvate kinase not only catalyses substrate-level phosphorylation yielding ATP (Clinical box 3.3), but it is also another regulatory enzyme of glycolysis, though its action is in direct contrast to the ATP-consuming reactions catalysed by the other regulatory enzymes, HK and PFK-1.

Clinical box 3.3 — Pyruvate kinase deficiency in red blood cells causes haemolytic anaemia

Pyruvate kinase deficiency is the second most common genetic defect of the glycolytic pathway (after G6PD deficiency, see Clinical box 3.2) known to cause haemolytic anaemia.

There is reduced production of the energy (ATP) necessary to maintain the integrity of the red cell membrane and the biconcave shape of the red blood cells. Damage to the cells results in haemolysis.

Pyruvate kinase deficiency results in a shift in the haemoglobin-oxygen dissociation curve

Within the red cell, pyruvate kinase deficiency results in a build-up of glycolytic intermediates, particularly 2,3 bisphosphoglycerate (2,3-DPG), which cause a right shift in the haemoglobin-oxygen dissociation curve such that more oxygen can be delivered to the tissues for each gram of haemoglobin. Patients therefore experience fewer symptoms from what appears to be a severe anaemia.

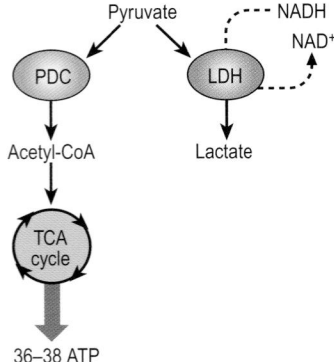

Fed state
When PDC is active, pyruvate can be converted to acetyl-CoA via PDC. Acetyl-CoA can enter the TCA cycle for complete oxidation. This generates far more ATP than glycolysis alone. Acetyl-CoA can also be converted to citrate (in the TCA cycle), and then can be transported to the cytosol to enter fatty acid synthesis.

Starvation
When PDC is inactive, pyruvate is converted to lactate, which is released into the circulation. This also regenerates NAD+.

Fig. 3.7 **Fate of pyruvate in the fed and fasted states.** LDH, lactate dehydrogenase; PDC, pyruvate dehydrogenase complex; TCA, tricarboxylic acid.

Kinetic studies have revealed three classes of pyruvate kinase isoenzymes, with qualitative differences in regulatory properties. For example, the pyruvate kinase isoenzyme found in liver is activated by the product of the PFK-1 reaction, F-1,6-BP, and shows allosteric inhibition by ATP. This links the regulation of pyruvate kinase with that of PFK-1. When glucose is abundant, conditions favour increased flux through PFK-1, and the level of F-1,6-BP increases. The rise in F-1,6-BP concentration acts as a feed-forward activator of pyruvate kinase.

Liver pyruvate kinase, like glucokinase, is induced by higher steady-state concentrations of glucose and insulin. This increase in enzyme concentration is a major reason why the liver of a well-fed person has a greater capacity for utilising carbohydrate than in a fasting person.

Fate of pyruvate

Pyruvate is metabolised in different ways, depending on the availability of glucose, as in the fed state or fasted state (Fig. 3.7).

In mitochondria-containing cells

Fed state

In the fed state, pyruvate is diverted into the more energy efficient metabolic pathway, the TCA cycle. The enzyme pyruvate dehydrogenase complex (PDC) converts pyruvate (a carbohydrate) to CO_2 and acetyl-CoA. Acetyl-CoA can then:

- Enter the TCA cycle for complete oxidation – this generates far more ATP than glycolysis alone
- Be converted to citrate (in the TCA cycle), and then be transported to the cytosol to enter fatty acid synthesis, where the first step is the conversion of acetyl-CoA to malonyl-CoA.

PDC activity can either determine or reflect fuel preference (carbohydrate versus fat), and therefore occupies a pivotal position in fuel homeostasis. Importantly, the initial decarboxylation of pyruvate catalysed by PDC begins a process that is physiologically irreversible, committing glucose-derived pyruvate to acetyl-CoA production (see Fig. 3.7).

Fasted state

In the fasted state, PDC is inactive, and, in liver and kidney, pyruvate is directed towards gluconeogenesis. Pyruvate is converted to:

- Oxaloacetate by pyruvate carboxylase (the water soluble vitamin biotin acts as coenzyme (see Ch. 16)).
- Alanine by alanine aminotransferase (ALT).

In cells that lack mitochondria, when oxygen is limited, and in starvation

In cells that lack mitochondria (e.g. RBCs) or tissues that contain relatively few mitochondria (e.g. cornea, lens, retina, kidney medulla and white muscle) pyruvate is converted by lactate dehydrogenase (LDH) to lactate as the principal end product. Conversion to lactate in other tissues also predominates when oxygen is limited or the activity of PDC is low.

Lactate production becomes important under conditions where dietary glucose is scarce (e.g. starvation) and glucose must be conserved for 'glucose-dependent' tissues. It is also important because lactate is used to synthesise glucose and regenerates NAD+ so that glycolysis can continue.

Lactate dehydrogenase

Pyruvate can be converted to lactate via LDH. In this process, NAD+ is regenerated from NADH. LDH catalyses a near-equilibrium reaction, and is not regulatory for glycolysis.

The regeneration of NAD+ by LDH is crucial under anaerobic conditions and in cells lacking mitochondria, because NAD+ is an essential cofactor for glycolysis. Lactate is moved out of the cell by facilitated diffusion. A family of membrane bound proteins, monocarboxylate transport proteins (MCT1–4), have been identified that transport lactate into and out of cells. The released lactate is transported to the liver and converted back to glucose for re-use in muscle (Cori cycle, see later).

The MCT system is a pH dependent antiport (see Ch. 2). When NAD+ is regenerated from NADH, lactate and H+ ions accumulate in the cell, leading to a fall in pH. This creates the pH gradient that activates the MCT system, and lactate diffuses out of the cell to enter the blood. Excessive accu-

Lactic acidosis occurs when there is excessive accumulation of lactic acid in the blood stream. It can be a metabolic emergency. The clinical features are those of metabolic acidosis. Tissue oxygen deprivation stimulates respiration, giving rise to 'air hunger' – Kussmaul respiration. Treatment should be aimed at the primary cause.

Lactic acidosis can be caused by:

- Severe exercise – the condition is self-limiting
- Defective tissue perfusion when cells are deprived of oxygen and undergo anaerobic glycolysis (type A lactic acidosis)
- Decreased enzyme activity for degrading lactic acid (type B lactic acidosis).

Type A lactic acidosis
- Clinically much more common than type B lactic acidosis.
- Occurs in shock – i.e. general circulatory insufficiency of any cause

Type B lactic acidosis
- This is less common, and occurs in the absence (at least initially), of circulatory failure, and may be caused by:
- Decreased pyruvate dehydrogenase activity in diabetes, sometimes after diabetic ketoacidosis
- Reduced lactic acid metabolism by the liver
- Drug-induced (e.g. biguanide accumulation in people with diabetes with chronic renal failure, some treatments for malaria).

PDC activity requires coenzymes from the B vitamin family, notably thiamine (B$_1$), but also riboflavin (B$_2$), pantothenic acid and nicotinamide (B$_3$). Dietary (beriberi) and alcohol-related thiamine deficiency leads to defective coenzyme synthesis so that PDC activity is impaired, and pyruvate entry into the TCA cycle is reduced (see Ch. 16).

PDC deficiency
PDC converts pyruvate to acetyl-CoA, needed for the production of citrate, which is essential for the TCA cycle. In PDC deficiency (PDCD), mitochondrial oxidation of pyruvate in the TCA cycle cannot proceed, so pyruvate is converted to lactate with consequent high blood pyruvate and lactate concentrations with or without overt lactic acidosis. Total PDCD is incompatible with life.

The extremely rare Leigh's and West's diseases are associated with an X-linked genetic PDC defect. Prenatal PDCD may lead to congenital brain malformations. Symptoms present early in infancy, including hypotonia, developmental delay, seizures and early death. Treatment is aimed to stimulate PDC activity with thiamine supplementation and to provide alternative metabolic fuels to glucose, e.g. low carbohydrate, ketogenic diet.

mulation of lactate leads to lactic acidosis (Clinical box 3.4). This can be caused by physiological lactate production, when there is inadequate tissue oxygen supply (as in intense exercise), or if there is defective pyruvate clearance or increased pyruvate production.

Under fasting conditions, even cells capable of oxidative metabolism produce lactate because PDC is inactivated (see above). In the fed state when PDC is active, cells (e.g. muscle cells) can take up circulating lactate derived from other tissues (e.g. the red blood cell) for conversion to pyruvate via the reversible LDH reaction and entry into the TCA cycle for energy (ATP) production.

OXIDATIVE GLUCOSE METABOLISM – AEROBIC GLYCOLYSIS

The conversion of glucose to CO$_2$ and water takes place in two stages: the anaerobic conversion of glucose to pyruvate, followed by the complete oxidation of pyruvate to CO$_2$ and water in two stages:

- In the TCA cycle, reduced coenzymes, such as NADH, are produced within the inner membrane of mitochondria
- NADH is then oxidised to NAD$^+$ in the electron transport system, coupled with the reduction of oxygen.

The ATP yield from glucose degradation is massively increased when pyruvate is oxidised completely through this process. Glycolysis produces two molecules of ATP for each molecule of glucose, whereas the complete oxidative metabolism of glucose can yield up to 36–38 molecules of ATP.

Acetyl-CoA is the molecule at the starting point of the TCA cycle and is a metabolite that is also common to the breakdown of fats and proteins. Entry of acetyl-CoA derived from carbohydrates is under the control of the PDC.

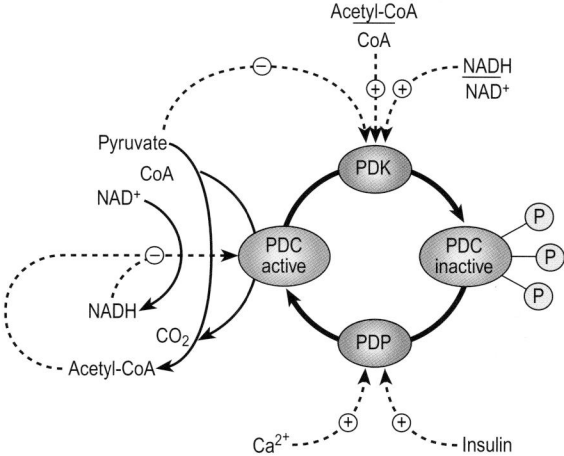

Fig. 3.8 **Mechanisms regulating pyruvate dehydrogenase complex (PDC) activity.** PDK, pyruvate dehydrogenase kinase; PDP, pyruvate dehydrogenase phosphate.

Pyruvate dehydrogenase complex

The PDC catalyses the entry of pyruvate into the TCA cycle. It is a tightly organised arrangement of polypeptides and cofactors working sequentially in the multienzyme complex catalysing a multi-step reaction in which pyruvate is converted to acetyl-CoA. The intermediate substrates and products remain bound to the complex, increasing overall efficiency. In this process, carbon is lost in the form of CO$_2$, and NAD$^+$ is reduced to NADH. This is oxidative decarboxylation.

Unlike the key controlling glycolytic enzymes HK, PFK-1 and pyruvate kinase, which are located in the cytosol, PDC is located in the mitochondria. Pyruvate produced by glycolysis must first be transported by a specific pyruvate transporter into the mitochondria for entry into the TCA cycle.

Regulation of PDC activity

Regulation of PDC activity (Fig. 3.8) is an important component of glucose homeostasis. Active PDC facilitates the entry of glucose carbon into the TCA cycle when fuel is abundant. When there is a lack of fuel (e.g. during prolonged starvation) suppression of PDC activity is crucial to glucose conservation.

PDC is inactivated through phosphorylation by pyruvate dehydrogenase kinases (PDKs). These are structurally related proteins of which four isoforms have been identified: PDK1–4. Most tissues contain at least two, and often three isoforms. Changes in tissue PDK isoform expression occur in response to:

- Starvation
- Variations in dietary composition
- Hormonal status: insulin increases PDC activity in adipose tissue.

The common products of glucose and fatty acid metabolism, acetyl-CoA and NADH, inhibit PDC activity. They also both activate PDK, which in turn inactivates PDC.

Intermediates of glucose and fatty acid metabolism have opposing effects on PDC and PDK:

- PDK is suppressed by pyruvate, generated via glycolysis or from circulating lactate.
- High mitochondrial acetyl-CoA/CoA and NADH/NAD$^+$ concentration ratios (which are generated when rates of fatty acid β-oxidation are increased) activate PDK.

PDC is re-activated by pyruvate dehydrogenase phosphatases (PDPs), of which two isoenzymes exist. One of these is activated by Ca^{2+}. Ca^{2+} activation of PDP increases PDC activity, leading to increased ATP generation from pyruvate. Cytoplasmic Ca^{2+} concentrations increase when there is increased demand for ATP (e.g. in muscle during exercise).

GLYCOGEN – THE STORAGE FORM OF GLUCOSE

Glycogen, a branched polysaccharide, is the principal storage form of glucose in mammalian cells. The two major tissue sites of glycogen storage are the liver and skeletal muscle. When carbohydrate is supplied in excess of tissue requirements, it is used for the synthesis of storage molecules:

- Glycogen, the storage form of glucose
- Triacylglycerol (TAG; also known as triglyceride), the storage form of fatty acids.

When the supply of metabolic fuels is restricted, tissue energy demands are met by the mobilisation of stored (endogenous) fuels. Metabolic stores can either:

- Provide substrates directly – glucose from glycogen (glycogenolysis), fatty acids from TAG, or
- Provide precursors such as lactate and glycerol for glucose synthesis via gluconeogenesis.

> ### Information box 3.7 — Liver and muscle glycogen have different functions
>
> - Hepatic glycogen is primarily directed towards glucose release to counteract a dangerously low blood glucose concentration (hypoglycaemia).
> - Muscle glycogen breakdown is primarily directed towards the provision of ATP for muscle contraction.

In the liver

In the liver, glycogen is mainly present as a glucose reservoir for other tissues, and the amount of glycogen stored in the liver changes constantly with changes in nutritional status.

During the post-absorptive state – between meals – glucose is produced directly from hepatic glycogenolysis. Hepatic glycogen is essentially depleted after overnight starvation because total hepatic glycogen stores (typically 50–100 g) are only sufficient to maintain blood glucose over a 12-hour fast.

In skeletal muscle

In skeletal muscle, glycogen cannot be broken down to glucose through glycogenolysis because it lacks the enzyme glucose-6-phosphatase (G6Pase). Glucose cannot therefore be supplied to the circulation by skeletal muscle.

SYNTHESIS OF GLYCOGEN

The general mechanism of glycogen synthesis is the same in all tissues. The first step is the conversion of G6P into glucose-1-phosphate (G1P) by the enzyme phosphoglucomutase. To be converted into glycogen, G1P has to be converted into a form that can be acted on by the next enzyme in the sequence, glycogen synthase.

G1P is combined with uridine triphosphate to form the sugar nucleotide, uridine diphosphate (UDP)-glucose, in an activation process catalysed by the enzyme UDP-glucose pyrophosphorylase. Apart from glycogen synthesis, UDP-glucose also takes part in the synthesis of other sugars, glycoproteins and glycolipids. Therefore it is the next enzyme in the pathway, glycogen synthase, and not UDP-glucose pyrophosphorylase, that is regulatory for glycogen synthesis (Fig. 3.9).

Glycogenin, the glycogen primer

A primer is required for glycogen synthesis when cells are totally depleted of glycogen: a protein called glycogenin. Glycogenin can attach glucose molecules to its own amino acid residues, a process called self-glucosylation.

- The 'C-1' of glucose is autocatalytically attached by glycogenin to one of its own tyrosine residues, using UDP-glucose to donate the glucose residue (UDP-glucose is a glucosyl donor). This forms the core glycogen sequence.
- Glycogenin then autocatalytically extends the 'glucan' chain by up to six or seven glucose residues to form the 'primed' glycogen. The glucose residues are joined together by α-1→4 links (Fig. 3.9).

Glycogen synthase

The 'primed' glycogen is further elongated by glycogen synthase, a member of the class of enzymes known as glycosyl transferases.

- Glycogen synthase elongates the primed glycogen by adding glucose molecules via α1→4 linkage.
- Glycogen branching enzyme transfers some of the α1→4-links to a α1→6 branch when the α1→4 chain

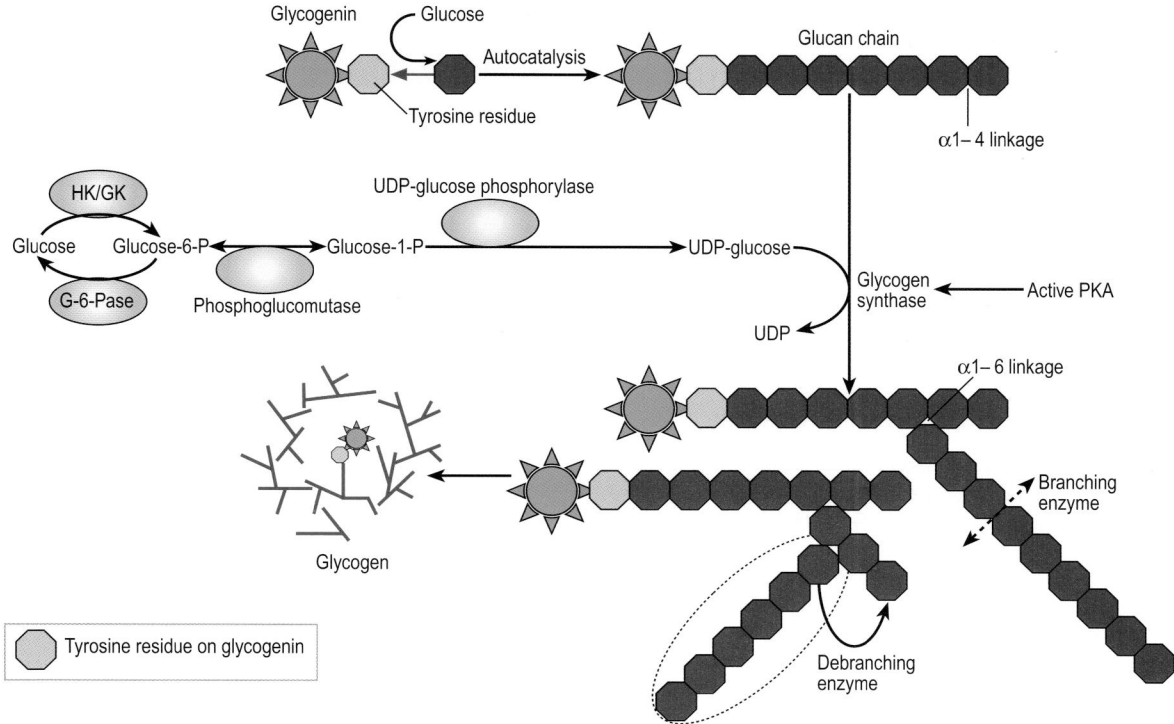

Fig. 3.9 **Glycogen synthesis and its regulation.** GK, glucokinase; G6Pase, glucose-6-phosphatase; HK, hexokinase; UDP, uridine diphosphate.

reaches 6–8 glucose residues, so that the glycogen molecule becomes tree-like (see Fig. 3.9).

Glycogen limits its own synthesis by end-product inhibition so that its accumulation in liver and muscle does not become excessive.

Structure of glycogen

A mature glycogen particle has a structure resembling the head of a cauliflower (see Fig. 3.9), with branches that form a left-handed helix with 6.5 glucose residues per turn.

About half of the glycogen mass is attributable to the external branches, which provide ready access to the glucose residues for the enzymes involved in their release from the glycogen polymer. The internal branches carry side chains separated by about four glucose units.

The cauliflower-like structure of glycogen accounts for the spherical shape of beta-particles (30 nm diameter, up to 60 000 glucose units), which are present in most cells. In the liver, about 20–40 beta-particles are associated into larger complexes known as alpha rosettes, which are visible under the electron microscope.

Control of glycogen synthesis

Glycogen synthesis occurs during and immediately following meals. In response to a rising blood glucose concentration, insulin is secreted from the β-cells of the pancreatic islets, lowering blood glucose concentration by promoting:

- Tissue glucose uptake,
- Cellular glucose metabolism
- Glycogen synthesis.

Insulin and glucagon are the main hormones concerned with controlling blood glucose concentration. Glucose stimulates the secretion of insulin and inhibits the secretion of glucagon. Insulin reverses the action of glucagon on phosphorylation, inhibiting glycogen phosphorylase and activating glycogen synthase, so initiating the metabolic processes that transform glucose to glycogen in liver and muscle, and glucose to lipids.

Glucose that is not stored in the liver proceeds to the peripheral circulation where it is taken up by:

- Muscle (for glycogen synthesis)
- Adipose tissue (to provide glycerol 3-phosphate for fatty acid esterification and fatty acid synthesis de novo).

Allosteric activation of glycogen synthesis

Because glucose can enter liver cells without insulin, the liver is responsive to the direct stimulus of a post-prandial rising blood glucose concentration, initiating glycogen synthesis before insulin concentration rises. This occurs by:

- Direct allosteric inhibition of glycogen phosphorylase by glucose, inhibiting glycogen breakdown (see Fig. 3.9),
- Secondary stimulation of protein phosphatase activity (dephosphorylation of phosphorylase; see below).

Covalent mechanisms regulating glycogen synthesis

Glycogen synthase is the key regulatory enzyme for glycogen synthesis. Acute regulation of glycogen synthase activity operates through covalent mechanisms achieved in part by a reversible phosphorylation (see Fig. 3.9).

- Glycogen synthase is activated by dephosphorylation, a reaction catalysed by protein phosphatases.

- Glycogen synthase is inactivated by phosphorylation, a reaction catalysed by protein kinases.

Glycogen phosphorylase, concerned with the breakdown of glycogen, is activated by phosphorylation and inactivated by dephosphorylation. By using common kinases and phosphatases, glycogen synthase can be activated when glycogen phosphorylase is inactivated, and vice versa.

There is an excellent linear correlation between the activity of glycogen synthase a (active form) and the rate of glycogen synthesis in liver. This positive correlation is also observed in fast-twitch skeletal muscle, where glycolysis from glycogen is a vital source of ATP for contraction.

Glycogen synthesis in the liver

The cell membranes of hepatocytes contain the glucose transporter GLUT2. Glucose is freely transported into the cells even when glucose is delivered at high concentration in the portal blood during the absorption of a carbohydrate-rich meal. Because the transport capacity of GLUT2 is not rate-limiting for hepatic glucose uptake, the liver functions as a blood glucose sensor.

The hepatocytes are rich in GK, which converts glucose into G6P. Unlike HK, GK is not inhibited by G6P, so the concentration of G6P increases rapidly in the liver cells following a carbohydrate-rich meal, leading to glycogen synthase activation by dephosphorylation. If liver glycogen concentrations are not at maximum, G6P is channelled into the glycogen synthesis pathway; as hepatic glycogen becomes replenished, excess G6P enters glycolysis.

Direct versus indirect pathway of hepatic glycogen synthesis

After a meal, ingested glucose is converted first into liver glycogen, stimulated by the secretion of insulin, which:

- Inhibits glycogen phosphorylase
- Activates glycogen synthase.

After fasting, however, when blood glucose falls and liver glycogen becomes the immediate source of glucose, liver glycogen can be replenished from the product of glycolysis – lactate – which is converted into G6P via gluconeogenesis.

Thus the liver has both direct (via glucokinase) and indirect (via gluconeogenesis) pathways for glycogen replenishment.

Glycogen synthesis in muscle

Skeletal muscle is a major tissue site for glucose disposal when insulin levels are elevated (e.g. after a carbohydrate-rich meal).

Glycogen synthesis represents the primary pathway for the non-oxidative disposal of glucose in normal healthy human subjects, and muscle glycogen synthesis is a major pathway of overall glucose metabolism (Information box 3.8). Impaired glycogen synthesis in muscle, due to defective insulin action or insulin resistance, is a major intracellular metabolic defect in type 2 diabetes mellitus (Clinical box 3.6).

The pathway for glycogen synthesis from glucose in muscle differs from that in liver. Muscle contains the glucose transporter GLUT4 (recruited to the cell surface following insulin stimulation) and the glucose phosphorylating enzyme,

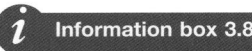

Information box 3.8 **Non-invasive techniques for studying the rate of glycogen synthesis**

Glycogen concentrations can be measured accurately with a time resolution of several minutes using carbon-13 nuclear magnetic resonance spectra of human muscle glycogen. Used in combination with indirect calorimetry, the rate of muscle glycogen synthesis during insulin stimulation can then be related to whole body glucose disposal.

Clinical box 3.6 **Insulin resistance in type 2 diabetes mellitus**

Diabetes mellitus is the result of disordered metabolism secondary to defects in the production and/or effectiveness of the hormone insulin, secreted by pancreatic β-cells.

In type 2 diabetes, resistance to insulin action is the major problem, but insulin secretion becomes impaired. Some β-cells are still active initially, but there is a suboptimal insulin response to glucose stimulation. Treatment would therefore be to stimulate the remaining β-cells to secrete more insulin, or to improve insulin sensitivity.

Insulin resistance results from inefficient glucose utilisation by target cells
Patients with type 2 diabetes often have hyperglycaemia despite the presence of plasma insulin, even at inappropriately high concentrations. The cause of this hyperglycaemia is uncertain, but has been postulated as the result of inefficient glucose utilisation by insulin target cells (insulin resistance), which may be due to:

- Defective insulin-receptor binding due to down regulation of insulin receptors.
- Gene mutation causing abnormality in insulin-receptor binding.
- Defective key enzymes, such as glycogen synthase or pyruvate dehydrogenase.
- Increased pyruvate dehydrogenase kinase (PDK) isoform expression in muscle leading to inactivation of muscle pyruvate dehydrogenase complex (PDC).
- Possible genetically determined post receptor defect, i.e. defective signal transduction.
- Defects in signalling pathway, due to defects in the insulin receptors (e.g. absence of tyrosine kinase) or in the post receptor cascade.
- Defects in insulin-induced glucose transport, such as defective translocation of GLUT4 to cell membrane.

HK. HK has a low K_m for glucose and is inhibited by G6P. Hence, efficient use of glucose by muscle for glycogen synthesis requires the continuous removal of G6P (unlike in the liver, which uses GK).

Intracellular glycogen content exerts a regulatory effect on glucose uptake in fast-twitch muscle (needed for short bursts of energy; Clinical box 3.7). However, in the period after prolonged and heavy physical activity, glycogen re-synthesis is of high priority and both glucose transport and glycogen synthesis are increased to replenish the depleted glycogen stores.

GLYCOGENOLYSIS – THE BREAKDOWN OF GLYCOGEN

Glycogenolysis is the process by which glycogen is broken down to glucose for use in energy metabolism. This is achieved not by simple hydrolysis, but by phosphorylation. Because of the branching nature of the glycogen molecule, separate enzymes are needed.

Clinical box 3.7   **Energy metabolism in muscles**

Skeletal muscles generally comprise two types of muscle fibre:

- Fast-twitch fibres in white muscle (as in chicken breast meat), are relatively low in mitochondria, blood flow (hence 'white') and fat, but rich in glycogen. These muscles contain a large number of fast-twitch fibres, which perform rhythmic contractions using glycogen stores and anaerobic glycolysis for short bursts of additional energy, since glycogen stores only last a short period of time.
- Slow-twitch fibres in dark muscle (as in red meat) are well perfused, have a high fat content and are rich in mitochondria. These muscles use aerobic (oxidative) metabolism of fatty acids for the energy required for prolonged, strenuous exercise.
- Cardiac muscle contracts continuously. It is has a rich blood supply and mitochondria, and relies mainly on oxidative fatty acid metabolism for ATP synthesis, similar to slow-twitch muscles.

Short-distance versus long-distance running
- Athletes specialising in short-distance running (e.g. 100 or 200 m sprinting) primarily use anaerobic metabolism for energy.
- Energy for long-distance running (e.g. 5000 m or marathon) is mainly obtained by aerobic metabolism.

Hitting the wall
Long-distance athletes sometimes 'hit the wall' when their glycogen stores are depleted. The popular high-carbohydrate diet before a race is intended to build up glycogen stores.

Glycogenolysis in liver

Liver glycogen is broken down to provide a rapid source of blood glucose as a short-term buffer to a fall in blood glucose concentration, and is particularly important between meals. The degradation of glycogen requires the concerted action of two enzymes:

- Glycogen phosphorylase, which breaks down the long chains of glucose molecules.
- Debranching enzyme, which lops off the branches.

The pathway of glycogenolysis begins with the removal of the terminal glucose residue of the abundant external $\alpha1\rightarrow4$ linked chains of glucose residues by glycogen phosphorylase, releasing G1P (see Fig. 3.10). G1P is converted into G6P by the enzyme phosphoglucomutase. G6P is then hydrolysed to glucose by G6Pase. Glucose is transported out of the cell by GLUT2 into the bloodstream.

Glycogenolysis in muscle

The breakdown of glycogen in muscle follows the same pathway as hepatic glycogenolysis, except that it lacks the enzyme G6Pase, so that G6P cannot be converted to glucose. Muscle G6P enters glycolysis to produce energy for muscle contraction (see Fig. 3.2). Although more of the body's glycogen is stored in muscle than in the liver, muscle cannot release glucose into the bloodstream.

REGULATION OF GLYCOGENOLYSIS

Regulation of glycogenolysis is achieved by:

- Hormones, mainly glucagon, adrenaline (epinephrine; sympathetic control), cortisol and to some extent human growth hormone (GH), that activate
- Intracellular enzymes to catalyse the breakdown of glycogen.

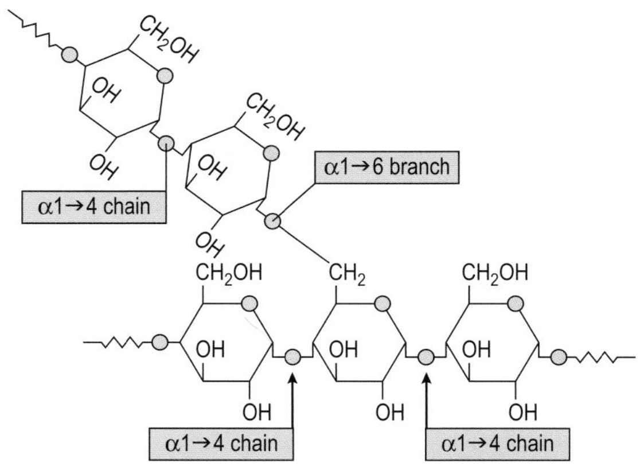

Fig. 3.10 **Pathways for hepatic glycogenolysis.**
Glycogen phosphorylase 'nibbles' at the external glucose residues until all external chains of the glycogen molecule have been shortened to four glucose units. At a branch point, debranching enzyme then removes a short segment of glucose residue by a glucose transferring activity (transglycosylase) and transfers the stub to the end of an adjacent chain. The remaining glucose molecule at the stub of the branch point is then liberated by the exo-α-glucosidase activity of the same debranching enzyme, which is bifunctional. The newly formed $\alpha1\rightarrow4$-linked glucose residues become available for phosphorylase to proceed with degradation until another branch point is reached. Adapted with permission from Baynes J, Dominiczak M 2005 Medical Biochemistry, 2nd edn. Elsevier Mosby, Edinburgh.

Because the production of glucose from glycogen serves different purposes in the liver and muscle, the presence of hormone receptors and enzymes in their cells are specific to their needs.

Regulation of hepatic glycogenolysis

A range of metabolic pathways have to be activated to mobilise glucose stores. Glycogenolysis in the liver is activated in response to falling blood glucose levels in the fasting state and in preparation for an increased demand for glucose, for example in response to:

- Physiological stress, as in increased or prolonged exercise
- Pathological stress, as in severe shock from blood loss
- Psychological stress as in fear and preparation for 'flight or fight'.

Hormone regulation of hepatic glycogenolysis

Hepatic glycogenolysis during fasting or moderate exercise is increased by the hormone glucagon, secreted by pancreatic α-cells in response to low blood glucose. Glucagon has the major function of activating glycogenolysis to maintain normoglycaemia. It has a half-life in the plasma of only a few minutes so the plasma concentration of glucagon fluctuates constantly in response to the body's need for glucose.

In severe acute stress and severe hypoglycaemia, adrenaline works in tandem with glucagon to amplify hepatic glycogenolysis. This may in part explain the symptoms of tachycardia, sweating and shaking in hypoglycaemia and fear. Glucagon and adrenaline (via β-adrenergic receptors) activate glycogenolysis through a mechanism resulting from their binding to their target cell surface receptors. Adrenaline has a second glycogenolytic pathway, via α-adrenergic receptors (see below).

In chronic stress (or in response to prolonged exposure to cold), plasma cortisol levels rise in response to the need for glucose, and stimulates glycogen synthesis. Cortisol is a glucocorticoid (see Ch. 2) that has a major role in glucose homeostasis. Like glucagon, the action of cortisol leads to increases in blood glucose concentration, but has a much slower effect. It acts through gene expression to stimulate the transcription of mRNA to synthesise enzymes that increase glycogenesis and gluconeogenesis. Cortisol is secreted by the adrenal glands, controlled by the hypothalamic–pituitary axis. Secretion varies according to circadian rhythm (see Ch. 10).

Mechanism of glucagon regulation of glycogenolysis – hormone signalling

Glucagon binds to a liver cell plasma membrane receptor, setting off a cascade of reactions to release glucose into the bloodstream. The glucagon receptor is coupled to the G protein, adenylate cyclase-cAMP second messenger system (see Ch. 4 and Fig. 4.11). The binding of glucagon to its receptor protein causes dissociation of a subunit from the G protein complex in the cell membrane.

G proteins are so named because they bind guanosine nucleotides and consist of three subunits – α, β and γ. In its resting state, guanosine diphosphate (GDP) is bound to G protein. Binding of glucagon to its plasma membrane receptor in the liver starts a cascade involving the G proteins as follows (Fig. 3.11):

- GTP loses one P to become GDP and the α-subunit dissociates from the other two subunits.
- Adenylate cyclase is activated by the stimulatory Gα-subunit, catalysing the conversion of ATP to cAMP and pyrophosphate.
- cAMP binds to protein kinase A (PKA), a tetrameric enzyme with two pairs of subunits, releasing its inhibitory R-subunits, thus activating PKA.
- PKA phosphorylates a series of enzymes (phosphorylase kinase and glycogen phosphorylase), which break down glycogen to form G1P, thus initiating glycogenolysis.

The activation of PKA by cAMP is instantaneous, thus providing very dynamic control of glycogenolysis.

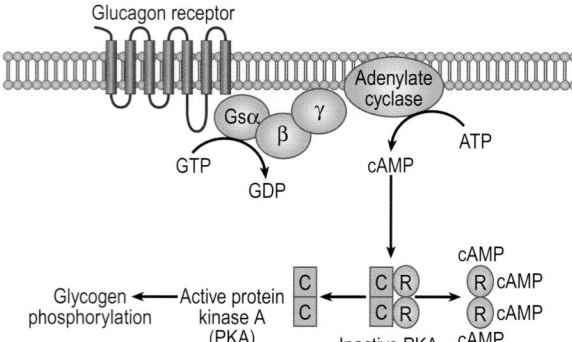

Fig. 3.11 **Signalling pathway from glucagon to cAMP-dependent protein kinase A.** PKA, cyclic AMP-dependent protein kinase A; GDP, guanosine diphosphate; GTT, guanosine triphosphate; C, catalytic; R, regulatory (inhibitory).

Sympathetic stimulation

Adrenaline is an important neurotransmitter acting through the sympathetic nervous system. Acute stress, regardless of its cause, activates glycogenolysis through the action of adrenaline, which is released from the adrenal medulla as part of a 'flight or fight' response or during prolonged exercise.

In both liver and muscle, binding of adrenaline to β-adrenergic membrane receptors, like glucagon, leads to a cAMP-mediated increase in glycogenolysis. The action of adrenaline can also be mediated via α-adrenergic receptors in a different process involving the phospholipase C-Ca^{2+} (PLC-Ca^{2+}) second-messenger system (see Ch. 4 and Fig. 4.11) as follows:

1. Binding to the α-receptor produces a conformational change in the G protein, which activates membrane bound PLC.
2. PLC splits a membrane phospholipid producing two second messengers: diacylglycerol (DAG, also known as diglyceride) and inositol trisphosphate (IP$_3$).
3. DAG activates PKC, initiating protein phosphorylation.
4. IP$_3$ promotes entry of Ca^{2+} into the cytosol where it binds to the cytoplasmic protein, calmodulin.
5. Ca^{2+}-calmodulin activates phosphorylase kinase, initiating phosphorylation to produce glucose via glycogenolysis.

Enzyme regulation of hepatic glycogenolysis

The rate-limiting step in glycogenolysis is catalysed by the enzyme glycogen phosphorylase. In the late 1930s, Carl and Gerti Cori discovered that there were two forms of the enzyme: a and b (Fig. 3.12):

- Phosphorylase-b is the inactive form and is activated to phosphorylase-a through phosphorylation. This reaction is regulated by a specific enzyme, phosphorylase kinase.
- Phosphorylase-a is the active form and is inactivated through reconversion to phosphorylase-b by dephosphorylation. Dephosphorylation is catalysed by a phosphate-releasing protein (phosphatase enzyme).

There are three mammalian glycogen phosphorylases, designated muscle, brain and liver isoenzymes according to the tissue in which they are preferentially expressed.

Regulation of hepatic glycogen phosphorylase

Activation of PKA sets off a series of phosphorylation reactions. In the liver, glycogen phosphorylase is very tightly controlled by phosphorylation (Fig. 3.12), as expected from an enzyme responding to extracellular signals involved in the maintenance of normoglycaemia, rather than responding to altered hepatic energy requirement. In addition, phosphorylase-a acts as a glucose receptor in the liver. When blood glucose concentration is high, direct binding of glucose to phosphorylase-a inactivates the enzyme by allosteric inhibition, which arrests glycogenolysis, a unique feature of the regulation of hepatic glycogenolysis.

Regulation of phosphorylase kinase by covalent modification – phosphorylation

Phosphorylase kinase is itself regulated by a phosphorylation-dephosphorylation mechanism:

- Dephosphorylation inactivates phosphorylase kinase, and is catalysed by a protein phosphatase that removes phosphate groups.

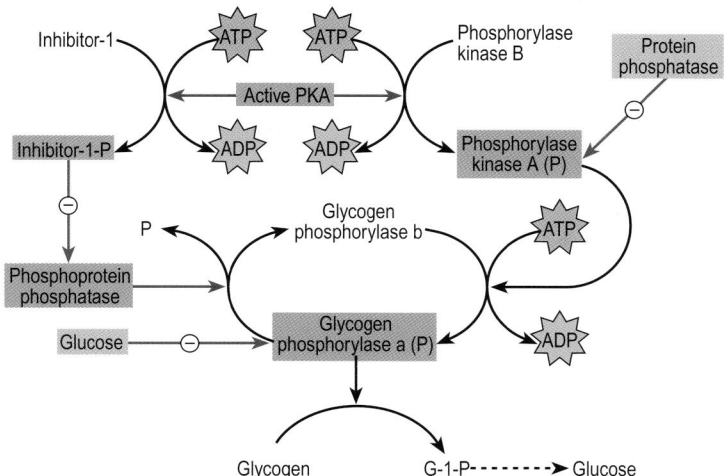

Fig. 3.12 **Regulation of hepatic glycogen phosphorylation.** Activated enzymes are shown in *red* and inhibitors are shown in *blue*.

- PKA catalyses the phosphorylation of hepatic phosphorylase kinase and activates it.

  PKA also phosphorylates glycogen-associated protein phosphatase 1 (PP1G), which inhibits the phosphoprotein phosphatases that would otherwise decrease the response to glucagon by reversing the phosphorylation of:

- Phosphorylase kinase
- Glycogen phosphorylase
- Glycogen synthase (see Fig. 3.9).

Amplification of the signalling cascade

Cyclic AMP regulates the activity of PKA, which is a key signalling enzyme in the interconversion of glycogen and glucose through the phosphorylation of phosphorylase kinase and glycogen synthase in the liver. PKA is very sensitive to small changes in cAMP concentration.

The activation of glycogen phosphorylase involves the phosphorylation and activation of many molecules of phosphorylase kinase by PKA (an example of a regulatory cascade).

Ca²⁺ as a second messenger

A subunit of phosphorylase kinase is functionally identical to the Ca²⁺-binding protein calmodulin (see Ch. 4). It acts as a Ca²⁺ receptor when there is an influx of Ca²⁺, activating phosphorylase kinase, and produces a conformational change.

Regulation of muscle and brain glycogenolysis

In contrast to liver, glycogenolysis in skeletal muscle is activated in response to increased energy requirement. Muscle cells lack glucagon receptors. Muscle glycogenolysis is activated by adrenaline via muscle β-adrenergic receptors acting via cAMP, mostly during 'flight or fight', but also during prolonged exercise.

Muscle glycogenolysis is also activated during short bursts of activity by two other mechanisms:

- In response to neural stimulation, Ca²⁺ enters the myocyte to activate unphosphorylated phosphorylase kinase by the Ca²⁺-calmodulin complex, which rapidly activates glycogenolysis. Muscle phosphorylase kinase

activity is thus coordinated with muscle contraction and associated with muscle calcium influx.
- Allosteric activation of phosphorylase by AMP: ATP is depleted during bursts of muscle contraction, leading to an accumulation of ADP. The enzyme myokinase (adenylate kinase) catalyses a reaction that converts part of the excess ADP to ATP and AMP:

$$2ADP \rightarrow ATP + AMP$$

The rapid rise in AMP concentration activates phosphorylase and the rate of glycogenolysis increases. Muscle and brain isoenzymes are allosterically:

- Activated by AMP, irrespective of whether they are phosphorylated or dephosphorylated.
- Inhibited by G6P.

Genetic defects in glycogenolysis

Disorders of glycogen metabolism occur when there are defects in the enzymes that enable glycogenolysis. These rare conditions, known as glycogen storage diseases (Clinical box 3.8), are inherited. All are autosomal recessive, presenting in childhood. The genes concerned may be expressed in either liver or muscle.

GLUCONEOGENESIS – GLUCOSE SYNTHESIS

- During starvation, hepatic glycogenolysis in the short term and gluconeogenesis in the longer term

Clinical box 3.8   Glycogen storage diseases

Glycogen storage diseases occur when liver or muscle enzyme defects lead to failure of glycogenolysis and excessive liver glycogen storage. Clinical features depend on the enzyme defect:

- Hypoglycaemia, in the absence of hepatic G6Pase, G6P cannot be converted to glucose and glycogen production will be promoted (fatal in neonates).
- Hepatomegaly results from excessive glycogen storage.
- Muscle weakness and cramps due to lack of glucose 1-phosphate for glycolysis and ATP production.

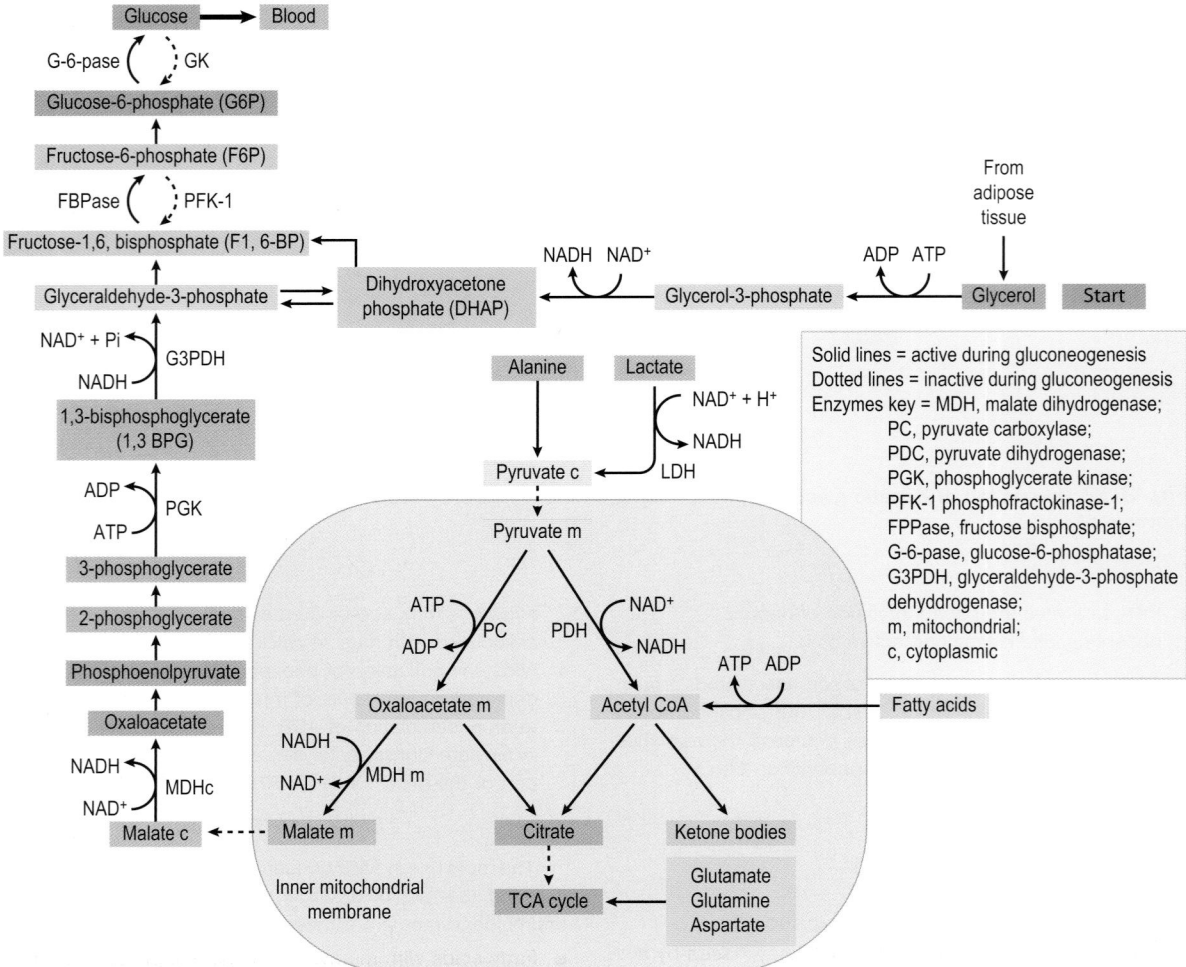

Fig. 3.13 Gluconeogenic pathway. Gluconeogenesis requires carbons to form the glucose skeleton and energy. The carbons are derived from lactose, alanine and glycerol. Energy is provided by the metabolism of fatty acids released by adipose tissue. Adapted with permission from Baynes J, Dominiczak M 2005 Medical Biochemistry, 2nd edn. Elsevier Mosby, Edinburgh.

compensates for the lack of glucose. Gluconeogenesis becomes increasingly important after hepatic glycogen is depleted.

These changes occur within 24 hours of fasting, depending on:

■ How well fed the individual was before the fast
■ How much hepatic glycogen was present
■ The amount of physical activity occurring during the fast.

Glycogenolysis cannot replace all the glucose oxidised by tissues in the post-absorptive period. Some new ('neo') glucose must be synthesised even at the expense of muscle protein breakdown. Gluconeogenesis is crucial for survival because of the continual fuel requirements of tissues that use only glucose as their primary energy substrate (e.g. brain in the short term, RBCs, kidney medulla, lens). For example, brain dysfunction occurs in hypoglycaemia; if severe, coma, death or (rarely) permanent brain damage may ensue. Therefore, even when fat may be supplying most of the energy requirements, a basal requirement for glucose has to be met. Furthermore, gluconeogenesis removes its products of metabolism from the blood (e.g. lactate). Lactate is generated in large quantities by glycolysis in RBCs and in anaerobically

exercising muscle. Elevated lactate concentrations are characteristic of impaired gluconeogenesis (Clinical box 3.9).

Precursors of gluconeogenesis

Gluconeogenesis occurs mainly in the liver and kidneys, requiring a source of carbon for the backbone of the glucose molecule and energy. Major carbon sources are (see Fig. 3.13):

■ Lactate from anaerobic glycolysis and exercising muscles
■ Gluconeogenic amino acids, including alanine from protein breakdown
■ Glycerol from triglyceride breakdown.

The main organs able to make glucose, by gluconeogenesis, are the liver and kidneys.

Gluconeogenesis from lactate

Gluconeogenesis from lactate is the reversal of glycolysis with three irreversible steps. Reversing the glycolysis pathway (see Figs 3.4 and 3.6), the irreversible steps are:

■ Last step in the generation of pyruvate, catalysed by pyruvate kinase

- Conversion of F6P to F-1,6-BP, catalysed by PFK-1
- First step in the conversion of glucose to G6P, catalysed by GK.

These reactions are all non-equilibrium, and therefore physiologically irreversible. The liver and kidney use four additional enzymes that bypass these reactions:

- Pyruvate carboxylase and phosphoenolpyruvate carboxykinase (PEPCK) bypass pyruvate kinase
- F-1,6-BPase bypasses PFK-1
- G6Pase bypasses glucokinase.

The pathway for gluconeogenesis from lactate involves both mitochondrial and cytosolic enzymes, and substrates have to be shuttled between the two intracellular areas.

Lactate is converted to pyruvate by LDH in the cytosol. NADH is generated from NAD^+ in this reaction, and this coenzyme is required for a subsequent step in the pathway (see Fig. 3.13).

1. Pyruvate enters the mitochondrion where it is converted into oxaloacetate by the intramitochondrial pyruvate carboxylase. Oxaloacetate is reduced to malate by mitochondrial malate dehydrogenase for export from the mitochondrion (see below, Malate shuttle, Fig. 3.25). Within the cytosol, malate is then reoxidised to oxaloacetate by cytosolic malate dehydrogenase. Cytosolic oxaloacetate is converted to phosphoenolpyruvate (PEP) by PEPCK.

   The high mitochondrial $NADH/NAD^+$ ratio generated from a brisk rate of β-oxidation of fatty acid facilitates the reduction reaction (see below, Lipid metabolism).

2. Gluconeogenesis proceeds in the reversal of glycolytic reactions to the next irreversible step, where F-1,6-BP has to be reconverted to F6P. PFK-1 is bypassed by a hydrolysis reaction catalysed by FBPase, without the production of ATP.

3. In the penultimate step, equivalent to the second step in glycolysis, phosphoglucose isomerase is freely reversible and functions in both glycolytic and gluconeogenic pathways. Finally, the irreversible GK is bypassed by the hydrolysis of G6P to glucose by G6Pase, again without the production of ATP. In the liver, the free glucose generated by G6Pase is then released into the blood by facilitated diffusion via GLUT2.

Gluconeogenesis from protein

The carbon atoms of gluconeogenic amino acids released by protein breakdown can be converted into glucose. The main amino acids used in gluconeogenesis are alanine and glutamine, from muscle protein hydrolysis. This protein breakdown is facilitated by low insulin levels when glucose is scarce.

The liver extracts alanine from blood, removes its amino nitrogen by transamination (see Fig. 3.17 below) to re-form pyruvate, and converts this via the gluconeogenic pathway to glucose, which is returned to the blood (as for gluconeogenesis from lactate; see above). Some of the glutamine released from muscle is used for energy by the gastrointestinal tract. The rest is converted to glucose in the renal cortex.

The carbon skeletons of amino acids can also be converted via TCA cycle intermediates to oxaloacetate, and malate is then released into the cytosol (see above – gluconeogenesis from lactate and Fig. 3.17 below).

| Clinical box 3.9 | **The rugby player who faints after three quick pints of beer has not fainted from alcohol excess but from hypoglycaemia** |

Hypoglycaemia after excessive alcohol intake can occur, and be severe, after prolonged and strenuous exercise, as in playing 80 minutes of rugby. At this stage, liver glycogen will have become depleted and blood glucose concentration is being maintained, in part, by gluconeogenesis from lactate accumulated during prolonged exercise. Dehydration and thirst after the game may, however, lead to the rapid consumption of pints, or litres, of beer containing alcohol. The alcohol is primarily metabolised in the liver, and competes with lactate for the coenzyme nicotinamide adenine diphosphate (NAD^+), needed for the conversion of lactate to pyruvate, before lactate can enter gluconeogenesis (see above). The metabolism of alcohol is poorly regulated, shifting the balance of metabolic reactions towards the metabolism of alcohol, reducing most of the available NAD^+ to NADH. Gluconeogenesis from lactate is inhibited, with an accumulation of lactate in the blood. Hypoglycaemia then ensues with sweaty, clammy skin, a rapid pulse and collapse.

Gluconeogenesis from glycerol

During nutrient scarcity, when glucose is in short supply, adipose tissue TAGs are broken down (hydrolysed) via lipolysis (see below). The products of adipose tissue lipolysis are fatty acids and free glycerol.

Most fatty acids in humans have straight chains with an even number of carbon atoms. Because acetyl-CoA and other intermediates of even-numbered fatty acid oxidation cannot be converted to oxaloacetate or any other intermediate of gluconeogenesis, it is impossible to synthesise glucose from such fatty acids. An exception to this general rule applies to:

- Fatty acids with methyl branches, e.g. phytanic acid, a breakdown product of chlorophyll
- Fatty acids with an odd number of carbon atoms – metabolism of these fatty acids yields the 3-C compound propionyl-CoA, which is a good, if minor, precursor for gluconeogenesis in humans
- Propionyl-CoA, which is also produced in the catabolism of the branched-chain amino acids valine and isoleucine, and in the conversion of cholesterol into bile acids.

Free glycerol liberated via activated lipolysis cannot be reutilised by adipose tissue to re-form TAG; it therefore diffuses out into the blood and can then be converted back to glucose by the liver and kidney. In times of nutrient excess, blood glucose entering glycolysis is the source of glycerol 3-phosphate, which is esterified in the synthesis of adipose tissue TAG. Glucose-glycerol cycling can therefore contribute to glucose homeostasis in starvation.

Glycerol enters gluconeogenesis at the level of the triose phosphates, with phosphorylation by glycerol kinase to form glycerol 3-phosphate. This is converted by glycerol 3-phosphate dehydrogenase to dihydroxyacetone phosphate (DHAP) for entry into the gluconeogenic pathway (see Fig. 3.13).

Peroxisome proliferator-activated receptors in energy homeostasis

From the foregoing, it seems clear that metabolism of the main metabolic fuels, glucose and fatty acids, follow dynamic, inter-related pathways in order to maintain energy balance. It has been shown that the associated chronic conditions hyperlipidaemia, insulin resistance, hypertension, obesity, athero-sclerosis and coronary heart disease (which make up the metabolic syndrome (also known as syndrome X), and can lead to type 2 diabetes) are the result of the interplay between changes in gene expression, nutrition and lifestyle. There is evidence to suggest that a family of nuclear receptors, the peroxisome proliferator-activated receptors (PPARs), have a major role in the control of glucose and fatty acid metabolism in energy homeostasis (see later Clinical box 3.22).

Energy for gluconeogenesis

Gluconeogenesis is an energy-requiring process. In the liver, oxidation of the fatty acids concomitantly generated by adipose tissue lipolysis provides most of the ATP required for gluconeogenesis. Metabolic conditions under which the liver is required to synthesise glucose favours the increased availability of fatty acids in the blood. Therefore prolonged fasting, malnutrition or starvation, whether voluntary or involuntary, are all characterised by loss of both adipose stores and muscle mass. Ketone bodies, the water-soluble products of fatty acids via hepatic ketogenesis, are an alternative source of energy during starvation.

Cori and glucose–alanine cycles

The Cori cycle refers to the inter-organ carbon recycling that takes place during hepatic gluconeogenesis from lactate. Lactate is formed continuously by tissues that lack mito-chondria or are anoxic. In addition, during prolonged fasting, skeletal muscle switches from the use of glucose to the use of lipid fuels as the primary oxidative fuel, and then it too releases lactate.

Alanine is a plentiful, simple amino acid. The glucose–alanine cycle moves carbon between tissues, like the Cori cycle, but also cycles nitrogen:

- Under conditions where muscle protein is being broken down (e.g. starvation), a proportion of available pyruvate is converted to alanine.
- Alanine, released from muscle into the blood, is converted in the liver to pyruvate, with removal of the amino group by transamination (see Fig. 3.17 below) to form urea for urinary excretion.

This prevents a build-up in muscle of nitrogen in the form of ammonium ions, which are toxic. Pyruvate can then enter gluconeogenesis and glucose can be returned to muscle for use in its various pathways.

Both Cori and glucose–alanine cycles depend on gluco-neogenesis in the liver, followed by glucose output and delivery to extrahepatic tissues. They can only operate between liver and tissues that can release either lactate (Cori cycle) or alanine (alanine cycle) as the end-products of glucose metabolism.

The Cori and glucose–alanine cycles are important because they ensure continued provision of substrate for gluconeogenesis. It should be emphasised that the Cori cycle does not provide carbon for net synthesis of glucose. Glucose formed from lactate merely recycles the carbon to the glucose to replace that which was converted to lactate by extrahepatic tissues.

Gluconeogenesis from sugars

Humans consume considerable quantities of fructose as one of the component sugars of the disaccharide sucrose (table sugar), which is composed of glucose and fructose. In the liver:

- Fructose is phosphorylated by an ATP-linked kinase, fructose kinase, to yield fructose-1-phosphate.
- A specific aldolase, fructose-1-phosphate aldolase, then cleaves fructose-1-phosphate to yield one molecule of DHAP and one of glyceraldehyde.
- Glyceraldehyde is reduced to glycerol for entry into gluconeogenesis via glycerol kinase.
  Two molecules of DHAP can either be converted:
- Into glucose via the gluconeogenic pathway, or
- Into pyruvate or lactate by glycolysis.

Gluconeogenesis also uses galactose as a precursor (Clinical box 3.10). Lactose (milk sugar), is a disaccharide composed of glucose and galactose. Galactose can be

---

> **Clinical box 3.10** **Some inborn errors of sugar metabolism**
>
> **Defects of fructose metabolism**
> Fructose is normally metabolised in the liver via glycolysis. Defects in fructose metabolism occur when essential enzymes in the metabolic pathway are deficient; such defects are inherited autosomal recessive conditions.
>
> - Fructose kinase deficiency leads to unconverted fructose being excreted in the urine – fructosuria, which is a benign condition, but carries a risk of early cataract formation, owing to high blood fructose concentrations.
> - In fructose intolerance, caused by fructose 1-phosphate aldolase deficiency, glycogenolysis and gluconeogenesis are decreased. This leads to hypoglycaemia; hepatomegaly and renal tubular damage may be associated features. This can be managed with a fructose- and sucrose-free diet. People with the genetic deficiency learn to avoid the discomfort caused by eating sweet food; children are very resistant to eating fruit and will not eat sweets. One advantage is that the incidence of dental caries is significantly reduced.
> - In F 1,6-BPase deficiency, failure of gluconeogenesis gives rise to hypoglycaemia, ketosis and lactic acidosis. This condition can cause death in infancy. About 50% present during the first few days of life with severe metabolic derangement. Early intervention with frequent carbohydrate feeds is the treatment of choice.
>
> **Galactosaemia**
> Galactosaemia, the accumulation of galactose in the blood, is an inherited, autosomal recessive condition in which there is deficiency in the enzymes that convert galactose to glucose. There are two main types, namely:
>
> - Galactokinase deficiency: this enzyme catalyses the first step in the conversion of galactose to glucose, when galactose-1-phosphate (Gal-1-P) is formed. Galactokinase deficiency leads to an accumulation of galactose in the blood, but causes less severe tissue damage.
> - Galactose-1-phosphate uridyl transferase deficiency: this mediates the conversion of galactose-1-phosphate (Gal-1-P) to G-6-P, a necessary step for the interconversion of galactose and glucose. Gal-1-P uridyl transferase deficiency leads to an accumulation of galactose and Gal-1-P in the blood.
>
> Galactokinase deficiency mainly causes cataracts. The transferase deficiency is much more severe. Feeding breast or cow's milk to infants with galactosaemia leads to vomiting and diarrhoea, failure to thrive, liver damage, cataracts and developmental delay. A galactose-free diet, as in formula milk containing sucrose instead of galactose, ameliorates the condition, but the child may still have poor growth, impaired speech and intellectual development, especially if diagnosis is delayed.

Clinical box 3.11   Metabolic defects in diabetes mellitus

The principal hormone defect in diabetes mellitus is a lack of insulin secretion from the pancreatic β-cells in type 1 diabetes, and insulin resistance and inadequate insulin secretion to combat hyperglycaemia in type 2 diabetes. Glucagon levels are inappropriately elevated for the increase in blood glucose. Knowledge of the defects in fuel metabolism due to insulin deficiency and the relative excess of glucagon is important for understanding the clinical features of diabetes mellitus.

Type 1 diabetes
- Results from the destruction of pancreatic β-cells due to the production of autoantibodies to β-cells, possibly related to an autoimmune reaction triggered by viral infection.
- No insulin, or only a trace amount, is secreted.
- Often diagnosed in childhood, but can be at any age. Latent autoimmune diabetes of adults (LADA) may be unrecognised and can develop in people with type 2 diabetes.
- Patients are dependent on exogenous insulin for survival.

Type 2 diabetes
- Insulin secretion is abnormal, but some β-cells are still active, with an inadequate response to glucose stimulation, relative to the degree of insulin resistance, which seems to be the primary defect.
- Normally diagnosed in middle age, but can occur in the young, even children.
- About half of the people with type 2 diabetes are unaware that they have the condition.

Clinical features of diabetes mellitus
The clinical features of type 1 and type 2 diabetes are similar, but with important differences. Some patients with type 2 diabetes may have no symptoms so that they are undiagnosed until they present with complications or are identified by incidental urine testing or blood glucose measurement. This is why some countries, such as the UK, recommend screening for type 2 diabetes so that patients can be identified before complications occur. The main clinical feature is a persistently elevated blood glucose concentration, hyperglycaemia. Increased glycogenolysis and gluconeogenesis are the major causes of hyperglycaemia.

Thirst and polyuria
Insulin deficiency leads to the inability of insulin-responsive tissues (e.g. muscle and adipose tissue) to take up glucose because transport into cells is impaired. Glycolysis and lipogenesis are thus inhibited; blood glucose concentration rises (hyperglycaemia). In addition, owing to inadequate insulin secretion by pancreatic β-cells, the insulin:glucagon ratio decreases, driving gluconeogenesis and further increasing blood glucose concentration. Hyperglycaemia in type 1 and many cases of type 2 diabetes causes the symptoms of:
- Excessive urination (polyuria) resulting from an osmotic diuresis caused by high blood glucose levels in blood and urine
- Thirst (polydipsia) due to loss of fluid.

Glucose tolerance curve in diabetes
In healthy subjects, blood glucose concentration rises sharply after a meal but falls to normal levels after 2 hours. In people with diabetes, this return to normal does not occur. Owing to insulin deficiency, glucose entry into cells is impaired, so that glycolysis cannot take place to maintain cellular energy. Hepatic glycogenolysis, lipolysis and gluconeogenesis are stimulated to generate increased levels of endogenous glucose. Together with impaired glucose transport, increasing amounts of glucose remain in the blood, leading to sustained hyperglycaemia after meals, characterised by the diabetic glucose tolerance curve. In the long term (after years), fasting hyperglycaemia occurs.

Metabolic ketoacidosis and ketonuria
The shift in the insulin:glucagon balance leads to unopposed lipolysis and fatty acid oxidation in the liver. This leads to the accumulation of excess acetyl-CoA, which stimulates the ketogenic pathway in the liver. When insulin secretion becomes inadequate to maintain anti-lipolysis in the fat stores, or under acute metabolic stress, the rising levels of ketone bodies (e.g. β-hydroxybutyrate and acetoacetate) lowers blood pH and causes life-threatening ketoacidosis. Ketonuria develops if renal function remains normal. Ketoacidosis is more common in type 1 diabetes, either at presentation or when insulin is omitted. Although less common in type 2 diabetes, metabolic acidosis can develop during stress, e.g. myocardial infarction.

Microvascular and macrovascular disease
Increased fat breakdown results in raised plasma lipoprotein concentration (either low-density lipoproteins (LDLs) or very-low-density lipoproteins (VLDLs), which eventually leads to atheroma formation and subsequent arterial narrowing. In diabetes with poor glycaemic control, the resultant ischaemic organ damage leads to the long-term vascular complications of diabetes, depending on the size and site of the arteries affected:
- Macrovascular disease (larger arteries) gives rise to peripheral vascular disease and a high risk of coronary arterial disease. Renal artery stenosis may lead to hypertension.
- Microvascular disease (arterioles, capillaries): damage to the glomerular basement membrane leads to renal damage and results in hypertension. In diabetic retinopathy, microaneurysms and haemorrhages lead to leaking blood vessels and new vessel formation; macula oedema and degeneration, and ischaemia can lead to visual impairment and eventual blindness. Restricted blood supply to peripheral nerves may be a factor in peripheral neuropathy.

Clinical features resulting from glycated protein
Glucose entry into some tissues is independent of insulin (e.g. red blood cells, lens). For some other tissues (e.g. liver, renal, peripheral nerves and brain), glucose entry can be insulin independent or dependent. The persistent, very high intracellular glucose level leads to non-enzymic attachment of glucose to proteins (protein glycation, the Maillard reaction). Protein structures become altered to form advanced glycation end-products (AGE). Typical sites of glycated protein are in:
- Lens, leading to opacities, the formation of cataracts and impaired vision
- Renal glomeruli, leading to albuminuria, glomerulosclerosis and eventually renal failure
- Vessels supplying peripheral nerves, a further contribution to peripheral neuropathy.

The glycated protein in haemoglobin is the basis for the measurement of glycosylated haemoglobin (HbA1c), which gives a guide to glycaemic control over the previous 6 weeks in both type 1 and type 2 diabetes.

---

enzymically converted to glucose by galactose kinase, and is an important source of glucose in the human diet, particularly for infants.

Regulation of gluconeogenesis

The pathways of hepatic glycolysis and gluconeogenesis are tightly controlled and counter-regulated by enzymes under the control of insulin and glucagon. This is to ensure that the glucose from gluconeogenesis is not used up by hepatic glycolysis but released into the blood stream for glycaemic control. A lowering of blood sugar concentration lowers insulin secretion, but increases glucagon secretion. Thus the insulin:glucagon ratio in the blood:

- Decreases with falling blood glucose, stimulating gluconeogenesis increases with rising blood glucose, and the shift in the insulin:glucagon balance in diabetes leads to unopposed lipolysis (Clinical box 3.10).

The glycolysis/gluconeogenesis pathways are antagonistic, so if they operated simultaneously at the same rate, there would be no net production of glucose for export from the liver. This situation would create a 'futile cycle' so called because the expended ATP is 'wasted'. However, normally one pathway prevails over the other.

AMINO ACID METABOLISM

In contrast to carbohydrates and fats, amino acids are not stored in designated sites in the human body. Although protein is not a major metabolic fuel under normal conditions, amino acids have key roles in human metabolism.

- Amino acids are a source of metabolic energy – in starvation, muscle protein can be broken down to keto acids for gluconeogenesis to maintain blood glucose concentration.
- The carbon skeletons of amino acids are the building blocks for the biosynthesis of all proteins and other important biomolecules (e.g. nucleotides) essential for cell growth, and haem.
- The carbon skeletons of amino acids are precursors of neurotransmitters, hormones and other important biomolecules (e.g. thyroxine, adrenaline (epinephrine), 5-hydroxytryptamine and melanin).
- Some amino acids are metabolised to form precursors of lipids and ketone bodies (see below, Lipogenesis).
- The carbon atoms of some amino acids may be used to produce energy via oxidative metabolism in the later stages of glycolysis and in the TCA cycle.

METABOLIC CLASSES OF AMINO ACIDS

Twenty amino acids are needed for human protein synthesis (see Ch. 2) (Fig. 3.14):

- Non-essential amino acids can be endogenously synthesised, using the carbon skeletons from metabolism.
- Essential amino acids cannot be endogenously synthesised. There are 10 of these amino acids, which have to be present in the diet (see Chs 2 and 16).

Another way of classifying amino acids depends on their ability to be converted to glucose or lipids. Because the body does not have protein stores, amino acid metabolism is dynamic. The carbon skeletons of amino acids are used in central metabolic pathways for energy production in oxidative metabolism. Any excess (and amino acids during starvation) is converted in one of two ways:

- Gluconeogenic amino acids are converted by gluconeogenesis to glucose, which may be released into the blood or stored as glycogen.
- Ketogenic amino acids are oxidised to acetyl-CoA or acetoacetate, and then converted to precursors of ketone bodies and lipids (see below, Lipogenesis).

ABSORPTION OF AMINO ACIDS

After a meal, dietary protein is hydrolysed to:

- Peptides (containing two or three amino acid residues)
- Free amino acids.

The peptides are transported into intestinal epithelial cells (enterocytes) by specific membrane transporters and then rapidly hydrolysed to free amino acids within the cells (see Ch. 15). The uptake of free amino acids from the gut is analo-

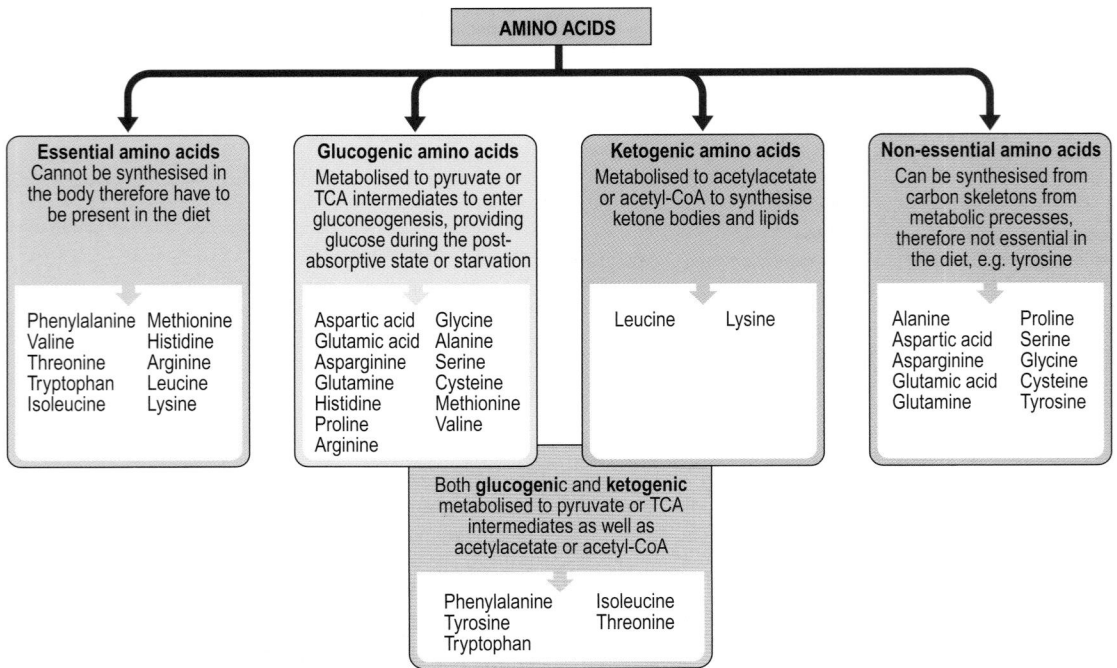

Fig. 3.14 **Metabolic classes of amino acids.**

gous to the uptake of glucose. It is worth noting that di- and tri-peptides are more rapidly absorbed than the amino acids themselves. Not all amino acids are released from the enterocytes into the portal vein blood.

■ Dietary glutamine, derived from glutamic acid, is the major fuel of the intestine and is oxidised by enterocytes in preference to glucose to provide the energy needed for the intestinal absorption of digestion products.
■ Dietary aspartate and glutamate are also used in enterocyte metabolism.

As aspartate, glutamate, and glutamine metabolism produce alanine, much more alanine appears in the portal vein blood after feeding than was originally present in the ingested protein. Thus, intestinally absorbed glucose is spared for the rest of the body and the alanine produced can be converted to glucose (see above, Gluconeogenesis).

NITROGEN IN AMINO ACID METABOLISM

The nitrogen component, the α-amino group of amino acids, has to be removed before the carbon skeleton can be metabolised (see Ch. 2). This is achieved by:

■ Transamination (Fig. 3.15) – the transfer of the amino group to a corresponding α-keto acid acceptor

or

■ Deamination, the oxidative removal of the amino group to give oxo acids, releasing ammonia (NH_3).

Transamination

Transamination is a reversible reaction catalysed by enzymes known as aminotransferases (transaminases) (Clinical box 3.12).

The process of transamination merely removes nitrogen in the form of an amino group from the amino acid donor to a suitable corresponding α-oxo acid acceptor. Conversely, amino groups can be added to the appropriate carbon skeleton to synthesise non-essential amino acids. This takes place through the transamination of the α-keto acid corresponding to that amino acid.

Aminotransferases are specific for particular amino acids, but most of them will transfer amino groups:

■ Most commonly to 2-oxoglutarate (α-ketoglutarate) to form glutamate
■ To a lesser extent to oxaloacetate to give aspartate.

In some skeletal muscle, pyruvate can act as an amino acceptor to form alanine, which is transported to the liver where it may either be used for protein synthesis or undergo transamination in the opposite direction to release NH_3 that enters the urea cycle. The liberated pyruvate then participates in gluconeogenesis.

Glutamine is synthesised from malate from the TCA cycle, when malate accepts amino nitrogen from skeletal muscle breakdown. Alanine and glutamine thus transport amino groups from the tissues to the liver.

Clinical box 3.12   **Transaminase enzymes as clinical markers of cell damage**

Plasma transaminase levels rise when there is liver cell damage, allowing the enzymes to leak into the blood.

● Aspartate aminotransferase (AST) is a mitochondrial enzyme.
● Alanine transaminase (ALT) is a cytosolic enzyme.

These enzymes are used as clinical markers of liver cell damage. Their serum levels are raised in various forms of cellular liver disease.

AST is also present in heart and skeletal muscle, kidney and brain cells, so high levels in blood plasma may also be seen in muscle damage, e.g. myocardial infarction or rhabdomyolysis (muscle injury).

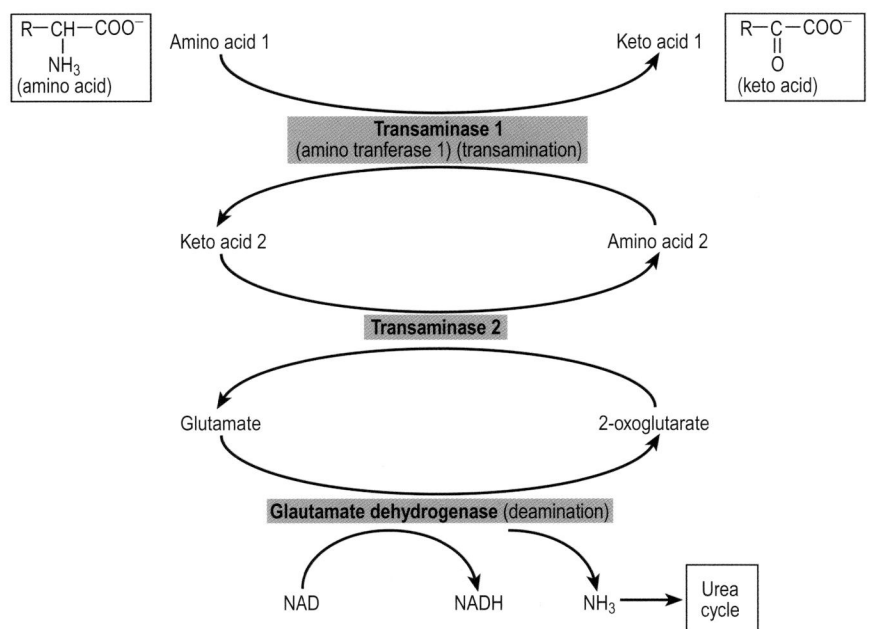

Fig. 3.15 **Conversion of surplus amino groups to ammonia (NH_3).**

Amino acid release by skeletal muscle in the post-absorptive state

In the post-absorptive state, two amino acids – alanine and glutamine – are released from skeletal muscle in large amounts (over 50% of the amino acid outflow). This does not reflect their relative concentration in muscle protein; rather, that other amino acid residues present in muscle protein are metabolised to give intermediates, pyruvate and 2-oxoglutarate, which accept amino groups to yield alanine and glutamine, respectively (see Fig. 3.17).

Branched-chain amino acids are a major source of nitrogen for the production of alanine and glutamine in muscle. They are oxidised within the muscles for energy, and the nitrogen is removed and trapped for disposal by this conversion of pyruvate to alanine. The alanine is released into the blood via amino acid membrane transporters.

Branched-chain α-keto acids produced from the branched-chain amino acids by transamination are partially released into the blood. These are taken up by the liver, which synthesises:

- Glucose from the keto acid of valine
- Ketone bodies from the keto acid of leucine
- Both glucose and ketone bodies from the keto acid of isoleucine.

Deamination

The α-amino group is finally removed from an amino acid molecule through deamination, although to a lesser extent than occurs with transamination. Deamination is the oxidative removal of the amino group from the amino acid molecule by amino acid oxidases. This activity results in the release of keto acids and NH$_3$. Glutamate (from hydrolysis of glutamine), the commonest intermediate in nitrogen removal, is oxidatively deaminated by glutamate dehydrogenase to form 2-oxoglutarate and ammonia (NH$_3$) (see Fig. 3.15). The NH$_3$ enters the urea cycle in the liver.

Glutamine in acid–base homeostasis

Maintaining blood pH at a constant 7.4 is a coordinated activity by the liver, kidneys and lungs (see Ch. 14). One of the mechanisms for acid–base homeostasis uses the products of amino acid breakdown. In an alternative pathway to the ones in liver and skeletal muscle, glutamine is hydrolysed by glutaminase to glutamate and ammonium ion (NH$_4^+$) in the proximal renal tubules. Glutamate is subsequently oxidised to 2-oxaloglutarate and more NH$_4^+$ is generated. NH$_4^+$ in these two steps is positively charged and water soluble. Some NH$_4^+$ is secreted into the tubular lumen, the rest is diverted to the liver, where one molecule of NH$_4^+$ and one of bicarbonate (HCO$_3^-$) combine to form carbamoyl phosphate,

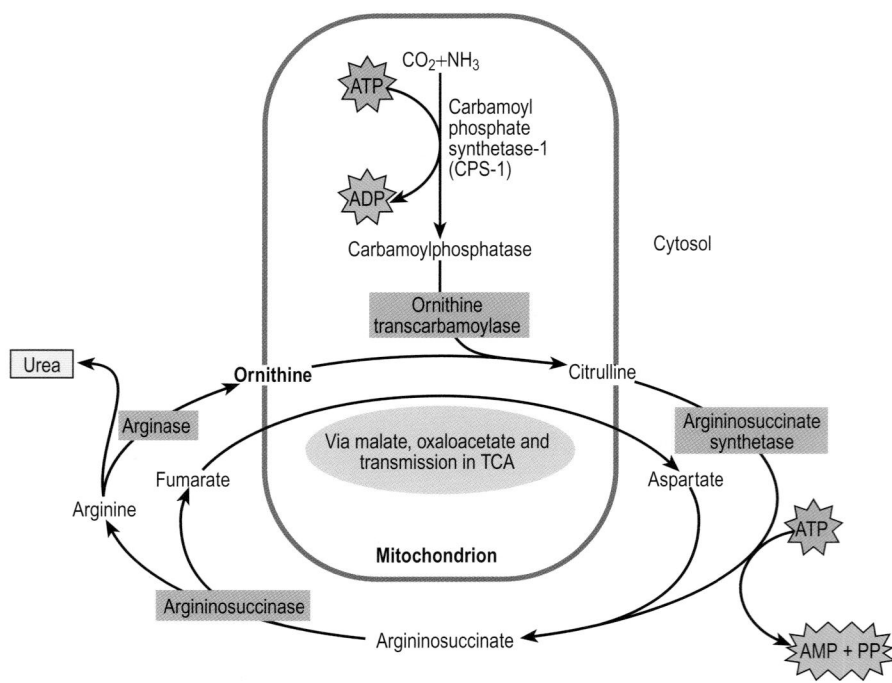

Fig. 3.16 **The urea cycle.**

In many forms of acidosis, glutaminase is upregulated so that more NH$_4^+$ appears. This excess NH$_4^+$ is diverted from the liver where it would normally be converted to urea. Urine has a minimum pH of 4.5 to be compatible with life. It is more acid than blood (pH 7.4), so a pH gradient is established between urine and blood. At the minimum urine pH of 4.5, the pH gradient is markedly increased, so increasing the NH$_4^+$ gradient between urine and blood. Urinary NH$_4^+$ excretion increases. In diabetic ketoacidosis, for example, urinary NH$_4^+$ excretion can increase from 50 mmol/24 h to 200–500 mmol/24 h (up to 10-fold). This urinary excretion of NH$_4^+$ deprives the liver of the opportunity to consume HCO$_3^-$ in urea synthesis. Thus, the HCO$_3^-$ derived from the peripheral oxidation of amino acid skeletons (see above) remains unconsumed, and tends to counteract the metabolic acidosis.

Clinical box 3.14   NH$_3$-induced encephalopathy

Although the mechanism is not well understood, NH$_3$ in the blood diffuses into cells and crosses the blood–brain barrier and is associated with encephalopathy (a brain disorder). Even low concentrations are neurotoxic. The uptake of NH$_3$ by the brain causes glutamate to be converted to glutamine, resulting in glutamate deficiency.

Glutamate is an important excitatory neurotransmitter and the encephalopathy is associated with glutamate deficiency. Decreased levels of γ-aminobutyric acid (GABA), which is synthesised from glutamate, also results. GABA is an important inhibitory neurotransmitter (see Chs 4 and 8).

Enzyme defects in infants leading to excessive accumulation of NH$_3$ result in life-threatening cerebral oedema requiring haemodialysis.

which starts off the urea cycle (see below and Fig. 3.16). The HCO$_3^-$ consumed in the liver in this way deals with the major quantity of HCO$_3^-$ derived from oxidation of amino acid carbon skeletons, thus regulating acid–base status.

Ammonia

The waste product of the deamination process is NH$_3$, which is associated with toxicity (Clinical box 3.14). NH$_3$ is usually rapidly converted to urea via the urea cycle.

Urea cycle

Urea synthesis takes place in the liver, involving both mitochondrial and cytosolic reactions. A key compound in the urea cycle (Fig. 3.16) is ornithine, which is derived from the dietary and endogenously derived amino acid arginine. Arginine is split by the enzyme arginase to yield ornithine and urea.

The urea cycle generates new urea molecules from recycled ornithine. Urea is excreted; all other intermediates in the urea cycle are recycled.

- Carbamoyl phosphate is synthesised from NH$_3$, CO$_2$ and ATP in the hepatic mitochondria, catalysed by carbamoyl phosphate synthetase 1 (CPS-1).
- Cytosolic ornithine is transported to the mitochondrion where it condenses with carbamoyl phosphate to form citrulline, catalysed by ornithine transcarbamoylase.
- Citrulline diffuses into the cytosol where it condenses with aspartate to form argininosuccinate, catalysed by argininosuccinate synthetase and requiring ATP.

Clinical box 3.15   Urea cycle defects

A number of enzyme defects in the urea cycle have been identified. Apart from ornithine transcarbamoylase deficiency, which has an X-linked dominant inheritance, they are autosomal recessive.

Carbamoyl phosphate synthetase (CPS-1) deficiency
- The most severe form of urea cycle defect (UCD)
- Symptoms (vomiting, poor feeding, convulsions, ataxia, coma) are due to the high levels of NH$_3$ (hyperammonaemia), and begin immediately after birth when the fetal and maternal circulations are separated.
- Invariably fatal within a few days if undiagnosed and untreated.

Deficiency in other enzymes of the urea cycle
- Deficiency in other enzymes of the urea cycle – ornithine transcarbamylase, argininosuccinate synthetase, argininosuccinase, arginase
- Give rise to varying degrees of hyperammonaemia.

Treatment of urea cycle defects
- Restriction of dietary protein
- Removal of NH$_3$ (e.g. antibiotics to eliminate NH3-producing intestinal bacteria, drugs such as benzoate and phenylacetate to promote the excretion of NH$_3$ nitrogen in faeces).
- Replacement of missing urea cycle intermediates by intravenous infusion.

- Argininosuccinate is split into arginine and fumarate by argininosuccinase.
- Arginine is split by arginase to give urea, regenerating ornithine, which re-enters the urea cycle.
- Aspartate, re-used for condensation with citrulline, is regenerated from fumarate.

The urea diffuses into the blood to be transported to the kidneys for excretion in urine. Note that ornithine and citrulline are amino acids that are not part of the set of 20 amino acids used for protein synthesis.

The urea cycle intersects with the TCA cycle at the point where fumarate branches off in the conversion of argininosuccinate to arginine. Some fumarate is converted to malate by the enzyme fumarase, then to oxaloacetate through the action of malate dehydrogenase. Oxaloacetate is then transaminated to aspartate by AST (see Fig. 3.16).

Regulation of the urea cycle

In the short term, the urea cycle is rate limited by the allosteric activator for mitochondrial CPS-1, N-acetylglutamate. The function of the urea cycle is to:

- Remove surplus nitrogen
- To consume bicarbonate generated in peripheral tissues (see above).

The urea cycle is controlled through regulation of the activity of its various enzymes via regulation of gene expression. For example, glucagon and glucocorticoids interact with various receptors to form complexes that interact with the promoter region of the CPS-1 gene (Clinical box 3.15). The enzyme CPS-1 concentration:

- Rises on high-protein diets and during starvation when proteins are degraded to provide carbon skeletons for energy, thereby increasing the amount of surplus nitrogen to be excreted
- Declines with more normal, balanced diets.

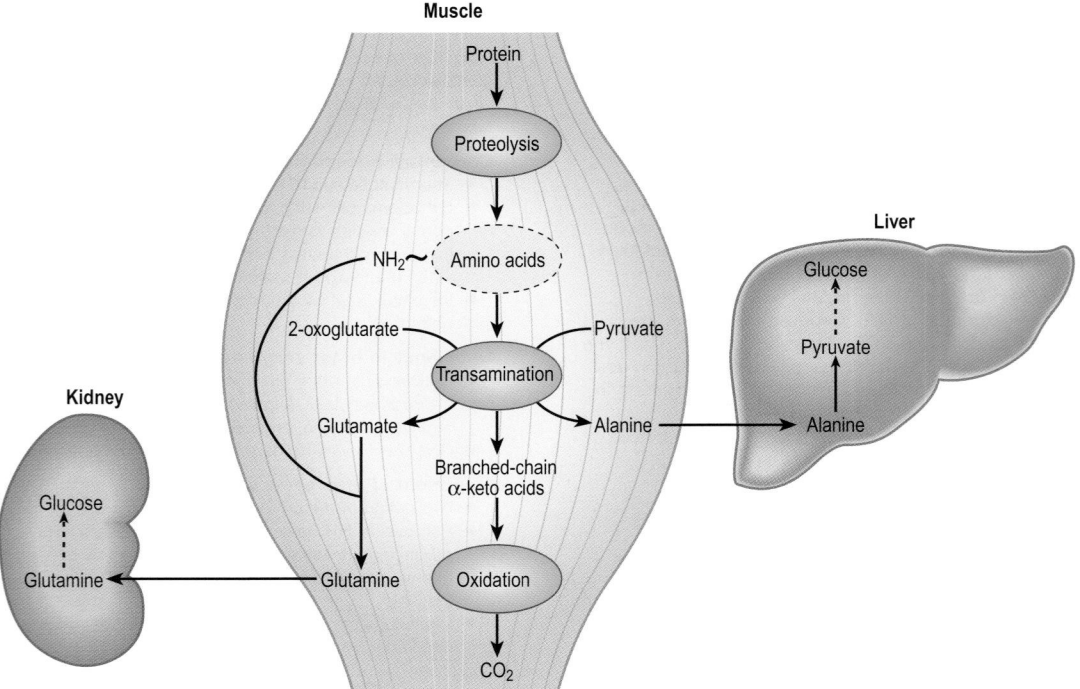

Muscle

Liver

Kidney

Fig. 3.17 Flux of key amino acids in relation to gluconeogenesis.

Nitrogen balance

The continuous turnover of amino acids, proteins and nucleic acids in healthy human beings underpins the concept of nitrogen balance, in which dietary intake and excretion of nitrogen are approximately equal (see Ch. 16).

- Positive nitrogen balance takes place when the body receives more nitrogen than it excretes, as in healing wounds, growth and pregnancy.
- Negative nitrogen balance occurs in protein malnutrition, severe exercise or starvation, when muscle protein is degraded to carbon skeletons for gluconeogenesis, so that more nitrogen is lost than is taken in.

AMINO ACIDS IN GLUCONEOGENESIS

Fig. 3.17 sets out the flux of key amino acids in gluconeogenesis. Nearly all the carbons can be converted to intermediates for entry into:

- Glucogenesis or ketogenesis
- The TCA cycle
- Lipogenesis.

There are complex inter-relationships between amino acid, glucose and lipid metabolism. Most amino acid nitrogen ends up in the liver (see Information box 3.10), having either been generated there or reached there from muscle or from intestinal cells, and is converted to urea for excretion by the kidneys in urine.

ESSENTIAL AMINO ACIDS

Some individual amino acids must be conserved for protein synthesis because, apart from collagen, all 20 of those that

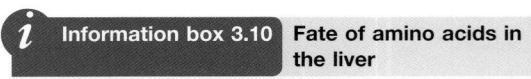

Information box 3.10 **Fate of amino acids in the liver**

In the well-fed state

- Carbon skeletons of excess amino acids are eventually used for ATP production.
- Glucogenic amino acids are converted to glucose, which may be stored as glycogen.
- Ketogenic amino acids are converted to lipids and transported to adipose tissue, ultimately to be stored as fat (see below).

In the fasting state

- Incoming amino acids are used for glucose production.

form proteins must be present together for protein synthesis. This applies particularly to the essential amino acids, which cannot be synthesised fast enough for requirements in the body and must be obtained from food (see Fig. 3.14 and Ch. 16).

The hepatic extraction of the branched-chain amino acids that cannot be synthesised by humans is less than the extraction of the other amino acids. Furthermore, although used for hepatic protein synthesis, these essential amino acids are not degraded to any great extent by the liver, and so they are found in higher concentrations in peripheral blood than other amino acids. Whereas they typically constitute about 15–20% of dietary protein, valine, leucine and isoleucine represent at least 70% of the total amino acids entering the general circulation after a meal.

Valine, leucine and isoleucine are, therefore, taken up by skeletal muscle to a greater extent than the other amino acids, accounting for 60–80% of the total amino acid uptake by muscle. Branched-chain amino acids that are not used

Clinical box 3.16   Inborn errors of amino acid metabolism

Inborn errors of amino acid metabolism can be due to:

- Enzyme defects in the urea cycle
- Deficiencies in the enzymes involved in the metabolism of the carbon skeletons of various amino acids.
- Inherited autosomal recessive disorders (most are this).

Phenylketonuria (PKU)
- Deficiency of phenylalanine hydroxylase, an enzyme required for tyrosine synthesis (see Ch. 2).
- Untreated individuals excrete phenylpyruvate and phenylacetate in the urine, and develop brain damage, mental retardation and epilepsy.
- The rate of incidence of around 1 in 20 000 births in the UK and USA is one of the reasons for screening infants soon after birth.
- Dietary control by restricting phenylalanine, and giving tyrosine supplementation, is successful, but there is generally some limitation of intellectual development.

Alkaptonuria (also known as black urine disease)
- Deficiency of **homogentisic acid oxidase**. Homogentisic acid is an intermediate metabolite in the breakdown of phenylalanine and tyrosine.
- Very rare condition, occurring in about 1:1 000 000 births.
- Homogentisic acid accumulates and is excreted in the urine, which turns a black-brown colour on standing.
- Deposition of the pigment in cartilage and other tissues causes distinctive (sometimes visible) brown discoloration (ochronosis), and tissue damage leading to arthritis.

Maple syrup urine disease
- Rare condition (1 in 300 000 births in the USA)
- Related to metabolism of branched-chain amino acids, leucine, valine and isoleucine.
- After transamination, the resulting keto acid is normally decarboxylated with a **keto acid decarboxylase**. A defect in this enzyme results in an accumulation of keto acids, giving a characteristic 'maple syrup' smell to the urine.
- Clinically, the infant suffers fits, neonatal acidosis and severe brain damage, leading to early death. There is no effective treatment.

Albinism
Albinism is a benign condition.

- Deficiency of tyrosinase, an enzyme catalysing the hydroxylation of tyrosine to dihydroxyphenylalanine (DOPA), a precursor of the skin pigment melanin.
- Results in amelanosis: a lack of colour in the skin, hair and irises (pinkish), and a risk of damage by sunlight.
- Although DOPA is an intermediate in the synthesis of neurotransmitters (see Ch. 2), there are no neurological defects.

Clinical box 3.17   Chinese restaurant syndrome

The Chinese restaurant syndrome, also known as Kwok's Quease, is a syndrome that occurs in some individuals after a meal. Only a very few individuals are susceptible. Symptoms include:

- Sudden onset of temporary headache, sweating and nausea after a meal in a Chinese restaurant.
- Attributed to the high content of monosodium glutamate (MSG) used in Chinese cuisine, and may be due to the action of glutamate or its derivative, GABA, on the CNS.
- No permanent damage has been demonstrated, although it can trigger bronchospasm in people with severe asthma.

Amino acids as neurotransmitters

Glutamate is an excitatory transmitter in the central nervous system (CNS), transported into neurons and glial cells. γ-Aminobutyric acid (GABA), the major inhibitory transmitter in the brain is synthesised from glutamate by glutamate decarboxylase (Clinical box 3.17). Glycine also acts as a neurotransmitter in the spinal cord.

Amino acids as precursors of neurotransmitters and hormones

The hormones adrenaline and noradrenaline (epinephrine and norepinephrine) are derived from the amino acid tyrosine. Their mode of action is described in Chapter 4.

- Dopamine is an intermediate metabolite in the synthesis of adrenaline and noradrenaline, and is also a neurotransmitter. It acts on the basal ganglia to control voluntary movement, and its deficiency is associated with the tremor and difficulties in the initiation and control of movement in Parkinson's disease.
- Tyrosine is also a precursor of thyroid hormones (see Ch. 10).
- Serotonin (5-hydroxytryptamine) is derived from the amino acid tryptophan and affects mood (see Ch. 8).

LIPID METABOLISM

Apart from cells that contain few mitochondria, such as red cells and neural cells, which can use only glucose as metabolic fuel, lipids are the major and immediate source of energy in liver, muscle, kidney and other tissues. The term 'lipids' includes triacylglycerols (TAGs; also known as triglycerides), phospholipids and glycolipids.

TAG is constructed from fatty acids and glycerol (a 3-carbon, sugar alcohol) by a process of 'esterification'. Non-esterified fats are known as 'free' fatty acids (FFA) and are the major fuel for metabolism (see Ch. 2). They are an immediate source of energy, and their importance as metabolic fuels arises because their oxidation yields much more ATP than the oxidation of either carbohydrate or protein (see below).

Lipids also contribute to the construction of cell membranes and intracellular membranes. Therefore, in addition to their functions as energy substrate, lipids are important for:

- Maintenance of the integrity of lung alveoli (surfactant, see Ch. 13)

for protein synthesis can be oxidised in the muscles to provide energy. The use of the branched-chain amino acids preferentially by muscle underlies their inclusion in parenteral feeding solutions for patients in situations of negative nitrogen balance (e.g. stress, trauma, burns), where there is excessive protein breakdown (see Ch. 16).

AMINO ACIDS AND SIGNALLING MOLECULES

Certain derivatives of amino acids are precursors for neurotransmitters and hormones. Some amino acids, notably glutamate and glycine, act directly as neurotransmitters. Others undergo metabolism to form neurotransmitters or hormones.

- Solubilisation of non-polar substances in body fluids
- Metabolic and cellular regulation (e.g. steroid hormones and the prostaglandins).

SOURCES OF FATTY ACIDS

In humans, most fatty acids are supplied as dietary TAG (90%), the remainder being made up of cholesterol, cholesteryl esters, non-esterified fatty acids and phospholipids. TAGs are broken down to fatty acids via lipolysis. Humans are unable to synthesise or desaturate polyunsaturated fatty acids (PUFA) with particular complex structures (e.g. linoleic and linolenic acids) (see Ch. 2). These PUFAs, known as essential fatty acids, are required for specific functions, including:

- synthesis of eicosanoids (biologically active derivatives of arachidonic acid, found in cell membranes, with hormone-like functions)
- actions as second messengers (diacylglycerol).

Essential fatty acids such as n-3PUFA and n-6PUFA, must be present in the diet or synthesised from other dietary fatty acids. They can be obtained from dietary plant or fish oils (see Ch. 16).

Dietary fatty acids

Dietary fats are digested by pancreatic enzymes (lipases) in the intestine to form free fatty acids, monoacylglycerols and glycerol, which are absorbed into the enterocytes. The enterocyte re-esterifies the free fatty acids and monoacylglycerols to synthesise TAG. Chylomicrons are then assembled from the TAG, together with cholesterol, apolipoproteins and phospholipids (see later).

Endogenously synthesised fatty acids

Humans can synthesise fatty acids from intermediates derived from the breakdown of sugars (glucose, fructose), some amino acids and other fatty acids. In general, the de novo synthesis pathway is primarily used under conditions of excess carbohydrate intake. Carbohydrate is converted to fatty acids in the liver and stored as TAG in adipose tissue.

- Fatty acids used for hepatic TAG synthesis are released from white adipose tissue TAG stores by lipolysis (see Storage of lipids below).
- In adipose tissue, lipoprotein-derived fatty acids are used almost exclusively for TAG synthesis (for storage). These are predominantly derived from dietary TAGs in circulating chylomicrons (Fig. 3.18).
- The liver is the major site of fatty acid synthesis.

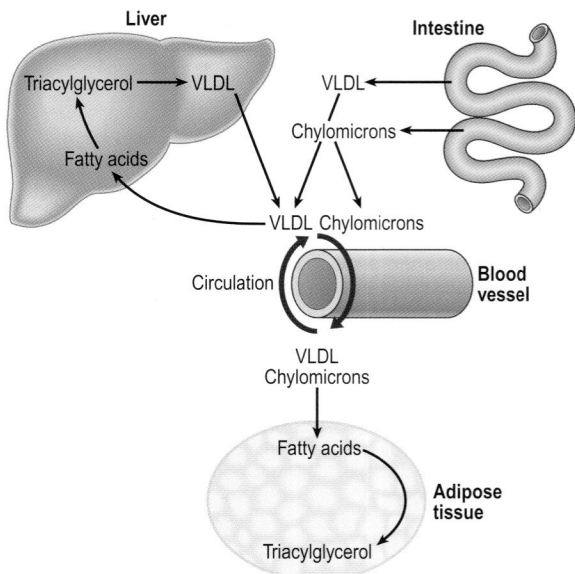

Fig. 3.18 Lipid homeostasis in the fed state. VLDL, very-low-density lipoprotein.

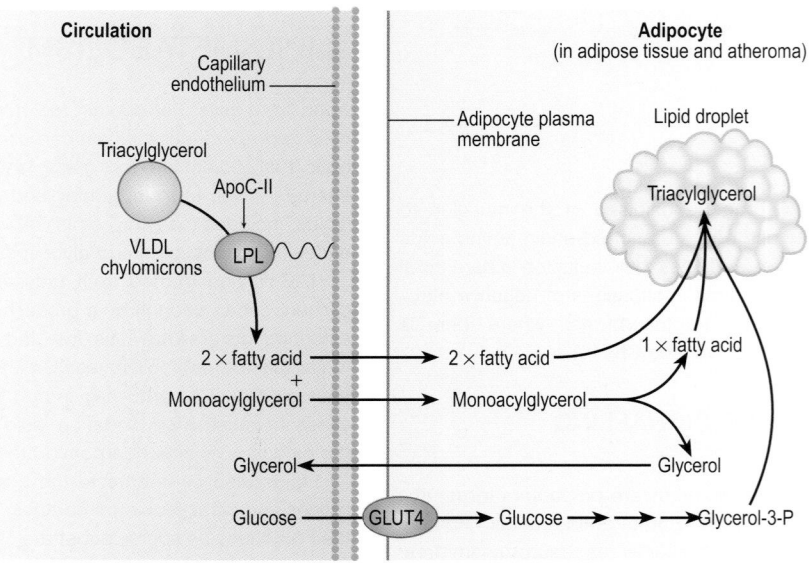

Fig. 3.19 Pathway of triacylglycerol uptake and storage by adipose tissue. LPL, lipoprotein lipase; VLDL, very-low-density lipoprotein; ApoC-II, apolipoprotein CII.

STORAGE OF LIPIDS

Fat metabolism is controlled primarily by the rate of stored TAG breakdown (lipolysis) although there is also local generation of fatty acids from circulating lipoproteins by the enzyme lipoprotein lipase (LPL) (Fig. 3.19).

The fatty acids used for adipose tissue TAG synthesis are derived from TAG contained in chylomicrons and very-low-density lipoproteins (VLDLs; see below), acted upon by LPL. Adipose tissue LPL is found attached to the basement membrane glycoproteins of capillary endothelial cells.

- LPL hydrolyses fatty acids from the 1 and/or 3 position of triacylglycerols and diacylglycerols present in VLDLs and chylomicrons.
- Apolipoprotein C-II must be present within the lipid particles to activate LPL. A deficiency in apolipoprotein C-II leads to increased plasma TAG levels (see below).
- Adipocyte LPL generates fatty acids locally for direct uptake and use by the adipocyte, without entering the general circulation.
- A rise in plasma insulin stimulates adipocyte LPL to release fatty acids from chylomicrons and VLDLs.

FATTY ACIDS

Lipids contain a mixture of fatty acids of different chain length, degree of saturation and branching (see Ch. 2). In contrast to carbohydrates, which are converted to water-soluble glucose, lipid fuels have to be transported by processes that are specific for varying chain lengths. In humans, lipids are catabolised only through oxidative processes, which take place primarily in the mitochondria and also occur in peroxisomes.

Non-esterified (or free) fatty acids (FFA), may be:

- Derived from dietary fats
- Endogenously synthesised de novo when there is energy excess (see below).

FFAs are not water soluble. Their soap-like detergent effect would dissolve lipid cellular and intracellular membranes. This is avoided as fatty acids are transported:

- Bound to albumin, in the blood
- Esterified as TAG for transport between tissues and organs, and for storage.
- In lipoproteins (TAGs are highly hydrophobic, i.e. insoluble in water; see below).

Protein-bound fatty acids

In plasma, fatty acids are bound to albumin for delivery to tissues. Each albumin molecule can bind up to eight fatty acid molecules and carry them to cells for metabolism.

In the small intestine, protein-bound short- and medium-chain fatty acids (<C-10) diffuse into cells directly and subsequently into the hepatic portal circulation (see Ch. 15). Long-chain fatty acids (≥C-12) are bound to fatty acid binding proteins to diffuse down a concentration gradient into cells, in proportion to their concentrations inside and outside the cells. The presence of fatty acid-binding proteins within the cell facilitates cellular fatty acid uptake by reducing intracellular FFA concentration.

TRIACYLGLYCEROLS (TRIGLYCERIDES)

Storage of fatty acids in the form of TAG is more efficient and quantitatively more important for energy production than the storage of glycogen. TAGs constitute the major transport form of fat.

Triacylglycerols are formed by the esterification of one molecule of glycerol with three molecules of fatty acids: the carboxylic acid terminals of fatty acid condenses with the hydroxyl terminal of glycerol (see Ch. 2, Fig. 2.11).

In both liver and adipose tissue, TAGs are produced by a pathway that involves the 3-carbon molecule glycerol 3-phosphate (gl-3-P). The gl-3-P is of different origin in the two tissues:

- In liver, glycerol provides the gl-3-P, catalysed by glycerol kinase.
- Adipose tissue lacks glycerol kinase, so glucose is the source of gl-3-P via glycolysis.

When there is plenty of glucose, insulin is secreted and stimulates glucose uptake by the adipocyte via GLUT4. The immediate precursor of gl-3-P in adipose tissue is dihydroxy-acetone-P (DHAP) (see Fig. 3.3). Fatty acid storage as TAG in adipose tissue can take place only when glycolysis is activated in the fed state.

The breakdown of adipose tissue TAG yields glycerol. The albumin bound glycerol is transported to liver for TAG synthesis. As a result of this adipo-hepatic axis, TAG stored in adipose tissue during times of dietary plenty can be transferred to the liver for metabolic remodelling to form VLDLs (see below) during times of nutrient scarcity.

Regulation of hepatic triacylglycerol synthesis

Triacylglycerols deliver fatty acids from adipose tissue stores to peripheral cells for catabolism. The hydrolysis of stored TAG is tightly regulated by the enzyme hormone-sensitive lipase, so-called because it is sensitive to a range of hormones (Fig. 3.20). Lipolysis is:

- Activated by glucagon and adrenaline (epinephrine)
- Inhibited by insulin.

Hormone-sensitive lipase removes the three fatty acids from TAG, stepwise. The liberated fatty acids and glycerol are then released to circulating blood.

LIPOPROTEINS

Lipoproteins are molecular combinations of lipids and protein components called apolipoproteins. Lipoproteins are classi-

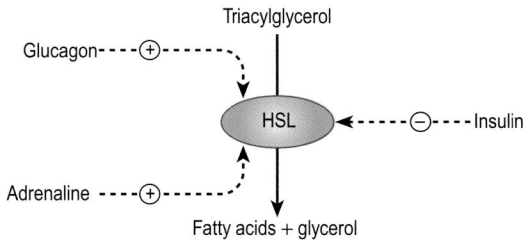

Fig. 3.20 **Hormonal regulation of hormone-sensitive lipase (HSL) activity.**

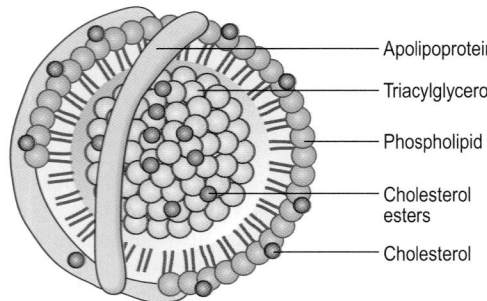

- Apolipoprotein
- Triacylglycerol
- Phospholipid
- Cholesterol esters
- Cholesterol

Fig. 3.21 **Generalised structure of lipoproteins.** The external monolayer contains phospholipids, cholesterol and apolipoproteins. Cholesterol esters and triacylglycerols are located in the particle core.

fied according to density. Apolipoproteins emulsify the lipoprotein particle to make it more stable in aqueous solution for carriage in plasma, and interact with cellular receptors that determine how and where lipoprotein particles are metabolised. Each lipoprotein particle has a specific set of apolipoproteins (see later).

Lipoprotein particles are constructed by hepatocytes and enterocytes from (Fig. 3.21):

- TAG
- Cholesterol
- Apolipoproteins
- Phospholipids.

The hydrophobic TAG and cholesteryl esters make up the 'core' of lipoprotein particles, with apolipoprotein strands, cholesterol molecules and phospholipids in the outer shells. Hepatocytes assemble VLDLs and high-density lipoproteins (HDLs). HDLs are also derived from the gut. These are distinguished by the difference in their size, density, lipid composition and apolipoprotein content.

Apolipoproteins

Apolipoproteins are protein strands embedded in the surface of lipoproteins (Fig. 3.21). They activate and inhibit enzymes in lipoprotein metabolism, and are ligands for the cellular apoB/E (LDL) receptors and scavenger receptors. ApoB/E receptors and scavenger receptors are responsible for LDL clearance (see below).

The important apolipoproteins are:

- ApoA (A-I and A-II) present in HDLs. Binding of apoA-I to cellular receptors mediates the efflux of cholesterol from peripheral cells, and the influx of cholesterol into hepatocytes (see below).
- ApoB: apoB-100 recognises apoB/E receptors and facilitates cellular uptake of LDL. ApoB-100 is derived from liver and forms part of LDL. ApoB-48 is derived from the gut and is found in chylomicrons.
- ApoC is made in the liver and is a peripheral activator of lipoprotein lipase (LPL). It is transferred between lipoproteins
- ApoE stabilises VLDL (and possibly intermediate-density lipoprotein (IDL) and remnant particles) for cellular uptake, and is a ligand for the apoB/E receptor.
- Apo(a) links with apoB-100 to oxidise LDL, giving Lp(a) lipoprotein particles.

On large particles, e.g. VLDLs, the apolipoproteins are stretched. As the particles shrink with increasing density,

apoB and apoE change conformation so that they can no longer bind to apoB/E receptors. However, apoE adapts to a shape that allows binding to apoE receptors for uptake into hepatocytes. As lipoprotein particles travel around in the circulation, apoC-II on chylomicrons and VLDLs allows TAG to be removed by LPL in the capillary endothelium.

Apolipoproteins are important because they control lipoprotein metabolism. Apolipoprotein and LDL receptor genes have been identified, sequenced and mapped to chromosomes. Apolipoprotein disorders are known to lead to defects of lipid metabolism.

Lipoprotein classes and functions

Lipoproteins vary in size and density, the denser being smaller. A high TAG content makes the lipoprotein particle less dense, and therefore larger in size. Intestinal, adipose and skeletal muscle lipoprotein lipase (LPL) and hepatic triacylglycerol lipase (HTGL), present in capillary endothelial cells, remove TAG from TAG-rich lipoproteins. Progressive removal of TAG increases the protein:lipid ratio and thus the density of the particle remnants.

Chylomicrons

The least dense and largest lipoproteins are chylomicrons, which are globules assembled by enterocytes following lipid digestion and composed principally of TAG, apoB-48, apoA-I and apoA-II, a smaller amount of cholesterol and cholesteryl esters. In the bloodstream, apoC-II and apoE are acquired from HDLs (see below). They transport products from dietary fat digestion to peripheral tissues (see Ch. 15). Progressive removal of TAGs by LPL leads to the formation of remnant particles, which are taken up and catabolised by the liver.

Very-low-density lipoprotein

VLDL is synthesised continuously in the liver. It is the main source of TAGs exported from liver to muscle and adipose tissues:

- TAG forms about 50% of the particle
- Contain apoB-100 as an essential component
- ApoC-II and apoE are incorporated by transfer from HDL.

Intermediate-density lipoprotein

IDL is a particle remnant derived from VLDL by the removal of TAG by LPL in extrahepatic tissues with loss of apolipoprotein. IDLs are precursors of LDLs. Some IDL particles are taken up by hepatocytes, when TAG is removed by HTGL:

- TAG content in the particle remnant is decreased, with a proportional rise in cholesterol
- Contains apoB-100 and apoE
- Loses apoC-II.

Low-density lipoprotein

LDL is also a particle remnant, resulting from further removal of TAG in liver and peripheral tissues when the molecule:

- Is depleted of almost all of its TAG, and mainly consists of cholesterol
- Contains a single apoB-100 molecule and some apoE

LDL is the main cholesterol carrier, delivering cholesterol to liver and peripheral tissues.

High-density lipoprotein

HDL particles are synthesised in both the liver and intestines. They carry cholesterol from adipose tissue directly to liver – reverse cholesterol transport – and to tissues that synthesise steroid hormones (e.g. adrenal glands, ovaries and testes). HDL also takes part in the metabolism of other lipoproteins by exchanging apolipoproteins, cholesteryl ester, TAG and phospholipids.

- HDL is rich in cholesteryl esters
- Only about 5% of the particle is TAG
- It contains apoA (A-I and A-II) and also apoC and apoE.

Lipoprotein receptors

Activation of membrane-bound lipoprotein receptors in hepatic and peripheral cells enables cholesterol entry. The main one is the apoB/E (also known as LDL) receptor, present on cell surfaces. ApoB/E receptors bind either apoB-100 or apoE, but not apoB-48 (cellular uptake of chylomicron remnants is mediated by apoE and apoB/E related receptors). Gene expression of apoB/E receptor is regulated by intracellular cholesterol concentration.

Binding of LDL to apoB/E receptors stimulates endocytosis (see Ch. 2). LDL is taken into hepatic (about 80% of total LDL) and peripheral cells, then broken down to cholesterol by lysosomes, destroying the LDL particle. The receptor is recycled back to the cell membrane.

Scavenger receptors

Scavenger receptors are membrane-bound receptors on phagocytic cells, e.g. macrophages. Unlike the apoB/E receptor, scavenger receptors do not bind intact LDLs, but rather the oxidised form – Lp(a) particles. The scavenger receptors (scavenger receptor type A) on macrophages are not regulated by raised intracellular cholesterol concentration, so they can be overloaded by the ligand – oxidised LDL – which can disrupt the macrophage, leading to atherogenesis (see Chs 11 and 16). Scavenger receptor type BI takes part in cholesterol removal in HDL metabolism (see below). Elevated Lp(a) concentration is associated with increased risk of atherogenesis.

Lipoprotein metabolism

Lipoprotein metabolism involves a series of processes:

1. Assembly of chylomicrons in enterocytes from TAGs, cholesterol, phospholipids and apolipoproteins.
2. Endogenous synthesis of VLDL in the liver from apoB-100, apoE, TAGs, cholesterol esters and phospholipids, but predominantly TAGs.
3. Fatty acids: LPL and HTGL catalyse the cleavage (by hydrolysis) of TAGs and fatty acids from chylomicrons and VLDLs to form remnant particles. IDLs, LDLs and HDLs (VLDL – IDL – LDL – HDL cascade) are delivered to peripheral cells for energy metabolism. LPL and HTGL are activated by apoC-II binding.
4. Cellular uptake of remnant particles through activation of membrane receptors by apoB/E binding.
5. The cell surface of an LDL particle has a single apoB-100 and some apoE.
6. Removal of cholesterol from cells by HDL particles – reverse cholesterol transport – for delivery to liver for VLDL synthesis or conversion to bile salts for excretion in bile.

Reverse cholesterol transport

HDLs are lipid-poor particles formed in the liver and intestine. Newly formed (nascent) HDL particles resemble flat, bi-layered discs, and mainly contain phospholipid and apoA-I. As they travel around the circulation, nascent HDL particles remove cholesterol from cells, mediated by the action of cholesterol efflux regulatory protein (CERP, also known as ATP-binding cassette transporter A-I; ABC1). CERP is activated by apoA-I, facilitating the movement of cholesterol out of cells to apoA-I.

ApoA-I also activates the enzyme lecithin-cholesterol acyl transferase (LCAT), which catalyses the synthesis of cholesteryl esters. The cholesteryl esters move deeper into the HDL particle to give it a more spherical shape (see Fig. 3.21). As HDL moves through the circulation, some cholesteryl esters are exchanged for TAGs from TAG-rich lipoproteins, and the HDL particle becomes larger as the space between the bilayer fills.

In reverse cholesterol transport, HDL transports cholesterol away from peripheral cells, delivering cholesterol directly to the liver and tissues that synthesise steroids. In the liver, binding of apoA-I to scavenger receptor type BI mediates the removal of cholesterol into the hepatocytes for excretion as bile salts and sterols. HDL is then released in the disc form to enter a new cycle of cholesterol transport.

ApoA-I is thus essential for both the efflux of peripheral cellular cholesterol into HDL, and the uptake of cholesterol from HDL into hepatocytes and steroid synthetic cells. Defects of apoA-I are associated with defective cholesterol excretion, and consequently hypercholesterolaemia.

Lipoprotein fuel transport and overflow pathways

The lipoprotein fuel transport pathway includes the VLDL – IDL – LDL – HDL cascade, cellular uptake of lipoprotein remnant particles and reverse cholesterol transport. Fatty acids, mainly in the form of TAGs, are transported to adipose tissue for storage and to peripheral tissues for energy metabolism.

TAG is depleted from lipoprotein remnants in the fuel transport pathway to generate LDL, which can no longer deliver TAG. The metabolic pathway of LDL is therefore unrelated to the supply of fuel, and may be considered an 'overflow pathway'.

FATTY ACID OXIDATION

The catabolism of fatty acids is entirely oxidative and requires both mitochondrial and cytosolic phases, metabolites being shuttled between the cytosol and mitochondrion. Fatty acids are delivered to cytosol bound to fatty acid binding proteins (see above), and have to be 'activated' to their fatty acyl-CoA derivatives in the cytosol before they can enter the mitochondrion for β-oxidation (see below).

Fatty acid activation and transport into mitochondria

Fatty acid activation is catalysed by the enzyme acyl-CoA synthetase (also known as acyl-CoA thiokinase), sited in the outer mitochondrial membrane (see Fig. 3.22). Two ATP molecules are used as the energy source.

Clinical box 3.18 **Disorders of lipoprotein metabolism – dyslipidaemias**

Disturbances of lipoprotein metabolism result in abnormalities in plasma lipoprotein concentrations, known as dyslipidaemias. Dyslipidaemias are associated with defects in either the fuel transport or overflow pathways, and in most cases will increase the risk for cardiovascular disease and atheroma. Clinical clues include family history of heart disease or acute pancreatitis, and physical signs in severe cases include xanthomata, lipaemia retinalis (specific for high VLDL), and retinal vein thrombosis. Available treatments include dietary control of fat intake, lipid-lowering diets, increased dietary fruit and vegetable content, exercise and lipid-lowering drugs (see Ch. 16).

Primary dyslipidaemia may be classified according to genetic/functional defects of lipoprotein metabolism.

Disorders of chylomicron and VLDL metabolism
Mechanisms for disordered chylomicron and VLDL metabolism are poorly understood.

- Polygenic hypertriglyceridaemia is a polygenic disorder possibly associated with a moderately elevated plasma VLDL concentration, with LPL or apoC deficiency, and is rare.
- Lipoprotein lipase (LPL) deficiency and apoC-II deficiency are rare conditions characterised clinically by high TAG levels and plasma chylomicrons persisting in the fasting state. The TAG in chylomicrons cannot be metabolised because either the LPL enzyme is absent, impairing TAG hydrolysis, or LPL cannot be activated owing to the absence of apoC-II.

Disorders of LDL metabolism – hypercholesterolaemia
- Heterozygous familial hypercholesterolaemia is the commonest disorder of LDL metabolism, more common is some racial groups (e.g. South Africans, Finns). It is an autosomal dominant, monogenic disorder, where there is defective gene coding for apoB/E receptor. Impaired apoB/E receptor production affects both fuel transport and overflow pathways, giving impaired LDL clearance.
- Homozygous familial hypercholesterolaemia is extremely rare, characterised by the absence of hepatic apoB/E receptors. Plasma LDL concentration is greatly elevated, and patients die in late childhood or adolescence from ischaemic heart disease. Possible treatments are LDL apheresis to remove LDL from the circulation or liver transplant. Research into gene therapy is ongoing.

- Mutations in apoB-100 is a single gene disorder, affecting LDL binding to hepatic clearance receptors, and results in hypercholesterolaemia. The condition clinically resembles heterozygous familial hypercholesterolaemia, but is less common.
- Polygenic hypercholesterolaemia is the most common type of hypercholesterolaemia that is not one of the monogenetic disorders. The nature of this condition is not well understood.
- Familial dysbetalipidaemia is a rare condition characterised by mutation of apoE gene to apoE isoforms (E2) that have a low affinity for apoB/E receptor, resulting in lipoprotein remnants not being taken into hepatocytes, with consequent cholesterol and TAG accumulation in blood.

Combined hyperlipidaemia – hypercholesterolaemia and hypertriglyceridaemia
Familial combined hyperlipidaemia is the commonest dyslipidaemia in which there is both hypercholesterolaemia and hypertriglyceridaemia, thought to be associated with an overproduction of apoB-100, leading to VLDL overproduction and consequent LDL overload. The high plasma concentration of LDL suppresses HDL synthesis. Both fuel transport and overflow pathways are overloaded. The inheritance is autosomal dominant.

Secondary hyperlipidaemia
Hyperlipidaemia can be associated with diabetes, hypothyroidism and liver disease (particularly alcohol related). Treatment of the underlying condition is essential.

In type 2 diabetes and metabolic syndrome, excess VLDL synthesis overloads the fuel transport pathway with increased remnant concentration which is accompanied by lowered HDL concentration. LDL concentration may be normal as the overload pathway is not compromised.

Disorders of HDL metabolism – Tangier disease
The role of HDL in cholesterol transport was elucidated from the study of the extremely rare dyslipidaemia, Tangier disease. Patients have almost no circulating HDL, with extrahepatic deposition of cholesteryl esters leading to corneal opacities and an orange discoloration of the tonsils, spleen and intestinal mucosa. Mutation in the CERP (also known as ABC1) gene prevents cellular cholesterol ester efflux. Plasma TAG and cholesterol concentrations are normal.

Clinical box 3.19 **Measurement of plasma lipoproteins and hyperlipidaemia**

The plasma concentration of lipoproteins can be diagnostically useful. Measurements of plasma cholesterol and TAG are commonly used as surrogates for lipoprotein concentration, and are often, but not always, sufficient for precise diagnosis. For example, because cholesterol concentration is highest in LDL, plasma cholesterol level reflects mainly LDL concentration. A fasting total TAG concentration reflects mainly the sum of VLDL and IDL levels. Total postprandial TAG concentration includes chylomicrons.

Fasting lipid profile
A fasting lipid profile (after a 14-hour fast) consists of the measurement of:

- Total plasma cholesterol (C)
- Total TAG
- HDL-cholesterol.

A formula, the Friedewald equation, provides an estimate of LDL-cholesterol concentration:

LDL-C = total C – [HDL-C + (TAG/2.2)] (all expressed in mmol/L)

A ratio of total plasma cholesterol: HDL-cholesterol above 5 has sometimes been used as an indicator of increased cardiovascular risk, although lower values have been shown to be associated with risk.

- The acyl-CoA derivatives of short- and medium-chain fatty acids enter the mitochondrion directly by simple diffusion across the mitochondrial membranes.
- Very-long-chain fatty acids (C22–24) have to be shortened to long-chain fatty acids in the peroxisomes.
- Long chain-fatty acids are converted to their acyl-CoA derivatives in the cytosol. Long-chain fatty acyl-CoA derivatives cannot cross the outer mitochondrial membrane by simple diffusion, and have to be transported across via the carnitine shuttle (Fig. 3.22).
- Very-long-chain and branched-chain fatty acids are oxidised in peroxisomes.

Carnitine shuttle

The carnitine shuttle is an antiport transport mechanism.

1. The large and polar long-chain fatty acyl-CoA molecule is transferred to the small carnitine molecule by carnitine palmitoyltransferase-I (CPT-I), located in the outer mitochondrial membrane.
2. Long-chain fatty acyl-carnitine is formed, releasing CoA. An acyl-carnitine carrier (a translocase) in the inner mitochondrial membrane then carries fatty acyl-carnitine

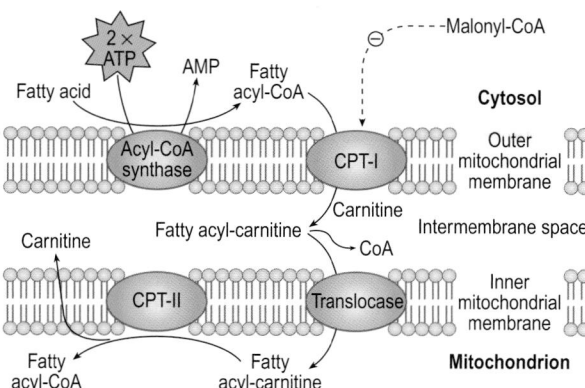

Fig. 3.22 Carnitine shuttle. The fatty acyl-CoA formed from short- and medium-chain fatty acids diffuse across the mitochondrial membranes into the mitochondrion. Fatty acyl-CoA from long-chain fatty acids have to be transported via the carnitine shuttle. CPT, carnitine palmitoytransferase.

into the mitochondrion. CPT-1 transports a range of long-chain acyl-CoAs.

3. On entry into the mitochondrion, a second transferase, carnitine palmitoyltransferase-II (CPT-II), regenerates the long-chain acyl-CoA and releases free carnitine, which diffuses out back through the inner mitochondrial membrane.

4. The entry of acyl-carnitine into the mitochondrion is obligatorily linked to the exit of carnitine from the mitochondrion (an antiport mechanism) for the shuttle to continue.

Carnitine shuttle in the regulation of fatty acid oxidation

The carnitine shuttle is an important site in the regulation of mitochondrial long-chain fatty acid oxidation. In the liver, inhibition of mitochondrial CPT-I by malonyl-CoA (see below) prevents the mitochondrial catabolism of newly synthesised fatty acids. Because long-chain fatty acids remain in the cytosol, their esterification to form TAG is favoured. Ultimately, this liver TAG will be exported as VLDL.

Regulation of CPT-I in muscle, which is not a major site of fatty acid synthesis from glucose, is an important aspect of metabolic fuel selection.

β-Oxidation of fatty acids in mitochondria

The β-oxidation of fatty acyl-CoA takes place in mitochondria, by the removal of two carbon atoms at a time from the fatty acyl-CoA molecule at the β-carbon position to form a ketone (C=O). The chain reaction finally releases:

- Acetyl-CoA
- Reduced nucleotides flavin adenine dinucleotide ($FADH_2$) and nicotinamide adenine dinucleotide (NADH). The reduced nucleotides are used directly for synthesis of ATP by oxidative phosphorylation.

Acetyl-CoA is oxidised either:

- In muscle, in the TCA cycle to CO_2 and water, releasing free CoA

- In liver, predominantly for ketone body formation (see Ch. 2).

The net ATP yield for the complete oxidation of such a fatty acid is far higher that the yield from glucose catabolism. The caloric value of palmitate is 37.6 kJ/g (9 kcal) compared with that of glucose 16.4 kJ/g (4 kcal).

Oxidation of acetyl-CoA in the TCA cycle

The oxidation of acetyl-CoA in the TCA cycle begins with the condensation of acetyl-CoA with oxaloacetate (OAA) to form citric acid (see Ch. 2) with the release of free CoA. This reaction is catalysed and regulated by citrate synthase.

Another key enzyme in the TCA cycle is isocitrate dehydrogenase, which catalyses one of the subsequent oxidative reactions when NAD^+ is reduced to NADH, releasing CO_2.

Inhibition of the β-oxidation spiral by excess CoA

Under fasting and starvation conditions, the balance of metabolic processes in the TCA cycle is shifted to favour gluconeogenesis. One of these shifts occurs through changes in OAA-malate equilibrium (see below, Malate shuttle, Fig. 3.25). Under physiological conditions, OAA is converted to malate in the mitochondrion in a ratio of 1:1. In starvation, the OAA-malate equilibrium shifts towards malate. Malate then leaves the mitochondrion and is consumed in gluconeogenesis. As a result, less OAA is available to take part in the citrate synthase reaction within the TCA, so less acetyl-CoA can be oxidised to free CoA. Excess acetyl-CoA then accumulates.

Free CoA is essential to the initiation and continuation of β-oxidation. When there is a deficiency in free CoA, an alternative pathway, the ketogenic pathway in the liver, is activated for the breakdown of acetyl-CoA to liberate free CoA.

Ketogenesis in the liver

Ketogenesis is a hepatic pathway for the metabolism of acetyl-CoA. The free CoA needed for the initiation and continuation of the β-oxidation spiral is generated in this process, which also results in the release of ketone bodies.

Ketone bodies are the water-soluble lipid derivatives:

■ Acetoacetate
■ β-Hydroxybutyrate
■ Acetone, a metabolic waste product formed by the non-enzymic decomposition of acetoacetate.

Under physiological conditions, only the liver is able to synthesise and export ketone bodies, the entire process taking place in the mitochondrial matrix.

Oxidation of acetyl-CoA in the ketogenic pathway

In the ketogenic pathway (Fig. 3.23), acetyl-CoA is converted to acetoacetate in the mitochondrion via the hydroxymethylglutaryl-CoA (HMG-CoA) pathway. Acetoacetate can decompose to acetone, or be converted to β-hydroxybutyrate enzymatically. Free CoA is liberated in this pathway for initiating and continuing the β-oxidation spiral.

There are three stages in the conversion of acetyl-CoA into ketone bodies:

1. Condensation of two molecules of acetyl-CoA to form acetoacetyl-CoA; releasing one CoA molecule.
2. Catalysis by mitochondrial HMG-CoA synthase (Information box 3.11), releasing a second CoA molecule.
3. Catalysis by HMG-CoA lyase. Together the synthase and lyase enzymes catalyse the conversion of acetoacetyl-CoA to acetoacetate.

Role of ketone bodies in fuel homeostasis

As well as enhancing hepatic ATP production by providing free CoA for continued β-oxidation, the formation of ketone bodies by the liver is vital to whole-body fuel homeostasis during starvation and uncontrolled diabetes.

In brief, fatty acids are converted, through hepatic ketogenesis, to water-soluble products, the ketone bodies, which, unlike fatty acids, can readily be transported in aqueous solution in the blood. Moreover, ketone bodies can be used for energy production by the brain during starvation (see below), whereas long-chain fatty acids are unable to cross the blood–brain barrier.

Ketone body utilisation

Although the liver is able to synthesise ketone bodies, it is deficient in the key enzyme needed for their metabolism. Thus, for further metabolism, ketone bodies are exported from the liver and taken up in extrahepatic tissues, including skeletal and cardiac muscle. In tissues other than the liver, ketone bodies appear to be used in proportion to their plasma concentration. They are, therefore, an efficient source of energy during starvation and in other conditions in which they are produced in large quantities (Clinical box 3.21).

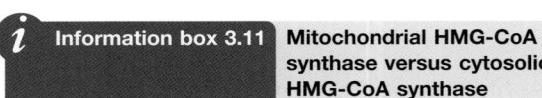

i **Information box 3.11** | **Mitochondrial HMG-CoA synthase versus cytosolic HMG-CoA synthase**

■ Mitochondrial HMG-CoA synthase is involved in the ketogenic pathway
■ Cytosolic HMG-CoA synthase is involved in cholesterol synthesis. This enzyme is inhibited by the statins used in the treatment of hyperlipidaemia.
■ Their modes of regulation are quite different.

Acetoacetate and β-hydroxybutyrate are inter-convertible by the mitochondrial enzyme, β-hydroxybutyrate dehydrogenase. Their relative concentrations therefore reflect the mitochondrial redox state, with β-hydroxybutyrate predominating when the NADH/NAD+ ratio is high due to brisk rates of β-oxidation. Thus, considerably more β-hydroxybutyrate than acetoacetate is released from the liver.

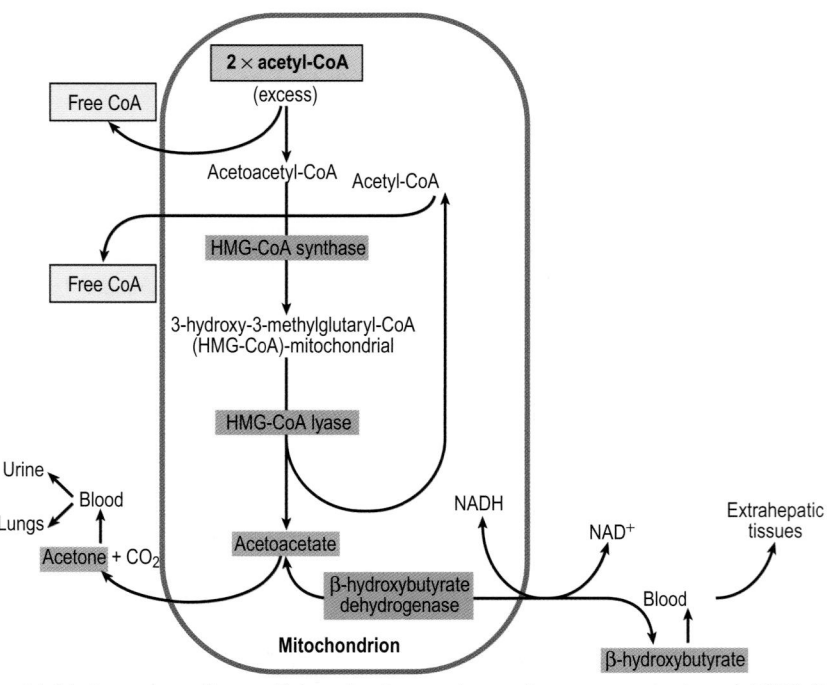

Fig. 3.23 Mitochondrial ketogenic pathway. Ketone bodies are in *purple*; enzymes are in *red*. HMG-CoA, hydroxymethylglutaryl-CoA.

Ketone bodies accumulate in starvation, uncontrolled type 1 diabetes mellitus and with serious loss of control in type 2 diabetes

- The ketone body level in the blood rises to 2–3 mM after a few days of starvation, increasing to 7–8 mM or more after prolonged starvation.
- Certain pathological conditions, notably diabetic ketoacidosis, are characterised by excessive accumulation of ketone bodies in the blood with acidosis, even if blood glucose levels are not much increased.

Diabetic ketoacidosis
- Blood ketone body levels can increase to up to 15–20 mM in uncontrolled type 1 diabetes mellitus.
- Blood pH falls because the ketone bodies are acid, giving rise to metabolic acidosis.
- In diabetic coma due to ketoacidosis, the β-hydroxybutyrate:acetoacetate ratio can rise to as high as 3 (from excessive adipose-tissue lipolysis, hepatic fatty acid oxidation and ketogenesis). Because a rapid 'dip stick' test for ketonuria detects only acetoacetate, the increased excretion of ketone bodies (ketonuria) may go unrecognised.
- Acetone, from acetoacetate decomposition, is expired by the lungs, producing a characteristic fruity (pear) odour on the patient's breath.

During short-term starvation (overnight fast, or up to 3 days), ketone bodies are important in providing a fuel for muscle, kidney and intestine. As the period of starvation is extended, the brain also converts to the use of ketone bodies for more than 50% of its energy. This metabolic switch allows considerable glucose conservation, reducing the demand for degraded muscle protein, which provides precursors for gluconeogenesis.

Ketone bodies are converted to CoA derivatives for oxidation as follows:

1. β-hydroxybutyrate is first oxidised to acetoacetate by NAD⁺ in a reaction catalysed by β-hydroxybutyrate dehydrogenase. This is a direct reversal of hepatic synthesis (see Fig. 3.23).
2. Activation of acetoacetate – its conversion to acetoacetyl-CoA – occurs by the transfer of CoA from succinyl-CoA, catalysed by the enzyme β-oxoacid CoA-transferase, which is absent in the liver.
3. Acetoacetyl-CoA is then split to acetyl-CoA by the reversal of the thiolase reaction, the direction of which depends on the concentration ratio of its substrates and products.
4. The major source of succinyl-CoA for the β-oxoacid CoA-transferase is the TCA cycle.

The increased production of succinate at the expense of succinyl-CoA allows increased production of oxaloacetate (via the TCA cycle), which facilitates the entry of more acetyl-CoA into the TCA cycle.

LIPOGENESIS – FATTY ACID SYNTHESIS

Whereas the degradation of fat, β-oxidation, occurs in the mitochondria, fatty acid synthesis occurs in the cytosol. Generally, palmitic acid (palmitate), a simple straight-chain saturated fatty acid containing 16 carbon atoms, is synthesised first; many other fatty acids are made by chain elongation and/or desaturation of palmitic acid. Not all fatty acids can be endogenously synthesised. The carbon atoms in the palmitate chain originate only from acetyl-CoA (see below). Insulin has a major role in promoting lipogenesis.

Fatty acid synthesis takes place in two stages (Fig. 3.24). Both stages use acetyl-CoA as the carbon source, and require multienzyme complexes. The acetyl-CoA units are derived from mitochondrial oxidative glycolysis via the pyruvate dehydrogenase pathway, then transported into the cytosol via the malate shuttle (see below).

- Stage 1: acetyl-CoA is converted to malonyl-CoA by acetyl-CoA carboxylase (ACC)
- Stage 2: fatty acid chain elongation, catalysed by fatty acid synthase (FAS) to form palmitate.

Stage 1: ACC – the committed step of lipogenesis

In stage 1, acetyl-CoA is converted, or 'activated', by the action of ACC to form malonyl-CoA. This reaction commits acetyl-CoA to fatty acid synthesis. The ACC enzyme is synthesised in an inactive single unit (protomer) form. The synthesis of ACC, like many enzymes that carry CO_2, requires the water soluble B vitamin biotin as cofactor (see Ch. 16). The protomer is activated to its polymeric form by citrate (or isocitrate). The ACC reaction takes place in two stages:

- Carboxylation (transfer of CO_2) of biotin, requiring energy in the form of ATP
- Transfer of the carboxyl group to acetyl-CoA to produce malonyl-CoA, releasing the biotin–carboxyl complex.

Regulation of ACC activity

In the short term, ACC activity is tightly controlled by two independent mechanisms.

Acetyl-CoA contains an allosteric site for the binding of citrate or palmitoyl-CoA
Citrate is a TCA cycle intermediate, which, on exit from the mitochondrion, acts both as:

- the immediate source of the cytosolic acetyl-CoA, required for the ACC reaction, and as
- a feed-forward activator of the ACC protomer.

When energy supply is high, storage of energy through lipogenesis is promoted by increased insulin secretion to prevent overproduction of fatty acids.
- Insulin acts indirectly to increase the availability of citrate through its promotion of glucose uptake, aerobic glycolysis and the TCA cycle.
- Palmitoyl-CoA, a product of stage 2 of lipogenesis, acts as an allosteric inhibitor of the ACC protomer, acting at the same site as citrate.

ACC control by hormone-dependent covalent modification
Independent of the citrate/palmitoyl-CoA mechanism, ACC is also controlled by hormone-dependent covalent modification, a phosphorylation-dephosphorylation mechanism. The phosphorylated ACC enzyme is less active than the dephosphorylated one. Under low-energy conditions, a cAMP-dependent protein kinase (AMPK) is activated by glucagon or adrenaline (epinephrine) to phosphorylate ACC. When cellular energy level is high (metabolic pathway moves towards fatty acid synthesis for storage), dephosphorylation is activated by a protein phosphatase stimulated by insulin.

The rate of ACC synthesis is highly regulated

Long-term regulation of ACC synthesis is exerted mainly at the level of changes in gene expression, induced by specific transcription factors.

Experimental data suggest that more ACC enzyme is produced by animals on high-carbohydrate or fat-free diets, whereas starvation and high-fat/low-carbohydrate diets

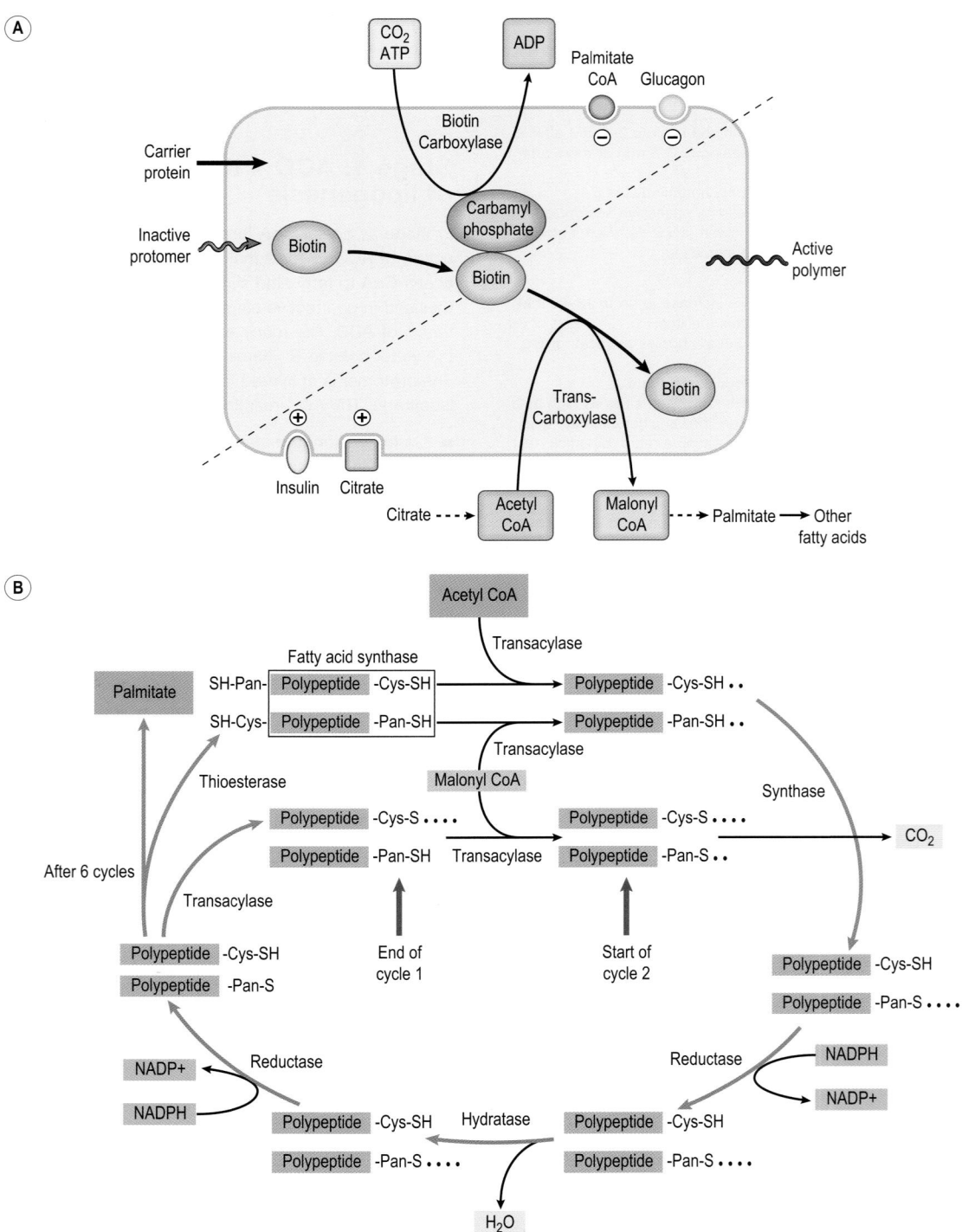

Fig. 3.24 **(A) The acetyl-CoA carboxylase (ACC) complex.** ACC converts acetyl-CoA to malonyl-CoA and exists as a small complex (protomer) in its inactive state, forming a polymer when activated. The diagram illustrates the molecule in its inactive and active states. Fatty acid synthesis is regulated by the activity of ACC in two ways: (i) allosteric binding of citrate (promotes ACC) or palmitate CoA (inhibits ACC) at one site; and (ii) hormonal binding by insulin (promotes ACC by dephosphorylating the enzyme) or glucagon (inhibits ACC by phosphorylating the enzyme) at a second binding site. **(B) The fatty acid synthase (FAS) enzyme.** FAS is composed of two identical polypeptides, placed head to tail. They each contain a carrier protein and a series of seven enzymes that catalyse the addition of four carbon units (•) at each end of the enzyme in the first step, then adding two additional carbon units in a cyclical set of reactions. Carbon units are added to both the cysteine (Cys) and pantetheine (Pan) ends of the enzyme and the growing fatty acid chain is transferred from one to the other between the two polypeptides. The diagram shows only the processes taking place on one end of the polypeptide pair. After six cycles there are 16 carbon units attached to the pantetheine-carrier part of the enzyme. At this point the enzyme complex is saturated and thioesterase cleaves off the 16-carbon fatty acid chain (palmitate) and FAS re-enters the cycle at the top of the diagram. ATP, adenosine triphosphate; ADP, adenosine diphosphate; Cys, cysteine; Pan, pantetheine; S, sulphur group; H, hydrogen; •, carbon unit; NADP, nicotinamide adenine dinucleotide phosphate (NADP+ oxidised, NADPH reduced).

decrease enzyme synthesis. A high insulin level therefore acutely increases ACC gene expression.

Stage 2: fatty acid synthase (FAS)

The second stage of fatty acid synthesis (Fig. 3.24B) is catalysed by FAS. Starting with acetyl-CoA as the carbon source, fatty acids are synthesised by the addition of two-carbon units, one at a time, to the activated carboxyl end of a growing chain, ending with an even number of carbon atoms.

FAS is a complex enzyme system in the cytoplasm containing seven enzymes and an acyl-carrier protein (ACP). Acetyl-CoA and malonyl-CoA are transferred to ACP, initiating the fatty acid synthesis cycle. All the reactions in the cycle are catalysed by fatty acid synthase. As the fatty acid chain grows, the carbon moiety is moved to a second site in ACP, freeing the original binding site, allowing the cycle to continue. The cycle is repeated six times until there is a saturated 16-carbon complex on the carrier protein, a palmitate molecule.

Thioesterase splits palmitate from the carrier protein to release the FAS molecule to restart synthesis.

Chain elongation

With the exception of the essential PUFAs, palmitate is the basis for synthesising other long-chain fatty acids. Chain elongation occurs by the addition of two-carbon units derived from malonyl-CoA by another enzyme complex, fatty acid elongase, located on the endoplasmic reticulum (mitochondrial membrane).

Short- and medium-chain fatty acids can also be elongated in mitochondria in a process that is the reversal of β-oxidation, using acetyl-CoA as the carbon source. Very-long-chain fatty acids (C22–24) are produced in the brain, which contains additional elongation systems. Elongation of stearoyl-CoA (C18) in the brain increases rapidly during myelination to generate the fatty acids required for the synthesis of brain-specific lipid (sphingolipids) (see Ch. 2).

Fatty acid elongation is greatly reduced during starvation, secondary to decreasing insulin secretion.

Desaturation

Chain elongation produces saturated fatty acids only. Desaturation takes place in the endoplasmic reticulum, catalysed by mixed function oxidases: desaturases. Oxygen and energy in the form of NADH are needed. The enzymes produce double bonds in the fatty acid chain.

An initial step in the formation of unsaturated fatty acids from palmitate (C16), or stearate (C18) is the introduction of a double bond between C-9 and C-10 atoms to produce palmitoleic or oleic acid, respectively. The desaturase system in humans cannot introduce double bonds between C-9 and the terminal methyl ω carbon atom. This is despite fatty acids with double bonds in this inaccessible region being necessary precursors of eicosanoids.

Regulation of fatty acid synthase and rate of lipogenesis

The regulation of FAS occurs primarily by long-term effects of changes in nutritional status on its rate of synthesis and degradation. Increased insulin secretion in the fed state stimulates ACC and FAS synthesis, starvation leads to decreased synthesis.

FAS levels are:

- High in individuals eating a high-carbohydrate/low-fat diet, promoting lipogenesis
- Low after starvation, or in individuals eating a high-fat/low-carbohydrate diet, inhibiting lipogenesis. The effects of consuming a high-fat diet to depress insulin secretion and inhibit lipogenesis is partly the basis for the 'Atkins diet'.

In the short term, substrate flux (the presence of phosphorylated sugars) causes allosteric activation of FAS.

Malate shuttle – production of acetyl-CoA for lipogenesis

Acetyl-CoA, the carbon source for lipogenesis, is produced from pyruvate, via glycolysis. Pyruvate is transported into the mitochondrion to undergo oxidative decarboxylation (losing CO_2) to form acetyl-CoA via the PDC (see Fig. 3.8) and oxaloacetate by pyruvate carboxylase (PC). PDC and PC are located in the mitochondrial matrix, whereas ACC and FAS are found in the cytosol. Acetyl-CoA does not readily traverse the mitochondrial membrane, and needs to be transported. This is achieved by the malate shuttle.

The malate shuttle is a complex antiport system. Acetyl-CoA combines with oxaloacetate in the TCA cycle to form citrate, catalysed by citrate synthase. Citrate is then translocated to the cytosol via the malate-citrate antiporter. At the same time, a molecule of malate is transferred to the mitochondrion (Fig. 3.25).

In the cytosol, citrate undergoes cleavage by citrate lyase to form acetyl-CoA and oxaloacetate. The action of ACC then converts acetyl-CoA to malonyl-CoA to enter lipogenesis.

Like acetyl-CoA, oxaloacetate does not readily cross the mitochondrial membrane. To re-enter the mitochondrion, oxaloacetate is converted to malate by cytosolic malate dehydrogenase. Malate is then transported back into the mitochondrion, via the malate-citrate antiporter, to be reconverted to oxaloacetate by mitochondrial malate dehydrogenase.

In starvation, malate is converted to pyruvate to enter gluconeogenesis.

FINE-TUNING OF FATTY ACID SYNTHESIS, OXIDATION AND KETOGENESIS

In the liver, inhibition of mitochondrial CPT-I by malonyl-CoA, the product of ACC reaction, prevents the catabolism of newly synthesised fatty acids, favouring their esterification to TAG, which is subsequently exported as VLDL.

With carbohydrate feeding (high insulin/low glucagon), the liver is actively engaged in fatty acid synthesis. Tissue malonyl-CoA content is high, and the capacity for mitochondrial long-chain fatty acid oxidation (and consequently ketogenesis) is depressed. Conversely, in starvation and uncontrolled diabetes mellitus, malonyl-CoA levels fall. Hepatic fatty acid synthesis is attenuated, and fatty acids reaching the liver from adipose tissue are efficiently oxidised.

The transition between normal and ketotic states is accompanied by marked shifts in the sensitivity of CPT-I to

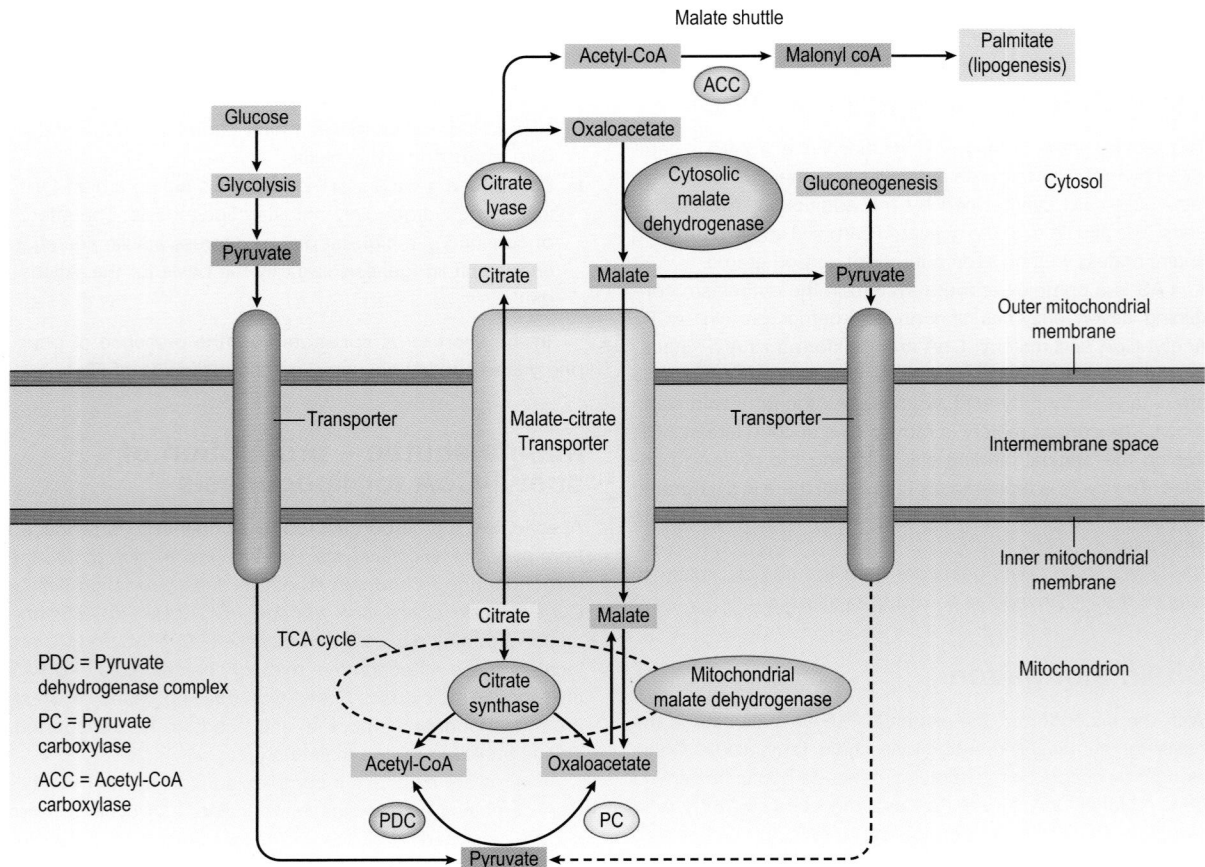

Fig. 3.25 The malate shuttle. Acetyl-CoA and oxaloacetate do not easily cross the mitochondrial membrane and are transported between the mitochondrion and cytosol via the malate-citrate antiporter. The malate shuttle is a method of transporting electrons (and reducing equivalents) from the cytosol to the mitochondrion. PDC, pyruvate dehydrogenase complex; PC, pyruvate carboxylase; ACC, acetyl-CoA carboxylase.

Clinical box 3.22   **Peroxisome proliferator-activated receptors**

There is evidence to suggest that the hyperlipidaemia, central obesity, insulin resistance, atherosclerosis and hypertension associations comprising the metabolic syndrome (syndrome X) are linked to an interplay of genetic propensity, nutrition and environmental factors (see Ch. 16). In this context, recent research has focused on a family of nuclear receptors, the peroxisome proliferator-activated receptors (PPARs), which may have a major role in glucose and fatty acid metabolism in relation to energy balance in humans. The discovery that PPAR activity can be modulated by certain drugs has prompted an increase in research effort into such drugs.

PPARs are transcription factors activated by the binding of specific ligands, usually hormones, to them. Three isoforms, PPARα, PPARβ (also known as δ) and PPARγ have been identified. More research is needed, but available data so far suggest that PPARγ promotes insulin sensitivity and lipid storage.

- PPARα is most abundant in liver cells and is also present in skeletal muscle, kidney and heart. It is actively involved in fatty acid catabolism in the peroxisomes, mitochondria and microsomes during fasting, when fatty acid oxidation and ketogenesis are strongly stimulated. PPARα also stimulates cellular uptake of fatty acids and lipoprotein synthesis.

- PPARα agonists are therefore hypolipidaemic. Fibrates, synthetic PPARα agonists, have been used for lipid lowering in the prevention and treatment of cardiovascular disease, for example.
- PPARγ is more active in the fed state, when glucose and chylomicrons in the circulation are abundant. It is lipogenic, stimulating the uptake of fatty acids and glucose and their conversion to TAG for storage in adipose tissue, and has hypoglycaemic properties.
- Decreased PPARγ expression in experimental animals may lead to increased leptin levels, which decreases food intake and weight gain (see also Ch. 16).

Thiazolidinediones (TZDs) are synthetic PPARγ agonists developed for the treatment of insulin resistance and type 2 diabetes. Increased PPARγ levels, however, can theoretically suppress leptin secretion, which could lead to weight gain.

- PPARβ is less well researched, but may be associated with colon cancer.
- PPARs have also been identified as anti-inflammatory transcription factors, so that they could be potential targets for the development of drugs in the treatment of the metabolic syndrome.

Clinical box 3.23 **Cushing's syndrome**

Increased cortisol secretion in Cushing's syndrome has a major long-term influence on fat metabolism by:

- Increasing gluconeogenesis
- Inhibiting glucose uptake and metabolism in peripheral tissues (insulin resistance)
- Stimulating glycogen synthesis and lipolysis.

Cushing's syndrome
High plasma cortisol concentrations result in:

- Hyperglycemia, which may lead to diabetes mellitus
- Muscle wasting
- Redistribution of adipose tissue from glucagon-sensitive depots to areas such the face, upper back and abdomen, giving the typical appearance of central obesity (apple versus pear shape, see Ch. 16).
- Osteoporosis.

The characteristic moon face and 'dowager's hump' in Cushing's syndrome is the result of facial fat deposition and thoracic spinal vertebral collapse from osteoporosis leading to kyphosis.

Although Cushing's syndrome can be the result of advanced adrenal or pituitary disease, it occurs more commonly because of long-term administration of therapeutic steroids.

inhibition by malonyl-CoA. As a result, the liver continues to oxidise fat on re-feeding after starvation, enabling gluconeogenesis to continue, and allows glycogen formation via the indirect pathway.

The suppressive effect of malonyl-CoA on CPT-I is not restricted to liver. Regulation of CPT-I in muscle, not a major site of fatty acid synthesis, appears to be an important aspect of metabolic fuel selection in muscle. Muscle malonyl-CoA concentrations fall with starvation, and also acutely in response to exercise, both conditions being associated with increased β-oxidation (when fatty acids become a major source of metabolic energy, ATP).

REGULATION OF FAT METABOLISM

Fat metabolism is controlled by the coordinated action of insulin, glucagon, adrenaline, cortisol and human growth hormone, and interacts with the regulation of carbohydrate metabolism. Insulin stimulates and regulates fatty acid synthesis and storage, promoting glucose uptake in both liver and adipose tissue. The rate of fat catabolism is controlled by the rate of TAG hydrolysis in adipose tissue, activated by rising concentrations of glucagon.

In the fasting (post-absorptive) state

As blood glucose concentration falls, glucagon activates hepatic gluconeogenesis, coordinating the release of amino acids and TAG hydrolysis. This results in increasing plasma concentrations of:

- Fatty acids
- Glycerol
- Ketone bodies.

Adrenaline secretion, in response to physiological or psychological stress, has a similar effect. Cortisol has a more long-term effect (over weeks) and may cause insulin resistance (see Clinical box 3.23).

In the fed (absorptive) state

When there is excess energy intake, especially excess dietary carbohydrate, the pathways for de novo fatty acid synthesis (lipogenesis) are activated by insulin. The carbohydrate is converted to fatty acids in the liver, then stored as TAG in adipose tissue.

4 Pharmacology

Walter Wieczorek and Jeannette Naish

INTRODUCTION

Pharmacology studies the effects of chemical substances on the function of living organisms. Initially, tissue and animal experiments enabled observation of the qualitative effects and measurement of quantitative effects of these chemicals. Therapeutic uses were discovered for human beings, and later, drugs were developed and even designed to exert specific effects. More recently, advances in the study of cell and molecular biology have moved the theoretical basis of pharmacology rapidly forward. Newer concepts have replaced the historical theories, and biotechnology now underpins the development of drugs.

The typing and cloning of the human genome has given further, exciting prospects for therapeutic development. The genetic makeup of individuals determines their response to drugs, and genetic variation is complex. Pharmacogenetics is an evolving subject, and although still theoretical, the future of pharmacogenomics could be far reaching.

There are, of course, therapies other than drug therapy. Surgical procedures and other forms of medicines are alternative approaches to ill health. These are beyond the scope of this chapter.

The components of pharmacology discussed in the following sections include:

- Pharmacokinetics – how drugs are taken into the body, distributed, metabolised and eliminated.
- Pharmacodynamics – the effects that drugs have on the functions of human organs, and the mechanisms through which these effects occur.
- The autonomic nervous system (ANS) – this controls nearly all the major human organs. Most clinically important groups of drugs act on this system.

Some drugs are selective, and work selectively on physiological processes. Others have a more diffuse action. Disturbance in absorption, distribution, metabolism and elimination can potentiate or inhibit the action of drugs. These lead to variation in the speed of onset and duration of action, drug interactions, toxic and other unwanted side effects. It is therefore important that these processes are understood when prescribing and dispensing drugs.

DIGOXIN – AN EXAMPLE IN CLINICAL PHARMACOLOGY

Digoxin is therapeutically the most important member of the family of cardiac glycosides, which are extracts from the foxglove plant (*Digitalis purpurea*). The general principles described here will be discussed in greater detail in later sections. Digoxin is an example of how a commonly prescribed and important drug works in the context of pharmacology.

Clinically, digoxin is used for its effects on the heart, which may be direct and indirect.

- Digoxin increases the force of contraction of cardiac muscle by a direct action on the myocytes, improving pumping efficiency in heart failure – **positive inotropic effect**.
- Indirect activity mediated through parasympathetic vagal stimulation reduces the rate of contraction of cardiac muscle, e.g. slows ventricular rate in atrial fibrillation – **negative chronotropic effect**.

Pharmacodynamics – how digoxin works

The positive inotropic effect of digoxin on heart muscle is probably caused by:

- Inhibition of the Na^+/K^+ pump in the membrane of the cardiac myocyte
- Intracellular Na^+ increases, while Ca^{2+} diffusion out of the cell via the separate Na^+/Ca^{2+} exchange transporter slows down
- The retained intracellular Ca^{2+} ions are stored, increasing the amount of Ca^{2+} released on muscle contraction
- The increased release of Ca^{2+} increases the action potential of the muscle and thus the force of contraction.

The negative chronotropic action of digoxin is due to central nervous system (CNS) effects that increase parasympathetic vagal activity (see later, ANS), potentiating the action of acetylcholine (ACh) to:

- Decrease the rate of firing at the sino-atrial (S-A) node to slow the heart rate
- Block conduction via the atrio-ventricular (A-V) node, increasing the intervals between ventricular contractions, allowing more time for ventricular filling in diastole, thus improving pumping efficiency.

Pharmacokinetics – how the body handles digoxin

Orally administered digoxin is well absorbed from the gastro-intestinal tract and excreted in the kidneys. The drug stays in the body for a long time, the half-life being about 1.5 days.

Unwanted effects

The unwanted effects of digoxin are related to the non-specific nature of some of its actions.

- Excessive accumulation of intracellular Ca^{2+} produces ectopic discharges at the A-V node, giving rise to tachycardia and ventricular ectopics. The clinical sign is known as coupled beats or **pulsus bigeminy**. Each normal pulse is followed by an ectopic beat. Fatal ventricular tachycardia may ensue.
- Excessive vagal activity at the S-A node can lead to atrial bradycardia and A-V block. Progressive A-V block leads to bradycardia and potentially fatal complete heart block. Excessive parasympathetic activity in atria will result in tachycardia.
- Excessive parasympathetic activity on the gastrointestinal tract causes nausea, vomiting, anorexia and diarrhoea.
- CNS effects include tiredness, vertigo, confusion and yellow vision. The precise mechanism for yellow vision is not known, but attributed to inhibition of the Na^+/K^+ pump in retinal cones.
- The steroid-like chemical structure of digoxin can lead to gynaecomastia.

Factors that contribute to digoxin toxicity

- Hypokalaemia – co-administration with K^+ losing diuretics leads to hypokalaemia, which potentiates the action of digoxin, causing toxic effects.
- Renal function impairment – common in elderly patients – slows down excretion, prolonging the half-life of digoxin as digoxin is eliminated unchanged. The drug accumulates with rising plasma concentrations, which could reach toxic levels.
- The toxic dose is only slightly higher than the therapeutic dose (very narrow therapeutic window).
- Drugs that displace digoxin from tissue (protein binding) sites increase plasma concentration with an increased risk of toxicity (e.g. verapamil, a Ca^{2+} channel blocking drug also used in the treatment of cardiac arrhythmias).
- Hypoxia – potentiates digoxin-induced cardiac arrhythmias.

PHARMACOKINETICS

Clinicians need to understand how the human body deals with drugs, the aim of drug therapy being to rapidly deliver and maintain therapeutic levels. Pharmacokinetics is a study of the interactions that determine the speed of onset, intensity and duration of drug action, which, following release from its formulation (see below) is the product of four simultaneous processes (Fig. 4.1):

- Absorption, into the body and into cells
- Distribution, around the different compartments of the body
- Metabolism, when the drug is broken down and inactivated, or sometimes transformed into an active form
- Elimination or excretion from the body.

These processes determine the most appropriate drug dosage, dosing interval and route for administration. Idiosyncrasies and disturbance of one or all these processes underlie overdose, toxicity and other adverse effects.

To produce a pharmacological response, a drug needs to achieve an adequate concentration at the site of action. The two fundamental processes that determine the concentration of a drug in any given part of the body are:

- **Absorption**, the process of transfer of a drug from its site of administration into the systemic circulation, and into tissues where the drug exerts its therapeutic effect. Both necessitate the transfer of a drug across cell membranes.
- **Distribution** of drug molecules from the site of administration to either their site of action or to storage depots.

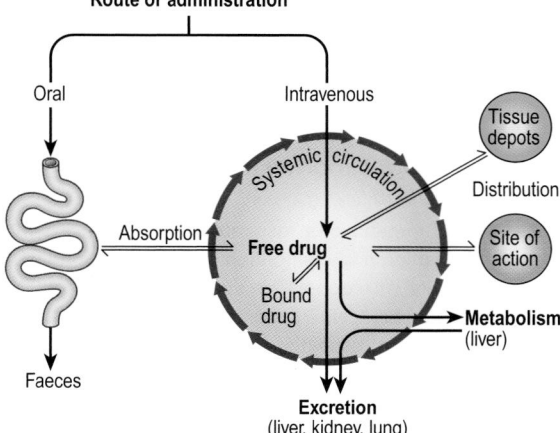

Fig. 4.1 **The relationship between absorption, distribution, metabolism and excretion of a drug.** The route of administration determines the degree of absorption, and thus the dose required for sufficient drug to enter plasma in the systemic circulation. The drug leaves the plasma to be distributed to its site of action and to storage sites (fat deposits). Finally, the majority of drugs are metabolised before excretion.

ABSORPTION – TRANSFER OF DRUGS ACROSS CELL MEMBRANES

Absorption is important for all routes of drug administration except intravenous injection. The degree of absorption depends on the route chosen and the physico-chemical properties of the drug. Cell membranes form barriers between intracellular and extracellular aqueous compartments in the body. A drug must cross at least one cell membrane to be absorbed, reach its site of action and eventually be eliminated.

The ways that drugs, nutrients and other substances (solutes) in aqueous solution cross a membrane barrier are by:

- Passive diffusion through cell membranes
- Carrier-mediated transport
- Endocytosis and exocytosis
- Diffusion through aqueous pores and intracellular pores.

PASSIVE DIFFUSION THROUGH LIPID MEMBRANES

The majority of drugs pass through cell membranes by the passive diffusion of molecules down a concentration gradient, which does not involve energy expenditure (see Ch. 2). There is no competition between compounds for the process, which cannot be saturated. As cell membranes are composed of a double layer of phospholipid molecules, the drug has to be lipid soluble to diffuse across them. The rate of diffusion across the membrane depends on:

- The lipid solubility of the drug
- The area over which absorption occurs
- The concentration gradient across the membrane.

Molecular size has little effect on diffusion because most drugs have a molecular mass of below 1000 daltons.

Lipid solubility

The human body largely consists of water, which forms the major part of extracellular and intracellular fluids (see Ch. 2). A drug must be water soluble to be distributed throughout the body. However, cell membranes that separate the extracellular from the intracellular compartments are mostly composed of lipids. The ability of a drug to enter or exit cells will depend on its lipid solubility. Some drugs are sufficiently lipid soluble to permeate the lipid membrane. Drugs that are not lipid soluble need to be transported across the cell membrane (Information box 4.1).

Ionised and non-ionised forms of a drug

Most drug molecules exist in solution as a mixture of ionised and non-ionised forms. The ionised form carries an electrical charge, has very low lipid solubility and cannot easily permeate lipid membranes. Most ionised drugs are weak organic acids. The non-ionised form of a drug molecule carries no

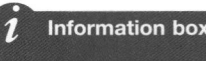

Information box 4.1   The relative ease with which drugs permeate cell membranes

The lipid solubility of a drug determines whether it can permeate cell membranes through passive diffusion.

- Aminoglycoside antibiotics are sufficiently lipid soluble for the whole molecule to permeate cell membranes.
- Thiopental, a general anaesthetic, is highly lipid soluble and can rapidly permeate cell membranes in the CNS and therefore has a rapid onset of action, making it useful as a general anaesthetic.
- Phenobarbital, of the same family of barbiturates as thiopental, used for its sedative and anti-epileptic action, is much less lipid soluble. Phenobarbital enters the CNS much more slowly, and is used in more long-term treatment.

Table 4.1   Variation in pKa of drugs and pH of body fluids

Variation in pH of drugs		Variation in pH of body fluids	
	Normal pKa		Normal pH
Acidic drugs			
Aspirin	3.5	Gastric juices	1.0–3.0
Thiopental	7.6	Intestinal fluids	4.8–8.0
Ethosuximide	9.5	Blood	7.4
Basic drugs		Cerebrospinal fluid	7.2
Diazepam	3.3	Urine	6.0–7.4
Codeine	7.9		
Amphetamine	9.8		

pKa, hydrogen ion dissociation constant.

charge, so less ionised drugs are weak organic bases. The non-ionised fraction of a drug is highly lipid soluble and easily diffuses across cell membranes.

The proportion of the drug that is non-ionised determines its lipid solubility. Since only this fraction is capable of passive diffusion across cell membranes, the amount of administered drug that reaches the interior of cells depends on the proportion that is non-ionised.

Degree of ionisation of a drug

A complication in the membrane permeability of a drug is the extent to which the drug may be ionised. This property is known as the **hydrogen ion dissociation constant** (pKa). The pKa values for different drugs vary widely (Table 4.1).

A further complication to membrane permeability is that the pH of the medium in which the drug is dissolved affects the degree of ionisation. The pKa of a drug is altered by the pH of the medium according to the Henderson–Hasselbach equation (see Ch. 2). Worse still, there is significant variation in the pH of different aqueous environments in the body (see Table 4.1). For example, the very acid gastric juices have a pH that varies between about 1.0 and 3.0, whereas plasma is normally maintained at a constant pH of 7.4.

Figure 4.2 shows the difference in the degree of ionisation between an acidic (A) and a basic (B) drug in the acid medium of the stomach and the basic medium of the plasma.

Passive diffusion across cell membranes

If the pH on either side of a cell membrane is different, the degree of ionisation of a drug on either side of the membrane will also be different (Fig. 4.2).

- Only the non-ionised form of the drug permeates lipid membranes readily.
- The pH in an aqueous compartment and the pKa of the drug determine how much of the drug is ionised (or remains non-ionised).
- The difference in pH on either side of the cell membrane gives unequal concentration of non-ionised drug on each side – known as **pH partitioning of drug molecules**. This is more pronounced where the pH difference is large, e.g. pH difference between gastric juices and plasma (see Fig. 4.2).
- The unequal non-ionised drug concentration on each side of the cell membrane gives rise to a concentration gradient. The non-ionised, lipid soluble form of the drug will passively diffuse down the concentration gradient across the cell membrane.
- The drive for passive diffusion is the concentration gradient, when the drug diffuses from an aqueous compartment with higher concentration to one with lower concentration. The rate of diffusion will be proportional to the concentration difference of the non-ionised form of the drug on either side of the membrane (Fick's Law, see Ch. 2).
- The distribution of the non-ionised form of the drug on each side of a cell membrane will reach equilibrium. This is known as the **steady state** distribution. Equilibrium is rarely achieved in vivo because the blood circulation and gastric motility constantly remove the drug. Also, the ionised form of the drug has some degree of permeability and can cross the lipid membrane down its concentration gradient.

Ion trapping

The effect of pH partitioning results in the accumulation of weak acids in compartments with relatively high pH (basic), and weak bases accumulate in compartments with a relatively low pH (acidic). This is the concept of **ion trapping**. Applying this principle, the degree of drug ionisation on one or other side of a cell membrane can be changed by increasing or decreasing intra- or extracellular pH, altering the concentration gradient of the non-ionised (lipid soluble) fraction of drug across the membrane, to increase or decrease the rate of passive diffusion into or out of the cell.

Effects of acidosis or alkalosis on absorption and distribution

The effects of metabolic or respiratory acidosis or alkalosis on drug absorption and distribution are of importance when treating patients with conditions such as respiratory failure and diabetic ketoacidosis. Restoration of acid–base balance in these patients is essential for avoiding ineffective drug treatment, adverse effects, overdose and toxicity.

Changes in plasma pH due to acidosis or alkalosis can have a significant effect on the pH partitioning or 'ion trapping' of drugs:

- In acidosis, blood pH falls so that the pH difference, or gradient, between the extracellular and intracellular fluids rises. An acidic drug would be retained in the cells.
- In alkalosis, blood pH rises so that indirectly, the difference between interstitial pH and intracellular pH

Gastric juices pH 2.4   Plasma pH 7.4

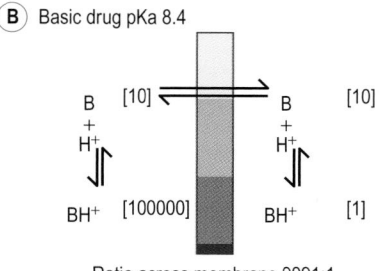

Ratio across membrane 1:9091

Ratio across membrane 9091:1

AH – an acidic drug is less ionised in an acid medium, so that a large proportion of the drug is the lipid soluble, non-ionised form in the stomach (pH 2.4). The non-ionised form crosses the cell membrane by passive diffusion into the plasma.

AH – the acidic drug in the more alkaline medium in the plasm (pH 7.4) is more ionised. The ionised form cannot diffuse back in the opposite direction.

At equilibrium, the concentration of non-ionised drug will be the same on both sides of the membrane, but the total concentration on the plasma side will be 9091 times higher.

BH – a basic drug is more ionised in the acid medium (pH 2.4) of the stomach so that very little of the non-ionised form of the drug can be absorbed by passive diffusion into plasma.

BH – in plasma, the basic drug is less ionised in the more alkaline medium. A high concentration of the non-ionised drug potentially could diffuse out of the plasma into the stomach.

In gastric juices at pH 2.4, the degree of ionisation for an acidic drug (pKa 3.4) is: 10
• for every 10 non-ionised molecules there is 1 ionised molecule (ratio 10:1)

The same drug in plasma (pH 7.4), the degree of ionisation is: 10,000
• for every 10 non-ionised molecules there are 100,000 ionised molecules.

The reverse happens for a basic drug.

Fig. 4.2 **Effect of pH partitioning on passive diffusion across the gastric cell membrane.**

Clinical box 4.1   **Therapeutic application of ion trapping: treatment of overdose**

Most drugs are excreted through the kidneys. If the pH gradient across the glomerular basement membrane can be increased, renal excretion is increased. This can be achieved by making the urine either more acid or more alkaline:

● Urinary acidification increases tubular excretion of weak bases and decreases excretion of weak acids.
● Urinary alkalinisation accelerates the excretion of weak acids and slows down the excretion of weak bases.

Therefore, in:

● **Aspirin overdose**: renal excretion of aspirin (weak acid) can be increased if urinary pH is increased (made more alkaline, i.e. basic) by the administration of Na^+ bicarbonate or a carbonic anhydrase inhibitor such as acetazolamide. Aspirin concentration in the more alkaline renal tubule could be increased fourfold.
● **Amphetamine overdose**: amphetamine is a weak base, so an acceleration in tubular excretion can be achieved by lowering urinary pH (making more acidic) by the administration of ammonium chloride.

decreases. Acidic drugs would tend to accumulate in the extracellular fluid.

CARRIER-MEDIATED TRANSPORT

Drugs that are ionised in plasma and will not diffuse into the cells, require specialist transmembrane proteins, **transporters**, to carry them across cell membranes. The ionised drug molecules combine with the protein on one side of the membrane, the transporter then changes its conformation and releases the drug on the other side. Drugs have been developed to facilitate or inhibit transporter activity.

Cells have two major classes of transmembrane proteins:

■ Transporters (carrier proteins)
■ Ion channel proteins.

Transporters (carrier proteins)

A given transporter is specific for a small group of related substrate molecules, which compete for the transporter. Protein transporters can be the sites of drug action, when the drug is similar to the substrate and competitively binds to the transporter. The process saturates when the number of drug molecules exceeds the number of transporter molecules. The drug then 'blocks' the action of the substrate (e.g. Na^+, K^+, neurotransmitter) on the cell.

There are three classes of transporters (see Ch. 2):

■ Uniporters
■ Symporters
■ Antiporters.

Uniporters are proteins of a specific size which allow specific compounds to be carried across the cell membrane, by **facilitated diffusion** down a concentration gradient, which does *not* require the expenditure of metabolic or electrochemical energy. **Ion channels** and glucose transporters are an example of uniporters where specific ions are allowed through. These are particularly important to the action of drugs (see below).

Symporters and antiporters are secondary active transporters, or **pumps**, requiring energy expenditure. Active transport can carry substances *against* a concentration gradient. Two substances are transported together across the cell membrane in the same direction by **symporters**, and in opposite directions (exchanged) by **antiporters**. For example, Na^+/K^+ ATPase is an antiporter ion pump, which removes Na^+ from the cytoplasm of the cell in exchange for K^+.

P-glycoproteins (PGPs) are antiporter transport proteins that use ATP to 'pump' noxious substances from cells. Recent research has shown that drugs may be expelled from

Clinical box 4.2	Drugs acting on protein transporters

- Probenecid competes for the transporter associated with the reabsorption of uric acid from the lumen of the nephron (facilitated diffusion). The resulting increase in uric acid excretion is exploited in the treatment of gout, a painful joint disease caused by deposition of uric acid in joints.
- Probenecid also competes for the transporter that is involved in the renal excretion of penicillin; competition reduces penicillin excretion, which helps to maintain plasma concentration.
- Digoxin inhibits the Na^+/K^+ pump in the membrane of cardiac myocytes so that Na^+ is retained in the cell. A related Na^+/Ca^{2+} symporter slows down in response to Na^+ retention. Intracellular Ca^{2+} increases, is stored, then released for muscle contraction.
- Omeprazole, a proton pump inhibitor of the benzimidazole group, irreversibly inhibits the H^+/K^+ ATPase pump (proton pump) in the last step in the pathway for acid secretion in the stomach. Omeprazole is prescribed for conditions in which excessive acid secretion causes gastritis, peptic ulceration and symptoms of gastro-oesophageal reflux (GORD).
- Amitriptyline and other tricyclic drugs used in the treatment of depression compete with noradrenaline (norepinephrine)/serotonin neuronal uptake transporters to produce their effects (see also The Autonomic Nervous System).

cells in the same way. If this occurs in the gut lumen then bioavailability of an orally administered drug is reduced, and PGPs effectively 'block' absorption. Some cancer cells overproduce PGPs, driving out anti-cancer drugs, effectively causing 'resistance'.

Ion channel proteins

Ion channel proteins are large proteins forming water-filled pores that span the lipid bilayer of cell membranes. These pores, or channels, allow ions of appropriate size and charge, that otherwise cannot permeate cell membranes, to be transferred across. The flux, or flow, of ions can be into or out of the cell.

All ion channel proteins allow solutes to cross membranes by facilitated diffusion without energy expenditure. The channel, or pore structure, is either open or closed and the conformational change is called gating, as in opening and closing a gate.

- With uncharged solutes, facilitated diffusion takes place down a concentration gradient without the expenditure of energy.
- If the solute carries a net charge then both its concentration gradient and the membrane potential influence the transport process. The concentration gradient and the membrane potential combine to produce the net driving force known as the **electrochemical gradient**.

ENDOCYTOSIS AND EXOCYTOSIS

Very large molecules (macromolecules), such as proteins, cannot be transported across the cell membrane by transporters, and have to be taken into or out of the cells through the processes of endocytosis and exocytosis. These are the most complex method of transport across a biological membrane (see Ch. 2). Drugs can facilitate or inhibit these processes.

- **Endocytosis**: a substance gains entry into a cell by first being captured into an invagination of the cell wall, which is then pinched off as a vesicle. The drug thus enters the cell without having to cross the cell membrane.
- **Exocytosis**: membrane-coated vesicles fuse with the plasma membrane to release their contents into the extracellular compartment, e.g. neuronal synapse (see Ch. 2). Examples are the vesicles associated with the storage of neurotransmitters (noradrenaline (norepinephrine), acetylcholine) and with pancreatic enzymes (see later).

DIFFUSION THROUGH AQUEOUS AND INTERCELLULAR PORES

Most biological membranes are relatively permeable to water that passes across the cell membrane via **aqueous pores**, either by diffusion or by bulk flow that results from osmotic differences across the membrane, carrying extremely small, water-soluble molecules of less than 100 daltons in diameter with it (e.g. lithium, urea, ethanol).

Gap junctions

Junctions between cells (intercellular pores) may allow the transfer of free, not protein bound, drug molecules in solution, a process known as **filtration**. These junctions are known as **gap junctions**. Other junctions prevent the transfer of molecules, and are known as **tight junctions**.

The ability of drugs to penetrate the endothelial membrane varies from one tissue to another. Gap junctions in vascular endothelium allow bulk transfer of drug molecules free in solution but not those bound to plasma proteins. In contrast, in the blood–brain barrier and the placenta, the capillary membranes are tightly joined together with only a few tight junctions, so that drugs can only pass through the membrane either by passive diffusion (lipid soluble molecules) or carrier-mediated transport. In the liver, the capillary endothelium is porous, allowing for free passage of large molecules.

DRUG DISTRIBUTION

Depending on pH, ionisation and lipid solubility, drugs can be moved for short distances by diffusion and membrane transport. Rapid transport over long distances around the body has to be done in the bloodstream, partly in solution as **free** (unbound) drug and partly **bound** to blood components (plasma proteins, blood cells). The bound and unbound forms are in **equilibrium**, and *only* the unbound drug is available for passive diffusion from the bloodstream to tissue sites where the pharmacological effects occur.

Drug distribution is the process by which a drug is transferred from the bloodstream (plasma) to tissues (interstitial fluid and cells). The rate and degree of drug distribution throughout the body depends on:

- Blood flow
- Capillary permeability
- Protein binding (affinity of the drug for various constituents of cells)
- Accumulation in and redistribution to other sites.

BLOOD FLOW

The rate at which a drug reaches different organs and tissues depends on the blood flow to those regions. Equilibration of free drug between plasma and tissue is rapidly achieved in well-perfused tissues, for example, the liver, kidneys, brain and skeletal muscle. Equilibrium in poorly perfused tissues, such as fat (adipose tissue), takes much longer.

CAPILLARY PERMEABILITY AND GAP JUNCTIONS

The ability of drugs to leave plasma and enter the interstitial fluid is determined by their physico-chemical properties (e.g. lipid solubility and ionisation) and via intercellular pores, the **gap junctions**, in the vascular endothelium. Gap junctions can be 4–10 nm in diameter, i.e. wide enough to allow the passage of ionised water-soluble drugs, even those as large as albumin, into the interstitial fluid. The capillaries in the liver are extremely permeable, with gap junctions that allow the passage of large protein molecules, whereas the vascular epithelium to the brain is the opposite, so that only drugs that are highly lipid soluble or have a selective transporter can enter the CNS.

Drug distribution to special organs

Central nervous system

Many drugs cannot gain access to the brain because of the **blood–brain barrier**. By virtue of tight junctions, much reduced number of aqueous pores in the cell membrane, the blood–brain barrier only allows drugs that are lipid soluble (e.g. thiopental, a general anaesthetic) or have a selective transporter protein (e.g. L-dopa for Parkinsonism) to enter the CNS. However, inflammation of the capillary epithelial layer, for example in meningitis, may increase the permeability of the blood–brain barrier and allow charged or polar drugs to attain therapeutic concentrations; this is exploited in the use of penicillin in the treatment of meningitis.

Fetus

Lipid-soluble drugs given to the pregnant mother can cross the placental barrier to the fetus by passive diffusion. Some drugs need active transport. Large, highly ionised molecules (e.g. heparin) do not cross the placental barrier easily. Compared with well-perfused organs such as liver and lungs, the placental circulation is slow, equilibrates slowly with maternal blood, and relies on maternal elimination for drug excretion. Although fetal plasma concentration of the drug will be much lower than in maternal blood, the fetus could still be affected:

- Serious fetal abnormalities can develop if the fetus is exposed during the first trimester, when the brain and major organs are developing. Thalidomide (α-phthalimido-glutarimide), marketed as Distaval and used to relieve symptoms of nausea in early pregnancy, caused an epidemic of severe birth defects.
- Toxic effects during the second and third trimesters are similar to those in the mother, but are exaggerated: tetracyclines can affect developing teeth and bones, warfarin can damage fetal brain.
- Drugs of addiction such as heroin or cocaine have a profound effect on the fetus, as can alcohol and nicotine (cigarette smoking).

- Drugs given just before delivery, e.g. analgesics and tranquilisers, can cause respiratory impairment in the newborn.

ACCUMULATION OF DRUG IN FAT AND REDISTRIBUTION IN OTHER TISSUES

When a drug is administered directly into the bloodstream, as in intravenous injection, the drug will rapidly reach well-perfused tissues, such as brain, liver and lungs, to reach equilibrium at high tissue concentrations. The drug will also be transported to, and enter, poorly perfused tissues, but at a slower rate, lowering the plasma concentration. If the concentration gradient between plasma and well-perfused tissue reverses, the drug will diffuse back into plasma for redistribution to poorly perfused tissues, terminating the action of the drug in well-perfused tissue (see Information box 4.2).

Fat, or adipose tissue, is poorly perfused. A few, highly soluble drugs can accumulate in body fat. Of importance to long-term administration are drugs such as benzodiazepine and some insecticides (e.g. DDT). The accumulation of long-acting benzodiazepine (e.g. diazepam) and their subsequent release can give cumulative effects.

BINDING OF DRUGS TO PROTEINS

At therapeutic plasma concentrations, many drugs bind extensively to plasma and intracellular proteins. This limits the amount of drug available for distribution outside the bloodstream. The protein-bound drug molecules cannot permeate cell membranes, be metabolised, excreted or produce their effect.

- Drug–protein binding has no pharmacological effect.
- Protein binding lowers the plasma free drug concentration.
- Protein binding reduces that amount of drug available for acting on receptors.

The major plasma proteins that bind drugs are **albumin**, **γ-globulin lipoproteins** and **α₁-acidic glycoprotein**. There are also binding sites on intracellular proteins. The ionic binding between drug and protein is competitive and readily reversible so that the protein acts as a reservoir for the drug. As the drug is eliminated, the ratio between bound and unbound drug is maintained by more drug dissociating from the proteins.

The degree of protein binding depends upon the drug and varies from almost 100% (warfarin, diazepam) to less than

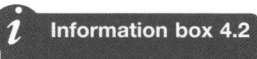

Information box 4.2   **Termination of the action of thiopental**

Thiopental, a highly lipid-soluble general anaesthetic, achieves equilibrium and a therapeutically effective concentration in the CNS in a matter of seconds. In muscle, which has a lower blood flow, it takes about 30 minutes to achieve equilibrium, and in adipose tissue it takes 4–8 hours. Thus, when the concentration of thiopental in the brain has reached equilibrium and may be declining due to redistribution, tissue concentration in muscle and adipose tissue is still rising. Thiopental will diffuse out of the brain to be redistributed to adipose tissue, lowering the concentration in the brain. The general anaesthetic effect of thiopental is terminated by redistribution of the drug into adipose tissue and not through metabolism.

Table 4.2	Examples of drugs that bind to plasma albumin. Those marked with an asterisk also bind to α_1-acid glycoprotein. The majority of drugs occupy less than 1% of the binding sites available to them. Drugs that occupy 50% or more of binding sites may induce displacement of other drugs		
Drug (chemical class)	% of drug bound	% of occupied binding sites on proteins	
Warfarin (acid)	99.5	<1	
Diazepam (base)	99	<1	
Digitoxin (neutral)	90–97	<1	
Propranolol (base)*	90–96	<1	
Phenytoin (acid)	90–94	<1	
Amitriptyline (base)*	82–96	<1	
Sodium valproate (acid)	80–90	50–60	
Imipramine (base)	80–95	<1	
Lidocaine (base)*	45–80	<1	
Salicylate (acid)	50–90	50	
Phenobarbital (acid)	50–60	<1	
Digoxin (neutral)	20	<1	
Lithium (ion)	0	<1	

30% (digoxin) (Table 4.2). This difference is of clinical importance because of its effect on the duration of action of the drug after administration. As the intracellular concentration of free drug falls, the drug will dissociate from its protein-binding site, sustaining drug concentration. If the proportion of bound drug is high, then a higher concentration of free drug will be maintained for longer, so that dosing intervals have to be adjusted to avoid overdose.

Competitive protein binding

Competition for binding sites can take place between drugs and between drugs and endogenous ligands. A drug with a high affinity for protein-binding sites (e.g. aspirin) can saturate its binding sites at therapeutic concentrations. This will displace a less highly bound drug (e.g. warfarin) from its binding site, increasing the concentration of free drug. If drug A is 98% bound then only 2% of this drug is available to give its therapeutic effect. If the binding is reduced to 96% through displacement by a second drug, the plasma concentration of drug A is doubled.

The importance of competitive interactions may sometimes be overstated because the number of binding sites occupied by any one of the majority of drugs is only a small

---

Clinical box 4.3	**Aspirin potentiates the action of warfarin**

Aspirin (salicylate), a non-steroidal anti-inflammatory drug, is highly protein bound, where up to 90% of the drug is bound, and occupies over 50% of the protein-binding sites. If warfarin is administered at the same time, the aspirin molecules will displace warfarin molecules so that less warfarin is protein bound, making more free warfarin available to exert its anticoagulant effect, thus 'potentiating' the effect of a given dose of warfarin. Spontaneous bruising, haematoma and prolonged bleeding after minor trauma will occur.

---

fraction of the total available for binding that molecule (i.e. the binding sites are not saturated).

Hypoproteinaemia

If the number of protein-binding sites in plasma are reduced, for example due to hypoalbuminaemia, drugs that are normally present in a predominantly bound form will be present in the free form at an elevated concentration, so that their therapeutic effect will be increased. Drug dosages need to be adjusted and reduced in these conditions to avoid adverse effects.

Hypoalbuminaemia can occur as a consequence of liver disease, nephrotic syndrome, malnutrition, burns, and renal failure, when less albumin is available to bind drugs. This is particularly important in elderly people, when dosages may have to be reduced to avoid overdose.

Sequestration of drugs in tissues

In addition to protein binding, a drug may bind to and accumulate within tissues, prolonging its duration in the body. This is because the stored (sequestered) drug is in equilibrium with drug in plasma, so as the drug is eliminated from the body, sequestered drug moves into plasma from the storage tissue. However, the binding between the drug and the tissue element may be so stable that the drug may not be readily available for release.

DISTRIBUTION OF DRUGS IN THE BODY

Distribution is the pharmacokinetic stage in which a drug in the plasma is transferred to tissues to exert its therapeutic action. Once a drug enters the body, it can be distributed between four major aqueous compartments (Fig. 4.3), which are separated by barriers composed of cell membranes:

- Plasma
- Interstitial
- Intracellular
- Transcellular.

Total body water, as a percentage of body weight, varies from approximately 50% to 75%, depending on age and sex.

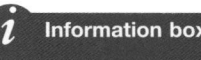 | **Information box 4.3** | **Consequences of drug sequestration** |

The antimalarial drug chloroquine only needs to be taken once per week: because of its binding to DNA, drug concentration in liver and white blood cells is several thousand times higher than its concentration in plasma. The sequestered drug in the liver and white cells is slowly released into the circulation as plasma concentration falls due to metabolism and excretion, prolonging the action and duration of chloroquine in the body.

- **'Bone seekers'** such as fluoride and strontium-90 may be deposited with bone salts in an insoluble form, making them difficult to remove. Fluoride deposition in teeth benefits mineralisation and prevents dental caries. Strontium-90, however, is harmful and can cause leukaemia.
- **Calcium chelators**, such as tetracyclines, are deposited with bone salts in an insoluble form, making them difficult to remove. Deposition in developing teeth causes discoloration. Tetracyclines should not be prescribed for pregnant women or young children.

Typical volumes of fluid compartments
in a 70 kg man

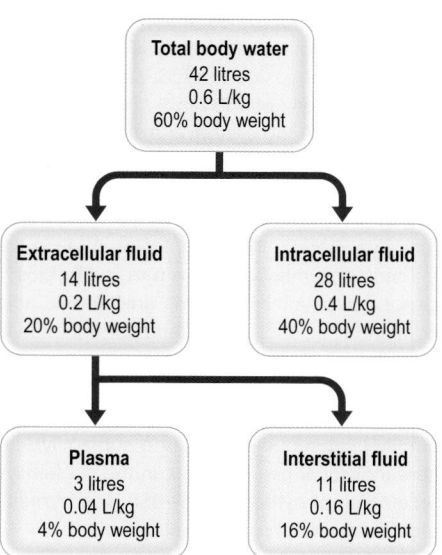

Total body water
42 litres
0.6 L/kg
60% body weight

Extracellular fluid
14 litres
0.2 L/kg
20% body weight

Intracellular fluid
28 litres
0.4 L/kg
40% body weight

Plasma
3 litres
0.04 L/kg
4% body weight

Interstitial fluid
11 litres
0.16 L/kg
16% body weight

Body water is distributed between three major compartments:

• **Extracellular fluid** (20% of body weight)
  composed of:
  – blood plasma (4–5% of body weight)
  – interstitial fluid (16% of body weight)
  – lymph (1%).
• **Intracellular fluid** (30–40% of body weight), the total
  amount of fluid in all the cells of the body.
• **Transcellular fluid** which includes synovial, cerebrospinal,
  peritoneal, pleural and intraocular fluids. These constitute
  approximately 2.5% of the total body weight.

Fig. 4.3 **The distribution of body fluids in a 30-year-old man weighing 70 kg.** (Expressed as total volume (L), volume per kg body weight (L/kg) and percentage of body weight.)

Women tend to have lower body water due to increased body fat.

Drug molecules also exist in free and protein-bound forms. Therefore, in each aqueous compartment, drug molecules may be:

■ Free in aqueous solution or bound to protein
■ In ionised and non-ionised form in equilibrium.

The degree of ionisation of free drug depends on whether the drug is a weak acid or weak base, and on the pH of the aqueous compartment.

Extent of drug distribution into aqueous compartments

Free drug is distributed between the four major aqueous compartments of the body, but most drugs are not exclusively associated with any one. The majority of drugs are:

■ Distributed into a number of aqueous compartments
■ Bound to cellular components, such as protein
■ Dissolved into lipid stores.

The **pattern**, or extent of drug distribution into the compartments depends on:

■ Permeability between cell membranes
■ Protein binding within compartments
■ pH partitioning
■ Accumulation in adipose tissue.

The estimated amount of drug that is distributed from plasma to other aqueous compartments is important, because the pharmacological effects of drugs are exerted in the interstitial, intracellular and transcellular compartments.

■ Some drugs remain in the plasma because their molecules are too big to cross capillary membranes into tissues (e.g. heparin).
■ Highly protein-bound drugs tend to remain in the plasma.

The amount of drug needed to reach a plasma concentration that enables adequate distribution to effector tissues depends on the extent of distribution from plasma. This will determine the therapeutic **dosage** that needs to be administered.

The concept of an apparent volume of distribution is an estimate of the extent of drug distribution from plasma to effector tissues.

Apparent volume of distribution

While it is possible to measure drug concentration in total body water in animal experiments, only plasma concentration is measurable in humans, as tissue biopsies merely to measure drug concentration would be impossible. The **apparent volume of distribution** measures the concentration of free and protein-bound drug remaining in the plasma after distribution is completed, and is used to predict distribution of the drug in the various compartments of the body.

The apparent volume of distribution of a drug is a calculated volume of fluid containing the total amount of drug in the body at the same concentration as plasma concentration, expressed as the ratio of the total dose of drug to plasma concentration and reflecting the amount of drug left in the plasma after distribution. It does *not* indicate where and how much drug has been taken up by effector tissues.

Apparent volume of distribution does have pharmacological importance. It:

■ Gives an estimate of total drug in the body in relation to plasma concentration, and the concept is useful for monitoring progress when treating drug toxicity and overdose.
■ Is related to drug clearance from the body (see later), and indicates the overall rate of drug elimination and thus the drug half-life (see below).
■ Can predict tissue drug concentration from the above two estimates.

DRUG METABOLISM

Drug metabolism is the process by which the body produces a change to the chemical structure of a drug molecule by enzyme activity to produce a new chemical with different pharmacological properties. Metabolic processes determine how long a drug is active in the body, drug interactions and toxicity.

The outcomes of drug metabolism may be:

- The inactivation of drug so that it no longer has any biological activity (by conjugation, see below)
- To produce metabolites with less biological activity
- To produce **active metabolites** that may be more potent and persist longer than the parent compound
- To convert an **inactive pro-drug** to the active form
- To produce toxic metabolites
- To produce inactive metabolites that are water soluble for excretion (by conjugation, see below)

The liver is the major organ for drug metabolism. After absorption from the gastrointestinal tract, orally administered drugs pass through the liver via the portal vein before distribution to other organs. The liver may extensively metabolise and inactivate some drugs. This is the concept of first pass metabolism (see later), which can make a difference to how much of the administered drug reaches the target tissues.

Metabolic reactions for drugs are classified as:

- **Phase I reactions**, or pre-conjugation consisting of oxidation, reduction and hydrolysis reactions followed by
- **Phase II reactions**, consisting mainly of conjugation but also including acetylation reactions.

These reactions are not always sequential. The enzymes involved in both phases have low substrate specificities and can metabolise a wide range of drugs. They are associated with the following cell constituents:

- Smooth endoplasmic reticulum (where the enzymes are called microsomal enzymes)
- Cytoplasm
- Mitochondria.

PHASE I METABOLIC REACTIONS (PRE-CONJUGATION REACTIONS)

Phase I reactions – oxidation, reduction, hydrolysis – mainly take place in the liver and are mediated by **microsomal enzymes**. The collective term, the **mixed function oxidase** (MFO) system, is used to describe the hepatic microsomal enzymes involved in phase I reactions.

Oxidation

Oxidation is the most important of the phase I reactions, mainly catalysed by microsomal enzymes.

Microsomal oxidation reactions

There are two types of microsomal oxidation reaction:

- One in which an oxygen molecule is added to the substrate
- One in which the primary oxidation leads to a loss of the oxygen atom in a small fragment of the original molecule – e.g. **deamination** and **dealkylation**.

Microsomal oxidation reactions require:

- Molecular oxygen
- NADPH (nicotinamide adenosine dinucleotide phosphate (reduced form))
- NADPH-cytochrome C reductase
- The haemoprotein cytochrome P-450 mono-oxygenase enzymes that bind both the drug and O_2 molecules.

Cytochrome P-450 system

Cytochrome P-450 is the most important enzyme system in the diverse group of enzymes that catalyse oxidation in humans. They are so named because cytochrome P-450 reacts with carbon monoxide to produce a pink (P) complex with an absorption peak at 450 nm.

The cytochrome P-450 system is a superfamily of related but distinct microsomal liver enzymes, subject to genetic variation (see below). Although drug metabolism by cytochrome P-450 takes place mainly in the liver, the enzyme also occurs elsewhere in the body, for example in the small intestine. These enzymes also take part in the biosynthesis of endogenous substances such as arachidonic acid, steroids, prostaglandins, cholesterol, and thromboxane (made by platelets and causing vasoconstriction).

For human beings, cytochrome P-450 enzymes are named as CYP in capitals (human), subsequent number (the isoform family), subsequent letter (the subfamily), and final number (the individual gene product in the subfamily). Table 4.3 lists examples of cytochrome P-450 isoenzymes. These enzymes differ from each other because of:

- Difference in amino acid sequence
- Specificity for the drugs that they metabolise
- The drugs that can inhibit or induce them.

Some drugs cause enzyme induction or inhibition, thereby reducing or enhancing the therapeutic effect of another, co-administered drug (Information box 4.4). These effects are discussed further in relation to enzyme induction and inhibition.

 Information box 4.4   **Examples of enzyme induction and inhibition**

- Some anticonvulsants (e.g. phenytoin) and rifampicin induce cytochrome P-450 enzymes, which increase the rate of metabolism and thus reduce the therapeutic effect of warfarin if administered at the same time. Patients on anticoagulant therapy being prescribed rifampicin or phenytoin will need a higher dose of warfarin.
- Cytochrome P-450 enzyme induction by rifampicin (and phenytoin) also increases the metabolism of oestrogens so that the efficacy of the combined oral contraceptive pill is reduced. Breakthrough bleeding or contraceptive failure may occur. Patients prescribed rifampicin (or anticonvulsants) need to be warned about this effect and advised to use alternative contraception.
- Components of grapefruit juice inhibit CYP3A4, slowing down the metabolism of substrates that use the same enzyme, such as simvastatin and atorvastatin, leading to elevated blood levels. The effect on calcium channel blockers, used for the treatment of angina, leads to elevated plasma levels with potentially disastrous consequences, such as hypotension and asystole.
- Grapefruit juice also enhances the effects of some antihistamines such as terfenadine, by inhibiting the action of CYP3A4 in the gut, reducing the breakdown of the drug and increasing bioavailability. Hay fever sufferers taking terfenadine should be cautioned about drinking grapefruit juice because they might become excessively drowsy, risking accidents when driving a car or operating machinery.
- Grapefruit juice is associated with a reduction in blood level of some drugs. This has been attributed to an interaction with p-glycoproteins in the gut, which pumps the drug out of the cells into the lumen, thus reducing absorption. Further research is needed to explain this phenomenon.

Table 4.3 Examples of drugs and their interaction with the isoenzymes of cytochrome P-450*

Isoenzyme	Substrate	Inducer	Inhibitor
CYP1A2	*Paracetamol*	Barbiturates	Cimetidine
	Amitriptyline		Erythromycin
	Clozapine	Nicotine	Grapefruit juice
	Diazepam		Diltiazem
	Methadone	Polycyclic aromatic hydrocarbons found in cigarette smoke and in the charred parts of charcoal-grilled meats	
	Caffeine		
	Calcium channel antagonists		
	Antihistamines		
	Tamoxifen		
CYP2B6	*Tamoxifen*	Phenobarbital	Orphenadrine
	Cyclophosphamide	Phenytoin	
CYP2C8	Diazepam	Phenobarbital	Omeprazole
	Diclofenac	Primidone	
	Tolbutamide		
CYP2C9	Amitriptyline	Carbamazepine	Amiodarone
	Diclofenac	Rifampicin	Cimetidine
	Indometacin		Fluvoxamine
	Phenytoin		
	Warfarin		
CYP2C19	Omeprazole	Barbiturates	Fluoxetine
	Phenytoin		Tolbutamide
	Valproic acid		
CYP3A4†	Amiodarone	Carbamazepine	Cimetidine
	Tamoxifen	Glucocorticoids	Diltiazem
	Paracetamol	Phenytoin	Omeprazole
	Diazepam	Rifampicin	Quinidine
	Dexamethasone		
	Imipramine		
	Oestrogens		
CYP2E1	*Paracetamol*	Ethanol	Disulfiram
	Enflurane	Isoniazid	Ritonavir
	Ethanol		
	Isoniazid		

*Drugs given in italics are substrates for a number of the isoenzymes.
†Involved in the metabolism of 50% of all drugs.

Non-microsomal oxidative reactions

Not all phase 1 reactions are carried out by the cytochrome P-450 system. Non-microsomal enzymes located in the cytoplasm, mitochondria of cells and in the plasma are capable of oxidation and the less common reduction and hydrolysis (see below). Important examples for drug therapy include:

- The soluble liver cytoplasmic enzyme, **alcohol dehydrogenase**, metabolises alcohol to acetaldehyde, which is further metabolised by aldehyde dehydrogenase to acetic acid (in addition to CYP2E1).
- **Xanthine oxidase** – also located in liver cytoplasm is important in the metabolism of purines to produce uric acid. Excessive accumulation of uric acid in joints leads to gout.
- **Allopurinol** – metabolised by xanthine oxidase, but also a competitive inhibitor of xanthine oxidase. This characteristic is exploited in the use of allopurinol in the treatment of gout to reduce uric acid production.
- **Tyrosine hydroxylase** and **tryptophan hydroxylase** are important neuronal cytoplasmic enzymes (see later, The Autonomic Nervous System). Tyrosine hydroxylase oxidises the amino acid tyrosine to levodopa in the sequence of reactions during the synthesis of the neurotransmitter noradrenaline (norepinephrine; see later). Tryptophan hydroxylase catalyses the oxidation of tryptophan in the synthesis of 5-hydroxytryptamine (5-HT, serotonin).
- Mitochondrial **monoamine oxidase** (MAO) is important in the metabolism of catecholamines, some sympathomimetic amines and 5-HT. Dietary 5-HT is completely metabolised by MAO in the intestines and liver (first pass metabolism, see below). MAO also metabolises 5-HT in the neuron (see later, The Autonomic Nervous System).

Reduction

Reduction is much less common, or important, than oxidation in drug metabolism, and can be performed by body tissues or intestinal flora. The enzymes catalysing reduction include both cytochrome P-450 and cytochrome P-450 reductase.

Hydrolysis – hydroxylation

Hydrolysis reactions involve the addition of a water (H_2O) molecule to the drug, and the process splits the drug. The reaction takes place in plasma, not mitochondria. This can occur spontaneously because of unstable groups in the drug molecule, or be catalysed by enzymes capable of hydrolysing amide and ester bonds in many drugs. Intestinal flora can also hydrolyse drug molecules, when metabolites are excreted in the bile or faeces.

A number of non-specific esterases and amidases are present in the endoplasmic reticulum of cells of the liver, intestine and kidneys, and in blood and other tissues. The alcohol and amine groups exposed following the hydrolysis of esters and amides are suitable for conjugation (phase II metabolism, see below), inactivating the drug and making it water soluble for excretion.

PHASE II METABOLIC REACTIONS (CONJUGATION REACTIONS)

Phase II reactions, known as **conjugation**, involve the synthesis of a covalent bond between a highly polar, normal substance in the body (endogenous) with a phase I metabolite or sometimes with the parent drug. Energy is needed for synthesising the bond. The conjugate is a less lipid-soluble, more water-soluble compound that is readily excreted in urine and/or bile and nearly always pharmacologically inactive. There are, however, exceptions, e.g. morphine 6-glucuronide has greater analgesic potency than the parent compound morphine.

Conjugation by glucuronidation

The most important phase II reaction is **glucuronidation**, when a molecule of glucuronic acid is transferred to the drug molecule. This is catalysed by microsomal uridine diphosphate (UDP)-glucuronyltransferase.

Other conjugation reactions

Other phase II reactions are catalysed by enzymes in the cytoplasm:

- **Sulphate conjugation**, catalysed by sulfotransferase
- **Methylation**, catalysed by transmethylase and
- **Acetylation**, catalysed by *N*-acetyltransferase.

Acetylation, in contrast to other forms of conjugation, sometimes produces metabolites that are less water soluble than the original substance. For example, the acetyl metabolites of some of the earlier sulphonamides (a class of antibacterial agents) produced crystalluria because they were precipitated in the renal tubules.

Drug detoxification

Conjugation with **glutathione** represents a major detoxification pathway for a number of drugs. Glutathione conjugates are cleaved to give cysteine derivatives, which in turn are acetylated to produce mercapturic acids. Many of the substrates for the enzyme glutathione-*S*-transferase are reactive metabolites, and depletion of the endogenous hepatic stores of glutathione can result in hepatotoxicity (Information box 4.6).

FACTORS AFFECTING DRUG METABOLISM

The ability of an individual to metabolise a drug can be influenced by a variety of factors including genetic factors, age, sex and disease. Exposure to a drug or environmental chemicals causing induction or inhibition of the enzymes associated with metabolism will also affect the way that patients metabolise drugs. These factors have an impact on the therapeutic effect of the drug and potential drug interactions that can give rise to adverse side effects, overdose and toxicity.

Genetic factors

When known, differences in the expression of metabolic enzymes in different groups of people need to be taken into account when prescribing. There is genetic variation in the ability of unrelated individuals to metabolise drugs. Most of the metabolic enzymes are under polygenic control. For some enzymes, however, there is polymorphism at a single gene. Although there is a 'normal' (Gaussian) distribution of enzyme activity in the general population, some people are 'fast' and some 'slow' metabolisers.

The earliest example to be identified of polymorphism at a single gene is the fast and slow acetylation of isoniazid (antituberculous drug). **Slow acetylator** status is an autosomal recessive trait that shows a race-dependent distribution. It is found in about 60% of Europeans but in only 5%

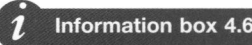

Information box 4.5　**Examples of drug hydrolysis by enzymes**

- Cholinesterase, which is found in plasma as well as in the cytoplasm of cholinergic neurones, is important in the termination of action of acetylcholine and a wide variety of drugs.
- Pethidine (US meperidine), an opiate analgesic, is de-esterified by a membrane bound microsomal esterase to meperidinic acid.
- Procaine, a local anaesthetic, is metabolised by both plasma pseudocholinesterase and a liver microsomal esterase.
- Suxamethonium, a neuromuscular blocker, is predominantly hydrolysed by plasma pseudocholinesterase.

Information box 4.6　**Hepatic failure in paracetamol overdose**

Although conjugation is a major detoxification pathway for many drugs, some reactions produce metabolites that are more toxic than the parent drug.

Paracetamol (US acetaminophen) undergoes conjugation with sulphate or glucuronide. However, in a phase I reaction, it is also metabolised by the P-450 mixed function oxidase to produce a reactive metabolite (*N*-acetyl-p-benzoquinone imine). This reactive metabolite then interacts with glutathione to produce mercapturic acid. In paracetamol overdoses, glutathione eventually becomes depleted. The reactive metabolite accumulates and interacts with cellular proteins causing hepatotoxicity and nephrotoxicity, resulting in cell death in the liver and kidneys.

of the Japanese population. Clinically, slow acetylators are more likely to develop peripheral neuropathies with isoniazid. Procainamide (used in cardiac arrhythmia) and hydralazine (antihypertensive) show a similar pattern of 'slow' metabolism. Slow metabolisers will show a high concentration of the parent drug with lower concentrations of metabolites.

Environmental contaminants and drugs

The activity of drug metabolising enzymes can be induced (increased) or inhibited (decreased) by chemicals contained in environmental contaminants and drugs.

- Organochlorine insecticides (e.g. DDT)
- Organophosphate pesticides (e.g. sheep dip)
- Polycyclic aromatic hydrocarbons (contained in cigarette smoke and the charred parts of char-grilled [broiled] meat).
- Alcohol in chronic alcohol consumption.

Enzyme induction

Repeated exposure of the liver to certain lipid-soluble substances can cause an increase in microsomal enzyme activity by increasing the de novo synthesis of cytochrome P-450 enzymes – **enzyme induction**. Examples of inducers of specific cytochrome P-450 enzymes are given in Table 4.3.

Induction can be non-specific: for example, phenobarbital and rifampicin are non-selective inducers that act on a number of cytochrome P-450 families (CYP1, 2 and 3). In contrast, chronic ethanol consumption induces a specific isoenzyme, CYP2E1. Enzyme induction has clinically important effects (Clinical box 4.4).

Induction by broad-spectrum inducers of cytochrome P-450, such as phenobarbital, leads to:

- Hepatic hypertrophy, proliferation of smooth endoplasmic reticulum
- Increased protein and phospholipid synthesis
- Increased synthesis of cytochrome P-450 isoenzymes and NADPH cytochrome P-450 reductase.

The induction occurs over a period of time (weeks) and is slowly reversible after the cessation of the drug. The mechanism of induction is not fully understood.

Enzyme inhibition

Enzyme inhibition slows down the metabolism of a drug so that it persists for longer periods in the body. Most cytochrome P-450 enzymes that metabolise drugs are not very specific. A single enzyme is usually capable of metabolising several different drugs, and two or more enzymes with overlapping substrate specificities can contribute to the metabolism of a single compound. As a result, two or more drugs may *compete* for the active site of a single cytochrome P-450 enzyme, interfering with the normal metabolism of a co-administered drug or endogenous compound. For example, imidazole-containing drugs, such as cimetidine (a histamine receptor agonist), bind competitively to a number of cytochrome P-450 enzymes, reducing the metabolism of endogenous steroids and co-administered drugs such as warfarin, phenytoin, quinidine. Plasma levels of these drugs will be elevated, and may contribute to adverse reactions or toxicity.

Enzyme inhibition by metabolites

Metabolites of cytochrome P-450 can form a complex with the enzyme that inactivates the enzyme. This process is reversible. Another form of enzyme inhibition, known as 'suicide' inhibition is irreversible. A reactive metabolite of cytochrome P-450 binds to the enzyme and destroys it. Furthermore, a drug may be an inhibitor of a specific cytochrome P-450 enzyme without necessarily being a substrate for that enzyme. For example, quinidine is a potent inhibitor of CYP2D6 but is metabolised by CYP3A4.

CONVERSION OF INACTIVE PRO-DRUG TO ACTIVE METABOLITE

Some drugs are inactive pro-drugs, only becoming therapeutically active after metabolism. The inactive pro-drug is sometimes designed to bypass problems with drug administration (see later).

Clinical box 4.4   Clinical importance of enzyme induction

Induction of a specific cytochrome P-450 will increase the metabolism of its substrate drugs; this will reduce the amount of drug that is available to give a therapeutic effect.

This is an important consideration in prescribing drugs that induce liver metabolic enzymes: dosages of other medication, e.g. oral contraceptives and antibiotics, may need adjustment. Alternative methods for contraception will be needed.

Examples

Rifampicin, phenobarbital, and many anticonvulsant drugs used in the treatment of epilepsy, increase the rate of metabolism of a wide range of drugs (e.g. phenytoin, warfarin, oral contraceptives). Their own rate of drug metabolism also increases, thereby reducing their therapeutic effectiveness.

The measurement of serum levels of hepatic enzymes is used as an indicator of liver disease. An elevated serum γ-glutamyl transpeptidase (γ-GT, a hydrolysing enzyme) could be an early sign of either alcohol- or drug-related liver enzyme induction.

Clinical box 4.5   Examples of pro-drugs designed for bypassing problems with drug administration

- Olsalazine, a member of the sulfasalazine family of drugs used to treat inflammatory bowel disease, is a pro-drug. Olsalazine is inactive until metabolised by colonic bacteria in the distal colon, the desired site of action.
- Azathioprine, an immunosuppressant drug, is inactive until metabolised to mercaptopurine. It is well absorbed in the gastrointestinal tract, so oral administration would not damage the intestinal mucosa.
- Enalapril, an angiotensin-converting enzyme (ACE) inhibitor used in the treatment of hypertension, has to be hydrolysed to enalaprilat to become active.
- Cortisone and prednisone are inactive pro-drugs that have to be converted to hydrocortisone and prednisolone respectively, in vivo, to be become active drugs.
- Cyclophosphamide, a cytotoxic agent, only becomes active after metabolism in the liver. Therefore, cyclophosphamide can be orally administered as the pro-drug that should not damage the intestinal mucosa.

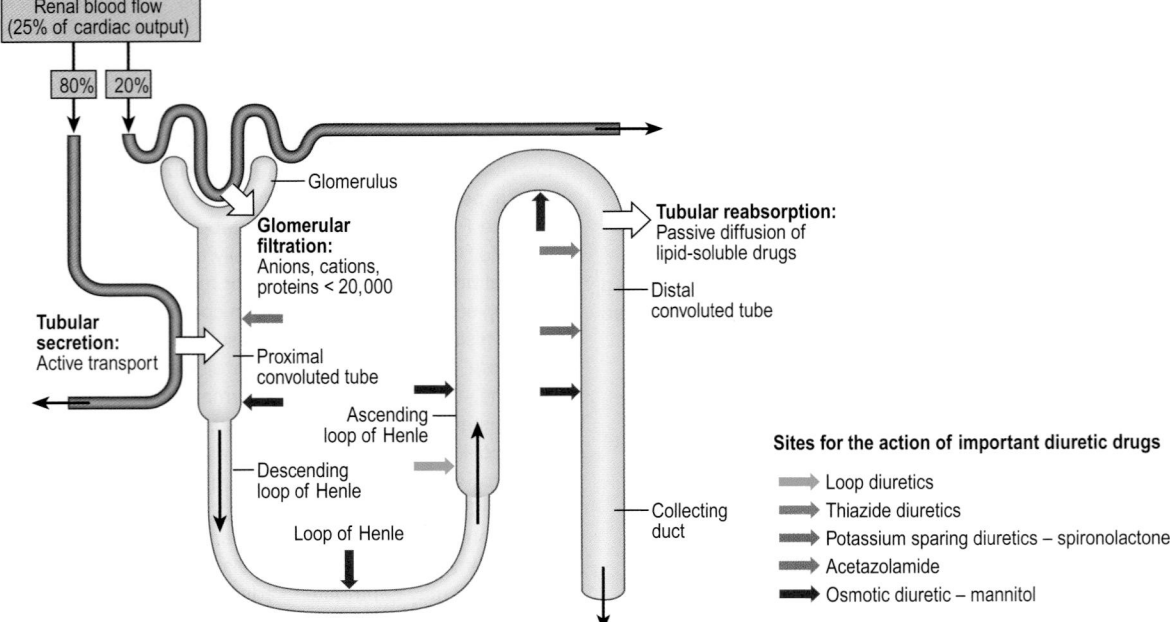

Fig. 4.4 **Renal excretion systems.**

EXCRETION OF DRUGS AND METABOLITES

Water-soluble drugs may be excreted unchanged, whereas metabolic inactivation makes drugs more soluble for excretion. The main routes of excretion for drugs and their metabolites are via:

- The renal system
- The hepatic/biliary system
- The lungs: this route is important in the excretion of gaseous anaesthetics; the lungs also have a role in the biotransformation of prostaglandins (see Ch. 13).

Losses of drugs via sweat and milk play only a small part in the overall excretion of drugs. However, excretion in milk is important because of the potential exposure of the breast-fed infant.

RENAL SYSTEM

Although the renal system is fully discussed in Chapter 14, renal functions concerned with drug excretion will be discussed here. Figure 4.4 is a schematic representation of the renal tubular system, where renal excretion mainly takes place. The processes are:

- Glomerular filtration
- Tubular secretion
- Tubular reabsorption

Glomerular filtration

Drugs and metabolites are excreted via renal glomeruli by filtration. The kidneys are highly perfused organs and receive about 25% of cardiac output of which 20% is filtered (180 L/day) to produce the initial urine. Glomerular capillaries allow the filtration of molecules with a molecular weight of below

20 000, irrespective of whether they are anions or cations, ionised or non-ionised. Plasma proteins, which have a molecular weight of 68 000 or more, and protein-bound drugs are not normally filtered. Therefore protein binding of drugs significantly affects their elimination via glomerular filtration.

Tubular secretion

Tubular secretion takes place in the proximal renal tubules, where the 80% of the renal blood flow that is not filtered by the glomerulus passes through to the peritubular capillaries of the proximal convoluted tubule. Here the tubule removes a wide variety of substances from plasma into the lumen of the tubule through **active transport** *against* a concentration gradient – tubular secretion. In the proximal tubule there are two non-specific carrier-mediated transport processes:

- A cation transporter for weak bases (e.g. quinine, morphine)
- An anion transporter for weak acids (e.g. penicillin, furosemide).

These two processes are rapid and saturable. In contrast to glomerular filtration, protein binding of the drug has no effect on drug clearance via tubular secretion. The affinity of drugs for the transporter is greater than that of the drug for plasma protein and results in maximum drug clearance. Substances that are transported by the same transporter compete with each other, resulting in drug interactions (Clinical box 4.6)

Tubular reabsorption

Tubular reabsorption of drugs takes place in the distal convoluted tubules of the kidney. There are specific transporters in the nephron for the reabsorption of essential constituents of tubular filtrate (e.g. amino acids, glucose, vitamins, water), but only very rarely are drugs reabsorbed in this way. The majority of drugs that are reabsorbed are lipid soluble and pass through the distal convoluted tubule membranes by passive diffusion.

The urine is concentrated during its passage to the distal convoluted tubule as water is reabsorbed. This increases the tubule to plasma concentration gradient for drugs that have been filtered or secreted into the lumen. While polar and ionised molecules (water soluble) remain in the urine, only the non-ionised (lipid-soluble) fraction of a weak acid or base contributes to the concentration gradient. As the degree of ionisation of a drug depends upon the pH of the urine and pKa of the drug, altering the pH of urine can promote drug excretion (see Clinical box 4.1).

Diuretic drugs

Diuretic drugs are used in the treatment of the conditions in which the retention of water and salt (NaCl) in the body severely interferes with normal function. Major clinical uses for diuretics include:

- Oedema in heart failure, nephrotic syndrome, hepatic cirrhosis
- Hypertension
- Acute renal failure
- Raised intracranial pressure (mannitol)
- Raised intraocular pressure (acetazolamide).

The complexities of the pharmacodynamic and pharmacokinetic processes of diuretics can, however, give rise to unwanted effects. Diuretic drugs act by:

- Inhibiting the reabsorption of Na^+ and Cl^- from the glomerular filtrate. Excretion of Na^+ and Cl^- ions increases, taking water with them.
- Opposing the antidiuretic action of aldosterone
- Increasing urine osmotic pressure to prevent tubular reabsorption of water
- Alkalinising the urine to promote excretion of bicarbonate, other ions and water.

Diuretics acting on the loop of Henle

Loop diuretics act on the loop of Henle (see Fig. 4.4). The main therapeutic example, furosemide, is a powerful diuretic, alleged to cause 'torrential urine flow'.

Pharmacodynamics

Loop diuretics promote Na^+ and Cl^- excretion by preventing reabsorption from urine in the ascending loop of Henle.

- Loop diuretics are actively secreted into the urine in the proximal convoluted tubule.
- Inhibition of the active symporter $Na^+/K^+/Cl^-$ ion pumps in the cell membrane of the ascending loop of Henle prevents the reabsorption of these ions.
- Urine passing into the distal convoluted and collection tubules is therefore hypertonic. The increased osmotic pressure prevents the reabsorption of water.
- 25% of glomerular filtrate passes out instead of the normal 1%, causing profuse diuresis.
- Increased Na^+ in the distal tubules increases the loss of K^+ and H^- ions, which may lead to hypokalaemia and metabolic alkalosis.

Pharmacokinetics

Loop diuretics are well absorbed when administered orally. In an emergency, e.g. acute heart failure or cerebral oedema, administration could be directly into the bloodstream by intravenous injection. The drug molecules are bound to plasma proteins and secreted into the urine in the proximal renal tubules by active, carrier-mediated transport.

Furosemide is metabolised in the liver by conjugation with glucuronide. Other loop diuretics, e.g. bumetanide, are metabolised by cytochrome P-450.

Unwanted side effects

The more common, unwanted side effects of loop diuretics include:

- Hypokalaemia due to potassium loss, which affects the contractility of heart muscle and may be life-threatening. Hypokalaemia may be avoided by giving K^+ supplements, or by concomitant administration of a K^+ sparing diuretic.
- Metabolic alkalosis due to H^- and Cl^- loss, which exacerbates hypokalaemia.
- Sodium and water depletion, particularly in the elderly, leading to collapse due to hypotension and hypovolaemia (from hyponatraemia).
- Urinary incontinence due to 'torrential urine flow'.

Diuretics acting on the distal tubule

Diuretics acting on the distal renal tubule include the thiazide diuretics, of which bendroflumethiazide (bendrofluazide) is the most commonly prescribed. Less commonly prescribed thiazides include hydrochlorothiazide and newer ones such as indapamide. The mechanism of their action is similar to loop diuretics, but their diuretic action is less powerful.

Pharmacodynamics

Thiazide diuretics act at the luminal surface of the distal convoluted tubules:

- Inhibition of Na^+ and Cl^- reabsorption by inhibiting the Na^+/Cl^- pump.
- Potassium is lost to a significant extent
- Onset of diuresis is slower than loop diuretics, but duration of action is longer
- Diuretic effect is reduced with impaired renal function (as in elderly people).

Unwanted side effects

The unwanted side effects of thiazide diuretics are similar to those produced by loop diuretics:

- Hypokalaemia
- Salt and water depletion
- Glycosuria – with long-term administration, a dose-related, progressive hyperglycaemia occurs. This is related to chronically low intracellular K^+ concentration, which inhibits insulin synthesis. This effect is reversible over time after cessation of the drug
- Impotence has been reported.

Potassium sparing diuretics

The main potassium sparing diuretic is spironolactone, which only has a weak diuretic action. Its main usefulness is as an adjunct to loop diuretics.

Pharmacodynamics

Spironolactone acts competitively on aldosterone receptors in the cells of the distal convoluted tubules, inhibiting its anti-diuretic effect by inhibiting the Na^+ retaining and the K^+ secreting actions of aldosterone, hence 'potassium sparing'.

Pharmacokinetics

Orally administered spironolactone is well absorbed, and is metabolised in the gastrointestinal tract and liver to active metabolite, canrenone, which has a long duration of action with a half-life of 16 hours. Its onset of action is slow, over several days.

Unwanted side effects

- Used alone, spironolactone can cause hyperkalaemia, which is life-threatening.
- Long-term administration may lead to metabolic acidosis.
- Gynaecomastia may occur, because the steroid structure of spironolactone has an oestrogen effect.

Osmotic diuretics

Osmotic diuretics act by increasing the osmotic pressure of urine in the renal tubules to limit tubular reabsorption of water. Mannitol is a pharmacologically inert substance. It is administered intravenously and filtered, unchanged, at the glomerulus, with little or no tubular reabsorption, and excreted unchanged. The most important uses are:

- Cerebral oedema and raised intracranial pressure
- Acute glaucoma.

Unwanted side effects

- Expansion of the extracellular fluid volume by osmotic diuretics can precipitate heart failure and pulmonary oedema.
- Side effects include headache, nausea and vomiting.

Diuretics acting on the proximal tubule

Drugs acting on the proximal tubules are not used as diuretics, except for acetazolamide, which is used for treating glaucoma. Acetazolamide inhibits carbonic anhydrase to increase the excretion of bicarbonate, together with Na^+, K^+ and water in the urine. The urine is alkaline, and there may be an accompanying metabolic acidosis.

HEPATOBILIARY EXCRETION AND ENTEROHEPATIC CIRCULATION

Drugs, and glucuronide conjugates formed in the liver, can be secreted into the **bile** by active transport processes

similar to those found in the renal tubules for anions and cations. Basic drugs (e.g. atropine) and non-ionised molecules (e.g. digoxin) can also be secreted into bile. Biliary secretion becomes more important as the molecular weight exceeds 300. Drugs and their metabolites with molecular weight exceeding 300 are released into the alimentary tract where, depending on the drug or conjugate:

- Either the drug or conjugate can be excreted via the **faeces**
- Or the bacterial flora of the lower intestine may hydrolyse the conjugated drug back to the original drug, which is then reabsorbed by the intestine (e.g. oestrogens, morphine). This is known as **enterohepatic circulation**.

ROUTES OF DRUG ADMINISTRATION

Choosing how any particular drug is administered depends on how quickly effective plasma concentrations must be achieved, and how the drug is absorbed into the systemic circulation, metabolised and excreted. The main routes of administration of a drug, and abbreviations for them, are:

- Oral (PO)
- Parenteral: intravenous (IV), intramuscular (IM), subcutaneous (SC)
- Buccal/sublingual
- Rectal (PR)
- Transdermal and topical (vaginal, nasal, ocular)
- Inhalation.

ORAL ADMINISTRATION

Oral drug administration is the most commonly used route. It is also the cheapest and most convenient. Its suitability for a specific drug depends on how well the drug is absorbed into the systemic circulation from the gastrointestinal lumen and on how it is metabolised. Oral administration may be used to produce local effects within the gastrointestinal tract or for systemic effects.

Factors affecting gastrointestinal absorption of a drug

The factors that affect absorption of a drug from the gastrointestinal lumen into the systemic circulation are:
- Drug formulation
- Physico-chemical properties
- Passage through the gastrointestinal tract.

Drug formulation

The active drug in an oral preparation (tablet, capsule, etc.) is only a small proportion of the preparation's constituents. The rest is made up of ingredients that influence the speed and site of absorption: excipients, disintegrating agents, diluents, lubricants, etc. These ingredients and their proportions – the **formulation** – vary among manufacturers, but with the aim of ensuring similar effects.

The formulation determines the rate at which a tablet or capsule disintegrates and dissolves. A drug cannot be absorbed until it is liberated into the gastrointestinal fluid to form a solution. Usually, this occurs rapidly, but there are special **modified-release** formulations that disintegrate more slowly to control the amount of drug available for absorption over time.

Drugs may be affected by the acid gastric juices and need to be protected by having a special **acid-resistant** coating on the tablet/capsule (**enteric coated**). For example, mesalazine, used in the treatment of inflammatory bowel disease, is enteric coated to protect the drug from the action of acid gastric juices and is transported to the colon where it is released.

Physico-chemical properties of the drug, the medium and surface area

Absorption of orally administered drugs is influenced by:

- Its solubility in water and lipid
- The characteristics (e.g. pH) of gastrointestinal contents from which it has to be absorbed into the systemic circulation
- The available surface where absorption takes place.

Drug solubility

Orally administered drugs have to cross cell membranes in the gastrointestinal tract to be absorbed into the systemic circulation. As drugs exist in the ionised and non-ionised forms, the non-ionised lipid-soluble form moves across cell membranes much more readily than the water-soluble, ionised form. Highly acid (ionised) and basic drugs are poorly absorbed from the gastrointestinal tract, and most of the dose is excreted in the faeces.

Acid–base considerations

As most drugs are weak acids or weak bases, they undergo pH partitioning between the lumen of the gastrointestinal tract and the mucosal cells. Acid drugs are least ionised in the stomach so that they are best absorbed there. Basic drugs are better absorbed in the small intestine, where the pH is higher. There is also a zone with neutral pH at the interface of the stomach contents and the gastric mucosa, which acts as a barrier limiting drug absorption.

Surface area for absorption

The **surface area** over which absorption can take place in the stomach is relatively small compared with the small intestine. The surface area in the small intestine is increased 600-fold by the presence of villi and microvilli so that the small intestine is the major site for absorption. This large area allows even ionised drugs to be absorbed.

The **time** taken for the drug to pass through the small intestine also influences absorption. Absorption increases the longer the drug stays in contact with the mucosal surface. Intestinal hurry, as in diarrhoea, will reduce absorption. Inflammatory bowel disease that destroys the villi will also prevent absorption.

Fate of drugs in the stomach

Apart from the high acidity of the gastric juices, the presence of food and other drugs could affect the eventual absorption of the drug:

- Formation of complexes with food or other drugs reduces absorption.

Clinical box 4.7   The stomach and drug administration schedules

When an administered drug forms an insoluble complex with food in the stomach, the drug is best given on an empty stomach, usually about 30 minutes before meals:

- For example, tetracyclines chelate with the Ca^{2+} or Mg^{2+} ions in antacids and in calcium-rich foods in the stomach to form a complex that is poorly absorbed in the small intestine. Tetracyclines are therefore better administered on an empty stomach. Dairy products (high in Ca^{2+}) should be avoided at the time the drug is taken.

Gastric emptying can be slowed by:

- Meals that are high in fat or carbohydrate content
- Co-administration of anticholinergic drugs (e.g. atropine) or opioid analgesics (e.g. morphine).

Gastric emptying can be hurried by:

- Reducing the temperature of food
- Fasting
- Drugs such as metoclopramide which increase gastric motility.

Usually, when a drug is taken with a meal, absorption from the intestine is delayed due to delayed gastric emptying, but some foods may improve absorption. For example:

- Griseofulvin is absorbed better in the presence of fatty foods.
- A higher plasma concentration of propranolol has been reported in patients after a meal.

The enhanced absorption is probably due to increased postprandial blood flow to the intestines. These drugs should be taken with or immediately after a meal.

- Gastric emptying determines the time that it takes for an oral dose of a drug to reach the small intestine where absorption takes place.

Metabolism of drugs in the gastrointestinal tract

How much of an orally administered drug actually enters the systemic circulation and exerts a therapeutic effect is called **bioavailability**. Because most drugs are, to some extent, metabolised in the gut and liver before reaching the systemic circulation, bioavailability is not the same as the amount administered. It is calculated by comparison with an intravenously administered equivalent dose.

Some orally administered drugs undergo metabolism in the gastrointestinal tract and are then transported to the liver by the hepatic portal vein for further metabolism before distribution throughout the body:

- The **lumen of the intestine** contains **digestive enzymes** that can split amides and esters.
- The **colon** contains a large number of **aerobic and anaerobic bacteria** that possess enzymes capable of catalysing a number of reactions, including hydroxylation (hydrolysis) and reduction.
- Phase I hydroxylation and phase II sulphate conjugation enzymes are also present in the intestines (see drug metabolism).
- P-glycoproteins 'block' absorption by extruding drug molecules into intestinal lumen, and may be part of the 'first pass' mechanism (see below).

Drug metabolism in the intestines reduces bioavailability. A normal oral dose of drug may not be therapeutically effective if much of the dose were inactivated in the intestine or first metabolised by the liver before reaching the systemic circulation (**first pass metabolism**).

Bioavailability and bioequivalence

Although bioavailability indicates the proportion of orally administered drug that reaches the blood, it does *not* indicate the extent of absorption. Regulatory authorities that approve the use of drugs on humans use the concept of bioequivalence, which is a comparison of the generic drug with the new, proprietary product to ensure that the new product is as effective as the generic.

First pass metabolism

Even if the orally administered drugs were absorbed intact, first pass metabolism reduces bioavailability to a greater or lesser extent.

- Some drugs are completely inactivated by first pass metabolism and therefore cannot be administered orally (e.g. glyceryl trinitrate). An alternative route, or a specific drug design, e.g. pro-drug, may be needed to bypass first pass metabolism.
- A larger dose of drug may be needed for drugs that are not entirely inactivated by first pass metabolism to achieve a therapeutic effect (e.g. propranolol, aspirin, morphine).

Impact of liver disease on first pass metabolism

Patients needing long-term medication may have coexisting impairment of liver function:

- The drug is not extensively metabolised by the liver before entering the systemic circulation.
- The usual dose of the drug could therefore become an overdose or toxic dose.
- Care must therefore be taken when prescribing for patients with liver failure, e.g. elderly or patients with pre-existing liver disease.

PARENTERAL ADMINISTRATION

Parenteral administration is to give a drug by injection. This could be through a variety of methods including intravenous, intramuscular, subcutaneous or intrathecal (into the cerebrospinal fluid) routes.

Drugs are administered by injection:

- When effective plasma concentrations are needed rapidly
- To bypass first pass metabolism
- When administration by the oral route is not possible, as in severe vomiting. Also, some drugs are **acid labile** and are destroyed by the low pH of the stomach contents or denatured by proteolytic digestive enzymes.

Intravenous

The intravenous administration of a drug produces a rapid onset of action. A known concentration of drug is administered into the blood stream, either as a **bolus** when the whole amount of drug is given as one dose, or by **infusion** when the total dose is given slowly over a period of time. Drugs that would otherwise act as irritants can be administered intravenously, because veins are insensitive and the drug is rapidly diluted by plasma, particularly if injected into a large forearm vein.

Factors that determine the rate of **systemic absorption** after intravenous injection are the solubility of the drug in interstitial fluid and intercellular pores (gap junctions) in the vascular endothelium that promote rapid diffusion, independent of the lipid solubility of the drug. **Toxicity** can be a problem because of the rapidity of drug administration and onset of therapeutic effect. It requires trained personnel. It is also expensive because of sterilisation requirements and storage costs.

Subcutaneous

Subcutaneous injection is when the drug is injected just under the skin (e.g. insulin). Absorption is relatively slow, but usually complete and can be improved by massage or heat at the site of injection. Highly ionised or high molecular weight drugs are absorbed by diffusion through large intercellular pores in the capillary endothelium. A vasoconstrictor may be co-administered to delay the absorption of a drug (e.g. adrenaline (epinephrine) and local anaesthetic agent), thereby prolonging its effect at the site of injection. Drugs that have irritant properties can cause local tissue damage if administered subcutaneously.

Intramuscular

Drugs administered intramuscularly are either specialised depot (the drug is in a solvent, or vehicle, that keeps it at the site of injection, to be absorbed gradually), or sustained release preparations. These are a suspension of the drug in a non-aqueous preparation called the **vehicle**. For example, fluphenazine decanoate used in the treatment of schizophrenia, depot progestogens used as a long-acting contraceptive.

Absorption from depot injection is sometimes erratic, especially for poorly soluble drugs. The vehicle may be absorbed faster than the drug causing precipitation of the drug at the injection site.

OTHER FORMS OF INJECTION

Other forms of injection are used to deliver drugs to their precise site of action. Trained personnel are needed to perform these techniques.

Intrathecal

Some drugs have to be delivered directly into the cerebrospinal fluid (CSF) because the blood–brain barrier prevents entry from the systemic circulation. This is done via an intrathecal injection – the drug is injected through the theca of the spinal cord into the CSF in the arachnoid space. A lumbar puncture is performed under local anaesthesia and the drug, for example a cytotoxic drug, is injected straight into the CSF.

Epidural

Epidural injections are delivered into the space surrounding the meninges (dura) and therefore not into the CSF. They are used as a form of local anaesthesia, producing selective nerve block. This can be temporary, using a local anaesthetic, for surgical procedures such as inguinal herniorrhaphy, childbirth and caesarean sections. More permanent nerve block, using phenol (which destroys the nerves), is sometimes used to relieve intractable pain.

Local injections into tendons/bursae

Cortisone injections directly into tendon insertions (tennis elbow, golfer's elbow) and bursae sometimes help to relieve pain, but delays healing.

Buccal/sublingual administration

Some drugs are taken as small tablets that are held in the mouth, in contact with the buccal mucosa (buccal) or under the tongue (sublingual) (Clinical box 4.8). This route facilitates rapid absorption of lipid-soluble drugs into the systemic circulation across the mucous membranes, thus avoiding extensive first pass metabolism.

Rectal

The rectal route is useful for patients who are unable to take drugs orally because of vomiting and for younger children. When given as a suppository or enema, more than 50% of the drug absorbed via the rectum bypasses the liver and so the effect of first-pass metabolism is reduced. However, absorption is often incomplete and erratic, and it may also cause irritation of the rectal mucosa.

Topical/transdermal

Some drugs are formulated for direct application to the skin for **topical** cutaneous application when a local effect is needed. Some absorption through the skin (transdermal absorption) can, however, take place to give systemic effects.

To produce local effects, some drugs are applied directly (topical application) to the mucous membranes of the conjunctiva, or vagina (pv).

Lipid-soluble drugs can be formulated as skin patches to allow absorption through the skin (dermis) for systemic effect, known as the **transdermal** route. The topical and transdermal routes of administration bypass first pass metabolism. Some drugs are formulated for topical application so that they can be absorbed through the skin to bypass possible adverse side effects on the gastrointestinal tract (Clinical box 4.8).

Intranasal administration

Some drugs are administered as a nasal spray, to be absorbed through the mucous membrane to act directly on the mucosa or on the pituitary gland. Examples include:

- vasopressin used in the treatment of diabetes insipidus
- bromocriptine used for the suppression of lactation, hyperprolactinaemic disorders and the down regulation of menstrual cycles in the treatment of infertility.

| **Clinical box 4.8** | **Examples for choice of route for drug administration** |

Selecting the appropriate route for the administration of a drug depends on the therapeutic indication of the drug and its physico-chemical properties.

- Glyceryl trinitrate (GTN), a drug widely used for the treatment of angina, is extensively inactivated by first pass metabolism in the liver, so that oral administration is contraindicated.

For the relief of angina:

- Oral tablet: GTN is inactivated by first-pass metabolism and so is not suitable for oral administration
- Buccal/sublingual tablet or spray: because of its high lipid solubility, GTN is absorbed rapidly through mucous membranes; effects last 20–30 minutes, so it is used for rapid relief of angina attacks in the patient who has occasional angina attacks.
- Transdermal patch: GTN is absorbed more slowly through skin, so patches are used for prophylaxis in the patient who has frequent angina attacks.

For chest pain due to myocardial infarction:

- Intravenous: rapid relief in emergency situations.

When oral administration is impossible:

- Diazepam is given rectally to epileptic patients who are fitting continuously (status epilepticus).
- Prochlorperazine, an anti-emetic, is administered rectally for patients with intractable vomiting.
- Penicillin G, a broad-spectrum antibacterial drug, is destroyed by the low pH of the stomach contents. It has to be given by intramuscular injection. The formulation of penicillin V, however, is not acid labile, and can be given by mouth.
- Insulin is denatured by proteolytic digestive enzymes, therefore cannot be given orally. Insulin has to be administered subcutaneously.

When oral administration leads to unwanted effects:

- Non-steroidal anti-inflammatory drugs have been formulated for topical application for a local action on joints via the skin. This is to avoid undesirable effects on the stomach – irritation, ulceration or bleeding.
- Timolol, a β-adrenergic antagonist, is formulated for direct application to the eye in the long-term treatment of glaucoma. Not only is the drug effective, it also avoids the troublesome side effects produced by the systemic action of β-adrenergic antagonists.

Inhalation

Gaseous and volatile drugs (e.g. the general anaesthetics nitrous oxide, halothane) are administered by inhalation. Absorption of drugs by the lungs is rapid because of the large surface area within the lung and the rich blood supply to the relatively thin pulmonary epithelium.

In the treatment of lung disorders (e.g. asthma) drugs can be inhaled as a powder or an atomised solution of a drug, which enables a high concentration of drug to be delivered directly to the target structures, for example mast cells or bronchial muscle, without significant systemic side effects.

Drugs can also be formulated for inhalation in a way that deliberately reduces their absorption across the cell membrane, to reduce side effects. The physical characteristics of the formulation, i.e. size of the particle, also determine the effectiveness of the drug. Particles greater than 20 μm in diameter stay in the mouth and throat and are swallowed, but 2–6 μm diameter particles penetrate deep into the lungs to produce a rapid local effect as well as being absorbed to produce a systemic effect.

THE MATHEMATICS OF PHARMACOKINETICS

The mathematical basis of pharmacokinetics seeks to analyse the drug concentration in different parts of the body, over time from administration to arrival at the site of action. The mathematics is complicated, attempting to synthesise the four basic processes of drug absorption, distribution, metabolism and excretion. These processes affect:

- The amount of drug that arrives at the site of action
- The intensity of action
- The duration of action.

Information about these variables informs the choice of appropriate drug dose and dosing regimen. This is a very simplified account of mathematical concepts that are relevant for understanding the relationship between drug dosage and the time it takes for the drug to reach target tissue sites and to be eliminated. Textbooks of pharmacology will give more details of the mathematics.

FIRST-ORDER KINETICS

Most physiological processes follow first order kinetics, for example, passive diffusion down a concentration gradient. Protein-mediated active transport also follows first order kinetics but only at low concentrations of the drug (see below).

When applied to the fate of drugs, first order kinetics states that: the rate of elimination of a drug is directly proportional to plasma concentration. If plasma drug concentration (C) is plotted against time, the reduction in drug concentration as it is eliminated describes an exponential curve (Fig. 4.5A). Using the logarithm of concentration ($\ln C$) gives a straight line (Fig. 4.5B). This gives the information on how long it takes for the drug to be eliminated from the time of administration. The angle of decline for the slope ($-k_e$) indicates how quickly the drug is eliminated.

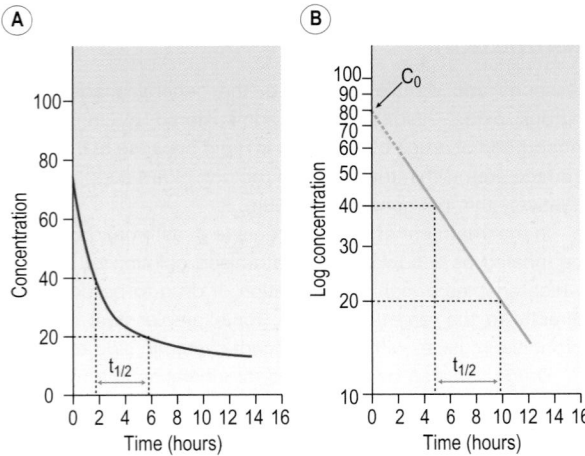

Fig. 4.5 First order kinetics: plasma concentration curves for the distribution of a drug. (A) A sigmoidal curve is obtained when plotting concentration (arithmetic) versus time. (B) A straight line is obtained when plotting log concentration versus time. C_0, concentration at zero time; k_e, rate constant; $t_{1/2}$, half-life.

Drug half-life

Drugs vary in the time that it takes for the body to eliminate them. An important parameter in first order kinetics is the time taken for the plasma concentration of a single dose of drug to decrease by 50%, the **half-life** ($t_{1/2}$). $t_{1/2}$ is independent of drug concentration at zero time, and the slope of the logarithmic curve is characteristic of the first order process. The rate of decline for the log concentration curve (k), or slope, is specific for each particular drug, so that different drugs have different half-lives. There is, thankfully, no need to know the $t_{1/2}$ of every drug. It is a useful indicator of how long a drug remains in the body.

Drug clearance

Clearance is an estimate of the volume of plasma completely cleared of drug in a unit of time (e.g. mL/min), and is a measure of the ability of the organs of elimination to remove drugs from the body:

- The kidneys (renal clearance)
- The liver (hepatic clearance)
- Other organs, such as lungs.

Total body clearance is the sum of renal, hepatic and other clearances, measuring the time it takes for the body to be totally cleared of drug. It is a function of the volume of plasma cleared per minute, and the total apparent volume of distribution.

For drugs that follow first order kinetics, clearance is constant over the therapeutic concentration range, so that a threefold increase in plasma concentration leads to a threefold increase in clearance.

Renal clearance

Renal clearance is important because it is the major process through which the body gets rid of foreign chemical compounds that might potentially be toxic. Renal clearance can be measured from the rate of excretion in the urine, or the amount of unchanged drug excreted in the urine over a fixed time period (e.g. 24 hours) (see also Ch. 14). Measuring renal clearance can be useful because:

- Comparing renal clearance with plasma clearance gives an indication of whether renal function is normal or impaired.
- Hepatic clearance can be estimated from the difference between plasma and renal clearance to give an estimate of possible liver disease.
- Comparing renal clearance with glomerular filtration rate gives an estimate of drug reabsorption or excretion by tubular secretion.
- Changing the pH of urine can increase renal clearance (see Fig. 4.2).

ZERO-ORDER (NON-LINEAR OR SATURATION) KINETICS

At low drug concentrations, protein mediated processes for some drugs, e.g. enzymes and receptors, exhibit first order kinetics. At high concentrations, however, binding sites on enzymes and receptors become saturated. The rate of reaction, e.g. drug elimination, can no longer respond to further increases in concentration, and can *only* proceed at a fixed

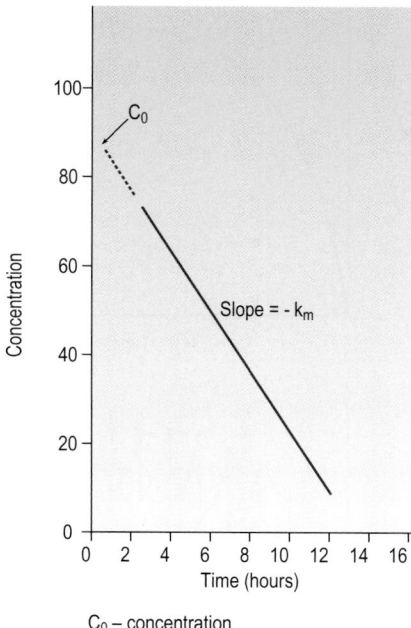

C₀ – concentration
kₘ – rate constant

Fig. 4.6 Time course of a hypothetical drug demonstrating zero order kinetics.

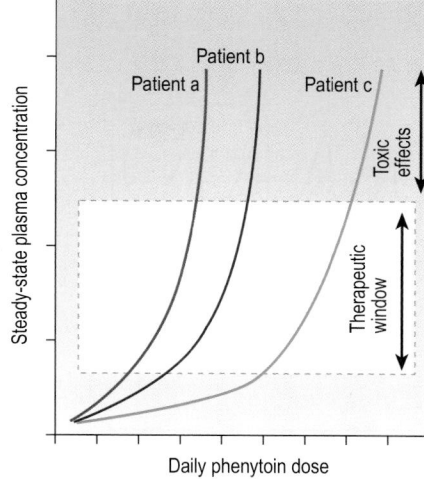

Fig. 4.7 Steady state plasma concentrations as a function of the daily phenytoin dose. Each curve represents a different patient receiving the same dose of phenytoin. In all three, initially the rise in plasma concentration is linear but it rises steeply to possibly produce toxic effects. The difference in the daily dose that produces therapeutic effects and the dose that produces toxic effects is small (very small in patients a and b), so that great care needs to be exercised when increasing daily dosage.

maximum rate. The mathematics of this phenomenon is known as **zero order kinetics**.

In zero order kinetics, the drug concentration over time during the processes of absorption, distribution, metabolism and excretion is a fixed amount per unit time, independent of the overall (protein-bound and unbound) drug concentration. A plot of concentration against time gives a straight line (Fig. 4.6).

Consequences of zero order kinetics

For zero order kinetics, the decline in plasma drug levels is not exponential, unlike first order kinetics, and therefore the duration of action is more dependent on the dose. The concept of half-life has no meaning. As the rate of elimination is constant, increasing the dose of the drug can result in a large and variable increase in plasma concentration. This can give exaggerated pharmacological responses and an increased risk of toxic effects.

Theoretically, if the rate of drug administration exceeds the rate of elimination then infinite accumulation of the drug would occur. However, this does not happen in practice because at high drug concentrations the relative contributions of other pathways of elimination (e.g. hepatic excretion) increase to achieve a steady state plasma concentration.

Steady state concentration of drugs

A **steady state concentration** of the drug is reached when the plasma and tissue concentrations (including target tissue) reach equilibrium. Long-term drug therapy aims to achieve a constant steady state plasma concentration. When a drug is given intravenously, the time needed to reach steady state depends on the elimination half-life. The steady state concentration of a given drug varies markedly between patients, which can be further influenced by drugs that change the

rate of metabolism, as in enzyme induction. Figure 4.7 shows an example of how the difference between a daily dose that gives therapeutic effects and one that gives toxic effects is very small.

Time needed to reach steady state plasma concentration

The decision about drug dosage and dosing regimen to achieve a therapeutically effective steady state concentration will depend on whether it follows first or zero order kinetics. A continuous intravenous infusion of a drug bypasses the absorption phase. The distribution phase is assumed to be constant, and anyway human tissue concentration cannot be measured easily. Therefore, elimination is the only measurable factor that affects the time needed for the drug to reach steady state plasma concentration. The rate of elimination is measured as the elimination half-life.

Figure 4.8 shows the log plasma concentration curve where steady state plasma concentration has been reached after several (usually five) elimination half-lives. However, the effect of oral administration of multiple doses will look different, if the elimination $t_{1/2}$ is shorter than the absorption $t_{1/2}$. The absorption phase now has an effect on the time to reach steady state. Figure 4.9B shows the time concentration graph of the logarithm of plasma concentration of repeated, fixed doses of a hypothetical, rapidly absorbed drug given at regular intervals.

- The rate of absorption will affect plasma concentration between doses.
- Bioavailability of the drug (extent of absorption of the administered dose) will affect the steady state concentration.
- Absorption has to be balanced by the rate of elimination, which is influenced by the function of the organs of elimination in the patient.

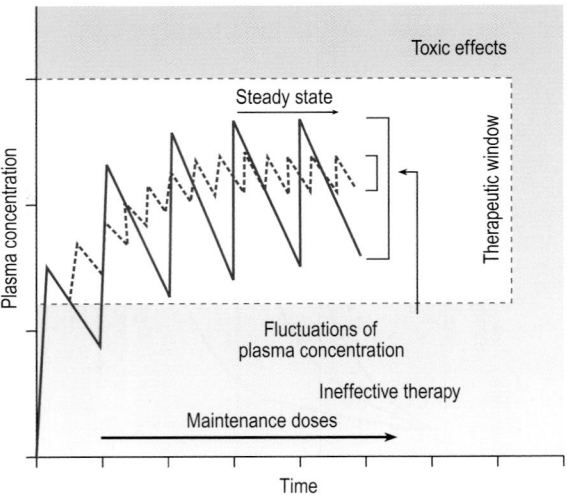

Fig. 4.8 Drug accumulation and steady state concentration. The diagram shows the effect of dividing the dose, and reducing the dosing intervals, on the accumulation and steady state concentration of a drug. The *dotted line* shows the effect of halving the time interval between doses: plasma concentration fluctuates less but the mean steady state concentration is higher. In both these cases, the dose and intervals achieve a steady state within the therapeutic window.

Safety margins of drugs: the difference between therapeutic and toxic doses

All drugs have some risk of toxicity. This risk always has to be taken into account in the context of disease severity. Patients have to be informed of this risk when being prescribed therapeutic agents, particularly those with a high risk of toxicity.

Therapeutic index

The **therapeutic index** is a useful indication of safety margins.

Therapeutic index (TI) = Dose giving toxicity / Dose giving therapeutic response

Some drugs, such as benzodiazepines, have a therapeutic index of about 50, so that it would be difficult to be poisoned by benzodiazepines. Digoxin only has a therapeutic index of about 2, so that the dose difference between toxicity and therapeutic effect is very small.

Therapeutic window

The **therapeutic window** (see Fig. 4.8) refers to a range of responses in relation to rising plasma drug concentrations that varies from giving no therapeutic (subtherapeutic) to therapeutic to toxic responses. The therapeutic window is the range of plasma concentrations in which the patient is more likely to gain therapeutic benefit, with least risk of ineffective or adverse effects.

MULTIPLE DOSING AND STEADY STATE

Very few drugs are administered as a single dose; most are administered serially with a fixed time interval between

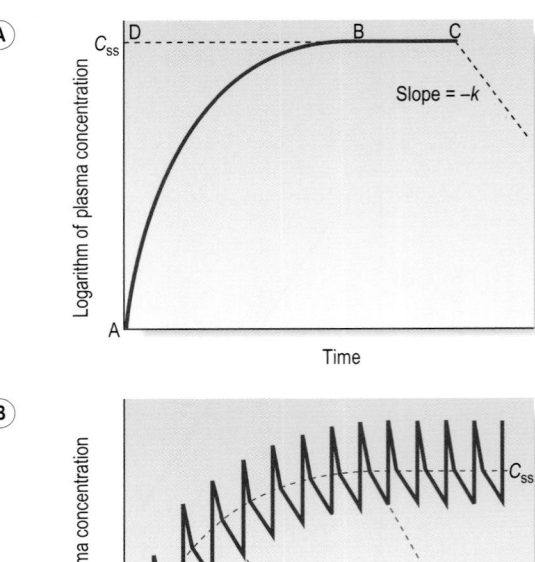

Fig. 4.9 Steady state plasma concentrations after intravenous (IV) infusion and oral administration of a drug. (A) Constant IV infusion (between A and C). Steady state concentration is reached at B. The steady state concentration C_{ss} is given by D. The slope on cessation of infusion C is the rate of elimination. (B) Regular oral therapy (——) compared with IV infusion (----) at the same dosage rate. The oral dose is rapidly absorbed and distributed followed by a slower elimination phase within each dosing interval. Cessation of therapy after any dose would produce the rate of elimination shown by the *blue dotted* slopes. Adapted with permission from Waller DG, Renwick AG, Hillier K 2001 Medical pharmacology and therapeutics. WB Saunders, Edinburgh.

doses. The objective of repeat dosing is to achieve a therapeutically effective plasma drug concentration by accumulation and to maintain a steady state (Fig. 4.9).

- If an intravenous dose (A) of a drug with a $t_{1/2}$ of 2 h is administered to give a maximum plasma concentration of 10 units/mL, the plasma concentration will be 5 units/mL after 2 h.
- If a second dose A is administered at this time, the maximum plasma concentration will be 15 units/mL.
- After another 2 h the plasma concentration will be 7.5 units, an increase of 2.5 units in the lowest concentration.

The drug is accumulating in that the minimum concentration it reaches between half-life intervals, the peak plasma concentration, will gradually approach the maximal value of 10 units. At this stage the plasma concentration has reached a **steady state or plateau** (C_{ss}) because the amount of drug being eliminated from the body is approximately equal to the amount injected.

The fluctuations between the maximum and minimum plasma concentration can be large. The time taken to reach the steady state is strictly dependent on the half-life of the drug and occurs within about five half-lives. A drug with a long half-life will take much longer to achieve a steady state than one with a short half-life. As a consequence, the final plasma concentration at which steady state occurs can be altered, as can the fluctuation between the maximum and minimum plasma concentrations, by altering:

- The time interval between doses
- The dose given

  or

- Both.

Dosing at time intervals greater than half-life results in greater fluctuation in the plasma levels (*solid line* in Fig. 4.8).

Dosing at intervals less than half-life results in smaller fluctuation in plasma concentrations but the mean concentration at steady state is much higher (*dotted line* in Fig. 4.8).

Dividing the dose and increasing dosing frequency can achieve a steady state within the therapeutic window and reduce the fluctuation of the plasma concentrations (*dotted line* Fig. 4.8). Above the therapeutic window, toxic effects of the drug may be observed while below the therapeutic window the drug may not produce its desired effect.

If the drug has a long half-life or it is therapeutically desirable to achieve a rapid steady state concentration, a **loading dose** can be given. This dose is greater than the normal maintenance dose, so that disadvantages might be:

- Toxicity in a sensitive individual.
- Delayed elimination (particularly after a toxic reaction).

PHARMACODYNAMICS

Pharmacodynamics is about how drugs work on living organisms; the qualitative and quantitative study of the biochemical and physiological effects of drugs on the body. Qualitative studies investigate the mechanisms of the action of drugs and endogenous molecules, while quantitative studies allow comparison of the relationship between drug **concentration** and **effect**. Quantitative studies include the measurement of drug effects at varying concentrations and this information is useful for estimating drug **potency** and **efficacy**.

DRUG TARGETS

For drugs to exert their pharmacological effect, they have to be bound to macromolecular components of a cell. The interaction of the drug molecule with the binding site on the cell elicits the therapeutic response from the cell. Because the amount of drug molecules relative to cellular macromolecules is small, binding has to be highly specific. Drugs are therefore designed to **target** specific macromolecules, most commonly proteins. Endogenous, naturally occurring, chemicals such as hormones and neurotransmitters act in the same way. There are four main regulatory proteins that are targets for drugs:

- Enzymes
- Transporter proteins.
- Ion channels
- Receptors.

Some specific classes of drugs target structural proteins and nucleic acids. For example, colchicine inhibits the assembly of the subunits that form microtubules, and anti-cancer drugs target DNA or RNA. Many drugs bind non-selectively to plasma proteins and other cell constituents without producing a biological response.

No drug is entirely specific in selecting its binding sites, giving rise to side effects if the drug binds to regulatory proteins that are not specific targets. For example, tricyclic antidepressant drugs are noted for producing the side effects of dry mouth and urine retention because they block receptors other than the monoamine transporters for which they were designed (see below, The Autonomic Nervous System). No drug is entirely without side effects.

In some texts, drug targets are sometimes referred to as receptors. Here, the term **receptor** will be used specifically for a protein molecule to which a drug or endogenous molecule binds selectively. The chemical substance, drug or naturally occurring molecule, is known as a **ligand** (tied or bound to the receptor). Binding of a ligand to a receptor may elicit a change in cellular function.

However, the binding of a ligand to a drug target does not necessarily induce a change in cell function: many proteins (enzymes, transporters and certain types of ion channel) do not act as receptors but do have **recognition sites** for ligands.

ENZYMES

Drugs may target enzymes as:

- Inhibitors – when normal enzyme action is inhibited
- False substrates – when an abnormal metabolite is produced

- Pro-drugs – when an inactive precursor is converted to an active drug by enzyme action.

Enzyme inhibitors

Enzyme **inhibitors** are drugs or their metabolites that inhibit enzyme activity. The inhibition may be:

- Reversible (e.g. anticholinesterase drugs such as neostigmine, the angiotensin converting enzyme inhibitor captopril)
- Irreversible (e.g. cyclo-oxygenase (COX) inhibitors such as aspirin): when the target enzyme is permanently altered so that a new enzyme has to be synthesised to replace the one bound to the drug.

The drugs produce their pharmacological effect by interacting with ligand recognition sites on enzymes by mimicking the substrate for that enzyme. The drug molecule may have a similar chemical structure to the natural substrate, competing with the substrate for recognition sites.

In non-competitive inhibition, the drug binds directly with the recognition site or to an allosteric site (another site on the enzyme to inhibit binding of the natural ligand), thereby inhibiting the action of the enzyme (Information box 4.7).

False substrates

Some drugs act as **false substrates**. The drug molecule is converted by endogenous enzymes to an abnormal substance that enters and disrupts normal metabolic pathways (Information box 4.8).

Pro-drugs

Inactive precursors of drugs, pro-drugs, can be converted by enzyme action to the active compound. Some drugs are designed to exploit this characteristic. Conversely, therapeutically active drugs can be converted to toxic, reactive metabolites e.g. paracetamol toxicity (see Clinical box 4.6).

CARRIER PROTEINS (TRANSPORTERS)

Carrier proteins, or transporters, transfer ions and small molecules that are not sufficiently lipid soluble, across the cell membrane. ATP-dependent transporters, also called pumps, are the sites of action of a number of therapeutic agents. Transport-mediated responses are slower than ion-channel-mediated ones.

ION CHANNELS

Ions cannot penetrate the lipid cell membrane and need ion channels to facilitate their diffusion across the membranes. Ion channels are large protein complexes that span the cell membrane. The intracellular concentration of important ions such as Na^+, Ca^{2+}, K^+ and Cl^- are controlled by the state of the channels, whether they are:

- Open, or activated, allowing selected ions to diffuse down a concentration gradient

Information box 4.7   **Therapeutic uses of drugs that inhibit enzymes**

- Angiotensin-converting enzyme (ACE) inhibitors are used in the treatment of hypertension. The kidney plays a very important role in the regulation of blood pressure (see Ch. 14). Renin is secreted by the kidney in response to reduced renal perfusion and/or increased sympathetic activity, and converts angiotensin (produced by the liver) to angiotensin I. ACE then converts angiotensin I to angiotensin II, which is a powerful vasoconstrictor and has a role in hypertension. ACE inhibitors (inhibit the conversion of angiotensin I to angiotensin II, e.g. captopril) are now used extensively in the treatment of hypertension.
- Acetylcholinesterase (AChE) inhibitors: skeletal muscles contract through the stimulation of acetylcholine on neuromuscular junctions. Myasthenia gravis is a rare, autoimmune disorder in which the number of acetylcholine nicotinic receptors at the neuromuscular junction is greatly reduced, giving rise to the characteristic drooping eyelids (ptosis), rapid muscle fatigue on exertion and weakness. AChE is an endogenous enzyme that breaks down acetylcholine and terminates its action. The objective for the treatment of myasthenia gravis is to prolong the action of acetylcholine by inhibiting its breakdown by AChE. Neostigmine is a reversible, competitive inhibitor of AChE used in the treatment of myasthenia, although pyridostigmine is used more commonly because of longer duration of action and fewer side effects. Some poisons, such as nerve gases and insecticides, irreversibly inhibit AChE.
- Disulfiram is used as an adjunct in the treatment of alcohol dependence, as aversion therapy. Alcohol is metabolised to acetaldehyde by the enzyme alcohol dehydrogenase, then to acetic acid by aldehyde dehydrogenase. Disulfiram irreversibly inhibits aldehyde dehydrogenase so that acetaldehyde accumulates in the blood causing nausea, flushing of the face, palpitations and throbbing headaches among other symptoms – collectively called the **antabuse effect**. Some other drugs, such as metronidazole (treatment of anaerobic bacterial and protozoan infections), also inhibit acetaldehyde dehydrogenase to produce the antabuse effect if combined with alcohol. Patients prescribed metronidazole need to be warned against taking alcohol.
- Penicillin is a bactericidal antibiotic. In the last step in the synthesis of bacterial cell walls, an enzyme, transpeptidase, catalyses the 'transition state' reaction. This is the crucial step in bacterial cell wall synthesis. Penicillin is a synthetic analogue of the transition state and binds to transpeptidase, irreversibly inhibiting the enzyme. Bacterial cell wall synthesis is inhibited so that the bacteria are thin walled and fragile, destroyed by plasma osmotic pressure.

Information box 4.8   **Therapeutic use of drugs as false substrates**

- α-Methyldopa is metabolised as a false substrate in the biosynthetic pathway for noradrenaline (norepinephrine), when α-methyladrenaline instead of noradrenaline is formed. α-Methyladrenaline is a peripheral vasodilator used in the treatment of hypertension.
- Fluorouracil, an anti-cancer drug, acts as a false substrate by replacing uracil in normal purine biosynthesis. The intermediate cannot complete the conversion to purine and blocks DNA synthesis so that cell division cannot then take place.

- Their selectivity for specific ions, for example, cation channels are selectively permeable to Na^+, K^+, or Ca^{2+}, or all three. Anion channels would be permeable to Cl^-. This property depends on the size of the ion channel and the difference in the proteins that line it.
- The molecular structure of the ion channel.

The gating mechanism of ion channels are:

- Voltage-gated – when the ion channel opens or closes in response to a change in the transmembrane electrochemical gradient.
- Ligand-gated – when ion channels change status in response to the binding of a ligand to a receptor site incorporated into the channel structure. Ligand-gated channels are also known as **ionotropic receptors**.

Voltage-gated channels

Voltage-gated channels are therapeutically the more important ion channels. Voltage gating, as the name implies, is when ion channels selective for cations or anions open or close, due to a change in the transmembrane electrochemical potential. For example, a change in transmembrane potential in response to nerve impulses will cause different channels to open selectively to Na^{2+}, Ca^{2+} or K^+. Na^{2+} and Ca^{2+} will diffuse into the cell, making the cytosol less negative and causing depolarisation of the membrane, and K^+ will diffuse out to make the cytoplasm more negative – repolarisation or hyperpolarisation.

Molecular structure of voltage-gated ion channels

Voltage-gated channels are made up of four subunits: an α subunit, a large glycoprotein (MW 270 000), and smaller β, γ and δ glycoprotein subunits. Although not yet understood, different combinations of the subunits determine the selectivity of the subtypes of ion channels. The main channel forming subunit, known as the α1 subunit, is responsible for gating (Fig. 4.10).

The α subunit of Na^+ and Ca^{2+} channels is a single polypeptide chain consisting of four homologous repeat domains (I–IV) that orientate themselves to form a pore. Each domain is made up of six transmembrane α helices (S1–S6). The polypeptide chain loops into the membrane to form the lining of the ion pore at the P-region, between S5 and S6. K^+ ion channels only have one domain. The S4 helix contains a set of positively charged amino acids (lysine and/or arginine) in a part of the protein that passes through the membrane. These charged molecules are thought to 'sense' the voltage

- Closed, or inactivated and unresponsive to stimulus
- Rested, closed but opening in response to stimulus.

The electrochemical gradient of an ion between the intra- and extracellular compartments determines the direction and rate that the ion passes through the ion channel. Ion-channel-mediated responses are extremely fast, being measured in milliseconds. Drugs are developed and designed to target ion channels.

Ion channels are classified according to:

- Their gating properties – many drugs target ion channels to exert a therapeutic effect by changing the status of the channel (i.e. open or closed).

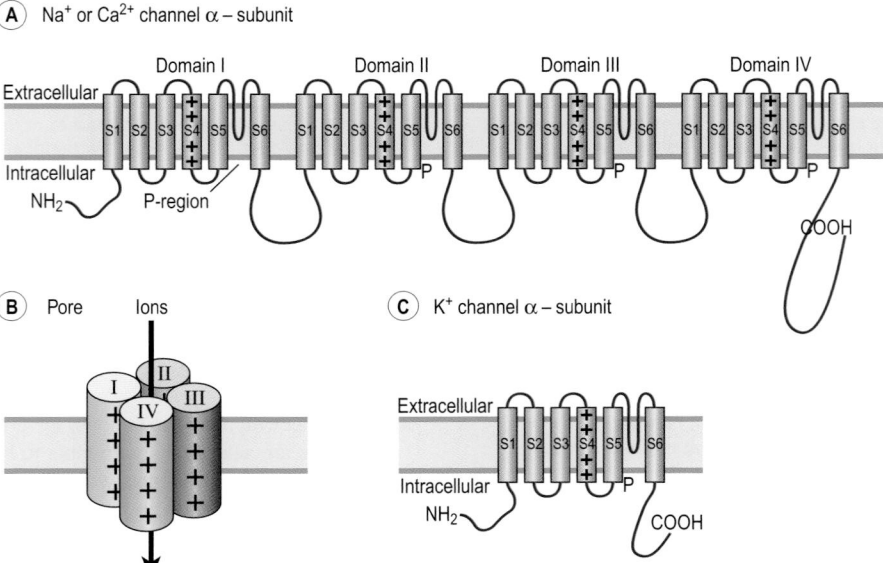

Fig. 4.10 **Voltage-gated ion channel.**

across the membrane, causing the channel to either open or close.

Calcium channel antagonists

Calcium channel (Ca^{2+}) antagonists (blockers) were designed to target voltage-gated Ca^{2+} ion channels. Examples include nifedipine, amlodipine, verapamil and diltiazem. They are commonly prescribed for angina and hypertension.

Pharmacodynamics

The Ca^{2+} ion is essential for cardiac muscle contraction. Free Ca^{2+} ions have to enter the cardiac myocyte through voltage-gated Ca^{2+} channels or be released from intracellular stores before the muscle can contract. Ca^{2+} antagonists target the gating mechanism to inhibit Ca^{2+} influx. The effects include:

- Coronary artery dilatation to relieve or prevent the arterial spasm that reduces myocardial blood flow (ischaemia), causing the symptoms of angina.
- Negative chronotropic effect by slowing the rate of firing at the SA node, and conduction in the AV node.
- Peripheral arterial dilatation lowers peripheral resistance and blood pressure, reducing the work of the left ventricle and oxygen demand, thus relieving ischaemia.

Pharmacokinetics

The Ca^{2+} antagonists are well absorbed from the gastrointestinal tract, undergoing variable first pass metabolism by the liver. They have short half-lives, so the duration of action is relatively short. Attempts are made to prolong the duration of action by using modified-release formulations.

Unwanted side effects

- Heart block and bradycardia occur if administered with other negative inotropic drugs, e.g. digoxin, β-adrenergic antagonists.
- Heart failure due to the reduced cardiac contractility in patients with poor ventricular function, e.g. elderly patients.
- Symptoms due to arterial dilatation – ankle oedema, dizziness, flushing.

Ligand-gated channels

Ligand-gated channels are complex. They incorporate a receptor site that needs to be bound by a ligand (agonist) to open or by an antagonist to prevent the action of a ligand. Because a ligand-gated ion channel has a receptor recognition site incorporated into its molecular structure, the ion channel plus the recognition site is known as an **ionotropic receptor** (see below).

Ion channels as drug targets

Drugs are designed to block ion channel activity by one of two methods.

- They enter the channel during the open state and bind to a recognition site, for example the Na^+ channel and the Ca^{2+} channel blockers.
- They diffuse across the cell membrane and bind to an intracellular recognition site when the channel is in the inactivated state (e.g. lidocaine, a local anaesthetic).

The faster the ion channels 'cycle' through the open, inactive and rested states, the greater the blocking effect of the drugs will be. This is called use-dependency, a property exploited in therapeutics when the drug is designed to selectively act on ion channel cycles that are fast.

RECEPTORS

The majority of receptors targeted by drugs are transmembrane proteins involved in chemical signalling in cells. As most water soluble drugs (ligands) do not cross cell membranes, they have to exert their intracellular effect from an extracellular location. A **transmembrane receptor**, a protein that traverses the width of the cell membrane, is the means of signalling their 'message' to intracellular sites.

Ligands that activate receptors to send signals across the cell membrane are known as **first messengers**: they activate an intracellular **second messenger** system that causes changes in cell function.

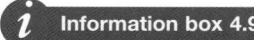

Information box 4.9   **Example of user dependency and drug action on ion channels**

Phenytoin is an important anti-epileptic drug despite having complex and sometimes serious side effects. Phenytoin produces user dependent block on voltage-gated Na^+ ion channels in neurons. It targets the abnormally fast firing neuronal tissue in the brain of patients suffering from epilepsy. Closing the ion channel prevents the influx of Na^+ into the neuron, thus 'damping down' the excessive neuronal discharge.

The unwanted effects of phenytoin are related to the effects of phenytoin on ion channels other than Na^+ channels. Its unpredictable toxicity is related to zero order kinetics.

A transmembrane receptor has a specific recognition site on the extracellular surface of the cell membrane for a given ligand – the **ligand binding domain**. The ligand–receptor interaction produces a small conformational change of the receptor protein, which in turn initiates a series of intracellular events via an intracellular **effector domain**. This is known as the **transduction mechanism**.

In a biological context, transduction means transforming a signal from one form to another. For example, light entering the eye (one form of signal) is transduced by rhodopsin, a protein in retinal rods, into nerve impulses (another form of signal) that are relayed to the brain. Transduction mechanisms can be the simple opening of an ion channel or the activation of a G protein (see below) by the effector domain, which in turn activates one of a number of enzymes, culminating in a physiological or biochemical response.

It is worth noting that some ligands are lipid soluble (e.g. steroid hormones, thyroid hormone). These readily diffuse through the cell membrane and bind to intracellular receptors to produce their effects, and so they do not need signal transduction.

Binding of a ligand to the receptor

A ligand is called a receptor **agonist** when it binds to a specific receptor, activates it and produces a cellular response. When a ligand binds to the receptor and produces no effect itself, but prevents the binding of an agonist acting at that receptor, it is a receptor **antagonist**.

- Binding is usually rapidly reversible, and the intensity and duration of the response depends on the continuing presence of the ligand.
- The interaction between ligand and receptor involves a combination of weak, but readily reversible, chemical forces such as hydrogen bonds, ionic bonds and Van der Waals forces.
- If the binding is **covalent**, the duration of the ligand–receptor association may be prolonged, if not irreversible.
- The effect of irreversible binding can only be overcome, in the long term, by the synthesis of new receptors to replace those bound to the ligand.

The number of receptors present in any cell is not static. There is a high turnover of receptors as they are continually formed and removed from the cell membrane. The number of receptors may be increased **(up-regulation)** or decreased **(down-regulation)** by drugs or disease. For example, during the treatment of infertility using artificial reproduction techniques, the woman's own ovulation cycle has to be suppressed so that ovulation can be stimulated by artificial means. A synthetic gonadotropin may be administered to inhibit the normal release of follicle-stimulating hormone and luteinising hormone, to 'down-regulate' normal pituitary control over ovarian follicle development (see Ch. 10).

RECEPTOR CLASSIFICATION

Receptors were traditionally classified according to the drugs that act on them to produce a pharmacological response. For example, histamine receptors are activated by histamine, muscarinic receptors by muscarine and nicotinic receptors by nicotine.

Newer techniques in molecular biology, however, have identified many more new receptor subtypes and biochemical pathways. These techniques include molecular cloning, and studies of ligand binding and transduction pathways for receptor activation. The classification discussed below is only one system, at a point in time. As experimental data proliferate, systems for receptor classification are under constant review, and a useful summary is published annually.

Receptor classification based on structure and signal transduction

Receptors can be characterised in terms of their molecular structure and signal transduction mechanisms. There are four known superfamilies (Fig. 4.11):

Type 1: **Ionotropic receptors** also termed **ligand-gated** or receptor-operated ion channels (Fig. 4.11A). These are membrane receptors coupled directly to an ion channel and are receptors on which 'fast' transmitters act. The tissue response occurs in a few milliseconds.

Type 2: **G protein-coupled receptors** (GPCR) also known as **metabotropic receptors** or 7 transmembrane spanning receptors (Fig. 4.11B). These are membrane receptors which are coupled to intracellular effector systems via a G protein. G proteins are so called because they interact with the guanine nucleotides GTP and GDP. The intracellular effector system is the second messenger (see below). The response to receptor activation occurs in 100 ms or seconds.

Type 3: **Enzyme-linked receptors** also termed kinase-linked receptors (Fig. 4.11C). These are membrane receptors that incorporate an intracellular protein kinase domain within their structure. Tissue response occurs in minutes.

Type 4: **Intracellular receptors** or DNA-linked nuclear receptors (Fig. 4.11D). These are receptors that regulate gene transcription and are located either in the cell cytoplasm or within the nucleus. The response to these receptors occurs in hours to days.

Ionotropic receptors (ligand-gated ion channels)

Ionotropic receptors are membrane bound proteins that are similar to other ion channels, but have a receptor binding (recognition) site on the extracellular domain. In some ionotropic receptors, the receptor protein is a G protein (see later).

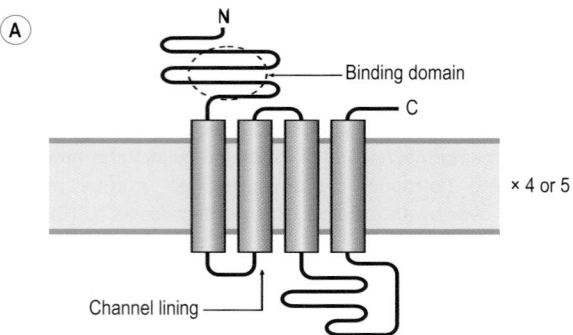

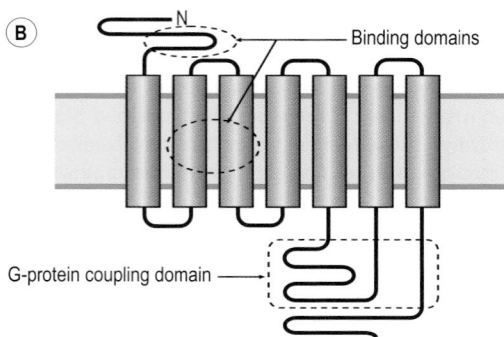

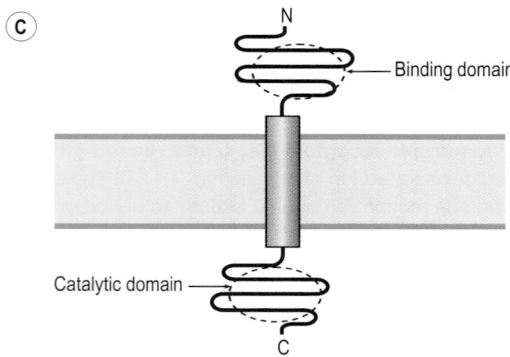

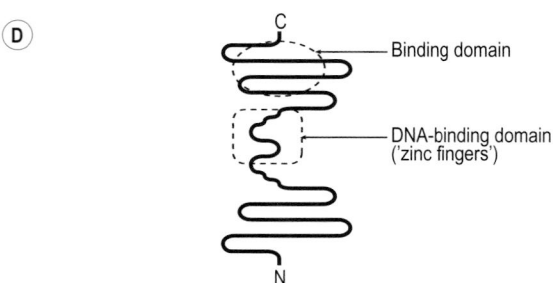

Fig. 4.11 General structure of four receptor families.
(A) Type 1 ionotropic receptors. (B) Type 2 G protein-coupled receptors. (C) Type 3 kinase-linked receptors. (D) Type 4 nuclear receptors. Adapted with permission from Rang HP, Dale MM, Ritter JM, Moore PK 2003 Pharmacology, 5th edn. Elsevier Science, Edinburgh.

Ionotropic receptors are usually the targets for fast neurotransmitters (see below, The Autonomic Nervous System). Important examples include:

■ Nicotinic receptors (stimulated by acetylcholine, nAChR): γ-amino-butyric acid A receptor (GABA$_A$-R), glycine

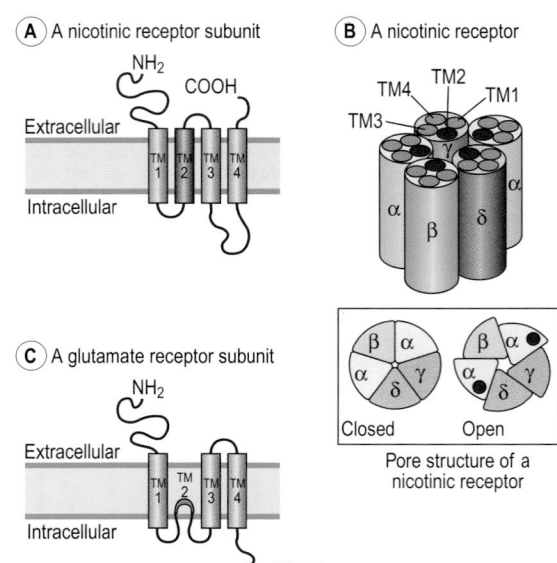

Fig. 4.12 Molecular structure of ionotropic receptors.
TM, transmembrane.

receptor (Gly-R) and one subclass of the serotonin receptors (5-HT$_3$).
■ Glutamate receptors (Glu-R).

Molecular structure of ionotropic receptors

The ionotropic receptor protein is a long peptide chain (Fig. 4.12A) that:

■ Forms loops on the extracellular side of the cell membrane to produce the ligand binding site, known as the N-terminal
■ The protein then loops through the channels in the cell membrane a number of times. The lining of the ion channels is made up of four subunits, α, β, γ and δ.
■ The subunits are membrane-bound proteins that congregate around a central, water-filled pore, thus forming a channel through the lipid bilayer of the cell membrane.
■ The gating and ion-selective properties of ionotropic receptors are determined by the combinations of the subunits.

Nicotinic receptors (nAChR)

The ion channel in the nicotinic receptor is made with five subunits around the central pore (Fig. 4.12B). These are termed α (which is duplicated, i.e. there are two copies) β, γ and δ subunits. Each subunit consists of four transmembrane loops (TM1–4) (Fig. 4.12A). ACh is the ligand that activates the nicotinic receptor. There are two binding sites on the receptor and both have to be occupied by ACh before the channel pore will open.

GABA$_A$ receptor

The molecular structure of the GABA$_A$ receptor is similar to a nicotinic receptor. The α-subunit contains the extracellular binding site, which has a high affinity for GABA$_A$. The central pore (channel) is selective for anions, particularly Cl⁻. Best examples of drugs that potentiate the binding of GABA$_A$ to its receptor are benzodiazepines and barbiturates.

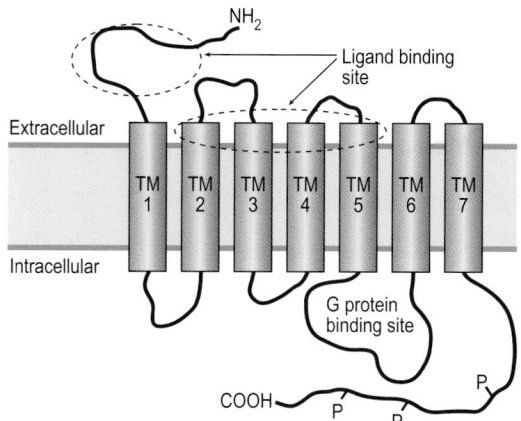

Fig. 4.13 The molecular structure of a G protein-coupled (metabotropic) receptor. Each of the seven transmembrane domains (TM1–7) is an α helix and consists of approximately 24 hydrophobic amino acids. Each domain is linked to the next one by an amino acid loop of varying length; three loops are intracellular and three are extracellular. The NH_2-terminal extends into the extracellular space and the COOH-terminal into the intracellular space.

Glutamate receptors

Glutamate is an excitatory amino acid neurotransmitter found in the central nervous system. There are two main classes of glutamate receptors: NMDA (*N*-methyl-D-aspartate), and non-NMDA receptors. The NMDA receptors are a family of ligand-gated ion channels that are also voltage dependent. For ions to flow, the receptor must bind glutamate and be depolarised. This receptor allows a significant influx of Ca^{2+}.

GPCR

GPCRs are a large family of transmembrane receptors. They are also known as metabotropic receptors because they initiate a chain of intracellular reactions known as the **second messenger system**. Over 250 GPCRs have been cloned.

Molecular structure

A GPCR protein is a single polypeptide chain, rather like a microscopic, very flexible electric wire (Fig. 4.13).

- The ligand binding site on the extracellular side of the cell membrane is a single polypeptide chain termed the N-terminal. The N-terminal is large, and extends into the extracellular space.
- From the N-terminal, the GPCR loops across the cell membrane seven times, the transmembrane domains of the receptor (TM1–7).
- After looping through the cell membrane, the GPCR terminates with the C-terminal on the intracellular side of the membrane.
- The loop connecting TM5 to TM6 contains the **G-protein coupling domain**, where the second messengers are produced.

GPCR (metabotropic receptors) and signal transduction mechanism

The major player in signal transduction by GPCRs is the **G protein**. G proteins are heterotrimers (trimers) consisting of three different subunits, α, β and γ. All three subunits are attached to the cell membrane by a fatty acid chain, coupled to the G protein. At the molecular level, the G protein is freely diffusible in the plane of the cell membrane, but bound to the intracellular surface. This allows the G protein to interact with a variety of enzymes and effectors in the cell in an apparently indiscriminate way.

However, ligands are particular about the receptors with which they interact. For example:

- The endogenous protein glutamate and neuropeptides, which are large molecules, will only bind to the large GPCR N-terminal.
- Smaller neurotransmitters, noradrenaline (norepinephrine) and ACh, bind to the smaller terminals in the transmembrane domain. In fact, all the adrenoreceptor subtypes belong to the GPCR superfamily.
- Muscarine ACh receptors and β-adrenergic receptors have opposing actions in cardiac muscle, yet the G proteins associated with the receptors can be selective.

G protein and signal transduction

When a ligand binds to a GPCR, through enzyme action:

- A change in conformation takes place in the αβγ trimer
- The trimer dissociates to α and βγ subunits

The α and βγ subunits are the 'active' forms of G protein that diffuse in the plane of the cell membrane and interact with various enzymes and ion channels, and initiate the production of second messengers.

Types of G protein

The specificity and selectivity of G protein is due to different characteristics in the α subunit, giving rise to three types that selectively produce different second messengers in the cell:

- G_s increases cAMP by activating the enzyme adenylate cyclase
- G_i (also G_o) inhibits adenylate cyclase
- G_q (also G_{12}) activates phospholipase C.

Second messenger systems

GPCRs control various cellular effector systems via the G protein. The G protein targets two key complementary pathways that initiate the production of second messengers:

- Cyclic nucleotide system:
  - **Adenylate cyclase** to synthesise cyclic adenosine monophosphate (cAMP) from ATP (adenosine triphosphate)
  - **Guanylate cyclase** to synthesise cyclic guanosine monophosphate (cGMP)
  - **Phospholipase C** catalyses the formation of inositol trisphosphate (IP_3) and diacylglycerol (DAG).

  G proteins can also target ion channels (see below).

Cyclic nucleotide system

A variety of drugs are designed to relax vascular smooth muscle by targeting the cyclic nucleotide system to increase intracellular cAMP or cGMP. Inhibition of the phosphodiesterase (PDE) enzyme systems that inactivate cAMP and cGMP has similar effects on non-vascular smooth muscle.

Adenylate cyclase and cAMP Different drugs stimulate (drug A) or inhibit (drug B) production of the second

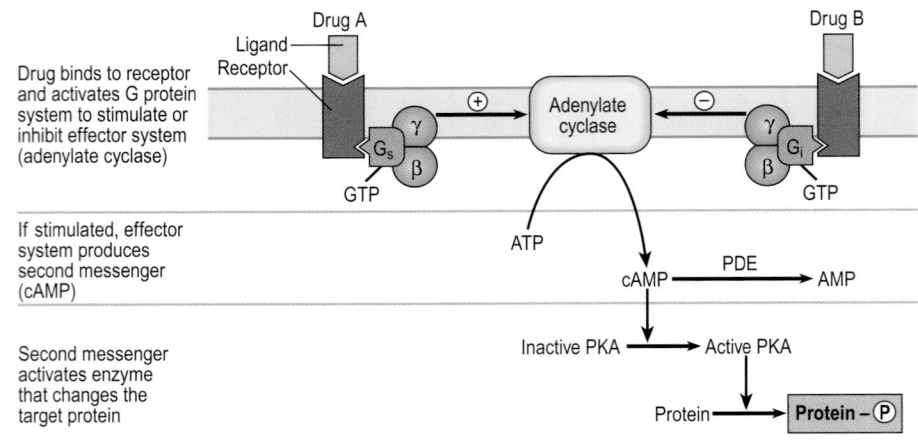

Fig. 4.14 Action of drugs to stimulate or inhibit cAMP as a second messenger. PDE, phosphodiesterases; PKA, protein kinase A.

messenger, depending on whether their receptor is linked to G_i or G_s (Fig. 4.14).

The synthesis of intracellular cAMP from ATP is a continuous process, catalysed by a membrane-bound enzyme, adenylate cyclase. cAMP is inactivated through hydrolysis by phosphodiesterases.

The cAMP formed from ATP activates **cAMP-dependent protein kinase** also known as **protein kinase A (PKA)**. PKA regulates a variety of cell functions including cell division and differentiation, muscle contraction, ion transport and energy metabolism.

Guanylate cyclase, cGMP and nitric oxide (NO) Two types of guanylate cyclase (membrane-bound and soluble) can synthesise cGMP from GTP in a reaction similar to the synthesis of cAMP from ATP.

- **Membrane-bound guanylate cyclase** is a transmembrane protein with a single α-helix domain, an extracellular binding site for neuropeptides (e.g. atrial natriuretic peptide), and a cytoplasmic **catalytic domain**. There are several isoforms of guanylate cyclase, each with a binding site for a distinct neuropeptide.
- Soluble guanylate cyclase is activated by nitric oxide (NO) to produce cGMP.

cGMP exerts its effects by:

- Altering the activity of a number of phosphodiesterases
- Direct binding to ion channels
- Activating cGMP-dependent protein kinase (PKG).

Phosphodiesterases hydrolyse cGMP to GMP to terminate its action.

Phosphodiesterase inhibition Phosphodiesterases are inhibited by naturally occurring methylxanthines and xanthine drugs. Clinically important phosphodiesterase inhibitors include theophylline, theobromine and caffeine found in tea, cocoa and coffee. Methylxanthines cause bronchial smooth muscle relaxation. The second line asthma drug aminophylline is a theophylline derivative used to relieve bronchospasm when the response to β-adrenergic antagonists is poor. Side effects include those of CNS

> **ℹ Information box 4.10   Activation of cGMP by NO**
>
> Organic nitrates (e.g. glyceryl trinitrate and some longer acting nitrates) donate NO, which activates soluble guanylate cyclase to stimulate cGMP synthesis from GTP. These are used as therapeutic muscle relaxants in the treatment of angina.
>
> Sodium nitroprusside, a NO donor activates cGMP causing arterial and venous vasodilatation. Sodium nitroprusside:
>
> - Is used in intensive care units to control hypertensive crisis
> - Has to be given by IV administration.
>
> Exposure to light converts nitroprusside to cyanide (poison!). The compound needs to be protected from light. Freshly made up intravenous solution is essential.
>
> Sidenafil (Viagra) is a selective phosphodiesterase inhibitor. This inhibits the breakdown of cGMP, and releases NO to activate cGMP to increase penile erection.

stimulation leading to wakefulness, alertness and tremor (c.f. excessive tea/coffee consumption).

Nitric oxide NO is derived from O_2 and L-arginine in a reaction catalysed by NO synthase to form NO and L-citrulline (Fig. 4.15). NO synthase is activated by Ca^{2+}-calmodulin complex (see below). NO is a gas which readily diffuses from its site of synthesis, across the cytosol or cell membrane, to act on targets in the same cell or in nearby tissues (Information box 4.10).

Calcium Calcium has a dual role as a carrier of electrical current and as a second messenger. The main mediator of Ca^{2+} action is the ubiquitous calcium-binding protein – calmodulin. Calmodulin has no intrinsic enzymatic activity but has a central regulatory role by modulating the activity of various cellular targets. Ca^{2+}-calmodulin complex activates more than 20 enzymes including Ca^{2+}-ATPase, adenylate cyclase, cyclic nucleotide phosphodiesterases, nitric oxide synthase and several protein kinases. Ca^{2+} also affects proteins and enzymes independently of calmodulin, for example PKC, K^+ and IP_3 channels, calcium-binding proteins.

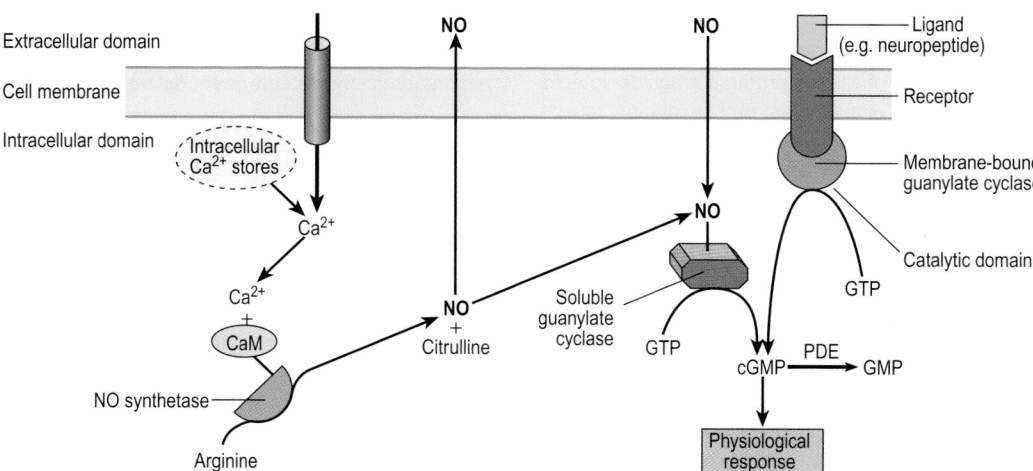

Fig. 4.15 cGMP and nitric oxide (NO) as second messengers. PDE, phosphodiesterases; cGMP, cyclic guanosine monophosphate; NO, nitric oxide.

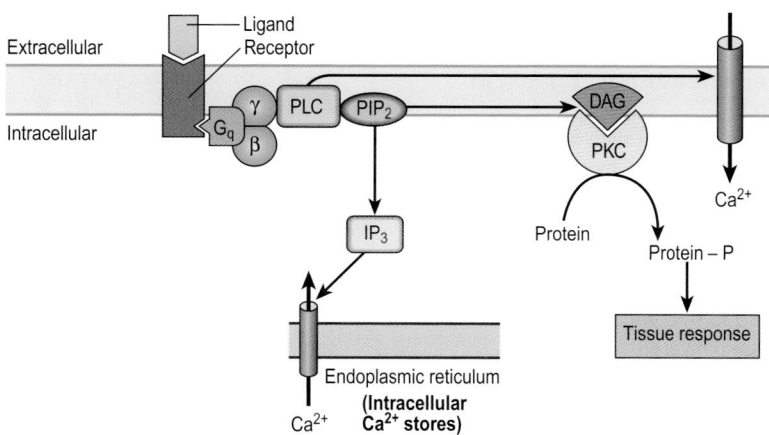

Fig. 4.16 The inositol trisphosphate second messenger system – IP$_3$ and DAG.

Phospholipase C

Phospholipase C (PLC) is a membrane-bound enzyme which, when activated by the binding of G protein, converts the membrane phospholipid, phosphatidylinositol 1,4-bisphosphate (PIP$_2$), into **inositol 1,4,5-trisphosphate (IP$_3$)** and **diacylglycerol (DAG)** (Fig. 4.16).

Inositol phosphates The main function of IP$_3$ is to control intracellular calcium. IP$_3$ is formed at the plasma membrane, diffuses into the cytoplasm and binds to IP$_3$ receptors on the membrane of endoplasmic reticulum to release intracellular Ca^{2+}. Activation of PLC also results in the influx of Ca^{2+} ions via Ca^{2+} ion channels. The IP$_3$ receptor, a macromolecular complex, thus functions as a Ca^{2+} channel as well as a receptor.

IP$_3$ is a transient signal, terminated by complete dephosphorylation back to inositol 1,4-bisphosphate, which is recycled into the phospholipid biosynthetic pathway.

DAG DAG is formed at the same time as IP$_3$, but unlike IP$_3$ is highly lipid-soluble and remains membrane bound. Its main effect is the activation of a PKC, which catalyses the phosphorylation of proteins.

Clinical box 4.9	Example of a drug targeting the phosphatidylinositol pathway

Lithium is used to stabilise mood in bipolar affective disorder (manic depressive psychosis). Although not entirely understood, the action of lithium is thought to be due to inhibition of the phosphoinositol pathway by blocking the dephosphorylation of IP$_3$ back to inositol. However, it also inhibits cAMP formation; one of the effects is to inhibit the response of the thyroid gland to thyroid stimulating hormone (TSH) with resulting hypothyroidism as an adverse effect.

- PKC is a cytosolic enzyme of which there are at least 13 different types with different tissue distribution and substrate specificities in terms of which proteins are phosphorylated.
- PKC is involved in the transduction of a wide variety of processes including inflammation, ion transport, modulation of neurotransmitter release and smooth muscle contraction.
- The action of DAG is rapidly terminated by conversion to phosphatidic acid and recycled to phospholipids.
- Raised intracellular Ca^{2+} concentration, also stimulated by GPCRs, can also activate PKCs.

Phospholipase A$_2$ and eicosanoids

Receptor-mediated activation of phospholipase A$_2$ (PLA$_2$) results in the hydrolysis of PIP$_2$ to produce arachidonic acid and its metabolites (the eicosanoids: prostaglandins, leukotrienes etc). These metabolites are released into the tissues as local hormones (e.g. insulin, glucagon).

Protein kinases in signal transduction

As a general rule, the protein kinases produced by the second messenger system have a central role in signal transduction. They control a number of different aspects of cell function, including:

- Enzymes, transport proteins
- Muscle contraction, to increase rate and force of cardiac muscle contraction, increase gut motility and secretion
- Energy metabolism via modulation of neurotransmitter release
- Ion transport via action on ion channels, particularly Ca^{2+} channels
- Cell division and differentiation
- Cytokine synthesis.

Amplification of transmembrane signals in signal transduction

The binding of a ligand to a GPCR activates a transmembrane signal that initiates a chain of events, which greatly amplifies the original signal to produce the tissue response.

Signal amplification takes place at a number of stages in a G protein-mediated signal:

- Ligand binding – at the point of binding, and as long as the ligand stays bound to the GPCR, as many as 20 G protein subunits will be activated.
- Each G protein subunit will activate an effector enzyme, e.g. adenylate cyclase.
- Each **effector** enzyme will produce a number of second messenger molecules.
- Each second messenger will activate a number of second enzyme systems e.g. protein kinase A.
- The second enzyme system produces many molecules of a third enzyme system which activates numerous reactions to produce the tissue response (e.g. opening ion channels).

Speed of GPCR transmembrane signalling

GPCR transmembrane signalling is slow (100 ms to seconds) compared with ion channel signalling (2 ms). The advantages of GPCR signalling are that:

- A single GPCR class can initiate a variety of signals to produce a cumulative response
- A GPCR initiated signal can reach a cellular process that may be some distance from the receptor
- Diffusion of the second messengers can extend the signal transduction through the cell and into the nucleus to alter gene expression.

Termination of GPCR transmembrane signals

Metabolism of cyclic nucleotides by hydrolysis terminates the signal.

- IP$_3$ is dephosphorylated to inositol.
- DAG is converted to phosphatidic acid.
- Inositol and phosphatidic acid are recycled to generate PIP$_2$.

Ion channel modulation by G proteins

In addition to regulation by voltage changes and phosphorylation, ion channels can be modulated by G proteins:

- Indirectly through the second messenger system, e.g. via IP$_3$ or cAMP, to change channel status
- Via direct action by the G protein subunits, bypassing the second messenger system. For example, muscarine ACh receptors have been shown to enhance membrane permeability to K$^+$ in cardiac muscle.

Enzyme-linked receptors (kinase-linked receptors)

Enzyme-linked, or kinase-linked, receptors are hormone receptors that are transmembrane proteins. They have an extracellular ligand-binding domain and an intracellular catalytic domain (see Fig. 4.12) that has enzyme activity when the ligand-binding domain is appropriately occupied.

The **extracellular ligand-binding domain** is very large because the endogenous ligands are large hormones such as insulin. The enzymic catalytic site of the intracellular domain is a protein kinase:

- **Tyrosine kinase**, which phosphorylates tyrosine (less commonly serine or threonine)

or

- **Guanylate kinase**, which synthesises the second messenger cGMP (see above).

The peptides that are ligands for this type of receptor are hormones that promote cell growth and proliferation. They include insulin, insulin-like growth factor, platelet-derived growth factor, cytokines, leptin and atrial natriuretic peptide. These receptors are the focus of much research as drug targets for the treatment of cancers, obesity and disordered immunity and inflammation.

Intracellular receptors and nuclear receptors

Intracellular and nuclear receptors are proteins that are mostly in the nucleus, but may be free floating in the cytoplasm. They act on DNA to regulate the expression of specific genes to:

- Alter the genetic expression of enzymes
- Alter the genetic expression of cytokines
- Alter the genetic expression of receptor proteins.

Their action, therefore, initiates different patterns of protein synthesis to give different physiological effects. Nuclear receptors have a ligand-binding domain and a DNA binding domain known as 'zinc fingers' (see Fig. 4.11D). The ligands are all lipid-soluble compounds.

Unlike non-lipid-soluble compounds, lipophilic drugs and hormones do not need signal transduction by transmembrane receptors. They simply diffuse across the cell membrane to interact with nuclear and intracellular receptors.

In its inactive form, the intracellular receptor forms a complex with a protein called the heat shock protein (HSP90).

- The receptor dissociates from HSP on hormone binding, forming a receptor/hormone complex.
- The receptor/hormone complex passes through pores in the nuclear membrane into the nucleus and interacts with hormone response elements (zinc fingers) on the DNA.

- Binding of the receptor/hormone complex with hormone response elements usually activates genes, but sometimes inhibits the transcription of a specific mRNA.

Different steroid hormones (or drug analogues) induce or inhibit specific genes, which determines the pattern of DNA expression that is affected.

- Often the hormone response element requires two receptor/hormone complexes to form a dimer in order to alter gene expression.
- Some receptor/hormone complexes bind to the same receptor/hormone complex to form homodimers.
- Others bind with a different receptor/hormone complex to form heterodimers.

Selectivity for a specific DNA is the function of the **DNA binding domain** of the receptor, which is responsible for DNA binding and transcription; hormone specificity is the function of the **ligand-binding domain**.

Drugs that target nuclear and intracellular receptors

Most steroid hormone analogues (drugs) act as agonists for the endogenous hormone, but have better pharmacokinetic properties. Some are antagonists, blocking the binding of the endogenous hormone. With drugs that activate intracellular receptors, there is a delay of several hours to days before the onset of the pharmacological effect, because this type of signal transduction requires new protein synthesis.

Examples of drugs that target nuclear and intracellular receptors include sex hormones, mineralocorticoids, glucocorticoids, thyroid hormones, vitamin D and the retinoids.

There are, however, two classes of drugs used for treating diseases in humans that need special mention:

- Anti-cancer drugs
- Antibacterial drugs.

Anti-cancer drugs

The origins of cancer cells and the theories for oncogenesis are beyond the scope of this chapter (see Ch. 6). The majority of drugs used in the treatment of cancer, cytotoxic drugs, act by inhibiting DNA synthesis in the cancer cells. Their clinical use would therefore be most effective on rapidly dividing cells, but less effective on slow growing, solid tumours.

Toxic and side effects of cytotoxic drugs are related to their action on rapidly dividing human tissue. The tissues most likely to be affected include:

- Gastrointestinal tract – giving rise to the symptoms of anorexia, nausea, diarrhoea and mucosal ulceration
- Bone marrow – myelosuppression leads to anaemia, neutropenia and thrombocytopenia
- Hair follicles – partial or complete hair loss (alopecia)
- Reproductive organs – sterility, loss of libido
- Growing tissue in children – growth retardation, arrested sexual development, risk of second malignancy.

Antibacterial drugs

This is an extremely brief summary of antibacterial drugs. Textbooks of pharmacology and drug formularies should be consulted for more detailed classification. Antibacterial

---

Clinical box 4.10	Therapeutic examples for drugs targeting nuclear receptors

Anti-cancer drugs targeting hormone nuclear receptors
Tamoxifen is an anti-oestrogen drug that competes with endogenous oestrogen for nuclear oestrogen receptors in order to inhibit the transcription of oestrogen-responsive genes in breast tissue. Tamoxifen is used in the treatment of hormone-dependent breast cancer. Cyproterone, an anti-androgen drug, is used in the treatment of prostate cancer.

Gonadotropin-releasing hormone analogues
Goserelin, for example, can inhibit gonadotropin release. These drugs can be used in the treatment of advanced pre-menopausal breast cancer and prostate cancer.

---

agents can be classified according to their mode of action on the invading microorganism:

- Inhibit bacterial cell wall synthesis so that the weak wall is ruptured by osmotic pressure, or activate enzymes that disrupt bacterial cell walls.
- Target bacterial DNA to inhibit bacterial cell division and growth.
- Inhibit bacterial protein synthesis. This is highly selective because bacterial protein is very different from human protein.
- Disrupt bacterial metabolism by blocking metabolic pathways.

Further classification of antibacterial agents is into whether the agent kills the bacteria (bacteriocidal), or merely stops it multiplying (bacteriostatic).

- **Bacteriocidal** drugs destroy the invading bacteria. They are more effective if the bacteria are not multiplying rapidly, and if the body's natural immune system is functioning normally.
- **Bacteriostatic** drugs are effective against rapidly multiplying bacteria, but rely on the immune system of the host to destroy the bacteria. They are much less effective in an immunocompromised patient.

The range of antibacterial action that the drug exhibits is also important when selecting the appropriate drug, known as the spectrum. A broad-spectrum antibacterial agent is effective against a wide variety of bacteria and protozoa, whereas as a narrow-spectrum antibacterial agent is selective for specific bacteria.

Resistance of bacteria to antibacterial agents occurs when a safe dose of the drug is no longer effective against the micro-organism. This occurs when:

- The microorganism produces enzymes that destroy the drug.
- The microorganism modifies itself so that the drug can no longer penetrate bacterial cell membranes.
- The microorganism changes its molecular structure so that the drug can no longer bind to bacterial receptors.
- The microorganism finds alternate metabolic pathways to bypass the ones blocked by the drug.

Classification of some common antibacterial agents Table 4.4 sets out a classification of some commonly used antibacterial drugs.

Table 4.4	Classification of some commonly used antibacterial agents		
Mode of action	**Bacteriocidal or bacteriostatic**	**Spectrum**	**Antibacterial agent**
Inhibits cell wall synthesis/ disrupts cell walls	Bacteriocidal	Broad	β-Lactams and penicillin and derivatives
	Bacteriocidal	Broad	Cephalosporins
	Bacteriocidal	Gram-negative bacteria	Other agents (glycopeptides e.g. vancomycin)
	Bacteriocidal	Gram-negative organisms	Polymyxins e.g. colistin
	Bacteriocidal on dividing cells, bacteriostatic on dormant cells	*Mycobacteria tuberculosis*	Isoniazid
Uncertain, probably on cell wall	Bacteriostatic	*Mycobacteria tuberculosis*	Ethambutol
Targets bacterial DNA	Bacteriocidal	Broad	Quinolones (fluoquinolone), e.g. ciprofloxacin
	Bacteriocidal	Anaerobic bacteria and protozoa	Metronidazole
	Bacteriocidal	Gram-negative cocci, *Escherichia coli*	Nitrofurantoin
	Bacteriocidal	Broad	Rifamycin, e.g. rifampicin
Inhibits bacterial protein synthesis	Bacteriostatic	Broad	Macrolides, e.g. erythromycin, azithromycin
	Bacteriocidal	Broad	Aminoglycosides, e.g. gentamicin, streptomycin
	Bacteriostatic	Broad	Tetracyclines
	Mainly bacteriostatic, bacteriocidal for some organisms	Broad	Chloramphenicol
	Bacteriostatic	Broad	Lincosamides e.g. clindamycin
	Bacteriocidal	Gram-positive organisms	Fusidic acid
Inhibits bacterial metabolism	Bacteriostatic	Broad	Sulfonamides
	Bacteriostatic	Broad	Trimethoprim
	Bacteriocidal to dormant cells	*Mycobacteria tuberculosis*	Pyrazinamide
	Bacteriostatic	*Mycobacteria leprae*	Dapsone

THE SAFETY AND EFFECTIVENESS OF DRUGS

Safety and effectiveness are essential considerations before a drug can be used to treat patients. Regulating authorities, such as the Committee on the Safety of Medicines (CSM) in the UK, the Food and Drugs Administration (FDA) in the USA and the European Medicines Agency (EMEA), are responsible for the approval of drugs for human use. Laboratory testing on tissues, and animal experiments, provide evidence of safety and potential effectiveness to the point when controlled testing on human populations may be permitted.

The properties that contribute to the safety and effectiveness of drugs are those that are also likely to give rise to unwanted side effects and toxic effects. These properties are exhibited as:

- Specificity
- Selectivity
- Potency
- Efficacy.

The parameters for potency and efficacy are measured by dose–response curves in laboratory experiments. It should be noted that other variable factors affect the performance of a given drug, and observations in the laboratory are not necessarily replicated in vivo.

GRADED DOSE–RESPONSE CURVES

Dose–response curves are constructed by measuring target tissue response in relation to the concentration of the drug or dose. In an experimental setting, if a strip of smooth muscle is suspended in an organ bath, then a drug is added to the bath to elicit muscle contraction. The dose (concentration) of the drug needed to elicit the maximal response is measured. The measurement is based on a graded response e.g. strength of muscle contraction.

The curve is produced by plotting the biological response on the ordinate (y) axis, and the drug concentration on the x axis. The resulting curve shows a rectangular hyperbola (Fig. 4.17A). By convention, the log of the dose (log[D]), giving a sigmoidal curve, is used for graded dose–response curves so that a wide range of concentrations can be displayed more easily (Fig. 4.17B). Both figures show the dose–response curve for a drug that is capable of a maximum response from the tissue.

The important features in a dose–response curve are:

- Increasing drug concentration produces an increasing response to reach a maximum that the tissue is capable of (E_{max}).
- The drug concentration that produces 50% of the maximal response (EC_{50}).
- The **slope** of the linear portion of the sigmoidal curve (between 20% and 80% in Fig. 4.17B).

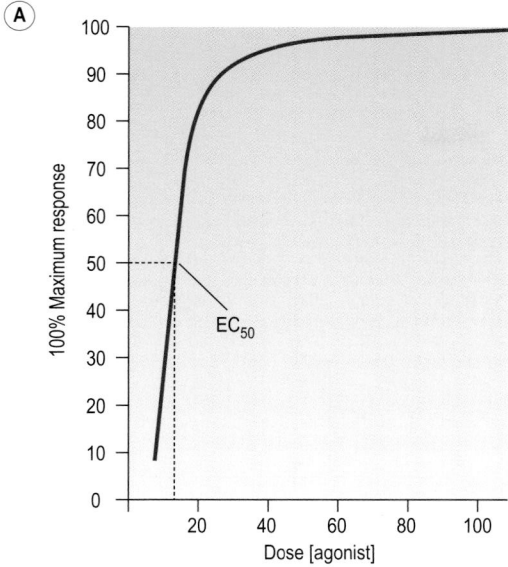

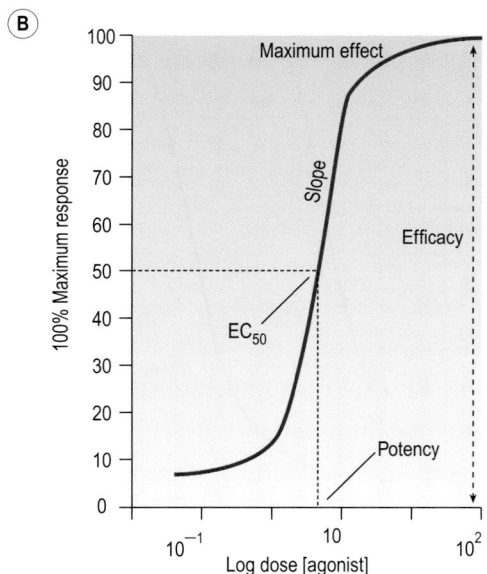

Fig. 4.17 Graded dose–response curves for an agonist drug.

Clinical box 4.11   **Example of drug selectivity**

- The non-selective β-adrenergic antagonist, propranolol, binds equally to β₁- and β₂-adrenoceptors.
- The effect of propranolol binding to β₁-adrenoceptors would be to decrease heart rate and decrease the force of cardiac muscle contraction due to noradrenaline (norepinephrine).
- Binding of propranolol to β₂-adrenoceptors, however, will block (antagonise) adrenaline (epinephrine) induced relaxation of bronchial smooth muscle, causing bronchoconstriction and precipitating acute bronchospasm in patients with asthma and COPD (chronic obstructive coronary disease).
- A selective β₁-adrenergic antagonist, atenolol, would be less likely to have this effect on β₂-adrenoceptors as it would bind more selectively with β₁-adrenoceptors.
- A selective β₁-adrenergic antagonist, when indicated, should therefore be prescribed if patients have a history of asthma or COPD.

Drug selectivity

Although many drugs are selective in binding to particular receptors, they tend to bind to different receptors to a greater or lesser degree, so that they may produce a variety of effects.

Drug potency

The **potency** of a drug depends on the strength of binding to its receptor targets – **receptor affinity**. Therefore:

- A drug has **high potency** if it has high receptor affinity. It will produce or block a tissue response at a low concentration.
- A drug with **low potency** has low receptor affinity. It will produce little or no response at low doses, and will need higher concentrations of drug to produce or block the tissue response.

Comparing potency between drugs

The concentration of a drug needed to produce 50% maximal response, EC_{50}, is used for comparing the potency of different drugs acting on the same receptors to produce similar therapeutic effects.

In Figure 4.18A, drugs A_1 and A_2 are both **agonists**, capable of producing maximal response. However, drug A_1 produces a maximal response at a lower concentration than drug A_2. Therefore, drug A_1 is more potent. Drug A_3, which is unable to produce a maximal response, is therefore a **partial agonist**.

The **potency ratio** is a comparative index of drug potency, and is derived by dividing the log EC_{50} of the test drug by the log EC_{50} of the comparator drug (Fig. 4.18B).

Drug efficacy

Efficacy is a measure of the ability of a drug, after receptor binding, to activate receptors, so that

- A **full agonist** is able to produce increasing responses with rising drug concentrations (doses) up to the maximal (drugs A_1 and A_2 in Fig. 4.18A)
- A **partial agonist** also produces increasing response to rising drug concentration, but cannot reach the maximal response (drug A_3 in Fig. 4.18A)

CLASSIFICATION OF DRUGS ACCORDING TO PERFORMANCE

Drugs are classified according to the type of response they produce in tissues:

- **Agonists** are drugs that produce maximal response from tissues.
- **Partial agonists** are drugs that are only able to produce submaximal response from tissues.
- **Antagonists** reduce the effects of agonists by reducing their action.

Drug specificity

Most drugs bind to specific receptors: proteins that are drug targets have ligand **specificity**. Drugs with low specificity would bind to a series of different receptors, thereby producing a variety of side effects, for example, chlorpromazine used in the treatment of schizophrenia.

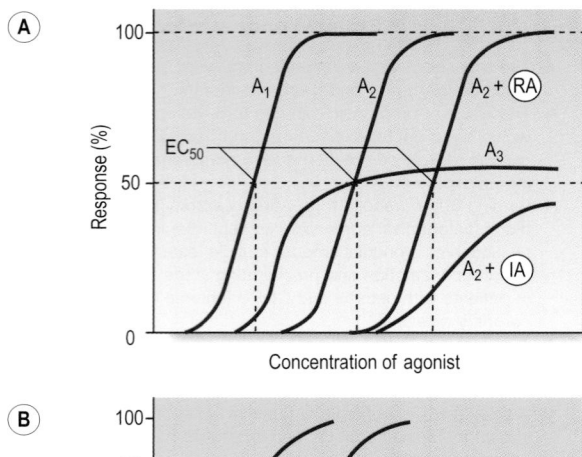

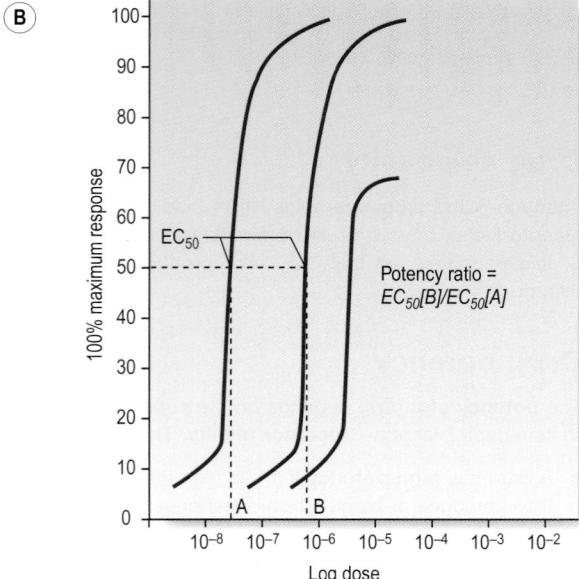

Fig. 4.18 **Dose–response curves for comparing potency.** RA, reversible antagonist; IA, irreversible antagonist. Figure 4.18A adapted with permission from Waller DG, Renwick AG, Hillier K 2001 Medical pharmacology and therapeutics. WB Saunders, Edinburgh.

- An **antagonist** drug is not shown in the figure, as it would produce a zero response, i.e. has no efficacy.

QUANTAL DOSE–RESPONSE CURVES

A **quantal response** is an all-or-none effect, such as death, and sometimes known as a **discontinuous** response. The outcome is a binary variable, 'yes' or 'no' to whether the specified response was observed. In animal experiments, the defined effect (e.g. death) will be produced in an increasing proportion of the experimental population as the dose of the drug increases. In humans, quantal responses to drugs are assayed on selected samples of the population. The relationship between the drug and the response is plotted as a graph of dose versus the number of subjects responding to that dose. As there will be individual variation in the response to the drug, the responses will follow the bell shaped, 'normal' distribution. The histogram is known as a **frequency distribution plot** (Fig. 4.19A). A more 'uniform' population will give a steeper curve.

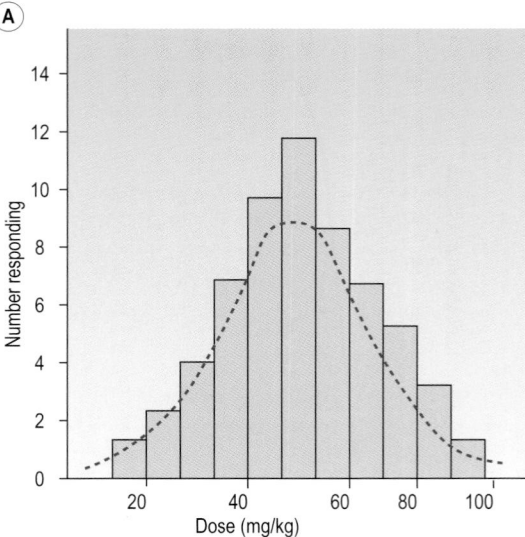

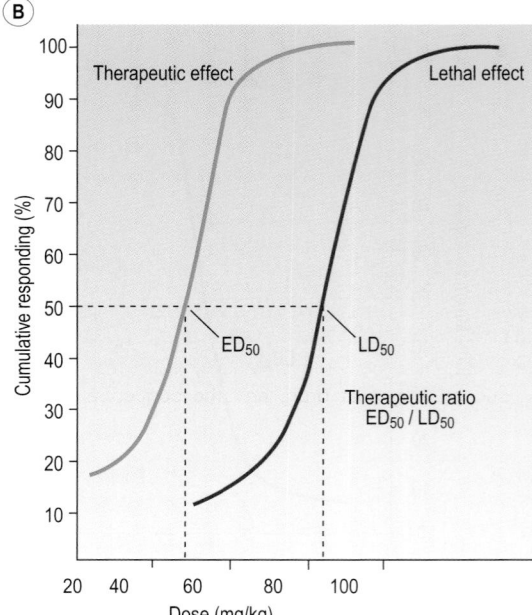

Fig. 4.19 **Quantal dose–effect curves.** In an experiment where a group of subjects were given an increasing dose until a required response was observed (e.g. pain relief), the results can be expressed as either: (A) a frequency distribution plot – each *bar* represents the minimum dose required for that number of subjects to respond (the *broken line* demonstrates a normal frequency distribution curve); or (B) a cumulative frequency distribution curve.

The bell-shaped frequency distribution plot is transformed into a sigmoidal curve by plotting dose against the cumulative percentage of subjects responding to the drug – a **cumulative frequency distribution curve** or **quantal dose–effect curve** (Fig. 4.19B).

Quantal dose–effect curves to measure the safety of drugs

All drugs produce at least two effects – **therapeutic** and **toxic (or side) effects**. Therefore each drug can have at least two quantal dose–response curves – one for the therapeutic effect and one for the toxic effect (Fig. 4.19B).

- The dose of a drug that produces the desired therapeutic effect in 50% of the population is the **median effective dose (ED$_{50}$)**.
- If the end point is death or toxicity, the median effective dose is called **the median lethal dose (LD$_{50}$)** or **the median toxic dose (TD$_{50}$)**, respectively.
- The relative safety of a drug can be determined by dividing the TD$_{50}$ or LD$_{50}$ by ED$_{50}$ to give the **therapeutic ratio**. The higher this ratio, the safer the drug.

FACTORS THAT AFFECT THE PERFORMANCE OF DRUGS

The factors that affect the specificity, selectivity, potency and efficacy of drugs relate to the nature of drug-receptor binding. A number of theories have been postulated in the attempt to quantify the relationship between a drug, or a natural ligand, and its receptors. These serve as a framework for interpreting experimental data. Advances in experimental techniques will uncover more and more surprises, so that some theories will be superseded.

Occupation theory

The binding of a drug to specific receptors to form a drug-receptor complex is governed by the Law of Mass Action, which states that the rate of any given chemical reaction is proportional to the product of the activities (or concentrations) of the reactants. In pharmacology, the effect of an agonist drug is directly proportional to the number of receptors occupied by that drug, and the concentration of the drug.

Agonist drugs

The action of an agonist drug on specific receptors mimics that of its natural ligand, so that the action is additive. The dose of drug needed to produce a response depends on:

- The **affinity** of drug molecules for binding to receptor
- The proportion of receptor binding site occupied by the drug molecules – **receptor occupancy**
- The concentration of the drug – **dose**.

A full agonist can evoke a maximal tissue response at low concentrations and low occupancy.

Spare receptors

Some drugs need to occupy all the receptors to produce a maximal response. Most drugs are able to produce a maximal response without occupying all the receptors, so that there are **spare receptors**. Many full agonists are able to achieve a maximum response while occupying only a small fraction of the receptors, so that the tissue has a **receptor reserve**. The existence of spare receptors provides biological systems with flexibility:

- The greater the number of receptors in a tissue, the more able it is to respond to lower concentrations of drug.
- If some receptors are inactivated or if the number of receptors decreases (down-regulation), spare receptors can come into play.

The response will depend on the extent of receptor occupancy required to produce the maximum response. The spare receptors in a tissue are all equally capable of interacting with the effector system to produce a response.

Partial agonist drugs

The ability of a drug to activate a receptor is graded. Partial agonists show:

- Agonist properties at low concentrations of natural ligand
- Antagonist properties at high concentrations of natural ligand by blocking the receptors.

The response by a partial agonist at any given occupancy is always less than the maximal evoked by a full agonist, and cannot produce a maximal response even if all the receptors are occupied.

Strength of drug–receptor binding

Most drugs bind reversibly to receptors. However, the duration of drug–receptor interaction could be prolonged, and even be irreversible, if the binding is with covalent bonds. This has been discussed earlier in this section.

Receptor activation and efficacy

Receptors exist in a resting state or an activated state – the so-called 'two state model'. Drug molecules have a relative affinity for either the activated or the resting state.

- Agonists have a higher affinity for receptors in the activated state. The efficacy of the agonist will depend on its relative affinity for the receptors in the activated state, so that a higher affinity will give greater efficacy.
- Antagonists show no selectivity for receptors in either the activated or resting state. They simply block the effects of agonists, and have zero efficacy.
- Some agonists have a higher affinity for resting receptors, so that they produce a change that is the opposite of an agonist. These are known as **inverse agonists**.

Inverse agonists are said to have 'negative efficacy', tending to reduce the basal level of activity by the natural ligand. A further complication arises when normal antagonists at some tissue sites become agonists at other sites. The real role of inverse agonists in therapeutics is yet to be discovered.

Allosteric modulation of drug–receptor interaction

A drug sometimes interferes with the natural ligand/receptor interaction not by binding to the ligand/receptor site, but elsewhere on the receptor to decrease ligand/receptor binding. This is known as allosteric modulation.

Drug antagonism

A drug is classified as an antagonist when it binds to a receptor but produces no response. However, when two drugs that target the same receptor are present in the system, the effects on one may be reduced, or abolished by the other. An antagonist drug may block access to receptors by:

- An agonist drug, thus diminishing or abolishing the effects of the agonist
- A natural ligand, reducing or abolishing its effects.

Mechanisms of drug antagonism

Antagonist drugs block access to receptors by natural ligands and other drugs without activating the receptor. The mechanisms can be classified as follows:

- Chemical antagonism/drug sequestration
- Receptor antagonism
- Non-competitive antagonism
- Pharmacokinetic antagonism
- Physiological antagonism.

Chemical antagonism/drug sequestration

Chemical antagonism occurs when drugs combine in solution to produce an inactive product, reducing the plasma concentration of free drug. Examples include chelating agents used as antidotes in heavy metal poisoning.

Receptor antagonism

Receptor antagonism occurs when the drug blocks access to the receptor, and involves two important mechanisms (see Fig. 4.18A):

- Reversible competitive antagonism
- Irreversible (non-equilibrium) competitive antagonism.

Reversible competitive antagonism

Reversible competitive antagonism has been discussed in the context of how antagonists can displace agonists from receptor binding sites. However, because a potent full agonist would only need to bind on a small number of drug–receptor binding sites to achieve maximal response, unless all the binding sites are occupied by the antagonist, the effect of reversible, competitive antagonism can be overcome by increasing the drug concentration: the curve for A_2 merely shifts to the right, in the presence of a reversible antagonist.

Irreversible, competitive antagonism

Irreversible or non-equilibrium, competitive antagonism occurs when the antagonist dissociates very slowly or not at all from the receptor. Irreversible antagonists are chemically reactive compounds that bind to the receptor via covalent bonds. The synthesis of new receptor protein may be required to make antagonist free receptors available.

Because an irreversible antagonist reduces the total number of available receptors, increasing the drug concentration would not restore full agonist activity. Spare receptors may come to the rescue. In Figure 4.18A the presence of the irreversible antagonist depresses the curve for A_2 so that it no longer reaches maximal response despite increasing agonist dose.

Non-competitive antagonism

Non-competitive antagonists block the chain of events leading to a tissue response at some point after the drug–receptor binding stage. As a rule, this turns a full agonist into a partial agonist.

Clinical box 4.12   **Clinical application of drug antagonism: therapeutic examples**

Chemical antagonism
Chelating agents form a complex with the drug, reducing the concentration of free drug – dimercaprol chelates mercury to reduce the plasma concentration of mercury. Dimercaprol is used as an antidote for mercury poisoning.

Receptor antagonism
- Irreversible, competitive receptor antagonists are only used experimentally. They have no clinical application. However, the irreversible, competitive COX enzyme inhibitors do have a clinical use (e.g. aspirin).
- **Non-competitive antagonism:** verapamil and nifedipine, which are Ca^{2+} antagonists, non-specifically block the influx of Ca^{2+} into cells, and can block smooth muscle contraction produced by other drugs.

Pharmacokinetic antagonism:
- Increasing the rate of renal excretion of aspirin by alkalinising the urine with bicarbonate.
- Enzyme induction to increase metabolism and reduce the effectiveness of other drugs: e.g. enzyme induction by rifampicin or barbiturates reduces the effectiveness of oral contraceptives and warfarin.
- Reduction of gastric motility, e.g. atropine reduces absorption in the small intestine.

Physiological antagonism:
- Clinically important in the treatment of conditions such as asthma. The effectiveness of bronchodilators (e.g. salbutamol) is related to the reversibility of the airways constriction produced by histamines and prostaglandins. If the constriction is produced by infection or scarring, as in chronic obstructive airways disease, the bronchodilator will be less effective.

Pharmacokinetic antagonism

Drugs that increase the rate of drug excretion or metabolism, or reduce the rate of absorption, may appear to act as antagonists by altering the pharmacokinetic parameters of the agonist.

Physiological antagonism

Physiological antagonism is an interaction between two drugs whose opposing actions (e.g. contraction and relaxation) via different receptors on the same tissue modulate each other's effect.

TOLERANCE, DESENSITISATION, TACHYPHYLAXIS

Receptors not only initiate physiological and biochemical responses but are themselves subject to regulatory controls. Continuous or repeated stimulation of receptors by an agonist can result in a diminished response.

Tolerance

Tolerance has occurred when the dose of a drug has to be increased to produce the same pharmacokinetic or pharmacodynamic effect, associated with continuous use over a prolonged period of time.

In **pharmacokinetic tolerance** the rate of drug metabolism changes primarily as a result of increased synthesis of hepatic microsomal enzymes (e.g. enzyme induction by barbiturates). Excretion of metabolised drug increases and concentration of active drug in the blood, and subsequently at the drug's site of action, decreases. **Pharmacodynamic tolerance** results from changes within systems affected by the drug so that the same dose results in a reduced response. It can be due to receptor down-regulation or reduced efficiency of receptor coupling to the signal transduction pathway.

Cross tolerance occurs when repeated use of a drug in a given class confers tolerance not only to its own actions but also to the actions of other drugs in that class (e.g. opioid analgesics).

Receptor desensitisation

Receptor **desensitisation** is a loss of receptor-activated response due to persistent exposure to an agonist. Desensitisation can occur within the course of a few minutes and is classified as short- or long-term:

- **Short-term desensitisation** is usually associated with phosphorylation of the receptor protein, followed by uncoupling from the signal pathway.
- **Long-term desensitisation** usually involves changes in the regulation of gene expression of the receptor and other proteins in the signalling pathway.

Tachyphylaxis

Tachyphylaxis is a form of desensitisation due to depletion of an essential intermediate substance. For example, repeat administration of indirectly acting sympathomimetic amines (e.g. tyramine) over a short period of time results in a loss of pharmacological activity due to depletion of the vesicular pool of noradrenaline (norepinephrine) released by tyramine from the nerve terminals, and not to receptor desensitisation.

THE AUTONOMIC NERVOUS SYSTEM

The human nervous system is divided into the **central nervous system** (CNS) and **peripheral nervous system** (PNS). The PNS consists of the **motor (somatic)** and **autonomic nervous systems**, which are anatomically distinct (Fig. 4.20).

The autonomic nervous system (ANS) is further divided into the parasympathetic and sympathetic systems. The cell bodies of the parasympathetic and sympathetic **preganglionic** neurones are in the spinal cord; the preganglionic nerve fibres carry their messages to a series of parasympathetic and sympathetic **ganglia** outside the spinal cord. Autonomic ganglia contain the preganglionic nerve endings that synapse with the cell bodies of the postganglionic neurons. The ganglia act like junction boxes, where signals are relayed from the preganglionic nerve endings to the postganglionic cell bodies. The adrenal medulla functions as one big ganglion.

NEUROTRANSMITTERS

Neurotransmitters are the chemical messengers that carry signals across synapses to stimulate postsynaptic receptors. They are synthesised in the neurons from precursors that are already present. There are systems for storage within the nerve terminals. The transmitters are released in response to sympathetic or parasympathetic stimulation to activate postsynaptic receptors, then removed by transport proteins or degraded to terminate their action. The most important neurotransmitters in the ANS are **acetylcholine** and **noradrenaline** (norepinephrine).

- The neurotransmitter associated with all **preganglionic** neurons (parasympathetic and sympathetic) is acetylcholine, which stimulates postsynaptic nicotinic receptors at the ganglionic synapse.
- In the parasympathetic system, the neurotransmitter at the short postganglionic neuron is acetylcholine, and the postsynaptic receptors stimulated by acetylcholine are muscarinic receptors.
- Nicotinic and muscarinic receptors are collectively known as **cholinergic** receptors and owe their names to historical experiments when their actions were reproduced by the injection of nicotine and muscarine. Muscarine is an extract of the poisonous toadstool *Amanita muscaria* (antidote is atropine).
- All sympathetic postganglionic nerves release noradrenaline at the **postganglionic** synapse, with the exception of sweat glands. Noradrenaline acts on **adrenergic** receptors.
- The postsynaptic transmitter for sweat glands is acetylcholine, which activates muscarinic receptors (see later).

FUNCTIONS OF THE AUTONOMIC NERVOUS SYSTEM

The ANS carries all the outflow from the CNS to the major organs of the body, with the exception of the motor outflow to skeletal muscles. The parasympathetic and sympathetic systems are entirely linked to the CNS. Although part of the

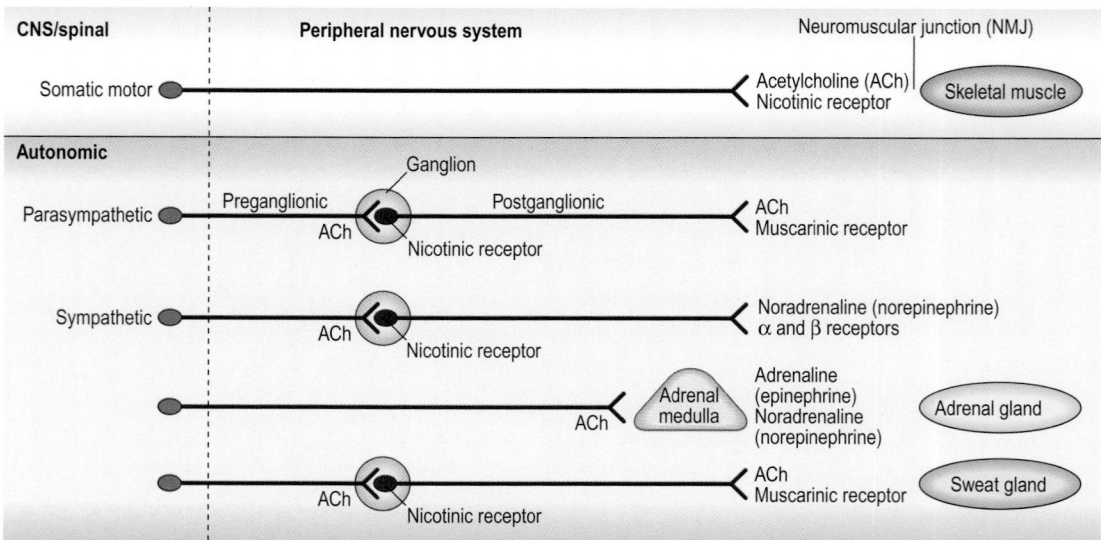

Fig. 4.20 **Simplified, diagrammatic representation of the anatomical and pharmacological subdivisions of the autonomic (peripheral) nervous system.** Somatic motor neurons convey signals from the spinal cord via efferent nerves to skeletal muscles. In the CNS, the cell body of each somatic motor neuron is in the spinal cord; the neuron terminates in close proximity to the effector muscle at a specialised site, the neuromuscular junction. The neurotransmitter released by the motor efferent at the neuromuscular junction is acetylcholine and the receptor stimulated by acetylcholine is a subclass of the nicotinic receptor.

enteric nervous system receives autonomic input, most of the enteric system has local networks that are independent of the CNS. The ANS is not under voluntary control and regulates essential physiological processes such as:

- Rate (chronotropic) and force (inotropic) of contraction of heart muscle (Ch. 11)
- Secretions of exocrine glands: bronchial, salivary, sweat, etc.
- Vascular smooth muscle and thus blood pressure
- Smooth muscle contraction and relaxation: bronchial, enteric, eye, etc.
- Energy metabolism, e.g. hepatic glycogenolysis, skeletal muscle glycogenolysis, fat cell lipolysis, pancreatic insulin secretion (see Ch. 3)
- Some endocrine secretion (see Ch. 10).

The ANS is important pharmacologically because:

- It controls the functions of almost all the major human organ systems.
- The relative simplicity of the ANS in terms of receptor subtypes and the fact that there are only two main transmitters – acetylcholine and noradrenaline – made study of the chemical transmission relatively easy.
- The action of neurotransmitters can be mimicked and modified by drugs, which are synthetic analogues.
- Diseases with ANS dysfunction are common.

OVERVIEW OF THE AUTONOMIC NERVOUS SYSTEM

The ANS is subdivided into parasympathetic (cholinergic) and sympathetic (adrenergic) systems, which can be distinguished anatomically and functionally:

- **Parasympathetic system**: maintains essential bodily functions, controls the gastrointestinal tract (secretions and motility), and controls defecation, urination and sexual function (genital erection). A complex system of neurons innervates and controls the function of glands, and smooth and cardiac muscles.
- **Sympathetic system**: primarily enables the body to adjust to stressful situations (exercise, fear, fight and flight) by acting to increase cardiac function, alter vascular tone (e.g. vasodilatation in skeletal muscle) and mobilise body energy stores.

At rest, most organs are under parasympathetic drive. This can be altered by increasing sympathetic drive when adrenaline (epinephrine) is secreted by the adrenal medulla, as in the exercise, fear and flight responses. The two branches of the ANS often have opposing organ effects (physiological antagonism). Parasympathetic and sympathetic activity have to be coordinated for normal physiological function; for example in defecation, there is increased muscarine drive to the colonic smooth muscle to increase motility, at the same time as decreased adrenergic drive to relax the anal sphincter muscle.

There are, however, exceptions. For example, the two systems produce similar effects in the salivary glands. In some organs, only one or the other of the sympathetic or parasympathetic system is present:

- Sweat glands and most blood vessels only have sympathetic innervation.
- Ciliary muscles in the eye only have parasympathetic innervation.
- Bronchial muscle only has parasympathetic innervation (constriction).

THE PARASYMPATHETIC SYSTEM

Long preganglionic neurons terminate at a ganglionic site or in close proximity to the effector tissue (see Fig. 4.22). Acetylcholine is the neurotransmitter for nicotinic receptors at the ganglionic synapse, and muscarinic receptors at the postganglionic synapse.

THE SYMPATHETIC SYSTEM

The sympathetic nervous system consists of short preganglionic neurons that terminate in the ganglionic **sympathetic chain** (see Fig. 4.22), where acetylcholine is the neurotransmitter stimulating nicotinic receptors. The postganglionic sympathetic neuron is long, synapses at the effector site and the neurotransmitter is noradrenaline (norepinephrine). The receptors stimulated by noradrenaline are adrenergic receptors, consisting of α and β receptors.

Adrenal gland

The adrenal gland is innervated by a sympathetic preganglionic neuron and the acetylcholine that is released stimulates nicotinic receptors associated with **chromaffin cells** of the adrenal medulla, containing the hormones adrenaline (epinephrine) and noradrenaline (norepinephrine), which when released into the bloodstream stimulate adrenergic receptors.

Sweat glands

The innervation of sweat glands is an exception in that although it is under sympathetic control, the postganglionic neuron of thermoregulatory sweat glands consists mainly of parasympathetic nerve fibres. Sympathetic stimulation results in the release of acetylcholine, activating muscarinic receptors. The pathways controlling nervous sweating (palms, armpits, etc.) release noradrenaline to activate α_1-adrenoceptors.

THE REFLEX ARC

In both the somatic and autonomic nervous systems, information from the periphery to the spinal cord and out to effector organs is relayed by simple reflex arcs. Although this chapter concerns the ANS, the somatic motor reflex arc is also described for comparison.

Autonomic motor reflex

The autonomic efferent pathway consists of two types of neuron – the pre- and postganglionic neurons in series (Fig. 4.21A). The neurons synapse in the autonomic ganglia. The autonomic reflex consists of:

- visceral sensory afferent neurons conveying information from interoreceptors (e.g. chemoreceptors or mechanoreceptors)

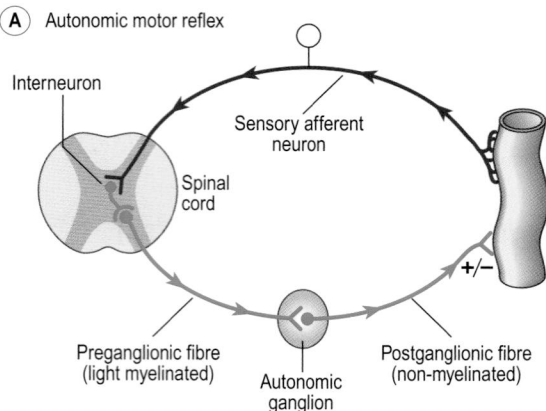

(A) Autonomic motor reflex

Interneuron

Sensory afferent neuron

Spinal cord

Preganglionic fibre (light myelinated)

Postganglionic fibre (non-myelinated)

Autonomic ganglion

+/−

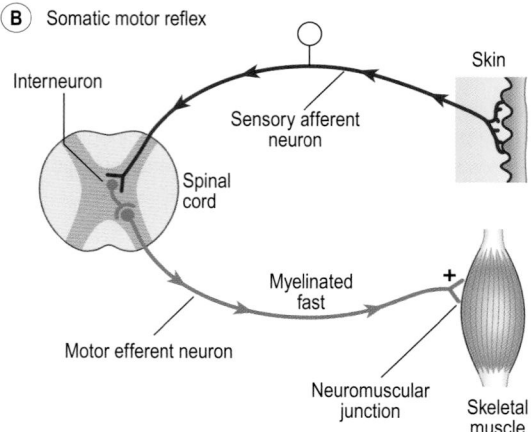

(B) Somatic motor reflex

Interneuron

Skin

Sensory afferent neuron

Spinal cord

Myelinated fast

+

Motor efferent neuron

Neuromuscular junction

Skeletal muscle

Fig. 4.21 **The reflex arc.**

- visceral motor efferent neurons, which regulate visceral activity either by excitatory or inhibitory activity on the effector tissue (cardiac, smooth muscles, glands, etc.). The efferent output from the spinal cord is composed of a two-neuron pathway, consisting of a slow conducting, lightly myelinated preganglionic fibre and a non-myelinated postganglionic fibre.

Most nerve bundles are mixed nerves carrying both sensory and motor neurons in different proportions.

Somatic motor reflex

The somatic nervous system regulates the voluntary control of skeletal muscle function (Fig. 4.21B). In contrast to the autonomic efferent pathway, which consists of two neurons, the somatic motor efferent consists of a single motor neuron. A simple somatic motor reflex arc is composed of:

- A sensory (afferent) neuron carrying information to the CNS from receptors, e.g. exteroreceptors (sight, sound, vision, taste, smell, pain, touch, thermal) and proprioceptors (muscle and joint position)
- A motor efferent neuron transmitting information from the CNS or spinal cord via a single motor nerve that is myelinated and fast conducting to the periphery. The absence of a ganglion body in the motor efferent increases the speed of conduction to the effector

(skeletal) muscle to cause a contraction. The junction between the motor nerve and the skeletal muscle is the neuromuscular junction (NMJ).

ANATOMY OF THE AUTONOMIC NERVOUS SYSTEM

The cell bodies of the preganglionic neurons in the ANS lie in the CNS; their nerve terminals synapse with postganglionic neurons in the ganglia. Most of the parasympathetic ganglia lie in or close to their effector organs. The sympathetic ganglia are either paired, and lie on either side of the spinal cord to form the paravertebral, sympathetic chains, or are unpaired (single) and lie in the midline to form the prevertebral chain (Fig. 4.22).

The nerve supply to the gastrointestinal tract is more complex. Enteric neurons lie in the walls of the intestine. Some receive parasympathetic and sympathetic input, while others form a plexus of local reflex arcs that function independently of the ANS.

THE PARASYMPATHETIC SYSTEM

The efferent parasympathetic pathway consists of cranial and sacral outflows. The cell bodies of cranial preganglionic neurons are in the brainstem. Preganglionic fibres synapse in ganglia that are close to the effector organ.

Nerve fibres from the sacral preganglionic cell bodies leave the spinal cord via the ventral roots of the spinal nerves S2–4 to synapse in scattered ganglia in the pelvis. Their postganglionic fibres innervate the distal colon, rectum, genitalia and urinary system.

THE SYMPATHETIC SYSTEM

The cell bodies of the preganglionic neurons are situated in the lateral grey horns of the 1st to 12th thoracic and 1st and 2nd lumbar segments of the spinal cord. The preganglionic fibres leave the spinal cord in the anterior roots of the spinal nerves. The ganglia of the postganglionic fibres of the sympathetic division are located at three sites:

- **Paravertebral ganglia** (sympathetic chain): 22 pairs of interconnected ganglia on either side of the spinal column. The output from any given segment of the thoracolumbar division of the spinal cord can stimulate a number of paravertebral ganglia. A single preganglionic fibre may travel through many ganglia and can synapse with up to 20 or more postganglionic sympathetic fibres. This accounts for the diffuse nature of the sympathetic response in humans. Postganglionic fibres innervate sweat glands and pilomotor muscle as well as blood vessels of the skin and skeletal muscle.
- **Prevertebral ganglia**: the unpaired coeliac, superior and inferior mesenteric ganglia which are in the walls of the main branches of the abdominal aorta. Preganglionic fibres associated with these ganglia pass through the paravertebral ganglia before synapsing with the prevertebral ganglia to innervate the gastrointestinal and urinary tracts.
- **Terminal ganglia**: the inferior hypogastric plexus ganglia associated with the urinary and rectal areas, and

Mammalian autonomic nervous system

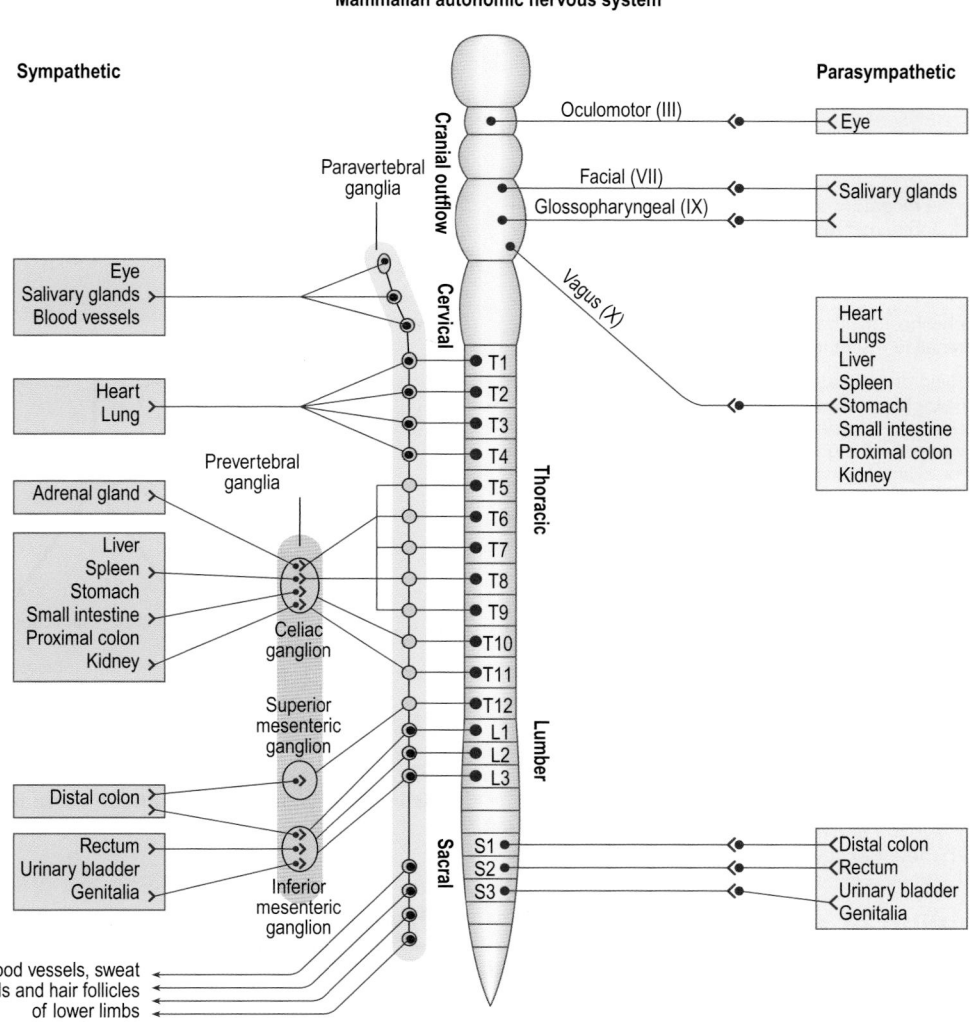

Fig. 4.22 **The autonomic nervous system.**

the cervical ganglia (superior, middle and inferior) innervating the eye, salivary glands and blood vessels of the head and neck.

NEUROTRANSMITTERS AND RECEPTORS OF THE AUTONOMIC NERVOUS SYSTEM

Acetylcholine and noradrenaline (norepinephrine) are the major neurotransmitters of the ANS. Therapeutic manipulation of their effects is mainly aimed at modifying the concentration of neurotransmitters at their site of action:

- Change rate of synthesis – increase or reduce concentration
- Change storage – deplete neurotransmitter
- Change rate of release – reduce concentration
- Block re-uptake (into presynaptic neuron) – increase concentration
- Block degradation of neurotransmitter – increase concentration
- Change number of receptors – up- or down-regulation.

PARASYMPATHETIC (CHOLINERGIC) SYSTEM

Acetylcholine (ACh) is the neurotransmitter at both pre- (nicotinic) and post- (muscarinic) ganglionic nerve terminals. The receptors are collectively known as cholinergic receptors (Fig. 4.23).

Synthesis of acetylcholine

ACh is synthesised from a precursor, choline, and acetyl-CoA (see Ch. 2) by the enzyme choline acetyltransferase (CAT). Choline is derived from the diet, ACh breakdown or synthesised by the liver and transported into the nerve terminal by a high affinity Na^+-choline co-transporter. Acetylcholine synthesis is inhibited by hemicholinium, a neuronal choline transporter inhibitor.

Storage of acetylcholine

Once synthesised, ACh is transported by a vesicular transporter to be stored in vesicles. The ACh vesicular transporter can be inhibited by vesamicol.

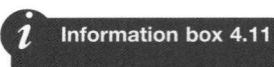

Information box 4.11   Potential sites of drug targets in the ANS (see Fig. 4.20)

Ganglion blockade:

- Postsynaptic ganglionic receptors (nicotinic receptors)
- Presynaptic receptors (auto- and hetero-receptors, see later)
- Muscarine receptors at the postganglionic synapse
- α and β adrenergic receptors at the postganglionic synapse.

The drug acts to facilitate or inhibit:

- Acetylcholine – synthesis, storage or release
- Noradrenaline – synthesis, storage or release.

The earliest drugs that were found to affect the ANS were **ganglion-blocking** drugs. They blocked acetylcholine receptors in both parasympathetic and sympathetic ganglia. They now have restricted clinical use because of the mixed effects. For example, ganglion blockers used in the treatment of high blood pressure (hypertension) are now obsolete (except for specialised indications) due to:

- Sympathetic blockade causing vasodilatation, leading to hypotension
- Parasympathetic blockade causing the side effects of dry mouth, urine retention, blurred vision, impotence and constipation.

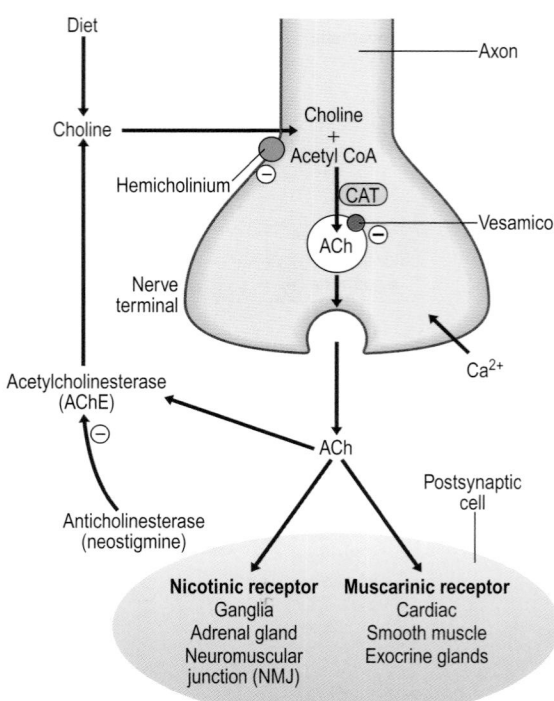

Fig. 4.23 Synthesis, metabolism and receptors associated with parasympathetic nerve terminal.

Release of acetylcholine

Acetylcholine in the vesicles is released into the synaptic cleft by Ca^{2+}-dependent exocytosis.

Inactivation of acetylcholine

ACh is rapidly hydrolysed by the enzyme **cholinesterase**, which is associated with the cholinergic synaptic membranes and also in a soluble form in plasma, to choline and acetic acid, which in turn is converted to water and CO_2.

There are two distinct types of the cholinesterase enzyme and they have different distributions and functions:

- **Acetylcholinesterase** is membrane bound and hydrolyses ACh released at cholinergic synapses. The function of the soluble form is not well understood.
- **Butyrylcholinesterase**, also known as pseudocholinesterase, is widely distributed in tissues such as brain, liver, gastrointestinal tract, and in the soluble form in plasma. The function of the synaptic membrane-bound form is not well known, but the soluble plasma enzyme inactivates a variety of circulating drugs including procaine, benzocaine (local anaesthetics) and suxamethonium (NMJ blocker). A subpopulation of patients is deficient in plasma pseudocholinesterase activity, resulting in prolonged activity of drugs such as suxamethonium, a muscle relaxant used during general anaesthesia for major surgery.

Anticholinesterase drugs

Anticholinesterase drugs are used therapeutically to increase cholinergic activity, but are also poisons. Anticholinesterase drugs may be reversible short- or medium-acting, or irreversible.

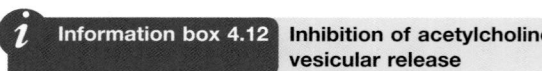

Information box 4.12   Inhibition of acetylcholine vesicular release

Substances that inhibit the influx of Ca^{2+} into nerve terminals prevent vesicular release of ACh (Fig. 4.23). Effects of inhibiting ACh vesicular release into the **synapse** include:

- Inhibition of sweating, giving symptoms of a dry, warm skin
- Inhibition of salivation with symptoms of dry mouth
- Pupillary constriction.

Inhibition of ACh vesicular release at the **neuromuscular junction** would lead to muscle paralysis:

- Aminoglycoside antibiotics such as streptomycin and neomycin block ACh vesicular release and occasionally produce muscle paralysis as an unwanted side effect.
- Botulism is a severe form of food poisoning with a high mortality rate, caused by the anaerobic bacillus *Clostridium botulinum*. *C. botulinum* can multiply in canned or preserved food, producing an exotoxin that inhibits the vesicular release of ACh. Blockade at the NMJ leads to voluntary muscle paralysis and fatal respiratory muscle paralysis. Botulinum poisoning also causes parasympathetic paralysis with symptoms of dry mouth and blurring of vision.
- β-Bungarotoxin is contained in the venom of a variety of cobras and the black widow spider, and has similar effects to botulism. The same venoms also contain α-bungarotoxin, which acts presynaptically, causing the rapid discharge of vesicular contents, followed by paralysis.

Blockade of cholinesterase enzymes results in increased autonomic cholinergic activity:

- At the postganglionic nerve terminal with increased stimulation of muscarinic receptors (see below), enhancing synaptic cholinergic activity, causing excessive salivation, bradycardia, bronchospasm and hypotension
- By increasing NMJ activity with muscle fasciculation and twitching, and may result in a depolarisation block and paralysis
- Anticholinesterase drugs that cross the blood–brain barrier have central effects due to increased muscarinic receptor activation, leading to excitation and convulsions followed by unconsciousness and respiratory failure. The antidote is atropine.

Short-acting, reversible anticholinesterase

The ionic bond formed between short-acting, reversible anticholinesterases is rapidly reversible, and the duration of action of the drug is very brief, measured in seconds. Edrophonium is the only clinically important one, used primarily in the diagnosis of myasthenia gravis. Muscle strength temporarily improves after the injection of edrophonium in myasthenia gravis, but not other conditions with muscle weakness.

Medium-acting, reversible anticholinesterase

Medium-acting, reversible anticholinesterases are carbamyl, instead of acetyl, esters. The carbamyl ester takes longer to hydrolyse than edrophonium so that the action can be long-lasting, although reversible. Physostigmine and neostigmine are clinically important in the treatment of glaucoma, reversal of a competitive NMJ block and the treatment of myasthenia gravis.

Irreversible anticholinesterase (organophosphates)

Irreversible anticholinesterases are phosphorus compounds with a labile fluoride (e.g. dyflos) or an organic group (e.g. malathione, used in preparations for the treatment of head lice) that binds covalently to the cholinesterase enzyme. The phosphorylated enzyme is stable, with no appreciable hydrolysis so that a new enzyme has to be synthesised to restore cholinesterase activity, which may take several weeks.

Cholinergic receptors

Acetylcholine, the neurotransmitter of the parasympathetic system, stimulates the two major classes of cholinergic receptor:

- Nicotinic receptors (nAChR)
- Muscarinic receptors (mAChR).

Nicotinic receptors

There are two subtypes of nicotinic receptor:

- **N_M receptors**, at the neuromuscular junction
- **N_N receptors**, at all autonomic ganglia, in the adrenal gland and in the CNS (neuronal nicotinic receptors)

The molecular structures of these receptors are similar. Both types are ligand-gated ion channels with varying selectivity for cations (Na^+, Ca^{2+}), which, when stimulated by ACh,

 Information box 4.13   **Chemical and biological weapons**

Irreversible anticholinesterases were developed as nerve gases for chemical warfare and pesticides (e.g. sheep dip used by farmers). These compounds have high lipid solubility and are readily absorbed through mucous membranes and unbroken skin. Poisoning by these agents requires the antidote pralidoxime and hospitalisation. Pralidoxime reactivates the enzyme by attracting the phosphate group away from the active site on the enzyme. Reactivation has to be done in the first few hours, because the enzyme cannot be reactivated after prolonged binding to the organophosphate.

The Geneva Protocol of 1925 banned the use of chemical weapons. In 1971, the Biological Weapons Convention (BWC) completed work on the Convention on the Prohibition of the Development, Production, Stockpiling and Use of Chemical Weapons and on Their Destruction. This should have banned all production and use of these weapons. The BWC was opened for signatures and ratification by all nations in 1972, and was entered into force in 1975.

produce rapid excitatory responses, owing to localised depolarisation of cell membranes. The differences between the two types are exploited pharmacologically. See Table 4.5 for examples and therapeutic effects.

Pharmacological effects of nicotinic receptor agonists

Acetylcholine and nicotine are N_N receptor agonists (Table 4.5). Stimulation of ganglionic N_N receptors by ACh causes complex peripheral responses due to generalised stimulation of all autonomic ganglia (i.e. increased sympathetic and parasympathetic activity). Ganglionic N_N stimulation also stimulates the adrenal medulla to release adrenaline and noradrenaline (epinephrine and norepinephrine). **Nicotine** initially stimulates N_N in the autonomic ganglia but produces a depolarisation block with prolonged use (i.e. becomes antagonistic).

Suxamethonium has a similar structure to ACh and acts as a N_M receptor agonist at the neuromuscular junction. In contrast to ACh, which is rapidly hydrolysed, suxamethonium remains at the NMJ for a long time. After initial stimulation of the NMJ leading to muscle twitching or fasciculation, muscle relaxation sets in due to depolarising block, when the muscle loses electrical excitability for the duration of the drug action.

Pharmacological effects of nicotinic receptor antagonists

The effect of blocking ganglionic nicotinic receptors results in a generalised decrease in postganglionic parasympathetic and sympathetic activity (see Table 4.5). The physiological response observed depends on which division of the ANS is dominant in any given organ. In the majority of organs the parasympathetic innervation is dominant (heart, eye, gastrointestinal tract, urinary tract, sweat glands, salivary glands). The vascular system is, however, solely under tonic sympathetic control and so ganglionic nicotinic receptor antagonists produce a fall in blood pressure, with ensuing postural hypotension. Some N_N antagonists, such as hexamethonium, have only experimental use but trimetaphan is used to lower blood pressure during surgery.

Table 4.5	Examples of drugs acting at cholinergic receptors and their clinical uses			
Receptor	**Agonists**	**Clinical uses**	**Antagonists**	**Clinical uses**
Nicotinic (ganglionic)	Acetylcholine	None	Hexamethonium	
	Nicotine	None	Trimethaphan	Orthostatic hypotension in surgery
Nicotinic (NMJ)	Suxamethonium	Muscle relaxant (depolarising block)	Tubocurare	
			Pancuronium ⎫	Muscle relaxants
			Atracurium ⎭	
Muscarinic	Acetylcholine	None	Atropine	Antispasmodic, causes CNS excitation, tachycardia
	Pilocarpine	Reduces intraocular pressure in glaucoma, contracts iris (smooth muscle)	Hyoscine	Anti-emetic, motion sickness
			Ipratropium	Bronchodilator (asthma, COPD)
			Trihexyphenidyl hydrochloride (benzhexol)	Anti-muscarinic action at NMJ: used to treat tremor and spasticity in Parkinsonism
			Tropicamide	Mydriatic: used to dilate pupils in ophthalmology
			Pirenzepine	Inhibits gastric secretions in peptic ulcers
	Carbachol ⎫ Bethanechol ⎭	Stimulate smooth muscle contraction in bladder and intestinal tract	Oxybutynin Tolterodine	Inhibits bladder contraction, used to treat urinary incontinence

Drugs that act as N_M receptor antagonists, such as tubocurare, competitively block the action of ACh on N_M receptors at the NMJ. The effects of these drugs are mostly to produce motor paralysis. They have very little or no antagonistic action at neuronal N_N receptors and vice versa.

Muscarinic receptors

Molecular biology has identified five different subtypes of muscarinic receptors (M_1–M_5). Each subtype couples to a second messenger system through an intervening G protein. M_1, M_3 and M_5 receptor stimulation results in increased levels of the second messengers IP_3 and DAG whereas M_2 and M_4 receptor stimulation results in reduced cAMP levels. The important functions are those of M_{1-3}. The tissue distribution differs for each subtype:

- M_1 – act at autonomic ganglia (where they produce depolarisation of the cell membrane). Mainly located in the hippocampus and cerebral cortex and on the parietal cells (where they increase HCl release) and in the gastrointestinal tract.
- M_2 – also known as 'cardiac' receptors, cause slowing of the heart rate and a decrease in the force of contraction. Mainly located in the heart, gastrointestinal smooth muscle, and CNS, they are also presynaptic autoreceptors (see later).
- M_3 – also known as 'glandular' receptors, stimulate secretion of exocrine glands (salivary, gastric, etc.) and visceral smooth muscular contraction. Receptors in vascular endothelium cause vasodilatation and a fall in blood pressure.

Pharmacological effects of muscarinic receptor agonists

Stimulation of muscarinic receptors has the following effects (Table 4.5):

- **Cardiovascular**: slowing of heart rate (sino-atrial node), reduction in force of contraction (atria) and reduction in atrio-ventricular node conduction.
- **Vascular endothelium**: mediation of the release of nitric oxide to produce vasodilatation.
- **Smooth muscle**: contraction of bronchial and bladder smooth muscle.
- **Gastrointestinal tract**: increase in smooth muscle tone, peristalsis and increasing gastric and pancreatic secretions.
- **Exocrine glands**: increased sweating, lacrimation, salivation and bronchial secretions; induction of histamine release from histaminocytes; increased HCl secretion from gastric parietal cells.
- **Eye**: contraction of pupillary muscle (constrictor pupillae) causing pupillary constriction in response to bright light, and contraction of ciliary muscles to change the shape of the lens in ocular accommodation.

Pharmacological effects of muscarinic receptor antagonists

Muscarinic receptor antagonists selectively block parasympathetic activity with the following effects:

- **Inhibition of secretions**: causing dry mouth and skin (dry and warm to the touch due to lack of sweating), inhibition of mucociliary clearance in lungs.
- **Heart**: initial slowing in rate (bradycardia) due to central stimulation, followed by tachycardia (vagus blocked and the sympathetic effect is unopposed).
- **Eye**: dilation of pupil (mydriasis), which becomes unresponsive to light; relaxation of ciliary muscles, resulting in loss of accommodation and blurred vision (cycloplegia).

- **CNS**: a dose-dependent excitatory effect (restlessness, disorientation), which can be reversed by physostigmine (anticholinesterase).

Table 4.5 shows some examples of muscarine receptor agonists and therapeutic uses.

SYMPATHETIC (ADRENERGIC) SYSTEM

With the exception of sweat glands, noradrenaline (norepinephrine) is the principal postganglionic neurotransmitter in the sympathetic nervous system. Noradrenaline belongs to a group of neurotransmitters known as catecholamines. They have the biochemical structure of a benzene ring joined to two adjacent hydroxyl groups (catechol), which forms a complex with an amine. Both the catechol and the amine groups are receptor binding. The main catecholamines are noradrenaline (norepinephrine), dopamine and adrenaline (epinephrine). Serotonin, or 5-HT, although not strictly a catecholamine, has catecholamine-like actions. Isoprenaline (US: isoproterenol) is a synthetic analogue of noradrenaline.

Sympathetic receptors are adrenergic, and drugs that activate adrenergic receptors (adrenergic agonists) are known as sympathomimetic amines, as they mimic the action of sympathetic stimuli.

Sympathomimetic amines

Sympathomimetic amines are developed by modifying the noradrenaline molecule. They may be directly or indirectly acting.

- **Directly acting sympathomimetic amines** have a direct action on adrenoceptors and mimic the action of noradrenaline and adrenaline.
- **Indirectly acting sympathomimetic amines** act weakly on adrenoceptors, but are taken into the nerve terminals by the monoamine transporter, displacing noradrenaline, which is released to act on postsynaptic receptors.

Noradrenaline (norepinephrine) synthesis

The sympathetic ganglion contains the cell bodies of noradrenergic neurons, whose postganglionic nerve terminals end in numerous varicosities (swellings or boutons) that contain many synaptic vesicles. Tyrosine is converted to dopamine in the cytoplasm of the nerve terminals and transported into the synaptic vesicles where it is converted to noradrenaline for storage and release. The last step in the catecholamine synthesis pathway is the catalysis of noradrenaline to adrenaline in the adrenal medulla (see later). The carbon skeleton of noradrenaline comes from the metabolism of the essential amino acid tyrosine or its precursor, phenylalanine (Fig. 4.24). Phenylalanine is converted to tyrosine by phenylalanine hydroxylase.

Noradrenaline synthesis pathway

Noradrenaline is synthesised from L-tyrosine in adrenergic neurons. Tyrosine is converted to dopa (levodopa) by the enzyme tyrosine hydroxylase, which requires a pteridine cofactor (Fig. 4.24). The activity of tyrosine hydroxylase is **rate-limiting** for catecholamine synthesis (i.e. the slowest acting enzyme in the series involved in the synthesis of

Sympathetic synthesis and receptors

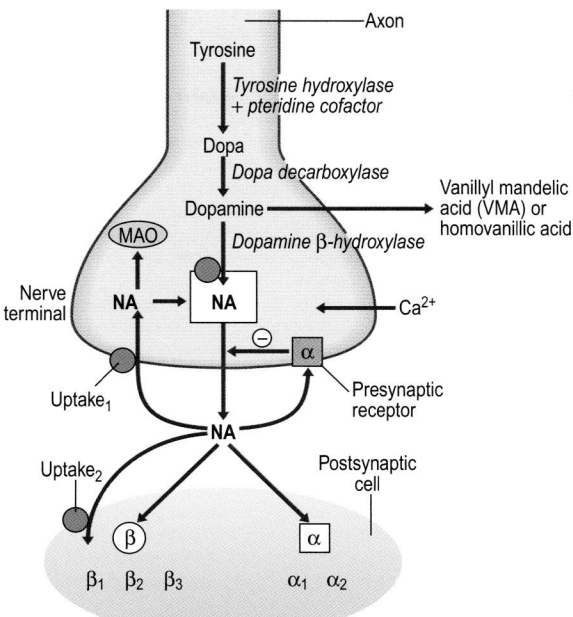

Fig. 4.24 **Synthesis and release of noradrenaline (norepinephrine) from sympathetic neurons.** MAO, monoamine oxidase; NA, noradrenaline; α, alpha-adrenoceptor; β, beta-adrenoceptor.

noradrenaline). Tyrosine hydroxylase activity can be regulated by a variety of signals within the nerve cell body or terminal:

- Increased cytoplasmic concentration of free noradrenaline inhibits the enzyme by competing for the cofactor, pteridine – known as **end-product inhibition**.
- Increased phosphorylation of tyrosine hydroxylase by elevated cAMP levels results in an increased rate of conversion and/or affinity of the enzyme for the cofactor.
- Increased intracellular Ca^{2+} levels due to increased neuronal activity increases the sensitivity of the enzyme.
- Increased neuronal firing rates or depletion of neuronal transmitter stores results in increased tyrosine hydroxylase activity, as indicated by increased levels of mRNA for the enzyme.
- Dephosphorylation of the enzyme by stimulating autoreceptors (α_2 resulting in reduced cAMP levels) reduces activity of tyrosine hydroxylase.

These changes in the synthesis and function of tyrosine hydroxylase, in response to neuronal activity, serve to maintain the rate of synthesis of noradrenaline relative to the requirement for the transmitter. The adrenal medulla contains an additional enzyme that converts noradrenaline to adrenaline (epinephrine).

Dopa is rapidly converted to dopamine by the enzyme dopa decarboxylase. In dopaminergic neurons, this is the end of the synthetic pathway. In sympathetic neurons, a proportion of the dopamine that is formed in the cytoplasm of the nerve terminal is actively transported by a vesicular transporter into the storage vesicle, where it is converted to noradrenaline by the enzyme dopamine β-hydroxylase. The remainder of the dopamine is converted to the metabolite vanillyl mandelic acid (VMA) also known as homovanillic acid, which is excreted in the urine.

Adrenal conversion of noradrenaline to adrenaline

Noradrenaline is further converted to adrenaline by the enzyme phenylethanolamine-*N*-methyl transferase in the adrenal medulla.

Noradrenaline storage

In the nerve terminal, cytoplasmic dopamine is actively taken into vesicles by a vesicular transporter and converted to noradrenaline. The vesicle is impermeable from inside to outside, under usual circumstances, preventing noradrenaline from leaking out. Inhibition of the vesicular transporter leads to the depletion of noradrenaline stores.

Noradrenaline release

Noradrenaline is released in response to sympathetic stimulation. The synaptic vesicles release their contents by Ca^{2+}-dependent exocytosis. Noradrenaline may be released by substances that are taken into the vesicles, where they displace noradrenaline into the cytoplasm. Noradrenaline is then released into the synapse by reversing neuronal uptake transport. Examples include tyramine, ephedrine and amphetamine. These substances are structurally related to noradrenaline, and are known as indirectly acting sympathomimetic amines. Prolonged, repeated use of these drugs produces diminishing responses (see Tolerance, desensitisation and tachyphylaxis, above).

Modulation of noradrenaline release

Noradrenaline release is modulated by substances that act on presynaptic receptors. Presynaptic modulation is an important control mechanism in the peripheral nervous system. A variety of nerve terminals are subject to this kind of control; different mediators can act on presynaptic terminals. For example, acetylcholine acting through presynaptic muscarinic receptors regulates cholinergic nerve terminals. Other presynaptic receptors include dopaminergic-D_2 and serotinergic-$5HT_{1D}$ receptors.

Presynaptic autoreceptors

Noradrenaline can modulate its own neuronal release by the stimulation of presynaptic **autoreceptors**. These autoreceptors can be either inhibitory or excitatory (Fig. 4.25).

- **$α_2$-Adrenergic receptors** are inhibitory receptors – reduce noradrenaline release.
- **$β_2$-Adrenoceptors** are excitatory autoreceptors – increase noradrenaline release.

Presynaptic / autoreceptors

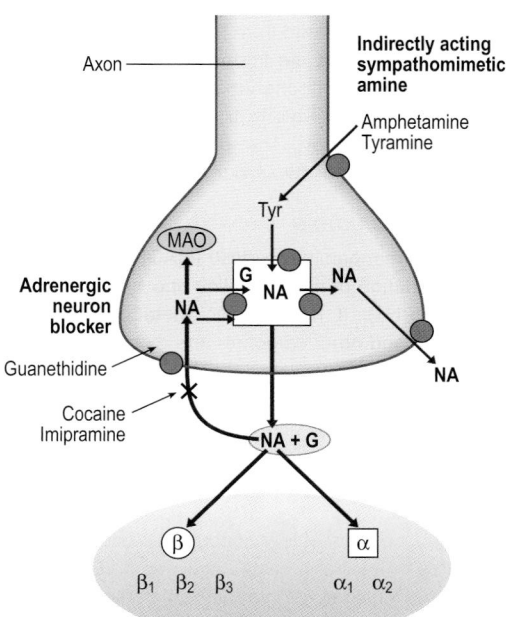

Fig. 4.25 **Inhibition of noradrenaline release.** MAO, monoamine oxidase; NA, noradrenaline; α, alpha-adrenoceptor; β, beta-adrenoceptor.

Presynaptic heteroreceptors

There are other receptors involved in controlling noradrenaline release. The neurotransmitter is released by a different neuron, and is different to the neurotransmitter released by the neuron itself. For example, dopaminergic D_2 and cholinergic M_2 receptors can also inhibit release of noradrenaline. These are called presynaptic heteroreceptors.

Adrenergic neuron blocking drugs (ANBs)

ANBs act presynaptically on noradrenaline release. ANB drugs, such as guanethidine and bretylium, enter the vesicle and replace noradrenaline. This reduces the concentration of noradrenaline released by exocytosis in response to sympathetic stimulation. These drugs are hypotensive, but are obsolete because of their unpleasant side effects. The effects of ANBs can be reversed or prevented by uptake$_1$ inhibitors (e.g. cocaine, tricyclic antidepressants).

Termination of action of neuronally released noradrenaline

The action of neuronally released noradrenaline is terminated by its re-uptake from the synapse into the presynaptic nerve terminal by two specific transporters (Fig. 4.26):

- neuronal uptake$_1$
- extraneuronal uptake$_2$

Neuronal uptake$_1$

Neuronal uptake$_1$ is the most important process for terminating the action of noradrenaline. About 70% of neuronally released noradrenaline is taken back into the nerve terminal, so that neuronal uptake can be considered as a mechanism of transmitter conservation. The uptake$_1$ transporter is a protein that is selective for the different types of neurotransmitter released from particular neurons, e.g. noradrenaline, dopamine, 5-HT. The more recently developed drugs exploit

Drugs and noradrenaline release

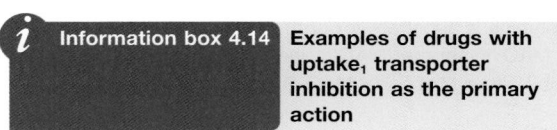

Fig. 4.26 **Drugs and noradrenaline release.** A diagrammatic representation of the site of action of an adrenergic neurone blocker (guanethidine), neuronal uptake$_1$ inhibitor (cocaine, imipramine) and indirectly acting sympathomimetic amines (tyramine, amphetamine). MAO, monoamine oxidase; NA, noradrenaline; α, alpha-adrenoceptor; β, beta-adrenoceptor; G, guanethidine.

> ℹ️ **Information box 4.14** **Examples of drugs with uptake$_1$ transporter inhibition as the primary action**
>
> - **Tricyclic antidepressants** exert their major action on the CNS. Blocking the action of uptake$_1$ increases noradrenaline concentration at the synapse. PNS effects, however, will give rise to the unwanted side effects of tachycardia and cardiac dysrhythmia.
> - **Cocaine** has a similar stimulant action to tricyclic antidepressants on the brain but causes excitement and euphoria, effects that make the drug liable to misuse. It also increases sympathetic transmissions leading to tachycardia and raised arterial pressure.
> - Other drugs that have an effect on noradrenaline synthesis, storage or release, may also have an uptake$_1$-blocking effect. Examples include amphetamine, guanethidine and phenoxybenzamine.

the differences between transporters so that the drugs are selective in their neuronal uptake inhibitory properties. The uptake$_1$ transporter has a greater selectivity for noradrenaline than adrenaline, so drugs that inhibit the transporter have no effect on the action of adrenaline. Other substrates for the transporter are dopamine, 5-HT and tyramine.

Extraneuronal uptake$_2$

The uptake$_2$ transporter effects the re-uptake of adrenaline from the bloodstream into extraneuronal tissue. It is unaffected by the drugs that inhibit uptake$_1$. Although not of major clinical significance, uptake$_2$ is inhibited by corticosteroids. This may be relevant in the treatment of conditions such as asthma.

Metabolism of catecholamines

Noradrenaline is eliminated from the body by metabolic degradation. Two enzymes are important in the metabolism of catecholamines: the mitochondrial monoamine oxidase and cytoplasmic catechol-*O*-methyltransferase. Both are widely distributed in the body. The degradation of adrenaline, dopamine and 5-HT follow similar pathways.

Monoamine oxidase

Mitochondrial monoamine oxidase (MAO) mediates the oxidative deamination of noradrenaline and other monoamines (dopamine, 5-HT). It is the main metabolic pathway for noradrenaline and other catechol- and monoamines. Deamination produces:

- A corresponding acid – 3,4-dihydroxymandelic acid (DOMA) or
- A corresponding alcohol – dihydroxyphenylethylglycol (DOPEG).

The highest activity of MAO occurs in catecholamine containing nerve terminals. It is also active in 5-HT nerves, liver and intestinal mucosa. A number of dietary amines (e.g. tyramine) are detoxified by MAO in the intestine and liver.

There are two main forms of MAO: MAO-A and MAO-B. They have different distributions in the brain and peripheral organs:

- MAO-A – most abundant in placenta, liver and intestines
- MAO-B – abundant in the brain.

The isoforms differ in their substrates specificity: noradrenaline and 5-HT are substrates primarily for MAO-A; dopamine is substrate for both.

MAO inhibitors (MAOIs) were developed to selectively inhibit either MAO-A or MAO-B to minimise side effects.

Clinical box 4.16 **Monoamine oxidase inhibitors**

MAOIs were developed to act as antidepressants by increasing the accumulation of neurotransmitters such as noradrenaline and 5-HT (serotonin). The original MAOIs were non-selective, and had many unwanted effects:

- Inhibition of the metabolism of other monoamine drugs administered at the same time (e.g. indirectly acting sympathomimetics in common cold and cough medicines): their accumulation, through not being degraded, increases their pressor effects and can lead to severe hypertension.
- MAOI prevents the destruction of dietary tyramine, potentiating the hypertensive effect of tyramine in foods (abundant in cheese, fava beans, meat and vegetable extracts): this causes severe hypertension.

The discovery of the two isoforms enabled the development of MAOIs that were selective for either MAO-A or MAO-B. MAO-A is abundant in the liver and gut, so inhibition of MAO-A is more likely to lead to the side effects due to interaction with tyramine. MAO-B is abundant in the extrapyramidal system in the brain, but not in gut or liver. The selective MAO-B inhibitor selegilin, which was developed for the treatment of Parkinsonism, does not have the interaction with tyramine containing foods and drugs.

MAOIs used for treating depression have to be prescribed with great caution and accompanying dietary advice. This is why they are used less frequently for depression than tricyclic antidepressants and selective serotonin re-uptake inhibitors (SSRIs).

Cytoplasmic COMT

Catechol-*O*-methyltransferase (COMT) is a widespread enzyme that occurs in neuronal and non-neuronal tissues. COMT is particularly active in the liver. It is an alternative, but relatively minor, pathway for inactivating noradrenaline and dopamine.

COMT methylates one of the catechol hydroxyl groups on the benzene ring to give a methoxy derivative (e.g. noradrenaline forms normetanephrine). It also methylates the deaminated products of catecholamines from MAO activity: DOMA and DOPEG to produce the major urinary metabolites of VMA and 3-methoxy-4-hydoxyphenylglycol (MOPEG), respectively. VMA is the predominant metabolite of peripheral noradrenaline metabolism whereas MOPEG is the main metabolite associated with noradrenaline turnover in the CNS. Urinary VMA and MOPEG are useful indicators of the amount of noradrenaline released peripherally and centrally.

COMT inhibitors, e.g. entacapone, that block the degradation of levodopa, are used with levodopa in the treatment of Parkinson's disease to prolong its action.

Adrenergic receptors

Adrenergic receptors (adrenoceptors) respond to stimulation by noradrenaline. It was originally thought that there were two types of adrenergic receptors: α and β types based on their pharmacological responses. It is now recognised that there are two main α-subtypes and three main β-subtypes. Adrenergic receptors are distributed in the CNS and the sympathetic branch of the ANS. The different subtypes vary in their affinity for adrenaline and noradrenaline. All α- and β-adrenoceptors are G protein-coupled receptors. Each receptor type is linked through the G protein mechanism to a specific second messenger system.

α-Adrenoceptors

α-Adrenoceptors are subdivided into α_1 and α_2: α_1 are postsynaptic; and α_2, although termed presynaptic, are also present postsynaptically. Each subtype has been further divided into three subtypes.

Clinically, the most important effects of α-adrenoceptors are on vascular smooth muscle. Generally, smooth muscle contracts in response to a stimulation, but gastrointestinal smooth muscle relaxes. Responses to α-adrenoceptor stimulation include:

- α_1-Adrenoceptors: vasoconstriction, gastrointestinal muscle relaxation, salivation, hepatic glycogenolysis.
- α_2-Adrenoceptors: smooth muscle contraction, inhibition of noradrenaline release, inhibition of insulin release, platelet aggregation.

β-Adrenoceptors

The β-adrenoceptors have been divided into β_1, β_2, β_3, and possibly β_4.

- β_1-Adrenoceptors are located mainly in the heart but are also present in the gastrointestinal tract and presynaptically.
- β_2-Adrenoceptors are located on a number of tissues including bronchi, blood vessels, gastrointestinal tract and mast cells.

- β_3-Adrenoceptors are present in adipose tissue.
- Recent evidence suggests that there may be a β_4-adrenoceptor associated with cardiac tissue.

β-Adrenergic stimulation generally causes smooth muscle relaxation. The most important clinical effect is cardiac stimulation. Clinically important physiological effects in response to β-adrenoceptor activation include:

- β_1-Adrenoceptors: increased heart rate and force of cardiac muscle contraction.
- β_2-Adrenoceptors: bronchodilation, vasodilation, visceral smooth muscle relaxation, hepatic glycogenolysis.
- β_3-Adrenoceptors: fat cell lipolysis.

Physiological and pharmacological effects of adrenoceptor agonists

Adrenaline and noradrenaline are not particularly selective in receptor binding. Directly and indirectly acting sympathomimetic drugs that activate, or drugs that block, adrenoceptors were developed by modifying the noradrenaline molecule. Their specificity for receptor binding and potency depends on their chemical structure, and this relationship is complex. The basic principles of receptor affinity and efficacy, and neuronal uptake and reaction with MAO and COMT, affect therapeutic response.

Cardiovascular and cardiac effects

Stimulating α- and β-adrenoceptors has a profound effect on both cardiac and vascular smooth muscle. These effects are the basis of drug therapy in angina, hypertension and some respiratory diseases. The net effect in the whole body will depend on the proportion of each class of receptor and the response at any given site.

Adrenoceptor agonists in cardiovascular disease

- **Anaphylactic** shock (type I hypersensitivity) is a life-threatening condition. Adrenaline (epinephrine), a non-selective α-adrenoceptor agonist, is used in anaphylactic shock caused by hypersensitivity reactions to drugs (e.g. penicillin), allergens (e.g. nuts) and bee-stings. A severe reaction results in airways obstruction from glossal and laryngeal oedema due to mucosal swelling, bronchospasm and cardiovascular collapse due to generalised vasodilatation. Adrenaline (epinephrine) produces vasoconstriction by stimulation of α-adrenoceptors and β_2-adrenoceptor mediated bronchodilatation. Adrenaline (epinephrine) is also used to restore cardiac rhythm in patients with **cardiac arrest**.

- The local vasoconstriction effect of adrenaline can be used to prolong the action of local anaesthetics (LA) by reducing tissue perfusion and preventing the dispersal of the LA.

- Non-selective β-agonists, e.g. isoprenaline, have positive chronotropic and positive inotropic effects on the heart. It is sometimes used in the treatment of cardiac dysrhythmias and in heart block while awaiting electrical pacing.

- The selective α_2-adrenoceptor agonist, clonidine, is used in the treatment of **hypertension**. Its action is thought to be primarily due to the activation of α_2-adrenoceptors in the lower brainstem resulting in a reduced sympathetic outflow to the periphery. Clonidine also has partial agonist effects.

- Dobutamine, a synthetic analogue of dopamine, is a selective β_2-adrenoceptor agonist, and a cardiac stimulant without vasoconstriction. It has a more pronounced inotropic than chronotropic effect on the heart so that tachycardia is less likely. It is useful in the treatment of impaired cardiac contractility due to **congestive heart failure** or **myocardial infarction**, and in open heart surgery.

Respiratory system

Although the respiratory system has very sparse sympathetic innervation it is populated by β_2-adrenoceptors. Circulating adrenaline and noradrenaline stimulate these receptors to produce relaxation of bronchial smooth muscle and maintain the patency of the airways. Stimulation of β_2-adrenoceptors decreases secretion by bronchial goblet cells but increases mucociliary clearance in the lumen of the airways. β_2-adrenoceptor agonists also inhibit histamine release from mast cells.

Adrenoceptor agonists in respiratory disease

β_2-adrenoceptor agonists are primarily used in the treatment of bronchospasm associated with asthma and chronic obstructive pulmonary disease (COPD).

- Selective β_2 agonists include salbutamol, terbutaline and salmeterol. Salbutamol by aerosol inhalation is still the mainstay of therapy but new longer acting agonists have been developed (salmeterol). Tachycardia and tremor have been reported as side effects. Chronic stimulation of β-adrenoceptors may result in receptor desensitisation, resulting in a reduced physiological response to subsequent β-adrenoceptor stimulation. The increase in reported asthma deaths in the 1960s was attributed to receptor desensitisation.

- β_2-Agonists can inhibit histamine release in the lung responding to allergic challenge.

ℹ Information box 4.15 | **Adrenergic effects on heart and blood vessels**

Cardiac tissue contains predominantly β_1-adrenoceptors. Stimulation of β_1-adrenoceptor in the sino-atrial node results in increased rate (positive chronotropic) and increased force of myocardial contraction (positive inotropic).

In blood vessels, sympathetic nerve stimulation produces either α-adrenoceptor mediated vasoconstriction or β-adrenoceptor mediated vasodilatation in both the arterial and venous systems. Distribution of α- and β-adrenoceptors and their subclasses on vascular smooth muscle determines the response of any given vascular bed:

- Vasoconstriction in skin and mucous membranes because the vascular bed contains predominantly α_1- and α_2-adrenoceptors.
- Coronary arteries dilate because β_2-adrenoceptors are dominant although α-adrenoceptors are present.
- Increased peripheral resistance due to stimulation of α-adrenoceptors on arteries, arterioles and veins. Both subclasses of α-adrenoceptors produce vasoconstriction.

- Selective α_1-agonists include ephedrine, phenylephrine and metazoline. They cause vasoconstriction and are used in nasal decongestants.

Gastrointestinal tract

Both α- and β-adrenoceptors cause gastrointestinal smooth muscle relaxation. The pyloric and ileocaecal sphincters are constricted by α-adrenoceptor stimulation. This effect often leads to chronic constipation in patients taking adrenoceptor agonists, particularly in elderly people. Administration of other drugs, such as a diuretic, can further exacerbate the problem.

Metabolism

Adrenoceptor stimulation mobilises energy stores for fuel metabolism.

- β_2-Adrenoceptor stimulation in the liver and muscle increases the conversion of glycogen and fats to glucose and fatty acids, causing a rise in plasma levels.
- β_2-Adrenoceptor stimulation in adipose tissue results in increased lipolysis.
- Insulin release is increased via stimulation of β_2-adrenoceptors but inhibited by α_2-adrenoceptor stimulation.
- Glucagon release is activated by stimulation of β-adrenoceptors associated with the α cells of the pancreatic islets.
- Anti-obesity drugs based on selective β_3-agonists are being developed.

Other effects

- β_2-Adrenoceptor stimulation in skeletal muscle increases the twitch tension of fast-contracting fibres, but shortens the active state of red, slow-contracting muscle. These two effects plus an increased discharge of muscle spindles are thought to be important in the production of tremor associated with β_2-adrenoceptor agonists (e.g. salbutamol).
- β_2-Agonists can cause long-term changes in skeletal muscle. Clenbuterol is a performance enhancing 'anabolic' drug that increases muscle bulk and force of contraction.

Adrenoceptor antagonists

Unlike adrenoceptor agonists, adrenoceptor antagonists are selective for either α- or β- adrenoceptors.

α-Adrenoceptor antagonists

α-Adrenoceptor agonists may be selective or non-selective. Their main clinical uses are in treating hypertension.

- Selective α_1-adrenoceptor antagonists, prazosin and the longer-acting doxazosin, are used in the treatment of essential hypertension as they produce less tachycardia than with phentolamine; they do not block the inhibitory presynaptic α_2-adrenoceptors.
- Selective α_1-adrenoceptor antagonists are used in the treatment of urinary retention in benign prostatic hypertrophy. Tamsulosin causes relaxation of the smooth muscles of the bladder neck and prostate capsule.

- Selective α_2-antagonists are mainly used experimentally. Presynaptic α_2-blockade will result in increased noradrenaline being released from sympathetic nerve terminals.
- Non-selective α-adrenoceptor antagonist, phenoxybenzamine, is used to treat hypertension associated with phaeochromocytoma. Phenoxybenzamine produces an irreversible antagonism and requires the synthesis of new receptor protein for cellular responsiveness to be restored. Phentolamine is a non-selective competitive antagonist at the α-adrenoceptor and is useful in the diagnosis of hypertension due to phaeochromocytoma. Neither of these drugs is used in the treatment of essential hypertension as the rapid fall in blood pressure due to inhibition of vascular α-adrenoceptors triggers reflex tachycardia.

Unwanted side effects of α-adrenoceptor antagonists
- Non-selective α-adrenoceptor antagonists may cause tachycardia, cardiac dysrhythmia and increased gastric motility.
- α-Adrenoceptor antagonists may cause impotence.

β-Adrenoceptor antagonists

β-Adrenoceptor antagonists can be classified according to a number of pharmacodynamic and pharmacokinetic properties.

- **Selectivity**. β-Adrenoceptor antagonists are classified as non-specific (propranolol, alprenolol) or specific β_1-adrenoceptor antagonists (atenolol). The specificity of the latter group of drugs is dose-dependent (increase the dose and β_2-adrenoceptors will also be blocked).
- **Membrane stabilising activity** (propranolol, alprenolol, oxprenolol, timolol). A number of β-adrenoceptor antagonists possess membrane stabilising effects. (Propranolol affects electrical conduction in the heart, similar to quinidine, but unrelated to its β-adrenoceptor antagonist properties. Propranolol increases atrio-ventricular conduction time and decreases spontaneous ectopics.)
- **Intrinsic sympathomimetic activity**. Several β-adrenoceptor antagonists (pindolol, alprenolol) have initial agonist activity at β-adrenoceptors before exerting an antagonistic action, but their intrinsic activity is less than that for a full agonist such as isoprenaline. These partial agonists are said to have intrinsic sympathomimetic activity. Whether there is a therapeutic value for this property is debatable.

β-Adrenoceptor antagonists can also be classified according to their route of elimination being either completely metabolised in the liver (alprenolol, propranolol, oxprenolol) or excreted predominantly unchanged (60–100%) by the kidneys (atenolol, sotalol). Care should be taken in patients with renal failure as these agents may accumulate.

Clinical uses of β-adrenoceptor antagonists

The β-adrenoceptor antagonists (β-blockers) are very important drugs used primarily for their effects on the cardiovascular system and on bronchial smooth muscle. The cardiovascular effects produced in humans are dependent on the degree of sympathetic activity. At rest, propranolol has little effect on heart rate, cardiac output or arterial pressure. During exercise, however, propranolol reduces heart rate and cardiac output, thereby reducing the exercise tolerance. In addition to the effect on the heart, skeletal muscle vasodilatation is also reduced.

Cardiovascular disease

A major role for β-adrenoceptor antagonists is in the treatment of **hypertension**. A fall in arterial pressure is only seen in hypertensive patients. The exact mechanism by which β-adrenoceptor antagonists produce their effect is complex and is probably a combination of the following effects:

- Reduction in cardiac output
- Reduction in renin release from the juxtaglomerular apparatus in the kidney. The relationship between renin and hypertension is unclear. Pindolol has little or no effect on renin levels but is an effective antihypertensive agent.
- Central action, which may reduce peripheral sympathetic activity. However not all β-adrenoceptor antagonists enter the CNS in significant concentrations (e.g. timolol).

In the presence of β-adrenoceptor antagonists, coronary perfusion is slightly reduced. There is, however, a significant fall in cardiac O_2 consumption due to the reduction in heart rate and force of contraction, resulting in improved myocardial oxygenation. This effect is important in the treatment of **angina pectoris**.

Propranolol is also used in the treatment of **cardiac dysrhythmias**, due to its ability to slow heart rate and decrease atrial and atrio-ventricular node conduction. It has proved particularly useful as an adjunct in the treatment of atrial fibrillation due to thyrotoxicosis.

Randomised controlled clinical trials have shown that β-adrenoceptor antagonists may prolong survival in stable **cardiac failure**.

Migraine

The mechanisms underlying the classic symptoms of migraine – the premonitory aura, momentary loss of visual field and unilateral, severe headache and vomiting – are not well understood. Blood flow studies in patients during migraine attacks have shown changes in blood flow during the different phases, but no consistent pattern. Many theories have been postulated over decades. There is a strong suggestion that 5-HT deficiency is implicated in some way.

For an acute attack, if simple analgesics (e.g. aspirin, paracetamol) together with an anti-emetic is insufficient, then 5-HT agonists are effective:

- Ergotamine is a 5-HT partial agonist
- Sumatriptan is a 5-HT agonist. Newer proprietary compounds are said to be longer and faster acting.

β-Adrenoceptor antagonists (e.g. metoprolol, propranolol) are effective for prophylaxis.

Other clinical uses

- β-Blockers are used as adjuncts in the treatment of hyperthyroidism where tachycardia, atrial fibrillation and tremor are due to increased sympathetic activity.
- Timolol is used in the treatment of glaucoma, as β-blockers reduce the production of aqueous humour.
- β-Blockers are used to treat acute anxiety states to control symptoms due to excessive sympathetic drive such as tremor and palpitations.

Unwanted effects of β-adrenoceptor antagonists

Side effects of β-adrenoceptor antagonists are caused by receptor blockade:

- Bronchoconstriction – β-blockers cause bronchoconstriction in patients with asthma or chronic obstructive pulmonary diseases. Normal subjects are not affected.
- Cardiac failure – patients with heart disease may depend on sympathetic drive to maintain their cardiac output. Blocking this drive with β-blockers could precipitate cardiac failure.
- Bradycardia – antidysrhythmic drugs (e.g. verapamil) impair cardiac conduction. Concomitant administration of a β-blocker can further impair conduction leading to bradycardia, progressing to complete heart block (atrioventricular block).
- Hypoglycaemia – β-blockers reduce the early warning signs of hypoglycaemia, mediated by the sympathetic nervous system (e.g. tachycardia). Non-selective β-blockers may worsen the effects of hypoglycaemia by inhibiting sympathetic nervous system and adrenaline-mediated glycogenolysis and lipolysis, prolonging the period of hypoglycaemia.
- Tiredness – β-blockers cause a reduction in cardiac output and muscle perfusion during exercise. This may account for the fatigue experienced by patients on this medication.
- Exacerbation of ischaemic heart disease – sudden cessation of long-term β-blockers can result in exacerbation of angina, increased ventricular arrhythmias, myocardial infarction and sudden death. These effects have been reported to be due to receptor supersensitivity which may be due to an increase in the number of β-adrenoceptors.
- Oculomucocutaneous syndrome – idiosyncratic reactions to practolol consisting of keratoconjunctivitis with scarring and loss of lacrimation, mucosal ulcerations in the nose and mouth, and rashes were reported, leading to its withdrawal from clinical use.

GENERAL ANAESTHETICS

General anaesthetics (GAs) enabled the development of modern surgical procedures, during which the patients need to be entirely unaware of all sensory input so that they are:

- Unconscious, therefore unaware and have no memory (amnesia) of the procedure.
- Unresponsive to painful stimuli (analgesia).
- Immobile, with complete skeletal muscle relaxation and loss of reflexes.

In the distant past, alcohol was the only help available to patients during surgery, for example amputations. Ether and chloroform, now obsolete, were the first volatile anaesthetics in clinical use. 'Laughing gas', nitrous oxide, was the first gaseous general anaesthetic, and is still in use today. Much progress has been made in the development of anaesthetic agents. The two most commonly used forms of general anaesthetic are:

- Inhaled anaesthetics, which may be volatile or gaseous
- Intravenous anaesthetics.

The administration of general anaesthetics needs to be controlled, to achieve **safe** blood and tissue concentrations that meet the main aims of unconsciousness, unresponsiveness to pain and immobility. Highly trained and skilled anaesthetists are required.

From the patient's viewpoint, rapid onset of anaesthesia and rapid recovery with minimal or no side effects would be most beneficial. Generally, a combination of the different forms of anaesthetics are used for surgery.

Inhaled anaesthetics

- Volatile anaesthetics are liquid at room temperature, they vaporise to produce enough partial pressure for inhalation. They are all non-flammable and non-explosive. (Examples: halogenated derivatives of ether, e.g. isoflurane, enflurane, sevoflurane; halogenated derivatives of alkanes, e.g. halothane, widely used.)
- Gaseous anaesthetics are simple gases. They may be explosive, and are usually administered in a mixture with air or oxygen. (Examples: the best example of a gaseous anaesthetic that is widely used is nitrous oxide (N_2O), administered as gas and air, and an effective obstetric analgesic during labour.)

Intravenous anaesthetics

Intravenous anaesthetics act much faster than inhaled agents.

- Barbiturates – e.g. thiopental, induces unconsciousness in 20 seconds.
- Benzodiazepines – e.g. diazepam, midazolam act directly on GABA receptors.
- Phenols – e.g. propofol.
- Cyclohexanes – e.g. ketamine.
- Opiates – e.g. fentanyl, remifentanil, used for sedation, analgesia and to reduce anxiety.
- Dopamine antagonists – droperidol (related to antipsychotics) used as an anti-emetic.

Because of their rapid action, intravenous GAs such as thiopental and propofol are used to induce unconsciousness before surgery, and anaesthesia is maintained by inhaled anaesthetics during surgery.

A combination of an opiate, e.g. fentanyl, and a dopamine antagonist, e.g. droperidol, is used to induce deep sedation and analgesia, **neuroleptanalgesia**, for minor surgical procedures such as endoscopy.

Pharmacodynamics of GAs

How GAs work is not well understood, as the agents can vary from simple gases to steroids. It is, however, generally agreed that at the cellular level, GAs act on signal transmitters at the **synapse**, rather than at the neuron. Several theories have been proposed to explain the action of GAs, of which two are discussed here.

Lipid theory

At the turn of the twentieth century, Meyer and Overton described a relationship between lipid solubility of anaesthet-

ics (i.e. olive oil : water partition) and their anaesthetic potency in which the more soluble the anaesthetic is in oil, the more potent it is. This theory suggested that dissolving anaesthetic agents into cell membranes altered cell function. It does not, however, explain how the entry of an exogenous substance into the cell membrane can alter cell function.

Protein theory

Recent research in cell biology has found evidence to show that anaesthetic drugs target proteins, e.g. intracellular enzymes, ion channels and membrane receptors. The example of the effects of GAs on ion channels illustrates the molecular mechanisms leading to the inhibition of synaptic transmission.

Laboratory research has found evidence that inhibition of synaptic transmission may occur at three processes:

- Inhibition of neurotransmitter release.
- Inhibition of the action of the neurotransmitter.
- Inhibition of the excitability of the postsynaptic cell (e.g. muscle).

Inhibition of the action of the transmitter is not thought to be important, so the significant mechanisms are the inhibition of neurotransmitter release and responsiveness of the postsynaptic cell.

- Inhibition of presynaptic ACh vesicular release by closing the ligand-gated (ionotropic) Ca^{2+} channel. The influx of Ca^{2+} into the presynaptic nerve terminal is prevented, inhibiting vesicular release of ACh by exocytosis.
- Most of the presynaptic receptors are GPCRs that control the status of ion channels either via a second messenger pathway or by the direct action of the G protein on the channel. Gating by ionotropic receptors (rather than GPCRs) also occurs.
- The ion channels in glutamate receptors are voltage gated as well as ligand gated.
- In the context of GAs, nAChRs in the autonomic nervous system facilitate the release of two important N_N receptors: $GABA_A$ and glutamate receptors (see below).
- In the somatic motor system, inhibition or activation of ACh N_M at the NMJ produces muscle relaxation.
- Inhibition of mAChRs causes temporary CNS excitation and amnesia, bradycardia followed by tachycardia and inhibition of secretions.

The effect of GAs on neurotransmitter release

- $GABA_A$ is an inhibitory receptor. Indeed, $GABA_A$-mediated inhibitory transmission is enhanced by most anaesthetics.
- GAs inhibit the action of excitatory receptors such as ACh, glutamate (NMDA) and 5-HT. This is why gaseous anaesthetics such as nitrous oxide produce CNS excitation and euphoria initially, before the onset of unconsciousness.

It has not yet been possible to identify the 'target' postsynaptic cells that are affected by GAs. Increasing the concentration of anaesthetic eventually leads to suppression of all brain function, including all autonomic control, respiration and reflex motor activity.

Pharmacokinetics

Inhaled, volatile and gaseous, GAs are absorbed through the alveoli into the bloodstream for distribution, and eliminated through the lungs. Intravenous anaesthetics bypass the absorption phase altogether, and are eliminated via hepatic metabolism and renal excretion. As both forms of anaesthetics are highly lipid-soluble, distribution by crossing the **blood–brain barrier** is no problem.

Inhaled anaesthetics

Inhaled anaesthetics are small, lipid-soluble molecules that easily permeate the alveolar membrane, and enter and leave the body via the lungs. Their kinetic behaviour is determined by:

- The rate of delivery from inspired air to the blood circulation – increasing alveolar ventilation (see Ch. 13) enables a faster equilibration between alveolar and blood concentration, whereas respiratory depression slows elimination.
- Solubility in blood
- The rate of delivery to brain
- Accumulation in fat and other tissues.

Elimination via metabolism is not problematic, except for the production of toxic metabolites.

The brain is well perfused, and the blood–brain barrier is easily permeable to GAs, so concentration in the brain rises rapidly, and equilibrium between the blood and brain is quickly achieved. Surgical anaesthesia is achieved when the patient no longer responds to pain, i.e. the first incision.

Halothane

Anaesthetic concentration in poorly perfused adipose tissue rises slowly, to equilibrate with blood concentration, and anaesthetic accumulates in the fat. At effective anaesthetic doses, halothane at equilibrium mostly accumulates in adipose tissue (95%), which is slowly released into the bloodstream after GA administration ceases. This prolongs the action of halothane to give the 'hangover' symptoms of drowsiness, confusion, amnesia and headache.

Hepatic metabolism of halothane produces bromide, trifluoroacetate and other metabolites that are hepatotoxic. Severe reactions can give rise to hepatic failure.

Nitrous oxide

Nitrous oxide (N_2O) was first used in the 1800s as a general anaesthetic to cause unconsciousness and analgesia. N_2O has a good analgesic effect but is of low potency and is therefore used in combination with other inhaled anaesthetics. It has the following properties:

- Although it has a low potency as an anaesthetic, it has a rapid onset of effect due to its low blood:gas partition coefficient and high inhaled concentration.

- Abrupt discontinuation results in a rapid transfer of N_2O from blood and tissues to the alveoli and a decrease in arterial tension of oxygen, i.e. diffusion hypoxia.
- Has a good analgesic property. Entonox (50%/50% with O_2) is used for pain control.
- By itself has minimal effects on respiratory drive, minimal skeletal muscle relaxation, minimal effects on the circulation.
- Causes euphoria.
- Anoxia will occur if it is used with less than 20% O_2.
- Thought to be free of adverse effects, but shown to oxidise cobalt in Vitamin B_{12}, required for synthesis of methionine which is essential in DNA and protein synthesis, leading to anaemia if used repeatedly.

Intravenous anaesthetics

Intravenous anaesthetics are administered directly into the bloodstream, so the onset of anaesthesia is much faster than inhalation: the time for the blood to travel from the injection site in an arm vein to the brain. Metabolism and elimination are rapid, so the duration of action is short. Intravenous anaesthetics are commonly used for induction of anaesthesia.

Anaesthetic from the brain is redistributed to fat, and accumulates in fat so that highly lipid-soluble drugs like thiopental could have their action terminated by redistribution (see Information box 4.2), shortening the duration of action. Release of the drug from fat prolongs the hangover effects.

Unwanted effects

The unwanted effects of general anaesthetics are related to:

- 'Hangover' effects
- Respiratory and cardiac depression
- Muscarinic inhibition of secretions leading to dry mouth, dry hot skin and lack of bronchial secretions
- Toxic metabolites
- Hypotension due to the rapid action of intravenous anaesthetics
- Allergic reactions to intravenous anaesthetics.

Muscle relaxants

The use of muscle relaxants to produce immobility enables lighter levels of anaesthetics to be used. They are given as premedication, and are similar in structure to acetylcholine (ACh). Acting on N_M receptors at the neuromuscular junction (NMJ).

- Suxamethonium is a N_M receptor agonist, but after initial stimulation of the NMJ, it produces a depolarising block to paralyse the muscle.
- Derivatives of curare, the active ingredient in the poisoned arrows of South American Indians, tubocurare and atracurium are competitive N_M receptor antagonists.

5

Human genetics

Denise Syndercombe Court and David P Kelsell

INTRODUCTION

HISTORICAL BACKGROUND

Genetics is a very new science, changing rapidly by the day with advances in technology. Although humans have long been aware of some form of heredity, the mechanisms have only recently become clear. Early philosophers talked about the male ripening the female, or seeds being produced in various organs to be transmitted to the child. In the early eighteenth century scientists were divided as to whether the sperm held the new child, the purpose of the female simply to provide the womb, or whether the egg held the child, already determined as male or female, growth being stimulated by the sperm.

The theory of **pangenesis** was a major early influence: pangenes were said to be developed in each organ and then passed to the child through blood. This is probably the origin of phrases such as 'royal blood' and 'blood line'. **Blending** was the most accepted theory at the time: a tall man and a short woman would tend to produce offspring of average height. This clearly did not always work, for example when two brown-eyed parents had blue-eyed children.

Although **Gregor Mendel's** experiments, over 8 years in the late nineteenth century involving thousands of garden pea plants, were perhaps all too perfect, his crossing of plants with different characteristics laid the foundation for modern genetics. Describing the appearance of simple characteristics, he used mathematical principles to show that these traits were passed from parents to offspring

through what became to be known as genes. Four fundamental principles of modern genetics were illustrated by his experiments:

- Each parent contributes only one of a pair of factors (tall or short, wrinkled or smooth in Mendel's experiments) – or **alleles** – of each trait (plant size or seed shape) through a process of separation, or **segregation**, when the gametes are formed.
- Factors can be **dominant**, while others can be hidden, or expressed when the dominant factor is not present (**recessive factor**), but remain unchanged when passed to their offspring (do not blend).
- Males and females contribute equally to their offspring.
- Different traits are inherited independently of each other – **independent assortment**.

The later recognition of **chromosomes** (see below), leading to the chromosomal theory of inheritance, and understanding of the process of **meiosis** when gametes are formed (see below) helped to explain these observations during the early twentieth century. Occasionally Mendel's prediction for what should be inherited in the next generation did not happen; these occurrences were described as **mutations**. Mendel's principles of inheritance and an acceptance of mutation provided scientific support for the theories put forward in **Charles Darwin**'s *On the origin of species* in 1869.

Although DNA had been isolated at about the same time as Darwin's publication, its recognition as the hereditary material, rather than a protein being responsible, was not proved until the 1950s. The publication in 1955 of the structure of DNA marked the start of modern molecular biology, to which the rest of this chapter is devoted.

BASIS OF MODERN GENETICS

The genetic code, located within DNA, provides the instructions for the complex development and organisation of the multicellular human. Genetics has become an essential component of medicine, extending our understanding of disease mechanisms to facilitate preventive, diagnostic, prognostic and therapeutic developments.

The understanding that disease can be caused by chromosomal abnormalities, or can be inherited, because of the segregation of mutant genes, has provided the impetus to the development of genomic medicine. Along with the association of specific gene mutations and disease comes a greater understanding of the molecular and cellular mechanisms required for normal human development and homeostasis. A key factor that has facilitated our current understanding of human genetics has been the technological developments that have enabled the complete sequencing of the human **genome** and led to the collection of vast amounts of data that can be 'mined' to produce useful information. Current sequencing technology can now sequence two individuals' genomes in 1 week.

- The **genome** is the complete collection of genetic material within an organism.

Three levels of genetic classification are used to enable the management of an enormous amount of information:

- **Genomics** – the DNA structure of genes and their localisation within the genome
- **Gene expression** – the mechanisms through which genes are 'switched on' and transcribed into **messenger RNA** (**mRNA**) to be translated into protein or other types of RNA
- **Proteomics** – the characterisation of biological processes from measurement of protein expression, localisation and post-translational modification.

These 'banks' of genetic data can be used to provide information for disease therapies. The variable responses to established drugs, and the effects of particular chemicals on gene transcription and protein expression (drug discovery), are collectively described as **pharmacogenomics**. The combination of pharmacogenomics and the traditional pharmaceutical sciences offers the potential for better and safer drugs and the ability to provide individualised therapies.

Profiling an individual's DNA for the presence of specific gene variants will enable the future understanding of the inherited basis of many **congenital** disorders (disorders present at birth) and the risk of developing particular **multifactorial** conditions (those with many causes) in later life, such as cancer and neurological disease. With more research, it is likely that our lifetime risks of developing a whole range of diseases could be predicted by our individual 'genetic barcode' and, of equal importance, what medicines and lifestyle changes will prevent the onset and early management of these diseases.

Most human disorders have a genetic component that is either inherited in the **germline** or acquired through **somatic** mutation.

- The **germline** refers to the **gonadal** cells that become eggs or sperm, and also to the genetic material that comes from them.

- **Somatic** cells are those that come from the body, but not directly from the gonads. A particular genetic variant (often termed mutation) underlies the **monogenic** disorders.
- **Monogenic** disorders are those controlled by a single gene, in contrast with **polygenic** disorders. In **polygenic** diseases, a complex genetic interaction of several genes and environmental factors predisposes to or protects an individual from a particular disorder.

Genetic disorders can be classified in a number of ways:

- **Single gene disorders** – a mutation in a single gene leading to disease (e.g. cystic fibrosis)
- **Chromosomal disorders** – a change, gain, loss or exchange of chromosome elements (e.g. trisomy 21 – Down's syndrome)
- **Polygenic disorders** – due to the combined effects of many genes, or in combination with environmental factors (multifactorial) (e.g. neural tube defects)
- **Somatic disorders** – disorders of body (non-germline) cells, such as uncontrolled cell growth, or cancer.

Individuals who are affected, or are at risk of being affected, by genetic disorders are likely to be offered **genetic counselling** and prenatal diagnosis – this is when a trained professional provides information, risk assessment and support to patients and their families.

Along with the rapid developments that are coming with the sequencing of the human genome and the associated advances in analytical technologies, there is also a proliferation of ethical, legal and social questions that must be considered by governments. This means that individuals are increasingly faced with important decisions; it is the role of the genetic counsellor to provide information and support to help affected individuals make informed decisions.

Clinical box 5.1   Trisomy 21

Trisomy 21 is seen in about 0.1% of live births, and produces the phenotype originally described by John Langdon Down in 1866. It was recognised to be due to the presence of an extra copy of chromosome 21 in 1959. The extra chromosome copy appears more often to originate from the mother and prevalence increases significantly with increasing maternal age from less than 1 in 1000 under the age of 30 years, to about 1 in 25 over the age of 45 years. Individuals with Down's syndrome have distinctive facial features: a small head, a flat nose bridge, misshapen ears, a broad and short neck, and narrow upward slanting eyes. These are often accompanied by a variety of medical conditions including intellectual disability, congenital heart defects, gastrointestinal obstruction and leukaemia.

Trisomy 21 accounts for about 95% of cases of Down's syndrome. The remaining 5% are due to other abnormalities:

- **Translocation and partial trisomy**: in this condition copies of parts of chromosome 21 are **translocated** to other chromosomes. Although there are no additional chromosomes in this case, there are still three copies of particular genes from chromosome 21 (partial trisomy).
- **Mosaics**: in which there is a mixture of cell lines in different tissues within one body, some displaying trisomy 21, others being normal.

Down's syndrome can be screened for in early pregnancy through the measurement of various proteins and hormones that are characteristically altered in this condition. Women at high risk are normally offered an examination in early pregnancy that samples fetal cells and allows a detailed examination of all of the chromosomes.

THE HUMAN GENOME

Genetic information is stored within **deoxyribonucleic acid (DNA)**, its sequence providing the 'blueprint' for all the proteins in the body. The **Human Genome Project** (HGP, see below) began formally in 1990, and the identification of the entire human genome sequence was completed in 2003.

The information is arranged in genes that code for the proteins. The genes are located on chromosomes. Forty-six chromosomes, arranged in 22 pairs of different chromosomes, plus two sex chromosomes, are found within each somatic cell in the body. The gametes (sperm or egg cells) contain just one sex chromosome and one of the pairs of each of the 22 **autosomal**, or non-sex, chromosomes.

DNA AND CHROMOSOMES

DNA is a double-stranded molecule (the **double helix**), the strands forming a twisted 'ladder' with sides of sugar and phosphate molecules, connected by 'rungs' of nitrogenous bases. The order of the nucleotide bases on the strand is called the DNA sequence; these specify the genetic instructions to produce and maintain an organism. There are four bases in DNA:

- Adenine (A)
- Cytosine (C)
- Guanine (G)
- Thymine (T).

The stands of DNA are joined by the specific pairing of these nucleotides, linked by phosphodiesterase bonds: A with T, and C with G to form a double-helical structure. Each of the strands is therefore complementary to the other. Each strand has a 3′ ('β prime') and a 5′ end and the complementary strand reverses these. There are 3 billion base pairs making up the human genome sequence. The majority of human DNA is packaged into different-sized chromosomes (Fig. 5.1) located within the nucleus of the cell, with an additional circular piece of **DNA** located in the **mitochondria**.

In a **diploid** human cell (having two sets of chromosomes), there are 46 chromosomes comprising 22 paired autosomal chromosomes (numbered 1–22). Each pair of chromosomes is homologous (very similar), and one of the pair is inherited from the father and the other from the mother (see Meiosis, below). The largest is known as chromosome 1 and consists of around 250 megabases (mb) of DNA, chromosome 2 has 240 mb and then chromosomes descend in size to the smallest autosomes, 21 and 22, which have 55 mb and 60 mb of DNA, respectively. The remaining two are the sex chromosomes, which are not homologous and are called the X and Y chromosomes.

In the gametes (egg and sperm cells), the genome is **haploid,** carrying only one copy of the 23 chromosomes. The Y chromosome (60 mb of DNA) is much smaller than the X chromosome (140 mb of DNA) (see Fig. 5.2).

- Males have an X and a Y chromosome. The Y chromosome is inherited from the father and contains the primary genetic information for determining some of the male characteristics. The Y chromosome is much smaller than the X chromosome and has very few genes: for this reason there are not very many diseases associated with defects in the Y chromosome, compared with those associated with the X chromosome.
- Females have two X chromosomes, although only one of the two X chromosomes is transcriptionally active in order that female cells do not express twice as much of the X chromosome genes as male cells. This random inactivation of one of the female X chromosomes is termed **X-inactivation** (or **lyonisation**) and occurs via a chromosomal/gene silencing mechanism involving **methylation** in early embryogenesis. Once this occurs, the same X chromosome is inactivated in all somatic cells.

Chromosome karyotypes (Fig. 5.2)

Chromosome karyotyping is the process of visually examining the chromosomes, arranged in pairs, for gross abnormalities. To see chromosomes under the microscope, dividing somatic cells (such as white blood cells) are exposed to spindle toxins, such as colchicine, which arrest the cell cycle in **metaphase** when the chromosomes are more condensed and thus easiest to see.

Each chromosome has a constriction at the middle (**metacentric**) or towards one end (**acrocentric**). This constriction is termed the **centromere** and joins the homologous chromosomes (**chromatids**) together during mitosis.

The centromere also divides the chromosome into two diagnostic parts, the shorter **p arm** and the longer **q arm**. The banding pattern seen across each chromosome is produced by nuclear staining that produces a characteristic light and dark banding pattern. The dark bands represent condensed supercoiled chromatin (**heterochromatin**) that is transcriptionally silent. The light-staining bands represent chromatin that is not so tightly coiled, and these are transcriptionally active regions of the chromosome. At the end of each chromosome arm are the **telomeres**, which do not contain any coding genes but numerous copies of the hexameric nucleotide sequence TTAGGG. Telomeres are thought to maintain the stability of the chromosome, promote complete DNA replication and aid chromosome pairing. Telomeres become progressively shorter as the cell divides and this has been linked to the regulation of cell longevity.

Mitochondrial DNA

The remaining DNA within the genome is packaged in circular DNA molecules (around 16.5 kb), found in the numerous mitochondria within the cytoplasm of the cell. The mitochondrial genome encodes 13 proteins, 22 **transfer RNA (tRNA)** and two **ribosomal RNA (rRNA)** molecules that are primarily involved in the generation of ATP to fulfil the cell's energy requirements. There can be hundreds of mitochondria within each cell. This DNA is always inherited from the mother, since at fertilisation only the nucleus of the sperm cell is transferred into the egg.

Cell division

Human cell division occurs by two processes, **mitosis** and **meiosis**.

- In **mitosis** the entire DNA content of the cell is duplicated and the cell divides into two identical **diploid** daughter cells.

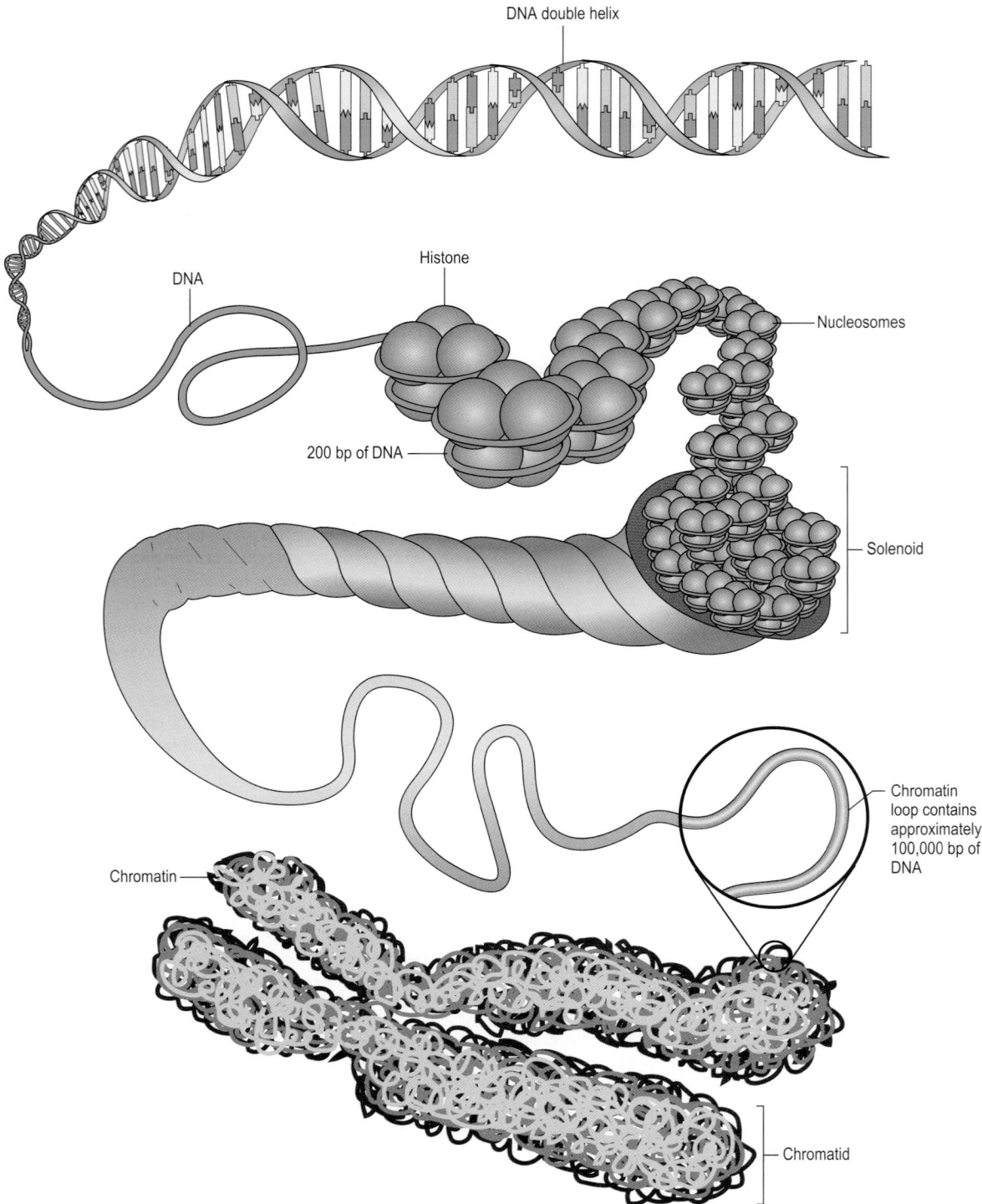

Fig. 5.1 Organisation of DNA within a chromosome. DNA strands are about 2 m in length and need careful packing to fit within a cell nucleus. The helical molecule is packaged into **nucleosomes** that consist of about 150 bp wrapped around a histone protein core, having a 'bead-on-a-string' appearance. Nucleosomes themselves wind in a helix, about six forming a **solenoid**. Solenoids in series are arranged in **chromatin loops**, each being about 100 kilobases (kb) in length. These chromatin loops pack themselves together in **chromatids** that form the familiar X-shaped chromosome, which has two short and two long arms. Redrawn with permission from Jorde LB et al. 2003 Medical genetics, 3rd edn. Elsevier, Edinburgh.

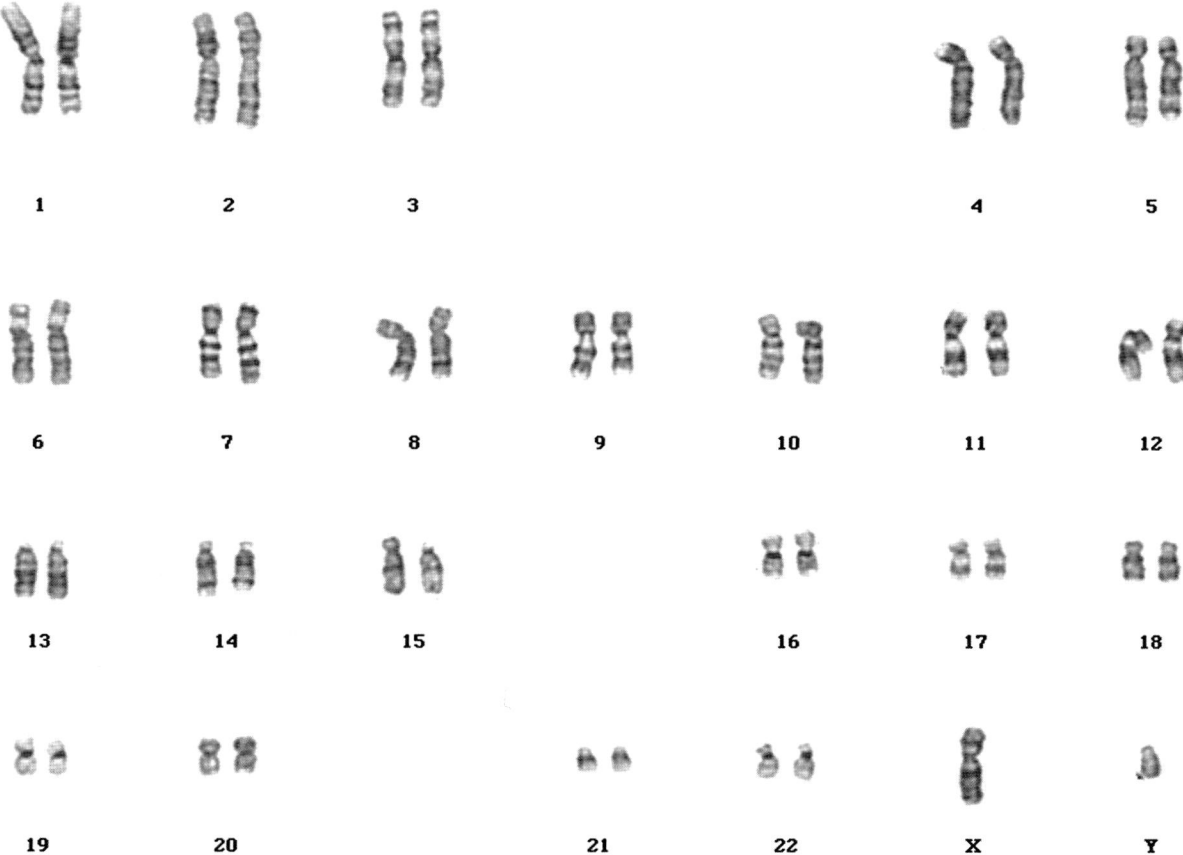

Fig. 5.2 **Human chromosome karyotype.** Paired human metaphase autosomes from a human male are shown from the largest to the smallest, followed by single X and Y chromosomes. The banding pattern is produced by Giemsa staining. Courtesy of Dr Debra Lillington.

■ **Meiosis** is a special form of cell division that maintains the correct number of chromosomes in the gamete cells. During fertilisation the egg and sperm cells merge to form a single cell with 23 pairs of chromosomes. To ensure that the gametes only have a single set of chromosomes, in meiosis the DNA content of the cell is halved and the daughter cells are referred to as being **haploid**.

The cell cycle

The cell cycle is the name given to the series of events by which cells duplicate their DNA and divide, in a process known as **mitosis**. This process is preceded by the longer **interphase** in which the cell prepares for the division, synthesising the necessary material (Fig. 5.3). DNA replication occurs once during each cell cycle and the process is tightly regulated to ensure that DNA is accurately copied and equally divided between the two daughter cells.

The length of the cell cycle varies depending on the cell type: epithelial cells in the human gut may divide every 12 hours, whereas neurons and muscle cells lose their ability to divide altogether. Key molecules in this regulation are the **cyclin-dependent kinases (CDKs)** that are produced and destroyed at key points in the cell cycle. An understanding of these and other proteins is an important focus of research into the causes of cancer.

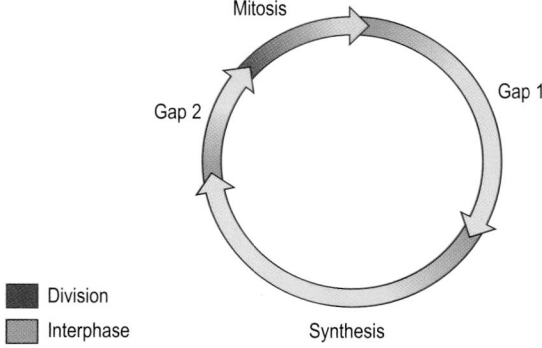

Fig. 5.3 **The cell cycle.** During the cell cycle, cells spend most of their time in interphase, during which synthesis of RNA and proteins occurs in the G1 (gap 1) phase, DNA is then replicated in the S (synthesis phase), and in G2 some DNA repair takes place and the cells, now containing 46 pairs of chromosomes, prepare to divide by mitosis.

Interphase

The time from a cell completing mitosis to the beginning of the next mitosis is referred to as **interphase**. Cells can remain in a nascent stage, the **G0** phase, until stimulated to enter the cell cycle by a variety of agents, such as growth factors or intracellular messengers. Three stages follow:

- G1 (gap 1) phase
  - The step between division and synthesis
  - Transcription factors activated
  - DNA synthesis initiated
- S phase (synthesis)
  - Chromosomes duplicated to form the 'sister' chromatids
  - Material may be exchanged between sister chromatids (**recombination**)
- G2 (gap 2) phase
  - The step between synthesis and division
  - DNA repair
  - Preparation for mitosis.

Each cycle starts with 46 (a pair of 23) chromosomes, and ends with a duplicated set by the end of G2.

Mitosis (Fig 5.4)

Mitosis is a continuous process during which the duplicated chromosomes are separated prior to the physical division of the cell into two daughter cells. The main physical events that occur during mitosis were first observed in the latter part of the nineteenth century and elucidated by Flemming in 1882. Flemming divided mitosis into four stages based on morphological changes in the nucleus and cytoplasm of the dividing cell:

- **Prophase**: chromosomes condense and become visible. Each chromosome comprises two chromatids lying side by side and attached at the **centromere** (Fig. 5.5). A bipolar **mitotic spindle** starts to form outside the nucleus, radiating out from the **centrioles** lying at opposite sides of the cell.

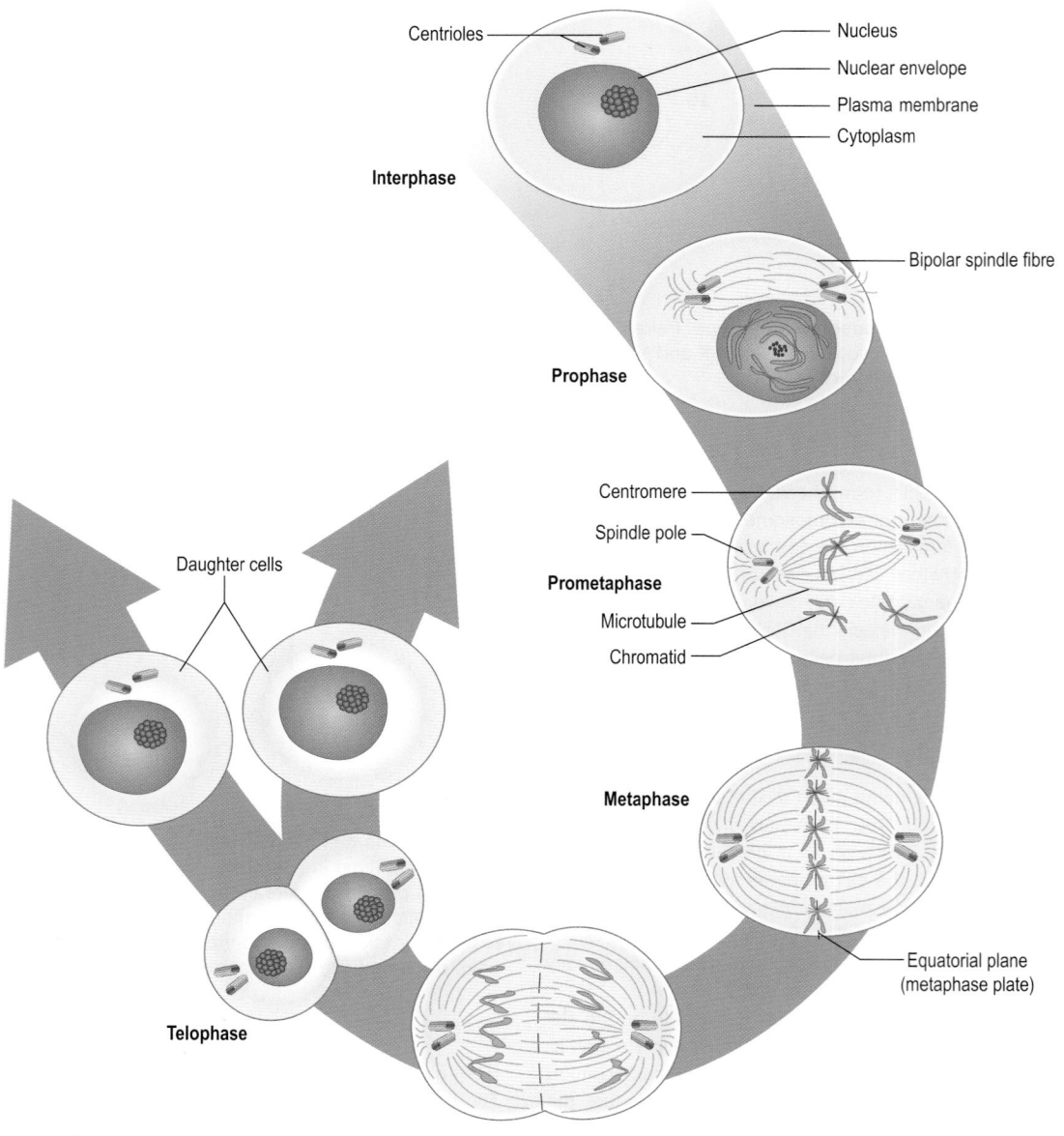

Fig. 5.4 **Mitosis.** A diploid cell undergoes mitosis to form two identical daughter cells. Redrawn with permission from Jorde LB et al. 2003 Medical genetics, 3rd edn. Elsevier, Edinburgh.

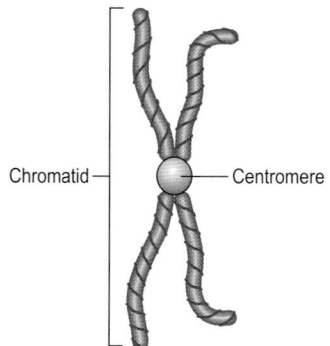

Fig. 5.5 Chromosome structure. The diagram shows a pair of sister chromatids joined at the centromere.

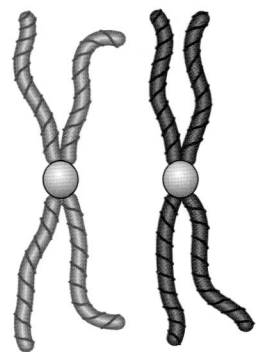

Fig. 5.6 Diploid chromosomes: homologous chromosomes, each containing paired sister chromatids.

- **Metaphase**: metaphase starts (**prometaphase**) with the disappearance of the nuclear membrane. Chromosomes become attached to the mitotic spindle via **kinetochore microtubules**. At the end of metaphase the chromosomes are aligned in a plate around the centre of the mitotic spindle apparatus, the **equatorial plane**. At this point the chromosomes are at their most condensed. Examination of chromosomes for clinical diagnostics is normally done on metaphase chromosomes.
- **Anaphase**: during anaphase the spindle fibres contract and sister chromatids are separated and pulled apart, apparently from the centromere, towards opposite spindle poles. This process typically lasts only a few minutes. At this point there will be 92 chromosomes, identical halves being located at opposite sides of the cell.
- **Telophase**: the daughter chromatids lie at the spindle poles. The kinetochore microtubules disappear and a nuclear envelope forms around each group of daughter chromosomes.
- **Cytokinesis**: cleavage of the cytoplasm starts during anaphase. The cell membrane around the centre of the cell is drawn in to form a cleavage furrow and then tightens until it reaches the remains of the mitotic spindle. This is known as the **midbody** and may persist for some time before it breaks to form the two daughter cells.

Meiosis

In meiosis (see Fig. 10.7) DNA replication is followed by two rounds of cell division and leads to the formation of four haploid cells, each containing a single set of chromosomes, i.e. half the normal chromosomal content. Like mitosis, each round of division in meiosis can be divided into four phases based on the nuclear and cell morphology.

The process begins with **interphase I**, in which, like mitosis, a single DNA strand duplicates to form a sister chromatid, joined with the other at the centromere. Because the cells are diploid for each chromatid, these are **homologues** (Fig. 5.6).

Meiosis I is the phase in which two haploid cells are produced from a single diploid cell. It is during this phase that genetic diversity takes place.

- **Prophase I**: this is a very different process from mitotic prophase and about 90% of meiotic time is spent in this phase. Prophase I can be subdivided into five stages:
  - **Leptonema** (thin): the diploid chromosomes condense to form long thin threads. Each

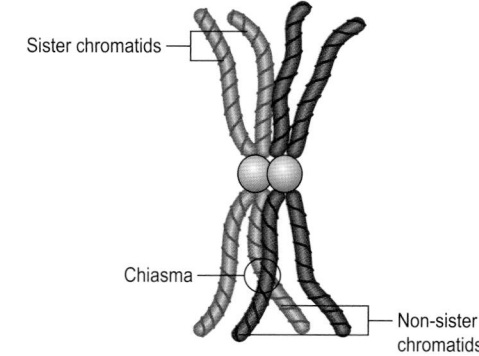

Fig. 5.7 Tetrad chromosome formation: the tetrad has four chromatids, with the non-sister chromatids joined at the **chiasma**.

chromosome attaches by both ends via an attachment plaque to the nuclear envelope. Individual chromatids are not visible at this stage.
  - **Zygonema** (yoke shaped): **synapsis** or intimate pairing marks the beginning of zygonema. Synapsis starts when the homologous regions of the two chromosomes come together, starting a zipper-like process during which the two chromosomes become aligned side by side. This process often starts at the nuclear membrane and proceeds inwards, but can also start in the centre of the chromosome and proceed out towards the ends. The paired chromosomes are known as **bivalents** (one from each parent) and have four chromatids. The whole is known as a **tetrad** (Fig. 5.7).
  - **Pachynema** (thick): cells enter pachynema when all the chromosomes are aligned. This stage can last several days. Recombination nodules become visible, which are thought to result in an exchange of chromosomal material between the two non-sister chromatids.
  - **Diplonema** (double): at this stage the two homologous chromosomes start to move away from each other. Each tetrad remains attached at **chiasmata**, which are formed at the point where crossover has occurred. In oocytes, this stage can last for several months or years, but it only takes about 24 days in the human male. The chromosomes de-condense and RNA synthesis starts, to provide storage materials for the egg.

- **Diakinesis** (across): RNA synthesis ceases, and chromosomes condense, thicken and detach from the nuclear membrane. The four chromatids can be clearly distinguished within each tetrad. Sister chromatids are joined at the centromere. Non-sister chromatids are joined by chiasmata.
- **Metaphase I**: in this phase spindles form between centrioles, at opposite **poles** of the cell, within the nuclear membrane, and the tetrads line up on the spindles on the equatorial plane (**metaphase plate**), with centromeres from the homologous chromosomes lying on opposite sides of the plate (Fig. 5.8).
- **Anaphase I**: the spindles pull the two homologous chromosomes apart, towards opposite ends of the cells. Unlike in mitosis, the chromosomes do not duplicate and so only half the original number will lie in each half of the cell, which will contain only one of a pair of autosomes (with crossed-over genetic material), and one sex chromosome.
- **Telophase I**: when the chromosomes reach the poles, a new nuclear membrane develops between each set of chromosomes (Fig. 5.9). Cytoplasmic division is about equal between the daughter cells in males, whereas in females there is unequal division. The daughter cell with the most cytoplasm goes on to form the egg, the other becoming a **polar body** that eventually degenerates.

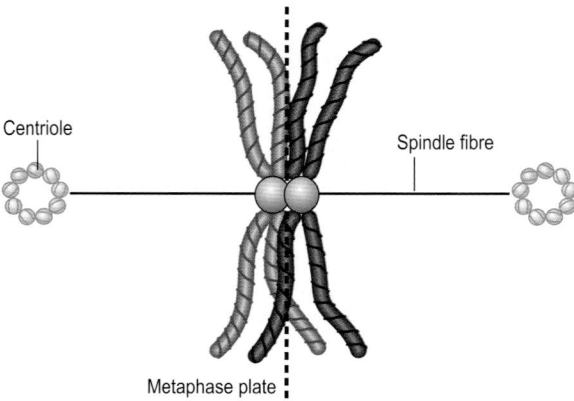

Fig. 5.8 **Metaphase I**: spindle fibres form between centrioles at opposite sides of the cell and tetrads line up on the metaphase plate.

Meiosis II is the phase in which each haploid cell produces four daughter haploid cells. Like in the previous phase, there are a number of similar stages:

- **Prophase II**: this is very similar to mitotic prophase, sister chromatids lying together, joined at the centromere, but the cell nucleus has only a haploid number of chromosomes.
- **Metaphase II**: spindle fibres line up the chromosomes on the equatorial plane.
- **Anaphase II**: this resembles mitotic anaphase – the centromeres split and sister chromatids are pulled towards separate poles. In meiosis, however, because of crossing over that has taken place in the first stage, the separated daughter cells may not be identical.
- **Telophase II**: this is like telophase I; nuclear membranes again form round each set of chromosomes. Again the cytoplasmic division is unequal in female gametes.

At the end of meiosis the result in males is four daughter cells, whereas in female cells, two daughter cells plus two polar bodies will form. Occasionally, polar bodies formed in stage 1 can divide and there will be three polar bodies.

Chromosome abnormalities

Abnormalities in number

Defects in fertilisation or meiosis can result in an additional or reduced number of chromosomes being detected. The body is better able to deal with small excesses of genetic material than a deficit.

- **Polyploidy** occurs when an additional set of chromosomes is present; this always happens as a multiple of 23 chromosomes. **Triploidy** results in 69 chromosomes, and **tetraploidy** leads to 92 chromosomes in each cell. These conditions are rarely compatible with life and triploidy is a common cause of spontaneous miscarriages.
- **Aneuploidy** occurs is when a multiple of 23 chromosomes is not present. There can be a gain or loss of chromosomes, which can affect either autosomal or sex chromosomes. These conditions are usually caused by non-disjunction during meiosis and can lead to **monosomy** (one copy of a chromosome in a

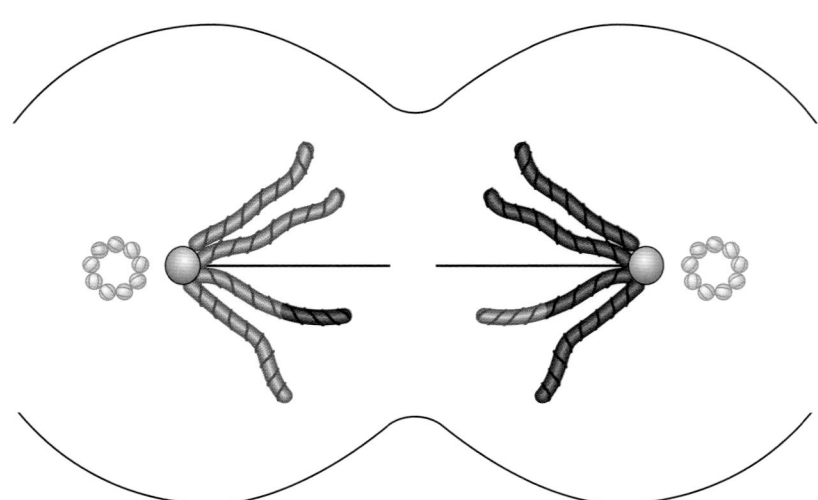

Fig. 5.9 **Telophase I**: The chromosomes reach the poles and a cytoplasmic membrane forms between the two halves.

normally diploid cell) or **trisomy** (three copies of a chromosome in a normally diploid cell).

- **Autosomal monosomy** – is rarely compatible with life.
- **Autosomal trisomy** – trisomy 21 (Down's syndrome) is the most common.
- **Sex chromosome monosomy** – because of normal X inactivation, the loss of a single X chromosome (Turner's syndrome) is compatible with life.
- **Sex chromosome trisomy** – XXY (Klinefelter's syndrome), XXX (trisomy X) and XYY syndrome have fewer problems than the above.

Abnormalities in structure

Sometimes, as gametes are formed, structural alterations can occur – pieces can be lost, moved to another chromosome or duplicated. These events can be the result of homologous chromosomes failing to line up properly during meiosis, causing an unequal crossover, or chromosome breakage with an imperfect repair. The alterations that can occur are:

- **Translocations** – where genetic material is exchanged between different chromosomes (**reciprocal translocation**), or where the short arms of two chromosomes are lost and the long arms fuse at the centromere to make a single large chromosome (**Robertsonian** translocation). In the latter, although there is the overall loss of one chromosome, this is usually only seen in chromosomes where the amount of genetic material in the short arm is limited, such as in chromosomes 14 and 21.

The **Philadelphia chromosome** involves a translocation between chromosomes 9 and 22, and is characteristically observed in chronic myeloid leukaemia (see Ch. 12).

- **Deletions** – a loss of genetic material can occur when breaks happen. Some of these deletions can lead to clinically important abnormalities:
  - **Cri-du-chat** syndrome, so called because of the child's distinctive cry, occurs because of the loss of part of the short arm of chromosome 5.
  - **Wolf–Hirschhorn** syndrome is because of the loss of part of the short arm of chromosome 4. This, and the previous example, are examples of a **microdeletion**.
  - **Ring** chromosomes occur when there is a deletion at both ends of the chromosome and the ends join, forming a ring. This often leads to the loss of that chromosome, resulting in a monosomy.
  - **WAGR** syndrome is due to a deletion of the p arm of chromosome 11, involving a series of genes, resulting in **W**ilms tumour (a kidney cancer), **a**niridia (no iris), **g**onad tumours or other genitou**r**inary abnormalities, and **r**etardation. This is an example of a **contiguous gene syndrome**.

    High-resolution banding techniques and **fluorescence in situ hybridisation** (**FISH**) (see Information box 5.1), and more latterly gene array molecular technologies, have enabled many microdeletions to be described, and more are likely to follow.
- **Duplications** – can occur as a result of unequal crossover, or in the children of someone with a reciprocal translocation.

> **ⓘ Information box 5.1** **Fluorescence in situ hybridisation** (Fig. 5.10)

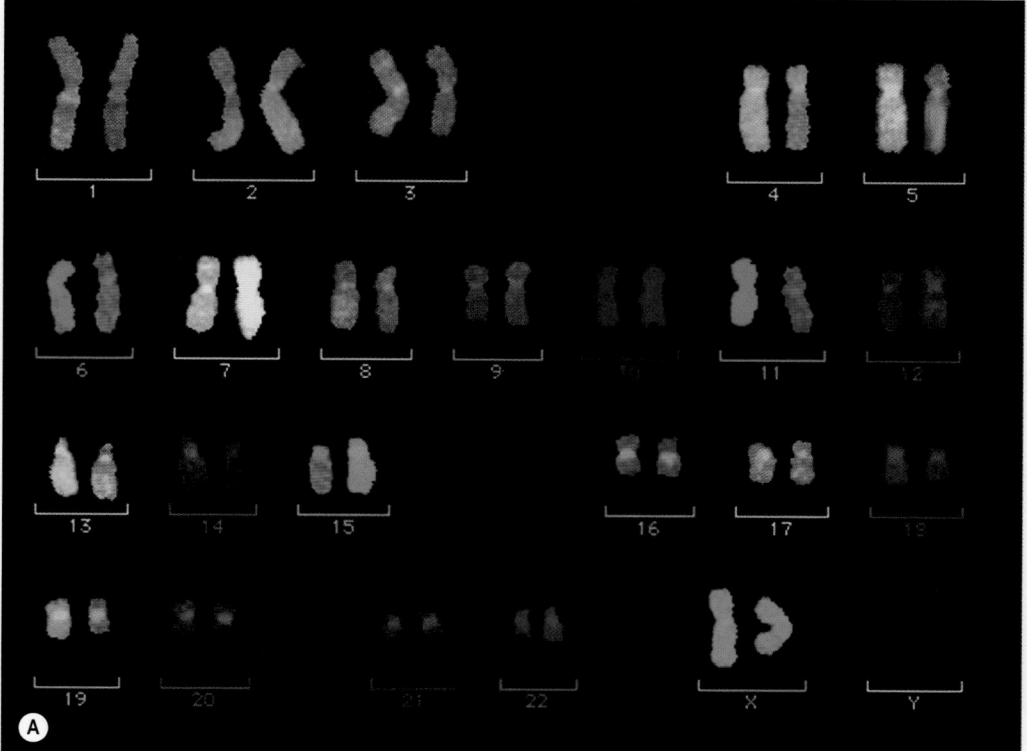

Fig. 5.10 **Fluorescence in situ hybridisation (FISH). (A)** M-FISH showing a normal human karyotype from a female.

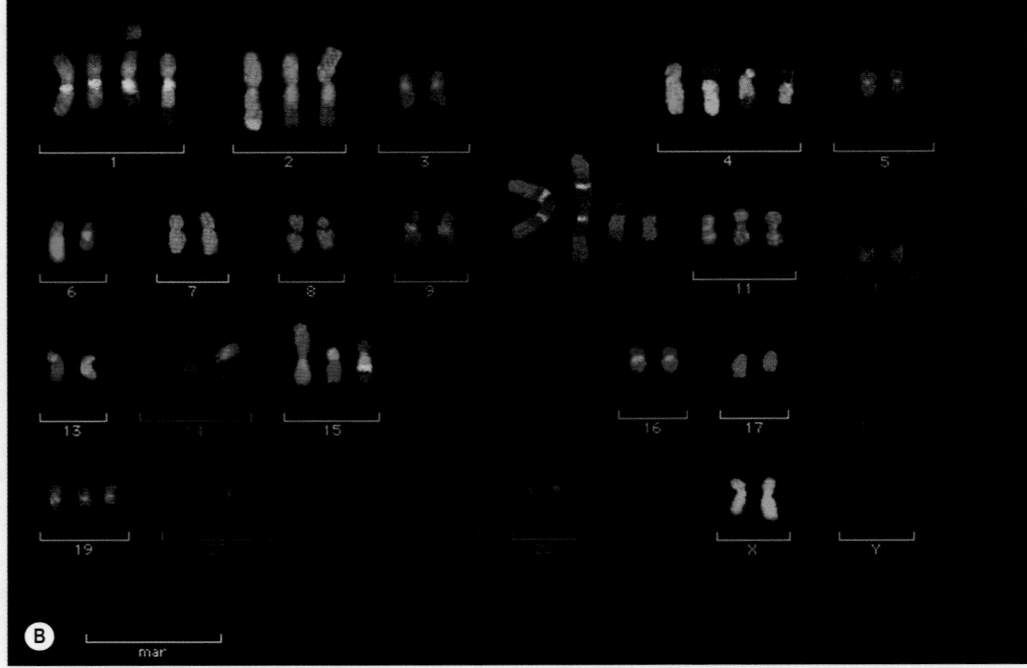

Fig. 5.10, cont'd **(B)** M-FISH showing an abnormal human karyotype with duplications and translocations in a female.

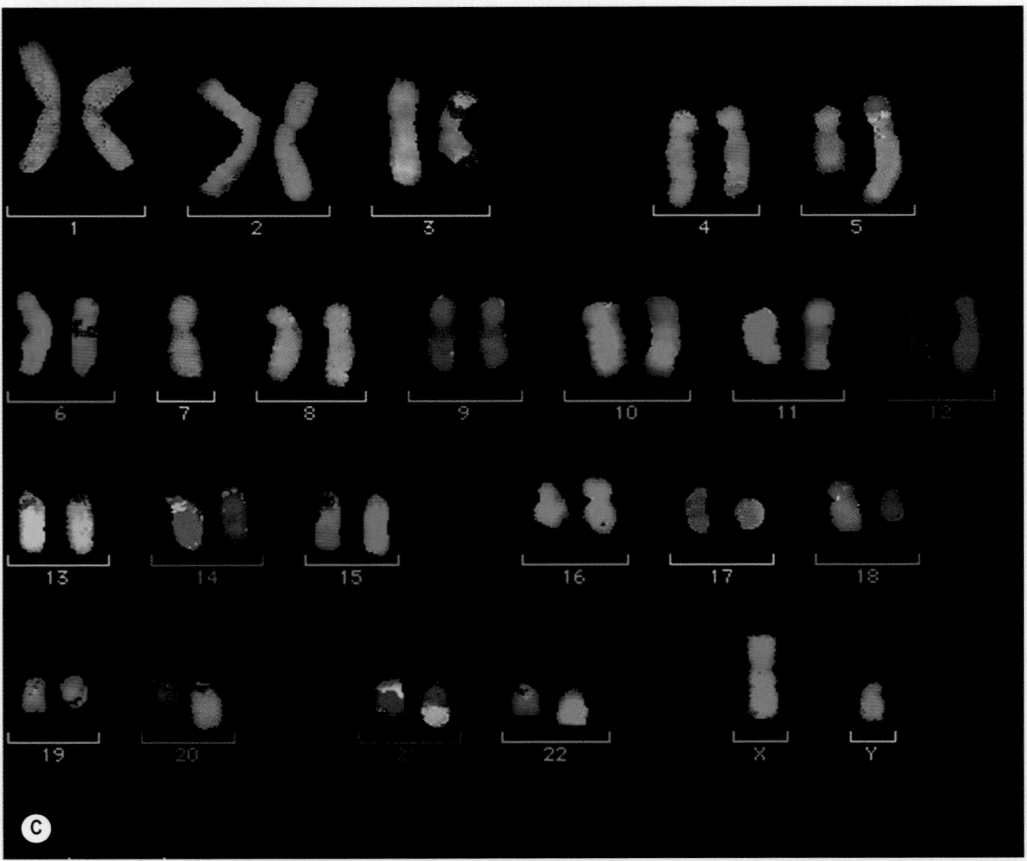

Fig. 5.10, cont'd **(C)** M-FISH showing an abnormal human karyotype with chromosome loss and translocations in a male. Courtesy of Dr Debra Lillington.

ℹ️ **Information box 5.1**   Fluorescence in situ hybridisation—cont'd

FISH is a technique that has been developed to map (locate) particular regions of a chromosome, or even whole chromosomes, regardless of whether or not the cells are actively dividing. The technique requires the use of a piece of single-stranded DNA that matches the genetic sequence in the area of interest – the **probe**.

Chromosomes prepared on a glass slide are **denatured** (the DNA complementary strands are separated) **in situ** (on the slide), allowing the probe DNA to **hybridise** (bind) to its complementary sequence on the separated strand. Fluorescent dyes are attached to the probes so that the results can be visualised under a fluorescent microscope.

FISH can be used in different ways:

- **Gene location**: the genetic sequence of every gene is known and a probe can be developed to show the chromosomal location of the gene. The technique is sensitive enough to identify deletions of very small amounts of DNA from a chromosome.
- **Centromeric probes**: probes can be used to identify the repetitive sequence found around the centromere. This can be used to check the number of chromosomes.
- **Spectral karyotyping**: this involves the use of a large number of probes, labelled with different coloured fluorescent dyes, in order to 'paint' a whole chromosome. This technique is particularly useful in detecting chromosomal translocations, in which a part of one chromosome is moved to another chromosome.

- **Inversions** – this can happen when there are two breaks in the chromosome and the free portion rotates. These changes are said to be **pericentric** if they involve the centromere, **paracentric** if they do not. While these abnormalities may not have severe consequences, they can interfere with the normal meiotic process and therefore they are at higher risk of producing offspring with deletions or duplications. Occasionally, the inversion can be very serious and is the cause of almost 50% of cases of severe haemophilia, where the inversion has interrupted the factor VIII gene, resulting in insufficient production of factor VIII for normal clotting processes (see Ch. 12).
- **Isochromosome** – chromosome pairs normally line up, joining and separating at the centromeres, but retaining their own long and short arms. An isochromosome occurs when the chromosomes split at the centromere to produce two chromosomes, one with only short arms, and the other with only long arms. Only isochromosomes involving the X chromosome appear to be compatible with life.

DNA AND GENES

Chromosomal DNA is located in the nucleus and is composed of regions that actively make proteins and those that are inactive. **Genes** are the active DNA sequences coding for proteins and are organised into:

- Regulatory regions (**promoters**, enhancer or repressor sequences)
- **Exons** – which encode the mRNA, and, in most cases, the protein
- **Introns** – which are not transcribed into proteins.

Some genes are only found only at a single **locus** (chromosome location). They are called **single copy** genes and share little or no DNA sequence homology with other genes. Other genes are part of large **gene families**. These families have occurred due to gene duplication, and gene members therefore share a high degree of DNA (and amino acid) sequence homology. They often cluster at specific regions of the genome and have similar but distinct functions in different tissues.

Homeobox (HOX) genes

Genes can also be classified into gene families based on the presence of highly conserved **domains**, with the rest of the gene sequence sharing no homology at all with other family members. **Homeobox (HOX)** genes are examples of these.

HOX genes are associated in clusters and control production of body parts. They are organised in similar ways throughout the animal kingdoms and are arranged along chromosomes in an order that reflects the body parts that they control. While a specific HOX gene from a fly can be identical with one from another organism, such as the chicken, reflecting their common ancestry, a small mutation can lead to fundamental changes in morphology – called **homeotic mutations**. For example, additional fingers on the hand are the result of a mutation in a specific HOX gene.

Non-coding DNA

Genes are also separated by repetitive non-coding regions. Despite not being used for making proteins, this DNA is not unimportant and has a number of gene regulatory functions.

Unlike human chromosomal DNA, all the mitochondrial DNA (MtDNA) sequence codes for protein. MtDNA is present in many copies in the mitochondria within the cytoplasm.

Two processes are involved in making proteins:

- **Transcription** – in which DNA is transcribed (copied) into mRNA, which then leaves the nucleus
- **Translation** – in which mRNA is used to specify the amino acids required to make the relevant protein.

These processes take place in one direction only along a nucleic acid strand. Nucleic acids are arranged in sequence along a strand and each end is named after the number of carbon atoms in the nucleotide sugar ring at the end.

- The **5′** end has a 5-carbon deoxyribose ring.
- The **3′** end has a hydroxyl group on the third carbon in the sugar ring.

The distinction between the two ends of the molecule is important because nucleic acid can only be synthesised in a 5′ to 3′ direction. By convention sequences are written in a 5′ to 3′ direction.

Transcription (Fig. 5.11)

The process of making mRNA is initiated when an RNA polymerase enzyme binds to a **promoter** site on the DNA. The promoter region is a sequence of DNA close to, but outside the gene. The position of the promoter determines which strand is used, because nucleotides can only be added to a 3′ end. Thus mRNA is only made in the 5′ to 3′ direction along the chromosome. Several different promoters can exist in different parts of the gene, and this results in slightly different proteins being produced in different locations in the body.

Transcription begins by the assembly of the basal transcription apparatus, involving transcription factors and associated proteins upstream of the start codon. In most promoters the assembly site is determined by the **TATA box** sequence. This is a conserved sequence of A:T pairs, usually located 25–35 bases upstream of the start codon. Other sequences are involved in determining the efficiency of the promoter, such as those found in the **CAAT box**, normally located further upstream. Many genes also have GC-rich

regions, or **CpG islands**, upstream of the transcription start site. CpG islands are unmethylated regions of the genome that are associated with the 5′ ends of many genes.

The polymerase enzyme pulls the DNA strands apart, exposing the DNA bases. This provides a template (**antisense** strand), with the enzyme moving from the 3′ to 5′ direction along this template, producing a complementary copy (**sense** strand), which eventually becomes the mRNA. Note that this molecule is identical to the other of the DNA strands that has not been used as a template, except in that the thymine base is replaced with a uracil base.

To the 5′ end of the developing mRNA molecule is added a modified guanine molecule – the **5′ cap**. This 'cap' appears both to protect the molecule from degrading and to act as a marker for translation to begin. Transcription continues, through a sequence of exons and introns, until a **termination sequence** signals the end. Before mRNA leaves the nucleus introns are excised and the exons sliced together.

Splicing can also happen in different ways: intentionally, resulting in different proteins being produced, or unintentionally, resulting in a **mutation** (error), which can produce genetic disease. A large number of adenine sequences are added to the 3′ end – **polyA tail** – close to this termination sequence and although transcription may continue, this tail is later lost. The mRNA finally separates from the polymerase enzyme and template DNA. Figure 5.12 illustrates the process. The sequence formed consists of a series of **codons** – three nucleotides that code for particular amino acids.

Regulation of transcription

The regulation of transcriptional processes is a vital component in the control of gene expression. Genes are normally transcribed in particular tissues at particular times. Thus, even though all cells have the same DNA sequence, only a few genes are actively transcribed in any one cell. For example only nucleated red cell precursors transcribe globin,

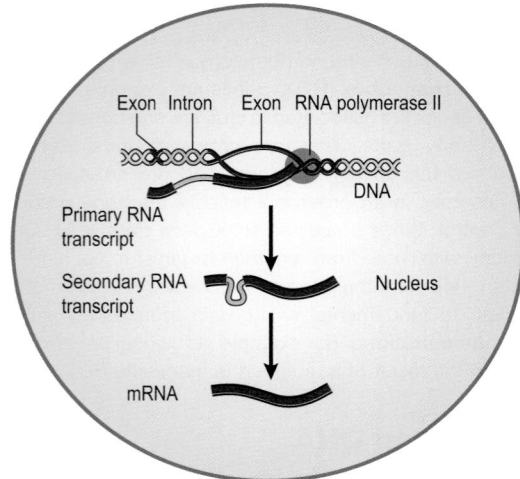

Fig. 5.11 **Transcription of DNA to messenger RNA (mRNA)**: the enzyme RNA polymerase II moves along the DNA strand separating the strands and assembling a strand of mRNA nucleotides that are complementary to the DNA.

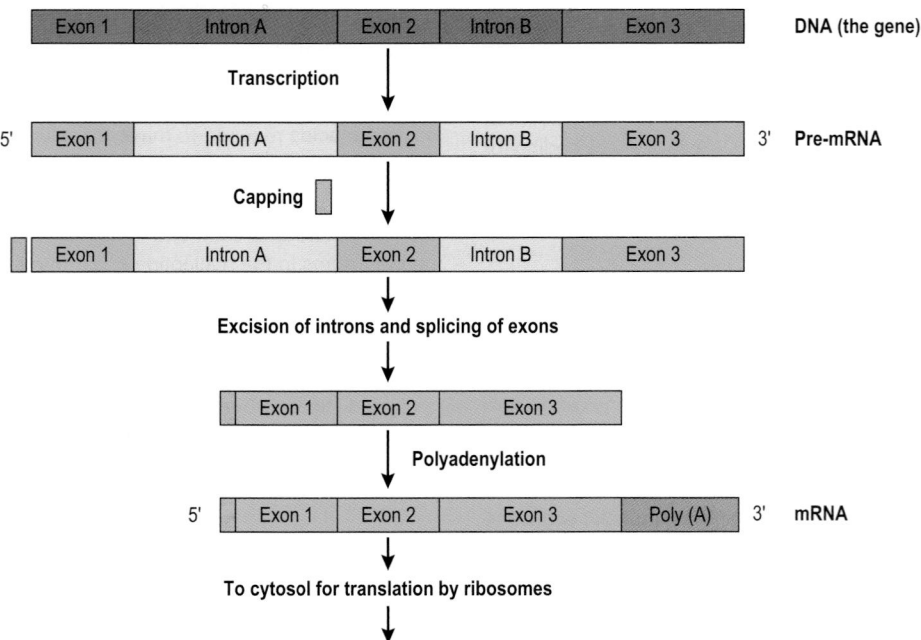

Fig. 5.12 **Production of messenger RNA (mRNA)**: after transcription from the antisense DNA strand, the growing mRNA molecule is capped at the 5′ end, introns are spliced and the exons joined. mRNA produces a tail of adenine nucleotides (polyA tail) at the 3′ end.

used in the production of haemoglobin. Other genes may be transcribed all the time, to maintain cell integrity (**housekeeping genes**), or at particular times to aid other processes. For example, RNA polymerase needs other proteins to stabilise the polymerase, to help it bind in order to initiate transcription.

Transcription can be modified by **enhancers**. These are sequences that do not interact with the relevant genes, and may not even lie close, but which bind to transcription factors, known as **activators**. The whole then binds to **co-activators**, increasing transcription. **Silencers** are analogous to enhancers but they repress transcription. The various transcription factors interact with their targets through **DNA-binding motifs**, particular protein configurations that fit with, interact and modify the secondary and tertiary structure of the target molecules. These are some characteristic motifs:

- Helix–turn–helix (hth):
  - Two α-helices lie in different planes, one fitting into the groove on the DNA molecule.
- Zinc finger:
  - Zinc ions are used to stabilise protein secondary structure in the form of α-helices and β-sheets, enabling the α-helix to bind with DNA in the major groove.
- Leucine zipper:
  - Two α-helices that form a y-shaped structure, being held together with amino acid side chains that also bind to the DNA molecule in the major groove.

Translation

This process takes place on ribosomes; mRNA provides the template, specifying the amino acid sequence, helped by molecules of **tRNA**. tRNA consists of about 80 nucleotides that have a clover-leaf structure (Fig. 5.13). There is at least one type of tRNA molecule for each amino acid, determined by the **anticodon** sequence in the loop of the molecule.

rRNA first binds to mRNA at the **start codon** at its 5′ end. This is the sequence adenine–uracil–guanine (AUG), which codes for the amino acid methionine. The stRNA that binds is determined by the nucleotide sequence of the mRNA: the three nucleotide codon binds to the complementary anticodon on the tRNA molecule. In the process, the ribosome provides specific enzymes (aminoacyl tRNA synthetases) that pick up and attach to the 3′ acceptor end the specific amino acid – matching the codon in the mRNA molecule. Ribosomes move along the mRNA sequence in a 5′ to 3′ direction and also provide enzymes that make covalent bonds between each of the amino acids, in order to produce the growing polypeptide chain. Translation continues until reaching a **stop codon** (a nucleotide triplet, normally UAG, UAA or UGA).

DNA DAMAGE (MUTATION)

DNA can be damaged by a variety of factors (**mutagens**), such as X-rays, and a large number of chemicals, but damage can also occur naturally during replication. The resultant changes are known as **mutations**. There are two main processes producing mutations.

DNA damage from environmental factors

- **Nucleotide base alteration**: non-ionising radiation, such as Ultraviolet light and certain chemicals can

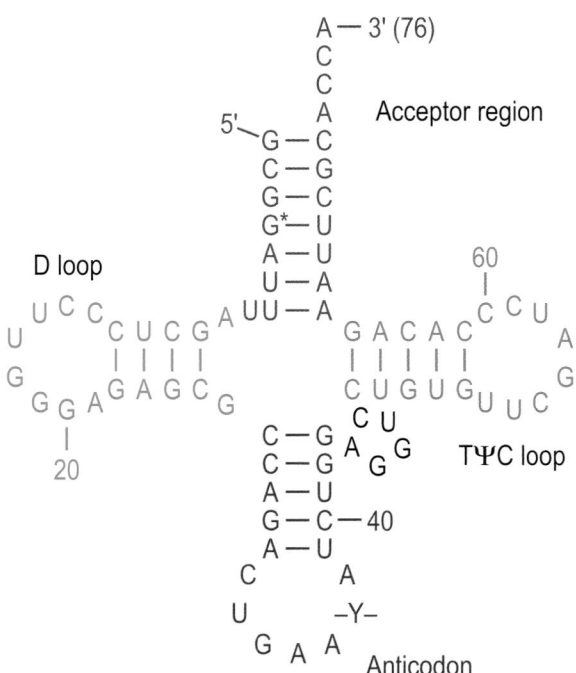

Fig. 5.13 Structure of tRNA: the diagram illustrates the secondary structure of the molecule which is composed of four base-paired stems and three non-base-paired loops: D loop (green); the anticodon (red); the TΨC loop (blue); as well as a variable region (black) and an acceptor region (purple). The 3′ end always terminates with the sequence CCA, with the 3′ hydroxyl of the ribose of the terminal A being the point of covalent attachment of specific amino acids, determined by the three nucleotide anticodon sequence.

damage DNA by altering nucleotide bases. When the DNA strands are separated and copied, the altered base will pair with an incorrect base. This may lead to altered proteins with different functions.

- **Phosphate backbone breakage**: environmental agents such as ionising radiation (X-rays) and nuclear radiation can damage DNA by breaking the bonds between oxygen and phosphate groups. Mechanisms exist to attempt to fix the broken ends, by joining to other pieces of DNA within a cell – a translocation. Where the translocation breakpoint is within or near a gene then the function of the gene may be affected.

Spontaneous damage (DNA replication mistakes)

During DNA replication, the polymerase very occasionally makes a mistake, about once every 100 000 000 bases, even after normal repair mechanisms.

Repair mechanisms

A series of genes are involved in producing enzymes that assist in repair mechanisms, recognising altered bases, excising them and replacing them. The process is highly efficient, correcting about 99.9% of errors.

Direct reversal of base damage

- Common damage involves the addition of a methyl group (alkylation) to a C, followed by deamination, changing the C to a T.

Xeroderma pigmentosum (XP) is a rare inherited disease that predisposes individuals to skin lesions (dry skin and freckles) and an increased incidence in skin cancer. The areas affected are particularly those areas exposed to sunlight. Several genes have been implicated, all involved in nucleotide excision repair. Patients are advised to avoid ultraviolet light exposure.

- **Glycosylase** enzymes reverse the process without breaking the DNA backbone.

Excision repair

- **Base excision repair (BER)**: first the glycosylase enzyme removes the damaged base and other enzymes remove the phosphate in the backbone. This is followed by **DNA polymerase beta (β)** replacing the correct nucleotide; then ligation enzymes mend the break.
- **Nucleotide excision repair (NER)** (see Clinical box 5.2): protein factors recognise the damage, and **transcription factor IIH** (also involved in normal transcription) unwinds the DNA to produce a 'bubble'. Cuts are made on the 3′ and 5′ side of the damage, removing a 'patch' of nucleotides. **DNA polymerases delta (δ) and epsilon (ε)** then synthesise the repair using the opposite strand as a template. Finally, DNA ligase binds the new piece into the backbone.
- **Mismatch repair (MMR)**: this process corrects mismatches of normal bases and uses enzymes involved in BER and NER. The **MSH2** protein recognises the mismatch and the **MLH1** protein cuts it out. DNA polymerase δ and ε repair the patch. Mutations in the genes *MSH2* and *MSH1* predispose to colon cancer and they are therefore referred to as **tumour suppressor genes**.

Breakage repair

- **Single-strand breaks**: these are repaired using the BER mechanism.
- **Double-strand breaks**.

Non-homologous end-joining (NHEJ)

This process enables the direct joining of broken ends – the nucleotides involved do not have to be complementary. The **Ku** heterodimer protein is needed for the process. Errors in NHEJ lead to translocations, e.g. the Philadelphia chromosome (see Ch. 12).

Homologous recombination

Broken ends can also be repaired using information from:

- the homologous chromosome in G1 phase
- the sister chromatid from G2 phase
- the same chromosome, if there are duplicate copies of the gene on the same chromosome in opposite directions. The process involves **BRCA1** and **BRCA2**; mutations in the genes encoding these proteins predispose to breast and ovarian cancers.

GENES AND DEVELOPMENT

The most common cause of infant death is due to a birth defect, and up to 3% of babies have a recognisable defect.

Many of these defects are due to mutations in developmental genes. The prevalence of genetic abnormalities is even higher among fetuses that miscarry.

After fertilisation the developing ovum not only undergoes simple multiplication but changes to form different cell types, tissues and organs in a highly coordinated fashion. Understanding how cells with identical genes (**stem cells**) develop into different cell types has been studied through the discipline of developmental biology.

Many of the genes and pathways involved in human development are the same across a large range of species and the function of many of these genes has been elucidated using non-human organisms, such as the roundworm, fruit fly, zebrafish, frog and mouse. Many of these organisms have fast generation times and so facilitate the research by being able to examine a large number of events in a short period of time.

Embryo development begins with defining the major axes of the body: ventral/dorsal, anterior/posterior, medial/lateral, left/right. Cells then are differentiated and arranged spatially to form the tissues; organs and limbs are then formed through organogenesis. These processes are driven through the production of proteins that provide signals and switches.

MEDIATORS OF DEVELOPMENT

Developmental genes code for a variety of proteins with differing functions, for example signalling, DNA transcription and extracellular matrix components.

Signalling molecules

Signalling molecules allow interactions between cells. A protein is secreted by a cell and diffuses across the extracellular space to bind to a receptor on the target cell. These molecules are called **paracrine** signalling molecules and include:

- Fibroblast growth factor (FGF) family
- Hedgehog family
- Wingless (Wnt) family
- Transforming growth factor β (TGF-β).

Fibroblast growth factor

The receptor for FGF (FGFR) is a glycoprotein consisting of peptides and immunoglobulin-type areas on the outside of the cell, with a protein that crosses the cell membrane and an intracellular **tyrosine kinase**. Different FGFs can bind to the receptor, leading to phosphorylation and activation of the tyrosine kinase. Many FGFs are involved in bone development, and mutations in the FGFR lead to a variety of skeletal problems in children.

Individuals with **achondroplasia (ACH)** have short limbs in comparison with the trunk and a prominent forehead (**macrocephaly**). ACH is usually caused by an amino acid substitution in the *FGFR3* gene, and has autosomal dominant inheritance, although 'new' mutations are very common. The gene produces a protein that controls **chondrocyte** (cartilage cell) proliferation; a mutation causes overactivation of the gene and leads to inhibition of chondrocyte growth, resulting in bone shortening.

Sonic hedgehog

The hedgehog family of genes were called after a mutant form of hairy fruit fly. Vertebrates have similar forms, the most common of which is called **sonic hedgehog** (**SHH**), involved in specifying the body axis. *SHH* binds to its receptor, a transmembrane protein called **patched** (**PTC**), which suppresses transcription of **Wnt** and **TGF-β** and inhibits cell growth.

- PTC *somatic* mutations affect the regulation of cell differentiation and cause cancer, such as basal cell carcinoma.
- PTC *germline* mutations cause birth defects – rib anomalies, jaw cysts and cancer in later life – **Gorlin's syndrome**.

Wingless (Wnt)

The **Wnt** genes were named after wingless mutant flies. A variety of different types are present in humans, and are involved in *dorsal/ventral axis* specification and development of various organs, binding to **frizzled** and low-density lipoprotein (LDL) receptors.

Wnt genes are involved in signalling processes throughout the cell and have been linked to the development of B cell and lymphoid malignancies. Different forms appear to act as both tumour suppressors and tumour activators in cancer formation. Mutations in **R-spondin** proteins that are involved in Wnt signalling have produced inherited defects such as **anonychia** (absence of nails) and Sex reversal.

Transforming growth factor β

TGF-βs are a large number of related genes that are involved with bone formation through the production of **bone morphogenetic protein** (**BMP**).

DNA transcription factors

There are many families of transcription factors. These are genes that produce proteins that activate or repress other genes. They often share a common DNA-binding domain but have a wide variety of effects (**pleiotropy**).

Transcription factor genes are important in human development: HOX, SOX and T-box are important examples of these.

SOX family genes

There are a large number of **SOX** genes that are involved in neuronal development and sex determination. SOX genes have much in common with the **SRY** (**sex-determining region on the Y chromosome**) gene found on the human Y chromosome.

- **SRY** produces DNA-bending proteins that promote events leading to male differentiation through:
  - **Sertoli cell** differentiation (these cells are found in the testes and aid sperm development)
  - Production of **Müllerian-inhibitiory factor** (embryonic Müllerian ducts develop into the female reproductive organs).
- *SRY* abnormalities can produce sex reversals:
  - XX males and XY females can be the result of a faulty crossover in meiosis between the X and Y chromosome, where the *SRY* gene is transferred to the X chromosome and the resultant affected offspring depends on the chromosome the father passes to his child.
  - XY females can also be the result of a mutation in the *SRY* gene.

Extracellular matrix proteins

These is a large collection of molecules, including collagens and glycoproteins, that form the extracellular matrix and allow for cell migration.

A mutation in the **fibrillin** gene, responsible for the development of microfibrils in connective tissue, results in **Marfan's syndrome,** with its multiple pleiotropic effects, leading to skeletal, cardiovascular and ocular defects.

PATTERNING

The position of organs and appendages are laid down in patterns defined during embryogenesis under the control of a series of genes. Important in this process are genes that specify the various body axes.

Most of the knowledge of pattern formation has come from experimentation with 'knockout' mice and tissue transplantations between regions in the early embryo (Fig. 5.14). Mutations in many of the early developmental genes are likely to be lethal in humans.

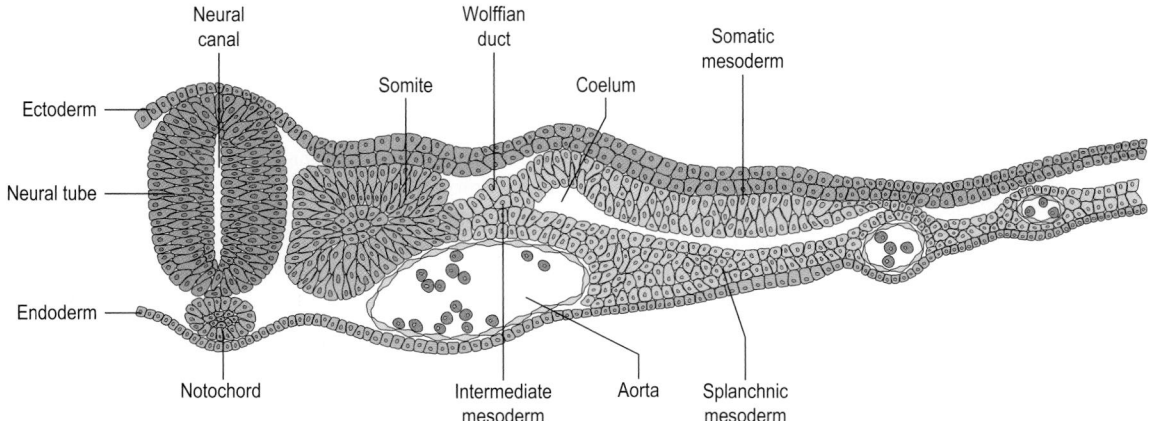

Fig. 5.14 Cross-**section of a chick embryo at 45 hours' incubation**, showing the principal anatomical features of the early embryo. Redrawn with permission from Standring S et al. (eds) 2008 Gray's anatomy, 40th edn. Elsevier, Edinburgh.

Anterior/posterior axis formation

The developing collection of cells in the fertilised ovum, or blastula, undergoes **gastrulation** in which the three embryonic layers, **ectoderm**, **mesoderm** and **endoderm**, are defined and an anterior/posterior thickening occurs, the **primitive streak**, under control of a series of **HOX** and other developmental genes.

There are a large number of HOX genes on different chromosomes and they are expressed at different times, in an order that specifies the positioning of cells and tissues along the anterior/posterior axis. A mutation in one of these genes results in the replacement of antennae by legs in the *Drosophila* fly; limb abnormalities have also been observed in humans.

Left/right axis formation

At the anterior end of the primitive streak lies the **node**, which is the source of the left-side-expressed **nodal** protein, stimulated by asymmetrical expression of **SHH** from the **notochord**.

Dorsal/ventral axis development

BMPs are growth factors influencing the development of bone and cartilage, and are also important in the embryonic development of the heart and central nervous system.

- **BMP-4**, excreted from the dorsal notochord in the mesoderm, along with SHH proteins, from the ventral notochord, establishes the dorsal/ventral axis and stimulates development of the overlying ectoderm.
- **Noggin** and **chordin** are **morphogens** (proteins that govern pattern development) that spread from a node and are expressed in a concentration gradient across a tissue. They *inhibit* BMPs. Noggin is needed in embryonic development to form the neural plate that lies opposite the primitive streak, allowing it to develop into the neural tube and subsequently to form the brain and spinal cord.
- Noggin and chordin bind directly to BMP-4, inhibiting its ventralising signal, promoting dorsalisation in the mesoderm region that experiences high concentrations of the proteins. Noggin and chordin are thus important in defining the back, as opposed to the front, of the developing embryo.

ORGANOGENESIS

Organogenesis occurs after gastrulation and involves many of the same proteins, expressed differentially.

Neuronal development

FGFs influence differentiation of the neural plate into the spinal cord. Absence of FGF towards the anterior part of the neural tube allows brain tissue to generate. HOX genes further control the development of the forebrain, midbrain and hindbrain from the neural tube. FGFs are also important in the development of the skull bones and limb formation.

Neural crest cells, located on the lateral edges of the neural folds and formed from ectoderm, are induced by BMP, Wnt and FGF signalling to migrate through the extracellular matrix. They are very important in development and there are four major types:

- **Cranial** – important in development of tissues in the facial region
- **Vagal and sacral** – forming parasympathetic neurons involved in gut peristalsis and blood vessel dilation
  - **Hirschsprung's disease** leads to severe constipation. It is commonly due to mutations in the *RET* (**rearranged during transfection**) gene that is important for neural crest cell migration into the distal bowel
- **Trunk** – forms two populations that influence the development of skin pigment cells and neurons of the sympathetic nervous system
- **Cardiac** – influencing the development of the great vessels supplying the heart.

The asymmetrical heart

While the developed heart shows left/right asymmetry, the embryonic heart is formed inverted and is bilaterally symmetrical. Various influences are needed to transform the heart tube into chambers and establish the asymmetry.

dHAND and **eHAND** are basic helix–loop–helix transcription factors that are expressed in different areas of the heart tube. Both factors are transcribed initially, but later dHAND predominates in the region due to become the right ventricle, and eHAND in the region that will become the left ventricle. This, along with the **right cardiac forward looping** produced by the **nodal** protein, changes the anterior/posterior orientation into the left/right asymmetry of the developed heart.

Organ formation

While the endoderm gives rise to the gastrointestinal tract, respiratory system, liver and pancreas, the mesoderm produces the circulatory, reproductive and urinary systems, the muscles and connective tissues, through complex interactions mediated by a variety of signalling molecules acting through complex interconnected networks.

Genes that are involved in the development of a particular organ are often also involved in the function of specialised cells within the organ, for example:

- Transcription of **insulin** from β-cells in the pancreas is stimulated by binding of **insulin promoter factor 1**.
- Mutations in the gene producing this factor prevent development of the pancreas.

Limb development

Much is known about genes that control limb development because, next to congenital heart defects, abnormalities of the limbs are the next most common birth defect. Many of the pathways and transcription controls involved in limb development are conserved throughout the animal kingdom and experimentation in model organisms, such as *Drosophila*, has helped in understanding the processes involved.

Limbs develop from the **lateral plate mesoderm**, which leads to bone and cartilage development, and the **somatic mesoderm**, which produces the muscles, nerves and blood vessels. The **intermediate mesoderm**, close to the Wolffian duct, is thought to be the origin of the signal that induces limb production from the **apical ectodermal ridge (AER)**

Thalidomide teratogenesis

Thalidomide was marketed in the late 1950s as an anti-sickness drug given to women in early pregnancy. Use within a particular gestational window led to multiple birth effects, predominantly characterised by an absence of arms.

Thalidomide has been shown to increase the production of free radicals, leading to oxidative stress. **Nuclear factor κB**, an anti-apoptotic transcription factor, is redox sensitive and it is proposed that a species-selective failure to bind to its DNA promoter, because of oxidative damage, leads to a failure of expression of fibroblast growth factor 10 (**FGF10**), which in turn attenuates expression of FGF8 in the apical ectodermal ridge, essential for limb development.

structure in the ectoderm under control of FGF and Wnt signalling proteins. The protein **FGF8**, for example, is capable of producing a limb if transplanted into mesoderm tissue (see Clinical box 5.4).

The AER, destined to produce the skin covering of the limb, sustains the limb formation within the **progress zone** in the mesoderm, where the limb develops. Both the AER and the progress zone of the mesoderm are needed for limb development. Three developmental axes are important:

- **Proximal/distal**. The length of time that cells spend in the progress zone will determine the proximal–distal axis. Removal of the AER will lead to a short limb with more distal elements, the actual elements depending on how late the AER influence was removed.
- **Anterior/posterior**. The AER provides signals to the **zone of polarising activity** (**ZPA**), at the root of the limb bud, and establishes the anterior/posterior axis (thumb/little finger) in the limb bud. **FGF8 is** needed to maintain the expression of SHH from the ZPA, which guides the anterior–posterior patterning through the asymmetrical expression of various downstream genes.

Apoptosis leads to separation of the fingers, stimulated by BMP signalling; noggin blocks cell death within the digits.

HUMAN GENETIC VARIATION

POLYMORPHISMS

EB Ford was a British ecological geneticist who defined genetic polymorphism in 1940 as a 'type of variation in which individuals with sharply distinct qualities co-exist as normal members of a population…', stating that they occur 'in such proportions that the rarest of them cannot be maintained merely by recurrent mutation.'

Polymorphisms are all the result of mutational events:

- Mutations in the germline cells that produce the gametes are inherited mutations. Some of the these will produce deleterious effects, leading to inherited diseases, while others will have no effect, and are therefore passed down the generations as a polymorphism that is maintained at a reasonable level, generally in more than 1% in the population.
- Mutations of somatic cells potentially result in cancer.

The different polymorphisms, or different sequences of DNA at a particular region (**locus**) of the genome, are referred to as **alleles** of a gene. Each person inherits half their DNA from one parent, and half from the other. Individuals sharing the same allele on both their chromosomes are said to be **homozygous** for that particular polymorphism; those having different alleles are therefore **heterozygous**.

Mutation or polymorphism?

The distinction between what is a pathogenic mutation and what is polymorphic variation is not always clear.

- A mutation can be defined as an alteration in the (normal) DNA sequence that affects protein function or expression.
- A polymorphism is defined as a locus where two or more alleles have been seen at a frequency greater than 0.01 (or 1%) in the population.

This implies therefore that a polymorphism is a mutation that is compatible with life in its **heterozygous** form.

Types of mutational events leading to polymorphisms

At the nucleotide level polymorphisms can be a **single base substitution**, the insertion or deletion of one or more bases, or **repeat length** or **copy number polymorphisms** and rearrangements. They are present through out the genome and can be subdivided into those alter a protein sequence (**coding polymorphisms**) and those which do not (**noncoding polymorphisms**).

Single nucleotide polymorphisms

The most common type of polymorphism in the human genome is the **single nucleotide polymorphism** or **SNP**. Each SNP will have two, or sometimes three, alleles. Approximately 10 million SNPs have been identified with a minor allele frequency of greater than 0.5%. SNPs are not homogeneous across the genome; the greatest diversity is found at the **human lymphocyte antigen** (**HLA**) locus, the least on the sex chromosomes. Less than 1% of SNPs are predicted to result in change in the composition of proteins and are therefore unlikely to be a major source of phenotypic variation. It is not currently known, however, to what extent SNPs in regulatory regions contribute toward phenotypic diversity.

Sequence variation that does not result in a change in the amino acid that is coded for are referred to as **silent** substitutions; those that produce an amino acid change, as **missense** mutations (e.g. **sickle cell disease**); and those that produce **stop codons**, as **nonsense** mutations.

Deletions and insertions

Deletions and insertions are defined as the loss or addition of one or more bases from a DNA sequence. Because of the

Sickle cell disease

Sickle cell disease is an example of a **missense** mutation in which A is replaced by T at the seventeenth nucleotide of the β-chain haemoglobin gene. The normal GAG codon for glutamic acid thus becomes GTG, which encodes the amino acid valine. When it is present in two copies it results in the **sickling** (a sickle shape) of red blood cells. The consequences of this are numerous, and include severe anaemia and tissue and organ damage due to the accumulation of the rigid red cells in small blood vessels (see Ch. 12).

Examples of deletions and insertions

Cystic fibrosis is a common inherited autosomal recessive genetic disorder among Caucasians, affecting as many as 1 in 2000 in northern Europe, leading to fibrotic lesions throughout the body, but particularly affecting the lungs, pancreas and intestines. The most common mutation involves a three-base deletion that removes the amino acid phenylalanine from the **cystic fibrosis transmembrane regulator** (**CFTR**) gene sequence, although more than 1300 mutations have been described involving several different mutational types.

The gene codes for a chloride channel protein controlling the movement of chloride from the inside to the outside of the cell, and from sweat into the cytoplasm in the sweat glands. The mutant gene needs to be present in two copies (recessive), inherited from both parents, to produce the disease. *CFTR* mutations lead to the negatively charged chloride ions being trapped and this accumulation also prevents the movement of positively charged ions, such as sodium. The ions combine to form salt, which is found in large amounts within sweat glands in this condition. This forms the basis of the **sweat test** for cystic fibrosis. The salt imbalance leads to loss of water and results in thick obstructive secretions, including mucus within the lungs. The thick mucus is an ideal environment for bacterial infections.

Huntington's disease results from increased numbers of repeated CAG (glutamine Q) sequences (polyQ) that produce a mutant Huntingtin protein (mHTT), which interferes with synaptic transmission in the brain. Neuronal transmission worsens with increasing size of the polyQ component.

PolyQ lengths involving more than 36 glutamines lead to increased neuronal death. An early age of onset and more rapid progression of the disease are associated with increased polyQ lengths. The autosomal dominant inheritance is also affected by 'dynamic' mutations, in which the number of repeats is not always exactly copied. The disease occurs at higher prevalence in the Afrikaner population of South Africa and is thought to be the result of a **founder** (see below), a Dutch man who arrived there in 1652 (see also Clinical box 5.7).

Fragile X syndrome results from stretches of CGG repeats in the X chromosome. Repeats can be many without obvious effect but the repeat stretch tends to get longer from generation to generation and several thousand repeats have been described. These very long repeats weaken the structure of the X chromosome and can lead to varied conditions including intellectual disability. Because females carry two X chromosomes, males are predominantly severely affected, though females can show variable clinical symptoms.

three-nucleotide code for a single amino acid, loss of bases that are not multiples of three is more likely to produce major detrimental effects (**frameshift** mutations).

Sometimes the proteins produced are truncated, or not produced at all. These types of mutation are often associated with recessive diseases. A four-base pair insertion in the *HEXA* gene results in low activity of an essential lysosomal enzyme, leading to Tay–Sachs disease when inherited in a recessive fashion. The mutation is prevalent in Ashkenazi Jews.

Some disorders are caused by insertions of nucleotides in multiples of three, preserving the **reading frame**. Several trinucleotide repeat diseases exist, such as **Huntington's disease**, and **fragile X syndrome**.

Gene duplications

In meiosis, when the sister chromatids line up, if there is a slight mismatch this can result in an unequal crossover, which can result in two copies of a gene. For example:

- Families showing two copies of the **aldosterone** gene suffer from high blood pressure and are at increased risk of stroke.

- **Charcot–Marie–Tooth** disease arises from a duplication on chromosome 17. One of the genes involved produces a protein involved in myelin formation; demyelination is one characteristic of this disease.

The unequal crossover can also interrupt the promoter region of the gene (**promoter mutation**), which may result in different gene expression.

Consequences of genetic mutation

Not all genetic variation is detrimental to the organism. SNPs can have positive or negative effects, or can be neutral. **Sickle cell disease** in its homozygous state is almost always lethal and one would expect the allele to be selected against, and therefore be very rare in all populations. The sickle gene is, however, present in about 15% of the black population. In its heterozygous state it causes mild anaemia but confers resistance to malaria. Thus the heterozygous individual is at an advantage in populations where malaria is present (Fig. 5.15). Comparison of African Americans with Africans has shown that the sickle cell gene is much reduced in African Americans, indicating that the gene is being eliminated where there is absence of positive selection pressure. This is an example of a **balanced mutation**.

Duplications lie at the core of evolution. Within single organisms there are many genes with similar sequences (**paralogous genes**) that have resulted from repeated duplications of an ancestral gene. In contrast, **orthologous genes** are homologous genes in different species – these are likely to have descended from a common ancestor. For example, there is about a 99% similarity between human and chimpanzee DNA, with the differences mostly being seen in those influencing the nervous system.

Paralogous genes can be beneficial by providing for **redundancy**. Removing a gene (such as in **knockout** mice) sometimes has little effect because the function has been taken over by a paralogue. Over time one of a pair of duplicated genes can also mutate and acquire a new and advantageous function (**adaptive evolution**).

Founder effects

The **founder effect** was defined by Ernst Mayr as 'The establishment of a new population by a few original founders (in an extreme case, by a single fertilised female) which carry only a small fraction of the total genetic variation of the parental population', and is recognised when a particular polymorphism can be traced back to a single individual.

The reasons for this phenomenon are twofold. First, a particular area may become populated with a small number of individuals, with all subsequent generations originating from these people while the particular population remains isolated (Fig. 5.16). For example, many individuals living in Tristan da Cunha originate from the original British settlement in 1816.

The second reason concerns the origin of a particular set of Y chromosome polymorphisms. The male Y chromosome is passed without change (other than rare mutations) through the generations. Thus males with the same paternal ancestors are very likely to share identical Y chromosome polymorphism (known as a **haplotype**, as there is only one Y chromosome).

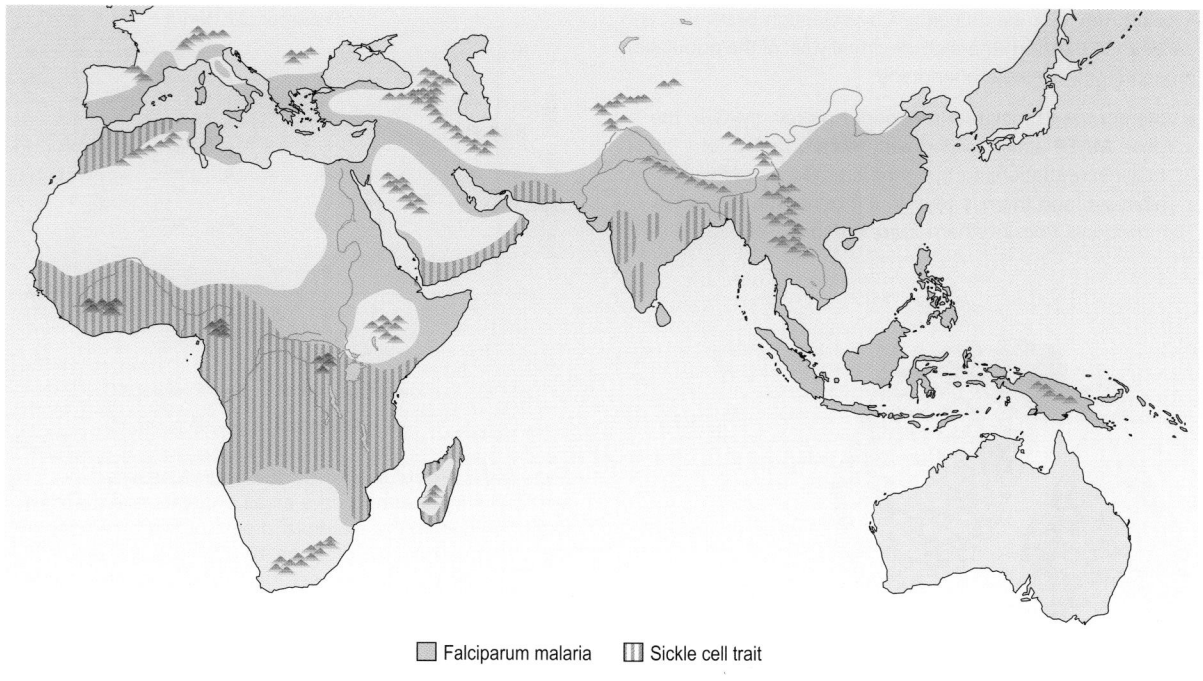

☐ Falciparum malaria   ⊞ Sickle cell trait

Fig. 5.15 **Map of the Old World showing regions where** *Plasmodium falciparum* **malaria and sickle cell trait are prevalent.** Source: www.ablongman.com/html/anthro/phys/databank/map2.18.html)

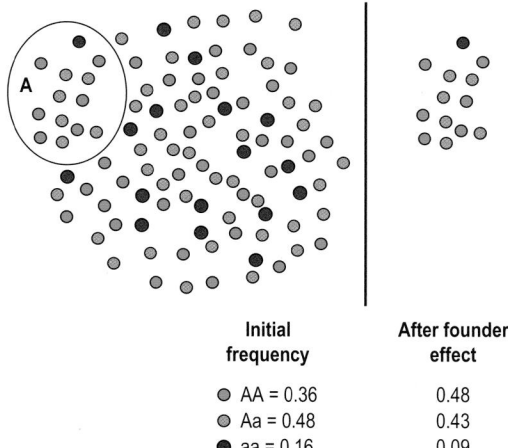

	Initial frequency	After founder effect
⬤ AA = 0.36		0.48
⬤ Aa = 0.48		0.43
⬤ aa = 0.16		0.09

Fig. 5.16 **Founder effect.** The relative frequencies of the different phenotypes in the population are shown on the left of the diagram. A small subpopulation that has become separated (area A) from the main population is shown on the right. The phenotype frequencies in this new population differ from the original by chance alone and as long as the founder population remains relatively isolated the founder frequencies will be propagated.

Genghis Khan and the founder effect

One particular Y chromosome haplotype is found in about 8% of the population in the former Mongolian Empire, and has spread throughout the world population. Although the success of this haplotype could be the result of it having some form of biological advantage, scientists have suggested that it could originate from the dynastic family of Genghis Khan and his male relatives in their predominance and subsequent spread of the Mongolian Empire across the whole of Asia. Social norms were very different at the time and Khan's male descendants appeared to have sired many sons from a high number of associations with women.

Bottlenecks

Sometimes the same effect can be the result of a **bottleneck**, where only a few individuals pass through, or survive, and then expand later. The individuals who pass through the bottleneck may have some polymorphisms that are rare in the original population, but proportionately are not so rare in the second new population.

A bottleneck is one possible reason for the very different mitochondrial sequences seen when comparing African and non-African populations. African mitochondrial DNA shows high divergence, whereas non-African lineages appear to be less divergent and originate from an African branch. This supports an **out-of-Africa** origin of humans and suggests that there might also have been a bottleneck some 80 000 years ago, with a relatively small population thereafter populating the whole of Europe and Asia (Fig. 5.17).

Population drift

Population drift has also resulted in populations in different areas possessing different polymorphisms. This has led to phenotypic variation in humans with respect to their race or geographical origin. Figure 5.18 illustrates this over a limited number of generations within a small population. In practice drift is seen to be inversely proportional to population size and so the frequency differences that we observe between populations are likely to have taken place over a considerable period of time.

Drift may also be influenced by selection pressures and can lead to **fixation** where all, or virtually all, of the population presents only a single phenotype.

■ Membrane associated transporter protein (MATP): the gene **MATP** is associated with the production of melanin (mutations in the gene are associated with albinism) and there is SNP in the gene that is fixed in individuals from northern Europe (Fig. 5.19).

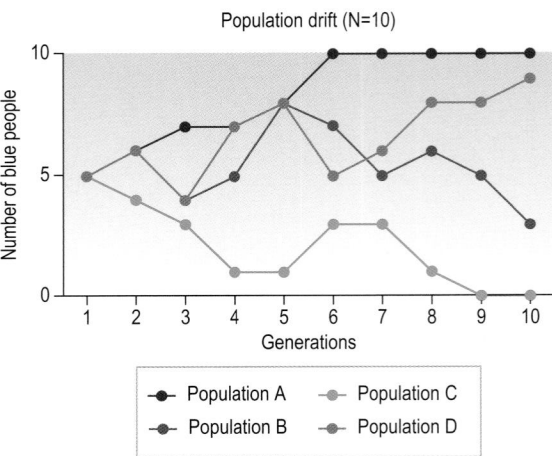

Fig. 5.18 Population drift: the figure illustrates the possible effects of drift on a small population that shows two phenotypes. For example, if sets of five blue people and five green people produce 10 offspring, the binomial theorem tells us that, on average, five will be blue. There will be some variation and it is quite possible that one of the sets will actually produce only four blue offspring (population C, for example). In the next generation of that set, on average, four will be blue. Not every set will produce four blue individuals: some, like population C, may have only three blue individuals; others may have more, or less. This results in **drift** of blue individuals. Eventually a population may end in **fixation**, with all individuals being all blue, or all green, as population A has after six generations (all blue people), and population C has after nine generations (all green people).

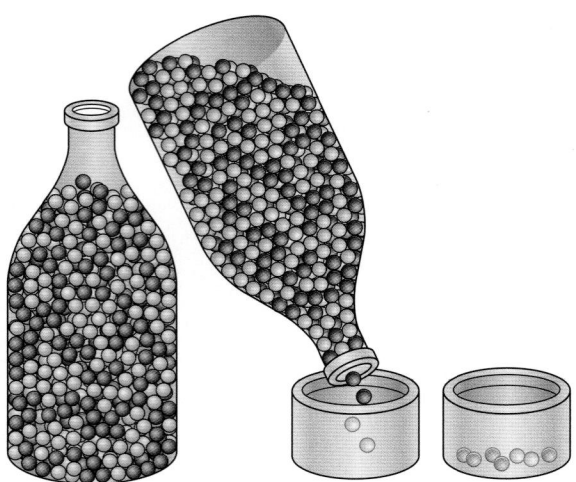

Fig. 5.17 Bottleneck effect. A 'bottleneck' that allows only a small proportion of the population through has the effect of reducing genetic variation in the new population. Bottlenecks could result from stringent conditions due to geography or climate.

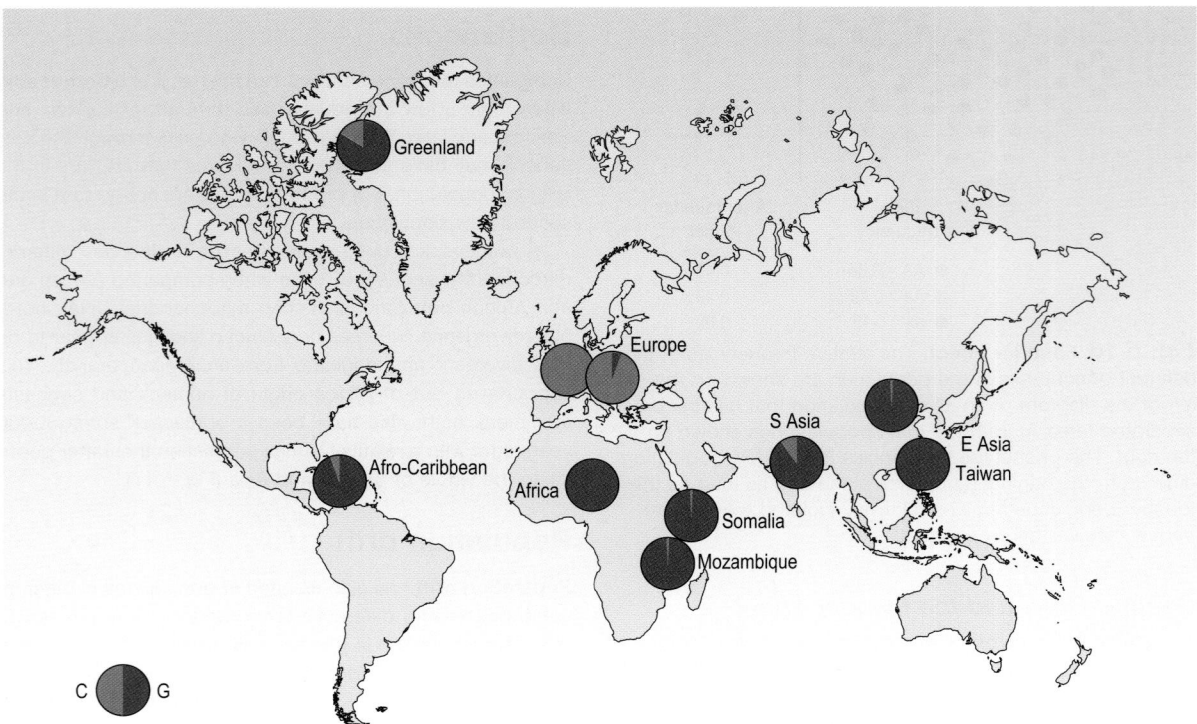

Fig. 5.19 Fixation in the MATP gene single nucleotide polymorphism (SNP). The C SNP (shown in blue) is almost universally found among white-skinned Europeans, although the G SNP (shown in red) does not identify individuals with a dark skin as the latter also predominates among the light-skinned south-east Asian populations.

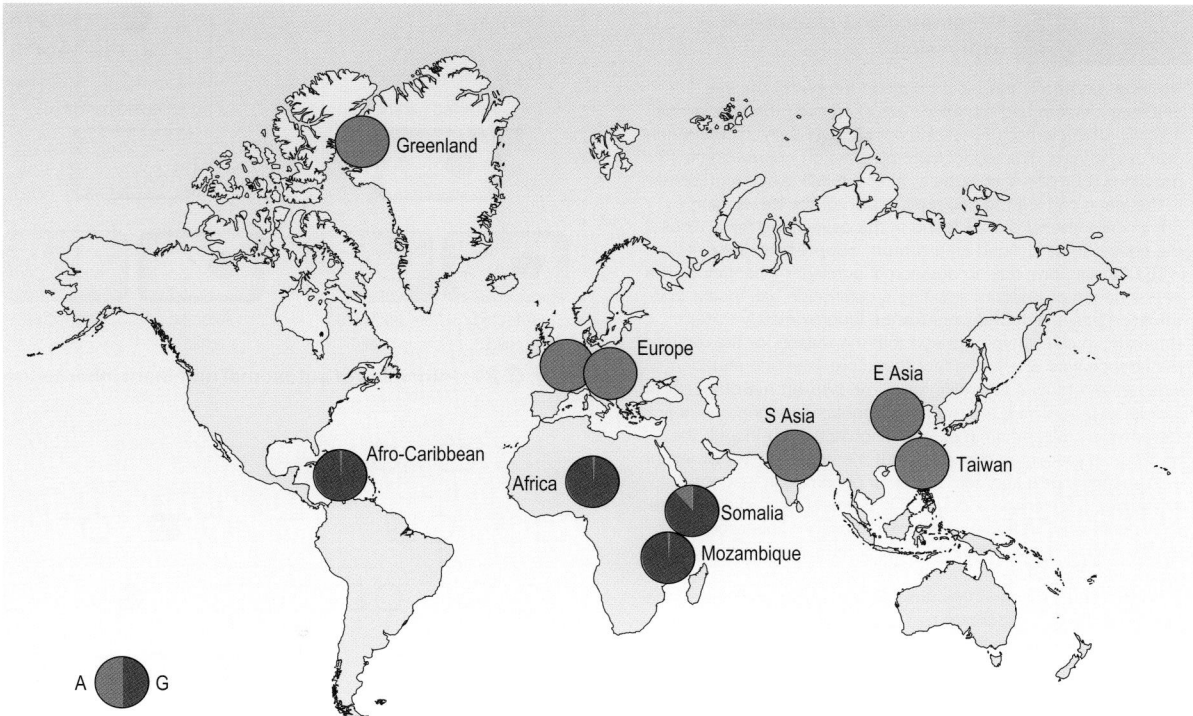

Fig. 5.20 Fixation in the *DARC* gene single nucleotide polymorphism (SNP). The G SNP (shown in red) is found among individuals of African origin that have originated from areas where malaria is prevalent. The more evident mixture of the two SNPs seen in the Somali population reflects the admixture in Somalia with the nearby Asian population.

- Duffy antigen receptor for chemokines (DARC): the *DARC* gene has a SNP that codes for a particular Duffy blood group polymorphism, Fy (a⁻b⁻) in which the DARC protein is not expressed. The G polymorphism has reached fixation among a large proportion of individuals of African origin (Fig. 5.20). Its predominance appears to be related to environmental pressure from the malarial parasite that uses the DARC as a receptor in order to infect the red blood cell.

Genotypes, phenotypes and genetic penetrance

A **genotype** is the allelic composition at a particular locus. Because autosomal chromosomes are present in pairs, inherited from an individual's parents, there are also pairs of alleles on these chromosomes. When the same allele is inherited from both mother and father, the individual is said to be **homozygous**, and when the alleles are different, the individual is said to be **heterozygous** at that locus.

- For example, an individual who is blood group O has inherited the O gene from both mother and father, and is therefore homozygous for the O allele.
- An individual who is blood group AB has inherited an A gene from one parent and a B gene from the other; therefore the individual is heterozygous for the A and B alleles.

Whereas the genotype details all the alleles present at a locus, the **phenotype** details the alleles that can be observed:

- For example, the *genotype* of someone who is blood group O is OO, whereas the *phenotype* is O.

Table 5.1	Phenotype series associated with cardiovascular disease
Phenotype	**Examples**
Healthy	Possessing none of the following
Possessing risk factors	Hyperlipidaemia, diabetes, smoking, hypertension, possession of certain haemostatic and inflammatory mediators
Subclinical disease	Coronary, carotid and peripheral atherosclerosis
Clinical complex disease	Coronary artery disease, peripheral vascular disease, stroke, death from cardiovascular disease, sudden death

- In blood group AB, both the genotype and phenotype are AB.
- Other ABO blood groups are more complicated because both the A and B alleles are dominant over the O allele. An individual who is blood group A (phenotype is A) may be homozygous with a genotype AA, or heterozygous with a genotype AO.

Sometimes, despite a particular genotype, the phenotype is not expressed. This extent to which the phenotype is expressed is known as **penetrance**, and alterations in penetrance can be a characteristic of certain disease processes. Penetrance may be reduced, or possibly age dependent. Phenotypic expression can also be variable, even though penetrance is 100%, due to allelic heterogeneity, modifier genes and environmental experience (see Clinical box 5.7) (Table 5.1).

Penetrance and phenotypic expression

Retinoblastoma is the most common tumour of the eye affecting children and mutations are expressed through familial (usually affecting both eyes) and sporadic (usually affecting only one eye) origins. The retinoblastoma gene on chromosome 13 produces a protein that helps control the cell cycle. Mutations in this gene can lead to cell proliferation of the developing retinal cells (retinal blasts) found in the developing fetus. Thus the gene can be defined as a **tumour suppressor gene**.

The familial form has an autosomal dominant inheritance. The phenomenon of tumours skipping a generation has meant that the gene has a **reduced penetrance** (approximately 90%). Knudson, in 1971, hypothesised that the reason for the reduced penetrance was due to the fact that more than one mutation was needed to lead to proliferation (the **two-hit hypothesis**). An individual possessing the mutant retinoblastoma gene does not experience proliferation in every retinoblast, even though the mutation is present in every cell, but the large number of retinal cells means that a sporadic mutation occurring in just one retinoblast, resulting in a double hit, is much more likely. Those individuals who do not, by chance, experience this second hit, remain free of disease, but still have a 50% chance of passing on the affected gene.

Huntington's disease (**Huntington's chorea**) is an autosomal dominant disease described by George Huntington in 1872. It is a neurological disease that usually becomes apparent in middle age and leads to progressive loss of motor control and dementia. The disease normally has 100% penetrance (all who inherit the defect will be sufferers) but is an example of **age-dependent penetrance**. The famous American folk musician Woody Guthrie died of the disease in 1967. Until the molecular defect was identified, children of affected individuals could only wait to see if they had inherited the gene from their parent. The defect is due to a trinucleotide expansion of CAG repeats within the HD gene, resulting in an accumulation of a neuronal transport protein (**Huntingtin**) around neuronal nuclei, leading to neuronal death. Paternal transmission of the disease tends to result in a higher repeat instability (**anticipation**), resulting in even greater expansions and earlier onset.

Osteogenesis imperfecta (**brittle bone disease**) is due to an inherited defect in collagen production and leads to affected individuals being particularly vulnerable to bone fractures. Some individuals have many fractures, others have few, and the degree of severity can be different within the same family (**variable phenotypic expression**). Several reasons have been proposed for the varying severity of this disease:

- **Allelic heterogeneity:** different mutations within the procollagen molecule, which is then further cleaved to form collagen, can result in different disease severity, depending on the end of the molecule the mutations occur.
- **Gene modifiers:** even where genes are inherited, individuals may experience different disease severity. This is thought to be due to the presence of genes at a different loci that interact with the gene, changing its expression.
- **Environmental factors:** an event that results in a bone fracture can mean that the damaged area is much more vulnerable to subsequent trauma.

MODES OF INHERITANCE

MENDELIAN DISORDERS

A **Mendelian disorder** is defined as a trait that is associated with one specific genotype, such as a mutation at a particular genetic locus. There are a number of different forms of single gene disorders, based on:

- The pattern of inheritance being either **dominant** or **recessive**
- Whether the mutation is **autosomal** or **sex linked**.

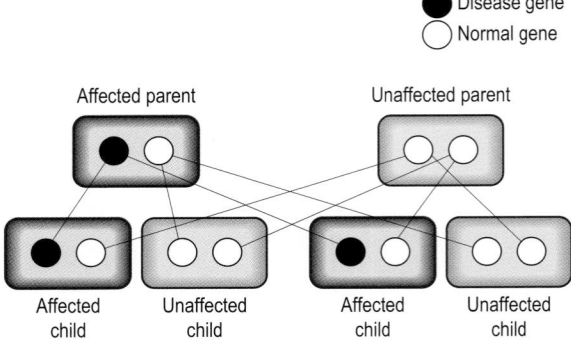

Fig. 5.21 **Principles of autosomal dominant inheritance.**

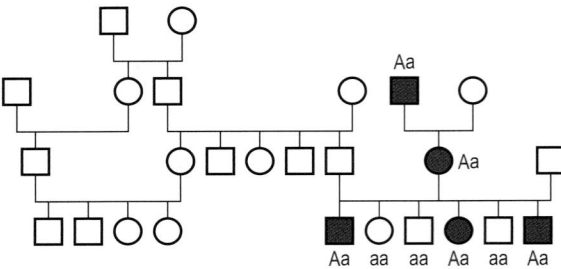

Fig. 5.22 **Pedigree illustrating the typical pattern in autosomal dominant disease inheritance.** Affected individuals are shown in solid red, with the normal gene being indicated by (a) and the disease gene by (A). Autosomal dominant inheritance typically results in the disease being seen in each generation, with about half the offspring being affected, regardless of their gender.

In reality, it is often very difficult to determine the mode of inheritance of the disorder in many families for a number of reasons (see below).

Autosomal dominant inheritance (Figs 5.21 and 5.22)

Autosomal dominant disorders are seen in around 1 in every 200 individuals. The main characteristics of autosomal dominant inheritance are:

- Sex-independent – that is, it affects both sexes and can be transmitted by either sex
- One of the affected child's parents will also be affected with the same condition
- A child with an affected parent has a 50% chance of inheriting the disease genotype
- The mutant genotype, when present on only one of the autosomes, is sufficient to cause the disorder.

Dominance is when the expression of the wild-type (normal) allele is not sufficient to prevent the manifestation of the disorder and is normally associated with a **gain of function**. Cellular mechanisms associated with dominant mutations are:

- Overproduction of a protein at the wrong time, or in the wrong place. For example, in **neurofibromatosis type II**, a deletion of a tumour suppressor gene leads to overgrowth of the Schwann cells that surround nerve cells. An example is an acoustic neuroma.
- **Dominant-negative effects:** the mutant protein inhibits the function of the normal protein produced by the wild-

type allele. For example, in **glucocorticoid resistance syndrome**, a mutation in the gene for GR decreases the activity of hGRα protein, which in turn leads to excessive secretion of androgen hormones.

- **Haplo-insufficiency** may also produce a dominant disorder. This occurs when loss of 50% of the protein product is not sufficient for normal function. For example, in **familial hypercholesterolaemia**, a gene mutation in the LDL receptor (*LDLR*) gene results in loss of half the receptors for transporting LDL, leading to a build-up in circulating cholesterol.

- **Anticipation** is seen in a small proportion of autosomal dominant disorders, including fragile X and Huntington's disease. It describes the phenomenon seen when the disease becomes progressively more severe and has an earlier onset through each generation, related to an increase in trinucleotide repeats as the gene is transmitted. A critical expansion size has an adverse effect on the RNA and protein production that it is associated with. For example, in Huntington's disease, greater than 36 repeats are associated with the disease, but repeats of between 10 and 26 are present among normal individuals.

Autosomal recessive inheritance

(Figs 5.23 and 5.24)

Autosomal recessive disorders are more rare, being seen in about 1 in 500 individuals and may appear as a sporadic mutation. Only when another affected child is born is the genetic nature of the disease recognised (unless it is an already known recessive disorder). Characteristics of autosomal recessive disorders are:

- Sex independent
- The affected child inherits the disease gene from both parents (the child will be homozygous for the disease gene)
- The affected child's parents appear normal (the parents will be heterozygous **carriers**, carrying a normal and a disease gene)
- A child with carrier parents has a 25% chance of inheriting the disease genotype and a 25% chance of inheriting a normal genotype
- 50% of children of carrier parents will also be heterozygous carriers
- Offspring of consanguineous relationships are more likely to have an autosomal recessive disorder because the disease gene, if present, will be present at a higher frequency within a family.

Recessive disorders are often characterised by **loss-of-function** mutations. The mutation results in a complete loss of protein production, but in the heterozygous individual protein continues to be produced at 50% of the normal level. Where this level continues to be sufficient for normal function (contrast with haplo-insufficiency), heterozygous individuals will be unaffected.

For example, in **oculocutaneous albinism**, there is a defect in melanin production, caused by a mutation on chromosome 11 that results in a lack of expression of the protein tyrosinase. When no tyrosinase is produced (in the homozygous individual) the lack of melanin results in the pale skin, white hair and pink eyes associated with albinism.

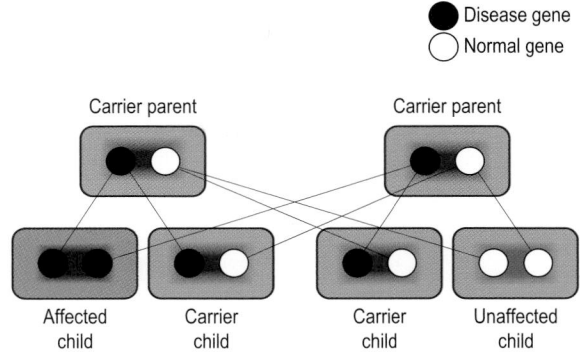

Fig. 5.23 **Principles of autosomal recessive inheritance.**

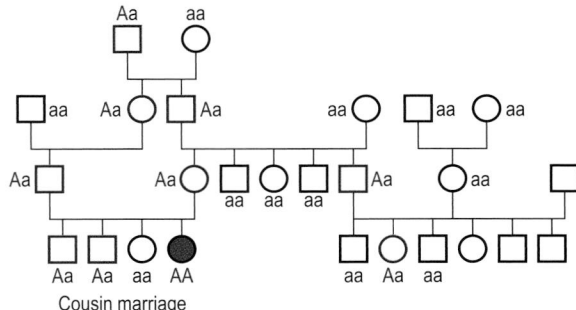

Fig. 5.24 **Pedigree illustrating the typical pattern in autosomal recessive disease inheritance.** The affected individual is shown in solid red, and carriers outlined in red, with the normal gene being indicated by (a) and the disease gene by (A). Autosomal recessive inheritance typically results in the disease being seen in siblings, regardless of their gender, but usually not in previous generations. Only about a quarter of the offspring of carrier parents are affected, and sibling expression is therefore only likely in larger families, although another 50% are carriers. In very rare disorders consanguinity is likely to be evident in the family.

Consanguinity and recessive disorders

The rate of transmission of recessive disorders increases dramatically with increased incidence of consanguineous matings, or relatively high frequency of recessive alleles in the population. The latter is often related to heterozygote advantage, whereby recessive alleles are maintained in the population as they offer some selective advantage in the heterozygous form. For example, carriers of the **sickle cell** gene appear to be protected against malaria, and mutations in the **cystic fibrosis** gene are thought to offer some protection against cholera and other diarrhoeal diseases.

Sometimes recessive disorders appear to occur at a relatively high frequency in the population because mutations in a number of different genes result in clinically similar disorders, for example **non-syndromic sensorineural deafness**.

Coefficient of relationship

Related individuals are more likely to share mutant genes that have been inherited from a common ancestor. The **coefficient of relationship (COR)** provides a measure of the probability of related individuals sharing a gene.

As a parent will pass half of his or her genes to their children then we can say that the probability that the parent and child share a particular gene is 0.5. As there are two parents,

Table 5.2	Coefficient of relationship values
Relationship	**Coefficient of relationship (probability of gene sharing)**
Full siblings	$\frac{1}{2}$
Half siblings	$\frac{1}{4}$
Grandparents	$\frac{1}{4}$
Uncles/aunts	$\frac{1}{4}$
First cousins	$\frac{1}{8}$
Second cousins	$\frac{1}{16}$

each parent will have a 0.5 chance of sharing a particular gene with their child, but together they have a $0.5 + 0.5 = 1.0$ (certain) chance of sharing a particular gene with their child. This makes sense as all genes present in a child must have been inherited from one or other parent, unless there has been a mutational event.

The COR can be calculated using the formula:

$$COR = \left(\frac{1}{2}\right)^N$$

- where *N* is the number of generation steps between individuals and a common ancestor.

For example, there are two generation steps between siblings through their common father:

$$COR = \left(\frac{1}{2}\right)^2 = \frac{1}{4}$$

- *and* an additional two generation steps between siblings through their common mother.

Therefore the combined COR for siblings is $\frac{1}{4} + \frac{1}{4} = \frac{1}{2}$. In other words, siblings will share half their genes, on average. Probabilities for gene sharing between other related individuals can be calculated in the same fashion. Table 5.2 gives these probabilities down to second cousins.

Rare disorders and consanguinity

Cystic fibrosis is one of the most common autosomal recessive disorders affecting northern Europeans. About 4% of individuals (1 in 25) are carriers, leading to a prevalence of affected children in the population of around 1 in 2500.

- Chance of two individuals having the cystic fibrosis gene = $\frac{1}{25} \times \frac{1}{25} = \frac{1}{625}$
- Chance of both parents passing the cystic fibrosis gene to their children = $\frac{1}{2} \times \frac{1}{2} = \frac{1}{4}$
- Chance of a newborn child having cystic fibrosis = $\frac{1}{4} \times \frac{1}{625} = \frac{1}{2500}$

Someone who is a carrier has a 1 in 25 chance of mating with another carrier if he chooses a partner from the general population. If the carrier chooses his cousin as a partner, the chance that his cousin is also a carrier is 1 in 8 (from the COR calculation). Mating of cousins is therefore about three times more likely to result in a child with cystic fibrosis.

Familial Mediterranean fever is a very rare autosomal recessive disorder where affected individuals suffer from acute fevers, but is generally seen only in a few restricted populations around the world. The highest number of cases are found in Israel where the frequency of cousin marriages approaches 50% among the Arabic population. A very rare autosomal recessive disorder therefore can become considerably more likely (in comparison with cystic fibrosis, for example) in a population with a high rate of consanguinity.

X-linked inheritance

The Y (male) chromosome is relatively gene-free and there are no significant disorders associated with mutations on the Y chromosome; if there were, they would only affect the males in the family. However, there are a large number of **X-linked** disorders that can be inherited either in a dominant or a recessive manner.

Lyonisation

Proteins produced by genes on the X chromosome are expressed at similar levels in males and females, whereas it might be expected that, because females have two X chromosomes, they may produce double the amount of protein. In the 1960s, Mary Lyon hypothesised that one of the two X chromosomes is inactivated, and that this happens at random, sometimes affecting the paternally derived X chromosome, and sometimes the maternally derived X chromosome. This is known as **lyonisation** or the **Lyon hypothesis**. Evidence supporting the hypothesis came from an observation made in the 1940s of interphase nuclei which showed densely staining chromatin material in females, but not in males. These have become known as **Barr** bodies, named after their discoverer, Murray Barr. Individuals who have variable numbers of X chromosomes will also have more or fewer Barr bodies. XXY male individuals will have one Barr body, XXX females will have two Barr bodies and X females will have none.

Biochemical evidence of the phenomenon was shown when individual cells in females heterozygous for variants of glucose-6-phosphate dehydrogenase were shown to express just a single variant type. The inactivation takes place very early on after fertilisation and is not complete, spreading down the long arm of the X chromosome. It must also be reversible in cells destined to become egg cells, which will only carry a single set of chromosomes.

Males are thus **hemizygous** for X (because they only have a half representative in the pair) and females are **mosaics** for the X chromosome because they have two different populations of cells, some carrying active maternal X chromosomes, and others having active paternal X chromosomes.

Dominant X-linked inheritance (Figs 5.25 and 5.26)

Dominant X-linked disorders can affect either sex, but predominantly affect females. This is because all female offspring of an affected male will inherit the mutation on the X, but male offspring will receive the affected man's Y chromosome and therefore be normal. Offspring of an affected female (carrier) will have a 50% chance of passing on the gene, to both males and females: hence the slight female imbalance.

Because females still have a normal X chromosome their disease may be milder. In certain conditions, males, having no normal X chromosome material, may die in utero. Dominant X-linked diseases are much rarer than the recessive forms.

- **Incontinentia pigmenti** is a single gene disorder of the X chromosome due to mutations in NF-κB essential

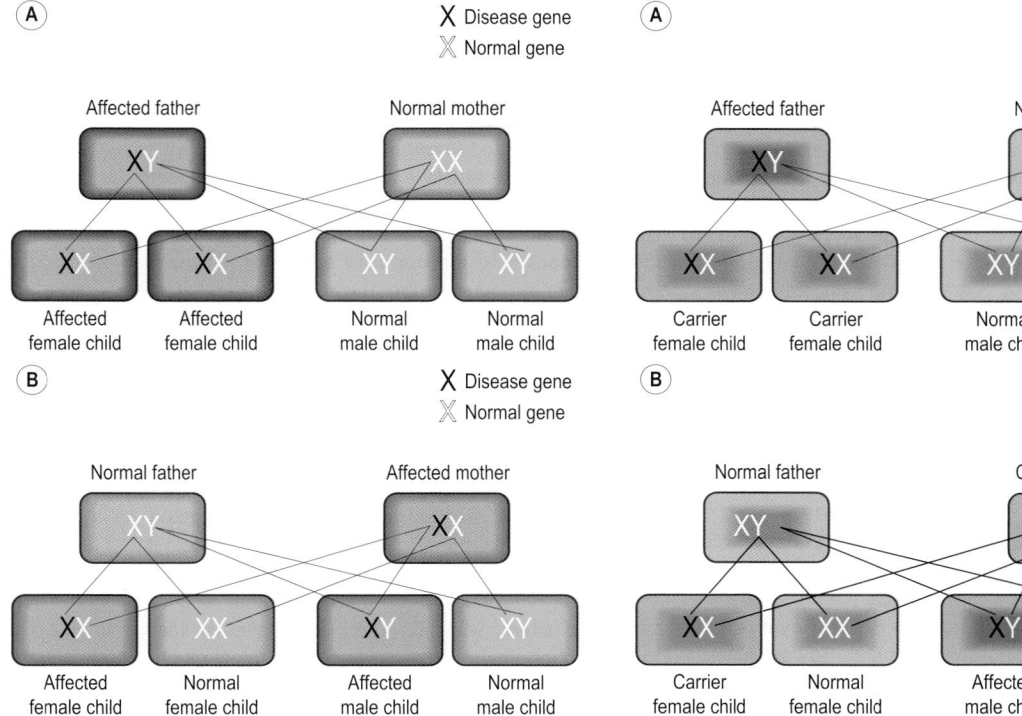

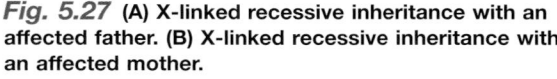

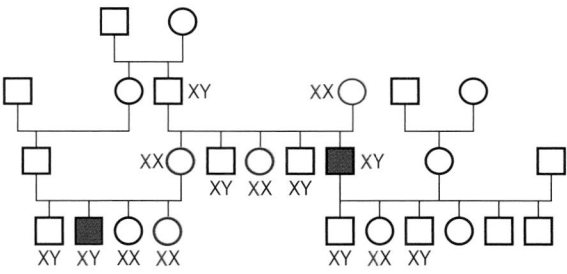

Fig. 5.25 **(A) X-linked dominant inheritance with an affected father.** When the father has the disease all of his female offspring will be affected, but males will be normal. **(B) X-linked dominant inheritance with an affected mother.** When the mother has the disease, half of her children will be affected, regardless of gender.

Fig. 5.26 **Pedigree illustrating X-linked dominant inheritance.** Affected individuals are show in solid red, with the normal X gene being shown in black, and the diseased X gene in red. X-linked dominant inheritance typically results in the disease being seen in each generation, like autosomal dominant disorders. In contrast, affected individuals are predominantly female. Males can only pass the disease to their daughters. Females pass the affected X chromosome to about half of their offspring, regardless of gender.

modulator (NEMO). The gene is also known as inhibitor of κ light polypeptide gene enhancer in B cells kinase gamma (IKBKG or IKK-gamma) and affects tissues derived from the embryonic ectoderm and neuroectoderm. As well as early skin involvement, which gets worse with age, there are often major developmental and other nervous system problems. Female carriers of the gene for NEMO are only mildly affected. There appears to be selective apoptosis as part of the X-inactivation process, promoting the normal X chromosome containing cells. Males usually die in utero.

Fig. 5.27 **(A) X-linked recessive inheritance with an affected father. (B) X-linked recessive inheritance with an affected mother.**

Fig. 5.28 **Typical X-linked recessive inheritance.** Pedigree illustrating the typical pattern in X-linked recessive disease inheritance. Affected individuals are shown in solid red, and carriers outlined in red, with the normal gene being shown in black and the diseased gene in red. X-linked recessive inheritance typically results in the disease being seen in some males only, with a sporadic appearance within the family. While the disease may be evident among male siblings and other relatives, it would not be seen in the parents, as affected fathers can only pass the disease gene on to their daughters, who will be carriers. Carriers will have a 50% chance of passing the affected chromosome on to their male offspring, who will show the disease, and a 50% chance of passing it to their female offspring, who will also then be carriers.

■ **Hypophosphataemic rickets** is an X-linked disorder where the reduced amounts of inorganic phosphate lead to problems in bone ossification. The disorder is milder in females because of the random X inactivation, leaving some of the cells carrying the normal X chromosome.

Recessive X-linked inheritance (Figs 5.27 and 5.28)
Recessive X-linked disorders are more prevalent than the dominant forms and, in the vast majority of cases, affect only the male offspring. This is because males with the disease

inherit an abnormal X chromosome from a female carrier (they are **hemizygous**), whereas females will generally only inherit one abnormal chromosome, the presence of the normal X chromosome being sufficient for normal life, despite having lower levels of the gene product. This leads to an inheritance that skips generations and is only evident in males.

Haemophilia A is the best known of the two haemophilic disorders, this one resulting from a defect in the factor VIII gene. Affected individuals produce very low levels (less than 1% normal) of factor VIII, which is a key component of the intrinsic clotting pathway. As well as severe external bleeds, sufferers experience bleeds into joints, resulting in joint deformities; intercranial bleeding used to be a common cause of early death before treatment options improved.

Other examples of X-linked recessive disorders are haemophilia B, red-green colour blindness, fragile X syndrome and Duchenne's muscular dystrophy.

Haemophilia A – the royal disease

One of Queen Victoria's nine children, Leopold, died at the age of 31, from an internal head bleed after a fall as a result of inheriting haemophilia A. He was the only one of four sons to suffer from the disorder. The British Royal Family, which stems from Queen Victoria's first son, Edward, has therefore remained free of the disease. Before Leopold died he married and produced a daughter, an obligate carrier, Alice, and one of her sons developed haemophilia.

Haemophilia A is found as a new, spontaneous, mutation in about one-third of cases. Before Leopold was born there was no history of the disease in the family, and his disease could have resulted from a spontaneous mutation in himself. Evidence that he inherited it from Queen Victoria, however, came from the marriages of two of Victoria's daughters, Alice and Beatrice.

■ Alice married into the Prussian Royal Family and one of her sons, and three of her grandchildren, including the famous Alexis, son of Czar Nicholas II of Russia, had the disease. Prince Philip, who was one of her great-grandchildren down a female line, would have been potentially vulnerable had the intervening females been carriers, but the disease has not developed in any male in that line.
■ Beatrice had two sons with the disease and her daughter married into the Spanish Royal Family, resulting in two more affected sons.

It is generally accepted that Queen Victoria received her carrier status as a new mutational event. Her father was old at her conception, suggesting that his age may have been instrumental. (Sperm are more vulnerable to mutations as they are continuously produced from a bank of primitive cells that may accumulate mutations with age; this is in contrast to egg cells which are essentially frozen in time until signalled to develop through fertilisation.) This theory has not stopped historians from speculating that she was the illegitimate child of a haemophilic man. It is also possible that Victoria inherited the disease from a carrier mother as several male children of her maternal antecedents died young.

Other modes of inheritance

Genetic imprinting

The expression of some mutant genes during development, and in diseases such as cancer, may be dependent on the parental origin. The mechanism that regulates the differential expression of two alleles of the same gene is termed **genetic imprinting**.

The imprinted locus follows a Mendelian pattern of inheritance. The first examples discovered were **Prader–Willi syndrome** and **Angelman's syndrome**, the former related to loss of the paternally expressed gene and the latter to loss of the maternally expressed gene. The mutations are only expressed when they are passed through the gametogenesis process leading to the opposite sex. Both disorders are related to genes found in the 15q11–q13 region of the genome. The region is about 5 Mb and consists of three regions:

■ Distal – non-imprinted genes
■ Central – maternally expressed genes
■ Proximal – paternally expressed genes

These regions appear to be under the control of an **imprinting centre**.

DNA methylation has been suggested as a possible mechanism for imprinting, as hypermethylated areas are associated with inactive chromatin regions. There is also an asynchronous DNA replication that occurs in these gene clusters, with non-imprinted alleles replicating earlier. This phenomenon is also seen in the female X chromosomes that are inactivated by the lyonisation process.

Mitochondrial disorders

Although most genetic diseases are associated with nuclear DNA, mitochondrial mutations lead to a significant number of inherited disorders. A feature of **MtDNA** is that it has a much higher mutation rate than nuclear DNA (5–10 times higher).

Mitochondrial inheritance of a disorder produces unique inheritance patterns because it is passed only by the mother but can affect offspring of either sex. During fertilisation the sperm cell contributes only nuclear DNA, the MtDNA being that present in the material egg cell.

Mitochondria are membrane-bound cytoplasmic organelles present in large numbers in a single cell and are essential for cell metabolism in the production of ATP. MtDNA has 16 569 base pairs in a double-stranded circular molecule. MtDNA has no introns (redundant genetic code); about 93%

Clinical box 5.8 Some clinical syndromes associated with gene deletion

Prader–Willi syndrome (PWS) is a common microdeletion causing genetic obesity and associated with neuro-behavioural disorders. It is caused by transmission of a maternal imprinting mutation, but is only expressed when passed from a female ancestor through a male during the gametogenesis process. The normal loss of the maternal epigenotype during male gametogenesis does not happen (the maternal–paternal switch is blocked) and maternal imprinting will therefore be transmitted to half of the gametes. Those individuals who inherit the abnormal epigenotype develop PWS.

Angelman's syndrome is characterised by particular behavioural features of intense happiness, associated with developmental delay, seizures, hyperactivity and severe intellectual disability. In most patients there is a large deletion in the maternally derived chromosome. It is caused by transmission of a paternal imprinting mutation when passed from a male ancestor through the female germline. It blocks the paternal–maternal switch, leading to the inheritance of an abnormal paternal epigenotype in about half the offspring, affected individuals developing Angelman's syndrome.

Clinical syndromes associated with mitochondrial DNA mutation

Leber's hereditary optic neuropathy (**LHON**) is an inherited form of blindness due to gradual atrophy of the optic nerve. It has a maternal inheritance and, although affecting both sexes, affects males more than females. In 1988, it was linked to several mitochondrial DNA mutations but the reason for the male predominance has not been explained.

Other conditions linked with mitochondrial mutations are:

- Kearns–Sayre syndrome – muscle weakness and heart failure
- Chronic progressive external ophthalmoplegia (CPEO) – paralysis of external eye muscles
- Myoclonic epilepsy with ragged red fibres (MERRF) – epilepsy and myopathy
- Mitochondrial myopathy, encephalopathy, lactic acidosis with stroke-like episodes (MELAS).

Mitochondrial mutations are also linked to common disease processes: diabetes, deafness and Alzheimer's disease and are associated with the ageing processes.

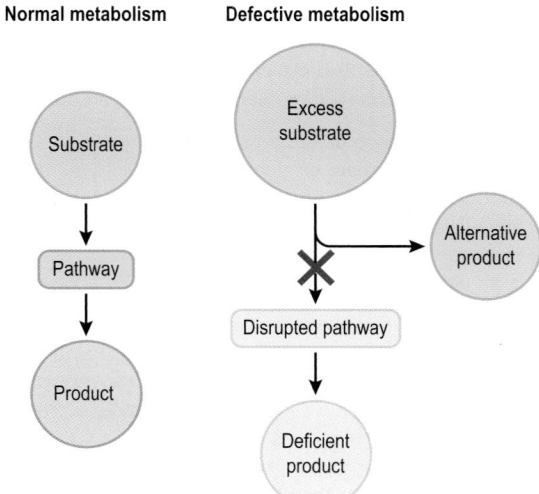

Fig. 5.29 Pathological mechanisms in inborn errors of metabolism. The defective enzyme or transporter within a metabolic pathway leads to a build-up of substances upstream and a loss of product downstream with clinical consequences being related to any potential toxicity of the excess material or alternative product, and effect of the lack of the intended product.

is coding (compared with about 3% of nuclear DNA). Mitochondria are thought to have origins as aerobic bacteria enabling oxidative phosphorylation.

Disease expression of a mitochondrial mutation also depends on whether all the mitochondria in a cell are identical (**homoplasmy**) or whether different populations of mitochondria exist (**heteroplasmy**) and, when heteroplasmy exists, what proportion carries a mutation. Because of the random segregation of mitochondria in cell division the proportion can vary between mother and child, leading to **variable penetrance**.

Mosaicism

Mosaicism is when more than one genotype contributes to the phenotype of an organism. An adult has approximately 10 trillion cells, and mutations occur at any given locus about once in every 50 000–1 000 000 cell divisions. It is, therefore, likely that we are all mosaics in some sense. The effect of these mutations will depend on how many cells are involved, where the cells are, and which genes are affected. There are three types of mosaicism:

- **Chromosomal mosaicism** occurs in all females, in that there is random, almost complete inactivation of one of the X chromosomes.
- **Somatic cell mosaicism** is a mutation that can occur in any body cell, rather than a germline cell, and may not be very apparent as they may only affect portions of the body. Somatic mutations that occur early in the embryonic process will have more wide-ranging phenotypic effects and can lead to gonadal mosaicism. Somatic cell mosaicism is a common event in the development of cancer; for example cancer might be the result of mutation in a tumour suppressor gene. All subsequent cancer cells will retain this mutation.
- **Gonadal mosaicism** occurs in the germ cells and may be present in a small or significant proportion of the germ cells. This form of mosaicism:
  - Leads to the observation of two or more affected children from normal parents with 'apparently' non-mutant genotypes. The pedigree would suggest an autosomal recessive inheritance
  - Often occurs in very severe disorders that would normally result in impaired reproduction. Thus the

only way the disorder can be transmitted is either by new mutation, or via a 'mosaic' germline from a phenotypically normal parent

- Is the cause of some incidences of osteogenesis imperfecta, epidermolysis bullosa, Ehlers–Danlos syndrome type IV and Duchenne's and Becker's muscular dystrophies

Inborn errors of metabolism (see Ch. 3)

The term 'inborn errors of metabolism' was used by Sir Archibald Garrod in 1908 to describe the genetically inherited amino acid disorder, **alkaptonuria**, or 'black urine disease'. Although individually rare, many disorders have been described, simply reflecting the vast numbers of metabolic reactions in the human, all of which have the potential for error. Overall they affect about 16 per 100 000 births and result in significant morbidity and mortality. They may present clinically in the prenatal environment, through to adulthood.

Traditionally inborn errors of metabolism are thought of as Mendelian traits caused by single gene mutations, normally inherited in an autosomal recessive fashion; however, greater understanding of many of these diseases has shown that they are often a more complex interaction between genes and nutrients. The primary defect is best considered in relation to an alteration in **metabolic flux**. In the classical sense only one metabolite flux is involved but in a more complex disease more fluxes might be involved, all leading to a particular phenotype, typical of the disease. Any metabolic pathway can be affected and may affect any organ or system. For example, fatty acid metabolism defects can result in low blood glucose (hypoglycaemia), loss of muscle (rhabdomyolysis), changes affecting heart muscle (cardiomyopathy) and liver disease.

The pathogenic mechanism is normally associated with a loss of function or a gain of function, of an altered protein, generally an enzyme or transporter (Fig. 5.29). The actual genetic change can be of any type – point mutation, deletion, insertion, rearrangement – and affect different regions of the gene. The clinical consequence of the defect is related to the changed metabolic flux and can be due to:

- Toxicity of excess upstream substrate
- Lack of downstream product
- Feedback activation or inhibition of this or other pathways
- Diversion of the metabolite to other pathways, resulting in an alternative product.

Treatment of inborn errors of metabolism depends on the particular defect but these conditions can often be treated through diet, whether restriction of a substrate, replacement of the enzyme, or supplementation of downstream products. For example, phenylalanine is an essential amino acid that is normally metabolised by **phenylalanine hydroxylase**. Where there are mutations in this enzyme **phenylketonuria** (**PKU**) results. The amino acid accumulates and disrupts cellular processes in the brain, causing intellectual disability. Restriction of phenylalanine in the diet can ensure development of children with normal intelligence.

POLYGENIC OR COMPLEX DISEASE

The main genetic contribution to human disease is found in relation to much more complex genetic interactions between different genes. **Polygenic disease** is defined as a disease thought to be caused by the effects of two or more genes. When environmental factors are also thought to influence the expression of the disease, then its cause is said to be **multifactorial**. As a consequence the presence of a genetic variant in the family is not sufficient to lead to the disease, but this may significantly increase the risk to family members (Fig. 5.30). There are many examples of multifactorial diseases, **hypertension** and **diabetes** being two examples.

CONTINUOUS EFFECTS MODELS

Polygenic diseases are influenced by a series of different factors to varying degrees; therefore they do not exhibit simple inheritance patterns that tend to suggest that a disease is either present or absent. Where the traits are expressed quantitatively they tend to follow a bell-shaped distribution. **Height**, for example, which is typical in this respect, may be influenced by a series of SNPs that collectively influence height. These genetic polymorphisms appear to act in an additive fashion, each adding or subtracting small amounts to the phenotype. They also interact with environmental factors, such as diet, to determine final height.

Diseases are often characterised by their phenotypes in series, from the healthy state, through a disease risk state and subclinical disease, ending with the clinical complex disease. Progression through the phenotypes is influenced by various environmental and genetic determinants. Clinical and scientific assessments can be used to define phenotypes. Phenotype determination is likely to become more sensitive over time with increasingly sensitive biomarkers and high-resolution imaging. Genetic tools offer more information by helping to define functional genomic phenotypes, such as:

- **Transcriptome** – the set of all active mRNA molecules (transcripts) expressed in a particular tissue under particular conditions
- **Proteome** – the set of all the proteins expressed in a particular tissue under particular conditions

---

Clinical box 5.10 | **Primary carnitine deficiency**

Primary carnitine deficiency (see Ch. 3) is a rare inborn error of metabolism seen in at most 1 in 40 000 newborns, and often will result in sudden death. The defect here is not in an enzyme, but in a *transporter* protein. This lack of transporter results in significant metabolic changes that illustrate all of the consequences of altered metabolic flux.

Carnitine is a naturally occurring hydrophilic amino acid derivative produced within the kidneys and liver, and ingested through the diet. Carnitine is utilised in ATP production from fatty acids within mitochondria. This is facilitated through the following normal process:

1. Fatty acids in the cytosol are esterified with CoA (coenzyme A) to form acyl-CoA.
2. Medium-chain fatty acids (8–10 carbon atoms in the chain) diffuse across the plasma membrane into the mitochondria.
3. An oxidation step releases acetyl-CoA to enter the TCA cycle and electron transport chain, releasing ketone bodies in the process.
4. Longer-chain fatty acids require a **carnitine transporter**.
5. This is facilitated through the carnitine palmitoyltransferase system in which CoA is exchanged for carnitine, which allows movement across the membrane.
6. Within the mitochondrial matrix, carnitine is exchanged for CoA and the process proceeds as for medium-chain fatty acids, carnitine being transported back to be reused.

Primary carnitine deficiency is due to a mutation in the *OCTN2* gene that leads to a lack of the plasma membrane carnitine transporter. The altered metabolic flux has considerable consequences:

- Carnitine cannot be transported from the cytosol and excess is lost in the urine.
  - Systemic secondary carnitine depletion means that this substrate is not available for use within muscle, leading to cardiac and skeletal myopathy.
- There is an excess of long-chain fatty acid substrate within the cytosol.
  - Excessive lipid accumulates in muscle, heart and liver.
  - Accumulated long-chain acylcarnitines are believed to cause cardiac arrhythmias.
- There is a reduction in products downstream: the long-chain fatty acids are not available to produce energy, nor are sufficient ketone bodies produced.
  - Energy loss leads to weakness.
  - Lack of ketone bodies leads to acute hypoketotic encephalopathy in the brain and liver.
- An imbalance in under-utilised CoA within the mitochondria leads to an accumulation of acyl-CoA.
  - Excess acyl-CoA interferes with all pathways requiring CoA – including the TCA cycle, amino acid oxidation and pyruvate oxidation.
  - Acute hypoglycaemia, secondary to the above, contributes to the encephalopathy associated with hypoketosis.
- Excess long-chain fatty acids are diverted into other pathways and lead to secondary inhibition of the urea cycle enzymes, resulting in excess toxic ammonia. Ammonia is normally metabolised to urea by the urea cycle and excreted in urine. Where it accumulates in the blood it can lead to encephalopathy and death (see Ch. 3).

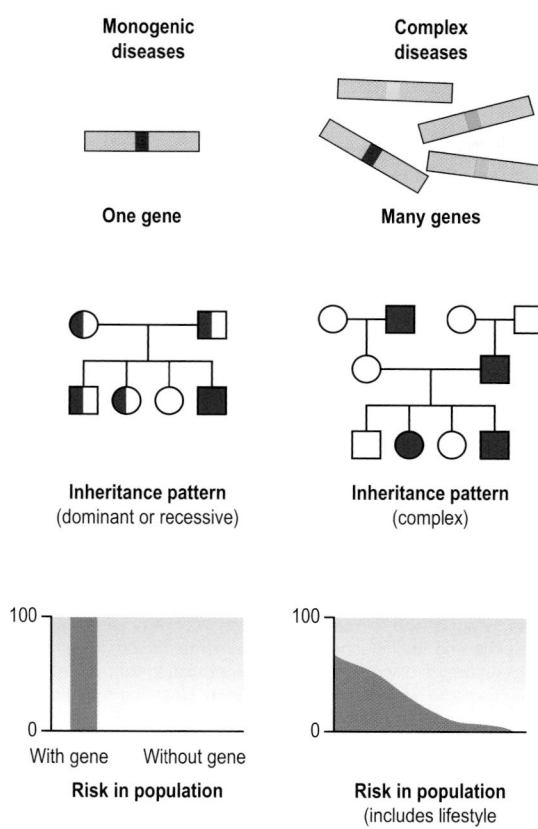

Fig. 5.30 Monogenic versus complex (polygenic) disorders.

- **Metabolome** – the set of metabolic pathways that are followed in a particular tissue under particular conditions.

THRESHOLD EFFECTS MODELS

Some diseases seem to be polygenic, but do not show the typical bell-shaped distribution with its associated severity of disease. Instead, disease symptoms seem to be related to a liability threshold within a distribution that must be passed before the disease is expressed. This threshold is sometimes different between the sexes, resulting in different risks between male and female siblings. An individual at the high end of the liability distribution is more likely to have more of the disease-causing genes and experience more of the environmental factors, and therefore be more likely to develop the disease. Conditions such as cleft palate, spina bifida, infantile autism and pyloric stenosis are considered to follow the threshold model of inheritance.

Clinical box 5.11 **Infantile autism**

Infantile autism is an example of the threshold model of inheritance. It is more common in males but, conversely, the risk of disease among siblings is greater among female family members with the disease. This is because females need to experience more of the disease genes and so families will, by definition, have experienced a higher proportion of the risk factors.

CHARACTERISTICS OF MULTIFACTORIAL DISEASES

Multifactorial diseases tend to show characteristic risks of the disease in family members, but there is no clear Mendelian pattern of inheritance and environmental factors can increase or decrease the risk of disease. It may occur more frequently in one gender and in particular ethnic groups, perhaps because they have more of the contributing 'bad' genes or are exposed to a more detrimental environment.

- Affected children may have apparently normal parents due to the variable penetrance of the disease genes, but parents who are related have children with a higher risk of disease. Although the parents may appear normal, they may have contributed some of the genes that are associated with an increased risk. For example, in cleft lip and palate, it may be that the parents have contributed some underactive genes that would be needed for normal development.
- There is often evidence that environmental factors influence the risk. For example, there is an association between nutritional deficiencies and maternal cigarette smoking and the cleft lip and palate birth defect. There is evidence from twin studies that risk is not simply associated with the genes that have been inherited (see **concordance** below).
- The risk in the family is higher if more than one family member is affected. This is because if you see more affected relatives, it is more likely that that these people have more risk factors (are at an extreme position on a liability distribution) than those in families that only have one affected family member.
- If the disease is severe in the patient then the risk in a family member is increased. This is because they are more likely also to have inherited some of the genetic factors that result in disease expression.
- The disease may occur more frequently in one gender than in the other, but is not a sex-linked disorder. The risk is higher in first-degree relatives of diseased individuals from the less commonly affected gender. This is because these affected individuals are likely to be from families with high liability.
- The risk decreases considerably as the degree of relationship decreases, because disease is the result of a combination of many genes and factors, all of which may not be uniformly present. This is unlike single gene disorders, where the risk is 50% in siblings, 25% in half-siblings, decreasing by half with each degree of distance.

Coronary artery disease has all of the characteristics of a multifactorial disease. For example, coronary artery disease can occur in isolation, and also runs in families and shows no clear Mendelian inheritance pattern. The risk is greater in males and in African Americans, in comparison with females and Caucasians or Asians, and there are a number of environmental and other factors that increase the risk, including obesity, high blood pressure, high levels of LDL-cholesterol and type II diabetes.

Heritability

Heritability is an estimate of the proportion of the variability in a trait that is due to genetic rather than environmental factors. Unlike single gene mutations, multifactorial diseases do not show complete heritability. For example, lipid levels vary across the population, but less so between family members. Assessments of heritability can be made by correlating biochemical levels in relatives of individuals with cardiovascular disease, in comparison with controls, such as spouse pairs. Different estimates of heritability are quoted in the literature. Table 5.3 presents these in terms of very high, high, median, low and very low heritability.

Complex diseases are influenced by both genetic and environmental factors and the balance between these affects how public health will target prevention. For example, where a disease has low heritability, such as lung cancer, changes in environmental exposure to tobacco smoke will be very important. In contrast, the environmental influences on the

Table 5.3	Examples of heritability estimates
Very high (>90%)	Bipolar affective disorder Autism Body fat percentage Fingerprints (ridge count) Idiopathic epilepsy Height
High (>65%)	Ankylosing spondylitis Asthma Body mass index Cleft lip or cleft palate Pyloric stenosis Schizophrenia Spina bifida
Median	Alcoholism Blood pressure Club foot IQ Multiple sclerosis Myocardial infarction (female)
Low (<35%)	Myocardial infarction (male) Peptic ulcer
Very low (<10%)	Contagious disease

i Information box 5.2   DNA databanks and the hunt for disease genes

An innovative approach to studying complex diseases has been set up by deCODE Genetics. This company, founded by an Icelander, aims to use the Icelandic community as a genetic resource in the hunt for disease genes. This population offers a number of advantages over other populations:

- The population is large (about 275 000) and genetically homogenous.
- Genealogical information goes back 1000 years.
- Good medical records are available.
- The population is cooperative.
- There is a large databank of DNA.

There are, however, a number of concerns with this approach. There is some doubt about whether the population is suitable, particularly because most diseases have an environmental component and these are currently not being studied. The main criticism from the international community is ethical. Individuals who do not wish to be involved in the study have to actively opt out and consent is not required for the deceased individual, or for children.

The approach has, however, made a number of significant advancements in relation to the risk for breast cancer, a link to the gene involved in nicotine dependence and the link between obesity and the onset of common disorders.

Clinical box 5.12   Heritability of diabetes

Diabetes, in which the body fails to produce enough insulin, occurs in two main forms (see Ch. 3):

- Type 1 diabetes is due to an autoimmune destruction of the cells that produce insulin.
- Type 2 diabetes occurs when there is an imbalance between the ability of the cell to produce insulin and the reduced effectiveness of insulin on a target tissue (insulin resistance).

Both forms of diabetes run in families. The risk for a sibling developing type 1 diabetes is between 10 and 100 times the risk in the general population, reflecting the high genetic contribution to this form of the disease.

Concordance is higher among monozygotic twins in type 2 diabetes, reflecting the high hereditability. However, environmental factors are also thought to be important in this form of the disease. Low birthweight is associated with subsequent development of type 2 diabetes, but another explanation could be that there are genetic factors that explain both. Studies of identical twins, in which only one twin has developed type 2 diabetes, show that this twin is more likely to be of lower birthweight, supporting an environmental contribution.

Diabetes is increasing in prevalence, especially among the middle aged, and mirrors the increase in obesity worldwide, emphasising the influence of environmental factors in accelerating a disease process in a population that is already at risk. Genome-wide studies have already identified mutations within genes that point to an increased risk of type 2 diabetes. One of these is in the zinc transporter gene that is involved in regulating insulin secretion; this may help identify people at risk at an early stage.

occurrence of breast cancer are not considered of importance in comparison with family history, because of the much higher heritability of breast cancer.

Genetic epidemiology

Multifactorial diseases may be caused by defects in one or more genes that seem to explain most of the disease seen, but influenced possibly by many other genes and environmental factors that have modifying influences. Twin and adoption studies are used to distinguish genetic and environmental influences. Identifying possible genes that may be involved is the role of genetic epidemiology.

Twin studies

Monozygotic twins originate from one embryo and the individuals are identical. In contrast, **dizygotic** twins are produced after fertilisation of two eggs at the same time, so they are no different from full siblings. Any differences observed between monozygotic twins must be due to environmental factors. Same-sex dizygotic twins form good controls for epidemiological studies, as they are more likely also to have been exposed to identical environments, particularly in the womb, whereas the same cannot be said for siblings.

Concordance – inheritance of a genetic factor – is 100% in monozygotes, in whom a trait is determined only by genes. Dizygotic twins are expected to be **discordant** as they will only share about half of their genes. Concordance is measured as either a rate or a correlation coefficient, and the difference between these in monozygotic and dizygotic twins is used to calculate heritability. Where heritability is high there is a large difference between concordance rates in the different twin types.

Infectious diseases, such as measles, are not expected to be influenced by genetic factors (although genetic factors can influence the course of the infection). Both twin types have high concordance (because they both tend to share the infectious experience) and the concordance rates are quite similar, leading to very low estimates of heritability.

Biases in twin studies

Studies of twins were once thought to provide a perfect model in order to tease out genetic and environmental influences. However, problems exist:

- It is assumed that monozygotic twins and dizygotic twins will share the same environment, but monozygotic twins will tend to show higher concordance because they are:
  - Treated more similarly
  - More likely to seek similar environments or experiences.
- Because of the polygenic nature of many behavioural traits, and the fact that the genes tend to act synergistically, the absence of just one gene in a dizygotic twin pair may produce a marked difference in behaviour, significantly overestimating the importance of the genetic contribution.
- Monozygotic twins are probably not completely identical, as there may be a small number of mutations (SNPs) that may have occurred early in the development of one or other of the twins.
- Uterine environments may vary among monozygotic twin pairs as they may or may not share amnions or chorions.

Because of the possible biases, studies of twins raised apart have been done. However, these also have problems:

- Sample sizes are small and so there may be a relatively high standard error of measurement (see Ch. 7)
- Recruitment bias may lead to volunteers with an interest in being twins
- Twins are likely to have contact before separation
- Separated twins are more likely to be placed in similar environments as social services aim to provide them with a background that reflects their heritage.

Adoption studies

In adoption studies, children with diseased parents, but brought up by adoptive parents who do not have the disease, can provide useful information. The likely genetic involvement of schizophrenia has been made more persuasive by the higher rates of disease among adoptive children of affected parents than in adoptive children of unaffected parents. Potential biases, however, also exist here:

- Prenatal environmental influence may be very strong.
- Children may be adopted after several years, retaining a parental influence.
- Children are likely to be placed in similar environments to those of their natural parents.

TOOLS TO INVESTIGATE POLYGENIC DISEASES

Twin studies cannot identify the genes responsible for disease, but can only provide as assessment of the genetic involvement. A variety of other tools (see also 'Identifying disease genes') are used in order to provide a better under-standing of these complex diseases. Information is gleaned from studies of candidate genes using:

- Information from single gene disorders
- Whole genome-wide scans using linkage and association studies
- Animal models
- Expression profiles.

Information from single gene disorders

The bulk of disease is polygenic and caused by the interactions of genes that are common in the population and the underling environment. Diseases caused by mutations in single genes are rare and usually exhibit extreme phenotypes. Where these monogenic diseases produce phenotypes that are similar to the polygenic disease, this can give clues to the more complex form and can help elucidate pathways in the disease and provide ideas for therapeutic targets.

Whole-genome association studies

Most disorders are influenced by a small number of genes spread across the genome that have major effects but underlying these are a comprehensive catalogue of genes that influence linked pathways and can provide useful predictive biomarkers in the future. These genes may be identified by chance through SNP analysis, but this is usually only achieved with any significant success through the use of high-sensitivity **whole-genome association SNP arrays**. These studies have already identified a series of important SNPs involved in the development of type 2 diabetes, for example, but are currently being applied to a large number of diseases.

Animal models

Animals that are inbred to develop a form of human disease (**animal models**) may be useful in the investigation of the molecular basis of the disorder. For example, research in mice with alopecia, a skin condition resulting in hair loss in adults and thought to be a defect of T lymphocytes that act on hair follicles, has identified areas on chromosomes 8, 9, 15 and 17 as associated with the condition.

Expression profiles

A large number of genes can be monitored in parallel using microarray technology, identifying clusters of genes that are over- or underexpressed in an **expression profile**. Although this technology can be used to study the whole genome, arrays can be customised to include sets of genes of interest.

Linkage studies

Linkage analysis looks for polymorphic areas of DNA or SNPs that are inherited along with a disease. **Microsatellites** are small pieces of DNA that are highly polymorphic. By using a selection of microsatellites across the genome, it may be possible to track a particular polymorphism within a family pedigree whose members have also developed the disease. This technique helps identify areas of a chromosome that are likely to contain the disease gene. One of the early discoveries using this methodology associated type 1 (insulin-dependent) diabetes with an area on chromosome 11, where the insulin gene is located.

CANCER GENETICS

CANCER AS A MULTI-STEP GENETIC DISEASE

Cancer is a collection of disorders that share the common feature of uncontrolled cell growth, leading to the formation of a mass of cells known as a **neoplasm** or **tumour**. Malignant neoplasms have the ability to invade adjacent tissues and often **metastasise**, or spread, to more distant parts of the body, a process that is the cause of 90% of cancer deaths. There are more than 100 distinct types of cancer, and each is classified according to the tissue type they arise in. In some families an inherited disposition has been shown to play a role in cancer formation.

There is strong evidence that a cancer arises from a single cell, as a result of clonal expansion. The model that fits best is that of **multi-hit carcinogenesis** (Fig. 5.31). There are two classes of mutations that cause a normal cell to develop into a cancer cell:

- Mutation types that enhance cell proliferation, so that there are more cells harbouring the somatic mutation
- Mutations that make the genome more unstable, either at the DNA level or at the chromosomal level.

Cell growth and differentiation are normally regulated by a series of external signals:

- Growth factors transmit signals from other cells acting through:
  - Growth factor receptors, resulting in
  - Signal transduction molecules (protein kinases), which, through a series of phosphorylations, interact with
- Nuclear transcription factors that regulate genes that influence cell growth and proliferation.

Although any mutations are rare, those that occur produce cells that fail to differentiate normally. Progressive mutations may lead to further deregulation and allow the cell, and its descendants, to escape the confines of normal cell regulation, leading to unrestricted growth.

INHERITANCE OF CANCER GENES

Mutations that occur in the germline may lead to cancers being seen more commonly within families. **Familial retinoblastoma** is a clear example of this. Many forms of breast and colon cancers also show evidence of a strong family history.

Colon cancer

Although most cases of colon cancer occur sporadically, about 25% show a family history of the disease. Particular genetic mutations have already been identified that account for about 8% of colorectal cancers:

- **Familial adenomatous polyposis** is due to germline mutations in the **APC** gene, which codes for a tumour suppressor protein
- **Hereditary nonpolyposis colorectal cancer**, caused by germline mutations in **MMR** genes.

Most of the mutations that predispose to colorectal cancer are inherited in an autosomal dominant fashion.

CANCER GENES

A number of genes have been implicated in carcinogenesis. They have been identified as having an important inherited component and/or are somatically altered during tumour formation. Cancer genes can be divided into three main groups:

- **Tumour suppressors** – inhibit proliferation
- **Oncogenes** – activate cellular proliferation
- **DNA repair genes**.

Tumour suppressor genes

The loss of specific chromosomal regions is a common event in the majority of tumours. These deletions may result in loss of function of a gene or genes which are involved in the aetiology of the cancer. Such genes are termed **tumour suppressors** and their subsequent inactivation removes the gene's inhibitory role in the regulation of cell growth and differentiation.

For example, the **retinoblastoma gene** (**RB1**) normally produces a protein that interacts with components in the cell cycle, blocking the uncontrolled proliferation of cells.

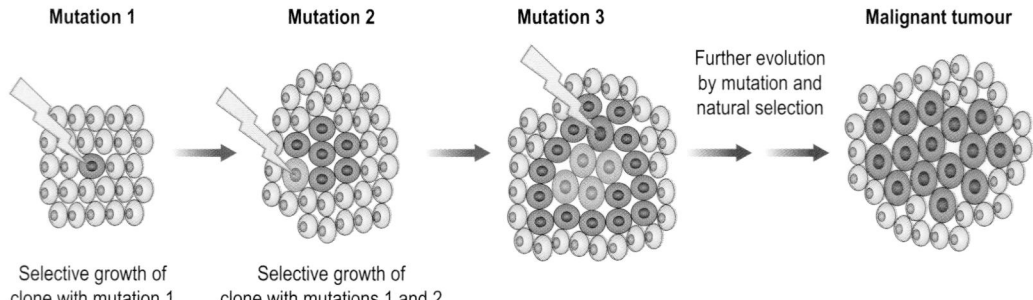

Mutation 1   Mutation 2   Mutation 3   Malignant tumour

Further evolution by mutation and natural selection

Selective growth of clone with mutation 1   Selective growth of clone with mutations 1 and 2

Fig. 5.31 **Multi-hit hypothesis of carcinogenesis.** Normal cells may experience a mutation after exposure to a genotoxic agent, or from random errors in DNA replication. Epigenetic influences may allow selective clonal growth of the mutated cell, which may also be more vulnerable to further mutating influences, forming a 'pre-cancerous' cell. Time and possible further epigenetic influences, enhancing the clonal expansion of altered cells, may result in some cells becoming cancerous, producing tumours of cells that lack the normal cellular mechanisms that inhibit uncontrolled proliferation.

- When the protein is active (unphosphorylated) it binds to a complex necessary for the cell cycle to enter into the S phase, therefore putting a 'brake' into the cycle.
- When the protein is inactive (phosphorylated by a **CDK**) the cell cycle continues.

A '**loss-of-function**' mutation in the *RB1* gene can lead to permanent inactivation, allowing cell division to continue uncontrolled. Other tumour suppressor genes may also produce inhibitors of CDK, preventing it from phosphorylating target proteins, providing a further brake in the cell cycle, or by inducing apoptosis.

Retinoblastoma and the two-hit theory of carcinogenesis

Knudson, in 1971, described the **two-hit theory of carcinogenesis** to explain the inheritance of **retinoblastoma**, the most common eye cancer in childhood. Retinoblastoma has two forms:

- Sporadic:
  - Parents are normal
  - No risk to offspring
  - Single tumour affecting only one eye.

The mutation rate for the retinoblastoma gene is 10^{-6} (1 in 1 000 000). If two events are needed for retinoblastoma then this will occur at a rate of 10^{-12}. There are around 10^8 retinoblasts in an individual, which would explain a sporadic rate of a single tumour in 1 in 10 000 cases, which is close to the observed rate of sporadic mutation.

- Inherited:
  - Parent is normally affected
  - 50% of offspring inherit the disease
  - Several tumours, affecting both eyes.

The multiple bilateral tumours are thought to be due to two mutations – **the two-hit theory**. A mutation to the retinoblastoma gene in the germline, if passed on to a child (50% chance), will show the mutation in every cell of the body (a **constitutional mutation**), including all retinoblasts. They will be heterozygous for the mutation. But not all of the retinoblasts form tumours.

A second mutation, within any of the retinoblasts in embryonic life, can then result in loss of the normal chromosome. Any retinoblast that carries two abnormal chromosomes, a homozygote, will develop a retinoblastoma. With a 1 in 1 000 000 chance of a second mutation, one might expect around 100 retinoblasts to experience a second hit, resulting in multiple tumours occurring in both eyes. A small minority of individuals will not experience the second hit and so will not inherit the disease.

Inheritance will therefore tend to be autosomal dominant in relation to the disease (because individuals that inherit the gene from an affected parent will be affected) but recessive as far as the cell is concerned as the cell must be homozygous for the abnormal gene for the tumour to develop.

Loss of heterozygosity

Loss of heterozygosity (LOH) can be used to investigate inherited cancers. In situations where surrounding normal cells are heterozygous for a genetic polymorphic marker, but tend to be homozygous for the marker within a tumour, familial cancer involving tumour suppressor genes may be implicated (Fig. 5.32). In the past, these genes have been identified using polymorphic microsatellite markers. The information provided by the HGP, however, has allowed whole-genome SNP array analysis, which provides a more sensitive analysis to help rapidly identify important target genes in a given cancer (see also Gene arrays, below).

Oncogenes

Proto-oncogenes are involved in normal cell growth regulation. If a mutation leads to unregulated growth it is said to be an **oncogene**, and the cell is said to be **transformed**. The presence of the single mutation in only one copy of the gene leading to the oncogene means that expression is dominant at the cellular level. Oncogenes promote cellular growth and proliferation and are thus characterised as **gain-of-function** mutations.

Unlike tumour suppressor genes, oncogenes are mainly found in sporadic tumours. The discovery of oncogenes has been helped through experimentation involving **retroviruses**, **transfection** and **tumour mapping** techniques.

Retroviruses

Oncogenes can also be induced through the action of a retrovirus. **Retroviruses** have an RNA genome and are common in animals. When they attack a cell the viral reverse transcriptase changes the viral RNA into DNA, integrating with the DNA of the host cell, referred to as **transduction**. The viral genome contains a powerful promoter of transcription that promotes the production of new viral particles and this will also give a growth advantage to the host cell – producing oncogenes and **transforming** the cell.

Studies of transforming retroviruses have identified many oncogenes involved in growth and proliferation. The **RAS** (rat sarcoma) oncogenes have been identified this way and are involved in about 25% of cancers.

Transfection

Transfection takes place when cellular proto-oncogenes are transferred from tumour cells into normal cells. Studies look at whether recipient cells are transformed as a result, and what changes have taken place. The first study to be done transferred human bladder cancer cells into mouse cells; examination of the transformed mouse cells revealed a mutated RAS oncogene. The RAS protein product produced by the mutated gene remained in an active form, stimulating cell growth.

Mapping

Mapping uses several techniques in order to find the chromosomal location of genes. Mapping can be **physical** to find the exact position of a gene on a chromosome, or **genetic**, which uses studies of human pedigrees to locate the relative position on a chromosome. Physical techniques may also reveal rearrangements in chromosomes associated with particular cancers. Many cases of chronic myeloid leukaemia are characterised by the presence of the **Philadelphia chromosome**, in which a translocation between chromosomes 9 and 22 activates the *ABL* proto-oncogene.

DNA repair genes

DNA repair genes exist to repair DNA to facilitate accurate DNA replication. In some inherited disorders and familial

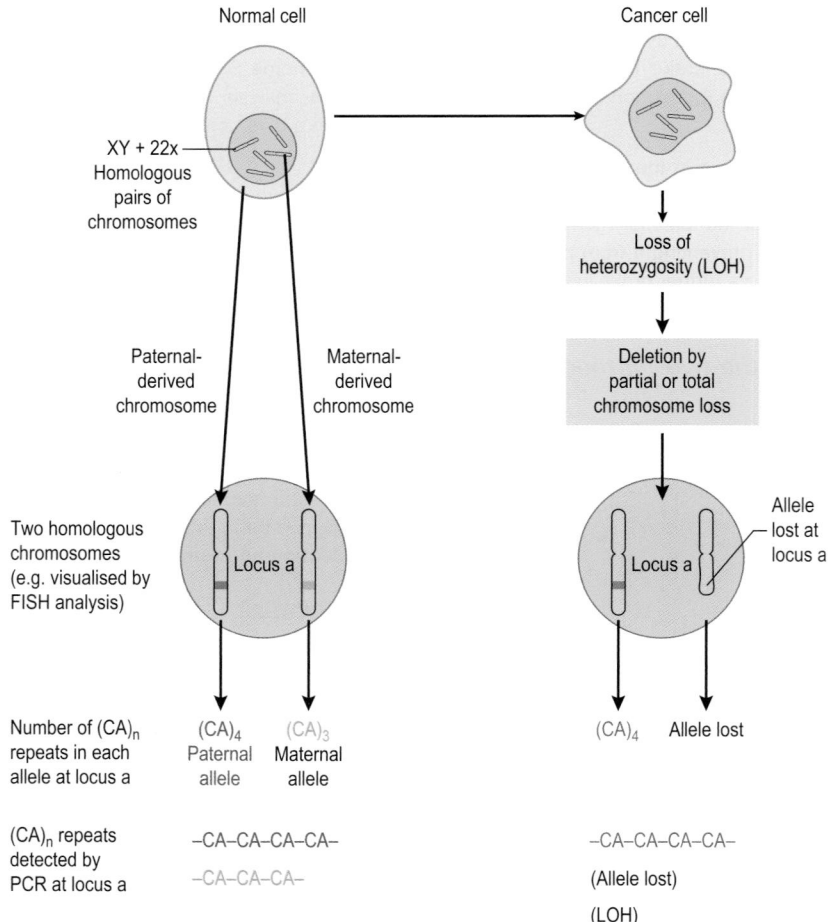

Normal cell

Cancer cell

XY + 22x
Homologous
pairs of
chromosomes

Loss of
heterozygosity (LOH)

Deletion by
partial or total
chromosome loss

Paternal-
derived
chromosome

Maternal-
derived
chromosome

Two homologous
chromosomes
(e.g. visualised by
FISH analysis)

Locus a

Locus a

Allele
lost at
locus a

Number of (CA)n
repeats in each
allele at locus a

(CA)4
Paternal
allele

(CA)3
Maternal
allele

(CA)4

Allele lost

(CA)n repeats
detected by
PCR at locus a

–CA–CA–CA–CA–

–CA–CA–CA–

–CA–CA–CA–CA–

(Allele lost)

(LOH)

Fig. 5.32 **Loss of heterozygosity observed in cancer cells.** The normal cell is heterozygotic at locus a, showing two alleles with three and four repeats, respectively, one paternal in origin, the other maternal in origin. In the cancer cell the a locus on the maternally derived chromosome, for example, has been lost through a deletion, leaving only the paternal allele. Cells originating from the tumour will appear to be homozygous. Adapted from Pharaoh PDP, Caldos C 1999 Molecular genetics and the assessment of human cancers (figure 2). Expert Reviews in Molecular Medicine, March 11, www.expertreviews.org/99000526h.htm

cancer syndromes, defects in these repair mechanisms lead to **genomic instability**. Genomic instability results in chromosomal abnormalities such as breaks, abnormal chromosome numbers and widespread mutations, these somatic changes often affecting genes important in proliferation and carcinogenesis.

Several gastric and breast cancer syndromes are known to have defects in the replication of short tandem repeat sequences (**microsatellite instability**). This indicates an **MMR** defect in which, for example, a single base change can lead to a DNA molecule where the base pairs are not complementary (Fig. 5.33). This replication error defect is caused by mutations in the MMR genes, leading to a cascade of secondary mutations in oncogenes, and tumour suppressor genes that give rise to cancer.

Gene arrays to identify oncogenes and tumour suppressor genes involved in cancer

Genes that are likely to be involved in the genesis of cancer include growth factors and their receptors; many of these will be oncogenes or tumour suppressors. Identification of muta-

tions and comparisons of gene expression between individuals with and without cancer, or between patients with different outcomes from cancer, are all vital techniques used in cancer research. This research has been facilitated using **gene arrays**, or gene 'chips'.

Gene arrays use a form of solid support, such a glass slide or nylon membrane, onto which a collection of nucleic acids, specific for a particular gene, are **spotted**. These **target** nucleic acids are **probed** with fluorescently labelled nucleic acids extracted from a sample, and those that **hybridise** to the spot are detected through the fluorescent label. The advantage of using an array is that many thousands of targets can be examined in a single experiment. Arrays can be used in different ways for a number of different purposes:

- Expression arrays: these can be used to compare different RNAs from, for example:
  - Different tissues
  - Normal and tumour tissue
  - Treated and untreated cell cultures.

RNA is converted to complementary DNA (cDNA) using reverse transcriptase before being hybridised onto the array.

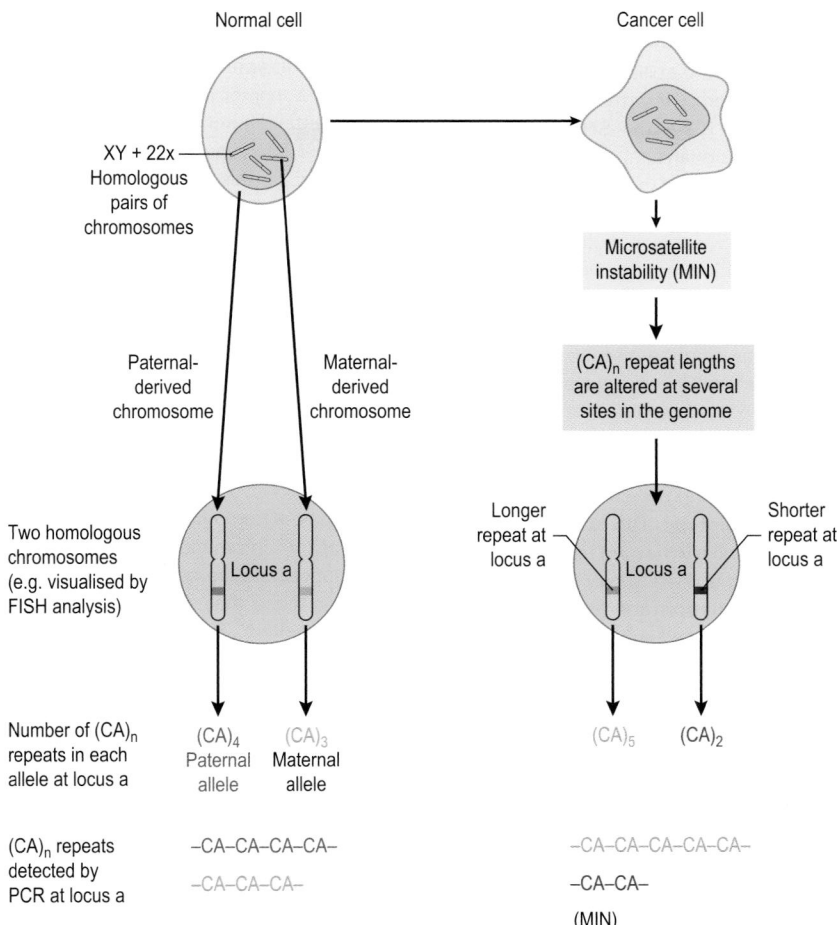

Fig. 5.33 **Microsatellite instability in cancer cells.** The normal cell is heterozygous at locus a has alleles with three and four repeats, respectively. In the cancer cell mutations in mismatch repair genes have led to an inability to repair nucleotide mismatches during DNA replication. This produces changes in the number of repeats observed (microsatellite instability). Adapted from Pharaoh PDP, Caldos C 1999 Molecular genetics and the assessment of human cancers (figure 2). Expert Reviews in Molecular Medicine, March 11, www.expertreviews.org/99000526h.htm

- SNP arrays: The accumulation of large numbers of SNPs through worldwide projects, such as the HapMap project, and their availability within databases has facilitated large numbers (up to one million) covering the majority of the human genome, to be spotted onto a single array offering a statistically very powerful approach to the identification of SNPs that are associated with particular diseases, as well as identifying chromosomal alterations in tumours.
- Copy number arrays: Copy number variation (CNV) is important in a number of different mechanisms and modern arrays include around one million known variants. Analysis of copy number has been used in:
  - Cancer – changes in copy number are associated with tumour initiation and progression, and analysis of copy number arrays can help identify new tumour suppressor genes and oncogenes.
  - Disease association – germline CNV is common but has also been associated with specific diseases and analysis of copy number is often done in association with SNP analysis.

IDENTIFYING DISEASE GENES

GENETIC MAPPING

Genetic mapping is the first step in identifying the position of where disease genes are located on a chromosome. The human genome has now been sequenced in a number of individuals, including James Watson, and this information is available in public genome databases.

Genetic linkage mapping of monogenic disease

Genetic linkage studies involve using families that have a number of diseased individuals and show evidence of Mendelian inheritance. These studies help identify disease genes by pinpointing the location of the disease-associated mutation in the genome. Linkage analysis depends on the presence of polymorphic markers near to the disease gene of interest. Until the variation in DNA sequences could be exploited there were very few polymorphic markers; those that existed (blood groups, red cell enzymes and serum protein polymorphisms) were of little use where they did not lie close to the gene of interest. The ability to utilise DNA has resulted in many more markers, and more polymorphic markers, including more than 10 million SNPs, becoming available for use as tools in the analytical process.

Linkage analysis has been used successfully to map numerous disease genes of either dominant or recessive inheritance with complete or variable penetrance and the density of the SNP map has added more power to the analysis. Genetic mapping of a disease or trait involves the identification of markers that are always inherited together. If the marker lies within the gene causing the disease then linkage will mean that the same marker allele will always be inherited along with disease. Figure 5.34 illustrates the principle of linkage mapping.

Genes that are physically very close to each other are rarely separated in this process and therefore sets of alleles are inherited as a block, or **haplotype**. The closer two genes are on a chromosome, the less likely they are to be separated during recombination. This fact is used to provide a measure of closeness, measured in **centimorgans** (**cM**). One cM is defined as a 1% recombination between two loci (a **recombination frequency** of 0.01). The maximum recombination possible is 50% (recombination frequency 0.5). Therefore loci that are more than 50 cM apart are considered to be unlinked.

Clinical box 5.13 | **Some clinical conditions identified by linkage analysis**

Glutathione reductase is an important enzyme as it protects haemoglobin, red cell enzymes and cell membranes from oxidative damage. **Glutathione reductase deficiency** can lead to a haemolytic anaemia in patients. The gene was located on the short arm of chromosome 8 when a child with anaemia and a deletion on chromosome 8 was also shown to have about 50% of the normal glutathione reductase activity.

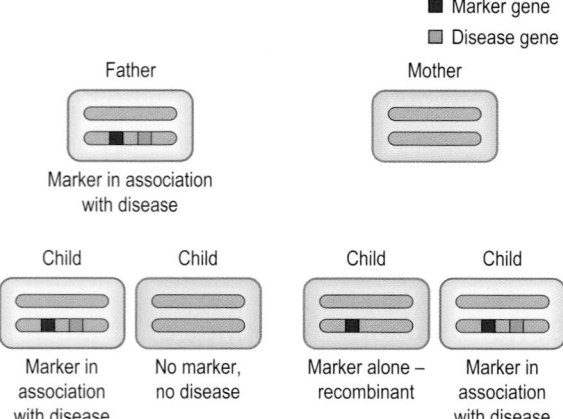

Fig. 5.34 **Linkage mapping.** The frequency of recombinant events between markers within a family pedigree provides a measure of relative proximity of the genes. The lower proportion of recombinants seen, the closer the marker is to the gene, and the higher the chance of linkage. The larger a family pedigree, the more accurate is the assessment.

Linkage disequilibrium

Linkage disequilibrium also looks at the association between a marker and a disease locus, but there are some fundamental differences. When the appearance of a particular marker allele is not influenced by the presence of the disease locus, this absence of association between the two loci is called **linkage equilibrium**. Some alleles, however, exhibit an association – **linkage disequilibrium**. This technique increases the resolution even further, down to 0.1 cM approximately.

The concept of linkage considers the locus, and recent recombination events, within a family pedigree. In contrast, linkage disequilibrium considers particular alleles seen within the population as a whole that co-segregate with a disease allele – an **association**. It is thus characterised by allele frequencies that do not match with those predicted by chance. As explained above, during meiosis, chromatids are formed from a pair of chromosomes and recombination occurs when parts of the chromatids exchange (cross over). Genes that are a long distance apart will tend to be separated in this process; those that are close together will tend to remain together (linked). The tighter the linkage, the longer the disequilibrium (association) will last.

During fertilisation, genetic material is swapped between paired chromosomes in the crossing-over process, known as **genetic recombination**. The position and frequency of crossover differs at each meiosis with, on average, one or two exchanges per chromosome per meiosis. Genetic recombination accounts for the differences seen between siblings.

LOD scores

An assessment of the strength of a particular recombination frequency is provided by comparing the likelihood that two loci are linked at a given recombination frequency versus the likelihood that they are not linked (recombination frequency 0.5). This likelihood is known as the **logarithm of the odds** (**LOD**) **score**. LOD scores with a likelihood ratio greater than 3.0 are said to be evidence of linkage; scores less than −2.0 are said to be evidence that the loci are not linked. Because LOD is a logarithm, a score of 3.0 means that the likelihood of linkage occurring at the particular genetic distance is 1000 times greater than there being no linkage.

Genetic linkage – a clinical example

One of the first chromosomal linkages identified in humans was between the locus for **nail–patella syndrome** (**NPS**) and the ABO blood group on chromosome 9. NPS is inherited as an autosomal dominant trait and individuals have abnormalities of nails and patella and other skeletal problems. Associated abnormalities of the basement membrane lead to renal problems, which are a significant cause of mortality among individuals with the disease.

Calculating the recombination frequency

The pedigree of a family with NPS (Fig. 5.35) allows one to make certain observations:

- All affected individuals have at least one parent with NPS, suggesting dominant inheritance.
- Both males and females are similarly affected with NPS, suggesting an autosomal defect.

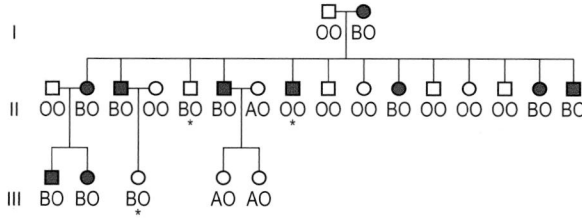

Nail–patella syndrome = ● or ■
Blood types = OO, BB, BO, AO

Fig. 5.35 Pedigree detailing nail–patella syndrome (NPS) phenotypes and ABO blood group genotypes. The pedigree shows a strong association between NPS and blood group B, suggesting that these genes are closely linked. Only three individuals show only blood group B, or have NPS, indicated with *. These individuals are the recombinants.

- Of the 19 related individuals:
  - 10 are affected and 9 of these carry blood group B, suggesting that NPS is linked to ABO blood type.
  - 9 are unaffected, but only 2 of these carry blood group B, suggesting that these two are recombinants.
- One affected individual is blood group O, suggesting that he too is a recombinant.

In the family there are 16 informative loci; 13 in the second generation, but only 3 in the third. The two children of the marriage with the group A woman have to be ignored; as the B group has not been transmitted, it is not possible to know whether recombination has taken place. Three in total are recombinant. The genetic distance can be calculated as follows:

$$\text{Genetic distance} = \frac{3}{16} \times 100 = 18.8\,\text{cM}$$
$$= 0.188 \text{ recombination frequency}$$

Calculating the LOD score

The example with NPS suggests that the genes for NPS and the ABO blood group may lie close together. The LOD score is calculated from:

$$LOD = \log \frac{\text{Probability of offspring with these genotypes if the genes are linked}}{\text{Probability of offspring with these genotypes if the genes are not linked}}$$

From the examined pedigree the following observations can be made:

- If the recombination frequency is 0.188, then the probability of seeing the recombination genotype is also said to be 0.188. But the chance of an individual child being a recombinant has to be half of this (0.094), as there are two parents and thus two parental types.
- The probability of *no recombination* is therefore $1 - 0.188 = 0.812$, and the chance of an individual child *not* being a recombinant is therefore 0.406.
- As there are 3 recombinant and 13 non-recombinants in the pedigree examined, the chance of seeing the genotypes in the children of the NPS pedigree can be calculated by multiplying each separate and independent probabilities for each child. This is the top part of the equation (the probability of offspring with these genotypes if the genes are linked):

$$(0.406^{13})(0.094^3) = 6.76 \times 10^{-9}$$

- If there is no linkage, then the recombination frequency is 0.5. It is 0.5, because there is a 50% chance of a particular allele being passed from a parent to child. The chance of possessing a particular genotype from a pair of parents is half of this (0.25).
- The probability of seeing the particular genotypes in the NPS pedigree can be calculated using the individual probabilities for each child. This is the bottom part of the equation (the probability of offspring with these genotypes if the genes are not linked):

$$0.25^{16} = 2.32 \times 10^{-10}$$

- The LOD score can be calculated as follows:

$$\log\left(\frac{6.76 \times 10^{-9}}{2.32 \times 10^{-10}}\right) = \log 29.05 = 1.46$$

- Note that the LOD score here has not reached the level of 3.0, the level where we can safely assume linkage, and therefore, from this family alone, it is not possible to be sure that the NPS and ABO blood group genes are linked, despite the pedigree appearing to be quite convincing in this respect. We can look at other families with NPS and calculate the LOD scores for each family. The LOD scores can then be added together, accumulating evidence until a convincing LOD score is achieved of either:
  - LOD > 3.0, supporting linkage
  - LOD < −2.0, against linkage.

It should be noted that, in other families, the link between NPS and the ABO blood group may not involve the B antigen. In other families it could be the A or O antigen that shows the apparent linkage. It is the gene linkage that we are interested here, not the particular allelic type.

Problems encountered in linkage studies

Locus heterogeneity

Locus heterogeneity is seen when mutations in different genes give rise to the same disease phenotype. This is more likely to be seen when a large number of families are examined. If evidence from several small families is used, rather than one or two large pedigrees, and locus heterogeneity is present, then simply combining LOD scores may suggest a lack of association.

Many diseases have been described that show locus heterogeneity, including **osteogenesis imperfecta type I**, which is due to mutations in genes on chromosome 7 and chromosome 17.

Incomplete penetrance

Even though an individual may have inherited a mutation in a susceptibility locus, other factors may affect the clinical presentation of the disease, such as environmental effects, chance and/or modifying gene loci, any of which may result in the individual appearing to be unaffected. This will cause a problem while doing linkage analysis as one cannot assume that unaffected people do not carry the disease allele.

Phenocopies

This occurs when individuals show the disease even though they are not carrying a susceptibility mutation. This sporadic disease may be explained by a non-inheritable occurrence, or by a distinct mutation in the same gene or a gene different from that inherited by the majority of affected cases in the family. For example, there is a very high rate of sporadic prostate cancer (a 1 in 5 lifetime risk in US males), thus making it difficult to find informative families for linkage analysis.

As long as the proportion of **phenocopies** to gene carriers in a family is low enough, linkage analysis models can cope with this problem. The same problem can occur if there has been a misdiagnosis. This underlies the importance of clinical confirmation of the affected status of each individual, which can be difficult in extended pedigrees.

Association studies

Association studies make use of particular study design methodologies (see Ch. 7):

- **Case–control studies:** individuals with the disease of interest are collected and controls are selected from the same population, except that they do not have the disease. The frequencies of possible predictors (genotypes) in each group are then compared.
- **Prospective cohort studies:** a group (cohort) of individuals representative of the general population is selected and divided into two subgroups, depending on whether the individuals have a particular genotype of interest. The cohort is then followed over a defined period of time in order to see whether the individuals develop the disease of interest and the possible association evaluated.

Molecular tools

Many of the methods used in the mapping techniques described below rely on the use of particular tools to manipulate DNA. Both restriction enzymes and the polymerase chain reaction (PCR) are utilised in many of the analytical processes to examine the DNA but these have been largely superseded by analysis of SNPs on array platforms. Now that the whole genome has been sequenced, many of these tools are now redundant. Nevertheless some key techniques have been described here as they provide a historical background to the complex nature of unravelling genetic material.

Restriction fragment length polymorphism

The endonuclease enzyme has the ability to cut DNA into separate pieces at a particular DNA sequence (**restriction site**). For example, the enzyme *Eco*R1 cuts DNA at GAATTC. If there is a mutation (base change, insertion or deletion) at the site (**restriction site polymorphism**), the enzyme will not cut the DNA. The cut, or uncut, fragments can be separated by placing the DNA in a gel and applying an electric current (**electrophoresis**). The charged DNA fragments will be pulled through the gel by the current, small fragments will move more easily and the fragments will be spread out by size.

The presence of a particular cut, or uncut, fragment is detected by using a DNA **probe**, which is a sequence of DNA that is complementary, and therefore binds, to the respective cut, or uncut, sequence type. Addition of a marker to the probe, such as a chemiluminescent tag, will mean that the relative position of the fragments on a gel can be detected when the gel is transferred to a membrane and then exposing the membrane to an X-ray film (**Southern blotting**).

These polymorphisms are called **restriction fragment length polymorphisms** (**RFLPs**) and have provided many thousands of new polymorphic markers, enabling major advances in gene mapping in recent years.

Variable number of tandem repeats

Historically, RFLPs were not sufficiently polymorphic or abundant for fine mapping of the genome (although many SNPs could be regarded as RFLPs). There are areas of the DNA with sequences that are repeated, one after the other (in tandem). The number of repeats in any particular area of the genome varies considerably.

- **Minisatellites** or **variable number of tandem repeats** (**VNTRs**) have repeated sequences that are tens of base pairs long.
- **Microsatellites** or **short tandem repeats** have repeated sequences that are much shorter – generally 2–6 base pairs.

A disadvantage of VNTRs is that they are found more often towards the ends of the chromosomes. In contrast, dinucleotide repeats (**CA repeat microsatellites**) – CACACACA… – are found spread throughout the whole genome and the number of repeats is very polymorphic.

There are no restriction sites within the repeats and so the restriction enzymes cut outside the repeat region, but the resultant fragments are very small – too small to be seen using a DNA probe on a gel – and the relative difference in the numbers of repeats requires highly sensitive detection. These problems have been resolved in two ways:

- The small amount of DNA has been resolved by the use of the **PCR** (Fig. 5.36) in which a sequence of DNA is copied many times.
- The resolution of small size differences, sometimes only by a single base, has been enabled by passing the fragments through very fine capillaries, and employing sensitive fluorescent probes in the PCR reaction that anneal to the DNA sequence just beyond the repeat region.

Single nucleotide polymorphisms

SNPs are simply those polymorphisms where a single base has changed. For example, one person may have a DNA base A, where another person might have a base C. There are estimated to be at least 10 million SNPs in the genome and many have been identified as part of the international HapMap project. SNPs that are close together will tend to be inherited together as a **haplotype** and most chromosome regions have only a few common haplotypes, with frequencies greater than 5%. Not all SNPs need to be analysed, however, as typing only a few SNPs (called tagging SNPs) can capture all the haplotype data for genetic association studies – they will define the haplotype.

Cloning vectors

Cloning vectors are another way that large amounts of DNA can be multiplied up. The vectors are artificial circular DNA molecules (**plasmids**), derived from a variety of cellular types: bacteria, bacteriophages, yeast cells. These **bacterial artificial chromosomes** (**BACs**) or **yeast artificial chromosomes** (**YACs**) are made by assembling all the essential parts of the natural bacterial or yeast chromosome and splicing in some human DNA (Fig. 5.37). The artificial plasmid is put back into its parent cell, such as a bacterium, where it behaves as through it were a normal constituent of the cell. The plasmid is copied many times during each cell cycle. The result is a colony of cells, each containing a many copies (**clones**) of the human DNA fragment.

A **genomic library** is made by using restriction enzymes to break up genomic DNA and cloning these in vectors.

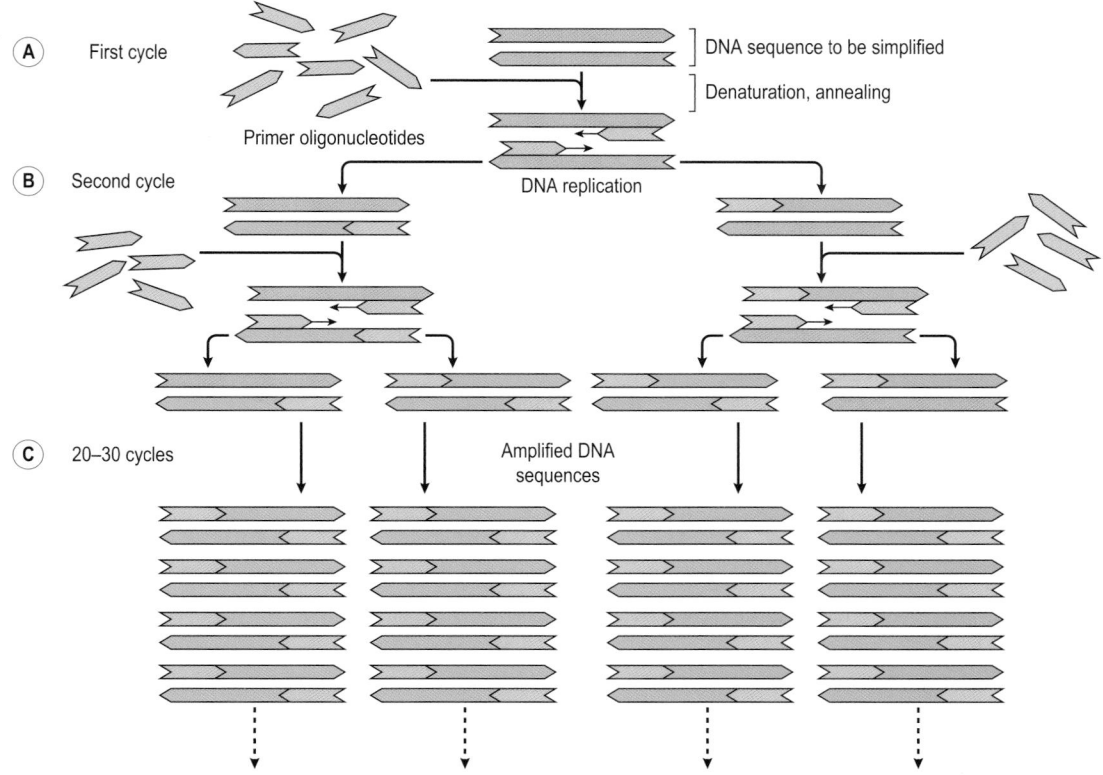

Ⓐ First cycle

DNA sequence to be simplified

Denaturation, annealing

Primer oligonucleotides

Ⓑ Second cycle

DNA replication

Ⓒ 20–30 cycles

Amplified DNA
sequences

Fig. 5.36 Diagrammatic representation of the polymerase chain reaction (PCR). PCR is a method of multiplying (**amplifying**) DNA. The process starts by heating the double-stranded DNA (in purple). Heating separates the two strands (**denaturation**) and allows **primers** (small pieces of DNA that are complementary to a specific location on the DNA) (in yellow) to stick (**anneal**) and provide a starting point for the DNA polymerase enzyme. A copy of each strand results (with new single-stranded DNA (in blue) and the new complementary strand pairs come together as the temperature is allowed to fall. At the end of the first cycle the DNA has doubled. Further heating and cooling sequences repeat the process. After 40 cycles, the DNA will have been amplified by about one trillion-fold.

These fragments will have fragments that overlap each other but will include all of the human genome: introns, exons, promoters, enhancers and non-coding (filler) DNA. A **cDNA library** is more limited as it contains only exons. It is made by taking mRNA and using the **reverse transcriptase** enzyme to produce cDNA to clone within a vector.

Bacteriophages can only carry small fragments of DNA, around 10–20 kb; in contrast YACs can hold 1000 kb of human DNA inserts. Use of different vectors allows the cloned DNA molecules to be made progressively smaller, until small enough to be sequenced. This technique, as well as providing material for sequencing, can also be used to produce large amounts of **recombinant** material for medical use – insulin (for treatment of diabetes) and erythropoietin (for treatment of renal failure) are produced in this way.

PHYSICAL MAPS

Physical maps are where the distances between particular features are measured in real units, such as numbers of base pairs, rather than genetic distances. Just like an atlas, a map can display the information at different scales or resolution.

Low-resolution mapping

Karyotyping

An example of a **low-resolution** map is a human chromosome **karyotype**, seen with standard microscopy, with characteristic banding. Low-resolution mapping can only resolve differ-

ences that are several million base pairs apart. Examination of a chromosome karyotype can identify translocations, such as the Philadelphia chromosome, where there is an exchange of material between two chromosomes, and additions, or losses, of whole chromosomes, but deletions large enough to be visible by light microscopy are likely to be lethal.

Dosage mapping

Gene associations with deletions may be broadly mapped by **dosage mapping** when they are seen in association with reduced levels of their protein product.

FISH

FISH utilises complementary strands of DNA, labelled with a fluorescent marker to find out on which chromosome, and where on the chromosome, a particular sequence lies (Fig. 5.38). This technique is useful for areas of repetitive DNA, which is not suitable for cloning. When the probe used is a copy of the mRNA, this cDNA identifies the area that enables the gene protein production.

High-resolution mapping

Sequence tagged sites

Key tools in fine mapping of the human genome were the use of BACs or YACs in libraries. **Contig maps** contain all the DNA from within a predefined region of a chromosome, in series of DNA fragments that partially overlap so that a contiguous series is available for analysis. The overlap is

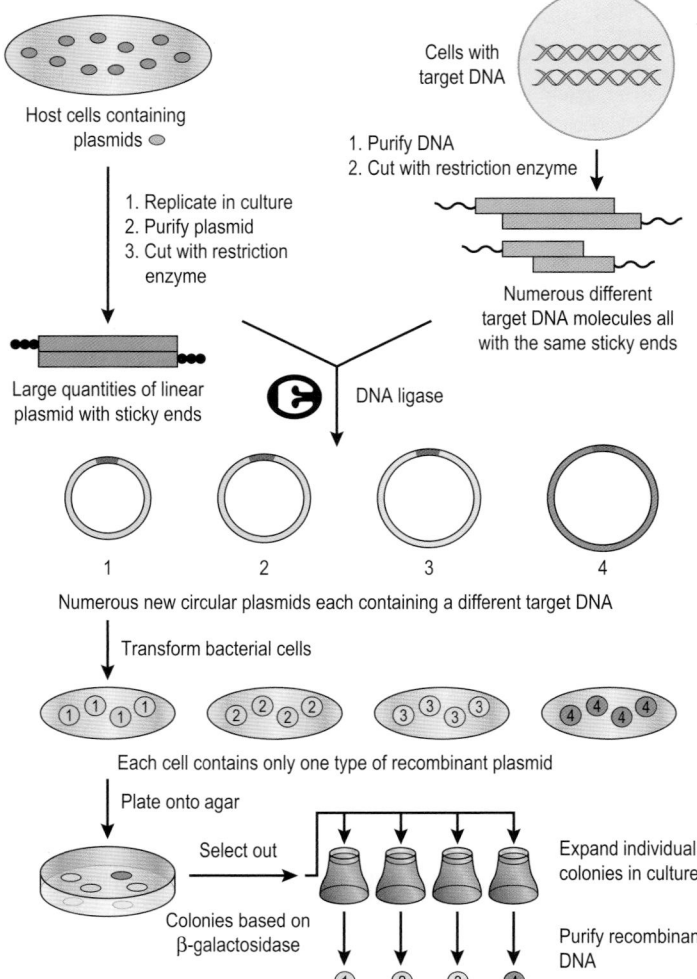

Fig. 5.37 **DNA cloning using bacteria.** One of the characteristics of bacteria is that the take up of plasmids is very inefficient and usually only one type of plasmid will enter each bacterium. Plating the bacteria onto agar will produce bacterial colonies, some of which will contain many copies of the original single plasmid, and particular piece of target DNA, originating from a single bacterium. Colonies that contain plasmids are selected using another molecular tool: the gene for β-galactoside. This is a marker gene placed within the plasmid but designed so that, if DNA is inserted, the β-galactoside gene becomes disrupted and non-functional. The normal gene product reacts with substrates in the culture to produce a coloured colony. Thus the *uncoloured* colonies will be those that contain the plasmid. In the diagram the 'uncoloured' plasmid-containing colonies are shown coloured to illustrate the different plasmid types containing the target DNA. Individual colonies can then be selected and separately cultured to produce large quantities of the target DNA. From Baynes J, Dominiczak M 2004 Medical biochemistry, 2nd edn. Elsevier, Edinburgh.

defined with the use of **sequence tagged sites (STSs)**, which are sequences of DNA of known chromosome location used as signposts throughout the DNA.

In order to define the whole sequence of interest it was important to be able to order the fragments using STSs. Using primers to the STS sequences, if two clones each produce the same PCR product they have sequences that overlap. A series of different STSs are used with several clones to order the sequences they contain. Thus, analysing Table 5.4 shows that the clones are in the following sequence of STSs: B C E D A on the DNA (Fig. 5.39).

The sequences defined by the STSs form the contig map, from which the overlaps can be identified and the molecular sequence of the DNA discovered and recorded.

Positional cloning

Positional cloning is the name given to the process of locating and cloning the disease gene once a process such as

Table 5.4					
CLONE	**STSa**	**STSb**	**STSc**	**STSd**	**STSe**
1	–	–	+	+	+
2	–	+	+	–	–
3	+	–	–	+	+
4	+	–	–	+	–

STS, sequence tagged site.

linkage has provided an approximate region on a chromosome. A primer is made to a known sequence in the area of the gene on a particular clone from a genomic library, and then a short complementary strand is synthesised. The complementary strand is then sequenced and its end used as the next primer. In this way it is possible to move down the chromosome (**chromosome walking**), systematically sequencing from between markers flanking the gene of interest (Fig. 5.40). Various approaches can be used to help define the position of the gene within this sequence.

- **Candidate genes**: candidate genes are possible disease-causing genes, identified because they produce a protein possibly associated with the disease profile and are therefore useful starting points to look for the gene.
- **Conserved sequences**: a large amount of DNA that codes for particular proteins required for life will be very similar (**highly conserved**) across species. This is

because any mutational changes may be lethal to the organism. Over time, some mutations may provide an advantage to the species and be maintained over others – an evolutionary change.

In contrast, the non-coding DNA may undergo mutational change without it being lethal and so it is reasonable that non-coding DNA will be more variable, especially between different species. This characteristic can then be used to define coding sequences.

- **GC islands**: GC dinucleotides are usually methylated, but in the 5′ end of many genes they are unmethylated. This may be to facilitate transcription. Identification of clusters of these unmethylated GC clusters (GC islands) may indicate the position of a gene.

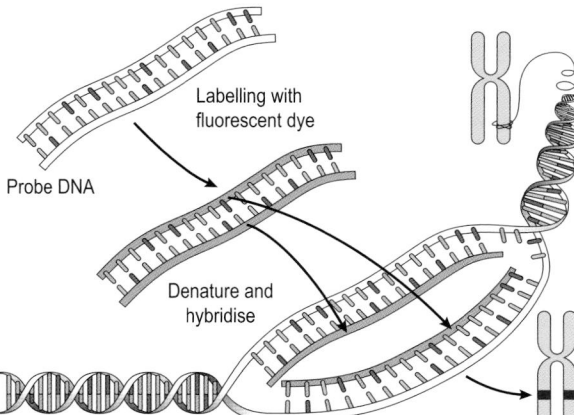

Fig. 5.38 Principle of fluorescence in situ hybridisation (FISH). Probes, complementary copies of the target DNA with a fluorescent marker, are hybridised with denatured metaphase chromosomes. The label indicates the position on the chromosome of the target DNA.

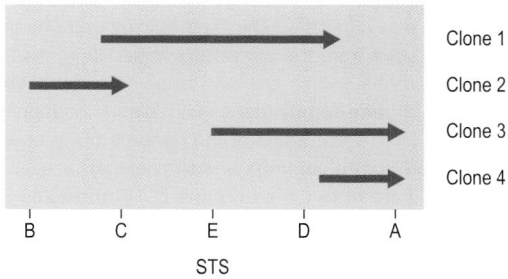

Fig. 5.39 Diagram showing order of sequences in clones according to the sequence tagged sites (STS). The order of overlapping DNA from each of the clone set can be defined by examining the PCR product shown in the table and knowledge of the STS. Sequencing all of the clones in this order will provide information for the whole of the functional area under examination.

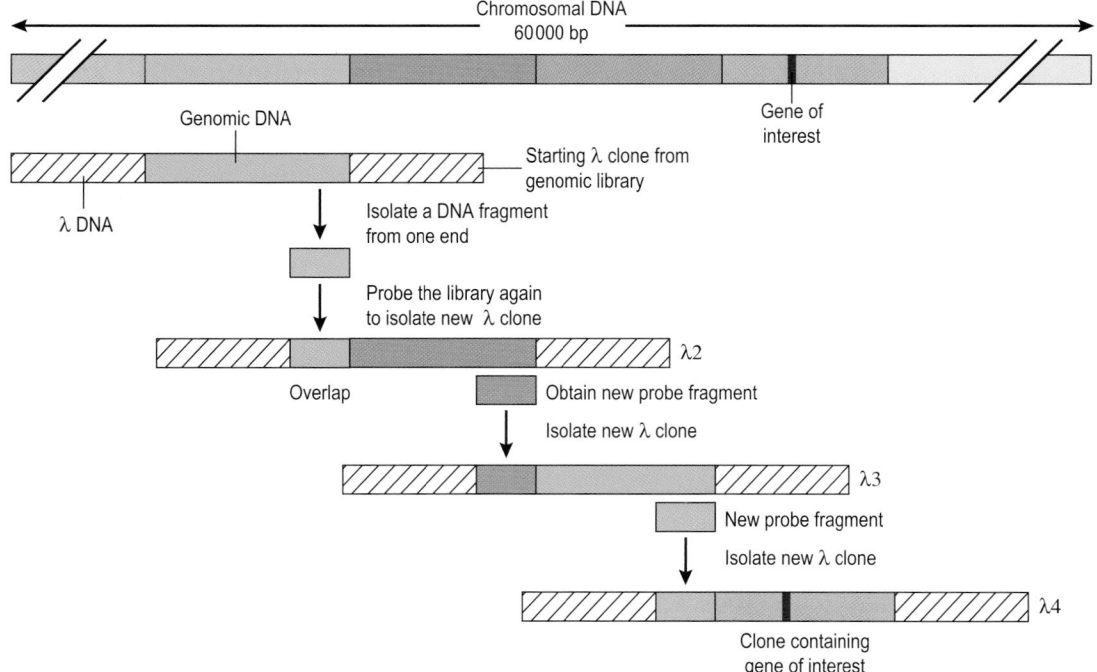

Fig.5.40 Chromosome walking. The region of λ DNA containing the genomic DNA sequence where the sequencing will start is selected from a library made within a bacteriophage and used to make a complementary strand, which is sequenced. The end of this sequence, closer to the gene of interest, is used as a probe to find a new clone from the library which contains this short overlapping sequence. The process is repeated, sequencing each complementary strand until the gene has also been sequenced.

- **cDNA selection**: a sequence of DNA is inserted into a YAC, which is then hybridised to clones from a cDNA library. cDNA is coding only and so will only hybridise with **exon** sequences (DNA that codes for proteins in a gene).
- **Trapping exons**: a sequence of DNA inserted into a vector that undergoes transcription will produce mRNA which is then processed to leave only exons. Therefore DNA containing exons will result in larger fragments after transcription than if there are no exons present.
- **Expressed sequence tags** (**ESTs**): ESTs are short sequences segments of DNA clones taken from a cDNA library. Because cDNA originates from mRNA, the sequenced must be expressed (protein-producing) regions of genes. These pieces are around 200–500 nucleotides long and are used as a tag with techniques such as FISH or radiation hybrid mapping. ESTs are normally sequences from each end of the cDNA molecule and can be synthesised quickly and cheaply.
  - 5′ ESTs are from the part of the molecule that codes for a protein and so will tend to be highly conserved within a **gene family** (genes with similar sequences found in different areas of the genome but probably evolved from a common ancestral gene).
  - 3′ ESTs are from the end of the cDNA molecule and much more likely to be from a non-coding region, or **untranslated region** – a region that is not translated into a protein. In consequence they are more liable to mutations and exhibit more cross-species differences. Because of their inherent variability, 3′ ESTs are often used as a source of STSs as they are both more identifiable and point directly to the gene.

ESTs have been used to identify the genes involved in Alzheimer's disease. Candidate genes are examined for areas of the DNA that match with the ESTs. Then the identified genes can be examined for mutations in affected individuals. Further family studies must be used to validate the link. Scientists contribute ESTs for public use to a database, **dbEST**, which is part of the National Institutes for Health (USA) **GenBank** gene sequence database.

- **Mutation screening**: identified genes are examined for mutations in affected individuals. This is usually performed by PCR amplification of the gene, followed by sequence analysis.
- **Gene expression**: possible disease-causing genes are further verified by looking at tissue expression. This is done by a technique called **northern blotting**, in which purified mRNA from tissue is hybridised with a probe made from the gene. If the gene is the disease gene, it would be expected to hybridise with mRNA from the tissue known to be affected by the disease. For example, a gene responsible for osteoporosis will be more likely to be expressed in the bone-forming cells than in other tissues.
- **Family studies**: further validation and verification associating a particular disease with a gene may be done by examining affected families and control populations to look for consistent patterns.

THE HUMAN GENOME PROJECT

The Human Genome Initiative was started by the US Department of Energy in 1986 and, with the National Institutes of Health, the **HGP** began in 1990, soon to be joined by major collaborators around the world. HGP's aim was to create a high-quality reference DNA sequence for the whole human genome, consisting of three million base pairs, and to identify all human genes. While scientists from China, France, Germany, the UK, Japan and the USA have all collaborated in the project, five institutions, four in the USA and one in the UK, have been the most productive:

- Baylor College of Medicine, Houston, USA
- Joint Genome Institute, Walnut Creek, USA
- Washington University School of Medicine, St Louis, USA
- Whitehead Institute/Massachusetts Institute of Technology Center for Genome Research, Cambridge, USA
- The Wellcome Trust Sanger Institute, Cambridge, UK.

The working draft of the human genome sequence was announced in June 2000, accompanied by separate publications in 2001 from both the publicly funded HGP and the private company Celera Genomics. Since then the sequence has been finished with over 99% of the gene regions being sequenced to an accuracy of 99.99%. What is left are small areas where the sequence has been technically difficult to resolve, due to the underlying structure. However, these regions are very repetitive in structure and not thought to contain genes.

Bioinformatics

Bioinformatics is the science that links biological information and information technology through computers. The construction of genetic databases is proving an invaluable tool to the investigator. These databases are complex and very powerful as they contain much linked information and must be updated on a regular basis.

Beyond the sequence

In addition to sequencing each chromosome to a high level of quality the project has been examining sequence variation at the level of single nucleotides (**SNPs**), as well as looking at variation in much larger chromosome segments. Already more than 10 million SNPs have been identified. The project will also examine genomes of many diverse organisms that will help the understanding of human evolution. For example:

- The **Japanese pufferfish** has the smallest known vertebrate genome, which makes it simpler to investigate, and comparison with the human genome will help identify those genes that have been preserved over some 450 million years.
- The **sea squirt** is the smallest organism with a spinal cord and over 80% of its genes are also found in the human genome. It will be particularly useful for the investigation of the evolutionary aspects of the nervous system.
- The **Western clawed frog** is being used as the major vertebrate model for embryonic development and cellular mechanisms.

Microbes are the oldest and most prevalent organisms on earth. Most have not been sequenced and it is hoped that knowledge of their molecular structure will enable scientists to use them for pharmaceutical, industrial, agricultural and environmental purposes.

What the HGP has already told us

Sequencing the human genome has been a major achievement but it is only the tip of the iceberg. Much work remains to be done, not only so that we can discover much more about particular organisms but also so that we can gain a better understanding of the more complex interactions involved within and between different life systems. Early analysis has already produced useful information.

Statistics

■ The human genome consists of over three billion nucleotide bases (A, C, T and G) and it is estimated that 99.9% of the order is identical between all individuals.
■ The total number of genes is estimated to be around 20 000–25 000, with each gene being composed of around 3000 bases. The number of bases in a gene is very variable, however.
■ The **dystrophin** gene is possibly the largest with 2.4 million bases. The highest number of genes on a chromosome are found on the largest chromosome 1 (almost 3000), whereas the small Y chromosome has relatively few (around 230).

Functions

The function of more than half of the genes are not yet known.

Structure

■ About 50% of the human genome is composed of repetitive short sequences of nucleotides. These repeated regions do not code for proteins and may have no direct function, other than as a separator between the genes.
■ While most of the gene-dense regions are rich in G and C nucleotides, the intervening gene-poor areas are characterised by being AT rich.

Variation

■ The genetic sequence of different humans is very similar but a SNP occurs in about 1 in 1200 bases and there are about 10 million common SNPs. Mutations are about twice as common in the male germline.
■ A second type of variation, copy number, has been shown to be a common occurrence.

Comparison with other species

■ The structure of the human genome is much more random than in other organisms, whose genes are also more evenly spaced. Humans have the same protein families as worms, flies and plants but proteins involved in development and immunity are more prolific.
■ Humans have about three times as many protein products as other organisms and about five times the number of repeat sequences as other organisms. The apparent evolutionary expansion of repeated sequences in humans over time seems to have halted about 50 million years ago, whereas the process seems to be continuing in rodents.

Using data from the HGP

The altruistic principles that have been embedded into the HGP, along with the ready worldwide access to information provided through the internet, have ensured that genetic information has been made widely available to the whole scientific community. This has led to the provision of databases of information, such as those of the International Nucleotide Sequence Database Collaboration, comprising:

■ The DNA Databank of Japan
■ The European Molecular Biology Laboratory
■ GenBank (part of the National Library of Medicine).

Investigating the human genome

The **National Centre for Biotechnology Information (NCBI) Human Map Viewer** can be accessed via a link on the NCBI website homepage (http://www.ncbi.nlm.nih.gov). As well as humans, the NCBI source also has maps of other mammals, other vertebrates, invertebrates, plants, fungi and protozoa. A particular gene can be entered as a search term and this will lead to a diagram of human chromosomes showing the gene location. Figure 5.41 shows a search for cystic fibrosis that identifies the *CFTR* gene on chromosome 7.

Maps available from the NCBI webpage provide different pieces of information:

■ UniGene clusters map shows ESTs that align, indicating the exons
■ A gene sequence map showing the introns and exons
■ A phenotype map shows the cytogenic position of the phenotypes associated with human genes
■ A morbid map shows the cytogenic location of disease genes (Fig. 5.42). Figure 5.42 shows a close up of part of chromosome 7. The map identifies the position of genetic disorders associated with particular genes. Cystic fibrosis is shown at position 7q31.2, associated with the gene 602421 – cystic fibrosis conductance regulator (*CFTR*) gene. Other diseases associated with genes nearby on the same chromosome are also shown.

Also available is a wealth of information that has already been gathered about the gene such as the nucleotide sequence, SNPs, known biological evidence available in the literature and sequences that are orthologous with the mouse genome, along with a vast amount of other information that can be used by scientists wishing to research the gene.

Other databases are also available that can be used to provide similar information, such as the University of California, Santa Cruz (UCSC) browser and Ensembl.

Gene families

The molecular basis of a disease can also be investigated by examining **homologues**. These are genes that share a common evolutionary history and so will have a similar sequence. There are two kinds of homologues:

■ **Orthologues** are genes with similar sequences in two different species that have evolved from a single gene in the last common ancestor.
■ **Paralogues** are genes with similar sequences within a single organisms that that have diverged because of gene duplication.

Figure 5.43 illustrates the differences.

Homo sapiens (human) genome view
Build 36.2 statistics Switch to previous build

Search results for query "cftr AND (gene[obj_type])": 5 hits

Chr	Assembly	Match	Map element	Type	Maps
7	reference	all matches			
		CFTR: cystic fibrosis transmembrane conductance regulator...	CFTR	Gene	Genes cyto I Genes seq
		CFTR: ENSG00000001626	CFTR	GENE	ensGenes
7	CRA_TCAGchr7v2	all matches			
		CFTR	GA0044	GENE	TCAG Genes
		CFTR: cystic fibrosis transmembrane conductance regulator...	CFTR	GENE	Genes seq
7	Celera	**CFTR:** cystic fibrosis transmembrane conductance regulator...	CFTR	GENE	Genes seq

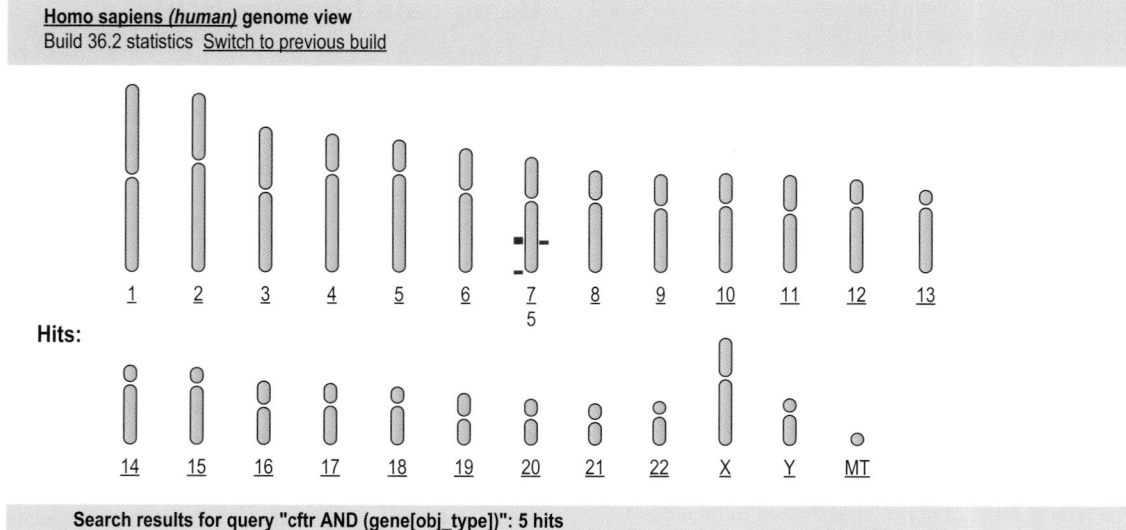

Fig. 5.41 **NCBI Human Map Viewer displaying information about cystic fibrosis** (www.ncbi.nlm.nih.gov/). A search for the cystic fibrosis gene *CFTR* has revealed references locating the gene on chromosome 7.

Chromosome: 1 2 3 4 5 6 [7] 8 9 10 11 12 13 14 15 16 17 18 19 20 21 22 X Y MT
Query: omim morbid [clear]

Master Map: OMIM Morbid Summary of Maps

Region Displayed 7q31.1–7q31.31

Morbid	MIM Number	Symbol	GeneID	Disease
	608391	AIS2	378426	Autoimmune disease, susceptibility to, 2
	603511	LGMD1D	9186	Muscular dystrophy, limb-girdle, type 1D
	607458	SCA18	94008	Spinal cerebellar ataxia 18
	601500	SMOH	6608	Basal cell carcinoma, somatic
	238331	DLD	1738	Maple syrup urine disease, type III, 248600; Leigh syndrome, 256000
	605646	SLC26A4	5172	Pendred syndrome, 274600; Enlarged vestibular aqueduct, 603545
	222800	BPGM	669	Hemolytic anemia due to bisphosphoglycerate mutase deficiency
	164860	MET	4233	Renal cell carcinoma, papillary, familial and sporadic, 605074
	603678	DFNB14	1706	Deafness, autosomal recessive 14
	605317	FOXP2	93986	Speech-language disorder-1, 602081
	603010	DFNB17	1709	Deafness, autosomal recessive 17
	602421	CFTR	1080	Cystic fibrosis, 219700; Congenital bilateral absence of vas deferens

Fig. 5.42 **Morbid map showing the position of the gene implicated in cystic fibrosis**: cystic fibrosis transmembrane conductance regulator on chromosome 7 (www.ncbi.nlm.nih.gov/). Online Mendelian Inheritance in Man (OMIM) Map showing the location of disease genes lying close to the *CFTR* gene on chromosome 7.

Molecular phylogenetics

Phylogenetics examines the evolutionary relationship between organisms. These relationships are depicted in **phylogenetic trees**, the relative position of branches representing the evolutionary time point at which species split from their common ancestor. Trees can be **rooted**, where a common ancestor is identified, or **unrooted**, in which case the trees only show the relationships between the species.

Patterns of DNA, the nucleotide and protein sequences are used to build trees using the observed patterns. Gene trees can be compared with species trees. Branches in gene trees occur at mutational events, whereas branches in species trees occur at the point at which a new species is

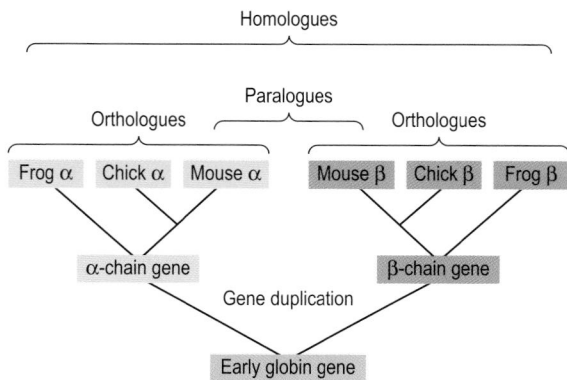

Fig. 5.43 **Difference types of homologues.**

identified. Therefore the trees are unlikely to be identical. Figure 5.44 shows an evolutionary tree predicted from mutational changes observed in the cytochrome c gene and corresponds reasonably, but not completely, with that expected in the evolution of vertebrates.

The **molecular clock hypothesis** assumes that mutations occur at a constant rate and so that the difference between two sequences can be used to date the time of divergence. The rate of change however differs between organisms and so must be calibrated against fossil DNA.

Protein modelling

The nucleotide sequence is not sufficient on its own to be able to understand how the proteins that are encoded are structured. Scientists need to be able to determine the two- and three-dimensional structures of proteins in order to be able to understand how they function. Different techniques are used to investigate the structure of proteins.

X-ray crystallography

Proteins must first be made into crystals having a regular lattice structure, which is done by slow precipitation and can be very difficult. When an X-ray is passed through a crystal, the ray will be deflected and split, dependent on the angle of the crystal surfaces that the ray encounters. The intensity and relative positions of the deflected rays reflect the protein structure, and the information can be collected and used to produce a computer model of the protein.

Nuclear magnetic resonance

Nuclear magnetic resonance has the advantage over crystallography as the proteins can be examined in solution. However, the technique cannot be used to examine very large proteins. The protein molecules are placed in a magnetic field and excited by bombarding them with radio waves. This causes the nuclei to spin (resonate) in a particular direction. At a certain frequency the nucleus will flip over and this frequency is associated with protein structure.

Homology modelling

This technique uses the genome and computers to predict the structure of a protein. There are various databases that assist in this process:

- The **Protein Data Bank (PDB)** is managed by the Research Collaboratory for Structural Bioinformatics (RCSB).

- The **Molecular Modeling DataBase (MMBD)**, managed by the NCBI, also has a three-dimensional view of the protein structure.
- **Clusters of Orthologous Groups (COGs)** attempts to classify proteins according to their phylogenetic, or evolutionary, links.
- **Basic Local Alignment Search Tool (BLAST)** is a tool to search for homologous sequences over large databases. Modifications of BLAST aid protein analysis.
- **Vector Alignment Search Tool (VAST)** is a tool to search for homologous protein structures.
- **Conserved Domain Database (CDD)** is a database of protein building blocks that have been retained throughout the evolutionary process.

Model organisms

Although enormous progress has been made towards identifying the genetic changes underlying many human disorders, there are still a large number of inherited conditions for which the gene or genes responsible have yet to be found. Even in cases where the underlying genetic lesions are well established the mechanism of the disease is often poorly understood.

A large proportion of the human genome shares many common elements, even with seeming disparate species, such as flies. An understanding of both the differences and similarities are critical to our understanding of biological processes in humans. Model organisms are those non-human species that have been chosen for laboratory research because they have particular characteristics:

- Rapid development
- Short lifecycle
- Small adult size
- Ready availability.

In addition, it is obviously an advantage of having many scientists working on just a few representative species so that all the genetic information can be pooled and made available to the whole scientific community. Model organisms are found among mammals, non-mammals and plants.

Mammals as model organisms

The mouse

The mouse genome is the closest model organism to humans (approximately 99% of mouse genes are present in humans) and this has already been invaluable in genetic, developmental and immunological research. Knowledge of the mouse genome will assist in our understanding of the genetic mechanisms of disease. This is particularly so because experiments can be carried out in animals with a uniform genetic background in a controlled environment, helping to tease out the disease variability that occurs in humans because of the greater genetic variation and the variable effects of the environment on humans.

Mice are also very economic models as maintenance is inexpensive, sexual maturity is achieved after 6 weeks, gestation is only 20 days and they have litters of 10 or more pups. Mutant strains of mice – mice with particular disease characteristics that have been bred for laboratory use – are particularly useful for studying these diseases. Mutations can be readily induced in mice using *N*-ethyl-*N*-nitrosourea (ENU).

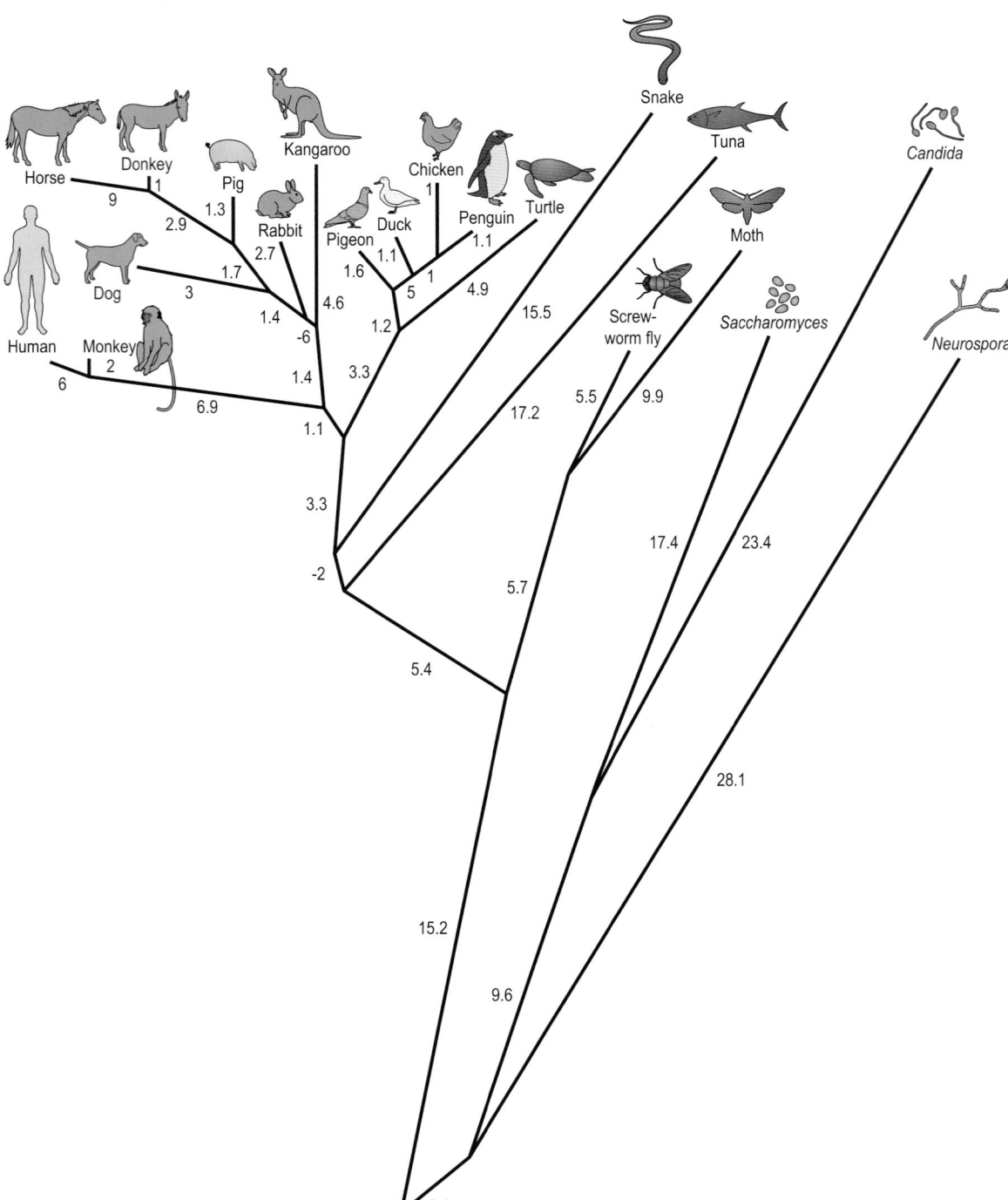

Fig. 5.44 A phylogenetic tree of 20 species developed by Walter Fitch and Emanuel Margoliash from observed changes in the cytochrome c gene between species. The numbers in the diagram relate to the average corrected minimum number of nucleotide substitutions to produce the different proteins seen in each species. Adapted from Fitch WM, Margoliash E 1967 Construction of phylogenetic trees. Science 155: 279–284.

Transgenic mice have their genome altered artificially. DNA sequences developed in the laboratory are introduced into mouse embryos which are then placed into foster mice until birth. The changes produced by these designed mutations can be researched in the quest for an understanding of human disease. **Knockout mice** have specific genes altered by engineering a change sufficient to make the gene non-functional.

Non-mammals as model organisms

Retroviruses

Retroviruses are important because they are the causative agent of many serious diseases, such as acquired immune deficiency syndrome (AIDS). They are different from other viruses as their transmission is horizontal by infection, and vertical through the genome. The infective particle does this by converting its RNA to DNA and incorporating this into the host genome. Retroviruses are important organisms in the study of DNA replication, transcription and RNA processing.

Bacteria and other microbes

Microbes make up a high proportion of the earth mass and have survived longer than most other living organisms. Microbes are also extremely diverse and can survive in many environments. Knowledge of the various genomes will aid the understanding of medical, industrial and environmental processes.

Saccharomyces cerevisiae (baker's yeast)

This was the first eukaryotic organism to be fully sequenced (as early as 1996). It is easy to manipulate genetically and the Saccharomyces Gene Deletion Project aims to produce deletion mutant strains for each of its 6000 genes.

Archaea

Archaea are very primitive, having some genes in common with bacteria (prokaryotes) and some in common with later organisms (eukaryotes), in addition to genes not found anywhere else. Because these organisms can survive in extreme environments their study is useful for biotechnology and studies on climate change and evolution.

Caenorhabditis elegans (round worm)

Caenorhabditis elegans is one the simplest multicellular organism comprising 959 cells with a full set of organs and a complex sensory system. The fate of each cell during the lifetime of the organism is known and its genome has been completely sequenced. The nematode can be rapidly grown and genetically modified.

Caenorhabditis elegans has approximately 20 000 genes of which many are orthologues of human genes. Recently it was discovered that previously unknown genes in the insulin signalling pathway of the worm have human homologues and that human insulin can function in the worm insulin pathway. Thus C. elegans is a viable system in which to model disorders of the insulin pathway.

Drosophila (fruit fly)

Drosophila has been studied over many years and has a biological system of similar complexity to humans. The fly has many human homologues and its genetic system is easy to manipulate. Its short reproductive cycle and its exoskeleton make it easy to screen for developmental abnormalities. Its genome was sequenced in March 2000, which is a further advantage.

Danio rerio (zebrafish)

Danio rerio has many advantages as a model organism. It is small, easily grown, has a short lifecycle and produces hundreds of eggs. It is a vertebrate, but with half the genes of humans, making it invaluable in identification of key vertebrate genes. Mutations are easily induced and embryonic development can be observed through its transparent coat and the use of fluorescent markers.

A large number of cardiovascular mutations have been identified and more than 100 genes are known to be required for normal heart development and function. The mutant 'pickwick' (pik) zebrafish are associated with dilated cardiac myopathy, and mutations of the same gene in humans results in a similar disorder.

GENETIC DISEASE, DIAGNOSIS AND THERAPY

GENE TESTING

Gene tests are undertaken in various ways:

- Direct examination of the DNA molecule, looking for mutated sequences
- Biochemical tests for gene products – abnormal, or abnormal amounts of particular enzymes or proteins
- Examination of stained chromosomes, looking for abnormal structures.

Gene tests may be used, for example:

- To identify **carriers** – individuals who are not affected because they carry only one copy of an aberrant gene that requires two copies for the disease (recessive) to be expressed
- To undertake prenatal testing
- To undertake presymptomatic or susceptibility testing
- To confirm diagnoses in symptomatic people.

Genetic tests can provide useful information, enabling therapeutic actions to be taken to improve the life of individuals thus affected. Identification of individuals who are currently healthy, but who are at high risk of developing a life-threatening disease, is more problematic, since not everyone who tests positive will develop the disease.

Certain diagnostic predictions may result in individuals being discriminated against, and the uncertainty about whether the disease may develop will lead to inevitable anxieties. These factors may outweigh any benefit of testing.

Genetic counselling

Genetic counsellors are health professionals with experience in the area of medical genetics, who are trained to provide information and support to families or individuals at risk of, or already affected by, genetic disease. The American Society of Human Genetics defines genetic counselling as 'A communication process which deals with human problems associated with the occurrence, or the risk of occurrence, of a genetic disorder in a family.' This process involves an attempt by one or more appropriately trained persons to help the individual or family to:

- Comprehend the medical facts, including the diagnosis, probable course of the disorder and the available management
- Appreciate the way heredity contributes to the disorder, and the risk of recurrence in specified relatives
- Understand the alternatives for dealing with the risk of recurrence
- Choose the course of action which seems to them appropriate in view of their risk, their family goals and their ethical and religious standards, and to act in accordance with that decision
- Make the best possible adjustment to the disorder in an affected family member and/or the risk of recurrence of that disorder.

Genetic counsellors often work as part of a multidisciplinary team that may include medical geneticists, physicians in the relevant speciality, nurses, psychologists, social workers and nutritionists. Support will also come from the primary care physician and disease support groups, the latter often set up by family members of sufferers.

CONGENITAL DISEASE

Congenital defects are those present, but not necessarily identified, at birth and are the most frequent cause of death in infants. Table 5.5 lists the most common congenital anomalies and their causes. Mostly there is no known reason for the malformation – this accounts for around 45% of all abnormalities, with multifactorial inheritance, familial causes and chromosome defects explaining a further 45%.

Different abnormalities can be defined as:

- **Malformation** – a primary defect due to abnormal development affecting part of the body, or an organ, such as a cleft lip
- **Dysplasia** – a primary defect of tissue formation, such as a vascular malformation
- **Sequence** – a primary defect that results in secondary structural changes, such as in oligohydramnios (reduced amniotic fluid) that leads to growth deficiencies, facial and limb deformities and pulmonary hypoplasia
- **Syndrome** – multiple primary malformations with a single cause, such as Down's syndrome
- **Deformation** – change in body shape due to external sources affecting the developing fetus, such as a mechanical force
- **Disruption** – a change due to the breakdown of an originally normal development, such as a limb not developing properly because a vascular problem has limited the blood flow.

Teratogens

Teratogens are external agents that produce birth defects. There are some well-established teratogens, of which thalidomide is one of the best known. Others include alcohol, isotretinoin (prescribed in the treatment of acne), phenytoin

Table 5.5	Some common congenital disorders
Congenital anomaly	**Cause**
Down's syndrome	Chromosomal
Trisomy 13	Chromosomal
Trisomy 18	Chromosomal
Turner's syndrome	Chromosomal
Prader–Willi syndrome	Microdeletion
Williams' syndrome	Microdeletion
Neurofibromatosis type I	Single gene autosomal dominant
Marfan's syndrome	Single gene autosomal dominant
Noonan's syndrome	Single gene autosomal dominant
Achondroplasia	Single gene autosomal dominant
Osteogenesis imperfecta	Single gene; heterogeneous
Oligohydramnios sequence	Heterogeneous
VATER	Unknown
Cornelia de Lange syndrome	Unknown
Fetal alcohol syndrome	Excess alcohol

Clinical box 5.14 | **Some birth defects caused by teratogens**

Fetal alcohol syndrome is a preventable teratogenic congenital abnormality. High alcohol consumption in the first trimester leads to children showing several facial abnormalities with a small head and accompanied by developmental delay, heart defects and intellectual disability.

Neural tube defect (**NTD**) is a malformation of the developing neural tube that leads to anencephaly (normally fatal because most of the brain is absent), encephalocele (when the skull plates do not seal) and spina bifida (where the spinal column does not seal). Individuals with NTDs have significant problems, including hydrocephalus (accumulation of spinal fluid in the skull that compresses brain tissue), leg paralysis and urinary obstruction. Ingestion of 4 mg folate has been shown to reduce the risk of NTD by 70%, and it is recommended that all pregnant women, and those planning pregnancy, should take folic acid daily.

(given to treat epilepsy), maternal infections (such as rubella), maternal disease (such as diabetes mellitus) and ionising radiation.

PHARMACOGENOMICS

No patients react in exactly the same way when given a drug and some will display dramatic differences when treated with a particular drug for the same condition. If we could predict which patients were going to react badly from a study of their genetic make-up then modifications could be made to the drugs, or alternatives prescribed, before the adverse events.

Pharmacogenomics is the study of the many different genes that determine drug behaviour. This is done by being able to define individual SNPs that predict a variable response to the particular drug. The hope for the future is that we will be able to provide treatment that is individualised to the individual. We must not lose sight, however, of the possibility that this personal genetic information will be misused and consideration of safeguards should be at the forefront of plans to utilise this approach more widely.

The best known examples of the potential of a pharmacogenomic approach are related to single gene traits that affect drug metabolism.

It is not only variations in drug metabolism that are observed; there is a growing collection of polymorphisms within genes that encode proteins involved in transporting and targeting drugs. Most of those that have been found are the ones that are easy to identify because they are associated with single genes and clearly recognisable effects. This

---

Clinical box 5.15 | **Examples of variation in drug metabolism associated with gene traits**

Thiopurine-S-methyl-transferase (**TPMT**) breaks down drugs used as immunosuppressants, such as mercaptopurine and azathioprine. There are, however, polymorphic variants in the enzyme that result in TPMT not working. For those people who inherit two inactive variants and need to be treated with these drugs, the result will be an excess level of the drugs, leading to high toxicity that may be life-threatening. Knowledge of the type of TPMT polymorphism that an individual carries may allow lower doses of the drugs to be used effectively, without the danger of increased toxicity.

is not how many drugs work, however, as multiple genes may be involved in determining the outcome of treatment. This has led to genome-wide approaches to identify genes that determine variant drug response. For example, between-family responses to the antihypertensive drug debrisoquine were used to identify the **CYP2D6** gene in the action of this drug and polymorphisms identified that were responsible for this variation. This gene has also been shown to be important in the metabolism of around 20% of described drugs, including sparteine and propafenone, both anti-arrhythmic drugs, amitriptyline, an antidepressant, and codeine, an analgesic, and this knowledge could be utilised to benefit individuals.

Even where a single gene variant appears to have a strong effect on drug action, much of the variation in patient response remains unexplained by the polymorphism alone. The reasons for this are that there may be many other polymorphisms within genes that are important in cellular pathways that are involved in the interaction between the drug and its subsequent effect. It is not only the direct effect on the gene itself, but there may be polymorphisms within, for example, the promoter and enhancer regions that affect the expression of the gene.

Future studies are likely to identify polymorphisms that interact with each other in different ways. For example, cytochrome P450 enzymes, including **CYP3A5**, are important in the metabolism of many drugs and a high expression of the latter enzyme, leading to more rapid drug metabolism, is seen more often in the black population. However, many of these same drugs are also metabolised faster if an individual possesses a particular p-glycoprotein polymorphism. These are more common among Caucasian individuals. Thus, customised treatment will have to consider all the polymorphisms that alter a drug's metabolism.

The identification of drugs that may have different efficacies in different racial groups may lead to questions of discrimination if some drugs are developed that benefit particular groups, even if no benefit ensues. Any approach is complicated by:

- False negatives – where there are differences between the tissue used in research and the tissue of action in the body
- False positives – simply because of the large number of areas that are being looked at, as areas will be identified by chance alone.

Identified regions in the genome will need to be confirmed through epidemiological association and biochemical functional studies, as well as in clinical models. The future hope for pharmacogenomics is the development of:

- New drugs
  - Genes identified with differing expression in cancer cells that are sensitive or resistant to anti-cancer drugs are candidates for the development of inhibitors of the gene product, reversing the drug-resistant phenotype.
  - Development of drugs, or drug combinations, targeted to particular tissues to maximise therapeutic benefits and decrease damage in healthy cells.
- Safer and better drugs
  - Instead of the current 'trial and error' approach, where a patient is treated and switched to another therapy if the first one does not work or has too many side effects, knowledge of the patient's genetic profile may allow the more appropriate treatment to be given from the start.
- Appropriate drug dose
  - Genetic response may be a better way to determine dose than a person's body mass in future.
- Susceptibility to disease
  - Most diseases are influenced by environmental factors and knowledge of risk may allow individuals to make important lifestyle changes and influence the timing of future drug therapies.
  - Genetic variants associated with increased risk of many common diseases are being identified.
- Better drug discovery
  - Many potentially useful drugs have been abandoned because of toxic side effects in some people. If this can be shown to be linked to polymorphic variations then individuals can be selected to receive, or not receive, the particular therapy.
  - For example, abacavir, an anti-HIV drug, produces extreme hypersensitivity reactions in a minority of patients. This has been linked to possession of the HLA-B*5701 genotype and prospective screening of individuals has led to a significant reduction in side effects of abacavir.
- Lower healthcare costs
  - The costs associated with getting a drug to market will be reduced if there is more information that allows the prediction of the likely response through knowledge of the genetic pathway involved.

Antibiotics and pharmacogenomics

The increasing resistance of bacterial pathogens to the current antibiotics has led to the need for new ways of identifying potential antimicrobial compounds. Traditional methods of identifying such compounds have involved whole-cell screening assays, with selection based on antibacterial activity. More recently biochemical assays have been used to screen compounds for their ability to target enzymes or specific cellular pathways. Neither approach, however, has resulted in many new antibiotics been developed.

A more rational approach in the identification of potential antibiotic targets has come from genomic sequencing. The genomes of more than 100 bacteria have been sequenced and this allows the identification of proteins that are conserved across pathogens. This approach produces better information about the likely spectrum of activity of an antimicrobial agent against a particular protein, and is an unbiased approach. Comparison with the human genome also allows the identification of homologues that could present toxicity problems. Using currently available data, around 300 potential drug targets have been identified.

Clinical box 5.16	Genomic sequencing and potential antibiotic targets

Peptide deformylase is a critical enzyme in the initiation of bacterial but not mammalian protein synthesis. Inhibiting the enzyme will lead to a reduction in bacterial growth and this therefore may provide a useful antibiotic target. Two compounds have been identified that inhibit the enzyme and show antibacterial activity with a potential for treating Gram-negative and Gram-positive infections.

Evidence-based treatment (see also Ch. 7)

We are some way off using pharmacogenomic approaches for making treatment decisions, despite there being clear candidates for their use. Current approaches in drug therapy use a trial and error approach, starting with a standard dose that will be modified by the results of biochemical tests or reporting of side effects. Changes in clinical practice will not come without proper randomised controlled studies that demonstrate a benefit in outcome. This will require a significant investment and there may be commercial pharmaceutical pressures that do not, necessarily, see the advantage of the approach. Despite the costs of essential clinical trials, others will point to the high cost of providing an individual genetic profile, although this will be offset by the reduced ongoing need to monitor deleterious effects through biochemical tests, and cost is already being driven down through the introduction of SNP genotyping arrays.

GENETIC MEDICINE

Greater knowledge of the human genome means that there is hope for significant breakthroughs in the treatment of hereditary diseases. To date there has been considerable success with some diseases using metabolic manipulation or protein augmentation; genetic strategies being researched use stem cells, gene transfer and RNA modification.

Metabolic manipulation

Metabolic manipulation has been used extensively to treat inborn errors of metabolism, but may also be used to prevent complications of other therapies. Examples are:

- Diet modification
  - **Galactosaemia**, caused by mutations in galactose-1-phosphate uridyl transferase, means that galactose cannot be converted to glucose and is metabolised to galactitol and galactonate. These metabolites lead to liver disease, intellectual disability and poor growth. Galactosaemia is the commonest disorder of carbohydrate metabolism and can be treated by restricting dietary galactose.
  - **Familial hypercholesterolaemia** can be treated with a low-cholesterol diet but this is best supplemented by drugs (**statins**) that inhibit hydroxymethylglutaryl co-enzyme A reductase.
- Protein substitution
  - **Hydroxyurea** given to sufferers of **sickle cell anaemia** stimulates production of fetal haemoglobin, which lowers the proportion of the abnormal sickle haemoglobin, thus limiting the occurrence of sickle cell crisis.
- Treatment of toxic therapies
  - The anaemia caused by **thalassaemia** is treated with repeated red cell transfusion. This leads to iron overload, leading to organ failure. **Desferrioxamine** chelates excess iron.
- Altering tertiary protein structure
  - Genetic mutations may result in a mis-folding of a protein that prevents its normal function. Research is underway to look for molecules that will modify these proteins, or their target sites, in order for normal function to progress.

Protein augmentation

Individuals with absence of particular proteins can be treated through external purification of the protein and delivery back to the patient. Because there are problems with proteins reaching particular sites, such as the brain, these treatments are more simply used in diseases where the protein only needs to be available within the extracellular milieu.

- Extracellular augmentation
  - **Cystic fibrosis** is due to mutation in the cystic fibrosis transmembrane receptor (**CFTR**) and leads to problems in sodium and chloride transport resulting in obstructive thick secretions and pancreatic insufficiency. Pancreatic enzymes are given as dietary supplements as part of the treatment.
- Intracellular augmentation
  - **Lysosomal storage diseases**, such as **Tay–Sachs** disease, are produced by accumulations of substrates, such as sphingolipids, mucopolysaccharides, glycoproteins or glycolipids, which are not metabolised because of deficiencies in lysosomal enzymes. Excess substrate leads to cell, tissue and organ dysfunction. Enzymes need to be delivered across the cell membrane and this has been achieved, for example, by modifying the enzyme to accept markers that recognise and bind to mannose-6-phosphate within the **lysosome** (organelles that contain enzymes that digest cellular waste, including worn-out organelles or engulfed viruses and bacteria).

Stem cell therapies

Stem cells are cells that have the ability to reproduce themselves and to differentiate along specialised lineages.

- **Embryonic stem cells** are derived from embryos in the blastocyst stage (around 100 cells) and are pluripotent.
- **Somatic stem cells** are derived from organs and are already partially differentiated along the lineage of the tissue from which they originate.

Embryonic stem cell transplantation

The pluripotent nature of embryonic stem cells makes them attractive propositions for the delivery of genetic medicine but science is not sufficiently advanced for trials to begin since human cells were first isolated and cultured only in 1998. Furthermore, there are considerable ethical considerations and public acceptability discussions to be had because of the requirement for 'unwanted' embryos. There are various ways in which it is proposed that embryonic stem cells are used:

- Cells may be differentiated in vitro and then transplanted to replace cells, or lineage-determined progenitors, in vivo
- These cells could be used to deliver genes to alter phenotype through gene transfer.
- In vitro research can use embryonic stem cell lines carrying particular genetic disorders, derived originally from pre-implantation genetic diagnostic procedures. These form models of the disease so that pathogenesis can be studied and drug screening to be tested in vitro.

Immune rejection of material from unrelated donors may be overcome by integrating normal gene material from the patient into autologous cells, then replacing the nucleus of an unrelated donor egg by the genetically correct nucleus from the patient. The egg is stimulated to develop to the blastocyst stage and corrected autologous pluripotent stem cells are removed and transplanted into the patient. This simple-sounding process, however, will depend on cells differentiating appropriately and being able to function properly when returned.

Haematopoietic stem cell transplantation

Bone marrow transplantation with haematopoietic stem cells has been used for many years to replace abnormal blood cell-forming lineages of the bone marrow in conditions such as leukaemia. This method has also been used to provide a presence of normal genes in diseases such as haemoglobinopathies, immunodeficiencies and lysosomal storage diseases.

Non-haematopoietic stem cell transplantation

Somatic stem cells have been identified in various organs and can be used to target particular deficiencies within the same lineage. Recent data demonstrate these cells can be reprogrammed to pluripotent cells similar to embryonic stem cells by overexpressing (by gene transfer, see below) a number of transcription factors such as Oct4 and Sox2.

Neuronal ceroid lipofuscinosis (Batten's disease) is due to a deficiency in **palmitoyl-protein thioesterase** and causes a neurodegeneration. Experiments in animals have shown that the transplantation of neural stem cells into the central nervous system has produced engraftment of normally differentiated cells and a reduction in accumulated pathogenic substances.

Gene transfer

The principle of gene transfer is simply the introduction of a normal gene into the cells of an affected individual. Animal models have been quite successful but correction of human disorders is proving more difficult. Of the large number of trials already in place only a few have shown phenotype correction and clinical improvement. These include adenosine deaminase deficiency and X-linked severe combined immunodeficiency. There are two main methods to achieve transfer: ex vivo and in vivo.

Ex vivo approach

Cells from the relevant population are removed from the patient, modified genetically and replaced. This process is useful where the cells can be easily obtained, such as from within bone marrow, or the skin. For example:

- Transfer of factor VIII gene into autologous fibroblasts to treat haemophilia A
- Transfer of a 'suicide' gene into T lymphocytes to treat the graft-versus-host disease associated with non-autologous bone marrow transplantation.

In vivo approach

This involves direct transfer of the gene in vivo within a **vector**. If the abnormal phenotype is due to a secreted (extracellular) protein, then the transfer only needs to be sufficient, and to any site, to correct any clinical phenotype. Organs that prevent protein transfer, such as the brain and eye, will require direct delivery. If the protein works intracellularly, then the gene has to be transferred to sufficient numbers of the appropriate cells.

- Genes for transfer consist of cDNA with a promoter site, a stop site and a polyadenylation site, known as the **expression cassette**.
- The genes are placed within a vector which may be **viral**, or **non-viral**, the aim being to deliver them into the nucleus but not into a chromosome in non-dividing cells, as that will result in dilution of effect as the cells divide, or integrate the gene directly into the genome.
- *Viral vectors* include DNA-based adenoviruses, adeno-associated viruses, retroviruses and lentiviruses. Only retroviruses and lentiviruses allow permanent insertion of the gene into the genome.
- *Non-viral vectors* are normally circular plasmids that incorporate the expression cassette and an antibiotic resistance gene within a liposome that helps transfer across the plasma membrane. There are, however, no mechanisms to direct the plasmid into the nucleus, and no trials involving this method have proven successful to date.

RNA modification

This method targets mRNA in order to suppress it, or add functions. Delivery of these therapies is dependent on successful delivery and advances in research in gene transfer methodology.

Four approaches have been suggested to modify mRNA: antisense oligonucleotides, RNA interference (RNAi), trans-splicing and ribozymes.

- **Antisense oligonucleotides** are short single-stranded DNA sequences, complementary to the mRNA sequence. Once bound, ribonuclease in the cell is upregulated and this cleaves the mRNA strand, thus reducing expression of the protein that the mRNA codes for. Research to influence pre-mRNA in **Duchenne's muscular dystrophy** using antisense oligonucleotides to stimulate skipping of exons leads to removal of the mutant material and production of a truncated protein with some function.
- **RNAi** is a natural mechanism that works on a double-stranded mRNA loop and is thought to provide protection against viruses. The Dicer enzyme removes the loop and creates short double-sided fragments with a small 3′ overhang. One strand forms a complex and activates a ribonuclease silencing complex, which cleaves complementary sequence mRNA. If this is the mRNA associated with the disease process then expression will be reduced. This process will require significant development in the future. It needs to be able to continuously deliver enough RNAi, because it can only correct the phenotype of the cell it reaches, and would also need to be incorporated into a vector to pass across plasma membranes. Combined gene transfer RNAi strategies have shown to work in a mouse model of **Huntington's disease**, leading to improved phenotype.
- **Trans-splicing** involves correcting mutant pre-mRNA. The pre-mRNA exon is attacked by a trans-splicer pre-mRNA which has a normal exon and is delivered by a gene transfer vector. It has a 5′ tail that is complementary to the RNA strand lying 5′ of the mutant form exon, with which it hybridises. Spliceosomes remove the between-exon RNA and the normal exon is incorporated into the resultant mRNA. Animal models

using this approach have been shown to correct **haemophilia A** and **cystic fibrosis**.

- **Ribozymes** are RNA constructs of the correct mRNA sequence, combined with an enzyme that recognises and cleaves the mutant mRNA, and allows ligation of the correct sequence. Specificity is provided by complementary flanking sequences. This process could replace mutant sequences, or reduce mutant mRNA levels. There are problems with ensuring efficient uptake into cells and ribozymes are not very stable. In vitro studies using ribozymes have been shown to correct the mutation associated with **familial amyloidotic polyneuropathy**.

Future of genetic therapy

Currently, no gene therapy has been approved for use in humans and there will be a significant time period before that can happen. There are many challenges to be met before any therapy is used:

- Any treatment must be shown to be safe and effective.
- The rarity of individual diseases means that it will be difficult to conduct randomised controlled trials.
- Government advisory bodies will need to consider the public view of genetic therapy, and this may require education to allay fear.
- The development of genetic therapies will be very costly and impossible without the involvement of the pharmaceutical industry and there may not be sufficient financial incentives to take these processes forward.
- Use of embryonic stem cells is potentially more problematic. Some groups consider that use of blastocyst cells is the equivalent of a destruction of human life. Only since the inauguration of US President Barack Obama in 2009 has the US food and Drug Administration approved the first clinical trial using human embryonic stem cells to treat patients paralysed through spinal cord injury.

Pathology and immunology

Denise Syndercombe Court, Paola Domizio and Nigel Yeatman

INFECTION

Denise Syndercombe Court, Nigel Yeatman

INTRODUCTION

Disease results from a failure of homeostasis within the body, which causes impaired function. Failure of homeostasis itself can be due to a multiplicity of causes, extrinsic and intrinsic, many of which are discussed in other areas of this book, and are summarised in Tables 6.1 and 6.2.

This section deals with biological agents that are the agents of infectious disease as well as the body's defence system, both immune and cellular, and the failure of cells to control their growth.

- Biological agents, such as bacteria and viruses, cause infections by entering the host body and are important causes of injury and damage. Often, but not always, specific organisms cause particular diseases. The defence system deals with the body's attempt to resist and repair injury. It includes inflammation, wound healing, non-immunological defence and the immune system.
- A disorder of cell growth, or neoplasia, is an abnormal proliferation of cells. Proliferation may be benign (non-progressive) or invasive (malignant).

Table 6.1	Extrinsic causes of disease	
Extrinsic factor	**Agent**	**Example**
Biological	Prions	Creutzfeldt–Jakob disease
	Viruses	Acquired immune deficiency syndrome
	Bacteria	Urinary tract infection
	Fungi	Candidiasis
	Protozoa	Malaria
	Helminths	Schistosomiasis
Chemical	Toxin	Bee sting
	Inflammatory substances	Asthma
	Poison	Tobacco smoke
Physical	Trauma	Fracture, laceration, crushed tissue
	Temperature	Burn, frostbite
	Radiation	Cancer
	Environment	Dehydration

Table 6.2	Intrinsic causes of disease	
Intrinsic factor	**Agent**	**Example**
Biochemical	Endocrine	Diabetes
	Nutritional	Obesity
	Metabolic	Phenylketonuria
Cellular	Autoimmune	Rheumatoid arthritis
	Degenerative	Alzheimer's disease
	Uncontrolled cell division	Cancer
Genetic	Single gene	Sickle cell disease
	Multifactorial	Hypertension
Structural	Congenital	Heart malformation, spina bifida
	Acquired	Osteoarthritis

BIOLOGICAL AGENTS

The burden of infectious disease

Infectious disease is the cause of almost 20% of deaths worldwide, but in Africa this increases to almost 50%. Figure 6.1 shows the relative contributions of the top six causes of death worldwide and separately within Africa in 2002, showing the higher relative contributions of human immuno-deficiency virus/acquired immune deficiency syndrome (HIV/AIDS) and malaria within Africa.

The variety of biological infectious agents

Organisms that cause infectious diseases can be grouped into the seven major categories: prions, viruses, bacteria, fungi, protozoa, helminths and arthropods. Many are **microbes** that need a microscope to be visualised. Each has its own classification system.

Prions are collections of protein molecules and are not considered living organisms. **Viruses** have genetic material, but no other cellular characteristics, depending on other cells for their survival. All other agents are single cells (most microbes) or consist of multiple cells. Early classification divided organisms into **prokaryotes** and **eukaryotes**.

Prokaryotes:

- Have no nuclear membrane
- Have DNA in the form of:
  - A single circular chromosome, forming a nucleoid
  - Plasmids, which are extracellular circular DNA molecules of varying size
- Have no membrane-bound organelles
- Have cytoplasm rich in ribosomes
- Transcription and translation can be carried out at the same time.

All **bacteria** are prokaryotes and they can be further sub-divided into **eubacteria** (true bacteria) and **archaebacteria** (archaea).

Archaea are prokaryotes, because they have no nucleus, but have introns within their genes and their ribosomal RNA (rRNA) sequence is similar to that found in eukaryotes. They

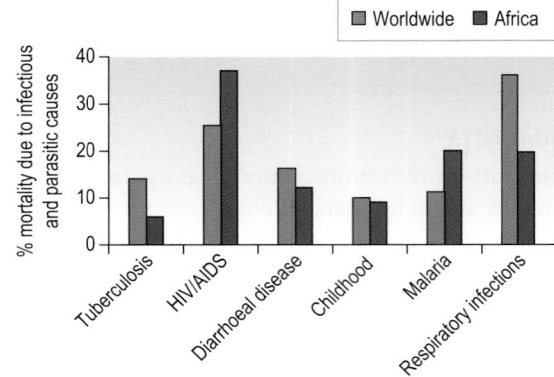

Fig. 6.1 **The burden of infectious disease worldwide.**

were originally discovered in extreme temperature and chemical environments but none are known pathogens and they will not be discussed further. Eukaryotes:

- Have a separate nucleus
- DNA is carried on several chromosomes within the nucleus
- Have membrane-bound organelles – mitochondria, ribosomes on endoplasmic reticulum, Golgi apparatus and lysosomes
- Transcription requires movement of messenger RNA (mRNA) from the nucleus to the cytoplasm
- Translation takes place on ribosomes.

Fungi, **protozoa** and **helminths** are eukaryotes.

Each organism can be further classified according to various characteristics and described as a species, within a genus. For example bacteria can be grouped according to how they stain, what their shape is, whether they need oxygen and how they group or reproduce.

PRIONS

Prions were named by the American neurologist, Stanley Prusiner, when he defined them as: '**pro**teinaceous **in**fectious particles that lack nucleic acid'. The unlikely concept of an infectious agent that lacks nucleic acid has meant that there continue to be scientists who believe that they could be acting with other agents, such as slow-acting viruses.

PrP^C is a normal protein found in cell membranes and consists of amino acids in a mainly α-helical structure. There is some evidence that the protein is involved in the maintenance of long-term memory within the part of the brain known as the **hippocampus**. PrP^{SC} is an atypical form in which a large proportion of the α-helical structure is replaced by a different type of secondary structure, the β-sheet. Its amino acid sequence is, however, no different from the normal form, although there are sequence differences in the protein between species. This sequence difference is thought to be the reason for resistance to cross-species infectivity.

An isoform of PrP^C appears to catalyse its transformation into the abnormal form, PrP^{SC}, resulting in a different struc-

Information box 6.1 General features of prions

- Not a living organism
- Protein molecule with atypical sheet structure that accumulates in tissues
- Resistant to denaturation by chemical and physical agents.

The potential infectivity of protein was demonstrated in 1996 when scientists were able to transmit the disease **kuru** to chimpanzees by injecting them with diseased brain extracts. Normal strategies used to destroy infective agents, such as bleach, heat or radiation, are ineffective. Prions have been implicated as the likely cause of the **transmissible spongiform encephalopathies (TSEs)**. Prions are composed principally of a protein which is expressed mainly in neurons of the central nervous system and encoded by the **PRNP (PRioN Protein)** gene. The protein has two different forms:

- Protein-resistant protein (common) or PrP^C
- Protein-resistant protein (scrapie) or PrP^{SC}.

ture and attracting, through aggregation, free proteins, to form **amyloid** that accumulates and is deposited locally in the tissues. Over 20 different strains of the infective agent have been described, resulting in variable incubation periods and pathology. It is thought that these strains arise through a conformational change that occurs on crossing between the species.

VIRUSES

The origin of viruses is unknown, but because they are dependent on host cells it seems unlikely that they are some form of precursor to life in its cellular form.

Viruses are metabolically inert; although they have genetic material they can only use this information to reproduce within host cells where they are assisted by enzymes and ribosomes from the infected cell. Outside the cell they are in the form of virus particles, or **virions**, and may lie within body fluids, within the body tissues or outside the body within the environment. Virions may sometimes be in the form of a

Clinical box 6.1 Human transmissible spongiform encephalopathies

Five different human prion diseases have been identified, including Creutzfeldt–Jakob disease (CJD), variant CJD (vCJD) and kuru.

- **CJD**: classic CJD is a fatal neurodegenerative disease that occurs sporadically in about 1 in 1 000 000 people each year, although inherited forms caused by a mutation in the prion gene also exist. It is more common with increasing age and patients experience dementia and show early neurological abnormalities. Sections of brain tissue have a 'sponge-like' appearance. Transmission has been shown within human growth hormone, through corneal implants, and on surgical instruments.
- **vCJD**: this was first described in 1996 and had a different clinical presentation from CJD, patients typically being young adults displaying marked behavioural symptoms and a marked accumulation of the abnormal protein.

There is strong evidence that the disease is causally linked to ongoing outbreaks of **bovine spongiform encephalopathy (BSE, or 'mad cow disease')** which is a prion disease occurring in cattle. BSE began in the 1970s after cattle were fed with a bone meal food probably from sheep infected with **scrapie**, another prion disease. BSE became more common in the UK when calves were fed with BSE-infected bovine material. By the end of 2005 more than 35 000 herds of cattle had been affected.

vCJD was linked to the BSE outbreak during which individuals ate beef contaminated with central nervous system material from infected cattle. Until the end of 2007, 166 patients have been identified in the UK, 163 of whom have died, with a peak in deaths in 2000. Although many individuals may carry the infection, only those who are homozygous for amino acid methionine at position 129 in the *PRNP* gene have so far been infected by this route. Although there are measures to prevent potentially infected tissues from entering the human and animal food chains, reducing the disease incidence, more recent cases have been associated with blood transfusions from individuals who themselves subsequently developed vCJD, suggesting that blood donation is a relatively efficient transmission route.

Kuru, meaning 'trembling in fear', was a fatal disease that occurred in the Fore people of Papua New Guinea in the 1950s and was associated with cannibalistic rituals in which the people ate human brain tissue. It is very similar to vCJD and is thought to have originated from scrapie-infected sheep.

- Dependent on a living cell (obligate intracellular pathogen)
- Nucleic acid core (DNA or RNA, and rarely both) with protein coat (the nucleocapsid)
- 10–300 nm in size
- Circular, elongated or segmented
- Surface binding protein to attach to cell.

- **Helical** – in which the capsomeres assemble around the genome to form a tubular capsid. Most human pathogenic viruses have an envelope, for example the **paramyxovirus** family.
- **Polyhedral** – in which the capsid forms a geometrical shape with a central cavity. **Icosahedral** viruses have 20 faces and are a common form, for example the **adenovirus**. Sometimes these too are enveloped, such as the **herpesvirus**.
- **Complex** forms are larger and more varied in their structure. The **bacteriophage**, for example, has an icosahedral head and helical tail and can have a hexagonal base with protein fibres coming from it. Other complex viruses are very different in form; the **poxvirus** may show an ovoid or brick shape.

nucleocapsid, but sometimes this may be surrounded by an outer envelope which is normally a lipid bilayer of host origin. These different forms influence how viruses survive and are transmitted.

NUCLEOCAPSID STRUCTURE

Genomic material

This may be DNA or RNA, single stranded or double stranded. It can be linear or circular and may, or may not, use enzymes that copy the viral genome once it enters the host cell. In addition, single-stranded RNA may be:

- **Sense** – used directly as mRNA to translate viral protein
- **Antisense** – the complementary strand must be produced within the host cell to be used as mRNA.

Capsid

The capsid is a protein shell made up of numerous subunits (**capsomeres**) that give the virus a particular shape. There are three main shapes:

HOST CELL INFECTION

Viruses enter the human body in a variety of ways:

- Inhalation – through infected droplets
- Ingestion – from contaminated food or drink, or from saliva
- Inoculation – through injection, trauma exposure or insect bites
- Transplacentally
- Sexual intercourse.

Viruses normally infect only one or a small range of species and, once within the body, the continued success of the virus will depend on its ability to attach to the host cell and then replicate. Although replication varies, there are six basic stages (Fig. 6.2):

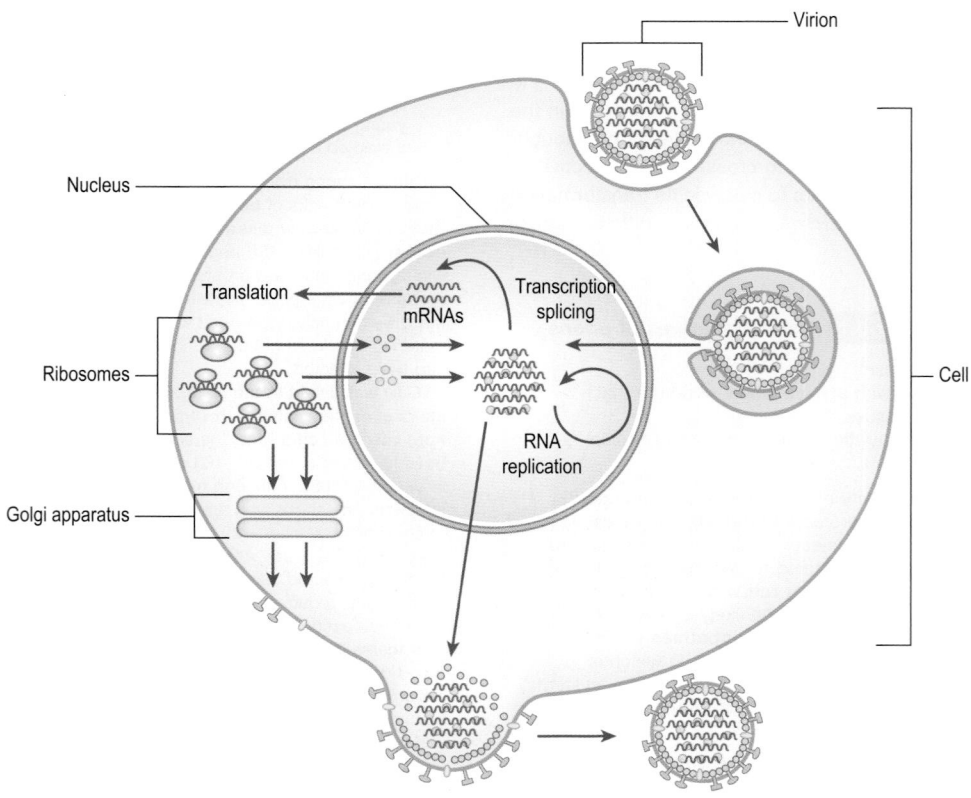

Fig. 6.2 **Viral replication.**

- **Attachment**: specific receptors on the host cell bind with the viral capsid:
  - HIV binds to human T cells through its surface protein **gp120** interacting with **CD4**, a glycoprotein found on the surface of T cells.
  - Influenza virus binds to **sialic acid** found on the surface of red cells and mucous membrane cells.
- **Penetration**: this can happen in two main ways in human infections:
  - **Fusion**: attachment to the receptor causes a change in the viral envelope allowing the membranes to fuse.
  - **Viropexis**: the virus is taken up in an endocytic vesicle and the virus enters the cytoplasm. If the virus has an envelope this fuses with the vesicle membrane, like the above process but this time from within the cell.
- **Uncoating**: enzymes from the virus or host degrade the capsid and release the genomic material into the host cell cytoplasm.
- **Replication**: this is a complex process and depends on the genomic material made available. The **Baltimore classification** proposes seven different schemes to deal with the different genomic structures. Important enzymes in these processes are:
  - **DNA-dependent DNA polymerase** which makes a complementary strand of DNA, converting a single strand into a double strand. Some viruses use the human enzyme, others use their own.
  - **DNA-dependent RNA polymerase** which uses viral DNA to produce mRNA, which can then be translated into proteins and other enzymes on host ribosomes. There are human and viral forms of this enzyme and different viruses will use different ones.
  - **RNA-dependent DNA polymerase (reverse transcriptase)** which makes a complementary strand of DNA from RNA strands. Humans do not have this enzyme and so these viruses (e.g. retroviruses) must use their own.
  - **RNA-dependent RNA polymerase** makes a complementary strand of RNA. Again humans do not have this enzyme, which must therefore be provided within the virion.
- **Assembly**: some of the mRNA produced through the above enzymes acting on the viral genomic material is translated on host ribosomes into viral proteins which, with replicated viral genomic material, are assembled into new nucleocapsids. This may be followed by modification (or maturation) of the viral protein, which may take place after the virus has been released from the host cell, such as in HIV.
- **Release**: although some viruses are released through lysis of the host cell, enveloped viruses **bud** off. New virions accumulate near the cell membrane which then envelopes them and then forms a bud which breaks off from the host cell, releasing the virions into the environment.

Viruses differ in how long they infect the host cell. Some are only present within the cell for a few days (such as that producing the common cold), others are present for a long time producing a chronic infection (for example, hepatitis B) and some may infect but not replicate for years, resulting in a chronic latent infection (such as HIV, or the chickenpox

---

Clinical box 6.2   Human immunodeficiency virus (HIV)

HIV is the cause of the acquired immunodeficiency syndrome (AIDS). The infection may be sexually transmitted, vertically transmitted from mother to baby, acquired through transfusion of contaminated blood, blood products and organ donation, or via intravenous drug misuse. Symptoms include fever, lymphadenopathy, sore throat, mucosal ulcers, joint and muscle pains and occasionally a transient rash. There is usually an incubation period of 2–3 weeks followed by HIV conversion lasting about 6 weeks after exposure, before symptoms develop. Clinical manifestations of AIDS cover a wide spectrum, and are related to either the direct effects of HIV infection or to immunodeficiency.

HIV infection directly affects nearly all the body systems, including neurological complications, eye disease, skin and mucus membrane complications, haematological complications and diseases relating to the gastrointestinal, renal, respiratory, endocrine systems and the heart. Immunodeficiency increases the risk of all types of infections, including tuberculosis, candidiasis, herpes simplex, pneumonias (those caused by *Pneumocystis carinii (P. jiroveci)* in particular), cytomegalovirus, toxoplasmosis and septicaemias. Tumours, such as lymphomas and Kaposi's sarcoma, may also develop.

The introduction of highly active anti-retroviral therapy (HAART) has improved prognosis greatly to the extent that AIDS has become a chronic disease in the developed world.

Clinical box 6.3   Influenza

Influenza is caused by a virus of the orthomyxovirus family, not to be confused with the common cold which is caused by a rhinovirus. The clinical features and normal course of the two conditions are also different, where influenza is more debilitating and has potentially more long-lasting complications, such as the postviral or chronic fatigue syndrome. After an incubation period of 2–3 days, influenza presents with an acute onset of fever, muscle pains, severe headache and sore throat. Secondary bacterial infection (*Streptococcus pneumoniae* and *Haemophilus influenzae*) may lead to pneumonia, particularly in vulnerable patients.

The influenza virus has two main forms, A and B. Influenza A has the ability to develop antigenic variants at irregular intervals and was the cause of the 1918 pandemic. A major change in the antigenic makeup of influenza A led to the emergence of the Hong Kong influenza type H3N2 in 1968, and the avian H5N1 strain in 1997 (see also Pandemics).

---

virus when it result in shingles). They also differ in their seriousness: Ebola, SARS (severe acute respiratory syndrome) and avian influenza are recognised as being very serious infections whereas the common cold virus and herpes simplex virus type 1 (producing cold sores) are not serious human infections (see also Clinical boxes 6.2 and 6.3).

VIRUS CLASSIFICATION

Although very varied, viruses are distinct from all other organisms. In biology a species is a population whose members can interbreed to form fertile offspring. Viruses do not undergo sexual reproduction; nevertheless the concept of species is still used, differentiating between them according to structure and genome sequence. Groupings within a species are called **strains** or **serotypes**, produced as a result of mutations that occur when the viral material undergoes replication. Table 6.3 gives examples of the classification of various clinically important viruses.

Table 6.3	Examples of clinically important viruses and their classification		
Species	**Baltimore class**	**Shape**	**Envelope**
Adenovirus	Double-stranded DNA (dsDNA)	Icosahedral	No envelope
Ebola, Marburg	Antisense single-stranded RNA (−ssRNA)	Complex	Enveloped
Hepatitis A, poliovirus	Sense (+) ssRNA	Icosahedral	No envelope
Hepatitis B	dsDNA and single-stranded DNA (ssDNA)	Icosahedral	Enveloped
Hepatitis C	+ssRNA	Icosahedral	Enveloped
Herpes simplex, Epstein–Barr virus, cytomegalovirus, varicella zoster	dsDNA	Icosahedral	Enveloped
Human immunodeficiency enzyme (HIV)	+ssRNA	Icosahedral	Enveloped
Influenza	−ssRNA	Helical	Enveloped
Measles, mumps	−ssRNA	Helical	Enveloped
Papillomavirus	ssDNA	Icosahedral	No envelope
Rabies	−ssRNA	Helical	Enveloped
Rotavirus	dsRNA	Icosahedral	No envelope
Rubella	+ssRNA	Icosahedral	Enveloped
Smallpox	dsDNA	Complex	Enveloped

VACCINES

History

Vaccination is the administration of antigenic material to a person in order to make them immune to a disease. It first became known about in Britain when Lady Mary Wortley Montagu wrote about the practice of people inoculating themselves with fluid from people suffering from smallpox when she was in Turkey and used it on her children. Edward Jenner (1749–1823) is regarded as the founder of modern vaccination: milkmaids who had been exposed to cowpox (vaccinia) were resistant to smallpox infection and he tested this hypothesis by experimenting on a young boy, first infecting him with cowpox. Subsequent inoculation with smallpox failed to produce the latter disease.

Aim of vaccination

The best that can be hoped for is that vaccination should be used so that a disease is eradicated. Smallpox was reported as being eradicated in 1977 and polio is close to being eradicated. Sometimes vaccination is used to prevent the symptoms of a disease, such as avoiding toxins produced by tetanus, or attempting to block transmission of a disease, such as malaria.

Types of vaccines

■ **Live attenuated**: these are the most successful vaccines and consist of live virus particles that are less virulent (attenuated), perhaps by passing them through cell lines, or adapting the virus to work best at low temperatures. Polio (Sabin), measles, mumps, rubella and yellow fever are all examples of diseases that are treated with live attenuated vaccines.
■ **Inactivated**: inactivated viruses have been killed by a process, such as heat, or exposure to formaldehyde. The virus capsid is still recognised by the immune system, thus protecting the individual, but because there is no replication an individual will need booster injections over time. Polio (Salk), rabies, hepatitis A and influenza are examples of these types of vaccine.

■ **Subunit**: These vaccines use parts of the virus, such as the capsid, or surface coat, or other viral proteins. This is not always very successful because the proteins are readily denatured and any antibodies that are produced may bind to the denatured protein, but not the viral protein itself. A development of this idea has led to **recombinant** vaccines in which the relevant protein gene is placed into another virus. Vaccination with the second virus will lead to expression of the harmful virus protein, stimulating antibody production protecting the patient from the harmful infection. Hepatitis B vaccination is an example of this type of vaccination.

Table 6.4 summarises the advantages and disadvantages of the different types of vaccine.

VIRUSES AND CANCER

Both RNA and DNA viral infections are associated with certain cancers and can lead to a malignant transformation in cells. Sometimes it is believed that other agents (**cofactors**) may also be implicated, such as malaria influencing Burkitt's lymphoma, or ultraviolet light stimulating skin cancer. Generally, but not always, the viral genome has been isolated within the cancer cells. Table 6.5 lists some viruses that are associated with particular human cancers.

PANDEMICS

Human pandemics have been recorded throughout history.

■ An **epidemic** is when the frequency of an infection or disease increases above the normal (**endemic**) levels.
■ A **pandemic** is a 'global' epidemic. The first recorded pandemic was thought to be smallpox in 430 BC, to be followed over the intervening years by outbreaks of bubonic plague (the Black Death) and, more recently, cholera. In the twentieth century, it was the viral infection influenza which produced three pandemics. The first 'Spanish' flu was estimated to have killed over 40 000 000 people and was followed by 'Asian' flu in 1957 and 'Hong Kong' flu in 1968. Pandemics occur when a new virus emerges (see also Clinical box 6.3).

Table 6.4 Advantages and disadvantages of different types of vaccines

	Advantages	Disadvantages
Live attenuated	Most successful as they produce all features of the infection in a mild form and protect over many years Attenuated strains may pass into the population, further protecting people	May revert to a more virulent form Produce severe disease in immunocompromised patients Hypersensitivity to proteins from the attenuation process, such as chicken eggs Danger of passing on animal viruses
Inactivated	Present no hazard as they are killed	Short acting
Subunit	Non-hazardous as do not contain whole virus	May only stimulate B cells, producing only a primary response, rather than producing the longer antigenic memory that is the result of T cell activation T cell activation may vary between people, depending on their inheritance of different polymorphisms of the class II human lymphocyte antigens (HLA-D)

Table 6.5 Viruses associated with particular human cancers

Virus	Cancer
Epstein–Barr	Burkitt's lymphoma Nasopharyngeal carcinoma
Hepatitis B and C	Liver cancer
Human papilloma	Cervical cancer Skin cancer
HTLV-1 (human T cell lymphotrophic virus)	T cell leukaemia
HSV-2 (human simplex virus)	Cervical cancer

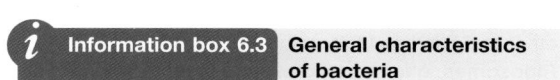

Information box 6.3 General characteristics of bacteria

- Prokaryotes – contain DNA, and RNA
- No nuclear membrane or membrane-bound intracellular organelles such as mitochondria, Golgi apparatus or endoplasmic reticulum
- Have ribosomes for protein synthesis but these are different structurally from eukaryotic ribosomes
- Have a plasma membrane, like eukaryotes
- Most also have a cell wall, which gives bacteria their distinctive shapes
- Divide by binary fission, but can exchange genetic material.

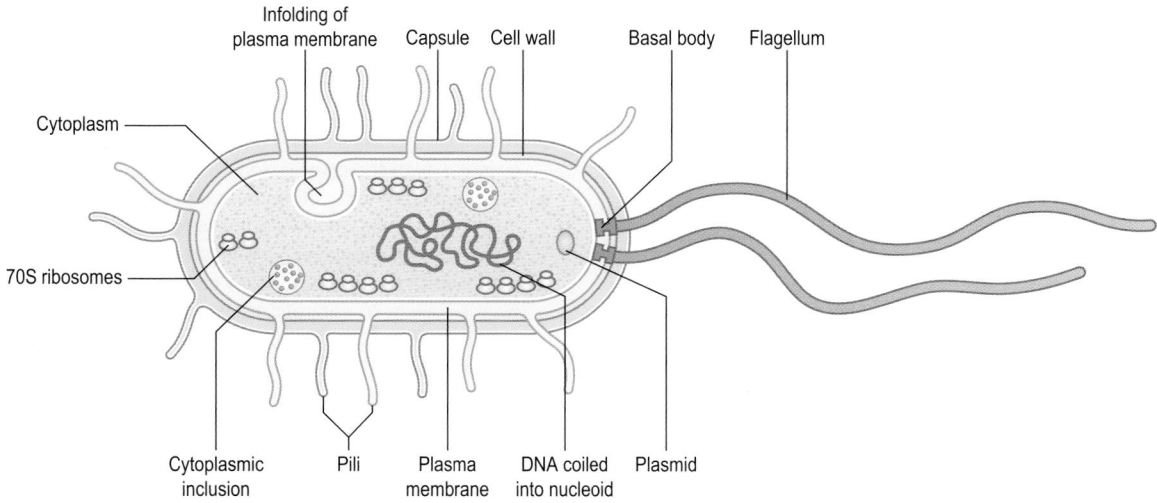

Fig. 6.3 **Illustration of a generalised bacterium.** Adapted with permission from Goering R et al 2007 Mims' medical microbiology, 4th edn. Mosby, Edinburgh.

H5N1 is a strain of avian flu that has the potential to become the cause of the next major pandemic. Most avian flu viruses do not affect humans but H5N1 has led to over 100 cases in Asia. The virus, in its present state, does not seem to spread readily but if it evolves into a more contagious form then it is expected that it will produce a truly global infection, because of increased and rapid travel across continents, and will result in many millions of deaths. Because of the danger that such a pandemic brings to the whole world community, both medically and economically, the World Health Organization has recommended that all countries prepare themselves, stockpiling vaccines and antiviral drugs, and having policies to deal with the unprecedented numbers of people who will need medical care.

BACTERIA

Bacteria are a large group of ubiquitous unicellular micro-organisms. They form much of the world's biomass and are vital components of the living world. Most, when they invade the human body, are destroyed by our immune system; some are beneficial, but others are harmful to humans and are described as **pathogens.**

STRUCTURE

The main cellular features of bacteria are illustrated in Figure 6.3.

Cytoplasm

Within the bacterial cytoplasm are:

- **The genome**: a single circular chromosome, plus or minus **plasmids**, which are independently replicating fragments of circular, double-stranded, DNA. The chromosome is located in the **nucleoid** but there is no nuclear membrane. The genetic material is coiled and supercoiled, under the control of the enzymes DNA gyrase and DNA topoisomerase. The DNA lacks introns and extragenic sequences, such as are found in eukaryotes – it is just a continuous coding sequence of genes.
- **Bacterial mRNA** is transcribed from DNA as in animal cells. There is no editing. Ribosomes can begin translation at one end of a mRNA molecule before the other end has been fully transcribed.
- **Ribosomes**: often a string of ribosomes is joined by a single mRNA molecule. Bacterial ribosomes are different from eukaryotic ribosomes:
  - Bacterial ribosomes are 70 S, and are composed of a 30 S portion and a 50 S portion.
  - 'S' refers to **Svedberg units**, which relate to how a particle behaves under ultracentrifugation.
  - Eukaryotic ribosomes are 80 S, although they do have 70 S ribosomes in their mitochondria.
- **Granules** – some bacteria have granules containing stored nutrients.
- **Mesosome** – an invagination of the cell membrane, involved in cell division.
- **Other constituents** – proteins, carbohydrates, messenger and transfer RNA, amino acids, etc.

Cell membrane (plasma membrane)

This is a phospholipid bilayer with embedded protein molecules and structures, similar to eukaryotic membranes. The membrane has four important features:

- Pores to control the entrance and exit of substances, such as nutrients, waste products and toxins
- Respiratory enzymes on the inner surface
- Enzymes involved in cell wall synthesis on the outer surface
- Is involved in binary fission.

Entry and exit of molecules through the membrane is controlled by permeases through a variety of mechanisms:

- Carrier-mediated down a concentration gradient
- Phosphorylation-linked transport
- Active transport.

Cell wall

This important structure surrounds the bacterium outside the plasma membrane. Animal cells do not have cell walls. The cell wall is strong, protects the bacterium from lysis in hypotonic solutions and from some physical trauma, and controls the access of some chemicals to the cell membrane. Different groups of bacteria have differently structured walls, determining the shape of the bacterium. They also cluster in different ways. Non-motile bacteria often stick to each other after replication.

- If they always divide in the same plane, they will end up forming long chains, like streptococci.
- If they divide in different planes, they form clusters, e.g. staphylococci.
- Some bacteria stick together more firmly forming long filamentous threads, such as those seen in *Actinomyces* or *Streptomyces* cultures.

The main bacterial forms are:

- Spherical (coccus) – cocci often occur in pairs (**diplococci**) or clusters like grapes (**staphylococci**), or lie in long chains (**streptococci**).
- Rod shaped (bacillus) – these too can be found in pairs (**diplobacilli**) chains (**streptobacilli**) or stacks (**palisades**)
- Comma shaped (vibrios)
- Spiral (spirochaetes) – spirochaetes are long thin spiral-shaped bacteria with an outer membrane. Between the cell wall and the outer membrane are 'internal flagella': filaments running the length of the bacterium. They are motile through a spinning action and the filaments flex the bacterium to achieve this.

BACTERIAL CLASSIFICATION

Gram staining, invented by a Danish scientist in 1884, remains the standard method for classifying bacteria dependent on the structure of the cell wall. Gram staining of a heat-fixed smear of bacteria is used to separate them into **Gram positive** or **Gram negative**. The process has four stages:

- Primary staining with crystal violet (CV) which penetrates the cell wall and plasma membrane, staining the cells purple
- A mordant, Gram's iodine (I), is added and forms a complex with the crystal violet (CV-I)
- Adding alcohol or acetone interacts with the cell membrane lipids, removing the outer layer and exposing the peptidoglycan layer. This layer is very thin in Gram-negative bacteria and the CV-I complexes are readily washed away. In contrast, the multilayered structure of Gram-positive bacteria retains the purple stain
- Counterstaining with basic fuchsin gives a red colour to the otherwise decolourised Gram-negative bacteria.

Some Gram-positive bacteria (mycobacteria, responsible for tuberculosis, for example) also have fatty acids and waxes within the cell walls, making it very difficult for materials to pass through the wall. While this means that they are very slow dividing, they are also resistant to Gram staining. Ziehl–Neelsen staining method uses an acid to allow fuchsin to penetrate the cell wall and colour the bacteria, making them visible under the microscope (see Clinical box 6.4).

OTHER BACTERIAL SURFACE FEATURES

- Some bacteria form **endospores** – tough, spherical forms that resist extremes of temperature. Spore formation is triggered by adverse environmental conditions. In this form they remain dormant, with the ability to survive for many millions of years.
  - Inhalation of endospores of *Bacillus anthracis* can lead to **anthrax**.
  - Contamination of wounds with endospores from *Clostridium tetani* leads to **tetanus**.

Clinical box 6.4 Tuberculosis

Tuberculosis is an infectious, airborne disease caused by *Mycobacterium tuberculosis* (less commonly *M. bovis*, *M. africanum* or *M. canetti*). Primary tuberculosis develops in response to the first infection by *M. tuberculosis*. This is usually subpleural, in the upper part of the lower lobe or the lower part of the upper lobe surrounded by the lobar fissure, know as the Ghon focus. The hilar lymph nodes draining the area may also be affected, and together with the primary lesion are known as the Ghon, or primary, complex. A delayed hypersensitivity reaction, an immune response, then takes place over 3–8 weeks after the initial infection, with exudate formation, and aggregations of neutrophils which are replaced by macrophages that react with T lymphocytes to form granulomas. The bacteria are not eliminated, but cell necrosis occurs to form the caseous (like soft white cheese) centre of the granuloma (tubercle) with variable amount of fibrosis. The caseous lesions heal completely, and may be calcified so that they are visible on X-ray. Some of these lesions still contain active tubercle bacilli that are dormant, but may be re-activated (usually years later) if the host immune system is compromised (e.g. in diabetes, immunosuppression, AIDS or malnutrition). Post-primary tuberculosis may then develop if the bacteria enter the blood stream and disseminate to other foci in the body causing infection. The commonest site of post-primary tuberculosis is the lungs. Other sites include lymph nodes, the brain, skin, gastrointestinal tract and kidneys. Diffuse blood-borne dissemination results in miliary tuberculosis, which is fatal without treatment.

A positive tuberculin test, an intradermal injection of a purified protein derivative of *M. tuberculosis* (tuberculin/PPD), indicates the development of cell immunity. The Mantoux test is used for testing in individual patients, and the Heaf test is used for population screening. The vaccine bacille–Calmette–Guérin (BCG), a live attenuated vaccine made from a bovine strain of tuberculosis (*M. bovis*), is effective in reducing the risk of developing tuberculosis. The public health policy of vaccination for school children in the UK had almost eradicated the disease. The AIDS pandemic, however, has led to the re-emergence of tuberculosis, particularly in the developing world where poverty and malnutrition combined with limitation of access to medicines compound the problem.

Successful treatment of tuberculosis entails continuous self-administration of a combination of anti-tuberculous drugs, rifampicin and isoniazid (see Ch. 4), over at least 6 months. A lack of compliance, misuse of therapy and inadequate treatment have led to the emergence of multidrug-resistant tuberculosis (MDR-TB). Direct supervision in special clinics – directly observed therapy short course (DOTS) – improves compliance. Hospitalisation for treatment may sometimes be necessary for persistently uncooperative patients or those with severe disease or social indications.

- Bacteria sometimes have extra material (**capsule**) outside the cells wall (Gram positive) or outside the outer membrane (Gram negative), composed of carbohydrates and/or proteins. This material hides the antigenic proteins, making them resistant to host cell phagocytosis. *Escherichia coli* bacteria commonly form capsules with a wide variety of constituents.
- **Flagella** are whip-like structures that move, making the bacterium motile and allowing them to respond to chemical stimulants. They are completely different from eukaryotic flagella in both structure and function.
- **Pili** (**fimbriae**) are long thin stiff structures, enabling bacteria to adhere to the cells of the host through specialised molecules, **adhesins**. Adhesins of *E. coli* allow these bacteria to interact with fucose and mannose molecules on the intestinal epithelial cells. Although the pili are immunogenic their antigens can

change (**antigenic variation**), leading to avoidance of immune recognition.

UNUSUAL TYPES OF BACTERIA

- **Chlamydia** are small Gram-negative bacteria, difficult to see, which can only divide within host cells. They have a 'lifecycle' with two forms: the **elementary body** and the **reticulate body**. Both forms have a cell wall and an outer membrane. They are reminiscent of viruses, in that they have to replicate in a host cell, but they encode all of their own material, obtaining only nutrients from the host.
- **Rickettsia** can also only replicate within a host cell, but they lack the special structures and lifecycle of chlamydia. They are just small fastidious bacteria with Gram-negative structure.
- **Mycoplasma** have no cell wall, are very small and of no definite shape. They can be seen only by immunofluorescence. rRNA sequences show them to be related to corynebacteria, but in medical classifications it is usual to consider them as a separate group because the lack of the cell wall means their survival, pathogenicity, detection, identification and treatment are all very different from those of the former. They are very susceptible to osmotic lysis and need to spend most of their time within a host.

REPLICATION

The rate at which bacteria grow and divide depends mainly on the nutritional environment. *Escherichia coli*, in a rich nutrient, can divide several times in an hour: others, due to structural differences, may only divide once every 24 hours. Bacteria when placed in a new environment grow according to a characteristic pattern:

- **Lag phase** – adjustment to the environment
- **Exponential phase** – rapid growth with constant doubling rate
- **Stationary phase** – induced as nutrients are depleted and toxic products accumulate
- **Death phase** – cell growth declines and the cells die.

Bacteria divide by binary fission. The circular chromosome replicates by using a DNA-dependent DNA polymerase, with the help of **DNA gyrase** and **DNA topoisomerase** to facilitate uncoiling. The plasmids (if any) replicate independently of the chromosome. The chromosomes attach to the plasma membrane on opposite sides of the mesosome, and binary fission takes place, dividing the cytoplasm where the mesosome invaginates.

Bacteria do not form gametes, but DNA can be exchanged between them by various methods:

- **Conjugation**: a conjugation tube forms between two bacteria, made by an outgrowth of the cell wall. Plasmids pass from one bacterium to the other along the tube.
- **Transduction**: bacteriophage viruses (complex DNA viruses) infect bacteria and replicate in the usual viral fashion. The new virions may incorporate bacterial genes from the chromosome or from plasmids, and transfer them to other bacteria.

■ **Transformation**: bacteria can pick up naked DNA molecules and transcribe and translate the genes thereon. This is useful in the laboratory, but it is not certain if it occurs outside.

DNA can also move within the genome of a single bacterium: to a different place in the chromosome, from the chromosome to a plasmid, or from a plasmid to the chromosome. This is mediated by **transposons**: sequences of DNA that can loop out and in again to the main DNA strand. This ensures that any gene can be transferred by conjugation.

FUNGI

Fungi are multinucleate or multicellular organisms and are eukaryotes, but quite distinct from plants and animals.

STRUCTURE

Fungal cells are eukaryotes, possessing a DNA genome, organised in linear chromosomes, with introns and extragenic material. There are no plasmids.

> ### Information box 6.4 General features of fungi
>
> ■ Possess DNA and RNA and have a nuclear membrane
> ■ Have complicated membrane-bound intracellular organelles: mitochondria, Golgi, endoplasmic reticulum
> ■ Have a cell wall outside the cytoplasm, different from bacterial cell walls
> ■ Can grow as filaments (**hyphae**) forming a mesh (**mycelium**).
> ■ Can be **syncytial** – having multiple nuclei in the same cytoplasm
> ■ May grow as single cells (**yeasts**) which divide asexually
> ■ Replicate asexually (**budding**) and sexually, with gamete formation.

■ The **chromosomes** are in a nucleus, with a nuclear membrane and nucleolus.
■ There are **ribosomes** typical of eukaryotes having mitochondria, endoplasmic reticulum, Golgi material, etc. within the cytoplasm.
■ Around the cytoplasm is a **cell membrane** which differs from those of other groups in using **ergosterol** instead of cholesterol. This is the main feature exploited by antifungal therapy.
■ Outside the cell membrane is a **cell wall**; although different from bacterial cell walls it stains Gram positive. There is sometimes a **capsule** outside this.

There are two main forms that fungi can take: yeasts and mycelia. Some species can take both forms:

■ **Yeasts** are individual cells, which divide by budding or binary fission.
■ **Mycelia** are long threads, in some cases divided by septa into cells, in others existing as syncytia.

CLASSIFICATION

There are over 250 000 species of fungi, which are classified by mycologists into four phyla according to the mode of sexual reproduction, or lack of it. Fewer than 200 species are pathogenic in humans. The mycologist's classification is not much use to the medical practitioner, and a strictly pragmatic classification is used instead, with the fungi being divided into groups depending on where the infection takes place:

■ Superficial infection of the skin or hair
■ Infection of the nails or subcutaneous layers of the skin
■ Systemic infections.

The first two groups generally produce mild infections. Systemic infections may be life-threatening and are often seen as opportunistic infections in patients who are immunocompromised.

Fungi enter the human body through inhalation, or through wounds, but others are part of the normal flora and only cause problems in individuals whose normal body defences are reduced. Table 6.6 lists some of the important fungal infections in humans.

Table 6.6 **Examples of fungal infections in humans**

Type	Region of infection	Disease	Characteristics
Superficial	Hair cells, dead skin	Tinea nigra	Produces brown macules on the hands or feet
Cutaneous	Epidermis	Tinea (ringworm)	Raised red area of skin, often looking like a ring, rapidly spread by contact
Subcutaneous	Dermis	Mycetoma	Caused by actinomycetes entering into abrasions and producing a granulomatous disfiguring infection of the skin
Systemic	Internal organs	Histoplasmosis	Fungal infection usually affecting the lungs through inhalation
Opportunistic	Internal organs	Cryptococcosis	Produces a type of meningitis in immunocompromised people. Normally found in soil and harmless otherwise.
		Candidiasis	A yeast infection generally symptomatic in superficial infections (e.g. thrush) but systemic infections occur in the immunocompromised
		Aspergillosis	The fungus is found widely and used in industrial applications (such as production of citric acid) but produces an aspergillosis infection of the lungs in immunocompromised patients and others with poor respiratory function
		Pneumocystis pneumonia (PCP)	Produces pneumonia in immunocompromised people but rare otherwise

PROTOZOA

Protozoa are single-celled animals, some of which affect humans. While the disease may be a direct consequence of the infestation, normally the symptoms are the result of the immune response.

CHARACTERISTICS

Protozoa form the bulk of the biomass and play a vital role in ecology. They can grow up to 1 mm in size and are easily seen under a microscope. They are predators of bacteria and microfungi, absorbing food through their cell membranes and digesting the food in vacuoles. Protozoa have complex life-cycles. Some alternate between growth, as **trophozoites**, and dormancy, as **cysts**. Cysts allow protozoa to survive extremes of environmental conditions outside the host.

Some protozoa are important parasites of humans, infecting them in an opportunistic fashion, or are only important in the immunocompromised. The AIDS epidemic has meant that new important human parasites have come to light. Parasitic protozoa can infect all major tissues and organs either as **intracellular** or **extracellular** parasites and are most prevalent in hot countries.

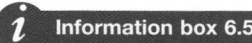

Information box 6.5	**General characteristics of protozoa**

- Are unicellular eukaryotic organisms, with DNA, RNA and a nuclear membrane
- Possess complicated membrane-bound intracellular organelles: mitochondria, Golgi apparatus, endoplasmic reticulum, etc.
- May form cysts with thick walls outside the plasma membrane, different from fungal or bacterial walls
- May have complicated lifecycles
- Replicate asexually (binary fission), and sexually, with gamete formation.

CLASSIFICATION

Although originally protozoa were classified according to their movement ability, as human parasites it is more useful to classify them according to their intracellular or extracellular location.

- **Intracellular** parasites obtain nutrients from the host by direct uptake or by ingestion of cytoplasm. They infect a wide variety of cells – epithelial cells, red cell, muscle cells, brain cells, macrophages. They are normally transmitted by insects (e.g. **malaria**), but can also be acquired through ingestion or in utero (e.g. *Toxoplasma*).
- **Extracellular** parasites obtain nutrients directly, or by ingesting host cells. This latter action can have serious implication, such as where the **malarial parasite** ruptures the infected human red cells. They are found in various locations – blood, intestine, urinogenital tract – and are normally transmitted by ingestion cysts in contaminated food and water. Other mechanisms are possible: insect vectors transmit **trypanosomes**, and *Trichomonas vaginalis* is transmitted through sexual activity.

Figure 6.4 shows the main sites of parasitic infections in the human body.

STRUCTURE

As single cell organisms protozoa vary in size from 2 μm up to 1 mm and have evolved in different ways in order to evade immune detection of their plasma membrane.

- Intracellular species, when within the cell, are removed from attack by antibodies, complement and phagocytes. In order to survive within macrophages (such as in **leishmaniasis**) they have developed a range of mechanisms to evade or inactivate harmful intracellular enzymes, reactive oxygen species and nitrogen

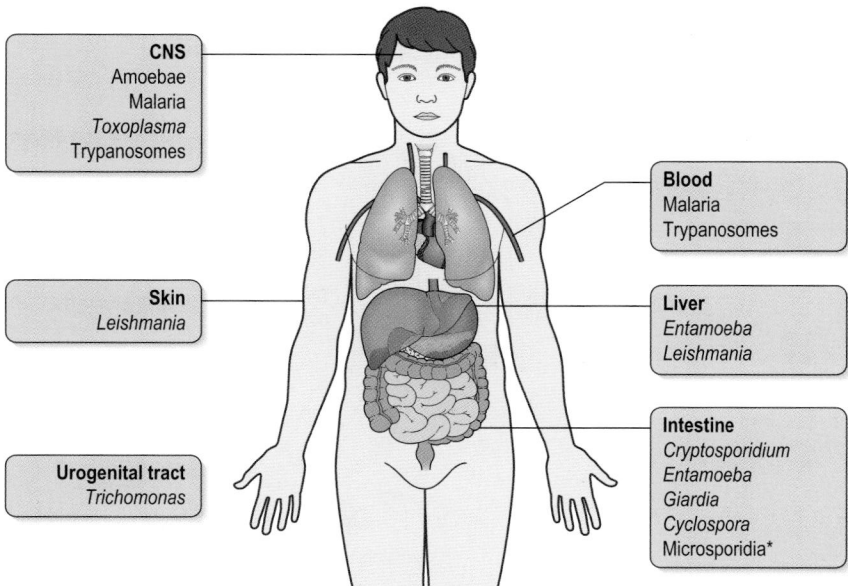

Fig. 6.4 **The occurrence of protozoan parasites in the body.** *Can also occur at other sites. CNS, central nervous system. Adapted with permission from Goering R et al. 2007 Mims' medical microbiology, 4th edn. Mosby, Edinburgh.

metabolites. Because their antigens may be expressed at the surface of the host cell, this has offered opportunities for therapeutic intervention.

- Extracellular species evade recognition through changes in their cell membrane, or through their fight against body responses:
  - **Amoebae** consume complement at the cell surface
  - **Malarial parasites** have polymorphic surface antigens
  - **Trypanosomes** undergo repeated antigenic variation, changing their surface antigens.

REPRODUCTION

In humans, reproduction of parasites is usually asexual, through binary division in trophozoite stages, which involves multiple divisions. Sexual reproduction is usually only seen within insect vectors but **Cryptosporidium** undergoes sexual and asexual reproduction in humans.

The complex nature of staged reproduction is illustrated by the lifecycle of the **malarial parasite** (Fig. 6.5) (see also Clinical box 6.5). The lifecycle of the malarial parasite involves a human and a mosquito host which is prevalent in tropical regions. The disease leads to the deaths of several million people annually, mostly in sub-Saharan Africa.

In the human host:

1. During a blood meal an infected **Anopheles** mosquito injects **sporozoites** into the human.
2. **Sporozoites** infect liver cells and grow into **schizonts**, which mature, rupture and release **merozoites** (**exo-erythrocytic schizogony**).
3. **Merozoites** infect red cells and undergo asexual reproduction, producing **ring stage trophozoites** that mature again into schizonts, rupturing to release more merozoites (**erythrocytic schizogony**).
4. Rupturing of the red cell produces the clinical manifestations of the human disease.
   Some parasites differentiate into male and female **gametocytes** (**sexual erythrocytic stage**).

In the mosquito host (**sporogenic cycle**):

1. During a blood meal the Anopheles mosquito ingests gametocytes from an infected human host.
2. In the mosquito stomach the male and female gametocytes fuse to make **zygotes**.
3. Zygotes become motile and elongate as **ookinetes**, invading the midgut, and develop into **oocysts**.
4. Oocysts develop and grow, rupturing to release **sporozoites**, which travel to the mosquito salivary glands

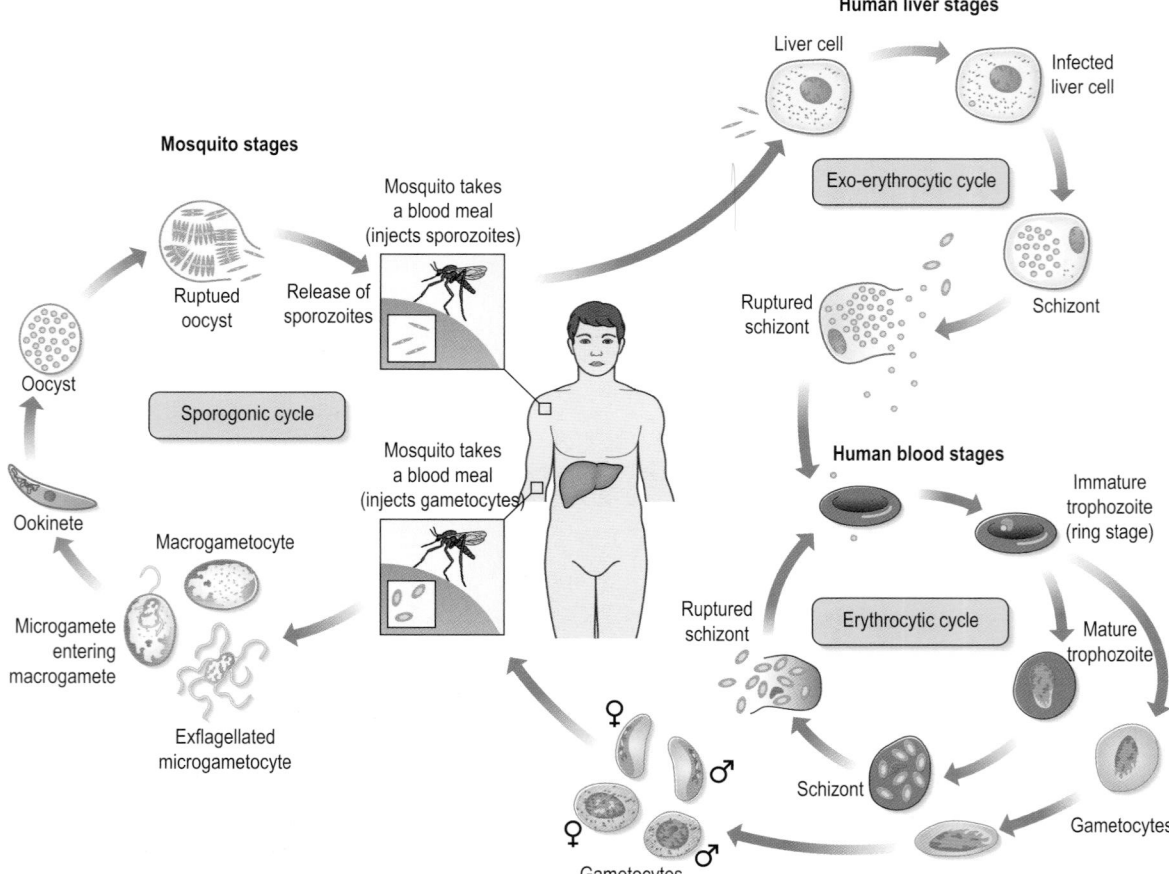

Fig. 6.5 **Lifecycle of the malarial parasite.** Adapted with permission from Centers for Disease Control and Prevention, National Center for Zoonotic, Vector-Borne, and Enteric Diseases (ZVED), Division of Parasitic Diseases. DPDx. Available at: http://www.dpd.cdc.gov/dpdx/Default.htm.

Malaria

Malaria is a parasitic, protozoal infection caused by *Plasmodium falciparum*, *P. vivax*, *P. ovale* or *P. malariae* in humans. The disease is transmitted by a vector, the female anopheline mosquito, but may also be transmitted by transfusion of contaminated blood and blood products. When the mosquito bites an infected individual, gametocytes, the sexual form of the malaria parasite, enters the insect. During an incubation period of 1–3 weeks in the mosquito stomach, fertilisation takes place and the infective malaria sporozoites develop and migrate to the salivary glands to be inoculated into the next victim bitten by the mosquito. Malaria then develops in non-immune individuals with fever, general malaise and sometimes gastrointestinal symptoms. The fever is usually severe with body temperature reaching up to 41 °C, sweating and rigors.

Once the immature parasites have entered the circulation, those that are not destroyed by the immune system are taken up by the liver where they multiply in the hepatocytes (merozoites). The hepatocytes rupture after a few days to release merozoites into the bloodstream where they invade the red cells and multiply and form new merozoites. The red cells then rupture, releasing the new merozoites which infect more red cells. Some species attack young red cells and reticulocytes. The subsequent course of the disease depends on the infecting *Plasmodium* species. Widespread organ damage may occur due to haemolytic anaemia resulting from the rupture of red cells, cytokine release and impaired microcirculation (*P. falciparum*). Cerebral, renal, metabolic, respiratory and endocrine complications may also occur. The genetic variation that resulted in the sickle cell gene evolved owing to the increased malaria resistance conferred by sickle cell disease (see Ch. 12).

Treatment of malaria with chloroquine is usually effective, but widespread resistant strains of *Plasmodium* have emerged. Personal protection (malaria prophylaxis) when travelling to endemic areas is preferable. Vector eradication is necessary, but not always feasible or desirable (e.g. use of insecticides). Protection from mosquito bites with treated bed nets is also effective.

 Information box 6.6 **General characteristics of helminths**

- Multicellular eukaryotic organisms, with DNA, RNA, and a nuclear membrane
- Lack backbones, notochords, and jointed exoskeletons: they are 'worms' in common parlance
- May form cysts with thick walls around the whole organism
- May have complicated lifecycles, with different forms in different hosts
- Replicate asexually and sexually, with gamete formation.

erythrocyte membrane protein 1) dependent interactions. These proteins are impaired in individuals with sickle cell haemoglobin, explaining why sickle cell disease has not been lost from the tropical world through natural selection.
- *Plasmodium ovale* (**tertian**):
  - Rarer than *P. vivax* and *P. falciparum*, it is found in west Africa and the extremes of south-east Asia.
  - Like *P. vivax* it can produce hypnozoites in the liver, allowing relapses.
- *Plasmodium malariae* (**quartan**):
  - Rare but found worldwide.
  - Produces a benign or chronic long-lasting disease.

HELMINTHS

Helminths are eukaryotic parasitic worms that live within and obtain nutrients from their hosts.

Worms are complex and often large organisms. Although the infecting larval forms are usually small (100–200 μm), the adults can be several metres in length. Infections are more common in warm countries, in children and in people working closely with animals because of the association with food. Intestinal infections, in particular, are seen worldwide, but worms can live in other tissues. Transmission occurs in four main ways (Fig. 6.6):

- Faecal-oral – ingesting infective eggs or larvae from an infected human host
- Intermediate – ingesting infective larvae from another infected host, such as eating uncooked infected meat
- Active – when larval stages penetrate the skin
- Bite – when insects suck blood.

CLASSIFICATION

There are three main groups of helminths important in human infections:

- Tapeworms (Cestoda)
- Flukes (Trematoda)
- Roundworms (Nematoda).

Flukes and roundworms feed on human tissues and the contents of the host intestine. Tapeworms have no digestive system and must absorb digested nutrients from their host. Both tapeworms and flukes have complex plasma membranes with mechanisms to protect themselves from a host attack. They release large amounts of soluble antigenic material that plays an important role in the disease and

5. Sporozoites are injected into the human host with mosquito saliva during a blood meal.

There are four main parasites that produce malaria, and the disease caused by each is usually characterised by the frequency of the fevers produced by the reproductive stages in the human. Fevers tend to occur at 2-day (tertian) or 3-day (quartan) intervals.

- *Plasmodium vivax* (**tertian**):
  - The most common malarial parasite and most widely spread and prevalent in Asia and Latin America and some parts of Africa.
  - Has a dormant phase in which **hypnozoites** persist in the liver and result in relapses, weeks or years later.
  - Generally the disease caused is non-fatal, but it can result in **splenomegaly** (enlarged spleen) which can cause complications that lead to death.
- *Plasmodium falciparum* (**tertian**):
  - The most dangerous malarial parasite, accounting for about 80% of infections and about 90% of deaths.
  - Prevalent in sub-Saharan Africa.
  - Trophozoites and gametocytes are often seen in the peripheral blood, unlike in other species.
  - Individuals with the abnormal **sickle cell** haemoglobin are protected from *P. falciparum* infection. Merozoites normally interact with red cells through two PfEMP-1 (*Plasmodium falciparum*

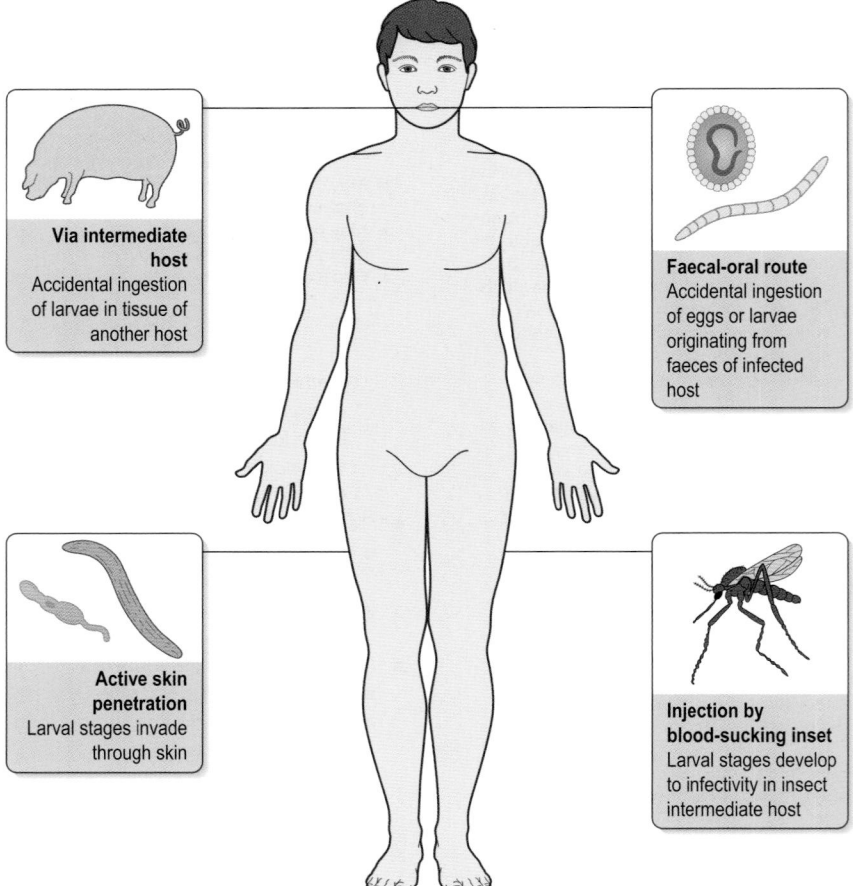

Via intermediate host
Accidental ingestion of larvae in tissue of another host

Faecal-oral route
Accidental ingestion of eggs or larvae originating from faeces of infected host

Active skin penetration
Larval stages invade through skin

Injection by blood-sucking inset
Larval stages develop to infectivity in insect intermediate host

Fig. 6.6 **How helminth parasites enter the body.** Adapted with permission from Goering R et al. 2007 Mims' medical microbiology, 4th edn. Mosby, Edinburgh.

subsequent immunity. Nematodes have a collagenous cuticle in the adult form, which makes them less vulnerable to immune attack.

Humans may also be infected by larvae from other hosts. *Toxocara canis* is a dog parasite that can also infect humans.

REPLICATION

Most helminths replicate outside the host. In the intestine sexual reproduction produces eggs which are released in the faeces and return to the human host as adults through faeces or injection.

- Nematodes:
  - Can develop to maturity within a single host. The *Strongyloides* nematode also hatches its eggs within the intestine producing an **autoinfection**
  - Have separate sexes
  - Some mature in the intestine: *Ascaris*, hookworms, *Strongyloides*, *Trichinella*
  - Some mature in deep tissues: filarial worms.
- Flukes and tapeworms:
  - Must pass through an intermediate host or hosts
  - Flukes are mainly hermaphrodites that release larva from intermediate hosts, such as fish, crustaceans or vegetation, which are subsequently ingested

Clinical box 6.6 | Schistosomiasis

Schistosomiasis is the most important of the helminth parasitic infections in humans. Also known as **bilharzia**, the disease is spread in water contaminated with infected freshwater snails. Common in many tropical developing countries it particularly affects children who may be playing or swimming in the water. Although it is not fatal, it produces a chronic disease that damages other organs and can impair development in children, and can increase the risk of some cancers.

- Schistosomes, whose larvae released from snails penetrate the skin, have separate sexes.
- Tapeworms have replicated reproductive organs along their body (**strobila**) that break off when filled with mature eggs, passing out through the faeces.

THE SYMBIOTIC RELATIONSHIP BETWEEN INFECTIOUS AGENTS AND HUMANS

An infectious agent may be able to live completely independently of its potential host, but usually it has to form some association with it. These associations are called **symbiosis**.

- **Parasitism** is when one member of the association gains an advantage, and the other is harmed. The harm ranges from some disadvantage without overt disease, to overt disease which may be lethal.
- **Commensalism** is where one member of the association gains an advantage, and the other is left unaffected. *Bacteroides* species are present in large numbers in the large intestine.
- **Mutualism** is where both members of the association gain an advantage, the popular meaning of symbiosis. *Bacteroides* infection in cattle rumen provides fatty acids as a nutrient for the host.

When an infectious agent causes disease it is acting as a parasite. However, there are many infectious agents that can exist in a commensal or even mutualistic relationship with their host, and become pathogenic in some special circumstances.

THE NORMAL FLORA

The normal flora consist of microorganisms, mostly bacteria, present on many of the body surfaces in the normal healthy individual. They may be beneficial, neutral or harmful to the host, and the role may change in different circumstances.

The whole body is normally sterile immediately before birth, but the surfaces rapidly become colonised after delivery. The skin, mouth, upper respiratory tract, gastrointestinal tract, and genitourinary tract acquire a variety of microorganisms from the environment and from contact with other people. Bacteria form a major component of faeces. Secretions such as saliva, sebum and tears are normally sterile within the glands but become contaminated as soon as they reach the mucous membrane or skin surface. Blood, cerebrospinal fluid, lymph, bones, joints and all internal organs are normally sterile in health.

Establishment of microorganisms at particular sites depends on several factors, including exposure of the site, availability of suitable receptor sites and ability of organisms to adhere to target receptor sites, to compete for nutrients and to evade or withstand host defence mechanisms. Figure 6.7 illustrates the common microorganisms found within the body as normal flora.

The normal flora offer humans several benefits:

- Colonisation leads to resistance to more virulent bacteria.
- Microorganisms may digest nutrients in the bowel (more important in animals).

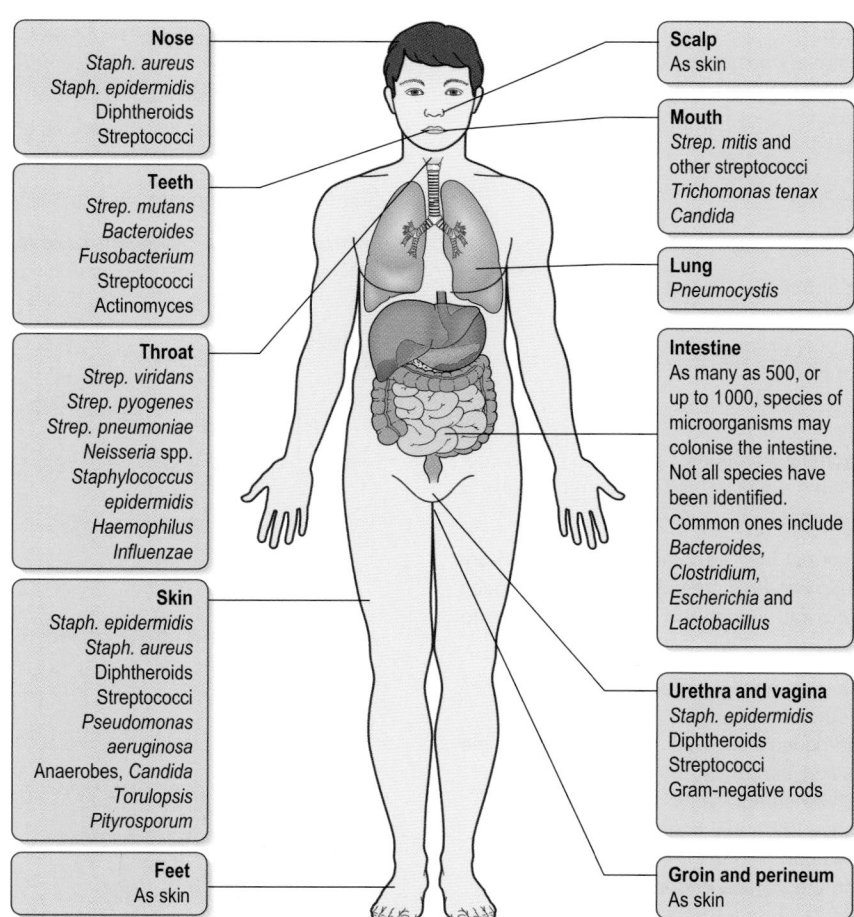

Nose
Staph. aureus
Staph. epidermidis
Diphtheroids
Streptococci

Teeth
Strep. mutans
Bacteroides
Fusobacterium
Streptococci
Actinomyces

Throat
Strep. viridans
Strep. pyogenes
Strep. pneumoniae
Neisseria spp.
Staphylococcus epidermidis
Haemophilus Influenzae

Skin
Staph. epidermidis
Staph. aureus
Diphtheroids
Streptococci
Pseudomonas aeruginosa
Anaerobes, *Candida*
Torulopsis
Pityrosporum

Feet
As skin

Scalp
As skin

Mouth
Strep. mitis and other streptococci
Trichomonas tenax
Candida

Lung
Pneumocystis

Intestine
As many as 500, or up to 1000, species of microorganisms may colonise the intestine. Not all species have been identified. Common ones include *Bacteroides*, *Clostridium*, *Escherichia* and *Lactobacillus*

Urethra and vagina
Staph. epidermidis
Diphtheroids
Streptococci
Gram-negative rods

Groin and perineum
As skin

Fig. 6.7 **Examples of organisms that occur as members of the normal flora and their location on the body.** Adapted with permission from Goering R et al. 2007 Mims' medical microbiology, 4th edn. Mosby, Edinburgh.

- Presence of the normal flora also resists other colonisation attempts through:
  - Competition for receptor sites involved in adhesion
  - Competition for essential nutrients for growth
  - Creation of unfavourable micro-environments that discourage colonisation
- Lactobacilli in the vagina produce acid from glycogen and maintain low pH which is unsuitable for many exogenous bacteria and *Candida*.
- Production of inhibitory substances. Some staphylococci on the skin produce antibiotics, which inhibit other bacteria.

Different groups of bacteria that are adapted to live as normal flora are found in different sites: the mouth, the gastrointestinal tract, the nose and oropharynx, the skin, the vagina. There are no simple criteria such as morphology, staining, biochemical characteristics or growth requirements that distinguish normal flora from pathogens. The normal flora may be disrupted through a variety of mechanisms:

- Suppression by antimicrobial agents allowing overgrowth with resistant organisms
- Changes in general health or immunity
- Hormonal changes
- Local trauma.

Particular sites of normal flora may be affected in certain circumstances, allowing overgrowth by more virulent organisms:

- Mouth:
  - Dietary changes
  - Reduction in salivary secretion
  - Dental disease, dental treatments and oral hygiene
- Gastrointestinal tract:
  - Dietary changes
  - Gut disorders
- Female genital tract:
  - Menstrual cycle
  - Pregnancy
  - Intrauterine contraceptive device
- Skin
  - Use of soaps, cosmetics, antiseptics
  - Moisture – wet or dry
- Respiratory tract
  - Viral infections
  - Secondary bacterial infections
  - Damage to ciliated epithelial cell function (through smoking, for example).

Sometimes the normal flora become **pathogenic**. There is considerable overlap between normal flora and pathogens and various situations can induce the change from one to the other:

- Breakdown in the local epithelium because of trauma (e.g. surgery) or other infection
- Introduction to an unusual site (e.g. gut organisms in the urinary tract, possibly introduced by medical interventions such as catheterisation)
- Alteration in balance of normal flora (e.g. use of antimicrobial drugs can also lead to suppression of *Lactobacillus* in the vagina, encouraging *Candida* growth)
- Immunodeficiency.

PATHOGENS: SUCCESSFUL BIOLOGICAL INFECTIOUS AGENTS

HOW PATHOGENS ENTER THE HOST

Microorganisms, in order to become pathogens, must attach to, or penetrate the **body surface** – a series of surfaces (Fig. 6.8) that is extensive, offering considerable opportunities for its penetration. All these surfaces offer a portal for entry and all are covered by some kind of epithelium; the keratinised stratified squamous epithelium of the skin is the toughest. Epithelia have both innate and adaptive immune mechanisms in place and are capable of mounting an immunological response (see below). For example:

- IgA in mucous membranes blocks pathogenic adhesion
- Lysozyme attacks bacterial peptidoglycan.

The epithelial surfaces are more easily breached if defence mechanisms are impaired. In untreated or uncontrolled diabetes mellitus, which impairs phagocyte activity, there is increased glucose available for pathogens, predisposing the patient to infection, especially of the skin and urinary tract. In AIDS, depletion of CD4 T lymphocytes and infection of dendritic cells allows opportunistic infections to gain access (see below). Other mechanisms that allow, or protect from, entry are described below.

Skin

The skin is a tough, multilayered membrane rendered waterproof by keratin, and more resistant to pathogenic invasion than internal membranes.

- Sebum from sebaceous glands has antibacterial action
- Clothing helps maintain integrity.

Some agents can penetrate intact skin:

- **Arthropods**: some pathogens have adapted to a lifecycle that is dependent on biting arthropods

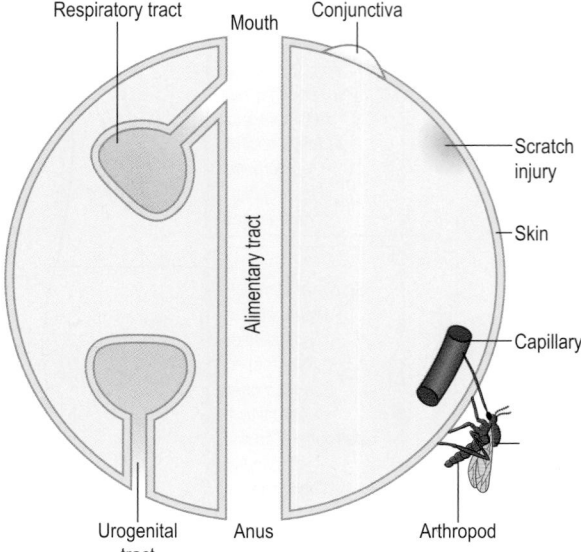

Fig. 6.8 **Body surfaces which are sites of infection and shedding.**

(e.g. mosquitos, flies, fleas, bugs, ticks and mites), penetrating the skin when they feed on human blood.

- **Needles**: any mechanism in which needles are introduced into patients (taking blood, setting up intravenous access, blood transfusion) may introduce a pathogen. A patient may be infected locally by skin flora, staff may be infected, or the agent that is being transmitted may carry a pathogen. Good hygiene, screening of donated blood and education of intravenous drug users can reduce this.
- **Surgical wounds** allow entry of any contaminating pathogens in much the same way: *Staphylococcus aureus* is a particular problem because of antibiotic resistance.
- **Abrasions and wounds**: apparently intact skin often allows entry through minor cuts and abrasions leading to conditions such as warts, from the **papillomavirus**, or impetigo from *S. aureus*.
- **Animal bites** enable a large variety of bacteria to infect the tissues. For example, **rabies** virus is present in the saliva of infected animals, and is passed on via bites.
- **Wounds of violence and war** allow infection by a wide variety of contaminating bacteria. Foreign bodies in tissues are associated with local anoxia, encouraging the growth of anaerobic bacteria.
- **Intact skin** can be penetrated by some larvae.

Respiratory tract

This is particularly vulnerable because it is a very large area of moist living cells which are exposed to pathogens that may be present in inspired air, or through the lachrymal duct in the eye. The fact that the barrier between air and circulation in the alveoli is only one cell thick makes the potential for infection high. The respiratory system offers various defences:

- Hairs in the nose trap large foreign particles.
- Sneeze and cough reflexes expel foreign bodies, excess mucus and infected secretions.
- Mucus, produced by goblet cells and subepithelial mucus glands, contains IgA and lysozymes and traps foreign particles.
- Cilia in the pharynx help remove particles so they can be swallowed (mucociliary escalator).
- Alveolar macrophages phagocytose and destroy small particles.

Other environmental factors may break these defences:

- Conditions that inhibit the mucociliary escalator – such as cystic fibrosis, or smoking
- Anatomical defects that allow mucus to collect, e.g. bronchiectasis
- Foreign bodies that might block bronchi, e.g. peanut inhalation
- Drugs that suppress the cough reflex
- Inhalation of food or vomit in the unconscious person.

Gastrointestinal tract

This is vulnerable because, in order to absorb nutrients, it has a very large surface area which is constantly being exposed to the environment through food and drink, which might be contaminated (see Clinical box 6.7).

Clinical box 6.7   **Bacterial causes of food poisoning**

Food poisoning (gastroenteritis) may be defined as 'usually either infectious or toxic in nature, caused by agents that enter the body through the ingestion of food (or water)'. Diarrhoeal diseases are among the leading causes of death in children under the age of 5 years, particularly in the developing world. Bacteria cause gastroenteritis in three possible ways, sometimes a mixture of all three:

- By adherence to specific receptors in the intestinal mucosa prior to invasion, to produce secretory diarrhoea as the direct result of adhesion.
- By invasion of the intestinal epithelium to produce bloody diarrhoea with abdominal pain (dysentery). Common infecting agents include *Campylobacter*, *Shigella*, *Salmonella* and enteroinvasive *Escherichia coli*.
- By producing toxins that cause excessive fluid loss into the intestinal lumen, causing profuse, watery diarrhoea. Organisms include *Salmonella*, *Vibrio cholerae*, verotoxin-producing *E. coli*, *Bacillus cereus*, *Staphylococcus aureus*, *Clostridium difficile*, *C. botulinum* and *C. tetani*.

The gastrointestinal tract defends itself through:

- Stratified squamous epithelium in the mouth and oesophagus, which is less easy to penetrate than the simple epithelium found below the stomach
- Low pH in the stomach and bile, both of which kill many pathogens
- Mucus traps microbes and impedes their transport
- IgA in saliva and digestive juices blocks the adherence of pathogens, and lysozyme attacks bacterial cell walls
- Normal flora in the small and large intestine compete with pathogens
- The vomiting reflex and diarrhoea void damaging contents through refection and increased turnover of gut epithelium.

Urogenital tract

Pathogens may pass up the urethra or vagina. Sexual intercourse is frequently involved. There are various defence mechanisms, which vary according to male or female anatomy:

- In the **urinary tract** the flow of urine, complete emptying of the bladder and functional integrity of the epithelium are important to resisting infection.
- In the **vagina** normal flora are important, competing with pathogens and maintaining an acid pH.

Most **urinary tract infections** come from the outside, via the urethra (**ascending**). Females are much more vulnerable because they have a shorter urethra and are more exposed through sexual intercourse, which can breach the intact epithelium. The entire urinary tract can also be infected through other routes: e.g. renal abscess, renal tuberculosis and bladder schistosomiasis offer opportunity for infection to enter the urinary tract other than the usual route, through the urethra.

The eyes

- The conjunctiva of the eye is formed of stratified, but not keratinised, epithelium and is protected by tears (containing lysozyme and IgA) and the cleansing action of the lids.

- **During childbirth**, neonates' conjunctivae are vulnerable to infections of the mother's cervix or vagina, such as those caused by *Neisseria gonorrhoeae* or *Chlamydia trachomatis.*
- The naso-lachrymal duct offers a possible route of infection from the eye to the upper respiratory tract.

Placenta

A variety of pathogens may cross from an infected mother to the fetus across the placenta, such as HIV and the rubella and hepatitis B viruses.

Childbirth

Childbirth offers further opportunities for exposing a newborn infant to infections through a variety of portals described above and it may not always be possible to determine which.

HOW PATHOGENS EXPLOIT THEIR ENVIRONMENTS

Pathogens are successful because they exploit the environments provided by a host, whether living within or outside cells. All pathogens need a supply of metabolic material, although viruses (which lack nuclei) need nuclear synthesis. This means that viruses can only live within host cells. Other organisms may flourish inside or outside the cell, or both, taking their nutrients from the cytoplasmic or extracellular fluid. The larger pathogens, such as **nematodes**, are almost always extracellular and some may gain their nutrients by ingesting host cells.

- **Intracellular pathogens**, while being vulnerable to intracellular killing mechanisms, are protected from many of the host defence mechanisms, as well as from therapeutic agents. The pathogens may also live within the same cells that are responsible for the host immune reaction, reducing the ability of the host to mount a defence against the infecting organisms. To succeed, however, these organisms must have an extracellular phase as they pass between cells, and this offers opportunities for host and therapeutic attack. Any attack, intracellular or extracellular, makes the host cells vulnerable and many will die, leading to tissue damage.
- **Extracellular pathogens** are exposed continuously to the host cellular defence mechanism. For this reason they tend to be larger and more complex: they are able to move rapidly and reproduce faster than others. They may also have a structure that means, for example, that they are not vulnerable to mechanisms such as phagocytosis. The **helminths** (worms) are typical of these organisms.

THE PROGRESS OF A PATHOGENIC INFECTION

Adhesion

Almost all pathogens have to adhere to host cells. The cells at the portal of entry are often the first target, but adhesion is essential later in dissemination round the body. Pathogens that are injected into the host do not have to adhere in order to invade, but they will probably have to adhere later.

- **Viruses** have docking proteins, e.g. haemagglutinins on the influenza virus. This may be at the portal of entry, or if they are injected in some way, they may travel to a site where they can bind.
- **Bacteria** exhibit various different adherence mechanisms:
  - **Non-specific** adherence: hydrophobic molecules in walls, capsules and slime all adhere non-specifically to host cells.
  - **Specific** adherence: many bacteria have adhesins, either on the cell wall, outer membrane or other wall structures, which bind to molecules on host cells
  - Carbohydrates, such as D-mannose, sialic acid and blood group carbohydrates
  - Proteins, e.g. fibronectin.
- **Helminths** may have specialised mouth parts, such as found in the tapeworm or hookworm, that enable the organism to be retained within the bowel.

Invasion

Some pathogens do not invade, but continue to adhere to the epithelium at the portal of entry, e.g. skin fungi, *Vibrio cholerae.* Others may invade the portal of entry, and spread no further, while others do spread further. Invasion may take the pathogen into the host's cells, or between the cells into the extracellular spaces, or both. It usually follows adhesion, but a pathogen may invade by being injected.

- **Viruses**: all viruses must invade (infect) a cell to reproduce after adhesion via the docking protein. Many viruses enter cells on mucous membranes and remain localised to the epithelium with disease developing within a few days. There is little or no invasion of underlying tissue, and the virus is shed directly to the exterior. These local infections offer only short-term immunity. Influenza viruses, rhinoviruses and, in the gastrointestinal tract, rotaviruses are all viruses of this type.
- **Bacteria**: Bacteria may move between cells, through the intercellular junctions, e.g. *Salmonella* spp., while others may invade the cells to which they have adhered. This can lead to host cell involvement: (a) host cell actin polymerisation may be induced, leading to pseudopod formation and bacterial engulfment within a vacuole, and (b) the vacuole disintegrates and the bacterium lies free within the cytoplasm.
- **Fungi** use enzymes to break down ground substance and matrix of epithelia and connective tissue.

Host organ dissemination

- **Viruses** that have the capacity to invade subepithelial tissues may enter the lymphatic system.
  - If the virus is quickly inactivated by macrophages from the lymph nodes sinuses, the immune response is initiated, resulting in a regional **lymphadenopathy**, but the infection does not progress.
  - If the virus is not inactivated, particularly if it can survive or replicate in macrophages or lymphocytes, the particles are passed through the lymph nodes into the bloodstream.

- The virus is likely to be distributed to distant parts of the body and establish infection in the reticulo-endothelial system (the **primary viraemia** – an asymptomatic event during the incubation period).
- Following a period of replication in distant sites, such as liver and spleen, large amounts of progeny virus may be released into the bloodstream, leading to the onset of clinical effect of a **systemic viral infection**, which can spread to other organs.
- If the virus lodges in skin capillaries, a rash may be a prominent feature, such as is seen in measles and chickenpox.

- The nature of viraemia depends on the virus. Those carried in monocytes or lymphocytes are more protected and can be disseminated more widely.
- **Bacteria** can be disseminated through:
  - Tissues, aided by enzymes such as collagenase, hyaluronidase and streptokinase
  - Blood through which bacteria can reach any tissue or organ. A **bacteraemia** is the presence of live bacteria in the blood; when the bacteria multiply in the blood this produces **septicaemia**.

See also Clinical boxes 6.8 and 6.9.

Clinical box 6.8 **Meningitis**

Meningitis, a serious inflammation of the meninges, is an important public health issue that is potentially preventable, but more prevalent in developing nations. The cause of acute bacterial meningitis (without immunisation) is estimated as:

- *Haemophilus influenzae* B: 32%
- *Neisseria meningitidis*: 21%
- *Streptococcus pneumoniae*: 24%
- Other bacteria: 23%.

Clinically, the classic triad of fever, headache and neck stiffness should give rise to suspicion of meningitis. A petechial rash may precede the symptoms, septicaemic shock may develop, and death may ensue. Bacteraemia may lead to multisystem/multiorgan infection.

The capsular polysaccharides of *N. meningitides* that inhibit destruction and clearance (phagocytosis) by the host defence mechanisms have been used to produce vaccines (meningococcal conjugate C vaccine), which were introduced into the UK routine vaccination of children programme in 1999. *Haemophilus influenzae* B (Hib) vaccine and a polyvalent pneumococcal vaccine are also available.

Viral meningitis is a more benign, usually self-limiting condition, although the patient may be left with a severe headache that persists for some time.

Clinical box 6.9 **Multisystem bacterial infection: *Escherichia coli***

Most bacteria target specific organs or systems, but some bacterial infections can lead to multisystem disease. One example is *E. coli*, which has an enterohaemorrhagic form (serotype 0157:H7), also known as verotoxin-producing *E. coli* (VTEC). The enteroinvasive form of *E. coli* causes bacillary dysentery, but VTEC not only causes bloody diarrhoea but also secretes a toxin that affects vascular endothelial cells in the bowel and kidneys, when the patient may develop thrombocytopenic purpura and/or haemolytic uraemic syndrome (HUS). Administration of antibiotics may exacerbate HUS by increasing toxin production.

Survival within the host

As soon as a pathogen reaches the portal of entry, it encounters the defence system. The **non-immune aspect** includes the integrity of the epithelium, chemical defences and normal flora. Agents of the innate and adaptive immune systems may be present at the portal, and will be further encountered if the pathogen invades or is disseminated. Survival of the pathogen depends on circumventing the defence system, which it does in several ways:

- **Stress survival**:
  - Host defences may damage the pathogen by denaturing proteins.
  - **Chaperonins** (heat shock proteins) protect against denaturing of other proteins.
  - **Free radicals**, such as superoxide and hydroxyl radicals, and hydrogen peroxide damage and kill pathogens. They may be produced by the pathogen's aerobic metabolism, or by host defences.
- **Scavenge for nutrients**:
  - Some nutrients, sugars, amino acids and fatty acids are freely available, but iron, in the form of Fe^{3+}, is not. This form of iron is important for bacterial survival and its inaccessibility is part of the non-specific defence provided by the body.
  - Bacterial siderophores bind iron avidly and capture it for the bacterium.
  - Fungi use sophisticated mechanisms to acquire nutrients as **saprophytes**.
- **Shelter**:
  - If the pathogen can enter host cells it will be protected from **antibody** attack. All viruses replicate within host cells, and some bacteria, fungi and protozoa shelter within cells.
  - Some survive within phagocytes, either by escaping from the phagosome into the cytoplasm, preventing phagosome–lysosome fusion (e.g. **toxoplasmosis**), or by being tough and resisting the phagocytic enzymes and radicals (e.g. *M. tuberculosis*).
  - When bacteria or virions are released from the cell they are fully exposed to the immune system, but viruses or bacteria that pass directly from one cell to another minimise this exposure.
  - Some pathogens survive in sites where the immune system is poorly represented, such as the lens of the eye, which can become infected in congenital rubella infection.
  - The pathogen is not completely protected from the immune system. The infected cell will present pathogen-derived antigens on class I human leucocyte antigen (HLA) molecules, and can be killed by CD8 T lymphocytes, destroying the shelter (see below).
  - Some viruses, however, can suppress the expression of HLA molecules (for example cytomegalovirus). Latent infections by viruses will not generate any viral proteins.
- **Stealth**: sometimes the pathogen is fully exposed but avoids a lethal encounter through disguise or deception. This can be done in a variety of ways:
  - **Shielding**: bacteria, for example, may have structures outside their cell walls, such as capsules and slime, which prevent recognition and subsequent

phagocytosis and complement activation that would destroy them.

- **Active action**: bacteria may also possess protein A, which blocks binding of the Fc portion of the antibody to its receptor, thus blocking **opsonisation**, the process through which a pathogen is prepared for phagocytosis.
    - IgA proteases within bacteria can also cleave IgA, which mediates transport of immune complexes across epithelial cells.
- **Antigenic variation**: some pathogens mutate and thus change their antigens. This may happen during an infection of a single individual, such as in **African trypanosomiasis**, or it may happen between outbreaks, such as in **influenza**, so that the pathogen remains one step ahead.
- **Antigenic mimicry**, or adsorption of host protein: for example, *S. aureus* adsorbs fibrin and IgG.
- **Ineffective antibody**: many pathogens elicit an antibody response, but it is ineffective because it is acting on unimportant determinants. Sometimes the antibody produced may even help the pathogen by enabling uptake into phagocytes where it can survive.
- **Forming a stronghold**: pathogens may create some form of sanctuary where the immune system cannot reach them, or which is too strong to be destroyed. For example:
    - Coagulase, e.g. *S. aureus*, causes coagulation of plasma proteins around the bacterium, hindering the immune system.
    - Abscesses are surrounded by fibrosis, isolating the contents.
    - Some helminths form cysts that are too tough to be destroyed.

Attacking the host

Inhibition or death of cells of the immune system, and damage or death of other cells, can inhibit the defence system.

- **Viruses** often kill the cells which they infect, and if they are cells of the immune system this will promote their own survival. For example, HIV infects CD4-positive T cells and causes profound immunosuppression.
- **Bacteria** make a variety of toxins, which make the patient ill, and promote bacterial survival by killing cells of the defence system, or by killing other cells and disabling tissue function, which indirectly damages defence:

- **Exotoxins** are substances produced by bacteria with a variety of functions.
- **Pore-forming** proteins lyse cells by assembling into pores in the cell membrane.
- Enzymes with **phospholipase** activity lyse cells by destroying part of the membranes.
- Toxins can enter cells and **inhibit protein synthesis**, e.g. **diphtheria** toxin.
- Toxins can also enter cells and **deregulate** their metabolism, e.g. cholera toxin stimulates adenylate cyclase in the gut epithelium, leading to massive electrolyte efflux, and copious watery diarrhoea.
- Toxins **stimulate nerves**, e.g. **staphylococcal enterotoxins**, that act on gut nerves, which signal to the brain to cause vomiting.
- Toxins also act as **superantigens**, activating many T lymphocytes, with the release of many cytokines, especially tumour necrosis factor (TNF), causing shock (see Clinical box 6.11).

Endotoxins are lipopolysaccharides from the cell wall, produced by Gram-negative bacteria in large quantities, particularly in Gram-negative septicaemia. They stimulate macrophages to release cytokines, especially TNF and interleukin (IL) 1. They also initiates intrinsic coagulation and alternative complement cascades that can lead to fever, hypotension, shock, disseminated intravascular coagulation, organ failure through poor perfusion, and death.

Some bacteria and protozoans **disable the phagocyte response** by living within phagocytes.

Clinical box 6.11   **Septic shock**

Bacterial endotoxins in the bloodstream due to severe infection promote the release of pro-inflammatory factors such as tumour necrosis factor (TNF) from phagocytic and non-phagocytic cells that mediate a systemic inflammatory response. At the same time, compensatory anti-inflammatory cytokines are released. This is part of the normal defence mechanism in response to the challenge of exogenous infection. However, when this response is disseminated due to overwhelming infection, shock and widespread tissue damage can occur, known as septic shock, which is clinically characterised by fever, hypotension and intravascular coagulation, and is potentially fatal. The initial overwhelming inflammatory response may be followed by immune suppression. Gram-negative bacteria that produce endotoxins are more likely to have this effect, mediated by the release of TNF.

Clinical box 6.12   **The virulence of microorganisms: example *Staphylococcus aureus***

Microorganisms can produce disease by direct invasion of tissues or by producing toxins. The bacterium *S. aureus* is a good example.
Diseases produced by invasion include:

- Skin infections such as impetigo, boils and cellulitis
- Bone infections such as osteomyelitis
- Brain abscesses, meningitis
- Pneumonia, lung abscesses.

Diseases produced by the toxins include:

- Staphylococcal food poisoning (enterotoxin B)
- Scalded skin syndrome
- Toxic shock syndrome (most commonly due to retained vaginal tampons).

Clinical box 6.10   **Versatility of microorganisms: example *Helicobacter pylori***

In order to invade the host, microorganisms have to evade normal protective physical or chemical barriers. One example is *H. pylori*, a Gram-negative spiral organism that causes gastritis and peptic ulcers, and is a predisposing factor for gastric cancers. *Helicobacter pylori* infects 50–90% of the world population with the highest prevalence in developing countries with poorer hygiene. In order to attach to and colonise the human gastric mucosa, *H. pylori* has to survive in the extreme acidic environment and overcome the mucous secretions in the stomach. This is facilitated by its motility and the secretion of the enzymes urease and catalase.

Exit

For a microorganism to be successful, it must leave the body and be transmitted to a fresh host. Most microbes leave from the body surfaces, but some have to be extracted by vectors. Examples of exit mechanisms are the:

- Gastrointestinal tract through faeces, vomit or anal intercourse
- Respiratory tract through coughing and sneezing producing droplets
- Genitourinary tract through sexual intercourse or in urine
- Conjunctival fluids entering water, such as when swimming, or going onto the hand
- Skin surfaces through touching or shedding of bacteria on skin
- Through normally intact skin by insect vectors, needles, donating infected blood, blood splashing after wounding.

Transmission

The ability for an organism to transmit its infection once it has exited the host depends on three main factors:

- The number of organisms shed and the route of shedding
- Its stability and survival outside the host within a wide variety of environments
- The number of organisms needed to infect a fresh host.

Infections are transmitted through a variety of routes and these are the focus for many public health initiatives (Fig. 6.9). Transmission can also be described, not only by the route, but by the mechanism:

- **Vertical transmission** occurs when infection is spread from mother to fetus, or breastfed infant:
  - The rubella virus, and HIV, for example, if present in the mother's blood, crosses the placenta, infecting the fetus, which will not be protected because of the lack of ability to produce antibodies.
  - During delivery, abrasions and wounds from the birth process can breach the skin, or infectious agents can enter through the conjunctiva or mucous membranes. Hepatitis B and streptococcal infections are both examples of this type of transmission.
  - During breastfeeding, if the infectious agent is present within breast milk, this may infect the child. human lymphotropic virus 1 (HTLV-1) and HIV can both be spread in this way.
- **Horizontal transmission** occurs between individuals or between species, other than mother and offspring. The transmission may be:
  - **Direct** – when the transmitter and recipient are close. For example, through infected skin or other **surface contact** with a portal of entry, or inhaled **droplet infection** from a sneeze
  - **Indirect** – where the transmitter and recipient can be distant from each other. Several mechanisms are

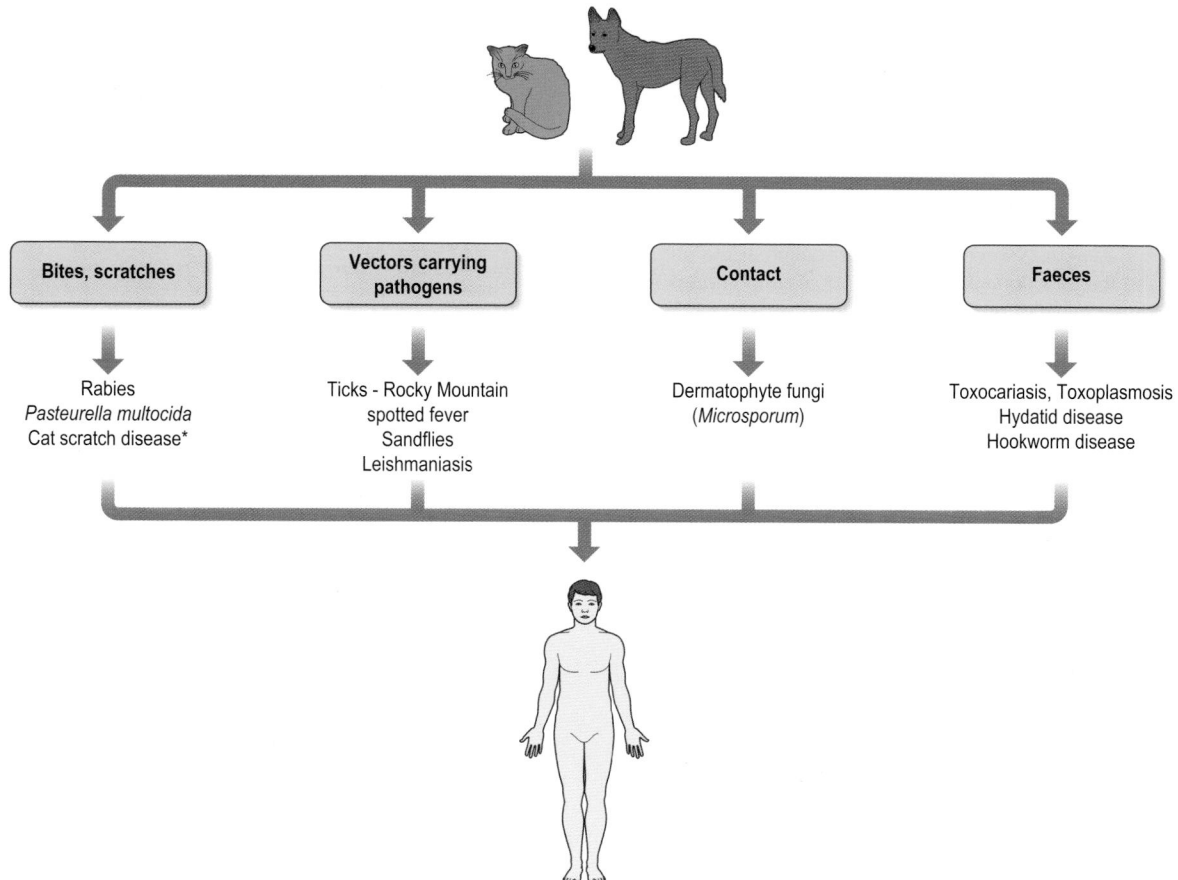

Fig. 6.9 **Zoonoses transmitted from dogs and cats.** *A benign infection, with skin lesions and lymphadenopathy, shown to be because of infection with bacteria of the *Bartonella* or *Afipia* species. Adapted with permission from Goering R et al. 2007 Mims' medical microbiology, 4th edn. Mosby, Edinburgh.

possible and involve some form of vehicle, for example: food – such as *Salmonella* being transmitted through eggs; water – sewage can infect water, and cholera can be transmitted this way; fomites – any agents that retain an infective agent, such as cytomegalovirus surviving on toys; surgical instruments – before the days of sterilisation, or if sterilisation fails (prions are not inactivated by heat sterilisation), or through needle-stick injury; and transfusion of infected blood – the transmission of HIV to individuals with haemophilia through factor VIII concentrate prepared from pools of individuals, some of whom were later found to have HIV, is an example of how large number of people were adversely affected by therapeutic intervention.

- Vectors, such as mosquitos, that transmit malaria or yellow fever, and the tsetse fly, that transmits trypanosomes.
- Airborne: such as dust from dried smallpox crusts, or water droplets from air conditioning transmitting legionnaires' disease.

THE PATTERN OF DISEASE

The disease experienced by a person will depend on the infecting agent, the status of the patient, the circumstances of the infection and its subsequent treatment. Treatment of microbial infections is too big a subject for this chapter and the reader should consult a specialist textbook on microbiology. Distinctions can be drawn between the various patterns, however, which help in describing what is observed.

LOCAL VERSUS GENERAL INFECTIONS

- Some viruses cause **local infection** at the portal and replicate, but do not spread.
- In some cases there is limited replication at the portal and the infection spreads to the local lymph nodes for a further cycle of replication, spreading subsequently to a target tissue, resulting in a **general infection**.

PERSISTENCE

- Some virus infections cause local or general infections but these do not persist.

- Those that persist, with continuous viral production, lead to a **chronic infection** (e.g. HIV and hepatitis C infections)
- Those that persist for long periods without virus production, but which can be reactivated, are called **latent infections** (e.g. herpes infection).

INCUBATION PERIOD

This is the time between infection and disease manifestation and can be short, medium, long or very long.

DISEASE MANIFESTATION

Sometimes diseases may first become evident as a result of a **prodromal** illness, or become evident, because of the appearance of specific symptoms which may or may not continue over time. Fever is a common feature of infections (see Clinical box 6.13).

Clinical box 6.13   Fever in response to infection

In healthy human beings, inflammatory cytokines are released to combat bacterial or viral infections. These cytokines stimulate the hypothalamic thermoregulatory centre in the brain to increase prostaglandin (PGE_2) synthesis, leading to an increase in body temperature (fever). Fever has an inhibiting effect on bacterial and viral proliferation, and thus a beneficial effect on the course of infection. The use of salicylates and non-steroidal anti-inflammatory drugs to reduce fever is based on their inhibitory effect on prostaglandin synthesis.

- A **prodromal illness** is one that produces non-specific symptoms, usually due to the release of cytokines, which usually occurs at the end of the incubation period of viral infections. For example, fever, malaise, myalgia, abdominal pain, anorexia and bowel disturbance may be observed several days before the patient becomes jaundiced in hepatitis B infection.
- **Acute** disease starts suddenly, lasts a few hours or days, and then ends in death or the person recovers (such as the bubonic plague, or the common cold, respectively). Some diseases have a more insidious onset (**subacute**), while others are **chronic**, lasting many years. The same disease can produce all of these patterns. For example, osteomyelitis can have an acute onset, but can then last a long time and eventually lead to death. Pulmonary tuberculosis has an insidious onset but it too leads to a chronic disease, which without effective treatment culminates in death.
- **Self-limiting** diseases are those in which the person recovers without treatment.

IMMUNITY

Denise Syndercombe Court, Nigel Yeatman

Everybody, to stay healthy, tries to keep other life forms outside. We are surrounded by a large variety of organisms, from viruses to insects, many of which try to subvert our cells, or live in our bowel, eat our food, frolic in our tissue spaces, breed in our bladders or brains, or lay their eggs under our skin. It has been known for a long time that such invaders are associated with disease. Koch, in 1890, defined four criteria that needed to be fulfilled to establish a causal relationship between a microbe and a disease (**Koch's postulates**). He later abandoned the italicised part of the first postulate, because of the finding that asymptomatic carriers existed.

Koch's postulates (the italicised part now having been abandoned):

- The microorganism must be found in abundance in all organisms suffering from the disease, *but not in healthy organisms*.
- The microorganisms must be isolated from a diseased organism and grown in pure culture.
- The cultured microorganisms should cause disease when introduced into a healthy organisms.
- The microorganisms must be re-isolated from the inoculated, diseased experimental host and identified as being identical to the original specific causative agent.

To keep these infecting organisms away, the body has defence mechanisms, which may be classified as:

- Non-immunological
- Immunological – innate or adaptive.

THE NON-IMMUNOLOGICAL DEFENCE SYSTEM

The body has various barriers, which have been more fully discussed in the previous section. Some examples are given here.

PHYSICAL AND FUNCTIONAL BARRIERS

- The skin acts as a barrier, preventing microorganisms entering the body fluids.
- The upward flow of mucus in the bronchi, propelled by the cilia, washes out microorganisms (see Ch. 13, the mucociliary escalator).
- Complete emptying of the bladder and the inhibition of urine flow up the ureters both inhibit infection of the urinary tract (see Ch. 14, the vesicoureteric reflux).

SIMPLE CHEMICAL AND BIOLOGICAL BARRIERS

- There is a low pH in the stomach and vagina. If the pH of the stomach rises, for example, infections of the bowel are more frequent (see Clinical box 6.10 above).
- The skin is constantly anointed with **sebum**, an oily secretion from the sebaceous glands which contains chemicals that do no harm to the human host, but are not liked by many pathogens.
- There is significant growth of bacteria in the lumen of the bowel, in the vagina and on the surface of the skin in the form of **normal flora**, which inhibit the growth of pathogens.

THE IMMUNOLOGICAL DEFENCE SYSTEM

Destructive agents, in the form of specialised cells and molecules – lymphocytes, macrophages, antibodies and complement – form the body's immunological defence mechanisms. To be successful they must be able to distinguish friend from foe – to recognise **non-self** – and to be able to tell the difference between **damaged** and **undamaged** tissue.

Activation of some of these cells and molecules is called an **immune response**. Some other definitions that will be useful at this point are:

- **Immunogen** – anything that provokes an immune response
- **Antigen** – anything that is recognised by the cells and molecules of the immune response
- Agents of the defence system recognise antigens through receptors and recognition sites. The part of the antigen that is recognised is called a **determinant**
- A **receptor** is a molecule or complex of molecules which has at least one recognition site, the molecular feature recognised being the determinant. Receptors are normally present on the surface of cells.

DETECTION AND DESTRUCTION OF THE INVADING IMMUNOGEN

The immune system needs:

- To detect the presence of **non-self** and, usually, to destroy and/or eliminate the invader
- To leave undamaged, as much as possible, the body's own components (**self**)
- Sometimes to allow **toleration** of some non-self substances where an aggressive immune response serves no useful purpose.

It does this by acting through receptors and antigenic determinants and applying mechanisms that assist in destruction of the immunogen.

Receptors

The recognition site on the receptor binds to the determinant not only because of their respective shapes, but also because of electrostatic forces. There are different types of receptor that aid in the detection of the invader and subsequent healing processes.

- **Antigen receptors** recognise determinants that are present on non-self substances, but are scarce or absent on self – distinguishing **self** and **non-self**.

- **Scavenger receptors** recognise determinants or features characteristic of dead or denatured material, but scarce or absent on healthy tissue – distinguishing **damaged** and **healthy** tissue.

Some elements of the defence system distinguish between these forms by recognising determinants characteristic of healthy self tissues. Cells and molecules of the immune system also interact and cooperate with each other through specialised receptors and determinants, such as:

- Receptors on macrophages for antibodies
- Interactions within the complement cascade.

Receptors can be **specific** or **non-specific**.

- A receptor is said to be very **specific** if it binds only to one particular kind of determinant. Some receptors are more specific than others.
- A receptor that is **non-specific** might, for example, bind to a variety of determinants with strong negative charges, because of its strong positive charge, in spite of there being differences in their shapes.

Specificity, on the other hand, is a different concept and refers to the identity of the determinant which it recognises. For example, the specificity of one receptor might be a determinant on *S. aureus*, and the specificity of another a determinant on tetanus toxoid. A **cross-reaction** occurs when a receptor binds to more than one kind of antigen. This may be because the same determinant is present on different antigens and the receptor is acting in a specific fashion, or because the receptor is acting in a non-specific way, binding to determinants of different shapes, as described above.

Antigens

Antigens are usually polypeptides or polysaccharides, sometimes with other chemical groups attached. The determinant size is probably only between three and 10 peptides or saccharides in length. Individual molecules may have several determinants recognisable by the receptors of the defence system. This allows tissues, cells (live or dead), cell fragments, molecular aggregates or single protein molecules (of eukaryotic, prokaryotic, viral or artificial origin) to be recognised, simply through the presence of a determinant that is foreign to the body.

Agents of destruction

Identification must be followed by destruction and elimination of the invader. The defence mechanism does this by acting through cells that use phagocytosis, lytic enzymes and strong oxidising agents, both inside and outside the cells. Some cells kill other cells by opening ion channels in their cell membranes. An important factor is that the destruction should be as localised as possible to minimise damage to healthy tissue.

While it is important that **self** is not a target of destruction, there are many molecules that are foreign, but not dangerous. There is evidence that the defence system can specifically **tolerate** such potential antigens. For example, pollen antigens probably cross the lung mucosa but do not produce significant damage: an inappropriate aggressive immune response might result in damage also to self.

Cells that are part of the immune response communicate with each other through:

- Cell surface molecules – cells touching each other may communicate through structures that allow them to fit or bind together to mediate communication
- Secreted molecules, or mediators – such as hormones, cytokines or lymphokines
  - Hormones are products of specialised endocrine cells
  - Cytokines are polypeptides
  - Lymphokines are cytokines secreted by, or acting on, lymphocytes.

In general, a cell must express a receptor for a mediator to be influenced by it: usually on the cell surface, but sometimes in the nucleus.

- In **autocrine** activity a mediator acts on the cell that secreted it.
- In **paracrine** activity a mediator diffuses from the secreting cell to neighbouring cells and acts on them.
- In **endocrine** activity the mediator is carried by the circulation all over the body, and acts on cells remote from those that secreted it.

THE INNATE IMMUNE SYSTEM

Some components involved in the body defence cannot readily distinguish self and non-self but, nevertheless, provide elements that protect the body. For example, all **lysozyme** molecules are the same and have the same specificity of attack, which is different from other defending molecules, such as **mannose-binding protein**. There are several other soluble factors that assist in the body defence:

- Lysosomes act by damaging bacterial cell walls, but do no harm to eukaryotic cells, which lack a cell wall.
- Mannose-binding protein acts through recognition of particular carbohydrate patterns found on the surface of many pathogenic microorganisms.
- **C-reactive protein** (**CRP**) binds to phosphorylcholine on bacteria, enhancing phagocytosis and assisting in **complement** binding.
- The **complement pathway** is a cascade system of enzymes reminiscent of the clotting pathway and is triggered by certain foreign chemical configurations found in endotoxins, and bacterial and fungal cell walls. It culminates in the activation of enzymes destructive to foreign organisms. It also produces chemotactic substances and adherent factors that promote the phagocytosis. It also acts to discriminate self and non-self as it is only stimulated by foreign material.
- **Chemotactic factors** are chemical substances that direct the movement of cells – human or invading – to particular locations.

All body cells play their part in the innate immune system. Any cell that is damaged or undergoes necrosis may release mediators, or material such as heat shock proteins that signal the damage to neighbouring cells. Many cells that are virally infected signal the fact by releasing mediators (**interferons** (IFNs)).

Basophils in blood and **mast cells** in tissues are motile and chemotactic, but not phagocytic. They are activated directly by physical and chemical stimuli, and also by nerves (collateral branches of afferent sensory nerves, which can detect damage through their receptors), complement and receptors, allowing them to interact with the **adaptive immune system**. **Phagocytes**, such as neutrophils, monocytes/macrophages, dendritic cells and eosinophils, deploy a variety of cell surface receptors which can detect non-self and damaged tissues. Some are also used in cooperation with other parts of the immune system. Examples of the different types of receptors are:

- **Toll-like receptors** – molecules which in various combinations recognise microbial molecules, molecules released from damaged self cells (heat shock proteins) and dead self material.
- **Collectins** – proteins which recognise sugar groups characteristic of microbes, e.g. the mannose receptor.
- **CD14** – a receptor for lipopolysaccharide, a component of Gram-negative bacterial cell walls. When an antigen engages these receptors, the cell will attempt to phagocytose and destroy it in the lysosomes.
- **C3b and Fc receptors** – mediate cooperation with complement and antibodies, respectively.

All these phagocytes can degrade the material that they phagocytose, and if they phagocytose microbes they are often able to kill them. These mechanisms involve enzymes, free radicals and exclusion of nutrients from the phagosome. The phagocytes, however, retain no memory of the attack to protect the body against repeat incursions. Secretion of mediators is an important function of phagocytes, mediating the recruitment of more phagocytes and inflammatory changes.

In summary, the innate immune system uses a relatively small number of receptors and recognition sites that detect components common on microorganisms, but not found within the human body. These mechanisms do not recognise all determinants and successful pathogens hide these. The body needs a more sophisticated defence mechanism to deal with these – the **adaptive immune system**.

THE ADAPTIVE IMMUNE SYSTEM

When the innate immune system fails to resolve an infection, the adaptive immune system comes into action. In contrast to the innate immune system, the adaptive immune system initiates and uses specific memory of the infection. This system is provided through the **lymphocytes**. There are different forms of lymphocytes: B lymphocytes, T lymphocytes and null lymphocytes. T lymphocytes can be further divided into:

- CD4-positive (helper T cells)
- CD8-positive (cytotoxic T cells)

Figure 6.10 summarises the difference between these two systems of body defence. Any one lymphocyte, and its **clone** from division of a single cell, will have receptors which are **specific** for an antigen, but different lymphocytes will have different specificities. After recognising an antigen the lymphocyte will divide to form a clone, which is generally stable. The body may produce receptors on lymphocytes specific for self components but these are deleted or inactivated, probably through **clonal deletion**. Thus lymphocytes are produced that have receptors for many different non-self specificities, producing a comprehensive defence system.

T lymphocytes

T lymphocytes originate in the bone marrow, but undergo further development in the **thymus** before they are mature. They have two-chain receptors on their surface which recognise antigen but which are *not* antibody. Like B lymphocytes, the receptors on the surface of any one T lymphocyte all have the same specificity.

The receptors on T lymphocytes are known as complementarity determining regions (**CDRs**). Highly variable, these regions interact with an **MHC** (**major histocompatibility complex**)–peptide complex to activate the lymphocytes.

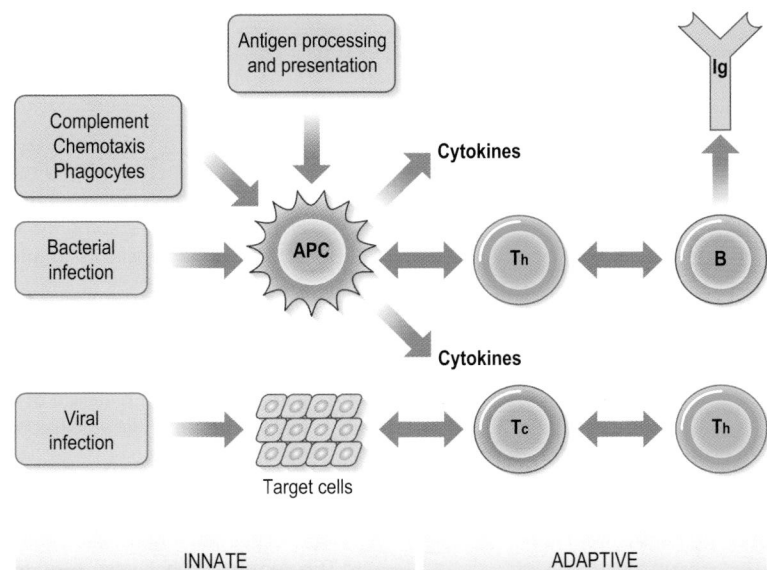

Fig. 6.10 **Innate and adaptive immunity.** Th, helper T cells; Tc, cytotoxic T cells; B, B cells; Ig, immunoglobulin; APC, antigen-presenting cell. Adapted with permission from Nairn R, Helbert M 2006 Immunology for medical students. Mosby, Edinburgh.

HLA refers to a subset of MHC genes that encode for cell surface antigen-presenting proteins.

Terminology

CD nomenclature
CD stands for **cluster of differentiation**. This is a classification system for the different antigenic determinants found on cells.

- Each cell surface molecule on a T lymphocyte must be recognised by a cluster of monoclonal antibodies developed in the laboratory before it is assigned a CD number.
- The surface molecules are different on different cells and so act as markers of differentiation. The different CD complexes are given a number to differentiate them.

Major histocompatibility complex
The MHC region is located on chromosome 6 and consists of about 140 genes, many having immunological functions. Proteins produced from fragmented microorganisms bind to various MHC molecules. The MHC molecule can be divided into three groups: class I, class II and class III.

- **MHC class I** molecules are present on the surface of virtually every cell. They present antigen fragments to T lymphocytes and bind to **CD8** receptors on cytotoxic T cells.
- **MHC class II** molecules are found mainly on macrophages and B cells and present antigen to helper T cells, binding to the **CD4** receptor.
- **MHC class III** genes encode for other immune components, such as complement, or cytokines such as TNF-α.

Human leucocyte antigen
HLA antigens are classified into nine divisions:

- HLA-A, HLA-B and HLA-C all belong to MHC class I.
- HLA-D consists of six genes, all belonging to MHC class II.

The HLA molecules, class I and II, are both two-chain glycoproteins. Class I molecules have a single transmembrane chain whereas class II molecules have two transmembrane chains. Both classes have an antigen-presenting groove where oligopeptides bind (Fig. 6.11).

Interactions with T lymphocytes
The interaction of a T cell receptor with an MHC-receptor indicates the presence of a cell with a foreign particle, such as an intracellular microbe. The binding stimulates the T lymphocytes, which become activated and release various cytokines, depending on what type of lymphocyte has been stimulated.

- **CD4 T lymphocytes** (having CD4 receptors) have a **helper function**. When a helper T lymphocyte encounters an antigen of the correct specificity, correctly presented, it responds by dividing and secreting cytokines. These lymphocytes cannot eliminate or kill antigen but the secreted cytokines initiate events that do.

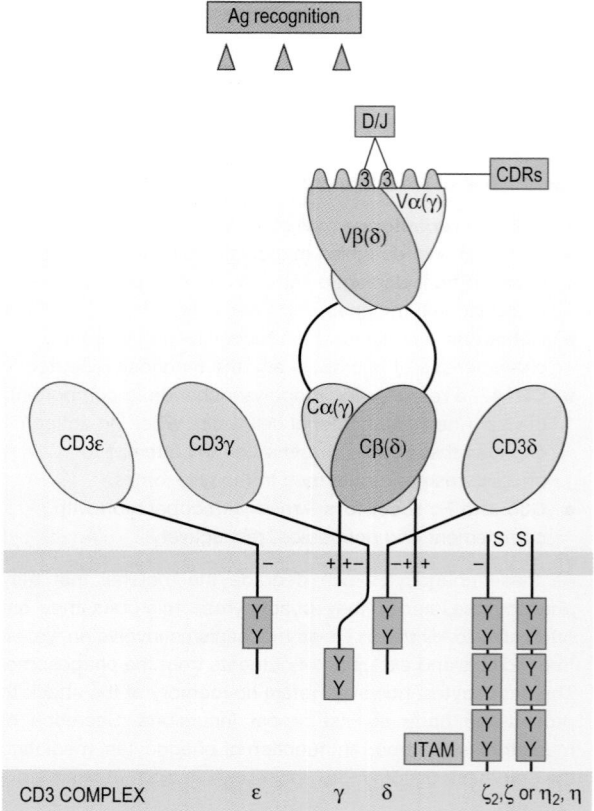

Fig. 6.11 **T cell receptor on αβ T cells** consists of an α- and a β-chain, each composed of a variable (V) and a constant (C) domain resembling the immunoglobulin Fab antigen-binding fragment in structure. The highly variable (complementarity determining) regions (CDRs) on the variable domains contact the major histocompatibility complex–peptide antigen complex. This produces a signal that is transduced by the invariant CD3 complex composed of γ, δ, ε and ζ or η chains, through their cytoplasmic immune receptor tyrosine-based activation motifs (ITAM), which contact protein tyrosine kinases. γδ T cells have receptors composed of γ and δ chains. Ag, antigen. Adapted with permission from Goering R et al. 2007 Mims' Medical Microbiology, 4th edn. Mosby, Edinburgh.

- CD4 cells have high affinity receptors for the viral gp120 glycoprotein, allowing HIV antigens to bind, along with a co-receptor, the CCR5 β-cytokine, activating these cells in an attempt to respond to the invasion. Around 1% of individuals have deletions in the *CCR5* gene which provides resistance to the infection. The subsequent failure of the immune response leads to a decline in CD4 counts, and their level is used as a measure of the patient's immune health and potential vulnerability in the fight against secondary infections.
- Most **CD8 T lymphocytes** (having CD8 receptors) are cytotoxic. They recognise antigens associated with intracellular pathogens, like viruses, when presented. This recognition activates them and also stimulates neighbouring cells. The activated cell induces signals that promote apoptosis of the infecting cells.

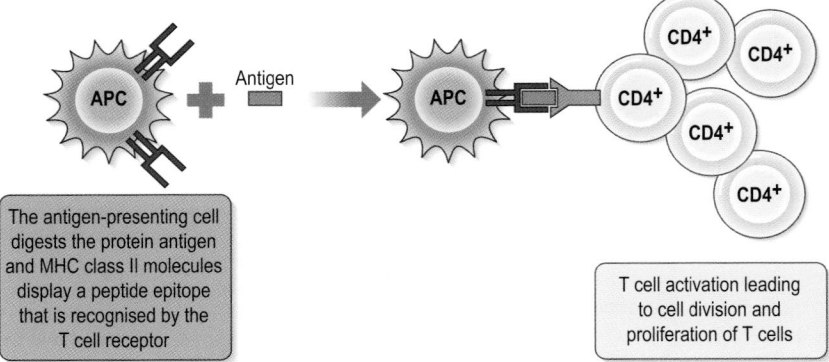

Fig. 6.12 **Antigen presentation to T cells by antigen-presenting cells (APCs).** MHC, major histocompatibility complex.

T lymphocytes cannot respond to antigen: it has to be presented to them by HLA molecules on cells such as dendritic cells, macrophages, B lymphocytes or other cells (**antigen-presenting cells (APCs)**) (Fig. 6.12). There are two possible sources for the antigen presented by APCs:

- **Exogenous antigen** – an antigen taken in by the APC. It may be self or non-self.
- **Endogenous antigen** – an antigen manufactured within the APC. It may be self (coded for by the APC's own genes) or non-self (derived from an intracellular pathogen infecting the cell).

There are various cells that act to present antigens:

- **B lymphocytes** recognise exogenous antigen (determinant) through their antigen receptors (antibodies). Unless there are many copies of the determinant on the same antigen molecule, the B lymphocyte cannot respond immediately. Instead, it endocytoses the antigen, processes (cuts) it into peptides, which it presents, on **class II HLA** molecules, to **helper CD4 T lymphocytes**. If the antigen is recognised, the T lymphocyte may become activated, and secrete cytokines (**help**) which complete the activation of the B lymphocyte. The B lymphocyte can now form a clone: antibody production follows after receiving 'permission' from helper T cells.
- **Macrophages** also pick up antigens because they have various surface receptors for foreign determinants. Although they can become activated and destroy what they have phagocytosed, in order to become fully activated, they must process and present antigen in a similar way to the B lymphocytes, the released cytokines activating the macrophage.
- **All nucleated cells** can become infected by viruses or other intracellular pathogens, which are then shielded from antibodies and macrophages while they remain in the host cells. However, cells process a sample of these proteins (endogenous antigen), and present the resulting peptides (on class I HLA molecules) to **cytotoxic CD8 T lymphocytes** which, if activated, can kill that cell.
- **Dendritic cells** are derived from blood cell precursors. Within different tissues the dendritic cells differentiate and become active, taking up and presenting antigens to MHC molecules. The activated cells migrate to lymphoid tissue where they act as APCs and interact with other cells to produce cytokines.

- **Langerhans cells** are specialised dendritic cells that can activate 'virgin' T cells. They are not themselves seeking to be activated through presenting antigen, but appear to be a determinant of T lymphocyte activation. The potential importance of these cells in HIV patients has been recently recognised. Dendritic cells can take up HIV via specific receptors. While they may have a role mopping up viral particles, they may also provide a reservoir of HIV.

Antigen recognition

Mature T lymphocytes are released from the thymus bearing antigen receptors. Each cell has many thousands of receptors and all on a single cell have the same specificity, but they are derived from the same set of genes by random genetic rearrangement. It is thought that the maturation in the thymus deletes any self recognition and commits the cells to either the CD4 or CD8 lineage.

T lymphocytes also have other receptors. CD3 is a molecular complex on all T lymphocytes. When antigen is recognised, a conformational change takes place in the lymphocyte which enables particular activation events to take place.

The HLA molecule is on the APC and presents an oligopeptide antigen bound within the groove of the molecule. The size of the oligopeptide differs between the two classes.

- **Class I HLA** molecules (on most nucleated cells) present **endogenous** antigen to **CD8** cytotoxic T lymphocytes.
- **Class II HLA** molecules (on B lymphocytes and macrophages) present **exogenous** antigen to **CD4** helper T lymphocytes.

A mnemonic

Extra Help for you **too** = **Exogenous** antigen, **Help**er T lymphocytes are CD**4**, and recognise antigen presented on class **II** HLA molecules.

It should be noted that there is not a 100% correlation between function and CD4/CD8 status: thus CD4 cells are not always helper cells, nor CD8 cells always cytotoxic cells. CD4 T cells that can activate macrophages, but cannot help B cells, are called Th1 cells, and CD4 T cells that can help B cells but cannot activate macrophages are called Th2 cells (T helper 1 and 2). CD4 T cells that retain both patterns of cytokine secretion are called Th0.

T cell activation and killing

Once antigen has been recognised, the T cell may be activated, or remain unresponsive (**anergic**). Various factors encourage activation:

- **Antigen presentation by dendritic cells**, probably because of their ability to stimulate 'virgin' T cells. T cells are likely to become anergic if their initial exposure to antigen is not through a dendritic cell.
- **Past memory**. Once a T lymphocyte has been activated, it and its mitotic descendents are memory cells, activation is more likely on re-exposure to the antigen, whatever the APC is.
- **Adhesion molecules**. There are several pairs of adhesion molecules that are important in T cell activation. For example, all T cells have CD2 molecules on their surface which interact with CD58 on APCs, promoting adherence and transmitting activation signals (positive or negative) to the T cell.
- **IL-1** is a polypeptide cytokine, secreted by APCs during antigen presentation. It lowers the activation threshold of CD4 T cells.

Once activated, the CD4 T cells, in particular, respond by expressing receptors for **IL-2**. IL-2 binds to receptors which continue activation, producing more cytokines which are different, dependent on the type of T lymphocyte. If there is insufficient IL-2, or if some of the other factors are lacking (dendritic cells, adhesion molecules, etc.), then the cells become anergic. CD8 T cells probably do not make enough IL-2 to induce activation without help from neighbouring CD4 T cells.

Table 6.7 compares the different cytokines released by activated CD4 and CD8 T cells and their actions.

Cell killing can take place in two ways:

- Perforin in the granules produces ion channels in the target cell membrane followed by osmotic lysis.
- Release of TNF interacts with receptors on the target cell and initiates programmed cell death (**apoptosis**).

The T cell can thus lead to the death of many cells, but is undamaged by this process.

Switching off activated T cells

Continued antigen presence continues to stimulate the T cells and so when the antigen disappears, the stimulus to release the activating cytokines is 's**witched off**'. Other substances appear to assist in this process:

- **Transforming growth factor β (TGF-β)** controls proliferation and cell differentiation and is released by many cells. Some cells not only secrete TGF-β, but also have TGF-β receptors, which means that this substance can suppress surrounding cells non-specifically (**autocrine signalling**).
- **Hydrocortisone**, a steroid hormone, interferes in various ways with antigen presentation.
- T cells might specifically suppress each other, not responding to consumed cytokines.

B lymphocytes

B lymphocytes originate from the bone marrow with receptors for antigen on their surface (**antibodies**) and circulate through blood and lymph to B cell areas in lymphoid tissues.

Clinical box 6.14   **Asthma**

Asthma is essentially an inflammatory disease of the airways, which is as yet poorly understood, but thought to be a type 1 hypersensitivity reaction (see below) (see also Ch. 13). The inflammation is due to an immune response to allergens (e.g. pollen, house dust mite faecal particles, fungal spores and some chemicals). Airway hyper-responsiveness in asthma is due to airway inflammation, but airway remodelling also takes place. The airway inflammation is initiated by an increase in immunoglobulin E (IgE) synthesis, stimulated by eosinophils and Th2-type T lymphocytes:

- Eosinophils produce interleukin 5 (IL-5), facilitating IgE synthesis.
- T lymphocytes are upregulated, and produce IL-4 to promote IgE synthesis.

Airway inflammation:

- Mast cells release histamine, prostaglandin D_2 and leukotriene C_4, powerful mediators that act on bronchial smooth muscle and blood vessels to cause the immediate bronchial constriction in asthma. Here, the β-adrenoceptor agonists (e.g. salbutamol, salmeterol) used in the treatment of asthma inhibit mast cell mediator release, but have no effect on airway inflammation (or hyper-responsiveness). Mast cell activation is inhibited by the anti-inflammatory agents sodium cromoglicate and nedocromil sodium. In susceptible patients, the inadvertent administration of drugs that inhibit prostaglandin synthesis leads to an overproduction of leukotrienes by eosinophils (see below) (e.g. aspirin, non-steroidal ant-inflammatory agents), and the administration of non-selective β-adrenoceptor antagonists (blockers) may thus precipitate an acute asthma attack.
- Eosinophils congregate at the airways under the influence of eosinophilopoietic cytokines (IL-3, IL-5) and chemokines. When activated, the eosinophils release leukotriene C_4 and other proteins (enhanced by cytokines and chemokines) that are toxic to the bronchial epithelium, triggering airway inflammation, when oedema and increased exudative secretions obstruct the airways. Inhaled or oral corticosteroids (the preventive and rescue treatments for asthma) inhibit eosinophil activation and decrease their number. Leukotriene receptor antagonists may also be effective in reducing inflammation. Eosinophil activations is also prevented by sodium cromoglicate and nedocromil sodium.
- Lymphocytes and dendritic cells: dendritic cells take up and present allergens to the lymphocytes, stimulating the lymphocytes to produce and release cytokines that promote the migration and activation of mast cells and eosinophils. Lymphocyte and macrophage activity is inhibited by corticosteroids, but not β-adrenoceptor agonists.

Airway remodelling:

- In chronic asthma, the structures of bronchial epithelium and smooth muscle are altered. When combined with the ongoing effects of inflammatory cells and mediators, the normal function is impaired. Damage to the epithelium causes thickening of the airway wall and makes it more vulnerable to infection. Hyperplasia of the bronchial smooth muscles increases hyper-responsiveness.

Antibodies are glycoproteins with a characteristic structure – two heavy chains and two light chains. Any one B lymphocyte has antibodies all of the same specificity.

When antigen interacts with the antibodies on the surface of a B lymphocyte, the cell responds by dividing. Some of the progeny change their appearance and become **plasma cells**, which continually **secrete antibody**. Antibodies cannot themselves destroy or eliminate non-self or antigen, but they interact with other agents that do, such as the classical complement pathway, null cells, macrophages, neutrophils, mast cells and eosinophils.

Table 6.7 Cytokines released by CD4 and CD8 activated T lymphocytes

Cytokine	CD4 cell	CD8 cell	Functions
Interleukin 2 (IL-2)	✓	Low	Maintains T cell activation Increases natural killer cell activity Help CD8 cytotoxic T cells Facilitates B cell antibody production
Migration inhibitory factor	✓	✗	Retains macrophages and activates them
α-Interferon	✓	✓	Activates macrophages Induces cells to become antiviral Amplifies TNF activity Increased expression of class I and class II HLA molecules
Tumour necrosis factor α (TNFα) (lymphotoxin)	✓	✓	Kills some tumour cells and some virally infected cells, amplified by TNF Increased expression of class I and class II HLA molecules Can activate eosinophils, neutrophils and macrophages
IL-3	✓	✗	Growth factor for pluripotent stem cells
Granulocyte-monocyte colony-stimulating factor (GM-CSF)	✓	✗	Stimulates growth and differentiation of monocytes and granulocyte precursors
IL-4	✓	✗	B cell growth factor promoting proliferation, antibody secretion and switch to IgE Mast cell growth factor Weak macrophage activator
IL-5	✓	✗	B cell growth factor Growth factor and activator of eosinophils
IL-6	✓	✗	B cell growth factor and promotes antibody secretion Stimulates acute phase protein release from liver
IL-8	✓	✓	Chemotaxis and activation of neutrophils, monocytes, eosinophils, basophils
Perforin	✗	✓	Pore forming protein, producing apoptosis with granzyme
Transforming growth factor β (TGF-β)	✓	✓	Switches off activated T cells

B cell activation

The first step in B cell activation is when the surface antibody binds to an antigen of the correct specificity. It the antigen is **T independent**, then this is sufficient to activate the B lymphocyte. T-independent antigens have many copies of the same determinant, cross-linked on the surface of the B cell, providing a strong enough signal to exceed the activation threshold. The capsule of **pneumococcus** is a clinically significant T-independent antigen. Most antigens do not have this repetitious structure and are **T-dependent antigens**. In this case the B lymphocyte must present the antigen to a helper T lymphocyte of the correct specificity:

1. The B cell endocytoses and processes the antigen.
2. Fragments of processed antigen are presented to the T cell on the B cell surface, in association with class II HLA molecules.
3. The helper T cell responds by secreting lymphokines – B cell growth factors (IL-2, IL-4, IL-5 and IL-6) which push the B lymphocyte over the activation threshold.

IL-1 from nearby macrophages can also contribute to the activation by reducing the activation threshold of B cells and helper T cells.

Antigen may also be trapped on the surface of macrophages or follicular dendritic cells in lymphoid tissue, making it more available to B cells (called **antigen presentation**). Antigen processing and HLA molecules are *not* involved. This antigen retention may be essential to the persistence of memory B cells. Following activation, B lymphocytes get bigger (**blast transformation**) and divide. Some members of this expanded clone differentiate to form plasma cells, which secrete the antibody into the surroundings.

Plasma cells are short lived, so for the clone to survive, some members must remain as B lymphocytes, eventually to become memory cells. Immediately following the first acti-vation, the B cell membership of the emerging clone will express IgM only, and the descendant plasma cells will secrete IgM. However, over time, individual B cells from the clone may switch production to a different immunoglobulin class. Plasma cells descended from such a B cell will secrete antibody of the new class. If the antigen exposure is repeated or prolonged, most of the B cells concerned will switch away from IgM antibody production. This class switching can only occur with T lymphocyte help.

B cell response

Primary responses, to an antigen never encountered before, are measured by detectable specific antibody in the serum that occurs after about 5 days, peaking after about 9 days. Initially the response is mainly IgM, but IgG may reach a comparable concentration after about 11 days. Antibody levels are often low again by about 3 weeks.

The **secondary response** to this same antigen is much more rapid, becoming evident in about 3 days and resulting in a higher peak of specific antibody concentration. The majority of the antibody is IgG and of a higher affinity. The plateau of response is longer and antibody production has a much slower decline (Fig. 6.13).

Antibodies may neutralise viruses and toxins by binding to active sites, but they cannot themselves destroy non-self. Instead they:

- Prepare antigens for phagocytosis (**opsonisation** – any molecule that allows cells to come together, such as coating negatively charged molecules on the membrane surface)
- Interact with killer cells
- Trigger the classical complement pathway.

All these processes lead to the destruction of non-self.

Switching off B cells

B cells may be switched off in several ways. Possible mechanisms include:

- Disappearance of antigen because of successful defence
- Withdrawal of T cell help through suppression
- Negative feedback from immune complexes.

Null lymphocytes

These cells do not make antibodies or produce T cell receptors. They kill some neoplastic and virally infected cells through two different mechanisms, both promoting apoptosis:

- **Natural killer (NK) activity** acts through recognising and inhibiting normal healthy cells, allowing the killing of cells without self (MHC class 1) markers (innate immunity).
- **Killer activity**. Null cells also bear receptors that enable them to interact with antibody that has bound to other cells (Fc receptors). Here it is the antibody that discriminates between non-self and self.

ANTIBODIES

Antibodies are glycoproteins. They are the antigen receptors on the surface of B lymphocytes and are secreted by plasma

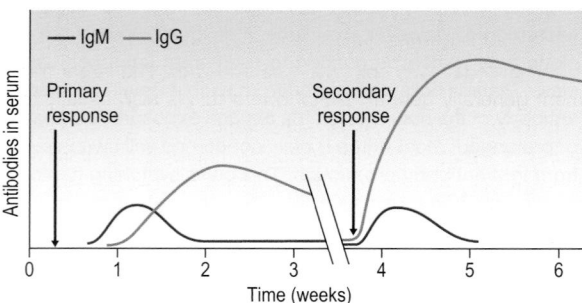

Fig. 6.13 Pattern of antibody production after initial and second exposure.

cells. Plasma cells are B lymphocytes that are in their final antibody-secreting phase. Each receptor binds a specific antigenic determinant, and all antibodies produced by a particular plasma cell clone have the same specificity as the antigen binding site. Between them, the many millions of plasma cells produce an enormous range of specificities.

Figure 6.14 illustrates the structure of a typical immunoglobulin molecule, or antibody. Each antibody has two identical light chains and two identical heavy chains.

- Each light chain consists of two domains: one **variable region** domain, and one **constant region** domain.
- Each heavy chain has one variable region domain, and either three or four constant region domains.

Variable regions have very wide variation between clones. In contrast, the constant regions are more or less the same between clones.

Light chains come in two types – lambda (λ) and kappa (κ) – but only one type of light chain is present per antibody, determined by the constant region domain. **Heavy chains** come in five different classes: alpha (α), delta (δ), epsilon (ε), gamma (γ) and mu (μ), determined by the constant region domains of the heavy chain. The type of heavy chain determines the class of antibody – IgA, IgD, IgE, IgG and IgM, respectively. Subclasses have also been defined. The λ and ε chains have four constant region domains; the remainder have three and a **hinge** region, which probably gives more flexibility to α, δ and ε chains.

- The **specificity**, determined by the variable region domains, is almost fixed, as is the type of light chain.
- The **class**, determined by the heavy chain constant regions is not fixed. A given clone can (and well may) produce antibodies of all the different classes and subclasses. Even so, each plasma cell is probably committed to a single class.

The 'arms' of the antibody form the **fragment, antigen binding (Fab) region**, composed of a constant and a variable domain from each heavy and light chain. At the tip is the **antigen-binding site**. The base region, composed of two heavy chains that contribute two or three constant domains, is called the **fragment, crystallisable (Fc) region**. This region is involved in modulating the *immune* cell activity by binding

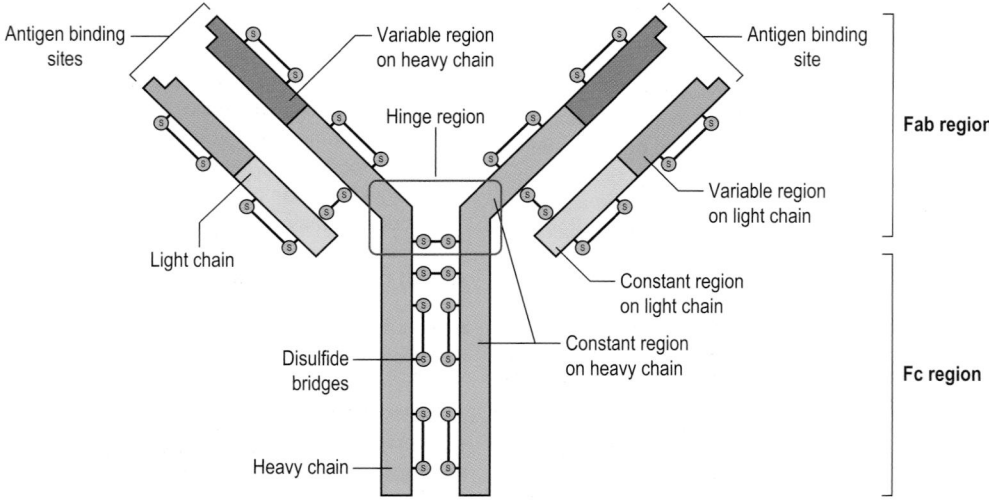

Fig. 6.14 Generic structure of immunoglobulins.

to specific proteins. The Fc region also binds to other cell receptors and molecules, such as **complement**, enabling various responses such as opsonisation and lysis of cells.

- Fc receptors for IgG on phagocytes and null lymphocytes are of low affinity, so these cells will only bind onto immune complexes where multiple Fc portions are available in an array, minimising the opportunity for the complex to dissociate by chance.
- Mast cells have a high affinity Fc receptor for IgE, so they are able to bind individual IgE molecules effectively.

Antibody complexes

While IgD, IgE and IgG exist as monomers, IgA forms a dimer, and IgM a pentamer (Fig. 6.15).

Antibody functions

Antibodies can be described according to their strength. **Affinity** refers to the strength of the antibody–antigenic determinant bond. **Avidity**, in contrast, is the strength of attachment between an antibody and antigen – different because antibodies have at least two antigen-combining sites and antigens may have many different determinants of the relevant specificity.

The different antibody classes have different functions, described below and summarised in Table 6.8.

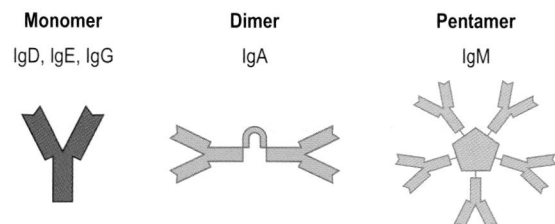

Monomer	Dimer	Pentamer
IgD, IgE, IgG	IgA	IgM

Fig. 6.15 **The different antibody complex shapes.**

- **Blocking and neutralisation**. IgG, IgM, and IgA are all present at significant concentration, and if they are specific for the appropriate molecule they may block the binding of microbes and toxins to human tissue.
- **Complement fixation**. IgM and IgG subclasses 1, 2 and 3 fix complement (classical pathway).
- **Opsonisation and killer activity**:
  - IgG mediates opsonisation and phagocytosis of bound antigen by neutrophils, macrophages, monocytes, dendritic cells and eosinophils, all of which possess Fc receptors for IgG.
  - IgG also mediates killer activity by null lymphocytes, which possess Fc receptors for IgG.
  - IgE mediates phagocytosis by eosinophils, which possess Fc receptors for IgE.
- **Mast cell activation**. Mast cells possess Fc receptors for IgE leading to granulation and release of mediators.

COMPLEMENT

The complement system is a triggered enzyme cascade. The components circulate in inactive forms, the first member of the series, once it is activated, activating the next. Each molecule can activate several molecules of the next component of the series, so the reaction is amplified. There is a complex collection of factors and controlling molecules that make up the complement system: C factors (C1 though to C9), factor B, factor D, MCP (membrane cofactor protein), DAF (decay acceleration factor), factor H, factor I, properdin and C1 inhibitor.

Activation of a component is often achieved by splitting, and the two products that result are labelled with the suffixes **a** and **b**: thus C4 is split into C4a and C4b. The larger fragment generally gets the suffix b and this is also usually the active part. Difficulty arises with the nomenclature of the C2 subunits because C2a and C2b are similar in size and, historically, C2a was the active unit. There has been a move to change C2a to C2b, because 'b' otherwise stands for the functional part, but there is no consensus on this and people

Table 6.8			
Class	**Serum concentration (g/L)**	**Functions**	**Comments**
IgM	0.6–2.0	Blocks binding of toxins and adherence of microbes	In secretions and on surface of B cells
		Activates classical complement pathway	Destroys pathogens in early stages of B cell-mediated immunity
		First antibody to appear in the immune response	
IgG	8.0–16	Blocks binding of toxins and adherence of microbes	Provides majority of antibody-based immunity
		Subclasses 1, 2 and 3 activate classical complement pathway	Can cross the placenta to protect the fetus
		Opsonises antigen for phagocytic cells	
		Mediates killer activity of null cells	
IgA	1.5–4.0	Blocks binding of toxins and adherence of microbes	Mucosal linings
		Transported across mucous membranes, including gut	Saliva, tears, breast milk
		Has a secretory piece to protect against digestion	
IgD	0.03	Function unclear but may act as an antigen receptor on virgin B cells. Very low concentration	
IgE	0.0003	Low serum concentration because adsorbed onto mast cells	Involved in allergy, triggering release of histamine from mast cells and basophils
		Cross-linking of IgE on mast cells by antigen mediates degranulation	Provides protection against parasitic worms
		Opsonisation of antigen for eosinophils	

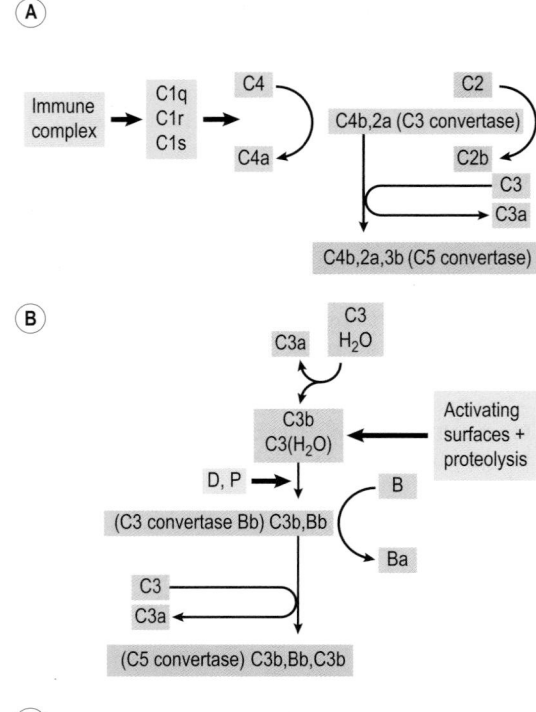

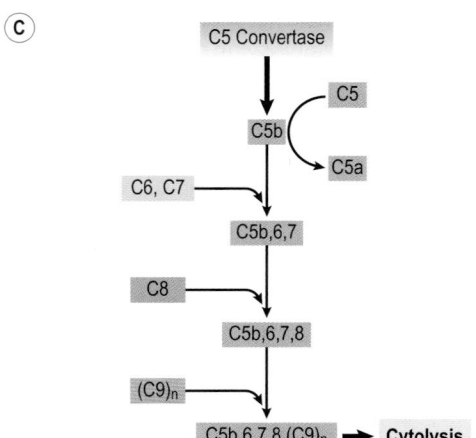

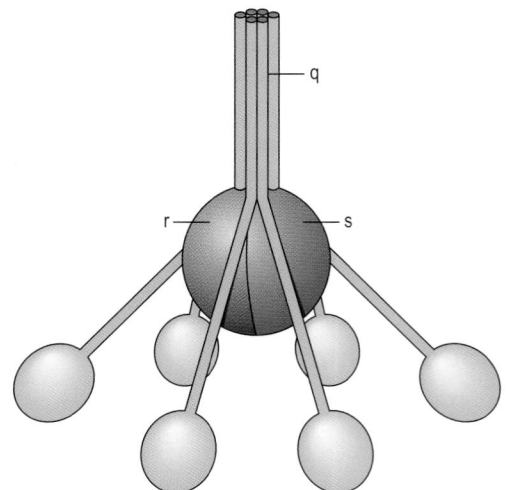

Fig. 6.16 The complement pathways. (A) The complement cascade in which C5 convertase is formed in the classical pathway. (B) The complement cascade in which C5 convertase is formed through the alternative pathway. (C) The complement cascade in which C5 convertase acts on other complement components to produce the membrane attack complex, which results in lysis of the cell to which it is bound. Courtesy of Professor Peter Schneider, University of Cologne, Germany.

working in complement genetics continue to use C2a to stand for the active part.

The aim of the complement cascade is to activate C3 by splitting it into C3a, C3b, C3c and C3d:

- C3a is a chemotactic agent
- C3b initiates the formation of a lytic structure and also binds to C3b receptors on macrophages, aiding phagocytosis.

There are two pathways leading to activation of C3: the **classical pathway** and the **alternative pathway**:

- The classical pathway is triggered by the interaction of an antibody with an antigenic determinant.

Fig. 6.17 Structure of the C1 complex.

- The alternative pathway is triggered by some bacterial cell walls, fungal cell walls and some endotoxins, and does not depend on a pathogen-binding protein.

The classical pathway (Fig. 6.16A)

The classical pathway is triggered when the C1q part of the C1 complex (C1q, C1r and C1s) binds to IgM or IgG complexed with antigen, or when C1 binds directly to a pathogen.

C1q has a bunched form (Fig 6.17) and each of the six subunits can bind to a constant region domain on the immunoglobulin. It is necessary for several of the subunits to bind for the pathway to be triggered: this ensures that activation does not simply occur when C1q happens to meet a circulating immunoglobulin molecule. Although a single IgM, in contrast to IgG, can initiate the pathway, because of its pentameric structure, the site to which the C1q binds is only revealed when most of IgM antigen-binding sites are actively binding antigen.

Activation leads to conformational changes in C1q, activating C1r and then C1s, cleaving it. C1r and C1s are controlled by C1 inhibitor, raising the triggering threshold.

- **Angioneurotic oedema** is due to a deficiency of C1 inhibitor so that triggering the complement cascade can lead to a dermal and submucosal oedema that can be life-threatening if the airway in involved.
- The C1 complex splits C4, and then C2 and the subunits C4b and C2a form a complex, **C4b2a**.
- C4b2a (**C3 convertase**) cleaves C3 and C3b joins the former to make **C5 convertase (C4b2a3b)**. C3a is chemotactic for leucocytes. The interaction between C5 convertase and C5 initiates the lytic sequence.

The alternative pathway (Fig. 6.16B)

The alternative pathway is activated when circulating C3 interacts directly with some pathogens or endotoxins. The activated classical pathway can also activate this pathway, amplifying the response. C3 is cleaved and C3b combines with factor B to form **C3b,B**. Factor B is split with factor D and **C3b,Bb** (**C3 convertase Bb**). C3 convertase Bb, located on the pathogen surface, activates more circulating C3, leading to more C3b adhering to C3 convertase Bb – positive feedback. The resultant complex on the pathogen, **C3b,Bb,3b** cleaves C5 to initiate the lytic sequence. C3b,Bb,3b from the alternative pathway is thus the equivalent of **C4b2a3b** from the classical pathway.

Factors that inhibit the alternative pathway

Some factors control the alternative pathway:

- C3b is inactivated by factors H and I in the blood, and the proteins DAF and MCP on cell surfaces.
- DAF and factor H compete with factor B for the C3b.
- MCP and factor I (**C3b inactivator**) together cleave C3b.
- C3 convertase Bb has a limited survival time and does not generate enough C3b to overwhelm the controlling factors.

Factors that encourage positive feedback of the alternative pathway

In addition to any disturbance of the presence of membrane factors DAF and MCP, or of circulating factors H and I, activation of **properdin** protects C3b from factors H and I. Properdin circulates in an inactive form and is inactivated by some non-self component.

The central role of C3

C3 is central to both the classical and alternative pathways and is the most abundant. It contributes to innate immunity and a deficiency of C3 leads to a susceptibility to bacterial infections. C3 cleavage results in:

- The activation of the lytic sequence
- The release of C3a, which activates mast cells, and is weakly chemotactic
- The release of C5a at the beginning of the lytic sequence. C5a activates mast cells, and is strongly chemotactic
- Opsonisation: macrophages and polymorphs have receptors for C3b. Using these they can interact efficiently with microorganisms to which the C3b has bound.

The lytic sequence (Fig. 6.16C)

C5 is cleaved by the C5 convertase from either the classical or the alternative pathway.

- C5a leaves the pathway but is also chemotactic and activates mast cells.
- C5b has a cell membrane binding site and normally attaches to the cell which has the activating complex attached to it. **Bystander lysis** occurs because sometimes innocent bystander cells may be affected and lysed. This is an important factor in **hypersensitivity** as, for example, if platelets are the innocent cells, their destruction and degranulation can lead to activation of the clotting system and lead to a thrombosis.
- C5b also binds to C6 and C7, to form **C5b,6,7** and then C8 and multiples of C9 are bound, forming the **membrane attack complex (C5,6,7,8(C9))**.
- C8 and C9 have hydrophobic components that incorporate into the membrane lipid but making, at the same time, an ion channel. This channel allows water to move, but not protein. As a result water enters somatically and the cell is lysed.

THE CELLULAR DEFENCES

Basophils and mast cells

Basophils are derived from the pluripotent stem cell in bone marrow via precursors (see Ch. 12). Found in blood, basophils move into tissue during inflammation. **Mast** cells are derived from the pluripotent bone marrow stem cell, like basophils probably from cells expressing CD34 cell surface markers, and are distributed throughout the tissues. Mast cells are heterogeneous, those in mucous membranes being different from those in connective tissue, but they have much in common with basophils and what follows generally applies to both cell types.

Both cells are rich in granules that contain **histamine** and other substances that are released by degranulation. The cells are also involved in the manufacture of leukotrienes, prostaglandins and other substances.

Mast cell activation

A number of different mechanisms lead to activation of mast cells and subsequent release of active components:

- **IgE meeting its antigen**: mast cells have Fc receptors for IgE molecules. The cells' different antigen-binding sites are exposed on the surface and bind to any antigen they encounter in the circulation. As the antibody sites become filled with antigen so the complexes become cross-linked and the mast cell degranulates. Helper T lymphocytes are required as IgE production is under their control. Even if the antigen is T independent, class switching to IgE can only take place with helper T lymphocyte approval through presentation by APCs. It is not known how helper T lymphocytes decide which specificities of B lymphocyte should switch to IgE but IL-4, secreted by Th2 T cells, is involved.
- **C5a and C3a components of complement** are chemotactic and cause mast cell degranulation.
- **Neurological factors**. Mast cells are frequently found near nerve endings. The neurotransmitter **substance P**, involved in pain recognition, activates mast cells.
- **Physical stimuli** such as pressure, heat/cold and products of tissue damage, possibly mediated through IL-8 cytokines.
- **Certain chemicals** can stimulate mast cells directly, for example substances in foods.

Substances released by mast cells

- **Histamine**: this is not chemotactic. Its release produces powerful and visible changes through acting on:
  - **H1 receptors** (blocked by antihistamines such as chlorphenamine) and slightly on
  - **H2 receptors** (blocked by cimetidine and ranitidine)

  to:

  - Increase venule permeability
  - Cause some arteriolar dilatation
  - Contract smooth muscle.

  This results in a local increase in blood flow and oedema. In the skin, the consequences can be seen as a weal (swelling), and flare (erythema), which appear within a few minutes of histamine release, peak within 30 minutes and are often accompanied by itching.

- **Leukotrienes**: these are metabolites of arachidonic acid and increase permeability of post-capillary venules over a longer period than histamine. They also contract smooth muscle and are chemotactic for various phagocytic cells. Macrophages and polymorphonuclear cells also produce leukotrienes, whereas these cells do not make histamine.
- **Other prostaglandins** from arachidonic acid: these are made in the cell membrane and released on degranulation. Many other cells also produce various prostaglandins that are released by the action of IL-1 and as a result of tissue damage. They act to:
  - Dilate arterioles, increasing local blood flow
  - Induce pain (by blocking **glycine**, which suppresses the transmission of pain signals in the dorsal root ganglion)
  - Cause fever (through their action on the hypothalamus).
- **Cytokines**: these include TNF, IL-1, IL-4, IL-5, IL-6, IL-3 and granulocyte-macrophage colony-stimulating factor (GM-CSF).

Neutrophils

Neutrophil granulocytes are circulating white cells that play an important role in the body's defence system. Along with eosinophils and basophils, these granulated cells originate from the same precursor in bone marrow and are part of the myeloid series of white cells. On their surface are class I HLA molecules, but not class II, which means that they cannot present antigen. They also have Fc and C3b receptors.

Neutrophils are the most common and most dynamic of all the polymorphs with large numbers being made available from bone marrow when stimulated by **chemotactic factors**, released from activated endothelium, mast cells and macrophages at sites of damage. Cell surface receptors on the neutrophils enable detection and movement up a concentration gradient, enabling their rapid relocation of these cells to the site of damage. Various chemical signals encourage neutrophil chemotaxis and include:

- Complement breakdown products, especially C5a
- Secretory products of inflammatory cells (polymorphs and macrophages) such as leukotrienes, platelet-activating factor (PAF) and IL-8
- Oligopeptides that contain a formylated amino acid, which are products of prokaryote metabolism. Response to these may indicate the capacity of neutrophils to recognise non-self.

Role of neutrophils in inflammation

Movement to site of damage
Neutrophils form the bulk of the early acute inflammatory cellular infiltrate at the site of damage and generally arrive before monocytes. In response to chemotactic agents they adhere to the endothelium of local capillaries and venules, and then their pseudopodia squeeze between the endothelial cells and dissolve basement membrane in order to move into the tissue space (**diapedesis**).

Phagocytosis
Neutrophils and other polymorphs have receptors for antibody (Fc receptors) and for C3b. Material coated with these opsonins is phagocytosed, if not too big. Some other mate-

rial, e.g. latex beads, can be phagocytosed without the aid of opsonins, perhaps indicating an ability of polymorphs to recognise the non-living. Polymorphs are activated mainly by:

- Either C5a and the engagement Fc or C3b receptors
- Or PAF and N-formylated peptides – metabolites from microorganisms.

Activation produces a **respiratory burst** in which oxygen is consumed and large quantities of reactive oxygen species (e.g. hydrogen peroxide) are released. Enzymic catalysis of the superoxide and subsequent products produces **hypochloric acid** (chlorous bleach), which is a potent killer of microorganisms and results in **degranulation**, releasing enzymes both into and outside the phagosome. These include proteases and hydrolases, myeloperoxidase, lysozyme and proteins:

- **Myeloperoxidase** is bactericidal in the presence of hydrogen peroxide and halide.
- **Lysozyme** breaks the bond between muramic acid and N-acetylglucosamine (key bacterial cell wall components).
- **Lactoferrin** (binds iron) and **vitamin B$_{12}$-binding protein** deprive bacteria of important nutrients.

The neutrophil response is continued through release of leukotrienes and PAF, which attract more polymorphs and macrophages and contract smooth muscle. Leukotrienes increase local vessel permeability and prostaglandin release dilates local arterioles and induces the pain and fever associated with inflammation.

Monocytes and macrophages

Monocytes are circulating white cells derived from precursors in the bone marrow, becoming macrophages when they leave the circulation. Like neutrophils they are chemotactic, although with a slower response, and have Fc and C3b receptors. In contrast they have both class I and class II HLA molecules and therefore they can present antigen.

Macrophages and monocytes respond to the following chemotactic agents:

- C5a, and (much more weakly), C3a
- Leukotrienes (from mast cells, polymorphs and macrophages)
- The IL-8 group cytokines, from other macrophages, and activated CD4 T cells
- Products of tissue damage (denatured proteins, etc.)
- Some non-self substances (e.g. formylated peptides, typical bacterial products).

Migration inhibition factor (**MIF**), released from activated helper T cells, prevents macrophages migrating away.

Role of macrophages in inflammation
Macrophages are versatile cells and act as the main scavengers of old cells and debris. Producing a wide variety of substances, they are important agents in the inflammatory response and are also the main APCs in the fight against pathogens. They are activated by a variety of agents including:

- **Macrophage-activating factors** (**MAFs**) from activated helper T cells are the most efficacious and include IFN, MIF and TNF

- Non-self substances engaging macrophage receptors
- Chemotaxins (the least efficacious).

Phagocytosis is initiated when cell surface receptors are engaged, leading to expression of class II HLA molecules and triggering of the respiratory burst, induced by MAF. Cytokines also assist in antigen presentation to T helper cells, enabling antibody production. Antibodies coating the pathogen makes it easier for the macrophage to stick and phagocytose the foreign body.

Activation also leads to the lysosomes being filled with strong oxidising agents (superoxide radicals), destructive enzymes (including those specifically to attack bacteria, such as lysozyme) and antibacterial agents (such as vitamin B_{12}-binding protein and iron-binding lactoferrin, removing substances needed by bacteria for their growth).

Highly activated macrophages may have their 'index of suspicion of non-self' raised sufficiently to attempt to destroy most neighbouring substances and cells discharging the content of the lysosomes outside the cell. Not all macrophage products are destructive. α_1-Antitrypsin and α_2-macroglobulin neutralise destructive proteases and also release factors that promote repair and cell division.

Macrophages may help cancer cells proliferate through their attraction to hypoxic tumour cells. TNF released by the macrophage activates a transcription factor, **nuclear factor-κB** (**NF-κB**), which enters the cancer cell and produces substances that inhibit apoptosis.

A functioning macrophage

Pneumocystis carinii (*jiroveci*) is a protozoon which we are exposed to continuously. The immune system, with assistance from macrophages, ensures that healthy people are not affected. People with pure B cell deficiencies are also not affected. Macrophages on their own do not become sufficiently activated but interaction with the helper T cell is key. Individuals who are T cell deficient can experience life-threatening pneumonia as a result of exposure to *P. carinii* (see Clinical box 6.2).

A struggling macrophage

Mycobacterium tuberculosis is phagocytosed by macrophages but is not killed. This is because macrophages lack a receptor for a particular component in the tough mycobacterial cell wall which inhibits the usual lysosome–phagosome fusion. This ensures that bacteria are retained within the cell, producing a prolonged chronic response that leads to widespread tissue damage; this **delayed-type hypersensitivity** (**type 4 hypersensitivity**) encourages the development of granulomas.

Eosinophils

Eosinophils are derived from the same precursors as neutrophils in the bone marrow and circulate as white cells in the blood. Precursor differentiation into eosinophils depends on particular stimulation from IL-3 and IL-5. Like neutrophils they are phagocytic, chemotactic, have Fc and C3b receptors and class I, but not class 2, HLA molecules. They differ particularly in their granule content.

Eosinophils may be activated by engagement of Fc or C3b receptors with specific IgG and C3b molecules, by formylated peptides (metabolites from microorganisms), and by cytokines (including IL-3 and IL-5).

Role of eosinophils in inflammation

Eosinophils have special roles in combating helminth parasitic incursion (such as in schistosomiasis) and are also important in the mechanisms involved in the control of allergy. They are less effective than neutrophils in destroying bacteria but play a role in fighting viral infections and in the removal of fibrin, deposited as part of the inflammatory process.

Toxins are released into phagosomes or, in the case of helminths, onto the surface of the parasite to which the eosinophil is attached. These toxins include:

- Superoxides from the respiratory burst
- **Eosinophil cationic protein** and **major basic protein**. These are toxic to helminths
- Peroxidases and neurotoxins (with antiviral activity).

Red cells

Some red cells have receptors for C3b and carry immune complexes that contain C3b, to be phagocytosed in the liver or spleen.

Platelets

While platelets are mainly involved in haemostasis, they are also involved in the inflammatory process where they interact with other cells through secretion of various inflammatory mediators. Substances released from the lytic sequence of complement activation and PAF from activated neutrophils stimulate the aggregation and degranulation of bystanding platelets, bringing about a local thrombosis. Platelets also have Fc receptors for IgG and so bind to antigen via specific antibody. They also secrete PAF and IL-8. While filarial and other worms release prostaglandins that inhibit platelet aggregation, the interaction between platelets and the parasite can induce cytotoxicity.

HYPERSENSITIVITY

Hypersensitivity refers to the undesirable side effects of the normal immune response, whether or not that response is directed against self or non-self. There are five types of hypersensitivity (Table 6.9).

Type 1 hypersensitivity

The interaction between antigen and IgE results in mast cell degranulation and the release of histamines, leukotrienes, prostaglandins and other substances that cause symptoms within minutes. Figure 6.18 summarises the process.

Local exposure can result in:

- **Hay fever** (due to pollen antigens)
- **Asthma** (pollens, house dust mite, fungal spores)
- Local **urticaria** (insect bites and stings).

In highly sensitised people, antigen exposure, trivial in most people, causes massive mast cell degranulation, with systemic effects: anaphylaxis, general urticaria, angioneurotic oedema of skin and mucosa, asthma, hay fever, gastrointestinal symptoms. Individuals who are **atopic** have an increased predisposition to form IgE antibodies against common environmental antigens, leading to conditions such as asthma or eczema. These conditions have a strong inherited component.

Type	Synonyms	Mediator	Example
	Table 6.9 **Different types of hypersensitivity and their manifestation**		
1	Allergic, immediate	IgE	Asthma; anaphylaxis; urticaria
2	Cytotoxic, antibody dependent	IgM or IgG (and complement)	Autoimmune haemolytic anaemia (AIHA), idiopathic thrombocytopenic purpura (ITP), haemolytic disease of the newborn
3	Immune complex	IgG (and complement)	Systemic lupus erythematosus (SLE), polyarteritis nodosa
4	Delayed type, antibody independent	T cells	BCG vaccination, transplant organ rejection, contact dermatitis
5	Subtype 2	IgM or IgG (and complement)	Graves' disease; myasthenia gravis

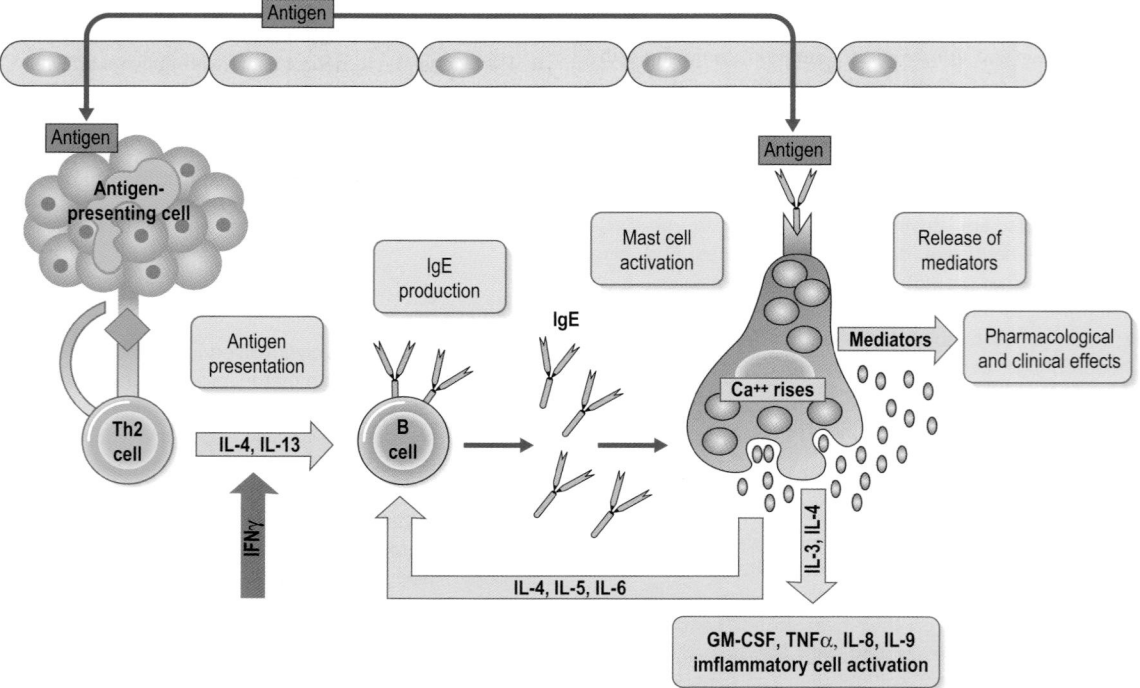

Fig. 6.18 **Type 1 hypersensitivity.** See text for abbreviations. Adapted with permission from Actor J 2006 Elsevier's integrated immunology and microbiology. Mosby, Edinburgh.

The **Prausnitz–Kustner (PK)** experiment showed that type 1 (immediate) hypersensitivity could be transferred by serum. Prausnitz was hypersensitive to a certain antigen and he injected this antigen into Kustner's skin. Subsequent injection of serum from Prausnitz injected into Kushner's skin showed an immediate flare and weal, mediated by specific IgE in the transfused serum. Other stimuli can lead to a type 1-like hypersensitivity resulting from mast cell degranulation:

■ Heat/cold/pressure leading to urticaria
■ Food allergy – although some foods may act as antigens for IgE, the effect is probably due to direct activation of mast cells from chemicals in the food
■ Complement mediated – often mixed with type 2 or type 3 hypersensitivity.

Type 2 hypersensitivity

This occurs when antibodies attach to determinants on self structures (auto-antibodies). The tissues are damaged by classical complement activation, phagocytosis and/or killer activity. Although originally used to describe antibodies against blood cells, it now includes antibodies against other

tissues that mediate damage. For example, **Goodpasture's syndrome**, in which antibodies develop against basement membrane in kidney and lung.

Type 3 hypersensitivity

Antigen–antibody immune complexes, with or without complement, cause damage to neighbouring tissue. The antigen may be self, e.g. nuclear constituents as in systemic lupus erythematosus (SLE), or non-self, e.g. streptococci. Effects can be local or systemic.

■ **Local form**: the Arthus reaction. In this model of the reaction, an individual is thoroughly immunised against an antigen, producing high titres of IgG. Antigen is then injected subcutaneously, producing localised inflammation of the skin, peaking several hours later. Clinically, inhaled fungal spores can cause **extrinsic allergic alveolitis** (farmer's lung).
■ **Systemic form**: serum sickness. Experimentally, when a large quantity of foreign (horse) serum is injected intravenously, antibodies build up. When the concentration equals that of the antigen, immune complexes precipitate resulting in rashes, joint pain,

Disordered immunological response to bacterial infection

Disease can result from disordered immunological responses to apparently minor bacterial infections. Examples include rheumatic fever (type 2 hypersensitivity) and glomerulonephritis (type 3 hypersensitivity) in children.

- **Rheumatic fever**: Rheumatic fever is a complication of throat infection by a group A *Streptococcus* (sore throat, scarlet fever) in children (aged 5–15). Although the precise mechanism is unclear, it is thought to be the result of a type 2 hypersensitivity reaction leading to an autoimmune response triggered by molecular mimicry between bacterial cell wall M proteins and cardiac myosin and laminin. All the tissues of the heart may be affected leading to pancarditis, but consequent damage to the heart valves is common. Associated inflammation of the synovial membranes of joints (flitting arthritis), subcutaneous nodules (Aschoff's nodules) and erythema marginatum may be present during the acute stage of the disease. Owing to the widespread prescription of antibiotics in the developed world, rheumatic heart disease is now rare, but it still occurs in developing nations.
- **Post-streptococcal glomerulonephritis** (PSGN): PSGN is thought to be due to a type 3 hypersensitivity reaction where immune complexes formed to combat a bacterial infection infiltrate the glomerular basement membrane. Activation of the complement cascade then destroys the basement membrane. A child may develop an acute nephritic syndrome, with proteinuria, oedema and hypertension (see Ch. 14), 2–3 weeks (the time taken for development of the immune complex) after a streptococcal infection (Lancefield group A β-haemolytic *Streptococcus*). Treatment with dietary salt and protein restriction, diuretics, antihypertensives and dialysis may be necessary. Prognosis is usually good.

fever, lymphadenopathy and hypotension, for example. Clinical examples are **SLE**, **glomerulonephritis**, **Henoch–Schönlein purpura**, and **polyarteritis nodosa**, but often the causative antigen is unclear.

Type 4 hypersensitivity

This is damage associated with the interaction between activated helper T cells and activated macrophages, or activated cytotoxic T cells and NK cells (**delayed type hypersensitivity**). It cannot be transferred through serum.

- BCG vaccination (injection of attenuated *M. bovis*: the causative agent of bovine tuberculosis and a relatively uncommon cause of human tuberculosis) in people who have previously been exposed to tuberculosis produces a lesion that is maximal after more than 2 days.
- Granulomas, T cell infiltrates, contact dermatitis and organ rejection are probably all results of this.

Type 5 hypersensitivity

This is a subtype of type 2 hypersensitivity – instead of the antibodies acting against cell surface components, this definition is used to describe situations when the antibodies act against cell receptors. For example:

- **Graves' disease**, where antibody to thyroid stimulating hormone receptors stimulates the thyroid, causing thyrotoxicosis

- **Myasthenia gravis** in which antibodies develop to acetylcholine receptors in postsynaptic neuromuscular junction, resulting in muscle weakness and fatigue.

TOLERANCE

Tolerance is a specific immune non-reactivity against a certain substance. Individuals should be tolerant of their own body components (**self-tolerance**). Experiments in newborn mice show that foreign antigens introduced within a few hours of birth are usually tolerated while the antigen persists (**neonatal tolerance**). In humans the exposure probably happens when the fetus is only a few months old. Particular immunisation schedules in adults may induce tolerance, rather than immunity (**acquired tolerance**). Variations in solubility, route of delivery, or concentration of antigen, and the ability of the person to launch a response are all factors that influence the development of tolerance.

Tolerance mechanisms

There are three main cellular mechanisms that lead to toleration.

Clonal deletion (central tolerance)

Clonal deletion occurs when developing B cells and T cells recognise self-antigen while in the bone marrow or thymus and are deleted before they become fully immunocompetent. Initiated in fetal life it will continue throughout life as new lymphocytes are produced.

Anergy

If a mature T cell or B cell recognises antigen in certain unfavourable circumstances, it will become anergic, or frozen, temporarily but not permanently refractory to activation.

- T cell anergy can occur in the absence of dendritic cells at the first encounter with antigen.
- B cell anergy may occur in the absence of T cell help.

Acquired tolerance

Acquired tolerance is where there is a specific non-reactivity to an antigen which would normally lead to an immune response. For example, in pregnancy, the fetus must be tolerated by the mother. There are several hypotheses that have been suggested to explain this phenomenon: Eu-FEDS is the best known.

- **Eu-FEDS (eutherian fetoembryonic defence system)** hypothesis states that glycoproteins and carbohydrate present in the reproductive system and expressed on gametes (for example α-fetoprotein and **CA125**) suppress the immune response that would otherwise reject sperm and eggs. The latter do not carry any HLA antigens allowing them to be recognised as self and so there must be another mechanism. Support for this model comes from the apparent acquisition of these substances by invading pathogens. The profile of the main oligosaccharides linked to CA125 and the major surface glycoprotein of HIV-1 (gp12) almost perfectly overlap.

The ability to produce acquired immunity is an important aim of medical treatment in organ transplantation. **Oral**

Crohn's disease (CD) and ulcerative colitis (UC) are the major recognised forms of inflammatory bowel disease. CD can affect any part of the gastrointestinal tract (including oral manifestations), whereas UC affects the colon. Clinically, they both present with diarrhoea, abdominal pain and weight loss (malnutrition), but a diagnostic distinction is important because they are managed differently. Clinical, radiological and histological information give the diagnostic clues. Extra-gastrointestinal manifestations include inflammatory arthritis.

Immunologically, the inflammatory process in CD and UC is similar. It is thought that susceptible patients have defects in the genetic regulation of the immune response so that both specific and non-specific inflammatory responses to endogenous antigens in the intestinal lumen are exaggerated. In CD, macrophages and T helper 1-type T lymphocytes are upregulated leading to an excess of pro-inflammatory mediators such as cytokines (interleukins and tumour necrosis factor-α). In UC, the Th2-type T lymphocyte response is altered with excess production of interleukins (interleukins-5 and 10). Activation of neutrophils, eosinophils, mast cells and fibroblasts leads to excess chemokine production, which can result in tissue damage, ulceration and inflammation in the wall of the bowel.

tolerance is important as the gut mucosa will be exposed to a variety of foreign antigens in food. **Inflammatory bowel disease** may be the result of a failure in oral tolerance (see Clinical box 6.16).

AUTOIMMUNE DISEASE

Autoimmune disease is a disease resulting from **autoreactivity**. Autoreactivity, a response to self, is common, but does not necessarily lead to autoimmune disease. There are also many diseases characterised by a lymphocyte/macrophage inflammatory infiltrate that have no detectable infection. They are often called 'autoimmune', meaning that they are caused by some breakdown in self-tolerance. This is often unproven. Examples of such conditions are where there is:

- **Covert viral infection** and the viral antigens manufactured by the body's cells are the targets of the immune response. No breakdown in self-tolerance is necessary.
- **Chronic tissue destruction** provokes a chronic inflammatory infiltrate, and this might be called 'autoimmune' if the real mechanism of tissue destruction is not detected.

Examples of true autoimmune disease are where there is a breakdown in B cell or T cell self-tolerance.

B cell self-tolerance breakdown

Autoreactive B cells that escape clonal deletion in the bone marrow and enter the circulation may avoid anergy in two ways:

- **Recognition of mixed self/non-self material**. Foreign infective material may have some determinants that resemble self which the autoreactive B cells process. The material will also have non-self determinants and presentation of these may gain help from a self-tolerant helper T cell population. For example, autoimmune disease can be initiated artificially by injecting self tissue in **Freund's adjuvant** (a suspension of mycobacteria in

an oily suspension) which can lead to the production of particular immunoglobulins.
- **Autoreactive B cells** may receive help from **autoreactive T cells**.

T cell self-tolerance breakdown

This may also allow breakdown of self-tolerance among B cells. There are several theories as to how this might happen:

- **Release of material from a privileged site**. Some structures, like the lens of the eye, contain self material that is not accessible to the immune system, and is only released in minute quantities and so there will have been no deletion or anergy of lymphocyte clones. A substantial release of this material, perhaps as a result of injury, may result in an autoimmune response against it.
- **Unusual expression of HLA molecules and/or other ligands**. If a specialised cell only expresses class I HLA molecules, for example, along with few other immunologically important adhesion molecules or ligands, T cells may not be deleted or anergised against peptides made only in that cell type. These active peptides become 'immunologically invisible'.
- **Cross-reaction of microbial peptide with uncommon self-peptide**. If a microbial peptide cross-reacts with an immunologically invisible self-peptide, or with a self-peptide that has elicited anergy but not deletion, then it may elicit an immune response. As it is the HLA molecules that present self and foreign peptides, and different HLA alleles select different peptides, then the HLA alleles that an individual possesses may determine whether or not an immune response is elicited.
- **Loss of suppression**. If autoreactive cells are being suppressed by other T cells, then this might change if the suppressing cells are eliminated, or the cytokine profile changes, as it might during a microbial infection.

OTHER SUBSTANCES IMPORTANT TO THE IMMUNE SYSTEM

Interferons

IFNs are natural proteins or glycoproteins that have non-specific antiviral activity acting through cellular metabolic processes involving synthesis of RNA and protein. There are three major classes of IFN, which depend on the type of receptor. Some are produced by virally infected cells and activated macrophages, others may be produced by activated T lymphocytes.

IFNs have an antiviral effect, repress cell growth (of both normal and tumour cells) and regulate the immune system through signals induced when they interact with cell surface receptors. They increase NK activity, increase expression of HLA molecules (synergistically with TNF) and are the main macrophage activator. Binding of IFNs to special receptors on the cell surface induces an **antiviral state**. They act by triggering a process in the cell that:

- Inhibits viral replication
- Upregulates class I HLA molecules, thus increasing presentation of molecules to cytotoxic T cells
- Increases activity of p53, a transcription factor that induced apoptosis of the infected cells.

Clinical box 6.17 | Inflammatory arthritis

Inflammatory arthritis is characterised by synovial membrane inflammation that ultimately leads to destruction of the joint. The large variety of inflammatory arthritides may roughly be divided into rheumatoid factor (RF)-seropositive (principally **rheumatoid arthritis**) and RF-seronegative types. Depending on the eventual condition, the initial inflammatory process is 'triggered' by an antigen that is sometimes infective (bacterial or viral) but not necessarily targeted at synovial membranes alone, but is often unknown. Other organs may be affected. **Molecular mimicry**, the phenomenon where antibodies against molecules of the attacking organism (antigen) mistakenly recognise similar host molecules for foreign molecules, sets off an autoimmune response when the antibodies destroy 'self' molecules and tissues. Once initiated, persistence of the condition (like most autoimmune diseases) is usually associated with genetic factors.

Rheumatoid arthritis (RA) is the commonest autoimmune inflammatory arthritis. It is a multisystem disease, but predominantly affects synovial membranes where inflammatory cytokines cause synovitis. Typically, symptoms and signs begin symmetrically (sometimes asymmetrically) in small, peripheral joints (fingers, toes, wrists); multiple joints may be affected. Presentation is variable, and may begin in early childhood. Non-articular manifestations may occur, including fibrosing alveolitis and other pulmonary manifestations, vasculitis, pericarditis, neuropathies, scleritis and episcleritis affecting the eyes, amyloidosis of the kidneys and anaemia, and other organs in the reticuloendothelial system may be affected (e.g. Felty's syndrome: splenomegaly and neutropenia).

- The triggering antigen is unknown; it has been postulated that abnormal glycosylation of immunoglobulins leads to antigen mimicry: the RFs are the circulating autoantibodies where the Fc part of IgG is the antigen. A high RF titre is diagnostic of RA, and patients are said to be seropositive. Potential bacterial and slow virus infections have also been suggested, but unproven.
- Molecular inflammatory mediators include tumour necrosis factor alpha (TNF-α), interleukins (the rationale for using TNF-α and interleukin-1 blockers to treat RA) and some growth factors.
- The persistence of synovial (and other) inflammation is thought to be related to continuing T cell activation. The genetic association with chronic inflammation is better understood than the triggering mechanism for RA. Defects in the genes that regulate the immune response are thought to be responsible for the persistence of the inflammatory response. For example, HLA-DR4 (and some other genes have been identified) is associated with a poor prognosis for RA (see also Ch. 5).

Seronegative spondylarthritis includes ankylosing spondylitis, reactive arthritis (e.g. Reiter's syndrome), crystal arthritis (e.g. gout), psoriatic arthropathy and enteropathic arthritis associated with inflammatory bowel disease.

Tumour necrosis factor

TNF is a polypeptide made by activated macrophages and activated lymphocytes. Its primary role is in the regulation of immunity. It activates and **enhances the ability of phagocytes** to destroy microbes and also **acts on vascular endothelium** to allow leucocytes to move out of the circulation.

TNF is also involved in the induction of **apoptosis** of tumour cells and virally infected cells, assisted by IFNs, and also interacts with cell surface receptors (different from IFN receptors) to elicit an antiviral state. Increased production of TNF has significant side effects. Chronically high levels are seen in malignancy, producing **cachexia**. Cachexia is an unwanted loss of weight and loss of appetite seen in some conditions, particularly end-stage cancer. Cachexia was named after a substance, cachectin, now called TNF. Acutely high levels produce shock (fever, hypotension, metabolic acidosis, disseminated intravascular coagulation and diarrhoea).

Acute phase proteins

Acute phase proteins are secreted by liver cells. They increase or decrease in concentration in response to inflammatory processes. Those that increase in concentration act to destroy or inhibit microbe growth (e.g. CRP) or provide negative feedback (e.g. α_2-macroglobulin – a damage limitation agent).

Transforming growth factor β

TGF-β is secreted by almost all cells in an inactive form but can be activated by proteases. Activated T cells and activated macrophages secrete the active form, which has a wide range of effects, positive and negative, on cell growth. It causes the growth of new blood vessels and inhibits T cell proliferation. It also induces **apoptosis** through two pathways:

- **SMAD** is a class of proteins that are altered and form complexes through TGF-β interacting with cell receptors. The complex enters the cell nucleus, where it acts as a transcription factor inducing apoptosis.
- **DAXX** (death domain-associated protein) plays a major role in apoptosis. It is involved with TGF-β as it interacts with its receptor. Binding of TGF-β induces the main DAXX apoptotic pathway.

INFLAMMATION AND REPAIR

ACUTE INFLAMMATION

Inflammation is the reaction of a vascularised living tissue to local injury. Its aim is to:

- Contain and isolate the injury
- Destroy invading microbes and neutralise toxins
- Heal and repair the damage.

There are five main signs of acute infection: **heat**, **redness**, **pain**, **swelling** and **loss of function**. These are the result of vascular and cellular events.

Vascular events

Substances released as part of the inflammatory response produce transient and rapid **vasoconstriction** of arterioles, followed by **vasodilation**, causing increased flow of blood through downstream capillaries. The increase in permeability leads to an **extravascular exudate**.

- An **exudate** is a fluid with a high protein content, approaching that of plasma. The combination of the increased intravascular hydrostatic pressure (because of the vasodilation) and reduced or absent osmotic gradient (because of the leakage of protein) contribute to the increased volume of the exudate.
- **Pus** is inflammatory exudate rich in leucocytes, especially neutrophils, living and dead, together with microorganisms.

Cellular events

Leucocytes need to move from the circulation to the site of infection (**extravasation**). They do this through a series of processes. In leaky capillaries, they **marginate**, moving to the vessel wall, **roll** along the endothelium and **adhere** to the wall. **Diapedesis (transmigration)** follows, in which the leucocytes insert pseudopodia through the endothelium at or near the intercellular junctions, then pass through the basement membrane into the tissues. Endothelial cells and leucocytes express mutually recognising adhesion molecules that are necessary for rolling, adhesion and diapedesis.

The leucocytes then **migrate** through the tissues, induced by **chemotaxis**, moving within tissues up concentration gradients of various chemicals and mediators, leading them to the site of the inflammation.

Phagocytosis and killing of microbes

A phagocyte must **bind** to material that is to be phagocytosed through its own receptors that recognise dead/denatured or non-self material, or use special receptor molecules that have been made by other cells in the body and are already bound to the microbe, such as acute phase proteins, complement or antibodies. The phagocyte extends pseudopodia around the material producing a vacuole, or **phagosome**.

Intracellular **lysosomal granules** fuse with the phagosome, introducing enzymes such as lysozyme, proteases and hydrolases that can destroy the cell. Other agents are also involved which are dependent on the **respiratory burst**: by generating NADPH, the phagocyte can generate toxic superoxides

Initiation of the inflammatory response

In the **plasma** there are three 'cascade systems' of proteins that help to mediate the inflammatory response:

- The **coagulation system** is activated in tissue damage by both intrinsic and extrinsic pathways, culminating in the production of fibrin which helps to contain the infection. When fibrin is broken down its degradation products act as chemotactic factors for leucocytes and increase endothelial permeability, bringing more cells to the site of the damage and increasing the blood flow in the area.
- The **kinin system**, activated through coagulation factor XII, culminates in the production of bradykinin. Bradykinin leads to vasodilation and sensitises sensory nociceptor peripheral terminals, reducing the pain threshold and allowing pain to be experienced.
- The **complement system** is activated by foreign substances. C3a and C5a activate leucocytes to express adhesion molecules. They are also chemotactic for leucocytes and activate mast cells. C3b also acts as a receptor for phagocytes. The system produces products that lyse microbes and cells.

In the **tissues**, various cells, especially **mast cells**, produce important **mediators of inflammation**:

Figure 6.19 shows the pathways that lead to the production of various inflammatory mediators. **Mast cells** are scattered throughout the tissues, especially near epithelia and

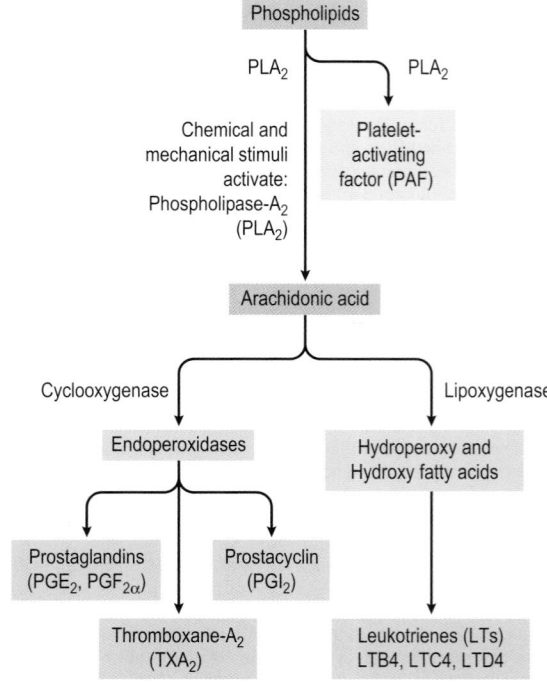

Fig. 6.19 Inflammatory mediators derived 'de novo' from cell membrane phospholipids.

blood vessels, and are important sources of mediators. They can be activated:

- Directly by **tissue damage** and agents causing tissue damage
- Through **nerves**, including the branch axons of sensory nerves, which secrete substance P
- Through the action of **C3a** and **C5a**, derived from complement
- Through foreign substances interacting with **IgE**.

Activated mast cells produce important mediators:

- **Histamine** causes arteriolar dilatation and an increase in vascular permeability.
- **Leukotrienes** cause an increase in vascular permeability and are chemotactic for leucocytes.
- **Prostaglandins** cause arteriolar dilatation and pain.
- **PAF** causes activation and aggregation of platelets, increases vascular permeability, activates leucocytes to express adhesion molecules, and is chemotactic for leucocytes.

Many body cells produce **prostaglandins** and **chemokines** when damaged, or exposed to the products of tissue damage, like denatured proteins.

- Chemokines activate **leucocytes** to express adhesion molecules, and they are chemotactic for leucocytes.
- **Macrophages** resident in uninflamed tissue become activated if exposed to the products of tissue damage or microbial products. They secrete **prostaglandins**, **chemokines**, **IL-1** and **TNF**, causing endothelial cells to express adhesion molecules, TNF increases vascular permeability.
- **Endothelial cells** are activated by direct damage, by IL-1 and TNF, and by interacting with activated leucocytes in the lumen. Once activated, expression of adhesion molecules increases, permeability increases,

and thrombosis is promoted, which prevents spread of infection. They also secrete **chemokines** and **nitric oxide**, which is toxic to microbes and cells, and is a powerful vasodilator.

Systemic effects of acute inflammation

Fever occurs through resetting the hypothalamic thermostat at a higher level. IL-1 and TNF release prostaglandins in the hypothalamus and prostaglandins act directly on the thermostat. Fever helps infection, but if the temperature increases too much it can lead to fitting and death. **Acute phase proteins** are released from the liver, stimulated by IL-1, some of which interact with microbes and aid phagocytosis.

Colony-stimulating factors stimulate the release of more leucocytes by the bone marrow causing a **raised white cell count**. Feelings of **malaise**, **lethargy** and **sleepiness** are due to cytokines acting on the brain, preventing behavioural excesses that might enhance the damage. Acute inflammation can also cause damage to self. The main dangers are through:

- The release of destructive lysosomal contents
- The action of complement
- Swelling in a confined space (e.g. brain)
- The excessive release of cytokines causing hyperpyrexia, shock and death.

Outcome of acute inflammation

Acute inflammation may be resolved in several ways. Resolution is the best outcome, the tissue returning to the state before the damage took place. Often, however, organisation and repair processes that lay down fibrous tissue lead to scarring. Abscesses can also form, in which pus remains trapped in the tissues and may, with time, become organised and persist as a chronic inflammation. Outcomes can be more serious. Local damage can result in death because important structures are involved, e.g. in meningitis. Uncontrolled infection may lead to septicaemia and excessive cytokine release can cause hyperpyrexia, shock and death.

| Clinical box 6.18 | Abscess and empyema |

Abscess formation is the result of an acute inflammatory response to bacterial or parasitic invasion. The body's defence mechanism isolates the inflammatory exudates, **pus**, from surrounding healthy tissues by thick fibrous tissue that encapsulates the pus, so that an abscess is a localised collection of inflammatory exudate containing mainly leucocytes and microorganisms. Perversely, owing to the relative avascular nature of the fibrous capsule, cellular inflammatory mediators and antibiotics are prevented from entering the abscess to destroy the invading organism. Antibiotics alone are therefore rarely effective in treating abscesses. Surgical incision for draining the pus and removal of necrotic tissue (debridement) are usually necessary. Abscesses may form as the result of bacterial or parasitic infections or foreign bodies. Common sites include superficial or deep skin abscesses (pustules, boils and carbuncles), dental abscesses, lungs, brain, renal or liver abscesses. Recurrent abscesses may occur due to infection by community-acquired methicillin-resistant *Staphylococcus aureus* (MRSA) infection.

Empyemas, unlike abscesses, consist of pus formation in existing body cavities such as the gall bladder, pleura, subdural space, joints and uterus.

CHRONIC INFLAMMATION

Chronic inflammation differs from acute inflammation in various ways:

- Longer time span (months/years rather than days/weeks)
- Tissue destruction, inflammation and healing all happen simultaneously
- The predominant inflammatory cells are different – macrophages, lymphocytes and plasma cells predominate, rather than polymorphonuclear leucocytes.

Initiation of chronic inflammation

Chronic inflammation can occur after, or in the absence of, an acute inflammatory process. An example of the former, where an initial acute inflammation does not resolve, is found in **chronic osteomyelitis**. In this disease there is an initial acute infection due to blood-borne bacteria seeding in the bone, possibly at the site of minor damage. Resolution is impaired because the tissues are rigid: pressure builds up, pus cannot drain, the blood supply is impaired and pus tracks under the periosteum, further impairing the blood supply. Some bone dies and acts as a foreign body, continuing the stimulation.

Chronic inflammation also occurs where an initial phase of acute inflammation is absent or not severe. This occurs if:

- A non-degradable foreign substance is present in the tissues (for example, talc, asbestos or silica)
- There is a persistent pathogen, often intracellular (for example viruses or mycobacteria)
- An immune response is made in the absence of any apparent pathogen – an **autoimmune** reaction.

| Clinical box 6.19 | Lung diseases associated with inhaled foreign bodies |

A number of lung diseases are associated with inflammation due occupational exposure to foreign bodies, giving rise to health and safety issues. These conditions may be caused by acute or chronic inflammation or allergy. They include:

- Acute bronchitis from inhalation of noxious, irritant gases such as chlorine, sulphur dioxide and ammonia
- Widespread pulmonary fibrosis from inhalation of mineral dusts, such as pneumoconiosis (miner's lung) from inhalation of coal dust, localised pulmonary fibrosis due to asbestosis from inhaling asbestos among shipbuilders and from the use of asbestos in insulation material in houses and even domestic appliances, and silicosis in glass foundry workers, stonemasons and sand blasters
- Occupational asthma and chronic obstructive pulmonary disease, due to inhalation of varnishes and paint sprays, cement dust, enzyme washing powders, and allergens from flour and grain
- Cryptogenic fibrosing alveolitis (idiopathic pulmonary fibrosis) of unknown aetiology may occasionally be associated with exposure to wood or metal dust. Some patients, however, may have autoimmune disease
- Allergic alveolitis (extrinsic) is associated with exposure to moulds and fungal spores, e.g. farmer's lung (mould from hay or vegetables), bird fancier's lung (bird feathers and excreta), and cheese washer's, mushroom worker's and wine maker's lungs
- Cancers associated with exposure to industrial substances such as asbestos (mesothelioma) and radon (miners).

Manifestation of chronic infection

The principal signs of acute inflammation (redness, heat, swelling, pain, loss of function) and inflammatory exudates are often less marked in a chronic infection. The tissues are infiltrated by many cells. In chronic infections this infiltration tends to be macrophages, with or without lymphocytes and plasma cells. In acute inflammation neutrophils predominate. Repair takes place through:

- New vessel formation
- Fibroblast accumulation
- Laying down intercellular matrix including collagen
- Remodelling.

   The repair has special features:

- **Granulomas** (granulomas). If there is non-degradable foreign matter, or persistent pathogenic presence, these special histological features may occur.
- **Eosinophils**, specialised phagocytes for fighting helminths, increase in these infections.

Granulomas

Granulomas differ in appearance depending on the cause. They are roughly spherical and macrophages are the essential ingredient. Granulomas have a distinctive architecture:

- A central zone of **necrosis** – not present in all granulomas.
- A zone rich in **macrophages** and cells derived from macrophages – if there is no necrosis, this will be in the centre; if there is central necrosis, the macrophages surround it. Macrophages may adopt an elongated shape to form **epithelioid cells**, or may join together to form **giant** cells.
- A zone of mainly **lymphocytes** and **plasma cells** develops surrounding the macrophages – these are not always present: they are scanty or absent in granulomas caused by non-degradable foreign material.

Old granulomas may become infiltrated with **fibroblasts** and **collagen**, ending as a fibrous scar. They may **calcify**.

Stimulants of granulomas

Foreign body granulomas are caused by non-degradable foreign substance within tissues, such as talc or asbestos.

- In granulomas there is no central necrosis and few or no lymphocytes, because there is no protein, carbohydrate or lipid antigen. Instead there are collections of **macrophages**, and **foreign body giant cells**, formed from macrophages, with nuclei scattered throughout the cytoplasm.
- Macrophages secrete IL-1, TNF and IFN-α, which are involved in the formation of the granuloma, and of giant cells. In the longer term they stimulate **fibrosis**. In conditions such as silica inhalation, granulomas develop widely throughout the lung tissue. The subsequent widespread fibrosis impairs lung function.

Tuberculosis

Mycobacterium tuberculosis most commonly enters the body by inhalation into the lungs, or through the gut, by swallowing (see Clinical box 6.4).

- After an initial neutrophil infiltrate, the mycobacteria are taken up by macrophages. Mycobacterial antigens are presented to T lymphocytes and the macrophages become strongly activated.
- Mycobacteria are resistant to this killing process, and the contents of lysozymes spill out and damage surrounding tissues before many mycobacteria are killed.
- Granulomas form, with a central zone of necrosis (caseous 'cheesy' necrosis).
- Beyond the granuloma is a macrophage-rich zone, containing epithelioid cells and **Langerhans giant cells**, surrounded by lymphocytes (T cells, B cells and plasma cells).

It is the secretion of cytokines, particularly IFN-α, which fully activates the macrophages. If the infection is contained, then the granulomas may eventually fibrose and calcify, though they may still contain viable mycobacteria.

Schistosomiasis

This is an important helminth infection with a complicated lifecycle. The adult forms live in mesenteric or bladder veins (depending on species), and the eggs are shed and may accumulate in the liver or bladder wall. Granulomas form around these, with eosinophils as well as macrophages and lymphocytes surrounding them.

   Many other **bacteria, fungi and helminths** induce granuloma formation, though only a few have central necrosis. The details differ from pathogen to pathogen.

Other granulomatous conditions

Sarcoidosis an immune system disorder of unknown origin and involves granuloma formation, mainly in the lungs. The granulomas are similar to those in tuberculosis, but with no central necrosis (see Clinical box 6.20). **Crohn's disease** affects the gut. The granulomatous chronic inflammation affects all layers of the bowel wall, with a lymphocytic infiltrate, and granulomas develop, similar to those in sarcoid, with no central necrosis (see Clinical box 6.16). **Rheumatoid arthritis** is a complicated disease, with many manifestations, including subcutaneous nodules at pressure points (at the elbows, for example) called rheumatoid nodules. These nodules manifest a central zone of fibrinoid necrosis, surrounded by a palisade of epithelioid cells, further surrounded by lymphocytes (see Clinical box 6.17).

   There are a number of diseases with **no apparent pathogen or foreign body** that manifest chronic inflammation. Some of them involve granuloma formation.

Clinical box 6.20   **Sarcoidosis**

Sarcoidosis is a granulomatous multisystem condition of unknown aetiology most often presenting as lung disease. Genetic and environmental factors, atypical mycobacterial, fungal and viral infections have been proposed as risk factors, but none has been proven. Diagnosis is commonly made on routine chest X-ray, which shows bilateral hilar lymph node enlargement and pulmonary infiltration. Ocular, neurological and skin (erythema nodosum) lesions may also be present. Myocardial sarcoidosis leads to cardiac failure. Rarely, hypercalcaemia may be presents. Young adults are more often affected, and African Americans appear to experience a more severe course of the disease. The condition may resolve spontaneously, and although controversial, corticosteroids may be used for treatment. Respiratory functions tests are used to monitor progression.

Granulomas and granulation tissue

Granulomas and **granulation tissue** have similar names. This is not a coincidence. They both play a part in chronic inflammation. Granulation tissue is the result of new vessel formation and fibrous connective tissue that replaces a fibrin clot as part of the tissue repair process. Both involve macrophages and fibroblasts, albeit in different roles, and both may end as fibrous scars. There are important differences, however, in:

- **Purpose**: granulation tissue repairs pre-existing defects. Granulomas destroy or isolate foreign material, but they may cause tissue destruction in the process.
- **Components**: new vessel formation is an important part of granulation tissue, but plays no part in granulomas.
- **Fibroblasts**: play an essential role in granulation tissue. In granulomas they are only sometimes involved at the end in healing.
- **Activity of macrophages**: in granulation tissue macrophages clear debris and fibrin, and direct new vessel formation and fibroblast accumulation through secretion of growth factors. In granulomas macrophages are trying to kill, eliminate or isolate microbes and foreign material through release of their lysosomal contents and cytokine secretion.

Complications of chronic inflammation

There are many complications of chronic inflammation that are the result of the immediate response to the inflammatory processes, or of longer-term changes to tissues.

- Consequences of fibrosis: contractures, stretching of tissues, and diffuse fibrosis in tissues (such as in the lungs) may compromise function. The lumens of nearby arteries and arterioles may be narrowed or blocked by fibrosis: **endarteritis obliterans**.
- Constitutional effects: fevers, sweating, anorexia, weight loss and chronic malaise are all symptoms of chronic inflammation.
- Anaemia of chronic disease.
- **Amyloid** formation: this is extracellular deposition in various organs (especially in the kidneys, liver, thyroid, adrenal glands and lymphoid tissue) of an acute phase protein, **serum amyloid associated protein** secreted by the liver. The tertiary structure of amyloid usually involves β-pleated sheets which form into long thin fibres (**fibrils**). Amyloid deposition can result in death through failure of the organs concerned.
- Reduction in growth, especially seen in children, is mediated by:
  - Increased energy requirements of inflammation
  - The influence of cytokines on cell division and on the systems that control growth.

Outcomes of chronic inflammation

The various outcomes of a chronic inflammatory process are **resolution** (rarely complete), **repair** (almost always present, culminating in fibrosis) or **persistence**. Chronic inflammation can persist indefinitely, even until death, to which it may contribute through tissue destruction, fibrosis, and amyloid deposition.

Clinical box 6.21 | **Amyloidosis**

Amyloidosis refers to a condition where amyloid protein is deposited in the tissues of various organs. The precise mechanisms are as yet unclear, and much research effort is given to it. The tendency to amyloid deposition may be secondary to chronic inflammation (acquired) or inherited. Amyloid deposits can only be identified histologically on tissue biopsy, which is not always feasible or possible (e.g. brain biopsy). Specific clinical signs and symptoms of amyloidosis related to chronic inflammation are few and uncommon, so that clinical suspicion related to some important clinical conditions need to be confirmed by tissue biopsy.

- Cerebral and cerebrovascular: amyloid deposits in the brain have been found in Alzheimer's disease, Down's syndrome, prion diseases (e.g. transmissible spongiform encephalopathies), Parkinson's disease. Cerebrovascular amyloidosis, although rare, can present as recurrent cerebral haemorrhages.
- Cardiomyopathies: the commonest form of restrictive cardiomyopathy is associated with amyloidosis.
- Type 2 diabetes: amyloid deposits have been found in the pancreas of some cases of type 2 diabetes.
- Chronic inflammatory conditions: e.g. inflammatory bowel disease, rheumatoid arthritis.
- Chronic infections: e.g. tuberculosis, osteomyelitis, bronchiectasis.
- Dialysis amyloidosis: amyloid protein is not adequately cleared by dialysis, and is deposited in a variety of organs giving rise to dysfunction and/or debilitating symptoms; e.g. carpal tunnel syndrome, bone cysts and fractures, gastrointestinal bleeds, joint stiffness and pain.
- Renal and hepatic failure due to amyloid deposits is associated with amyloidosis elsewhere in the body. There may be renal and liver (hepatomegaly) enlargement and treatment of the underlying condition is essential.

REPAIR

If tissue is lost through damage, there are four possible outcomes: regeneration, repair (healing) with fibrosis, persistence of a gap, immediate death, or some combination of these.

Regeneration

Regeneration implies that the tissues grow back to look the same as they did before the damage, in contrast to **resolution** in which acute inflammatory changes ebb away, leaving the tissue the same as it was before. If acute inflammation leads to some cell death and then the tissue returns to its former appearance, the combination of *regeneration* and *resolution* is called **restitution**.

Only labile and stable cells can regenerate. **Labile cells**, such as epithelial cells and bone marrow stem cells, are dividing all the time; **stable cells** only divide intermittently but can divide faster if the cells need to be replaced. **Permanent cells**, such as neurons, cardiac and skeletal muscle cells, cannot regenerate. Even if the constituent cells are labile or stable, the tissue or organ may not be able to regenerate, because the architecture cannot be rebuilt. For example:

- If a burn kills epithelial skin cells, the basal cells can regenerate more basal cells, but if the destruction penetrates through the basement membrane into the dermis over a significant area, the original structure cannot be achieved, and there will be fibrotic repair.

- In lungs, alveolar cells, and in the kidneys, renal tubular cells, can regenerate, but only if the basement membrane remains intact.

There are only three organs which can regenerate all the cell types, and the structure: the liver, bone and bone marrow.

Liver

If some liver tissue is excised or destroyed, it can be regenerated from the remaining tissue. If liver cells scattered throughout the liver are destroyed they can also be replaced. Although this regeneration can occur repeatedly, after many such episodes, some fibrous tissue gets laid down. This distorts the structure with regeneration creating nodules of new tissue, surrounded by fibrous tissue, known as **cirrhosis** (see Ch. 15).

Bone

Regeneration of bone is limited to a particular situation – where there has been a **fracture**. Following the fracture of a bone, there is bleeding at the fracture site, and clot forms. The bleeding lifts the periosteum, allowing the clot to extend around the bone fragments.

As part of the **healing** process that occurs in all tissues, neutrophils and then macrophages move into the clot and remove the debris. New blood vessel formation follows, fibroblasts accumulate and collagen is deposited forming **granulation tissue**. This is well developed as early as 4 days after the fracture. Differing from wound healing, cartilage cells now appear within the granulation tissue and islands of cartilage form, initially mostly round the outside of the bone where the periosteum has been elevated. The fractured ends of the bone are united by a fusiform sleeve of granulation tissue and cartilage, the **provisional callus**.

About a week after the fracture, calcification starts within the cartilage, and new osteoblasts appear, which produce new seams of osteoid. Over the next week calcification of the callus occurs prolifically, both subperiosteal and within the marrow cavity. It forms **fibrocartilaginous callus**, and then **bony callus**, which is mostly woven rather than lamellar bone, bulging out around the fracture site and extending into the marrow cavity.

The callus is then remodelled by osteoclasts and osteoblasts working together, guided by the stresses on the bone. By 7 weeks the bone is once again lamellar, and the normal architecture and strength is restored. Fractures in bone will not always heal perfectly. This will depend on factors such as the blood supply, relative movement and subsequent placement of the bone ends, relative splintering of the bone and presence of infection. The final result may be an angulation, twisting or shortening of a limb.

The regeneration of granulation tissue in bone is unique. In all other tissues the presence of granulation tissue leads to repair, with fibrous tissue, rather than regeneration.

Bone marrow

All the elements of blood and bone marrow are derived from pluripotent bone marrow stem cells, which divide constantly to produce all the derived cells (see Ch. 12). If blood or bone marrow is removed in haemorrhage or donation, the rate of replication increases to make up the loss. If there is extensive haemorrhage or destruction of blood cells, the marrow may colonise bone spaces previously unused. Bone marrow is semi-liquid and its cellular constituents are motile; thus when new marrow is laid down the structure is easily achieved. If regeneration cannot take place, there may be **repair**.

Repair

The body repairs itself through regeneration of dermal and epidermal tissue. It does this by initiating a complex cascade of different biochemical processes: inflammation, proliferation and remodelling.

Inflammation

The first response in inflammatory repair is **blood clotting**, in which platelets are activated by contact with subendothelium. They aggregate to form a platelet plug and this is strengthened by production of fibrin, either as a result of activation of the clotting cascade, or directly as a result of thrombin released from platelets when the damage is minor, catalysing fibrin production from plasma fibrinogen. Fibrin cross links with plasma fibronectin, forming a structural support until collagen is deposited.

In addition to producing the platelet plug, **platelets** release a variety of factors, such as serotonin, prostaglandins, thromboxane and histamine, which increase blood vessel permeability and stimulate cell proliferation and migration to the site of damage. Initial **vasoconstriction**, to reduce blood flow, is followed by **vasodilation** that assists

---

Clinical box 6.22 **Ulcers**

An ulcer (from Latin *ulcus*) is produced by the shedding (sloughing) of necrotic tissue from the surface of an organ. The tissue necrosis is the consequence of an inflammatory response to injury (e.g. skin abrasions, lacerations or burns), ischaemia or infection, and the sloughing results in a surface defect (an ulcer) from excavation of the slough. Secondary bacterial infection exacerbates the condition. Ulcers may be acute or chronic. Healing takes place from the base of the ulcer by granulation, new vessel formation and laying down of new fibrous connective tissue. Ulcers can form on the surface of any mucous membrane, e.g. mouth ulcers, peptic ulcers, colonic, bronchial and others. The skin, however, is the largest organ of the body where ulceration may be relatively common in vulnerable patients, such as people with diabetes, other circulatory problems or compromised immune systems.

Common skin ulcers encountered in the community include venous or arterial ulcers (mostly on the lower limbs) and pressure (decubitus) ulcers mainly in elderly, bed-bound and immobile patients. Distinction between venous and arterial ulcers needs to be made because the underlying conditions that led to the ulceration are different, and healing requires different management strategies.

Venous ulcers occur mainly in the lower legs. Although the precise mechanism is uncertain, it is postulated that incompetence of venous valves (e.g. varicose veins) give rise to venous hypertension (increased blood pressure in the veins), which can exceed arterial blood pressure, resulting in the failure of tissue perfusion and transudation of inflammatory mediators into extravascular tissues with consequent tissue necrosis in the skin and ulcer formation. Logically, compression and elevating the leg would lower the venous pressure below arterial pressure to improve tissue perfusion and thus help healing.

Arterial ulcers are caused by ischaemia of the affected tissues. Narrowing of medium to small arteries by atherosclerosis (peripheral vascular disease), intravascular coagulation (as in thalassaemia or sickle cell disease) and vasculitis are some examples. Leg ulcers in diabetes mellitus may be due to atherosclerosis or be neurogenic, where sensory loss due to peripheral neuropathy increases the risk of injury, but often a mixture of both. Here, good glycaemic control is essential.

in facilitating the movement of leucocytes to the area and through the vessel wall locally into the local tissue.

Neutrophils arrive at the site within an hour by chemotaxis. They phagocytose debris and any bacteria and secrete proteases that break down damaged tissues. **Macrophages** follow, removing dead neutrophils, assisted by **helper T cells** that secrete cytokines to maintain the inflammatory process. The macrophages attract cells involved in the proliferative process that follows, stimulating **angiogenesis** and the creation of **granulation tissue**, used as a foundation for a new **extracellular matrix** (ECM) in the next phase.

Proliferation

As the granulation tissue gets laid down, columns of **endothelial cells** grow in from the nearest intact capillaries, attracted by released growth factors and relative local hypoxia. These columns are initially solid, but then they hollow out to form new, patent, fragile, leaky capillaries which loop into the macrophage-infested clot, then loop back, so that blood can flow through: **angiogenesis** or **neovascularisation**. As the tissue becomes perfused so the angiogenic stimulation declines.

If the wound is a simple incision and the edges can be brought together, basal epithelial cells of the skin proliferate and meet at the surface of the wound, while granulation tissue forms in the clot underneath. This is healing by **primary intention**. If there is a large wound space this is filled by a mass of granulation tissue and the epithelial basal cells grow across the top. This is termed healing by **secondary intention**.

Fibroblasts begin to enter the wound as the inflammatory phase is ending. Fibroblasts are the main cells in the wound from about 1 to 4 weeks, migrating there from normal tissue, forming part of the granulation tissue laid down in the wound. They add glycoproteins, glycosaminoglycans and other substances to form a provisional **ECM**. Growth factors, such as **platelet-derived growth factor** (**PDGF**), TGF-β and fibronectin, stimulate the development of a more permanent ECM. The production and deposition of **collagen** by fibroblasts is important in the healing process, strengthening the repairing tissues. Collagen is also broken down by collagenases. Initially collagen predominates until production of more has no added benefit.

Once the open wound has been sealed, **re-epithelialisation** takes place with epithelial cells migrating in sheets across the wound from the outer edge, meeting in the centre. This process takes much longer if the basement membrane has also been penetrated. The faster the process, the less likely there is to be a scar. **Keratinocytes** (the main epidermal cell) migrate to the site and anchor to the ECM with transmembrane proteins. They secrete **plasminogen activator**, which activates **plasmin** to dissolve the fibrin scab. New epithelial cells follow, growing from the edge of the wound and replacing the keratinocytes. Cells re-establish desmosomes and anchor to the basement membrane. **Basal cells**, lying at the base of the epidermis, divide and differentiate to form the different strata found in normal skin.

Around 1–3 weeks after the wound is initiated the fibroblasts differentiate into **myofibroblasts** (smooth muscle cells) and the repair begins to **contract**, pulling in from the wound edge and laying down more collagen to reinforce the structure. As the provisional ECM breaks down so hyaluronic acid (a glycosaminoglycan which is a main component of the ECM) decreases, its place taken by chondroitin sulphate (a sulphated glycosaminoglycan which attaches to protein in the ECM where it forms proteoglycans and becomes the main component of the ECM), triggering the fibroblasts to stop proliferating, and the contraction phase ends.

Remodelling

As this phase of the healing process starts the macrophages will have phagocytosed all of the fibrin and moved away. Type III collagen, prevalent in the proliferation phase, is replaced by the stronger type I collagen. The new blood vessels are no longer needed and are removed by apoptosis, changing the tissue colour from pink to white. This is now **fibrous tissue**. As collagen fibres are resorted and new ones laid down there is a cross-linking and increase in fibre size. This causes the fibrous tissue to shrink and strengthen, producing a **fibrous scar**. The larger the wound, the more myofibroblasts form, and the potential for contraction is increased. Sometimes the contraction is substantial, reducing the size of the wound by more than 50%. This phase can continue for longer than 1 year after the initial wound.

Repair complications

Following a wound, granulation tissue may grow too exuberantly, and when fibrosis takes place the scar is thick and bulges out above the level of the skin: **keloid** formation. This is seen more commonly in people of African origin. **Contractures** occur when scars contract as part of remodelling, distorting the surrounding structures. This can lead to restriction of movement, or disfigurement. Sometimes, internally, important structures may be entrapped or squeezed. **Stretching** of the scar occurs if it is under constant strain after remodelling has taken place.

Repair following operations within the peritoneal cavity may leave bands of fibrous tissue round which the bowel may become entangled – **adhesions**. These can be very painful for the patient where nerves are involved. Sometimes there is neither regeneration nor repair, and a **cavity** persists in the tissues. It may be filled with pus, forming an **abscess**, or with fluid, forming a **cyst**. These may become organised later but, otherwise, the tissue is less bulky than normal. This can happen in skeletal muscle if a significant number of fibres have been destroyed.

The **brain** is a special case. Neurons do not regenerate, and granulation tissue is not formed. Instead, there is proliferation of astroglia: **gliosis**, without new vessel formation or fibroblast ingrowth. This often does not fill the space left by the damage, leaving a fluid-filled cavity. Problems also occur if **peripheral nerves** are damaged. Neurons cannot divide, and if a neuron dies it cannot be replaced. Schwann cells, however, can divide and damaging the axon does not usually kill the neuron. If a nerve is crushed, but the endoneurial channels are preserved, the axons peripheral to the injury will die, but will grow back down the appropriate channels. If a nerve is severed, the axons will try to regrow, but may not find the appropriate, or any, endoneurial channel.

Factors that hamper tissue repair

Healing is a complex process that marshals many resources in order to repair damaged tissue. It is not unexpected, therefore, that there is a long list of factors that may lead to the process taking much longer than expected and not having a perfect outcome. Some of the more important factors that can delay the process are:

- A poor blood supply
- Poor nutrition: protein, calories, vitamins (especially vitamin C) and zinc
- The presence of infection
- The presence of a foreign body
- Movement: wounds heal better if closed as well as possible, then not disturbed
- Low numbers of white cells
- Steroid therapy (anti-inflammatory)
- Radiation and cytotoxic therapy (inhibit cell division)
- Diabetes mellitus, which impairs white cell function
- Rare genetic defects of white cell function, affecting extravasation, chemotaxis, phagocytosis and the respiratory burst.

LYMPHOID ORGANS

LYMPH NODES

Lymph nodes are found throughout the body and form part of the lymphatic system. Several hundred are distributed around the body with clusters in the neck, chest, abdomen, under the arms and in the groin. They are important organs in the successful functioning of the immune system as they act as traps for foreign material.

Naïve lymphocytes enter the nodes through specialised venules and are stored in the lymph nodes where they are exposed to antigen delivered to the site on macrophages and other specialised cells. B lymphocytes proliferate in the area as they respond to the need to produce antibodies. This is often experienced by the patient as a swollen gland.

Structure

Figure 6.20 illustrates the structure of a lymph node. Nodes range in size from a few millimetres to about 2 cm in the healthy individual. It is a kidney-shaped organ with a surrounding **fibrous capsule**. Inside the node, the fibrous capsular material extends in as collagenous **trabeculae** that divide up the outer part of the internal space.

Lymph circulates through the node, entering through **afferent lymph vessels** that penetrate the capsule and open into the **subcapsular sinus**. Underneath the sinus lies the **cortex** on the outside, which surrounds the **medulla**, the latter opening into the medullary sinus at the **hilum**. The **efferent lymph vessel** drains lymph from this sinus, leaving the node at the hilum

Afferent and efferent lymph vessels

The **afferent vessels** collect lymph from other lymph nodes or from tissue spaces where it has drained from blood vessels. The vessels have valves that prevent back flow. Lymph leaves the node via the **efferent lymphatic vessel** travelling to more lymph nodes and eventually draining into the large lymph ducts and central subclavian vein.

Cortex

The **cortex** consists mainly of B cells, particularly in the outer zones. The cells are arranged in **follicles**. The **primary follicle** contains B cells, follicular dendritic cells, tingible body macrophages and a few helper T cells, but no cytotoxic T cells.

- **Follicular dendritic cells** are unique to follicles and unlike any other dendritic cells, even those also found in lymph nodes. They retain antigen and are recognised by particular antibodies.
- **Tingible body macrophages** are different from other macrophages (tissue macrophages). They possess CD4 but not CD2 or CD3 and have unique cytoplasmic tingible bodies.

Secondary follicles in the cortex are like the primary follicles except they also contain a **germinal centre**. This is

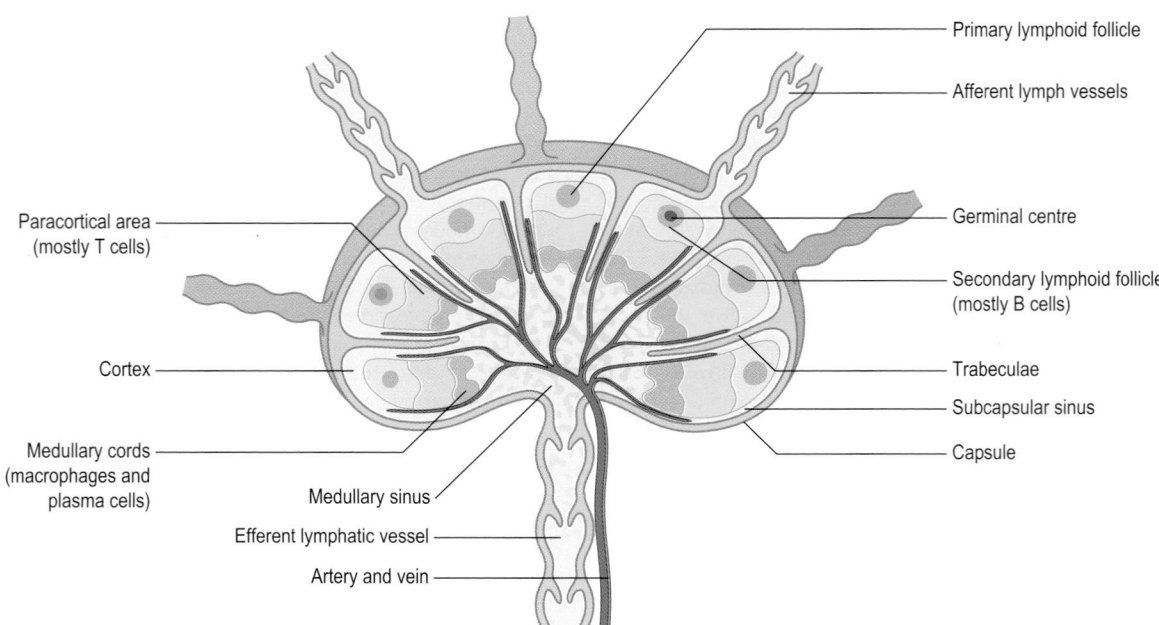

Paracortical area
(mostly T cells)

Cortex

Medullary cords
(macrophages and
plasma cells)

Medullary sinus

Efferent lymphatic vessel

Artery and vein

Primary lymphoid follicle

Afferent lymph vessels

Germinal centre

Secondary lymphoid follicle
(mostly B cells)

Trabeculae

Subcapsular sinus

Capsule

Fig. 6.20 **Schematic drawing of a section through a lymph node.**

an area of B cell proliferation, stimulated by contact with an antigen, and is surrounded by a **mantle zone** of quiescent B cells with surface IgD and IgM. Areas between the follicles are filled with mixtures of T cells and B cells. Deeper in the cortex is the **paracortex** in which T cells predominate, with helper T cells, cytotoxic T cells and many interdigitating dendritic cells.

Medulla

The medulla is composed of **sinuses** with intervening **medullary cords** of lymphoid tissue, mainly plasma cells and tissue macrophages.

Reticular network and sinuses

Fine fibres form a **reticular network** within the nodes, providing the support for the tightly packed follicles of lymphocytes, along with the dendritic cells and macrophages. The reticular cells are lined with endothelial cells which enable a smooth flow of lymph. The meshwork provides a large contact surface with the lymph node cells (macrophages and lymphocytes) enabling an efficient filtering process and an easy exchange of material with blood flowing through **high endothelial (post-capillary) venules** in the paracortex.

Blood is supplied to the lymph node though an artery and vein that enters through the hilum. Lymphocytes continuously circulate between the blood and the nodes, entering through the venules and moving into the sinuses by diapedesis. Lymph flows in through afferent vessels into the macrophage-lined **subcapsular sinus**. This sinus is continuous with **cortical sinuses** that are found on either side of the trabeculae and joins with the **medullary sinuses**, which are also lined with macrophages, into which the lymph drains before leaving the node through the efferent vessel at the hilum. Antigens and immune cells carried in the lymph are phagocytosed by the sinus wall macrophages and presented to lymphocytes within follicles. The number and composition of the follicles change when exposed to antigen as they form a **germinal centre**. Plasma cells, producing antibody, are formed and migrate to the medullary cords.

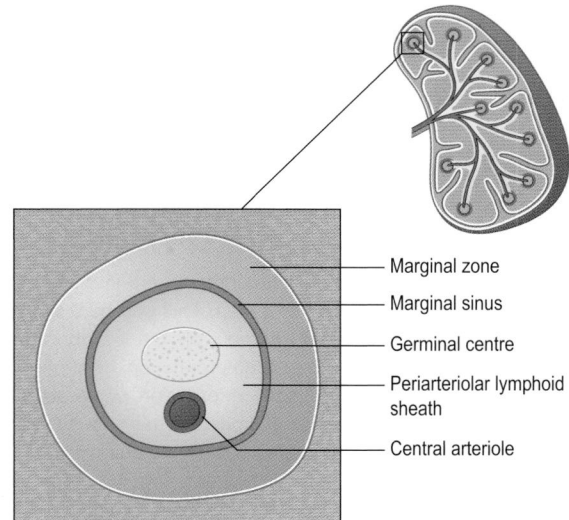

Fig. 6.21 **The spleen and its main functional regions.** Adapted with permission from Actor J 2006 Elsevier's integrated immunology and microbiology. Mosby, Edinburgh.

Labels:
- Marginal zone
- Marginal sinus
- Germinal centre
- Periarteriolar lymphoid sheath
- Central arteriole

THE SPLEEN

The spleen functions in a similar way to lymph nodes, filtering blood instead of lymph. It is located in the abdomen, under the ribcage and above the stomach. It has two main regions: red pulp and white pulp (Fig. 6.21).

Red pulp is so called because it is mostly composed of sinuses filled with blood. The sinuses are lined by macrophages and phagocytes that filter the blood, removing material, including effete red cells. **White pulp** is composed of follicles rich in B cells and **periarticular lymphoid sheaths** rich in T cells. After antigen stimulation, germinal centres form in the follicles. The sheaths form a cuff around arterioles with the B cells at the periphery in the follicles, the whole sheath being surrounded by a marginal zone of macrophages. Blood flows into the sheaths from arterioles via capillaries and can also leave through capillaries, passing into the red pulp.

NEOPLASIA

Paola Domizio

INTRODUCTION

GROWTH, DIFFERENTIATION AND DEVELOPMENT

Changes in cell growth and differentiation are implemented by the switching on and off of genes. This can be a normal event in response to certain stimuli, or can be abnormal, leading to defective growth and differentiation. The interaction of cellular signals and gene expression permeates all biology, and its discussion is not limited to this section. Most chapters discuss this material, especially Chapter 5.

The cell cycle

The cell cycle is discussed in detail in Chapters 2 and 5, and consists of two processes of cell division: mitosis and meiosis.

- **Mitosis** takes place in dividing somatic cells, where the entire DNA content of the cell is duplicated in distinct physical stages to produce two identical daughter cells, known as diploid cells (see Fig. 2.38 and Fig. 5.4).
- **Meiosis** occurs in germ cells, producing daughter cells with half the DNA content, where the entire chromosome complement is halved, known as haploid cells (see Fig. 2.39 and Figs 5.6–5.9). The process is divided into stages depending on nuclear and cell morphology.

Between the end of one phase of mitosis or meiosis and the beginning of the next is the interphase. The cell cycle is driven through its stages by **cyclin-dependent kinases** (CDKs) that phosphorylate specific proteins. The CDK molecules and cyclins are specific for each stage of the cell cycle.

Control of cell proliferation

During the quiescent, G0 (gap) phase in **interphase**, the cells are dormant until activated by a variety of stimuli towards cell growth, differentiation or proliferation. These stimuli are receptor-mediated actions of various growth factors from other cells transmitted via intracellular second messengers to the nucleus, where interaction with nuclear transcription factors initiates DNA synthesis, which in turn will initiate another phase of mitosis or meiosis. These nuclear transcription factors regulate the genes that control cell growth and proliferation (see Ch. 5).

In cancers, a common feature is uncontrolled cell proliferation leading to the formation of a tumour or **neoplasm**, a 'new growth'. Mutations in the genes that control cell proliferation can lead to the development of cancer cells for normal cells by:

- Enhancing cell proliferation so that there are more cells with the mutant gene
- Loss of the ability to repair minor abnormalities in the gene thereby destabilising the genome at DNA or chromosome levels.

Cell death

Cells die either through **necrosis** or **apoptosis**:

- **Necrotic cell death** occurs as the result of external injury, such as hypoxia due to the sudden reduction in blood flow to tissues (embolism, thrombosis, infarction), or toxins which may be externally administered chemicals or endogenous (e.g. free radicals). The cell disintegrates as the result of damage to its normal physiology, and sets off an inflammatory response.
- **Apoptosis** is 'programmed' physiological cell death when specific genes are activated to cause the cell to die. Apoptosis is necessary for normal physiology, which may occur with ageing (as with shedding the superficial layer of skin or the epithelial lining of the gastrointestinal tract), the removal of apparently healthy but superfluous cells, tissue and organ formation in embryogenesis, wound healing and many other examples. Apoptosis also occurs as the result of injury by external agents such as viruses, toxins and genetic mutation. This does not, however, lead to an inflammatory response.

In the treatment of cancers, the aim of radiotherapy or chemotherapy is to trigger the cancer cell's apoptotic pathway.

Variation in cell growth and differentiation

Cellular growth and proliferation can vary under physiological and pathological influences.

Increased growth

Increased growth occurs in a tissue or organ due to increased functional demand. It can be the result of **hyperplasia**, **hypertrophy** or a **combination** of both. Hyperplasia is an increase in cell number by cell division, while hypertrophy is an increase in cell size without cell division. Both lead to an increase in the size of an affected tissue or organ. In tissues that cannot divide, such as cardiac muscle, hypertrophy is the only adaptive response possible.

The stimuli for hyperplasia and hypertrophy are very similar and include hormones, growth factors and work against

---

Clinical box 6.23	**Examples of physiological hyperplasia and hypertrophy**

Physiological hyperplasia
- The breast undergoes hyperplasia during puberty, pregnancy and lactation, stimulated by hormones such as oestrogens, progesterone and prolactin.
- Red cell precursors in the bone marrow undergo hyperplasia at high altitude, in response to erythropoietin release stimulated by hypoxia.
- The thyroid undergoes hyperplasia in puberty and pregnancy, stimulated by increased metabolic demand.

Physiological hypertrophy
- Skeletal muscle undergoes hypertrophy stimulated by increased muscle activity on exercise.
- Cardiac muscle undergoes hypertrophy stimulated by sustained outflow increase in athletes.
- The myometrium undergoes hypertrophy in pregnancy stimulated by oestrogens.

Examples of pathological hyperplasia and hypertrophy

Pathological hyperplasia
- The prostate undergoes hyperplasia, stimulated by relative oestrogen excess in elderly men. This causes the syndrome of urinary outflow obstruction.
- The adrenal cortex undergoes hyperplasia in response to adrenocorticotropic hormone (ACTH) produced by either a pituitary adenoma or as a paraneoplastic syndrome by a small cell bronchial carcinoma. This results in Cushing's syndrome.
- The thyroid undergoes hyperplasia in Graves' disease, stimulated by auto-antibodies.
- The parathyroid undergoes hyperplasia in chronic renal failure, stimulated by hypocalcaemia.
- The endometrium undergoes hyperplasia as a result of excess oestrogen exposure. This results in abnormal uterine bleeding.

Pathological hypertrophy
- Left ventricular myocardium undergoes hypertrophy in systemic hypertension and aortic valve disease due to increased outflow pressure (Fig. 6.22).
- Right ventricular myocardium undergoes hypertrophy in conditions such as pulmonary hypertension and pulmonary valve disease, also due to increased outflow pressure.
- Arterial smooth muscle undergoes hypertrophy in hypertension due to increased work against resistance.

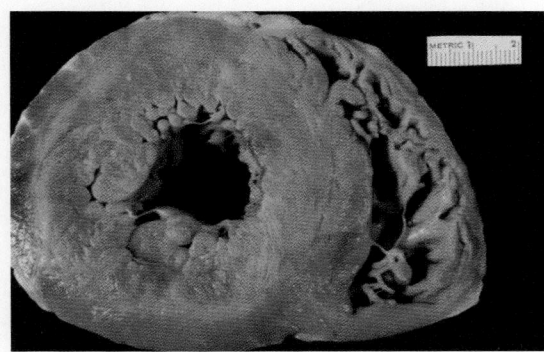

Fig. 6.22 **Cross-section through a heart showing concentric hypertrophy of the left ventricle.**

Examples of physiological atrophy
- In the embryo and fetus, the notochord and branchial clefts undergo atrophy.
- In the neonate, the umbilical vessels and ductus arteriosus undergo atrophy.
- In early adulthood, the thymus undergoes atrophy.
- In old age the uterus, testes, brain and bone all atrophy (Fig. 6.23).

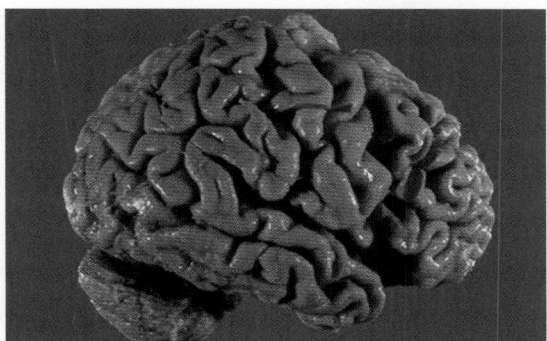

Fig. 6.23 **Atrophy of the brain in old age. There is widespread shrinkage of gyri with widening of sulci.**

Examples of pathological atrophy
- In immobilised patients, loss of function causes muscle atrophy and osteoporosis.
- In patients with nerve transection or poliomyelitis, loss of innervation causes muscle atrophy.
- In patients with peripheral vascular disease or bed-bound patients, reduction in blood supply causes skin atrophy or pressure sores.
- In patients with hypopituitarism, loss of hormonal stimulation causes atrophy of the adrenal cortex, thyroid and gonads.
- In patients on corticosteroid therapy, prolonged use causes skin atrophy.

resistance. Both hyperplasia and hypertrophy can occur as a normal physiological response or they can be 'pathological', which usually results in clinical consequences.

Decreased growth

A tissue or organ can be reduced in size either as a result of developmental failure, or as a consequence of atrophy. **Atrophy** is a decrease in cell size and/or number in a previously normal tissue or organ. Decrease in cell number is mediated by apoptosis, decrease in cell size by a reduction in cell growth. As with hyperplasia and hypertrophy, atrophy can be a normal physiological event or it can be pathological.

Abnormal differentiation

Under certain conditions, mature tissues can differentiate abnormally, undergoing metaplasia, dysplasia or both. **Dysplasia**, which literally means disordered growth, is used in two contexts. The more common usage is to describe the abnormal maturation that often occurs before the development of malignancy but it can also be used to describe abnormalities of developmental differentiation.

Metaplasia

Metaplasia is defined as the transformation of one fully differentiated cell type into another. It is an adaptive response to environmental stress, usually chronic irritation or inflammation, as the metaplastic tissues are better able to withstand the adverse environmental changes than their normal counterparts. Metaplasia is caused by activation and/or derepression of groups of genes involved in the maintenance of cellular differentiation. Unlike dysplasia and neoplasia, there is no intrinsic gene defect; therefore metaplasia is reversible. Metaplasia per se does not progress to neoplasia, but because the metaplastic tissues are less genetically stable than their normal counterparts, they are prone to undergo further transformation to dysplasia and neoplasia. Metaplasia can affect epithelial or connective tissue cells.

Epithelial metaplasia
Epithelial metaplasia can be:

- Squamous – when there is transformation to squamous epithelium
- Glandular – when there is transformation to glandular epithelium.

Clinical box 6.27 Examples of squamous metaplasia

- Ciliated pseudostratified columnar epithelium of the respiratory tract changing to squamous epithelium as a result of mucosal damage caused by smoking, bronchiectasis or chronic bronchitis
- Simple columnar epithelium of the endocervix changing to squamous epithelium due to changes of pH, injury or chronic inflammation
- Transitional cell epithelium of the bladder changing to squamous epithelium secondary to chronic inflammation caused by long-standing schistosomal infection or bladder calculi.

Clinical box 6.28 Examples of glandular metaplasia

- Stratified squamous epithelium of the oesophagus changing to simple columnar epithelium as a result of mucosal damage caused by gastro-oesophageal reflux. This is termed Barrett's oesophagus (Fig. 6.24).
- Simple columnar epithelium of the stomach changing to intestinal epithelium due to persistent chronic inflammation caused by *Helicobacter pylori* infection. In this example, one type of glandular epithelium (simple columnar) transforms into another (intestinal).

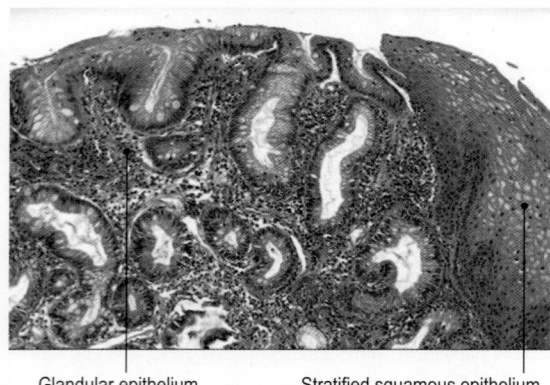

Glandular epithelium   Stratified squamous epithelium

Fig. 6.24 Oesophageal biopsy showing glandular metaplasia of stratified squamous oesophageal epithelium (Barrett's oesophagus).

(A)

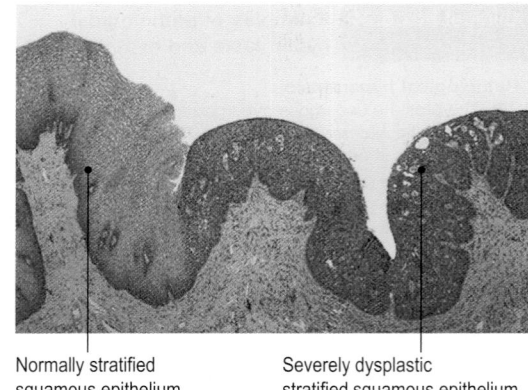

Normally stratified squamous epithelium

Severely dysplastic stratified squamous epithelium

(B)

Mitoses

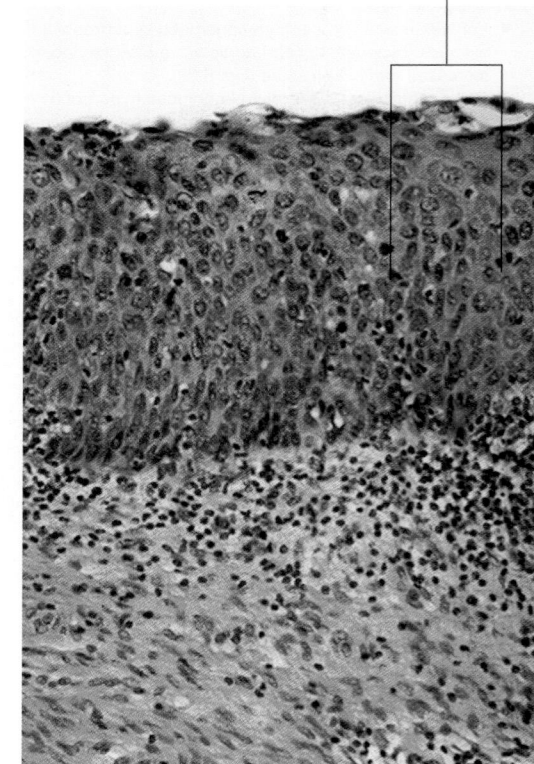

Fig. 6.25 Cervical biopsy. (A) Low-power view of a cervical biopsy sample showing an abrupt change between normal stratified squamous epithelium on the left and severely dysplastic squamous epithelium on the right. (B) High-power view of cervical biopsy sample showing severe dysplasia of the stratified squamous epithelium (equivalent to CIN 3 or carcinoma in situ). There are several mitoses visible and the nuclei are enlarged, hyperchromatic and atypical throughout the entire thickness of the epithelium.

Connective tissue metaplasia

Connective tissue (mesenchymal) metaplasia is much less common than epithelial metaplasia. The main type involves formation of cartilage or bone in old scars, known as chondroid and osseous metaplasia, respectively, such as tuberculous scars in the lungs, in atheromatous plaques and in chronically damaged muscle. The term **myeloid metaplasia** is sometimes used to describe extramedullary haemopoiesis that occurs in the spleen, liver and lymph nodes in patients with myeloproliferative diseases.

Dysplasia

In this context, **dysplasia** refers to a failure of normal maturation that occurs prior to the development of malignancy. Dysplasia is often preceded by metaplasia, but in contrast to metaplasia, it is usually irreversible. The features of dysplasia are more easily recognised in epithelia than in mesenchymal or other tissues. Such features include nuclear enlargement and atypia, loss of nuclear polarity and increased mitoses (Fig. 6.25). Nowadays, the term intraepithelial neoplasia is commonly used instead of dysplasia, reflecting the fact that this is a premalignant process. The term is most often applied to stratified epithelia, for example **cervical intraepithelial neoplasia (CIN)** and **anal intraepithelial neoplasia (AIN)**, though pathologists are trained to recognise the changes even in glandular epithelia.

In the most severe form of intraepithelial neoplasia, the entire epithelium is replaced by cells showing all the features of malignancy, but the basement membrane separating the epithelium from the underlying stroma has not yet been breached. This pre-invasive lesion is termed **carcinoma in situ** (Fig. 6.25B). The prognosis of carcinoma in situ is much better than that of invasive carcinoma because the neoplasm is not yet capable of metastasis. Detection of carcinomas at the stage of carcinoma in situ or intraepithelial neoplasia forms the basis of the breast and cervical cancer screening programmes. Other screening programmes to detect dysplasia before the development of invasive malignancy include screening for colonic mucosal dysplasia in patients with long-standing ulcerative colitis and screening for glandular dysplasia in patients with Barrett's oesophagus.

Defects of development

Failure to achieve normal development occurs because of a wide spectrum of disorders including inherited genetic defects, acquired lesions and environmental events. **Inherited genetic defects** include chromosomal abnormalities, such as Down's syndrome or Edward's syndrome, which affect many aspects of development, and **single gene disorders** such as cystic fibrosis. **Acquired lesions** include early events in embryological and fetal development, with many possible causes. Organs may be completely absent, as in renal aplasia, incompletely formed, as in spina bifida, renal hypoplasia and cleft palate, or wrongly sited, as in situs inversus. In some cases there may be extra tissues, as in polydactyly.

Environmental events affecting the embryo or fetus include maternal illness or placental dysfunction, birth hypoxia causing central nervous system damage, and infections or injuries in childhood that can have serious sequelae, such as meningitis. Malnutrition during infancy and childhood, and child neglect or cruelty, will also have an adverse effect on development.

Anomalies of organ development

Anomalies of organ development can occur at any stage during development but often begin during fetal life, when the structure concerned is being formed.

Aplasia (or agenesis) is the complete failure to develop an organ or structure. Examples include:

- Di George syndrome, when the thymus (and sometimes parathyroid glands) is absent due to defective development of the third and fourth branchial arches
- Renal aplasia, when one or both kidneys are completely absent due to failure of development of the metanephric blastema
- Anencephaly, when there is absence of the cerebrum and often the cerebellum due to failure of development of the neural tube.

Hypoplasia is the failure in development of the normal size and/or shape of an organ. Examples include:

- Thalidomide-induced limb hypoplasia
- Failure of neuromuscular development after poliomyelitis, resulting in a hypoplastic limb
- Failure of normal development of the acetabulum due to hypoplasia of the osseous nuclei, resulting in congenital dislocation of the hip.

Atresia is the failure in development of a normal lumen or orifice in the body. These conditions are always congenital. Examples include:

- Oesophageal atresia, in which the lumen of the oesophagus is narrow or absent. This is often associated with tracheo-oesophageal fistula
- Biliary atresia, in which there is obliteration of the biliary system leading to obstructive jaundice.

Dysplasia (or dysgenesis) used in this context is the failure of normal differentiation of an organ, often with the retention of primitive embryological structures. Examples include:

- Cystic renal dysplasia, in which islands of mesenchyme and/or cartilage are present within the kidney and cysts develop, possibly because of obstruction
- Fibrous dysplasia of bone, in which there are irregular masses of woven bone embedded in vascular fibrous tissue affecting predominantly the ribs, femur, tibia and skull.

Tumour-like developmental lesions

Some developmental abnormalities form tumour-like masses that can be difficult to distinguish from true neoplasms. Though they are usually present from childhood, such lesions may not present until later in life or may only be discovered incidentally.

Heterotopia is the displacement of part of an organ from its normal position. Examples include:

- Endometriosis, in which islands of endometrium are found outside the endometrial cavity
- Rests of pancreatic tissue in the wall of the stomach
- Foci of gastric tissue lining a Meckel's diverticulum.

Choristoma is a particular type of heterotopia in which one or more histologically mature tissues form a discrete mass at an abnormal site. An example is conjunctival choristoma, arising in the eye, which often contains masses of cartilage, bone, smooth muscle and adipose tissue. **Hamartoma** is a tumour-like malformation composed of mature tissues native to the organ in which the lesion arises. Hamartomas represent the borderline between developmental lesions and neoplasms. Like neoplasms, the tissues in a hamartoma are haphazardly organised and grow excessively but, unlike neoplasms, they do not proliferate autonomously. Examples of hamartomas are:

- Bronchial hamartoma, composed of bronchial epithelium and cartilage
- Juvenile polyp composed of an overgrowth of lamina propria
- Peutz–Jeghers polyp, composed of an overgrowth of muscularis mucosae (Fig. 6.26)
- Bile duct hamartoma, composed of haphazardly organised bile ductules
- Telangiectasia, composed of haphazardly organised, dilated blood vessels.

There has been disagreement in the literature as to whether lesions such as haemangiomas, lymphangiomas and pigmented naevi represent benign neoplasms or hamartomas. Though they are not neoplastic per se, in some cases hamartomas contain defective tumour suppressor genes and are consequently at higher risk of developing malignancy than are normal tissues. This is particularly true when hamartomas occur as part of clinical syndromes, such as Peutz–Jeghers syndrome and tuberous sclerosis.

PATHOLOGY OF NEOPLASIA

Neoplasm literally means new growth but the usual definition is 'a mass formed by the autonomous proliferation of cells that persists after cessation of the stimulus that provoked the change'. The word tumour has come to be used synonymously with neoplasm despite the fact that the literal meaning of tumour is 'abnormal swelling'. Compared with their normal counterparts neoplastic cells have disordered phenotype, function and behaviour. They can also have a damaging effect on the host – the more disordered the cells, the greater the adverse effect.

Benign neoplasms show the least cytological variation from their parent tissue, they do not invade surrounding structures and are not usually harmful to the host. Malignant neoplasms, on the other hand, usually show substantial cytological changes, they invade surrounding tissues and are frequently harmful to the host. The word cancer is synonymous with malignant neoplasm.

EPIDEMIOLOGY OF NEOPLASIA

Malignant neoplasms cause 26% of all deaths in the UK (154547 deaths in 2003). Bronchial carcinoma is the most common cause of death from neoplasia, accounting for 22% of cases, followed by carcinoma of the colorectum (10% of cases). Though carcinoma of the breast is rare in men, the high incidence in women means that it is the third most common cause of death from malignancy in all persons (8% of cases). Carcinomas of the lung, large bowel, breast and prostate together account for almost half (46%) of all deaths from malignancy (Fig. 6.27).

Death rates from malignancy rise with increasing age, more than 75% of deaths occurring in persons aged 65 and over. Although there are fewer deaths from malignancy in people aged under 65, the proportion of deaths from malignancy in this group is greater (37%) than in the population as a whole. This proportion is even higher for women, in whom almost half (47%) of deaths in the under 65 age group are due to malignancy compared with 31% of deaths in men of the same age.

Despite the increasing incidence of malignant neoplasms in the UK, overall mortality from malignancy is decreasing. Between 1993 and 2002 the age-standardised mortality rates for all malignancies fell by 13.5% for men and 9.8% for women. The largest falls were seen for carcinomas of the cervix, stomach, lung, bladder, breast and large bowel, largely due to earlier diagnosis and better treatment. In contrast, death rates from a few malignancies have increased in the past 10 years, particularly carcinomas of the oesophagus and kidney and malignant melanoma. This rise has been attributed to a large increase in the incidence of these neoplasms caused by increased exposure to predisposing factors – ultraviolet radiation leading to malignant melanoma and gastro-oesophageal reflux leading to Barrett's metaplasia and oesophageal adenocarcinoma.

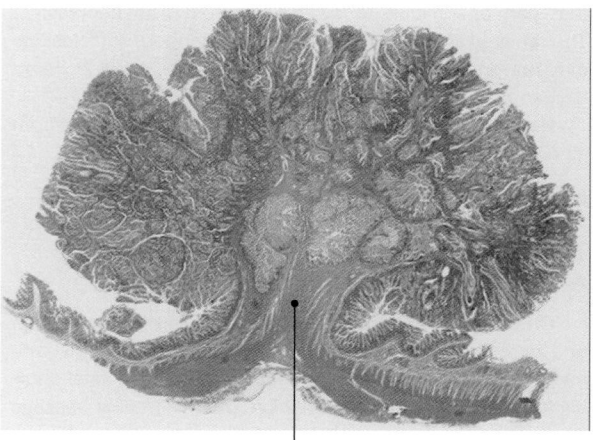

Overgrowth of muscularis mucosae

Fig. 6.26 **Peutz–Jeghers' polyp in the ileum.**

	Males	Females	Total
Other	10252	12356	22608
Body of Uterus		1059	1059
Cervix		1098	1098
Malignant Melanoma	934	832	1766
Mesothelioma	1524	270	1794
Liver	1551	1015	2566
Multiple Myeloma	1332	1291	2623
Head and Neck	1941	924	2865
Brain and CNS	1946	1441	3387
Kidney	2076	1337	3413
Leukaemia	2453	1886	4339
Ovary		4617	4617
NHL	2472	2202	4674
Bladder	3218	1710	4928
Stomach	3744	2273	6017
Pancreas	3421	3619	7040
Oesophagus	4740	2610	7350
Prostate	10164		10164
Breast	82	12614	12696
Bowel	8564	7543	16107
Lung	19806	13630	334360
Total	80220	74327	154547

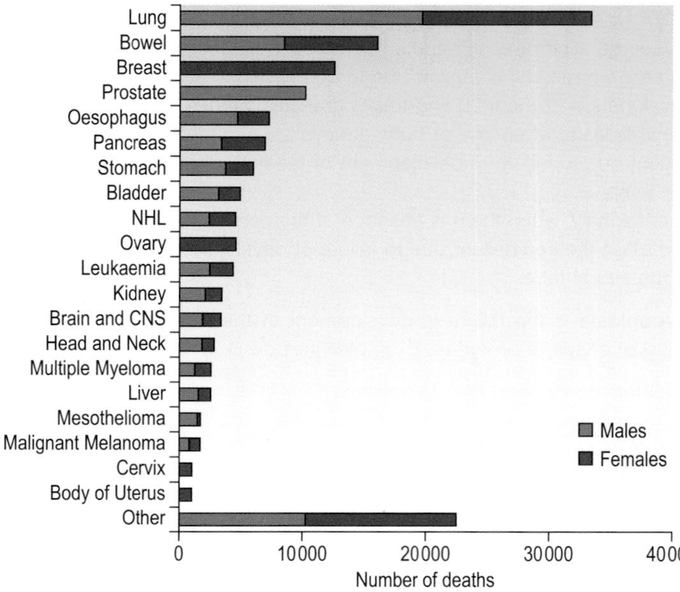

Fig. 6.27 **Mortality from the 20 most common cancers in the UK, 2003.** NHL, non-Hodgkin's lymphoma. Adapted with permission from CRC UK.

NOMENCLATURE AND CLASSIFICATION OF NEOPLASMS

Neoplasms are named according to whether they are benign or malignant, and also by their cell of origin (**histogenesis**). Accurate classification of neoplasms is vitally important for tailoring treatment and assessing prognosis. The major histogenetic categories of neoplasm are:

- Epithelial neoplasms, derived from epithelia or glandular structures
- Mesenchymal neoplasms, derived from tissues descended from mesenchyme: muscle, fibroblasts, bone, cartilage, fat, etc.
- Haemopoietic neoplasms, derived from cells descended from the pluripotent bone marrow stem cell
- Nervous system neoplasms, derived from cells of the central and peripheral nervous system
- Primitive embryonal neoplasms, derived from immature cells
- Germ cell neoplasms, derived from germ cells in the ovary and testis.

All neoplasms have the 'surname' -oma, though it should not be forgotten that several other non-neoplastic lesions have similar ending names, e.g. hamartoma, haematoma, granuloma. The 'forename' of neoplasms depends on the specific tissue of origin, as described below.

Epithelial neoplasms

Benign epithelial neoplasms are either **adenomas** or **papillomas**. Adenomas are derived from glandular or secretory epithelium, such as that of the gastrointestinal tract, breast and endocrine glands, while papillomas originate from nonglandular epithelium, such as stratified squamous or transitional cell epithelium (Table 6.10).

All malignant epithelial neoplasms have the suffix carcinoma. Carcinomas of glandular or secretory epithelium are termed adenocarcinomas, while those of non-glandular epithelium are named according to their cell of origin, e.g. squamous cell carcinoma, transitional cell carcinoma, basal cell carcinoma (Table 6.11).

Carcinoma in situ is a term used to designate an early, pre-invasive phase in the development of epithelial malignancy. It is closely related to epithelial dysplasia and is discussed more fully above.

Mesenchymal neoplasms

All benign **mesenchymal neoplasms** end in -oma and are prefixed by the name that indicates the cell or tissue of origin (e.g. leiomyo- for smooth muscle, rhabdomyo- for striated muscle). Malignant mesenchymal neoplasms keep the same prefix but the ending becomes -sarcoma (Table 6.11).

Haemopoietic neoplasms

Haemopoietic neoplasms arise in the bone marrow and lymph nodes. The features that allow distinction between benign and malignant neoplasms are not so easily applicable to haemopoietic neoplasms since, apart from lymphomas, they rarely form solid masses. While some neoplasms behave less aggressively than others, it is difficult to classify any of

Table 6.10	Nomenclature of epithelial neoplasms	
Epithelial cell type/ normal tissue	Benign neoplasm	Malignant neoplasm
Stratified squamous, e.g. skin	Squamous cell papilloma	Squamous cell carcinoma
Basal cell, e.g. skin	Basal cell papilloma	Basal cell carcinoma
Transitional cell, e.g. urogenital tract	Transitional cell papilloma	Transitional cell carcinoma
Glandular, e.g. gastrointestinal tract	Adenoma	Adenocarcinoma

Table 6.11	Nomenclature of mesenchymal neoplasms	
Cell type or normal tissue	Benign neoplasm	Malignant neoplasm
Fibroblast	Fibroma	Fibrosarcoma
Fat	Lipoma	Liposarcoma
Striated muscle	Rhabdomyoma	Rhabdomyosarcoma
Smooth muscle	Leiomyoma	Leiomyosarcoma
Cartilage	Chondroma	Chondrosarcoma
Bone	Osteoma	Osteosarcoma
Endothelium	Haemangioma	Angiosarcoma

Table 6.12	Nomenclature of nervous system neoplasms
Cell type	Neoplasm
Glial cell	Glioma
Arachnoid cell	Meningioma
Nerve sheath cell	Schwannoma, neurofibroma

them as truly benign. There are four main groups of haemopoietic neoplasms:

- Leukaemias, derived from myeloid (white blood cell) precursors
- Myeloproliferative disorders, derived from myeloid cells, with differentiation to mature forms. This group of neoplasms includes thrombocythaemia, polycythaemia rubra vera and myelofibrosis
- Myeloma, derived from plasma cells in the bone marrow
- Lymphomas, derived from B and T lymphocytes or their precursors.

The -oma suffix of lymphoma and myeloma should not lead to the assumption that these are benign neoplasms.

Nervous system neoplasms

As with epithelial and mesenchymal lesions, neoplasms of the nervous system are classified according to their cell of origin (Table 6.12). The nomenclature does not differentiate between benign and malignant; for example, **gliomas** are always malignant, while **meningiomas** and **schwannomas** are usually benign. In order to distinguish the small number of meningiomas and schwannomas that show atypical cytology and/or aggressive behaviour, the word 'malignant' is used as a 'forename', e.g. malignant schwannoma. Gliomas and meningiomas arise only in the central nervous system whereas schwannomas can arise in both the central and peripheral nervous systems.

Primitive embryonal neoplasms

These neoplasms arise from primitive cells and so resemble the embryonic form of the tissue in which they arise. They end in -blastoma and are prefixed by the name of the cell or tissue of origin (Table 6.13). All are malignant and occur in children below the age of 5.

Germ cell neoplasms

Neoplasms derived from germ cells are called **teratomas**, from the Greek for 'little monster'. Reflecting the pluripotent nature of germ cells, teratomas have the capacity to differentiate into tissues from any of the three germ cell layers (ectoderm, mesoderm and endoderm) and often contain derivatives of all three layers admixed haphazardly. Teratomas can be benign or malignant depending on the degree of differentiation of their component tissues. In benign teratomas, the tissues are mature and easily recognised. Such teratomas are common in the ovary, where they are often cystic and contain teeth, hair, cartilage, skin and sebaceous material. In malignant teratomas, the tissues are immature and resemble fetal or embryonic tissues; these teratomas are more common in the testis.

CHARACTERISTICS OF BENIGN AND MALIGNANT NEOPLASMS

All solid neoplasms, whether benign or malignant, are composed of neoplastic cells and variable amounts of supporting connective tissue (stroma). The neoplastic cells of individual neoplasms differ in the extent to which their morphology, growth pattern and synthetic activity resembles that of their parent tissue. Those that closely resemble their parent tissue

Table 6.13	Nomenclature of embryonal neoplasms
Cell type/normal tissue	**Malignant neoplasm**
Kidney	Nephroblastoma
Liver	Hepatoblastoma
Primitive neuroectodermal cell	Medulloblastoma
Neural tissue	Neuroblastoma
Retina	Retinoblastoma

continue to synthesise and secrete cell products such as mucin, keratin and collagen so that the histogenesis of the neoplasm is easily recognisable. Neoplasms that bear little resemblance to their parent tissue are often difficult to classify histogenetically.

The stromal component of neoplasms provides not only mechanical support but also nutrition to the neoplastic cells. Fibroblasts and myofibroblasts are the predominant cells found in stroma, though chronic inflammatory cells are also common. Neoplasms that contain many stromal fibroblasts are rich in collagen and are consequently firm and rigid to the touch; such neoplasms are said to show a desmoplastic reaction. Myofibroblasts are contractile, so neoplasms that have abundant myofibroblasts show puckering and retraction of adjacent tissues.

Neoplasms produce their own vascular supply (a process known as angiogenesis) by elaboration of angiogenic factors such as fibroblast growth factor, TGF-α, epidermal growth factor, PDGF and vascular endothelial growth factor. The signal for angiogenesis probably results from the same genetic events that underlie formation of the tumour itself. Lack of vascular supply causes tumour necrosis and infarction.

Macroscopic features and growth pattern

Benign neoplasms are mostly slow growing, always remain localised and never spread to distant sites. They grow by expansion and typically have a pushing margin that does not infiltrate adjacent tissues (Fig. 6.28). In solid organs, benign neoplasms are well circumscribed and often encapsulated (Fig. 6.29). Their cut surface can be soft or firm, but is not usually rock-hard; necrosis is rare. Benign neoplasms that arise in mucosal surfaces such as the bowel or skin usually take the form of a polyp, which may be pedunculated (with a stalk), sessile (without a stalk) or papillary (with seaweed-like fronds).

Malignant neoplasms are mostly fast growing, invasive and commonly spread to distant sites through the process of metastasis (see below). They grow by destroying adjacent tissues and have an infiltrative margin (Fig. 6.28). In solid organs, malignant neoplasms are typically poorly circumscribed and tethered to surrounding tissues – the exception

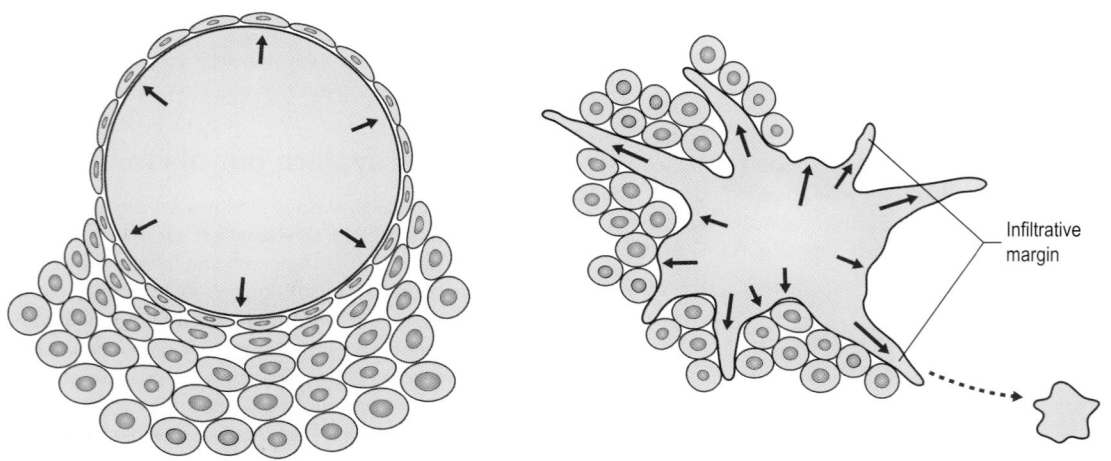

Benign neoplasm   Malignant neoplasm

Fig. 6.28 **Growth patterns of benign and malignant neoplasms.**

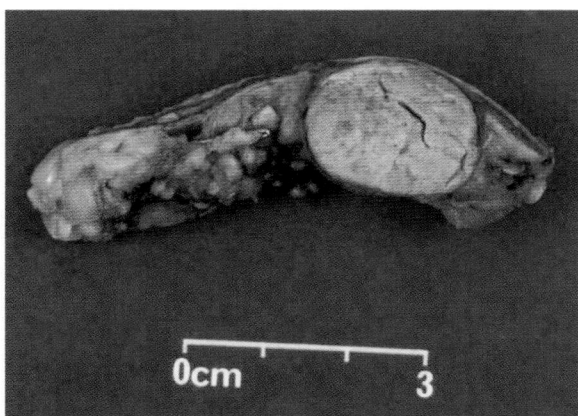

Fig. 6.29 Benign neoplasm of the adrenal cortex showing a well-circumscribed margin. The cut surface is homogeneous and lacks necrosis.

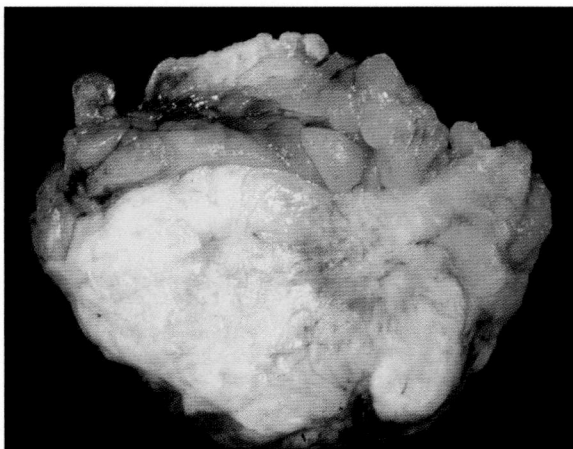

Fig. 6.30 Lumpectomy from the right breast showing a poorly circumscribed spiculate mass tethered to the surrounding tissues.

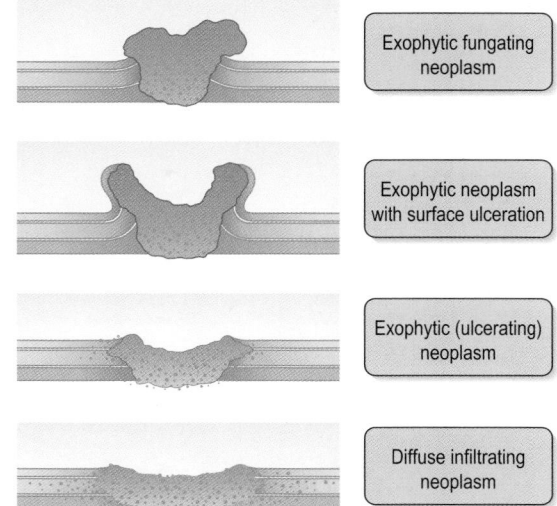

Exophytic fungating neoplasm

Exophytic neoplasm with surface ulceration

Exophytic (ulcerating) neoplasm

Diffuse infiltrating neoplasm

Fig. 6.31 Macroscopic appearance of neoplasms arising in mucosal surfaces.

being malignant mesenchymal neoplasms, which can sometimes be circumscribed. The cut surface is often heterogeneous with areas of haemorrhage and necrosis. Some malignant neoplasms, breast carcinomas in particular, have a rock-hard (scirrhous) surface and show spiculate extensions of neoplasm into the peritumoural tissues (Fig. 6.30). This growth pattern, which has been likened to the way a crab runs along the sand, gave rise to the word 'cancer' (Latin for crab).

Malignant neoplasms that arise in mucosal surfaces can be exophytic and fungating or endophytic and ulcerating (Fig. 6.31). In addition, those that occur in the bowel can be 'annular stenosing', which means that they involve the whole circumference, causing luminal obstruction, or they can be 'diffuse and infiltrating' with little intraluminal growth. Even neoplasms that do not have a predominant ulcerating growth pattern can show areas of surface ulceration leading to blood loss.

Histological features

Histological features that distinguish neoplasms from their parent tissue include:

- Loss of normal architecture
- Loss of cell cohesion

- Nuclear pleomorphism (variability in size and shape)
- Nuclear enlargement with increased nuclear:cytoplasmic ratio
- Increased mitotic activity.

In malignant neoplasms the extent and severity of these changes is greater than in their benign counterparts (Fig. 6.32). Consequently, malignant tumours show less resemblance to their tissue of origin than do benign neoplasms. The main features used in distinguishing benign from malignant neoplasms are listed in Table 6.14.

Differentiation and grade of malignant neoplasms

The extent to which the morphology, growth pattern and synthetic activity of a malignant neoplasm resemble that of its parent tissue determines its differentiation. Neoplasms that closely resemble their parent tissue are termed well differentiated while those that show little resemblance are known as poorly differentiated (Fig. 6.33). Some neoplasms are so poorly differentiated that it is impossible to establish their cell of origin at all; such neoplasms are termed anaplastic. Because benign neoplasms tend to resemble their parent tissue closely, it is convention not to assign a differentiation to them.

The differentiation of a malignant neoplasm is useful not only in determining the histogenesis of the neoplasm but also in assigning a grade. The grade of a malignant neoplasm is a reflection of its histological features and is correlated with behaviour. High-grade neoplasms tend to be poorly differentiated and behave aggressively while low-grade neoplasms are usually well differentiated and behave less aggressively. Consequently, the grade of a malignant neoplasm is important in deciding which treatment to offer a patient and also gives an indication of prognosis.

BEHAVIOUR OF MALIGNANT NEOPLASMS

The distinction of benign from malignant neoplasms is usually possible on morphological criteria alone. In a few cases,

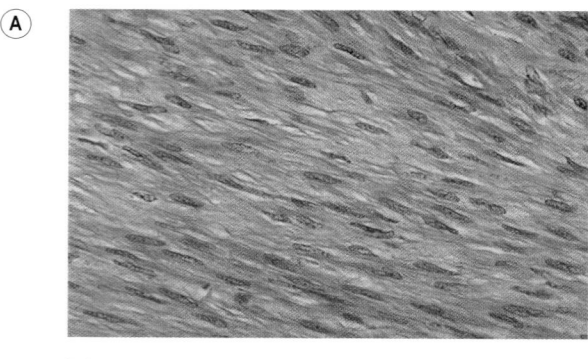

Leiomyoma

Mitotic figure

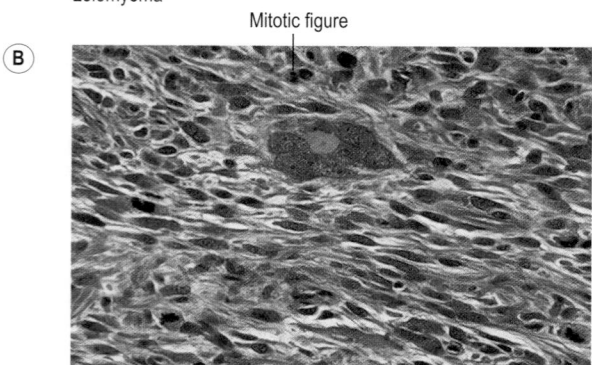

Leiomyosarcoma

Fig. 6.32 **High-power photomicrographs contrasting (A) a leiomyoma with (B) a leiomyosarcoma.** In the leiomyosarcoma, the nuclei are much more atypical; there is pleomorphism, hyperchromatism and multinucleation. Mitotic figures are easily visible.

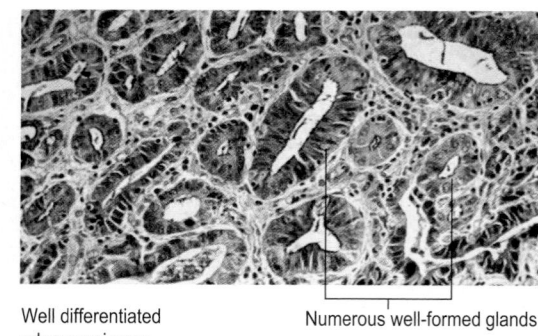

Well differentiated adenocarcinoma

Numerous well-formed glands

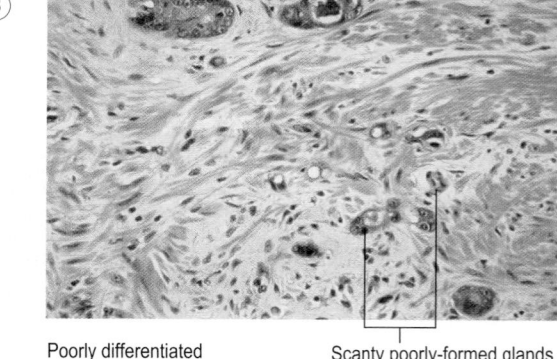

Poorly differentiated adenocarcinoma

Scanty poorly-formed glands

Fig. 6.33 **High-power photomicrographs comparing (A) a well-differentiated with (B) a poorly differentiated adenocarcinoma.** In the former there are many well-formed glands whereas the latter contains only a few poorly formed glands.

Table 6.14	Characteristic features of benign and malignant neoplasms	
Feature	**Benign neoplasm**	**Malignant neoplasm**
Macroscopic appearance	Well circumscribed, often encapsulated	Poorly circumscribed, rarely encapsulated
Cut surface	Homogeneous	Heterogeneous
Margin	Blunt, pushing	Infiltrative, invasive
Nuclear:cytoplasmic ratio	Usually normal	Often high
Nuclear pleomorphism	Uncommon	Common
Necrosis	Uncommon	Often present
Mitotic rate	Very low, normal mitoses	Usually high, abnormal mitoses frequent
Metastases	Never	Often

Local invasion

Secretion of collagenases and elastases by neoplastic cells facilitates growth into surrounding connective tissue, vessels and nerves. This results in the poorly circumscribed margin typical of malignant neoplasms and also causes fixation of the tissues, pain and haemorrhage in the host.

Metastasis

Metastasis is secondary growth of a neoplasm at one or more locations distant from the primary site (Fig. 6.34). It only occurs with malignant neoplasms. Spread may occur:

- Via lymphatics
- Via blood vessels
- Across coelomic cavities
- Within cerebrospinal fluid
- Through implantation of neoplastic cells following biopsy or surgery.

Patterns and sites of metastasis

The route of metastasis taken by a neoplasm and the eventual site of metastasis can be predicted according to the type of neoplasm, its location and its drainage pathways. Typically, carcinomas first metastasise via lymphatics to regional lymph nodes and only via the bloodstream later in the disease. Sarcomas characteristically metastasise via the bloodstream early in their course, usually to the lung.

however, the distinction can be difficult or even impossible. In such neoplasms, the defining feature of malignancy is the ability of the neoplasm to invade locally and/or metastasise. Benign neoplasms never undergo local invasion or metastasis.

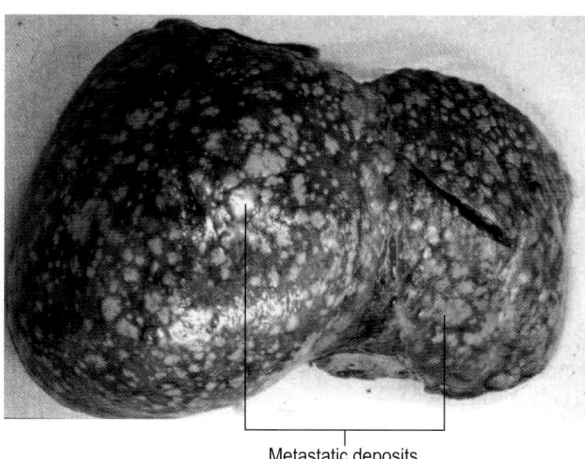

Metastatic deposits

Fig. 6.34 **A liver full of metastatic deposits from a primary carcinoma of the colon.**

Clinical box 6.29	Mechanism of invasion and metastasis

Metastasis is a complex process involving the following sequence of events, shown diagrammatically in Figure 6.35:

1. Detachment of neoplastic cells from each other (through down-regulation of cadherin expression)
2. Attachment to ECM via specific receptors
3. Degradation of the ECM through secretion of collagenases and proteases
4. Locomotion through the ECM via secretion of motility factors
5. Vascular intravasation
6. Interaction of tumour cells with host lymphocytes
7. Formation of tumour embolus
8. Adhesion to endothelium at a distant site via adhesion molecules
9. Vascular extravasation
10. Regrowth of the metastatic clone.

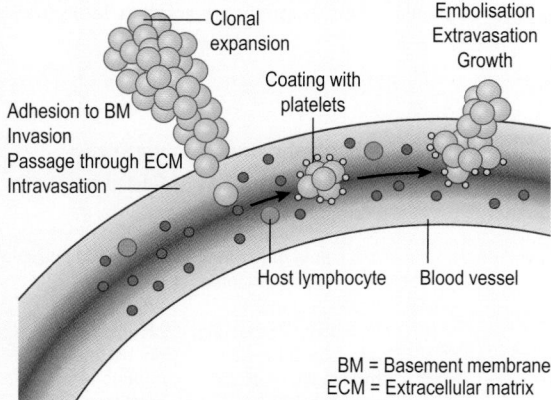

Clonal expansion

Embolisation
Extravasation
Growth

Coating with platelets

Adhesion to BM
Invasion
Passage through ECM
Intravasation

Host lymphocyte   Blood vessel

BM = Basement membrane
ECM = Extracellular matrix

Fig. 6.35 **The stages involved in metastasis.**

Some tumours (prostate, lung, thyroid, kidney and breast) metastasise preferentially to bone. Certain sites of metastases are preferred by individual malignancies, for example prostatic carcinoma metastasises to the skeleton, serous adenocarcinoma of the ovary metastasises to the peritoneum, bronchial carcinoma metastasises to adrenal and brain, and neuroblastoma metastasises to the liver. The reasons for this specificity are obscure but may be related to chemoattractants produced by the involved organ or to adhesion molecules produced by the neoplasm, which 'fit best' with a ligand on the epithelial cells of a particular organ.

Clonal evolution

Additional mutations frequently occur within monoclonal malignant neoplasms, resulting in subclones that differ from the original phenotype in terms of metastatic ability, proliferative activity and resistance to therapeutic agents. This is known as clonal evolution and results in **tumour heterogeneity**.

EFFECTS OF A NEOPLASM ON THE HOST

Neoplasms do not benefit the host. Indeed, many malignant neoplasms shorten the lifespan of the host significantly. Even benign neoplasms, which are not usually harmful to the host, can sometimes have serious consequences.

The multitude of clinical effects produced by a neoplasm can be classified into local effects, metabolic effects, immunological effects or the effects of metastases. Some malignant neoplasms cause symptom complexes that cannot be explained by local or distant spread or by hormone production from the tissue in which the neoplasm has arisen. Such complexes are called paraneoplastic syndromes. The specific effects of a neoplasm on the host will depend on its histological type, its site of origin and its behaviour.

LOCAL EFFECTS

Neoplasms occupy space alongside normal tissues, which can lead to pressure effects or obstruction. In a large organ such as the liver, pressure effects are usually minimal, but if the neoplasm is close to a vital structure or there is little space for expansion, the consequences of even a benign neoplasm can be life-threatening. For example, a meningioma arising in the cranium can cause raised intracranial pressure, as there is no room for the underlying brain to expand. An adenoma arising in a main bronchus can cause the bronchus to become obstructed leading to bronchiectasis or atelectasis in the distal lung.

Malignant neoplasms infiltrate the adjacent normal tissues due to secretion of collagenases and proteases, thus destroying their structure and interfering with their function. Invasion of nerves around the neoplasm often causes considerable pain, while erosion of blood vessels causes local haemorrhage. Ulceration of neoplasms arising in mucosal surfaces can cause significant blood loss. Consequently, malignant neoplasms of the gastrointestinal tract are often associated with iron deficiency anaemia. Some malignancies, such as basal cell carcinoma of the skin, cause substantial local destruction with significant disfigurement, but rarely metastasise.

IMMUNOLOGICAL EFFECTS

Many neoplasms, particularly malignant ones, stimulate an immunological response in the host. Lymphoid infiltrates, usually cytotoxic T lymphocytes, are present at the invasive margin of many malignant neoplasms. Indeed, lack of such an infiltrate is often a poor prognostic factor. Infiltration of a malignant neoplasm by host NK cells can (very rarely) lead to spontaneous regression.

Certain malignant neoplasms, particularly of haemopoietic origin, cause down-regulation of the immune system. This can lead to relative immunodeficiency, which is later compounded by the effects of chemotherapy. The consequence of this immune depression for the patient is predisposition to infection, particularly with opportunistic organisms. Haemopoietic neoplasms can also stimulate other immunological processes such as auto-antibody formation against erythrocytes, resulting in haemolytic anaemia. Formation of auto-antibodies against the acetylcholine receptor occurs with some thymomas, resulting in myasthenia gravis. Some malignancies, particularly bronchial carcinoma and melanoma, cause immune complexes to be formed, which, when deposited in the glomerular basement membrane, lead to membranous glomerulonephritis.

METABOLIC EFFECTS

Most malignant neoplasms disrupt the host's normal metabolic function to some degree, though the severity of the disruption varies from minimal to profound. The metabolic effects can be specific to individual neoplasms, usually resulting from hormone secretion, or non-specific resulting from release of cytokines and other metabolic products.

Specific metabolic effects

Neoplasms that arise in endocrine organs are (not surprisingly) associated with hormonal effects. Benign neoplasms produce such effects, as do well-differentiated malignant neoplasms that retain the synthetic activity of their parent tissue. Examples include acromegaly, resulting from secretion of growth hormone by a pituitary adenoma, and Cushing's syndrome, resulting from secretion of cortisol by an adrenocortical adenoma or well-differentiated carcinoma. Some neoplasms that arise in non-endocrine organs can also produce hormones, surprising in view of the fact that their parent tissue does not normally do so. This 'inappropriate' hormone secretion is discussed fully in the section on paraneoplastic syndromes below.

Substantial necrosis within a malignant neoplasm, which can occur spontaneously but which more usually occurs following treatment with chemotherapy, results in the breakdown of neoplastic cells. The purine component of nuclear DNA is broken down to uric acid, so the net result of extensive tumour necrosis is the generation of large amounts of uric acid. Unless this hyperuricaemia is prevented by the use of prophylactic treatment, the likelihood of developing clinical gout is high.

General metabolic effects

Weight loss, anorexia and weakness are common in patients with advanced malignancy. This state of catabolism, debilitation and poor nutrition is known as **cancer cachexia** and is the source of considerable distress since affected patients are often little more than 'skin and bone'. The probable cause of cancer cachexia is secretion of cytokines such as TNF-α,

IL-1 and IFN-γ, either by the neoplasm or by reactive host cells, though the underlying metabolic changes are obscure. Other causes of anorexia and weight loss in patients with malignancy include intractable pain, depression and side effects of chemotherapy.

PARANEOPLASTIC SYNDROMES

As outlined above, **paraneoplastic syndrome**s are symptom complexes that cannot be explained by local or distant spread of the neoplasm or by hormone production from the tissue in which the neoplasm has arisen. They are associated with 5–10% of malignant neoplasms but not with benign neoplasms. Their recognition is important as they can cause significant clinical problems and in a small number of patients they may be the presenting feature of the neoplasm. The most common type of paraneoplastic syndrome is endocrinological, though haematological, neurological, dermatological and rheumatological syndromes are also recognised.

PARANEOPLASTIC ENDOCRINOPATHIES

Some malignant neoplasms that arise in non-endocrine organs secrete hormones, even though their parent tissue does not normally do so. One of the most common examples is the production of adrenocorticotropic hormone (ACTH) by about 10% of small cell anaplastic carcinomas of the bronchus. The ACTH secreted by the neoplastic cells stimulates the adrenal glands to produce cortisol, resulting in Cushing's syndrome. Because the lung does not normally produce ACTH, when neoplasms that arise from the lung do so, the ACTH production is termed 'ectopic' or 'inappropriate' and the Cushing's syndrome is termed 'paraneoplastic'.

Another common example is the production of parathyroid-hormone-related peptide by squamous cell carcinoma of the bronchus and adenocarcinoma of the breast. This results in non-metastatic hypercalcaemia. Other types of paraneoplastic endocrinopathy are listed in Table 6.15.

Table 6.15	**Paraneoplastic endocrinopathies**	
Clinical syndrome	**Most common tumour type**	**Causal mechanism**
Cushing's syndrome	Small cell anaplastic carcinoma of the lung; pancreatic carcinoma	Production of adrenocorticotropic hormone
Hypercalcaemia	Squamous cell carcinoma of the lung; adenocarcinoma of the breast; renal cell carcinoma	Production of parathyroid-hormone-related peptide or cytokines TGF-α, TNF-α and IL-1
Polycythaemia	Cerebellar haemangioblastoma; hepatocellular carcinoma	Production of erythropoietin
Hyponatraemia	Small cell anaplastic carcinoma of the lung	Production of vasopressin

TGF, transforming growth factor; TNF, tumour necrosis factor; IL, interleukin.

Table 6.16	Other types of paraneoplastic syndrome	
Clinical syndrome	**Most common tumour type**	**Causal mechanism**
Eaton–Lambert myasthenic syndrome	Bronchial carcinoma (all types)	? Immunological
Clubbing	Bronchial carcinoma (all types)	Unknown
Hypertrophic osteoarthropathy	Bronchial carcinoma (all types)	Unknown
Acanthosis nigricans	Gastric carcinoma; bronchial carcinoma (all types)	? Immunological
Dermatomyositis	Adenocarcinoma of the breast; bronchial carcinoma (all types)	? Immunological
Migratory thrombophlebitis	Pancreatic carcinoma; bronchial carcinoma (all types)	Tumour products that activate clotting
Non-bacterial thrombotic (marantic) endocarditis	Advanced malignancy	Hypercoagulability

OTHER TYPES OF PARANEOPLASTIC SYNDROME

The most common examples of non-endocrine paraneoplastic syndromes are finger clubbing and hypertrophic osteoarthropathy. The former is hypertrophy of the soft tissues under the nail bed and the latter is subperiosteal new bone formation presenting with pain in the wrist and arm. Both of these usually occur in patients with bronchial carcinoma. A fuller list is given in Table 6.16.

DIAGNOSIS, STAGING AND PROGNOSIS OF NEOPLASMS

There may be a strong clinical suspicion that a patient is harbouring a neoplasm from the history and clinical examination. Systematic investigation, however, is needed to confirm the suspicion, assess the neoplasm to formulate treatment, and attempt to predict the future course of events (prognosis).

DIAGNOSIS OF NEOPLASMS

The presence of a neoplasm can be suspected clinically, radiologically or by the use of tumour markers (see below) but ultimately, diagnosis depends on visualising the neoplastic cells under the microscope. Histology (the study of tissues) and cytology (the study of cells) are the cornerstones of microscopic diagnosis. Biopsies for histological examination can be obtained by the use of cutting needles, which produce core biopsies, or by the use of forceps during endoscopic procedures. If the neoplasm is inaccessible externally, a laparoscopy or open operation is necessary to obtain diagnostic tissue.

Samples for cytological examination can be obtained by aspiration of a cystic or solid mass with a thin needle (known as fine needle aspiration cytology) or by retrieving cells shed from a luminal surface or into a cavity (known as exfoliative

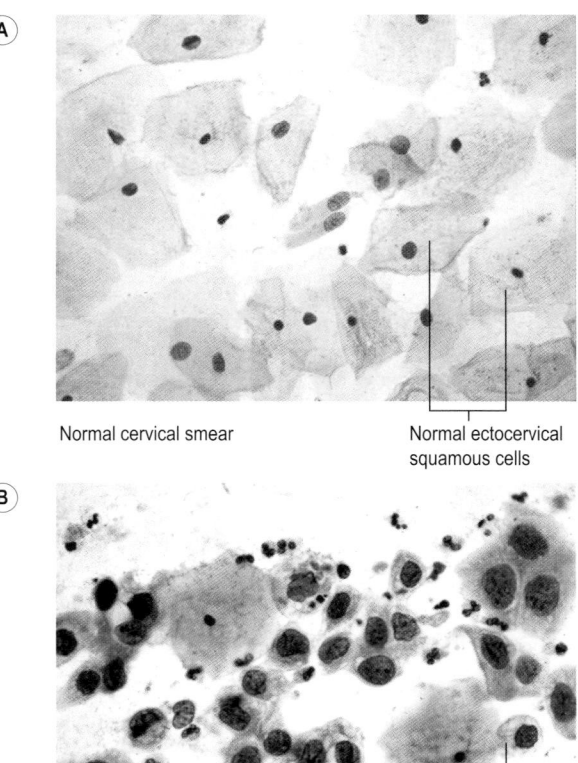

(A)

Normal cervical smear   Normal ectocervical squamous cells

(B)

Smear showing severe dyskaryosis   Severely dyskaryotic squamous cells

Fig. 6.36 **High-power photomicrographs of cervical smears**: (A) a normal smear, and (B) a smear showing severe dyskaryosis.

cytology). Examples of the former include aspiration of a breast or thyroid lump; examples of the latter include cervical smear (Fig. 6.36), bronchial brushing, sputum cytology and examination of ascitic fluid.

Cells and tissues must be stained in order to be visible microscopically. Most neoplasms can be diagnosed by the use of routine stains alone, haematoxylin and eosin (H&E) for histology and Papanicolaou stain for cytology. Histochemical stains are useful for demonstrating substances such as mucin, which do not stain with H&E. Immunohistochemistry, which uses labelled antibodies to detect specific antigens, is particularly useful for determining the histogenesis of a neoplasm when this is not apparent on H&E- or Papanicolaou-stained sections. Molecular biological methods such as in situ hybridisation and polymerase chain reaction are used in the diagnosis of haemopoietic neoplasms.

Tumour markers

Tumour markers are compounds (proteins, antigens or hormones) that can be detected in higher than normal amounts in the blood, urine or tissues of patients with certain types of malignant neoplasm. A tumour marker can be produced by the tumour itself or by the body in response to the neoplasm. The main uses of tumour markers are in:

- Screening for malignancy, either random screening of general populations (e.g. PSA) or targeted screening of high-risk populations (e.g. CA125)
- Diagnosis of suspected malignancy
- Assessment of prognosis (e.g. HER-2)
- Allocation of patients to therapeutic subgroups (e.g. HER-2)
- Detection of recurrence following completion of therapy (e.g. carcinoembryonic antigen).

A diagnosis of malignancy should not be based on the presence of a raised tumour marker alone. Not only are none of the available markers specific to a particular malignancy but most marker levels can also be raised secondary to benign conditions, leading to false-positive results. False negatives are common because not every malignancy will cause elevated levels of its associated tumour marker, particularly in the early stages.

The most frequently used tumour markers are listed in Table 6.17.

STAGING OF NEOPLASMS

Staging is an indication of how far a malignant neoplasm has spread. The stage of an individual neoplasm is determined using several modalities – clinical assessment, imaging and histopathological assessment of the resected neoplasm. The purpose of staging is to decide which treatment to offer a patient and to give an indication of prognosis.

The first staging system to be widely applied was **Dukes' system** for colorectal carcinoma, first described by Cuthbert Dukes in 1932. This uses only histopathological analysis of the resected neoplasm to place a carcinoma into one of three staging groups:

- Dukes' A – invasion into, but not through, the bowel wall
- Dukes' B – invasion through the bowel wall into the mesentery without lymph node metastases
- Dukes' C – invasion of any part of the bowel wall with lymph node metastases.

Dukes' stage D was added later to describe carcinomas with distant metastases.

Nowadays, the most widely used staging system is the **TNM** (Tumour, Node, Metastasis) system based on the size or local extent of the primary tumour (represented by T), the number and site of involved lymph nodes (represented by N) and the presence or absence of extra-nodal metastases (represented by M). The TNM score is denoted as Tx Ny Mz where x, y, and z are numbers allocated according to specified criteria for each neoplasm site. An example of the TNM system for staging of adenocarcinoma of the breast is shown in Clinical box 6.30. For some neoplasms, particularly gynaecological malignancies, staging groups (e.g. stage I–IV) are used instead of the TNM system.

Clinical box 6.30 **TNM staging for adenocarcinoma of the breast**

Stage 0: carcinoma in situ, where there is no local invasion of surrounding normal tissues.

Stage 1: T ≤ 2 cm, has not metastasised to the axillary lymph nodes (N = 0) and there are no metastases to other sites (M = 0).

Stage 2: is considered in two categories:
- Stage 2A where:
  - T < 2 cm, N positive, but nodes are not stuck together, M = 0
  - T are < 5 cm, N = 0, M = 0, **or**
  - T = 0 (i.e. presence of tumour not detected in the breast, but N positive but not stuck, M = 0.
- Stage 2B where:
  - T < 5 cm, N positive but not stuck to each other, M = 0
  - T > 5 cm, N = 0, M = 0.

Stage 3 breast cancer is in three categories:
- Stage 3A where:
  - T = 0, axillary N positive and stuck together, M = 0, **or**
  - T ≤ 5 cm, axillary N positive and stuck to each other, M = 0, **or**
  - T > 5 cm, axillary N positive and may be stuck together, M = 0.
- Stage 3B where:
  - T attached to skin or chest wall, N positive or negative, M = 0.
- Stage 3C where:
  - T = any size, axillary and other (neck, internal mammary) N positive, M = 0.

Stage 4 where:
- T = any size
- N positive or negative
- M positive to distant sites.

Table 6.17   Frequently used tumour markers

Tumour marker	Compound	Primary malignancy	False positives
α-Fetoprotein (AFP)	Protein produced by the yolk sac and fetal liver	Hepatocellular carcinoma; germ cell neoplasms of the testis and ovary	Cirrhosis; hepatitis; inflammatory bowel disease
β-Human chorionic gonadotrophin (β-HCG)	Peptide hormone produced by trophoblast cells in the placenta	Hydatidiform mole; choriocarcinoma; germ cell neoplasms of the testis and ovary	Pregnancy
Carcinoembryonic antigen (CEA)	Glycoprotein found on the apical surface of normal intestinal epithelium	Adenocarcinoma of the colon and rectum; some adenocarcinomas of the stomach, pancreas, breast and thyroid	Pancreatitis; hepatitis; inflammatory bowel disease; biliary obstruction
CA125	Cell surface glycoprotein found on mesothelial cells	Adenocarcinoma of the ovary; some adenocarcinomas of the breast and pancreas	Pregnancy; endometriosis; pelvic inflammatory disease
Calcitonin	Hormone secreted by C-cells of the thyroid	Medullary carcinoma of the thyroid	
HER-2	Cell surface receptor	Adenocarcinoma of the breast – used to predict response to therapy	
Prostate-specific antigen (PSA)	Serine protease secreted into seminal fluid by prostate gland	Adenocarcinoma of the prostate	Benign prostatic hyperplasia; prostatitis

PROGNOSIS OF NEOPLASMS

The prognosis for a patient with malignancy is given in terms of the 5-year survival rate. Neoplasms with good prognosis usually have a 5-year survival of 80% or greater while those with poor prognosis have a 5-year survival of 20% or less. The main indicators of prognosis are the type of neoplasm, its grade and its stage at presentation. Some types of neoplasm, for example small cell anaplastic carcinoma of the bronchus, behave aggressively and have a poor prognosis irrespective of stage. Others, such as seminoma of the testis, have a good prognosis, even if they present at a high stage.

As discussed above, the grade of a neoplasm is based on an assessment of its histological features and differentiation. The histological features most useful in assigning a grade are mitotic activity, nuclear size and nuclear pleomorphism. High-grade neoplasms behave more aggressively and so have a worse prognosis than low-grade neoplasms. For most neoplasms, the greater the stage, the worse the prognosis. For example, Dukes' stage A colorectal carcinoma has a 5-year survival of 80–90% while a Dukes' stage C neoplasm has a 5-year survival of 30%.

Prognostic factors in pathology reports

Every pathology report on a malignant neoplasm should include an indication of the type and grade of a neoplasm, and (if appropriate) the stage. In addition, the pathologist should report on other factors that have also been shown to give prognostic information. These include completeness of excision, presence or absence of vascular invasion and presence or absence of premalignant lesions in adjacent tissues.

SCREENING FOR MALIGNANCY

From the foregoing discussion, it is evident that if a malignant neoplasm can be diagnosed early, the chances of successful treatment and cure will be maximised. This is best achieved by screening asymptomatic individuals in the population at risk with the aim of detecting neoplasms at the premalignant stage or, in the unfortunate event that a malignancy has already developed, before it has had the chance to metastasise. The criteria for a screening test are described in Chapter 7. In the UK, two national screening programmes have been ongoing for several years:

- Screening for carcinoma of the breast by mammography. This is followed up in suspicious cases by clinical examination, ultrasound and cytology or needle biopsy.
- Screening for carcinoma of the cervix by cervical smear. When a severe abnormality is detected, further investigation by colposcopy and biopsy is offered.

Other screening strategies involve targeting specific populations at high risk of developing malignancy, for example patients with Barrett's oesophagus and long-standing ulcerative colitis. Patients with these diseases are at high risk of developing adenocarcinoma of the oesophagus and colorectum, respectively. Although there is no national screening programme for these patients, because the risk of developing malignancy is so high, local screening programmes for the detection of epithelial dysplasia have been developed in most regions.

Screening programmes have considerable financial and organisational implications, so the cost-benefit analysis is continually under review. The reasons why screening programmes may not be as effective as anticipated are beyond the scope of this discussion, but there is no doubt that results are improving as experience grows. Currently in the UK, discussions are progressing with regard to the development of screening programmes for prostatic carcinoma, using levels of the tumour marker prostate specific antigen (PSA), and for colorectal carcinoma through the detection of faecal occult blood. Trials are also well advanced of a screening programme for ovarian carcinoma using ultrasound and/or the tumour marker CA125. Ultimately, the success of screening programmes will depend on public education and investment of sufficient resources.

Why do patients die from neoplasia?

Evolution has not yet managed to create a symbiotic relationship between malignant neoplasms and their host, with the result that many malignancies remain fatal. Preventing death from malignancy is one of the main challenges to medicine in the twenty-first century. There is no single reason why malignant neoplasms are so harmful. Death can occur from a number of factors related to the behaviour of the neoplasm or to the effects of therapy:

- Widespread disease in multiple organ sites (**carcinomatosis**)
- Metastatic disease in vital sites such as the brain, lung or heart
- Immunosuppression, either due to the neoplasm or to chemotherapy, leading to opportunistic infections
- Organ failure
- Haemorrhage exacerbated by anaemia and thrombocytopenia
- Late second malignancies, either due to inherited genetic abnormalities in the patient or to the effects of previous therapy.

Benign neoplasms do not generally cause significant harm to the host, though rarely they can be fatal. The most common neoplasms that cause death of the host are meningiomas, due to pressure effects inside the cranium, and insulinomas of the pancreas, which can cause profound hypoglycaemia and coma.

CARCINOGENESIS

Carcinogenesis is the process by which a normal cell becomes a cancer cell. Cancer cells are characterised by uncontrolled proliferation, invasion of adjacent tissues and often metastasis or spread to distant organs. Transformation of normal cells into cancer cells may be triggered by:

- Alteration of the genes that control cell proliferation and differentiation: gene mutation caused by mutagens
- Alteration of gene expressions by changes in the chemical structure of DNA (e.g. DNA methylation) where there is no gene mutation, known as the epigenetic theory for carcinogenesis.

Cancers are classified according to the type of tissue from which they originate (see above).

BIOLOGY OF NEOPLASTIC CELLS

Multiple genetic changes take place over time before a normal cell becomes cancerous. During the pre-neoplastic stage (precursor), the cells appear different from normal, with variable sizes of nuclei, variable shapes and increased numbers of dividing cells. Dysplasia is characteristic of pre-malignant cells, and classified as carcinoma in situ when severe (see above). There is evidence to suggest that a cancer can arise from a single cell due to clonal expansion or clonal evolution (see Ch. 5 and above), when the aberrant gene due to damaged DNA enhances the cell's survival and reproduction despite the disorderly growth that would normally lead to apoptosis. Progressive gene mutations lead to properties of neoplastic cells that may be summarised as follows:

- Deregulation of normal cell growth and loss of sensitivity to anti-growth signals leading to unchecked cell proliferation
- Cell proliferation continues because cancer cells do not respond to the normal stimuli leading to apoptosis (genetic errors, ageing and external anti-growth signals)
- Ability to sustain growth beyond its blood supply
- Ability to invade surrounding tissues and metastasis to distant sites
- Inability to repair genetic errors with an increased mutation rate (genomic instability).

GENES ASSOCIATED WITH CANCER AND ONCOGENESIS

Three main groups of changes in genes that control cell proliferation and death, involving specific target genes, have been implicated in carcinogenesis (see Ch. 5):

- Oncogenes are normally silent (proto-oncogenes), but may gain expression in excessively high levels, or be genetically altered to activate cell proliferation through chemical messengers (hormones) between cells, the signal conducted to the nucleus causing an alteration in gene transcription that promote mitosis. Oncogenes also inhibit cell death.
- Inactivation (loss of function mutation) of tumour suppression genes that inhibit cell proliferation or promote cell death by deletion of specific chromosomal regions (alleles). Mutations in tumour suppression genes in germ cells may be inherited (hereditary cancer syndromes).
- Defects in DNA repair genes lead to genomic instability, resulting in chromosomal abnormalities with widespread mutations in genes that affect cell proliferation and accelerates carcinogenesis.

CHEMICAL CARCINOGENS

Chemical carcinogens may be mutagenic (causing mutation in genes) or non-mutagenic. The best researched mutagenic carcinogen is tobacco smoke, linked to cancers in many sites, particularly lung cancer. Asbestos is also mutagenic and associated with mesothelioma of the lung. Alcohol is not mutagenic, but is a chemical carcinogen that stimulates the rate of mitosis, reducing the time available for DNA repair and increasing the risk of genetic error (**aneuploidy**, see Ch. 5).

INFECTIVE CARCINOGENS

Epidemiological data suggest that viruses may be the second most important cause of human cancers (second to tobacco). Some viruses (acutely transforming viruses) carry an active viral oncogene that acutely transforms an infected cell into a cancer cell. Slowly transforming viruses insert a virus genome near a host proto-oncogene leading to up-regulation of cell growth so that the proto-oncogene is transformed to an oncogene, inducing uncontrolled cell proliferation (see Ch. 5).

The main viruses associated with human cancers are the human papillomavirus (HPV) (cervical cancer), and hepatitis B and C viruses (liver cancer). The combination of alcoholic cirrhosis and chronic viral hepatitis represents the highest risk for liver cancer. Some virus infections, such as HIV infection, are associated with defects in immunity, which in turn is a possible aetiology for cancer. Kaposi's sarcoma and non-Hodgkin's lymphoma are associated with AIDS. It has also been postulated that the link between HPV and anal and cervical cancer is immunodeficiency. Some bacteria have a link with cancer, for example *H. pylori*, a bacterium that causes peptic ulceration, is linked to stomach cancer.

EFFECTS OF RADIATION

Ionising radiation occurs as electromagnetic rays (X-rays, γ-rays) or as particles (α- and β-particles). Exposure to ionising radiation has known associations with the development of cancer. Some occupations have a higher risk than others depending on the nature of the work and environment, with implications for health and safety at work. For example, ionising radiation from radon (radon 222), a naturally occurring gas usually found in enclosed underground spaces, is recognised as a cause of lung cancer.

Non-ionising radiation, of which ultraviolet rays from the sun is best known, can also cause cancers. Prolonged exposure to ultraviolet radiation has a known association with skin cancers.

EFFECTS OF HORMONES

Some hormones stimulate excessive cell proliferation, acting as a non-mutagenic carcinogen. Examples include excessive oestrogen secretion and endometrial cancer.

GENES AND INHERITED CANCER SYNDROMES

Although most cancers occur sporadically, there are some well-described cancer syndromes that have a hereditary component (see Ch. 5), including:

- Inherited genetic mutations associated with increased risk of breast and ovarian cancers (*BRCA1* and *BRCA2*)
- Familial adenomatous polyposis (FAP) and hereditary nonpolyposis colorectal cancer
- Retinoblastoma
- Increased risk of leukaemia in people with Down's syndrome (trisomy 21).

The development of genetic techniques for diagnosing hereditary cancer syndromes is clearly important for affected people and their families.

HOST FACTORS

The lifestyle and behaviours of individuals may increase their risk of exposure to carcinogens, so that modification of these factors may give a better chance for avoiding the development of cancers. The major potentially modifiable risk factors for carcinogenesis related to lifestyle include:

- Smoking tobacco
- Excess intake of alcohol
- Inadequate dietary intake of fibre as fruit and vegetables
- Limited physical exercise
- Obesity.

These bear a remarkable resemblance to risk factors for coronary heart disease. Other behavioural factors include:

- Prolonged exposure to ultraviolet radiation
- HPV infection
- Intravenous drug use (increasing the risk of hepatitis B and C)
- Unprotected sexual intercourse.

The above host risk factors may be amenable to targeted health education or strategies for prevention such as vaccination against HPV infection. Other risk factors that may be related to the environment, such as the risk of exposure to ionising radiation, could be reduced through health and safety controls.

Some cancer risk factors are not modifiable, as in the hereditary cancer syndromes. Here, the possibility of early diagnosis using genetic techniques could be important, particularly if the technology for gene therapy becomes a practical reality.

MULTISTEP THEORY OF CARCINOGENESIS
(see also Ch. 5, Cancer Genetics)

Many neoplasms progress from normality to malignancy in a stepwise fashion. This usually starts with histologically invisible changes followed by the development of dysplasia or a benign neoplasm such as an adenoma. This can then develop into a locally invasive malignancy, which eventually acquires the ability to metastasise. Each of these steps is associated with changes in proto-oncogenes and/or tumour suppressor genes and, in an established malignancy, with clonal evolution.

This model of tumour progression is well illustrated by the adenoma–carcinoma sequence, which occurs in the development of colorectal adenocarcinoma (Fig. 6.37). The

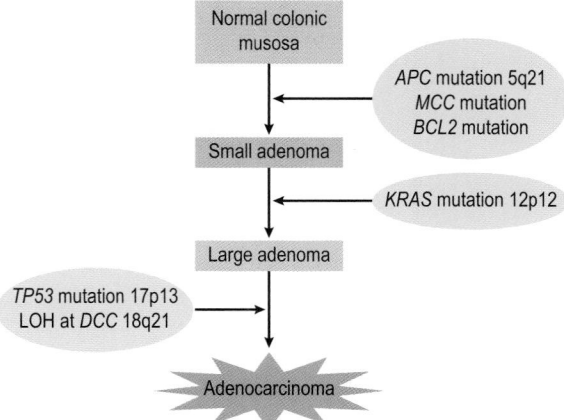

Fig. 6.37 Adenoma–carcinoma sequence for colorectal cancer. *APC*, the adenomatosis polyposis coli gene, a tumour suppressor gene mutated (inactivated) in people with familial adenomatous polyposis and early onset colorectal cancer; *MCC*, mutated in colorectal cancers, a colorectal tumour suppressor gene that inhibits cell proliferation, inactivated in colorectal cancer; *BCL2*, a gene that promotes apoptosis, loss of function mutation occurs in response to carcinogens in intestinal lumen; *KRAS*, a proto-oncogene mutated to oncogene; p53, a tumour suppressor gene that encodes the transcription factor p53 in response to DNA damage, delays DNA synthesis (S phase of cell cycle) to allow time for DNA repair. Loss of function mutation in colorectal cancer; *DCC*, deleted in colorectal carcinoma (cancer), a tumour suppressor gene. DCC is also the protein product of DCC (interchangeable name), a single transmembrane receptor; LOH, loss of heterozygosity.

changes from normal to cancer cells begin in the epithelial stem cells at the bottom of the colorectal crypts. In sporadic colorectal cancer, epigenetic changes take place in response to carcinogens in the lumen so that the cells escape the control of normal signalling for cell proliferation, apoptosis and DNA repair. The presence of the mutated adenomatosis polyposis coli (*APC*) gene in hereditary colorectal cancer syndrome is responsible for the changes in hereditary colorectal cancer. Premalignant lesions, small adenomata, form, and further exposure to luminal carcinogens leads to mutations in pro-oncogenes, such as *KRAS*, to oncogenes, when the cells no longer respond to appropriate signalling. Large adenomata form, to eventually become malignant through further mutations in tumour suppressor genes (e.g. p53). Clonal evolution, when the cells acquire the ability to proliferate despite the normal controls for cell growth and cell death, then enables the cells to invade local tissues and to metastasise.

7

Epidemiology: science for the art of medicine

Jeannette Naish and Denise Syndercombe Court

INTRODUCTION

The term **epidemiology** has its roots in Greek words meaning, very roughly, 'a discourse about something visited on the people'. While it is clearly a close cousin of 'epidemic', it is important to understand how the two relate to each other. **Epidemic**, though commonly understood to mean an outbreak of infectious disease, is more strictly defined as the prevalence of a disease among populations or groups of people at a particular time, and produced by special causes not usually present in the affected locality. The realm of epidemiology, however, is wider and more complex than the mere study of epidemics.

In clinical medicine, the focus is on the individual, on the **symptoms** and **signs** of the illness, on its diagnosis, and on subsequent decisions about therapy. Epidemiology, on the other hand, investigates patterns of disease among populations or groups of people, in order to understand causation and determine appropriate responses. Definitions and explanations of many of the terms that are used throughout the chapter are given in Table 7.1.

THE EPIDEMIOLOGICAL APPROACH

In diagnosing and managing the illness of particular patients, clinicians rely not only on their own experience, but also on knowledge and understanding derived from other clinicians' observations of patients with similar signs, symptoms and laboratory findings. For example, the observation of groups of children with **whooping cough** led to the understanding of how this disease develops.

The selection of effective treatments depends on an understanding of how similar patients fared on different treatments in the past. Epidemiology provides a scientific framework for understanding how health problems occur, how diseases behave and whether interventions are effective. In a clinical context, epidemiology also provides a better understanding of the issues that can inform the development of

---

> ### *i* Information box 7.1 Whooping cough
>
> Whooping cough begins with symptoms similar to a common cold. After an incubation period of 7–10 days, an irritating cough progresses to spasms, or paroxysms, of coughing, sometimes accompanied by a characteristic 'whoop', particularly in young children. The coughing spasms may be followed by vomiting, and could last for 2–3 months – hence the term '100-day cough'. Severe complications such as dehydration, brain damage or death may occur, particularly in infants under 6 months old. The disease is transmitted by droplets and is highly infectious. Diagnosis is usually made from the history and symptoms, but may be confirmed by isolating *Bordetella pertussis* from the sputum. The problem for clinicians can be that their own direct experience of whooping cough is limited, so that they will need to draw on the collective story. The rarer the condition, the more important this is.

more effective strategies to reduce disease incidence (see below) and improve health.

EPIDEMIOLOGY AS THE DETECTIVE

By careful and accurate descriptions of observed phenomena and by logical comparisons of these phenomena, epidemiology seeks to describe the natural progression of disease and epidemics, and identify factors that may have a causal relationship with diseases. This knowledge contributes to the understanding of how diseases and epidemics arise so that strategies for controlling and preventing epidemics and for treating disease may be formulated.

The Broad Street pump

In 1855, Dr John Snow published his treatise on the mode of communication of **cholera** (Greek *cholé bilea*; highly infectious disease characterised by profuse vomiting and diarrhoea). The 'cholera morbus' was first described near Jessore, India, in 1817. In 1823, it had spread to Russia; by 1831 it was in Hamburg, and the first case in east London was identified on 12 February 1832. Variously called 'Asiatic', 'spasmodic', 'malignant', 'contagious' and 'blue', cholera was also confused with 'common' or 'English' cholera, dys-

Table 7.1	Terms used in epidemiology
Allele	Genes exist in different allelic forms defined by differences in nucleotide sequence
Allocation concealment	The inability to predict or discover the potential random allocation group until the point of assignment
Alternative hypothesis (H_1)	A statement that is different from the null hypothesis and that is true if the null hypothesis is false
Bias	A systematic difference between the observed and true effect
Binary data	Have two possible values. For example yes or no, up or down. These data are represented mathematically by the binomial distribution
Case–control study	A study where diseased individuals (cases) are identified and compared with individuals who are as similar as possible as the cases except that they do not have the disease (controls)
Clinical trial	An experiment involving humans used to evaluate a new treatment in relation to a particular clinical outcome
Cohort study	A study in which a group of individuals without the outcome of interest (disease) is followed over time (usually prospectively) to investigate the effect of their exposure to a risk factor on outcomes in future
Collinearity	When two factors are very strongly associated
Confidence interval	A range in which we are confident (to a specified extent) that the true population parameter lies
Confounding	Occurs when we are looking at a relationship between two factors and a third factor (the confounding variable) masks or exaggerates the observed relationship between the two because that third factor is associated with *both* the other factors
Contingency table	A table which contains frequencies in 'cells'
Correlation coefficient	The extent of the relationship of the points to a straight line
Crude rate	A measure made without adjustment for other factors, such as age, that otherwise may be misleading
Degrees of freedom	A measure of how many numbers in the table are free to vary without affecting the totals. In a 2×2 table, provided the totals remain the same, only one number at a time is free to vary. As soon as this number is changed in *one* cell, the numbers in the other cells are forced to change. There is therefore *one* degree of freedom in a 2×2 table
Fisher's exact test	A method that evaluates all possible tables with the same totals as if the null hypothesis was true
Histogram	A graphical display of frequencies in separate categories of data. Frequencies are represented as bars, the area under the bar denotes the frequency (unlike bar charts where the height of the bar denotes the frequency). (Greek origin: *histos*, upright as in a vertical ship's mast, *gramma* a record or writing)
Incidence	Measure of the number of *new* cases of a disease, occurring during a specified period of time in a specified location
Interdecile range	The central 80% of the ordered data (between the 10ths, or 10th percentile and 90th percentile)
Interquartile range	The central 50% of the ordered data (between the quarters or 25th percentile and 75th percentile)
Kappa	The proportion of agreement in a classification beyond that due to chance in relation to the potential agreement beyond chance, where a value of 1 implies perfect agreement and a value of 0 no better than chance alone
Likelihood ratio (LR)	A ratio of two likelihoods, for example a ratio of the chances of getting a particular test result in those having and not having the disease
Matching	A process of selecting individuals who are similar in characteristics known to be associated with the outcome but which are not of interest. Most common are age and sex which are known to be associated with many diseases.
Mean or arithmetic mean	A measure of the centre of the data obtained by summing the individual values and dividing the total by the number of data points
Median (or fiftieth percentile)	When data are put into rank order the median divides the data into two equal parts. For example, if there are 9 data points the fifth in rank order will be the median, four datum points being below, and four above. If there are 10 datum points then the fifth and sixth, in rank order, will be in the middle. Traditionally, the median of those two numbers is given by their mean
Minimisation	Selection of an individual based on minimising the chance that the selection will unbalance the group for a particular factor
Mode	The item that is the most common in the data set
Null hypothesis (H_0)	A statement that assumes no difference or effect
One-tailed	Where the alternative hypothesis specifies a direction to the effect
Outcome or dependent variable	The characteristic or outcome of interest that is affected by one or more variables
Percentile	Division of ordered data into 100 equal parts. The median is the fiftieth percentile
PPV or positive predictive value of a test	The probability of actually having the condition when the test for the condition is positive. Sometimes referred to as the OAPR (odds of being affected given a positive test result)
Predictor or independent variable	An attribute that can have an effect on the outcome
Prevalence	Measure of the number of *existing* cases of a disease at a particular point in time (point prevalence) or over a specified period of time (period prevalence), in a particular place, divided by the total population

Table 7.1	Terms used in epidemiology—cont'd
Prospective study	One where individuals are followed forward in time
Random	Selection of a subject or item from a population such that the chance of being selected is the same for all subjects or items within that population
Randomised controlled trial	A clinical trial in which individuals are allocated to the different treatment groups in a randomised fashion
Retrospective study	A study in which what has happened in the past to individuals enrolled in the study is investigated
Sample	A subgroup of a population being studied
Sampling frame	A list of all individuals within a population
Scattergram	Plot of one variable against another with each pair of measurements represented by a point
Selection bias	Bias that occurs when the individuals being studied are not representative of the population of interest
Sensitivity	The proportion of people *with* a disease who are correctly identified by the diagnostic test (true positives). Sometimes referred to as the 'detection rate'. If a test is not 100% sensitive then there will be false positive results
Sign	Manifestation of a target disorder perceived by the clinician during an examination
Specificity	The proportion of people *without* a disease who are correctly identified by the diagnostic test (true negatives). If a test is not 100% specific then there will be false negative results
Standard deviation	A measure of the spread of numerical (continuous or discrete) data
Standard error	A measure of how precise the summary statistic is. The standard error of a proportion is a measure of how sure we are about an observed proportion
Standardise	To adjust a rate to allow comparison between different populations
Standardised mortality ratio (SMR)	Ratio between observed and expected number of an event (such as death) multiplied by 100 and computed by indirect standardisation
Stratification	Selection of a subgroup that has similar characteristics
Symptom	Manifestation of a target disorder perceived by the patient, spontaneously or on questioning
t-distribution	A continuous distribution with a shape similar to the normal distribution. It is used to make inferences about means
Two-tailed	A test in which the alternative hypothesis does not specify a direction to the effect

entery and food poisoning. Although the general populace believed the disease to be contagious, its exact nature was much debated among the medical profession. A large proportion actually thought that the disease did not spread from person to person but could arise spontaneously, as a result of bad air. The popular *London Medical Gazette* agreed that there was a serious problem but simply discussed its prevention and cure, rather than the origin of cholera or its causes.

John Snow was prompted to study 'The most terrible outbreak of cholera which ever occurred in this kingdom'. This took place in Broad Street, Golden Square, in the centre of London's West End in 1854. Within the space of 10 days more than 500 people had died and most others had fled the area (Table 7.2).

Snow had already published a report suggesting that cholera was spread by contaminated water. Cholera, he noted, 'always commences with disturbances of the functions of the alimentary canal', and he suggested that it was spread by a poison passed from victim to victim through sewage-tainted water. Neither the authorities nor other members of the medical profession were persuaded by his theories, but the 1854 outbreak gave him a further opportunity to prove his thesis.

Since most of the deaths appeared to have occurred close to the water pump in Broad Street, Snow took the view that this was the source of the problem. He examined the water and at first saw nothing suspicious, but over a few days noted that the quality of the water varied, and that it seemed to have small white flocculent particles floating in it. At this point he decided to undertake a systematic survey of the deaths in the vicinity. Eighty-three deaths, mapped accord-

ing to place of residence, had occurred within 3 days at the beginning of September in the three sub-districts that surrounded the Broad Street pump (Fig. 7.1).

In virtually all cases the Broad Street pump was the closest to the victims' home. Where this was not so, affected individuals were regular users of the Broad Street pump in preference to others closer to where they lived. Only two cases were exceptions to this pattern and these might in any case have been examples of the low incidence of cholera that was normally to be expected in London at this time. Within the area, however, were industries, breweries and workhouses where the workers were generally shown not to have developed the disease. Snow questioned the owners and found that each establishment had its own separate source of water, or, in the case of the brewery, the workmen only drank the malt liquor, made using deep well water. The pump had a reputation for 'better' water and 'was widely used for mixing with spirits in all the public houses around. It was used likewise at dining-rooms and coffee-shops'.

After presenting his evidence, Dr Snow persuaded the authorities to remove the pump handle. The pump well was examined, but there was no defect that would suggest the reason for the contamination of the water, and the local sewer was too far away. The whitish particles that Snow saw were examined under the microscope by Dr Arthur H Hassall, a contemporary physician, who thought they were just decomposition of another matter. The water, however, even when clear, smelt offensive and Dr Hassall noted 'a great number of very minute oval animalcules in the water', which he declared to be of no importance.

It would be some years before the agent, bacterium *Vibrio cholerae*, was formally identified, but Snow did unearth the

Table 7.2	Reported attacks of cholera in Broad Street, Golden Square in Soho, in the West End of London, published by John Snow in 1854; 545 deaths occurred between 1 and 11 September		
Month	**Date**	**Number of fatal attacks**	**Deaths**
August	19	1	1
	20	1	0
	21	1	2
	22	0	0
	23	1	0
	24	1	2
	25	0	0
	26	1	0
	27	1	1
	28	1	0
	29	1	1
	30	6	2
	31	56	3
September	1	143	70
	2	116	127
	3	54	76
	4	46	71
	5	36	45
	6	20	37
	7	28	32
	8	12	30
	9	11	24
	10	5	18
	11	5	15
	12	1	6
	13	3	13
	14	0	6
	15	1	8
	16	4	6
	17	2	5
	18	3	2
	19	0	3
	20	0	0
	21	2	0
	22	1	2
	23	1	3
	24	1	0
	25	1	0
	26	1	2
	27	1	0
	28	0	2
	29	0	1
	30	0	0
Date unknown		45	0
Total		616	616

Birth defects are distressing, but thankfully rare. A single example can appear to a clinician to be nothing more than an isolated and random occurrence. The following story illustrates the importance of clinicians reporting unusual events such as these in order to contribute to a broader epidemiological understanding.

Thalidomide (α-phthalimido-glutarimide) was produced by the German company Chemie Gruenthal and supplied under the name Distaval in the UK, originally as an anticonvulsant, but later as a sedative, and was widely prescribed to women to combat symptoms common in early pregnancy. An apparent advantage – that overdoses did not result in death – led to its wide promotion, not only as a sedative, but in combination with other drugs for a wide range of common medical conditions.

In Germany, where thalidomide was available over the counter, two apparently similar cases of **amelia**, an unusual congenital absence of long bones in a limb or limbs, were first reported at a paediatric meeting in 1960. A year later, a clinician described 13 cases that had been referred to him over the previous 10 months, describing a variety of severe malformations seen in these children and remarking that the occurrences had the appearance of an epidemic. By the end of 1961 Lenz had reported that a common factor in these cases was that the mother had taken thalidomide. The same suggestion was reported from Australia and later confirmed throughout many Western countries. Fewer cases were seen in the USA because, as a result of early side effect reports from Europe, the drug had not been passed for general use there. Thalidomide was withdrawn from use in the UK in November 1961.

probable cause of the outbreak. Just before the epidemic, a child living in Broad Street had been taken ill with symptoms of cholera. The nappies had been steeped in water to be washed, and the water was subsequently tipped into a leaking cesspool, just 3 ft from the Broad Street well.

PATTERNS OF LIFE AND DEATH

In order to understand the 'health' of populations, observation and recording of events relating to ill health or death provide the information that is needed. These events arise naturally, rather than as the result of experimentation; for example, to see if a vaccination programme for whooping cough actually reduces the incidence of whooping cough. Descriptions of the information (data, statistics) collected through observation are the cornerstone of public health, where:

- **Morbidity** refers to the incidence (see below) of a disease or all diseases in a population
- **Mortality** refers to the death rate in a population, which may be from all causes, i.e. the ratio of all deaths to the total population, or for a specific population, e.g. infant mortality rate refers to the ratio of the number of deaths of infants under 1 year of age to the total number of live births in a population in a particular year, or for a specific condition.

Descriptive studies

The essential components of descriptive epidemiology are concerned with people, time and place. Epidemiological

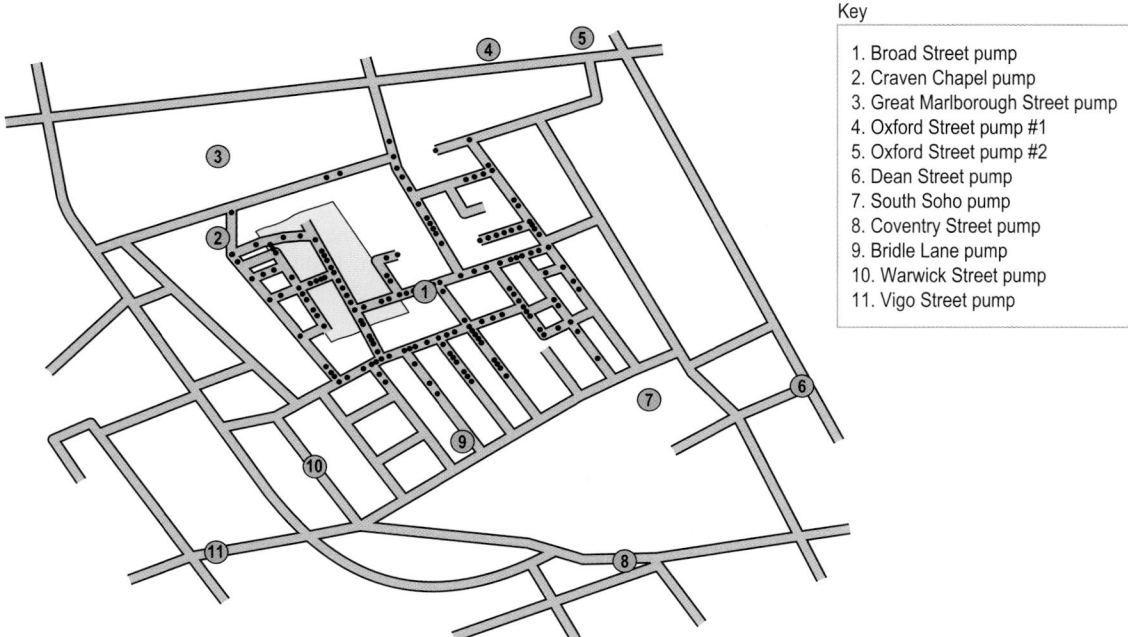

Key
1. Broad Street pump
2. Craven Chapel pump
3. Great Marlborough Street pump
4. Oxford Street pump #1
5. Oxford Street pump #2
6. Dean Street pump
7. South Soho pump
8. Coventry Street pump
9. Bridle Lane pump
10. Warwick Street pump
11. Vigo Street pump

Fig. 7.1 **Map of deaths in Soho showing that reported deaths from cholera clustered around the Broad Street pump.**

methods are used to make inferences based on descriptions of groups of *people*, or populations, rather than individual patients. These groups have shared characteristics, which could be geographically defined (e.g. living within 2 km of pylons or nuclear power stations, or living in the vicinity of the Broad Street pump); defined by a common condition (such as coronary heart disease, childhood leukaemia, cholera); associated with possession, or lack, of a particular gene (such as in Alzheimer's disease) or share personal attributes such as age, sex, racial origins, occupation, social class or lifestyle behaviour (e.g. tobacco smoking, alcohol consumption). Such characteristics may be used to identify and investigate differences in patterns of disease, and generate hypotheses about causal association, evaluate the effectiveness of treatment, plan health service provision or ask further questions.

Descriptive studies use collected information to examine a population, either at a single point in time, or over a period of time, looking at long-term trends, cyclical change or the kinds of sudden change associated with epidemics.

Measuring disease occurrence

Epidemiological methods make it possible to estimate the risk within a group of people of the disease developing. To define disease occurrence, two important concepts are used: **incidence** and **prevalence**.

Disease incidence

Incidence is concerned with the new cases of disease. The number of events (e.g. heart attacks) that are new cases occurring during the specified time (5 years) in a defined population (e.g. overweight male smokers aged 45 to 55), and resident in a particular geographical location is referred to as the **incidence**.

Disease prevalence

Prevalence is concerned with the number of people having the problem at one time and is another way of measuring disease occurrence. It is the total number of people with the disease (heart attack, new or old) over the specified time (5 years) in the population (overweight male smokers aged 45–55).

Rates and relationship between incidence and prevalence

A simple count of the kind described above does not really describe the size of the problem, however, since the same number will have different significance in populations of different sizes. Five cases in 50 is clearly very different from 5 in 5000. This is why it is more useful to think in terms of rates:

$$\frac{\text{Number of new events}}{\text{Population at risk of event in a specified time period}}$$

= **incidence rate**

Prevalence is related to both the incidence and duration of a disease. A chronic condition such as rheumatoid arthritis would have few new cases in a year (low incidence) but a higher total number of cases (high prevalence), as there will be many more cases diagnosed in previous years. Prevalence of a particular condition therefore varies with incidence and the likely duration of the condition:

Prevalence = incidence × duration

Measuring disease outcome

With the exception of death, which is usually unequivocal, measuring health outcomes can be difficult because of individual differences in the understanding of health-related terms. The assessment of causes of death and the diagnosis of stroke are just two examples that may be recorded differently by different clinicians. In these circumstances, different estimates of disease incidence may simply reflect differences in definition rather than in the frequency of events. This means that case definition becomes important when collecting information, so that there is unequivocal shared understanding of the way a case is defined. A case of high blood

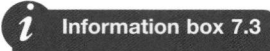

- **Absence of information**: important information from individuals, such as occupation, which may be relevant to the presence of a particular disease, may often not be reported, or not reported in sufficient detail.
- **Inconsistent information**: in countries where death registration is standard practice, mortality measures can be reliable, but measures of morbidity can be more difficult because different points of reference may be variously recorded, such as onset of symptoms, onset of disease, first diagnosis, first hospital admission.
- **Case ascertainment**: information about numbers of people with a particular disease may be influenced by the extent to which the condition comes to the attention of the medical profession, and this may also be related to the availability of medical services. Also, some debilitating chronic conditions may not always be managed medically, and so not brought to the attention of general practitioners, and if a condition does not directly cause death, it will not be recorded on the death certificate.
- **Diagnostic criteria**: diagnosis produces many difficulties that can lead to inaccuracy in data collection – inadequate definitions, inadequate diagnostic facilities and diagnostic procedures not being carried out routinely, or not applied to the whole population. In addition there may be changes in the International Classification of Diseases (ICD). For example, in 2001, WHO lowered the threshold for the diagnosis of diabetes mellitus in pregnant women (gestational diabetes mellitus (GDM)). While this made little difference in the UK population as a whole, in the London borough of Newham, where South Asians at high risk of GDM form over 30% of the population, the numbers diagnosed almost doubled.
- **Variable formats for data**: some data may be presented in records that are not suitable for classification because of lack of information or detail. Some data may be inaccessible for confidential reasons.

pressure, for example, may be defined as 'a person with an average blood pressure >160/100 mmHg from three readings over a period of no more than 2 years'.

If patterns of morbidity and mortality are to be established, the collection of data needs to be reliable and accurate, and this is not without its difficulties (see Information box 7.3). Much data depends on clinicians' vigilance, recording of observations and diligence in notification. Mandatory systems for reporting disease, birth and death are in place in all developed nations. The World Health Organization (WHO) publishes and updates morbidity and mortality information worldwide (http://www.who.int/en/). In the UK, some notifications of disease are required by law, while others are voluntary. Other types of data result from large-scale surveys and government initiatives such as the General Household Survey and the decennial population census. Individual clinicians are mainly involved with reporting on births, congenital anomalies, abortions, deaths, cancers, communicable diseases and adverse drug reactions. This information is vitally important for understanding the trends and patterns of diseases, and, in the UK, it is also used to monitor the performance of the National Health Service (NHS).

Births and deaths

The civil registration of births and deaths is compulsory in the UK, as in many countries, where someone (usually parent or relative) has to register the event with local registrars. Births have to be registered within 42 days in England, Wales and Northern Ireland, and 21 days in Scotland. Other information required in birth registration includes the date and place of birth and occupation of the father, mother, or both parents depending on circumstances.

Deaths have to be reported within 7 days. Infants born dead after 24 weeks' gestation are registered as **stillbirths**. Infants born alive who die have to be registered as both a birth and a death. Death certificates are filled in by the attending doctor, who has to give accurate details of each death.

Terminations of pregnancy under the 1967 Abortion Act have to be reported on a prescribed form to the chief medical officers of England, Wales and Scotland within 7 days. The Act does not apply in Northern Ireland (as the law on terminations is different there). Data are published by the Office of National Statistics (ONS) (www.statistics.gov.uk/statbase). Enquiries into deaths in some special categories are made through **confidential enquiries**, when information from anonymised case notes and reports from the professionals who looked after the deceased are reviewed by panels of relevant experts. The panels try to determine whether the deaths were 'avoidable', whether the quality of care given was of an acceptable standard and whether lessons can be learned. In the past, there was no attempt to compare the standards of care in the 'cases' with standards for people who did not die. The four main panels in the UK are the Confidential Enquiry into Maternal Deaths (CEMD), the National Confidential Enquiry into Peri-operative Deaths (NCEPOD), the National Confidential Inquiry into Suicide and Homicide by People with Mental Illness (CISH) and the Confidential Enquiry into Stillbirths and Death in Infancy (CESDI).

Disease surveillance

Collection of data on the incidence of some specific conditions has to rely on general practice consultations or hospital admissions. Asthma is a good example in which accurate diagnosis (case definition) and coding are important, and where a universally agreed system of case definition and coding (e.g. ICD) would be even more useful. Specific notification or registration systems are in place for monitoring **communicable diseases**, cancers and congenital anomalies.

Communicable disease surveillance

In the UK there is a statutory requirement to notify certain infectious diseases (Information box 7.4). The lists of diseases change over time and the Communicable Disease Surveillance Centre of the Public Health Laboratory Service (PHLS) in the UK is responsible for the administration of the notification system. The PHLS was re-established as the Health Protection Agency in 2003 (www.hpa.co.uk).

Cancer registration and congenital anomalies notification

Cancer registration is voluntary and undertaken by regional registries in the UK. The national system tries to record information on every patient with a diagnosis of cancer. Topics include diagnosis, tumour stage, treatment, place of treatment, consultant and place of death. Data are published by the ONS, giving direct and indirect measures of incidence, mortality and survival. Cancer registration data are also used for epidemiological research into healthcare outcomes.

Information box 7.4 | **List of notifiable infectious diseases in the UK (2002)**

- Acute encephalitis
- Acute poliomyelitis
- Anthrax
- Cholera
- Diphtheria
- Dysentery
- Food poisoning
- Leprosy
- Leptospirosis
- Malaria
- Measles
- Meningitis
- Meningococcal septicaemia
- Mumps
- Ophthalmia neonatorum
- Paratyphoid fever
- Plague
- Relapsing fever
- Rubella
- Scarlet fever
- Smallpox
- Tetanus
- Tuberculosis
- Typhoid fever
- Typhus
- Viral haemorrhagic fever
- Viral hepatitis
- Whooping cough
- Yellow fever

Notification of **congenital anomalies** is also voluntary, and linked to birth notifications. The ONS keeps track of any trends and reports to the relevant health authorities if necessary. Information from death and stillbirth registrations is also used.

Examining data from different sources

Putting data from different sources together can be very informative. For example, in the early 1980s in the UK, when the public health policy of rubella immunisation of 11-year-old schoolgirls had been in operation for about 12 years, the first cohort of immunised girls were having their first babies. It was noted that notification of congenital rubella remained high, as did therapeutic abortions on the grounds of rubella in the first trimester. Rubella infection in the early stage of pregnancy results in fetal damage in about 90% of infants, and the lack of a major policy effect was disappointing. Immunisation of girls only, and not boys, had allowed the disease to continue to circulate. The partial immunisation of the population raises the average age at which the unvaccinated catch the disease, causing those women who had missed immunisation, or who were poorly protected, to remain vulnerable. With the introduction of the measles, mumps and rubella (MMR) vaccine in 1988, the policy was changed to rubella immunisation for girls *and* boys before the age of 2.

Infectious disease surveillance and information sources

Most developed countries have systems for reporting and monitoring communicable diseases. The WHO was established on 7 April 1948 by the United Nations. The objective was to enable all peoples of the world to attain the highest level of health – defined as a state of complete physical, mental and social well-being, and not merely the absence of disease or infirmity. The WHO vision is that every country should have the means to identify, verify and respond to epidemics and emerging infectious diseases as they arise, in order to minimise their impact on the health and economies of all nations. Globalisation, climate change, the growth of huge cities and the explosive increase in international travel are increasing the potential for rapid spread of infections.

Aims of global infectious disease surveillance

The WHO Department of Communicable Disease Surveillance and Response (CSR) was set up in 2001 with three strategic aims:

- **To contain known risks**: focusing on the leading epidemic and emerging diseases, CSR develops and strengthens specific global surveillance and response networks for diseases associated with poverty such as cholera, dysentery, influenza, meningococcal meningitis, plague, viral haemorrhagic fevers (Ebola, Lassa), 'mad cow' disease, avian flu, anthrax and others.
- **To respond to the unexpected**: rapid, effective response to disease outbreaks relies on timely alert and response mechanisms. CSR's epidemic intelligence system gathers and verifies outbreak information daily from around the world and coordinates international responses to outbreaks of global importance.
- **To improve preparedness**: focusing particularly on poorer countries, CSR aims to strengthen national capacity for alert and response through a multi-disease or integrated approach. It provides tools, expert assistance and carefully tailored training to enhance skills in laboratory diagnosis, field epidemiology and public health mapping.

These strategic aims underpin all public health strategies for the surveillance, prevention and control of infectious diseases. The overall framework for the CRS strategy is the International Health Regulations (IHR), which is the only global regulatory framework agreed by the international community to support surveillance of global infections. Its website publishes health statistics on a wide variety of infectious diseases worldwide (http://www.who.int/csr).

Notification of infectious diseases

In the UK, **communicable disease surveillance** relies on notification of new cases by clinicians, and on information from a network of microbiological laboratories which, since 1939, have been required to report to a national centre. A cohort of 80 general practices distributed across England and Wales reports diagnoses of infectious diseases to the Royal College of General Practitioners' (RCGP) weekly returns service (Information box 7.5).

The diagnoses are made clinically, without laboratory confirmation, using 'diagnostic guidelines' provided by the RCGP. These are not strict diagnostic criteria, but do represent an attempt to achieve some standardisation in the diagnoses. Information on influenza in this context can be found on the UK Health Protection Agency (HPA) website (www.hpa.co.uk). The HPA also collects data from the microbiology laboratories in district and other general hospitals.

Notification of infectious diseases was first established in the late nineteenth century, when it was based on clinical suspicion and the reports of alert clinicians, with or without microbiological confirmation. The Communicable Disease Surveillance Centre (CDSC) of the Public Health Laboratory Service (PHLS) set up in 1977 and now known as the Health Protection Agency, is responsible for the collection, verification, collation and dissemination of information in England and Wales. Similar systems and regulation are in operation in Scotland and Northern Ireland.

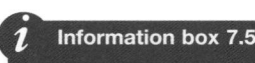

Information box 7.5 **Common infections reported by the RCGP weekly returns service**

- Infectious intestinal disease
- Whooping cough
- Scarlet fever
- Chicken pox
- Herpes zoster
- Measles
- Rubella
- Infectious hepatitis
- Mumps
- Infectious mononucleosis
- Scabies
- Meningitis
- Hand, foot and mouth disease
- Other (e.g. warts, candida).

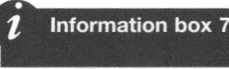

Information box 7.6 **Aims of communicable disease surveillance**

The objectives for communicable disease surveillance are to:

- Identify risk factors and their distribution
- Monitor levels of infection
- Inform targeting of health promotion and monitor its effects
- Monitor effects of prevention and treatment
- Forecast care needs
- Allow comparison with other countries
- Increase professional and public awareness
- Inform policy makers and service providers
- Detect new problems promptly.

Special surveillance systems

The UK has a **special surveillance system** for acquired immune deficiency syndrome (AIDS). Genito-urinary specialists, dermatologists and microbiologists supply confidential reports to the HPA. In Europe, information from European communicable disease surveillance schemes of interest to the European Union is published in *EuroSurveillance* weekly. Similar surveillance and monitoring systems are in place in North America.

Monitoring adverse reaction to drugs

A system for monitoring adverse reactions to medicines is in place in most countries. In the UK, a **yellow form** is used to report all suspected reactions to new medicines, and serious suspected reactions to established medicines; even if the reaction is already well recognised, or the causal association is uncertain. The completed forms are returned to the Medicines Control Agency, to be reviewed by the Committee on Safety of Medicines.

Measures for health of populations

Mortality and morbidity statistics are published by the WHO, and mortality statistics such as child (deaths in children under the age of 5 years) and infant (deaths under 1 year of age) mortality rates are used as measures of the health of nations, using comparisons between high-, medium- and low-income countries.

Mortality and life expectancy

The ONS in the UK regularly publishes mortality statistics that are used extensively for monitoring the health of populations. They are also used in resource allocation, in planning and monitoring services, and in describing and monitoring patterns of disease. For example, the number of deaths from AIDS and influenza epidemics is used to monitor the patterns of those conditions.

Mortality rates are often used as proxy measures for morbidity in the population; for example, using deaths from suicide to monitor psychiatric morbidity and the effectiveness of health interventions on mental health. The appropriateness of the way measures of performance are chosen and applied is open to debate. Mortality statistics are derived from notification and civil registration of death, where the doctor performs the vital role of death certification. Accuracy and standardisation of case definitions are clearly essential.

Years of life lost refers to the number of years of life lost due to premature death, taking age 85 as the 'cut-off', and years of working life lost is the number of years of life lost if death occurs before the end of working life, taken as age 65. These statistics are useful in comparing mortality in different parts of the world and in evaluating the effectiveness of policy and service innovations (e.g. accident prevention, legislation for compulsory car seat belts).

Other official statistics relating to health outcomes include life expectancy, maternal and perinatal mortality, child and infant mortality, communicable disease surveillance, cancer registration, congenital abnormalities and abortion notifications.

Morbidity

True morbidity, in terms of incidence and prevalence, is often difficult to measure. **Service activity**, such as Hospital Episode Statistics (HES), is sometimes used as another proxy measure for morbidity, or to assess the need for services.

The population census and health surveys

General measures of health (and sickness) are obtained from the population census held every 10 years in the UK, and from a variety of health surveys. The GHS is an annual survey of a stratified random sample (see below) of households, carried out by the ONS since 1971. The survey aims for a sample of 17 000–20 000 different households every year, and is intended as a continuous longitudinal survey which can detect trends. Financial constraints have meant that there are some years missing. A large range of questions are asked, covering health and sickness (including long-standing illness or disability, acute illness and general health), life style and health behaviours. Additional questions have been included on mental health.

Some other health surveys have focused on specific conditions, such as cardiovascular disease. The annual Health Survey for England was commissioned by the Department of Health and started in 1991, aiming to monitor progress on *Health of the Nation* targets in obesity and high blood pressure. Occasional ad hoc surveys cover psychiatric morbidity and other subjects, such as the health of prisoners.

General practice morbidity statistics

Morbidity statistics from general practice are published at about the same time as the population census, every 10 years. These are based on consultations from 40 'sentinel' British general practices, out of about 30 000. These practices are not randomly selected, and the information may not be representative of practices in any health district at any given time.

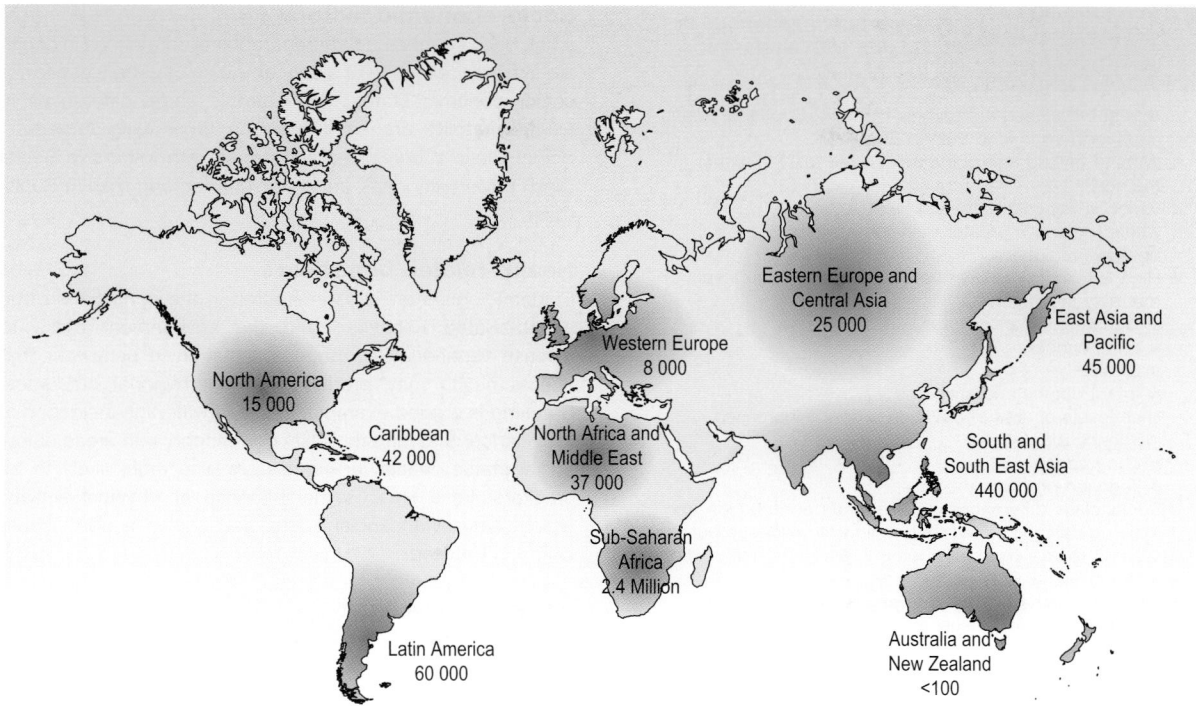

Fig. 7.2 **Global variation in health outcomes:** mortality from human immunodeficiency virus (HIV)/AIDS infection in 2002.

Measures for quality of life (QALYs)

With the aim of measuring health in terms of 'quality of life', a series of instruments for measuring socio-medical indicators of positive health and well-being have been developed. The Nottingham Health Profile was among the first and has been well validated.

Health inequalities

There are clear differences in health as measured by death rates, or incidence and prevalence for particular diseases. For example, there were 42 million people living with AIDS worldwide at the end of the year 2002, of whom 29.5 million were in sub-Saharan Africa, and under 600 000 were in western Europe (Fig. 7.2). Of the 3.1 million deaths from AIDS in that year, 2.4 million were in sub-Saharan Africa and 8000 in western Europe.

There are many factors that could contribute to this wideranging variation. As a general rule, consideration of the impact of social, economic, environmental and political influences, as well as access to medicines and medical services, on the health of populations gives an indication of how improvements might be achieved. Not all these factors are amenable to medical intervention.

Health inequalities in the UK

Since the passing of the New Poor Law Act in 1834 in the UK, there has been much interest in the patterns of health and disease, led by the General Register Office, which was founded in 1837. The Poor Law Commissioners commented on the 'filthy, close and crowded' housing, the 'want of drainage' and the 'putrefying matter' where the 'industrious poor are obliged to take their abode'.

Socio-economic differentials in health still persist today, and the UK government has launched a number of initiatives to reduce polarisation in society. The Social Exclusion Unit Report (2001) *A New Commitment to Neighbourhood Renewal* aims to ensure that 'within 10–20 years, no-one should be seriously disadvantaged by where they live'. Throughout the UK, strategies have been developed for the improvement of health, with the reduction on inequalities within different regions being an important integral part of the proposals: *The NHS plan* for England, *Toward a Healthier Scotland, Better Health Better Wales* and, from Northern Ireland, *Investing for Health*.

The decennial supplement produced by National Statistics, *Geographic Variations in Health* (2001), reviews the current position, looking at regional and social inequalities. The key findings are given in Information box 7.7.

Changes in health outcomes over time

Although mortality rates are generally declining, reviewing the changes over time has shown that the areas where health is poorer show the lowest reduction in mortality. Certain areas stand out as unchanged over many years. Examples are the high infant mortality in urban districts, such as Whitechapel in 2003 and in 1964, and similarly, low levels of life expectancy in Manchester and Liverpool in 1911–1912 and in 1995–1997.

In contrast, since 1950, deaths from heart disease, stroke and infectious diseases have all declined greatly. Not so cancer, which has now become the most common cause of death for both sexes in the UK, where survival rates in 2005 were lower than in other western European countries and the USA. The National Cancer Plan in the UK aims to reduce the rate of death from cancer in people under 75 by 20% over the years to 2010. Improvements in treatment have already led to reductions in mortality for many cancers over the preceding 30 years, but the incidence of some cancers appears

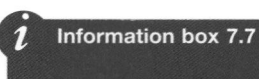

Information box 7.7 | *Geographic Variations in Health*, 2001 in the UK – key findings

- Age-standardised mortality is higher in Scotland, Wales and Northern Ireland than in England
- Within England age-standardised mortality is higher in the north
- Variation in health between local authorities within regions is greater than the variation between regions
- High levels of area deprivation produce higher levels of mortality in relation to:
  - Ischaemic heart disease
  - Lung cancer
  - Stroke
  - Infant deaths and stillbirths
- High levels of area deprivation produce increased incidence of:
  - Lung cancer
  - Teenage pregnancy
- Social class differences make a larger contribution to male mortality variation than region of residence but the latter is still an important determinant of mortality among those in Social Class V
- London has the highest rate of mortality from infectious and respiratory diseases.

to have increased considerably, along with consequent mortality (Fig. 7.3).

Interpretation of data

An important part of the study of epidemiology is the understanding and detection of **bias** (see below). For example, are the increases in incidence or mortality of certain cancers over time real, due to improved diagnosis, or the result of better cancer registration? While births and deaths are collected by national registration and considered to be high-quality data, much else is of very poor or variable quality, including factors such as registration of cause of death where there has been little regulation over the years.

Data inadequacies

The inadequacy, incompleteness and inaccuracy of much available data have already been referred to. For example, abortion statistics may be influenced by non-residents moving into temporary accommodation, or policy differences in different parts of the UK. Administrative boundary changes and postal code changes also produce problems of data interpretation over time. The latter is being improved with the use of map grid referencing.

Clustering

Clustering of risk factors in areas where health outcomes are poor may encourage the suggestion that one causes the other. The strong association, or **collinearity**, may in fact be due to clustering. Areas where health outcomes are poor are usually areas of multiple deprivation. Careful analysis of the data is required before one can conclude that specific deprivation might cause one or more of the poor outcomes. For example, sick people are more likely to be out of work and hence poorer than those who are well, so they may end up living in poor areas because of their ill health, rather than the reverse.

Socio-economic factors

It has been suggested that geographical differences in health are simply a reflection of a concentration of people of a lower socio-economic status. For example, large differences in infant mortality are seen between those with fathers in Social Class V compared with those with fathers in Social Class I. Mortality rates are also higher among men in Social Class V.

Health-related behaviours

Epidemiologists are also interested in the contribution that health-related behaviour and the environment make to disease variation. Geographical variation in behaviour that affects health may produce different regional outcomes. Smoking is a good example, as areas with high incidence of lung cancer and high mortality correspond with areas of low social status, where individuals are also more likely to be smokers. Less clear is the influence of physical activity, which varies with social status and shows a north–south divide in England.

Healthcare facilities

The aim of the NHS, established in 1946, was to have healthcare facilities evenly spread throughout the population. In the 1970s, Tudor Hart saw that those most in need of healthcare were the least likely to receive it, and proposed the 'inverse care law' that led to the introduction in 1976 of formula resourcing. This should have made things equitable. Nevertheless expansion of private services remains concentrated in the south of England and poverty and poor educational skills both reduce appropriate access.

Environmental factors

Environmental factors are also likely to produce different geographical patterns in, for example, the incidence of various congenital anomalies. Ischaemic heart disease has been shown to be correlated with rainfall, water hardness, temperature, manual employment and car ownership, but questions about the environmental contribution to disease have proved controversial as in, for example, the role of electric power lines in the incidence of leukaemia. In contrast, atmospheric pollution is strongly associated with excess mortality from respiratory disease. The industrialisation of Britain resulted in a major increase in air pollution, when smoke from coal burning mixed with mist and fog to produce smog, which then contributed to increased mortality and morbidity (Fig. 7.4).

Migration

When health differences at a single point in time are considered, another effect that needs to be taken into account is that of migration. A 'healthy migrant effect' has been observed: this occurs because younger people in good health and with, consequently, lower mortality rates, tend to move longer distances and into more affluent areas or countries. This can affect the average mortality rate of the area they move into. When migrants become ill, they may return home to die, and it is the place of death, not the place where they became ill, that is registered. Migration effects may obscure real health differences caused by locality and disadvantage. Migration may also influence birth rates and fertility.

Genetic factors and international migration also probably play an important part in disease incidence, producing

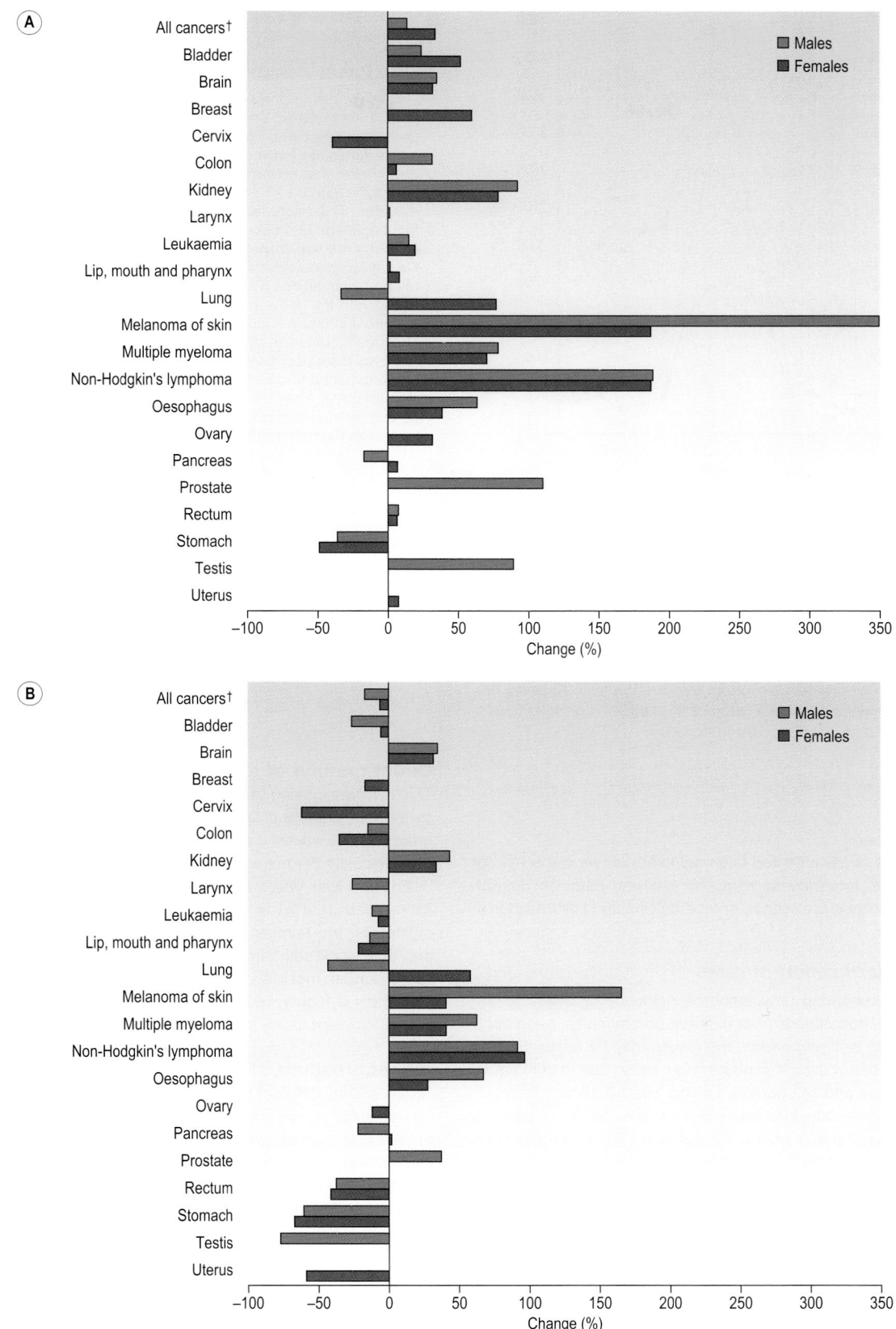

Fig. 7.3 **(A) Percentage change in age-standardised incidence of cancers by sex and site, England and Wales 1997 (provisional) compared with 1971. (B) Percentage change in age-standardised mortality from cancers by sex and site, England and Wales 1999 (provisional) compared with 1971.** †All malignant neoplasms excluding non-melanoma skin cancer.

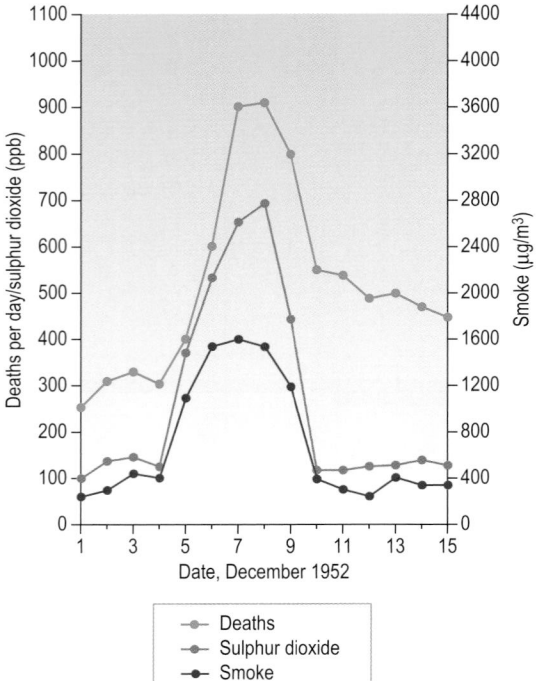

Fig. 7.4 **Deaths associated with pollution.** On 4 December 1952 an anti-cyclone formed and smog settled over London. The levels of sulphur dioxide were seven times of normal, and the smoke three times of normal. Four thousand deaths occurred in under a week and peaked at the time of greatest pollution. Information from Reports of Public Health Medicine Subject 95, HMSO, London, 1954 (available at: www.doc.mmu.ac.uk).

Information box 7.8 | **Example of confusing factors in migration: confounding**

Unless we have appropriate knowledge about our population make-up and the way it changes over time, our understanding can be confused. For example, in a study of native American Indians in 1988, a very strong **negative** association was seen between a particular genetic haplotype (Gm3;5.13.14) and non-insulin dependent diabetes. This might lead to speculation that **absence** of this haplotype is a risk factor for the disease; but in fact, although the haplotype is very common among the Caucasian population, it was rare among American Indians. Migrant populations (in this case the Caucasians) have mixed with the native population over time and once the genetic admixture is taken into account, the particular relationship between the Gm haplotype and not having diabetes disappears. What has happened in this example is a phenomenon known as **confounding**. The study does also illustrate, however, that there is likely to be another genetic component present in American Indians that increases their susceptibility to diabetes.

Table 7.3	Is Bournemouth bad for your health?	
	Bournemouth	**England and Wales**
Deaths per 1000 people in 1971	17.4	11.1
Standardised mortality ratio 1971	87.4	100

pockets of the inherited haemoglobinopathies in the UK, for example. International migration has had much to do with the increased prevalence of tuberculosis and HIV infection in London.

Standardisation of rates

When comparing prevalence or incidence of death or diseases in populations from different communities, geographical areas or time periods, the results may be misleading, as differences in overall (**crude**) rates may be due to differences in the age and sex structure of the populations.

One way to standardise rates would be by comparing rates in age bands of, say, 10 years, but this is laborious and cumbersome, and does not give a summary rate. The more usual way is to **standardise** the rates for age and sex. This would be the rate for a population of a specific age and sex structure. It must be borne in mind that standardised rates are simply mathematical manipulations, undertaken to allow comparison, and the resultant numbers are not the same as the crude rates.

There are two ways of standardising rates – direct and indirect (Information boxes 7.9 and 7.10). Both have the same objective – to get round the problem of different (age and/or sex) structures when comparing populations. Comparisons are normally made using a reference, or **standard** population.

Direct method of standardisation

This involves looking at the age-specific (death) rates in the *study* population and applying these rates to the same age groups in the *standard* population. In our example we could then calculate the number of deaths we would expect to see in England and Wales if the country was experiencing the same death rate as in the study populations. This number divided by the number of deaths actually seen in England and Wales (the standard population) multiplied by 100 is the **comparative mortality index** (**CMI**). Results greater than 100 imply a higher death rate than expected in the study population than in the standard population.

Indirect method of standardisation

This is slightly different from the direct method and takes the age-specific (death) rate of the standard population and applies it to the same age groups in the study population to calculate expected deaths. The ratio of observed deaths to expected, multiplied by 100 gives us the **standardised mortality ratio** (**SMR**). Again values above 100 imply the death rate in the study population is higher than the death rate in the standard population.

Table 7.3 shows that in 1971, the death rate was higher in Bournemouth than in the country as a whole. Bournemouth is a coastal resort in the south of England, which has a large elderly population, so it is not unreasonable to suppose that this may be the cause of the increased death rate. Only by adjusting the numbers in the table to take the different age structures into account can we make an attempt to answer the question (see Information box 7.10). In our example we

Information box 7.9   **An example of direct standardisation**

The crude death rate for England and Wales in 1949 was 12.24 per 1000 and in 1979 was 12.41 per 1000. Is it possible that health advances have made no impact on the rate of death or are differences in the population age structure over time giving a false impression? In order to examine this we can use direct standardisation and calculate what the likely death rate would have been in 1949 (study population) if the population had the same age structure as that of 1979 (standard population). In other words, apply the rate in the study population to calculate the rate for the standard population. The age-standardised death rate for 1949, based on the 1979 population structure, can be

calculated from the totals in Table 7.4. Numbers in italics in the table are those calculated.

$$\text{Age-standardised 1949 death rate per 1000} = \text{Expected deaths/population in 1000s}$$
$$= 339868.4/23202 \times 1000$$
$$= 14.65 \text{ per 1000}$$

Thus it seems that the death rate has fallen between 1949 (standardised at 14.65 deaths per 1000) and 1979 (actual 12.41 deaths per 1000).

Table 7.4   **Death rate in 1949 if the population had the same age structure as in 1979**

Age group (years)	Deaths (1949)	Population in 1000s (1949)	Crude death rate per 1000 (1949)	Population in 1000s (1979)	Expected deaths
	A	B	A/B	C	C × A/B
0–9	17 643	3417	5.16	3339	17 229.2
10–19	2345	2869	0.82	4063	3331.7
20–29	5031	3339	1.51	3534	5336.3
30–39	6839	3189	2.14	3326	7117.6
40–49	16 062	3178	5.05	2020	10 201.0
50–59	32 097	2335	13.75	2924	40 205.0
60–69	60 580	1727	35.08	2257	79 175.6
70–79	77 127	957	80.59	1384	111 536.6
80+	42 218	228	185.17	355	65 735.4
Total	259 942	21 239	12.24	23 202	339 868.4

 Information box 7.10   **An example of indirect standardisation**

In 1988, 516 men were diagnosed with stomach cancer in Wales. Since Wales had a male population of 1.39 million at that time, the crude incidence rate of the disease in that region was 372 per million of the male population. We may wish to compare that figure with incidence in the whole of the UK. Table 7.5 shows how to estimate the expected incidence of stomach cancer in Wales, if Wales was experiencing the same incidence as the UK as a whole, i.e. applying the rate in the standard population to the rate in the study population.

The incidence we would expect in Wales, if Wales were experiencing the same rate as the whole UK, is 402 per million of the population. This can be directly compared with what has been observed.

$$\text{Age-standardised incidence ratio} = \text{Observed rate/expected rate}$$
$$= 516/402.07$$
$$= 1.28$$

Standardised mortality ratio $= 1.28 \times 100 = 128$

A ratio of 1.28 implies that the risk of stomach cancer in Welsh men is 1.28 times the risk in men in the UK in general. This could also be expressed as a 28% increase in risk.

Table 7.5   **Incidence of stomach cancer in Wales in 1988 if the incidence was the same as in UK as a whole**

Age group (years)	Incidence per million in reference population (UK)	Population of Wales in millions	Expected incidence per million
	A	B	A × B
0–24	0	0.5	0
25–34	5	0.19	0.95
35–44	42	0.16	6.72
45–54	182	0.16	29.12
55–64	558	0.15	83.70
65–74	1478	0.11	162.58
75 +	2380	0.05	119.00
Total			402.07

could calculate the number of deaths we would expect to see in Bournemouth if the people there were experiencing the national death rates for England and Wales in 1971. When we do this we would expect to see 1664 deaths, but in fact only 1454 deaths actually occurred. This difference is expressed as the:

$$SMR = (number\ of\ observed\ deaths/expected$$
$$number\ of\ deaths) \times 100$$
$$= (1454/1664) \times 100$$
$$= 87.4$$

If the SMR were equal to 100 it would mean that the expected mortality rate in the study population was the same as the reference population. Because the SMR is less than 100, as it is in Bournemouth, this means that Bournemouth has a comparatively low mortality rate even though the actual death rate is higher. The true association between death and living in Bournemouth has been confounded by the age structure of the population. The indirect method (SMR) is the one more commonly used when comparing mortality in different geographical areas.

Choice of method for standardisation

Why do we need both ways of standardising? Each has its advantages and disadvantages. If we wanted to compare the death rates in two study populations, one of which has an elderly population and the other a relatively young population, then it is best to take a ratio of the two CMIs obtained from the direct method. Ratios of SMRs can be misleading in this situation.

The direct method has a disadvantage when the study group is small – because the numbers of people in the different age groups may be very small. Applying the death rates from these small groups to a large population can mean that a small change in the numbers of deaths in the study population can produce a large variation in calculated numbers of deaths from one year to the next. This increases the possibility of error in the measurement. For example, if in one year you were to observe just one death in 50 people in the 20–25-year age group, and in the next you observed two or three deaths in the same group, you might put that down to a chance finding and not be too concerned. But the increase is from a 2% death rate to 4% or 6%. Applying these proportions to a large population produces large differences in expected deaths, which may be very misleading. Using the indirect method is better, because we apply the death rate in the standard large population to the smaller study population.

Sometimes it is just not possible to use the direct method. In our example we would need to know not only the number of people who had died in Bournemouth, but also the number of people who had died within each of the age groups that we used for the standardisation. This sort of information is generally available for the standard population but is more difficult to find easily or collect for a small study population.

The **SMR** can be calculated for all causes of death, or for a specific cause (e.g. cancers), or for a particular age (e.g. >65), or for an occupational group. A similar principle can be applied to activities such as hospital admissions, in which case the index becomes a standardised admission ratio (SAR).

EPIDEMIOLOGICAL ENQUIRY

As has been discussed, analyses that use routinely collected data may not give accurate results. We can, however, also undertake specific studies for specific purposes, which include understanding the natural history of diseases, some causes of disease and the effectiveness of interventions. A variety of methods are used, each selected to answer a specific research question. Understanding the principles underlying the epidemiological approach not only enables a critical appraisal of research evidence, as when reading research papers in the medical journals, but also helps towards understanding research methods.

SOME BASIC CONCEPTS IN EPIDEMIOLOGY

Some basic concepts used in epidemiology have already been discussed, e.g. incidence and prevalence, standardised mortality and morbidity rates. Other important basic concepts concern the distribution of data collected for epidemiological enquiry and statistical methods employed for analysing the data. The meaning of basic concepts rather than the mathematical calculations will be discussed.

The distribution of data

The distribution of actual data can be represented by a **histogram**. Distributions can be symmetrical, e.g. height, where the tails of the distribution are symmetrical (Fig. 7.5A). Some distributions are asymmetrical, where there are more instances of extreme values at either small values (negative skew) or high values (positive skew) (Fig. 7.5B). Adult weight is positively skewed, in that the proportion of very heavy people is greater and further away from the most common value than is the proportion of very thin (light) people. Gestational age is negatively skewed, most babies being born at 39 or 40 weeks, very few born after 42 weeks, but a high proportion born below 36 weeks. Most distributions are unimodal in that they have only 1 peak, but Figure 7.5C is bimodal (two peaks). Only very rarely are distributions U shaped.

The normal or Gaussian distribution curve

Frequency distributions can be thought of as smoothed curves through the appropriate large sample histogram. The **Gaussian (or normal) distribution curve** is bell shaped, symmetrical with certain fixed properties. Its shape is uniquely defined by the mean and standard deviation of the data. Figure 7.5A is an example of a Gaussian distribution, and adult height is very close to a Gaussian distribution. Much of theoretical statistics is based on the properties of the Gaussian distribution.

Some numerical data vary continuously, such as the height and weight of growing children, and are known as **continuous variables**. Other numerical data are **discontinuous**, such as the numbers of people in defined populations. The numbers of people are variable, but differ at different points in time.

Measures of centre

In describing data, the concept of 'average', or **centre**, is important. Commonly used to mean 'normal', 'regular' or

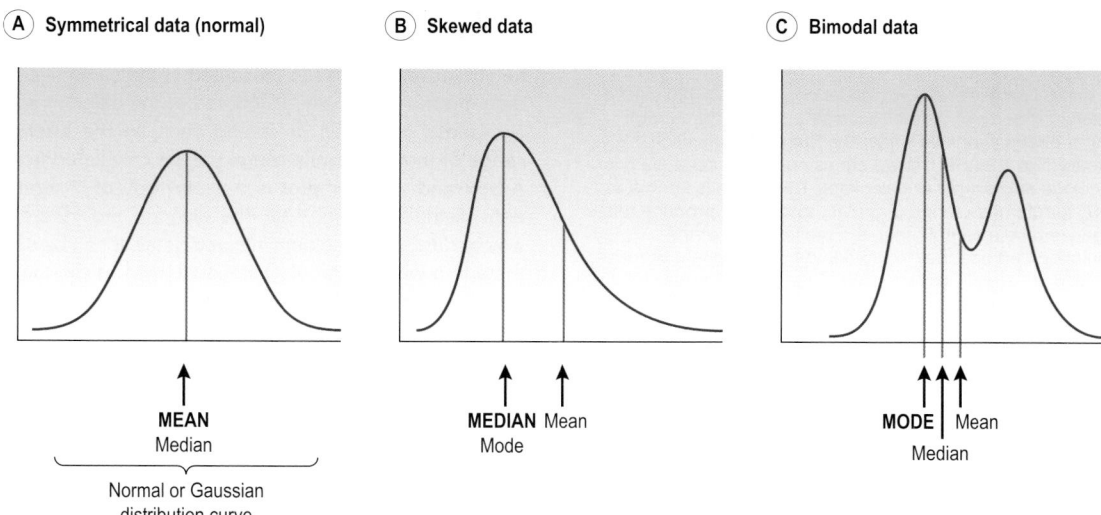

(A) Symmetrical data (normal)   (B) Skewed data   (C) Bimodal data

MEAN
Median

Normal or Gaussian
distribution curve

MEDIAN Mean
Mode

MODE | Mean
Median

Fig. 7.5 **Data distributions and measures of centre.** The most appropriate measure of centre is shown in bold for each of the distributions.

'middling', for statistical purposes 'average' needs to be more precisely defined. There are three main measures of average that are useful; the **mean**, the **median** and the **mode**. The best one to use in describing the data will depend on the shape of the data. In making the choice of which measure to use, it is very important to look at the data graphically. Because the mean is better than median (because it is a summary of a greater amount of information), and median is better than mode for statistical analysis, medians tend to be used only for quite skewed data while mode would be restricted to bimodal or other oddly shaped distributions.

The mean

The mean for the data, sometimes called the arithmetic mean, is what we normally think of when we say 'average'. The mean of a set of values is found by adding up all of them and dividing by the total number in the set. The mathematical formula for this is:

$$\bar{x} = (\Sigma x_i)/n$$

where $\bar{x}$ is the mean, x_i is one of the observations in the set, Σ means the sum of all the individual values, and n is the number of observations in the set. The mean is best used for data that are unimodal and not strongly skewed (Fig. 7.5A).

The median

The median is the value that lies in the middle of a set of values, once they are put in order (Fig. 7.5B). For example, if we have five babies with birth weights:

   3100 g, 3300 g, 3100 g, 3200 g and 3800 g

   The order would be: 3100, 3100, 3200, 3300, 3800

   Thus 3200 g would be the middle value, or median. The median is slightly less obvious if there is an even number in the set. For example, if the set of birth weights were:

   3100, 3100, 3200, 3300, 3300, 3800

   There are two middle values, 3200 and 3300. In this case the arithmetic mean of the two middle numbers is calculated to give the median = 3250 g. The median is sometimes also referred to as the fiftieth percentile since half the data will lie at or below it and half at or above. The median is best used for data that has a substantial skew, or for data where the measurements are ordered (**ordinal data**) rather than arithmetical (e.g. pain scores). In this type of data the difference between adjacent categories is not usually the same (e.g. the difference between mild and moderate is almost certainly not the same as between moderate and severe).

The mode

The mode represents the observation that is the most frequent. In Figure 7.5C, there are two peaks, and the mode is the higher peak. In this case, however, the distribution would be better described as **bimodal** and it would not be appropriate to simply report the first peak. The mode is often used when dealing with data that are in categories and cannot be put into an order (**categorical data**). For example: among the four blood groups O, A, B and AB, blood group A is the modal category in London because it occurs more frequently in this population.

   Data from surveys about attitudes often use what is known as the **Likert scale**, which is a three to five point scale of responses that ranges from 'strongly disagree' to 'no idea' to 'strongly agree.' Medians can be used with these type of data as they are ordinal (ranked and ordered), and if the data can be sensibly aggregated, means are sometimes used.

Measures of spread: standard deviation from the mean

In describing data, if the distribution is symmetrical enough to be described by the mean then it is appropriate to describe the variability – a measure of spread of data from the mean – by the **standard deviation** (SD). The standard deviation is arrived at using a formula (which it is not necessary to describe here, especially since every scientific calculator has a key to provide that number when a set of data are entered). Where data are normal (Gaussian), 95% of the data will lie between the mean ± 1.96 times the SD. For practical purpose we can usually assume that for data that are approximately Gaussian, 95% will lie within the mean ± 2 SD. This is often

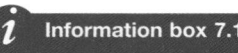

Information box 7.11 | **Standard deviation of normal platelet counts**

The normal range for blood platelet count is 150–400 × 10⁹/L. A useful property of the normal distribution is that about 95% of observations lie within the range, mean ± 2 SD. (Actually it is 1.96 SD but we are using 2 here because it is very close and simple to calculate). This range is known as the 95% reference range (Fig. 7.6). In order to produce this range we take a sample that is representative of the population and use that to provide our assessment of mean and SD.

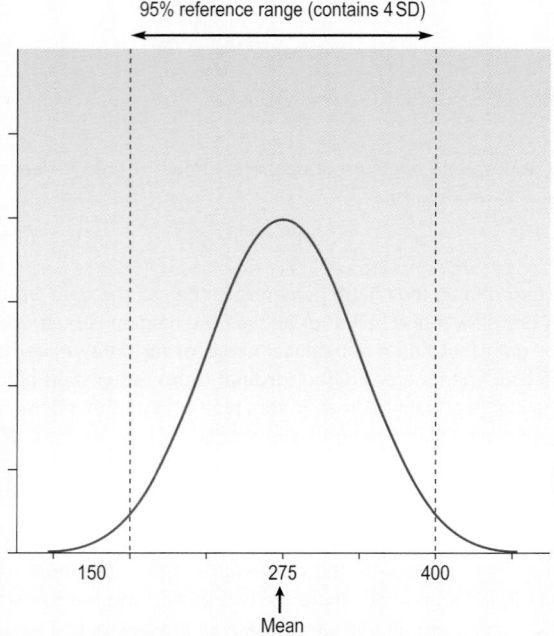

Fig. 7.6 **Distribution of *all* platelet counts in a normal population.** 95% of the platelets lie within the mean ± 2 SD, where SD is the standard deviation. The range 150–400 (×10⁹/L), is referred to as the reference (or normal) range of platelet counts in the population and individuals would normally be expected to have a platelet count within this range. The value of the standard deviation of the sample should be contrasted with the standard deviation shown in Figure 7.9.

the range that is considered 'normal' in clinical medicine, i.e. not of concern or not unusual. (See Information box 7.11).

Outliers

Sometimes, an isolated value will stand out from the rest of the data set. This is known as an outlier and checks are needed to see whether this is a mistake in measurement or transcription, or even consistent with life. If wrong it can be excluded, but if it is real then other methods of dealing with the data may be required, particularly if the data set is small.

Ordered data and the interquartile range

Some data do not follow a normal distribution and so a standard deviation (although it can be computed) is not appropriate. Instead the data can be described in terms of

percentiles, or percentage points. Paediatric weight growth charts are examples of skewed data (Fig. 7.7), Paediatric height growth charts are presented in the same way but the data are more normally distributed at the different ages.

Various measures of spread such as the **interquartile range** or the **interdecile range** can be calculated from data. A **box and whisker plot** is a useful way of illustrating the data distribution (Fig. 7.8). The diagram provides a simple way of describing the data in some detail. It can be seen that there is a wide range of gestational ages at the lower end, with 50% of gestational ages ranging between 32 and 40 weeks, whereas at the top end the data are very tight, with 50% of gestational ages being between 40 and 41 weeks, showing a very skewed distribution.

How accurate is the distribution summary?

Measurements in epidemiology are usually taken from samples of the population, as it would be too difficult to take measurements from the whole population. But even when the whole population is measured we are often interested in how representative it is of an unknown underlying rate. An estimated mean from one sample is unlikely to be the true mean in the population. However, if we could take an infinite number of random samples of the same size from the population, the distribution of the potential sample means will be normal or Gaussian with a mean equal to the true mean, provided that the sample size is not too small for distributions that are not Gaussian. The standard deviation of the distribution of potential sample means is the **standard error** (SE) of the mean (SEM). The standard error represents the uncertainty in the sample mean as a representative of the true mean (Fig. 7.9).

While in clinical medicine we may be interested in an individual measurement, in epidemiology we are often more concerned with the true; i.e. population or underlying mean. We can never find the true mean because people are dying and being born every second, so we have to find a way of estimating where the true mean might lie. We could take the means of a number of samples of data, thus creating a set of means, and calculate the mean and standard deviation of the means. However, it is possible to estimate the standard error from one sample and from that infer the range in which the true mean is likely to lie.

Because the distribution of all potential sample means of given size is normal with a standard deviation equal to the standard error, 95% of all sample means will lie within the true mean ± 1.96 × SE. The one sample mean that we have calculated is within the true mean ± 1.96 × SE with 95% probability, hence the sample mean ± 1.96 SE will include the true mean with 95% probability. The sample mean ± 1.96 SE is referred to as the **95% confidence interval** (Information box 7.12) of the mean.

Standard errors and hence confidence intervals can be calculated for most summary measures including difference in means, proportions, differences in relative risks, odds ratios and SMRs.

Differences in **non-symmetrical** distributions are often better described by mean differences and 95% confidence intervals of mean differences rather than differences in medians. For example, it is more sensible to describe gestational age by median and percentiles, but if describing the difference in gestational age for babies born alive between

Name.. Date of birth..................... Reg. No...............

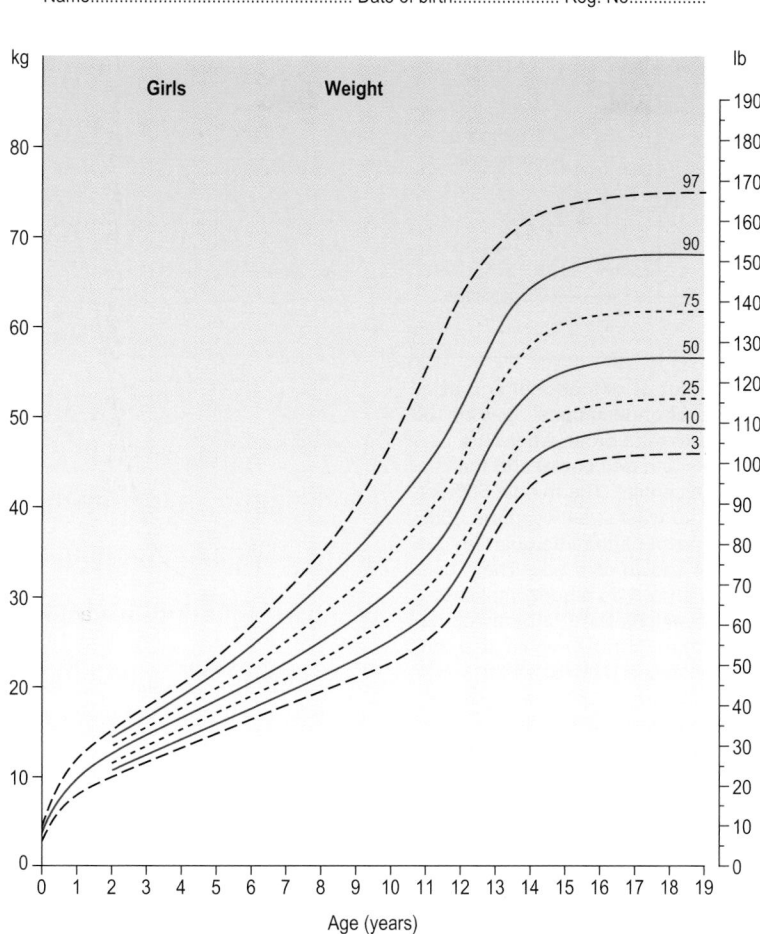

Fig. 7.7 Growth centile chart for girls, showing weights for girls aged up to 19 years of age. Weights lying between the 3rd and 97th centile are considered 'normal', with the 50th centile considered the 'median' or average. The girls' weight is measured at different ages, beginning at birth. Growth in weight is considered 'normal' as long as a child stays on the centile at which she was born.

Information box 7.12 | **Calculating confidence intervals**

Confidence intervals are calculated from the standard error. The formula for estimating the standard error from one sample is:

SE = SD/$\sqrt{n}$, where n is the number of observations.

The 95% confidence interval, the parameters (limits) of the range of means in which the true mean lies, is the sample mean ± two standard errors (rounding up 1.96 to 2). For example, if the sample we took to find the normal range of platelet counts consisted of 100 people, with a mean of 275 and SD of 63, then we can calculate the SE and 95% confidence interval as follows:

SE = 63/$\sqrt{100}$ = 6.3
95% CI = 275 ± 2 × 6.3 = 262.4 to 287.6.

1970 and 2000, it would be better to describe this by a mean difference in gestational age.

Contingency tables

Some data cannot be expressed numerically but have to be grouped into descriptive categories. If a variable has only two values it is known as binary (e.g. dead/alive) and if there are more it is known as categorical data (e.g. blood group). If we are interested in comparing proportions that died by blood group, we would construct a **contingency table** where each cell in the table contains the number in each of the mutually exclusive categories. The percentages and differences can also be shown but it is the number of cases in each cell which is used to calculate statistical significance using a chi-squared test (see below). A commonly encountered form is the 2 × 2 contingency table (Table 7.6).

Some statistical concepts used in epidemiological enquiry (hypothesis tests and *p* values)

The purpose of clinical epidemiological enquiry is to reach a plausible and valid conclusion from observations, most often about cause and effect, which contributes to the body of knowledge about disease so that strategies for disease prevention and management may be formulated. This necessitates the generation of a theory, or **hypothesis**, about a disease, e.g. what caused it and how it progresses, before further hypotheses for what constitutes effective management and prevention can be developed. The **validity**, or truth,

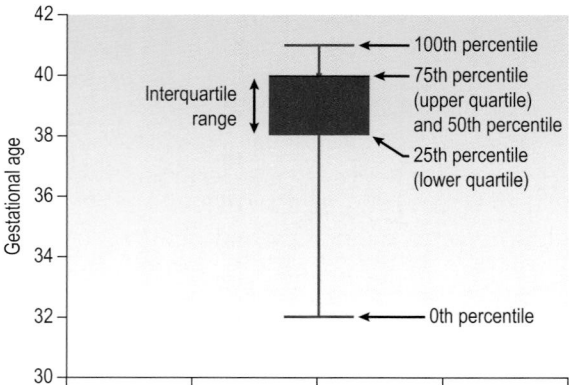

Fig. 7.8 Box and whisker plot of gestational age at birth. This figure relates to a set of gestational ages of 100 live births. The data are put into rank order, where the shortest gestation is 32 weeks (0th percentile) and the longest is 41 weeks (100th percentile). The middle 50% of births occur between 38 and 40 weeks, between the 25th and 75th percentiles – also known as the interquartile range, which by convention is shown as a box. The median, or 50th percentile, is shown as a horizontal line across the box (40 weeks' gestation); 25% of births occur between 32 and 38 weeks (0th to 25th percentile) and 25% between 40 and 41 weeks' gestation (75th to 100th percentile). These ranges are shown as lines, or whiskers, above and below the box. In this particular example, the 75th percentile (upper quartile) and 50th percentile (median) occur in the same place (and so we cannot see the median line within the box). This simply means that 25% of births occurred at 40 weeks in the data set.

of the hypotheses is tested employing good study design and valid statistical methods. Both of which are employed to limit the possibility of the results being affected by bias. When carried out logically and carefully, statistical analysis is 'an aid to clear thinking with regard to the meaning and limitations of the original records' (Bradford Hill 1977). Hypotheses are difficult to prove as being true or false, but whether they are considered to be acceptable or not is based on the available evidence, and tested by statistical analysis.

Hypothesis tests

Statistical tests involve the examination of two alternative hypotheses. The **null hypothesis H_0** is one that assumes no effect in the population. For example if we wanted to examine the prevalence of smoking in teenagers and see if there is a difference between girls and boys the null hypothesis might be:

- H_0: there is no difference in smoking rates between teenage girls and teenage boys in the population.

An **alternative hypothesis H_1** is what holds if the null hypothesis is not true. Different alternative hypotheses can be examined. For example:

- H_1: smoking rates are higher in teenage boys than in teenage girls in the population.

This hypothesis only considers a change in one direction and would not examine the possibility that smoking rates were lower in the boys than in the girls, so it would not allow us to discover whether smoking were more prevalent in the girls.

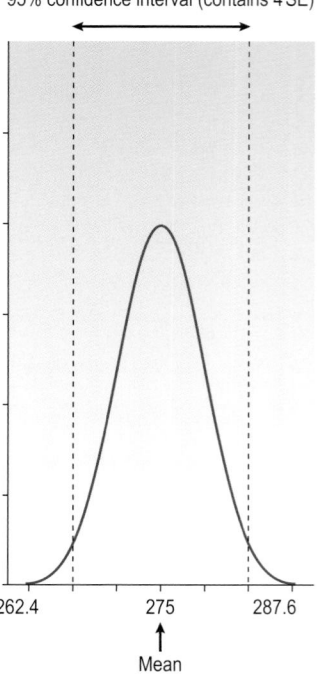

Fig. 7.9 The *sampling* distribution of mean platelet counts in a normal population. 95% of sample means lie within the mean ± 2 SE, where SE is the standard error. In a normal population you would expect that the mean platelet count is between 262.4 and 287.6 (×10⁹/L). Note that in this figure, in comparison with Figure 7.6 above, the mean is the same, but the range is considerably reduced because the distribution relates to what the average might be, not what platelet count an individual healthy person might have.

Table 7.6	A 2 × 2 contingency table		
Characteristic	**Group 1**	**Group 2**	**Total**
Present	*a*	*b*	*a + b*
Absent	*c*	*d*	*c + d*
Total	*a + c*	*b + d*	*a + b + c + d*

One subcategory of characteristics is tabulated in rows, e.g. brown eyes (present or absent). Another subcategory of characteristics is tabulated in columns, e.g. Asian (Group 1), Caucasian (Group 2). The letters *a–d* represent numbers or observations, not percentages or proportions, and each letter is in a **cell**. Any data in the column under the heading 'Total', as well the bottom row, would be called **marginal totals**.

The statistical test that is undertaken in such a case is said to be **one-tailed**. However, we are rarely sure that a difference will only ever be seen in one direction, and it is always advisable to construct an alternative hypothesis to allow for that possibility by undertaking a **two-tailed** test. For example:

- H_1: there is a difference in smoking rates between teenage boys and girls in the population.

Evaluating these two hypotheses involves looking at the evidence for each in order to obtain a test statistic. The particular statistic will depend on the type of test done, but generally the larger its absolute value (ignoring whether the number is positive or negative), i.e. the bigger the difference, the stronger the evidence against the null hypothesis.

Tests of probability: p values and confidence intervals

Probability is a concept inherent to all descriptive and comparative statistics. The only way to say that there is likely to be a difference (i.e. we reject the null hypothesis) is by finding that it is unlikely that the results from the study are consistent with there being no effect in the populations (i.e. the null hypothesis is true). It is of course always possible that we obtained this 'unlikely' result if the null hypothesis is true (often referred to as by chance). This probability is known as the **p value**.

- By convention, if the probability of getting the result we did (or one more extreme) if the null hypothesis is true is <0.05 (<1 in 20), we infer that there is a real effect.
  - If $p < 0.05$, we *reject* the null hypothesis and say that the result is statistically significant – unlikely to be due to chance. Further evaluation of the hypothesis can then be done.
- By convention if the probability of getting this result if the null hypothesis is true is ≥0.05, we say the result is not statistically significant.
  - If $p \geq 0.05$ (no *statistically* significant difference between one set of observations and the other) this does not necessarily mean that the null hypothesis is true, but the null hypothesis cannot be rejected.

All test statistics have a mathematical probability function that describes the distribution of possible test results from a series of observations. Commonly used distributions (cited in medical journal articles) are those of the normal (Gaussian) and associated *t*-distribution (see below *t*-tests) and the χ^2 (chi-squared, pronounced ki-squared) distribution (see below χ^2 tests). Examination of where the test statistic value lies in relation to the appropriate distribution provides the probability of the test result, or one more extreme, occurring if there is no difference in the populations, or the *p* value.

An alternative to calculating the *p* value to establish the probability that a particular observation arose by chance or not, is to calculate a **confidence interval** (see above). Because it gives information about where the `true or under-lying' result lies, it is used to assess whether or not clinical importance can be established for the range of possible results. It also gives information about the precision of the observations. The narrower the confidence interval, the more precise is the observation.

AN OVERVIEW OF EPIDEMIOLOGICAL ENQUIRY

To understand how disease occurs and progresses, observation of people at a particular point in time or over longer periods of time is required to see what factors are associated with incidence of disease. These are known as **observational studies**, the cornerstone of epidemiology (see Information box 7.13).

Studies are also done to investigate the effectiveness of a procedure, such as a particular surgical procedure. These are **experiments**, rather than simple observations of process and are known as **clinical trials**.

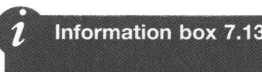 **Information box 7.13** **Observational studies and experimental studies used in epidemiology and clinical medicine**

The designs for **observational studies** include:

- **Cross-sectional** studies: these are carried out with a defined population at a point in time at a specified geographical location. The information (data) of interest about individuals in the selected population are carefully collected, then analysed using the appropriate statistical method (see below). The conclusions are usually descriptions of population characteristics, such as 'at a moment in time, in the London Borough of Tower Hamlets (or Brooklyn New York), there are more cigarette smokers among teenage boys than girls'. **Surveys** are a form of cross-sectional study.
- **Case–control** studies: these compare two groups of people – those with disease (the **cases**) with those without disease (the **controls**), to investigate potential causes for the disease. The groups have to be carefully matched to avoid the results being dominated by known associations with incidence such as age and sex (e.g. teenage boys). The data collected might lead to conclusions such as 'cigarette smokers are more likely to develop lung cancer than non-smokers'. The **retrospective-type of case–control study** looks at the relevant histories of the individuals comprising the study population, to identify factors known as **risk factors**. These are factors that may be associated with the development of disease. Occasionally, matched cases and controls are taken from cohort studies (see below) for analysis. As in such a study (nested case–control study) data will have been collected prospectively, it will be a **prospective study**.
- **Cohort studies**: these identify a group of individuals at some risk of the disease(s) of interest (e.g. civil servants, newborn infants), at a particular time (e.g. 1984) and a specified place (e.g. England and Wales, Whitehall in London). The individuals in this group, known as the **cohort**, are then followed up over time, i.e. **prospectively**, to record the incidence of disease as well as measuring, at the start and intervening periods in the study, potential risk factors. The follow-up period varies, and could be very long, for up to 15–40 years or more, and thus these studies are costly. The purpose would be to identify factors in the individuals' lives that may have a causal association with disease. An example of the kind of conclusions that can be drawn from a cohort study is 'civil servants of a lower administrative grade are more likely to develop ischaemic heart disease and chronic bronchitis'.
- An **experimental study** design is adopted for investigating the effectiveness of an intervention, be it a pharmaceutical therapy, surgical procedure or population vaccination or screening programme to prevent disease. Preventive programmes, however, are less commonly subject to experiment for establishing effectiveness.
- The **randomised controlled trial (RCT)** is an experimental clinical trial to see if a new intervention is more effective than an established one or no intervention if none currently exists. Individuals, usually patients, are selected according to particular characteristics and randomly assigned to the experimental group (new intervention) or the control group (established or no intervention), then followed up over time to compare the effects in the two groups. Here, **randomisation** has a very specific meaning (see below).

Investigation by observation: causation or association?

Much of epidemiology is about inferring causation. How does the observer then infer that the relationship is one of **causation** rather than mere association, and further, that the association was not the product of chance? In the words of Sir Austin Bradford Hill (1977) 'the interpretation of statistical data turns, it should be seen, not so much on the technical methods of analysis but on the application of common sense to figures and on elementary rules of logic.' It is unlikely that absolute proof of cause and effect can be found statistically, and what needs to be demonstrated is the most reasonable interpretation of the association. Some basic questions have to be addressed:

- Is the difference observed in the two groups a real difference, or did it occur by chance?
- If we are satisfied that the difference was not by chance, then what inferences can be drawn from this difference?

The first question is relatively straightforward. Statistical tests of significance could be applied to the numbers for each sample to show whether the results were due to chance, or were 'significant' (see above). However, a statistically significant difference is not necessarily a sufficiently important difference from which to draw inferences about causality or about the effectiveness of clinical interventions. The second question is very much more complex and difficult, and cannot be simply answered with statistical tests. Bradford Hill formulated a set of nine criteria for inferring causation; these were modified by Wald in 1996 (Information box 7.14).

It would serve the reader well to consider these criteria when presented with assertions such as 'whooping cough vaccination causes brain damage' or 'MMR [measles, mumps, rubella] vaccine causes autism in children' as media headlines. (Autism is a condition starting in childhood with symptoms of delayed speech and communication being typically noticed between the first and second birthday.) It would be impossible to gather irrefutable evidence for (or against) a causal hypothesis. The evidence can, however, help us to decide whether there is any other explanation that is more likely than cause and effect.

Observational studies

Observations of a population may take place either at a particular *point in time*, or over a *period of time*. The monitoring of changes in disease patterns and behaviour over time (say 15 or 50 years) could yield clues to the aetiology and the impact of prevention. In a clinical context, knowledge of the incubation period of an infectious disease can help in its diagnosis, although we cannot always know when the exposure took place. Observation of other factors over time may, however, help the diagnosis, as in the example of whooping cough at the beginning of this chapter.

Where the observations took place could also be important. Differences in incidence or prevalence may be observed between countries (e.g. the prevalence of malaria) or within a country (e.g. higher prevalence of coronary heart disease in the north of England), giving further clues to the risk factors associated with particular conditions. The effect of population interventions, such as a vaccination programme, on

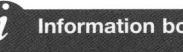

Information box 7.14 | Criteria and evidence for inferring causality between an exposure and a disease (from Wald 1996)*

Essential criteria
- A real association between exposure and the disease, that is, an association that is unlikely to be due to chance.
- The exposure precedes the occurrence of the disease (*temporal relationship of the observed association*).
- The association cannot be reasonably explained by bias (e.g. through systematic measurement error) or through the effect of one or more confounding factors.
- The causal explanation makes good biological sense (*biological plausibility depending on the biological knowledge of the day; coherence of the evidence with generally known facts about the natural history and biology of the disease*).

Additional evidence
- Strength of the association: a relative risk as high as 3 or 4 is less likely to be due to bias than a relative risk of 2 or less (*strength of the association; the relative incidence of the condition investigated in the populations contrasted must show a pronounced excess in the exposed population*).
- Consistency in the evidence from several studies that is unlikely to share the same bias (*consistency of the observed association repeatedly observed by different people, in different places, different circumstances and times*).
- Demonstration of a dose–response relationship between the exposure and disease in studies of individuals (*the association reveals a biological gradient*).
- The demonstration of reversibility; elimination or reduction in the intensity of exposure is associated with a reduction in the risk of disease.
- The distribution and frequency of the disease in different places and in different groups and over time follows the distribution and intensity of exposure (as for additional evidence 2).
- Support from animal or in vitro experimental evidence (*evidence from experimental or semi-experimental evidence, which can include experimental evidence from humans*).

Other Bradford Hill criteria:
- *Specificity of the observed association*: it would be preferable if the association were limited to specific people in particular places and particular types of disease. However, as diseases may have more than one cause, a specificity in the magnitude of the association would strongly support a causal relationship.
- *Reasoning by analogy*: in some circumstances, such as the known association of congenital amelia with the administration of thalidomide during early pregnancy, similar, but slighter, evidence about another drug may be acceptable.

*Original Bradford Hill concepts are in *italics*.

disease incidence could be monitored. One example is immunisation against whooping cough (Fig. 7.10).

The variation in the distribution of risk factors could suggest explanations for the difference in disease patterns, and may also suggest a hypothesis for causation. Here, attention to the criteria for inferring causation is extremely important. For example, differences in the rates of type 2 diabetes between south Asian and indigenous white people in the UK could suggest genetic factors for developing the disease, whereas variation in rates between south Asian people living in the UK and those living in rural communities in south Asia might suggest environmental and lifestyle

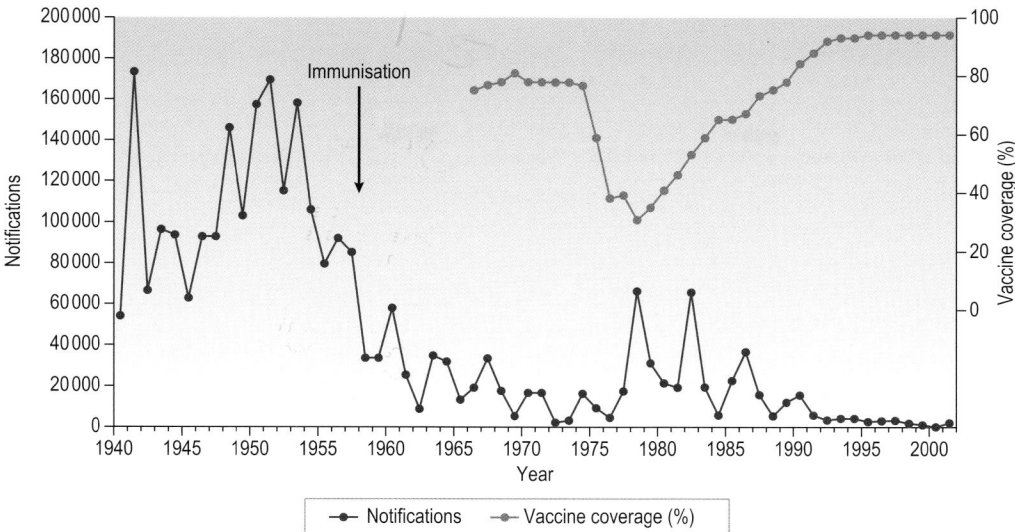

Fig. 7.10 Notifications and immunisation rates for whooping cough for England and Wales 1940–2001. The policy for immunising babies against whooping cough was initiated in the UK in 1958. The graph shows the incidence of whooping cough in England and Wales from 1940 to 2001, and how this came down once an immunisation programme was instituted. However, there was a 'scare' in 1974 that the whooping cough vaccine could cause brain damage, resulting in a dramatic fall in immunisation rate from over 80% coverage to under 30%. This was attended by a rise in whooping cough notifications. As the immunisation coverage improved, the incidence of whooping cough reduced. Source: Public Health Laboratory Service disease facts: whooping cough, www.hpa.org.uk

associations. The identification of risk factors is useful in the development of strategies to reduce disease and promote health, but conclusions drawn must be supported by evidence conforming to the criteria for inferring causation.

Cross-sectional studies

The commonest types of cross-sectional study are health surveys that collect data from a defined population in a particular way at a particular point in time. Table 7.7 sets out the design of cross-sectional studies that are commonly carried out and their uses.

Sampling for cross-sectional studies

A **sample** of the population is collected for a health survey, and this can be done by various means. Such studies are susceptible to a variety of biases, depending on the survey method used. For the results of a study to be useful, it is important that the sample should be representative of the population of interest. Although desirable, a truly random sample of the population is almost impossible to obtain and deliberate efforts must be made to ensure that the sample is as similar as possible to the population of interest. The way the sample was chosen must be described explicitly. For convenience, systematic sampling is often used in field studies – perhaps by collecting every tenth person in an alphabetical list. Lists that are compiled in other ways, such as the electoral roll, may also be used.

Sometimes a group of people will be selected instead of individuals. An example would be the General Household Survey carried out by the Office of Population Censuses and Surveys (OPCS). This has the advantage of concentrating fieldwork in a particular area, thus making the study cheaper and simpler. The assumption is made that people in a group are there for reasons unconnected with the reason for the study – although that of course might not be the case. Undertaking a survey is not without its problems. The minimisation

---

> *i* **Information box 7.15**   **Problems with data collection by survey: bias**
>
> Bias in samples collected by survey can occur in several ways:
>
> - Not using proper random selection. Volunteers are likely not to be representative of the population.
> - Not being able to identify certain groups within the population sampled. Some people are hard to identify or include, for example: people who do not often leave their homes, people without official residences, children frequently absent from school.
> - Selecting people who will not cooperate. Loss of information from large numbers of selected people will result in the study being unrepresentative and therefore meaningless. Leaving them out is not an answer but the process should be one that is most likely to engage their cooperation in the study.
> - Replacing people in surveys. If people originally selected cannot be found, or refuse to cooperate, replacement with others who are more easily traceable or are more compliant will result in bias.
> - Using an out-of-date list (sampling frame). Populations may change over time. For example, where there is movement in and out of a local authority, the area may change its demographic characteristics significantly, but out of date list will not reflect this.

of bias is an essential step in the design of any study that aims to infer causation (Information box 7.15).

Interpreting the data from cross-sectional studies

Often we will be interested, not just in making observations about one set of data, but also in making comparisons between different sets. The scientist first addresses the question: is the difference observed in the two groups a real difference, or did it occur by chance, using the process outlined below?

Table 7.7 Cross-sectional study design

Study type	Time	Definition	Past action	Starting point	Future action	Typical use for study
Cross-sectional	Present	Observation	None	Collect all information	None	Prevalence; current health status; reference ranges
Repeated cross-sectional	Present and future (longitudinal)	Observation	None	Collect all information	Collect all information again on several occasions	Changes over time

Table 7.8 Case–control study design

Study type	Time	Definition	Past action	Starting point	Future action	Typical use for study
Case–control	Present and past (longitudinal retrospective)	Observation	Record risk factor exposure	Collect cases and controls	None	Aetiology; rare disease aetiology

- The data are examined first, to determine the type of distribution.
- Statistical tests are then rigorously applied to ensure that the observed differences did not arise by chance (probabilities see above). We may be examining differences in proportions observed in different groups, but could also be looking at differences in the average value (mean) of a particular measurement.
- If the values are to be assessed more formally, then hypothesis tests and calculation of test statistics are required (see above).
  Only then may conclusions be drawn.

Case–control studies

The classic epidemiological enquiry is by observation. The examples of John Snow's Broad Street pump and cholera, and the thalidomide story were both case–control studies. **Case–control studies** may look back into the histories of affected persons (cases) and unaffected persons (controls) for evidence of exposure to the substance in question (Table 7.8). In other words, they are retrospective. By painstaking inquiry, the observer in each case found that appreciably more patients than unaffected people had consumed (or were exposed to) a particular substance.

Selecting the sample for case–control studies

In selecting a sample for a case–control study, as for *any* study, careful attention must be paid to the possibility of introducing bias, which would affect the ultimate outcome (see Information box 7.16).

A case–control study involves a comparison of the rate of exposure to a potential risk factor in groups with a disease with the rate of exposure in a group that is disease free. Cases are identified first, then suitable controls are selected. Ideally, in order to concentrate on a particular factor, the controls need to be as similar as possible to the cases in every respect (**specificity**, as referred to in the criteria for causation), except that they do not have the disease. Often this is achieved by rules which would result in cases being able to be controls if they did not have the disease, and vice versa. This selection also involves **matching** individuals, or groups, identifying and matching people for factors such as age, sex, ethnicity, etc., who have the potential to become cases, but without reference to the risk factor. However, care must be taken not to overmatch, in case the matching

i Information box 7.16 Potential biases in case–control studies

Minimising bias in studies designed to infer causation is extremely important. While it might be impossible to eliminate all bias, careful reflection about the potential sources of bias would help to avoid bias in the study design.

- Selection bias
  - Control selection: although controls are matched with cases, differences may sometimes be present that render them atypical. One reason could be overmatching: for a chest physician studying the relationship between smoking and lung cancer, the easiest source of controls may be other patients without lung cancer in his or her care. These controls, however, are likely to be patients who have other conditions related to smoking. Community controls are preferable but not so easy to recruit.
  - Case selection: a disease may vary in its causes and its association with other diseases. For example, lung cancer in a particular person may or may not have been caused by smoking, and may be accompanied by other conditions (co-morbidity). This will influence the extent to which any conclusions from the study can be generalised: a study based, for example, on elderly people without any co-morbid conditions is unlikely to be of wide value.
- Recall bias: in retrospective case–control studies, cases are more likely to recall the risk factors to which they have been exposed. The controls, on the other hand, may under-report their exposure. The discrepancy is likely to lead to bias. Historical information may also be inaccurate; while not biasing the results it will increase uncertainty.
- Ascertainment bias: also known as 'detection bias', ascertainment bias can occur when there is an association between an individual characteristic and the likelihood of detecting the event. For example, women taking the contraceptive pill may have more frequent cervical smears, so that cervical cancer may be detected sooner in this group.

variable is associated with the factor of interest. Having identified individuals we then enquire as to their exposure to that factor in the past (**temporality**). For example, if there is a group of cases of gastroenteritis after a wedding party, and a particular food preparation is suspected to be the cause, we would want to select our controls from the people who attended the party but did not suffer from gastroenteritis, since they had the potential to become cases, but without

Table 7.9	Case–control study: lung cancer and cigarette smoking among men (Doll and Hill 1950)			
Exposure	**Disease status**			**Total**
	Cases (lung cancer)	**Controls (no cancer)**		
Cigarette smokers	647		622	1269
		a	b	$a + b$
Non-smokers		c	d	$c + d$
	2		27	29
Total	649		649	1298
	$a + c$		$b + d$	$a + b + c + d$

taking into account what they ate when they were selected. We then see whether eating a particular food at the party was associated with people who become ill after the party.

Case–control studies have a number of practical advantages, principally because they are done at one point in time and so are quick and cheap. They are, however, difficult to do properly and there are a number of inherent biases that are difficult to overcome (Information box 7.16). Nevertheless where a condition is rare, this may be the only type of study that can be done that affords a sufficiently large number of cases. The study strength can be increased in particularly rare conditions by having more than one control for each case.

Analysing and interpreting data from case–control studies

The basic questions that need to be addressed by research studies are reiterated here:

- Is the difference observed in the two groups a real difference, or did it occur by chance? This question is about hypothesis testing.
- If we are satisfied that the difference was not by chance, then what inferences can be drawn from this difference? (This requires understanding of potential confounders and biases.)

Again, the data must be examined to look at the distribution, and the appropriate statistical tests applied to test the probability that the observed differences arose by chance.

The seminal work of Doll and Hill in 1950 and later Doll and Peto in 1994 (the British Doctors' Study) are classic examples of investigation by observation. The scientific rigour and principles inherent in these studies apply to all studies seeking to demonstrate cause and effect, and should always be borne in mind when considering claims of causality. Here the criteria for inferring causation are used to help distinguish probable cause from a chance association.

Strength of the association

The stronger the association, the more likely it is to be causal. The original study of cigarette smoking and lung cancer by Doll and Hill (1950) was a case–control study. A sample of patients in hospital with lung cancer (cases) was matched with patients without lung cancer (controls). Their case notes were reviewed for factors that may have influenced the development of carcinoma of the lung, and the subjects were interviewed about other social, environmental and occupational factors. A significant difference in whether the participants smoked cigarettes was found when comparing the groups with and without lung cancer ($p < 0.05$) (Table 7.9).

Doll and Hill showed that cigarette smokers were 14 times more at risk of developing lung cancer than non-smokers. Despite this large difference, a causal relationship between cigarette smoking and lung cancer cannot yet be presumed, as many other factors need to be considered.

Results of observational studies can be expressed in the form of a comparison of risks (see Information box 7.17).

In a case–control study, cases and controls are selected according to outcome (given in the columns) and the influence of various exposures (in the rows) is then investigated.

Odds of outcome (lung cancer) in smokers is a/b

Odds of outcome (lung cancer) in non-smokers is c/d

Odds ratio (OR) of outcome in smokers compared with non-smokers is:

$$\frac{a/b}{c/d}$$

or

$$\frac{a \times d}{b \times c}$$

In the above example the OR = $(647 \times 27)/(622 \times 2) = 14$

When the outcome that defines the cases is rare, then a/(a+b) (calculated when working out a risk) will be similar to a/b (calculated when working out odds) and so we can use the odds as an estimate of **relative risk** and interpret it in the same way as relative risk (see below). Otherwise, as in the case of the calculated example, we have to get to grips with odds. In tossing a coin, for example, the risk or chance of getting a head is 0.5, or 50%, whereas the odds are 1, or 50:50. An interest in betting often helps. In this above case the odds are 14, or 14 to 1.

Consistency of findings

Has the observed association been found by different observers, in different places and at different times? The same association between a causal agent and the disease should be observed in studies in different populations. If no such association is seen, it is important to compare methodologies in conflicting studies, and to know whether the selection of cases would have resulted in similar people being in all the separate studies.

At the time that Doll and Hill found the strong association in their sample between smoking and lung cancer, an Advisory Committee to the Surgeon-General of the United States Public Health Service reported the same finding in 29 retrospective and 7 prospective studies. It was then justifiably inferred that this association was a true one.

Specificity of the association

In 1951, Doll and Hill began a 20-year prospective study of smoking and mortality in male British doctors (Doll and Peto 1994), a **cohort study** (see below). Questionnaires on smoking habit were sent to all male doctors on the medical register at the time, and the respondents became the cohort for the study (34 440 men). Observations on mortality began in 1951, finishing in 1971. Details about doctors' deaths were obtained from the Registrar General and death notifications to the General Medical Council. Further follow-up questionnaires were sent in 1956, 1966 and 1972, including questions about stopping smoking (more doctors joined the study as they joined the medical register after 1951). During those 20 years, 10 072 men died. The death rate for smokers was higher than non-smokers, but from a number of causes of

Information box 7.17 **Comparing risks (odds ratio and relative risk)**

When estimating the risk of a particular outcome (e.g. developing a disease), the concepts of **odds ratio** or **relative, risk** are used. People who have been exposed to risk factors (such as cigarette smoking, excessive alcohol consumption), or who possess particular defining characteristics (e.g. employment, raised serum cholesterol) are compared to those without such exposure or characteristics. These statistics (summary statistics) are calculated from study data.

- In **case–control studies**, the outcome is already known, since cases are selected according to outcome, such as death or having lung cancer, and the influence of various exposures, the risk, (e.g. smoking, alcohol) is then investigated.
  - Risk is assessed using the concept of **odds**, referring to the likelihood, or odds, of developing a disease if exposed to a 'risk' factor. For example, if 4 people (cases and controls) have been exposed to a risk and 3 develop the disease and 1 does not, then the odds of disease in the exposed group are $3:1$.
  - Groups are compared by calculating the **odds ratio** (**OR**). If, for example, there are another 20 people who have not been exposed to the risk, but 4 of them develop the disease (and 16 do not), then the odds of disease in the non-exposed group are $4:16$, or $1:4$. The odds ratio is calculated as:

OR = Odds in exposed group/odds in non-exposed group (see also Table 7.9)
$$= (3/1)/(4/16)$$
$$= 12$$

It is important to be aware that in these studies the number of selected controls can be varied and the assessment of risk OR does not change. (Indeed, for rare outcomes, it would be usual to increase the number of controls several-fold in order to minimise bias and to have more precision for confidence intervals.) In the above example, there are 7 cases in total and 17 controls. If there were twice as many controls (34) then we would expect twice as many to have been exposed to the risk.

OR = (3/2)/(4/32) = 12 (identical to that above)

- In **cohort studies**, subjects are selected according to a defining characteristic, such as exposure to a factor, and subsequent outcomes (e.g. disease, death) are then investigated. The cohort is a defined (exposed) population. There is no concept of 'control' here, since the investigation is to observe the incidence of an outcome, such as heart disease, in this defined population. The overall number of people in the cohort (denominator) is more or less fixed (depending on loss to follow up).
  - Risk in this population is the proportion of people with the defining characteristic who develop the disease, and is compared with the proportion of people who develop the disease without the defining characteristic, known as the **relative risk (RR)**.
  - For example, suppose in a cohort of 24 people, 4 have been exposed and 3 of them subsequently develop the disease then the proportion of people who develop the disease in the exposed group is 3/4.
  - If, in the group of 20 people who have not been exposed, 4 of these subsequently develop the disease, then the proportion of diseased people in the non-exposed group is 4/20.

The RR = (3/4)/(4/20) = 3.75

- Note that if one applied relative risk calculations to the two case–control calculations above then very different estimates of risk would be obtained in the two situations.
- Relative risk does not provide an indication of the extent of a problem and calculation of the **absolute risk reduction (ARR)** or **absolute risk increase (ARI)** can be useful.
- **Absolute risk reduction (ARR)** is defined as the difference in proportions between the populations with and without the defining characteristics who develop the outcome. While this could lead to a *reduced* risk, looking at it in reverse would mean an *increase* in risk.
- In 1995 the UK Committee on Safety of Medicines reported a doubled risk (RR = 2) of deep vein thrombosis in women taking the third generation contraceptive pill (containing desogestrel and gestodene) in comparison with the second generation pill. As a result many women stopped taking the pill; there was a large increase in unwanted pregnancies and the number of legal abortions increased by about 6000, remaining at that level for the next 6 months.
- Although the risk had doubled with the use of the new pill, the actual risk had increased (ARI) by about 15 cases of deep vein thrombosis in every 100 000 women per year. This number of adverse events due to women continuing on the third generation pill is clearly very low in comparison with the marked increase in unwanted pregnancies.

death (heart disease, other cancers, Parkinson's disease, cirrhosis, etc.). Smoking was not *specifically* associated with lung diseases or cancers. By looking at the associations in age-standardised death rate for each cause of death, the excess in deaths among smokers was estimated. The magnitude of the excess mortality in cigarette smokers by cause of death (between 22% and 52%) led to the inference that deaths from cancer of the lung, oesophagus or other respiratory sites, chronic bronchitis and emphysema and pulmonary heart disease (cor pulmonale) were caused by cigarette smoking.

The observed association between smoking and many diseases other than lung cancer warrants more detailed examination. For example, mortality from cirrhosis of the liver was five times greater in current cigarette smokers than in non-smokers, but adjustment for a potential confounder in this association (alcohol) accounts for the excess deaths. Alcohol consumption may also be confounding the association between smoking and ischaemic heart disease in a different way. Alcohol, in moderation, appears to be associated with a reduced risk of ischaemic heart disease and so its action as a confounder is to mask what is probably a higher risk of ischaemic heart disease in smokers.

Relationship in time

It may seem obvious that there needs to be a temporal aspect in the observed association, since, in order to demonstrate causality, the exposure needs to precede the effect. This temporal relationship is not always easily observed, particularly in chronic, slowly developing conditions, and where multiple environmental factors could contribute to the development of disease. The prospective nature of a cohort study aims to avoid this difficulty.

In the 40-year follow-up of the British Doctors' Study, the excess mortality in smokers was almost twice as high in the second half of the study as in the first half (Fig. 7.11). This seems to be due to an improvement in survival in non-smokers, probably because of preventive measures, therapeutic improvements and environmental changes in the intervening years that have not been translated into improvements in smokers. Another reason for the non-improvement in smokers may be that those smokers who reached middle or old age in the 1970s and 1980s had a longer history of cigarette consumption than those who reached middle or old age in the 1950s and 1960s.

The biological gradient

The evidence for a causal relationship between cigarette smoking and lung cancer can be strengthened by demonstrating a biological gradient, or dose–response curve. In the study this was shown by dividing the data into categories for those who had never smoked, and those who smoked 1–14, 15–24, and more than 25 cigarettes per day. Doll and Peto (1994) demonstrated that with the exception of 4 out of over 20 conditions positively associated with smoking, mortality increased progressively from light to moderate to heavy smokers (Fig. 7.12).

Demonstration of reversibility

What effect did removal of the hazard have, if any? The smoking and mortality cohort study demonstrated this effect beautifully. As the study progressed, some doctors in the cohort stopped smoking, and after a period the rate of death from lung cancer in this group dropped compared with those who continued smoking, but the rate of death from some other cancers did not, underlining the causal relationship between cigarette smoking and lung cancer (Fig. 7.13). The statistical methods used for analysing effects over time are usually correlation and regression, with multivariable analyses when more than one predictor (independent variable) is studied (see below).

Biological plausibility

The evidence for causation is more acceptable if it is biologically plausible. This depends on the currently available

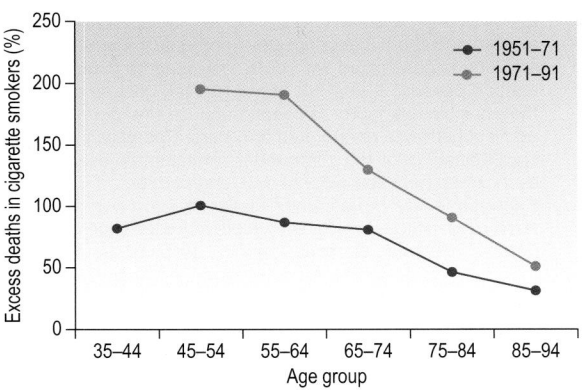

Fig. 7.11 Excess age-specific mortality in cigarette smokers in first half of study compared with second half. Source of data: Doll R, Peto R 1994 Mortality in relation to smoking: 40 years observation on British male doctors. BMJ 309: 910–11.

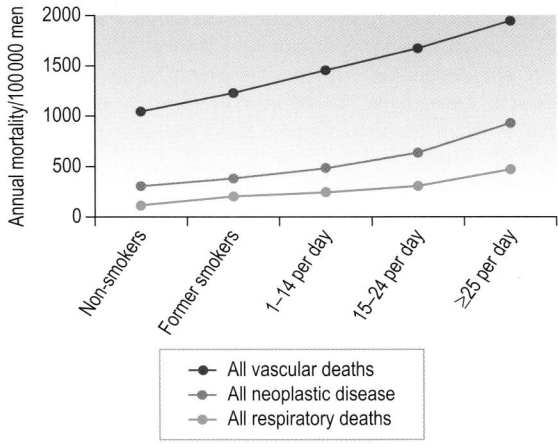

Fig. 7.12 Mortality in non-smokers and cigarette smokers. Analysis of data such as this may involve the use of a test for trend, such as a modification of the χ^2 test. Source of data: Doll R, Peto R 1994 Mortality in relation to smoking: 40 years observation on British male doctors. BMJ 309: 910–11.

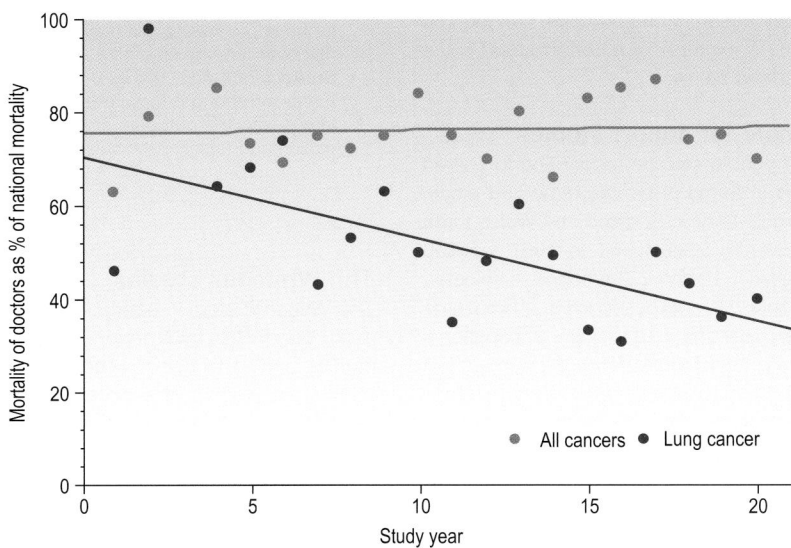

Fig. 7.13 Trends in deaths of male doctors certified 1951–1971. The doctors in the cohort reduced their cigarette consumption considerably; deaths from lung cancer grew less common, but not from other cancers. Source of data: Doll R, Peto R 1994 Mortality in relation to smoking: 40 years observation on British male doctors. BMJ 309: 910–11.

Table 7.10	Cohort study design					
Study type	Time	Description	Past action	Starting point	Future action	Typical use for study
Cohort	Present and future (longitudinal prospective)	Observation	None	Define cohort and assess risk factors	Observe outcomes	Aetiology; prognosis

biological knowledge, which is added to continually. Even where an observed association may be new to science, if the causal explanation makes biological sense it may deserve serious consideration.

Smoking tobacco causes cancer not only of tissues of the upper respiratory tract and lungs with which the smoke has direct contact, but also of the oesophagus, bladder and pancreas. Tobacco smoke contains many carcinogens that induce oxidative damage (see Ch. 16) to DNA, and many of these carcinogens also interact with DNA, forming DNA adducts that modify proteins and DNA itself, with potential mutagenic consequences. Techniques to demonstrate their presence have led to their detection in blood and in tissues not in direct contact with cigarette smoke, but associated with smoke-induced cancer. Increased levels of protein adducts have been found in non-smokers exposed to tobacco smoke, compared with those not so exposed.

Coherence of the evidence

To infer that an observed association strongly suggests cause and effect, the evidence should not seriously conflict with what is generally known about the natural history and biology of the condition. The association of lung cancer with cigarette smoking was coherent with the increase over time of cigarette smoking and the rise in deaths from lung cancer among men. We are now seeing more women smoking, and in almost all developed countries lung cancer rates in women are beginning to increase.

Cohort studies

The other main category of observation is the **cohort** study. This starts with an unaffected sample of the population: a cohort. Each member of the cohort is characterised by a number of features and enquiry made at intervals over a period of time to see if a particular outcome has occurred. The association between a feature and outcome can then be examined (Table 7.10). An example of a cohort study is the Whitehall I study described below.

Selecting the sample for cohort studies

A cohort is a group of people selected according to shared defining characteristics in terms of people, time and place, such as all babies born in 1942 in England and Wales (birth cohort), male civil servants aged 40–64 in 1967 working within 2 miles of Whitehall in London. The cohort is selected knowing that some people will be exposed to various hazards and others not. While selecting a particular occupational group can be useful as an aid to long-term follow-up, it will also mean that the cohort may not reflect the average health in the population. In addition, any cohort will be slightly healthier than the general population because it is composed of people who are free of disease on entry. Like any other study, it is important to be aware of bias (see Information box 7.18). When reading reports of cohort (and other) studies, the reader should always think about whether the investigators had done their best to minimise bias when they designed and carried out the study.

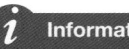 **Information box 7.18**   **Potential biases in cohort studies**

- **Selection of subjects**: the sampling frame, the population from which the cohort was drawn, can give rise to bias, especially if a high-risk group is chosen and the expected length of follow-up is intended to be short. If the study outcome was death, then a hospital-patient-based selection will be biased towards those patients likely to be at higher risk of death. More optimistic results for some conditions may be observed because the sample will not include individuals who have already died.
- **Association does not imply causation**: evidence for causation needs to be assessed against a number of criteria to be convincing (see above 'inferring causation'). Various biases can be introduced, but in particular, potential confounders need to be considered. For example, if an association is observed between drinking alcohol and the subsequent development of lung cancer, smoking is associated with both the outcome (lung cancer) because it *is* a risk factor for lung cancer, and the possible risk factor (alcohol) because they tend to occur together in restaurants and bars. Reanalysis of the data adjusting for the confounder (smoking) reveals no association between alcohol and lung cancer.
- **Expense**: even with common diseases, large populations need to be studied to detect significant differences in outcome between exposed and non-exposed groups. If the incubation period for a disease is long, many years of study may be required.
- **Loss to follow-up**: it is not unusual to be unable to record the outcome for every individual in a cohort, given that this may occur several years after inception of the study. Large numbers lost to follow-up, particularly if associated with a predictor, can produce significant bias. Studies need to be designed carefully so that this effect is minimised. It may be possible to provide ways in which some basic information can still be collected, such as, for example, information from death certificates.
- **Changes over time**: analytical methods and diagnostic criteria change over time, and information collected early in the study may not be comparable with later information. Individuals may change their exposure to risk over time by changing their occupation or lifestyle.
- **Surveillance**: this should be the same for all participants; if a group thought to be at high risk is studied more intensively, the outcome of interest may be detected earlier, and falsely associated with the risk.

The Whitehall studies

The Whitehall studies (Whitehall I in 1984 and Whitehall II in 1991) conducted by Marmot et al were **prospective** cohort studies aiming to see whether disease occurred more frequently in some civil service employment grades than in others. The subjects were all non-manual workers, not 'poor by any absolute standard', in stable employment, and living in one area (London), so that many of the socio-economic factors that affect health were controlled for. A clear gradient in mortality, and rates of non-fatal disease and sickness was demonstrated, inversely related to employment category.

It could be inferred that although there is an association between poverty and poorer health, other factors might be

Table 7.11	Cohort study: initial cholesterol level and death from coronary heart disease (Rose and Shipley 1986)		
Characteristic	Death from coronary heart disease at 10 years		Total
	Yes	No	
Cholesterol at or above median	421	8530	8951
	a	b	a + b
Cholesterol below median	c	d	c + d
	282	8485	8767
Total	703	17015	17718
	a + c	b + d	a + b + c + d

important from the public health perspective. To reduce mortality and morbidity in the lower employment grades to a level comparable with those in the higher grades would need strategies to address early environment, social environment, job design and the consequences of differences in income, as well as to encourage healthy behaviours. This kind of study does not help with the treatment of coronary heart disease, but can identify risk factors that may be amenable to modification as a preventive measure.

A well-designed and conducted cohort study provides the most valid evidence among the observational study types because it makes it possible to separate out prior causes from present associated factors, and although both suffer from potential confounding it is usually less likely to be biased than a case–control study. It can also be used to study several outcomes of the exposure to the same potential risk factor. Also, because the cohort is derived from the population, risk can be quantified (see Table 7.11).

Assembling the cohort
The Whitehall I study began in 1967, when a very large (17530) cohort of male civil servants aged 40–64 and working in various departments within 2 miles of Whitehall in London were invited to participate in the study, and classified according to employment grade. At the start of the study, they were surveyed about their family and past medical history (specifically in relation to cardiorespiratory disease), lifestyle (including smoking history) and symptoms of diabetes. They also attended a screening examination, where blood pressure, height and weight were recorded, and a two-lead electrocardiogram (ECG) was taken.

The prospective follow up
The assembled cohort of male civil servants was subsequently followed up for 10 years. Annual screening for illness and physical examination were undertaken and mortality was recorded.

It was found that there was a steep inverse relationship between employment grade and mortality. Compared with the highest administrative grade, the lowest grade had three times the mortality rate, not only from coronary heart disease but also from a range of other causes, and from all causes combined. The difference was partly accounted for by smoking, diet and other lifestyle gradients within each factor. Differences in height (higher grades were taller), relating to environmental factors in early childhood, suggested that early life may affect adult death rates, though height also has a genetic component.

Whitehall II
Twenty years later in 1985, a new, very large (10314) cohort of civil servants aged 35–55 was established, this time including women, and followed up for 3 years. The inverse association between employment grade and morbidity, angina, ECG evidence of ischaemic heart disease and symptoms of chronic bronchitis, remained. Self-perceived health status and symptoms were worse in the lower employment grades. There were employment gradient differences in lifestyle (as in smoking, diet and exercise) and in factors affected by early life (reflected in height), and in social position, social support and circumstances at work (monotony, hostility, low control and low satisfaction).

Analysing and interpreting data from cohort studies
Because some of the factors of interest will be confounded by other factors, depending on the outcome, either multivariable regression or multivariable logistic regression will be used to analyse the data (see below). As for case–control studies, the strength of the association between exposure to risk factors and developing disease needs to be explored in cohort studies before any inference of causation may be attempted (Information box 7.18).

Part of the Whitehall study of male civil servants in London examined the effect of cholesterol levels on the risk of death from coronary heart disease. Data in Table 7.11 have been extracted from this study.

$$\text{Relative risk (RR)} = \frac{a/a+b}{c/c+d}$$

The risk of death in the subsequent 10 years in those with above average cholesterol levels is 421/8951 = 0.047 whereas the risk in those with below average cholesterol levels is 282/8767 = 0.032, providing a relative risk of 0.047/0.032 = 1.47.

To interpret relative risk, if the risk (of death from coronary heart disease) in the lower cholesterol group was the same as that in the higher cholesterol group, then the ratio of the two risks (RR) would be 1.0. If being in the higher cholesterol group doubled the risk of death then RR would be 2.0. In the Whitehall study the relative risk is 1.47, meaning that the risk of death in the higher cholesterol group is about 1.5 times greater than the risk in the lower cholesterol group. We could also say that the risk was around 50% higher (150% − 100%) in the higher cholesterol group.

How the ratio is analysed will influence the way a risk is interpreted. We could say that the risk of death in the lower cholesterol group was 0.032/0.047 = 0.68 of the risk in the higher cholesterol group. While a concept such as doubling the risk may seem intuitive, it is probably more difficult to conceptualise 0.68 of a risk, so we might choose to invert the equation as above. Alternatively, we could talk about a 32% reduction in risk (100%–68%), or a 32% benefit. Although in the mathematical context, 'risk' does not necessarily imply something bad, for the sake of clarity, it is often useful to talk about relative benefit instead.

The role of genetics in observational studies
Possession of the ε **allele** of the apolipoprotein E gene is a major risk factor for late-onset Alzheimer's disease. Possession alone does not appear to be sufficient, and so combinations of several risk factors may be involved. When determining the importance of an association between the

gene and the disease we must also be aware of the various biases that occur when this kind of study is undertaken. **Selection bias** may occur in clinical or autopsy series of patients with Alzheimer's disease and misclassification may influence population studies. A further problem is that many people suffering from Alzheimer's disease are at a higher risk of dying because of their age. Bias can also occur when, for example, geneticists identify disease-associated genes within single blood samples. Since a **statistically significant** interaction will be found in about 1 in 20 comparisons, by chance alone, false positives will abound.

Association between genotype and risk factor

In the early stages of studying the prevalence of Alzheimer's disease, a strong association was found between presence of the ε apolipoprotein E genotype and vascular factors that indicate the presence of atherosclerosis. It was thus thought possible that the gene may exert its effect because of its possible role in the latter disease. When a later prospective study was done, this association with atherosclerosis was no longer evident. Confusion also arose between different populations, no relationship being seen in a Japanese autopsy series, while a clinical study in Americans showed an association. Differences in ethnicity and age of the many groups being studied, and also in the associations found, further add to the difficulties that epidemiologists face when trying to find the causes of a disease.

Interaction with environmental factors

A second example illustrates the interaction between genetic make-up and environmental factors. Colorectal cancer in Japanese migrants to the USA is among the highest in the world, and considerably higher than in the indigenous Japanese. Between 1880 and 1920, a large Japanese workforce was imported into Hawaii to work on the sugar plantations. Unlike the example involving Native American Indians and the immigrant Caucasian population, the Japanese did not mix, and today, people of true Japanese descent form about 30% of the Hawaiian population. Could the rise in incidence of the disease be due to their exposure to American lifestyle factors, or could there have been some form of change to their genetic susceptibility to the disease? These later migrants have, however, retained many of the elements of their ethnic diet, and although their fat intake is consistently lower than that of the Caucasian American population, their beef intake was higher.

Figure 7.14 illustrates the importance of possession of both a family history (genetic factor) and eating a large amount of red meat (environmental factor) in a study conducted by Marchand in 1999. The possible reason for this interaction lies in the high prevalence of a 'fast' acetylator N-acetyltransferase (NAT2) gene, present in 90% of the Japanese population compared with 45% of Caucasians. When meat is cooked at a high temperature or for a long time, the burning of the creatine/creatinine produces heterocyclic aromatic amines (HAA), which have been found to be carcinogenic in rats. In order to be toxic, however, HAA needs to be activated; two genes are involved and one of them is NAT2.

Investigation by experiment

When selecting the most appropriate and effective treatment or intervention, the clinician needs to know how these worked

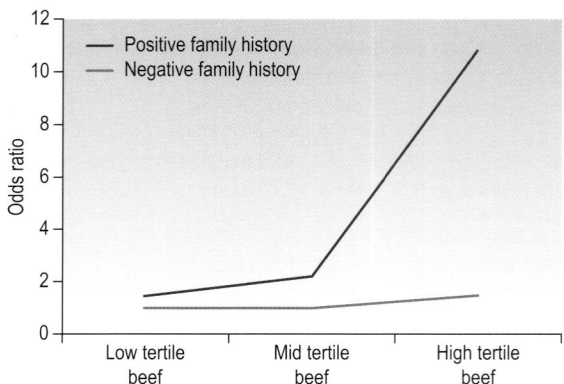

Fig. 7.14 Beef intake and colorectal cancer in people of Japanese origin, resident in Hawaii. A strong family history of colorectal cancer in the migrants increased the risk of disease (odds ratio of 3.0), and the Japanese migrants were found consistently to eat more red meat than the local Caucasian population. Source of data: Marchand LL 1999 Combined influence of genetic and dietary factors on colorectal cancer incidence in Japanese Americans. Journal of the National Cancer Institute Monograph 26: 101–105.

previously for similar patients. New treatments will need rigorous testing to see how effective they are and whether they cause harm. Experimental intervention of some kind is required, followed by observation of the effects of intervention: **clinical trials** are the usual method of study:

■ The intervention is administered to the experimental group.
■ The outcomes are observed and compared with those in a control group, which is not given the intervention.
■ The experiment has to be conducted in such a way that any difference that might be observed between the two groups is real, and not due to chance.

A second important question is whether the experimental treatment is the most likely cause of the difference: the two groups must, therefore, be similar in characteristics that could have a bearing on their condition at the start of the trial. A third question is that, apart from the experimental treatment, the groups are treated in the same way. If a difference in the two groups is observed, and this difference is deemed not to have occurred by chance (is statistically significant), it may be inferred that the difference was the outcome of the intervention.

Medical treatment and surgical procedures are not the only interventions that can be tested experimentally. In public health policy, for example, some preventive action is taken as the result of an observed association. Does such action, in fact, prevent, or at least reduce, risk or frequency of associated events? In this context, experimental trials could be the means of testing for cause and effect.

Evaluation of clinical effectiveness: RCTs

To illustrate the processes for evaluating clinical effectiveness of a medical treatment, the Scandinavian Simvastatin Survival Study (4S), a randomised trial of cholesterol lowering in 4444 patients with coronary heart disease published in 1994, is used as an example. The effectiveness of drug treatment to lower serum cholesterol concentration, in order to improve survival for people with coronary heart disease, had been in question because of insufficient clinical evidence of benefit. The 4S trial was a study of secondary prevention of the complications of established coronary heart disease, by the use of a drug that is known to reduce serum cholesterol. An RCT was done.

Selecting the sample: experimental and control groups

The first task here is to define the population of interest; what is meant by people with established coronary heart disease? The inclusion criteria for the 4S trial were men or women aged between 35 and 70 years, with a history of angina or acute myocardial infarct. There were also some exclusion criteria, which addressed the likelihood of pregnancy, severe disease or co-morbidity. Here, the idea is to eliminate, or at least minimise, bias and reduce any unknown risk to potentially vulnerable patients (pregnant or co-morbid) (see Information box 7.19). Patients were recruited from 94 centres. In many cases, participants became eligible for a trial when they were first diagnosed with a problem or disease (incident cases). This resulted in patients being recruited over a period of time and then followed up for either a specific period of time or until a specific time point.

Ethical considerations during the planning stage of clinical trials

The major ethical considerations when inviting patients to volunteer to take part in a clinical trial are:

- Respect for the autonomy of the volunteer
- No harm must be done to the volunteer.

Volunteers must consent to participate, but informed consent cannot be given without having all the information needed to understand the issues involved in the study, and the information must be fully understood and considered.

The Declaration of Helsinki (World Medical Association 1960, revised 1975) outlines the ethical considerations when undertaking clinical research.

- The first principle is that the study should be preceded by a careful assessment of risk and benefits and states that the interests of the subject must always prevail over the interests of science and society.
- Secondly, a potential subject, or their legal guardian, must be adequately informed of the aims, methods, possible benefits, potential hazards and possible discomforts of the proposed intervention.

Sometimes it is difficult to provide an adequate definition of the risk, as for example during pregnancy. Some subjects, such as those with mental disability, may not be legally competent. However, such people are more likely to meet exclusion criteria and will therefore rarely be represented in these experiments.

Another ethical consideration is that of coercion. This could be bribery, if the 'volunteers' to the trial were paid excessive sums of money to take part, or in the case of a family doctor inviting a patient to take part in a trial, consent could be influenced by the relationship between the patient and doctor, or consideration that any existing treatment might be withheld if consent was refused.

Achieving similar groups for comparison: randomisation to minimise bias

Only when the participants have been selected according to the inclusion and exclusion criteria and given informed

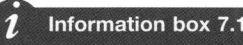

Information box 7.19 | **Potential bias in clinical trials (1) planning stage**

As with observation studies, introducing bias during the planning stage of an RCT must be avoided as far as possible. Factors that could affect the eventual outcomes of the trial may be introduced during the planning stage when selecting the sample.

- **Inclusion and exclusion criteria**: these need to be clear and unambiguous so that there is no possibility of excluding patients after randomisation is performed. The criteria need to be applied before randomisation to avoid any deliberate or inadvertent attempt to exclude or include once the result of randomisation is known.
- **Informed consent**: This should be taken before randomisation for ethical reasons and to minimise the chance of patients leaving the study once randomisation is known.
- **Allocation concealment**: if the researcher is aware of which group (treatment or control) subjects will be allocated to, subjects may be allocated to the treatment group in order to gain access to the new treatment. This may be an unconscious action, but nonetheless the result will be biased. The converse could also happen. It can be avoided by the randomisation being performed by a third party and the analysis being performed on the group according to how they were randomised.
- **Study sample size**: to ensure that any difference in outcome detected between the treatment and control groups reaches statistical significance, the power of the study to demonstrate this difference depends on calculating a large enough sample to do this (see below). A sample that is too small, or is underpowered, is unlikely to show a significant result even if, in truth, there is one, thus biasing the study. Medical literature is full of studies that suggest there is no difference between two treatments when the study samples have not been large enough to reveal a difference in effect by as much as 25%. Similarly, there must be a large number of negative studies that have not made it to publication because they did not show a positive effect that was statistically significant (**publication bias**).
- **Control treatment and blinding**: As far as possible the control treatment should be as similar to the intervention in looks, taste and follow-up from the health professionals in the study so that any 'inherent' placebo effects of taking a tablet are as similar as possible in both groups. If either the patient or the health professional is unblinded, this knowledge can affect the placebo effect, or the attitude of, or interpretation of results by the health professionals. Any of these could introduce bias between the groups.

consent can they be allocated to either the control or intervention group. The best method of ensuring that the two groups are as similar as possible for both known and unknown characteristics is random allocation. This is done using a random numbers table or a computer programme (see Information box 7.20). The only reason the groups may differ is then chance.

Selecting the sample for the 4S trial

In the 4S trial, potential subjects fulfilling the selection criteria were invited to take part and be screened for exclusion criteria. After final informed consent was obtained, they were randomly assigned to the treatment group taking 20 mg of simvastatin, or to the control group taking placebo. In this process, **allocation concealment** was provided so that it was impossible to predict the group an individual would have been randomised to until the point of randomisation. Because

Information box 7.20 **Random allocation**

Only when volunteers have been selected, and informed consent is given, can subjects be allocated. A variety of methods are employed for allocating subjects to treatment or control groups in an RCT:

■ **Simple random**: random, in this context, does not mean haphazard. Subjects are selected so that every individual has the same chance, or probability, of being chosen. A simple method could be by tossing a coin, but usually a computer is used.

■ **Blocking**: blocking, also known as restricted randomisation, is done to ensure that the numbers are balanced between different treatment groups, and kept balanced at all times throughout the life of the study to increase the **power** (see below). To facilitate this, subjects are allocated in two small 'blocks' in random order, ensuring that each block contains a balance of the treatments. In a block of six used to allocate treatments A and B, each block will contain three subjects receiving treatment A and three receiving treatment B, and the order in which they are allocated will be randomised.

■ **Stratified**: to overcome chance differences in important predictive characteristics arising from simple randomisation, subjects are defined by common characteristics which affect the outcome, e.g. cancer stage, and are then randomised within each stage to ensure similar proportions of cancer stage within the treatment and control groups. This is known as **stratification**. This is particularly useful for relatively small or multicentre studies where randomisation is usually stratified by the centre. **Minimisation** is another statistical technique that can be used to achieve very similar groups.

■ **Cluster randomisation**: it may be impossible to randomise individual subjects, for example in a study of a particular health promotion, when outcomes may be biased by **contamination** (see below). In these cases groups of people (families, schools, GP practices, hospitals, etc.) are identified, and each group (or cluster) is randomised to be in the intervention group or the control group.

treatment is more effective than the old or no treatment. In the case of opinion or attitude surveys, the difference would be in the proportions of people agreeing or disagreeing with something.

■ The study needs to be large enough to have a strong likelihood of showing a statistically significant difference if the true effect is the one decided on. This likelihood is known as the **power** of the study.

■ Knowing the required effect, the power and the *p* value that is to be taken as statistically significant, the sample size can be calculated.

■ Usually the *p* value is 0.05 and the power would be at least 80% although 90% is often used.

■ With the sample size required for an 80% power calculation, we can be 80% certain that *p* will be <0.05 if the underlying effect is that used in the calculations.

Some idea of the likely difference in clinical outcomes between the two groups is needed before a power calculation for sample size can be undertaken. In practice, it may not be possible to know what this difference will be, unless there is information from a pilot or other studies. Past experience could give an idea of what the outcome in the untreated, control group should be from the natural history of the disease. A decision then needs to be made about what constitutes a clinically important change in outcome. For example, the 4S study was planned to detect a 30% reduction in total mortality in the treatment group. The numbers required to give a 'statistically significant' result were then calculated using a 'power calculation' (see below). The research protocol specified 4400 patients to be followed up until there were 440 deaths.

Power calculations

To estimate the number of subjects needed in a trial, a power calculation is used. Before doing the power calculation you will have to decide what is to be achieved by the trial – what you want to measure as the main outcome (see below). This may be categorical, for example how many subjects are dead or alive at the end of the study (Information box 7.21), or numerical, for example the change in blood pressure measured in mmHg (Information box 7.22). Power calculations may be applied for sample sizes for surveys as well as clinical trials.

You will also need to decide what sorts of results you would expect from the standard treatment. For example, you may know that not giving treatment results in about 10% of patients dying each year, or that the standard treatment lowers mean systolic blood pressure by 5 mmHg. In the latter situation we also need to know how much the change in blood pressure can vary between individuals (measured by the standard deviation); publications may provide relevant information.

Although mathematical formulae can be used to decide the number of subjects needed, it is simpler to use the nomogram developed by Altman (1982) (Fig. 7.15), or talk to a statistician. There are also computer packages that can do power calculations.

patients have already fulfilled the selection criteria and consented, there is no opportunity to bias the selection process by leaving people out, as there would be if the randomisation details were available earlier. In the 4S study, a further refinement in randomisation was added by stratifying the subjects for geographical area and history of previous myocardial infarction. The eventual sample was almost perfectly balanced, and at the start of the trial the two groups were very similar.

Baseline characteristics for randomised patients are usually shown in the first table in reports of randomised clinical trials. Sometimes statistical tests are also done to indicate that the groups are balanced, though this should not be necessary if the patients have been properly randomised, and it should be remembered that in any series of statistical tests about 1 in 20 comparisons will be statistically different by chance alone (*p* = 0.05).

Calculating sample size

The size of a sample is chosen during the planning stage of a trial and is not an educated guess. Logical thinking at this stage of a study is needed:

■ First, a decision has to be made about how large a difference needs to be detected between the treatment and control groups to show that the experimental

Measuring the outcomes during a trial

As well as bias in the planning stage of clinical trials, events that occur during the trial can also distort the eventual findings. Information box 7.23 outlines some potential biases during a trial.

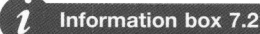

Information box 7.21 — Example of a power calculation (1) – using proportions

In the Medical Research Council/British Heart Foundation Heart Protection Study of cholesterol lowering with simvastatin in high-risk patients (age 40–80 years with coronary disease, or occlusive arterial disease, or diabetes) it was estimated that around 1500 out of 20 000 similar patients would die from coronary causes within 5 years. The aim of the study was to see whether this cholesterol lowering therapy could reduce coronary mortality by around 25%. A high level of power (90%) and a high level of statistical significance ($p < 0.01$) were set in order that the study should stand a high chance of being successful and convincing.

For this the standardised difference was calculated:

$$\text{Standardised difference} = \frac{p_{control} - p_{simvastatin}}{\sqrt{\bar{p}(1 - \bar{p})}}$$

where $p_{control}$ is the proportion of deaths expected in the control group (1500/20 000 = 0.075), and $p_{simvastatin}$ is the proportion of deaths expected in the treatment group (25% less – 1125/20 000 = 0.056) and $\bar{p}$ is the average of the two proportions (0.066).

$$= \frac{0.075 - 0.056}{\sqrt{0.066 \times 0.934}} = 0.076$$

See Figure 7.15. Draw a line between the standardised difference (0.076) and a power of 0.9, reading off the sample size (N) on the significance level 0.01 line. The nomogram gives a sample size of around 7000 in total so the researchers' plan to randomise over 20 000 patients gave them confidence not only to detect a 25% reduction in coronary deaths, but also to detect less pronounced differences associated with other non-coronary deaths or serious events.

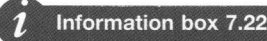

Information box 7.22 — Example of a power calculation (2) – using means

The aim of a randomised clinical trial for a new antihypertensive drug is to demonstrate that the new drug can lower systolic blood pressure by more than 10 mmHg in comparison with the standard treatment. Looking at published data we discover that the standard deviation of average systolic blood pressure is about 15 mmHg. We need to be sure that if a difference of 10 mmHg is found between the treated and control groups, the difference is measured at the 5% level of significance or lower, so the significance level is set at 0.05, with 80% certainty (80% power).

To use the nomogram we calculate a **standardised difference**:

$$\begin{aligned}\text{Standardised difference} &= \text{clinically relevant} \\ &\quad \text{difference/standard} \\ &\quad \text{deviation} \\ &= 10/15 \\ &= 0.67\end{aligned}$$

Draw a line between the standardised difference (0.67) and a power of 0.8, reading off the sample size (N) on the significance level 0.05 line. This gives a total sample size of about 70 subjects, 35 per group. Increasing the power of the study (the ability to detect a real difference) will increase the number of people needed for the study, as will reducing the size of the difference we want to be able to detect.

Information box 7.23 — Potential bias in clinical trials (2) – during the trial

Care should be taken when making observations during a trial. Bias may be introduced during the process of a clinical trial, which needs to be avoided.

- **The placebo effect**: the mere fact of taking a tablet (which could be a dummy, and therefore a **placebo**) can give a subject a sense of psychological well-being. Spontaneous events can also occur as part of the natural history of the disease. The placebo effect can account for up to 30% improvement in symptoms in some studies. Unpleasant effects can be ascribed to placebos, as in the 4S trial, where roughly the same number in the placebo group as in the treatment group stopped taking the tablets because they thought they were having adverse effects from the tablets.
- **Contamination**: individuals in the control group may intentionally or inadvertently receive the experimental intervention. This is more common in health education interventions, where news of a particular health-orientated approach being tested in one GP practice may become known throughout the community and be taken up by others who were within a control group. The bias will be towards the null, making it more difficult to detect a difference between the two groups.
- **Compliance**: subjects may not always comply with the allocated treatments in a trial, and this also occurs in the population at large. It is usual when planning the size of the study to take account of the proportion who may not comply with treatment and the proportion who may drop out (i.e. not have outcome measures). If non-compliance is larger than expected, the study may be compromised.
- **Intervention bias**: if a particular treatment is thought to have possible adverse effects in a particular subgroup of participants, it may be tempting to follow these subjects more carefully, thus adding an additional difference between the groups, beyond the experimental treatment. Bias may also occur in double-blinded trials in cases where it is possible to detect an active treatment because of an observable systemic effect. Both of these biases can make the two groups appear more different than they really are.
- **Cross-over**: if a particular treatment appears to be too aggressive for a particular subject then a medical decision might be made to treat them according to the other therapy. Depending on whether the new treatment is generally better or worse than the standard treatment, crossing over may bias either towards the null or towards a false impression of a difference (this is why we do intention-to-treat analysis).
- **Loss to follow up**: loss to follow-up occurs when a subject who enters the trial moves away or otherwise cannot be traced, so that they are unavailable for outcome assessment. This is more likely to occur in longer studies. Subjects in studies involving patients who are seriously ill (e.g. acute leukaemia) are more accessible for assessment than subjects in studies of primary prevention, where they are well and not so motivated to continue treatment. In such cases more rigorous ways of maximising follow up should be introduced into the study methodology at the design stage. (This is why all-cause mortality is usually an end-point, because provided permission to access these data was part of the inclusion criteria, it is generally possible to find out if someone has died or not even if they are lost to follow-up.)

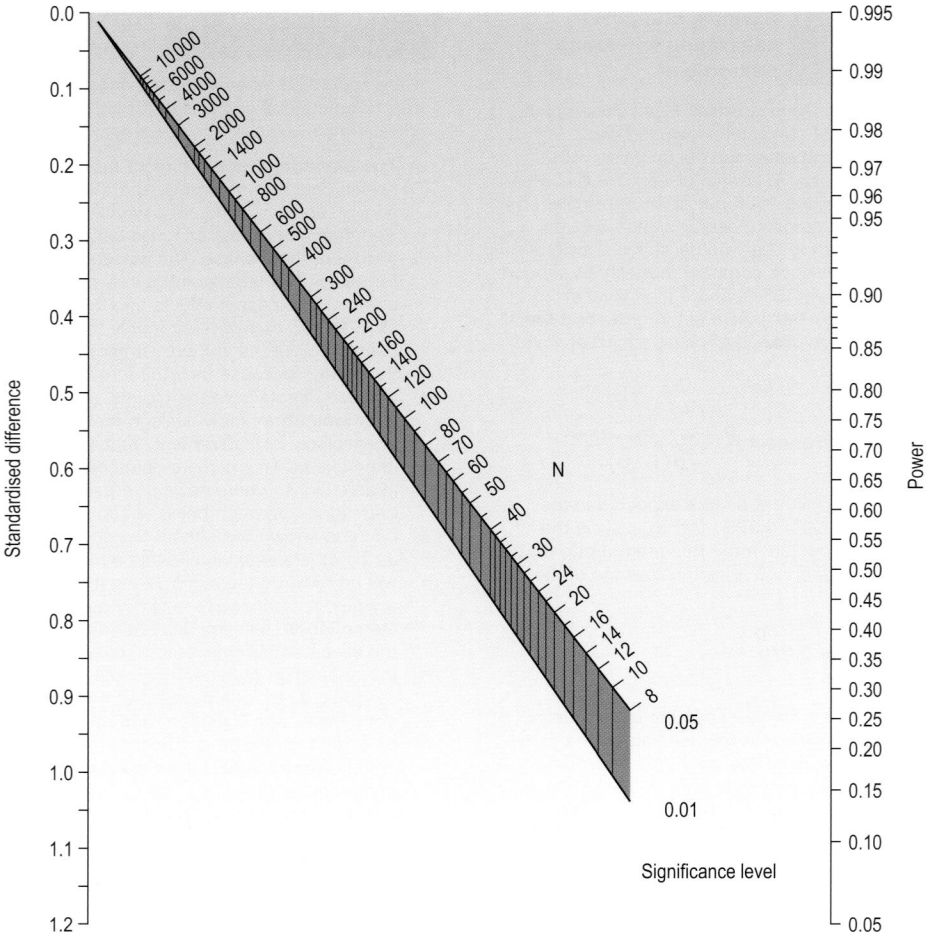

Fig. 7.15 **Nomogram for power calculations.** Source: Altman DG 1982. How large a sample? In: Gore SM, Altman DG, eds. Statistics in practice. British Medical Association, London, pp 6–8.

'Blinding' to avoid bias during a trial

To minimise **bias**, the subjects in each group to which they are allocated are **blinded**, so that they are not aware of whether the tablet they receive contains the active drug or the dummy. A trial in which the patient is blind to the treatment given is a **single-blind** trial.

The researcher (the doctor) could also introduce bias by favouring (or not) the treatment group, for example by assuming that someone not receiving an active treatment (in the placebo group) is more likely to experience a cardiac event. For this reason, the researcher also needs to be blinded to the nature of the tablet given to the patient, and the 4S trial was a **double-blind** trial in this sense. Studies that have not been double blinded, in comparison with those that have, have shown an overestimate of benefit of up to 17%. In the event that the patient is experiencing harm, the blinding is broken to establish the cause of this harm.

In some trials, for example in a trial of the effectiveness of a surgical procedure, it would be impossible to blind the patient who has to consent to the procedure or the surgeon who has to perform the procedure. It is therefore necessary to conceal the patient allocation from the observer, who takes measurements during the follow up period, as to whether the subject had one or other procedure under investigation. For example, in a trial of myringotomy versus grommets in children with impaired hearing as a consequence of 'glue ear', the follow-up audiometry would be performed by a technician 'blind' to the procedure the child received.

Outcomes of interest: end-point definition

There are few unequivocal objective health outcomes. How the patient feels must be subjective, and might depend on a whole series of factors not necessarily related to disease. It is important that outcome measures provide a valid assessment of the effects of intervention, and are not determined by what is easily measurable.

The duration of follow-up will also affect outcome, because treatment effects, whether beneficial or harmful, may not be evident if the follow-up is too brief. For example, the drug clofibrate, known to reduce serum cholesterol levels in those patients who had high levels, was used in a clinical trial published by the Committee of Principal Investigators, to examine its benefit in the primary prevention of ischaemic heart disease. The earlier publication in 1978 revealed that fewer people in the clofibrate group experienced non-fatal heart attacks, but the later follow-on publication from 1980 revealed that mortality from all causes was higher in the clofibrate group, underlining the importance of considering all relevant outcomes (in this case death from all causes) and for continuing a trial for long enough to reveal these differences, or at least undertaking follow-up studies to find out whether an apparently promising treatment might be detrimental.

Defining outcomes is made easier if the research question is clearly focused. The question in the 4S trial was 'Does a reduction in serum cholesterol concentration reduce the incidence of complications in people with coronary heart disease?'. The primary end-point was total mortality, secondary end-point was defined as 'major coronary events', and tertiary end-points included any coronary event and related atherosclerosis events such as stroke. The effective follow-up time for the 4S study was calculated in the power of the study, as when 440 deaths had occurred. Median follow-up was 5.4 years, and both subjects and controls had the same regimen of tests, such as annual electrocardiograms, observations and so on.

Ethical principles during a trial: stopping a trial and interim analyses

It has already been mentioned that trials that are too small are unethical. In addition, many people would consider a trial unethical if it had not been properly planned and organised. Furthermore, it is a fundamental principle that patients should not be exposed to any treatment if it is known to be harmful. The Declaration of Helsinki states that 'Doctors should cease any investigation if the hazards are found to outweigh the potential benefits'.

Unfortunately, there are probably many situations where trials have not been stopped in such circumstances, not necessarily by intention, but because of a lack of understanding of the principles behind an ethical trial. An understanding of the reasons for stopping an ongoing trial highlights these principles (see below). These reasons may become clear before the planned end of a trial, where **interim analyses** of the data can be useful. Interim analyses are only possible if follow-up is fairly long or recruitment is spread over a fairly long period.

In the UK, all ethical committees that give approval for trials to go ahead will consider the need for a data monitoring and ethics committee (DMEC) for the trial. Its members will determine whether interim analyses are required and approve any stopping rules.

Interim analyses

If decisions are to be made about stopping a trial, the reasons must be clear and valid, and the process should not bias the outcome of the trial.

What outcomes should be considered in an interim analysis? Outcomes relevant to a trial involve gathering large amounts of data about death, cause of death, morbidity, change in biochemical measurements, patient satisfaction, etc. If the interim analysis includes an assessment of all this information, the risk is increased of finding statistical differences between the treatments by chance alone. It may therefore be appropriate to have a p value much below 0.05 for each of them, otherwise multiple comparisons arising from the different outcomes would not be appropriate (because it would be desirable for all or most of them to be significant). The addition of an interim analysis itself increases the chance of getting $p < 0.05$ from 1 in 20 to 1 in 10. The reason that many outcomes are not considered

at interim analyses initially (but they would be if it appears likely that the trial might have to be stopped) is probably because it is important to do it quickly after the appropriate time or number of patients have been followed up for long enough.

In any comparison, a difference is considered to exist (be statistically significant) if it is likely to occur less than 5% of the time by chance alone ($p < 0.05$ or less than 1 in 20 occasions). This definition of statistical significance implies that in about 1 in 20 comparisons, a difference considered to be significant will occur by chance alone. Doing an interim analysis doubles the chance of getting a significant result to 1 in 10 so smaller p values would be used before stopping a trial.

How should the information be obtained? Usually, the data are collated and analysed and presented by the trial statistician to the DMEC blinded so the DMEC does not know if the results indicate better or worse outcomes.

In managing an interim analysis, it is important to have made a plan and then to keep to it. It is difficult not to be influenced when, for example, researchers in multicentre trials send in unscheduled and possibly incomplete information about patients who have died, or suffered bad side effects, as a result of one arm of a clinical trial. Only by a proper evaluation of all patients at a planned interim time in their treatment can doubt be avoided.

How should the information be treated? It is vital that the results of any interim analyses are kept confidential. The leaking of information about possible differences may result in investigators or subjects dropping out, or lead to a fall off in recruitment.

How should the decision be made to stop a trial? The decision to stop a trial is usually made by a monitoring committee (DMEC) set up as part of the trial management process. The committee should set up a formal stopping rule, although that will not necessarily be the only basis on which the trial might be stopped, since other factors, such as cost, acceptability, newer treatments, unacceptable rate of side effects, etc., may influence whether the trial should continue, and might also change over time.

The stopping rule should account for the size of the difference, the number of interim analyses and its statistical significance. Occasionally, the stopping rule will apply if the results cross a particular threshold for the number of data points analysed. The p value for stopping will be considerably less than $p = 0.05$. If a statistical difference of $p < 0.05$ is used, then there is around a 1 in 20 chance that the trial will be stopped without there being a real difference between the experimental treatments – a risk that increases with more interim analyses. Setting a more rigorous p value (e.g. <0.005) would reduce the likelihood of a trial being stopped because of a false-positive result.

Measuring outcomes: follow-up

Subjects in the study have to be carefully followed up to observe the effects of intervention. All the patients entered into the trial have to be properly accounted for and attributed at the end. If patients cannot be traced they will be 'lost to follow-up', and it will be impossible to tell what outcomes they may have experienced, whichever group they were allocated to (see Information box 7.23).

Analysing and interpreting the results

When analysing the results of a clinical trial, particularly one that has a long follow up period, all subjects have to be accounted for. The results may be biased by what happened to certain patients (Information box 7.23). To avoid distortion of the final result, patients are analysed by **intention-to-treat**, and it is important for the reader of reports of clinical trials to know that this was undertaken.

Analysis by intention-to-treat

Some patients in the treatment group may stop taking the tablets because of adverse effects, or illness severity may require that a subject in the control group has to take active treatment. In which group should these patients be accounted for? For example, in a trial of two different revascularisation procedures for coronary heart disease (the Randomised Intervention Treatment of Angina (RITA trial, 1989), some patients assigned to one procedure had to undergo the other because of disease severity.

The statistical analysis for randomised clinical trials works by comparing outcomes between patients receiving the experimental intervention and patients not receiving the experimental intervention. **Intention-to-treat** analysis means that all patients are analysed in the group to which they were originally assigned. Therefore, those patients who were intended for the treatment group, but failed to complete treatment are included in the treatment group. While this may seem obtuse, any other action will bias the result because it breaks the randomisation.

At the start of the 4S trial, the subjects in each group were well balanced and similar. The patients who stopped taking the tablets may have been more (or less) severely ill than the ones who completed the trial. Leaving them out of the treatment group, or putting them with the controls, would have introduced bias by distorting the profile of the treatment group and consequently the outcomes. The same applies if patients in the control group were analysed in the treatment group for some reason.

Another good reason for analysis by intention-to-treat is that, in real life, there will be some patients who stop taking tablets because of side effects (nausea, other gastrointestinal upset, etc.) so that retaining them in the analysis would be a more realistic reflection of what would happen in a practical way (pragmatic approach). The data for the 4S trial were analysed by intention-to-treat.

Sensitivity analysis

A **sensitivity analysis** should be done to determine whether the loss to follow-up is likely to bias the results. Subjects lost to follow-up are likely to be different from those who remain available, and research has shown that their prognosis is probably also different. If a study loses a large proportion of its subjects (say over 20%), or if the loss is significantly unbalanced, then the resultant study can either be importantly biased, or the certainty of the observations sufficiently compromised to limit the value of the study. The relative importance of the loss can be investigated by undertaking a sensitivity analysis, consisting of:

- An analysis based on a reasonable, possible poor outcome for the missing individuals
- An analysis based on a reasonable, possible good outcome.

If the conclusions derived from the two analyses are different, then it is clear that the loss to follow-up has been so large that the study is no longer valid.

Measures of treatment effect

Various methods can be used to describe the results and these are illustrated in Table 7.12. The quoting of a relative risk reduction alone can be misleading because it does not take into account the baseline risk. The absolute reduction in risk is sometimes a more useful concept. Converting an absolute risk reduction into a number needed to treat is useful because it provides a whole number, rather than a decimal proportion, that is easier to remember.

Statistical significance

It must be remembered that the nature of statistical significance being set at the $p = 0.05$ level means that there is a 5% chance of obtaining a p value <0.05 where there is truly no difference. This also highlights the importance of not over-interpreting significant differences where large numbers of comparisons have been made. Statistical methods exist to help in the interpretation where there are multiple comparisons.

Statistical significance, or not, does not necessarily imply that the result obtained is important, or not, clinically. For example, a small but statistically significant difference in blood pressure may be so small as to not be clinically important, either in terms of the size of the difference or other clinical end-points. In contrast, a large and potentially important clinical difference, which does not reach statistical significance, suggests that the study may have been underpowered. Careful examination of the position of the 95% confidence interval in relation to the point of no difference can help in the interpretation (Fig. 7.16).

Clinical significance: the number needed to treat

Whether a statistically significant finding has clinical meaning is largely dependent on the clinician's common sense. There is, however, a test that can give some clues: the **number needed to treat** (NNT). With reference to the 4S trial and its primary outcome, it means 'How many patients with

Table 7.12	Calculations for treatment effect						
Control event rate (CER)	Experimental event rate (EER)	Relative risk (RR)	Relative risk reduction (RRR)	Absolute risk (AR)	Absolute risk reduction (ARR)	Number needed to treat (NNT)
Event/control numbers	Event/experimental numbers	EER/CER	|CER − EER|/CER or (1 − RR)	EER for experimental group; CER for control group	|CER − EER|	1/ARR rounded to the next whole number quoting associated time

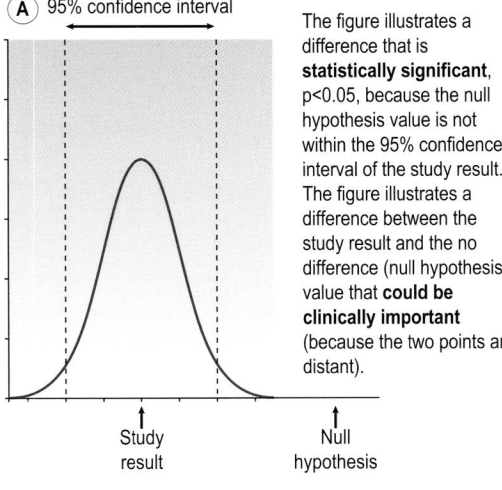

A 95% confidence interval

| Study result | | Null hypothesis |

The figure illustrates a difference that is **statistically significant**, p<0.05, because the null hypothesis value is not within the 95% confidence interval of the study result. The figure illustrates a difference between the study result and the no difference (null hypothesis) value that **could be clinically important** (because the two points are distant).

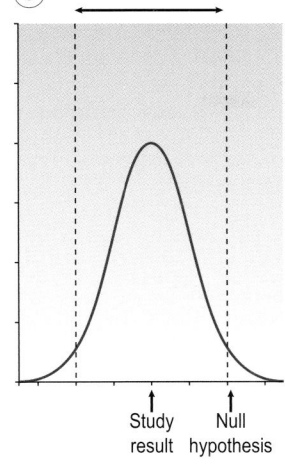

C 95% confidence interval

| Study result | Null hypothesis |

The figure illustrates a difference that is **statistically significant**, p<0.05, because the null hypothesis value is outside the 95% confidence interval of the study result. The figure illustrates a difference between the study result and the no difference (null hypothesis) value that **may, or may not be clinically important** (depending on the context).

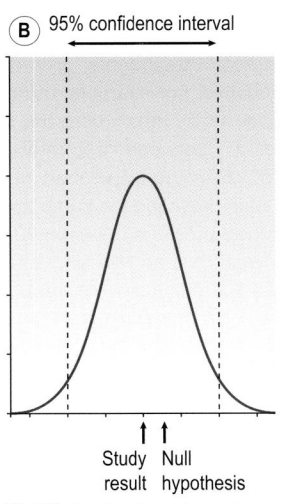

B 95% confidence interval

| Study Null | result hypothesis |

The figure illustrates a difference that is not **statistically significant**, p>0.05, because the null hypothesis value is within the 95% confidence interval of the study result. The figure illustrates a difference between the study result and the no difference (null hypothesis) value that **may not be clinically important** (because the two points are close).

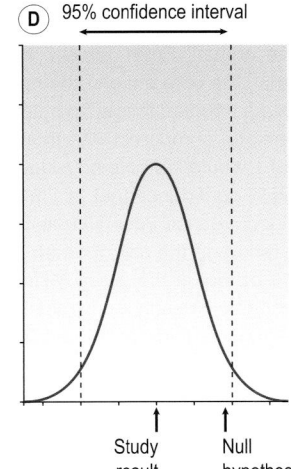

D 95% confidence interval

| Study result | Null hypothesis |

The figure illustrates a difference that is **not statistically significant**, p>0.05, because the null hypothesis value is within the 95% confidence interval of the study result. The figure illustrates a difference between the study result and the no difference (null hypothesis) value that **may, or may not be clinically important** (depending on the context).

Fig. 7.16 **Clinical and statistical significance.**

established ischaemic heart disease (IHD) do we need to treat with simvastatin for 5 years in order to avoid (or defer) one death?' In practice, this number is the inverse of the **absolute** reduction in risk. Table 7.13 uses data about deaths taken from the 4S trial, showing that this number is 30. The smaller the NNT is, the more effective the treatment.

The confidence interval for NNT from the 4S trial, however, ranges from 20 to 64. The sorts of issues that a clinician (or a public health director) with a prescribing budget might think about include:

- Does the number needed to treat (30) to avoid 1 coronary death, give sufficient benefit to *my* patients with IHD?
- From the result of the 4S trial, I will need to treat 30 patients with IHD for 5 years to prevent or avoid one death (without considering the prevalence of IHD in my area).
- Given the confidence interval, at best, I will have to treat 20 patients with IHD for 5 years to avoid, or defer, one death. At worst, it will be 64.
- Should I include the prescription of simvastatin in my treatment protocol for the secondary prevention of

ischaemic heart disease? In addition to the proven benefit of the treatment I will need to consider the increase in my prescribing budget, which will also depend on the prevalence of IHD in my population. The Health Protection Study Collaborative reported in 2006 that costs were less than £2500 per life year gained across a wide age range, which has led to the wide use of this treatment within the adult population.

Interpreting the results

Evidence of the effectiveness of treatment (or any intervention) has to be evaluated based on:

- Whether there was an effect that did not happen by chance, i.e. a reduction in the risk of death (or some other outcome of interest) in the treated group.
- How large the effect was clinically and statistically (magnitude of the difference).
- Whether the results apply to patients generally (i.e. 'my patients'), or only to a highly selected group of subjects in the experiment.
- Whether the likely benefits of the new treatment are worth the potential harms and costs.

Table 7.13   Results from 4S Trial

	Simvastatin		Placebo	
No of patients	2221		2223	
No of deaths	182		256	
Death rate (absolute risk, AR)	8.2% (experimental event rate)		11.5% (control event rate)	
				95% CI
Absolute reduction in risk (ARR)		3.3%		1.6% to 5.1%
Number needed to treat (NNT)		100 ÷ ARR = 30		20 to 64
Relative risk (RR)		8.2% ÷ 11.5% = 0.71		0.59 to 0.85
Relative risk reduction (RRR)		1 − RR = 0.29 (or 29%)		15% to 41%

Source: Scandinavian Simvastatin Survival Study Group. Randomised trial of cholesterol lowering in 4444 patients with coronary heart disease: the Scandinavian Simvastatin Survival Study (4S). Lancet 1994: 344: 1389–1399.

Tests of significance

The same statistical concepts apply to experimental studies as to observational studies (see above). From Table 7.13, showing death rates in the 4S trial, the difference in the risk of death (relative risk) within 5 years (median follow up study period) of subjects taking simvastatin compared with those taking placebo is 0.71 (a value of 1 would indicate no reduction in risk). It can be said with 95% confidence that this falls within the range of 0.58 to 0.85 (confidence interval) reflecting the 'true' relative risk. While reporting the risk of death in the simvastatin group being 0.71 of that in the group taking placebo, a more easily understandable explanation would be to say that risk was reduced by an average of 29% (1 − 0.71 = 0.29) in the simvastatin group.

The range of estimates for a confidence interval could be wide or narrow. If the confidence interval is wide, then the result is less conclusive. In the above example, if the range of values for relative risk (a ratio) included 1, then we would say that there was no statistical reduction in risk. Similarly, if in comparing the effect of two interventions and the result was expressed as a difference in rates, the range of possible differences included 0, there would be no statistical difference. This is sometimes referred to as the 'precision' of the result and the size of the sample has an effect, with larger samples giving more precise results (narrower confidence intervals).

The observed effect in a sample (a result) could happen by chance, and not as the outcome of an intervention. In the 4S trial, the probability (p) that the relative risk of 0.70 was a chance observation was 0.0003. The result was therefore highly significant, very probably related to the treatment with simvastatin, and not a chance finding.

Presenting the results

Having decided that the result of the study is statistically important, and relatively precise, there is a need to consider whether the result is clinically important enough to use the treatment generally for all patients with established coronary heart disease. Although the relative risk reduction (RRR) is more commonly cited, and here the RRR is 29%, it is worth thinking about absolute risk reduction (ARR) (Table. 7.13). In clinical terms, the reduction in the risk of death related to coronary heart disease if the patient takes simvastatin in the required dose for at least 5 years is 3.3%.

The 'numbers needed to treat' (NNT) calculation is sometimes presented as a measure of the clinical significance of the effects of intervention, and has already been discussed. The smaller number suggests more effective treatment. Comparison of NNTs for different treatments, or in different patient groups, can be educative. For example, using drugs to lower blood pressure over 18 months where the starting diastolic blood pressure is between 115 mmHg and 129 mmHg has an NNT of <5 in the prevention of death, stroke or heart attack, whereas providing the same treatment for those with a diastolic blood pressure between 90 mmHg and 109 mmHg for over 5 years has an NNT of >100.

We do not always want to refer to a risk reduction. It may be important to refer to a risk increase (where an experimental treatment is detrimental) and it may then be more appropriate to quote a number needed to harm (NNH). Other ways of wording the comparison can be used in order to express the result effectively and 'benefit' is often used instead of 'risk' in certain circumstances. Nevertheless the formulae remain the same, even though the interpretation differs.

Statistical assessment of data

There will be occasions when the data for a study do not follow a 'normal' distribution. Such data may be able to be ordered (ordinal data) or ranked. All of these data, whatever their distribution, are **quantitative** – the measurement being given in numerical format.

- **Parametric** statistical tests are done on data that follow a particular mathematical distribution. The 'normal' distribution is one such example. Statistical tests are used to compare sets of data. Parametric tests are the most powerful statistical tests because they use all of the information in the numbers.
- **Non-parametric** statistical tests are used when the data do not follow a particular distribution but can be ordered.

Some data are **qualitative**, describing, for example, the frequency of an observation within a category – **categorical data**. The frequency of particular blood groups is one such example. Sometimes it may be possible to order the categories in order to provide more detailed information. Numbers of responses within categories of pain can be better analysed if the categories are also ordered in degrees of severity.

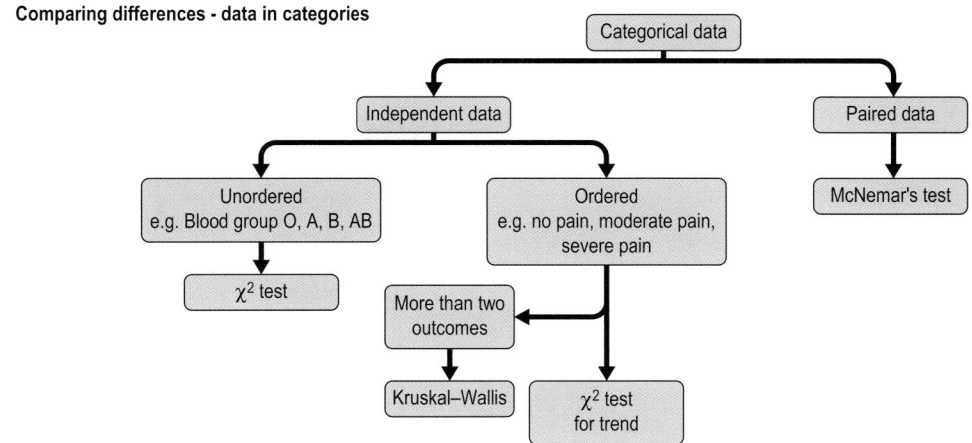

Fig. 7.17 **Statistical analysis of quantitative data.**

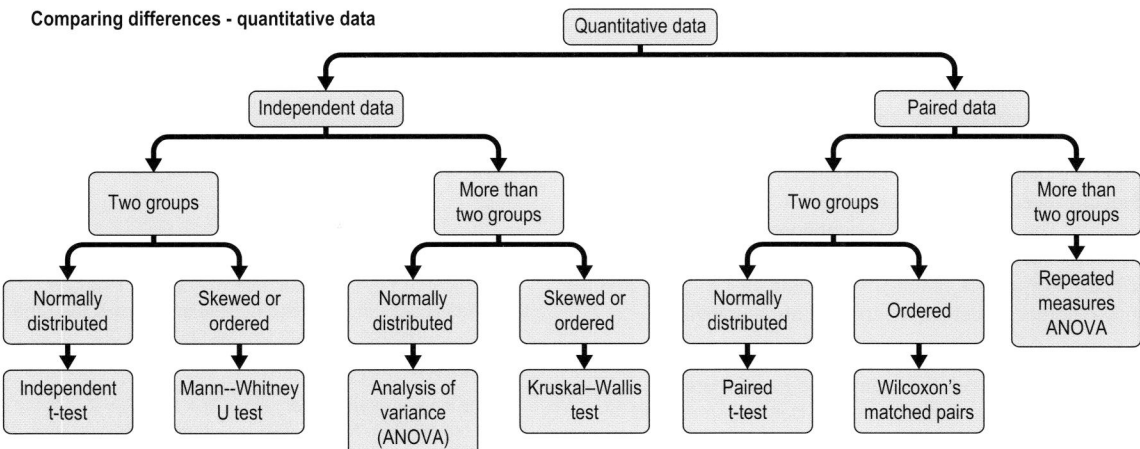

Fig. 7.18 **Statistical analysis of categorical data.**

Choosing a statistical test

Different types of data will need to be analysed by different statistical tests and the flow charts above can be used to help decide which test is the most appropriate.

Looking for differences in quantitative data
(Fig. 7.17)

- **Independent** data comes from sets of data that are not linked – for example the heights of men and women.
- **Paired (dependent)** data comes from sets of data that are linked – for example measurements of blood pressure in women, ante-natal and post-natal.

Both parametric (where the data are normally distributed) and non-parametric tests (where the data are skewed or is simply ranked) are shown in the figure. Sometimes it may be possible to mathematically transform skewed data so that parametric tests can still be used.

Statistical tests also need to be capable of being modified in order to deal with comparisons between more than two groups.

Looking for differences in categorical data
(Fig. 7.18)

Categorical data can also be independent or dependent. For example the reporting of pain in two groups, treated or untreated, would be independent, whereas the report of pain in two groups, before and after treatment, would be described as paired data, because the two measurements would be linked by coming from one person.

Looking for patterns in data (Fig. 7.19)

Sometimes we are interested in looking for patterns or associations within the data and different tests can be applied depending on the type of data. For example we may want to see if there is an association between current and past smoking, and lung cancer. Where we want to examine associations between sets of data that are continuous, for example height and weight, it is more powerful to use all of the data, rather than dividing the data into categories.

Degrees of freedom

In statistical tests of significance, such as the χ^2 test or the *t*-test, the concept of **degrees of freedom** is used. In a

Looking at relationships

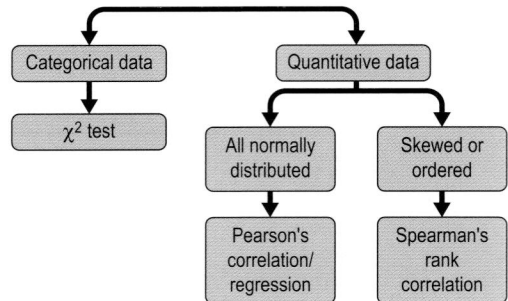

Fig. 7.19 Statistical analysis of association.

contingency table, the degree of freedom refers to the minimum number of cells in the table that need to be measured in order to complete the other cells. It is assumed that the totals for the rows and columns are known (Information box 7.24).

The t-test

A *t*-test is employed to evaluate a difference in means, and is particularly important for small samples of fewer than 30 observations, because the measured standard deviation may not be very close to the population standard deviation and hence the calculated standard error of the mean may be inaccurate. The *p* value and 95% confidence intervals calculated from *t*-tests allow for this uncertainty.

Depending on the nature of the data being compared, slightly different statistical techniques are employed:

- An **independent group *t*-test** is used if different groups are being evaluated, for example to see if there is a difference in mean blood pressure between men and women at a particular point in time and, if a difference has been observed, is that just due to chance, or is there a real difference between the two populations?
- A **paired *t*-test** is used when the individuals being observed are matched for characteristics, e.g. age, sex, or when the same individuals are observed over a period of time. For example we may be interested in whether there is a difference in blood pressure before and after dietary advice to lower blood pressure and, if a difference has been seen, is that due to chance or is the difference likely to be real?

The procedure to calculate a *t*-test will not be given here but it is useful to understand the basic principles of all statistical tests which simply contrast a summary statistic, such as a mean, with the error in that summary statistic. For example in a *t*-test:

- T-statistic = difference in means between the two groups / standard error in the difference in means.

Most statistical software can calculate the appropriate *t*-statistic much less laboriously and more accurately than by hand.

Evaluating probability for *t*-values

To look up the *p* value or to calculate the 95% confidence interval requires knowing the degrees of freedom. For the paired test it is the number of pairs minus 1, for an unpaired

---

 Information box 7.24 **An example of degrees of freedom**

This example is of fictitious data of a survey of 100 men and 100 women asking which of them would be more likely to use a particular product for cleaning carpets, to which the answers were 'yes', 'no' and 'don't know' (Table 7.14).

Assuming we know the totals in the table, we need to be told all except a minimum of any two of the numbers within the table in order to calculate the remainder. For example, in the samples of individuals questioned, if the observed numbers of 'yes' and 'no' were known, then the 'don't knows' calculated by simple subtraction must be:

Sample A : 100 − 32 − 12 = 56

Sample B : 100 − 25 − 15 = 60

We say that the table has 'two degrees of freedom'. If a table has R cells in rows and C cells in columns then the degrees of freedom (df) can be calculated from:

df = (R − 1) × (C − 1)

In the above example, df = (3 − 1) × (2 − 1) = 2

In a set of data divided into two independent groups, one would need to know all of the data except one in each group (df = 2). Where data are paired and the total known, then all of the data must be known except one data point (df = 1).

Table 7.14	Contingency table of the survey data			
Characteristic	**Answers**			**Total**
Sex	Yes	No	Don't know	
Male (A)	32	12	56	100
Female (B)	25	15	60	100
Total	57	27	116	200

---

test it is the total number of data points minus 2. For each degree of freedom, the *t*-statistic will correspond to a specific *p* value. The *p* value will be larger for the same *t*-statistic with smaller degrees of freedom.

The distribution can be shown as a graph (Fig. 7.20). The larger the degrees of freedom, the more closely does it resemble a Gaussian distribution. The *p* values are typically looked up in tables.

The *t*-distribution differs from the Gaussian or normal distribution in that the proportion of points that lie within the

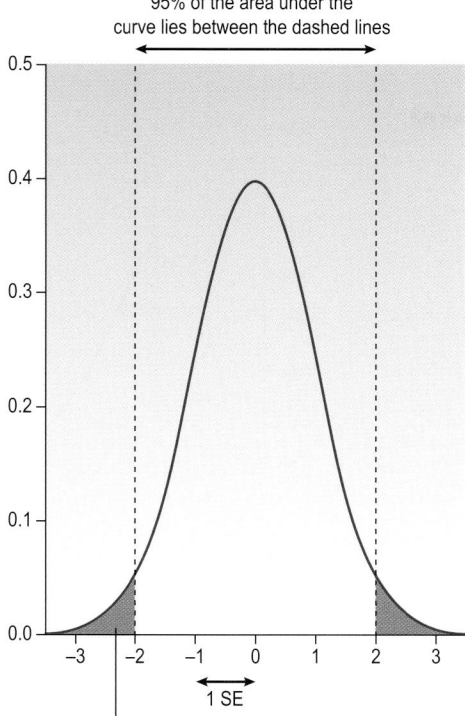

95% of the area under the curve lies between the dashed lines

1 SE

2.5% of area under the curve is found in each tail of the curve. The two 'tails', one positive and one negative, cover 5% of the distribution

Fig. 7.20 **The *t*-distribution.** The *t*-distribution is statistically derived from tables of *t*-values calculated from numerous sample means to approximate what would happen in a universal population of means. The centre, 0, is the 'true' mean. Each vertical blue line represents 1.96 standard errors from the centre (mean). The area of the curve of *t*-values within about 2 (actually 1.96) standard errors from the mean covers 95% of all means, if they were taken from samples of the universal population. The areas of the curve outside 2 standard errors are known as 'tails', covering 2.5% of all the *t*-values in each, 5% of the total.

central 95% varies according to the degrees of freedom. Hence the 95% confidence interval for results with 5 degrees of freedom would be much wider than a confidence interval of 10 degrees of freedom. The larger the study, and hence the larger the degrees of freedom, the more sure we will be about where the true value might lie within the confidence interval we have given, as that interval will increasingly narrow. When we do a *t*-test calculation and get a value for *t*, we see where the value for *t* lies on the *t* distribution for the particular degree of freedom, according to our test. The *t* distribution has a value of 0 at the centre.

The *p* value is the probability of the particular *t* value, or something further away from 0, by chance alone, if in truth there is no difference. On the *t*-distribution curve the *p* value is given by the area under the curve that is further away from the centre and beyond the *t* value. The larger the *t* value is, the further away from the centre it will lie and the smaller will be the area under the curve beyond it, and thus the lower the *p* value, or the less likely it is that what we have seen is due to chance.

When the degrees of freedom are large (above a sample size of about 30) then the *t*-distribution becomes more like the normal distribution in that 95% of all estimates of the mean will lie within the mean ± 1.96 standard errors (**the 95% confidence interval**). As we have discussed above, with smaller samples the number we need to multiply the standard error by will increase and the 95% confidence interval will increase.

Whatever the actual *t* distribution we use, a *t* value that falls into one of the two tails outside the confidence interval is unlikely to be due to chance. By convention we say that if the probability of something happening is less than 5% (*p* <0.05) then it is unlikely to be due to chance.

One- and two-tailed tests of significance

From the above discussion, it is clear that *t*-values may be positive or negative (Fig. 7.20). In a trial of the effects of a new drug for lowering blood pressure, for example, the effect could be beneficial or detrimental. As in calculating *p* values for the Gaussian distribution, we are interested in the probability of a result as extreme or more extreme in either direction, so *p* value corresponds to the proportion under the curve for values greater than +*t* and less then −*t*. This is known as a **two-tailed** test of significance and is the conventionally used approach.

Very occasionally, however, we are only interested in either a positive or negative difference in effect. For example, although we may be interested in the beneficial effects of a drug and are looking to get a large *t* value that lies within the 5% (*p* <0.05) area in one tail of the curve (a one-tailed test) then this would be equivalent to the 90% confidence interval for the two-tailed test and a lower *t* value would be needed to declare that the treatment was effective, in comparison with using a two-tailed test. There will be situations, therefore, where statistical significance could be declared using a one-sided test, but not two-sided, and this must be made clear and the significance of the result must be reported as being **one-tailed**. Rarely, however, should we be doing a one-sided test. Even though we may only be expecting beneficial effects of a drug, clearly if the drug had the opposite effect and the *t* value was in the opposite tail of the distribution, should we not think that was also important?

Criteria for applying the *t*-test

Certain criteria must be met if a *t*-test is to be used:

- The spread of the data in the two groups (the **variance**) should be similar and similarly shaped, although there are special *t*-tests for when the variances are known to be different.
- If the groups are small (degrees of freedom <15) the separate groups (in independent tests) or the differences (in paired tests) should have an approximately normal distribution. Sometimes the data are skewed (asymmetrical) but often a mathematical transformation, such as taking logs of the data and using those values in the test, will make it suitable for a *t*-test. If the data cannot be made relatively 'normal' then other tests based on the rank ordering of data should be used, such as the Mann–Whitney U test (for independent samples) and the Wilcoxon Matched Pairs test (for paired samples).

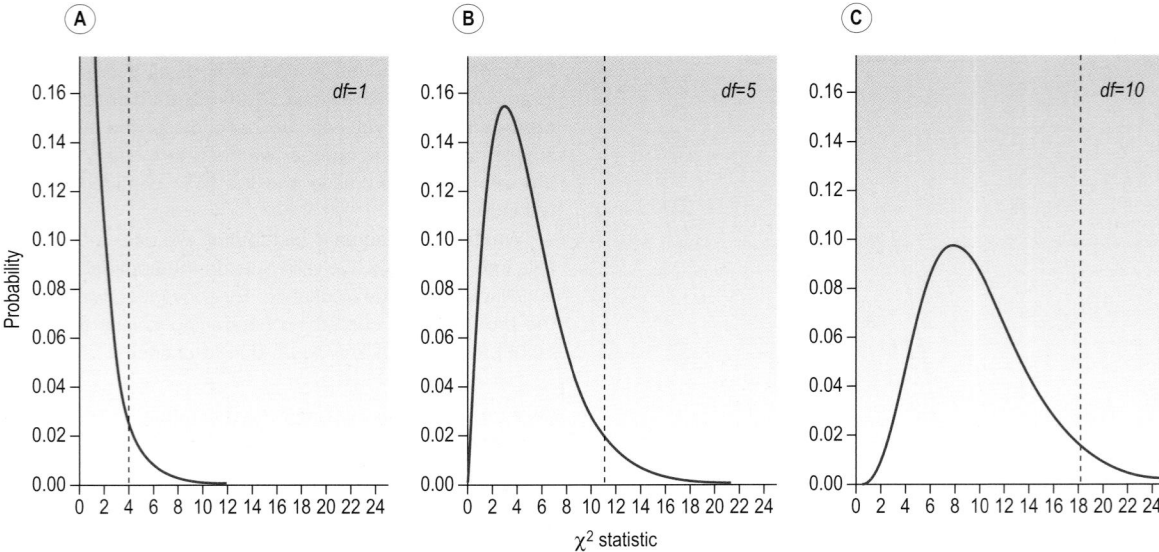

Fig. 7.21 **The χ² distribution.** (A) Data from a 2 × 2 contingency table and (B, C) data from tables with greater numbers of cells within the table. The *dashed lines* show the point on the distribution where the $p <0.05$ value lies. The area under the curve to the right of the line is 5% of the total area under the curve in each distribution. The p value is best obtained from χ² tables that show p values for different degrees of freedom. For example, from a table of the χ² distribution (A), a χ² value of 3.84 with 1 degree of freedom (shown by the *dashed line*) has a p value of 0.05 and, for any value larger than 3.84 ($p <0.05$), we can say that the distribution of numbers in the table is unlikely to have arisen by chance. A χ² value that is smaller than 3.84 will be not statistically significant ($p >0.05$). Looking up a table for χ² distributions, in part B, a χ² value of more than 11.07 with 5 degree of freedom, gives $p <0.05$, statistically significant. The degrees of freedom in any table is calculated as: df = (number of cells in rows − 1) × (number of cells in columns − 1).

■ If the samples are large, it is not necessary that the distributions are near normal, but for purposes of interpretation it is often better to use simple transformations to make the data more normal.

The χ² test

We might often be interested to see if people with particular attributes, for example having blue or brown eyes, might be differentiated in some other way, e.g. more or less likely to develop heart disease. We will need to randomly select a sample of people with blue eyes and another with brown eyes (a **predictor variable**), and then ascertain the proportions in the samples that have heart disease (an **outcome variable**). These (binary) data are best displayed in a contingency table. Such data do not follow a normal distribution curve when plotted graphically, and are said to follow the χ² distribution (Fig. 7.21). The χ² distribution is equivalent to the *t*-distribution squared so only has positive values. As the number of degrees of freedom increases it approaches the squared Gaussian distribution (see Fig. 7.20).

Even if eye colour and high blood pressure were not associated (null hypothesis), by chance there are likely to be differences in the proportions of people with heart disease in the two samples (Information box 7.25 comparing proportions). The χ² test was developed to test the null hypothesis for this type of enquiry, and is usually applied to a contingency table.

The purpose of the χ² test is to:

■ Establish whether the proportions of outcome in each category of predictor are inconsistent with each other. For example, does blood group differ by ethnicity?

■ A non-significant p value would imply that we cannot tell whether the proportions are the same or not.
■ A significant p value would imply that the proportions are unlikely to be the same in each predictor but cannot tell us which pair of groups might be different.
■ A χ² test is not appropriate if the outcome or predictor data are ordered.

There is a simple formula for calculating the follow-up value for 2 × 2 tables, but most statistical packages will also give information such as confidence intervals of differences in proportions and are therefore to be preferred.

Evaluating probability for χ² values

Once the χ² statistic has been calculated, the value is evaluated for probability at the 5% level ($p <0.05$) for statistical significance. The p values for χ² values are displayed in tables, adjusted for degrees of freedom. These are the proportions to the right of the *dashed* line shown in the χ² distribution (Fig. 7.21).

Criteria for applying the χ² test

There are certain criteria that must be met if the χ² test is to be used:

■ Each individual studied must be in one cell and only one cell.
■ Cells must contain frequencies (numbers of observations), not percentages or proportions.
■ No cell should have an expected value of less than 5 (it does not matter what the observed value is). If this condition cannot be met a **Fisher's exact test** can be used.

Information box 7.25 Comparing proportions

Quite often we will want to know whether the proportions of individuals with a particular characteristic are the same in two separate (independent) groups. For example, in a group of adolescents, 12% of those from a white European background were found to be regular smokers compared with 8% of those from an Asian background, and it would be of interest to see whether that reflects a real important difference. In order to determine this, a contingency table is drawn containing the different values. The proportional value (percentage) on its own tells you nothing about how good an estimate is and so it is essential that the table contains the actual observed numbers of people, or frequencies (O). This must be done in such a way that each individual is represented in one cell of the table only. If two characteristics in two groups are being compared, then the table will be a 2 × 2 table with four cells and marginal totals (Table 7.15). From the table it is possible to calculate the expected frequencies (E) given these values.

The proportion of regular smokers altogether in the study (the **prevalence**) is:

$(a+b)/n = 55/505 = 0.109 \ (10.9\%)$

As there are 344 White Europeans in the study, if there were **no difference** between the two racial groups we would *expect* to see, in the regular smokers' cell: 344 × 0.109 = 37.9.

The expected numbers are those given in brackets in the table, and the same reasoning can be used to work out the expected values for each of the cells. It will become evident when doing this that a simple way of thinking about the calculations is to use the formula:

Expected value (E) = [Row total ($a+b$ or $c+d$)
× column total ($a+c$ or $b+d$)]/
Overall total ($a+b+c+d$)

If there is a large difference between observed and expected values, then that would suggest that the two groups differ in respect to the characteristic under consideration (e.g. regular smoking).

For a 2 × 2 table the formula for χ^2 is:

$$\chi^2 = \Sigma \frac{(|O-E|-\frac{1}{2})^2}{E}$$

where O = observed value, E = expected value, Σ means 'sum' or add up and the '|' means make the answer positive. This is known as a χ^2 with Yates correction, which allows for the fact that the distribution is continuous, but the numbers in the cells are discrete (whole numbers). This can be translated into a formula that is easier to calculate if doing it by hand:

$$\chi^2 = \frac{N(|ad-bc|-N/2)^2}{(r_1 \times r_2 \times c_1 \times c_2)} = 1.53$$

Assuming 1 degree of freedom the p value given in a statistical table can be seen to lie between 0.1 and 0.25. Results from a statistical package, however, gives the p value more accurately at 0.22, which is clearly not significant as it is >0.05.

Table 7.15 Distribution of smoking habits in two populations

Characteristic	Group 1 White European	Group 2 Asian	Total
Present: regular smoker	42 (37.9)	13 (17.5)	55
	a	b	$a+b \ (r_1)$
Absent: non-smoker or occasional smoker	c	d	$c+d \ (r_2)$
	302 (310.1)	148 (143.5)	450
Total	344	161	505
	$a+c \ (c_1)$	$b+d \ (c_2)$	$a+b+c+d=n$

Source of data: Croghan E et al 2003 The importance of social sources of cigarettes to school students. Tobacco Control 12: 67–73.

Linear association: correlation and regression

In any investigation of the relationship between two variables it is important to produce a **scattergram** of the two measurements that usually come from an individual.

Scattergrams can show:

- Whether there is any linear relationship between the variables
- Whether a straight line can be roughly drawn between the lines
- If a more complex form, such as a curve is more appropriate.

In order to obtain valid results from the simple linear regression or correlation each data point on the scattergram must be independent (i.e. usually from separate individuals) and have the same weight (e.g. to have each point representing different sized towns would be wrong).

Correlation and regression are mathematically related but are used for different purposes.

- **Correlation** is used to measure the linear association between two variables whereas regression is used to predict one variable (**outcome** or **dependent variable**) from the other (**predictor** or **independent variable**).
- **Regression** is usually more appropriate than correlation. If we are interested in prediction, conventionally the predictor or independent variable is plotted on the x axis and the dependent or outcome variable is plotted on the y axis.

Because they are mathematically related, a correlation and linear regression on the same data points will give the same p value.

In analysing the data the **correlation coefficient** (r) measures degree, or strength, of the linear relationship between two variables, and can range from −1, where all the points lie on a straight line which slopes downwards, to 0, where there is no linear relationship at all (as in Fig. 7.22A) to + 1 where all the point are on an upward sloping line (Fig. 7.22C). It is always important to look at the distributions graphically because an apparently strong correlation may disappear once it becomes evident that this is the result of an outlier in the scattergram, or due to different subgroups within the data. **Linear regression** of an outcome or

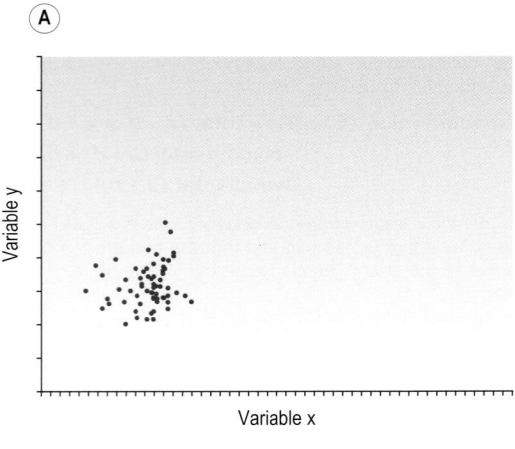

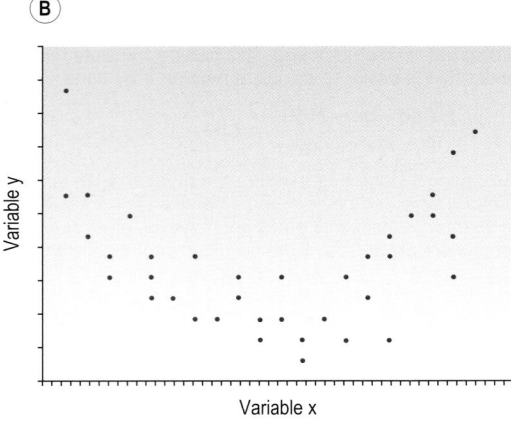

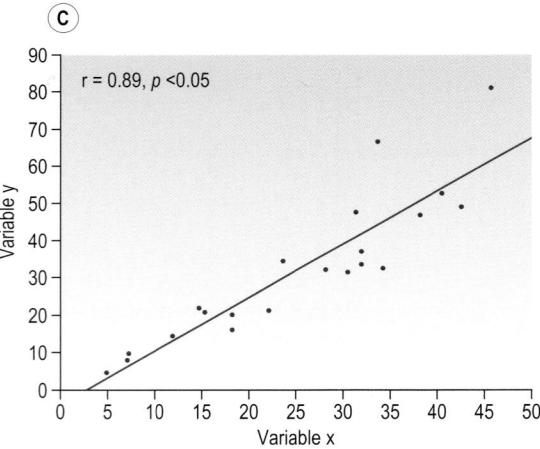

Fig. 7.22 **Various scattergrams.** (A) No linear relationship. (B) Curvilinear relationship. (C) Linear relationship. The direction of the slope indicated by the *red line* of best fit through the data shows a strong positive relationship, where as one variable increases, so does the other. In contrast, the slope for deaths from lung cancer in Figure 7.13 shows a negative relationship depending on the year of the study. The later the study, the lower the rate of death from lung cancer.

dependent variable (*y*) with a single predictor or independent variable (*x*) produces a prediction equation of the form:

$$y = a + bx$$

where *y* is the predicted value of the outcome variable, *a* is the predicted value at *x* = 0, and *b* is the predicted change in *y* for a unit change in *x* (this is the slope of the line of best fit).

Figure 7.22C is a plot of car speed on the *x* axis against particle emission in the environment from a study in an urban area of London and shows that particle emission increases as the average car speed increases. From the graph it is possible to read off an average speed and predict what the environmental pollution is likely to be. This estimate is likely to be useful in health outcome planning in the future.

Statistical packages will give confidence intervals for *b* and its associated *p* value. The null hypothesis is that *y* does not change with *x* and hence *b* = 0 (the best fit line will be horizontal, or not significantly different from the horizontal). In the case of Figure 7.22C we can see that *y* does change with *x* and $p < 0.05$.

Logistic regression is a useful method of statistical analysis used widely for studies. It is used where the outcome is binary, e.g. dead or alive, or got the disease or not. The results are given as **odds ratios** and the predictors can be binary or numeric. In the former case the odds ratio could be of death if male rather than female, and in the latter the odds ratio would be of death given a unit change in, for example, a biochemical test result. **Conditional logistic regression analysis** is similar but takes account of paired data, and is therefore commonly used in case–control studies. It also adjusts for the situation where there is more than one control for a case, but not every case has the same number of controls.

Multivariate analysis

When investigating observational data, we are often interested in more than one predictor of outcome. Usually it is already known that one or more factors may be associated with the outcome (age and sex are obvious examples), and if they are also associated with the predictor as well then they could confound the results by either masking or exaggerating them.

If we use only **univariate** analysis, for example for investigating whether alcohol might have a causal association with lung cancer, the positive and statistically significant association that we are likely to find, while being correct, will probably be inaccurate in terms of predicting the effect of changing the prevalence of alcohol use on the risk of contracting lung cancer. In other words, reducing alcohol consumption only in the population is unlikely to reduce, or significantly reduce, the risk of getting lung cancer. This is because alcohol use and lung cancer are each **independently** associated with smoking (the definition of a **confounding factor**). Including both alcohol use and smoking in a **multivariate** analysis will give us the effect of alcohol after adjustment for smoking (the alcohol effect will probably be weak or non-existent and not significant), and this will reflect better the (limited) causal effect of alcohol on lung cancer.

■ In cohort studies, age and gender are usually adjusted for as they both are generally associated with risk of death or with being diagnosed with a specific disease and they may also be associated with potential risk factors.

■ In case–control studies, where cases and controls are often matched according to age and gender, any factors that are matched for will not be considered in the analysis. Thought has to be given to what factors may need to be included and therefore measured in the studies.

INVESTIGATION BY REVIEW

A review of a series of experiments is productive, not only because it gives credence to a single, apparently beneficial, treatment, but also because it can be a device for accumulating evidence over time and revealing effective treatments where individual studies had not been so convincing. In order to be sure that the review is free from bias it must be systematic in nature, the principle being to have a systematic and unbiased methodology to collect and evaluate all the available evidence, both published and unpublished.

The Cochrane Collaboration consists of a network of interested parties with a commitment to prepare systematic reviews of the evidence produced by RCTs. The collaboration is named in memory of the epidemiologist, Archie Cochrane, whose forward-thinking idea it was in the 1970s. In 1979 he stated 'It is surely a great criticism of our profession that we have not organised a critical summary, by specialty or subspecialty, adapted periodically, of all relevant randomised controlled trials.' The collaboration began publication in 1993, forming the *Cochrane Library*, which includes the *Cochrane Database of Systematic Reviews*.

Meta-analysis

The Cochrane logo was developed from a systematic review, published in 1989, of trials of corticosteroids given to women at risk of giving birth prematurely (Fig. 7.23). Between 1972 and 1982, seven RCTs had been published. Figure 7.23 shows the results obtained in each study. Only two show a statistically significant effect (because the confidence interval does not cross the no effect line, where the odds are equal to one), but combining of information from all the studies increased the power and provided a significant effect estimate, the uncertainty of the combined measure being shown by the diamond at the base of the graph. The statistical method used to produce the combined effect is called a **meta-analysis**.

Cumulative meta-analysis

The review of treatment over time can be followed by constructing a cumulative meta-analysis, and can help avoid the continuation of RCTs where there is sufficient evidence of an effect. An early example, published by Antman and his colleagues examined 33 trials of the effect of intravenous streptokinase on death of people in hospital after a heart attack. These trials had been carried out over a period of time from 1959 to 1988, during which about 37 000 individuals had been randomised to receive streptokinase or a placebo (or no treatment).

Only six of the 33 trials reached statistical significance in favour of streptokinase but the meta-analysis (Fig. 7.24) revealed a highly significant odds ratio that was less than 1, reflecting an approximate 20% reduction in risk of death for those on treatment in comparison with those not given streptokinase. Had a cumulative analysis been done as each study was published, the meta-analysis would have revealed a statistically significant difference ($p < 0.05$) as early as 1971 when around only 1000 individuals had been randomised, and would have reached $p < 0.01$ two years later after a total of only 2500 individuals had been randomised. This has major ethical implications since about 35 000 patients had been unnecessarily randomised, of whom about half would

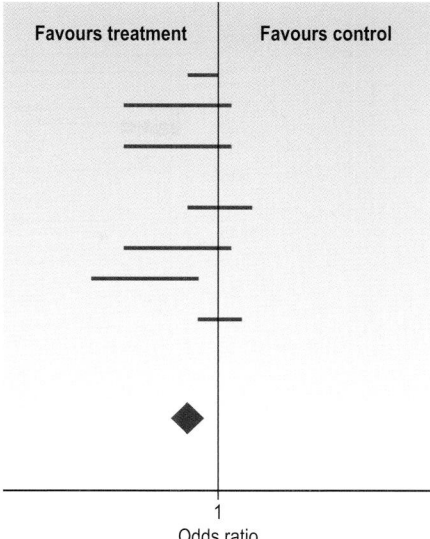

Fig. 7.23 **Systematic review of the first seven trials investigating the use of corticosteroids to reduce risk of infant death from complications of giving birth too early.** The horizontal line at the base shows the odds ratio scale with a vertical line being where the odds are equal to one (1 : 1, or no difference between treatment and control). The individual horizontal lines depict the 95% confidence intervals for the treatment effect for each of the seven published studies. Source: Crowley P et al. 1990 The effects of corticosteroid administration before preterm delivery: an overview of the evidence from controlled trials. British Journal of Obstetrics and Gynaecology 97:11–25.

not have had a treatment that would have reduced their risk of death by about 20%. Possibly an additional 3500 individuals died as a result of this lack of a cumulative review. Even after the meta-analysis was published, randomised trials of thrombolytic therapy continued for some time.

Experiment or review?

Studies that are small in size run the risk of producing a false negative conclusion, suggesting that a treatment is of no value because the study was not powerful enough to detect a difference. The meta-analysis makes use of these underpowered experiments to improve the power by considering the totality of the evidence. In around 10% of comparisons, conclusions based on the results of meta-analysis sometimes appear at odds with those looking at the same question but undertaken in large, sufficiently powered, clinical trials.

Differences between reviews and RCTs

There are several possible reasons for conflicting findings from systematic reviews and randomised clinical trials, some real and some spurious. One difficulty is **publication bias**, where published trials may not truly be representative of the truth since journals are more likely to publish those with statistically significant results, and leading journals may be more likely to publish those where the results differ from before. On the other hand, single large clinical trials are probably not as representative of the whole population as a large collection of small clinical trials. Sometimes the criticism that the

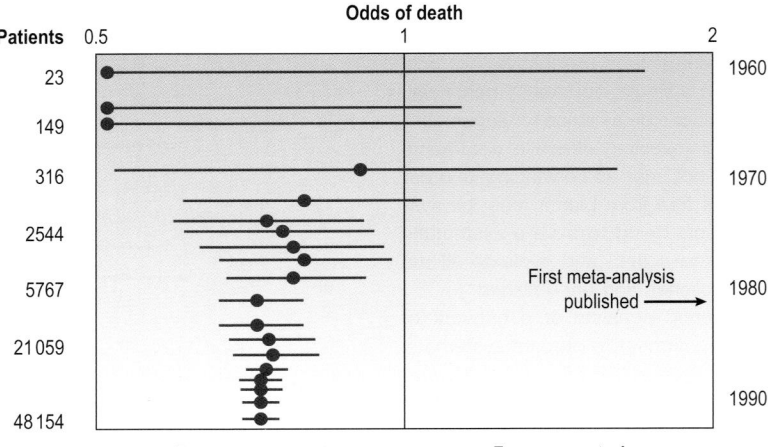

Fig. 7.24 **Cumulative meta-analysis of thrombolytic therapy.** Source: Lau J et al 1992 Cumulative meta-analysis of therapeutic trials for myocardial infarction. New England Journal of Medicine 327:248–254.

two methods are producing different results has been simply based on the fact that one method detects a statistical difference, while the other does not, when in fact the point estimates of effect measured in the two methods are very similar.

Other differences may be related to differences in the populations in the two methodological groups. Der Simonian and colleagues in 1999 looked at differences in recommendation for calcium supplementation in pre-eclampsia (characterised by high blood pressure, protein in urine and oedema, seen in the second and third trimesters of pregnancy) between a meta-analysis and a subsequent large clinical trial, the latter suggesting that there was no benefit to treatment. The clinical trial was undertaken in healthy women and when the trials involved in the meta-analysis were stratified according to risk, those at low risk also showed no treatment benefit, like the clinical trial, but a definite benefit was observed among the high-risk groups. Thus, what appeared to be a contradiction at first was due to a difference in the populations being studied.

What best evidence is

While both the clinical trial and meta-analysis are perceived as being the best forms of evidence, because of their methodological design focusing on the intervention of interest and avoidance of biases, it is important to remember that, in the best of all possible worlds, a clinical trial is always likely to be more convincing than the truth. People who consent to take part in a clinical trial are likely to be different from those who do not, and because this is an experiment, they are more likely to be compliant in undertaking their assigned treatment.

HEALTH EDUCATION AND PROMOTION

As well as doing the best for patients with disease (effective interventions), medical students and doctors in the twenty-first century need to understand the principles of disease prevention and the natural history of diseases to effectively

practise the art of clinical medicine. An important role for doctors (and all health professionals) is in providing patients with information and support that enables them to make appropriate choices for either staying healthy or to be restored to an approximation of their previous state of health. Choices for making changes in behaviour and lifestyle may be necessary. It must, however, be remembered that the decision to make changes is for the patient to make, and their ability to change depends not only on their motivation and their individual skills, but also on their environment. However well motivated an individual is, it is more difficult to follow a healthy lifestyle if they have an inadequate income, poor housing and work in a dangerous environment. The aim in providing health education is to help people to understand what is at stake and take control over decisions that affect their health, not simply providing information and expecting a change in behaviour.

Clinical medicine concerns the understanding of how a disease progresses and how best to treat a person who has already developed the disease, whereas epidemiology tries to identify the factors that contribute to the development of the disease, its causes, and how to prevent it. Epidemiology also addresses the likely consequences of a disease process, the complications, in order to understand how these may be avoided or minimised for people who have developed the condition. Thus prevention is about reducing the risk of disease, illness, injury or disability. Services include immunisation and screening, preventive health education, such as advice about sensible drinking, and preventive health protection, such as legislation for compulsory car seat belts, taxing tobacco and fluoridating water.

HEALTH EDUCATION

Agencies involved in health education include government, schools, local health promotion units and the media. For the doctor, the areas in which health education is most likely to be relevant are where there is evidence from epidemiological studies that particular diseases can be avoided, that the risk of developing a condition in a particular individual may be reduced, or that the risk of complications in a particular disease can be reduced by a particular action.

Approaches to health education

Three approaches to health education are often described:

- Disease orientated
- Risk-factor orientated
- Health orientated.

In disease-orientated health education there is a focus on a particular disease, e.g. cardiovascular disease, and the action is focused on the risk factors, e.g. providing dietary advice. There is often an overlap in risk factors for many types of disease (e.g. smoking for coronary heart disease and lung cancer) in this approach, and it reflects the perspective of the healthcare provider. The expert (the doctor) focuses on an area of expertise (disease) and imparts information to the patient. This focus also emphasises the prevention of disease rather than promotion of health. An alternative approach is to focus attention and action on risk factors rather than on the associated disease, for example focusing on smoking as a risk factor for carcinoma of the lung and coronary heart disease. This process recognises that single risk factors can be linked to more than one disease and therefore there is less duplication. But the approach is still from the expert's perspective and the emphasis is again on disease prevention rather than health promotion.

The health-orientated approach focuses attention and action on behaviours that contribute to positive health and prevent ill-health. For example, it can be pointed out that a healthy diet can be enjoyable, contributing to well-being in a positive way rather than just being a way of preventing diseases. On any occasion when there is interaction and communication with patients, some, or all, of the above approaches may be called into play.

Strategies for disease prevention and health promotion

There are two possible strategies for disease prevention and health promotion. The population strategy aims to reduce the risk of the whole population, usually by public health measures. The high-risk strategy focuses on the individual who is considered to be at high risk.

Population strategies

The rationale behind the population strategy is that the bulk of the morbidity and mortality of a disease in a population is contributed by those who have a moderate degree of risk. For example, the British Regional Heart Study about 'Who dies in a heart attack?' published in 1995 found that 60% of middle-aged British men have elevated total cholesterol levels, which carries at least a twofold risk of major coronary heart disease. Only one-third of all the heart attacks, however, occur in the 20% of men with the highest level of cholesterol. The most effective way, therefore, of reducing morbidity and mortality from heart disease would be to lower the population mean cholesterol level, thus reducing the risk of the majority. In the case of cholesterol this would be mainly by dietary means, by reducing the proportion of calories from saturated fat. This is most likely to be achieved by public health measures such as general health education, food and pricing policy, labelling of foods and so on.

Another example of a population strategy is the reduction of alcohol-related morbidity and mortality. Reducing the number of people drinking at moderate risk levels (14–35 units/week in women and 21–50 units/week in men) would have a greater effect than identifying and offering treatment to those drinking at harmful levels (>35 units/week for women >50 units/week for men).

High-risk strategy

While public health measures – dietary recommendations, raising the taxes on cigarettes and alcohol – are the most effective population strategies at a national level, the high-risk individual approach comes more naturally to the clinician. This approach aims to identify and treat individuals with a high risk of developing a disease (for example, those with familial hypercholesterolaemia, individuals with high alcohol consumption). A combination of these two approaches is often the case, so that 'healthy eating' advice is given to everybody (through the media, schools and in primary care) together with screening and, when indicated, specific treatment (e.g. with lipid-lowering drugs) of those at particularly high risk.

Two concepts of 'risk'

A risk factor may be thought of as a factor that has been shown to have a **causal** association with a disease. For example:

- Cigarette smoking has a strong causal association with lung cancer (see above). Reducing this risk, by quitting smoking, reduces the 'risk 'of this individual developing lung cancer.

Alternatively, characteristics of an individual that may be **prognostic** markers for an increased likelihood to develop a disease are 'risk' factors that identify a person as being at high 'risk' for a disease.

- A middle-aged man who leads a sedentary life, is overweight, has a family history of coronary heart disease and smokes 30 cigarettes a day has a higher risk of coronary heart disease than a woman of similar age, but with none of the other characteristics. These factors, or a combination of factors, could be used for screening to identify individuals who would or would not have a coronary event within the next 5 years.

These two concepts of 'risk' should not be confused, nor are they interchangeable. Some risks, e.g. tobacco smoking, alcohol consumption, are modifiable, whereas others, e.g. genetic makeup, age, sex, are not modifiable.

Essentials for effective health education

Health education involves exchanging (not just giving) information between patient and doctor. This means that there must be good and effective communication between the patient and the person involved in providing health education. Effective communication – using the skills of active listening, open questioning and picking up verbal and non-verbal cues – is essential. Tuckett in 1985 provided evidence that patients' recall of information given during a consultation is significantly improved if some simple rules are followed. When talking to patients about health education information and giving advice on healthcare, the following check list could be helpful:

- Find out what the patient already knows (may be inaccurate)
- Use short words and short sentences
- Organise the information into clear categories
- Give instructions and advice early in the interview
- Stress the importance of the advice and the instructions you give
- Check patient understanding
- Repeat the advice during the course of the interview
- Give specific advice.

Besides using good communication skills, it is essential when giving information to ensure that there is an exchange of information and ideas between patient and educator. A **health education interview** can be conveniently divided into four phases:

- **Elicit** the person's health beliefs.
- **Information phase**: this is a two-way process with the educator seeking information from the patient and at the same time providing information.
- **Negotiating phase**: if the patient decides to make a change, an achievable and realistic target must be discussed, choices offered and action agreed. The desirability for continued support is then discussed.
- **Promote change**: ways of promoting change include support from family and friends, ways in which the individual recognises the achievement by rewarding him/herself, and perhaps general changes in lifestyle.

Studies have shown that reinforcing the verbal advice with appropriate written material helps the patient to retain information and make choices. Health education resources, such as leaflets and DVDs, are usually available from local health promotion units.

Ethical considerations in prevention and health promotion

A detailed discussion of the ethics of prevention is beyond the scope of this chapter. Remember that in prevention, just as in the treatment of disease, we have a duty to:

- Ensure that the benefit of any procedure outweighs any possible harm to the patient
- Respect the patient's autonomy
- Distribute our resources fairly.

Furthermore, as will be seen from the section on screening, identifying people as being 'at risk' of a condition when there is no effective treatment for the condition is unethical. It is extremely important to follow these basic ethical principles in preventive activities when it is usually the health professional, rather than the patient, who initiates the activity.

Case scenario: a new diagnosis of diabetes

Mr Tate comes to see you, highly embarrassed because of an itchy rash around his genitalia, which turns out to be *Candida* infection. He is aged 51, married, with a daughter at university and a son in his final year at secondary school. He has worked in a warehouse since his early twenties. You find that he has developed type 2 diabetes with no detectable complications; he is moderately obese with a body mass index (BMI) of 32 (see Ch. 16), but his blood pressure is normal. His fasting cholesterol is raised at 6.8 mmol/L (desirable <5.2 mmol/L) with triglycerides of 2.8 mmol/L (desirable <2.3 mmol/L). He does not smoke, and only drinks moderately on social occasions. You decide to try him on diet alone for glycaemic control.

Elicit the person's health beliefs

You discover that Mr Tate's mother died of a heart attack when she was 64 years old, and she was diabetic. On enquiry, he tells you that he thinks diabetes is something to do with sugar in the blood. His mother had taken tablets for her sugar for many years, but from about her mid-fifties, she had high blood pressure and trouble with her eyesight. You find that he is very anxious and upset about the diagnosis of diabetes, afraid that he might also have a heart attack or lose his eyesight.

Information phase

You ask if Mr Tate knows how his mother managed her medication and if he understands how they worked. He tells you that he had no idea of how she really managed her condition other than having to take different sorts of tablets, and he is worried that the tablets may not be effective.

Explanation of the diagnosis

You explain to Mr Tate that he is correct to think that diabetes is to do with sugar in the blood. It is characterised by persistently high levels, which can lead to complications by damaging other organs in the body. This is caused by a relative deficiency of, or resistance to, insulin, the hormone that regulates sugar metabolism. Diabetes also runs in families. Much of the longer-term complications of diabetes is related to the increased risk of atherosclerosis leading to hardening and narrowing of relatively large (macrovascular disease) and very small (microvascular disease) arteries. These in turn could result in coronary heart disease (macrovascular) and damage to the vessels in the eye (diabetic retinopathy, microvascular) as may have happened to Mr Tate's mother. There is also a risk of damage to kidney tissues, which could lead to high blood pressure. Mr Tate has normal blood pressure, which is very good news.

Information

It is, however, important to remember that these complications can be avoided, or at least minimised, by keeping the blood sugar levels within normal limits and keeping a very close eye on Mr Tate's blood pressure. The type of diabetes that Mr Tate has is known as non-insulin dependent and can be treated with diet alone, or medication to lower his sugar levels. He does not smoke, which is another risk factor for heart disease and high blood pressure, and only drinks alcohol (a risk factor for hypertension) occasionally in moderation, although his cholesterol is a little high. It may only be necessary, therefore, to use dietary control to get his weight down, to keep his blood sugar within normal limits and to bring his cholesterol down to desirable levels.

Negotiating phase

You ask Mr Tate to describe the meals that he takes on an average day. He has always had a good cooked breakfast as his work is physically quite hard. His wife usually cooks bacon and two eggs, sometimes with a sausage or two, and of course toast and marmalade. She also does a packed lunch of three rounds of sandwiches, usually with cold meat of some sort and a large flask of sweet tea to keep his energy up. The evening meal is usually meat with two vegetables, although lately she has taken to grilling the meat and using 'oven chips' instead of frying, which is supposed to be less fattening. She makes a dessert only for lunch on Sundays since the children have grown up, and she is trying to lose a bit of weight herself. He tells you that they have only full cream milk in the house as he dislikes semi-skimmed milk.

Information

You tell Mr Tate that the main principles of healthy diet for diabetes include:

- Low sugar intake (although not sugar free), sugar-free drinks
- High intake of starchy carbohydrates (up to 50% of total energy) which are slowly absorbed, e.g. pasta, long-grain rice, wholemeal bread, cereals such as oats, pulses, fruit
- High intake of dietary fibre, to include five portions of fruit and vegetables per day. This helps to smooth the post-prandial peaks in blood glucose
- Low intake of dietary fat, particularly saturated fat.

Mr Tate should try to reduce salt intake and avoid special 'diabetic' food, which may be expensive and is not of any real benefit. You also refer him to a specialist dietitian for further advice, and draw his attention to the website for Diabetes UK, advising him that they have excellent information on diabetes. He should also see the nurse for monitoring his blood glucose and weight, and be taught how to monitor his sugar himself. You suggest that Mr Tate should try to lose 0.5 kg per week until you see him again.

You understand that there is a great deal to take in, and think about. Mr Tate wants to discuss all this with his wife, and also talk to his daughter, who is studying nutrition at university. You arrange to see him again in four weeks.

Promoting change

Mr Tate comes with his wife on the next appointment. You are very interested in how he is getting on. He tells you that the nurse has weighed him, he has lost 3 kg, his sugar is normal and so is his blood pressure. He is learning to keep a diary for self-monitoring. You congratulate him, and enquire how he is getting on, and is his wife also coping? Mrs Tate had been to see the dietitian with her husband, and they later talked over the difficulties of changing their eating habits with their daughter. Breakfast now consists of porridge (oats) and fruit, and only skimmed milk is used in the house. Lunch is two sandwiches, but made with wholemeal bread and a low-fat spread, and tea with no sugar, and also an apple and a banana. They have reduced their intake of red meat to twice per week, with more fish and chicken. Although they are finding it very hard to give up butter, most of the cooking is done with oil. It is taking a little time to get used to this, but they are getting there. The most difficult part has been with shopping, as the labels on the supermarket shelves are confusing about food values. Mrs Tate produced some food labels and asks your advice. You are very pleased to advise her (see Ch. 16).

PREVENTION

Preventive measures can be taken at different stages of a disease, often classified as **primary**, **secondary** or **tertiary**. This classification has been criticised on the grounds that it focuses on disease and includes a consideration of treatment, and also that there is no standard definition of the terms primary, secondary and tertiary. For example, the term secondary prevention is sometimes used to describe interventions that aim to prevent reoccurrence of an illness, such as the use of aspirin after myocardial infarction. All classifications draw boundaries that at times seem artificial, but they are useful as long as the reservations are borne in mind; the classification of prevention is no exception to this. Other terms that have been used with reference to prevention are health promotion, health education, health protection, emphasising the dual role of preventing ill health and promoting positive health.

Primary prevention

Primary prevention includes all activities aiming to remove the cause of disease in individuals, or to reduce the susceptibility of the individual to the causative agent. Some are general social or economic measures that may be part of national strategy. The example of the Broad Street pump led to the national public health policy of clean water, thereby removing a major cause for the transmission of infectious diseases. Although a direct link between environmental, social and economic determinants of health and specific diseases is difficult to demonstrate, and may not be amenable to medical intervention, government policies to reduce poverty, improve housing conditions, living standards and nutrition are important strategies for reducing the risk of mortality and morbidity in vulnerable population groups.

Current examples of primary prevention are:

- Immunisation programmes
- Legislation by Parliament (e.g. car seat belts) and fiscal policies (e.g. increased taxation of tobacco and alcohol)
- Helping patients to avoid coronary heart disease and to promote their well-being, e.g. providing dietary advice, sensible drinking, how to stop smoking
- Promoting information to patients about the appropriate use of health service resources; for example, giving advice about childhood immunisation, or about influenza vaccination for older people during the winter months.

Immunisation

The discovery of the cowpox vaccine by Edward Jenner in the early 1800s led to the widespread use of vaccination to prevent and eradicate infectious diseases by reducing individuals' susceptibility to the infecting agent. Compulsory vaccination against smallpox was introduced by British governments from the mid-nineteenth century onwards through Acts of Parliament. Although immunisation programmes are taken for granted in developed and developing countries, the original laws were seen as a violation of civil liberty and later changed to voluntary immunisation.

The World Health Organization (WHO) used a strategy of surveillance and containment to control smallpox. Reporting of cases elicited a reward and suspected cases were isolated while known contacts in the previous 2 weeks were traced and vaccinated. WHO declared the world free of smallpox in 1980.

Immunisation is an example of primary prevention where the aim is to eliminate the risk of the infectious disease in the individual occurring through reducing the susceptibility of the whole population. The WHO set out the aims of eliminating polio, diphtheria, tetanus in the newborn, measles and congenital rubella by the year 2000. To achieve this, all chil-

Table 7.16	Mortality and incidence of infectious diseases in the UK before and after introduction of an immunisation policy					
	Last year of no immunisation			**After immunisation**		
Disease	**Year**	**Deaths (all ages)**	**No of cases**	**Year**	**Deaths (all ages)**	**No of cases**
Diphtheria	1939	2133	47061	1996	0	12
Tuberculosis	1952	10590	48093	1996	420	5859
Whooping cough	1956	92	92410	1996	2	2387
Tetanus (not notifiable until 1968)	1960	32	?	1996	0	8
Measles	1967	99	460407	1996	0	5613
Congenital rubella syndrome	1971	–	162	1996	–	21
Haemophilus influenzae meningitis	1991	22	417	1996	0	38

Source: Immunisation against infectious disease 2006. By Joint Committee on Vaccination and Immunisation, D Salisbury, M Ramsay, Great Britain: Department of Health, K Noakes. The Stationery Office, London.

dren (at least 95%) needed to receive the appropriate vaccine before the age of 2. The European Region was certified free of poliomyelitis in 2002, at which time it had been free of indigenous poliomyelitis for over 3 years. Europe's last case of indigenous wild poliomyelitis occurred in eastern Turkey in 1998, when a 2-year-old unvaccinated boy was paralysed by the virus. To sustain this status of being free of indigenous infection, maintenance of immunisation, surveillance and the ability to respond to imported virus are essential. The best way of ensuring a polio-free Europe would be to reduce the susceptibility of children to poliomyelitis worldwide.

The efficacy of vaccination is shown in Table 7.16, which illustrates the reduction in mortality and incidence of infectious diseases after the introduction of immunisation.

Public perception and immunisation coverage

A combined vaccination for measles, mumps and rubella (MMR) was introduced in 1988, resulting in significant reduction in the incidence of these diseases. Table 7.17 shows the rate of serious complications of these diseases.

In the 1970s, there was a loss of confidence in the whooping cough vaccine, when it was suggested that the vaccine was a significant cause of brain damage. As a result there were three major whooping cough epidemics; there were over 300000 disease notifications, a large number of children were admitted to hospital and an estimated 100 died unnecessarily. More recently, there were concerns over a possible association between the MMR vaccine, autism and bowel problems. MMR is given routinely to babies aged between 12 and 15 months, with a pre-school booster to increase coverage and protection. Reports of an association between the measles virus and Crohn's disease (a chronic inflammatory bowel disease), and between MMR and autism (associated with intestinal symptoms), has led to widespread public concern over the vaccination policy. While the bulk of the reported evidence is against a causal association in either case, this has not prevented the decision by some parents not to vaccinate their children with MMR, or choosing to have the vaccines given separately, spaced over 1 year.

There is considerable public health concern over the reluctance of parents to allow their children to be vaccinated, or vaccinated on time, because, once immunisation rates fall below 75%, community outbreaks of MMR will occur, along with the serious complications reported in Table 7.17.

Primary prevention of coronary heart disease

The Joint British Societies' evidence based guideline (JBS 2) on the prevention of cardiovascular disease was published

Table 7.17	Serious complications of measles, mumps and rubella	
Disease	**Complication**	**Incidence**
Measles	Ear infection	1 in 20
	Pneumonia/bronchitis	1 in 25
	Convulsion	1 in 200
	Diarrhoea	1 in 6
	Hospital admission	1 in 100
	Meningitis/encephalitis	1 in 1000
	SSPE	1 in 8000 under 2 years
	Death	1 in 2500–5000
Mumps	Painful testicles in older males	1 in 5
	Central nervous system symptoms: meningitis/encephalitis	1 in 200
	Pancreatitis	1 in 5000
	Deafness (with full or partial recovery)	1 in 30
	Spontaneous abortion	1 in 25
Rubella	Encephalitis	1 in 6
	Bleeding disorders	1 in 3
	Joint symptoms	
	Spontaneous abortion	
	Congenital rubella syndrome resulting in babies born with:	
	■ Deafness	
	■ Blindness	
	■ Heart problems	
	■ Brain damage	
	■ Other serious problems	

Source of data: MMR fact sheets 1–4, Department of Health 2002. Crown Copyright.
SSPE, sub-acute sclerosing pan encephalitis (a rare degenerative neurological disorder developing some years after measles infection, causing brain damage and resultant death).

in 2005 and offers the current best advice on coronary heart disease prevention. Their priorities are to focus on healthy individuals who are at high risk of developing coronary heart disease or other major atherosclerotic disease and they have produced 'Coronary Risk Charts' that can assess the risk of developing coronary heart disease over the next 10 years using information about an individual's gender, age, smoking status, whether they are diabetic or not, systolic blood pressure and total cholesterol (Fig. 7.25).

High risk strategy for the prevention of coronary heart disease

At every level of risk the total coronary heart disease risk of a diabetic patient is much higher than that of a comparable non-diabetic and separate risk charts are available for these

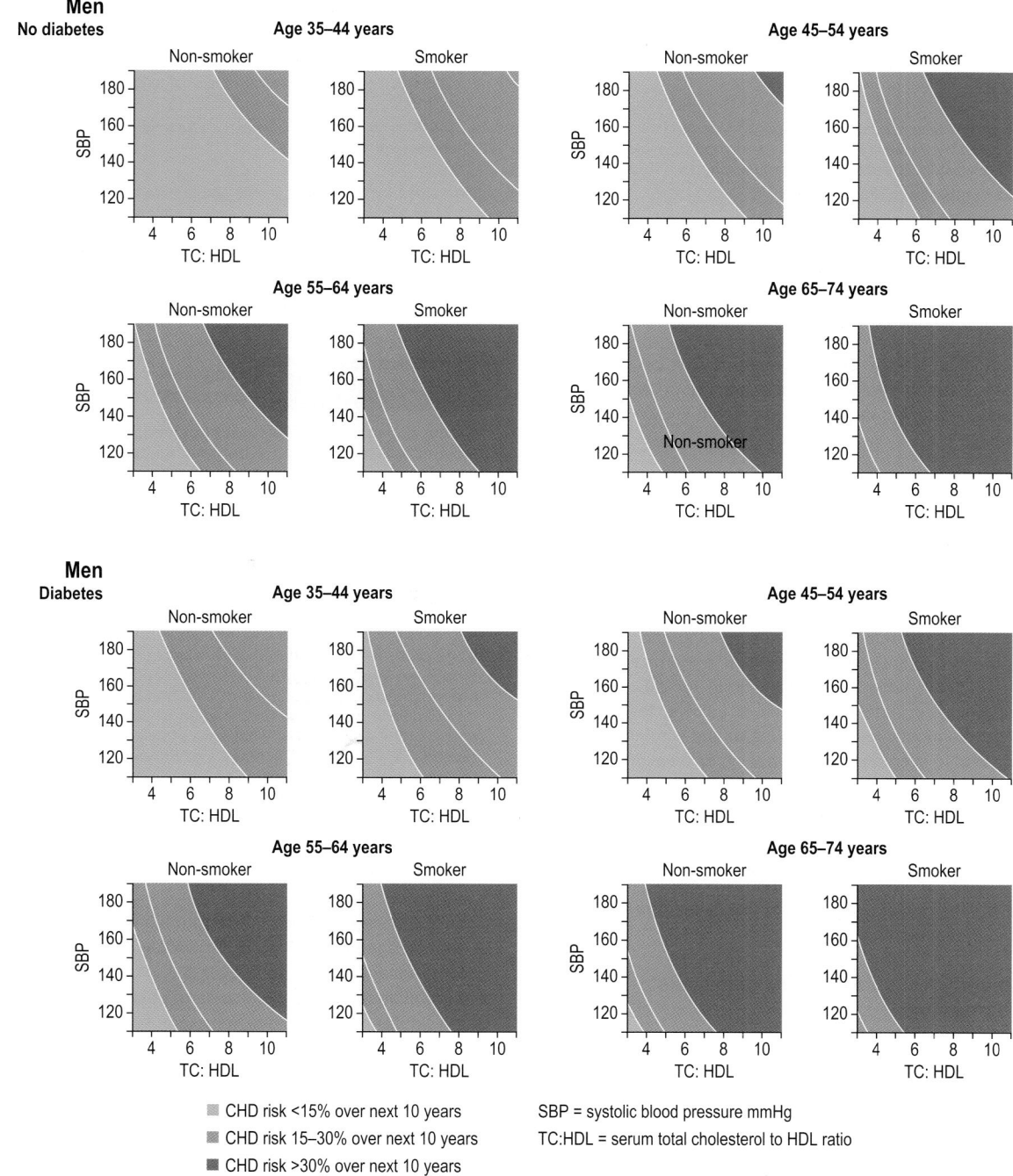

Fig. 7.25 **Chart for calculating risk of coronary heart disease.** © University of Manchester.

patients. Where the absolute risk for an individual is judged to be more than 20% over the next 10 years then intensive risk factor modification is recommended including, where appropriate, proven drug therapies. Lifestyle interventions, such as stopping smoking, making healthier food choices and becoming physically active, are particularly important in this context (Table 7.18).

Secondary prevention

Secondary prevention concerns the detection and treatment of disease before symptoms or disordered function develops, or before irreversible organ damage occurs as the consequence of the disease process. The possibility of being able to detect and treat pre-symptomatic disease and thus prevent or at least reduce morbidity and mortality has, in the past, generated considerable enthusiasm.

The finding of hidden morbidity among the people screened at the Peckham (London, UK) pioneer health centre, and the description by Last in 1963, provided the impetus to an expansion of screening activities. Last used epidemiological methods to estimate the expected numbers of individuals with particular conditions within an average general practice and compared these numbers with actual numbers known to the practitioners. Last referred to the diseases being picked up by general practitioners as being only the 'tip of the iceberg'. Screening is perhaps the best example of secondary prevention, with different programmes

Table 7.18	Lifestyle and therapy goals for healthy individuals at high risk of coronary heart disease (CHD)
Definition of a healthy person at high risk of CHD	Absolute risk of 20% or more over 10 years, or over 20% risk if projected to age 60
Lifestyle change goals	Stop smoking; healthy food choices; increased physical activity; achieve ideal weight
Other desirable risk factor changes. If these are not achieved by the lifestyle changes then blood pressure and cholesterol lowering drug therapies should be used	Blood pressure <140/90 mmHg; total cholesterol <5.0 mmol/L; low-density lipoprotein (LDL)-cholesterol <3.0 mmol/L
Other prophylactic drug therapies	Aspirin (75 mg) in treated hypertensive patients and in men at particularly high risk of CHD (in the top 20% of a risk score, or living in the top 25% of regions with the highest CHD mortality rate)
Other actions	Screen close relatives if familial hypercholesterolaemia or other inherited dyslipidaemia is suspected

for detecting disease before symptoms develop, as in population screening strategies in a healthy population, or more targeted screening of populations with a known high risk of disease.

Screening or diagnosis

Screening could be defined as the systematic application of a test (or enquiry) to identify individuals at risk of a specific disorder, who would benefit from further investigation or preventive treatment, among people who have not sought medical advice on account of symptoms of that disorder.

The main difference between screening and diagnosis is that the former is used to assess risk in the healthy population while the latter is normally done for the purpose of establishing an actual diagnosis. It follows, therefore, that when a diagnostic test is inexpensive and without risk, it can be offered to everyone, thus screening to select those at high risk is pointless. For example, the 'Guthrie' test is a routine screening test of newborn babies done in the UK on a blood spot card. The test detects high levels of thyroid-stimulating hormone (TSH), an indication of primary hypothyroidism and, if the replacement thyroid hormone T_4 is given within the first few months of life, it will prevent the development of cretinism in those infants.

Clinical versus laboratory diagnosis or screening

In many ways, the 'medical interview' is an enquiry, clinical 'screening' by the doctor, into the likelihood of an individual having a particular condition. The suspicion that there may be a condition is normally prompted by the presence of symptoms and/or signs of disease, which is then confirmed (or refuted) by further investigation with screening or diagnostic tests (Information box 7.26).

Screening strategies

Various screening strategies have been described using confusing definitions such as:

- **Population or mass screening**: this applies to a screening procedure which is offered to a whole population (Information box 7.27).
- **Multiple or multiphasic screening**: this means a variety of screening tests are carried out simultaneously, often adopted by private healthcare organisations offering screening packages. Some national health services have also adopted this policy from time to time.
- **Selective screening** (or targeted screening): this is the offering of a screening procedure to selected groups in a population that are considered to have an increased

---

ℹ Information box 7.26 **Diagnosis of pleural effusion**

A clinical diagnosis of a **pleural effusion** (an excessive amount of fluid in the space between the two connective tissue layers that cover the lungs (the pleura)) can be made simply and reliably by being able to distinguish, through clinical examination, a characteristic loud, sharp sound from a soft dull sound when tapping the chest wall and listening through a stethoscope (**auscultatory percussion**).

To confirm the diagnosis of pleural effusion and ascertain its precise cause, a chest radiograph is first performed, which may be considered a **screening** test, to confirm (or refute) the presence, and site, of fluid in the pleural cavity. If the presence of pleural effusion were confirmed, a pleural biopsy, an invasive and technically demanding diagnostic procedure to obtain a sample of fluid and pleural tissue, will be needed for laboratory examination to determine the cause of the effusion, i.e. what type of cells (blood, cancer, bacteria) the fluid might contain, and if there is disease of the pleura.

When a diagnostic procedure is hazardous or expensive, it would be appropriate to limit access to this procedure by identifying, through screening, those at high enough risk of the disorder to justify the hazard and expense of diagnosis.

risk of having the condition, e.g. mammography for women aged over 50 years, Down's syndrome screening for pregnant women aged over 35.
- **Surveillance**: this is the long-term observation of individuals or populations, for example developmental screening for pre-school children.
- **Case finding** is the screening of patients already in contact with the health services and is the same as opportunistic screening such as the 'new patient check' in UK general practice. The contact, but not always the screening activity, is usually patient initiated.

Important characteristics of all types of screening are that the person being screened is asymptomatic for the condition being sought and that the procedure is usually initiated by the medical authorities.

Criteria for population screening strategies

Criteria that should be fulfilled before screening for a particular condition is adopted were defined by Wilson and Jungner in 1968, and adopted by the WHO as **principles for screening**. These principles are still applicable today:

- The condition should be an *important health problem*.
- The *natural history* of the disease should be adequately understood.
- There should be a *recognisable latent* or *early symptomatic stage*.

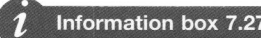

Information box 7.27 | **Examples of 'mass' screening**

Table 7.19 sets out the purpose of population screening.

Ideally, the person or team responsible for the care of the individual should carry out the screening procedure. Any intervention or treatment which is required is then an integral part of the individual's overall care. Screening carried out by a group or organisation which does not have responsibility for the overall care of the individual is an example of the separation of prevention from care and cure.

Table 7.19	Reasons for mass screening	
	Description	Who benefits
Determining the prevalence of a disorder	Surveillance	Community at large
Keeping an eye on a situation, ready to act if necessary	Monitoring	Community at large
Identifying high risk people early enough to help them	Screening	Individuals
Testing employees' fitness for work (e.g. food handlers)	Occupational testing	Customers/employers

- There should be a *suitable test or examination*, i.e. simple to perform and interpret, acceptable to those taking part, accurate and repeatable, and *sensitive and specific (*see below).
- Treatment started at an early stage should be of more benefit than treatment started at a later stage.
- There should be *accepted treatment* for patients with recognised disease. This principle is extremely important, but not always adhered to.
- There should be an agreed *policy* on who should receive treatment.
- Diagnosis and treatment should be cost-effective.
- Case finding should be a continuing process.

Ethical considerations about screening

It behoves all planning and policy-makers to consider each and every one of the Wilson–Jungner criteria for ethical implications before implementing screening programmes. 'Do no harm' is the ethical principle that applies. Some of these will be discussed here.

Screening or early diagnosis resulting in the 'labelling' of a person as being at high risk of developing a disease, or indeed having the disease, can hurt people, especially if there is no known effective intervention to ameliorate the condition. Often only a small proportion of those people screened as being at high risk will go on to develop the disease and so it is important to consider if there is a benefit to early labelling. If an early diagnosis is made, is there available a treatment that will benefit the individual if started early and which will outweigh the negative effects of loss of 'healthy time'? Several recent studies have examined the question of whether a breast mammography screening programme, leading to diagnosis and treatment, actually results in reduced mortality from breast cancer.

False positive (see below) screening tests can only harm, even if further tests prove negative. Macdonald and colleagues in 1984 in a review of the consequences of disease 'labelling' reported a series of studies showing that individuals who were told they had high blood pressure (were hypertensive), and who were not subsequently treated, had higher levels of absenteeism from work. Psychological well-being was also shown to be lower in those with high blood pressure and in those with normal blood pressure (were normotensive) but who had been wrongly labelled, compared with unaware normotensives. The adverse impact of screening on vocational and economic opportunities (e.g. life insurance, mortgages) have also been cited as 'doing harm'.

Screening and diagnostic test characteristics

Ideally, a screening test should select only those people who, on further (diagnostic) testing, are found to have the disease (the diagnostic test should ideally be 100% **sensitive**, with no false positives). All people without the disease should produce a negative screening test (the screening test should be 100% **specific**, with no false negatives). In reality such an ideal test does not exist but sensitivity and specificity (see below) should both be as high as possible for a test to be useful (Table 7.20).

In some cases it may be important to trade sensitivity in favour of specificity (for example if it is more important to detect as many people as possible who truly do not have the disease (true negatives)) because the available treatment for the disease is particularly toxic, or to trade specificity in favour of sensitivity (for example if it is more important to detect as many people as possible with the disease (true positives)) because, when treatment is available, lives will be saved.

Screening and diagnostic tests use these factors, in addition to the feasibility, cost and invasiveness of a particular test, to determine the actual test to be used in each particular circumstance. Often they will be used sequentially, screening tests being designed to work best in the asymptomatic population, with diagnostic tests working better in a situation where the disease is more prevalent (in the screen-positive population).

Diagnostic tests and non-dichotomous values

In many branches of medicine, a diagnostic test will often be something that gives a range of values (e.g. biochemical tests, haemoglobin estimates, blood pressure) rather than a dichotomous answer (yes/no). For tests of sensitivity and specificity, a dichotomous (or binary) concept, such as 'true' or 'false' is used. In such cases we need to convert the range into a binary answer by deciding on a **cut-point**. A cut-point is the limits of the range within which normal values lie. Outside of these limits, the value would be deemed 'abnormal', and thus the values can be dichotomised into normal/abnormal. In psychological tests for intelligence, for example, the range of intelligence quotients (IQ) follow a normal distribution curve. The 'cut-point' for normality is 2 standard deviations below the mean, below which the IQ is impaired. As these limits can vary, thus varying the cut-point, what might have been a positive test indicating an actual abnormality may become a false positive (a type I error).

Receiver operating characteristic (**ROC**) curves were first used during World War I for testing the sensitivity of radar receivers to detect objects such as aircraft. ROC curves

Table 7.20	Characteristics of screening and diagnostic tests		
Test	**Ideal**	**Purpose**	**Problem**
Screening	High sensitivity (ability to detect true positives). They will, therefore, have a low false-negative error rate (low type II error)	To detect as many people as possible who definitely have the disease (true positives). Ensures that not many true cases are missed. Those screening as negative are very likely not to have the disease. If the test is highly sensitive, it can be used to 'rule out' the diagnosis	Will also include people who do not have the disease (false-positives). Further (diagnostic) tests may be needed to deal with a high number of false-positives
Diagnosis	High specificity (ability to detect true negatives). They will, therefore, have a low false-positive error rate (low type I error)	To detect as many people as possible who definitely do not have the disease (true-negatives). Ensures that not many cases are misdiagnosed, and inappropriately treated. Those screening positive are very likely to have the disease. If the test is highly specific it can be used to 'rule in' the diagnosis	Will also exclude people who do have the disease (false negatives). Prior (screening) tests may be needed to deal with a high number of false negatives

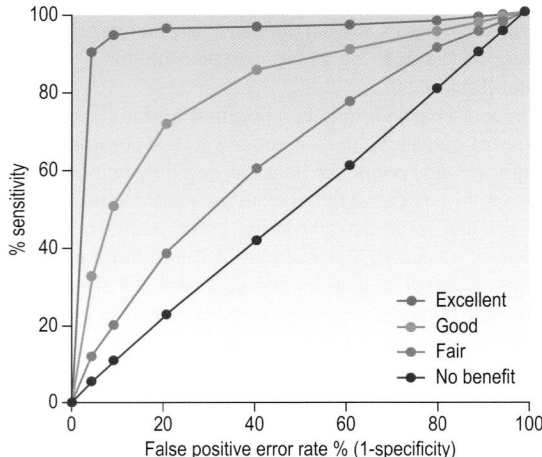

Fig. 7.26 Receiver operating characteristic (ROC) curves.

are used to plot different levels of sensitivity (to detect something) against the false-positive error rate (1 − specificity) produced by different cut-points in order to decide on the optimum cut-point (Fig. 7.26). The curves can also be used to compare the usefulness of a test between different subgroups, or to compare different tests. The closer the curve approaches the top left-hand corner of the graph the better the test.

Sensitivity and specificity

The **sensitivity** of a screening test (e.g. the cervical screening test) is the ability of a test to identify correctly those individuals who have the disease, as determined by a reference diagnostic test (e.g. cone biopsy), also known as the **gold standard**. It is a measure of the true positive rate, and is also referred to as the **detection rate**. A highly sensitive test will have a low false-negative rate (see Information box 7.28). Therefore, a screening test with high sensitivity would suggest that those testing positive are extremely likely to have the condition and should progress to having a diagnostic test.

It is important to understand that the predictive value of a test depends on the prevalence of the disease (i.e. the total number of cases in a population) that is being screened for, unlike sensitivity and specificity. If a disease is common in the population that is being screened, then the proportion of true positives and thus the positive predictive value is greater than when the prevalence is low (see below).

The **specificity** of a screening test is the ability of the test to identify correctly those who do not have the disease. It is a measure of the true-negative rate. A highly specific test will have a low false-positive rate (see Information box 7.28). A screening test with low specificity would give rise to a high rate of false positives, causing alarm and anxiety among those testing positive, and necessitating a great number of additional diagnostic tests on patients without disease. Table 7.21 shows how the results of screening and diagnostic tests can be set out in order to assess their usefulness.

The other important characteristics of a test are its positive and negative predictive values (Table 7.21). The values are not the same as sensitivity and specificity, although related, because a positive screening test identifies the risk of developing disease, when the disease may not actually be present. It is relevant when you have a test result from your patient and want to determine from that the chance that your patient has, or has not, the disease in question.

- The **positive predictive value** (**PPV**) is the proportion of people with a positive screening test who actually have the disease. Another way that this can be expressed is by the odds of being affected given a positive result (OAPR).
- The **negative predictive value** (**NPV**) is the proportion of people who screen negative and who do not have the disease.

Calculations for evaluating screening and diagnostic tests

Screening and diagnostics tests both identify the likelihood that a condition is present or absent. A diagnostic test, however, must give much more certainty so that a positive test has to identify the presence of a condition with close to 100% certainty, i.e. a sensitivity of 100% and, equally, if the test were negative, then the specificity should be as close to 100% as possible. In contast, the performance of screening tests are likely to be less sensitive and less specific, because they can be backed up by diagnostic tests. Because, as

Information box 7.28 | **True and false in screening and diagnostic tests**

When evaluating the characteristics of screening and diagnostic tests, the concepts of 'true' and 'false' refer to whether or not the outcome of the test indicates the presence or absence of the condition or disease that is being tested for:

■ True positive: positive test when the disease or condition is present

■ True negative: negative test when the disease or condition is absent

■ False positive: positive test when the disease or condition is absent. Also known in statistics as a type I error

■ False negative: negative test when disease or condition is present. Also known as a type II error.

Table 7.21 | **How to calculate important statistics in screening and diagnosis**

		Condition screened for (as determined by a reference, diagnostic test, the 'Gold standard')		
		Present	**Absent**	
Test result	Positive	True positive *a*	False positive *b*	Positive predictive value *a/(a + b)*
	Negative	*c* False negative *a/(a + c)* Sensitivity	*d* True negative *d/(b + d)* Specificity	*d/(c + d)* Negative predictive value

outlined above, the predictive value of these tests depends on the prevalence of a condition, the concept of pre-test probability comes into play. **Pre-test probability** is the judgement of the clinician about whether, based on symptoms, signs and personal characteristics such as age, sex, occupation etc., the patient is likely to have a particular disease. If nothing is known about the patient then disease prevalence might be the only clue.

Calculating and evaluating the functions of diagnostic and screening tests follow similar procedures. The following example illustrates how this is done.

Diagnosis of pulmonary embolism

This example for evaluating a diagnostic test for pulmonary embolism (PE, where a thrombus has broken away from its source and lodges in the pulmonary arteries) is taken from an article by Qanadli SD et al published in the journal *Radiology* in 2000. The authors wanted to see if dual-section helical computed tomography (CT; involves an X-ray tube rotating round the patient to provide a series of cross-sectional images) scanning functioned as well as pulmonary arteriography, the 'gold' standard diagnostic test that diagnosed pulmonary embolism with certainty. Pulmonary embolism is a life-threatening condition needing a reliable diagnostic test, but pulmonary arteriography is highly invasive, technically difficult and expensive to perform. The alternative tests were chest radiographs, which are usually normal in PE, or lung scans that are sensitive (high proportion of true positives) but not specific (high proportions of false negatives).

The study was carried out with 157 patients admitted as emergencies with suspected pulmonary embolism. Table 7.22 shows the results of pulmonary arteriography and dual CT scans. Of the 157 patients, 65 were tested positive for PE on dual CT scan, of which 59 were positive on pulmonary arteriography ('gold' standard). The disease prevalence in this population was calculated as the proportion of 'disease positives' in the sample (39.5%). Of the 92 patients who were negative on dual CT scanning, 3 were positive on arteriography. The sensitivity, specificity and predictive values can now be calculated to show that the dual CT scan has a:

■ Sensitivity of 0.952: the dual CT scan can pick up 95.2% of patients that have PE

■ Specificity of 0.937: of the patients who do not have PE, 93.7% will test negative

■ Positive predictive value of 0.908, meaning that 90.8% of patients who test positive on dual CT scanning actually have PE

■ Negative predictive value of 0.967, meaning that 96.7% of patients testing negative on dual CT scanning do not have PE.

The dual helical CT scan can therefore be reliably used to diagnose pulmonary embolism accurately for *patients suspected of PE on clinical grounds*, as examined in this study. The dual CT scan, however, is expensive, and needs an experienced radiologist for interpretation. There are now quicker and cheaper tests, and quicker biochemical tests may be preferred, but will need assessment in an analogous fashion.

The effect of prevalence on sensitivity and predictive values

To show how prevalence affects the functions of diagnostic and screening tests, a hypothetical prevalence of 10% has been attributed to a hypothetical 157 patients admitted with suspected PE. Table 7.23 shows the results.

At the hypothetical prevalence of 10% (instead of the original 39.5%) and the same total of 157 (hypothetical) patients, there will be a calculated 16 patients testing positive on pulmonary arteriography. If the dual CT scan performed as expected, 95.2% of the patients with PE will be picked up, resulting in 15 (actually 15.2 patients but this number has been reduced to 15) testing positive. Similarly, if the specificity stayed the same at 93.7%, 132 of the 141 patients testing negative on dual CT scanning will not have PE on arteriography. From Table 7.23, by reducing the prevalence to 10% from 39.5%, the sensitivity and specificity is unchanged (in fact the levels of these have changed a bit because 15 patients have been put into the cell, instead of

Table 7.22 Test results from 157 patients admitted as an emergency with clinical suspicion of acute pulmonary embolism

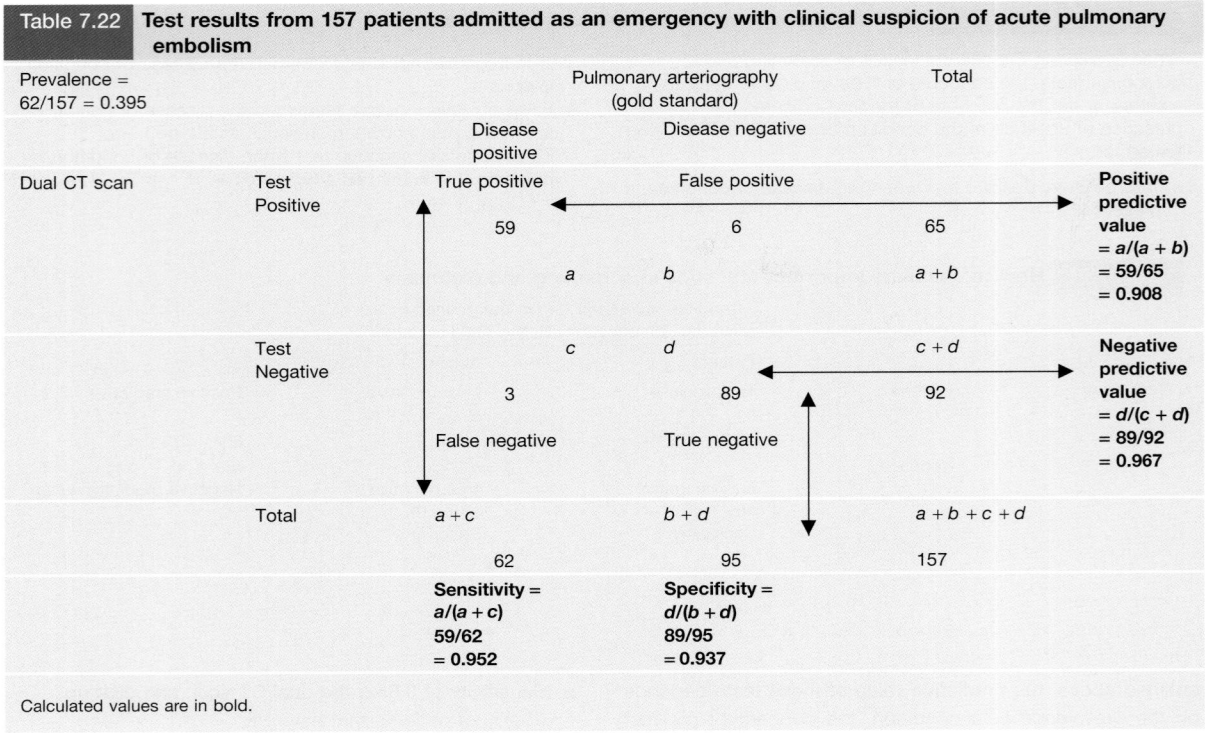

Prevalence = 62/157 = 0.395

		Pulmonary arteriography (gold standard)		Total	
		Disease positive	Disease negative		
Dual CT scan	Test Positive	True positive 59 *a*	False positive 6 *b*	65 *a + b*	**Positive predictive value = *a/(a + b)* = 59/65 = 0.908**
	Test Negative	*c* 3 False negative	*d* 89 True negative	*c + d* 92	**Negative predictive value = *d/(c + d)* = 89/92 = 0.967**
	Total	*a + c* 62	*b + d* 95	*a + b + c + d* 157	
		Sensitivity = *a/(a + c)* 59/62 = 0.952	**Specificity = *d/(b + d)* 89/95 = 0.937**		

Calculated values are in bold.

Table 7.23 Test results from 157 hypothetical patients among whom the prevalence of the condition is only around 10%, instead of about 40% in the previous example

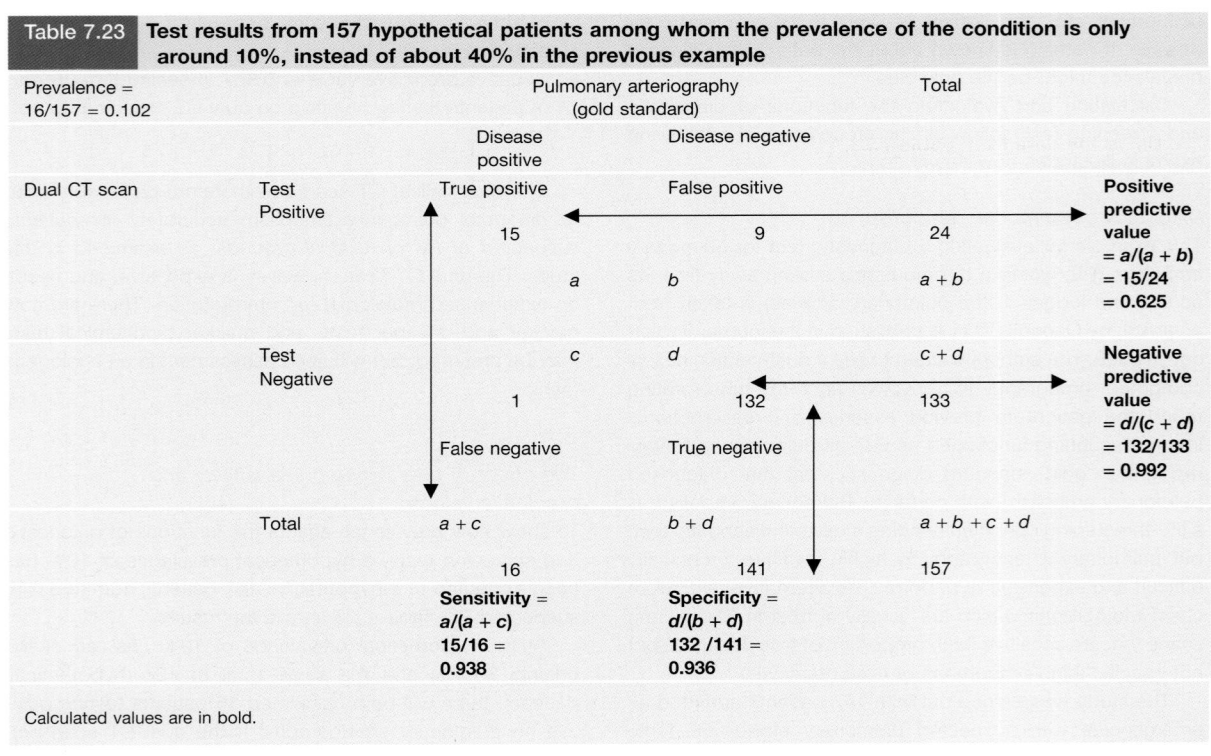

Prevalence = 16/157 = 0.102

		Pulmonary arteriography (gold standard)		Total	
		Disease positive	Disease negative		
Dual CT scan	Test Positive	True positive 15 *a*	False positive 9 *b*	24 *a + b*	**Positive predictive value = *a/(a + b)* = 15/24 = 0.625**
	Test Negative	*c* 1 False negative	*d* 132 True negative	*c + d* 133	**Negative predictive value = *d/(c + d)* = 132/133 = 0.992**
	Total	*a + c* 16	*b + d* 141	*a + b + c + d* 157	
		Sensitivity = *a/(a + c)* 15/16 = 0.938	**Specificity = *d/(b + d)* 132 /141 = 0.936**		

Calculated values are in bold.

an impractical 15.2 patients). With both values at over 90%, it would be safe to say that this is a 'good' diagnostic test.

The calculated predictive values, however, are different if the prevalence of PE is reduced to 10% (Table 7.23). Although the negative predictive value is very high at 99.2%, the posi-

tive predictive value is reduced to 62.5%. In other words, only 62.5% of patients testing positive on dual CT scanning for PE will actually have the disease, although if the test is negative, we are now even more sure that a particular patient would not have PE in these particular circumstances of low prevalence.

Likelihood ratios

In relation to screening and diagnostic tests, likelihood ratios (LR) refer to the likelihood of a positive test from a patient with the condition of interest (LRpos), or the likelihood of a negative test from a patient without the condition (LRneg), and obtaining the same result from a patient without, or conversely with, the condition.

Although likelihood ratios are not commonly used, they offer a very simple way of evaluating a test result in the context of a particular patient. Understanding these concepts helps with interpreting the utility of diagnostic tests. Sometimes they may show that doing the test adds nothing and it is almost certain that the patient either already does or does not have the condition. Unfortunately many laboratory tests are done in such circumstances, simply because of the 'litigation' culture. In contrast, there are tests, where a negative test result can be very useful. For example, a positive D-dimer test is not very useful in telling whether or not patients with a suspected deep vein thrombosis (DVT) actually have the condition, and further tests must be done to diagnose DVT, but where the result is negative, the patient is almost certain *not* to have the condition.

Likelihood ratios are related to the sensitivity and specificity of a test. With reference to Table 7.23, the likelihood of a positive test result in someone who has the disease, using the table convention, is $a/(a + c)$, which is the same as the sensitivity. The likelihood of a positive test result in someone who does not have the disease is $b/(b + d)$, the proportion of false positives, or $1 -$ proportion of true negatives or, in other words, $1 -$ specificity.

Thus LR positive test result = sensitivity/1 − specificity.

Using the data from Table 7.23, this is $0.938/(1 - 0.936) = 14.6$

We can interpret this by saying that a positive test result is about 14–15 times more likely to be seen in someone with the disease than in one without.

The LR negative test result = 1 − sensitivity/specificity

Using the data from Table 7.23, this is $(1 - 0.938)/0.936 = 0.066$

We can interpret this by saying that a negative test result is 0.066 times more likely to be seen in someone with the disease, than in one without or, in other words, is less likely. As we discussed before when talking about risk and benefit, it might be simpler to invert this figure for easier interpretation: $1/0.066 = 15.2$ – interpreted as a negative result being about 15 times more likely to be seen in someone *without* the disease, than in someone with.

In addition to the diagnostic test that has been performed, the clinical examination of the patient, or simply knowledge of the prevalence of the condition in your setting, will provide an idea of how likely it is that the patient has the condition (the pre-test odds) before you do any diagnostic tests. Putting these two pieces of information together – the usefulness of the diagnostic test and your best clinical assessment – produces a better estimate of whether or not your patient has the condition (the post-test odds). The calculation is simple:

Post-test odds (of having the condition) = Pre-test odds (clinical odds of having the condition) × LRpos (likelihood ratio of a positive test).

Many people prefer to think in terms of 'probability' of a condition, instead of 'odds'. Although they are mathematically linked it is easier to use a nomogram (Fig. 7.27) to determine the post-test probability after seeing your patient and doing a test.

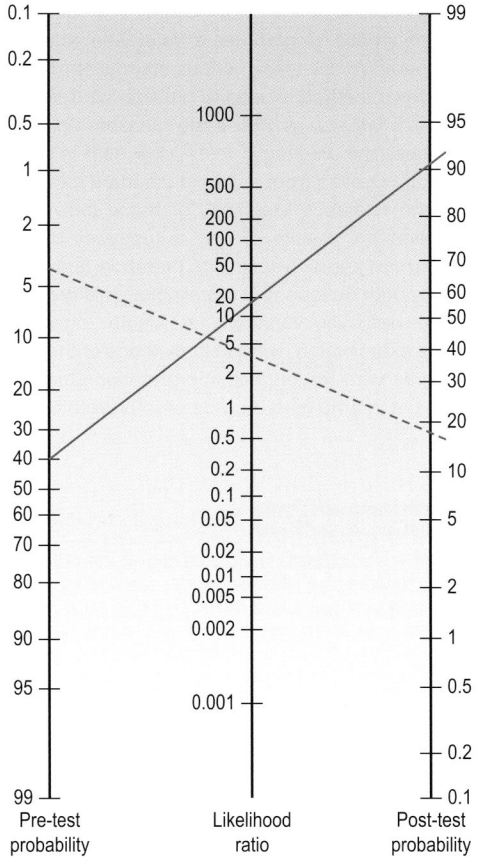

Fig. 7.27 Updating a diagnostic test result with clinical information. Using this diagram we can draw a straight line between the pre-test probability (clinical assessment or prevalence) of a condition, through the LRpos point, in order to assess the post-test probability. Using the example in the text, which had a LRpos of about 15 for the computed tomography (CT) scan test and considering that the patients being admitted had a pre-test probability (prevalence in this example) of PE of 40%, the fact that this patient had a positive test result would result in a post test probability of PE of over 90%, converting doubt into almost certainty, shown by the *solid line*. It will be clear from this diagram that, depending on the LRpos value of the test, and the prevalence of the condition (the pre-test probability), finding a positive test result may not result in any significant change in opinion. A hypothetical example is shown by the *dotted line* in the figure where doing the test and getting a positive result has increased the chance that the patient has the condition by less than 5%. In these circumstances doing a test will often be a waste of resources. Source: TJ Fagan 1975 Nomogram for Bayes' theorem [letter]. New England Journal of Medicine 293:257.

Evaluating a diagnostic test

If a diagnostic test is to prove itself, it must be assessed against the 'truth', and undertaken without knowledge of that truth, avoiding the problems of conscious and unconscious bias. Knowing the truth is, of course, problematic, but we aim in clinical diagnosis to get as close as possible to the truth by direct examination of the gross and cellular pathology with the use of autopsy or biopsy. The former can only be done after the patient has died and so evaluation in this way can be severely delayed. Biopsy, where tissues are taken for microscopic examination by a pathologist, is inevitably an invasive process and its use in the evaluation of screening tests (see below, breast cancer screening example) can be problematic. Sometimes a 'reference' standard may be developed. We call these various standards 'gold' standards. Whatever method is used to provide the truth, we must be sure of its validity, as this is the measure against which we will assess the diagnostic test – how gold is gold?

The 'truth' derived from any gold standard can only be as good as the reference standard, or those individuals who may interpret the results of any autopsy or biopsy. Two individuals may agree in their interpretation and be correct (reliable), or both be incorrect (unreliable), or differ from each other (inter-observer variation). A single individual who repeats the examination, without knowledge of the repetition, may disagree with the original interpretation (intra-observer variation). For example, in a study of interpretation of chest radiographs for progression of tuberculosis, Yerushalmy and colleagues in 1950 showed that pairs of individuals frequently disagreed, and individuals disagreed with their own interpretation almost as frequently.

Measuring clinical agreement

It is possible for two examinations to be interpreted in the same way just by chance alone and so we need to know how good the agreement is beyond chance. This is measured by 'kappa' (see Information box 7.29). Kappa levels are often disappointingly low. For example, an article published in 2002 by Speciale et al on the assessment of lumbar spine stenosis into categories of normal, mild, moderate or severe stenosis, reported an average inter-observer kappa of only 26%, and intra-observer kappa of 11%, although they were increased when the scales were combined to produce just two categories (to 33% and 43%, respectively), or when the observers were particularly experienced (to 32%), or in particular occupational groups (radiologists to 40%).

The surgical management of lumbar spine stenosis, by decompression, can produce excellent results in many patients, but a substantial number of those who seem to be good candidates do not benefit. Magnetic resonance imaging (MRI) has become the gold standard for evaluating lumbar spine stenosis, but with poor agreement between observers about the extent of the problem, it may be that there is significant misdiagnosis and inadequate surgical

---

Information box 7.29   The kappa statistic

Suppose two radiologists are asked to review radiographs from 100 patients and decide whether there were degenerative changes in the lower spine. In 60 patients, they agreed that there were no changes, and in another 20 they agreed that degenerative changes were present. They disagreed about the changes in the other 20 and their observations (fictitious data) are recorded in Table 7.24.

The radiologists agreed about 80% (20 + 60)/100 of their patients, as shown in cells 'a' and 'd'. But some of this agreement could just be due to chance. What would happen if the radiologists were to each toss a coin and record that outcome instead? If we applied the χ^2 test, we can calculate what each cell would be expected to contain by chance alone, assuming the totals were to remain the same (which they would because the average totals reflect the prevalence of the condition in the population).

Expected value = row total × column total/overall total

These expected values are shown in parentheses in the table. The agreement by chance is:

(8.91 + 48.91)/100 = 57.82%

The actual agreement beyond chance is:

80 − 57.82 = 22.18%

The potential further agreement beyond chance is:

100 − 57.82 = 42.18%

Kappa is the ratio of the actual agreement beyond chance and potential further agreement beyond chance:

22.18/42.18 = 53%

Kappa values have been given qualitative labels according to the ranges:

- 0–20% – slight agreement
- 20–40% – fair agreement
- 40–60% – moderate agreement
- 60–80% – substantial agreement
- 80–100% – almost perfect agreement.

Table 7.24   Observations of lower spine degenerative changes by two radiologists

		Radiologist 1 (first observation)		Total
		Present	Absent	
Radiologist 2 (second observation)	Present	20 (8.91)	13 (24.09)	33
		a	*b*	*a + b*
	Absent	*c*	*d*	*c + d*
		7 (18.09)	60 (48.91)	67
	Total	*a + c* 27	*b + d* 73	*a + b + c + d* 100

Expected values in brackets.

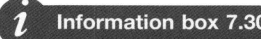

Information box 7.30 | **Six strategies for preventing or minimising clinical disagreement**

- Match the diagnostic environment to the diagnostic task.
- Seek collaboration of key findings:
  - Repeat key elements of your examination
  - Corroborate important findings with documents and witnesses
  - Confirm key clinical findings with appropriate tests
  - Ask 'blinded' colleagues to examine your patients.
- Report evidence as well as inference, making a clear distinction between the two.
- Use appropriate technical aids.
- 'Blind' your assessments of raw diagnostic test data.
- Apply the social sciences, as well as the biologic sciences, of medicine.

decompression, resulting in a poorer than expected prognosis. Information box 7.30 provides a summary of strategies, suggested by Sackett et al in *Clinical Epidemiology*, to reduce clinical disagreement.

Consider the prevalence of disease

A second important consideration when evaluating a diagnostic test is to make sure it has been used in a patient sample that contains the same spectrum of disease that would be found within the population of interest. The population of interest will, for example, be different between primary care and secondary care because the prevalence of the condition will be different. For example, a particular test for myocardial infarction that works well in patients admitted to hospital with chest pain, e.g. electrocardiogram (ECG) (where the proportion of patients experiencing chest pain due to a myocardial infarction is likely to be high) may be completely useless within the setting of general practice (where the proportion of patients experiencing chest pain due to a myocardial infarction is likely to be very low). Prevalence affects the predictive value of the diagnostic test (see above).

Clinical suspicion: pre-test probability

A diagnostic test may readily distinguish between people that definitely do, or do not have the disease, and may in fact be a biochemical test that does no better than consideration of a patient's signs and symptoms. A test will only be useful if it can discriminate in cases where there is some doubt about the clinical diagnosis, in the spectrum between these two extremes. For example, many conditions may exhibit symptoms of irritability, anxiety, trembling and sweating. These are also symptoms of mild hyperthyroidism (thyroid overactivity, also called thyrotoxicosis). In hyperthyroidism, measurement of the level of thyroid-stimulating hormone (TSH) can be a very useful diagnostic test as it is normally low in this condition (see Ch. 10).

Harming the patient

If the gold standard test is invasive, involving a risky clinical procedure, there may be some reluctance on the part of the evaluators of the test to submit all their patients to both tests. Nevertheless, the evaluation depends on both assessments being made in every case. An alternative has been proposed in order to rule out the disease that involves the absence of any adverse health outcome in a patient after long-term follow-up without that patient being treated for the condition.

Consistency of findings

Finally, as in all situations, a finding may be due to chance alone and it is important always to be able to evaluate the performance of a test in a second, independent, group of patients.

Screening for breast cancer

In the UK, there is a free, 3-yearly national breast screening programme for women aged between 50 and 64. Policies for the secondary prevention of breast cancer vary in developed countries, depending mainly on the way that health services are funded.

Case scenario: how effective is breast screening?

You are a general practitioner in the UK. Mrs A has just passed her fiftieth birthday, and was invited to attend the local unit for mammography screening. She comes to see you because although she has a general idea of what mammography is for (the letter inviting her to attend explained the procedures (the test involves a small dose of X-rays) and the reasons for screening), she is undecided about whether or not to attend. She is perfectly well in herself, has no history of breast cancer, and is not aware that anyone in her family has suffered from breast cancer. She wants to know what benefits and harms there are of having a mammogram in order to balance these against the inconvenience and discomfort.

There are several questions and other matters that both the patient and clinician might want to consider in this context (Wilson–Jungner criteria, see above). Some examples are discussed below.

How effective is breast cancer screening for preventing death from breast cancer?
Breast cancer is the leading cause of death from malignant neoplasm for women in England. The national screening programme aims to reduce deaths from breast cancer. Mammography screening is the most effective tool for the early detection of cancer at a stage when effective treatment is possible. Combined mortality data from various developed countries worldwide, from randomised controlled and case–control studies over 7–12 years, published by Blamey et al in 2000, has shown that breast screening does reduce deaths from cancer, and is most effective in the over-50 age group, in which the reduction in the screened population may be up to 29%.

Will the X-rays be harmful, as the screening test has to be repeated every 3 years?
There is a minute possibility (if two million women aged over 50 were screened, there might be one extra cancer after 10 years) of the radiation causing cancer, which is far outweighed by the incidence of 2000 cases per million women aged 60.

Is the test acceptable?
There is evidence to show that psychological problems such as anxiety are not associated with invitation and attendance for mammography, but awaiting the results could be anxiety provoking.

What happens after the mammogram? How accurate is mammography at early diagnosis of cancer?
Mammography is a screening test, which detects abnormalities including cancer. However, the sensitivity and specificity

of the test is not known, because they are not directly measured. The gold standard for mammography is breast biopsy, a painful, hazardous procedure. It would be ethically unacceptable to subject women with normal mammograms to breast biopsy.

From data from all the basic or first screening tests (**prevalent screening**) performed in the UK in 1997–8, 8.3% (23 637/286 184) were reported as abnormal in a publication in 2000 (Table 7.25). Those women with abnormal mammograms are recalled for repeat screening (**incident screening**), and about two-thirds will be shown to be negative after further mammography or ultrasound scan. The remaining third who are still positive on the retest will then be referred for clinical assessment and fine needle aspiration or core needle biopsy.

In 1997–8, a total of 1800 (1800/23 637 testing positive on the first test = 7.6%) were diagnosed with breast cancer (Table 7.25). We refer to the 7.6% as the positive predictive value (PPV). About 8 (7.6) women in 100 with an initial positive mammogram will end up being diagnosed with breast cancer. Thus the PPV is also referred to as the 'odds of being affected given a positive result – OAPR'. Even if the repeat screening is positive (one-third of 23 637 = 7879) of which 1800 will be diagnosed with breast cancer, the positive predictive value is still below 50% (1800/7879 = 22.8%), meaning that even if a woman has two positive screening tests it is still more likely that she does *not* have breast cancer.

Tertiary prevention

Tertiary prevention is the monitoring and management of established disease in order to prevent disability or handicap. In many ways, the practice of medicine, whether managing chronic or acute episodic conditions, could be thought of as tertiary prevention. In a person who presents with symptoms of coronary heart disease: stable angina (chest pain ranging from a central mild ache to a severe pain that may radiate to the jaw and/or arms and may cause sweating and breathlessness, often provoked by exertion), unstable angina (recent onset severe angina, worsening angina or angina at rest), or acute myocardial infarction (a thrombotic occlusion of one of the heart blood vessels resulting in loss of blood and therefore of oxygen delivery to a significant area of heart muscle), the aim of treatment would be to slow the progression of coronary artery disease, if possible, to induce disease regression, and to reduce the risk of thrombotic complications. As a result it is hoped that, not only will the risk of a further non-fatal or fatal event be reduced, but the patient will also have a better quality of life and longer life expectancy. Here, knowledge of the effectiveness of diagnosis and

Table 7.25	Results from a UK breast screening programme in women aged 50–64 (1998–9), first screening
No of women screened	286 184
No of women referred	23 637 (8.3%)
No of cancers detected	1800
Cancer detection rate	6.29 per 1000
Positive predictive value (%)	7.6

Source: Blanks RG, Moss SM, Patnick J 2000 Results from the UK NHS breast screening programme 1994–1999. Journal of Medical Screening 7:195–198.

treatment discussed above is essential for good clinical practice.

Components for tertiary healthcare delivery

Components for effective tertiary healthcare delivery have been formulated. For example, cardiac rehabilitation programmes are evolving to include a wide range of activities, therapies, lifestyle changes, psychologies and networks supported by a multidisciplinary team of healthcare professionals, integrated between hospitals and the community (Table 7.26). The WHO has defined such a programme (Needs and priorities in cardiac rehabilitation and secondary prevention in patients with coronary heart disease. WHO Technical Report Series 831, Geneva, 1993) as: 'The rehabilitation of cardiac patients is the sum of activities required to influence favourably the underlying cause of the disease, as well as the best possible physical, mental and social conditions, so that they may, by their own efforts preserve or resume when lost, as normal a place as possible in the community. Rehabilitation cannot be regarded as an isolated form of therapy but must be integrated with the whole treatment of which it forms only one facet.'

These components are essential for delivering the best care for any patient after any acute, major event.

Evidence-based medicine

Central to the practice of medicine as an art based in science is the integration of individual clinical expertise and the best external evidence. Clinical expertise is built on basic clinical skills, then derived from experience, and expressed as judgement (**clinical acumen**). Making clinical judgements is about the skill to make the best clinical decision for the patient, and to help the patient to make choices about their treatment. There are many components to the process of making clinical decisions. Some have good external scientific evidence in support. Of importance to how we present choices to the individual patient are her/his personal circumstances, social, psychological and educational background and, to some extent, public policy.

The best available external evidence is clinically relevant research. This covers the accuracy of diagnostic and screening tests, identifying risk factors and prognostic markers, and evaluating the efficacy and safety of therapeutic, preventative and rehabilitative interventions. The 'evidence' in support of evidence-based medicine is mostly quantitative, in the form of RCTs, emphasising the quantifiable and measurable aspects of medical practice. In the real-life situation, there may be areas of clinical uncertainty. The less easily measured factors that influence clinical decisions, such as the psychological and social condition of the patient, and the patient's own concerns and expectations are equally, or more, important and only to be ignored at the doctor's peril. It would be worthwhile to reflect upon these aspects and their relevance to the preferences of the patient sitting in front of you.

The epidemiologist, David Sackett, has described the discipline of evidence-based medicine as 'the integration of best research evidence with clinical expertise and patient values'. While much epidemiological research may relate more to an overall strategy for managing a population of patients, for example all people with diabetes, the practice of evidence-based medicine encourages individual learning and fosters important research by the health professional in order to offer the best possible care to the individual patient.

Table 7.26	Main components of a cardiac prevention and rehabilitation programme*
Component	**Activity**
Lifestyle and cardiovascular risk assessment	Assessment of: smoking, diet, physical activity, blood pressure and lipid levels. Integration of all these factors is needed to shape a programme according to the particular needs of the individual
Educational	Education about: the disease, its causes, how causes can be modified, medical and surgical treatments and resuscitation. Education is provided to patients and their families
Behavioural	Behavioural 'stages of change': preparation – preparing and advising change; action – assisting change; maintenance – providing follow-up. Done in partnership with patient and doctor and tailored to the needs and level of understanding of the patient
Health promotion	Promoting a healthy lifestyle: avoiding tobacco, making healthy food choices, becoming physically active
Family-based intervention	Assisting the patient by the family or partner: being tobacco free, participating in healthy diet changes, supporting leisure time exercise in the household, participating in programmes that address psychosocial and sexual problems
Risk factor management	Monitoring: weight, blood pressure, lipids, blood glucose. The monitoring is used to set goals, suggest lifestyle changes and introduce drug therapies as necessary
Drug therapies and compliance	Ensuring that: treatment and dose are the most appropriate, according to the best available evidence. The importance of sustained therapies should be emphasised with the patient
Psychology	Emotional response to development of disease by: stress management and relaxation
Screening of first degree blood relatives	In patients with premature disease (men under 55 and women under 65) screening of: parents, siblings and offspring (over 13) for blood pressure, lipids and glucose
Vocational	Advice on: preparations for return to work, seeking alternative work, driving licence considerations
Quality assurance	Audit of, for example: which patients take up and adhere to the programme, the quality and accessibility of information provided to the patients, the ability of the programme to make changes in factors such as blood pressure and cholesterol. Audit of a programme is necessary for any programme to evolve and improve in order to achieve the stated objectives

*Information taken from 1998 Prevention of coronary heart disease in clinical practice. Recommendations of the Second Joint Task Force of European and other Societies on Coronary Prevention. European Heart Journal 19:1434–1503.

8 The nervous system

Alan Longstaff

WHAT THE NERVOUS SYSTEM DOES

OVERVIEW

Self-organisation

The nervous system is made up of **neurons** or nerve cells whose function is to process and transmit information. They can do this because they are interconnected with each other to form **networks** which perform computations ensuring that an individual's behaviour is appropriate to current circumstances, in the light of what has happened in the past.

Both the outside world and internal physiology are continuously monitored by sense organs to provide input; the output, in the form of particular actions and responses, is carried out by nerve cells acting on effector organs such as muscles and glands. The nervous system is self-organising, being built and continually remodelled throughout life by the interplay of gene expression and environmental signals.

Uniqueness

The adult human nervous system contains between 300 billion and 500 billion neurons. Although most neurons prob-

ably only connect with a modest number of others, and connections are targeted rather than random, the number of possible ways in which a nervous system can wire up is immense. The complexity this affords is a basis for human individuality.

Input

Most human action is guided by sensory input. The extent to which this input is processed before it produces an action varies hugely. When speed is crucial the number of processing steps is small, as in **reflexes**, but the consequence of this is that the output options are limited.

Reflexes

In reflex circuits (**reflex arcs**), **sensory neurons** connect **directly** or via just a few intervening cells (**interneurons**) with **motor neurons** that produce some sort of output, e.g. muscle contraction or glandular secretion. The sensory input generates a stereotyped response that does not engage consciousness until after it has happened, neither can it be suppressed by effort of will. More complex reflexes can be altered by experience (learning) but simple reflexes – for example, the withdrawal of a limb in response to a painful stimulus – are essentially immutable.

Sensation

Raw sensory input, even that used initially to drive reflexes, is subject to extensive processing. Sensory systems detect change (e.g. boundaries between light and dark regions in the visual field) or the unexpected (e.g. a sudden noise), while largely ignoring regions or events that are constant in space or time. In this way they achieve high degrees of data compression. This means the brain can economise on the number of components it needs to run a given task.

Sensory systems also save time by **parallel processing**. This means breaking up a sensory task (e.g. vision) into several subroutines (form, colour, motion), all of which are analysed by separate neural pathways, but at the same time. Information in these separate channels must eventually be recombined. How this is done is not certain and is called the **binding problem**. One idea is that the nerve cells representing all the subroutines for a particular object are made to fire in synchrony.

The sensations that humans experience are limited by the capacities of sense organs. If judged by the volume of brain devoted to it, vision is the pre-eminent human sense, although we are blind to all but a tiny part of the electromagnetic spectrum, the rainbow of visible light with wavelengths from 400–700 nm.

Perception

To interpret the environment (e.g. to identify an object in the visual field) the brain compares incoming sensations to pre-existing internal representations of objects. In this way the nervous system makes hypotheses about the identity of the sensory patterns. This process is termed **perception**. Some internal representations are hard-wired; that is the neural circuits which run them are genetically specified and built during development. Many internal representations are learnt, however, as is indicated by cultural differences in susceptibility to optical illusions. Percepts are not faithful representations of what exists. They are selective and highly interpreted **models**.

Output

- The **autonomic nervous system** (Ch. 4) acts on smooth muscle, cardiac muscle and glands.
- The output of the **central nervous system** (CNS) is via skeletal muscles.

The motor neurons in the spinal cord that bring about the contraction of muscle fibres are regarded as a final common path by which motor systems in the brain bring about movement. Motor systems calculate variables such as the trajectory of a limb required to perform some action, and then signal to motor neurons the pattern of timing and force of muscle contraction needed to make the movement.

Much movement is executed unconsciously by reflexes (e.g. to maintain balance). Even voluntary movement, which we initiate intentionally, is generally performed unthinkingly by the actions of motor programmes that have been previously acquired. But, while routine motor tasks can be done automatically, a new task (learning to ride a bicycle or, when we were about one year old, learning to walk) requires conscious effort, and the brain improves its performance by reducing the perceived error between the action that was intended and what has actually been achieved. In this remarkable fashion, motor systems are self-training.

Cognition

Cognition is behaviour based on **knowledge**. Cognitive functions include planning, problem solving and language – attributes which we often regard as quintessentially human.

Semantic networks

Knowledge is stored in the brain as networks that allow associations to be forged between all the disparate elements that make up the mental image of an object or abstract concept; for example, what type of thing it is (e.g. face, animal, rock), its visual image, its name and the motor sequence needed to pronounce it. These **semantic networks** learn and store the internal representations of objects and concepts. They can be continually added to without disrupting any of the prior knowledge.

Association areas

About half of the **cortex** of the **cerebral hemispheres** – a thin rind that covers much of the brain's surface – is dedicated solely to a single sense or the direct planning and execution of intentional movements. The rest, termed **association cortex**, is concerned with the information processing that goes on between perception and action. Association cortex receives input from multiple senses and has access to the brain's knowledge base in the form of semantic networks. Integration of these information sources is thought to underlie multi-sensory perception and cognitive functions.

Consciousness

One of the greatest problems in contemporary neuroscience is the nature of **consciousness**. No unambiguous definition exists, although wakefulness is a pre-condition and self-awareness a component. In some sense, consciousness is about having access to certain categories of information. We are aware of the shape, colour and location of a cup in our field of view, but no amount of **introspection** informs us about the computation our brain has performed to make it look three-dimensional or to produce the muscle contractions we have used to grasp it. Hence information processing happens in two compartments. One we have access to in that we can dredge it into consciousness, the other is denied to us even though it governs our perceptions and actions.

The subjective experiences (e.g. the quality of redness) that we have by virtue of being conscious must be generated by particular brain states, but how this is done is not known. Moreover, although we can agree on the labels, i.e. ripe tomatoes and blood are both red, there is at present no experiment that can demonstrate that one person's experience of red is the same as another person's.

Consciousness is assumed to be a property of the cerebral cortex on the basis of studies of rare individuals with cortical damage who have deficits in consciousness. For example, patients with **blindsight** (Information box 8.19) lack a primary visual cortex but can navigate their way round obstacles, despite being completely unaware of their presence.

Consciousness is accompanied by the overwhelming subjective experience that there is a single **executive self** that is feeling, making decisions and acting. This is the basis for the belief in free will. Decision-making circuitry exists in the cerebral cortex, and the extent to which it may be at the top of a brain command hierarchy, or just one network among equals, is not known. Much of consciousness appears to be a stream of language over which we have some control. We cannot imagine what it is like to be conscious without language although we assume human infants and at least some animals are.

CELLS OF THE NERVOUS SYSTEM

There are two principal cell types specific to the nervous system:

- **neurons** (nerve cells), excitable cells which process and transmit information, and
- **glial** cells, which serve a variety of supporting roles.

NEURONS

There are many types of neuron, which differ in size and shape, but all adult nerve cells have two features in common, a cell body (soma) and neurites (Fig. 8.1):

- The **cell body** houses the nucleus and all the subcellular organelles seen in other cells, and is responsible for 'housekeeping' metabolic functions. Neurons have particularly high rates of protein synthesis and this is reflected by structures found in the cell bodies called **Nissl bodies**, which are densely packed with rough endoplasmic reticulum.
- **Neurites** are elongated processes that project from the cell body and are of two types: **dendrites** and **axons**.

A neuron may have many dendrites but only a single axon, and in general dendrites are thicker, shorter and more highly branched than axons. All neurites have mitochondria.

In functional terms, the cell body and dendrites receive and process inputs from other neurons, the axon hillock determines the outcome of the processing and the axon transmits the output as nerve impulses.

Dendrites

Dendrites are extensions of the cell body and they too contain rough endoplasmic reticulum and Golgi apparatus so they can manufacture and process proteins. Most dendrites are short, but as they are often numerous they collectively provide most of the surface area of a neuron. So a majority of the connections from other neurons are made on the dendrites.

Axons

The **axon** usually emerges from the cell body at a region termed the **axon hillock**. Axon diameters vary from about 0.2 μm to 20 μm, and the larger ones are covered by a **myelin sheath** made by glial cells (see below). Human axons vary hugely in length from a few micrometres to over a metre. Axons branch to form collaterals, at the end of each of which is a swollen **nerve terminal** or **bouton**. In some cases the axon has swellings, **varicosities**, at intervals along its length. Both terminals and varicosities form the presynaptic part of chemical synapses and contain mitochondria. Axons are not

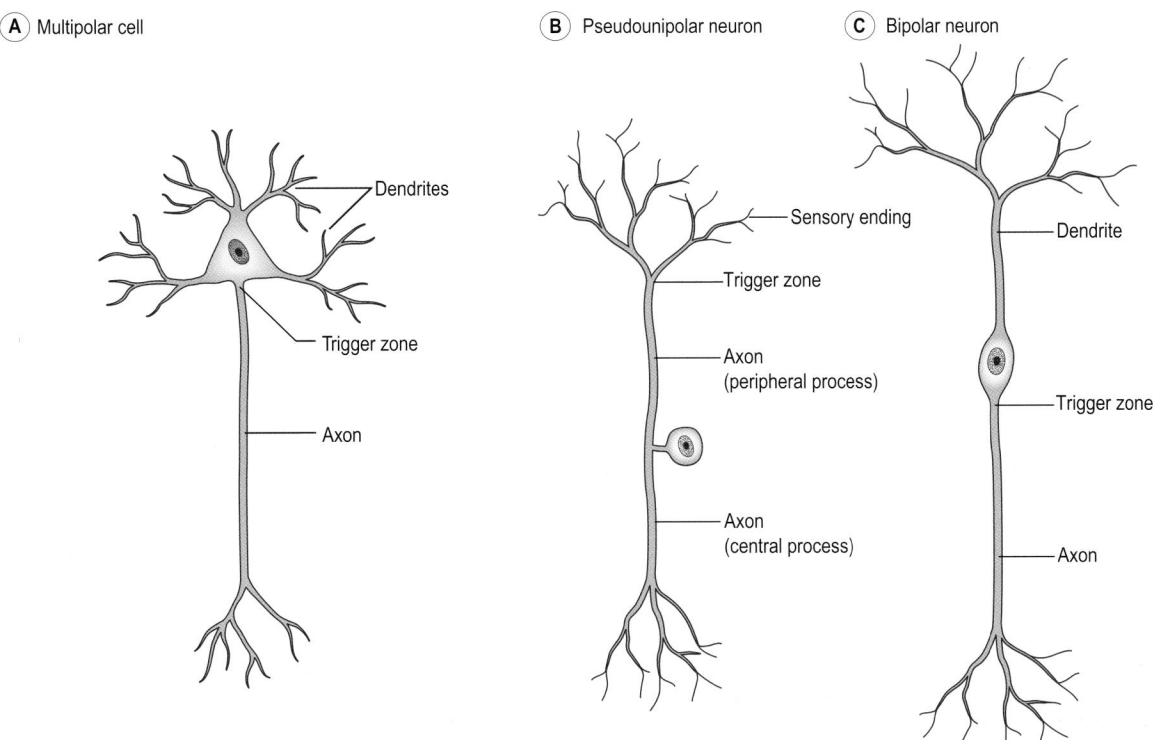

Fig. 8.1 **Three common neuron types:** (A) Multipolar neuron. (B) Pseudounipolar neuron. (C) Bipolar neuron. Redrawn with permission from Michael-Titus A, Revest P, Shortland P 2006 The nervous system. Churchill Livingstone, Edinburgh.

capable of protein synthesis so proteins needed in the axon and nerve terminals are manufactured in the cell body and carried along the axon by axonal transport.

Classification of neurons

Neurons can be classified in a variety of ways, including their size, shape (morphology), how they are connected, and by their chemistry.

Size

The cell bodies of neurons vary in diameter from about 6 μm to 8 μm for the granule cells of the cerebellum to 50 μm or more for α-motor neurons of the spinal cord. The most common type of nerve cells in the cerebral cortex, the pyramidal cells, have cell bodies 12–20 μm across.

Morphology

There are several morphological distinctions between the different types of neuron (see Fig. 8.1A–C).

Number of neurites

- The majority of vertebrate neurons are **multipolar** with an axon and multiple dendrites.
- Primary sensory neurons are **pseudounipolar**. These have no dendrites but they have a single axon that bifurcates within a short distance of the cell body. One branch of the axon goes to a sense organ in the periphery, the other enters the CNS.
- **Bipolar** neurons have two neurites – an axon and a dendrite – which project from opposite poles of the cell body. They are found in the retina, and in the cochlear and vestibular ganglia.
- **Unipolar** neurons have a single neurite. They are rare in the human nervous system and include retinal amacrine cells, which have a single dendrite.

Arrangement of dendrites

The dendrites of a neuron make up its **dendritic tree**. The size and geometry of the dendritic tree is important because it determines the number of synapses a neuron can accommodate, and how it processes the signals they deliver. Neurons are **spiny** if their dendrites have small projections called dendritic spines, or **aspiny** otherwise.

Connectivity

Classifying nerve cells by how they are connected is useful because it says something about their functions.

- **Afferent neurons**, which transmit signals towards the CNS, provide the nervous system with input. Afferents connected to sense organs or afferents that are directly responsive to sensory stimulation are **sensory neurons**.
- **Efferent neurons**, which transmit signals towards the periphery, are the vehicles for nervous system output. Efferents that synapse with muscles are **motor neurons**, a term also applied to some efferent neurons in motor pathways that do not synapse directly with muscle. The term **secretomotor** is sometimes used for efferents that drive glandular secretion.
- **Interneurons** make up the networks between afferent and efferent neurons and transform input to output. The vast majority of nerve cells are interneurons.

Chemistry

Different nerve cells release different chemical transmitters so they can be distinguished by the different enzymes and precursors they contain. For example, all neurons that use acetylcholine (ACh) as a transmitter contain:

- The enzyme choline acetyltransferase (CAT) which catalyses ACh synthesis
- The choline transporter
- In some cases the acetylcholinesterase (which catalyses the degradation of ACh).

Just as these proteins can be diagnostic of cholinergic (acetylcholine-using) cells, different markers allow other neurons to be classified by their transmitters. The importance of this is that the neurotransmitter provides clues about nerve cell function and about the pharmacology of the synapses they make; for example cells that use glutamate as a transmitter are usually excitatory.

Glia

Glial cells are generally smaller than neurons and outnumber them by at least 3:1. They have long processes which give them a resemblance to neurons, but they can be distinguished from neurons by staining for specific proteins and by their lack of Nissl bodies. There are three main types of glia, each of which has its own functions.

Astrocytes

The most abundant cell type in the nervous system are **astrocytes** (Fig. 8.2), the cell bodies of which are about 8 μm in diameter. Astrocytes are present only in the brain and spinal cord. Their processes closely surround nerve cells, other types of glial cell, synapses and capillaries (which they surround with swellings termed **endfeet**), leaving extracellular spaces only about 20 nm across.

Functions of astrocytes

Astrocytes maintain the appropriate environment for neuron functioning in several ways.

- **Ion homeostasis**. When neurons are active K^+ accumulates in the extracellular space, which makes neurons more excitable. To offset this, astrocytes move

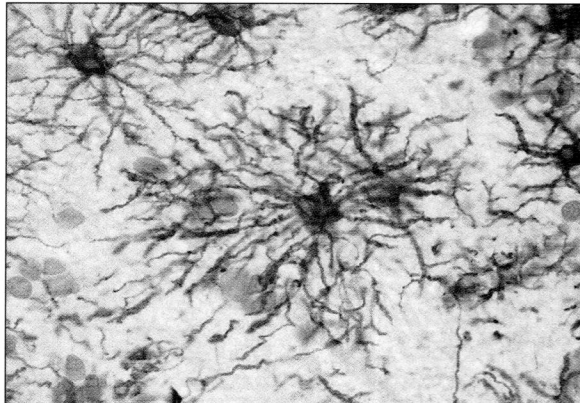

Fig. 8.2 Astrocytes: these glial cells are stellate (star-shaped) because of their branching processes. They are stained by an immunoperoxidase method to show glial fibrillary acidic protein (GFAP). Redrawn with permission from Stevens A, Lowe J 2004 Human histology, 3rd edn. Mosby, Edinburgh.

K^+ from regions of high concentration to regions of low concentration, particularly into the capillaries. Adjacent astrocytes are connected by gap junctions, so they form a syncytium through which K^+ ions can rapidly diffuse large distances.

- **Glucose metabolism**. Astrocytes take up glucose from blood and use it to synthesise lactate which is then exported to neurons (see Lactate shuttle, below). They also store glycogen.
- **Neurotransmitter metabolism**. Astrocytes have a crucial role in metabolism of the brain's major neurotransmitters, glutamate and γ-aminobutyrate (GABA) (see Metabolism of GABA).
- **Neurotransmitter inactivation**. Astrocytes have transporters which remove transmitters from the synaptic cleft. Furthermore, because astrocyte processes surround synapses, they act as barriers to the diffusion of peptide transmitters, the actions of which are thereby prolonged. (See Neurotransmitter systems, below)
- **Growth factors**. Astrocytes secrete a large number of growth factors which regulate the differentiation, proliferation and survival of neurons and other astrocytes. This is important during development and in inflammation and repair. Hypertrophy and mitosis of astrocytes (astrogliosis), due to secretion of growth factors from astrocytes, is seen in viral infections, neurodegenerative diseases and trauma.
- **Neuron guidance**. In early development, newborn nerve cells migrate to their proper destinations along astrocyte precursors called **radial glial cells**.

Oligodendrocytes and Schwann cells

Oligodendrocytes and **Schwann cells** both form **myelin sheaths** (Fig. 8.3) around axons of neurons. Oligodendrocytes are found in the CNS and can myelinate several axons whereas in the peripheral nervous system each Schwann cell only myelinates a single axon.

During myelination, glial cells wrap a process called a **mesaxon** around the axon 8–12 times. The mesaxon contains very little cytoplasm, so the myelin sheath consists mostly of concentric layers of glial cell plasma membrane. This has a high electrical resistance and the result is to increase the speed with which nerve impulses are conducted along the axon. Each glial cell covers a 0.15–1.5 mm length of axon, leaving a 0.5 μm gap, the **node of Ranvier**, between neighbouring stretches of myelin sheath. The myelination of long axons involves several hundred glial cells. However, **non-myelinated (or unmyelinated) axons** are not naked but lie in cylindrical invaginations of the mesaxon plasma membrane.

Schwann cells are involved in the regeneration of peripheral nerve axons. Disorders of myelin are responsible for diseases such as multiple sclerosis (see Clinical box 8.5) and some hereditary peripheral neuropathies.

Microglia

These are the smallest of the glial cells and have cell bodies containing many lysosomes and numerous fine processes. They are the **immune cells** of the nervous system. Many originate from monocytes formed in the bone marrow that migrated into the brain early in development, but there is

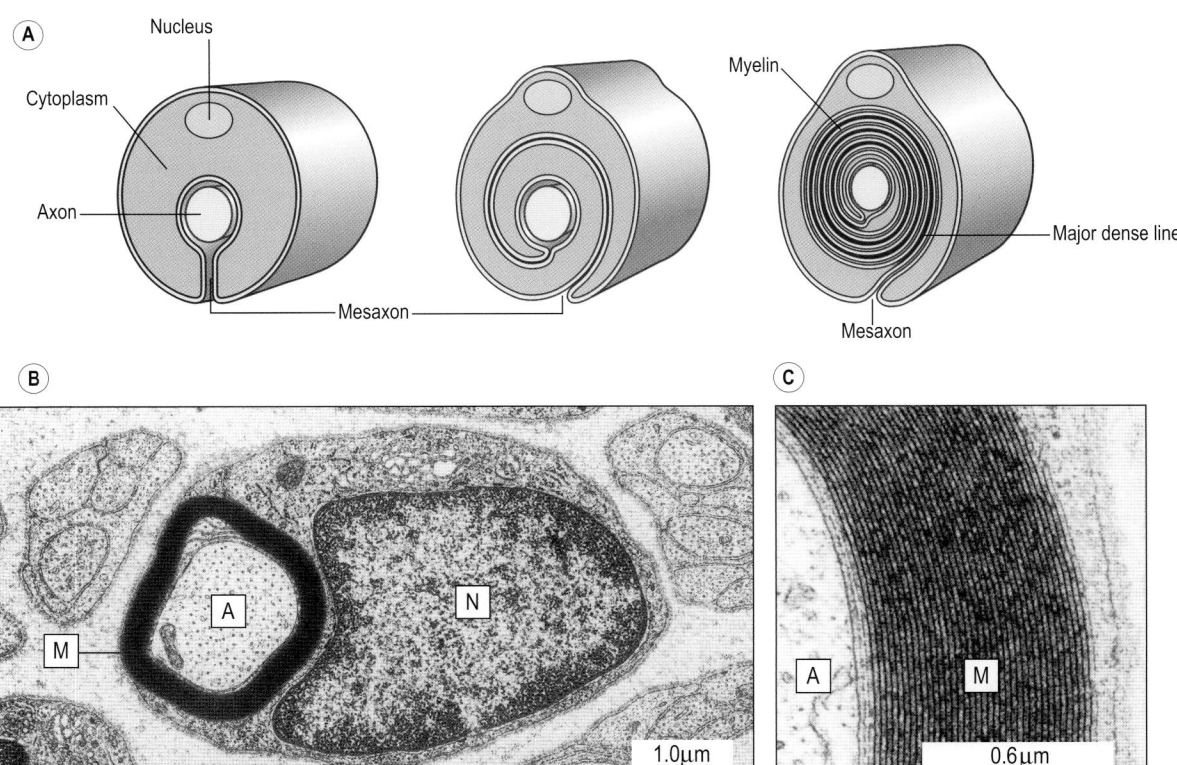

Fig. 8.3 **Transverse section of a myelinated axon.** (A) Myelination. (B) Low power electron micrograph (EM) of Schwann cell with myelin sheath. (C) High power EM of myelin. N, nucleus; M, myelin sheath; A, axon. Reproduced, with permission, from Young B, Lowe JS, Stevens A, Heath JW 2006 Wheater's Functional histology, 5th edn. Churchill Livingstone, Edinburgh.

evidence that some may be formed in the nervous system. Their functions are wide ranging:

- During development they secrete growth factors important in axon guidance, differentiation of glial cells and **angiogenesis** (the formation of new blood vessels). Acting as macrophages they phagocytose debris resulting from the high level of programmed cell death that is normal at this time.
- Towards the end of development and in the adult, they cease to be amoeboid, come to rest and extend their processes into a territory of surrounding grey or white matter. At this time they have as yet undefined homeostatic functions.
- During most types of injury to the nervous system – trauma, toxins, infection, autoimmunity or neurodegenerative disease – they revert to being macrophages and their numbers rise. These reactive microglia are important in the repair of injury.

ORGANISATION OF THE NERVOUS SYSTEM

The nervous system is divided into:
- The peripheral nervous system
- The central nervous system – composed of the brain and spinal cord.

PERIPHERAL NERVOUS SYSTEM

The **peripheral nervous system** consists of the nerves which carry afferent and efferent fibres to and from the central nervous system and the networks of nerve cells and glia in systems such as the gut. The peripheral nervous system is subdivided, somewhat artificially, into:

- **Somatic** nervous system (see below)
- **Autonomic** nervous system (see Ch. 4)
- **Enteric** nervous system (see Chs 15 and 16).

Somatic nervous system

The somatic nervous system consists of sensory and motor nerves which receive signals form sensory organs and innervate skeletal muscle. The organisation of the **somatic nervous system** shows bilateral symmetry (nerve trunks are paired) and segmentation (nerve roots emerge at regular intervals along the long axis of the nervous system) which is obvious for spinal nerves though less clear in the cranial nerves.

Spinal nerves
The **spinal nerves** convey information between the peripheral tissues and nerves in the spinal cord. There are 31 pairs of spinal nerves (Fig. 8.4), each arising from a single segment of the spinal cord and leaving the vertebral column via an intervertebral foramina. Spinal nerves are **mixed**; that is, all contain both afferent and efferent nerve fibres. Each nerve is formed by the union of two nerve branches, a dorsal and a ventral root which carry sensory and motor fibres (both somatic and autonomic), respectively. Primary afferent fibres are pseudounipolar (having a single axon with central and peripheral branches and no dendrites (Fig. 8.1)) and have their cell bodies in the **dorsal root ganglia**.

Cranial nerves
The **cranial nerves** transmit peripheral information directly to and from the brain. There are 12 pairs of cranial nerves (Table 8.1) of which only four contain both sensory and motor fibres; the others are either purely sensory or purely motor. Four also contain autonomic (visceral efferent) fibres. Most of the cranial nerves originate from or terminate in the brainstem (see below). By developmental criteria the optic nerves and retinas can be regarded as part of the central nervous system.

Structure of peripheral nerves
Peripheral nerves contain the axons of neurons. Nerve fibres consist of the axon and its associated mesaxon. Nerve fibres may be myelinated or unmyelinated and in the latter case the outer Schwann cell layer is known as the **neurolemma**. Nerve fibres are held together by connective tissue, the **endoneurium**, and are gathered into bundles called **fascicles** surrounded by more connective tissue, the **perineurium**. A peripheral nerve contains one or more fascicles along with blood vessels ensheathed in an **epineurium** (Fig. 8.5). The largest nerves are sometimes termed **nerve trunks**.

Nerve fibre classification
Nerve fibres in the peripheral nervous system are classified according to their diameter (Table 8.2). This is closely linked to their conduction velocity, the speed with which nerve impulses spread along them, and allows fibres to be crudely characterised as to function. The fastest fibres are the myelinated large diameter motor neurons and the slowest are small C fibres which transmit pain impulses.

CENTRAL NERVOUS SYSTEM

The CNS consists of the **brain** and **spinal cord** (Fig. 8.6). The brain has a **hindbrain**, a **midbrain** and a **forebrain**, divisions that are apparent very early in its development. The hindbrain and midbrain taken together (but excluding the cerebellum) are often referred to as the **brainstem**.

Spinal cord

The **spinal cord** contains about 100 million nerve cells. A transverse section of the cord shows that their cell bodies are contained in a butterfly-shaped central region of grey matter (Fig. 8.8). This is surrounded by white matter in which axons ascend and descend in tracts. A **central canal** runs the length of the spinal cord and is continuous with the **ventricles** (see The ventricular systems and cerebrospinal fluid) of the brain but in most adults the central canal is closed so cerebrospinal fluid (CSF) does not flow through it. The spinal cord proper terminates at the level of vertebra L2 and the roots for spinal nerves emerging below this level form the **cauda equina**.

Rexed's laminae
The spinal grey matter is organised into columns that extend the length of the cord. They are distinguished by differences in their neuron populations and how they are connected. In

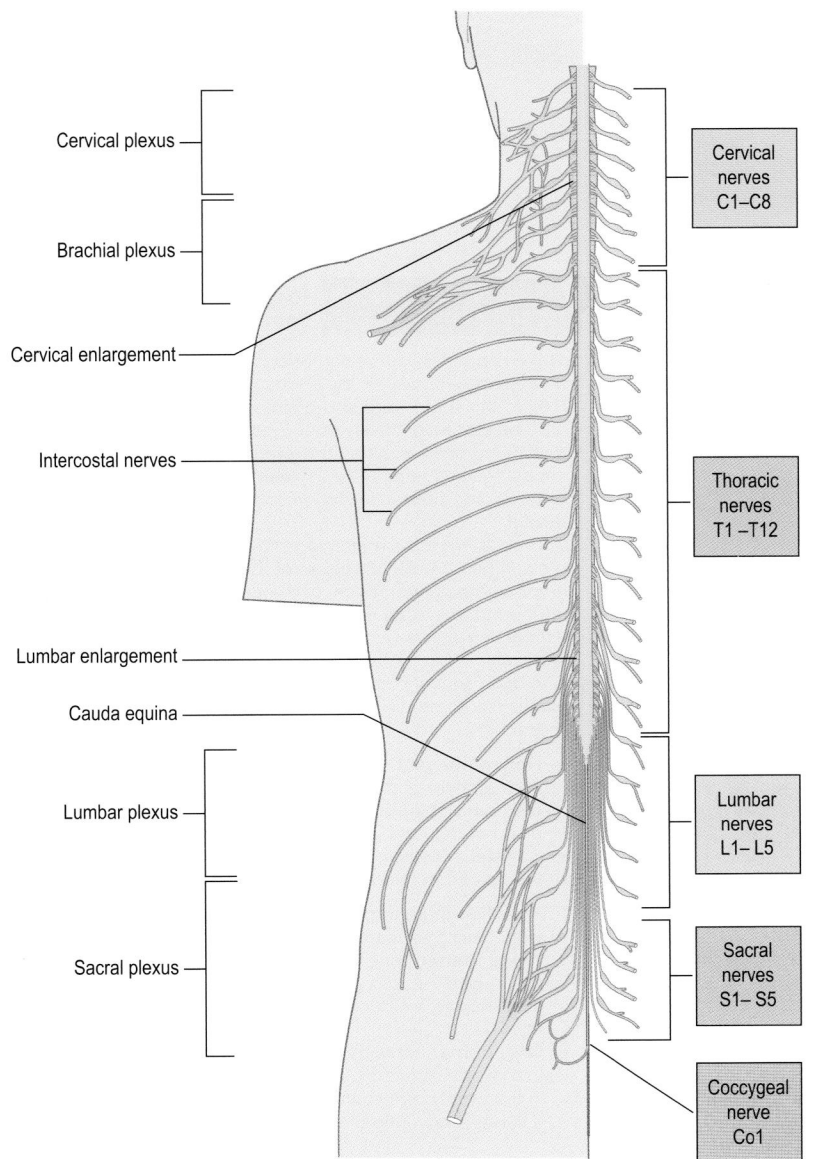

Fig. 8.4 Peripheral nerves.
Redrawn with permission from Marieb
EN, Hoehn K 2006 Human anatomy
and physiology, 7th edn. Benjamin
Cummings, San Francisco.

Table 8.1	**Cranial nerves**		
Nerve	**Type (motor/sensory/both, parasympathetic)**	**CNS origin/destination**	**Function**
I Olfactory	Sensory	Olfactory bulb	Smell
II Optic	Sensory	Thalamus	Vision
III Oculomotor	Motor, parasympathetic	Midbrain	Eye movements
IV Trochlear	Motor	Midbrain	Eye movements
V Trigeminal	Both	Midbrain and hindbrain	Sensory from head and face, motor to jaw
VI Abducens	Motor	Hindbrain	Eye movements
VII Facial	Both, parasympathetic	Thalamus (sensory), hindbrain (motor)	Taste, sensory from palate, motor to face, secretomotor to salivary and lachrymal glands
VIII Vestibulocochlear	Sensory	Thalamus (auditory division), hindbrain (vestibular division)	Hearing and balance
IX Glossopharyngeal	Both, parasympathetic	Thalamus (sensory), hindbrain (motor)	Taste, motor to pharynx, secretomotor to salivary glands
X Vagus	Both, parasympathetic	Thalamus (sensory), hindbrain (motor)	Taste, sensory from viscera, motor to pharynx and larynx, visceral motor
XI Accessory	Motor	Medulla, spinal cord C1–C5	Motor to palate and some neck muscles
XII Hypoglossal	Motor	Medulla	Motor to tongue

Table 8.2	Erlanger/Gasser classification of nerve fibres		
Fibre type	**Diameter (μm)**	**Conduction velocity (m/s)**	**Functions (example)**
Aα	12–20	72–120	Motor neurons
Aβ	6–12	36–72	Skin touch afferents
Aγ	2–8	12–48	Motor to muscle spindles
Aδ	1–6	4–36	Myelinated skin temperature and pain afferents
C	0.2–1.5	0.4–2.0	Unmyelinated skin pain afferents

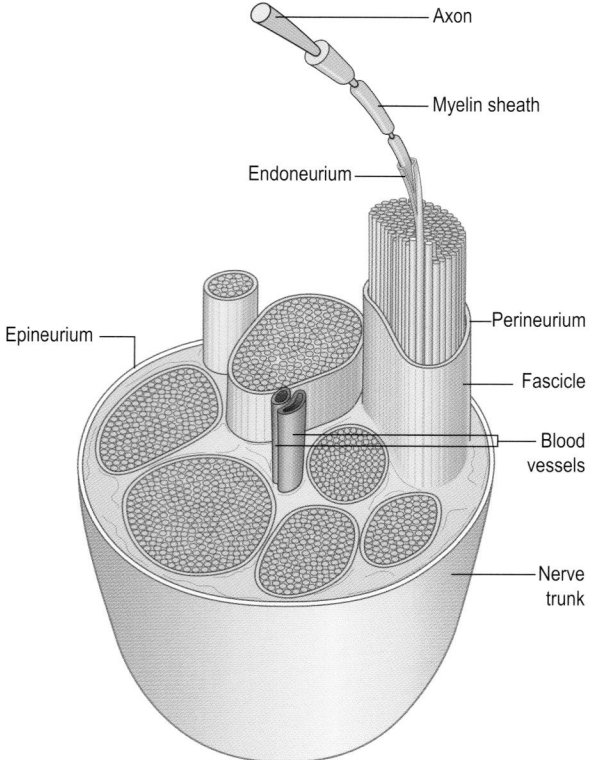

Fig. 8.5 Structure of a peripheral nerve. Source: Marieb EN, Hoehn K 2006 Human anatomy and physiology, 7th edn. Benjamin Cummings, San Francisco; Stevens A, Lowe J 2004 Human histology, 3rd edn. Mosby, Edinburgh.

---

i Information box 8.1 Central nervous system anatomical terms

There is possibly some confusion in describing the anatomical relations of the central nervous system (Fig. 8.6). In the spinal cord and brainstem the terms **superior** and **inferior** respectively refer to above and below in describing position along the long axis of the body. These are sometimes referred to as **rostral** and **caudal**, while **anterior** and **posterior** are synonymous with **ventral** and **dorsal**.

In going from the midbrain to the forebrain the entire brain is bent by 90°. Because of this flexure the anterior (front) and posterior (back) of the forebrain are then also referred to as rostral and caudal, respectively. Equally, ventral and dorsal become synonymous with inferior and superior.

In brain sections or imaging, three mutually orthogonal planes (i.e. three planes at right angles to each other) are defined.

- **Horizontal sections** are parallel to the plane that cuts both anterior and posterior commissures.
- **Coronal** or **frontal sections** are made parallel to the plane of the face.
- **Sagittal sections** lie in a plane parallel to the division of the cerebrum into left and right hemispheres.

A section through the CNS reveals distinct areas of white and grey matter:

- **White matter** consists of large numbers of nerve fibres assembled into discrete tracts, each with specific connections and functions. Its colour is conferred by myelin.
- **Grey matter** contains neuron cell bodies and dendrites. In the brain, it occurs either in discrete masses embedded in the white matter called **nuclei** (singular: **nucleus**), or as a thin rind covering the surface termed **cortex**.

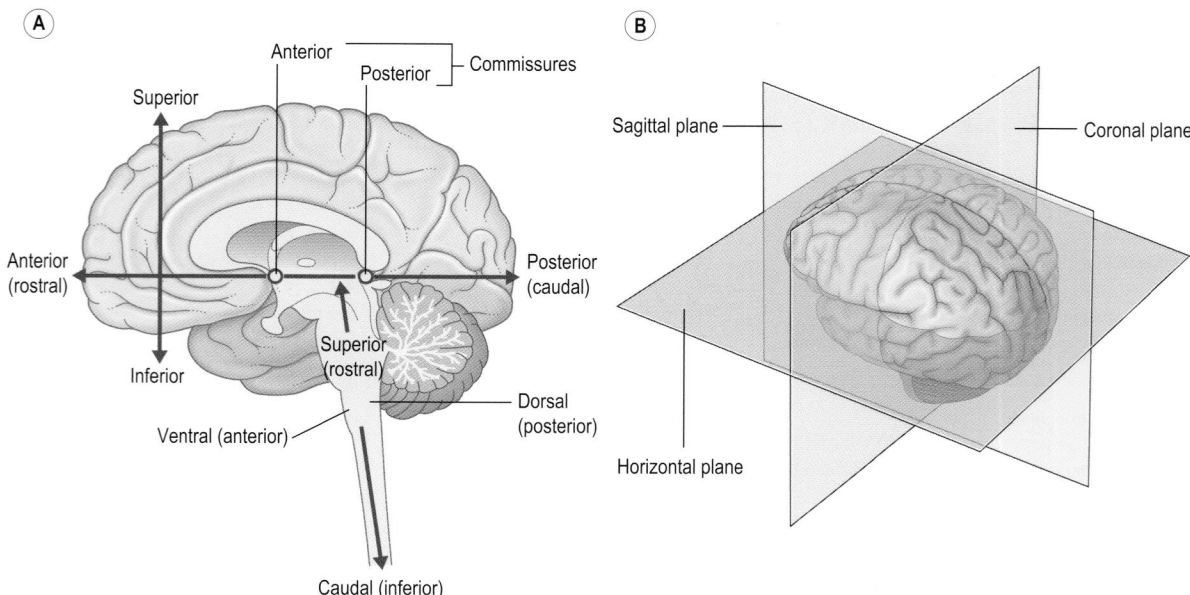

Fig. 8.6 Anatomical axes (A) and principal planes (B) of the human nervous system.

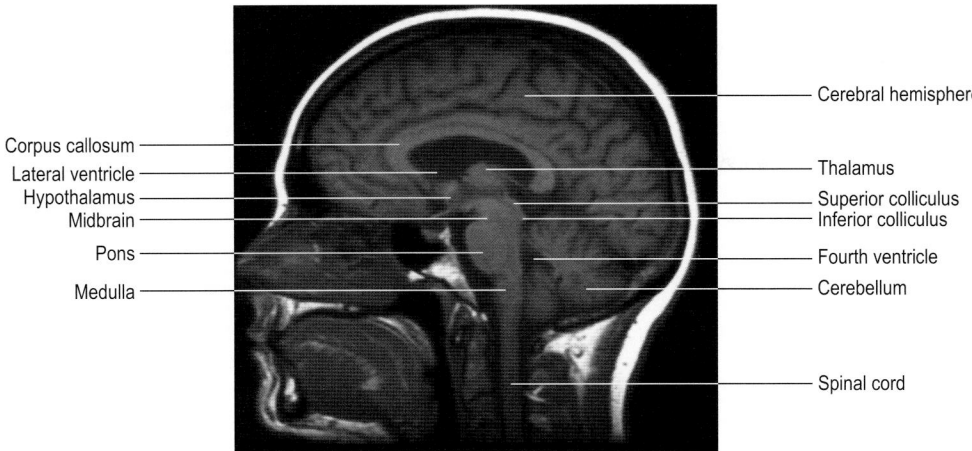

Fig. 8.7 **Magnetic resonance (MR) image of the midsagittal section of the brain and spinal cord.**

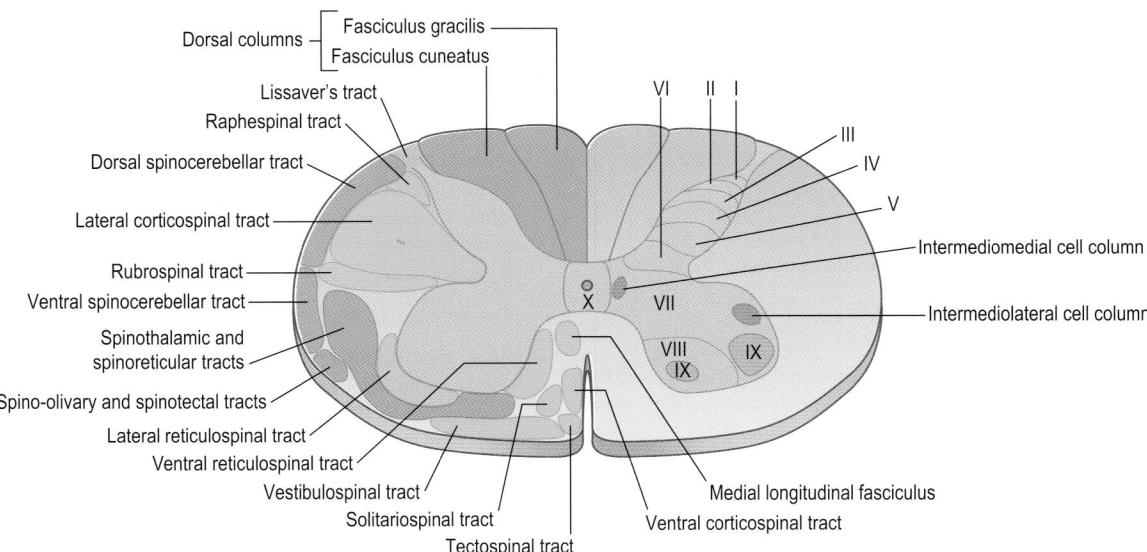

Fig. 8.8 **Transverse section through cervical spinal cord.** White matter pathways are shown on the *left*, descending in *blue*, ascending in *green*; rexed laminae are depicted on the *right*.

transverse sections through the cord these column appear as **Rexed's laminae.**

- The dorsal horns (**lamina I–VI**) contain the termination zones for primary afferent sensory neurons, and house **dorsal horn cells** which are involved in reflex circuits. **Lamina VI** is seen only in spinal segments C5–T1 and L2–S3 and receives sensory input from joints and muscles, providing information about limb position and movement.
- **Lamina VII** houses the **lateral column** which is most prominent in thoracic segments and contains the cell bodies of the preganglionic autonomic fibres.
- **Laminae VIII and IX** constitute the **ventral horns** of the spinal grey matter and contain the cell bodies of motor neurons whose axons innervate skeletal muscle.

White matter tracts

Tracts of nerve fibres enter and leave the white matter tracts at all levels of the cord, running to and from the brain. They are often named according to their origin and destination. For example, an ascending tract which projects to the cerebellum is a spinocerebellar tract, whereas a descending pathway starting in the vestibular nucleus (in the brainstem) is a vestibulospinal tract. The axons of neurons entirely within the spinal cord that run between different segments are termed **propriospinal fibres.**

Brainstem

The **brainstem** (Fig. 8.9) consists of:

- The **hindbrain**, minus the cerebellum
- The **midbrain**.

It contains the nuclei of all but the first two cranial nerves, plus numerous other discrete nuclei, many of which are part of the reticular formation (see below). Much of its bulk is taken up by ascending and descending fibre tracts going to and from higher levels of the **neuraxis**, the long axis of the central nervous system.

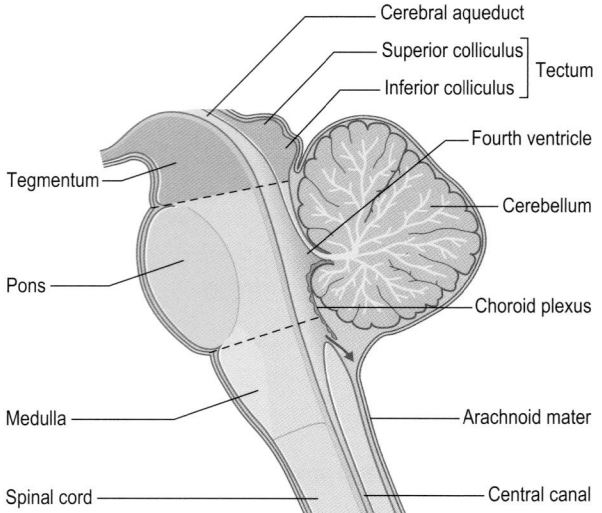

Fig. 8.9 **Brainstem anatomy; sagittal section through the brainstem.**

Hindbrain

The hindbrain consists of:

- The **medulla** and **pons** ventrally and
- The **cerebellum** dorsally.

  Ventral and dorsal structures are separated by the fourth ventricle.

Medulla and pons

The medulla and pons have neural networks that serve 'life support' functions including autonomic control of the cardio-vascular system, ventilation and airway reflexes, and gut reflexes (e.g. swallowing, vomiting). The hindbrain contains the **cranial nerve nuclei** for cranial nerves V–XII.

Cerebellum

The cerebellum (little brain) comprises about a quarter of the mass of the brain but contains about half of its neurons. In contrast to the rest of the hindbrain, the cerebellum is concerned with high level functions. It is associated with control of the precise timing and execution of voluntary movement and with learning new motor skills, and has a role in cognition.

Midbrain

The midbrain is by far the smallest division of the brain in adults and consists of:

- The **tegmentum** ventrally
- The **tectum** dorsally.

Tegmentum

The tegmentum contains the nuclei of cranial nerves III–V, dopamine-secreting neurons that project rostrally to form part of a brain system concerned with motivation, and several nuclei concerned with movement (e.g. **substantia nigra** and **red nucleus**). Surrounding the aqueduct of Sylvius (cerebral aqueduct) that traverses the midbrain is the periaqueductal grey (PAG) matter. This has a role in dampening the transmission of pain signals.

Tectum

The tectum is made up of paired **superior colliculi** (singular: **colliculus**) and **inferior colliculi**. These receive input from optic and vestibulocochlear nerves, respectively, and mediate visual and auditory reflexes, e.g. altering the gaze or orienting the head towards an object in peripheral vision, or a sound source.

Reticular formation

The reticular formation is situated within the core of the brainstem. It is a complicated ensemble of neural circuits that extend through the medulla, pons and brainstem. The cell bodies of reticular neurons are clustered into a number of discrete **reticular nuclei** that are distributed throughout the fibre tracts of the reticular formation.

  Reticular neurons are small and fall into two classes:

- Large, medially placed cells that use monoamine transmitters, and project axons into the forebrain. These are involved in activities such as sleep-wakefulness, arousal and motivation.
- Small, laterally placed cells that are arranged into local networks responsible for reflexes involving cranial nerve nuclei, e.g. emotional facial expressions (smiling, crying), chewing, and eye movements. Other networks involving the nucleus of the solitary tract (NST) coordinate visceral functions; gut reflexes (swallowing, vomiting), cardiovascular (e.g. baroreceptor) reflexes and airway reflexes (sneezing, coughing). The motor side of many of these reflexes has an autonomic as well as a somatic component.

  The reticular formation also:

- Generates the rhythmic output that drives **ventilation** and basic **locomotor** patterns
- Contributes to the control of **posture**
- Dampens the transmission of **pain** signals into the forebrain.

  The activities of the reticular formation are highly integrated. For example, swallowing and breathing must be precisely timed if we are not to choke.

Forebrain

The forebrain consists of:

- The **diencephalon**, the central core of the forebrain
- The **telencephalon** or **cerebrum**, made up largely of the conspicuous, cerebral hemispheres.

Diencephalon

The diencephalon comprises a ventral **hypothalamus**, which lies just above the brainstem, and a dorsal **thalamus** overlain by the **epithalamus**, and beneath which is the **subthalamus**. The third ventricle runs through the diencephalon.

Hypothalamus

The small size of the hypothalamus belies its importance. It is involved in thermoregulation and in triggering sleep. As part of the **limbic system** (see below), it is crucial for goal-directed behaviours (drinking, eating and sexual behaviour) and controls many endocrine functions, e.g. hormone involvement in reproduction, growth and stress, by way of both neural and vascular connections to the **pituitary gland**.

Table 8.3	Thalamic nuclei		
	Nuclei	**Connections**	**Function**
Anterior group	Anterior nucleus	Limbic system	Emotion
Medial group	Mediodorsal nucleus	Basal ganglia and amygdala	Memory
		Frontal cortex	
Ventral group	Ventrobasal nuclei	Basal ganglia	Sensory and motor
		Cerebellum	
		Motor cortex	
		Somatosensory systems	
Posterior group	Medial and lateral geniculate nuclei	Auditory and visual input	Pain perception
	Posterior nucleus		Visual attention
	Pulvinar		
Non-specific	Intralaminar nuclei	Widespread and diffuse	Sleep/wakefulness and arousal
	Midline nuclei		
	Reticular nuclei		

Thalamus

The thalamus is an aggregate of many distinct nuclei. All sensory input goes into the cerebrum by way of the thalamus with the exception of smell. It also has massive connections with parts of the cerebrum concerned with movement, emotion and cognition. Thalamic nuclei are named after their position in relation to a rostro-caudal sheet of fibres (the **internal medullary lamina**) that runs through the structure, and they fall into five groups (Table 8.3).

Epithalamus

The smallest part of the diencephalon, the **epithalamus** contains the **pineal gland**. It receives visual input and regulates circadian rhythms on the basis of hours of light and dark.

Subthalamus

The subthalamus lies at the junction of the diencephalon and midbrain and is a component of the **basal ganglia**, a set of five interconnected nuclei involved in movement.

Cerebrum (telencephalon)

The cerebrum, which is highly developed in humans, envelops and dominates the diencephalon. It is made up of two **cerebral hemispheres**. The two hemispheres are interconnected by axons which cross the midline in tracts called **commissures**, the largest of which is the **corpus callosum**. Each cerebral hemisphere has four lobes, named after the cranial bones which lie above them (Fig. 8.10). Within the hemispheres lie numerous nuclei, components of the **basal ganglia** and **limbic** system.

Cerebral cortex

The surface of the cerebral hemispheres is covered by **cerebral cortex**, a 2–4 mm thick layer of grey matter, densely packed with neurons. Its surface area is maximised by being thrown into folds, called **gyri**, with intervening grooves, called **sulci** (see Fig. 8.10). Most cerebral cortex in humans is composed of a six-layered **neocortex** (new cortex) which is found only in mammals.

The cerebral cortex is crucial for sensory perception, the planning and execution of voluntary movement, memory, language, and all cognitive functions. Consciousness and self-awareness are all functions attributed to the cerebral cortex.

Different areas of the cerebral cortex are concerned with specific functions and these areas have been mapped on the basis of function (Fig. 8.11) which can be correlated with differences in structure (see below). The most commonly used map is **Brodmann's** where the cerebral cortex is divided into 52 different functional areas (see Fig. 8.11).

Some areas of the cerebral cortex are purely sensory or motor in function. However, most is **association cortex** that has an integrative function, combining inputs from diverse sources and performing the transformations needed to generate outputs. Regions of cortex are heavily interconnected by **cortico-cortical fibres** that run through the white matter of the cerebral hemispheres.

At a cellular level the neocortex is divided into six layers on the basis of the populations of neurons they house and their connectivity (Fig. 8.12 and Table 8.4). The layers are not homogeneous across the hemispheres, which can be divided into regions based on differences in their histology, such as the relative thickness of the layers, which correspond to functional specialisations. For example, in the sensory cortex layer IV is particularly well developed whereas in the motor cortex layer V is predominant.

Cortical circuits and connectivity

The cerebral cortex appears to consist of the same basic circuit copied many millions of times (Fig. 8.12B). Moreover, the cortex is a mosaic of columns that extend through all the layers. Cells within a column are heavily interconnected but connections between columns are sparse. How the cortical circuits operate to produce behaviour is not understood.

Inputs to the neocortex are from two major sources.

- The thalamus sends input to layer IV.
- The majority of cortical inputs are **feedforward connections** that arise from layers II and III of the source cortex to enter layer IV of the target cortex. These target regions also send **feedback connections** to their input source from their cortical layers V and VI and input to layer I and VI. Some cortical input is from the corresponding region in the opposite hemisphere and arrives by way of **commissural fibres**, most of which cross in the corpus callosum.

Typically inputs to layer IV terminate on the **spiny stellate cells** which make excitatory synapses on the apical den-

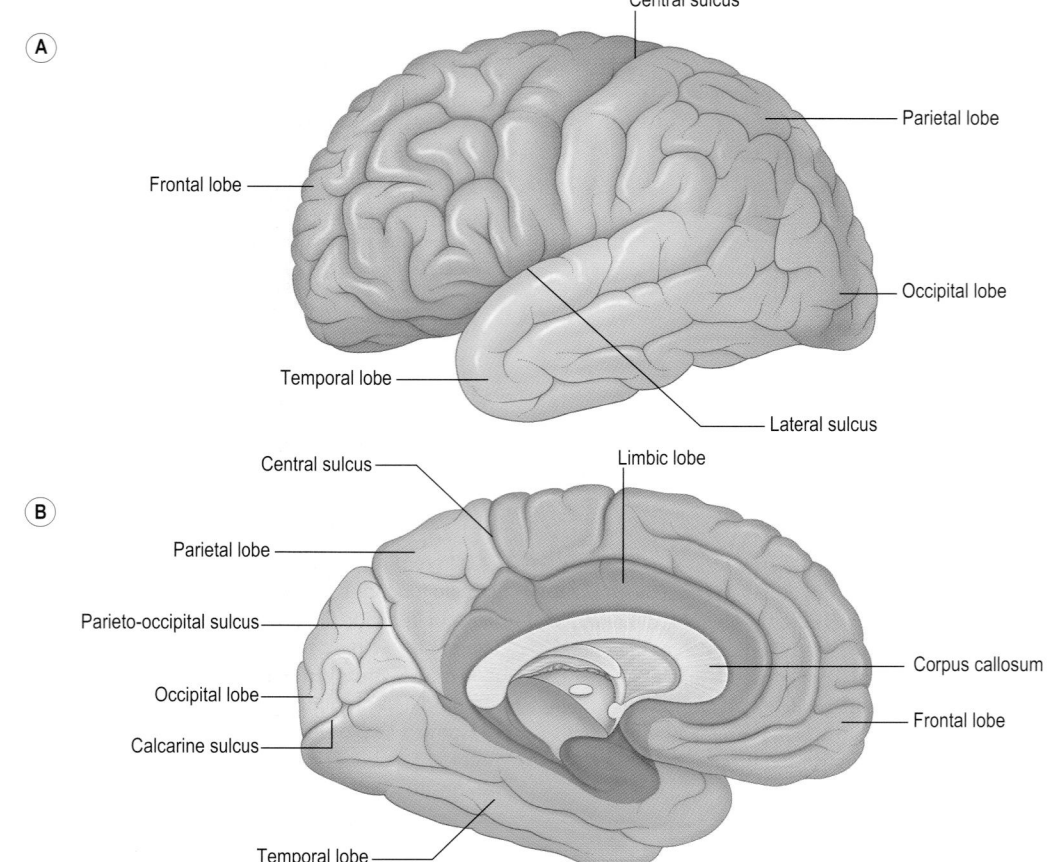

Fig. 8.10 Left cerebral hemisphere: (A) lateral surface; (B) medial surface, showing lobes, principal gyri and sulci.

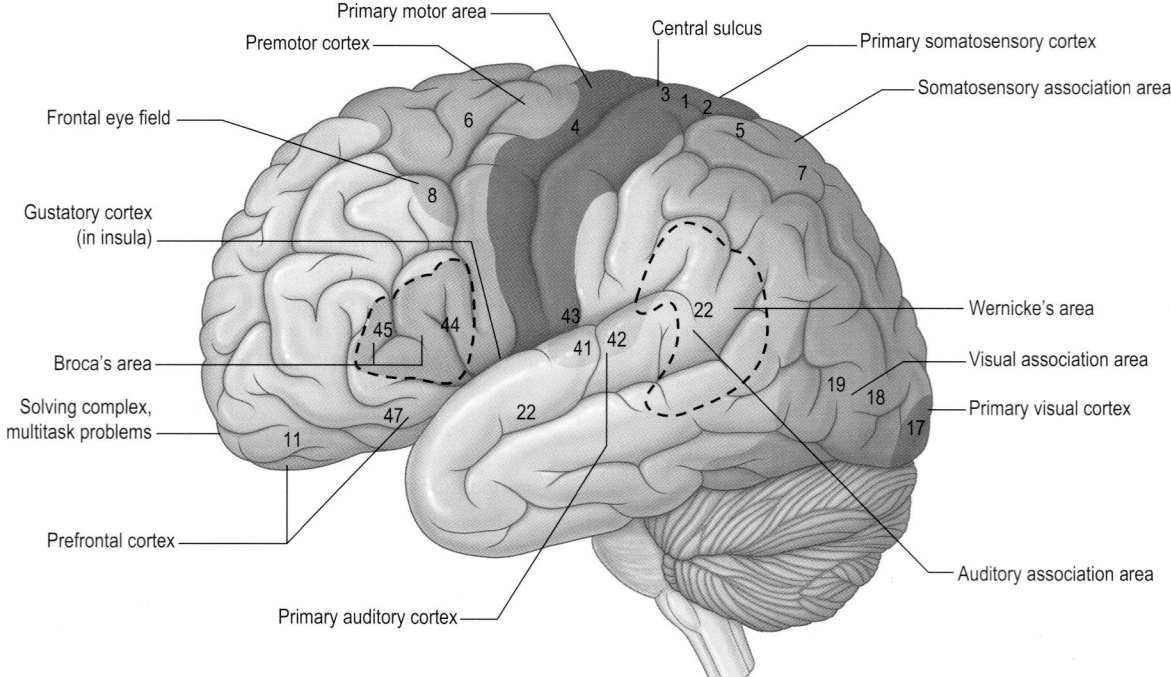

Fig. 8.11 Functional areas of the cerebral cortex, including Brodmann's areas (numbered). *Red*: motor cortex; *blue*: sensory cortex; *pale blue* and *pale red*: association cortex. Redrawn with permission from Marieb EN, Hoehn K 2006 Human anatomy and physiology, 7th edn. Benjamin Cummings, San Francisco.

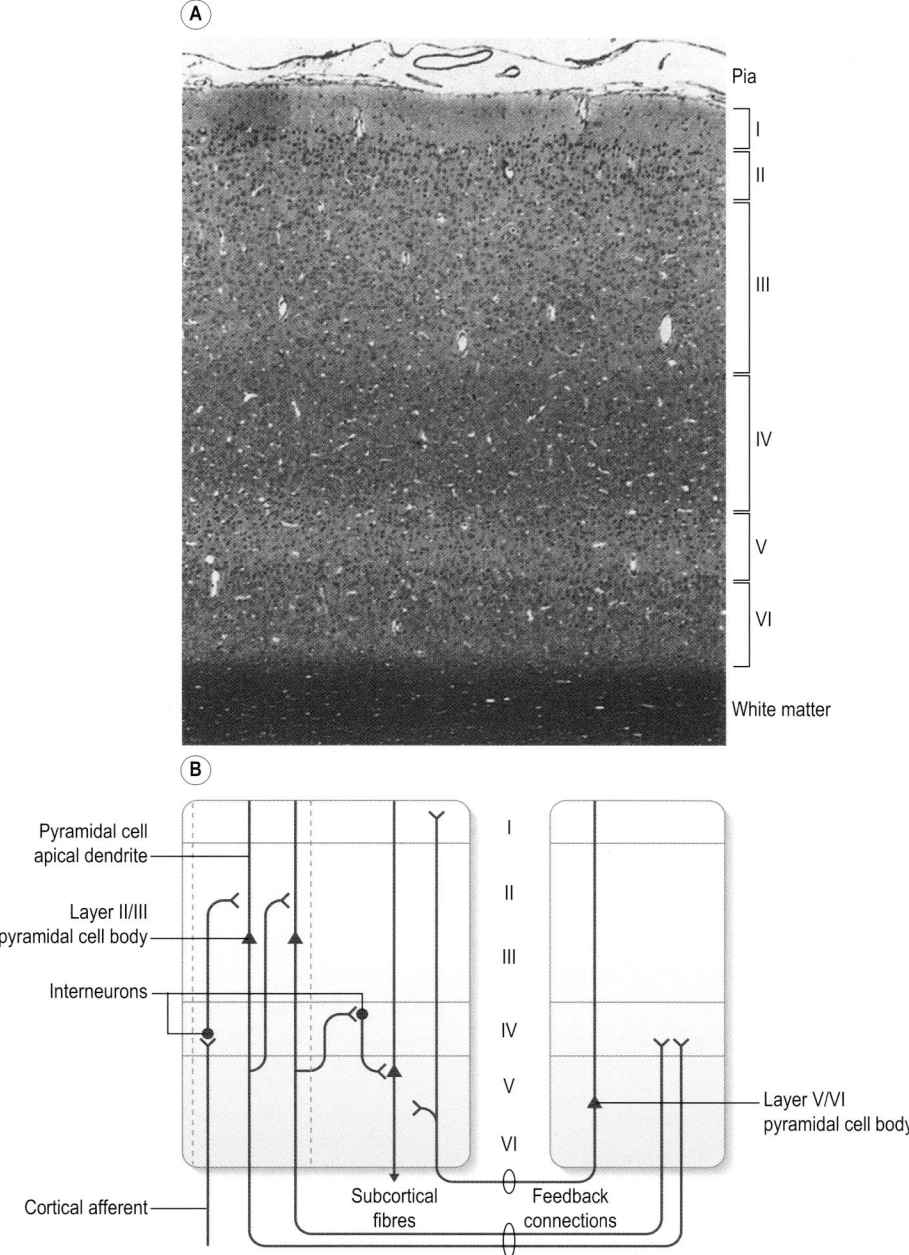

Fig. 8.12 Cerebral neocortex: (A) laminar structure; (B) cortical connectivity. Redrawn with permission from Young B, Heath JW 2006 Wheater's functional histology, 5th edn. Churchill Livingstone, Edinburgh.

Table 8.4	Features of the neocortical layers			
No	**Layer**	**Principal cell type**	**Input from**	**Output to**
I	Molecular layer	Apical dendrites of pyramidal cells	Cortex	
II	Outer granular layer	Small pyramidal cells		Ipsilateral cortex
III	Outer pyramidal cell layer	Medium-sized pyramidal cells		Contralateral cortex
IV	Inner granular layer	Spiny stellate cells (many interneurons)	Thalamus	
V	Inner pyramidal cell layer	Large pyramidal cells		Striatum, brainstem, spinal cord
VI	Fusiform layer	Modified pyramidal cells	Cortex	Thalamus

drites of pyramidal cells. The pyramidal cells in turn excite their nearest neighbours (those in the same column) by way of axon collaterals. However, pyramidal cells further away are inhibited by **smooth stellate cells**. Numerous other cells modulate the operation of the cortical circuit, including other types of inhibitory neurons and bipolar cells.

All cortical output is via the axons of excitatory pyramidal cells. The destinations of the principal outputs are to the:

- Ipsilateral and contralateral cortex
- Feedback connections to the cortex
- Subcortical nuclei
- Thalamus.

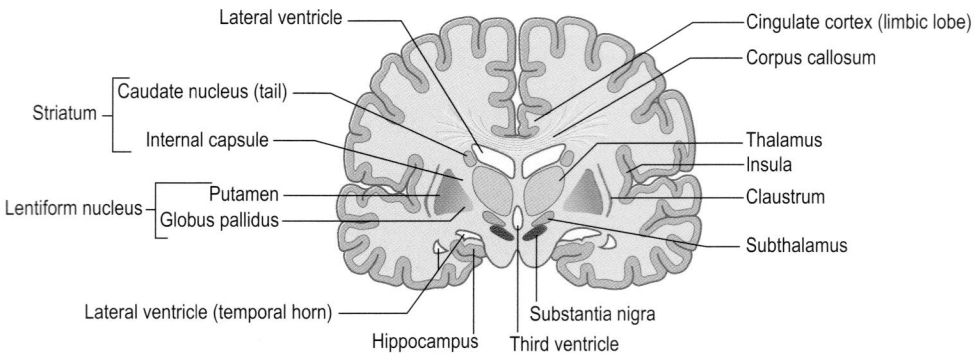

Fig. 8.13 Coronal section of brain showing structures of the basal ganglia and the limbic system.

Basal ganglia

Lying deep within the white matter of the cerebral hemispheres are subcortical nuclei, the **basal ganglia** which consists of five extensively connected structures (Fig. 8.13):

- Caudate nucleus
- Putamen
- Globus pallidus
- Subthalamus
- Substantia nigra.

The **putamen** and **globus pallidus** make up the lentiform nucleus, which is separated from the **caudate nucleus** by the internal capsule. Despite their anatomical separation the caudate and putamen are functionally homologous and collectively termed the **striatum**. The neostriatum interconnects with the **subthalamus** (diencephalon) and the **substantia nigra** of the midbrain and the whole ensemble is referred to as the basal ganglia. Together with some thalamic nuclei and regions of cerebral cortex, the basal ganglia make up the extrapyramidal motor system, which programmes the execution of voluntary movements.

Limbic system

The **limbic system** (Fig. 8.13) is involved in emotions and their expression. It is composed of:

- Cerebral cortical regions comprising the **orbital prefrontal cortex**, **cingulate cortex** and **hippocampus** and
- A number of nuclei: the mamillary bodies, amygdala, ventral striatum and medial dorsal thalamus.

On midsagittal section, these structures appear to form a rim (Latin *limbus*) around the corpus callosum. Although limbic structures are heavily interconnected, it is possible to attribute specific functions to some of them. For example, the hippocampus consolidates some forms of long-term memory, while the amygdala recognises important stimuli (such as facial expressions) and learns about fearful situations.

Meninges

The CNS is ensheathed by three connective tissue membranes, collectively called the **meninges** (Fig. 8.14), which serve to protect the brain.

Dura mater

The outermost and toughest of the meninges is the **dura mater**. It consists of two layers: the periosteal layer, which lies close to the periosteum (the inner surface of the skull),

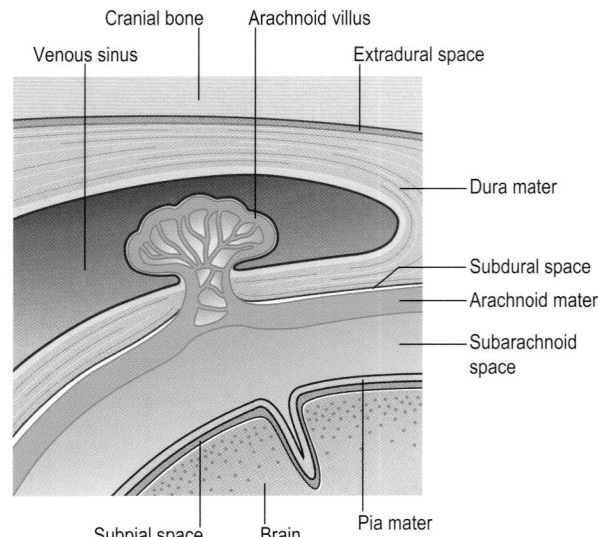

Fig. 8.14 The meninges.

and the meningeal layer, which lies closer to the brain. In most areas of the brain these two layers are fused but in some regions they enclose blood filled cavities called dural sinuses which collect venous blood, eventually draining into the internal jugular vein.

In two places the dura mater is thrown into folds which help support the brain:

- **Falx cerebri**, a midline sickle-shaped vertical fold which extends into the longitudinal fissure that separates the two cerebral hemispheres, arching over the corpus callosum.
- **Tentorium cerebelli**, a tent-shaped arching fold which divides the cranium into a **posterior fossa**, below, containing the brainstem and cerebellum, and **middle and anterior fossae**, above, occupied by the forebrain.

The cranial compartment and structures above the tentorium cerebelli are described as **supratentorial**, those below as **infratentorial**. A space-occupying lesion within the skull (e.g. a tumour or haemorrhage, Clinical box 8.1) or cerebral oedema compresses brain, cranial nerves or blood vessels against the free edges of these folds and so can wreak havoc on neural function.

In the vertebral canal the dura extends as a blind-ending sac. The **dural sheath** is not attached to the bony vertebrae and the resulting **epidural space** is filled with fat and blood vessels.

Arachnoid mater

The **arachnoid mater** is a fibrocellular layer which lines the dura. Tight junctions between its cells form a fluid-tight compartment, the **subarachnoid space** between the arachnoid and the pia mater, which contains **CSF**. Larger spaces within the subarachnoid space are termed **cisterns**. Arachnoid

---

Clinical box 8.1   **Intracranial haemorrhage**

Intracranial haemorrhage may occur at the brain surface or within the brain itself and is classified by the compartment into which the bleed occurs. It is usually caused either by head injury or cardiovascular disorders such as aneurysm or hypertension.

- **Extradural haemorrhage**. Bleeding from the meningeal arteries that run between the endosteum and the skull can open up an extradural space. The resulting extradural haematoma can cause brain compression. The raised intracranial pressure (ICP) reduces cerebral blood flow producing ischaemia. Vasomotor neurons in the medulla drive increased sympathetic vasoconstriction, which raises mean arterial blood pressure, **Cushing's reflex**. Baroreceptor reflexes (see Ch. 11) then cause a slowing of the heart rate (bradycardia). The combination of a rise in blood pressure and bradycardia in a head-injured patient is prima facie evidence for extradural haemorrhage.
- **Subdural haemorrhage**. Bleeding into the subdural space between the dura and the arachnoid is usually from superficial cerebral veins going from the cerebral cortex to the venous sinuses. The clinical picture depends on the time elapsing between the injury and presentation (hours to months). Chronic subdural haemorrhage can occur in the elderly as a result of brain shrinkage rupturing superficial cerebral veins.
- **Subarachnoid** and **intracerebral haemorrhage**. Bleeding into the subarachnoid space or brain constitutes a cerebrovascular accident or stroke (see Clinical box 8.4 and Information box 8.7).

---

trabeculae extend across this space to provide support for superficial cerebral vessels.

Pia mater

This is a thin fibrocellular layer that closely covers the surface of the brain and spinal cord; there is a small gap, the **subpial space** between the pia and surface of the brain. Because the pia allows the passive exchange of water and small molecules, metabolites can diffuse from brain extracellular fluid into the CSF.

The ventricular systems and the cerebrospinal fluid

The tissues of the brain surround a series of fluid-filled cavities called the **ventricles** which are derived from the lumen of the neural tube. The five ventricles are connected to each other, the central canal of the spinal cord and the subarachnoid space. This is filled with **cerebrospinal fluid (CSF)** (Fig. 8.15) which acts as a cushion, supporting the weight of the brain and protecting it from damage caused by movement.

Secretion of CSF

CSF flows continually from the ventricles to the spinal cord and subarachnoid space (Clinical box 8.2). About 500 mL of CSF is secreted each day, mostly by the choroid plexuses in the lateral, third and fourth ventricles. The **choroid plexus** is made up of cuboidal epithelium derived from the ependymal lining of the ventricles, together with a highly vascular region of pia. The vessels are quite permeable, so CSF secretion starts with the formation of an ultrafiltrate of plasma. However, the ependymal cells are coupled by tight junctions and so act as a **blood–CSF barrier**, selectively absorbing some substances while secreting others, so that CSF has a different composition from blood (Table 8.5). In health, CSF contains no red blood cells and only a few white blood cells,

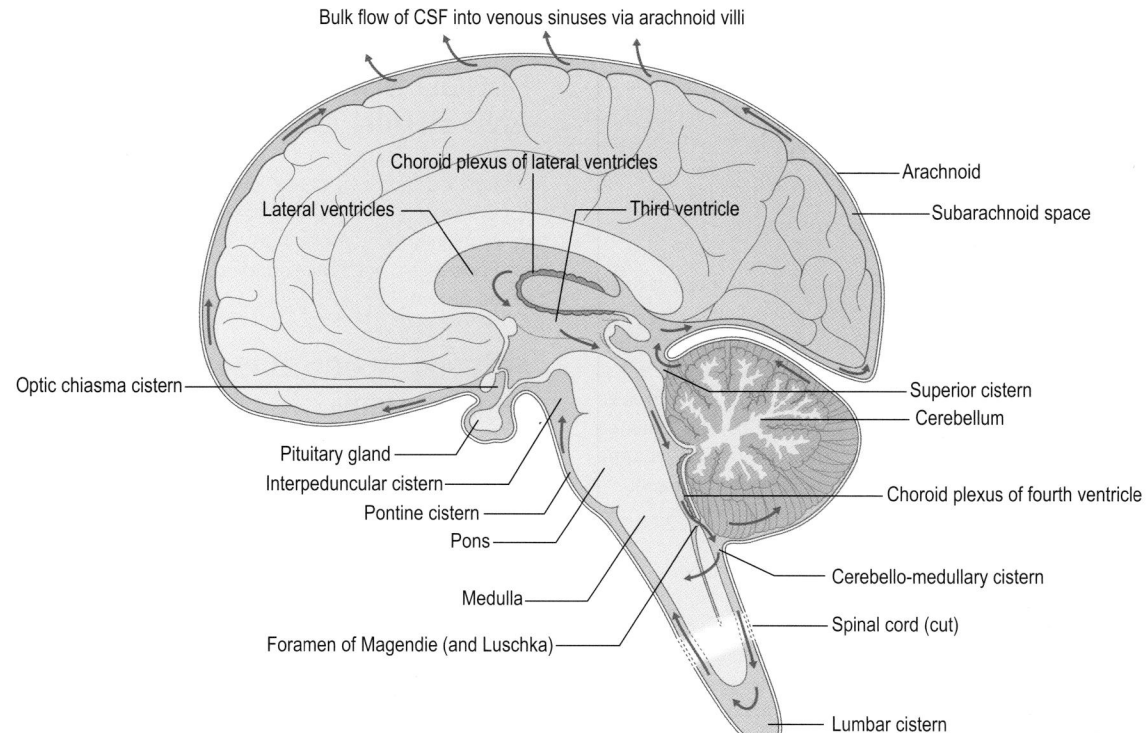

Fig. 8.15 **The ventricular system of the brain and circulation of the cerebrospinal fluid (CSF).**

Very little CSF flows through the central canal of the spinal cord, which is not patent in most adults, but some CSF flows within the subarachnoid space through the foramen magnum towards the lumbar region, reaching the end of the spinal meninges in about 12 hours. The spinal cord meninges extend as far as the second sacral vertebrae (S2) but the spinal cord only extends as far as the first or second lumbar level (L1, L2). Thus the space below L2 forms a large lumbar cistern containing CSF which can be sampled by lumbar puncture. The freely floating spinal nerves are not at risk of damage as they will drift away from the point of the needle. However, lumbar puncture should not be performed under circumstances of raised intracranial pressure as this can cause herniation of the brain.

Table 8.5   Composition of CSF compared with blood plasma

	CSF	Plasma
Protein (mg/dL)	35	7000
Glucose (mmol/L)	3.3	5
Na$^+$ (mmol/L)	138	138
K$^+$ (mmol/L)	2.8	4.5
Ca^{2+} (mmol/L)	2.1	4.8
pH	7.33	7.41

An obstruction to the circulation of CSF, due to a developmental abnormality, a tumour or in meningitis, causes fluid to accumulate in the space between cells (**interstitial cerebral oedema**); ventricles become progressively dilated, leading to brain compression and cerebral ischaemia.

In infants in whom the cranial sutures are unfused increased volume is partly accommodated by enlargement of the head; however, neural damage may happen very early in development in congenital hydrocephalus.

Some types of hydrocephalus can be treated by the insertion of a shunt which can divert the flow of excess CSF into a neck vein.

but in bacterial meningitis, for example, CSF glucose is reduced by the bacterial metabolism and white cell count is raised. About 30% of CSF is derived directly from the blood by Starling's mechanism (see Ch. 11). There is no lymphatic system in the CNS.

Absorption of CSF

The arachnoid mater has numerous tiny projections termed **arachnoid villi** (**granulations**) which project into the dural venous sinuses (see Fig. 8.14). These contain tubes that act as one-way valves which allow CSF to flow into the blood whenever the pressure in the subarachnoid space is greater than in the venous sinus (Clinical box 8.3). The balance between secretion and absorption gives a total CSF volume of 100–150 mL, of which about 30 mL is in the ventricles.

Functions of CSF

CSF has both metabolic and mechanical functions.

Metabolic functions

Because CSF equilibrates with brain extracellular fluid it contains unwanted metabolites or their catabolites. These are removed by a combination of selective absorption by the choroid plexuses and being dumped into venous blood via arachnoid villi.

Depriving a brain region of its blood supply for longer than a few minutes results in a region of damaged tissue called an **infarct**. This consists of **core**, in which hypoxia is so profound that cells undergo **necrotic cell death** in minutes, surrounded by a **penumbra** in which low oxygen concentration causes excessive release of the excitatory transmitter glutamate and cell death occurs partly by apoptosis (see Ch. 2). Because death of cells in the penumbra is not inevitable, treatment is aimed at salvaging them.

Neurological consequences depend on infarct size and location.

- Even small infarcts in the **brainstem** can be devastating because here neural structures are densely packed.
- Blockages (occlusions) in the **circle of Willis** or the principal cerebral vessels are often **circumvented** by flow through alternative routes so infarction is avoided.
- Because distal deep **end arteries** in the brain lack anastomoses, the deep brain regions they supply (**end zones**) are almost completely deprived of their blood supply by a bleed from, or occlusion of, these vessels.

Mechanical functions

- The weight of the brain is effectively reduced from about 1350 g to 50 g because it floats buoyantly in a 'pool' of CSF.
- The CSF and meninges dampen forces produced by head movement.
- The volume of the CSF compartment can undergo minor adjustments to resist the changes in intracranial pressure (ICP) that occur due to alterations in cerebral blood flow (CBF). When CBF rises, the subarachnoid space around the spinal cord can expand to accommodate CSF displaced by the increase in intracranial blood volume.

BLOOD SUPPLY TO THE BRAIN AND BRAIN METABOLISM

Although it comprises only 2% of the body mass, the brain uses 20% of the body's total oxygen consumption, a reflection of its high metabolic rate. This is matched by a high blood perfusion rate corresponding to 15–20% of the resting cardiac output.

ARTERIAL BLOOD SUPPLY

Circle of Willis

Blood is supplied to the brain by the circle of Willis, an arterial circle which lies beneath the base of the forebrain (Fig. 8.16). It is fed by four major arteries:

- A pair of **vertebral arteries** which then fuse to form the **basilar artery**, which traverses the underside of the pons
- A pair of internal carotid arteries.

The circle of Willis ensures that, should flow be obstructed to any one of these vessels, blood can still be delivered to all regions of the brain (Information box 8.2). The anatomy of this arterial circle varies greatly between individuals.

The circulation can be divided into the:

- **Anterior circulation**, comprising the:
  - Direct branches of the internal carotid arteries
  - Anterior cerebral arteries which are joined by the anterior communicating artery
  - Middle cerebral arteries.

- **Posterior circulation**, comprising the:
  - Vertebral arteries
  - Basilar artery
  - Posterior cerebral arteries.

The anterior and posterior circulation are connected by way of the narrow **posterior communicating arteries**. Three-quarters of strokes originate in the anterior circulation (see Information box 8.2).

Anterior cerebral arteries

The **anterior cerebral arteries** form an arch over the corpus callosum and supply the medial part of the frontal and parietal lobes of the cerebral hemispheres (Fig. 8.17). Occlusion of this vessel can cause damage to the contralateral motor nuclei of the V, VII and XII cranial nerves, affecting movement of jaw, lips and tongue, respectively.

Middle cerebral arteries

The **middle cerebral arteries** are the major branches of the internal carotid arteries and supply the lateral parts of the cerebral hemispheres except that of the occipital lobe and inferior temporal lobe. They give rise to the **lateral striate arteries**, which supply the corpus striatum and internal capsule. The **anterior choroidal arteries**, although small, supply important forebrain regions including the globus pallidus, caudate nucleus, parts of the thalamus, hypothalamus, amygdala and hippocampus, and the red nucleus and substantia nigra.

Posterior circulation

The **posterior cerebral arteries** supply the occipital lobe, medial and inferior parts of the temporal lobes, and the mid-

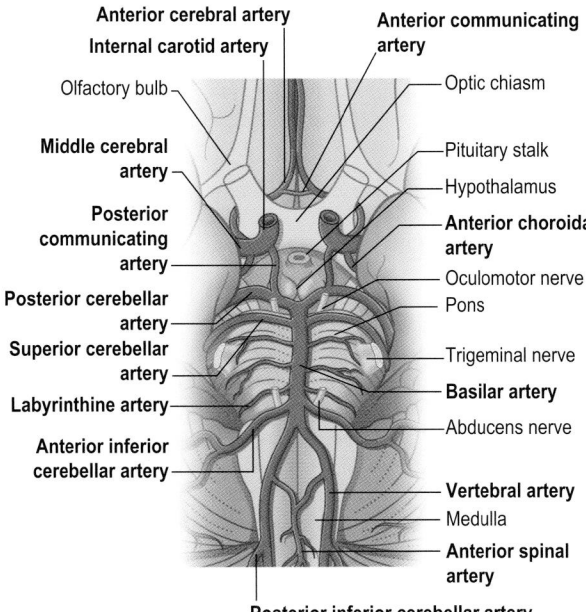

Fig. 8.16 Circle of Willis and principal arterial blood supply to the brain.

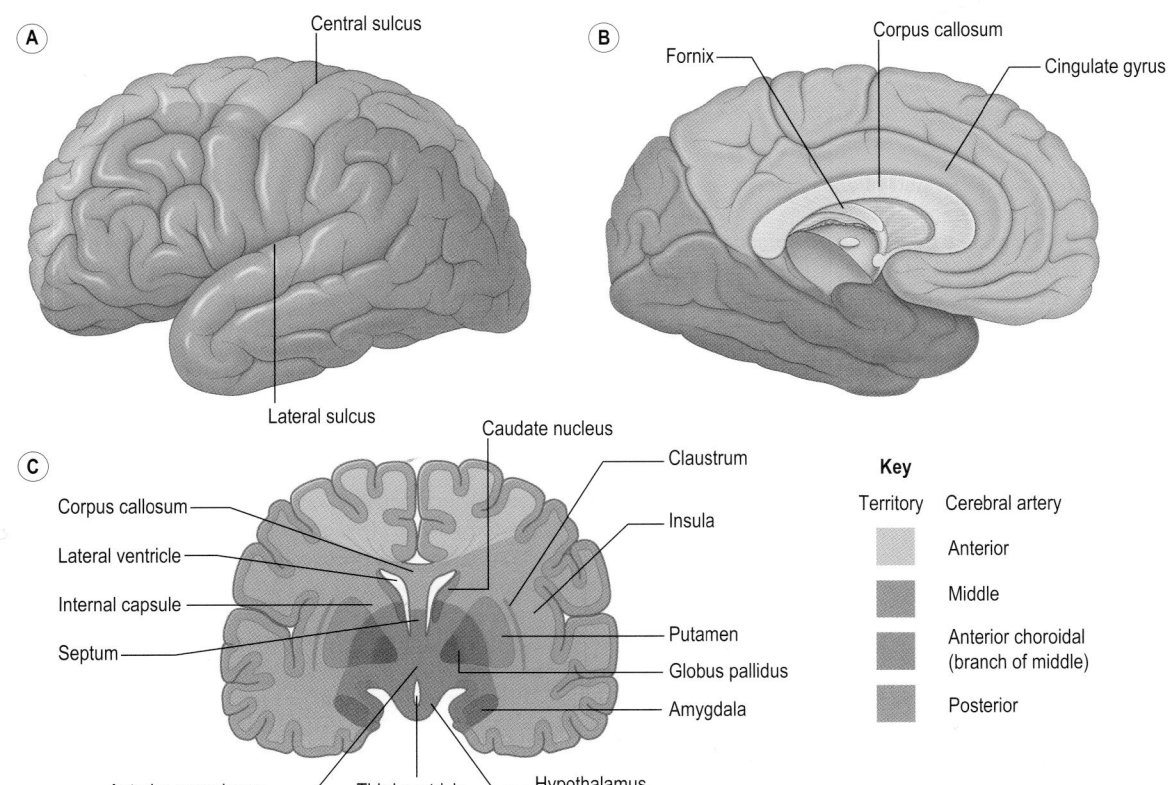

Fig. 8.17 **Territories of the cerebral arteries**: (A) lateral view; (B) medial view; (C) coronal section through the brain at the level of the anterior commissure.

brain. The hindbrain receives its blood supply from branches of the basilar and vertebral arteries. The **superior** and **anterior inferior cerebellar arteries** supply the lateral pons and cerebellum and the **posterior inferior cerebellar arteries** supply the lateral medulla and cerebellum. The medial parts of the pons and medulla are served by the small **pontine arteries**, which branch off from the basilar artery and the **anterior spinal artery**, respectively.

Venous drainage

The cerebral hemispheres are drained by superficial and deep cerebral veins. The superficial cerebral veins lie in the subarachnoid space and drain into venous sinuses as follows:

- Veins from the upper part of each hemisphere empty into the **superior sagittal sinus**.
- Those of the middle part of the cerebral hemispheres drain into the superficial middle cerebral veins and then into the **cavernous sinus**.
- Veins of the lower part of each hemisphere drain into the **transverse sinus**.

Deep veins drain blood from the thalamus and striatum on each side into an internal cerebral vein. The two internal cerebral veins join under the corpus callosum to form the **great cerebral vein**. This unites with the **inferior sagittal sinus** to form the **straight sinus**, which empties into the left transverse sinus. Finally, the transverse sinuses drain into the internal jugular veins by way of the **sigmoid sinuses**.

Control of the cerebral circulation

Large cerebral vessels are innervated by **sympathetic vasoconstrictor fibres** which release noradrenaline. However, there are few α-adrenoceptors on these vessels so constriction is probably brought about by co-released serotonin or neuropeptide Y. Vasodilation of large vessels is mediated by the co-release of ACh and vasoactive intestinal peptide. But this **autonomic control** of cerebral vasculature is weak.

Primarily, cerebral vessels show **autoregulation**. This is a negative feedback mechanism ensuring that over a wide range of pressures blood flow remains almost constant. This is important during postural adjustments, such as going from a standing to a lying position. As the pressure in a vessel rises it stretches the smooth muscle cells, opening Ca^{2+} channels in their plasma membranes. The rise in intracellular calcium concentration causes the smooth muscle to contract, constricting the vessel and limiting the rise in flow rate.

Cerebral arterioles are regulated by local factors. Neural activity causes **reactive hyperaemia**, a local rise in blood flow due to vasodilation, so that oxygen and glucose supply matches the metabolic demand. The vasodilation is brought about by:

- Increased carbon dioxide concentration causing a rise in $[H^+]$
- Adenosine and K^+ liberated by highly active nerve cells.

ENERGY SUBSTRATES AND THEIR UTILISATION

Glucose

The usual energy substrate for brain is glucose; lactate and pyruvate enter the brain at rates that are 20-fold and 50-fold lower than glucose, respectively. Glucose is transported into the brain mostly via glucose transporters on capillary endothelial cells, neurons and astrocytes. Brain glucose consumption slightly exceeds its oxygen consumption because not all of the glucose taken up is completely oxidised. Some glucose is diverted for:

- Anaerobic glycolysis to form lactate
- Synthesis of glycogen, mainly in astrocytes
- Incorporation into glycoproteins and glycolipids
- Synthesis of the neurotransmitters: glutamate, GABA and acetylcholine.

Lactate shuttle

Neurons can take up both glucose and lactate from the extracellular space. The glucose is transported directly into neurons from the blood but lactate comes via astrocytes where it is formed by anaerobic glycolysis from glucose that has been taken up by astrocytes. This is referred to as the **astrocyte–neuron lactate shuttle**. Astrocytes store glycogen which can be used as a source of lactate during periods of high neural activity.

Ketones

Ketones (acetoacetate and D-3-hydroxybutyrate) can substitute for glucose. This occurs naturally in breastfed infants in whom lipids provide over half of the brain's total calories. Ketones can be used by both neurons and astrocytes, but the β-oxidation of fatty acids (see Chs 2 and 3) which generates them occurs only in astrocytes. In starvation and diabetes mellitus, when blood glucose is unavailable, the brain can revert to its neonatal adaptation and use ketones.

Energy budget of the brain

Almost 90% of the brain's energy consumption goes to maintain the ion transport processes needed for neural sig-

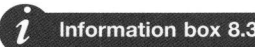

i Information box 8.3 | Functional brain imaging techniques

The development of techniques for imaging the living brain, in situ, in ways that provide information about its activity in real time, has revolutionised both basic research and clinical practice. There are two major techniques.

Positron emission tomography (PET)

Molecular markers of neural function are injected into the circulation or inhaled. These are labelled with short half-life radionuclides (e.g. ^{15}O, ^{18}F and ^{11}C) which emit positrons, allowing them to be tracked. The molecules include:

- $^{15}O_2$ to measure oxygen consumption
- **2-Deoxyglucose**, an analogue of glucose which is transported into cells but not metabolised, to study glucose uptake
- Radiolabelled water to determine cerebral blood flow
- Neurotransmitters or drugs that bind to receptors to assess transmitter system function.

Functional magnetic resonance imaging (fMRI)

- **fMRI** relies on detecting the magnetic properties of protons (hydrogen nuclei), which depend on their chemical environment, to visualise brain structure and function.
- MRI offers better resolution than PET in both space and time and it does not require the administration of radioisotopes.
- MRI can be used to map blood vessels (since flowing blood has distinctive magnetic properties), show changes that accompany trauma or inflammation, localise infarcts and tumours, and diagnose and follow the progress of some diseases (e.g. multiple sclerosis).
- **Blood oxygen level detection** (**BOLD**) is an important type of fMRI. The BOLD signal depends on the ratio of oxygenated to deoxygenated haemoglobin – which have different magnetic properties – and this ratio varies with blood volume flow rate, metabolism and other variables. BOLD can map increases in blood flow to active brain regions and can follow changes in activity with a time resolution of a few seconds.

nalling, and of this only a very small amount is needed for nerve impulses. Cerebral cortex glucose use reflects mostly presynaptic activity, largely that needed for glutamate transmission (80% of cortical neurons are glutamatergic) (see Information box 8.3).

BLOOD–BRAIN BARRIER

The blood–brain barrier controls what ions and molecules can enter or leave the brain and so is crucial for brain homeostasis and protection from noxious substances. It is formed by brain capillary endothelial cells that are linked by **tight junctions** (Fig. 8.18), thus the movement of water and ions into and out of the brain between endothelial cells is extremely low. Astrocyte endfeet surround the endothelial cells and secrete factors that maintain the tightness of the blood–brain barrier.

Transport across the blood–brain barrier

Only water, some water- or lipid-soluble gases (such as O_2, CO_2 and volatile general anaesthetics) and lipid soluble molecules (e.g. steroids), are able to traverse the blood–brain barrier by passive diffusion across the plasma membranes of endothelial cells. Brain endothelial cells have only low levels of pinocytosis, so there is little bulk flow of fluid across the barrier.

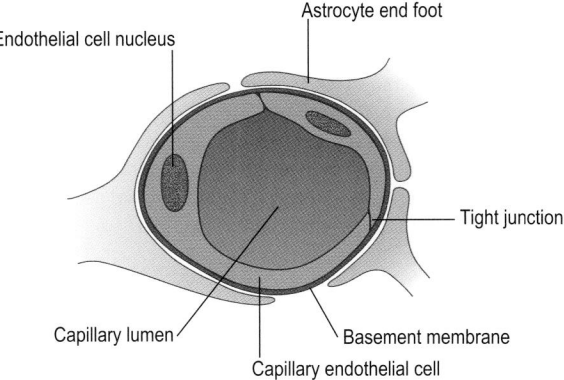

Fig. 8.18 **Blood–brain barrier.** Endothelial cells line the lumen and are joined by tight junctions. These are surrounded by a basement membrane and astrocytic endfeet.

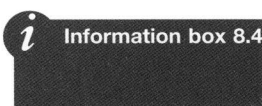

i Information box 8.4 | Cerebral oedema – inappropriate distribution of water between brain fluid compartments

Cerebral oedema, (swelling of brain tissue) can be generalised or localised around lesions, such as infarcts or tumours. Because the brain is encased within a rigid cranium, as it swells there is distortion, herniation and compression of brain structures. There are several types:

- **Vasogenic oedema** – breakdown of the blood–brain barrier allows proteins to enter the brain and Na^+ and water follow by osmosis.
- **Cytotoxic oedema** – occurs in hypoxia. Loss of ATP (adenosine triphosphate) production causes failure of the Na^+/K^+-ATPase and a rise in intracellular $[Na^+]$. Subsequent osmotic shift of water into brain cells causes them to swell. Water intoxication or hyponatraemia (low blood sodium) can also cause cytotoxic oedema by changing the concentration gradient of water across cell membranes.
- **Interstitial oedema** – seen in hydrocephalus.

Ions and charged or polar molecules enter only by specific **carrier-mediated transport mechanisms**, for example:

- Facilitated diffusion of glucose, mostly via GLUT1 transporters (see Ch. 2),
- Secondary active transport of amino acids.

Receptor-mediated endocytosis allows entry for some large molecules such as iron-transferrin, insulin and leptin. Breakdown of the blood–brain barrier can increase permeability to protein and lead to cerebral oedema (Information box 8.4).

Role of P-glycoprotein

A wide range of potentially toxic, lipophilic, molecules which diffuse into brain capillary endothelial cells are actively transported out again by **P-glycoprotein (Pgp)** (see Ch. 2). This transporter which carries a wide range of substrates thus protects the brain. Unfortunately many intracranial tumours also express Pgp, thus exhibiting **multi-drug resistance** in being able to exclude a variety of chemotherapeutic agents. Pgp on brain endothelial cells also hinders the entry of many potentially therapeutic drugs into brain tissue.

Circumventricular organs

Circumventricular organs are brain regions situated on the blood side of the blood–brain barrier by virtue of the fact that their capillaries are fenestrated. By being in direct contact with the blood these organs can monitor the concentrations of blood components or secrete large molecules into the blood. For example, the posterior pituitary gland secretes the hormones oxytocin and vasopressin (see Ch. 10).

NEURAL SIGNALLING

Almost all cells in the body have a small difference in electrical potential (tens of millivolts) across their plasma membranes called the **membrane potential**. In **excitable cells** (neurons, muscle cells of all types, and some endocrine and exocrine cells), in response to stimuli, this potential is rapidly reversed, producing an **action potential** which spreads at high speed over the surface of the cell. In neurons, action potentials are often referred to as **nerve impulses** and are signals which code information. In muscle cells, action potentials trigger contraction and in glands they bring about secretion.

Action potentials trigger the release of chemical messengers, **neurotransmitters**, from junctions between neurons termed **chemical synapses**. Neurotransmitters alter the excitability of the target cell on the receiving side of the synapses making it either more or less likely to fire action potentials. Since a given neuron may have hundreds of its synapses activated at any time its output (how many action potentials it generates each second) is determined by the overall effect of all these inputs. The firing pattern of all the neurons in a **neural network** determines the output of that network and so contributes to overall behaviour.

The transmission of information by neurons, which relies on the propagation of action potentials, and the processing of information by neurons, which depends on their synaptic inputs, constitutes **neural signalling**.

GENERATION AND PROPAGATION OF ACTION POTENTIALS

Excitable cell membranes

Ion distributions

The fluid inside cells has a different composition to the fluid surrounding them (see Ch. 2, Table 2.15). While extracellular fluid is essentially dilute sodium chloride, the major cation of intracellular fluid is potassium and a wide variety of substances within the cell (organic acids, phosphates) act as anions that exactly balance the charge of the potassium ions.

Resting membrane potentials

It is the asymmetrical distribution of ions and the selective permeability of the plasma membrane that causes the membranes of cells to have potential difference across them. In unstimulated excitable cells this is termed the **resting membrane potential** (V_r). The polarity of the resting potential is always inside negative. The magnitude of this potential varies somewhat depending on the tissue. For example, for neurons V_r ranges between about –60 mV and –80 mV, while skeletal muscle and ventricular heart muscle have V_r = –90 mV.

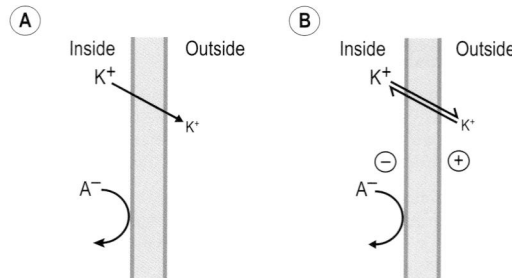

Fig. 8.19 **The origin of the resting potential.** (A) Initially K⁺ ions leak down their concentration gradient; the membrane is impermeable to large anions. (B) At equilibrium a small potential difference is established by the separation of charges.

How resting potentials are generated

Most of the resting potential arises because of the uneven distribution of K⁺ ions across the plasma membrane. To see this, consider a model system in which a cell membrane separates two aqueous compartments, one representing the inside of a cell, the other the outside. The inside compartment contains K⁺ ions, their positive charges completely balanced by an equal number of anions. Cell membranes are quite permeable to K⁺, but are impermeable to the much larger anions (Fig. 8.19A).

Because there are no K⁺ ions outside the model cell a concentration gradient exists for potassium across the cell membrane. Hence a **diffusion force** acts to drive K⁺ ions down this gradient. However, as soon as K⁺ ions leave the intracellular compartment an equivalent number of negative charges on anions are unmasked. This creates an **electrical force** which attracts the K⁺ ions and so acts in the opposite direction to the diffusion force. With time the system will go to an equilibrium which can be described by:

Diffusion force = Electrical force

At equilibrium there will be a small deficit of K⁺ ions on the inside of the cell membrane and a corresponding excess on the outside of the membrane; a potential difference is created (Fig. 8.19B).

Equilibrium potentials

The potential that arises due to the distribution of K⁺ across a semi-permeable membrane at equilibrium is termed the potassium **equilibrium** (or **reversal**) **potential**, E_K. This is because at E_K the number of potassium ions leaving the cell is exactly balanced by the number entering. The resting membrane potential of excitable cells is largely an equilibrium potential for potassium. However, each of the other permeable ions, Na⁺, Cl⁻ also produce their own equilibrium potentials and these make a small contribution to the resting membrane potential of excitable cells.

The equilibrium potential for any ion can be quantified using the **Nernst equation**, which allows the equilibrium potential E to be calculated from the concentrations of an ion outside, C_o, and inside, C_i, a membrane:

$$E = (RT/zF)\ln([C_o]/[C_i])$$

where R is the gas constant, T is the temperature in Kelvin, z is the oxidation state of the ion, and F is Faraday's number (the amount of charge carried by one mole of a monovalent ion).

For a monovalent cation at 37 °C and changing to base 10 logarithms the Nernst equation can be simplified to:

$$E = 61\log_{10}([C_o]/[C_i])$$

Using the values for extracellular and intracellular K⁺ concentration given in Table 2.15 gives a potassium equilibrium potential $E_K = -94$ mV. Equally the sodium equilibrium potential $E_{Na} = +62$ mV. This is the membrane potential that would result if sodium ions *only* were allowed to partition themselves across the membrane.

How resting membrane potentials are calculated

The resting potential in neurons is not as large as the potassium equilibrium potential because Na⁺ ions also contribute to the resting potential. It is clear that the actual membrane potential lies between E_K and E_{Na}. But it is much closer to E_K because the resting membrane has a much lower permeability for Na⁺ than K⁺, hence the sodium ions make a much smaller contribution to the resting membrane potential. Typically, neuron resting potentials are between −60 mV and −85 mV.

Because the resting potential is not at the equilibrium potential of either K⁺ or Na⁺, at rest there are electrochemical gradients (a combination of diffusional and electrical forces) for both of these ions. Consequently there will be a tendency for these ions to leak down their gradients, especially if the permeability of the membrane to these ions increases. The operation of the Na⁺/K⁺-ATPase offsets the effects of such leaks. In contrast, Cl⁻ gradients are not maintained by active transport in neurons. Chloride is passively distributed across the cell membrane according to the potential established by K⁺ and Na⁺ and the permeability of the membrane for Cl⁻. Given the concentrations of K⁺, Na⁺, and Cl⁻ and their relative membrane permeabilities, the resting membrane potential can be accurately calculated.

Action potentials

Depolarisation and hyperpolarisation

If some positive charges (e.g. Na⁺ ions) enter an excitable cell – equivalent to an inward current – its membrane potential decreases (becomes less negative), i.e. it will move a little closer to zero. The cell is said to be **depolarised**. Conversely, entry of negative charges such as Cl⁻ ions (or efflux of positive charges such as K⁺) – equivalent to an outward current – causes its potential to increase (become more negative), in which case the cell is **hyperpolarised**. When the flow of charges stops in either of these situations the potential returns within a few milliseconds to the resting value, because the ions redistribute themselves across the membrane according to their equilibrium potentials and permeabilities. In essence, the membrane resists attempts to change the potential across it; clearly negative feedback is at work here (see Ch. 1).

Generation of action potentials

If a sufficiently large inward current is injected into an excitable cell, the resulting depolarisation becomes big enough to drive the membrane into a positive feedback mode in which its potential rapidly drops to zero and overshoots to

become inside positive (Fig. 8.20). The normal resting potential is restored within a few milliseconds (in neurons and skeletal muscle). This is an **action potential**.

Changes in sodium permeability

The upslope of the action potential (Fig. 8.20, *A*) is caused by a rapid increase in the Na⁺ conductance (Information box 8.5). Because Na⁺ ions are far from their electrochemical equilibrium (recall $E_{Na} = +62$ mV), they rush into the cell. The entire upslope is referred to as the depolarisation phase of the action potential, even though it includes the **overshoot** in which the potential is actually increasing from 0 to +30 mV (i.e. polarising).

The influx of Na⁺ cannot continue for ever because:

- As the membrane potential approaches E_{Na}, the electrochemical gradient driving the sodium ions inwards reduces
- The increased Na⁺ permeability switches off.

Changes in potassium permeability

The falling phase of the action potential (Fig. 8.20, *B*) results from a rise in potassium conductance (gK) which occurs later than the increase in Na conductance (gNa). During the overshoot of the action potential the K⁺ ions are far from their equilibrium potential so they leave the cell causing it to **repolarise**. As repolarisation proceeds, the driving force for K⁺ efflux gets less and gK falls. For a brief period after the action potential spike the continuing potassium efflux, uncompensated by any sodium influx, causes the cell to hyperpolarise (*C* in Fig. 8.20). This is the **after-hyperpolarisation** phase of the action potential.

> ### *i* Information box 8.5 — Permeability and conductance
>
> Both permeability and conductance are measures of the extent to which a substance can diffuse across a membrane. Both are determined by the chemistry and size of the substance and the chemistry and thickness of the membrane. **Permeability** is the more general term that applies to both uncharged molecules and ions. In contrast, **conductance** (*g*) is used only to describe the ease with which ions flow and depends on the potential difference across the membrane. It is the reciprocal of the electrical resistance offered by the membrane to the flow of ions (*g* = 1/*R*), so the lower the resistance, the higher the conductance.

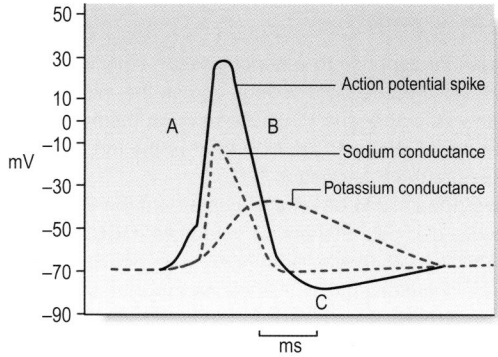

Fig. 8.20 Potential and conductance changes during a neural action potential.

Properties of action potentials

Action potentials have several key properties, determined by the exact behaviour of the ionic conductances that cause them, and these are crucial to how they encode and transmit information:

- Threshold voltage. Typically, neurons must be depolarised to between about −60 and −50 mV, the **threshold voltage**, before they fire an action potential. For a given cell, the threshold voltage depends on its recent firing history. The stimulus that makes a cell fire on 50% of the occasions in which it is applied is the **threshold stimulus**.
- Constant amplitude. In a given cell all action potentials have the same amplitude. The size of action potentials carries no information about the size of the stimuli that produced them. Together with the threshold property above, this means that action potentials obey an **all-or-none rule**: cells either fire or they don't.
- Latency. The stronger a stimulus the quicker it depolarises a membrane to the threshold voltage and so the shorter the **latency** – the time lag between start of the stimulus and onset of the action potential. Hence the action potential latency does carry information about the strength of stimulus.
- Refractory period. About 0.5–1.0 ms into the spike of the action potential, neurons become completely resistant (refractory) to further stimulation. This **refractory period** is important because:
  - Action potentials cannot be summated (added), so in a given neuron they are always the same size. This makes them **digital** signals, which are much less prone to transmission errors than analogue signals.
  - It limits the **firing frequency**, the maximum number of action potentials a neuron can fire in a second.
  - It means action potentials are only propagated **one way**; they cannot go the 'wrong' way because the membrane just upstream of the active region is inexcitable. Over the next few milliseconds they gradually reacquire their ability to respond.

Other excitable cells have refractory periods, though they vary with cell type; for example heart muscle cells have a refractory period two orders of magnitude longer than nerve cells.

Voltage-dependent ion channels

The ion conductance changes that underlie the action potential arise from the presence in the plasma membrane of several populations of integral transmembrane proteins called **voltage-dependent** (or **voltage-gated**) **ion channels** (see Ch. 4), which:

- Open in response to a depolarisation sufficient to exceed the threshold voltage across the membrane.
- Allow selected ions to diffuse through them when they are open; channels are named after the ion to which they are most permeant.
- Two populations of voltage-dependent ion channel are involved in neuronal action potentials – sodium and potassium channels. Both open in response to a depolarisation sufficient to exceed the threshold voltage.

Voltage-dependent sodium channels

The rise in gNa is due to the opening of a few hundred **voltage-dependent sodium channels**. On sensing the depolarisation, each channel goes from the closed to the open state, a transition that takes only a few microseconds, stays open for about a millisecond and then goes into a third, **inactivated**, state in which it is 'locked' shut. It is largely because the sodium channels inactivate that the sodium conductance falls to low resting levels by the end of the spike of the action potential. Inactivation also accounts for the **absolute refractory period** when the cell cannot be stimulated a second time.

Voltage-dependent sodium channels recover from inactivation – that is, go from the inactivated to the closed state – at a rate that depends on both time and voltage and means that within 2–3 ms neurons are able to respond to further stimuli, albeit with a higher threshold.

Voltage-dependent potassium channels

The same depolarisation that opens the sodium channels also triggers the opening of **voltage-dependent potassium channels** but, because they take longer to respond, their opening is delayed. Unlike the sodium channels the type of potassium channel involved in neuronal action potentials does not inactivate: it has only two states, open and closed. The fall in potassium conductance that accompanies repolarisation simply results from the reduced driving force on K^+ to leave as the membrane potential approaches the potassium equilibrium potential.

The after-hyperpolarisation, caused by the continuing efflux of K^+ ions, briefly carries the membrane potential further away from the threshold voltage than when the cell is at rest. Hence, during the after-hyperpolarisation larger than normal threshold stimuli are required to make the cell fire. This is the **relative refractory period**. The normal threshold is gradually restored as the after-hyperpolarisation wears off.

Propagation of action potentials

Action potentials are conducted along axons at a speed that depends on the diameter of the axon: the larger the axon diameter, the higher the conduction velocity. The speed also depends on whether the axon is nonmyelinated, in which the speed is proportional to the square root of the diameter, or myelinated, in which the speed is proportional to the diameter, and hence faster.

Local circuit currents

Propagation occurs because local circuit currents are generated in front of the action potential. At the spike of the action potential there is a slight excess of positive charge inside the axon and a corresponding excess of negative charge outside. This is the converse of the normal resting region of axon just ahead of the action potential. Thus a potential difference builds up between the region of axon undergoing an action potential and the region ahead. This causes local circuit currents to flow from A to B intracellularly (and from B to A extracellularly), which depolarises the membrane just ahead of the action potential, opening sodium channels so that the action potential advances (Fig. 8.21A). Local circuit currents also flow behind the action potential but because the sodium channels here are inactivated, the action potential cannot travel backwards.

Myelinated axons

Because the myelin sheath has a high electrical resistance, local circuit currents can flow only between adjacent, low

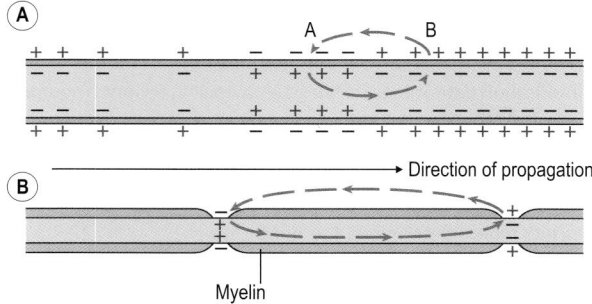

Fig. 8.21 Propagation of the action potential in **(A) unmyelinated and (B) myelinated axons.** Redrawn with permission from Pocock G, Richards CD (eds) 2004 Human physiology, the basis of medicine. Oxford University Press, Oxford.

Clinical box 8.5   Multiple sclerosis

Multiple sclerosis is a relatively common autoimmune disorder (see Ch. 6) in which T cells inappropriately target myelin proteins, producing demyelination of axons in the brain and spinal cord. It is of unknown cause but is possibly triggered by a viral infection.

In myelinated axons, although sodium channels are confined to the nodes of Ranvier, potassium channels are expressed all along the axon. Demyelination uncovers these potassium channels which can then be inappropriately activated by local circuit currents. Increased K+ efflux hyperpolarises the axon, rendering it less excitable. This causes **conduction block**, which accounts for the paralysis and sensory losses. Demyelination also results in the expression of a type of voltage-dependent sodium channel that does not inactivate readily in the exposed and previously internodal membrane. If these channels are activated, bursts of improperly conducted action potentials are generated; these cause **paraesthesias** ('pins and needles') and **fasciculation** (spontaneous motor unit discharge).

Treatment for multiple sclerosis is aimed at curtailing the autoimmunity. For example, a number of cytokines which curb T cells are currently being evaluated, including β-interferon.

---

resistance, nodes of Ranvier. Hence action potentials jump between successive nodes, a process known as **saltatory conduction** (Fig. 8.21B). Because local circuit currents can spread in less time than it would take for ion channels along the entire membrane to respond successively, conduction is faster in myelinated fibres than non-myelinated fibres. Multiple sclerosis is a disease caused by demyelination of axons in the CNS (Clinical box 8.5).

Local anaesthetics

Voltage-dependent sodium channels are the targets for **local anaesthetics** and several other clinically important classes of drugs such as type I antidysrhythmics (Table 11.8) and certain anti-epileptics. Local anaesthetics reversibly block the conduction of action potentials by entering the pore of open sodium channels and stabilising them in the inactivated state so it can take up to 1000 times longer than normal for inactivation to wear off.

Use-dependent blockade

Most local anaesthetics consist of a lipophilic group linked via an ester or amide to an ionisable amine group. They are weak bases which, at the normal pH of the tissues, are mainly but not entirely in the form of positively charged cations. This charged molecule cannot penetrate the hydrophobic walls of an ion channel, so can only enter the channel pore when it is opened. Moreover, the open and inactivated states of the sodium channel have a greater affinity for local anaesthetics than the closed state. Thus local anaesthetics demonstrate **use-dependent blockade**: the sodium channel block, and hence effectiveness of the anaesthetic, increases as more channels open.

In their uncharged form, anaesthetics are more able to permeate cell membranes, for example of the covering glial cells, to gain access to neurons, so the effectiveness of local anaesthetics is diminished in ischaemic or infected tissues, in which pH is low and almost all the drug is in the cationic form.

Ester-linked local anaesthetics are broken down rapidly in the plasma by plasma cholinesterases whereas the amide-linked anaesthetics are metabolised in the liver.

Pain blockade

Pain sensation, rather than other nerve function, is preferentially blocked by local anaesthetics because small diameter nerve fibres are more susceptible. This is due to two factors:

- The smaller the diameter of the axon, the shorter the distance that local circuit currents can passively spread to propagate an action potential, so fewer sodium channels need be blocked to curtail conduction.
- Smaller diameter fibres fire at higher frequencies and have longer action potentials so, they are more likely to suffer use-dependent blockade.

Myelinated fibres are more sensitive than non-myelinated fibres of the same diameter because the nodes of Ranvier create fewer barriers to drug access.

Motor fibres are generally in the outer mantle of nerve trunks, so they encounter the drug first and therefore motor block precedes sensory block. Also, sensory fibres that innervate distal regions are located in the core of a nerve trunk, whereas those innervating proximal regions are further out, so the analgesia starts proximally and spreads distally as the drug penetrates the nerve trunk.

SYNAPSES AND NEUROTRANSMISSION

A synapse is a specialised junction between a neuron and a target cell (e.g. another nerve cell or a muscle cell). Synapses allow individual neurons to interact, forming networks which process information that is ultimately encoded by action potentials. There are two types of synapse:

- **Electrical:** Transmission via pores at gap junctions between cells
- **Chemical:** Uses chemical signals.

Electrical synapses

Electrical synapses allow the rapid flow of currents (in the form of small ions) and metabolites between adjacent neurons or glial cells. They are also found extensively in cardiac and smooth muscle. However, overall, electrical synapses are far outnumbered by chemical synapses.

Structure

Electrical synapses are formed by **gap junctions**, where the plasma membranes of adjacent cells are only 3.5 nm apart. Pore proteins called **connexons** in each membrane form a channel with a diameter of 1.5 nm which provides continuity between the cytoplasm of the two cells.

Transmission

The size of the channel and its non-selectivity allows the flow of Na^+, K^+, Ca^{2+} and other ions, and small molecules (<1000 Da). The latter include ATP and second messengers such as cAMP; i.e. electrical synapses permit both **electrical and metabolic coupling** of neurons. Transmission across electrical synapses is bi-directional.

Functions

Electrical neurotransmission is important in some regions of the nervous system. For example, gap junctions between interneurons in the retina enable these cells to produce a signal that represents average light levels. Potentials cross electrical synapses with a delay of only about 0.1 ms, so they are able to synchronise firing of groups of neurons. This is important for ensembles of hormone-secreting neurons in the hypothalamus in which near-simultaneous firing brings about a burst of hormone secretion. Electrical synapses are abundant in embryonic tissue where they are involved in guiding development.

Regulation

Electrical synapses are subject to some regulation. At high concentrations of Ca^{2+} or H^+, the connexons can close. This isolates cells with abnormally elevated calcium concentrations or low pH, which are the ubiquitous hallmarks of damage.

Chemical synapses

Chemical synapses are concerned with information processing. With the exception of the neuromuscular junction (the specialised synapse between a motor neuron and skeletal muscle), synapses do *not* invariably relay action potentials from one neuron to another. Rather, synapses provide the inputs which a neuron integrates, and the outcome of this integration determines its firing behaviour. In essence neurons can be regarded as decision-making devices, deciding at each instant whether or not to fire, on the basis of the current state of *all* its synapses. Most neurons receive inputs from a large number of neurons and it is the integration of all these inputs which determines the firing rate.

Structure

A **synaptic cleft**, a gap 30 nm wide, separates the **presynaptic membrane** and **postsynaptic membrane** (Fig. 8.22). Within the presynaptic terminal lie two types of **synaptic vesicles** that contain neurotransmitter. The presynaptic membrane has an **active zone** where synaptic vesicles can dock and release transmitter. The postsynaptic membrane opposite the active zone has a **postsynaptic density** packed with receptors capable of binding transmitter.

Neurotransmission

Neurotransmission is an example of **excitation-secretion coupling**. A summary of the sequence of events during neurotransmission at a synapse (see Fig. 8.22B) is:

a. An action potential arrives at the presynaptic terminal.
b. Depolarisation opens voltage-dependent calcium channels in the presynaptic membrane allowing Ca^{2+} to enter the terminal.
c. The influx of and rise in Ca^{2+} concentration triggers the release of transmitter from a synaptic vesicle that has already docked at the active zone into the synaptic cleft.
d. The transmitter diffuses across the cleft, and binds to its receptors on the postsynaptic membrane.
e. Binding of transmitter and receptor alters the conductance of the postsynaptic cell to ions, producing a postsynaptic potential – precisely which ions depends on the nature of the transmitter and on which of its receptors is involved.
f. Transmitter is transported back into the neuron.

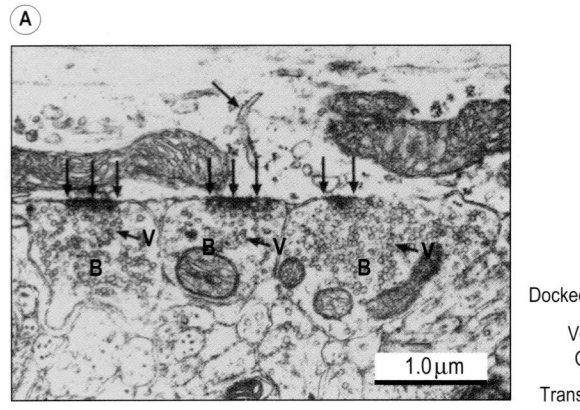

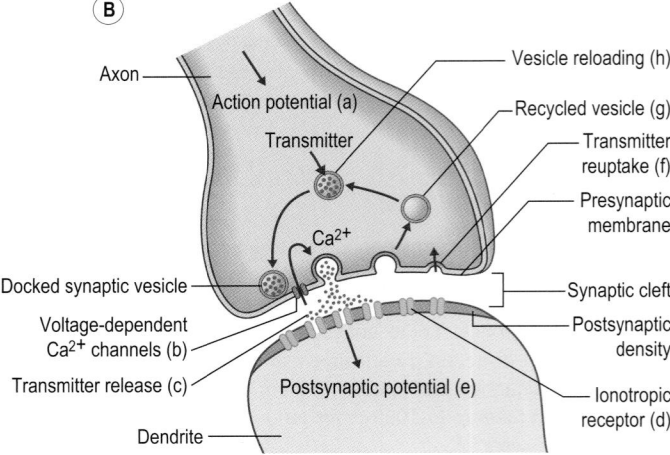

Fig. 8.22 **(A) Electron micrograph of a central synapse.** Arrows indicate active zones with postsynaptic densities; B, bouton; V, vesicle. From Young B, Lowe JS, Stevens A, Heath JW 2006 Wheater's Functional histology, 5th edn. Churchill Livingstone, Edinburgh. (B) Diagrammatic illustration of events in chemical transmission at central synapses. For explanation of the steps please see the text.

g. The synaptic vesicle is recycled and reloaded with transmitter (h).

The outcome is either to increase or decrease the probability that the postsynaptic cell will fire action potentials. A transmitter acting to increase the chance of firing is described as **excitatory** whereas if it decreases the firing probability it is **inhibitory**. A given transmitter might be excitatory at one synapse but inhibitory at another, depending on which of its receptors is present.

Neurotransmitters

There are two broad categories of neurotransmitters (Table 8.6).

- Small molecules such as amino acids and monoamines, often described as **classical transmitters**.
- Large peptides that are collectively referred to as **neuropeptides**.

The release of neuropeptides is typically slower than that of the classic transmitters and their effects are much more prolonged.

Vesicle filling

Small synaptic vesicles – clear, spherical, membrane-bound organelles about 50 nm across – are filled with amino acid or monoamine transmitters by specific secondary active transport in the vesicle membrane. This uses a proton (H^+) gradient which is maintained by a proton ATPase.

Peptide transmitters are synthesised on ribosomes, secreted into the rough endoplasmic reticulum and packaged into large (120–200 nm) vesicles by the Golgi apparatus. The neuropeptide-filled vesicles are moved from the cell body to axon terminals by fast axonal transport. In the synapse they appear as dense-core vesicles, usually found further away from the active zones than the small clear ones.

Neurotransmitter receptors

Generally neurotransmitter receptors fall into one of two of the receptor superfamilies:

- Ligand-gated ion channels (**ionotropic** receptors)
- G-protein-coupled (**metabotropic**) receptors (see Ch. 4).

Ionotropic receptors

Ionotropic receptors are transmembrane ion channels with neurotransmitter-binding sites on their extracellular face, which protrudes into the synaptic cleft. Transmitter binding opens the channel, thus permitting ions to flow. This produces a **postsynaptic current** which changes the membrane potential, generating a **postsynaptic potential**.

The current that passes through an ionotropic receptor is governed by intrinsic properties of the channel itself and by the electrochemical gradients across the membrane. The size of the channel and the chemistry of its walls determines two of its characteristics:

- The **ion specificity**, i.e. which ions can flow through it.
- The **single channel conductance**: the more channels that are open, the bigger the overall conductance, and therefore the larger the postsynaptic current and postsynaptic potential.

The electrochemical gradients determine the direction in which particular ions will flow. The flow of ions through ion channels in the postsynaptic membrane sets up **postsynaptic potentials** in the target cell. These are either excitatory or inhibitory. Because ionotropic receptors combine the functions of receptor and channel in a single molecule, there is only a short time between transmitter binding and channel opening – transmission is fast. Most fast transmission is mediated by two transmitters, **glutamate** and **GABA**, which to a first approximation act as on and off signals, respectively.

Excitatory postsynaptic potentials

If activation of a receptor causes a net inward current, the postsynaptic membrane depolarises. This brings the cell closer to the threshold for firing action potentials so it is termed an **excitatory postsynaptic potential** (EPSP).This is the case for the many ionotropic receptors that are relatively non-selective cation channels, for example, those for glutamate and acetylcholine, which are major excitatory transmitters (Fig. 8.23A).

Inhibitory postsynaptic potentials

If activation of a receptor produces a net outward current to flow through the postsynaptic membrane (i.e. K^+ efflux or Cl^- influx), the effect is to make the membrane potential more negative, producing an **inhibitory postsynaptic potential** (**ipsp**). This reduces the probability that the postsynaptic neuron will fire. Almost invariably ipsps are brought about by ion channels selective for chloride or potassium. GABA and glycine are the principal inhibitory neurotransmitters and their ionotropic receptors are chloride channels (Fig. 8.23B).

G-protein-coupled receptors

G-protein-coupled receptors, e.g. catecholamines and peptides, modulate the activity of ion channels indirectly (see Ch. 4) so transmission via these is slower. Many classic transmitters have both ionotropic and G-protein-coupled receptors and hence are both fast and slow transmitters.

Table 8.6	**Major neurotransmitters**		
	Classical transmitters		**Peptide transmitters**
Amino acids	**Monoamines**	**Purines**	
Glutamate	Acetylcholine	Adenosine	Substance P
γ-Aminobutyrate (GABA)	Dopamine	ATP	Vasoactive intestinal peptide (VIP)
Glycine	Noradrenaline		Somatostatin
	Adrenaline		Cholecystokinin
	Serotonin		β-Endorphin
	Histamine		Met-enkephalin

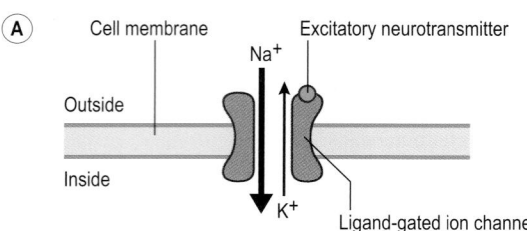

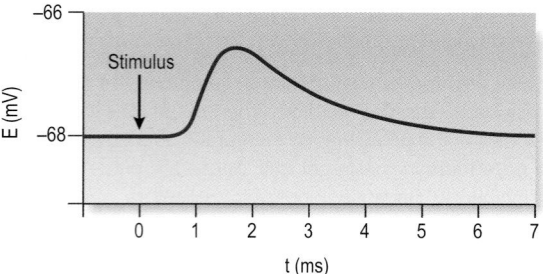

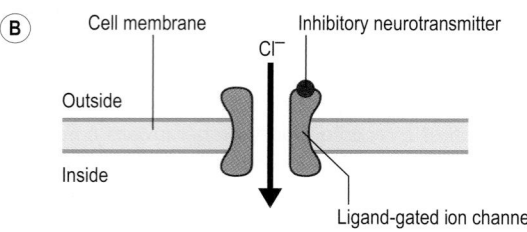

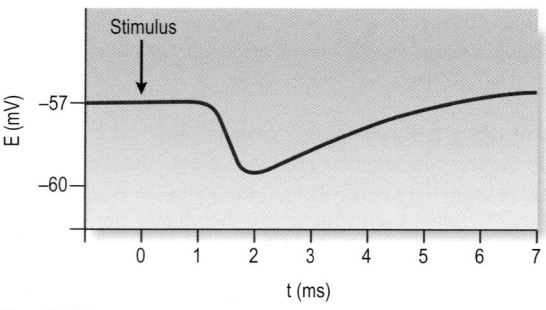

Fig. 8.23 **Ligand-gated ion channels and synaptic potentials.** (A) Glutamate and acetylcholine produce excitatory postsynaptic potentials (epsps); (B) γ-aminobutyrate (GABA) and glycine produce inhibitory postsynaptic potentials (ipsps). Redrawn with permission from Longstaff A 2005 Instant notes in neuroscience, 2nd edn. Taylor & Francis, Abingdon UK.

Neurotransmitter release

Excitation-secretion coupling

Calcium enters the presynaptic terminal via voltage-gated Ca^{2+} channels that are activated by action potential depolarisation. The concentration of Ca^{2+} in the vicinity of the active zone then reaches about 10^{-4} M. This high level is achieved in two ways:

- The resting concentration of free ionised calcium inside cells is about 10^{-7} M whereas the Ca^{2+} concentration in the extracellular fluid is of the order 10^{-3} M, so there is a large inward driving force for calcium.
- The calcium channels are localised close to the sites where synaptic vesicles are docked.

However, this sharp rise is restricted to within about 50 nm of the calcium channels and is rapidly curtailed by calcium

buffering mechanisms in the terminal. The calcium signal is thus localised and brief.

Voltage-dependent calcium channels

There are several populations of Ca^{2+} channel. Three of these (N, P, and Q types) are involved in the release of small molecule transmitters from the active zone. L-type channels are implicated in the release of neuropeptides and in the regulation of excitability of some neurons. L-type channels are also the major routes for the entry of calcium ions into cardiac and smooth muscle cells and they are the only type for which therapeutic drugs have so far been developed.

Quantal and probabilistic nature of release

Postsynaptic potentials at synapses, including neuromuscular junctions, are multiples of fixed discrete units termed **quanta**. Each quantum corresponds to the release of the transmitter from a single vesicle. Low level release of single quanta occurs even from resting cells and produces miniature postsynaptic potentials or miniature endplate potentials with an amplitude of order 0.5 mV. Postsynaptic potentials and muscle endplate potentials result from the simultaneous release of several quanta, the effects of which are additive.

The release of transmitter is stochastic. In response to the arrival of an action potential a given quantum may or may not be released. If there are several releasable quanta, the probability of any one being released is independent of what happens to the others.

CNS synapses are very different to the neuromuscular junctions between motor neurons and skeletal muscle fibres. Many central synapses seem to have only a single releasable quantum, which is liberated with low probability. In contrast, neuromuscular junctions operate at quite high probability and can have as many as 1000 releasable quanta, so are adapted for high fidelity transmission.

Vesicle recycling

Classical neurotransmitter secretion occurs via cycles of vesicle exocytosis followed by endocytosis. There are two distinct recycling pathways that differ in their time course.

- **Slow release:** the vesicle membrane completely flattens to become incorporated into the plasma membrane. Recovery of vesicle membrane requires its encasing in a clathrin coat, which is slow (about 30 s) and this operates at neuromuscular junctions.
- **Fast release:** ('kiss-and-run cycle'), operates at synapses in the CNS. The vesicle membrane fuses with the presynaptic membrane to open a pore through which transmitter is discharged, after which the pore closes and the vesicle disengages. This is fast (about 1 s) so it is able to support long periods of high synaptic activity.

Biochemistry of release

Exocytosis of transmitter from **small synaptic vesicles** has several steps, most requiring Ca^{2+}. Vesicles are normally anchored to the cytoskeleton by **synapsin I**. Calcium-dependent phosphorylation of this protein frees vesicles into a releasable pool. These vesicles dock with specific sites at the **active zone** by interactions of proteins termed **SNARES**. SNARES in the vesicle membrane recognise others in the presynaptic membrane, allowing the vesicle to attach to a docking site. Neurotransmitter release is inhibited by the **botulinum toxins** and **tetanus toxin**, the enzyme activities of which disrupt SNARES and other proteins involved in docking. Hydrolysis of ATP now causes partial fusion of vesicle and presynaptic membranes so that the vesicle is now ready to release its contents.

Release of transmitter is triggered by the sudden rise in intracellular calcium brought about by action potential depolarisation and involves the rapid opening of a pore where the vesicle and presynaptic membranes are fused. The subsequent method of vesicle recovery (**endocytosis**) depends on which cycle is operating.

Neuropeptide release

Neuropeptide release (secretion) is different from that of classical transmitters. Dense core vesicles are similar to secretory granules of non-neuronal cells and can liberate their contents from anywhere in the terminal membrane, in contrast to small synaptic vesicles that discharge their classic transmitters only from the active zone. This means that higher concentrations of calcium are required to trigger exocytosis of large dense-core vesicles, hence higher firing frequencies are needed to liberate neuropeptides.

Many synapses can release more than one transmitter. This is termed **co-transmission** and often involves the secretion of a classic transmitter in response to a modest firing frequency, supplemented by release of a neuropeptide at higher frequencies.

Presynaptic receptors

Neurotransmitter synthesis and release at many peripheral and central synapses can be regulated by presynaptic receptors either for the transmitter released at the synapse, **autoreceptors** (see also Ch. 4), or for transmitter released at neighbouring synapses, **heteroceptors**. Usually activation of autoreceptors results in a reduction of transmitter release. This can be thought of as a negative feedback mechanism to limit the degree of postsynaptic receptor activation or desensitisation. Autoreceptors are not confined to the presynaptic membrane but can also be found on the cell body and dendrites. Here they can regulate neuron firing rate.

Neurotransmitter inactivation

Several mechanisms exist to clear released transmitter from the synapse. This allows the synapse to alter its information processing on short timescales so that rapid changes in behaviour are possible. It also helps synapses to remain sensitive to transmitter by curtailing receptor desensitisation, which occurs if receptors are exposed to agonists for prolonged periods. There are three methods of transmitter inactivation.

- Reuptake: Classical transmitters are taken up by neurons or glia (amino acid transmitters only). This is achieved by specific high affinity, saturable, secondary active transport mechanisms (see Ch. 2). These harness the energy stored in ion gradients (Na^+, K^+ or Cl^-) to drive the neurotransmitter from the cleft into the cell. Some of the transporter proteins – e.g. those for noradrenaline and serotonin – are important targets for drugs used to treat depression (see Information box 8.25; Ch. 4).
- Diffusion: Diffusion away from the active zone is the method of peptide inactivation. However, because peptides are large and synapses are surrounded by glial cell processes, peptide diffusion is slow, which is why their actions can last for several minutes. It is also important for the inactivation of glutamate and GABA at central synapses.

- Enzymes: Acetylcholine is inactivated by **acetylcholinesterase (AChE)** hydrolysis to produce acetate and choline. A specific high affinity transporter in neurons removes the choline from the synaptic cleft where it is used to resynthesise ACh. A number of drugs act on AChE (see Chs 4 and 9). ATP, a co-transmitter at some synapses, is also inactivated by enzyme action.

NEUROTRANSMITTER SYSTEMS

There are more than 50 known neurotransmitters, which fall into four main groups (Table 8.6) based on their structure.

Amino acids

Excitatory amino acids

Glutamate is the major CNS excitatory amino acid transmitter. The two most numerous neurons in the nervous system, pyramidal cells of the cerebral cortex and granule cells of the cerebellum, are glutamatergic, and most cells in the cerebral cortex respond to glutamate. Pathways using glutamate are found throughout the brain, especially in sensory systems, in the hippocampus and within the cerebellum.

Glutamate receptors

Glutamate acts at both ionotropic and metabotropic receptors. There are two populations of ionotropic receptors which mediate glutamate fast transmission (Information box 8.6). Named after abbreviations of their preferred agonists, they are:

- AMPA receptors
- NMDA receptors.

Both are permeable to Na^+ and K^+ but NMDA receptors and one subtype of AMPA-kainate receptor are also permeable to Ca^{2+}, a property crucial to their physiological roles. While AMPA-kainate receptors are implicated in standard excitatory transmission, NMDA receptors have a more specialised role in the rewiring of neural circuits that occurs during development and during learning. Excessive activation of glutamate receptors contributes to several pathologies (Information box 8.7).

NMDA receptors are remarkable in several ways including:

- They require both glutamate and depolarisation for their ion channel to be open. At normal resting membrane potentials the ion channel is blocked by Mg^{2+} ions.

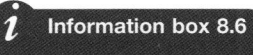

Information box 8.6   Drugs acting at ionotropic glutamate receptors

The NMDA receptor harbours the **sigma opioid binding site**, so named because it is responsible for the **psychotomimetic** – schizophrenia-mimicking – effects of some opiates. It also binds the psychotomimetic phencyclidine and the basal anaesthetic ketamine. Binding of these agents blocks activation of the receptor.

Ketamine produces **dissociative anaesthesia**, a state of analgesia and paralysis but without loss of consciousness. It is used mostly for minor paediatric procedures since children seem less affected by the hallucinations that commonly accompany recovery.

These leave the glutamate-activated channel when the membrane is depolarised. This property is crucial to its role in excitotoxicity.

■ It has a binding site for glycine, which although an inhibitory transmitter in its own right, is additionally a **co-agonist** of NMDA receptors.

Metabolism of neurotransmitter glutamate

Neurotransmitter glutamate is synthesised in neurons from glutamine, a reaction catalysed by **glutaminase**. It is then pumped into vesicles. After release it is removed from the cleft by glutamate transporters in neurons and glia (Fig. 8.24). In neurons the glutamate is probably metabolised although some may be re-used as a transmitter. However, in glia the glutamate is converted by **glutamine synthetase** to glutamine which is then liberated into the extracellular space for uptake by neurons. This closes the **glutamate-glutamine cycle**. This cycle allows glial cells to export transmitter glutamate back to the neurons in a form (glutamine) which cannot spuriously activate glutamate receptors (Information box 8.7).

Inhibitory amino acids

GABA and **glycine** are the predominant inhibitory amino acids in the CNS. Glycine is confined to the spinal cord but GABA is ubiquitous. GABAergic neurons form the major output of the basal ganglia and the sole output of the cerebellar cortex. A large number of CNS interneurons use either GABA or glycine.

GABA and glycine receptors

The ionotropic receptors for GABA (GABA$_A$ receptors, see Information box 8.8) and glycine are both selective chloride channels. The inhibitory nature of these receptors comes about because they 'clamp' the membrane potential at about −60 mV, the chloride equilibrium potential. When the chloride channel associated with these receptors is open, both depolarisation and hyperpolarisation are opposed as chloride flows across the membrane.

ⓘ Information box 8.7 **Excitotoxicity and strokes**

Cell death that occurs in the outer regions of a stroke infarct are caused by the excessive release of glutamate from neurons. This phenomenon is termed **excitotoxicity**. The sequence of events is as follows:

1. Hypoxia, resulting from the lack of blood flow, causes a fall in ATP concentrations, starving the Na$^+$/K$^+$-ATPase of its energy supply.
2. Consequently there is a rise in intracellular Na$^+$ and Cl$^-$, dragging water osmotically into cells, which swell (**cytotoxic oedema**; Information box 8.4), at the expense of the extracellular fluid volume (ECF), which falls.
3. Potassium ions accumulate in the ECF, depolarising neurons, opening voltage-dependent calcium channels and the resulting Ca^{2+} signal drives the release of glutamate, which stimulates glutamate receptors.
4. Large scale activation of AMPA receptors lifts the Mg^{2+} block on NMDA receptors, allowing more calcium influx.
5. In the absence of energy to power transport, mechanisms that keep cytoplasmic Ca^{2+} concentrations low are overloaded.
6. Intracellular calcium rises to pathological levels, triggering apoptosis or necrotic cell death.

ⓘ Information box 8.8 **Drugs acting at GABA$_A$ receptors**

GABA$_A$ receptors are the target for several important classes of drug, for example, benzodiazepines and barbiturates. Ethanol acts on GABA$_A$ receptors and this contributes to the intoxication and ataxia of drunkenness.

The barbiturates (e.g. phenobarbital) and benzodiazepines (e.g. diazepam) both bind to (different) sites which allosterically alter the affinity for GABA binding. Binding of the drug and GABA produces a greater flux of chloride through the GABA$_A$ receptor than does GABA alone, thereby enhancing inhibition.

All barbiturates and benzodiazepines produce sedation. Some barbiturates (e.g. phenobarbital) have a specific anticonvulsant action and are used in the long-term management of epilepsy. Highly lipophilic barbiturates, such as thiopental, cross the blood–brain barrier very fast and so are used intravenously for rapid induction of anaesthesia.

Benzodiazepines used orally for short periods are useful in reducing anxiety. Given intravenously before minor surgery the short-acting benzodiazepines act as basal anaesthetics, and will terminate life-threatening seizures of status epilepticus or eclampsia. However, most benzodiazepines are too sedative for maintenance therapy in epilepsy.

Flumazenil, an antagonist of the benzodiazepine binding site on the GABA$_A$ receptor, reverses the effects of benzodiazepine overdose and the CNS effects of acute ethanol intoxication. There are compounds which bind to the GABA$_A$ benzodiazepine site which reduce the GABA-evoked chloride flux. These **inverse agonists** have the opposite pharmacological profile to the usual agonist benzodiazepines; they are proconvulsants and anxiety-producing.

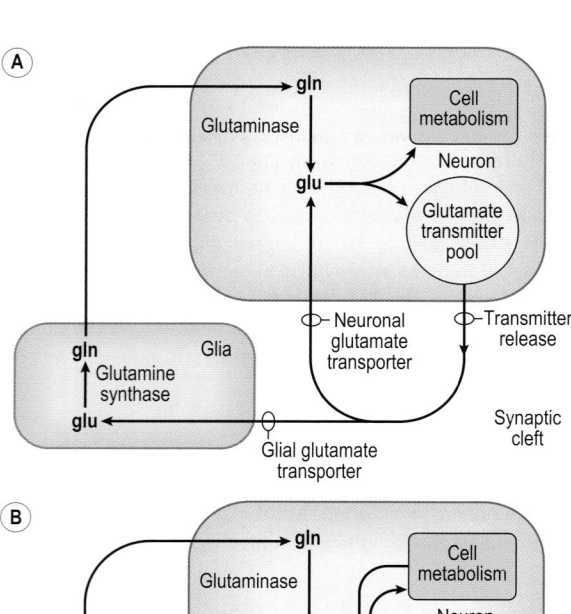

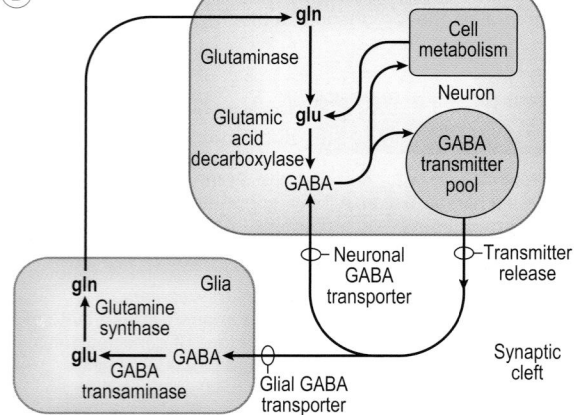

Fig. 8.24 **Metabolism of glutamate and GABA.**

Table 8.7	Major cholinergic pathways	
Origin	Destination	Role
Pontine reticular formation	Forebrain (thalamus) and spinal cord	Sleep and wakefulness
Forebrain	Cerebral cortex	Cortical arousal
Septum	Hippocampus	Learning and memory
Ventral horn of spinal grey matter	Skeletal muscle	Movement

Table 8.8	Major dopaminergic pathways	
Origin	Destination	Role
Substantia nigra (nigrostriatal)	Striatum	Intentional movement
Tegmentum (mesolimbic)	Limbic system	Reward, motivation
Tegmentum (mesocortical)	Prefrontal cortex	Working memory Cognitive tasks
Hypothalamus (tuberoinfundibular)	Median eminence	Pituitary secretion of prolactin
Hypothalamus	Spinal grey matter	Sympathetic

Metabolism of GABA

GABA is synthesised from glutamate by **glutamic acid decarboxylase** (**GAD**), an enzyme present virtually exclusively in GABAergic neurons. After release GABA is taken up by specific transporters into both neurons and glia. It is then catabolised to succinic semialdehyde by the mitochondrial enzyme **GABA transaminase**. The GABA analogue anticonvulsant vigabatrin is an irreversible competitive inhibitor of GABA transaminase and is thought to act by increasing the neurotransmitter pool of GABA (see Fig. 8.24).

Metabolism of neurotransmitter glycine

Neurotransmitter glycine is synthesised from serine by the mitochondrial isoform of **serine transhydroxymethylase**. After release, glycine transporters remove it from the cleft.

Monoamines

The major brain monoamines are:

- Acetylcholine
- The catecholamines: dopamine, noradrenaline and adrenaline
- Serotonin
- Histamine.

Monoaminergic neurons in the brainstem or basal forebrain send their axons forward along the neuraxis to many parts of the forebrain. In many cases their axons have swellings along their lengths, called **varicosities**, which act as presynaptic terminals and contain small dense-core vesicles. The synaptic clefts can be very wide (up to 500 μm), so released transmitter can diffuse widely to influence numerous cells. The synthesis and release of transmitter from many catecholaminergic neurons and serotonergic neurons is regulated by **autoreceptors**.

Monoaminergic transmission brings about widespread modulation of forebrain nuclei and cerebral cortex, producing the global changes necessary for sleep and wakefulness, arousal, attention and motivation.

The metabolism and receptors for acetylcholine, noradrenaline, adrenaline and serotonin are dealt with in Chapter 4. Histamine receptors are discussed in Chapter 6.

Acetylcholine

Although many cholinergic axons run through the brainstem reticular formation, most cholinergic neurons are found in the forebrain. In the CNS there are four major groups of cholinergic neurons (Table 8.7). In addition, cholinergic interneurons are found in the cerebral cortex, striatum, and limbic system. Loss of cholinergic neurons (among others) is seen in Alzheimer's disease. Both nicotinic and muscarinic receptors are found in the CNS.

Dopamine

The majority of dopaminergic neurons are localised to a few nuclei in the midbrain and send their axons further up the neuraxis (Table 8.8). A large majority (80%) of the dopaminergic neurons are in the nigrostriatal pathway and their loss is responsible for the motor defects of Parkinson's disease. Dopaminergic interneurons are important in the olfactory bulb, the retina (amacrine cells) and in sympathetic ganglia.

Dopamine metabolism

Dopamine is synthesised from L-tyrosine, the common precursor for all catecholamines, via L-dihydroxyphenylalanine (L-dopa) (see Fig. 4.24 in Ch. 4). L-dopa is a mainstay in the treatment of Parkinson's disease. Dopamine is synaptically inactivated by reuptake into neurons by a process similar to uptake$_1$ for noradrenaline (see Ch. 4). Dopamine that has been taken up and not used to refill vesicles is degraded in a similar manner to the other catecholamines. Inhibitors of one of the enzymes involved, monoamine oxidase (MAO), have a place in the treatment of Parkinson's disease (see under Basal ganglia below) and as antidepressants (see Ch. 4).

Dopamine receptors

Dopamine receptors are G-protein-coupled receptors and fall into two families:

- **D1** family (includes D1 and D5) – coupled to G$_s$ so they increase cAMP synthesis
- **D2** family (includes D2, D3 and D4) – G$_i$ linked and so they reduce cAMP.

D1 agonists are used in Parkinson's disease and in some endocrine disorders (Ch. 10). D2 antagonists are used in schizophrenia, which is associated with defects in dopamine neurotransmission in the mesolimbic and mesocortical systems. They also act as anti-emetics because they block D2 receptors in the **chemoreceptor trigger zone** of the medulla, which initiates vomiting.

Noradrenaline and adrenaline

The cell bodies of noradrenaline (NA) and adrenaline (AD) secreting neurons are found in several clusters in the medulla and pons and lie in two columns, one ventral and the other dorsal (Table 8.9). The largest group of noradrenergic cells are in the **locus coeruleus** and project widely throughout the brain, but most extensively to the cerebral cortex. The firing rate of locus coeruleus cells is very low during sleep and increases with arousal.

The cortical actions of noradrenaline are to enhance the effects of both excitatory and inhibitory inputs. Hence,

Table 8.9	Noradrenergic and adrenergic pathways	
Origin	**Destination**	**Role**
Locus coeruleus (dorsal pons)	Widely throughout brain but especially cerebral cortex	Sleep and arousal
Nucleus ambiguus (ventral medulla)	Hypothalamus	Endocrine and cardiovascular functions
Nucleus of the solitary tract	Hypothalamus Parabrachial nucleus	Effects on visceral and ventilatory networks
Motor nucleus of vagus nerve (dorsal medulla)		
Pons	Spinal cord	Pain perception (AD) Tonic vasoconstriction (NA)

Table 8.10	Major serotonergic pathways	
Origin	**Destination**	**Role**
Medulla and ventral pons	Spinal cord	Pain perception
		Autonomic modulation
		Modulation of motor output
Dorsal pons and midbrain	Medial forebrain bundle, especially hypothalamus	Cardiovascular and thermoregulatory homeostasis
Dorsal pons and midbrain	Cerebral cortex	Cortical modulation
Dorsal pons	Pons (cholinergic neurons)	Termination of rapid eye movement (REM) sleep
Several raphe nuclei	Cerebral blood vessels	Regulation of cerebral blood flow
	Choroid plexus	Secretion of cerebrospinal fluid

noradrenergic transmission widens the dynamic range of cortical cell responses, effectively turning up the signal-to-noise ratio of cortical processing.

Serotonin

Most **serotonin** (**5-hydroxytryptamine**, **5-HT**) secreting neurons are located in the **raphe nuclei**, which lie along the midline of the brainstem. Their targets are very wide ranging and serotonergic neurons project to virtually all parts of the CNS (Table 8.10).

Serotonin metabolism

Serotonin is synthesised from the essential amino acid **tryptophan**. This is transported across the blood–brain barrier and then into neurons via specific amino acid transporters. Tryptophan is hydroxylated by **tryptophan-5-hydroxylase** and subsequently decarboxylated by **aromatic L-amino acid decarboxylase** to form serotonin. The first of these reactions is the rate limiting step in serotonin synthesis. Since transport across the blood–brain barrier can be elevated by high plasma tryptophan concentration, serotonin synthesis may vary with dietary tryptophan. The major metabolite of serotonin, **5-hydroxyindoleacetic acid (5-HIAA)** is formed by the oxidative deamination of the transmitter by monoamine oxidase.

Serotonin released into the synapse is removed by a specific transport system. This is the target for the **selective**

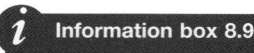

Information box 8.9 **Serotonin, GABA and anxiety**

Serotonin neurotransmission is implicated in anxiety:

- In animal experiments, destruction of serotonergic neurons reduces behaviours associated with anxiety.
- There is an association between anxiety and a long version of the gene for the serotonin transporter that clears serotonin from the synaptic cleft faster than the short version.
- Serotonin 5-HT$_{1A}$ receptors are inhibitory metabotropic autoreceptors of serotonergic nerve terminals which decrease serotonin secretion. Partial agonists of 5-HT$_{1A}$ receptors (e.g. buspirone) – which reduce serotonin release – have proved to be clinically potent **anxiolytic** (anxiety-reducing) agents.
- Antagonists of 5-HT$_3$ receptors (ondansetron) are anxiolytic.

GABA transmission is implicated in anxiety because high numbers of GABA$_A$ receptors are found in the limbic system, particularly in the amygdala, and benzodiazepines (Information box 8.8) are anxiolytic. Benzodiazepine inverse agonists are actually **anxiogenic** (anxiety-generating) agents. It is possible that there are endogenous inverse agonists which are mediators of anxiety.

Serotonergic neurons are inhibited by GABAergic neurons so indirect actions on serotonin transmission may contribute to the anxiolytic actions of benzodiazepines.

serotonin reuptake inhibitors (**SSRIs**) that are used in depression. This treatment is based on possible correlations between reductions in serotonergic transmission and clinical depression. The widely misused psychostimulant 'Ecstasy' (3,4-methylene-dioxymethamphetamine) competes with serotonin for the reuptake system, which may partly account for the euphoria it produces (see also Information box 8.9).

Histamine

Histaminergic neurons are concentrated in the tuberomamillary nucleus and project ubiquitously in the CNS. Histaminergic transmission is implicated in switching from sleeping to waking states and with cortical arousal. This accounts for the sedative effects of those antihistamines (H2 antagonists) which cross the blood–brain barrier. Brain blood flow could be affected by histamine release from mast cells associated with cerebral vasculature.

Purines

Both **ATP** and its catabolite, **adenosine**, are purine transmitters.

Adenosine

Adenosine is an atypical transmitter in that it is not stored in vesicles or released in a Ca^{2+}-dependent way. It is generated locally by enzyme-catalysed breakdown of released ATP and ADP. Synaptic actions of adenosine are inactivated by a nucleoside transporter. **Adenosine receptors** are all G-protein-coupled receptors which modulate cAMP (Table 8.10).

A$_1$ presynaptic receptors reduce the release of a number of transmitters in the peripheral and central nervous system. When brain metabolism is very high (e.g. during an epileptic seizure), or during ischaemia, adenosine concentrations rise. By inhibiting glutamate release, adenosine may naturally curtail seizure activity and be neuroprotective in ischaemia. Adenosine A$_1$ agonists are being developed for potential use in strokes.

Table 8.11	Receptors for purine neurotransmitters		
Receptor	Transduction	Endogenous agonists	Antagonists
A$_1$	G-protein-coupled receptor, increases cAMP	Adenosine	Caffeine, theophylline
A$_2$	G-protein-coupled receptor, decreases cAMP	Adenosine	
P$_{2X}$	Ligand-gated cation channel	ATP	Suramin
P$_{2Y}$	G-protein-coupled receptor	ATP, ADP	

Table 8.12	Opioid receptors		
Receptor	Location	Endogenous ligand	Preferential agonists*
μ	Ubiquitous	β-Endorphin dynorphin	Morphine and analogues (e.g. fentanyl)
δ	Spinal cord	β-Endorphin enkephalins	
κ	Peripheral nervous system	β-Endorphin dynorphin	Benzomorphans (e.g. pentazocine)

*All receptors are blocked by opioid antagonists (e.g. naloxone).

A$_2$ receptors mediate the pain of angina. Present on the terminals of nociceptors in the heart, they respond to the high adenosine levels produced in cardiac ischaemia.

ATP

ATP is stored in synaptic vesicles and co-released with classical transmitters from postganglionic autonomic fibres and central synapses.

The **P$_{2X}$ purinergic receptors** for ATP (Table 8.11) constitute a family of ligand-gated ion channels that is distinct from either the nicotinic receptor family or the ionotropic glutamate receptors. They are permeable to Na$^+$, K$^+$ and Ca^{2+} and their actions are excitatory.

Examples of ATP transmission include:

- The fast phase of smooth muscle contraction in response to sympathetic stimulation.
- Excitation of dorsal horn cells and motor neurons in the spinal cord by ATP release from primary afferents.
- Pain signalling by stimulating P$_{2X}$ receptors on unmyelinated visceral nociceptors, e.g. of urinary bladder.

ATP is inactivated in the synapse by a nucleotidase enzyme.

Peptides

Over 50 small peptides are thought to be neurotransmitters. Some are also hormones or neuroendocrines (released from a neuron into the blood) (see Table 8.6). They can be grouped into families on the basis of:

- Similarities in their amino acid sequences.
- Being derived by cleavage of a common precursor polypeptide encoded by a single mRNA molecule. Often the peptides generated from a common polypeptide have related functions. Different cells may process the same precursor or its mRNA in different ways.

Two prominent groups are the **tachykinins** and the **opioids**.

Processing of peptide neurotransmitters

As the mRNA encoding a peptide neurotransmitter is translated on ribosomes, the **prepropeptide** is transported across the membrane of the rough endoplasmic reticulum into the lumen with the aid of a hydrophobic signal sequence at the N-terminal end (see Ch. 2). The secreted prepropeptide is then cleaved to remove the signal sequence, giving the **propeptide**. Further proteolysis generates the functional peptide.

Tachykinins

The most well known of the tachykinins is **substance P** (**SP**). It is an excitatory transmitter in several brain regions including the cerebral cortex, striatum and substantia nigra. Their receptors are all G-protein-coupled receptors linked to phospholipase C. SP is released by both central and peripheral terminals of C fibre primary afferents:

- The central terminals synapse with dorsal horn cells to convey information about pain and temperature.
- Release from the peripheral terminals results in **neurogenic inflammation**.

SP-containing terminals are found adjacent to cerebral blood vessels, and abnormal release of SP may play a role in migraine and other headaches.

The gene which codes for SP also encodes other transmitters of the **tachykinin** family (so called because they are rapidly acting), such as **substance K** and **neurokinins A** and **B**.

Opioids

The opioids are a group of peptide neurotransmitters which act on opioid receptors, the targets for opiate drugs such as morphine. They are generally co-released with classical transmitters, typically GABA and serotonin, and are usually inhibitory. Opioid transmission is thought to be important in analgesia pathways in the CNS and is also implicated in sexual and aggressive/submissive behaviours. Opioids are encoded by three precursor genes:

- The enkephalin precursor encodes **met-enkephalin** and **leu-enkephalin** (so called because they differ in just one amino acid) and is expressed mainly in short interneurons throughout the brain.
- Pro-opiomelanocortin encodes **β-endorphin** and is expressed in neurons of the hypothalamus which project to the thalamus or brainstem.
- The dynorphin precursor codes for leu-enkephalin and **dynorphins**.

Opioid receptors

There are three populations of opioid receptors, the properties of which are summarised in Table 8.12. They are **G-protein-coupled receptors** that allow direct coupling of G proteins to ion channels. By opening K$^+$ channels and closing Ca^{2+} channels they hyperpolarise neurons.

The μ opioid receptors are responsible for the euphoria, dependence and respiratory depression of opiate drugs. However the μ-selective **weak agonists** do not produce dependence, so methadone is used to counter withdrawal in patients being weaned from addiction to strong opiate agonists such as heroin. A number of opiates have a complicated pharmacological profile, being **partial agonists** at one receptor subtype and antagonist at another. The major use of the pure **opiate antagonists** is in the treatment of agonist overdose.

NEURAL INTEGRATION AND INFORMATION CODING

The nervous system is, above all else, an information processor. Each neuron sums all its synaptic inputs and either fires or does not in consequence. The firing pattern of all the neurons in a neural network determines the output of that network and so contributes to overall behaviour. The way in which neurons integrate their synaptic inputs depends on their electrical properties and geometry.

Electrical properties and geometry of neurons

Unlike action potentials, which are actively propagated without loss of amplitude, **synaptic potentials** and the local circuit currents involved in propagation of the action potential get smaller (decay) both with time and with distance as they are conducted. Potentials which behave in this way are called **electrotonic potentials**. They are passively conducted, and because this depends only on the physics of the neuron, it can be modelled by treating the nerve cell as if it were an electrical cable.

Generally, the smaller the diameter of a neuron or a neurite (axon or dendrite) the shorter the distance over which an electrotonic potential will decay and the faster this will happen. In small diameter neurons with short axons (e.g. retinal bipolar cells) the synaptic potentials can reach the end of the axon with sufficient magnitude to affect neurotransmitter release. Large diameter neurons conduct electrotonic potentials more swiftly than small diameter ones. However, in neurons with long axons, synaptic potentials will have decayed to zero before they can reach the end of the axon, hence the need for regenerating action potentials. Distal synapses, which are further away from the axon hillock where action potentials are generated, have less of an influence on a nerve cell's behaviour than proximal ones because distal synaptic potentials decay more.

Summation

A crucial property of synaptic potentials is that they summate, i.e. combine to form a potential with an amplitude that depends in some way on the size of the individual potentials. This is an important distinction between synaptic potentials and action potentials, which are of fixed size.

Summation can be a straightforward algebraic addition (two 2 mV epsps summate to produce a combined potential of 4 mV), but in many instances the combined potential is less than the sum of its parts. This non-linear behaviour adds considerably to the complexity of the computations that nerve cells can do.

When ipsps sum they produce a larger hyperpolarisation and will tend to cancel epsps; i.e. the result of linearly combining an epsp of 4 mV with an ipsp of 2 mV is a summed potential of 2 mV.

There are two types of summation (Fig. 8.25):

■ **Spatial summation** describes the summation of potentials generated at the same time at different places on the nerve cell.

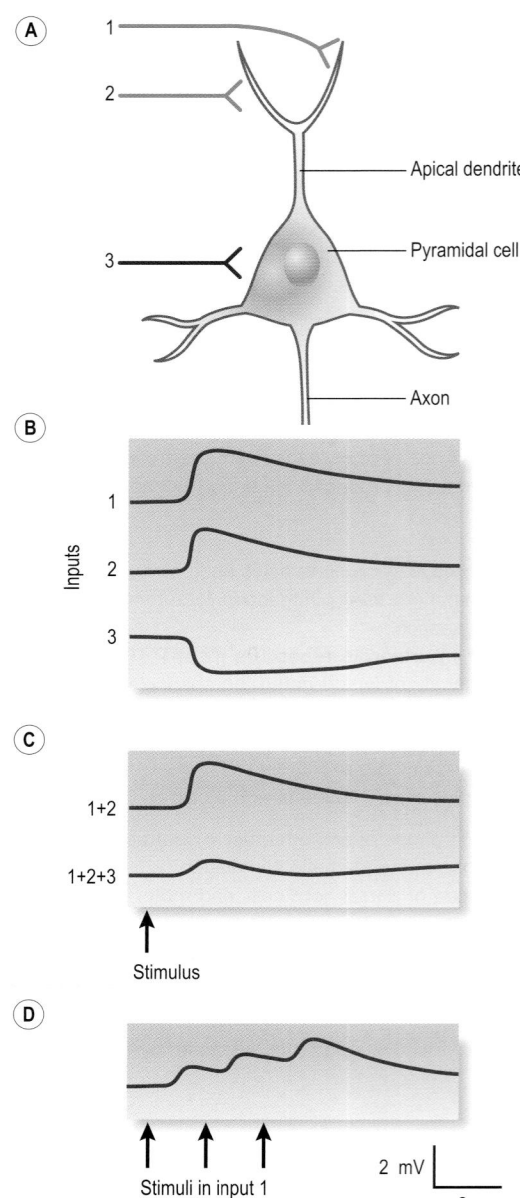

Fig. 8.25 Summation. (A) Three inputs onto different regions of a cortical pyramidal cell. 1 and 2 are excitatory, 3 is inhibitory. (B) Postsynaptic potentials recorded from the cell body after stimulating each of the inputs individually. (C) Spatial summation: postsynaptic potentials caused by stimulating pairs of inputs at the same time. (D) Temporal summation: the postsynaptic potential generated by repeated stimulation of an excitatory input.

■ **Temporal summation** occurs when several synaptic potentials are generated within a short space of time because a presynaptic cell fires a high frequency train of action potentials.

Although described separately, both spatial and temporal summation occur together when a neuron is stimulated. It is the summation of inputs which determines the firing behaviour of a neuron.

Integration of synaptic inputs

A neuron may have many hundreds or even thousands of synaptic terminals impinging on its surface. For example, pyramidal cells – the most numerous neuron of the cerebral cortex – may have as many as 10 000 incoming synapses. These are not randomly distributed. Excitatory contacts are made mostly on the dendrites while inhibitory synapses, of which there are far fewer, are located preferentially on the cell body.

A neuron processes information by 'deciding' at every instant whether or not to fire an action potential. This it does on the basis of the size of the **summed potential** that arrives at the axon hillock. This region, known functionally as the **trigger zone**, has the lowest threshold for firing action potentials because it has the highest density of sodium channels. If the summed potential – which is the combined effect of all the epsps and ipsps at that instant – exceeds the threshold the cell will fire. If the threshold is not crossed the cell remains silent.

The length of time the neuron is depolarised beyond threshold, and by how much, determines the duration of the train of action potentials and the firing frequency, respectively. It is estimated that activation of a minimum of 100 excitatory synapses is needed to make a pyramidal cell fire.

The effect that a given synapse has on the final outcome depends on the location of the synapse. The location of inhibitory synapses on the cell bodies of pyramidal cells makes them especially powerful as only a modest number of inhibitory inputs need be active to silence the cell even, in the face of a large barrage of excitation.

Neural networks

Neurons connect together to form neural networks. How they operate is poorly understood. This is a central problem for neuroscience because large regions of the nervous system (e.g. the cerebral cortex) apparently consist of the same network repeated millions of times. How the same circuit serves functions as diverse as those of the cerebral cortex is currently a mystery. However, some patterns of neural organisation are comprehensible.

Divergence

Divergence involves few cells connecting with many to disseminate information to a wide variety of targets, for example: in the autonomic nervous system preganglionic neurons connect to many postganglionic autonomic neurons, where the divergence may be 100-fold.

Convergence

Convergence funnels connections from many cells to few. It is the means by which target cells are able to integrate information from several sources. Convergence must involve data compression. Examples include: the retina, which has 100 million photoreceptors but only one million output neurons.

Feedforward and feedback

Feedforward circuits have input neurons which establish connections (either excitatory or inhibitory) with cells that are closer to the output, i.e. with higher order neurons than themselves.

In **feedback** circuits, higher order cells establish connections to lower order cells. The connections can be excitatory but are more usually via inhibitory interneurons to cause feedback inhibition.

A neuron may feedback on itself by making recurrent connections. **Recurrent excitation** by axon collaterals is important in the hippocampus, while **recurrent inhibition** of motor neurons in the spinal cord is crucial (see below).

Feedback inhibition is an example of negative feedback (Ch. 1). For example, α motor neurons which excite skeletal muscle inhibit each other by way of glycinergic interneurons called **Renshaw cells**. The purpose of this is to constrain activation of muscles. The glycinergic synapse is functionally blocked by both **tetanus toxin**, which prevents glycine release, and **strychnine**, a glycine receptor antagonist. These agents produce convulsions.

Central pattern generators

Neural networks that produce cyclical patterns of activity autonomously are called **central pattern generators** (**CPGs**). They mediate, for example:

- The inspiratory–expiratory cycle of ventilation
- Limb movements during locomotion, which involves alternate activation of flexors and extensors.

The basic operation of CPGs can be modified or overridden by extraneous pathways.

Information encoding

Afferent neurons encode information about sensory input whereas **efferent** neurons encode the motor output necessary to activate muscles and glands. The general principles involved in this neural coding are quite well understood. However, the transformations that occur to the input within the CNS to produce a particular output are not understood in most cases.

The information encoded by a neuron depends on its firing frequency and how it is connected at either end.

- Frequency modulation: The frequency of action potentials carries information about the intensity of stimuli or force of contraction and about the rate at which these variables changes.
- Connectivity coding: How the neuron is connected encodes the location and quality (also called **modality**) of stimuli or the precise form of motor response (see below).

SENSORY SYSTEMS
OVERVIEW

There are several distinct sensory systems. These may be conveniently divided into:

- Skin senses. These result from mechanical, thermal and chemical stimulation of the skin and give rise to touch, pressure, temperature and pain sensations. Skin sensory pathways from the body and limbs run in peripheral nerves to the dorsal horn of the spinal cord. Those from the face and head enter the brain via one of the cranial nerves; most through the trigeminal (V) nerve.
- Body senses. Receptors responding to mechanical forces are found in muscles, tendons and joints. These produce **proprioception**, the sense of how the body and limbs are positioned in space and the forces they are experiencing. Receptors for mechanical forces and/ or irritant chemicals are located in hollow organs (e.g. gut, airways, urinary bladder) which provide the

sensations which guide a wide variety of basic behaviours such as feeding, defecation, sneezing, coughing, micturition, etc. Proprioceptor pathways run in peripheral nerves to the dorsal horn of the spinal cord. Sensation from internal organs is relayed through peripheral nerves (e.g. gut and urinary bladder sensation) or cranial nerves (e.g. upper airways). In autonomic reflexes, although the efferent neurons are located in the autonomic nervous system, the afferent neurons run in the somatic nervous system; i.e. there are no sensory autonomic fibres.

- Special senses centred in the head are responsible for vision, hearing, smell, taste and the vestibular sensations of balance, body orientation and movement. The pathways of the special senses run in cranial nerves to the brain.

GENERAL PRINCIPLES OF SENSORY SYSTEMS

While each sensory system has its own characteristics there are general principles of sensory coding which apply to all systems.

Receptor transduction

All sensory receptors convert the energy of the stimulus into a change in membrane potential termed a **receptor potential**. This is called **transduction**. The transduction mechanism is receptor-specific. Receptor potentials have the same properties as synaptic potentials; they spread passively, decay with time and distance, and summate.

In some sensory cells, such as skin mechanoreceptors, if the receptor potential is sufficiently large it will cause the cell to fire action potentials. Sensory cells that are not excitable (e.g. retinal photoreceptors) transmit information further into their sensory pathway by means of the receptor potential.

Transduction in **mechanoreceptors** involves distortion of the afferent terminal which opens stretch-sensitive ion channels. The resulting flow of ions sets up the receptor potential, always depolarising, which can then trigger action potentials. The precise nature, extent and timing of the transduction are determined by the structure of the sensory receptor surrounding the nerve terminal. This acts as a filter that constrains the terminal to respond to a particular set of stimuli. This confers the specificity and type of adaptation shown by the afferent.

Most sensory receptors show some loss of sensitivity (**adaptation**) to a constant stimulus, reflected by a drop in firing frequency with time.

- Slowly adapting receptors adapt only over a long time, if at all; their afferents fire with a frequency which is a function of the stimulus intensity.
- Rapidly adapting receptors fire only transiently to a constant stimulus. These are sensitive to changes in stimulus intensity, usually in a specific direction.

Receptive fields

The region of sensory space (e.g. area of skin) which when stimulated changes the firing rate of a neuron is the neuron's **receptive field**. Receptive fields for particular neurons vary in size and structure.

Size

A sensory space served by many neurons, each with small receptive fields (i.e. where each afferent is responsible for only a small region), will be able to resolve the position of a stimulus better than a sensory space mapped by a few neurons with large receptive fields. For example, the ability to resolve two adjacent points of a divider touching the skin (the **two-point discrimination test**) is very much better on the hands than the trunk. This is because the skin of the hand is served by many sensory afferents with small receptive fields.

Structure

Many receptive fields have two (in some cases more) regions with different effects on the firing of the neuron.

- **On-centre cells** have an inner region where stimulation increases the firing rate of the afferent and an outer annulus where stimulation decreases the afferent's firing frequency.
- **Off-centre cells**, in which the zones are reversed, are just as common.

These cells exhibit **surround (lateral) inhibition** and are found, for example, in visual, auditory and touch pathways.

Surround inhibition

Surround inhibition is seen in many sensory systems. Excitatory input into a cell is accompanied by a zone of inhibition in surrounding cells, produced by inhibitory GABAergic interneurons. Hence any given cell is activated by direct stimulation but inhibited by peripheral stimulation. This enhances contrasts in neural activity, contributing to the ability to locate stimuli in space, and to **selective attention**, the facility to attend to one stimulus in preference to others.

Stimulus localisation

The location of a stimulus in space is related to the particular group of cells that is stimulated. Neurons in a sensory pathway that are stimulated by adjacent regions in sensory space (i.e. neighbouring regions of skin or retina) often maintain an anatomical relationship between each other throughout the pathway so that sensory space is mapped onto brain structures in the sensory pathway in an organised manner. This **topographic organisation** of pathways preserves information about the location of a stimulus, essentially creating **sensory maps** in the brain. For example, retinotopic maps are found at different levels throughout the visual system that preserve spatial relationships in the visual fields.

Stimulus modality

Modality is the **quality** of a sensation. It depends on the nature of the energy source providing the stimulus: electromagnetic, air pressure, chemical, etc. Submodalities can be defined by the stimulus that excites a homogeneous population of receptors (Table 8.13). Most sensory experience involves the activation of several classes of receptor. For example, when eating we engage not only vision, smell and

Table 8.13 Stimulus modalities

Modality	Stimulus	Physiological receptor
Vision	Light	Retinal photoreceptors
Hearing	Sound	Cochlear hair cells
Balance	Head acceleration and velocity	Vestibular hair cells
Somatosensory: touch, pressure, vibration	Mechanical forces acting on skin	Skin mechanoreceptors
Proprioception	Mechanical forces acting on joints and muscles	Muscle and joint mechanoreceptors
Temperature	Heat	Cold and warm thermoreceptors
Pain	Mechanical force on skin and viscera, heat on skin, chemical on skin, mucous membranes and viscera	Mechanical, thermal and polymodal nociceptors
Itch	Chemical on skin and mucous membranes	Itch receptors
Smell	Chemical	Olfactory sensory neurons
Taste	Chemical	Taste cells

Table 8.14 Properties of non-hairy skin mechanoreceptors

Receptor	Location	Adaptation*	Sensation
Meissner's corpuscle	Superficial	RAI	Touch, stroking, flutter
Pacinian corpuscle	Deep	RAII	Vibration
Merkel's disc	Superficial	SAI	Light pressure
Ruffini's corpuscles	Deep	SAII	Stretch

*RA, rapidly adapting; SA slowly adapting; type I, high resolution; type II, low resolution.

Colour vision requires comparisons to be made of the activation of three cell types differing in wavelength sensitivity, in different regions of the visual field.

SKIN MECHANOSENSORY SYSTEMS

Skin is a sensory organ that responds to mechanical stresses, changes in temperature and the presence of a variety of chemical substances. When stimuli are sufficiently intense as to threaten to damage tissue, they are described as **noxious**, are perceived as painful, and motivate defensive behaviours.

Touch and **pressure** sensation, often in concert with other skin sensations (e.g. temperature), serves a variety of functions.

Mechanoreceptors

Mechanoreceptors in the skin respond to mechanical forces that displace the skin, giving rise to the sensations of touch, pressure, vibration, tickle and stretch (see Ch. 9). They are low threshold, i.e. they have high sensitivity because they can be excited by weak stimuli. They are the specialised endings of large diameter (Aβ) myelinated fibres with their cell bodies in the dorsal root ganglia or brainstem.

Non-hairy skin mechanoreceptors

There are four types of mechanoreceptor in non-hairy skin at different depths below the epidermis (Table 8.14). The superficial receptors have small, well-defined receptive fields, which optimise the spatial location of low mechanical forces. Deep receptors have larger, less well-defined receptive fields and respond to more intense mechanical forces. The receptors are either rapidly adapting (RA), which respond to brief or quickly changing forces, or slowly adapting (SA), which respond to longer lasting pressure or stretch.

Hairy skin mechanoreceptors

Hairy skin has mechanoreceptors analogous to those of non-hairy skin, except for Meissner's corpuscles. In addition it has a variety of **hair follicle receptors**, which are rapidly adapting and respond to hair displacement. They produce the sensation of light stroking and are sensitive enough to detect small insects crawling across the skin.

Mechanoreceptor pathways

The two principal afferent pathways for the conscious experience of mechanoreceptor sensation, including proprioception, are:

Clinical box 8.6 Synaesthesia

Synaesthesia, a condition in which people have perceptions that are out of step with their sensory experience (e.g. 'seeing' colours in response to sounds), presumably occurs via neural circuitry which allows cross-talk between different sensory modalities.

taste but also somatosensory submodalities to assess the temperature and texture of food.

Modality is conferred by whichever neurons are being stimulated (Clinical box 8.6). Experiments in which visual pathways were surgically redirected to auditory cortex resulted in animals which behaved as if they treated input into the re-routed pathway as light, not sound. Two profound implications follow if this work can be verified:

- Modality is conferred by sense organs, not by specialisation of brain circuitry
- The cerebral cortex is a rather general purpose machine; common processing mechanisms may underlie several sensory modalities.

Population coding

Not all the properties of the sensation conferred by a given submodality arise from the stimulation of a single afferent. Some sensory attributes are coded by firing of many neurons; this is called **population coding**. Thus:

- Stimulus intensity is not always encoded by firing frequency. The intensity of vibration depends on the number of vibration-sensitive skin receptors activated.
- Skin temperature sensation is based on the relative firing rates of two populations of neurons, each of which is most sensitive to a particular temperature.

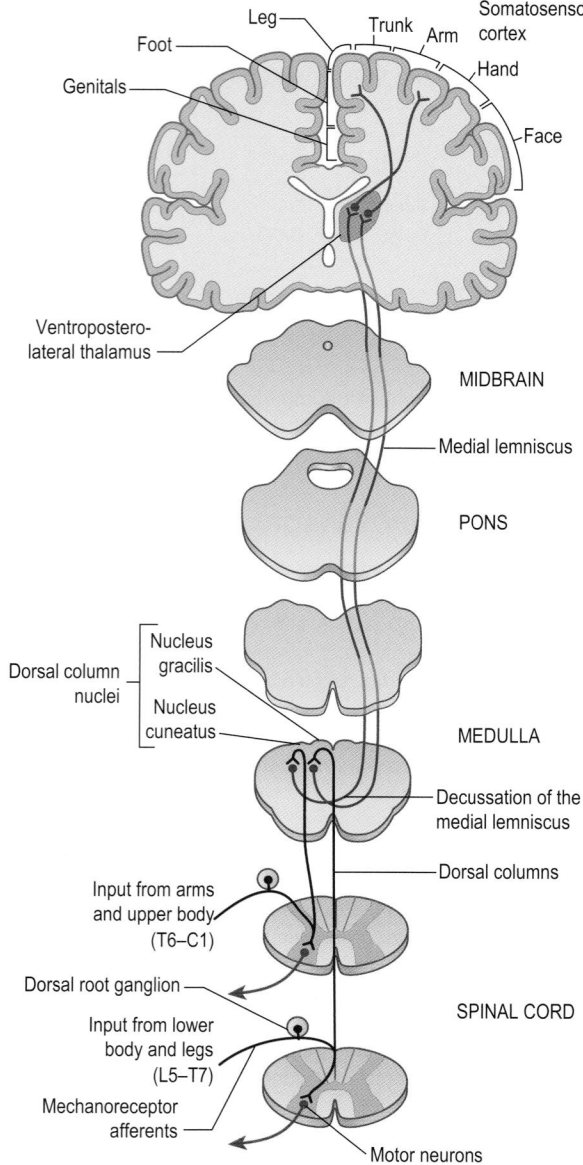

Fig. 8.26 Dorsal column–medial lemniscal pathways for transmitting skin mechanoreceptor sensations.

- The **dorsal column-medial lemniscus pathway**, for the limbs, trunk and posterior third of the head.
- The **trigeminal lemniscus pathway**, serving the face and anterior regions of the head.

However, mechanoreceptor afferents also go to the **anterolateral pathways**, which are responsible for temperature and pain sensation (see below).

Dorsal column–medial lemniscus pathway

When the sensory endings in the skin are stimulated, the large diameter primary afferents carry this information to the spinal cord. These first order neurons have their cell bodies in the dorsal root ganglia. Their axons enter the spinal cord and bifurcate into ascending and descending branches. The major branch ascends in the dorsal columns of the spinal cord (Fig. 8.26) to the **dorsal column nuclei** in the lower medulla where they synapse with second order neurons (Information box 8.10).

Each spinal nerve carries information from a specific region of the skin called a **dermatome** (Information box 8.11). Collateral branches of the ascending and descending branches form synapses in the spinal cord with **dorsal horn cells** (DHCs) of the same or adjacent spinal segments. DHCs are interneurons involved in spinal segmental reflex circuitry, so these connections permit the reflexes to be modified by incoming mechanosensory information (see reflexes section below).

Nerve fibres in the dorsal columns are sorted topographically. Those entering from lower spinal segments are medial and fibres entering successively higher spinal segments are added laterally. At high spinal segments this segregation resolves into two tracts: the medial **gracile tract** carrying fibres from L5 to T7 entering the **gracile nucleus**, and the lateral **cuneate tract** conveying fibres from T6 to C1 projecting to the **cuneate nucleus**. Proprioceptor afferents are located in the ventral dorsal columns, segregated from the tactile afferents, which lie laterally.

When they leave the dorsal column nuclei, the axons of the second order neurons cross to the opposite (contralateral) side of the spinal cord. This crossing over is called decussation and means that signals arising from one side of the body are represented in the brain on the other (contralateral) side. The axons travel in a ribbon-like tract, the **medial lemniscus**, to the **ventral posterior lateral** (**VPL**) **nucleus** of the thalamus in this pathway. As the medial lemniscus ascends, the topographic arrangement of fibres is reversed and in the thalamus the upper part of the body is represented medially, the lower body more laterally.

Trigeminal lemniscus pathway

The primary afferents responsible for low threshold, tactile and proprioceptor sensation of the face and most of the head have their cell bodies in the **trigeminal ganglion**. The centrally directed axons then go via the trigeminal (V) nerve to the **principal nucleus** in the pons, which is homologous to the dorsal column nuclei. From the principal nucleus axons of second order neurons cross the midline and project to the **ventral posterior medial** (**VPM**) **nucleus** of the thalamus by way of the **trigeminal lemniscus**, which runs parallel to the medial lemniscus.

Somatosensory thalamus

With inputs from both the medial and trigeminal lemniscus there is a complete representation of tactile sensation in the ventral posterior lateral and ventral posterior medial nuclei of the thalamus. This topographic map is projected to the somatosensory cortex in the parietal lobe by third order neurons with their cell bodies in the thalamus.

The region of skin innervated by a spinal nerve is called a **dermatome** (Fig. 8.27). By mapping which dermatomes have normal sensation and which do not, it is possible to estimate at which level the spinal cord is injured. However, the following provisos should be noted:

■ Dermatomes vary from one person to another.
■ Dermatomes overlap, and the overlap is more extensive for touch, pressure and vibration than it is for pain and

temperature, so pain sensation is the best guide to the level of cord injury.
■ Proprioceptor fibres follow the distribution of muscle innervation rather than dermatomes.

Because in **herpes zoster** (shingles) specific dorsal roots are infected with the virus, the resulting skin lesions and pain follow dermatomes.

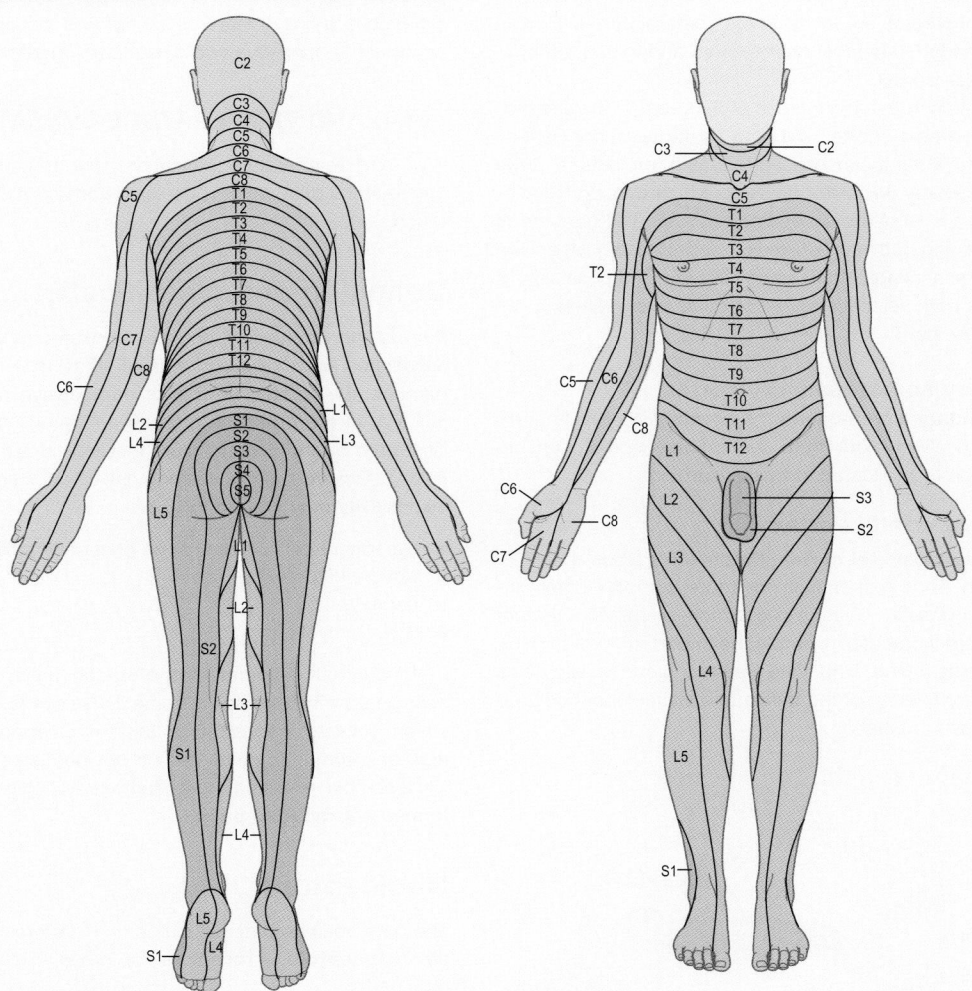

Fig. 8.27 **The dermatomes.** Redrawn with permission from Marieb EN, Hoehn K 2006 Human anatomy and physiology, 7th edn. Benjamin Cummings, San Francisco.

Somatosensory cortex

Primary somatosensory cortex

Neurons in the ventral posterior thalamus send their axons to the **primary somatosensory cortex** (SI) which lies on the post-central gyrus of the parietal lobe, in Brodmann's areas 1, 2, 3a and 3b (see Fig. 8.11). Each of these four areas is dominated by particular submodality (Table 8.15).

Clearly cells in 2 and 3b are implicated in **stereognosis**, the tactile perception of the three-dimensional shape of things. In humans, lesions of a single area almost never occur, so mixed deficits are found. Major lesions of SI lead not only to the expected losses in tactile discrimination and position sense but also to problems with hand movements, and altered (but not abolished) temperature and pain sensations.

Table 8.15	Functions of the primary somatosensory cortex	
Brodmann area	**Submodality**	**Input from**
1	Perception of surface texture	Cutaneous mechanoreceptors
2	Shape and size of a grasped object	Joint proprioceptors
3a	Position and direction of movement	Muscle proprioceptors
3b	Perception of surface texture and shape discrimination	Cutaneous mechanoreceptors

Each area also contains a complete representation of the body, a **somatotopic map**, from foot to face, in a medial to lateral arrangement. The different areas of the body are not represented proportionate to their size: areas that need more inputs, because their function demands high sensitivity (such as the fingers), or complexity (such as the face), are represented by a correspondingly larger area of the cortex (Fig. 8.28). On the other side of the post-central gyrus a similar map exists for the motor cortex (see below). Four other maps of the body surface are found in the cerebral cortex. Two lie in the secondary somatosensory cortex and two in the posterior parietal cortex.

Information from all four areas of SI is sent to the secondary somatosensory cortex (SII) and to the posterior parietal cortex. The somatosensory cortex also projects a large number of axons down the neuraxis which can exert inhibition to each level of the ascending pathway. The purpose of this descending pathway, which is topographically organised to match the ascending one, is not known. One possibility is that it acts as a selective attention mechanism, filtering out unnecessary input.

Secondary somatosensory cortex

The **secondary somatosensory cortex** (SII, Brodmann's area 40) receives input from the primary somatosensory cortex which is implicated in tactile learning.

Posterior parietal cortex

The **posterior parietal cortex** (Brodmann's areas 5 and 7), adjacent to SI, is responsible for more complex differentiation in response to variation in direction, orientation, texture or shape and would, for example, be important in manipulation of objects by the hand. One area of the cortex also deals with the coordination of the tactile and visual inputs needed in hand–eye coordination.

Many neurons in the posterior parietal cortex are feature-detecting cells specifically responsive to differences in direction, orientation, texture or shape. Posterior parietal neurons get convergent input from several submodalities and this provides the clue to their function, the sensory guidance of movement. Area 5 integrates proprioceptor input from muscles and joints, which informs about the position and trajectory of a limb, with tactile information. These cells are thought to be engaged when performing complicated arm and hand manipulations. Area 7 receives tactile and visual input and is important in hand–eye coordination (Information box 8.12).

PAIN AND TEMPERATURE SENSATION

Pain and temperature sensations are transmitted by the anterolateral pathways. These also transmit a crude sense of touch.

Definition and classification of pain

Pain is the unpleasant sensory and emotional experience associated with **noxious stimuli** that may cause tissue damage. The protective role of **nociceptive pain**, which is felt only in the presence of acute injury or inflammation, is illustrated by the serious injury that individuals with insensitivity to severe pain unwittingly inflict on themselves. Pain insensitivity may be due to:

- Hereditary disorders such as channelopathies
- Severe diabetes
- Leprosy
- Syringomyelia.

In contrast, **clinical (pathological) pain**, such as that associated with chronic inflammatory states (e.g. arthritis), or which persists long after an injury has apparently healed (e.g. phantom limb pain), has no obvious physiological role. Clinical pain resulting from damage to pain pathways is termed **neuropathic pain**.

Nociceptors

The bare endings of small diameter, high threshold afferents are **nociceptors** – receptors for noxious, pain-producing

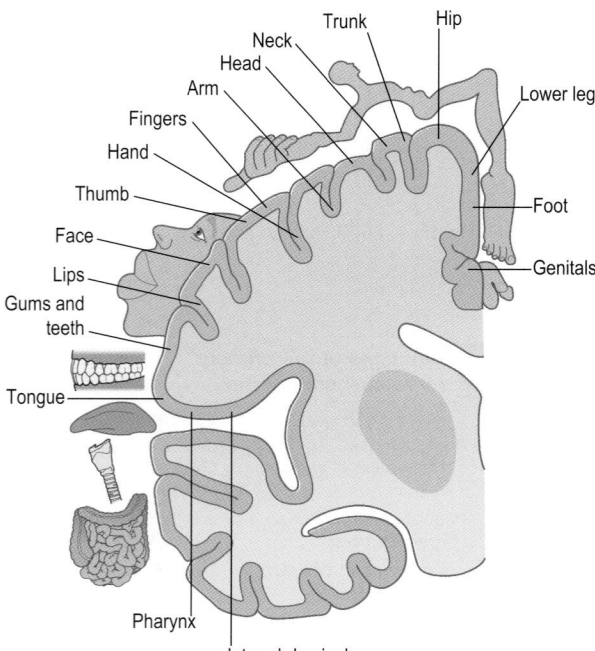

Fig. 8.28 **Somatotopic map of the primary somatosensory (SI) cortex.** Redrawn with permission from Michael-Titus A, Revest P, Shortland P 2006 The nervous system. Churchill Livingstone, Edinburgh.

Labels on figure: Trunk, Hip, Neck, Head, Arm, Lower leg, Fingers, Hand, Thumb, Foot, Face, Lips, Genitals, Gums and teeth, Tongue, Pharynx, Intra-abdominal

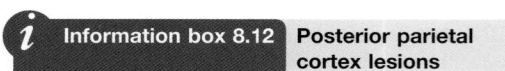

Information box 8.12 **Posterior parietal cortex lesions**

Lesions of the posterior parietal cortex occur most commonly as a result of a stroke. These do not affect the ability to detect a stimulus but affect the ability to know what the stimulus means. This can result in:

- **Astereognosis**, the inability to recognise the shape of objects by touch.
- **Sensory neglect syndrome**, in which sensory information from a part (often one half) of sensory space is not perceived. In patients with astereognosis this can manifest itself as a bizarre failure to recognise one half of their own body. A variant of sensory neglect syndrome, **spatial neglect**, involves a failure to perceive one half of the visual field.

Sensory neglect syndrome implies that the posterior parietal cortex has two **cognitive maps** (representations of where things are in space): one for body self-image and a second for extrapersonal space.

These problems are more likely to occur if the injury is on the right side as this part of the cortex is larger on the right.

stimuli. Unlike thermoreceptors, normally they have no background activity. They are classified into several groups by what excites them.

- **Mechanical nociceptors** are stimulated by intense mechanical forces, and those in the skin give rise to sharp, pricking pain. Their afferents are fast conducting myelinated Aδ fibres.
- **Thermal nociceptors** fall into two groups, one excited by temperatures greater than 45 °C, the other by temperatures less than 5 °C. They also respond to intense mechanical stimuli. Their afferents are Aδ fibres.
- **Polymodal nociceptors** respond to mechanical and thermal stimuli as well as to a wide variety of molecules liberated as a result of tissue damage. Stimulation of these nociceptors causes burning or aching pain. Their afferents are C fibres which conduct at less than 1.0 m/s. Polymodal nociceptors are also responsible for toothache and visceral pain.
- **Itch receptors** belong to a separate class of C fibres that respond to histamine released from mast cells.

Because conduction by Aδ nociceptor afferents is so much faster than that of C fibre polymodal nociceptors, a painful blow produces a sharp **fast (first) pain** initially, followed by an aching or burning **slow (second) pain**.

Primary nociceptor afferents, like mechanoreceptors, have their cell bodies in the dorsal root ganglion and their axons enter the spinal cord. There, they co-release **glutamate** (which acts as a fast transmitter) and **peptides**, most notably substance P. The peptides enhance and prolong the effects of glutamate because they diffuse away from their site of release to increase the excitability of neighbouring dorsal horn cells.

Glutamate and peptides are also released from the peripheral nerve terminals and from the central endings of the nociceptor afferent axon. This gives rise to neurogenic inflammation (Information box 8.13).

Nociceptor pharmacology

Substances released at the site of an injury, including inflammatory mediators, either activate nociceptors directly or sensitise them to other agents (see Ch. 6). Substances include:

Information box 8.13 | **Neurogenic inflammation**

Action potentials triggered by exciting polymodal nociceptor terminals are not only conducted centrally but, in what is termed an **axon reflex**, can also travel the 'wrong way' along side branches of the axons (axon collaterals) to stimulate secretion of **substance P** from their peripheral terminals. This contributes to the classic signs of inflammation at an injury site in what is termed **neurogenic inflammation**. Substance P vasodilates post-capillary venules, which produces heat and redness. It increases capillary permeability, which causes swelling and pain and can cause itching by liberating histamine from mast cells, which excites itch C fibres.

Capsaicin, the active compound responsible for the hot taste of chilli peppers, acts on **vanilloid receptors** in thermal and polymodal nociceptors. Vanilloid receptors transduce noxious heat stimuli (burning sensations). Capsaicin causes pain by releasing substance P from nociceptors, but repeated application causes depletion of the transmitter and hence a reduced sensitivity to nociceptor stimuli. Recovery takes days to weeks. Vanilloid receptor ligands are being explored as potential novel analgesics.

- **H^+ and K^+**: extracellular concentrations increase during ischaemia.
- **ATP** and **prostaglandins**: leak from damaged cells.
- **Serotonin** and **histamine**: released by platelets and mast cells, respectively.
- **Bradykinin**: a potent excitant of nociceptors. It is cleaved from its precursor, plasma kininogen, by the protease kallikrein, which is activated by tissue damage. Competitive antagonists of bradykinin (B_2) receptors are analgesic and anti-inflammatory and have potential as novel analgesics.
- **Arachidonic acid**: produced in response to cell damage. **Cyclo-oxygenase enzymes** act on arachidonic acid, producing prostaglandins which sensitise nociceptors to inflammatory mediators such as serotonin and bradykinin. **Aspirin** and other **non-steroidal anti-inflammatory drugs** (**NSAIDs**) work by inhibiting cyclo-oxygenases. Aspirin produces an irreversible inhibition by acetylating the enzymes (i.e. a covalent modification), whereas many NSAIDs are reversible competitive inhibitors.
- **Substance P**: this peptide is co-released with glutamate from primary afferents and is involved in pain neurotransmission.

Thermoreceptors

Temperature in the innocuous range is sensed by **thermoreceptors** which are the terminals of non-specialised small diameter afferent neurons. They fire continuously at rates that are a function of skin temperature but are slowly adapting and are more sensitive to changes in temperature. There are two populations of thermoreceptors:

- **Warm receptors** fire in the range 29–48 °C, with peak frequency at 42 °C. Noxious heat is not sensed by warm receptors.
- **Cold receptors** are sensitive to skin temperatures between 5 °C and 40 °C and have maximal activity at 25 °C.

Perceived skin temperature is given by comparing the relative activities of the warm and cold receptors. Thermoreceptors also signal the direction in which temperature changes. If the skin is cooled, warm receptors are briefly silenced and cold receptor firing rates rise rapidly and then drop as they adapt to the firing frequency that codes the new temperature. In a like manner, skin warming silences the cold receptors and boosts warm receptor firing.

Pain and temperature pathways

The Aδ and C fibre nociceptor afferents enter the dorsal horn where they bifurcate into ascending and descending branches, forming the dorsolateral tract of Lissauer. They terminate on the cell bodies of the second-order projection neurons in Rexed's lamina I, II and V within one or two spinal segments. The projection neurons in lamina I convey fast pain, slow pain or itch; these are separate submodalities and are processed in parallel but differently.

Anterolateral columns

The **anterolateral columns** contain the axons of the second-order neurons. These axons cross over to the opposite side (**decussate**) within one or two spinal segments.

In the anterolateral columns there are:

- Axons conveying temperature and pain sensations.
- Axons involved in crude touch sensation, in which localisation is preserved but modality is compromised.
- In contrast to the effect on the dorsal columns, compression of the spinal cord on one side which damages the anterolateral columns will lead to a loss of pain and temperature sensation below the level of the injury on the opposite (contralateral) side. This is because these fibres have crossed across the cord, while those of the dorsal columns ascend on the same side. This pattern of sensory losses along with losses of motor function is called **Brown–Séquard syndrome** (see below).

Spinothalamic and spinoreticular tracts

The projection neurons in lamina I are **nociceptor specific**; that is they respond only to high threshold afferent activity. The lamina I projection neurons enter the lateral **spinothalamic tract** STT. Those conveying fast (Aδ fibre) pain cross the midline within one or two spinal segments to ascend on the contralateral side to terminate in the **posterior nucleus** of the thalamus (Fig. 8.29).

Projection neurons transmitting slow (C fibre) pain send their axons (together with axons from laminae VII and VIII) into the **spinoreticular pathway**, which makes extensive

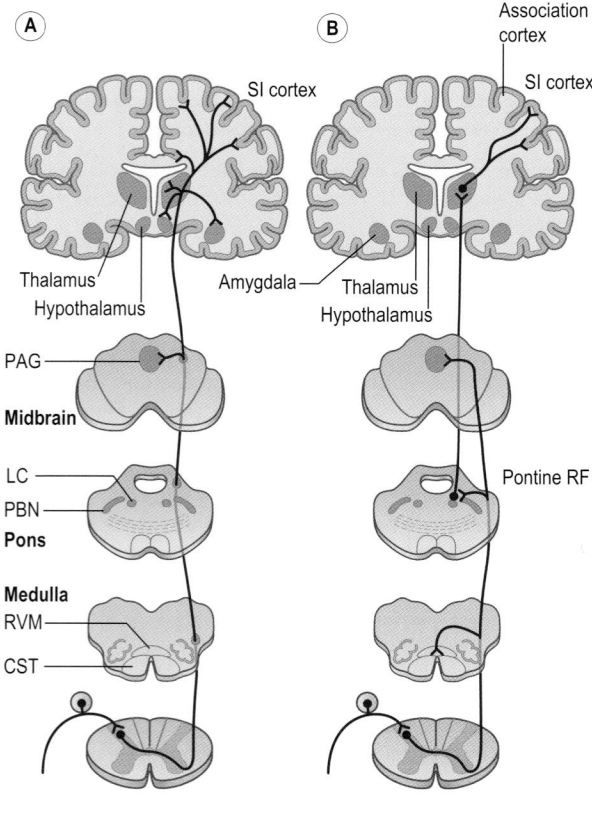

connections in the reticular system of the brainstem and the **reticular nuclei** of the thalamus. Many spinoreticular axons do not cross the midline but ascend ipsilaterally.

The largest number of STT cells is in lamina V. The dendrites of these neurons extend into lamina I and receive inputs from nociceptor afferents (both Aδ and C fibres). But lamina V neurons also receive connections from large diameter (Aβ) mechanoreceptor afferents so are said to be **wide dynamic range (WDR) cells**, because they get inputs from low threshold and high threshold afferents. Hence most spinothalamic tract neurons can be excited by both innocuous and noxious stimuli. Their axons cross the midline to enter the spinothalamic pathway and terminate in the **ventral posterior lateral (VPL)** and **posterior** nuclei of the thalamus.

The equivalent neurons in the **spinal nucleus of the trigeminal nerve**, which get their inputs from the primary afferents of the face and head, go to the **ventral posterior medial (VPM)** and posterior nuclei of the thalamus.

Crude touch sensation

When lamina IV and V cells are activated only by large diameter low threshold afferents, they convey crude touch sensation to the ventral lateral nuclei of the thalamus. These cells have small receptive fields and their projections are organised topographically so are able to localise stimuli. However, the ability of the spinothalamic system to discriminate between the different mechanoreceptor submodalities is poor.

Heightened pain responses

At the site of an injury, including surgical incisions, a number of different pain responses can occur:

- **Hyperalgesia**: noxious stimulation becomes more painful than usual.
- **Allodynia**: stimuli that are normally innocuous become painful.
- **Spontaneous pain**: pain which occurs in the absence of any stimulus.

When they are transient, these responses have a protective role in that they encourage guarding of the site of injury. However, when they outlast their usefulness they become pathological pain. Both peripheral and central mechanisms are implicated.

Primary (peripheral) hyperalgesia is due to the sensitisation of nociceptors by substances produced at the injury site. For example, prostaglandins enhance nociceptor excitability while glutamate released as a result of injury increases mechanical nociceptor excitability so as to cause **mechanical allodynia**.

Secondary (central) hyperalgesia arises partly from changes in the behaviour of dorsal horn cells (DHCs), termed **central sensitisation**. This is induced by tissue or nerve injury, so it occurs secondary to activity in primary nociceptor afferents and increases spontaneous (background) firing, and causes hyperexcitability to low threshold (Aβ fibre) primary afferent input.

Injury causes persistent firing of primary nociceptor afferents and continual release of glutamate, neuropeptides and inflammatory mediators. All play a role in setting up secondary hyperalgesia. DHCs become hypersensitive to glutamate so their firing rate progressively increases, a phenomenon called **wind-up**. Over a longer time-scale there are

Fig. 8.29 Pathways for transmission of pain, temperature and crude touch sensations. (A) Spinothalamic tract. (B) Spinoreticular tract. CST, corticospinal tract; LC, locus ceruleus; PAG, periaqueductal grey; PBN, parabrachial nucleus; RF, reticular formation. Redrawn with permission from Michael-Titus A, Revest P, Shortland P 2006 The nervous system. Churchill Livingstone, Edinburgh.

persistent increases in excitability that resemble long-term potentiation.

Wind-up can be blocked by **ketamine**, and by **opioid receptor (µ and δ) antagonists** given pre-emptively. Analgesic cover after surgery is optimal if given immediately and topped-up frequently: this curtails central sensitisation, dramatically reducing post-operative pain.

Discriminative pain perception

Any noxious stimulus will activate both lamina I and V cells (stimuli exciting only lamina V cells are perceived as innocuous). Lamina I cells signal pain, but because they have large receptive fields, and relay to thalamic nuclei which do not have topographic projections to the cortex, they cannot localise it well. The localisation of painful stimuli depends on the simultaneous firing of lamina V cells, which have somatotopic projections to thalamic nuclei. These thalamic nuclei project to the primary somatosensory cortex.

Brain imaging studies reveal that activity increases in a number of brain areas when human volunteers experience pain. These regions are collectively termed the **pain matrix**. Clinical ablation of large parts of the primary somatosensory cortex does not alter pain perception, hence discriminative aspects of pain may be conferred elsewhere, perhaps by the secondary somatosensory cortex. Other cortical (limbic) areas are concerned with emotional responses to pain.

Autonomic, arousal and emotional aspects of pain

The connectivity of the spinoreticular pathway brings about autonomic and arousal responses to painful stimuli.

1. **Medullary** and **pontine reticular system** connections mediate autonomic responses to pain.
2. Direct connections with the **hypothalamus** are responsible for activation of the hypothalamic–pituitary–adrenal axis stress response.
3. Activation of pathways in the **brainstem reticular system** contributes to the increased arousal experienced during pain.
4. Connections run to **midbrain reticular structures** including the PAG and the parabrachial nucleus. The PAG is part of a system for modulating nociceptor input, and the parabrachial nucleus projects to the amygdala and so is presumably involved in learning to fear situations associated with pain.
5. The **thalamic targets of spinoreticular neurons** establish widespread connections with the basal ganglia, influencing motor activity, and with the cerebral cortex.
6. All of the **thalamic nuclei** that receive nociceptor input send direct connections to the insula cortex, which is involved in emotional responses to pain.

Central control of nociceptive input

The perception of pain is modified by both non-noxious sensory inputs and by inputs from other brain areas. Mechanisms to reduce nociceptor input operate at both the spinal and supraspinal level. These are exploited in treating pain in the clinic.

Gate control theory

At the level of the spinal cord, whether a stimulus is considered painful or innocuous depends on the relative activity of large and small diameter afferent fibres. Patrick Wall and Ronald Melzack sought to explain this with the **gate control theory**.

The wide dynamic range projection neurons in lamina V transmit excitatory impulses to the cortex, where pain is experienced. These receive their stimulation from both large mechanoreceptor afferents (Aβ) and small nociceptor (Aδ and C) afferents. The projection neurons are also inhibited by interneurons in lamina II. These lamina II neurons receive input from both the large and small afferents. They are stimulated by collaterals of the large diameter mechanoreceptor afferents but are inhibited by collaterals of the small nociceptor afferents (Fig. 8.30A).

So how does this work?

When there is a noxious stimulus, small nociceptor afferents directly stimulate the dendrites of the lamina V projection neurons and indirectly excite the same cells by inhibiting the lamina II interneurons (inhibiting an inhibition is excitation). This opens the pain gate.

However, large diameter afferent activity offsets the effect of nociceptor input, reducing the firing of lamina V cells by increasing the inhibitory drive from the lamina II interneurons. Hence co-activation of low and high threshold afferents closes the pain gate.

Gate control-mediated analgesia

The gate control theory accounts for **counter-stimulation analgesia** in which pain is reduced by stimulating low threshold afferents. We reflexly rub the site of a painful blow, which stimulates mechanoreceptors. This will begin to inhibit the projection neuron, and pain will diminish. This mechanism is the basis for a technique called transcutaneous electrical nerve stimulation (TENS), which is purported to reduce pain (Clinical box 8.7).

Supraspinal pain modulation

Brainstem nuclei that receive connections from the spinoreticular pain pathways give rise to descending supraspinal analgesia systems which reduce nociceptor input in the spinal cord.

1. Axons of the **nucleus raphe magnus (NRM)** in the medulla terminate in the dorsal horn, releasing serotonin which reduces all somatosensory transmission, not just that of nociceptors.

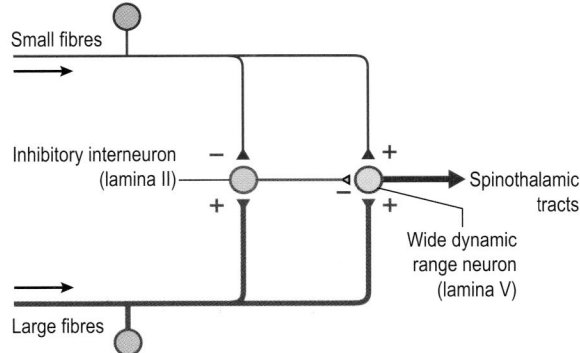

Fig. 8.30 **Gate control theory of pain.** The neurons which transmit pain signals are stimulated by both small pain fibres and large mechanoreceptor afferents. Collaterals from both of these inhibit and stimulate, respectively, lamina II interneurons.

Transcutaneous electrical nerve stimulation delivers high-frequency, low-intensity currents, sufficient to stimulate Aβ and Aδ fibres and hence close the pain gate. However, it may work by stimulating the production of endorphins (endogenous opioids) as the analgesia produced by TENS can be blocked by opioid receptor antagonists.

Although TENS is used in the treatment of acute pain, chronic pain and in labour, evidence-based reviews of randomised studies have failed to show benefit over placebo or sham TENS.

Stimulus-induced analgesia involves stimulation of the PAG by long-term implantation of electrodes. It is used for intractable pain.

Information box 8.14 **Opioid analgesics**

Opioids are ligands of opioid receptors. Analgesia is attributed to agonist or partial agonist activity at opioid receptors, mimicking the actions of the endogenous opioids in the pain-modulating pathways. The effects of opioid analgesics can be rapidly reversed by their competitive antagonists. There are a number of unwanted side effects of opioid analgesics:

- Respiratory depression (which occurs at therapeutic doses) and vomiting are due to activation of opioid receptors in the medulla.
- Increase in tone but reduced motility in the gastrointestinal tract is due to the stimulation of peripheral opioid receptors in visceral smooth muscle.
- Morphine and some other opioids may cause tolerance and dependence.

2. Noradrenergic neurons of the **locus coeruleus** in the pons project to the superficial dorsal horn and their activation reduces nociceptor input. This might account for the analgesia seen during intense arousal.
3. The **periaqueductal grey (PAG)** matter surrounds the cerebral aqueduct in the midbrain. Stimulation of the PAG in rats causes a powerful suppression of pain responses, a phenomenon termed stimulus produced analgesia (Clinical box 8.7). The PAG exerts its anti-nociception effects by activating the raphe nuclei and locus coeruleus.

Opioid peptides and opiates in analgesia systems

Some neurons in pain-modulating pathways use opioid neurotransmitters (Information box 8.14):

- **Met-enkephalin** is used by interneurons in lamina II which are responsible for mediating inhibitory effects of serotonin and noradrenaline on pain transmission.
- **β-Endorphin** and **met-enkephalin** are transmitters of neurons in the PAG. These cells inhibit GABAergic interneurons that normally tonically suppress the anti-nociception neurons.

Natural analgesia

The descending pain-modulating pathways appear to be brain analgesia systems. In the event of injury they produce the natural counterpart of stimulus-induced analgesia.

Emergency analgesia, seen in individuals who have sustained severe injuries when they are in threatening or highly arousing situations (e.g. during warfare or sport), is rapid in onset and wears off after a few hours. The analgesia is localised to the injured area, and autonomic reflexes and emotional responses reflect a typical defence reaction. The selective advantage of emergency analgesia is that it allows individuals to continue to function so that they can remove themselves from danger.

Stress analgesia occurs in individuals recovering from a stressful encounter. Here the analgesia is generalised, the individual is relaxed and has low levels of sympathetic activity. These two behaviours may be organised by different parts of the PAG (Information box 8.15).

Placebo effect

This refers to the therapeutic efficacy of agents or procedures that are without any physiological or pharmacological action. In general, the more elaborate the placebo treatment the better its effectiveness. There is evidence that the placebo effect, at least when harnessed to reduce post-operative pain, can be blocked by naloxone and so depends upon endogenous opioid neurotransmission.

fMRI shows that placebo analgesia is associated with decreased activity in pain-sensitive regions (such as the thalamus) but increased activity in the dorsal lateral prefrontal cortex (DLPFC), an area thought to be involved in cognitive control. A working hypothesis is that the expectation of pain relief activates a top-down control over pain perception in the DLPFC which acts by recruiting supraspinal opioid pathways that block pain transmission.

Effective **acupuncture** relies on stimulation of small diameter (group II and III) afferents from skeletal muscle and joints. This is thought to activate a descending endorphinergic pathway from the arcuate nucleus of the hypothalamus to the ventrolateral PAG, the midbrain region thought to be responsible for stress analgesia. Acupuncture produces a state similar to stress analgesia, and both can be reversed by the opioid receptor antagonist naloxone.

Visceral sensation

Mechanoreceptors respond to **tension** in the walls of hollow viscera (e.g. urinary bladder and gut), while nociceptors are responsible for visceral **pain**. This arises from excessive distension or contraction against an obstruction (e.g. kidney stone), ischaemia (e.g. as a result of myocardial infarction) or inflammation. ATP released from subepithelial cells of hollow viscera (e.g. urinary bladder) mediates the pain of distension.

Visceral afferents run in the autonomic and somatic divisions of the PNS. Most are the afferent side of autonomic reflexes (e.g. baroreceptor reflex) but some visceral afferents allow conscious visceral sensation. Visceral afferents project to the nucleus of the solitary tract (NST) in the medulla. This structure, apart from organising a number of gut, respiratory and vasomotor reflexes, sends outputs to the PAG and the parabrachial nucleus. The widely distributed outputs of the parabrachial nucleus, including connections to the hypothalamus and cingulate cortex, allow complex behavioural responses to visceral sensation.

Referred pain

Convergence of visceral and somatic nociceptor afferents in a given spinal root onto common spinothalamic neurons means that stimulation of nociceptors in internal organs is often perceived as pain in distant superficial regions. This is termed **referred pain** and the areas to which it is referred are called **Head's zones** (Fig. 8.31). These are useful in diagnosis. For example, pain in the heart due to poor perfusion of the coronary arteries (angina) is referred to the shoulder and arm. Another example is the pain from an inflamed appendix, which is referred to the area around the umbilicus.

Phantom pain

After amputation of a limb almost all patients experience the sensation that the limb is still present, and for some this is painful. Phantom sensations can also follow loss of other body parts (e.g. mastectomy). Children born without limbs have powerful phantom limb sensations. This implies that complete somatotopic representations can exist in the absence of peripheral inputs, and this is the situation in amputees. However considerable rewiring of the somatosensory cortex occurs after the amputation so that neurons that have lost their original inputs acquire connections from neighbouring cells. Phantom limb sensations can now be elicited by touching other parts of the body, commonly the face. With continuing cortical reorganisation phantom sensations usually fade over time.

VISION

Vision is a complex set of processes:

1. Detection of light photons by an array of light-sensitive cells on a two-dimensional sensory surface.
2. Transformation of the two-dimensional representation to a three-dimensional representation of the visual field.
3. Segregation of information on form, colour, depth perception and motion into quasi-separate streams for processing at the same time (**parallel processing**).

4. Recombining the separate data streams to create a unified percept (**binding**).
5. Comparing objects in the visual field with stored representations so they can be identified (**pattern recognition**).
6. Localisation of objects in the visual world.

These steps lead to conscious visual perception and involve the thalamus and much of the cerebral cortex of the occipital, parietal and temporal lobes. Highly transformed visual information is sent to motor systems for visual guidance of movement, and to the limbic system which assesses the significance of the visual world; having sight of a snake or a friend will produce very different behaviours. In addition sensory input is abstracted at an early stage to drive visual reflexes such as pupil, eye movement and orienting reflexes. These are organised by the tectum.

The eye

Anatomy

The eye has three layers (Fig. 8.32).

- The outer sclera
- The choroid
- The retina, the light-sensitive and innermost layer.

The outer **sclera** is composed of tough connective tissue which helps to maintain the shape of the eyeball and serves as an attachment for the extraocular muscles. Anteriorly it forms the transparent **cornea**, while posteriorly it becomes the dura of the optic nerve. The cornea is covered by a layer of epithelium, the **conjunctiva**, which also lines the eyelids. Corneal xenografts can be done without fear of rejection because the cornea has no blood supply.

Choroid

The highly vascular **choroid**, the middle layer of the eye, is pigmented dark brown by melanin so that it absorbs light reflected within the eye. Anteriorly the choroid gives rise to the ciliary body and the iris.

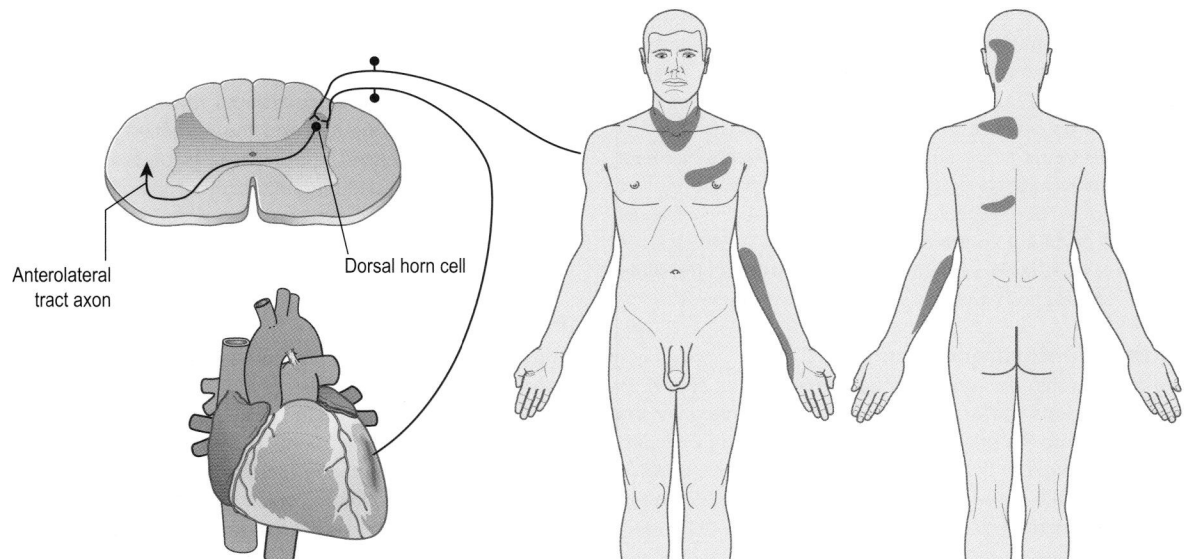

Fig. 8.31 **Referred pain**: in the case of the heart the pain is classically referred to the chest, neck and left shoulder and arm. Head's zones are shown in *red*.

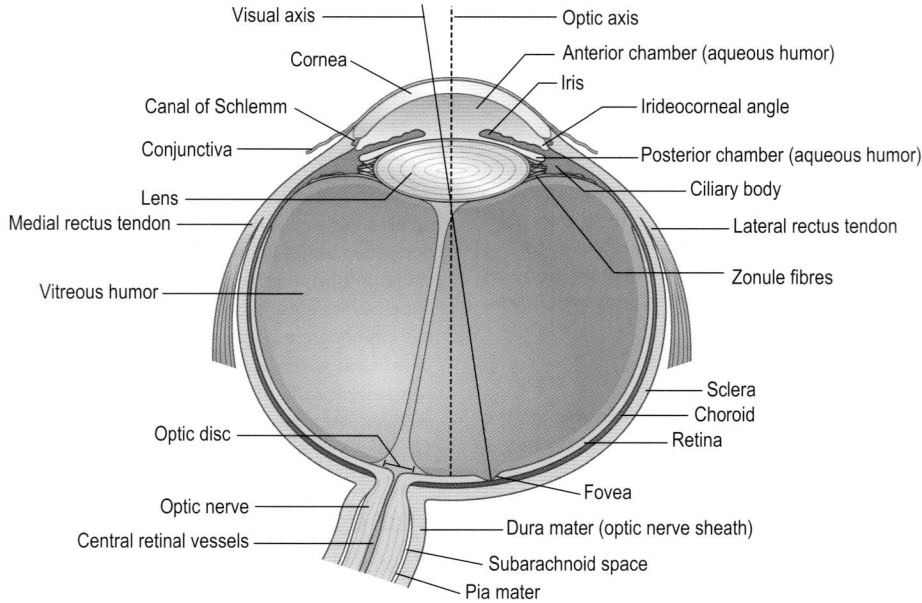

Fig. 8.32 Horizontal section through a human eye.

Labels (clockwise):
Visual axis — Optic axis — Anterior chamber (aqueous humor) — Iris — Irideocorneal angle — Posterior chamber (aqueous humor) — Ciliary body — Lateral rectus tendon — Zonule fibres — Sclera — Choroid — Retina — Fovea — Dura mater (optic nerve sheath) — Subarachnoid space — Pia mater — Central retinal vessels — Optic nerve — Optic disc — Vitreous humor — Medial rectus tendon — Lens — Conjunctiva — Canal of Schlemm — Cornea

---

Clinical box 8.8 **Cataract**

A variety of factors can result in the lens becoming opaque, causing a **cataract**.

● UV-B radiation destroys proper crystallin folding. The risk of developing cataracts is greater in low latitude (nearer the equator) and high altitude countries where solar radiation is more intense.
● Hyperglycaemia that attends poorly controlled diabetes mellitus. The lens contains **aldose reductase** which catalyses the synthesis of sorbitol from glucose. The osmotic action of excess sorbitol causes fluid to accumulate in the lens.

The **lens** of the eye is held by a **suspensory ligament** attached to the encircling **ciliary body**, the smooth **ciliary muscles** of which enable the shape of the lens and hence its refractive power to be altered. The lens is avascular and composed of concentric layers of lens fibres, cells with few organelles but packed with **crystallins** – proteins that are normally transparent by virtue of their precisely ordered folding. Lens fibres are generated by a proliferative epithelium on the anterior surface of the lens (Clinical box 8.8).

The **iris** forms a ring surrounding the pupil, the diameter of which is controlled by the balance of contractile tone in two sets of smooth muscle fibres in the iris. A ring of fibres forms the **pupillary sphincter**, contraction of which reduces pupil size, while radially oriented fibres make up the **pupillary dilator**, contraction of which increases pupil diameter.

Aqueous and vitreous humour

Two fluids within the eyeball help to maintain its shape. In front of the lens the **aqueous humour** is secreted by the ciliary body into the posterior chamber, from where it passes through the pupil to the anterior chamber. Aqueous humour perfuses into the **canal of Schlemm**, which encircles the eye at the **iridocorneal angle** (Fig. 8.32 and Clinical box 8.9). There are no valves between the canal and the venules into which it drains, so aqueous humour is driven into the venous circulation by the higher pressure in the eyeball (~3 kPa).

Clinical box 8.9 **Glaucoma**

In glaucoma the drainage of aqueous humour is compromised, so the intraocular pressure rises and this reduces blood flow through retinal capillaries. Untreated, this can cause blindness. Muscarinic agonists, by causing pupil constriction, open the iridocorneal angle and improve the drainage of aqueous humour.

Behind the lens lies a collagenous gel, the **vitreous humour**, which supports the lens and retina.

Optics of the eye

Most of the **refractive power** of the eye (its ability to bend light rays so they can be brought to focus) is due to the cornea and is fixed. However, the refractive power of the lens is important because it can be altered (Clinical box 8.10).

When the ciliary muscles are relaxed, the suspensory ligament is taut, making the lens relatively flat. In this state parallel rays of light from objects at infinity are brought to focus on the central part of the retina. This is the default state of the eye. However, for close objects rays of light are diverging as they enter the eye and the refractive power of the lens must be increased if the light is to be focused on the retina. This is achieved by contraction of the ciliary muscles (supplied by parasympathetic fibres) which relaxes the suspensory ligament so that the lens recoils into a more spherical shape. This is termed the **accommodation reflex**.

Pupillary light reflex

The amount of light entering the eye is proportional to the square of the pupil diameter. In young adults pupil diameter ranges between about 1.5 mm and 8 mm, depending on the intensity of the ambient light, corresponding to a 30-fold change in the light entering the eye. Pupil size is controlled by **pupillary light reflexes**, which operate over the range of light intensities experienced in moderately bright daylight.

Light intensity is signalled by optic nerve axons which synapse in the pretectum of the midbrain (Fig. 8.33). Pretectal axons relay to the **Edinger-Westphal nuclei**, which contain preganglionic parasympathetic neurons that run in the oculomotor nerves to the ciliary ganglia. From here postganglionic fibres run to the pupillary sphincter. An increase in light levels causes pupil constriction. Both pupils constrict, even if light is shone into one eye only, because there are reciprocal crossed connections between the pretectum and oculomotor nuclei (Clinical box 8.11).

Pupil constriction also occurs during accommodation and involves different central circuitry than that used to constrict the pupil in high light levels. Its function is to improve acuity when looking at close objects, by ensuring that the only light to reach the retina comes through the central regions of the cornea and lens where optical distortions are minimal.

Retina

The retina consists of a light-sensitive **neural retina** which sits on a single layer of **retinal pigmented epithelium** (**RPE**). The neural retina contains five basic types of neuron:

Photoreceptors are the light responsive elements and lie in close contact with the RPE, while the **ganglion cells**, the axons of which enter the optic nerve, provide the output of the retina.

Three populations of interneurons – **bipolar cells, horizontal cells** and **amacrine cells** – complete the retinal circuitry.

The retina has a high level of **convergence** overall – some 10^8 photoreceptors feed input to 10^6 ganglion cells – implying that the retina is responsible for a great deal of visual processing. Light must pass through almost the entire thickness of the retina before reaching the photoreceptors; however, the retina is extremely thin (0.1 mm) and highly transparent.

The region of retina where the optic nerve and retinal vessels emerge is termed the **optic disc** (Clinical box 8.12).

Clinical box 8.10	Refractive errors

Refractive errors can result in a failure to bring light from distant objects to focus at the retina. They may be due to a defect in the lens or in the shape of the eyeball or both.

Myopia (**nearsightedness**): The light is focused in front of the retina so distant objects are blurred. Because of the greater refractive power the eye can view close objects with less accommodation. Correction is with a concave lens of appropriate power. Myopia is extremely common and may be a modern disease. It is thought that an eye mechanism which regulates eyeball growth to ensure light is focused on the retina is disrupted by the large amount of near vision children engage in when they read, write and use computers.

Hyperopia (**farsightedness**): light is focused behind the retina. The accommodation reflex is in play continuously to bring distant objects to focus, but the lower refractive power of the hyperopic eye is unable to focus nearby objects. It is corrected with convex lenses.

Presbyopia: With age the lens becomes less elastic and less able to relax into the high-refractive-power spherical shape needed to focus close objects. Hence the closest point that can be clearly focused, the **near point**, recedes with age. The increased stiffness of the lens, and its tendency to become more convex with time because of the continual activity of the proliferative epithelium, also means it may not be so effectively flattened by tension in the suspensory ligaments. The result is a loss in the ability to focus on distant objects with age.

Astigmatism: the radius of curvature of the surface of the cornea or the lens is not the same in all radial planes, so that points of light are focused as lines. Presented with a starburst of lines the patient sees only one orientation of lines in focus.

Clinical box 8.11	Clinical utility of pupillary reflexes

Pupillary light reflexes can be used to diagnose visual system lesions. Normally, light shone into one eye causes constriction of the pupil of the same eye (direct reflex) and of the other eye (consensual reflex). **Optic nerve lesions** abolish the direct, but not the consensual, reflex. **Oculomotor nerve lesions** result in a fixed dilated pupil on the afflicted side, together with a characteristic defect of gaze, with the affected eye looking downwards and outwards and **ptosis** (drooping of the eyelid).

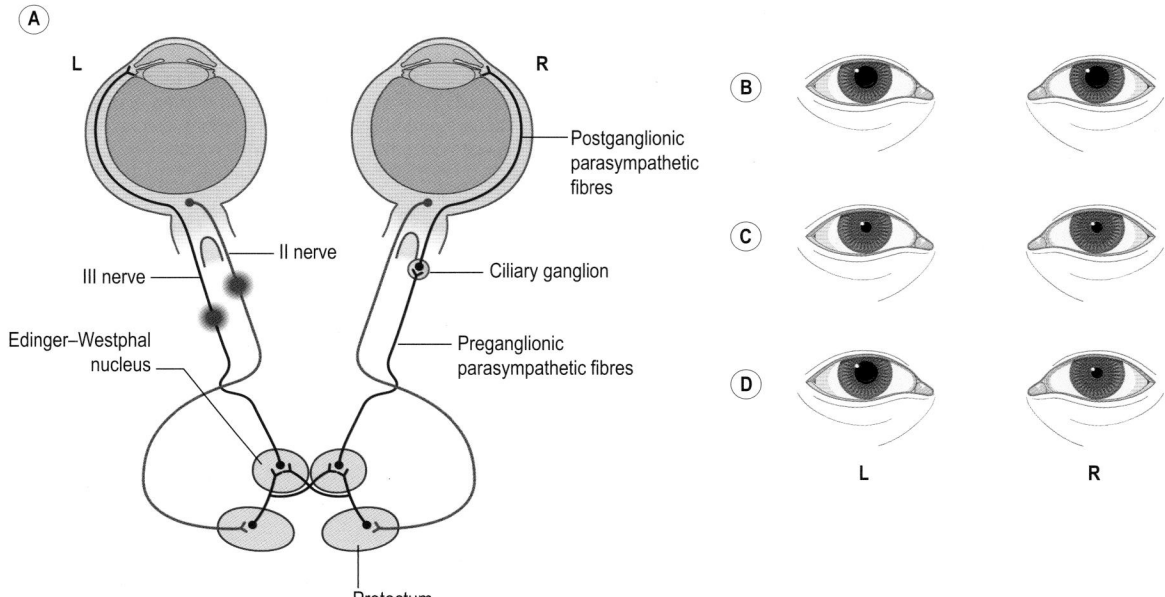

Fig. 8.33 **Pupillary light reflexes following damage to either optic (II) or oculomotor (III) nerves on the left side**: (A) reflex pathway; (B) optic nerve damage, left eye stimulated; (C) optic nerve damage, right eye stimulated; (D) oculomotor nerve damage, either eye stimulated.

The examination of the retina with an ophthalmoscope, called **funduscopy** (Fig. 8.34), is an important part of the neurological examination, for example:

- Because the optic nerve lies within the meninges, a rise in intracerebral pressure is transmitted through to the optic disc and can be diagnosed by **papilloedema**, a swelling of the disc.
- Characteristic alterations of retinal blood vessels, such as retinal haemorrhages, allow the diagnosis of a number of conditions, e.g. hypertensive and diabetic retinopathy.

Trauma can cause a **detached retina** where the neural retina peels away from the retinal pigmented epithelium. The loss of contact causes the death of the photoreceptors because they rely on the epithelium for metabolic support.

Macula degeneration is a failure of central vision that accounts for almost half of visual impairment in patients over 65. There are two types, both resulting from the functional disconnection of photoreceptors from the pigment epithelium.

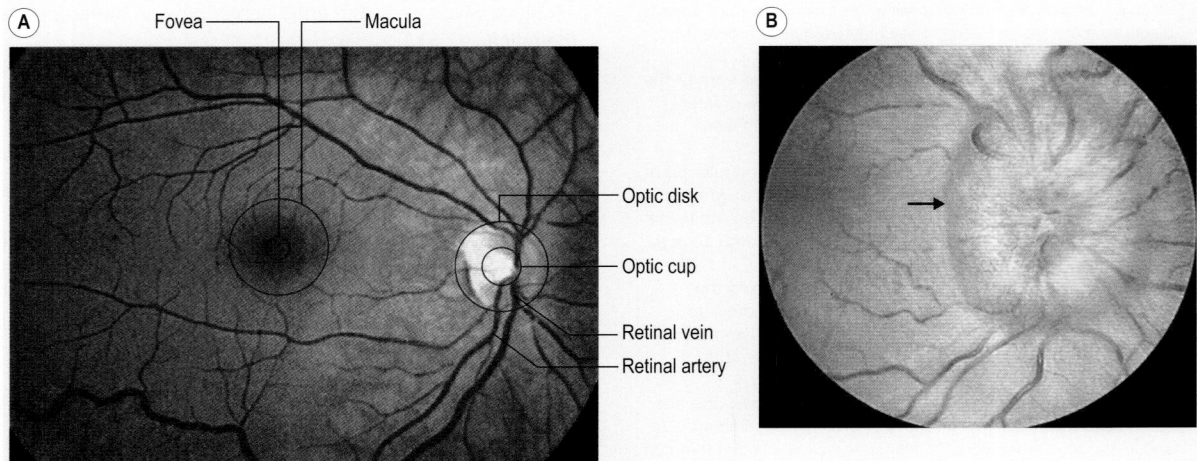

Fig. 8.34 Funduscopy. (A) Normal eye showing optic disc and retinal arteries. Redrawn with permission from Kumar P, Clark M. Clinical medicine, 6th edn. Elsevier, Edinburgh, 2006.
(B) Papilloedema with bulging of the optic disc. Redrawn with permission from Haslett C, Chilvers ER, Boon NA, Colledge NR, eds 2002 Davidson's principles and practice of medicine, 19th edn. Churchill Livingstone, London.

There are no photoreceptors here so it constitutes a functional blind spot. It is not noticeable in normal vision. Lateral to the optic disc lies the **macula lutea**, a region 2 mm across, within which lies a conical pit 0.4 mm in diameter, the **fovea centralis**.

Photoreceptors

There are two populations of photoreceptors – cones and rods. In different combinations they are responsible for vision in different light conditions:

- **Photopic vision** is the high acuity colour vision experienced in high light levels (daylight). It is mediated by **cone cells**. Each eye has five million cones and their density is highest at the fovea centralis and falls off very steeply away from it (Information box 8.16).
- **Mesopic vision** is needed for the moderate light intensities seen at dusk. **Rod cells**, which are unable to function in high light levels, come on-stream and operate alongside cones, boosting their ability to perceive colour as the light fails.
- **Scotopic vision** operates in the low light levels typical of a moonless night. Cones fail and rods, which are about 1000-fold more sensitive to light than cones, mediate low acuity, grey scale, dim light vision. Each eye has about 120 million rod cells. They are absent from the fovea centralis but their densities rise sharply

High acuity vision is achieved by the fovea centralis because it:

- Has the highest density of cones
- Lies at the optical axis where light comes through the optically best central parts of the cornea and lens
- Has all retinal layers above the cones displaced laterally so light does not have to pass through them
- Has a low number of blood vessels, thus minimising diffraction.

Only about 1/1000 of the visual field is seen by the fovea centralis at any instant and it is the only part in sharp focus, hence gaze must be frequently and rapidly shifted to view a significant portion of the visual field clearly. This is the purpose of **saccades**. These are rapid movements of both eyes simultaneously which jump around the visual field allowing the gaze to be fixed on one point after another.

just beyond it and the peripheral retina is populated almost entirely by rods.

Remarkably, rod cells can register a hit by just a single photon. Their high sensitivity is because they collect light for a longer time than cones before generating an integrated signal, but this means they cannot detect flicker frequency faster than 12 Hz. In contrast, cones can detect a flicker frequency up to about 50 Hz, the effective rate at which images are presented in TV systems.

Photoreceptor structure

Photoreceptors (Fig. 8.35) have an **outer segment** packed with discs of plasma membrane in which the visual pigment sits. The **inner segment** houses the nucleus and has a presynaptic terminal. The two segments are joined only by a thin cytoplasmic bridge.

Because light energy degrades the outer segment it has to be continuously regenerated. New discs are generated at the end of the outer segment closest to the nucleus, while the older discs are shed at the far tip. The damaged segments are then removed by phagocytosis by cells in the RPE.

Phototransduction

The visual pigment of rod cells is rhodopsin. It consists of the protein **opsin**, a member of the G-protein-coupled superfamily of receptors, plus a prosthetic group, **11-*cis* retinal**. When a light photon is absorbed by 11-*cis* retinal it is isomerised to **all-*trans* retinal** (photoisomerisation). This triggers a sequence of events termed **phototransduction** (Fig. 8.36).

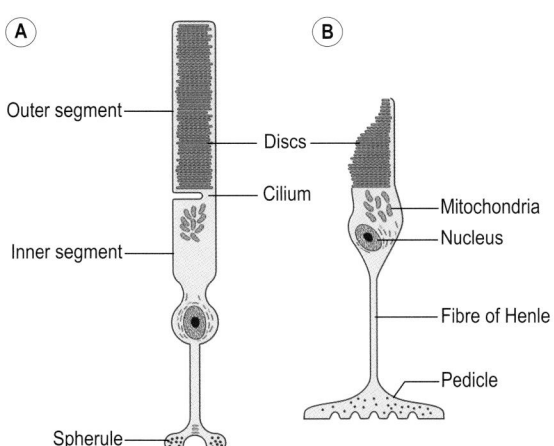

Fig. 8.35 **Photoreceptors**: (A) rod cell; and (B) cone cell. Redrawn with permission from Longstaff A 2005 Instant notes in neuroscience, 2nd edn. Taylor & Francis, Abingdon UK.

Photoreceptors in the dark

Rod cells are depolarised in the dark (their resting membrane potential is −40 mV), because a current called the **dark current** flows between their outer and inner segments. The plasma membrane of the outer segment contains a type of cation channel which is activated directly by high concentrations of cyclic guanosine monophosphate (cGMP) which are present in the photoreceptor. These channels allow Na⁺ (and Ca²⁺) to enter the photoreceptor. Sodium ions diffuse into the inner segment from which they are pumped out by the cation pump. This closes the circuit. Ca²⁺ ions are extruded by Na⁺–Ca²⁺ exchange.

Photoreceptor response to light

The photoisomerisation of retinal (Fig. 8.36) causes the rhodopsin to undergo a series of conformational changes to an activated state. This binds a G protein called **transducin (G$_t$)** which operates in a precisely analogous way to G proteins of metabotropic receptors (see Chs 2 and 4). The α-subunit of G$_t$ activates a phosphodiesterase which catalyses the conversion of cGMP to 5′-GMP. In consequence, the concentration of cGMP in the outer segment falls and the cation channels close. The fall in sodium entry into the outer segment causes a hyperpolarising receptor potential. The amplification of the transduction process is so great that a single photon can produce a 1 mV hyperpolarisation.

Ending the light response

Termination of the transduction cascade is due to:

- The intrinsic GTPase activity of transducin
- Phosphorylation of photo-excited rhodopsin by rhodopsin kinase, followed by binding of a molecule called **arrestin**, which prevents coupling to transducin.

Within a few seconds of light activation the non-covalent bonds which stabilise retinal in rhodopsin are broken and all-*trans* retinal is transported via a protein carrier from the outer segment to the pigment epithelial cells. Lacking its prosthetic group the rhodopsin is said to be **bleached**. This is the normal state for rhodopsin in daylight, during which time rods are unresponsive. In the RPE 11-*cis* retinal is regenerated by ATP-requiring catalysis from all-*trans* retinal, and is transported back to the outer segment; this process

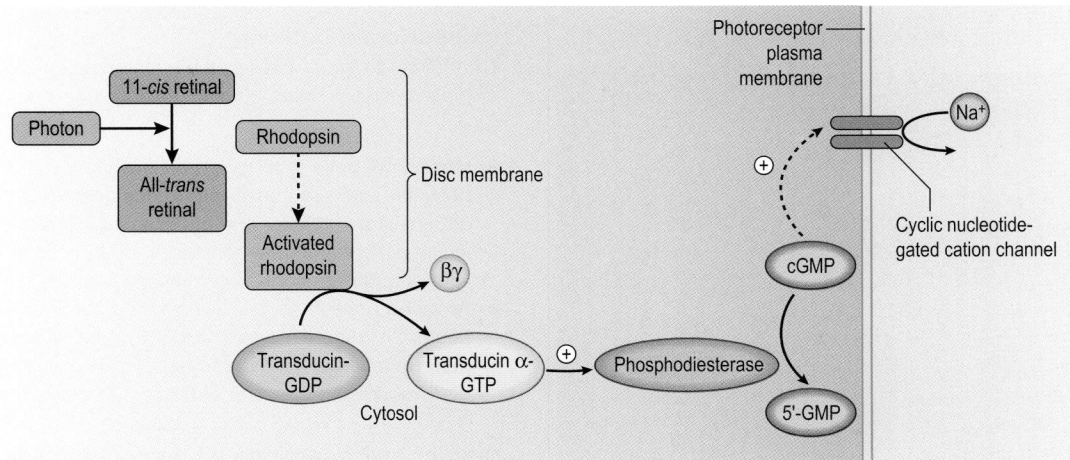

Fig. 8.36 **Rod cell phototransduction.** Light stimulates a cascade of events which results in the breakdown of cGMP. This closes cation channels, which reduces the dark current and hyperpolarises the rod. Redrawn with permission from Longstaff A 2005 Instant notes in neuroscience, 2nd edn. Taylor & Francis, Abingdon UK.

underlies **dark adaptation**, a rise in sensitivity to light that occurs in low light intensities. To achieve maximum sensitivity takes 40–50 minutes.

Cone responses

In cones much the same processes are thought to operate as in rods although the opsins are different (Clinical box 8.13). There are three distinct populations of cones, referred to as **short (S, blue)**, **medium (M, green)** and **long (L, red) wavelength cones**, each with a distinct opsin having different absorption curves (Fig. 8.37). It is by comparing the relative intensities of the signals from the different cones that colour vision is possible. Rod vision is monochromatic (grey scale) because all rods have identical absorption curves.

Only about 10% of cones are S cones and they are completely missing from the fovea centralis. So, colour vision at the fovea is **dichromatic** (it compares signals from only two cone populations) whereas elsewhere in the macula it is **trichromatic**.

Clinical box 8.13   Photoreceptor dysfunction

Abnormalities of cone opsins
Inherited defects in colour vision occur mostly as a result of abnormalities in one or more cone opsins. By far the commonest is **red-green colour blindness**, an X-linked recessive trait that afflicts up to 8% of European males and 0.4% of females. It arises because of mutations in M or L cone opsins which renders red and green indistinguishable from each other (and from grey). The S opsin gene is located on chromosome 7 so **blue colour blindness** is a rare autosomal dominant trait.

Lack of cones
More rarely defects in colour vision occur because of the lack of one, two or all three populations of cone. Patients missing two types of cone have no colour vision and those completely without cones are completely blind in daylight when their rods are saturated, but have scotopic vision at night.

Loss of both rods and cones
Retinitis pigmentosa is a blanket term for a set of heritable disorders characterised by progressive loss of both rods and cones, accompanied by disruption of the pigment epithelium and abnormal migration of pigment into the neural retina where it forms clumps. Most retinitis pigmentosa involves mutations of the various photoreceptor-specific proteins.

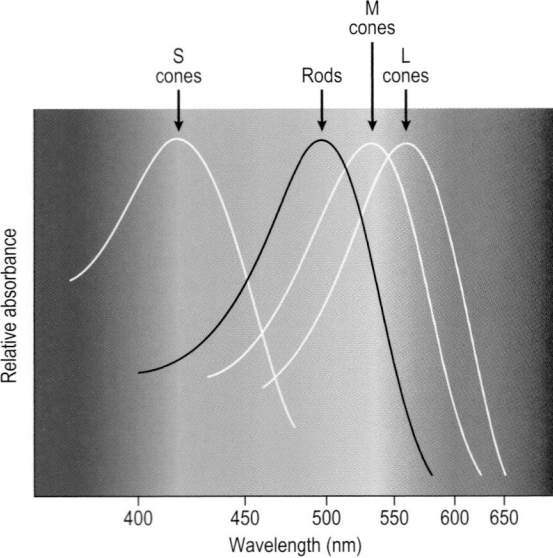

Fig. 8.37 Absorption curves for photoreceptors.

Retinal circuits

All photoreceptors synapse with bipolar cells which then signal to ganglion cells. The most striking difference between cone and rod pathways is in the extent of their convergence:

- **Rod pathways.** Input from numerous rods is fed into a bipolar cell, so rod pathways lose spatial information but gain in sensitivity.
- **Cone pathways** can have convergence ratios as low as 1:1, accounting for the high acuity of photopic vision, but by the same token are low sensitivity.

Visual information is relayed from cones to ganglion cells via both direct and indirect pathways.

Direct cone pathway

The direct pathway goes straight from photoreceptor to bipolar cell to ganglion cell. In the dark, because photoreceptors are depolarised they tonically release their transmitter, glutamate. Hyperpolarisation in response to light causes a reduction in glutamate release.

There are two populations of bipolar cell which have opposite responses to photoreceptor stimulation because they have different glutamate receptors:

- **On-centre** cells are hyperpolarised in the dark and depolarise in the light.
- **Off-centre** cells are depolarised in the dark and hyperpolarise in response to light.

Each cone is thought to drive one on-centre and one off-centre bipolar cell. Cone bipolar cells form excitatory synapses with **retinal ganglion cells (RGCs)** that provide the output of the retina. Over 90% of RGCs serve cones. RGCs are the only retinal neuron to fire action potentials; all the others can signal effectively by way of electrotonic potentials since the distances involved are very short. RGCs are never silent but fire with a background rate that is modified by light stimulation.

Each population of bipolar cells is connected to the equivalent population of RGCs. On-centre ganglion cells (which get their input exclusively from on-centre bipolar cells) increase their firing frequency, while off-centre ganglion cells decrease their firing rate, in response to light. In effect, on-centre cells signal brightening over time, while the off-centre cells signal dimming of light intensity with time.

Indirect cone pathway

The indirect pathway involves the transmission of information by means of retinal interneurons: the horizontal and amacrine cells.

- **Horizontal cells** form reciprocal inhibitory synapses between adjacent cones to produce centre-surround antagonism in bipolar and ganglion cells (see below) which accentuates the contrast at boundaries between light and dark regions, and between colours.
- **Amacrine cells** are very diverse, and numerous neurotransmitters are associated with these cells. Some perform a similar function to horizontal cells, others can discriminate the direction of motion of a stimulus.

Bipolar and ganglion cell receptive fields

The receptive fields of retinal bipolar and ganglion cells are circular and show centre-surround inhibition (Fig. 8.38). They fall into two classes:

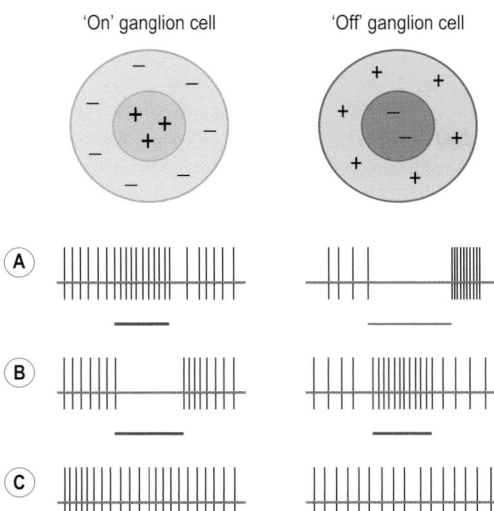

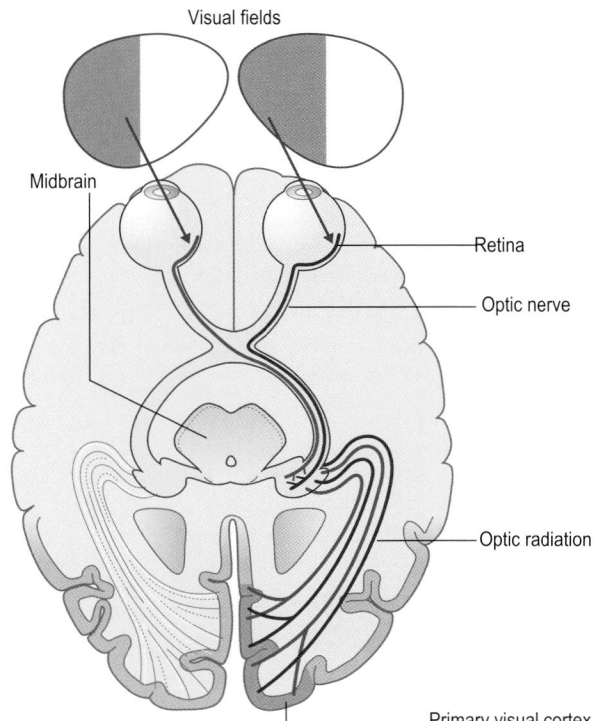

Fig. 8.38 **Surround antagonism in an on-centre ganglion cell.** *Top*: Receptive fields. Responses to: (A) central illumination; (B) surround illumination; and (C) overall illumination. Redrawn with permission from Michael-Titus A, Revest P, Shortland P 2006 The nervous system. Churchill Livingstone, Edinburgh.

■ On-centre cells have a central region of retina that is excited by light, surrounded by an annulus of retina where light stimulation inhibits the cell.

■ Off-centre cells have a central inhibitory region circumscribed by an excitatory annulus.

This surround inhibition is partly mediated by horizontal cells which can inhibit glutamate release from photoreceptors. Inhibition of glutamate release from a photoreceptor onto an on-centre bipolar cell by horizontal cells occurs when light is shone on the centre of the receptive field and ceases when the illumination is in the surround. Because on-centre bipolar cells depolarise and increase their firing in the light, this has the effect of enhancing the bipolar cell's response to central illumination and decreasing it to surround illumination.

Rod pathways

Rods have a direct pathway via dedicated on-bipolar cells which signal to rod on-ganglion cells by way of amacrine cells. This is the only circuit to operate in scotopic (low light) vision. However, there are extensive gap junctions between rods and adjacent cones and it is thought that at moderate light levels (mesopic vision) rod signals are routed into the cones, boosting their signals so that cone pathways are kept active for as long as possible as the light fades.

Retinal processing

Retinal output, transmitted by ganglion cell axons, essentially consists of information about small differences in light intensity and colour. Centre-surround antagonism, which acts particularly to produce contrasts of colour and at dark/light boundaries, signals differences in space, giving rise to the perception of form, while the parallel on- and off-channels signal changes in time. Correlating the differences in space and time gives movement perception.

There are two major populations of retinal ganglion cells. P ganglion cells are responsible for transmitting form and colour, whereas the M ganglion cells relay movement. These

Fig. 8.39 **Visual pathways.** Redrawn with permission from Fitzgerald MJT, Folan-Curran J 2002 Clinical neuroanatomy and related neurosciences, 4th edn. WB Saunders, London.

feed into two anatomically distinct visual pathways, the P and M pathways. The segregation of information into multiple streams that can be analysed independently but simultaneously is termed **parallel processing**. It is seen in many nervous system functions and its major advantage is that it increases the speed of computations.

Central visual pathways

All of the retinal output travels down the axons of the retinal ganglion cell that run down the **optic nerves** (cranial nerve III). Most (>90%) of these end up in the thalamus from where visual input is relayed to the visual cortex in the occipital lobe (Fig. 8.39). This route gives rise to conscious visual perception. Some RGC axons enter the superior colliculus and tectum where there are structures responsible for visual reflexes.

Anatomy of the visual pathways

Optic chiasma

At the **optic chiasma** just over half of the nerve fibres, those serving the nasal half of each retina, **decussate** (cross over). This means that after the optic chiasma each optic nerve carries information from the lateral ipsilateral hemiretina and the medial contralateral hemiretina. Fibres that contribute to the pathway for conscious visual perception terminate in the **lateral geniculate nuclei** (**LGN**) of the thalamus. From here the optic radiations project to the occipital cortex, mostly to the **primary visual cortex** (V1) in the striate cortex (Brodmann's area 17).

The projections at each level are mapped according to their positions on the retina (retinotopic) but there are several idiosyncrasies:

- The projection of the visual fields onto the retina are inverted and left-right reversed because the eye acts like a pinhole camera.
- Because of the optic decussation, each half of the visual field is mapped to the contralateral side; i.e. the entire visual field is mapped over the visual cortex of both sides.
- The fovea has a much greater representation in proportion to its retinal area than the peripheral retina, so retinotopic maps are greatly distorted.

When there are visual field deficits it is possible to determine at which point in the visual pathways damage has occurred because the retinotopic mapping is preserved at each level (Information box 8.17).

ⓘ Information box 8.17 | Visual field mapping and deficits

Accurate mapping of the visual fields is done by **perimetry**, in which the patient's head is held fixed facing a quadrant (marked in degrees) that can be oriented in any plane between vertical and horizontal. Coloured markers can be slid round the quadrant and the largest angle at which the patient reports seeing the marker is plotted as a point on the perimeter of their visual field. The mapping the areas of a visual field deficit gives information about the site of lesions in the visual system (Fig. 8.40). For example, compression of the optic chiasma by a pituitary tumour affects the axons which are decussating, producing a bilateral deficit affecting both temporal visual fields (Fig. 8.40C, a bitemporal hemianopia). Lesions posterior to the optic chiasma are bilateral due to the crossing of fibres from the nasal halves of the retinas at this level.

Visual fields

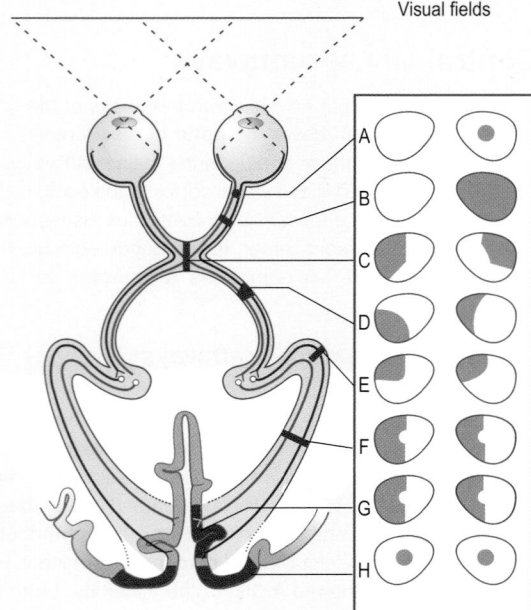

***Fig. 8.40* Visual field deficits.** Visual pathway lesions A–H result in the visual field deficits (*grey*) shown in the box. Redrawn with permission from Fitzgerald MJT, Folan-Curran J 2002 Clinical neuroanatomy and related neuroscience, 4th edn. WB Saunders, London.

Lateral geniculate nucleus

Axons from the retinal ganglion cells terminate in the **LGN** in the thalamus. Each LGN is a six-layered structure and each layer receives input from only one eye. Two magnocellular layers are supplied by M ganglion cells (one from each eye) while four parvocellular layers get input from P ganglion cells. Like retinal neurons, LGN cells have centre-surround receptive fields and respond optimally to spots of light.

Primary visual cortex

After leaving the LGN, the axons of the optic radiation take two slightly different routes to the **primary visual cortex** (V1, Brodmann's 17) which lies at the rear of the occipital lobe around the calcarine fissure (Fig. 8.41A). One route, which carries information from the fovea and the lower part of the visual field, passes directly through the parietal lobe, while the other fibres travel more laterally through the temporal lobe. This is called **Meyer's loop** and tumours arising in the temporal lobes may affect these fibres which represent the upper part of the visual field (Fig. 8.40E).

Axons from the LGN synapse in layer 4 of V1 but magnocellular and parvocellular inputs go to different sublayers. This maintains the separate **M pathway** and **P pathway** for analysing movement and form/colour respectively that continues into the cortex (Fig. 8.42). Cortical cells fall into three categories on the basis of their receptive field properties:

- Many driven by parvocellular LGN cells respond to lines or edges with a particular orientation and these are regarded as fundamental elements in the perception of shape.
- Others driven by parvocellular inputs are wavelength selective.
- Those driven by magnocellular input are movement sensitive and completely insensitive to wavelength.

Secondary visual cortex

V1 makes extensive connections to the extra-striate cortex (areas 18 and 19) where there are additional representations of the visual world (V2–V5). Projections from these higher visual areas go to both parietal and temporal cortex. Each of the three V1 cortical cell populations are anatomically segregated within V1 and project to distinct regions of the secondary visual cortex V2. In turn V2 funnels these different streams of visual information to distinct higher regions of visual cortex.

Visual perception
Depth perception

V1 is the first place in the visual system in which cells that can be driven by both eyes (cells with binocular receptive fields) are found. These allow **depth perception** by comparing the images from each eye, **stereopsis**.

Retinal images are two-dimensional yet the brain is able to reconstruct the relative positions of objects in three-dimensional space. This is done by using a combination of monocular clues and stereopsis.

However, **monocular clues** must be used for objects further than about 30 m away where binocular vision does not work. The types of clue include:

- **Parallax**, the greater apparent movement of near objects with respect to more distant ones brought about by head movement

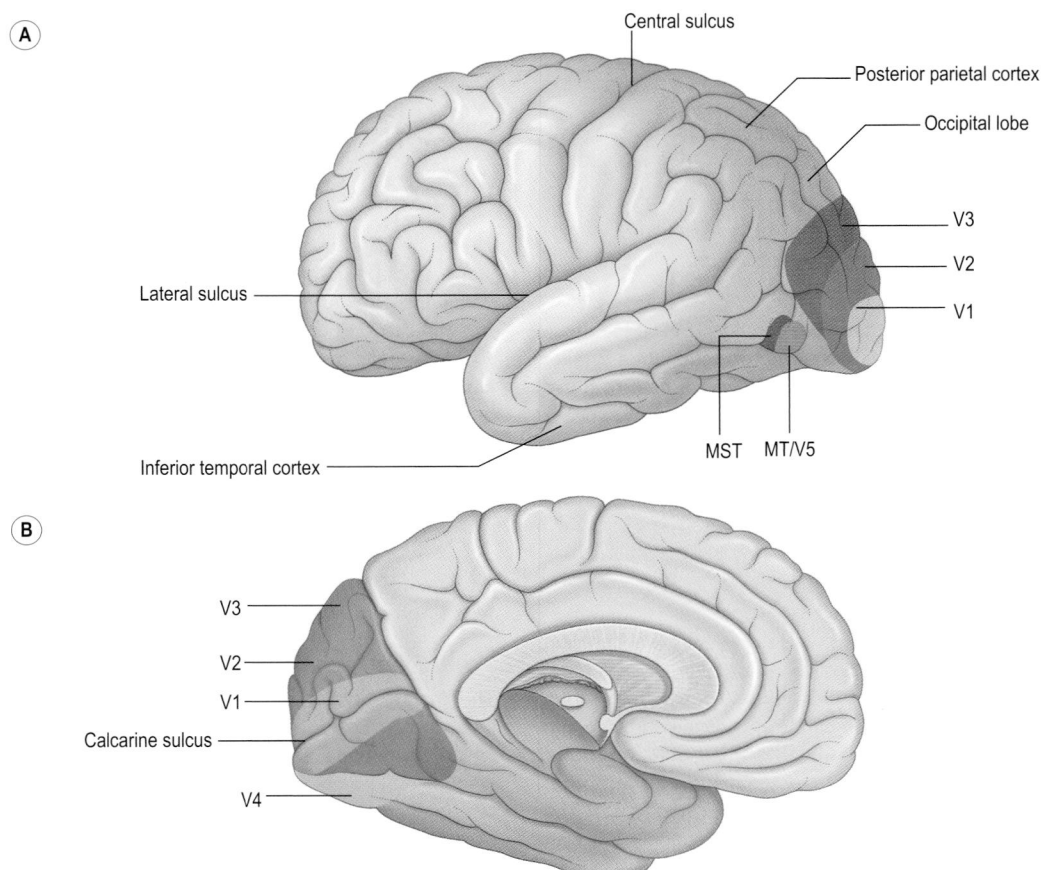

Fig. 8.41 Visual cortex. Location of visual cortical areas in the left hemisphere: (A) lateral aspect and (B) medial aspect. MT, middle temporal area; MST, medial superior temporal area.

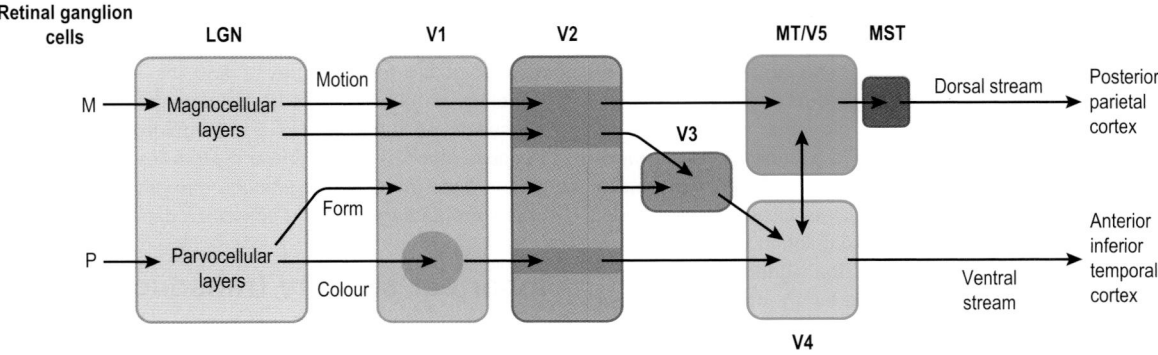

Fig. 8.42 Processing pathways in the visual system. LGN, lateral geniculate nucleus; MT, middle temporal area; MST, medial superior temporal area.

■ **Perspective**, parallel lines converge with distance
■ **Size disparity**, familiar objects appear smaller at greater distance
■ **Velocity disparity**, familiar moving objects (e.g. cars) appear to have higher velocities when they are nearer
■ **Occultation**, distant objects are hidden by closer ones
■ **Chiaroscuro**, closer objects cast shadows over more distant ones.

For objects closer than 30 m monocular clues are supplemented by **stereopsis** to compute depth. When viewing a close object both eyes are turned inwards so that the optic axes converge on the object at the fixation point. This is termed the **vergence reflex**. The image of the object is now precisely focused on the fovea in both eyes. The amount of vergence needed to fixate an object probably acts as one cue to its depth. However, the principal cue arises because the eyes are about 6.3 cm apart so that images of objects closer to, or further from, the fixation point will fall onto slightly different horizontal positions on the two retinas. The relative displacement of the two images is termed **retinal (binocular) disparity** and is sufficient for stereopsis; form, movement or colour information are not required. (Information box 8.18).

Movement perception

Movement in the visual field is monitored in the following ways:

- Gaze is altered to track a moving object
- Gaze is held fixed and retinal pixels are activated sequentially as the object moves through the visual field.

The visual system can differentiate between these because it receives copies of the motor commands to alter gaze. In addition, objects in the visual field appear to move as an individual moves through the environment. This is termed **optic flow** and its precise pattern is used by the visual system to assess distance (stationary objects that are closer appear to move faster than more distant ones as we approach them), direction (objects directly ahead do not move as we approach but peripheral ones do), and for posture.

The **M (magnocellular) pathway** is responsible for movement perception. Its signals come either from retinal ganglion cells that get input from all three types of cone, or from rods; the M pathway is colour blind. The M pathway is faster than the P pathway so its signals arrive earlier in the cortex. From V2 it projects via the dorsal stream to the **medial temporal area** (**MT, V5**) which relays via the **medial superior temporal area** (**MST**) to the posterior parietal cortex (Fig. 8.42). The first signals to arrive at the MST are those concerned with optic flow. Lesions of the MT cause loss of movement perception but not loss of visual acuity for stationary objects.

During saccades, the brief, rapid changes of gaze made to explore the visual field, the M system is shut down. This ensures that saccades do not confuse the movement system.

Colour perception

The colours of objects do not depend simply on the wavelengths of light they reflect since colours can remain remarkably constant even when the spectral makeup of the illuminating light is very different (e.g. sunlight versus tungsten filament bulb). This property is referred to as **colour constancy**. It has evolved to facilitate easy identification of objects, despite changes in ambient lighting.

Colour vision occurs because the signals from the three populations of cones are compared by **colour opponent cells**. These are parvocellular (P) retinal ganglion, lateral geniculate or cortical cells with surround-antagonist receptive fields in which centre and surround get input from different cones. They fall into two types:

- Cells with opposed signals from M and L cones
- Cells with opposed signals from S and some combination of M plus L input.

When light covers the entire receptive field (RF) of a colour opponent cell it produces a colour signal. When it strikes only the centre of the RF the signal is derived from just a single type of cone and it can only signal brightness variations. Hence P cells produce coarse scale colour vision but can respond to fine scale variations in brightness.

Many cells in the cortex that are wavelength sensitive have even more complex receptive fields and are able to account for colour constancy, which requires wavelength comparisons over large areas of retina.

P pathway neurons relay to **V4** where there seems to be some segregation of those carrying chromatic and form signals. Lesions of V4 results in **achromatopsia**, an inability to perceive colours, often, but not always, associated with deficits in form vision. Area V4 projects via the ventral stream to the **anterior inferior temporal cortex** (**AIT**).

Where and what systems

The final destination of the M pathway is area 7a in the parietal cortex. Lesions of this area result in **optic ataxia**, in which visuospatial skills are compromised but object recognition is unharmed. In contrast, lesions of the anterior inferior temporal cortex cause **visual agnosia**, a failure to recognise objects including once familiar faces (**prosopagnosia**), while retaining the ability to appreciate where objects are in space. These two routes for visual information have been described as **where** and **what** systems, respectively (Information box 8.19).

BALANCE

The sense of balance measures the position of the head with respect to the force of gravity, and the accelerations and velocities produced by head movements. This information is used in postural reflexes and to guide eye movements. Because much of the vestibular system lies in the brainstem, simple tests of vestibular function can provide insights into brainstem damage, even in comatose patients.

Inner ear sensory transduction

The inner ear subserves the senses of balance and hearing. Both require the detection of mechanical forces and use hair cells, which act rather like strain gauges to transform force into electrical current.

---

i   **Information box 8.18**   **Double vision**

Stereopsis requires that the images on the two retinas are perceptually fused. The visual system can only do this if the retinal disparity does not exceed about 2° of arc. If it does the result is **double vision** (**diplopia**). This occurs physiologically if an object lies too far away from the current fixation point for the retinal disparity to be smaller than 2° and is usually ignored. Clinically, double vision most commonly results from defects in the control of the extraocular muscles, which means that the visual axes of the eyes are not properly aligned. Hence images on the retinas that would normally be fused fall outside the range of binocular disparity cells and so cannot be fused.

   Information box 8.19   **Loss of conscious visual perception**

Bilateral loss of V1 causes a complete loss of conscious visual perception. However, a few humans with this damage are able to move through space avoiding obstacles far better than they would by chance, even though they are not consciously aware of them. This **blindsight** is thought to be mediated by connections from the magnocellular LGN to the where system that bypass V1. Interestingly, visual stimuli that result in action without visual awareness have been reported for normal individuals.

Hair cell structure

Hair cells (Fig. 8.43) are modified columnar epithelial cells with neuron-like characteristics. On their apical membrane they have a single long cilium, the **kinocilium**, and a hair bundle that consists of 20–300 rigid, cylindrical organelles called **stereocilia**. The stereocilia vary in length so the top of the hair bundle is bevelled. The base of a stereocilium is very thin so that a force applied to its tip causes the stereocilium to pivot. Each stereocilium is connected to the tip of its next longest neighbour by a 3 nm wide elastic protein filament, a **tip link**.

Mechano-electrical transduction

The tips of the stereocilia contain transmembrane ion channels. The ion channels in adjacent stereocilia are connected by the tip links. Under resting conditions about 15% of these channels are open and this allows an inward flow of K^+ ions. This happens because the fluid (endolymph) in which the apical membrane of the hair cell is bathed has a higher concentration of K^+ than the hair cell intracellular fluid. Deflection of the hair bundle by a mechanical force towards the kinocilium tenses the tip links, opening the ion channels to which they are connected. The increased K^+ flow into the hair cell causes it to depolarise. A force which deflects the hair bundle in the opposite direction closes the ion channels and hyperpolarises the hair cells. Hair cells form glutamatergic synapses with primary afferents.

Vestibular system

The **vestibular apparatus** or **vestibular labyrinth** is the part of the inner ear concerned with balance. It consists of a set of bony canals (the **bony labyrinth**) enclosing membranous sacs (the **membranous labyrinth**) filled with **endolymph**, which has ionic concentrations similar to that of intracellular fluid (high K^+ and low Na^+ concentrations). Endolymph is continuously secreted and drains into the endolymphatic sac from where it is absorbed into the CSF (Clinical box 8.14). Between the bony and membranous labyrinths is **perilymph**, a fluid similar in composition to CSF, secreted by the periosteum. Each vestibular apparatus consists of two otolith organs, the **utricle** and **saccule**, and three **semicircular canals**: lateral, posterior and anterior (Fig. 8.44).

Detection of linear accelerations

The **otolith organs** contain a sensory structure, the **macula**, which consists of numerous hair cells. The tips of the hair bundles are inserted into a collagen gel matrix, the **otolith membrane**, in which is embedded a large number of calcite (calcium carbonate) particles termed **otoconia**. When the head undergoes linear acceleration the inertia of the otolith membrane causes the hair bundles to deflect. As the acceleration ceases the hair bundles are deflected in the opposite direction by the inertia of the otolith membrane, which continues to move after the head has stopped. Hence the outcome of a transient acceleration will be hair cell depolarisation followed by hyperpolarisation or vice versa. Because of their orientations the saccule detects acceleration due to gravity while the utricle detects translational horizontal acceleration.

Clinical box 8.14 | **Ménière's disease**

In Ménière's disease endolymph reabsorption is impaired and the increase in endolymph volume damages the membranous labyrinth and hair cells in the vestibular inner ear and the cochlea. The result is:

- Intermittent, relapsing **vertigo** (loss of balance sensation often accompanied by nausea and vomiting)
- **Tinnitus** (ringing in the ears)
- Progressive hearing loss.

The disorder is usually unilateral and what triggers it is unknown. In severe cases surgical destruction of the afflicted labyrinth alleviates the vertigo. The vestibular system adapts to receiving unilateral input, so normal vestibulo-ocular reflexes and sense of balance are restored.

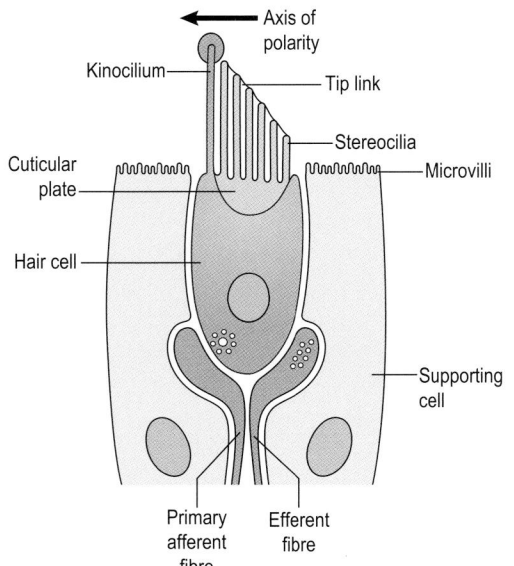

Fig. 8.43 Vestibular hair cell. Redrawn with permission from Longstaff A 2005 Instant notes in neuroscience, 2nd edn. Taylor & Francis, Abingdon UK.

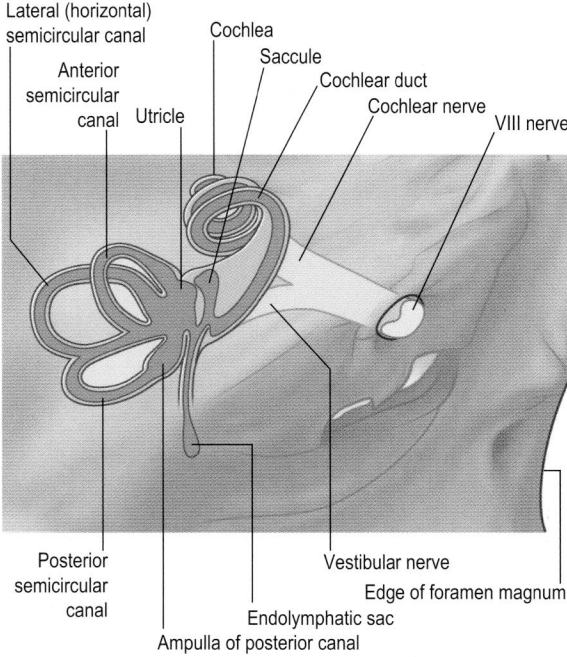

***Fig. 8.44* The left vestibular apparatus and cochlea viewed from above.** The membranous labyrinth is shaded. Redrawn with permission from Longstaff A 2005 Instant notes in neuroscience, 2nd edn. Taylor & Francis, Abingdon UK.

The otolith organs also measure stationary head position. Tilting the head forwards or backwards allows the utricles to respond to a component of the gravitational force which they do not feel when the head is upright. Tilting the head sideways has the same effect but in this case the saccules no longer respond to the full gravitational force they feel in the upright position.

The orientation of the hair cells in the two vestibular labyrinths are mirror images of each other; i.e. a head movement that causes a group of hair cells on one side to depolarise will make the corresponding hair cells on the other side hyperpolarise. So the brain can unambiguously measure accelerations in any direction or any static head position.

Detection of head rotation

Each vestibular labyrinth has three **semicircular canals**, aligned at 90° to one another, that are responsible for detecting head rotation around the *x* axis (roll), *y* axis (pitch) and *z* axis (yaw). A small swelling at the base of each semicircular canal – the **ampulla** – is lined with sensory epithelium, the **crista**, which contains hair cells. The hair bundles extend into a gelatinous **cupula** that forms a barrier to the movement of endolymph in the canal.

The semicircular canals work in pairs, one in each ear, that lie in the same plane. Any component of rotation in the plane of the pair causes their cupulas to be distorted by the inertia of the endolymph. This results in depolarisation of the hair cells for the semicircular canal on the side towards which the head is turning and hyperpolarisation of the hair cells on the opposite side. Between them the three pairs of semicircular canals can signal the plane and direction of any head rotation.

Vestibular pathways

Vestibular hair cell afferents are bipolar cells with their cell bodies located in the **vestibular (Scarpa's) ganglion**. Their processes run in the vestibular branch of the vestibulocochlear nerve (VIIIth cranial nerve) to the **vestibular nuclei** in the rostral medulla.

The **vestibulo-ocular reflex (VOR)** allows the eyes to be kept fixed on a particular point while the head moves. It relies on connections that run from the **medial vestibular nuclei** to the oculomotor and abducens nuclei, which control the oculomotor muscles which control eye movement. The semicircular canals signal the rotation and bring about equal and opposite rotation of both eyes by modulating the contraction of the extraocular eye muscles (Fig. 8.45). As the head rotates the eyes first slowly track an object in visual space and are then rapidly reset by a saccade to central gaze. Repeated sequences of these eye movements is termed **nystagmus**, which may be physiological or pathological (Clinical box 8.15). The direction of nystagmus is defined by the direction of the rapid saccade.

Inputs from the otolith organs go to the **lateral vestibular nuclei** which relays to the lateral vestibulospinal tract. This pathway powerfully excites ipsilateral motor neurons in the ventral horn driving antigravity (extensor) muscles, and hence enables an upright posture to be maintained (see below).

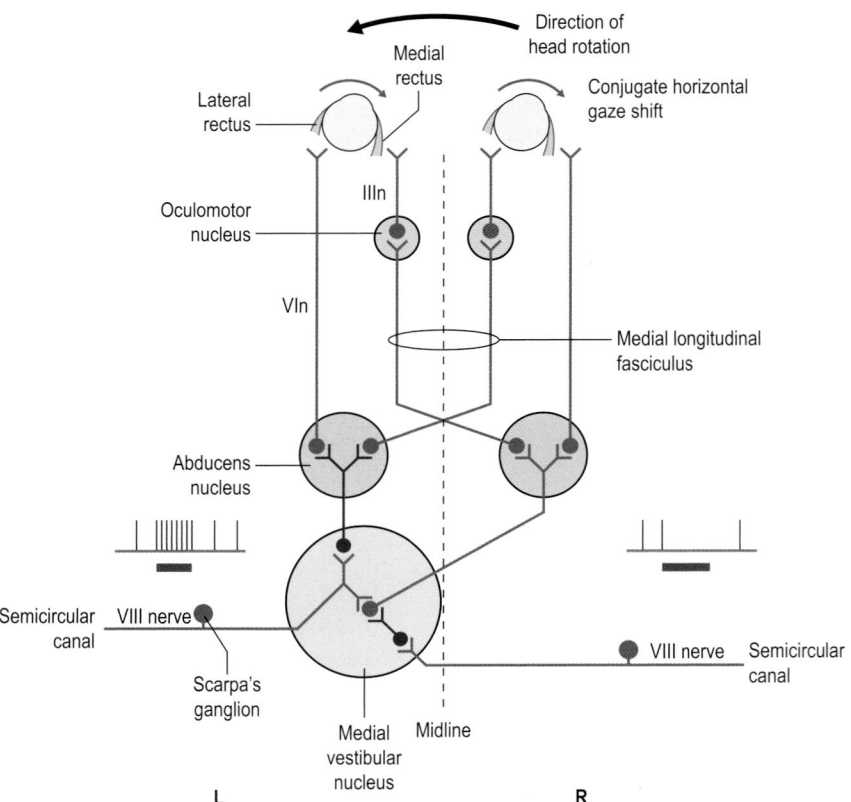

Fig. 8.45 **The circuitry of the rotational vestibulo-ocular reflex.** Stimulation of the horizontal semicircular canals by leftward head rotation (*red bars*) excites motor neurons to ipsilateral medial rectus and contralateral lateral rectus muscles. Motor neurons to the antagonists are silenced by inhibitory (*red*) neurons.

Brainstem lesions can often be assessed by examining the performance of the vestibular system because its circuitry lies in the medulla, pons and cerebellum. Hence, unilateral damage to the vestibular system can result in pathological nystagmus in the absence of head rotation.

Damage to the brainstem can be tested by examining the vestibulo-ocular reflex (VOR) in response to stimulating the semicircular canals using the **caloric test**. With the head at an angle of 30° the horizontal canals lie vertically, and irrigating one ear with cold water causes convection currents in the endolymph which mimic head rotation. In a normal subject this causes a nystagmus with a slow component towards the irrigated ear and a fast saccade away from it. Unconscious patients cannot make saccades, so only the slow component is normally visible. A low brainstem lesion abolishes the slow component in both eyes while a lesion to the medial longitudinal fasciculus abolishes the slow component in the eye on the non-irrigated side.

Axons of neurons in vestibular nuclei cross the midline and ascend adjacent to the medial lemniscus to the ventral posterior and ventral lateral thalamus. From here projections go to several cortical (mainly parietal and temporal) areas where vestibular information is integrated with other sensory modalities, e.g. proprioceptor and visual information. This allows for the conscious perception of body orientation in space and cortical control of postural reflexes (see below).

HEARING

Hearing requires two processes to occur in parallel:

- Localising the direction of a sound source
- Deconstructing a complex incoming pressure waveform into a series of pure frequencies.

By comparing combinations of pure frequencies with pre-existing representations of sounds, and by assigning each to a source, the brain identifies each of the different sounds in the auditory stream. Auditory input is sampled at an early processing stage to drive reflexes that allow orientation to the direction of a sound source.

Sound

Sound is pressure waves transmitted through a medium such as air or water. The frequency of the wave is the **pitch** of the sound. The **amplitude** of the wave is the difference in pressure, P, during the passage of the waveform. Because P covers such a large range it is expressed on a logarithmic scale as the **sound pressure level** (SPL), which is measured in **decibels** (dB). So a 10 dB increase in sound levels is a 10-fold increase in intensity. Normal speech is about 65 dB but prolonged exposure to sounds greater than 90 dB causes permanent damage and sounds above 130 dB cause pain.

Differences in SPL are heard as differences in **loudness**, although loudness also depends on frequency, since sensitivity is maximal around 3000 Hz, falling away at higher and lower frequencies.

The human ear is sensitive to pure tones at frequencies of between 20 Hz and 20 000 Hz, but there is a loss of high frequencies with age, termed **presbycusis**. Speech uses frequencies between 300 Hz and 4000 Hz.

Middle ear

The middle ear converts pressure waves in air to oscillations of the **perilymph**, a liquid within the inner ear. This is done by means of a lever system of three bones, the **ossicles**, which transmit vibrations of the **tympanic membrane** (eardrum) to the **oval window** (Fig. 8.46). It takes more energy to move the perilymph than the air but the area of the oval window is only 1/20 that of the eardrum, so the force per unit area acting on the perilymph is 20-fold higher. This, together with the mechanical advantage of the lever system, not only offsets the different energy requirements but produces a 20–30 dB amplification of the sound pressure level (Clinical box 8.16).

Inward motion of the tympanic membrane is transferred by the ossicles to an inward motion of the oval window which moves the perilymph in the cochlea. The **round window** bulges in response to relieve the pressure. The movements are reversed as the tympanic membrane moves outward.

Two muscles, the **tensor tympanum** and **stapedius**, reduce sound transmission by about 20 dB when they contract, by reducing the movement of the ossicles. This may offer some protection from prolonged loud sounds, but not for brief ones because the reflex time is too long.

Auditory inner ear

Hair cells are responsible for sensory transduction in the auditory inner ear, which occurs in a similar manner to transduction by the vestibular inner ear.

Anatomy of the cochlea

The **cochlea** is the auditory part of the inner ear (Fig. 8.47). It is a snail-shaped bony canal with 2¾ coils which spirals around a central pillar. The **base** of the cochlea is the widest end, nearest the middle ear, while its **apex** is the pointed end. Running through it is a wedge-shaped, blind-ending membranous **cochlear duct** enclosing a space, the scala media filled with endolymph.

Superior to the cochlear duct lies the **scala vestibuli**, and inferior is the **scala tympani**. These spaces are filled with

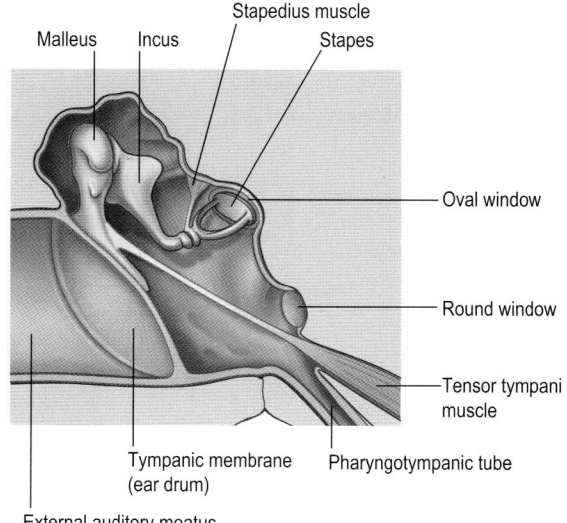

Fig. 8.46 **The anatomy of the middle ear.**

perilymph and are continuous at the apex of the cochlea. The roof of the scala media is the **vestibular membrane** while its floor, which lies above the scala tympanum, consists of the **basilar membrane** on which sits the **organ of Corti**.

Clinical box 8.16 **Clinical investigation of deafness**

There are simple tests for the two forms of hearing loss:

- **Conduction deafness** – a middle ear defect prevents sound reaching the inner ear
- **Sensorineural deafness** – the defect is cochlear or more central.

Rinne's test and Weber's test exploit the fact that sound is conducted by bone, albeit less well than by air.

In **Rinne's test**, the base of a ringing tuning fork (frequency 256 Hz) is applied to the mastoid bone:

- If the sound can be heard, even though it cannot be heard when simply held close to the ear, this demonstrates that sensory transduction in the inner ear has been activated, bypassing a defect in the middle ear, i.e. it implies **conductive deafness**.
- If the patient is unable to hear a tuning fork normally, or by bone conduction, this implies **sensorineural deafness** in which the inner ear is defective.

The most common cause of conduction deafness is **otosclerosis**, a disorder in which the ossicles fuse so that energy transfer from eardrum to oval window is compromised. **Weber's test** investigates sensorineural deficit. The base of a tuning fork is placed on the middle of the patient's forehead:

- If the sound is located more on one side, then either conduction deafness exists on that side, or sensorineural deafness exists in the other. The test is repeated by covering the ear in which the sound was faintest. Normally the closed ear hears best by bone-conduction.
- If no sound is heard in the covered ear sensorineural deafness is confirmed.

The frequency response and dynamic range of hearing can be tested by **audiometry**. Tones with different SPL and frequency are transmitted to one or other ear through headphones, and the patient says when they can hear them.

Sensory function of the cochlea

For audible sounds, oscillations of the perilymph in the scala vestibuli are transmitted through the vestibular membrane, causing oscillations of the endolymph, which in turn cause a travelling wave to move along the basilar membrane from its basal end to the apical end. The basilar membrane is narrow and stiff at the base of the cochlea, becoming wider and less stiff at the apex, and in consequence the place where it vibrates maximally is frequency dependent. At the basal end it is tuned to high frequencies, while its apical end resonates in response to low frequencies (Fig. 8.47). This mechanism allows frequency coding of sounds.

Organ of Corti

The **organ of Corti** (Fig. 8.48) has about 16 000 sensory hair cells, each with a bundle of stereocilia whose tips are close to, or inserted into, a cell-free collagen gel, the **tectorial membrane**. The hair cells form synapses with axons of the cochlear division of the vestibulocochlear nerve, the cell bodies of which lie in the **spiral ganglion**. When the basilar membrane vibrates in response to a sound, the stereocilia

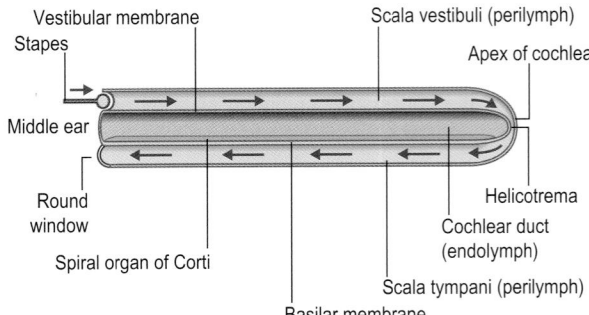

Fig. 8.47 **The propagation of sound through the cochlea** (depicted uncurled). The base is tuned to high frequencies while the apex is more sensitive to low frequencies.

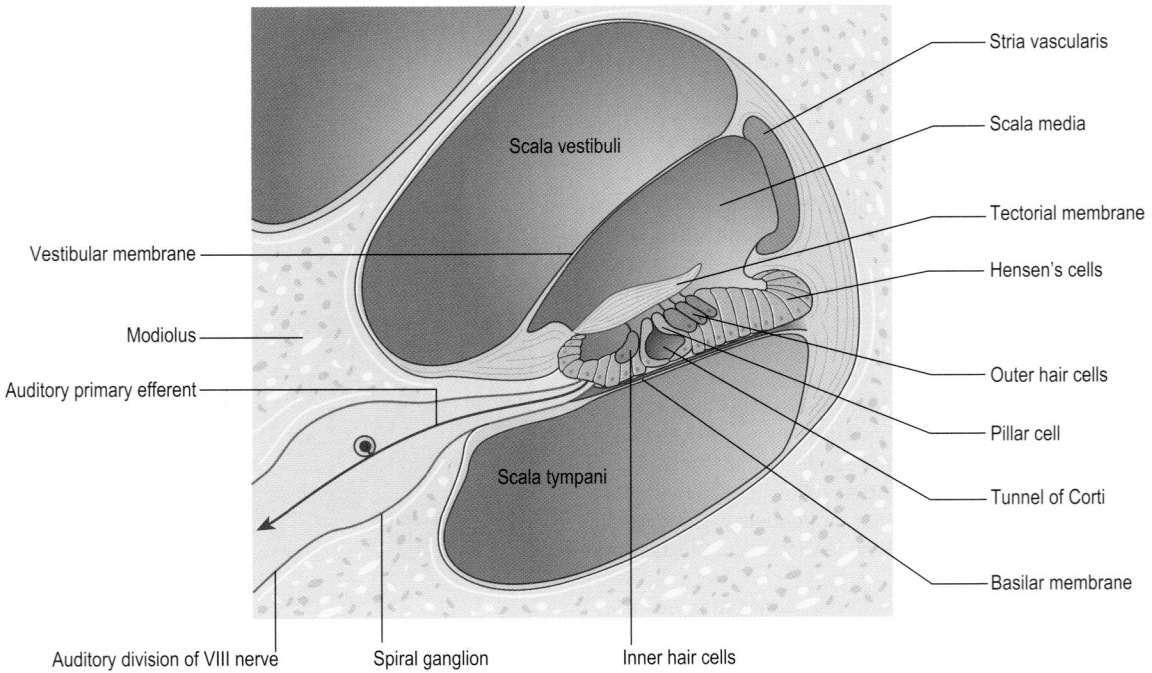

Fig. 8.48 **Transverse section through the cochlea to show the organ of Corti.**

bend first one way and then the other. This translates into depolarisation followed by hyperpolarisation of the hair cells and so periodic fluctuations in the release of their transmitter, glutamate. The end result is periodic firing of the cochlear afferents.

The precise location of a hair cell along the basilar membrane determines the frequency of sound to which it is maximally sensitive, its **characteristic frequency**. Adjacent hair cells differ in characteristic frequency by only 0.2% on average, compared with 6% for neighbouring notes on a piano.

Hair cells are arranged into two groups:

- Inner hair cells: There is a single row of about 4000 **inner hair cells**, each of which is innervated by about 10 afferents (high divergence) which transmit sound information.
- Outer hair cells: There are three rows of **outer hair cells** (12 000 in total), supplied by only about 3000 afferents (high convergence) of unknown function. The outer hair cells (OHCs) contain proteins which change in length, contracting on depolarisation and lengthening with hyperpolarisation, and this increases the amplitude of basilar membrane vibrations. This **cochlear amplifier** raises the sensitivity of the inner hair cells.

The sensitivity (gain) of the cochlear amplifier can be altered by inputs from the superior olivary nuclei in the medulla. The efferents release ACh which hyperpolarises the OHCs, dampening the cochlear amplifier. Sensitivity falls with increasing sound pressure level. For example, the sensitivity of inner hair cells to an 80 dB sound is only 1% of their sensitivity to a 10 dB sound. Excessive exposure to aminoglycoside antibiotics (e.g. streptomycin, kanamycin) causes selective loss of outer hair cells and deafness (Information box 8.20). This illustrates the importance of the cochlear amplifier.

Otoacoustic emissions

Movements of the basilar membrane generated by the outer hair cells can be transmitted through the cochlea in the reverse direction to vibrate the oval window. This excites the ossicle lever system of the middle ear to move the tympanic membrane so the ear emits sounds. These **otoacoustic emissions** may be spontaneous or evoked by sound input and are usually pure tones. They are inaudible to the individual. Evoked otoacoustic emissions are not seen with a sensorineural deafness greater than 30 dB and this forms the basis for testing of infants, in whom audiometry is difficult.

Central auditory pathways

Cochlear afferents in the spiral ganglion run in the auditory part of the VIIIth cranial nerve to the ipsilateral **cochlear nuclei** which lie in the rostral medulla (Fig. 8.49). These nuclei project to the **superior olivary nuclei** (not shown) on both sides, with some fibres crossing the midline. Bilateral auditory pathways ascend to the **nuclei of the lateral meniscus** and the **inferior colliculi** (**IC**) of the midbrain. Extensive reciprocal connections across the midline between the nuclei of the lateral meniscus and inferior colliculi provide for integration of information from both ears. Neurons in the inferior colliculus project to the **medial geniculate nuclei** (**MGN**) from where fibres go via the **acoustic radiation** to the primary auditory cortex.

The **primary auditory cortex** (**A1**) is on the surface of the superior temporal lobe (Brodmann's areas 41 and 42), which forms the floor of the lateral sulcus. Lying posterior to A1 and extending to cover the lateral surface of the superior temporal gyrus (Brodmann's area 22) is the **secondary auditory cortex** (**SAC**).

ⓘ Information box 8.20 | **Cochlear implants**

A cochlear implant is able to restore limited but useful sound sensation in patients with deafness due to cochlear damage, provided that there is still a functioning auditory nerve. The implant itself is a linear array of 22 electrodes, inserted through the mastoid bone and round window into the scala tympanum at the basal end of the cochlea, so that it follows the first 1.5 turns towards the apex. At its distal end is a radio receiver, and externally there is a microphone, speech processor and radio transmitter.

Sounds picked up by the microphone are analysed by the speech processor – a computer that filters sounds into frequency bands optimal for understanding speech – and the processed signal transmitted to the implant. This crosstalk between the electrodes, which are spread along the cochlea, degrades the quality of the perceived sound, but with experience patients can follow a conversation.

As well as being used for acquired deafness, cochlear implants are useful in congenital deafness. Because maximum plasticity of the auditory system occurs in the first two years of life, the implants are given as early as 12 months, optimising the conditions for language acquisition.

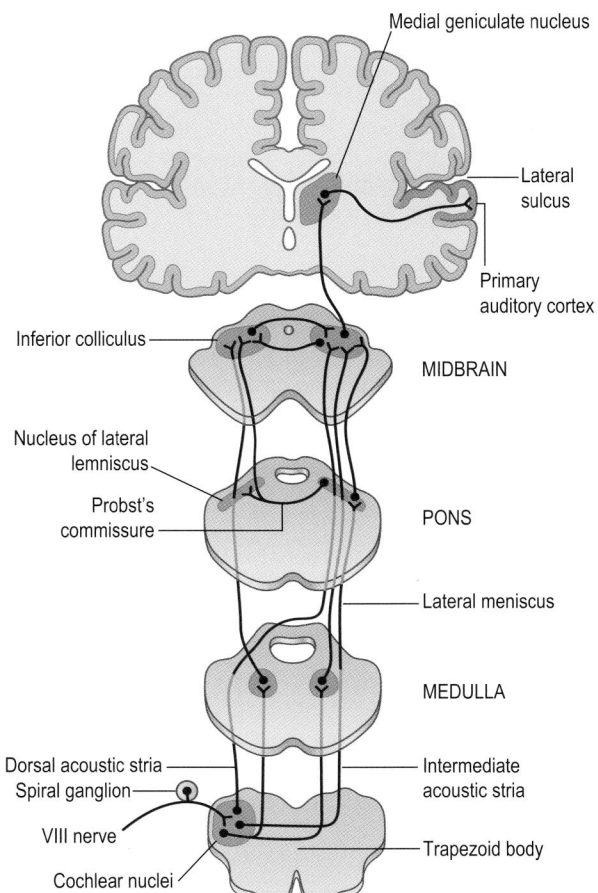

Fig. 8.49 Central auditory pathways.

Auditory processing

Sound frequency coding

The frequency of sounds is encoded in two ways. Because of the properties of the basilar membrane, the characteristic frequencies of hair cells vary systematically along its length. This provides **place coding:** a hair cell's position along the membrane specifies the frequency. However, for frequencies lower than 1–3 kHz temporal coding operates. Here afferents fire with greater probability during a particular phase of a sound wave. This is termed **phase locking**. Groups of cells fire at different phases so their integrated signal is a complete representation of the waveform and the population encodes the frequency.

Tonotopic maps (frequency maps) are found at every level in the auditory pathways. In A1 increasing frequencies are mapped in a rostrocaudal direction with all frequencies allotted a fair proportion of the map.

Coding of sound level

The range of sound levels that individual auditory afferents are sensitive to is only about 30 dB. In order to represent the full range of sound pressure levels (SPLs) there are different afferents that respond to different SPLs.

Localisation of sound

The ability to be able to localise the source of a sound has obvious survival value. Circuits responsible for sound localisation enable brainstem reflexes to alter gaze and head orientation to the direction of a sound. Signals specifying the localisation of sound are relayed from the inferior to the superior colliculi, generating an **auditory space map** that lies in register with a visual map. The superior colliculi organise auditory reflexes for gaze and head rotation towards the sound source.

Distinct mechanisms are involved in locating the **elevation** of a sound (how high it is with respect to the local horizon) and its **azimuth** (the angle, to the left or right, of the source in relation to the direction in which a person is facing).

Finding elevation

The complicated shape of the pinna of the outer ear means that sound waves are reflected from it in a manner that depends on the height of the sound source. From the time delays between the reflected waves and those which enter the ear canal directly the brain computes the elevation of the source.

Finding azimuth

Azimuth is found by comparing the input into the two ears and is sufficiently accurate to allow the source of the sound to be located to within a minute of arc. Two processes are at work.

- **Interaural level differences (ILDs)** compare the sound level in the two ears.
- **Interaural time differences (ITDs)** compare the time at which a sound enters the two ears.

Auditory perception

Electroencephalographic and brain imaging studies show the **SAC** is responsible not just for sound perception but is also involved in language (see under Language, below). The simultaneous mix of sounds that arrive at the ears are sorted into coherent streams, each of which is an independent sound object. This **auditory stream segregation** occurs at an early stage of auditory processing and is the basis of the 'cocktail party effect' by which we can recognise one voice among a babble.

The SAC has access to permanent representations of sound categories with which incoming sound streams can be matched. This allows voice and music recognition. Brain imaging implicates a network involving the SAC in the right hemisphere and the frontal cortex in **music perception**. In the left hemisphere the SAC is associated with Wernicke's area, which constructs transient representations of **speech sounds**, either heard or retrieved from lexical memory.

Two output streams leave the SAC. Sound object information is passed to the adjacent **temporal cortex** for semantic processing, while information about sound position is relayed to the inferior **parietal lobule**.

SMELL

A sense of smell has obvious survival value. Infants use their sense of smell to recognise their mother and to find her nipples. Noxious airborne molecules are avoided. The aroma of appetising food stimulates salivation, the secretion of gastric juice and increases gastric motility, whereas the stench of rotting food triggers nausea. Smell may also affect reproductive behaviour, as there is some evidence that humans secrete **pheromones**, small volatile molecules that, for example, act as sexual attractants or synchronise the menstrual cycles of women living in closely knit groups.

Olfactory epithelium

About half of the nasal cavity is lined by a sheet of epithelium which contains olfactory receptor neurons, the primary afferents subserving smell, plus basal cells, supporting cells and mucus-secreting cells. Because olfactory receptor neurons are continually exposed to potentially damaging materials in the air they are replaced by new neurons derived from basal stem cells.

Olfactory receptor neurons

The nasal mucosa contains about 100 million bipolar **olfactory receptor neurons (ORNs)**. Their apical neurites branch to form **olfactory cilia** which are embedded in the mucus layer. The central processes of ORNs are small diameter, unmyelinated axons that pass through the cribriform plate of the ethmoid bone, forming numerous bundles that together constitute the **olfactory nerve**, which enters the olfactory bulb.

Odorants and odorant receptors

There are a large number of **odorant** molecules. Their chemical structures are diverse, but all are volatile, fairly small molecules that are either fat or water soluble. Each group of chemically related odorants is bound by one of the approximately 1000 **odorant receptors**. These constitute the huge G_{olf} family of G-protein-coupled receptors that, like the G_s family, activate adenylyl cyclase (see Chs 2 and 4).

On dissolving in mucus, the odorants bind to G_{olf} receptors in the plasma membrane of the olfactory cilia. Adenylyl cyclase is activated and the resulting rise in cAMP opens cyclic nucleotide-gated ion channels that allow Ca^{2+} and Na^+ to enter and depolarise the olfactory cilia (cf. transduction in rod cells, above). The depolarisation is a receptor potential which spreads passively across the ORN, triggering action potentials on arrival at the axon hillock if it is sufficiently big.

Odorant coding

Each olfactory receptor neuron expresses just a single type of odorant receptor. The firing frequency of an ORN increases with the concentration of an odorant, but the ORNs sensitive to a given odorant have different thresholds; i.e. some require higher concentrations to excite them, because they have different numbers of odorant receptors. ORNs with the same odorant receptor are clustered in several zones of olfactory epithelium so damage to one part does not cause the loss of a particular smell.

Each **olfactory bulb** has several thousand **glomeruli**. These contain the apical dendrites of 25 **mitral cells**, which receive input from about 25 000 ORNs, a high degree of convergence which maximises the signal strength. Mitral cells provide the output of the olfactory bulbs. Each glomerulus receives input from a specific odorant receptor and responds only to its set of odorants, but any given odorant excites numerous glomeruli. As the concentration of an odorant rises, so the number of glomeruli responding increases because the odorant binds to receptors with progressively lower affinities. The glomeruli that get input from a given type of odorant receptor appear in the same place in the olfactory bulb in different individuals. The reason for this place coding is not understood, because it does not produce a mapping of smells by any property so far identified (e.g. systematic variations in chemical structure).

Central olfactory pathways

The axons of the mitral cells run through the lateral olfactory tract to a variety of forebrain destinations (Fig. 8.50). Odorant information is the only sensory input that is sent to the cortex directly, all others relay via the thalamus.

Connections to the hypothalamus and the amygdala are concerned with physiological responses to smells, emotional responses to odours in relation to feeding and mating, and learning to associate specific smells with unpleasant situations. Output to the hippocampus may be responsible for encoding the olfactory component of episodic memories (see under Learning and memory, below). The major target of the olfactory tract is the **pyriform cortex** may be involved in odour discrimination. Higher-order connections either directly or via the thalamus to the frontal cortex are required for the conscious perception of smell.

TASTE

Taste sensation (**gustation**) is crucial for determining whether potential foods are accepted or rejected, but palatability also depends on smell and on texture (see Ch. 16), which is signalled by proprioceptor and mechanoreceptor input from the mouth. In addition, polymodal nociceptors from the oral and nasal mucosa respond to substances that are palatable at low concentrations but irritants at high concentration, such as ethanol (drinking alcohol), H^+ ions from acetic acid (vinegar) and carbonic acid (carbonated drinks), and capsaicin (hot peppers). Irritants in high concentration trigger salivation, crying, mucus secretion, bronchoconstriction and sweating.

Although five different taste submodalities are traditionally recognised – sweet, salty, sour, bitter and umami (L-

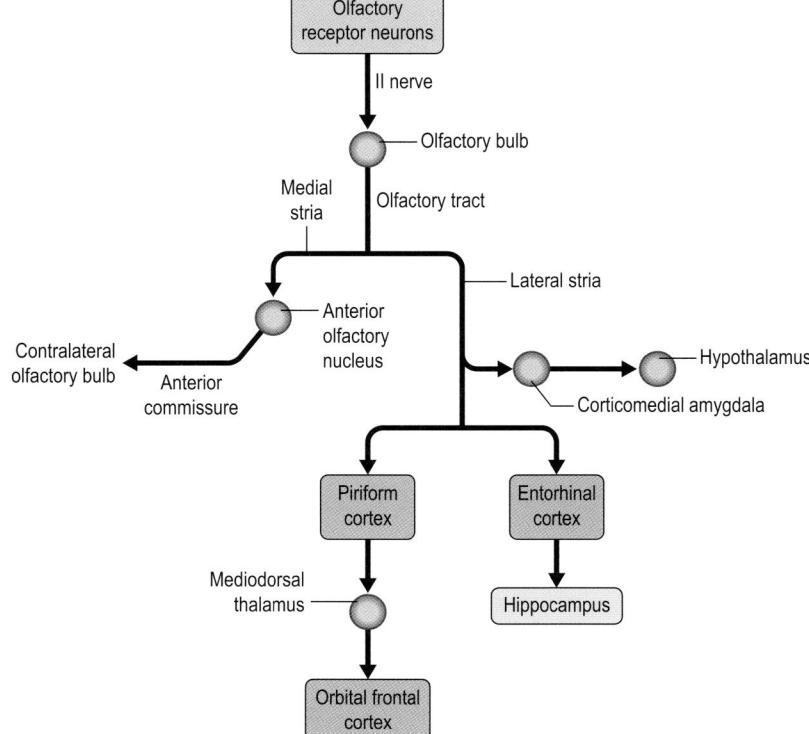

Fig. 8.50 **Central olfactory pathways.**

glutamate) – there are several others (e.g. fatty, pungent, metallic) that are less well defined. Foods high in salt, fat and sugar generally have a high energy content and are highly palatable. In contrast, foods tasting sour or bitter are usually rejected by infants as these tastes are markers of potential microbial spoilage or toxicity. Preferences for specific sour and bitter foods (e.g. yoghurt or beer) are learnt, but adults reject foodstuffs that are unexpectedly acidic or bitter. Taste sensations trigger appropriate physiological as well as behavioural responses. In hungry individuals palatable food triggers salivation whereas unpleasant tastes stimulate gagging.

Taste buds

Humans have about 4000 **taste buds** on the tongue, in the oral mucosa, pharynx, larynx and upper oesophagus. Most are found on the dorsum of the tongue in small projections called **papillae** which come in a variety of shapes. Taste buds are lined with taste cells: epithelial cells with microvilli on their apical border that have specific receptors for tastant molecules. Taste cells form serotonergic synapses with primary taste afferents. Taste cells have a lifetime of about 2 weeks and new ones are continually regenerated from stem cells at the base of the taste bud.

Tastants (ions and molecules that activate gustatory neurons) dissolve in saliva and reach taste cell microvilli through a small **taste pore** in the top of the taste bud. Specific tastes are *not* localised to particular parts of the tongue as is often claimed.

Transduction

Tastants bind either to ion channels or to G-protein-coupled receptors (GPCRs). All cause the taste cell to produce a depolarising receptor potential which triggers a rise in intra-cellular Ca^{2+} and the release of serotonin, but the exact mechanisms differ with the stimulus:

- **Salty** taste is due to the flow of sodium through an amiloride-sensitive Na^+ channel.
- **Sour taste** is due to the flux of H^+ through a proton-specific ion channel.
- **Sweet**, **bitter** and **umami** (L-glutamate) tastes are all produced by activation of GPCRs, many of which are linked to a taste-specific G protein called **gustducin** that triggers the same sequence of events in taste cells as transducin does in photoreceptors (see above).

In general, individual taste cells respond to several types of tastant but they do show considerable selectivity, so taste afferents have preferred stimuli. This allows for taste discrimination.

Central gustatory processing

Primary taste afferents have their cell bodies in the ganglia of three cranial nerves. Input from the anterior two-thirds and posterior one-third of the tongue run in the VII and IX nerves, respectively. Taste buds in the palate are also innervated by the facial nerve. The X nerve receives input from the epiglottis and oesophagus.

The afferents terminate in the rostrolateral **nucleus of the solitary tract (NST)** of the medulla (Fig. 8.51). This nucleus is responsible for integrating visceral sensory information from most of the gut with taste information. It projects to:

- **Preganglionic autonomic fibres** in the medulla and spinal cord which mediate autonomic responses to visceral sensations (e.g. salivation)
- **Reticular system networks** responsible for gastrointestinal reflexes (e.g. swallowing and vomiting) and respiratory reflexes (e.g. coughing and sneezing)

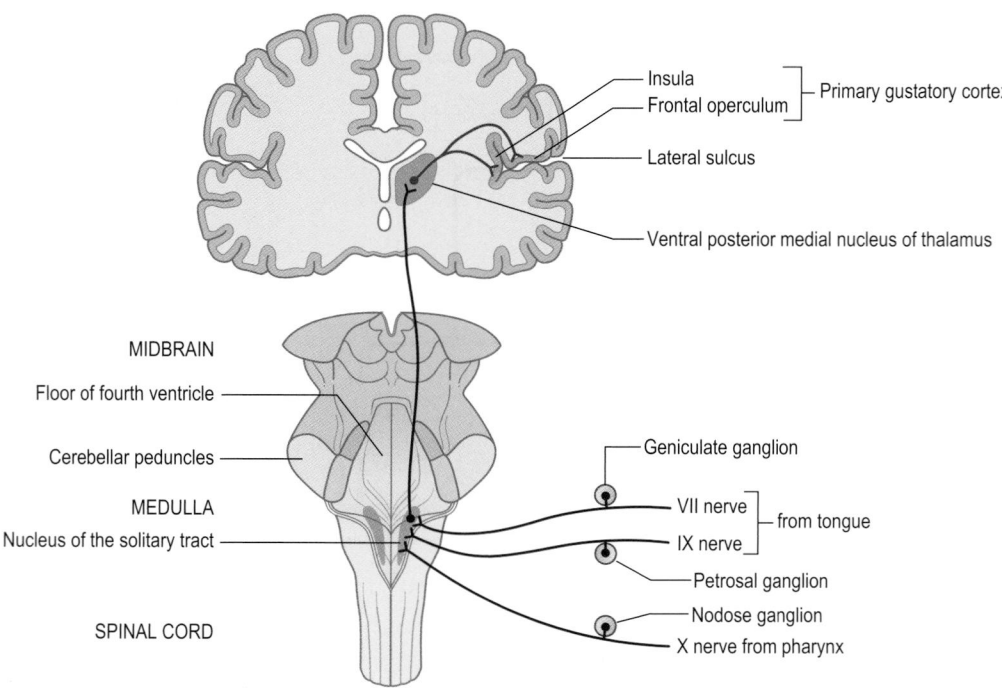

Fig. 8.51 Central taste pathways.

- **The parabrachial nucleus**, which makes reciprocal connections with the hypothalamus and amygdala, structures important for learned responses to tastes.

Taste perception

The pathway for taste perception consists of second order neurons from the NST which terminate on specific dedicated neurons in the ipsilateral **ventral posterior medial thalamus**. Hence taste information in the thalamus is segregated from other tongue sensory modalities. Third order neurons project to several cortical areas concerned with taste discrimination and perception and areas which control the motivation to eat on the basis of hunger.

MOTOR SYSTEMS

Motor systems control the pattern of skeletal muscle contraction in time and space needed to execute movements. The planning of movements requires sensory input. This includes vestibular and proprioceptor input about the position of the body in space, allowing movements to be made without losing balance. Movements are usually **goal-directed** (i.e. purposeful), often guided by vision and other sensory modalities, but frequently initiated without reference to any sensory stimulus.

Although the intention to make voluntary movements is done consciously, their execution, if routine (e.g. walking), can be done quite automatically. However, acquiring a new motor skill (e.g. learning to ride a bike or play the piano) requires conscious effort.

Motor systems are organised **hierarchically**. Sensory input occurs at each level of the hierarchy. Successively higher levels of the hierarchy are capable of organising increasingly complex motor activities and have access to more sophisticated sensory information. Stereotyped movements (e.g. stepping) can be executed using just lower levels of the hierarchy, but voluntary movements require higher levels also.

There are four separate but integrated systems which are involved in movement:

- Motor cortex
- Brainstem and spinal cord motor networks
- Basal ganglia
- Cerebellum.

High level motor function

Before a movement can be performed an **internal representation** of a voluntary movement is constructed at the highest level by the **premotor cortex**, based on sensory input from the posterior parietal cortex. This is necessary because achieving a specific outcome can involve choosing from several motor strategies (e.g. driving an articulated lorry or a small car uses different motor patterns to achieve the same aims).

This internal representation is then transformed into a **motor programme** which specifies the trajectory of the movement and the forces needed to execute it. This is done by the **motor cortex** which recruits two subsystems, both of which relay via the **thalamus** back to the motor cortex, thus forming two loops (Fig. 8.52):

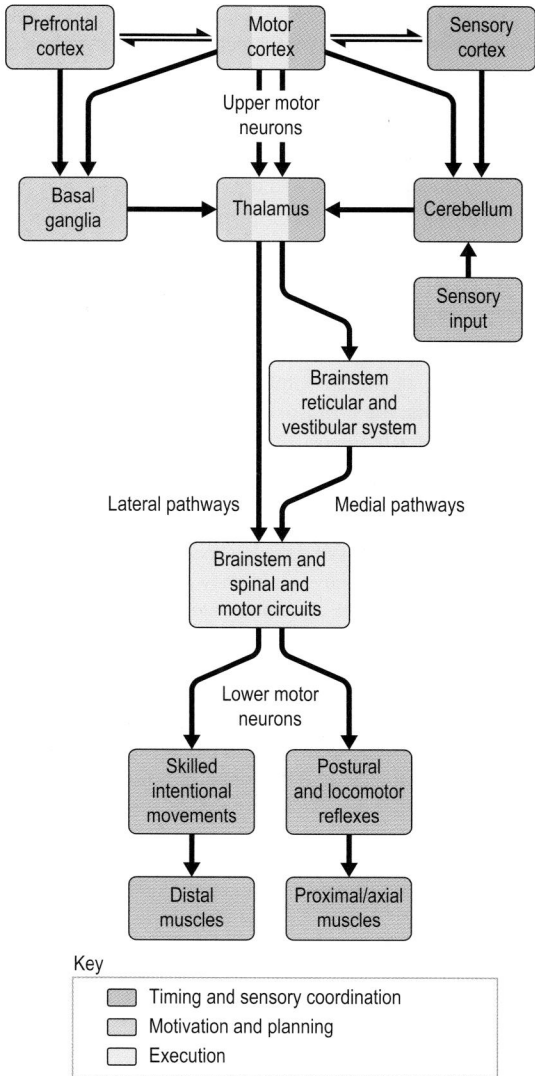

Fig. 8.52 **Motor system hierarchy.**

- The **basal ganglia** motivates a movement by activating the motor cortical networks required for it to occur, while inhibiting unwanted networks.
- The **cerebellum** ensures the precise timing and coordination of a movement and learns new motor skills.

The basal ganglia and cerebellum do not provide significant output to the brainstem and spinal cord; their effects on movement are brought about by via the motor cortex.

Low level motor function

The **output** of the motor cortex goes to **brainstem nuclei** that rise to the **medial motor pathways**. These pathways get input from the vestibular system and reticular system. They mediate postural reflexes by influencing motor units of trunk extensor and proximal limb muscles, and activate spinal cord locomotor circuitry.

In addition, the motor cortex gives rise to the **lateral motor pathways**. The most important in humans is the **corticospinal tract**, the axons of motor cortex neurons which go directly to lower motor neurons for head and distal limb muscles.

The lowest level in the hierarchy is occupied by the neural networks intrinsic to the motor nuclei of the brainstem and in the spinal cord. These circuits can act autonomously to produce stereotyped **involuntary movements** but they are activated by higher levels of the hierarchy during the execution of **voluntary movements**.

Acting alone these circuits are responsible for two types of movement:

- Rhythmical output, e.g. limb movements in locomotion; the circuits involved are called **central pattern generators**
- Reflexes.

Ultimately all motor output converges onto the **lower motor neurons**, the α **motor neurons**, that innervate skeletal muscle (see Ch. 9).

Reaction times

The time taken to make a movement depends on its complexity and the amount of decision-making needed. The simplest motor reflexes have a latency (the interval between stimulus and response) of 35 ms, determined by conduction time, delay at synapses and how long it takes the muscle to contract. By comparison it can take almost a second from the first electroencephalographic (EEG) signal of the intention to make a complicated sequence of finger movements and its execution. Reaction times are faster if the necessary response is known ahead of time than if choices must be made.

Motor control modes

The execution of voluntary movements can be controlled in two ways.

1. **Feedback** control. In motor feedback (Fig. 8.53) sense organs (e.g. limb proprioceptors) get signals about limb movement. The nervous system compares this information about the actual trajectory of a movement with that intended. Whenever there is a mismatch (i.e. the movement is not the desired one) an error signal is generated which goes to the motor system to correct its output. It allows a movement to be corrected if unexpected forces operate, but only during the execution (not the planning) of a movement. Feedback is not quick enough to correct fast movements. Feedback also allows **training** of motor skills, i.e. motor learning, by which the execution of motor tasks is improved with practice. The resulting motor programmes can then be used for feedforward control.

2. **Feedforward** control. Essential for fast movements, feedforward works by anticipating what is required of the motor system (see Fig. 8.53). Any given movement depends on a pre-existing motor programme that has previously been learnt, e.g. playing a fast passage on a musical instrument. Its disadvantage is that it cannot compensate for unexpected changes.

Many movements (e.g. catching a ball) use a combination of feedforward (running a motor programme appropriate to the flight of the ball and current posture) and feedback (to fine-tune the arm trajectory as the ball approaches).

SPINAL MOTOR FUNCTION

Reflexes

Motor reflexes generate a **stereotyped** pattern of muscle contraction in response to sensory stimulation. A reflex circuit consists of sensory neurons, motor neurons and, generally, interneurons linking them. Reflexes can be characterised by the number of central synapses in their circuits:

- Reflexes with no interneurons (i.e. the sensory neurons synapse directly with the motor neurons) are **monosynaptic** because there is only one central synapse in the reflex arc.
- Reflexes with exactly one set of interneurons are **disynaptic**.
- Reflexes with many interneurons are **polysynaptic**.

The more synapses, the greater the opportunity for information processing and the more sophisticated the reflex.

Motor neurons receive input from both excitatory and inhibitory interneurons so a stimulus which activates one group of muscles can silence others. This means even apparently simple reflex circuitry is capable of a large and sophisticated repertoire of outcomes, each shaped by the exact context. In addition, reflexes can be altered by experience, that is, their circuits are capable of simple learning. Neurons involved in reflexes are shared by the circuits of central pattern generators (CPGs) responsible for locomotion and are also recruited by descending motor pathways to participate in voluntary movement.

Stretch reflex

Muscle stretch (synonyms: **spindle**, **myotatic**) **reflexes** are referred to by clinicians as **tendon reflexes**. A sharp tap to a tendon stretches the attached muscle and elicits a reflex contraction that restores the muscle to its original length. At its simplest level, this is a negative feedback mechanism that defends muscle length. It is important in posture and locomotion and is modified during voluntary movement.

Muscle spindles

In the stretch reflex, sensory information comes from the **muscle spindle** (Fig. 8.54A), which is a connective tissue capsule containing about seven modified muscle fibres called **intrafusal fibres**. The spindles lie in parallel to the ordinary **extrafusal** (outside the spindle) muscle fibres so they feel the same forces as the muscle. This means that muscle spindles are proprioceptors which measure the length and rate of change of length (velocity) of the muscle. There are two morphological types of intrafusal fibre: **nuclear bag fibres** and **nuclear chain fibres**. The intrafusal fibres have contractile ends (poles), but non-contracting middle

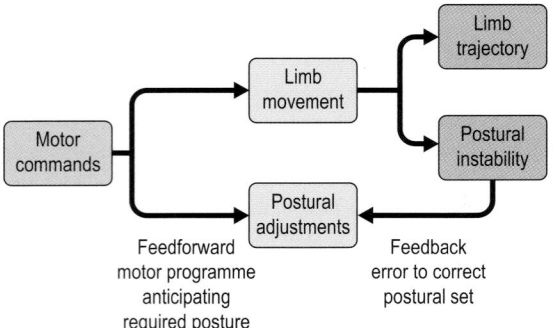

Fig. 8.53 **Feedforward and feedback motor control strategies.**

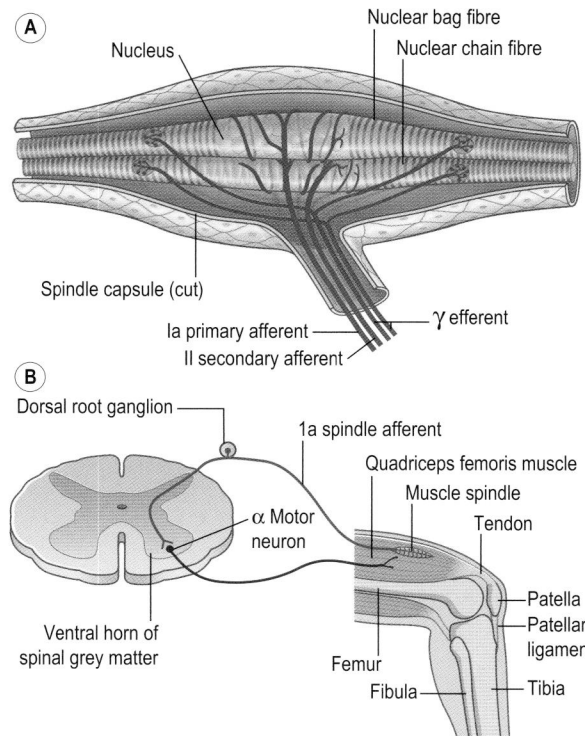

Fig. 8.54 **Stretch reflex**: (A) Structure and innervation of a muscle spindle; (B) myotatic reflex circuitry. Redrawn with permission from Longstaff A 2005 Instant notes in neuroscience, 2nd edn. Taylor & Francis, Abingdon.

regions innervated by two types of myelinated sensory fibre: large diameter **Ia afferents** which innervate both types of muscle spindle, and smaller diameter **II afferents** which are mainly restricted to nuclear bag fibres. The nuclear chain fibres are more numerous.

When the spindle is stretched the central regions of its intrafusal fibres are stretched, which increases the firing of the afferents. When a muscle shortens the spindle relaxes and afferent firing rate drops. The stretch reflex is monosynaptic: the afferents synapse directly with a pool of motor neurons which supply extrafusal muscle fibres in both the same (**homonymous)** muscle and synergist muscles (Fig. 8.54B). The afferents excite the motor neurons so muscle stretch causes contraction that restores the muscles to their pre-stretch length. The overall effect is to bring a limb back to its original position.

The Ia and II afferents convey slightly different sorts of information. So while both types of muscle spindle respond to muscle stretch, the nuclear bag fibres are also sensitive to the rate of muscle stretch.

The contractile poles of the intrafusal fibres are innervated by small diameter myelinated **γ efferents**. Firing of the γ efferents causes the poles of the intrafusal fibres to contract. This permits their central regions to remain taut and sensitive to stretch even as the muscle contracts, so that the stretch reflex works over a wide range of muscle lengths. During a voluntary movement both the γ and α motor neurons are fired simultaneously – **co-activation**. This does two things:

- It prevents the stretch reflex from inhibiting the voluntary movement
- It allows the stretch reflex to continue to operate during the movement and in the new position that results.

Increasing the activation of γ efferents raises the sensitivity of the spindles to stretch and reduces the response time (i.e. it increases the gain of the reflex). This is done when executing movements that are particularly difficult or fast.

Golgi tendon organ reflex

The **Golgi tendon organ reflex** is a negative feedback mechanism which maintains a set point in muscle tension. For example, it allows spinal cord control over the force of contraction.

Golgi tendon organs are proprioceptors which lie in series with muscle fibres and so are able to measure tension in the muscle. The Golgi tendon organ is an encapsulated network of collagen fibres which links a cluster of muscle fibres to their tendon. Interwoven between the collagen fibres are the branches of a **Ib afferent**. An increase in tension straightens the collagen fibres, squeezing the Ib terminals, raising their firing rate.

The **Ib inhibitory interneurons** inhibit α motor neurons to the homonymous and synergist muscles. They also receive input from muscle spindle, joint and cutaneous afferents. These are thought to be important for the spinal control of reaching and grasping. As the hand makes contact with an object the sensory input converging from several sources onto the Ib inhibitory interneurons reduces the force of contraction to give a 'soft landing'.

Flexor reflexes

A variety of afferents (group II and III muscle afferents, joint afferents, skin mechanoreceptors and nociceptors) are collectively known as **flexor reflex afferents** because when stimulated they elicit flexor reflexes of the ipsilateral limb. These reflexes are disynaptic or polysynaptic and their circuitry is also harnessed for normal locomotion, with the exception of that driven by nociceptors. One such flexor reflex is the **flexion withdrawal reflex** made in response to a painful stimulus. It is a protective reflex which involves contraction of limb flexors and inhibition of ongoing locomotion.

Spinal cord circuits

In the spinal cord most of the neural circuits, or networks, that are responsible for reflexes and locomotion depend on a variety of inhibitory mechanisms for their operation. **Glycine** and **GABA** are the major inhibitory neurotransmitters of the spinal cord (see Neurotransmitter systems, above).

Reciprocal inhibition

Many spinal cord circuits involve antagonist pairs of muscles. Sensory Ia afferents also synapse with Ia inhibitory interneurons of the motor neurons of antagonist muscles. Consequently stimuli which activate one set of muscles, suppress the contraction of their antagonists. This is termed **reciprocal inhibition**. It is seen most dramatically in the **crossed extensor reflex** that accompanies the flexion withdrawal reflex. However, most commonly it operates to assist in controlling voluntary movements.

Each movement of a limb involves a sequence of muscle activation: **agonist – antagonist – agonist**. Antagonist activation provides the brake for the movement initiated by the agonist, and the final burst of agonist activation slows the braking. The end result is that the intended limb position is attained without any undershoot or overshoot. Although descending signals trigger each of the phases in the sequence, reciprocal inhibition makes the movement smooth.

Reciprocal inhibition can be suppressed by descending pathways. This allows agonist and antagonist muscles around a joint to be contracted at the same time (**co-contraction**) so as to increase joint **stiffness**. This allows heavy loads to be supported.

Recurrent inhibition

A recurrent connection is one by which a neuron feeds its output back to itself. Where that is done via an inhibitory interneuron the term **recurrent inhibition** is applied. The best studied example in motor systems is mediated by the **Renshaw cells** of the ventral horn.

Renshaw cells are excited by collaterals of α motor neurons and make inhibitory synapses with both the same motor neuron and with motor neurons to synergist muscles. In addition, Renshaw cells inhibit the Ia inhibitory interneuron with the result that antagonist muscles are disinhibited. This has the effect of suppressing weakly firing α motor neurons and dampening strongly firing ones. In this way they modify the descending motor commands to produce an economical movement. Thus, Renshaw cells produce the motor equivalent of surround inhibition in sensory systems.

The importance of this recurrent inhibition is reflected in the convulsions that result from **tetanus** (due to infection with *Clostridium tetani*), or **strychnine** poisoning, both of which disable Renshaw cell glycine neurotransmission.

Presynaptic inhibition

GABAergic inhibitory neurons form axo-axonal synapses on the terminals of Ia, Ib, and II primary afferents. This is called **presynaptic inhibition**. This presynaptic inhibition of Ia afferents influences the muscle spindle reflex by reinforcing the reciprocal inhibition produced by Ia inhibitory interneurons. However, during a movement, presynaptic inhibition is reduced to Ia terminals synapsing with the motor neurons to activated muscle but increased to motor neurons of inactive muscle. In this situation muscle spindle activity enhances contraction, and the presynaptic inhibition flicks from agonist to antagonist and back to agonist.

The existence of separate presynaptic inhibition between Ib afferents allows control of feedback from Golgi tendon organs to be independent of feedback from muscle spindles. This means the CNS can switch between operating in response to muscle length or tension.

Spinal cord injury

Injuries to the spinal cord are most commonly caused by trauma, which can lead to combinations of sensory, motor and autonomic dysfunction that are dependent on the extent and position of the lesion (Clinical box 8.17). Paralysis of the lower limbs (**paraplegia**) results from damage at the thoracic or lumber levels. Depending on the number and level of segments involved, damage at the cervical level can causes paralysis of all four limbs (**quadriplegia**). Spinal cord injuries can also be caused by infections, degenerative diseases such as multiple sclerosis, vitamin B_{12} deficiency, spinal artery occlusion and tumours (primary and secondary).

Complete transection of the spinal cord results initially in **spinal shock** – a general hyperpolarisation of neurons

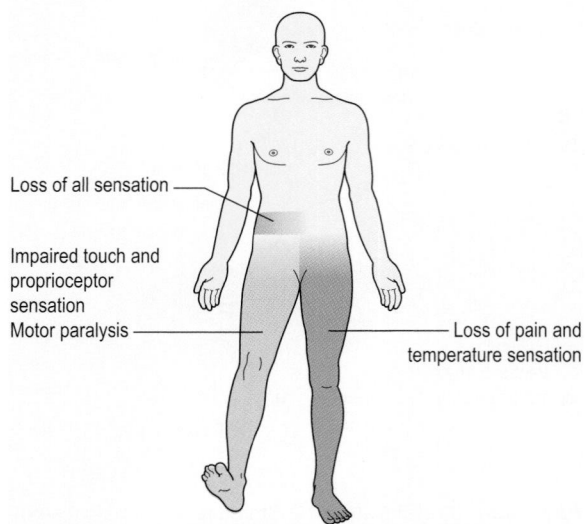

Clinical box 8.17   **Brown–Séquard syndrome**

Lesions confined largely to one side of the spinal cord are surprisingly common and give rise to a characteristic pattern of sensorimotor loss, the **Brown–Séquard syndrome**. There is ipsilateral paralysis, loss of touch and position sense, but contralateral loss of pain and temperature sense because the anterolateral pathway decussates within a couple of segments of the primary afferents (Fig. 8.55).

Loss of all sensation

Impaired touch and proprioceptor sensation

Motor paralysis

Loss of pain and temperature sensation

Fig. 8.55 **Brown–Séquard syndrome.** Cord hemisection on right side at level of T10. The ipsilateral motor deficit is largely an upper motor neuron syndrome.

below the lesion, possibly due to disinhibition of glycinergic interneurons. There is:

- A flaccid paralysis of denervated skeletal muscles
- Loss of muscle tone (**hypotonia**)
- Areflexia
- Loss of all sensation.

In addition, loss of drive to the preganglionic autonomic neurons results in paralysis of bladder and rectum, and loss of vasomotor output causes postural hypotension. After a few weeks, reflexes return with appearance of signs of a lower motor neuron syndrome (see Clinical box 8.20).

Damage to the **cauda equina**, the paired dorsal and ventral roots of spinal nerves L2–C0 which extend caudally from the end of the spinal cord, produce loss of sensation from the perineum, buttocks, bladder and rectum, combined with motor signs in the legs (if the lesion involves S4 or higher), and loss of autonomic control of the bladder and rectum.

Locomotion

Locomotion is movement from one place to another. On land the basic motor pattern is termed stepping and the precise form – or **gait** – this takes (e.g. walking, jogging, running) depends on the intended speed.

The **step cycle** has two phases:

- The **swing phase** starts with bending (flexion) of hip, knee and ankle followed by knee and ankle straightening (extension) in preparation to take the body weight.
- The **stance phase** begins with the foot touching the ground and flexion of the knee and ankle, despite contraction of all limb extensors, due to weight transfer to the limb, and finishes with extension about all joints to provide forward movement.

The step cycles of the two legs are out of phase: when one leg is in the swing phase the other is in the stance phase. When walking, the stance phases overlap, but with increasing speed the stance phases shorten and the overlap vanishes as running speed is attained.

Central pattern generators

The pattern of muscle activity needed for locomotion is orchestrated by **CPGs** (neural networks which produce oscillating output) which are:

- Located in the spinal cord
- Capable of autonomous action though they can be activated by supraspinal signals
- Modulated by proprioceptor input.

Each limb has a CPG and each CPG consists of two circuits called **half-centres**, one driving flexors and the other driving extensors, that reciprocally inhibit one another. While a CPG delivers the basic rhythm to each limb, neurons in the intermediate grey of the cervical spinal cord coordinate the CPGs of the individual limbs, and a **patterning network** between the CPGs and descending motor neurons maintains the appropriate gait.

The output of the half-centres is regulated by input from muscle proprioceptors to determine the length of the stance phase and hence the timing of the swing phase. Activity from muscle spindles determines the end of the stance phase but feedback from Golgi tendon organs can extend it by sensing the load carried by the leg.

Locomotion is normally initiated by the **mesencephalic locomotor region** (MLR). Its output goes to brainstem reticular nuclei that in turn relay to the spinal cord by way of the **reticulospinal tracts**.

BRAINSTEM POSTURAL MECHANISMS

Posture and movement

In order to maintain a stable body position, both at rest and during movements, postural mechanisms operate when forces shift the centre of mass. Posture is maintained largely by muscles which work against gravity, the **anti-gravity muscles**. These are **axial** muscles (trunk extensors), some proximal limb muscles, leg extensors and arm flexors. The required neural networks lie in the medulla, pons and cerebellum and have their outputs via the medial motor pathways.

Postural feedforward

Complex patterns, called motor programmes, run by the motor cortex include commands which drive the postural adjustment necessary during the execution of a movement. For example, for a standing dancer to raise her leg to the side she must shift her centre of mass to above the other leg so that it will continue to support her. This requires feedforward postural adjustments to trunk and arms, which anticipate the unbalancing forces that will act during the movement. The adjustments, termed the **postural set**, depend precisely on the intended movement, and they must be learned.

Postural feedback

Postural adjustments can be corrected during execution by negative feedback, using sensory input, principally vestibular, proprioceptor and visual.

POSTURAL REFLEXES

Postural adjustments are made by three types of reflexes:

- Stretch reflexes, triggered by muscle stretch
- Vestibular reflexes, triggered by gravity
- Tonic neck reflexes, triggered by neck stretch and visual and proprioceptor input.

Vestibular reflexes

Sensory input from otolith organs and semicircular canals is used to stabilise the head relative to space by activating motor neurons to neck muscles (**vestibulocollic** reflexes) or to limb muscles (**vestibulospinal** reflexes) that oppose any disturbance to head and limb positions. Vestibular reflexes are elicited by tilting or rotating head and body as one. By moving limbs, vestibulospinal reflexes shift the centre of mass to help maintain balance, and in falling humans they contract antigravity (extensor) muscles in the legs to prepare to support the body on landing.

Tonic neck reflexes

Proprioceptors in the neck, e.g. muscle spindles, are used to stabilise the head relative to the trunk. Turning the head triggers reflex contraction of neck (**cervicocollic** reflexes) and limb (**cervicospinal** reflexes) musculature. Neck reflexes are elicited by passively moving the trunk while the head is kept motionless in space.

Vestibulospinal reflexes and cervicospinal reflexes are antagonistic. For example, if the head and trunk are tilted to the left, vestibulospinal reflexes extend the left arm, while if the trunk alone is passively tilted to the left, the cervicospinal reflexes flex the left arm. However, in the more usual situation where the head is tilted to the left while the body remains stationary, the two opposing reflexes cancel out.

Righting reflexes use input from a wide range of sensory modalities including the visual system, the vestibular system, proprioceptors and skin mechanoreceptors and muscle spindles. They control trunk, limb and neck muscles to restore the body and head to an upright position from a lying position.

Medial motor pathways

Postural adjustments are made through the medial motor pathways which control the anti-gravity muscles (Fig. 8.56). The medial pathways consist of two separate pathways:

- Vestibulospinal tract
- Reticulospinal tract.

The pathways and their muscle targets are shown in Table 8.16.

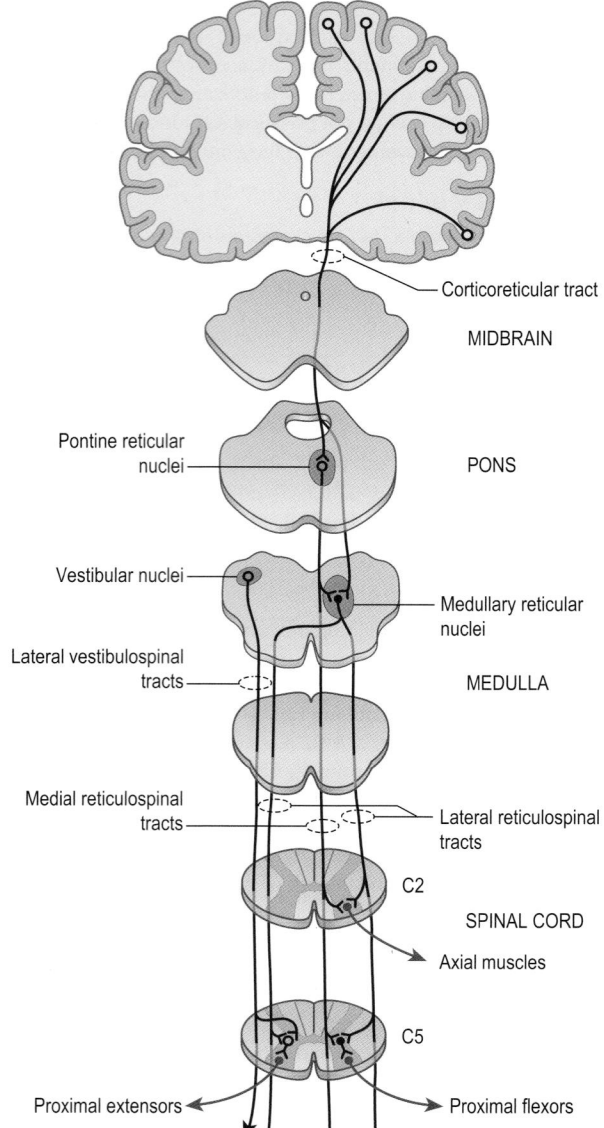

Corticoreticular tract

MIDBRAIN

Pontine reticular nuclei

PONS

Vestibular nuclei

Medullary reticular nuclei

Lateral vestibulospinal tracts

MEDULLA

Medial reticulospinal tracts

Lateral reticulospinal tracts

C2

SPINAL CORD

Axial muscles

C5

Proximal extensors ◄———— ————► Proximal flexors

Fig. 8.56 Medial motor pathways. The medial vestibulospinal tract is omitted for clarity. *Black filled* neurons are inhibitory, *black open* neurons excitatory. *Red* neurons are lower motor neurons. Redrawn with permission from Longstaff A 2005 Instant notes in neuroscience, 2nd edn. Taylor & Francis, Abingdon UK.

Table 8.16	Medial motor pathways		
Tract	**Distribution**	**Main effect* on α-motor neurons**	
		Excitatory to:	**Inhibitory to:**
Lateral vestibulospinal	Ipsilateral	Axial and proximal limb extensors	Axial and proximal limb flexors
Medial vestibulospinal	Bilateral	Ipsilateral axial muscles	Contralateral axial muscles
Pontine (medial) reticulospinal	Ipsilateral	Axial and proximal limb extensors	Proximal limb flexors
Medullary (lateral) reticulospinal	Bilateral	Proximal limb flexors	Axial and proximal limb extensors

*Both direct and indirect (i.e. via interneurons)

Vestibulospinal tracts

The **lateral vestibulospinal tracts** are uncrossed pathways from the **lateral (Deiter's) vestibular nuclei** to spinal segments controlling the limbs. The pathway excites both α and γ motor neurons to proximal limb extensors. Tonic activity in the lateral vestibulospinal tracts provides the extensor tone needed to stay upright. Transient activity in these pathways mediates vestibulospinal reflexes.

The smaller **medial vestibulospinal tracts** are bilateral and originate from the **medial and inferior vestibular nuclei**. They descend via the medial longitudinal fasciculus to terminate on excitatory and inhibitory interneurons in the cervical spinal cord that relay to neck muscle motor neurons. The medial vestibulospinal tracts mediate vestibulocollic reflexes. In general the pattern of muscle activation keeps the head upright when the body is tilted forwards or to the side.

Reticulospinal tracts

The **pontine (medial) reticulospinal tract** is ipsilateral and facilitates extensor motor neurons while the **medullary (lateral) reticulospinal tract** is partly crossed and is excitatory to flexor motor neurons. Damage to reticulospinal pathways can lead to an increase in muscle tone known as spasticity (Clinical box 8.18).

For axial and proximal limb muscles the two reticulospinal tracts synapse with interneurons shared with the corticospinal tract. A single axon may branch to influence motor neurons in several, widely separated, spinal segments. Hence they are probably involved in coordinating the activities of axial muscles and limb central pattern generators during tasks that use muscle groups throughout the body, such as locomotion. The reticular nuclei from which they originate are driven by corticoreticular neurons from the motor cortex. Hence the reticulospinal tracts convey postural instructions from the highest level of the motor hierarchy. They also contain fibres mediating some vestibular and neck reflexes.

CORTICAL CONTROL OF INTENTIONAL MOVEMENTS

Motor cortex

Primary motor cortex

The primary motor cortex (M1, Brodmann's area 4) lies in the frontal lobe immediately rostral to the central sulcus (see Fig.

Clinical box 8.18   **Spasticity and its treatment**

Spasticity is one of the consequences of damage to cortical motor neurons that regulate **muscle tone**, the background level of activity in skeletal muscles. Muscle tone depends on discharge of α motor neurons, but this is established by firing of the γ efferents to muscle spindles.

Normally a rise in muscle tone is brought about by increasing the gain of the muscle spindle reflex, i.e. increasing γ efferent firing rate. However, in spasticity the enhanced muscle tone (**hypertonus**) is not the result of enhanced γ efferent activity but exaggerated drive on α motor neurons from Ia primary afferents. This is due to the loss of presynaptic inhibition on the Ia terminals.

Normally, reticulospinal neurons synapse with presynaptic inhibitory interneurons that release GABA. This acts on both GABA$_A$ and GABA$_B$ receptors to reduce glutamate release from the Ia terminal. The reticulospinal neurons in the brainstem are in turn driven by **corticoreticular axons** that descend with the corticospinal tract (see also Clinical box 8.19).

8.11). It receives input from the somatosensory cortex and contributes the bulk of the corticospinal tract. It has a somatotopic map of body movements in which the hand and face have a very large representation compared with their size (Fig. 8.57). The map explains the pattern of excitation often seen in **Jacksonian epilepsy** in which the seizure often first affects the fingers or face and spreads to other muscles in a defined sequence as the seizure spreads across the motor cortex.

The somatotopic maps in the motor cortex can reorganise as a result of experience. This **cortical plasticity** can be followed using MRI. This could prove useful in studying and improving the rehabilitation of stroke patients.

Motor coding

The motor cortex does not control the activation of single muscles, but instead represents movements. Motor cortex neurons that project directly to lower motor neurons, called **corticomotor neuronal (CM)** cells, have axons that diverge to activate motor neurons for several muscles. This is the case even for neurons which control very fine movements such as the hand. Individual muscles can be activated from several cortical sites, hence many CM cells drive a given muscle. However, individual CM cells only fire in the context of a specific movement; that is, not all CM cells fire whenever their target muscle contracts. For example, a different set of CM cells fire depending on whether a power grip or a precision grip is made with the hand, despite the fact that both sets of CM cells innervate the same muscles.

The motor cortex encodes the magnitude and direction of the force required to produce a given movement. Individual neurons fire preferentially when the limb movement is in a particular direction. However, the cells are very broadly tuned and it is the average firing of a whole population of cells that encodes the precise direction. For individual cells,

the firing frequency also increases with the force needed to perform the task.

Premotor cortex

The **premotor cortex** (Brodmann's area 6) gets sensory – particularly visual – input from areas of the parietal cortex (areas 5 and 7) which is thought to help in guiding movements. Premotor cortex contributes axons to the corticospinal tract; indeed the premotor cortex can control hand movements independently of M1, although its major role is in planning movements. PET scans show that there is activity in the premotor cortex when mentally rehearsing a movement even when it is not actually executed.

There is functional specialisation within the premotor cortex:

- The **pre-supplementary motor area** is responsible for learning new motor sequences.
- The **supplementary motor area**, to which it inputs, sets up movements based on these sequences.
- The **lateral premotor area** learns to make specific movements in response to sensory stimuli and to trigger such movements when the appropriate cue occurs. It also transforms sensory information into signals that can specify the appropriate movement to reach for and grasp objects.

Reaching (which is determined by the object's location) and grasping (which depends on the object's shape) are controlled by different premotor cortex circuits, presumably because they depend on different types of visual information.

Lateral motor pathways

There are two lateral motor pathways for controlling limb movements (Fig. 8.58):

- The **corticospinal tracts** innervate distal muscles and bring about fine movements.
- The **rubrospinal tract** drives proximal limb muscles; it is relatively small in humans and so is not further discussed in this chapter.

Corticospinal tracts

The **corticospinal (pyramidal) tract** contains the axons of CM neurons from the motor and premotor cortex, and fibres from the somatosensory and superior parietal lobe cortex. It descends through the **corona radiata** and **internal capsule** to the brainstem, where **corticonuclear (corticobulbar) fibres** peel off to supply motor nuclei of the cranial nerves supplying face, jaw and tongue muscles (Clinical box 8.19).

At the level of the medulla it forms a ventral swelling termed the **pyramid**, at the lower end of which about 80% of the fibres cross the midline as the **pyramidal decussation**. Most of the contralateral axons descend the length of the spinal cord as the (crossed) **lateral corticospinal tract (LCST)**, the remainder run down the anterior funiculus of cervical and upper thoracic segments as the **anterior corticospinal tract**. The ipsilateral fibres run in the LCST.

All voluntary movement ultimately depends on just one million α **motor neurons (lower motor neurons)** in the brainstem and ventral horn of the spinal cord (Clinical box 8.20).

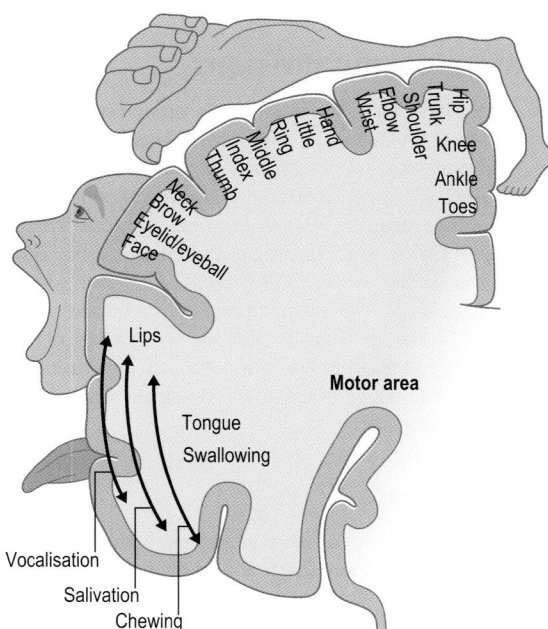

Fig. 8.57 Somatotopic mapping in the primary motor cortex. Compare it with the sensory somatotopic map in Figure 8.28.

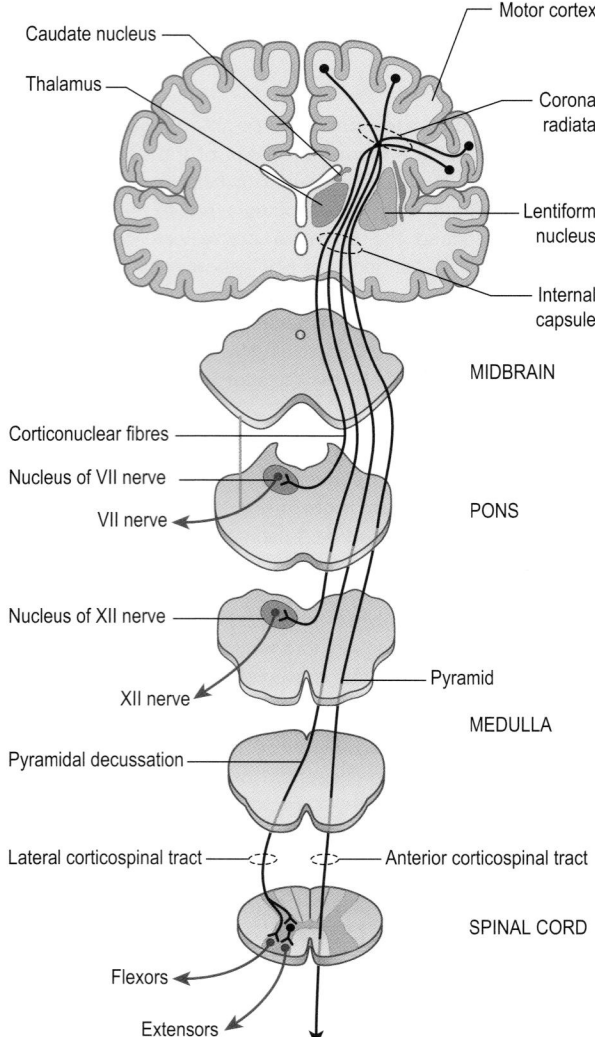

Fig. 8.58 **Lateral motor pathways: the corticospinal and corticobulbar pathways.** The rubrospinal tract is not shown. Only two cranial nerve motor nuclei, facial (VII) and hypoglossal (XII), with their corresponding corticonuclear fibres are depicted.

Clinical box 8.19   **Upper motor neuron syndrome**

Pure lesions of the motor cortex, or of corticospinal fibres above the medulla, initially cause a contralateral flaccid paralysis that is most severe in the limbs. Axial muscles are relatively spared because they are controlled by medial motor pathways. Subsequently there is some return of muscle tone but the ability to make fine movements with distal muscles (e.g. muscles of the hand) is lost. There is no spasticity.

However, generally, lesions (most commonly the result of strokes) damage corticoreticular fibres that descend along with corticospinal fibres so the final clinical picture is of an **upper motor neuron (UMN) syndrome** characterised by:

● **Spasticity**; increased muscle tone (**hypertonus**), hyperactive stretch reflexes and **clonus** (rhythmic, 3–7 Hz contractions of muscle triggered by muscle spindles).
● Hypoactive superficial reflexes (e.g. corneal and superficial abdominal reflex).
● Extensor plantar reflex (**Babinski's sign**), which is extension of the toes on hard stroking of the sole of the foot. Babinski's sign is normal in neonates, in whom the corticospinal tracts are immature.

Clinical box 8.20   **Lower motor neuron syndrome**

Loss of lower motor neuron function results in:

● **Paralysis** (lack of movement) or **paresis** (weakness) of muscles
● Loss of reflexes (**areflexia**)
● **Disuse atrophy** of the affected muscles after just 3 weeks
● **Fasciculations**, contractions of all the muscle fibres in a motor unit caused by spontaneous firing (injury potentials) of damaged α motor neurons
● **Fibrillation**, the spontaneous contractions of individual muscle fibres.

Fibrillation is due to **denervation supersensitivity**; the massive upregulation of nicotinic receptors in denervated skeletal muscle is enough to make the muscle responsive to circulating acetylcholine.

CEREBELLUM

Overview

The cerebellum receives a large number of inputs but produces many fewer outputs, with 40 inputs for every output, and is concerned with ensuring the precision of movements in space and time. It operates in two modes:

■ Feedback mode to correct ongoing movements
■ Feedforward mode, the same corrections are also used to train the feedforward operation in order to perform an improved version of the movement next time, i.e. motor learning.

The basic structure of the cerebellum is relatively simple. The surface of the cerebellum is covered with a three-layered laminar cortex which contains the same basic neural circuit repeated millions of times. Its input comes from the cerebral cortex, via the pons, and from brainstem and spinal cord, conveying both motor and sensory information. The output of the cerebellar cortex is exclusively inhibitory and goes to deep cerebellar nuclei that project predominantly to the cerebral cortex by way of the thalamus (see Fig. 8.52).

Anatomical subdivisions

The cerebellum lies in the posterior fossa and is connected to the dorsal brainstem by three **cerebellar peduncles**. It has two **hemispheres** linked by a midline **vermis**. It is divided into three **lobes** – anterior, posterior and flocculonodular (Fig. 8.59) – by two deep transverse fissures, and further subdivided by shallower fissures into several **lobules**. The surface area of the cerebellar cortex is increased by being thrown into numerous parallel convolutions termed **folia**. Buried within the cerebellar white matter are three pairs of deep cerebellar nuclei that provide the output of the cerebellum, except for the flocculonodular lobe, the output from which is via the vestibular nuclei.

Connections

The cerebellar cortex receives inputs sent from the lateral vestibular nucleus, spinal cord and inferior olive by way of the **inferior cerebellar peduncle**, and from the frontal (motor and premotor) and parietal (sensory) cortex, relayed through **pontine nuclei**, via the **middle cerebellar peduncle** (Fig. 8.60). Most of the output of the cerebellum from the deep cerebellar nuclei leaves by the **superior cerebellar**

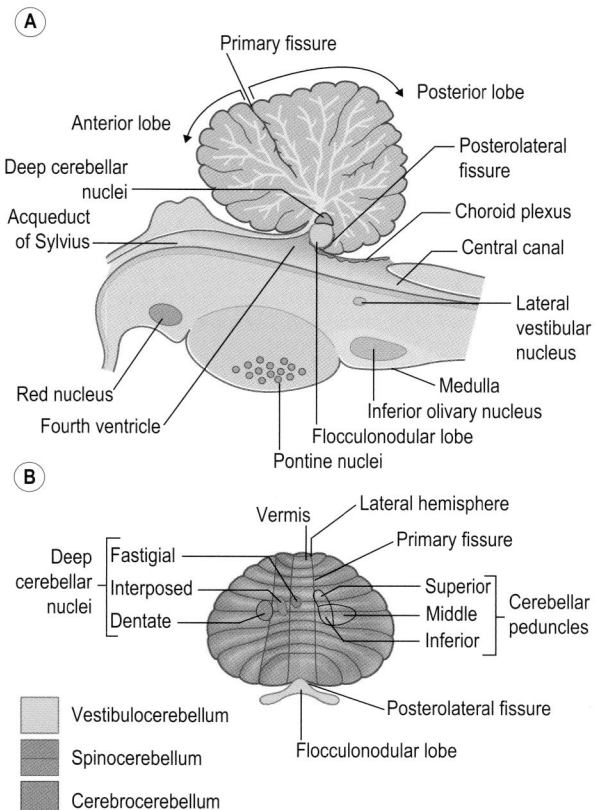

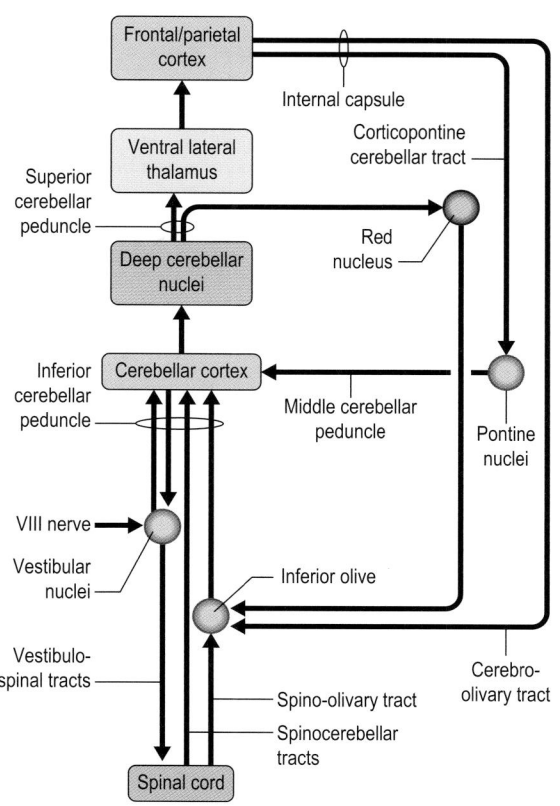

Fig. 8.59 Anatomy of the cerebellum: (A) midsagittal section; (B) flattened view of the cerebellar surface with location of intracerebellar nuclei.

Fig. 8.60 Schematic anatomy of the connections of the cerebellum.

Table 8.17	Input–output relations of the cerebellum				
Input	**Origin**	**Tract**	**Subdivision**	**Output nucleus**	**Destination**
Balance	Inner ear	Cranial nerve VIII	Vestibulocerebellum	Vestibular nuclei	Vestibulospinal tracts
Proprioceptive from face and jaw	Cranial nerve V	Trigeminocerebellar	Spinocerebellum	Globose and emboliform nuclei	Ventral lateral thalamus → cerebral cortex red nucleus (hence lateral motor pathways)
Proprioceptive from neck and arm	Accessory cuneate nucleus	Cuneocerebellar			
Proprioceptive from trunk and leg	Clarke's column	Dorsal spinocerebellar			
Proprioceptive	Ventral horn	Ventral spinocerebellar			
Vision, hearing	Tectum	Tectocerebellar		Fastigial nucleus	Reticulospinal tracts
Sensorimotor	Cerebral cortex → pontine nuclei	Pontocerebellar	Cerebrocerebellum	Dentate nucleus	Ventral lateral thalamus
Motor error signal	Inferior olivary nucleus	Olivocerebellar*	All		

*Climbing fibres, all other inputs are mossy fibres.

peduncle to go to the cerebral cortex via the ventral lateral thalamus, or to the red nucleus.

Functional subdivisions

The cerebellum has three subdivisions (Fig. 8.59B) which can be distinguished on the basis of function and their inputs and outputs:

- Vestibulocerebellum
- Spinocerebellum
- Cerebrocerebellum.

The input–output relations of the functional subdivisions of the cerebellum are summarised in Table 8.17.

Vestibulocerebellum

The **vestibulocerebellum** corresponds to the flocculonodular lobe. Its inputs come from the otolith organs and the semicircular canals. The flocculonodular lobe cortex relays directly with the lateral vestibular nucleus, controlling trunk and proximal limb extensors for posture (via the vestibulospinal tracts), and the medial vestibular nucleus which controls eye movements (Information box 8.21).

Spinocerebellum

The spinocerebellum is concerned with locomotion and posture. The vermis and two paramedian strips, one in each hemisphere adjacent to the vermis, constitute the **spinocerebellum** because it is the only region to get proprioceptor input and information about motor signals from the spinal cord. Additionally, the vermis gets vestibular, visual and auditory input.

Two pathways ascend the spinal cord to provide proprioceptor input to the spinocerebellum:

- The **dorsal (posterior) spinocerebellar tract** originates in the **dorsal (posterior) thoracic nucleus (dorsal nucleus of Clark)**. This receives proprioceptor input from muscles and joints, particularly from muscle spindles, and in addition gets collaterals of cutaneous mechanoreceptor afferents. The dorsal spinocerebellar tract, which serves the legs and trunk, ascends uncrossed to enter the ipsilateral cerebellum through the inferior cerebellar peduncle.
- The **cuneocerebellar tract** comes from the **accessory cuneate nucleus**. It is like the dorsal spinocerebellar tract but serves the arms and neck.

Two pathways supply copies of motor signals driving spinal motor circuits to the cerebellum:

- The **ventral (anterior) spinocerebellar tracts** from the lower part of the cord cross each other, ascend to enter the superior cerebellar peduncle, then cross again so the tract provides input to the ipsilateral cerebellar cortex.
- The **rostral spinocerebellar tract** from the upper cord is uncrossed and goes through the ipsilateral inferior cerebellar peduncle.

The vermis projects to the **fastigial nucleus** which controls trunk and proximal extensor muscles, while the rest of the spinocerebellum relays via the **interposed (globose and emboliform) nuclei** which project to the limb regions of the motor cortex by way of the ventral lateral thalamus. Because the fibres from the interposed nuclei cross the midline and most corticospinal fibres cross back, control by the spinocerebellum is largely ipsilateral.

Motor maps

The spinocerebellum has somatotopic maps in which sensory input and motor output lie in register. Somatotopic maps are also found in the deep cerebellar nuclei and in their targets, namely, the ventral lateral thalamus, red nucleus and inferior olivary nucleus.

Cerebrocerebellum

The largest functional subdivision in humans is the **cerebrocerebellum**, which consists of the lateral parts of

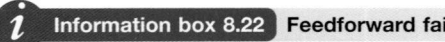

the hemispheres and the **dentate nuclei** which provide its output to the contralateral ventral lateral thalamus and red nucleus.

The cerebrocerebellum is so named because of the massive input it gets exclusively from the cerebral cortex. About 20 million fibres descend widely from the cerebral cortex (alongside the million or so fibres of the corticospinal tract) to terminate in nuclei in the pons. Axons leaving the **pontine nuclei** cross over to enter the cerebellum through the middle cerebellar peduncle. This pathway, the largest in the CNS, is termed the **corticopontinecerebellar tract**.

The cerebrocerebellum coordinates highly skilled limb movements (Information box 8.22) and (together with the vermis) speech. The cerebrocerebellum is also involved in cognitive functions, particularly associated with language.

Cerebellar circuitry

The cerebellar cortex has three layers, which from the inside out are:

- Granule cell layer
- Purkinje cell or piriform layer
- Molecular layer.

In these three layers there are five cell types arranged in a circuit that is copied millions of times (Fig. 8.61).

Granule cells: small (5–8 μm), excitatory (glutamatergic) and the most numerous type of neuron in the human nervous system (estimated approximately 10^{11} cells). Their cell bodies are in the **granule cell layer** and their axons ascend to the **molecular layer**, where they bifurcate to form **parallel fibres** that run for about 6 mm along the long axis of folia.

Purkinje cells: large (50 μm), inhibitory (GABAergic) neurons which are the output neurons of the cerebellar cortex. Their cell bodies are in the **Purkinje cell layer** and they have planar dendritic trees oriented at right angles to the parallel fibres. Each parallel fibre forms a single synapse with each of about 400 Purkinje cells arranged in a row along a folium termed a **microzone**. The effect of one parallel fibre on Purkinje cell firing is minimal but every cell receives synapses from about 200 000 parallel fibres.

The cerebellar cortex also has three types of inhibitory interneuron, all of which are GABAergic.

Basket cells and **stellate cells**, located in the molecular layer, get input from parallel fibres and inhibit adjacent rows

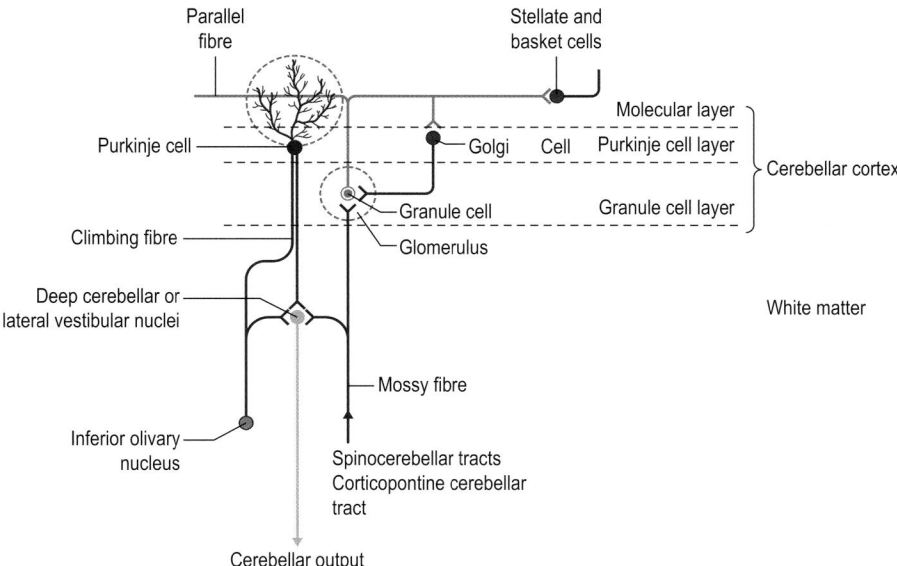

Fig. 8.61 Cerebellar cortical circuitry.

of Purkinje cells. Hence they focus the output of the cerebellar cortex by a sort of motor equivalent to surround inhibition.

Golgi cells which also get input from parallel fibres and synapse in the glomeruli with granule cells. This curtails the firing of Purkinje cells in response to protracted mossy fibre stimulation so Purkinje cells fire only transiently.

Two principal classes of afferent go to the cerebellar cortex – mossy fibres and climbing fibres.

Mossy fibres

The majority of inputs are **mossy fibres** conveying sensory information or motor signals, either from the cerebral cortex or spinal cord and brainstem. Mossy fibres branch at their tip and each branch has a swollen terminal which synapses with the dendrites of several cerebellar granule cells in a structure known as a **glomerulus**.

Climbing fibres

Climbing fibres arise from the inferior olivary nuclei and transmit the error signals needed for negative feedback and motor learning. Each climbing fibre winds its way up a single Purkinje cell, branching to make about 300 excitatory glutamatergic synapses. Every climbing fibre serves about 15 Purkinje cells, but each Purkinje cell gets input from just one climbing fibre. Stimulation of a climbing fibre triggers a burst of action potentials in its host Purkinje cell that is so powerful that for some time afterwards the effect of parallel fibre stimulation is reduced.

Cerebellar role in movement

The length of parallel fibres (6 mm) is sufficient to drive Purkinje cells that serve muscles across several joints. After cerebellar lesions, movements that use several joints are less accurately executed than movements across a single joint. Hence the cerebellum is particularly concerned with multijoint movements.

Generating the feedforward command

Mossy fibres carry either sensory input, informing about the execution of a movement, or copies of motor commands. Mossy fibres have two opposing effects:

- They excite their target cells in deep cerebellar nuclei as they ascend towards the cortex
- They synapse with granule cells whose parallel fibres excite specific microzones of Purkinje cells, which in turn inhibit their target cells in the deep cerebellar nuclei.

At rest the low tonic firing rate of mossy fibres means that excitation of deep cerebellar nuclei dominates inhibition. However, mossy fibre firing increases during voluntary movement and then inhibition of deep cerebellar nuclei cells predominates, which reduces the activity in corresponding cells in the thalamus and motor cortex (Information box 8.23). This pattern of neural activity, a negative image of the input activation, is the feedforward command.

Feedback error correction and motor learning

Climbing fibres come from the contralateral **inferior olivary nucleus** via the **olivocerebellar tract**. The inferior olivary nucleus gets inputs from the sensorimotor cortex via corticospinal collaterals. This brings both sensory information, and motor commands from the premotor area and M1. In addition, the spino-olivary tract sends tactile information to the inferior olivary nucleus.

The inferior olivary nucleus performs two calculations:

- It transforms the sensory signals – which provide information about what movement is actually being executed – into the motor signals that would have been needed to produce them.
- It compares the motor signals derived from the actual movement with the motor commands about the intended movement coming from the motor cortex. If there is a mismatch between them, the inferior olivary nucleus generates a **feedback error signal**.

Climbing fibres are activated when an unexpected force disturbs an ongoing movement, e.g. when lifting an object that is much heavier or lighter than anticipated. Climbing fibres reduce the effectiveness of parallel fibres in activating Purkinje cells, resulting in a pattern of disinhibition of neurons in the deep cerebellar nuclei which corrects errors in execution of ongoing movements. A similar but long-term depression of neurotransmission at the parallel fibre–Purkinje cell synapses occurs when learning new motor skills, e.g. learning to walk or play a musical instruments.

Motor learning writes new feedforward programmes. In learning a new motor skill conscious effort is required to begin with. Here the sensorimotor cortex, acting through the inferior olivary nucleus, is training the cerebellar cortex. Once the cerebellum has learnt the new task it can be executed with no conscious effort.

The inferior olivary nucleus is also involved in precise timing of movements. Olivary nucleus neurons discharge synchronously so that climbing fibres drive their Purkinje cell targets simultaneously.

Red nucleus

The role of the red nucleus is not clear. But it is thought that the red nucleus may generate error signals in response to a mismatch between motor commands at different levels in the motor hierarchy. Brain imaging studies suggest that a loop, which includes the cerebral cortex, cerebellar cortex, the red nucleus and the inferior olivary nucleus, is involved in both motor learning and the mental rehearsal of movements. Mental rehearsal is clearly closely allied to motor learning because it reduces the amount of time needed to perfect a motor skill by practising.

Cerebellar role in cognition

In addition to its role in movement, the cerebellum is implicated in cognitive functions; perhaps acting to detect and correct errors in thought. Evidence for this includes:

- The cerebellum forms multiple closed loop circuits with cortical areas serving cognitive (including language) and affective functions. The 'where' (but not the 'what') visual pathway feeds into the cortico-pontinecerebellar tract, which implies that the cerebellum has a role in spatial cognition and visual guiding of movement.
- A variety of cerebellar lesions may result in cognitive defects and altered mood (Information box 8.24).
- Brain imaging studies have revealed that the neocerebellum is activated during explicit memory and language tasks.

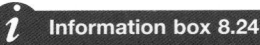

Information box 8.24 | **Cerebellar cognitive deficits**

Cerebellar lesions such as infarcts, olivo-pontinecerebellar atrophy and trauma, as well as surgery, can cause:

- Impaired estimation of elapsed time and poor judgement of the relative speeds of moving objects or relative lengths of tones
- Degraded frontal cortex functions such as abstract reasoning, planning and working memory
- Loss of visuospatial skills, particularly with left-sided damage
- Defects in language, especially with right-sided lesions
- Flattening of affect, particularly associated with vermis lesions.

A constellation of the last four items on this list is called the **cerebellar cognitive-affective syndrome**.

BASAL GANGLIA

The basal ganglia consist of several highly interconnected nuclei that motivate movement and enable specific motor sequences. This is accomplished by modulating the output of the motor cortex; the basal ganglia have no direct output to motor neurons (see Fig. 8.52). While some of the motor sequences are stereotyped, most are learnt. The basal ganglia form part of the extrapyramidal system for motor control, so called to distinguish it from the pyramidal (corticospinal) system, but they are also implicated in cognitive and affective functions.

Functional anatomy

For the gross anatomy of the structures discussed here, see Figure 8.13. The striatum is functionally a single structure split anatomically into the caudate and putamen by the internal capsule. These nuclei receive somatotopically organised, excitatory (glutamatergic) input from the cerebral cortex via the **corticostriatal tract** (see Fig. 8.62). The great majority (>90%) of striatal neurons, called **medium spiny neurons**, use GABA as their classic transmitter and provide the inhibitory output of the striatum. They can be divided into two populations on the basis of their connections and neurochemistry:

- One group of neurons, which have dopamine D1 receptors on their surface, project to the **internal part** of the **globus pallidus** (**GPi**) and **reticular part** of the **substantia nigra** (**SNpr**), which are functionally homologous. The GPi and SNpr relay to the motor cortex and frontal eye fields (prefrontal cortex), respectively, by way of the thalamus, thus forming a circuit – the **direct pathway** (Fig. 8.62 *black arrow*).
- The second group of neurons, which have dopamine D2 receptors, send axons to the **external part** of the **globus pallidus** (**GPe**). The GPe also makes a circuit, the indirect pathway (Fig. 8.62 *red*), via the GPi/SNpr, thalamus and cerebral cortex, but by way of the subthalamic nucleus (STN). The STN gets input directly from the motor cortex and its output to the GPi/SNpr is excitatory.
- Medium spiny neurons receive projections from the largest dopaminergic pathway in the brain, the **nigrostriatal pathway**, which emerges from the **compact part** of the **substantia nigra** (**SNpc**) (Fig. 8.62 *blue*).

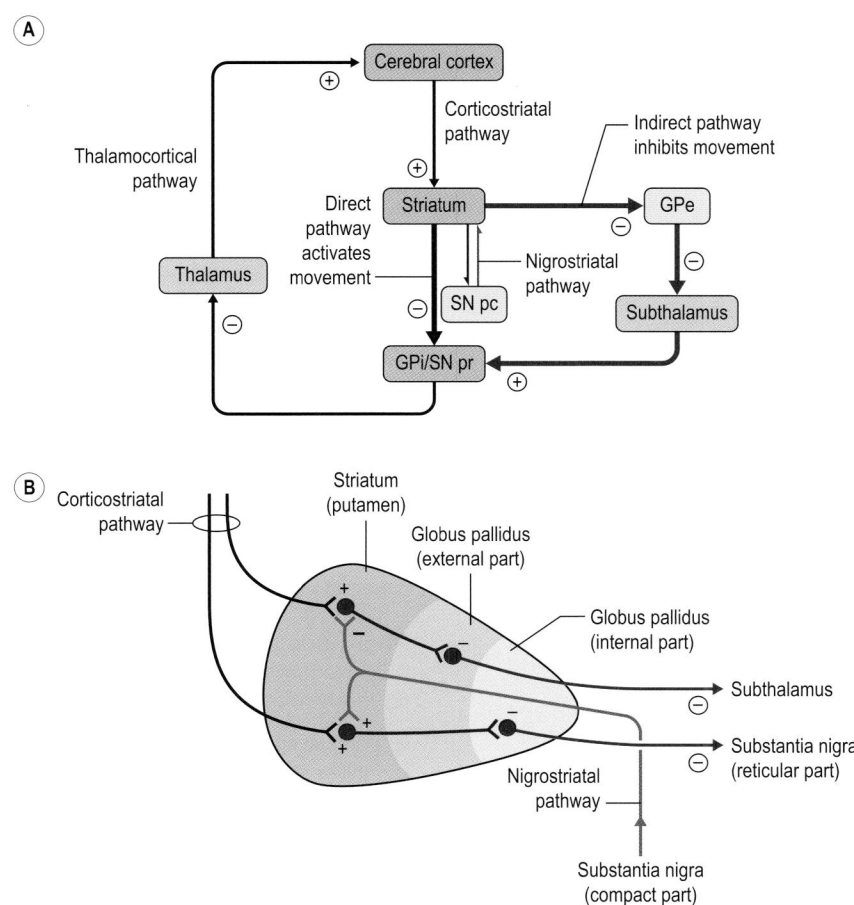

Fig. 8.62 Basal ganglia. (A) Schematic organisation. (B) Differential modulation of direct (*thick black arrow*) and indirect (*red*) pathways by dopaminergic neurons from the compact part of the substantia nigra (*blue*). Excitatory connections, +; inhibitory connections, −. GPi, globus pallidus (internal part); GPe, global pallidus (external part); SN pc, substantia nigra (compact part); SN pr, substantia nigra (reticular part).

Basal ganglia function

The direct and indirect pathways have opposite effects on the firing of neurons in the thalamus and cortex. The direct pathway excites thalamocortical neurons whereas the indirect pathway inhibits them (Clinical box 8.21). It is not clear what the outcome of this differential activity is, but there are two possibilities.

- A movement sequence requires input from direct and indirect pathways to the same set of GPi and SNpr neurons and corresponding thalamic and cortical neurons. In this model the balance of activity in the two pathways determines the amplitude and velocity of movements. Decreased firing of GPi and SNpr neurons permits movements to be produced by the motor cortex. By contrast, increased firing of GPi and SNpr neurons inhibits unwanted movements.
- The direct pathway facilitates a movement sequence by driving one set of thalamocortical neurons, whereas the indirect pathway projects to separate sets of neurons to inhibit conflicting, unwanted motor sequences. This would be the motor homology to surround inhibition seen in sensory systems.

Huntington's disease (HD) is an inherited (autosomal dominant) progressive neurodegenerative disorder in which motor and cognitive symptoms appear in the fifth decade. Medium spiny neurons of the indirect pathway are preferentially killed, so HD can be viewed as a failure of the indirect pathway to suppress unwanted motor sequences (Fig. 8.63A).

The mutation in HD is an excessive number of trinucleotide (CAG) repeats on the huntingtin gene which codes for a long sequence of glutamine (gln) residues on the mature **huntingtin (Htt)** protein. Normal Htt has 9–35 gln residues. The greater the number of CAG repeats in excess of 40 the earlier the age of HD onset. Moreover, above 40 the number of repeats tends to increase from one generation to the next. Hence successive generations of an afflicted family tend to get sick earlier. This pattern implies that the abnormal protein is toxic, i.e. HD is a **gain of function** mutation. However, why striatal medium spiny neurons are selectively killed, when huntingtin occurs in many cell types, is currently a mystery (see also Ch. 5).

Nigrostriatal modulation

The activity of the striatal medium spiny neurons is modulated by the dopaminergic projections from the **nigrostriatal pathway**. Because the two groups of medium spiny neuron have different dopamine receptors they respond differently to this input.

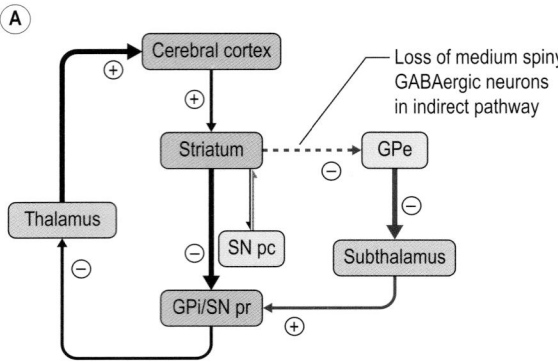

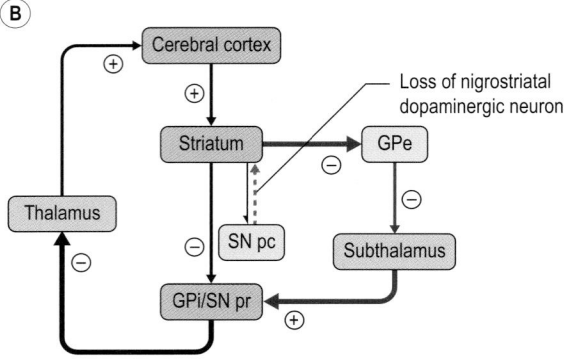

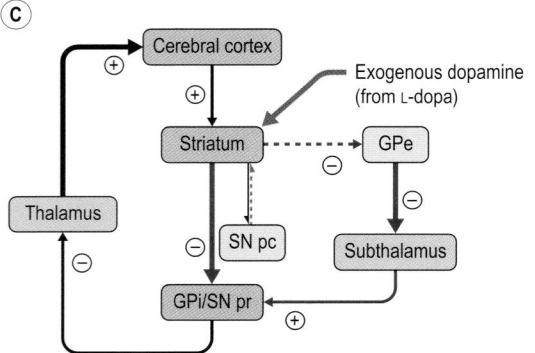

Fig. 8.63 Functional derangements of basal ganglia circuitry: (A) Huntington's disease; (B) Parkinson's disease; (C) L-Dopa-induced dyskinesia. Compare with the normal state shown in Figure 8.62. GPi, globus pallidus (internal part); GPe, global pallidus (external part); SN pc, substantia nigra (compact part); SN pr, substantia nigra (reticular part).

- Direct pathway cells with D1 receptors are made more responsive to cortical inputs.
- Indirect pathway neurons with D2 receptors are inhibited by dopamine release.

Hence activation of nigrostriatal neurons enhances the direct pathway but suppresses the indirect pathway, in effect increasing the chance that a given motor sequence is triggered. In this sense dopaminergic modulation of the basal ganglia motivates movement.

Parkinson's disease

Parkinson's disease (PD) is the commonest of the **hypokinesias** – disorders characterised by a poverty of spontaneous movement. The cardinal features of PD are:

- **Tremor** due to alternate activation of agonist and antagonist muscles, particularly around distal limb joints
- **Rigidity** due to an increase in passive muscle tone in extensors and flexors
- **Bradykinesia** (slowness in executing movements).

Pathophysiology

PD is caused by a loss of the dopaminergic neurons of the nigrostriatal pathway. This causes a failure in dopaminergic inhibition of medium spiny neurons in the striatum that comprise the indirect pathway. This results in excessive inhibition of the GPe by the striatum and disinhibition of the subthalamic nucleus (Fig. 8.63B). The increased excitatory drive from the STN to its targets (GPi and SNr) reduces the activity of the thalamocortical neurons and this is assumed to account for the bradykinesia.

The origin of the tremor is less clear since rhythmical, synchronised firing of several structures (GPe, GPi, STN and thalamus) is associated with it. Both thalamic and STN neurons are capable of spontaneous, periodic burst firing under appropriate conditions.

Pharmacological treatment

Drug treatment for PD is targeted at a number of neurochemical mechanisms (see also Ch. 4):

- Stimulating dopamine release (amantadine)
- Inhibiting dopamine catabolism by blocking monoamine oxidase B (selegiline)
- Providing a dopamine precursor (L-dopa)
- Activating dopamine D2 receptors (e.g. bromocriptine).

The most commonly used drug is **L-dopa** (L-3,4-dihydroxyphenylalanine), the precursor of dopamine, which readily crosses the blood–brain barrier. In early stages of the disease L-dopa is transported into remaining nigrostriatal terminals and decarboxylated to dopamine, which is released in a physiologically appropriate manner (Fig. 8.63C). This provides good control for the first few years of treatment. However, the drug does not curtail continuing loss of SNpc cells, so that eventually, in the absence of dopaminergic terminals, it is taken up by serotonergic terminals, which decarboxylate it, but from which the dopamine leaks.

Within two years of starting treatment the majority of patients develop **dyskinesia** (involuntary writhing movements of face and limbs) at L-dopa doses needed to completely suppress the PD symptoms. The precise cause of dyskinesia is uncertain but probably results from longlasting synaptic changes which alter the balance of activity in direct and indirect pathways in the basal ganglia.

Long-acting **dopamine agonists**, which mimic more closely the tonic exposure of dopamine receptors to transmitters that occurs physiologically than does L-dopa treatment, do not cause dyskinesia.

Surgical treatment

Hyperactivity of the STN is an essential feature of PD. This drives GPi and SNr cells to excessive inhibition of their thalamic and cortical targets. These observations form the basis for surgical treatment which involves making selective lesions of the STN or GPi, or producing functional blockade of these structures by **deep brain stimulation**, in which currents are delivered through chronically implanted electrodes. Brain imaging reveals increased cortical activation after these treatments, in parallel with clinical improvement. It is thought that the surgery is effective because under normal circumstances it is silencing of GPi and SNr neurons that, by disinhibition of their thalamocortical target cells, allows movements to be generated by the motor cortex.

A promising approach is the injection of dopaminergic cells (e.g. produced from immortalised neural stem cells) into the striatum; these survive to form synapses with striatal neurons and secrete dopamine.

Parallel circuits

As well as the motor loop described above, the basal ganglia have other non-motor **basal ganglia circuits** which, operating as described above, run in parallel through the basal ganglia. Each has inputs from several functionally related cortical regions which converge and project back to a much more limited part of the cortex. This pattern presumably provides for integration of several different types of information.

One of these circuits, called the **oculomotor loop**, is concerned with the control of saccades. In PD, neuronal degeneration in the substantia nigra causes oculomotor hypokinesia where some saccades are slow or inadequate. Other loops are involved in executive motor planning (**cognitive loop**) and the expression of emotions (**limbic loop**). Damage to these non-motor areas of the basal ganglia have been hypothesised in disorders such as Tourette's syndrome, obsessive compulsive disorders and schizophrenia.

Control of eye movements

Eye movements either **stabilise** the gaze during head rotation, or shift the gaze so as to track a moving object or jump to a different part of the visual scene.

Control of gaze
Gaze stabilisation
Gaze stabilisation during rapid head rotation is controlled by **vestibulo-ocular reflexes** on the basis of signals from the semi-circular canals, whereas gaze stabilisation during slow head movements is monitored visually and activates **optokinetic reflexes**. The eye movements are in the opposite direction to the head movement and matched for velocity so that the image does not shift on the retina.

Gaze shift
There are three types of **gaze shift**:

- **Saccades** are extremely rapid eye movements that bring new targets onto the fovea where vision is most acute.
- Shifting the gaze to follow a moving target is termed **smooth pursuit** and is a voluntary movement much slower than saccades.
- In the **vergence reflex**, required for stereopsis, the gaze of both eyes is changed to see an object that is getting closer or receding.

In saccades and smooth pursuit the eye movements are **conjunctive** in that both eyes move in the same direction. However, in the vergence reflex they are **disconjugate** – the eyes move in opposite directions – either converging or diverging.

Extraocular eye muscles and eye movements
Each eye is moved by three pairs of **extraocular (skeletal) muscles**:

- Lateral and medial rectus
- Superior and inferior rectus
- Superior and inferior oblique.

The rectus muscles originate from the annular tendon fixed to the rear of the orbit and insert into the sclera in front of the equator of the eyeball (Fig. 8.64). The oblique muscles have attachments behind the equator of the eyeball.

Eye movements
Working together the extraocular muscles rotate the eye about three **principal axes**:

- Rotation about the vertical axis produces motion in the horizontal plane, adduction (towards the nose) or abduction (away from the nose).
- Rotation about the horizontal axis produces movement in the vertical plane, elevation or depression of the eyeball.
- Rotation about the anteroposterior axis brings about intorsion (a rotation of the top of the eyeball towards the nose) or extorsion (rotation of the top of the eyeball away from the nose).

The extraocular muscles are arranged in six complementary pairs which, except for vergence, move the two eyes so that their visual axes point in the same direction. Thus when looking to the left, the left eye is abducted by its lateral rectus while the right eye is adducted by its medial rectus. In vergence that switches gaze to a nearer object, the medial rectus muscles are used to adduct both eyes. The actions of the four remaining muscles are more complicated because they pull in directions that are a combination of vertical and torsional components, and the relative size of these components depends on the horizontal position of the eye.

Innervation of extraocular muscles
The extraocular muscles are innervated by motor neurons of the oculomotor (III), trochlear (IV) and abducens (VI) cranial nerves (Table 8.18). Damage to these nerves causes typical

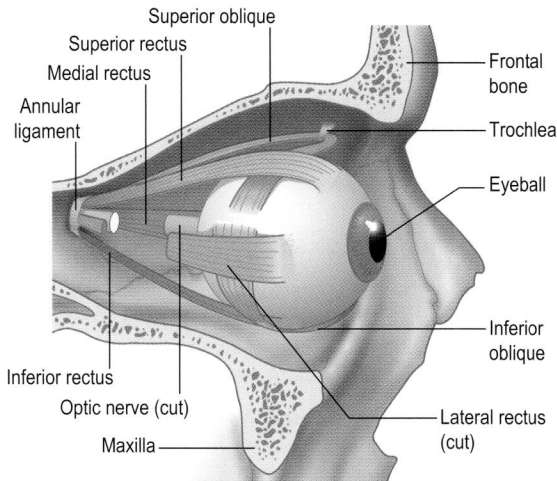

Fig. 8.64 **Extraocular muscles of the right orbit.**
Redrawn with permission from Longstaff A 2005 Instant notes in neuroscience, 2nd edn. Taylor & Francis, Abingdon UK.

Table 8.18 Innervation and actions of extraocular muscles

Muscle	Nerve	Movement	Direction of weakness after nerve injury	Direction of gaze causing double vision	Complementary muscle in contralateral eye
Lateral rectus	VI	Abduction (out)	In (convergent squint)	Out	Medial rectus
Medial rectus	III	Adduction (in)	Out (divergent squint)	In	Lateral rectus
Superior rectus	III	Elevation after abduction (up and out)	Down and in	Up and out	Inferior oblique
Inferior oblique	III	Elevation after adduction (up and in)	Down and out	Up and in	Superior rectus
Superior oblique	IV	Depression after adduction (down and in)	Up and out	Down and in	Inferior rectus
Inferior rectus	III	Depression after abduction (down and out)	Up and in	Down and out	Superior oblique

Clinical box 8.22 **Oculomotor disorders**

Squint (strabismus) is convergent if the visual axes cross or divergent if the visual axes diverge.

- **Paralytic squint** is an acquired defect in an extraocular muscle or its innervation and causes double vision.
- **Non-paralytic squint** is a developmental defect, manifesting early in childhood, in which the deviating eye moves so that the squint is the same for all directions of gaze, and there is no double vision.

If non-paralytic squint is not corrected very early – usually surgically by functionally shortening the appropriate muscle – the visual system wires itself to ignore the signals from the affected eye (unless the normal eye is closed) resulting in a functional blindness in the squinting eye termed **amblyopia**, in which stereopsis is permanently impaired.

Double vision (diplopia) generally accompanies paralysis of a cranial nerve controlling eye movements and is caused by the inability of the visual system to implement stereopsis when the visual axes of the two eyes are misaligned. Diplopia occurs when attempting to look in the direction that compensates for the eyeball deviation caused by the damage (see Table 8.18).

changes in gaze and/or double vision (Clinical box 8.22). The gaze stabilisation and gaze shift pathways terminate in several nuclei in the brainstem reticular formation. One nucleus organises horizontal eye movements while another is responsible for vertical eye movements. The trajectory of an eye movement is specified by the relative activation of these two nuclei. These innervate cranial nerve nuclei which give rise to lower motor neurons which go to the extraocular muscles.

CENTRAL CONTROL OF AUTONOMIC MOTOR SYSTEMS

The output pathways of the autonomic nervous system (Ch. 4) are modulated by sensory input and coordinated with other behaviours by **central autonomic networks** in the brainstem and forebrain.

Autonomic reflexes

The nucleus of the solitary track receives visceral (e.g. chemoreceptor, baroreceptor) and gustatory afferents in the facial (VII) and glossopharyngeal (IX) and vagus (X) cranial nerves (Fig. 8.65). Its principal outputs are to:

- **Medullary reticular formation** vasomotor and cardio-accelerator neurons that project to preganglionic sympathetic neurons.
- **Dorsal vagal nucleus** and **salivary nuclei**, which send parasympathetic output via the VII, IX and X cranial nerves to the gut.
- **Nucleus ambiguus** which sends parasympathetic output to the oesophagus, heart and airways and which also has special visceral motor neurons supplying striated muscle in the pharynx and larynx for controlling swallowing.

Integration of autonomic responses and behaviour

The visceral sensory input is also relayed to the **parabrachial nucleus**, which has reciprocal connections to structures that generate the autonomic components of more complex behaviours, including:

- Periaqueductal grey matter – which organises vasomotor 'fight and flight' responses
- **Visceral thalamus** – which projects to **limbic cortex** for conscious visceral perception
- Amygdala – which is concerned with learned responses to visceral and taste stimuli
- Hypothalamus.

The hypothalamus organises the autonomic and endocrine aspects of goal-directed behaviours such as feeding, drinking, sexual and reproductive behaviour, and thermoregulation, largely by way of feedback mechanisms, many of which are homeostatic. To accomplish this it has inputs from the viscera, olfactory system and retina, responds to a multitude of circulating signals which convey information about the metabolic state (e.g. osmolality, Na^+, angiotensin II, glucose, leptin) and has outputs to preganglionic autonomic neurons in the brainstem and intermediolateral columns of the spinal cord. The hypothalamus is also responsible for autonomic and endocrine correlates of emotion.

Examples of central autonomic control

Thermoregulation

The core of the body, the contents of the cranium, thorax and abdomen, and limb tissue inside the insulating subcutaneous fat layer, is maintained at about 37°C by behaviour and homeostatic physiological mechanisms (see Ch. 1). A naked resting adult is in thermal equilibrium at an ambient temperature of about 28°C in still air at 50% relative humidity. Any deviation from this condition requires thermoregulation.

There are two ways in which humans thermoregulate:

- Changes in behaviour, such as seeking sun or shade, are required to protect against large swings from thermoneutrality.

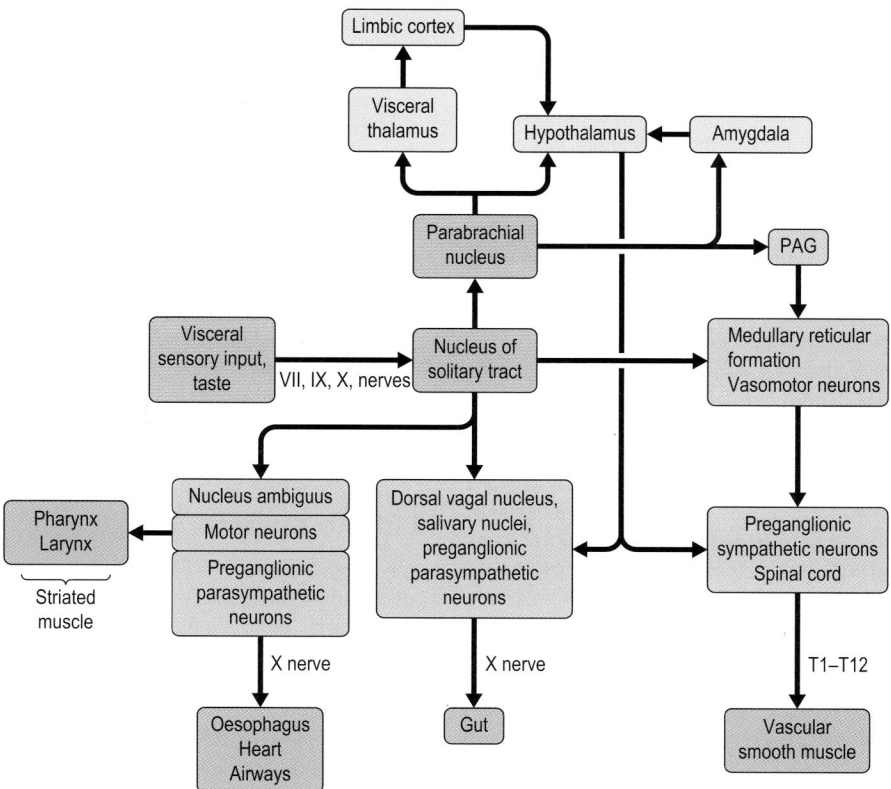

Fig. 8.65 **Central autonomic networks.** PAG, periaqueductal grey.

- Physiological adjustments, such as autonomic regulation of skin blood flow and sweating, and shivering can defend the core temperature against more modest deviations.

The central control of thermoregulation depends on integration of signals from two types of thermoreceptors.

- **Cutaneous thermoreceptors** – which convey information about skin temperature via the anterolateral pathways (see Thermoreceptors, above).
- **Internal warm thermoreceptors** – located in the preoptic nucleus of the hypothalamus and cervical spinal cord, which monitor core temperature.

Both of these sources send input to the posterior hypothalamus. This structure acts as a thermostat. It has temperature-insensitive interneurons, the signal from which is a set point, the core temperature which the thermoregulatory mechanisms attempt to maintain. The thresholds for triggering thermoregulatory responses are functions of the set point, core temperature and skin temperature. For example, during exercise, core temperature (monitored by internal warm thermoreceptors) will rise above the set point, but the degree of sweating for a given core temperature is proportionally less when the skin is colder.

In health the set point is altered by:

- **Circadian rhythm**, with lowest core temperature at night
- **Hormone status**, e.g. it increases about 0.5 °C due to the rise in progesterone during the luteal phase of the menstrual cycle (see Ch. 10)
- **Chronic exposure** to heat or cold.

The fever that can accompany infections is caused by re-setting of the set point by cytokines; e.g. macrophages challenged by bacterial endotoxins secrete interleukin 1 and virus-infected cells release interferons (see Ch. 6). The rise in core temperature – if not excessive – is adaptive as it:

- Raises metabolic rate, increasing the rate of immune responses, e.g. antibody synthesis
- Compromises growth of microorganisms.

Regulation of sexual function

The neural organisation of sexual responses in men and women appear to be broadly similar (see also Ch. 10). Initially the physiological effects of sexual arousal rely on parasympathetic activation which can be reflex, due to stimulation of erogenous zones (e.g. external genitals, breasts), or brought about by psychological arousal.

Erection of the penis or clitoris results from activation of sacral parasympathetic neurons to arteriolar sphincters. ACh triggers the synthesis of nitric oxide, which promotes relaxation of the vascular smooth muscle by raising cGMP concentration, increasing blood flow into the corpora cavernosa. As these structures swell they compress the veins that drain them and the erection becomes self-sustaining. Sildenafil (marketed as Viagra), used for erectile dysfunction in men, works by inhibiting the cGMP phosphodiesterase responsible for degrading cGMP.

In women, parasympathetic activation contributes to two additional responses:

- Vasocongestion, increased blood flow into pelvic tissues, most noticeably the labia minora and walls of the vagina, so that they become swollen

- Transudation, the secretion of a lubricating fluid through the squamous vaginal epithelium.

As the level of excitement rises, sympathetic neurons in the thoracolumbar cord are activated. In men, these generate contractions of smooth muscle of the epididymis, vas deferens, prostate and seminal vesicles. This drives sperm-laden seminiferous tubule fluid and glandular secretions into the posterior urethra (ejaculatory duct). This process is termed **emission**. In addition, sympathetic stimulation closes the internal urethral sphincter to prevent back flux of semen into the bladder. Sympathetic activity probably also plays a part in vasocongestion and transudation in women.

Emission excites afferents in the posterior urethra, prostate, seminal vesicles and vas deferens which drive motor neurons to the pelvic floor muscles so that they produce a series of clonic contractions, causing **ejaculation**. During this time, which corresponds to the orgasm, there is maximum parasympathetic and sympathetic outflow to the genitals. In women, clonic contractions of pelvic muscles also accompany orgasm and the trigger is afferents in the clitoris. In addition, the high sympathetic activity causes uterine contractions which open the cervix.

Reflex erection can usually be elicited after spinal cord transection. Even destruction of the sacral cord does not eliminate it in about 25% of men. In these individuals psychogenic erection might be driven by a cholinergic sympathetic supply. Spinal transection above T6 generally abolishes emission, ejaculation and orgasm, whereas they are often preserved with transections at lower levels.

BRAIN STATES

Behaviour, be it moving or thinking, is not just determined by current sensory input. Crucially, it also depends on emotions (affect), motivation, level of arousal (sleep-wakefulness), and prior experience (learning and memory). These can be thought of as global brain states in the sense that they are brought about by mechanisms that engage much of the nervous system.

EMOTION

Emotion may be defined as the unconscious evaluation of a situation as potentially harmful or beneficial. A **feeling** is the conscious experience that corresponds to an emotion. Emotions arise in response to changes in the state of the world that could have important consequences. Some emotional responses (e.g. fear of snakes) are hard-wired but most are probably learnt. Note that hard-wired responses need not be forever fixed.

Emotional states have three components:

- A visceral sensory component caused by autonomic and endocrine events
- A motor component, particularly involving the facial muscles
- A cognitive component.

Feelings encompass the perception of changes in the viscera and conscious analysis of the situation (cognition). It is likely that these two aspects of the emotional state are self-reinforcing because there are learned associations between visceral sensations and emotional states. Realisation of just how bad or good a situation is drives visceral changes, while conscious efforts to stem visceral sensation (e.g. controlled breathing) lessens emotional intensity.

Emotions have survival value for several reasons:

- They are arousing and direct attention to important aspects of a situation so that it can be assessed as threatening or beneficial.
- Emotions are goads to useful action – we usually avoid scorpions but try to spend time with those we love.
- Motor components of emotions (e.g. laughing or crying) communicate our emotional state to others, altering their behaviour. This is crucial for social interactions. Before they acquire language infants can only communicate needs and desires by expressing their emotions.

Limbic system

The limbic system is the part of the brain most closely associated with emotion. It is evolutionarily old; it is found in fish, amphibians, reptiles and mammals. It controls emotional behaviour, including goal-directed behaviours, and the formation of memories.

Affective basal ganglia loop

The core of the limbic system consists of the affective basal ganglia loop and its connections with the amygdala, which is responsible for fear learning (Fig. 8.66). The striatal component of the affective loop is termed the **nucleus accumbens (ventral striatum)** and is a major target of the dopaminergic mesolimbic brain reward system. The output of the nucleus accumbens goes to the compact part of the substantia nigra. This allows the activity of the other basal ganglia loops to be modified, providing for some of the motor and the cognitive aspects of emotional states (Clinical box 8.23).

Affective motor pathways

Facial expressions engendered by emotions, e.g. smiling, frowning, crying etc., are brought about by extrapyramidal motor pathways that run in the brainstem reticular formation (Clinical box 8.24).

Clinical box 8.23   Obsessive-compulsive disorder

Obsessive-compulsive disorder (OCD) is a chronic condition in which obsessions (intrusive thoughts) and compulsions (repetitive actions such as hand washing) occupy much of the time. Individuals with OCD recognise that their behaviour is irrational, but feel irresistibly compelled to continue with it and experience great anxiety if they cannot.

PET scans of patients with OCD show hyperactivity of structures (e.g. the head of the caudate) that form the **orbitofrontal basal ganglia circuit**. Lesions of the orbitofrontal cortex cause primates to persevere with actions long after they have ceased being rewarded.

Clinical box 8.24   Expressing emotion

Patients with unilateral damage to corticobulbar fibres descending from the motor cortex have voluntary motor paresis on the opposite side. When asked to smile on demand their smile is lopsided. However, when genuinely amused their smile is natural and bilateral (**Duchenne smile**) because different emotion-driven motor pathways are engaged.

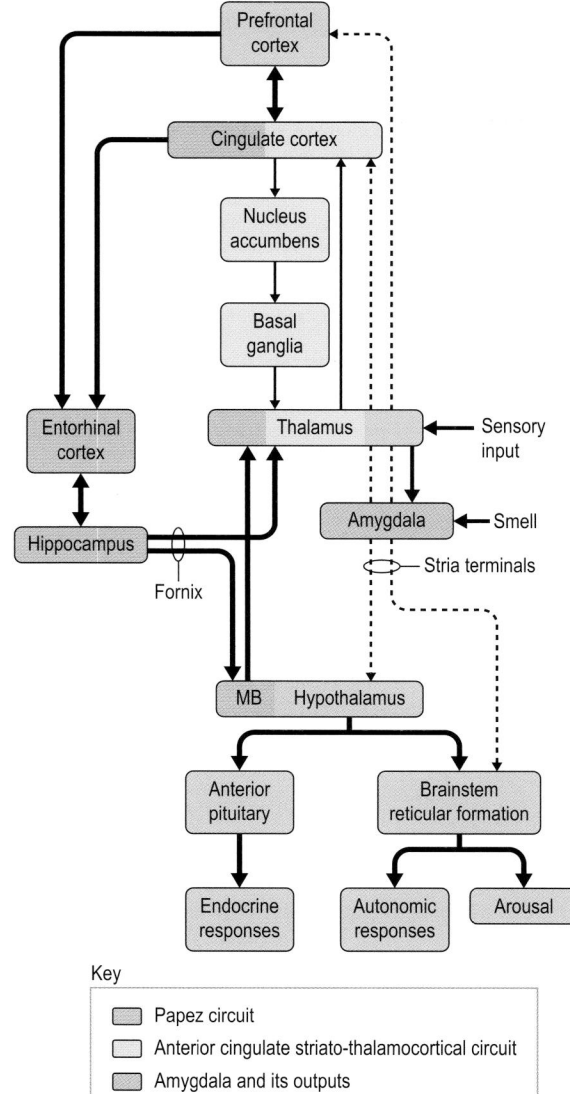

Fig. 8.66 Circuitry involved in emotions. MB, mamillary bodies.

Key
- Papez circuit
- Anterior cingulate striato-thalamocortical circuit
- Amygdala and its outputs

Table 8.19	Functions of amygdala outputs
Output target/pathway	**Effect**
Periaqueductal grey/raphespinal tract	Decreased pain transmission
Periaqueductal grey/reticulospinal tract	Fear responses
Nucleus coeruleus	Arousal
Noradrenergic cells in medulla/preganglionic sympathetic neurons	Cardiovascular fear responses (e.g. tachycardia)
Hypothalamus/dorsal vagal nucleus	Bradycardia (vasovagal syncope)
Hypothalamus (arcuate nucleus)	Release of corticotropin-releasing hormone
Parabrachial nucleus/medulla respiratory neurons	Hyperventilation

Amygdala

The amygdala is a limbic system structure concerned with innate and learned fear responses and avoidance behaviour, along with recognition of emotions in facial expressions.

Functional anatomy and connections

The **amygdala** is a cluster of nuclei in the white matter of the temporal lobe, lying anterior to the tail of the caudate nucleus. Sensory information enters the **basolateral nuclei** from the specific thalamic nuclei and their corresponding areas of sensory cortex. The basolateral nuclei also receive input from other limbic structures. Olfactory input occupies a separate stream running from the olfactory bulb to the **corticomedial nucleus**.

The output of the amygdala is from its **central nucleus** and follows two anatomical pathways. Efferents to the hypothalamus, septum, and several brainstem nuclei go via the **stria terminalis**, while the **ventral amygdalofugal pathway** conveys connections to the nucleus accumbens. The functions of these outputs in the expression of emotions is summarised in Table 8.19.

Fear learning

The amygdala can produce automatic fear responses to universal aversive stimuli (e.g. snakes) which seem to be hardwired, that is established before birth and not requiring experience and learning. It also learns associations between new aversive stimuli and the visceral arousal and motor responses of fear states produced by them. Thus armed, the amygdala can trigger fright, flight and fight responses to a threatening situation before there is conscious recognition of the situation. Emotional memories are not stored in the amygdala but in the cerebral cortex with which it is connected. Presentation of fear-evoking stimuli activates visual association cortex and orbital prefrontal cortex as well as the amygdala.

Development of fear learning

In the amygdala, fear learning is unconscious (implicit, see Procedural (motor) learning, below), which means that it cannot be consciously recalled, although presentation of the appropriate stimulus will generate fear responses. In infancy and early childhood the amygdala develops more rapidly than the hippocampus (responsible for explicit memory). During this time fearful memories may be acquired which

Papez circuit and learning

The affective loop is wired into a second (**Papez**) circuit.

1. The anterior cingulate cortex projects to the entorhinal cortex that acts as a gateway for all neocortical input to the hippocampus.
2. Efferents leave the hippocampus by way of the **fornix** for the hypothalamus.
3. Output from the mamillary bodies (by way of the **mamillothalamic tract**) goes via the **anterior thalamic nuclei** back to the anterior cingulate cortex.
4. The hypothalamus also has connections with the prefrontal cortex.

The Papez circuit was originally thought to be the circuit for emotion, but the well-established function of the hippocampus in memory consolidation shows its role to be more restricted, being largely involved in explicit learning during emotional states.

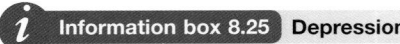
cannot later be consciously accounted for. This could underlie some specific phobias (Clinical box 8.25).

Emotion recognition

An important role of the amygdala is recognising emotions in facial expressions. Activity is increased in the amygdala in subjects shown fearful faces, and in the left amygdala the extent of the response increases the more fearful the expression. In patients with damage to the amygdala the ability to recognise fearful expressions is impaired, even though they are still able to identify individual faces. This confirms that the neural system for emotional memory is distinct from that for explicit memory of faces.

Neocortex and emotion

Extensive interconnections between different parts of association neocortex allows cognition to influence emotional states (despite feeling anxious we do sit the examination, because we recognise that in the longer term it will bring benefits), and vice versa (we know that the chance of our child being harmed on walking to school alone is negligible, but we feel sufficiently anxious to accompany her anyway).

The prefrontal cortex has extensive connections with brain structures implicated in emotion, including the amygdala, nucleus accumbens and hypothalamus. PET scans show decreased activity in the **prefrontal cortex** in patients suffering from depression (Information box 8.25). Lesions of the same region make it difficult for people to express emotions and they have abnormal autonomic responses to emotive stimuli.

Lesions of the orbital prefrontal cortex reduce emotional responses (e.g. aggression) in primates, while in humans lesions of the anterior cingulate cortex reduce the emotional distress of chronic intractable pain.

MOTIVATION AND GOAL-DIRECTED BEHAVIOURS

A variety of internal states that are intimately linked to emotions drive **goal-directed behaviours**. The process that leads from internal state to such behaviours is termed **motivation**. Goal-directed behaviours are purposeful actions aimed at achieving a specific outcome. The term is used to characterise behaviours that fulfil well-defined physiological needs (e.g. drinking and feeding), but also those which encompass more abstract and long-term goals, such as being successful at work.

Some motivated behaviours, such as drinking and feeding, are clearly homeostatic, and normally self-limiting in that the internal states that drive them, thirst and hunger, are sated by consumption. Others are not so straightforward:

sexual behaviour leading to copulation, although not homeostatic, does have an internal state (libido) which can be sated, whereas parenting behaviour is neither homeostatic nor self-limiting and almost nothing is understood about the internal state that motivates it.

Motivation: the brain reward system

The motivation of behaviour is thought to come about by modulation of the affective basal ganglia loop by a brain reward system. This consists of dopaminergic neurons in the **ventral tegmental area** (**VTA**) which project their axons to the nucleus accumbens, striatum and other limbic structures as the **mesolimbic system**, and to the frontal cortex as the **mesocortical system**. The brain reward system is responsible for the positive reinforcing properties of natural rewards (such as food, drink and sex). Natural rewards, self-stimulation (through implanted electrodes), and addictive drugs all increase dopamine release from mesolimbic terminals in the nucleus accumbens, and the reinforcing properties of these stimuli are blocked by dopamine receptor antagonists.

Firing of mesolimbic neurons in response to a natural reward depends on the predictability of the reward. Unexpected or novel rewards elicit a strong response which declines with repeated presentation. Predicted rewards have only modest effects.

Drugs and the brain reward system

Current theories suggest that many addictive drugs act on the brain reward system to enhance dopamine transmission, perhaps mimicking the effect of natural rewards (Information box 8.26). Cocaine is a well-studied example (see Information box 8.27).

Information box 8.26   Drugs that act on the mesolimbic system

- **Cocaine** – see Information box 8.27.
- **Nicotine** enhances the synthesis and release of dopamine by acting on cholinergic receptors on the dopamine cell bodies in the VTA.
- **Cannabinoids** act on excitatory cannabinoid receptors on dopamine terminals to increase dopamine release.
- **Opioids** (e.g. **morphine** and **heroin**) act on δ and μ opioid receptors to hyperpolarise GABAergic interneurons in the VTA that normally tonically inhibit the dopaminergic cells, so disinhibiting the mesolimbic system.
- **Ethanol** decreases the activity of the GABAergic interneurons, although the exact mechanism is unclear. The relationship between alcohol addiction and the mesolimbic system is not as clear cut as that seen with cocaine, but hypofunction of the mesolimbic system is seen in long-term alcohol abusers, the severity of which correlates with the amount of alcohol consumed.

Information box 8.27   Cocaine – a model of addiction

Cocaine blocks the **dopamine transporter** in the presynaptic terminals of mesolimbic neurons, limiting dopamine reuptake so that the concentration of transmitter in the synaptic cleft is raised. Cocaine administration in addicts causes transient activity in the VTA and nucleus accumbens (nAc) as recorded by brain imaging. However, a stronger nAc signal is seen in addicts who are craving the drug. This implies that the nAc is more important for learning contextual cues associated with drug taking than with the reinforcement and euphoria.

A single dose of cocaine can make the neurons of the VTA more sensitive to the drug by inducing long-term potentiation. This may be important in the early stages of addiction by enhancing the learning that leads to craving.

Tolerance develops later because the increase in synaptic dopamine concentration causes down-regulation of postsynaptic dopamine receptors. Higher amounts of transmitter, and hence drug, are needed to achieve the same level of dopamine transmission.

During **withdrawal**, dopamine concentrations drop back to baseline, but because there are fewer postsynaptic receptors, dopamine transmission in the mesolimbic system is decreased. This rebound drop in the effectiveness of the brain reward system is probably responsible for the **anhedonia** (lack of pleasure), reduced activity, depression and anxiety seen with drug withdrawal.

Brain imaging shows that cocaine causes an enduring reduction of dopamine synthesis in mesolimbic neuron terminals that gets worse the longer the period of abstinence. These long-term alterations seem to underlie persistent craving and provide a serious challenge to the treatment of drug addiction.

Some drugs that are both positively reinforcing and addictive (e.g. **barbiturates** and **benzodiazepines**) do *not* activate dopamine transmission, so not all addiction can be ascribed to the classic brain reward system.

Addictive drugs are generally positively reinforcing – that is, they become the object of goal-directed behaviours – and addiction is characterised by:

- **Tolerance** – in which repeated administration of a drug causes it to become progressively less effective, so the dose has to be increased if the original action (e.g. euphoria) is to be maintained.

- **Dependence** – which occurs when biological changes brought about by the drug are such that normal functioning is only possible when the drug is present.
- **Withdrawal** (**abstinence**) **syndrome** – which is seen when a drug is withheld after dependence is established. It is extremely unpleasant and lasts until the long-term biological changes that brought about dependence have abated. Hence, addiction can be driven as much by the aversion to withdrawal as by the positive reinforcing qualities of the drug.
- **Craving** – the intense desire for a drug that long outlasts the withdrawal (abstinence) syndrome. It is a learned response and involves different neural structures than those responsible for other aspects of addiction. Addicts form memories which associate the pleasure produced by the drug with the environment and cues that accompany the drug taking. Subsequent exposure to these contextual cues stimulates craving. This is accompanied by increased metabolic rate in the dorsolateral prefrontal cortex (implying involvement of cognition circuitry) and medial temporal cortex (explicit learning) as well as the nucleus accumbens (part of the 'reward' circuitry).

Goal-directed behaviours

Central control of feeding and satiety

Food intake is regulated in both the short and long-term by satiety signals. Both humoral and neural signals, such as **cholecystokinin** (**CCK**) secreted by the duodenum and activity of stretch receptor afferents conveying gastric distension, inhibit further feeding. In the long term, **adiposity signals**, such as **leptin** secreted from adipose tissue, reflect the size of the fat store and regulate it homeostatically by means of mechanisms that balance food intake and energy expenditure (see also Ch. 16).

Food intake is regulated in the CNS by two parallel brain pathways which originate in the **arcuate nucleus** of the hypothalamus. An **orexigenic** (anabolic) **pathway** promotes feeding while an **anorexigenic** (catabolic) **pathway** reduces feeding (Fig. 8.67). Leptin reduces food intake by inhibiting the orexigenic and stimulating the anorexigenic pathways.

Orexigenic pathway

Cells in the arcuate nucleus cells that use **neuropeptide Y** as a transmitter are the first order neurons in the orexigenic pathway. They project to the **lateral hypothalamus**, synapsing with second order neurons that secrete peptides termed **orexins** (**hypocretins**). These synapse on neurons in the **nucleus of the solitary track** (NST) decreasing their sensitivity to satiety factors (e.g. glucose).

Anorexigenic pathway

First order cells in the anorexigenic pathway contain **pro-opiomelanocortin** (**POMC**), the precursor protein for several biologically active peptides, one of which, **melanocortin**, is a neurotransmitter of these neurons. POMC cell axons run to the **paraventricular nucleus** (**PVN**) of the hypothalamus which contains neurons that use oxytocin, thyrotropin-releasing hormone or corticotropin releasing hormone as transmitters. These molecules suppress feeding by increasing the sensitivity of neurons in the NST to satiety factors. Stress probably reduces appetite by exciting the

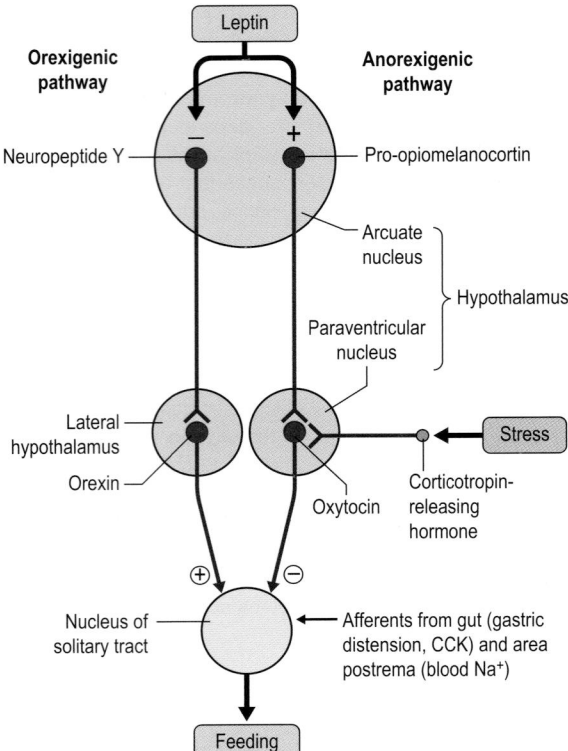

Fig. 8.67 Central pathways involved in feeding. CCK, cholecystokinin.

Clinical box 8.26   Anorexia nervosa

In anorexia nervosa, the patient deliberately opts to maintain extremely low food intake, often accompanied by very high levels of physical activity. Socio-cultural factors are very important, though there is evidence for a genetic pre-disposition, and there may be an underlying brain deficit, as evinced by evidence for reduced cerebral blood flow localised to specific limbic structures.

Anorexia is probably a constellation of related disorders and is often associated with depression or obsessive compulsive disorder. There are numerous psychological theories for the origin of the disease, all hard to test. Neurobiology-based ideas must distinguish cause from the effect of starvation, which is also difficult to do.

Anorexics have heightened secretion of corticotrophin releasing hormone and glucocorticoids, a stress response perhaps caused initially by anxiety about eating, and subsequently reinforced by the normal stress response to starvation. Whatever the reason, raised corticotrophin-releasing hormone secretion in the anorexigenic pathway could lead to suppression of appetite, though it is not clear why this is not overridden by the low leptin concentrations that are seen in untreated anorexics. The orexigenic pathway also appears to be defective in anorexia nervosa because the low leptin concentrations do not result in increases in neuropeptide Y. Leptin concentrations rise in weight-recovering anorexics in an apparently physiological fashion, but are higher than in normal women with the same body mass index (BMI).

---

corticotropin-releasing hormone neurons in the anorexigenic pathway. This may be a factor in the eating disorder, **anorexia nervosa** (Clinical box 8.26).

Central control of drinking

Provided that a minimum quantity of water is consumed there is little need for precise regulation of fluid intake because excess is renally excreted. Drinking is initiated whenever either tissue osmolality rises or blood volume decreases. If the sodium concentration in the extracellular fluid (ECF) falls, water shifts osmotically from the ECF into cells and blood volume drops (Ch. 1). Therefore the control of salt intake and water homeostasis are intimately intermeshed.

Vasopressin and water homeostasis

Cells in the supraoptic and paraventricular nuclei of the hypothalamus have their axon terminals in the posterior pituitary from where they release **vasopressin (antidiuretic hormone, ADH)** in response to water deprivation. The actions of ADH in the kidney conserve water (see Ch. 14).

Lack of water is signalled by **osmoreceptors**, osmotic pressure-sensitive neurons in the hypothalamus that are separate from the cells that produce ADH. Osmoreceptors act as osmometers, shrinking or swelling in response to changes in plasma osmolality. The set point is 280 mOsmol/kg; a rise in osmolality above this stimulates ADH release. ADH-secreting neurons also receive afferents from receptors in the low pressure side of the heart, the right atrium and great veins, and the high-pressure arterial baroreceptors (see Ch. 11) by way of the glossopharyngeal and vagus nerves.

Thirst and drinking

Increase in plasma osmolality produces a much greater sensation of thirst than low blood volume. Osmoreceptors distinct from those responsible for releasing ADH mediate hypertonicity thirst whereas **angiotensin II** is the signal for low-volume thirst. Angiotensin II in blood stimulates neurons in the **subfornical organ**, a circumventricular organ with fenestrated capillaries. A neural pathway between the subfornical organ and the preoptic nucleus of the hypothalamus, which itself uses angiotensin II as a neurotransmitter, conveys the blood volume signal. Pathways from the hypothalamus to the NST enable drinking behaviour.

Thirst is temporarily sated by the activity of afferents in the mouth, pharynx, oesophagus and stomach long before deficits in blood osmolality and volume are corrected. This means that several small drinks are taken at intervals until the loss is made up. This pattern of drinking is thought to prevent dilution of extracellular fluid and hypotonicity (**water intoxication**).

SLEEP AND WAKEFULNESS

Sleep is found in all mammals and birds, as well as many other animals. Sleep is thought to be essential for most humans, although there are a few individuals who seem to have survived without sleep for long periods without deleterious sequelae.

The function of sleep is not known, but the two strongest hypotheses are that:

- Rapid eye movement (REM) sleep has a role in memory consolidation
- Non-rapid eye movement (NREM) sleep serves some anabolic function needed for proper energy homeostasis.

During sleep humans experience dreams, the function of which are also not known.

Sleep states

There are two types of sleep, **non-rapid eye movement** and **rapid eye movement** sleep, which can be characterised by EEG (Information box 8.28) and other features.

- The awake state and REM sleep are both characterised by low voltage, high frequency waveforms (>12 Hz); this similarity is why REM sleep is sometimes called **paradoxical sleep**.
- NREM sleep has high voltage, low frequency waveforms (<3 Hz).

Brain blood flow and glucose utilisation are reduced in NREM sleep, but in REM sleep the brain is as active as it is when awake. Most dreaming occurs during REM sleep.

Timing

NREM sleep is divided into stages 1–4, in which the frequency of the EEG waveform drops and the arousal threshold increases. As a person falls asleep they drop progressively through these stages. During a normal night the amount of time in deep **delta** or **slow wave sleep** (stages 3 and 4) becomes less and NREM sleep is interrupted by progressively longer intervals of REM sleep.

Ontogeny

Human fetuses spend almost all their time asleep, mostly in REM sleep. At term, this falls to 17–18 hours sleep of which 50% is REM sleep. In infants, sleep is distributed throughout the 24 hour day, but by 4–5 years a child's 10 or so hours of sleep is restricted to night time. The amount of time spent in stage 4 sleep falls exponentially with age, with most of the decline in the first 20 years. Between 10 and 70 years the proportion of REM sleep is constant at about 25% of total sleep time and declines in elderly people.

Information box 8.28 Electroencephalography

EEG is a non-invasive method for measuring the surface electrical activity of the brain. Large numbers of cerebral cortical cells fire in synchrony and consequently their summed activity produces field potentials large enough to be recorded with electrodes attached to the scalp. An array of electrodes allows activity of different brain areas to be examined.

The EEG is a sensitive indicator of behaviour and shows characteristic patterns when a person is alert, drowsy or asleep. It is possible to analyse the patterns of activity to assess changes in amplitude and frequency of the waveforms. A frequency that is too fast or too slow is indicative of impaired cortical function. In addition, the presence of unusual waveforms such as sharp spikes, spike-and-wave potentials or unusually slow waves indicates a brain lesion or seizure disorder.

Although the EEG pattern of every individual is unique, there are a number of common patterns which can be related to specific brain states. The EEG waveform ranges in frequency from 1 Hz to 30 Hz and frequency ranges are conventionally grouped:

- Alpha (8–13 Hz) – typically seen in relaxed wakefulness
- Beta (13–30 Hz) – seen when an individual is alert or engaged in intense mental activity
- Delta (0.4–4 Hz) and theta (4–7 Hz) – seen during drowsiness and NREM sleep.

Generation of sleep–waking cycles

Arousal system

Monoaminergic neurons in the **ascending reticular formation** act as an **arousal system** (Fig. 8.68). This generates the awake state and increases the responsiveness of the cortex to sensory input. It has two branches:

- Axons of noradrenergic and serotonergic neurons in the brainstem that project through the lateral hypothalamus to the cerebral cortex. These are **wake-on/REM-off** cells; they fire at the highest rate in wakefulness, have low firing rates during NREM sleep and go silent during REM sleep.
- Axons of **pontine cholinergic neurons** (**PPT**) that project to the thalamus. These are **wake-on/REM-on** cells because they are active during wakefulness and REM sleep but go quiet during NREM sleep.

Reciprocal inhibition operates between these two groups of cells. However, during the waking state this is overridden by intense excitation of both groups. Interruption of these pathways can lead to loss of consciousness (Information box 8.29). **Thalamic relay cells** are directly excited by sensory input and excite cells in the cerebral cortex and in turn get reciprocal connections from the cortex.

NREM sleep

In NREM sleep mode:

- Sensory information is no longer transmitted from the thalamus to cortex
- The EEG becomes synchronised.

The sedative effect of antihistamines which cross the blood–brain barrier is due to reduced excitation of thalamic relay neurons. Burst firing of thalamic neurons is responsible for a type of epilepsy known as absence seizures.

The triggers for NREM sleep are not well understood but include a biological clock in the **suprachiasmatic nucleus** (**SCN**), which is entrained by light so normally has a 24-hour period, and elevated core temperature detected by warm receptors in the hypothalamus.

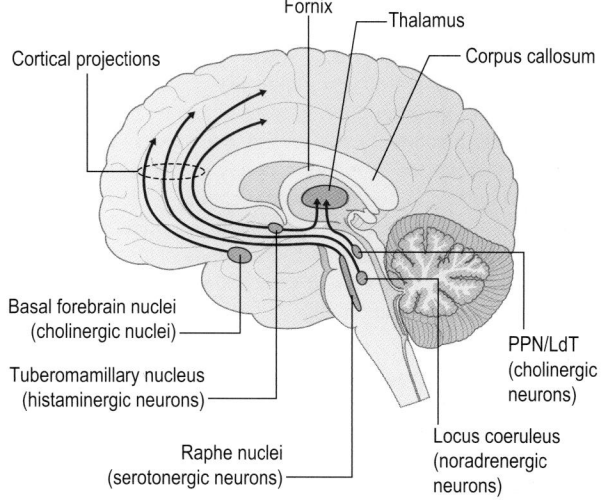

Fig. 8.68 Brain arousal systems. PPN/LdT, pedunculopontine nucleus/lateral dorsal tegmental nucleus.

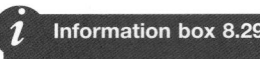

Cerebral cortical arousal can be impaired either by metabolic disturbance or structural damage (e.g. trauma, haemorrhage, infarct, tumour), which affect either the cortex itself or the ascending arousal system for generating consciousness. The most extreme case is **coma**, in which a patient cannot be aroused and does not make any purposive responses to stimuli. Usually cortical dysfunction is metabolic whereas impairment of the ascending arousal system is due to localised damage.

Interrupting either of the two branches of the ascending reticular formation impairs consciousness. Injuries above the level of the rostral pons may lead to loss of consciousness. Lesions of the posterior lateral hypothalamus or thalamus prevent EEG desynchronisation and arousal.

Loss of large numbers of cortical neurons can result in **persistent vegetative state**. In this state a patient has sleep–wake cycles, may eat food placed in their mouth and show some emotional responses. However, they show no evidence of self-awareness and only minimal responses to their environment.

Melatonin is synthesised by the pineal gland during the hours of darkness and is one factor involved in setting the period of the SCN clock. Flying across several time zones, or shift work, takes the SCN clock out of phase with light/dark cycles, resulting in **jet lag**. This disturbance can be shortened by appropriately timed administration of melatonin.

REM sleep

During REM sleep sensory input is relayed to the cortex and the EEG is desynchronised.

Although sensory input is transmitted from thalamus to cortex it cannot be acted upon because the body is effectively paralysed by neurons which suppress muscle tone.

Other REM-on cells in the pons are responsible for the rapid eye movements and muscle twitches, and for **pontine-geniculate-occipital (PGO) spikes**. These are brief high voltage spikes on the EEG which correlate with rapid eye movements.

LEARNING AND MEMORY

The acquisition of new knowledge or skills is **learning**. The fact that this information can subsequently be recalled shows that it must be stored as a **memory**. Learning occurs by alterations in the strengths of synaptic connections, changing the architecture of the neural network to which they belong. Learning is probably a nearly universal attribute of neural circuits: the nervous system should be thought of as hardware that is continually modified throughout life as a result of experience. Several distinct types of learning can be distinguished on the basis of time course, context, stimulus requirements and outcomes.

Categories of learning

There are two categories of learning: declarative and procedural. Many tasks have components of both. Sight-reading a new piece of music from the score requires knowing how to read music (declarative) and the correct sequence of finger movements to produce the notes (procedural).

Declarative (explicit) learning

Declarative or explicit learning is the acquiring of new facts about the world. It needs few trials, requires conscious recall and may be forgotten. There are two types:

- **Episodic memory** is autobiographical since it relates to specific events such as a particular evening in a particular place.
- **Semantic memory** is memory for facts, unrelated to any particular event (London is the capital city of the United Kingdom). Semantic memory includes memory for objects, concepts, and the meaning of words, so it is essential for verbal reasoning.

Episodic memories are stored in specific locations in association areas of the frontal cortex. In contrast, semantic memories are **distributed** since they are assembled from multiple representations in the cortex, each of which deals with a particular characteristic of the object. For example, semantic knowledge about people will be represented by neurons in the visual cortex, auditory cortex, olfactory cortex and probably other locations as well. Damage to the infero-temporal cortex causes a failure to recognise familiar faces or learn new ones, while leaving other ways of recognising people intact. Semantic knowledge is category specific; the lexicon for naming a specific class of object – fruit, animals, tools or whatever – is localised to a particular, discrete cortical region.

Procedural (motor) learning

Procedural or motor learning is the acquisition of a skill (e.g. learning to walk, ride a bike, play a musical instrument). It is slow and requires lots of rehearsal, and improvements are gradual. Like emotional learning mediated by the amygdala (see above), procedural learning is **implicit**. Performance does not need conscious recall and once mastered the skill is not forgotten even after years without practising. Motor learning is a feature of the cerebellum (see under cerebellum, above.

Declarative memory

Declarative memory has at least two phases that differ in the length of time that information is stored:

- **Long-term (remote) memory (LTM)** – which may last for many years and is not limited in capacity
- **Short-term (recent) memory (STM)** – which is temporary, limited in capacity, requires continuous rehearsal to retain it and is disrupted by distracting information.

Short-term memory

Short-term memory acts as a temporary buffer for holding ongoing streams of information. STM is often tested by asking a person to recall a random string of numbers after a single presentation. If they remember these correctly the next trial repeats the string but adds one extra number. This is continued until the person makes an error. The number of successful trials is plotted against the length of the string. Normal subjects show **primacy**, better recall of material at the beginning of the list because it is rehearsed most often, and **recency**, better recall for numbers at the end of the list because there has been less time to forget them.

Long-term memory and consolidation

It is clear that most new information to which we are exposed does not end up in long-term memory. A process termed **consolidation** selects certain items to be incorporated into long-term store, on the basis of current arousal levels and attention, which of course depend on our emotional state, motivation and the significance of the information.

STM and LTM seem to be separate parallel processes. Usually **amnesias** (loss of memory) are confined to LTM and leave STM untouched but in a few patients the reverse is true, showing that information can enter LTM even if STM is compromised.

Circuitry implicated in declarative (explicit) memory

Studies of patients who have suffered lesions to specific brain regions have played an important part in defining the circuitry involved in LTM (Fig. 8.69).

Role of the hippocampus

Damage to the **hippocampus** causes both severe **antero-grade amnesia** in which new long-term memories cannot be laid down (although STM and procedural learning are unaffected) and **retrograde amnesia** in which LTM established in the period about 6 months prior to the injury cannot be recalled. This pattern implies that the hippocampus is concerned with consolidation of long-term memory, and that the final storage site for LTM is elsewhere, in the neocortex, with which the hippocampus has extensive reciprocal traffic (Information box 8.30).

Highly processed sensory information from the association neocortex provides the major input to the hippocampal

> ### i Information box 8.30   Hippocampal cognitive maps
>
> PET scans of London taxi drivers show increased activity in the right hippocampus while they are recalling familiar routes. This, and considerable work with rats, suggests that the hippocampus houses a **cognitive map** which facilitates navigation through the environment. However, it is likely that the hippocampus is not restricted to the consolidation of spatial memories, but involved in an eclectic range of episodic memories, at least in humans.

formation which has a highly ordered structure. It is funnelled by way of the entorhinal cortex and subiculum into the perforant pathway. This pathway terminates on granule cells of the dentate gyrus and on CA3 pyramidal cells in the hippocampus proper (see Fig. 8.70).

CA3 cell axon collaterals form synapses with other CA3 cells, including those in the contralateral hippocampus. This remarkable architecture is crucial to the way the hippocampus learns. The main branch of CA3 axons project as Schaffer collaterals to synapse with CA1 pyramidal cells.

CA1 cell axons project back via the subiculum and entorhinal cortex to the neocortical regions that generated the original hippocampal input. The functions of this back projection are:

- To transfer the learning to the neocortex
- For recall.

Diencephalon and memory

The **anterior nucleus** of the thalamus receives a major output of the hippocampus, the **fornix**, by way of the mamillary bodies, and projects to the anterior cingulate, while the **mediodorsal nucleus** projects to the prefrontal cortex. Damage to the mamillary bodies and mediodorsal nucleus

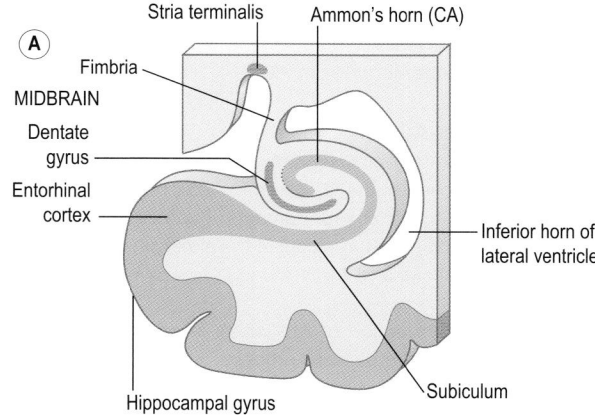

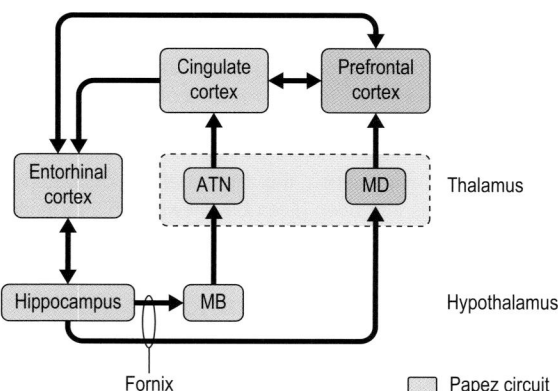

Fig. 8.69 Forebrain circuitry implicated in explicit learning and memory. Compare with Figure 8.66. ATN, anterior thalamic nuclei; MD, mediodorsal thalamic nucleus; MB, mamillary bodies.

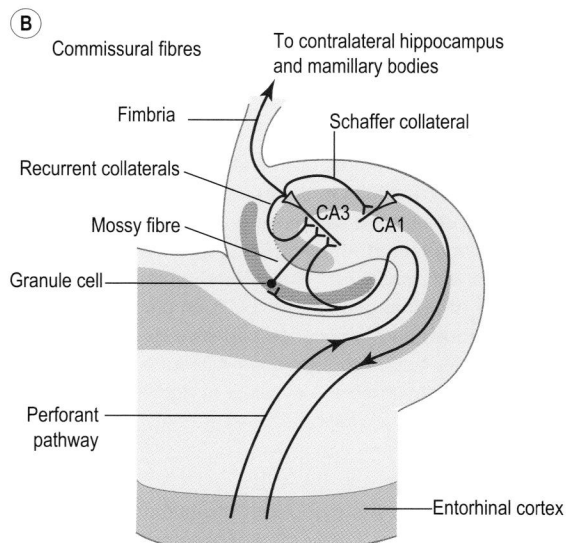

Fig. 8.70 Hippocampus. (A) Coronal section through the temporal lobe at the level of the hippocampus. (B) Excitatory connections of the hippocampus.

are seen in **Korsakoff's syndrome**, a dementia seen in chronic alcoholism and characterised by severe amnesia.

Dementia and Alzheimer's disease

Dementia is a progressive decline in cognitive function due to damage or disease in the brain which is not attributable to normal ageing. Most forms of dementia are irreversible.

The commonest form of dementia is **Alzheimer's disease** (AD) and memory impairment is a central feature of AD. The inability to retrieve semantic memories occurs early and manifests as difficulty in finding the words to formulate or follow speech, failure to recognise or identify people or objects and being unable to navigate through once familiar surroundings. The ability to make new declarative memories and retrieve motor skills (e.g. dressing) is subsequently eroded.

There is massive neuronal death in AD. Loss of cortical pyramidal cells occurs, together with the degeneration of the monoaminergic subcortical (most notably cholinergic) projections to them. One possibility is that the ascending projections die because they have been deprived of neurotrophic factors from their cortical targets. The loss of dopamine and serotonin neurons accounts for the lack of motivation, Parkinsonism and depression that are often part of AD.

CAT scans show cortical and subcortical atrophy with enlargement of the ventricles. Brain mass may be reduced by 30–40%. Two lesions, plaques and tangles, are invariably found in the cerebral cortex in AD.

Plaques and AD

Plaques are extracellular deposits of **amyloid**, an aggregate of fibrils composed of the 40–42 amino acid residue **amyloid β protein (Aβ)**, together with damaged neurites and reactive glia. However, plaques can occur in the elderly in the absence of cognitive deficits and Aβ is found in low levels in healthy individuals.

Excessive production of Aβ, which is neurotoxic, might be the trigger for the disease process. Aβ is formed from a membrane glycoprotein **amyloid precursor protein (APP)**, which can be enzymatically cleaved in two ways, by different secretase enzymes, to produce either Aβ or a soluble peptide, **sAPPα**, which is a neuroprotective trophic factor produced in healthy individuals.

Evidence for the involvement of plaques in AD comes from various sources:

- Patients with early-onset **familial Alzheimer's disease (FAD)** have mutations in the genes for APP or presenilin 1 (a component of a secretase enzyme) which results in greater amounts of Aβ being cleaved off.
- Patients with trisomy 21 (Down's syndrome) over-express APP (the gene for which is on chromosome 21), have plaques and experience cognitive decline.
- Several risk factors for acquiring AD, such as head injury, ischaemia and the ε4 allele of apolipoprotein E, promote plaque formation.

Tangles and AD

Tangles, located in the cytoplasm of neurons, are bundles of filaments made of highly phosphorylated **tau**, a protein which normally regulates the polymerisation of microtubules in the cytoskeleton (see Ch. 2). The number of tangles correlates with the severity of the dementia.

The link between Aβ and tangles is not clear. Mice with the same APP mutations as those in FAD have more Aβ and form plaques, but they do not develop tangles, neither do they lose neurons. Moreover, tangles occur in the absence of plaques in **frontotemporal dementias** in which there are tau gene mutations.

Possible therapeutic strategies

A number of possible therapeutic strategies are under investigation, although there is no current cure and drug treatments offer little relief of symptoms.

- The non-steroidal anti-inflammatory drug indometacin has been reported to halt the cognitive decline, implying that inflammation may contribute to AD.
- Active vaccination against Aβ clears plaques in animals and humans, but this does not seem to improve cognition.
- Treatment with cholesterol-lowering **statins** dramatically reduces the risk of developing AD. These may lower brain Aβ production directly or selectively affect the secretase enzymes so APP is cleaved to make sAPPα rather than Aβ.

Development of explicit memory

The human brain undergoes important changes at the end of the first year and into the second, including differentiation of cortical pyramidal cells and synaptogenesis in the hippocampus. These developments are presumably responsible for the improvements in memory retrieval seen during this time. At 6 months, infants can recall events for up to 24 hours. This extends to 1 month by 9 months of age and 4 months by 21 months old.

Arousal and learning

Only a tiny fraction of incoming information ends up in long-term memory. A major factor in determining what is consolidated is the ongoing arousal level.

Moderate plasma concentrations of noradrenaline and adrenaline enhance subsequent recall of emotionally neutral tasks, but low or high concentrations have deleterious effects. Although the catecholamines cannot cross the blood–brain barrier they exert their effects centrally by stimulating β-adrenoceptors on visceral afferents that run in the vagus nerve. These drive the noradrenergic neurons of the locus coeruleus that are part of the CNS arousal system.

The hippocampus has a very high density of steroid receptors which bind glucocorticoids. The high concentrations of glucocorticoids secreted in response to stress impair learning. Conversely, low glucocorticoid concentrations improve learning. A number of peptides released during stress (e.g. β-endorphin) have similar effects. Attempting to revise for an examination the night before, or loading a patient who has just been given bad news with information, is not sensible because of the high stress in both cases.

Cellular basis of learning

Learning involves the strengthening or weakening of connections between neurons. This occurs over a number of timescales, with permanent storage associated with de novo synthesis of proteins, morphological changes to synapses and growth or loss of neurites. The cellular events that strengthen or weaken synapses thought to underpin learning are long-term potentiation and long-term depression, respectively. The same synaptic mechanisms are thought to underlie the development of epilepsies (Clinical box 8.27).

Long-term potentiation

In **long-term potentiation** (**LTP**), brief high frequency firing of the inputs to a neuron makes its response to subsequent inputs larger, i.e. epsps have a bigger amplitude. This is mediated by an influx of Ca^{2+}, which switches on a variety of biochemical processes that increase synaptic transmission in response to subsequent low frequency input. LTP was first discovered in the hippocampus but has subsequently been shown in the neocortex, amygdala and other structures.

Two phases of LTP are defined. **Early LTP** does not require protein synthesis and decays within 3 hours. **Late LTP** requires synthesis of RNA and proteins and persists for at least 24 hours. The important lesson to be learnt from this is that experience changes gene expression. Both post- and pre-synaptic changes are implicated in the maintenance of LTP but the end result of LTP is that new synapses are formed by splitting of pre-existing ones.

Long-term depression

A persistent weakening of synaptic strength, **long-term depression** (**LTD**) is seen in the structures which show LTP. In addition, it occurs alone in the cerebellar cortex where it is thought to underpin motor learning. Here, LTD occurs at the synapse between parallel fibres and Purkinje cells in response to high activity in climbing fibres that represent error signals. It causes the parallel fibre–Purkinje cell synapses to become less responsive to glutamate released by the parallel fibre. In other words, the error signal weakens the synapses responsible for the erroneous movement.

COGNITION

Cognitive functions are those that involve planning and problem solving. Cognition depends upon being able to manipulate mental representations, not just of existing visual images and motor actions, but of abstractions (ideas, relations) that must be represented by symbols (e.g. words, mathematical forms). **Thinking** is the ability to manipulate these symbols to generate new ideas and relations. Although much thinking is done using language, infants must use non-linguistic modes of thought. Functional brain imaging shows that cognitive tasks are orchestrated by the prefrontal cortex. Cognitive tasks tend to be lateralised in the brain:

- **Language** is predominantly a left hemisphere function
- **Visuospatial** tasks engage the right hemisphere.

There are sex differences in the extent and nature of this lateralisation of cognitive functions.

PREFRONTAL CORTEX

The **prefrontal cortex** is all of the frontal lobe cortex other than premotor and motor cortices. It has three main areas. The medial prefrontal and orbitofrontal areas are connected to limbic structures and involved in decisions with an emotional content, whereas the lateral prefrontal area is engaged by purely cognitive tasks that leave the other regions unaffected.

Clinical box 8.27 Epilepsies

Epileptic seizures are self-limiting episodes of abnormal, synchronised firing of large populations of neurons. What causes **epileptogenesis** – the development of the hyperexcitable state that predisposes to seizures – is unclear in the majority of epilepsies, which are acquired, but it seems to involve synaptic changes similar to those that underlie learning.

Much of our understanding of epilepsy comes from animal models which are thought to emulate human **temporal lobe epilepsy** (**TLE**). Susceptibility to seizure activity is thought to be due to a hyperexcitable state of mossy fibre/CA3 synapses in the hippocampus (see above). CA3 cells have three features that contribute to their ability for prolonged synchronised firing.

- Like pacemakers, they fire bursts of action potentials spontaneously. In epilepsy this burst activity becomes abnormal **paroxysmal depolarising shifts** that cause **interictal spikes** seen in the EEG between seizures.
- They are heavily interconnected by recurrent axon collaterals by which each cell excites its neighbours and re-excites itself.
- There are gap junctions which allow adjacent CA3 cells to be electrically coupled for rapid spread of activity throughout the entire hippocampus. These electrical synapses are opened by a rise in pH. This is interesting for several reasons:
  - Seizures are often induced in the clinic by asking patients to hyperventilate, which produces a respiratory alkalosis
  - Ketogenic diets which produce metabolic acidosis reduce seizure frequency
  - The local fall in pH produced by high neural activity during a seizure may act to limit it.

In contrast, CA1 cells are only sparsely interconnected with each other and normally CA1 cells cannot be driven to burst fire by CA3 cells because they are inhibited by GABAergic interneurons. However, in epilepsy CA1 cells do burst fire, which implies a weakening of the GABAergic inhibition, and this allows the seizure to spread out of the hippocampus into the neocortex of the temporal lobe.

Individual seizures may be terminated by adenosine. Neural activity is very high during a seizure and intracellular adenosine concentration rises in consequence. It is transported out of the cell where it acts as part of a normal physiological response to increase local blood flow. In addition it binds adenosine receptors in neurons to bring about hyperpolarisation, which curtails firing.

Causes of epileptogenesis

Inherited epilepsies have been linked to mutations in voltage-dependent sodium or potassium channels or in ionotropic receptors (nicotinic receptor α subunits) that increase neural excitability.

Epileptogenesis in acquired epilepsies is far more difficult to account for. One thing is clear, however, seizure activity makes future seizures more likely, i.e. seizures are themselves epileptogenic. A possible mechanism for this is that seizures induce the expression of growth factors which enhance glutamate transmission but dampen GABA transmission (i.e. promoting excitatory transmission while suppressing inhibitory transmission) or trigger the formation of new synaptic connections between cells.

The pharmacological treatment of epilepsy is predicated on the notion that epilepsy is a matter of too much neural excitation or too little inhibition.

Principal modes of action of anti-epileptic drugs are:

- Blockade of voltage-dependent sodium channels (e.g. phenytoin), or calcium channels in absence seizures
- Increasing GABAergic inhibition by blocking GABA reuptake (e.g. tiagabine) or inhibiting GABA transaminase, the enzyme responsible for inactivating GABA (e.g. vigabatrin)
- Mimicking GABA inhibition with GABA$_A$ receptor agonists (barbiturates and benzodiazepines).

Working memory

Short-term memory for information needed for ongoing behaviour, planning and problem solving is called **working memory**. It can store incoming new information and explicit knowledge recalled from long-term memory; about 7–9 items can be held at any instant. Functional brain imaging and studies of patients with cortical lesions show that there are at least two subsystems to working memory.

- **Verbal working memory** allows **phonemes** (fundamental speech sounds that individually have no meaning) to be held for long enough to give continuity to phrases and sentences so that speech can be understood. It is localised in the left cerebral hemisphere.
- **Non-verbal working memory** is a transient store for spatial information provided by the visual system; when it is engaged increased activity in the inferior parietal cortex of the right hemisphere is seen.

Executive attention system

The **dorsolateral prefrontal cortex**, an area that surrounds the principal sulcus, is a component of the cognitive basal ganglia circuit and constitutes an **executive attention system**. This regulates the flow of information into various components of working memory (Clinical box 8.28). It does this by focusing attention on whatever is important at the time and by directed recall of specific items from long-term memory. The executive attention system is able to search for specific memories in a context-driven manner and keep track of what it has done recently. Switching attention from one item or task to another is attributed to the executive attention system.

Semantic memory networks

One of the resources the executive attention system has access to are **semantic memory networks**. These store representations of words, ideas and objects in such a way that those with similar or related meanings are most readily associated during recall. For example, the word 'bread' is quite likely to evoke 'butter' or 'jam', while 'headlight' or 'Mars' are highly improbable responses. The associations in semantic memory networks are learnt, and so are peculiar to the individual. Semantic memories are located particularly in frontal and temporal lobes. Evidence for these networks is provided by category-specific deficits that are seen in patients with brain injuries. For example, a patient has been reported who, when shown objects, cannot name vegetables but can name fruit.

LANGUAGE

Structure

Any language has two components:

- A **lexicon** – words and their modifiers (e.g. articles, auxiliaries, suffixes, etc.), which are symbols, arbitrary associations between a sound and a meaning that is an agreed convention for users of the particular language.
- **Grammar** – a set of rules for manipulating the symbols into larger units which communicate meaning.

Clinical box 8.28   **Schizophrenia**

Schizophrenia is a psychotic illness, affecting about 0.5% of the population, characterised by disordered thoughts and speech, hallucinations and delusional behaviour.

It is associated with a reduction in the size of the thalamus, thinner frontal cortex, medial temporal cortex and hippocampus, particularly in the left hemisphere, and less change in cerebral blood flow in the frontal cortex during working memory tasks than normal individuals. These abnormalities are thought to reflect inappropriate apoptosis of neurons in utero, leading to:

- Abnormal migration into white matter of neurons destined for the cortex, resulting in aberrant patterns of cortical connections.
- Loss of thalamocortical axons and dopaminergic projections in the cortex, and reduced number of distal dendrites on cortical pyramidal cells.

Interestingly, although schizophrenia is apparently a developmental defect, the young brain seems incapable of becoming schizophrenic; symptoms rarely occur until after puberty and drugs that can precipitate psychotic episodes in adults, such as amphetamines and ketamine, do not do so in children.

One hypothesis for the development of schizophrenia is centred around dopamine pathways in the cortex. In schizophrenia there is increased activity in the mesolimbic pathway but a decreased activity of the mesocortical system that may be due to a developmental defect in the frontal cortex.

Functional brain imaging studies suggest that excessive activation of a basal ganglia circuit involving the inferotemporal cortex underlies hallucinations. The thought disorder may be explained by a joint dysfunction of semantic memory and working memory. Normally dopamine enhances the signal-to-noise ratio in neural networks responsible for semantic memories. Psychological studies indicate that in schizophrenia semantic networks are less focused (lower signal-to-noise ratio), presumably as a result of decreased mesocortical activity. This explains why schizophrenics make looser or more unusual associations between words and ideas than normal subjects. Working memory is thought to be maintained by reverberating circuits stabilised by recurrent excitation via NMDA receptors and these circuits are predicted to be less stable in schizophrenics.

Most of the drugs used to treat schizophrenia are dopamine receptor antagonists. However, although dopamine receptor blockade is immediate, the therapeutic effects of antipsychotics may not be seen for several weeks. The key to their actions may be long-term adaptive changes which follow treatment with antipsychotics, such as reduced activity of dopaminergic neurons, upregulation of dopamine receptors and down-regulation of $5-HT_2$ receptors.

There are two broad categories of **antipsychotic** drug:

- **Typical** antipsychotics have high affinity for dopamine D2 receptors (see under Neurotransmitter systems, above). D2 receptors located in limbic structures and parts of the cortex are presumably responsible for the antipsychotic actions, but D2 receptors are also found in the striatum where they are responsible for unwanted extrapyramidal effects (e.g. tardive dyskinesia).
- **Atypical** antipsychotics act preferentially on D3 and D4 receptors. They are found in the limbic system and cortex but not in the striatum and so atypical antipsychotics are relatively free of extrapyramidal side effects. Most atypical antipsychotics act at serotonin $(5-HT_2)$ receptors as well as at dopamine receptors.

Ontogeny

Initially, infants learn to discriminate the fundamental sound units (**phonemes**) of their native tongue. Children speak their first words at about 18 months, begin to utter phrases when they are around 2.5 years old, and are speaking fluently with quite low grammatical error rates by 4 years. The nature of the errors shows that children are not just mimicking the sounds they hear but are learning the rules of their local grammar.

It is thought that children have neural circuits dedicated to learning language. Evidence for this is that early language acquisition requires no formal training and a number of pathologies show that language acquisition and other types of semantic learning are separate; e.g. some patients with hydrocephalus have compromised general intelligence but can construct grammatical speech and have normal speech comprehension.

Children growing up in multi-lingual households learn to discriminate individual languages and become multi-lingual, speaking each with a perfect accent. There is a critical period for learning language which ends by about 8 years old. Before this time brain imaging shows that the brain loci for learning other languages overlap extensively with those for the native language. Later in life brain regions involved in learning a second language do not overlap those for the first. Evidence for this is that in adults focal lesions can selectively disrupt either the native language or the foreign one while leaving the other relatively intact. Adults take many years to learn a foreign language well and rarely acquire a perfect accent.

Lateralisation of language

Language functions are lateralised, with the left hemisphere being dominant in 90% of people, and the right hemisphere in 7.5%. Cerebral dominance for language and motor function are independent; many left-handed individuals have left hemispheric language dominance. Infants who have their left cerebral hemisphere excised to treat neurological disease learn to speak fluently (although they do have deficits in speech comprehension), whereas adults treated in the same way have permanent, near total, loss of language. This reflects the huge plasticity of the infant brain. Brain imaging studies of normal individuals show that some aspects of language are less lateralised in women than men.

Neuroanatomy of language

A considerable volume of brain is involved in language (see Fig. 8.71).

- The superior temporal cortex is involved in sensory functions associated with speech and reading. It includes the auditory cortex and Wernicke's area (area 22). Bordering Wernicke's area lies the angular gyrus (area 39), which receives extensive visual input from the extrastriate cortex (area 19).
- The frontal and parietal cortex adjacent to the lateral sulcus is concerned with the motor aspects of reading and writing, and contains Broca's area (Brodmann's areas 44 and 45) that is reciprocally interconnected to Wernicke's area.

Speech

Two brain regions, usually located in the left hemisphere, are particularly active during speech:

- **Broca's area** is the premotor area for speech, sending its output to the face and tongue area of the neighbouring motor cortex. The **insula**, which forms the floor of the lateral sulcus, is responsible for planning the articulatory movements needed for speech on the basis of verbal working memory input from the prefrontal cortex, and projects to Broca's area. Lesions that include Broca's area cause **motor (anterior) aphasia**, in which speech is laboured and lacks fluency.
- **Wernicke's area**, which receives extensive connections from the auditory cortex, is concerned with understanding speech. **Sensory (posterior) aphasia**

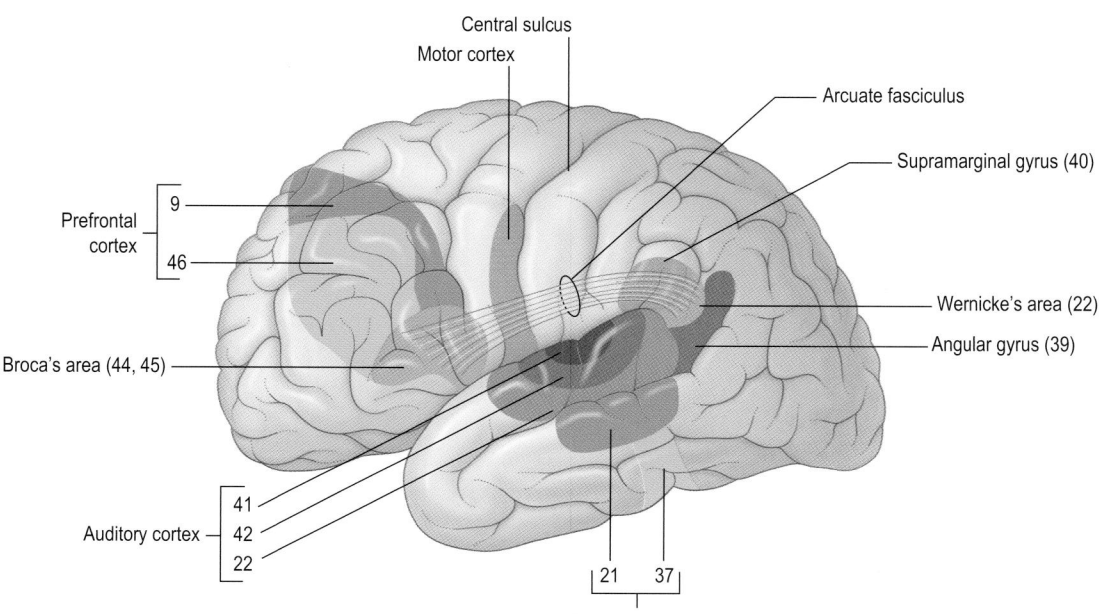

Fig. 8.71 **Cortical areas implicated in language by functional brain imaging studies.** *Green* regions show increased blood flow when listening to words (active listening). The auditory cortex (*red*), but not other regions, is also activated by tones (passive listening). *Blue* regions are, in addition, engaged during reading aloud.

results from lesions to Wernicke's area and is a deficit in auditory comprehension. Because patients cannot monitor their own speech it becomes unintelligible, albeit fluent.

Listening to speech

Brain regions specifically implicated in listening to the spoken word (active listening) have been identified on MRI by subtracting the signal from regions (such as the auditory cortex) that are engaged when listening to random tones (passive listening) from the total signal produced by listening to speech. Listening to speech activates:

- Wernicke's area on the left side, which is thought to permit discrimination of verbal from non-verbal material.
- The angular gyrus, which identifies phonemes.
- The middle temporal gyrus (area 21) and area 37, which identify words from phoneme strings, and tap into semantic networks located in the left dorsolateral prefrontal cortex (areas 9 and 46) that must be searched to traduce the meaning of speech.
- Broca's area, because when listening to speech we covertly rehearse the articulatory commands needed to pronounce the words, a process referred to as **subvocal articulation**.

Reading

Clearly reading requires visual processing. Subsequently, two pathways operate in parallel:

- The angular gyrus projects through Wernicke's area to area 21 to transform written syllables to phonemes.
- Activation of a network that links the supramarginal gyrus (area 40), and area 37, to the anterior part of Broca's area (area 45), via the insula, allows access to semantic networks in the dorsolateral prefrontal cortex so that the meaning and pronunciation of the words represented by the phonemes can be retrieved.

Clinical box 8.29   **Developmental dyslexia**

Difficulty in reading, writing and spelling in people who match their peers in other intellectual fields and have no apparent sensory deficits, is termed **developmental dyslexia**. It is probably a cluster of disorders. Three hypotheses are currently in vogue.

- The **magnocellular deficit** hypothesis is based on the finding that there are abnormally small cells in the magnocellular layers of the lateral geniculate nuclei and medial geniculate nucleus. This could impair the ability to process fast visual input and the speech perception, respectively, and so accounts for the reading difficulty and poorer speech discrimination.
- The **phonological deficit** hypothesis is that dyslexics have difficulty decomposing speech into its constituent phonemes and hence find it hard to learn the specific associations between phonemes and letters. PET shows that the insula is inactive, suggesting that the link between the supramarginal and angular gyri (the presumed locus of the phonological representation) and Broca's area, is not engaged in dyslexics.
- The **cerebellar deficit** hypothesis argues that phonemes come to be recognised not by their sounds but by the articulations that are needed to produce them, and that the cerebellum is important in learning this association. It is supported by behavioural evidence for impaired cerebellar motor functions in dyslexic children, and by PET scans which show reduced activation of the cerebellum during a motor learning task in dyslexic adults.

These pathways are not independent because of the heavy interconnection between Wernicke's area and Broca's area.

Finally, either subvocal articulation or reading aloud is accompanied by activation of the whole of Broca's area, the medial supplementary motor area (area 6), motor areas subserving the face and tongue (area 4), and the contralateral cerebellar hemisphere (Clinical box 8.29).

9 Bones, muscle and skin

Lesley Robson and Patricia Revest

INTRODUCTION

The **musculoskeletal system** is composed of the skeleton, the muscles and accessory tissues, which together allow movement of the body.

The bones of the **skeleton** are living tissue, and they can be found in a variety of shapes and sizes depending on their function. The skeleton is composed of 206 individual bones that articulate with each other via a network of joints. **Joints** vary in their structure and function, with some joints allowing a wide range of movements while other joints are virtually immovable and are designed for stability.

The **skeletal muscles** are the power houses that move the skeleton and most of them are attached to the skeleton via **tendons** which transmit the muscular contraction to the skeleton, and move the joints. The skeletal muscles of the face attach not only to the skull but also to other facial muscles and the skin, and contraction of these muscles changes the facial expression. The muscles that act on the skeleton are all under voluntary control and contain the contractile proteins, actin and myosin.

Knowledge of the musculoskeletal system is vital for medical practitioners as a third of general practitioner (GP) consultations involve the musculoskeletal system in some way. Conditions that affect the musculoskeletal system include osteoarthritis, which affects two-thirds of individuals over 75 years of age, and back pain, which affects 2.5 million people everyday in Britain. Musculoskeletal disorders therefore cost the UK health service considerable sums each year.

The **integumentary system** (integument means covering) is formed by the skin plus associated glands, hair and nails. It covers the entire body and has four main roles:

- Protective: it protects the body from the external environment
- Homeostatic: in the control of body temperature (see also Ch. 11)
- Perceptive: the skin contains receptors for pain, temperature and touch (see Ch. 8)
- Metabolic: synthesis of vitamin D (see Ch. 9).

THE SKELETAL SYSTEM

The skeleton is mainly composed of bones which form a rigid framework for the rest of the body tissues. Bone is a complex and dynamic living tissue. It is continually being broken down and replaced by new bone. The adult skeleton also contains cartilage, which is more elastic than bone and forms a semi-rigid part of the skeleton and a protective layer at many joint surfaces.

CARTILAGE

Cartilage, which consists largely of water, contains two cell types:

- Immature **chondroblasts** which secrete the components of the cartilage
- **Chondrocytes**, which are mature cartilage cells, derived from chondroblasts that are trapped within spaces called **lacunae,** surrounded by the extracellular matrix (see Ch. 2).

Cartilage does not contain blood vessels so all metabolites are exchanged by diffusion. Although cartilage has a low metabolic rate, diffusion limits the possible thickness of cartilage and prevents rapid repair following injury. The high water content of cartilage ensures that it is resilient and retains its shape under pressure, as water is virtually incompressible.

Three types of cartilage are found in the adult body:

■ Hyaline (glassy) cartilage: covers the ends of synovial joints (articular cartilage, see below), connects the ribs to the sternum (costal cartilages), forms the larynx and part of the nose and reinforces the trachea and bronchi.
■ Fibrous cartilage: has less matrix and more collagen than other cartilage, which makes it more compressible and able to resist high pressures. It is found in discs in areas of high stress such as between the vertebrae (intervertebral discs) and in the knee joint (meniscus).
■ Elastic cartilage: is found in only two places: the external ear, where it forms the **pinna** and the external auditory canal, and the epiglottis. Elastic cartilage contains high levels of elastic fibres, which gives these tissues a large degree of flexibility.

Both hyaline and elastic cartilages are surrounded by a layer called the perichondrium, which consists of a fibrous layer, containing fibroblasts, type I collagen and chondroblasts. It is continuous with the periosteal bone and the surface of surrounding connective tissue.

In the embryo (6 weeks) the skeleton is composed of hyaline cartilage and fibrous tissue formed by mesenchymal cells. These are then converted to bone by endochondral ossification and intramembranous ossification, respectively (see below).

BONE MICROANATOMY

Bone is classified as a connective tissue, and as such shows the basic arrangement of all connective tissues in that it is relatively acellular, with the osteogenic (bone generating) cells widely separated by an abundant matrix (see Ch. 2).

Bone matrix

In bone, the matrix is composed of approximately:

■ 25% water
■ 25% organic protein fibres
■ 50% crystallised mineral salts.

Most of the organic component of bone consists of **collagen fibres**, which form between 90% and 95% of the organic part of bone. Type I collagen is the most abundant type in bone, making up to 90% of the total collagen.

Between 50% and 70% of the bone is composed of **inorganic crystals** made up of the mineral **hydroxyapatite**, which itself is composed of calcium phosphate, calcium carbonate, calcium fluoride, calcium hydroxide and citrate.

Cellular content of bone

There are four types of cells in bone (Fig. 9.1):

■ Osteogenic progenitor cells
■ Osteoclasts
■ Osteocytes
■ Osteoblasts.

The **osteogenic progenitor cells** are the precursors of the osteoblasts and are derived from mesenchymal cells.

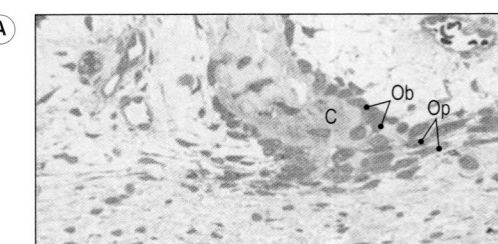

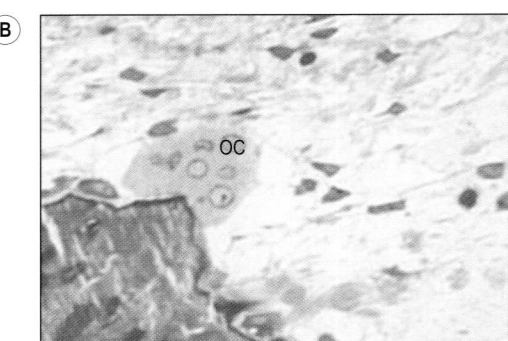

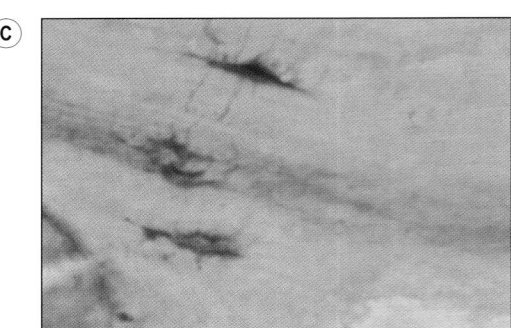

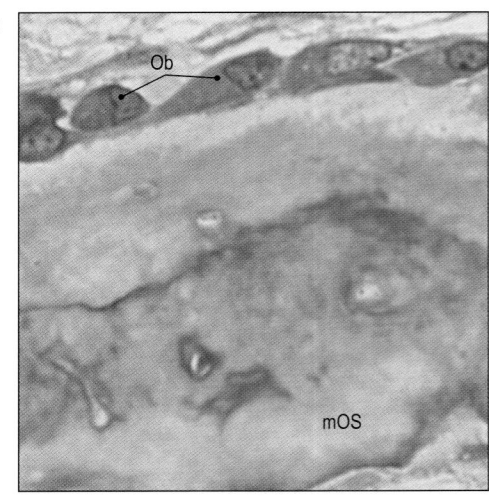

Fig. 9.1 **Bone cell types:** (A) osteogenic progenitor cells, (B) osteoclasts, (C) osteocytes and (D) osteoblasts. C, osteoid collagen (unmineralised osteoid); mOs, mineralised osteoid; Ob, osteoblast; OC, osteoclast. With permission from Stevens A, Lowe J. Human histology, 3rd edn. Mosby, Edinburgh, 2004.

They are the only cells that are able to undergo cell division, with the resulting daughter cells differentiating into osteoblasts. The osteogenic progenitor cells are found in the periosteum and endosteum of the bone and also in the canals within the bone that contain blood vessels (see below).

Osteoblasts are the cells that make new bone matrix. They synthesise and secrete collagen fibres and other organic components, and they initiate the calcification of the matrix.

Osteocytes are found in the more mature bone and were once osteoblasts, but have now become surrounded and entrapped in their own matrix. They no longer secrete matrix, and their role is to maintain the daily cellular activities of the bone tissue. These activities include the exchange of nutrients and waste products with the blood.

The final type of cell found in bone is the **osteoclast** whose role is the removal of old bone. These are not derived from the osteogenic progenitor cells but are formed by the fusion of up to 50 monocytes, and so are derived from white blood cells. They are very large and are concentrated in the endosteum. The plasma membrane of the osteoclast facing the bone surface is deeply ruffled and it releases powerful lysosomal enzymes and acids that digest and dissolve the protein and mineral matrix. The removal of old bone matrix is usually kept in balance with the osteoblasts production of new bone (see below).

BONE FORMATION

The bone matrix is unlike other connective tissues because it contains lots of inorganic salts, the main one being **hydroxyapatite** (calcium phosphate) but there is also some calcium carbonate. The bone matrix also contains small amounts of magnesium hydroxide, fluoride and sulphate. These are all deposited on the framework of collagen fibres secreted by the osteoblasts. As the minerals crystallise they harden the tissue, in a process called **ossification**.

The hardness of the bone depends on the amount and type of the crystallised salts. Bone must remain slightly flexible to be able to withstand the forces it is subjected to daily and this is dependent on the presence of collagen fibres which provide the bone with tensile strength. Calcification only takes place in the presence of the collagen fibres, with mineral salts first crystallising in the microscopic spaces between the collagen fibres (see Clinical Box 9.1). Once these spaces have been filled, more mineral crystals accumulate around the collagen fibres.

Bone is not completely solid and contains many small spaces, some of which provide space for blood vessels to supply the bone cells with nutrients and remove waste products. Other spaces are filled with bone marrow. Bone can be divided into two categories, compact and spongy, depending on the distribution of the spaces. Overall 80% of the total skeleton is **compact bone** and 20% is **spongy (cancellous) bone**, although bones in the axial skeleton are 70% spongy bone.

TYPES OF BONE

There are many different types of bone and they can be classified according to their shape (Fig. 9.2):

- **Long bones** are longer than their width and are the most common. They are mainly formed from compact bone with spongy bone in their centres and at their ends (see below). Examples include the long bones of the arms (humerus, radius and ulna) and legs (femur, tibia and fibula) as well as the small bones of the fingers and toes.

Clinical box 9.1 **Osteogenesis imperfecta**

Osteogenesis imperfecta, also known as brittle bone disease, is a genetic disease that affects the production of collagen type I. This collagen is important in forming the organic scaffold of bone. The inheritance pattern indicates that osteogenesis imperfecta is a dominant genetic mutation that causes either less collagen type I or an abnormal collagen type I protein to be made. New spontaneous mutations account for 25% of cases.

Four types of osteogenesis imperfecta have being identified: type 1 is the most common form of the disease and also the mildest, whereas type 2 is the most severe, with types 3 and 4 having intermediate severity. The main symptom is that the bones fracture easily so that X-rays of an affected person usually show evidence of multiple fractures that have or are in the process of healing. As collagen type I is found in other tissues besides bone, osteogenesis imperfecta also affects other tissues and organs. For example, in the eyes, the sclera (the whites of the eye) have a tendency to be blue rather than white, the joints tend to be loose or lax as tendons and ligaments are partly composed of collagen type I, and patients often have low muscle tone, brittle teeth and may suffer from hearing loss. Other features include increased perspiration and they tend to bruise very easily, as their skin tends to be thin and smooth, as collagen type I is found in the dermis of the skin.

Osteogenesis imperfecta is usually diagnosed during infancy, as babies with type 2, 3 or 4 are often born with fractures and babies with type 1 often have their first fracture in the first year of life; some milder forms are not diagnosed until teenage or even in adulthood.

- **Short bones**: these are cuboidal and contain mainly spongy bone with a surface layer of compact bone. Examples of these are the bones of the wrist and ankles, as well as the **sesamoid** bones such as the patella (kneecap), which are found within some tendons.
- **Flat bones**: these are flat, thin and usually slightly curved. They consist of two thin layers of compact bone, surrounding a thin layer of spongy bone. The skull, ribs, sternum (breast bone) and scapula (shoulder blade) are all flat bones.
- **Irregular bones**: these are bones that do not fit the other categories. They are made from spongy bone covered with compact bone. The bones of the vertebrae and pelvis are irregular bones.

The skeleton can also be divided into two parts:

- **Axial skeleton**, which forms the long axis of the body and contains the skull, vertebral column and ribs
- **Appendicular skeleton**, which consists of the limb bones and their attachments or **girdles**, the pelvis and scapula and clavicle.

STRUCTURE OF BONE

A typical long bone (Fig. 9.3) consists of the following regions:

- The **diaphysis**, which is the shaft of the long bone and is the main portion of the bone.
- The **epiphyses**, which are the distal and proximal ends of the bone.
- The **metaphyses**, which are the regions in a mature bone where the diaphysis joins the epiphysis. In a growing bone the metaphysis is the region occupied by the **epiphyseal growth plate**.

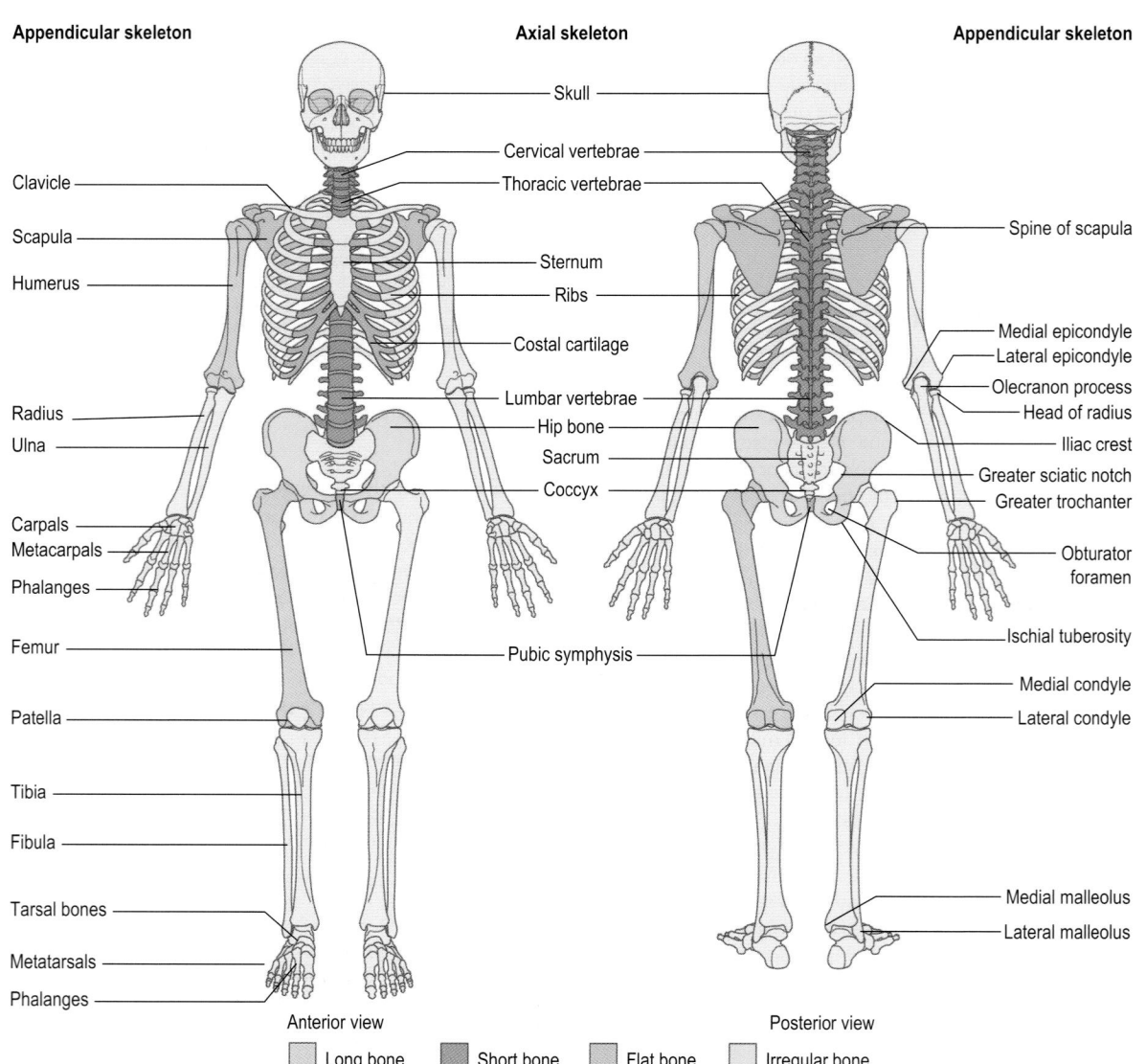

Fig. 9.2 The adult skeleton showing the types of bone.

Anatomy box 9.1 **The vertebral column**

The **vertebral column** is a rigid yet flexible structure that extends from the base of the skull to the tip of the coccyx (Fig. AB1). The vertebral column allows trunk movement, helps to maintain an upright posture, supports the weight of the body and head and allows the head to pivot. The vertebral column protects the spinal cord, which runs down through a canal formed by the vertebrae.

The vertebral column is composed of 24 moveable **vertebrae**:

- 7 in the **cervical** (neck) region (C_1–C_7)
- 12 in the **thoracic** region (T_1–T_{12})
- 5 in the **lumbar** region (L_1–L_5).

There are also two immobile composite vertebrae, the **sacrum** which is composed of five fused segments (S_1–S_5) and the **coccyx**, which is composed of three to five fused vertebrae. This gives a total of 33 ± 1 vertebrae. This number is fairly constant, with an estimated 5% of the population having a variation in the number of vertebrae.

The movements that the vertebral column can perform are:

- Anterior, posterior and lateral flexion
- Extension
- Rotation.

The movement between any two vertebral segments is relatively small, but added together there is a considerable range of movement possible.

The length of the vertebral column is 72–75 cm in adults and three-quarters of the length of the vertebral column is made up by the **vertebral bodies**, with the rest of the length made up by the **intervertebral discs** that lie between the vertebrae.

Curvatures
In the adult there are four curves in the vertebral column (Fig. AB1).

- Two primary curvatures: the **thoracic** and **sacral** curves. These curves develop in utero and give the newborn a single concave 'C' shaped curve to their backs.
- Two secondary curves: the convex **cervical** and **lumbar** curves. The cervical curve develops when the baby starts to hold up their head, and the lumbar curve develops when the infant starts to stand up and begins to walk.

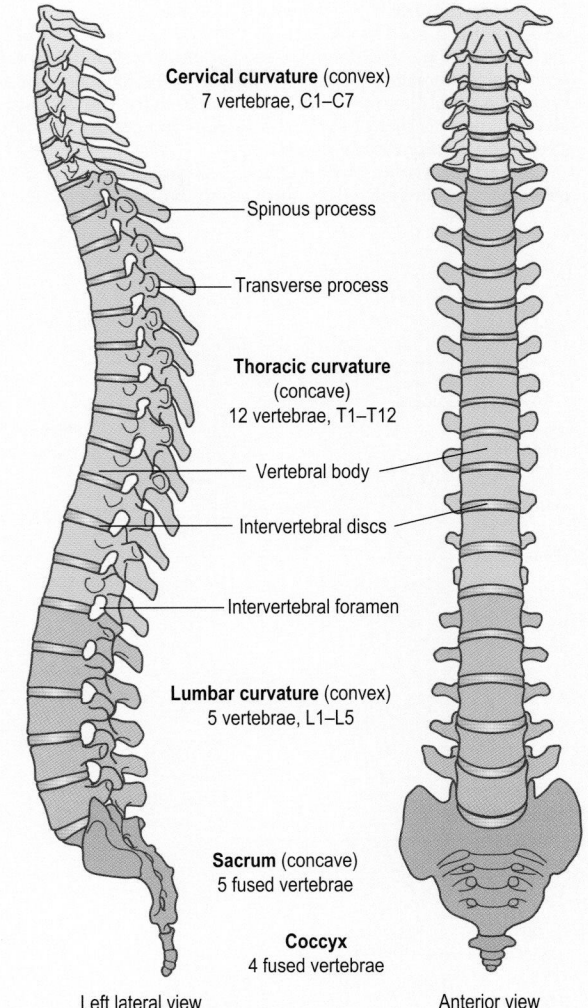

Cervical curvature (convex)
7 vertebrae, C1–C7

Spinous process

Transverse process

Thoracic curvature
(concave)
12 vertebrae, T1–T12

Vertebral body

Intervertebral discs

Intervertebral foramen

Lumbar curvature (convex)
5 vertebrae, L1–L5

Sacrum (concave)
5 fused vertebrae

Coccyx
4 fused vertebrae

Left lateral view   Anterior view

Fig. AB1 **The vertebral column.**

Clinical box 9.2 **Abnormal curves**

Scoliosis is a lateral curvature of the vertebral column. Most cases are idiopathic but some are due to a developmental defect. The lateral curvature of the spine often results in one shoulder and possibly one side of the pelvis being higher than the other. If the curvature is slight there may not be any significant defect when standing but the abnormal curve becomes more noticeable on bending over. Severe curves may restrict the lungs and the other internal organs, leading to the need for surgery to prevent any further advancement of the curve.

Kyphosis, also known as 'dowager's hump', is an increased thoracic curvature; this can form because of osteoporosis, where the thoracic vertebral bodies collapse. The progressive erosion and collapse of the vertebral bodies can result in an overall loss of height. In severe cases it may restrict breathing by reducing the capacity for the lungs to expand within the thoracic cage.

An increase in the lumbar curvature is called **lordosis** and is often associated with weakened trunk muscles. Lordosis can also result from obesity or during the latter stages of pregnancy, where the increase in weight anterior to the vertebral column pulls the lumbar vertebrae forwards. This abnormal curvature tends to be temporary and the vertebral column will revert to its normal curves after the baby is born or if the individual loses weight. If the abnormal curvature is severe enough then it can cause problems, again by restricting the internal organs, or by impinging on the nerve roots as they leave the spinal cord.

Anatomy box 9.2 The 'typical' vertebra

The **vertebral body** is the weight-bearing part of the vertebra; it is a solid block of bone that is the anterior part of the vertebra (Fig. AB2). Inferiorly the vertebral bodies become progressively greater in size, especially from T_4, reflecting the increased weight that the vertebrae have to carry; the largest vertebral body is that of L5. In the sacrum and coccyx, the size of the vertebral body decreases.

The **vertebral arch**, or **neural arch**, is composed of the **pedicles** and **laminae**, which form a ring through which the spinal cord passes called the **vertebral foramen** (spinal canal) (Fig. AB2). There are notches in the superior and inferior borders of the pedicles called the **vertebral notches**. These form an **intervertebral foramen**, through which the nerve roots exit and enter the spinal cord.

Each vertebral arch has seven processes which are attachment sites for muscles and ligaments:

- Four articular processes
- Two transverse processes
- One spinous process.

The vertebrae from different regions show a number of modifications, especially the atlas (C1) and axis (C2) vertebrae of the neck which form a specialised pivot joint (see below).

Joints and ligaments of the vertebral column

Between C2 to S1 adjacent vertebrae articulate at three joints:

- Two synovial (zygapophyses) between the vertebral arches
- One symphysis between the vertebral body and the intervertebral disc.

The **zygapophyses** are synovial joints of the planar kind and allow limited gliding movements between the vertebrae. Osteoarthritis may attack these joints, and the bony growths that form in this condition may reduce the size of the intervertebral foramen, leading to pressure on the spinal nerves.

The pivot joint between C1 and C2 allows the head to tip forward (the 'no' joint), and the atlanto-occipital joint between C1 and the base of the skull is the flexion/extension joint and therefore is the 'yes' joint.

Ligaments strengthen and stabilise the vertebral column and stop any excessive movements. The **anterior and posterior longitudinal ligaments** prevent hyperextension and hyperflexion, respectively. There are also short ligaments joining adjacent vertebrae: the **ligamentum flavum**. There are also **interspinous** and **supraspinous** ligaments and some specialised ligaments around the atlantoaxial joint.

Intervertebral discs

The joints between the vertebral bodies are secondary cartilaginous joints or symphyses designed for weight bearing and strength. The articulating surfaces of the adjacent vertebrae are connected by an **intervertebral disc**.

The intervertebral disc is composed of two parts: the **annulus fibrosus** is a fibrous ring consisting of alternating layers of obliquely orientated collagen fibres surrounding the central gelatinous **nucleus pulposus**, which is a turgid gel composed of 70–90% water, proteoglycans and some collagen fibres which allows compression between adjacent vertebrae. When weight is applied to the disc the nucleus becomes flattened and the annulus fibrosus bulges between the vertebrae.

The water content of the intervertebral discs declines with age so the intervertebral discs are better shock absorbers in the young than in the elderly and this also accounts for some of the loss of height that is experienced with age. If the intervertebral discs reduce in height, the intervertebral foramen also reduces in size, which may lead to entrapment of the spinal nerves.

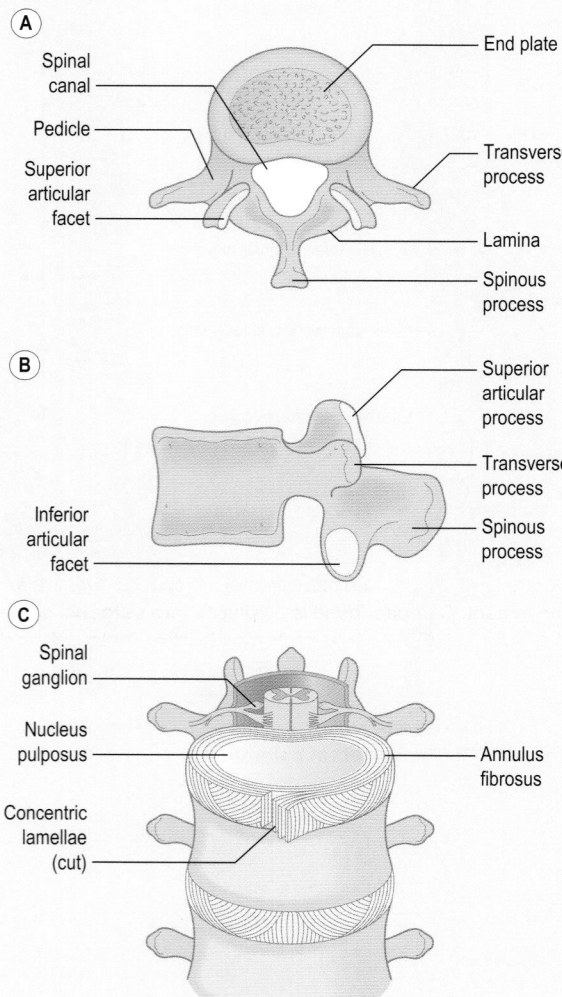

(A)
Spinal canal
Pedicle
Superior articular facet
End plate
Transverse process
Lamina
Spinous process

(B)
Inferior articular facet
Superior articular process
Transverse process
Spinous process

(C)
Spinal ganglion
Nucleus pulposus
Concentric lamellae (cut)
Annulus fibrosus

Fig. AB2 **A typical vertebra:** (A) cross-sectional view; (B) lateral view (showing vertebral body, pedicles, laminae, spinal cord, processes, intravertebral disc and ligaments); and (C) section showing intervertebral discs.

Slipped disc (herniation of the intervertebral disc)

A **slipped disc** is a protrusion of the nucleus pulposus through the annulus fibrosus. The protrusion can press on the spinal nerve roots, causing referred pain. This commonly takes place in the lumbar region, leading to **sciatica**, where the pain is felt in the lower back, posterior thigh and leg, which is the course of the sciatic nerve. Approximately 95% of herniations of the nucleus pulposus in the lumbar region take place at the L4/5 or the L5/S1 levels.

Muscles of the vertebral column

There are superficial, intermediate and deep muscles around the vertebral column. The superficial muscles are located around the back of the neck and shoulders and act to help move the shoulders. The intermediate group of muscles is located in the lower neck and thoracic level and may be related to inspiration. The deep back muscles maintain posture and move the vertebral column.

Extreme movements of the vertebral column may lead to back strain. The term strain is used to indicate some degree of stretching of the muscles and or ligaments of the back.

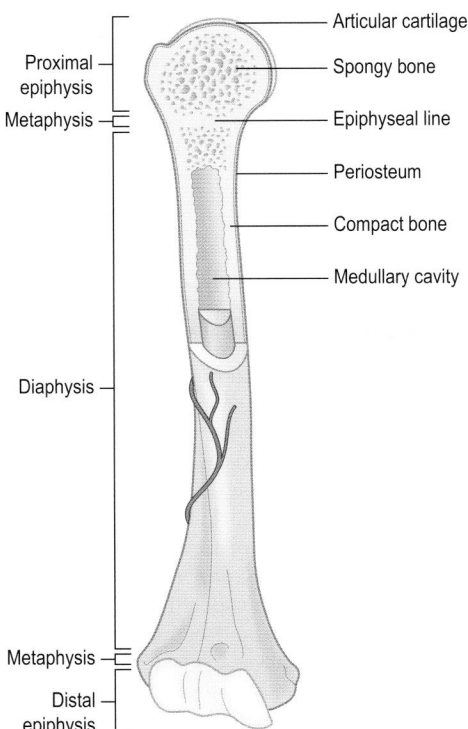

Fig. 9.3 Structure of a typical long bone.

Articular cartilage is a thin layer of hyaline cartilage that covers the epiphyses. The articular cartilage reduces the friction at the joints and acts as a shock absorber at freely moveable joints.

The **periosteum** is a tough layer of dense irregular connective tissue surrounding the bone surface where it is not covered by the articular cartilage. It contains the osteogenic progenitor cells and as these differentiate into osteoblasts they allow the bone to grow in thickness. The periosteum also helps to protect the bone, assists in fracture repair, helps nourish the bone tissue and serves as an attachment point for tendons and ligaments.

The **medullary cavity** in the centre of the bones is sometimes called the **marrow cavity** and is the space within the diaphysis that contains the bone marrow. Two types of bone marrow are found in the medullary cavity:

- **Red marrow**, which produces red and white blood cells and platelets
- **Yellow marrow**, which contains fat and connective tissue and produces some white blood cells.

The two types of bone marrow are interconvertible. At birth there is only red bone marrow present and as the person grows the red marrow in many of the bones is replaced by yellow marrow. By adulthood, only about half of the bone marrow is red. The change from red to yellow is due to a decrease in the levels of **erythropoietin**, the hormone that regulates erythrocyte mitosis and differentiation, and means that in bones of an elderly individual only 30% of the bone marrow is red bone marrow. Red bone marrow is found mostly in the ribs, sternum (breastbone), scapulae (shoulder blades), clavicles (collarbones), pelvis (hip bones), skull and vertebrae.

The **endosteum** is a membrane that lines the medullary cavity and contains bone-forming cells; it is the equivalent of the periosteum surrounding the outside of the bone. It serves as the site of formation for new bone and contains the osteogenic precursor cells.

Compact bone

Compact bone forms the outer layer of all bones, where it provides support and protection to the spongy bone in the centre and resists the stresses produced by weight and movement. Compact bone is organised into **osteons**, sometimes called **Haversian systems**. In the centre of each osteon there is a **central canal (Haversian canal)** which runs longitudinally through the bone; running through this central canal are blood and lymph vessels and nerves. Around the central canal the bone is arranged into concentric **lamellae** which are rings of calcified matrix in which osteocytes have become embedded, forming small lacunae. Radiating away from the osteocytes are small finger-like projections which form small channels called **canaliculi**. The canaliculi connect the lacunae with one another and also with the central canal. They therefore form a complex branching network for blood–borne nutrients and oxygen to diffuse through the bone and for waste products to diffuse back to the blood vessels. The blood vessels of the central canal are connected to the periosteal vessels on the surface of the bone by **perforating (Volkmann's) canals**, which also connect with the medullary cavity (Fig. 9.4A).

The osteons in compact bone are all aligned in the same direction along the lines of stress. In the diaphysis of a long bone, for example, they run parallel to the long axis of the bone. This allows the diaphysis to resist bending or fracturing even when considerable force is applied from either end. The stresses on bone are not constant and the organisation of the osteons is dynamic in response to these new stresses made on the bone, and is part of the normal destruction of old bone and the formation of new bone matrix. The response of bone to new stresses can be seen by the presence of interstitial lamellae between the osteons, these are the remnants of old osteons that have been partly broken down.

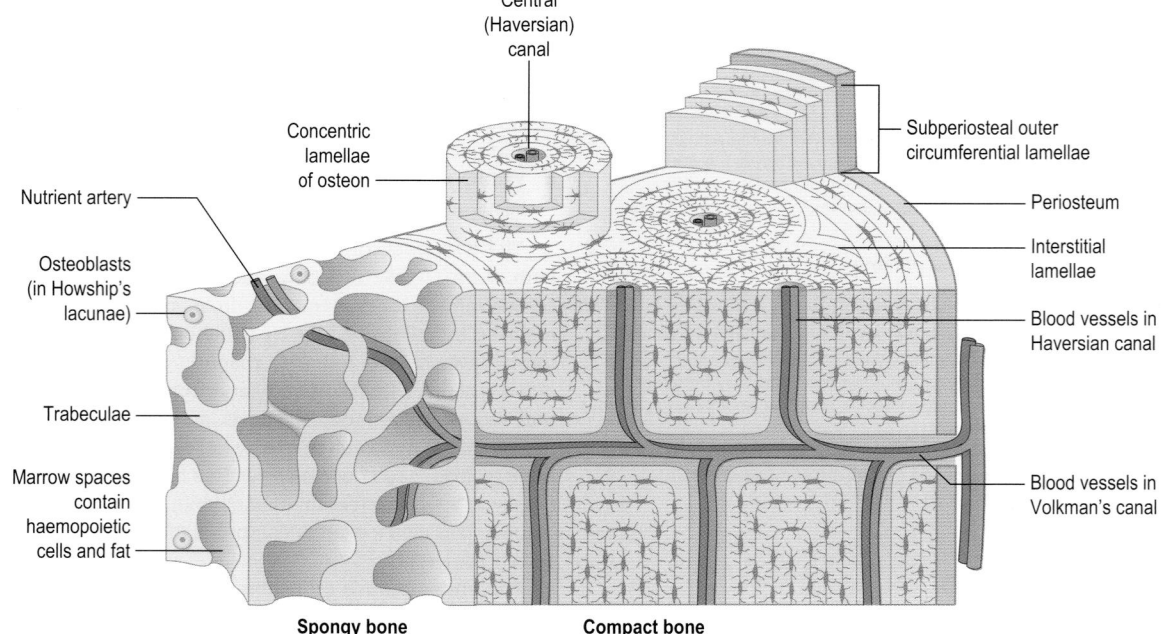

Fig. 9.4 **Compact and spongy bone.**

Spongy bone

Spongy bone does not contain true osteons and consists of lamellae arranged into an irregular lattice of **trabeculae**. The spaces between the trabeculae are filled with red or yellow bone marrow, which is responsible for the production of blood cells. Within each trabeculae osteocytes lie in lacunae with radiating canaliculi, much like in the osteons of the compact bone. The osteocytes in the spongy bone trabeculae receive their nutrients directly from the blood circulating through the medullary cavity (Fig. 9.4B).

Spongy bone makes up the majority of bony tissue in the short, flat, and irregularly shaped bones and the epiphyses of the long bones, and lines the medullary cavity of the diaphysis of the long bones.

The orientation of the trabeculae in spongy bone is along the lines of stress, like the osteons in compact bone. This characteristic helps bone resist stresses and the transfer of force without breaking. Spongy bone is located where bones are not heavily stressed or where the stresses are applied from many directions, as this type of bone has both flexibility and strength. Spongy bone has a higher rate of turnover than compact bone, and so responds to the changing stresses placed on it faster than compact bone does. For this reason osteoporosis is more evident in the spongy bone compartments than in compact bone.

Spongy bone reduces the weight of the skeleton, so that the muscles acting on the skeleton do not have to work as hard. In the adult the spongy bone and its red bone marrow is the only site of haemopoiesis, especially the spongy bone of the pelvis (hip), ribs, sternum (breast bone), vertebra and the ends of the long bones.

Blood and nerve supply to bone

Certain regions of bone contain large quantities of red bone marrow and these regions have a very good blood supply that passes from the periosteum into the interior of the bone. The **periosteal arteries** are accompanied by nerves and they enter the diaphysis through the perforating Volkmann's canals. They supply the periosteum and the compact bone. Near the centre of the diaphysis there is a large **nutrient artery** that passes obliquely through the compact bone through a hole – the **nutrient foramen**. When the nutrient artery reaches the medullary cavity it divides into proximal and distal branches, which supply both the inner layers of compact bone and spongy bone of the diaphysis and the red marrow as far as the epiphyseal growth plates (or lines). The number of nutrient foramina varies from bone to bone, the tibia has only one nutrient artery while the femur has many; this variation is due to the size of the bone and the relative amounts of red bone marrow that the bone has. The ends of the bone are supplied by the **metaphyseal** and **epiphyseal arteries**. These arteries arise from the arteries that supply the joint. Both the metaphyseal and epiphyseal arteries also enter the bone and supply the red bone marrow in their respective regions.

There are usually one or two **nutrient veins** that accompany the artery in the diaphysis, and there are many **epiphyseal** and **metaphyseal veins** which also exit with the respective arteries. Finally, there are also **periosteal veins** that drain blood from the periosteum.

Nerves accompany the blood vessels of bone. The periosteum has a rich supply of sensory nerves, some of which transmit pain sensations. These nerves are sensitive to tearing or tension and explain the severe pain from a fracture or a bone tumour.

BONE DEVELOPMENT

Bony tissue is formed by one of two processes during embryonic development:

- **Endochondral ossification**: the replacement of hyaline cartilage with bone tissue
- **Intramembranous ossification**: the direct ossification of the mesenchymal cells.

Ossification begins during the sixth or seventh week of human development; once they are fully formed the bones produced by these two processes are indistinguishable in structure.

Endochondral ossification

The majority of the bones in the body are formed from cartilage by **endochondral ossification**. Hyaline cartilage forms an initial model of the future bone from mesenchymal cells that differentiate into chondroblasts. Once the hyaline model of the bone has formed, osteoblasts gradually replace the cartilage with bone matrix, which is then ossified. The process is most clearly seen in the long bones of the arms and legs (Fig. 9.5).

The process begins with mesenchymal cells at the site of the future bone condensing into a rough approximation of the bones. These mesenchymal cells differentiate into **chondroblasts** (precursors of cartilage) under the influence of various factors in the environment. The chondroblasts then begin to secrete a cartilage matrix around themselves, with a membrane called the **perichondrium** forming around the cartilage model containing the chondroblast precursors. As more cartilage matrix is produced the chondroblasts become buried in the matrix, and they become **chondrocytes**.

As the fetus grows so does the cartilage model. The chondrocytes can divide and the new chondrocytes produce more cartilage matrix, causing an increase in the *length* of the cartilage bone model. This is called **interstitial** growth. The increase in the *thickness* of the bone is from new chondroblasts differentiating from the precursors in the perichondrium and becoming incorporated into the cartilage bone model, which is called **appositional** growth.

As the cartilage model grows, the chondrocytes in the centre of the model hypertrophy. Some of the hypertrophied cells burst and release their contents into the cartilage matrix around them. This changes the pH of the matrix and it is this change in pH that triggers the calcification of the cartilage matrix. As the cartilage begins to calcify, chondrocytes begin to die as their nutrients can no longer diffuse through the calcifying matrix. Where the chondrocytes had been, spaces called **lacunae** form and these eventually merge together forming small cavities within the calcifying matrix.

For bone formation or ossification to begin a nutrient artery must pierce the perichondrium and the calcifying matrix in the mid region of the cartilage model. This stimulates the osteogenic precursor cells in the perichondrium to become osteoblasts. Initially these remain just under the perichondrium and secrete a thin shell of compact bone called the **periosteal bone collar**. Once the perichondrium starts to produce bone rather than cartilage it becomes the **periosteum**. Osteoblasts are carried into the disintegrating calcified matrix by the nutrient artery and its capillaries. Once these are within the cartilage model they begin to form bone and the **primary ossification centre** is formed. **Spongy bone** is formed as osteoblasts deposit bone matrix on the remains of the calcified cartilage. As the ossification centre enlarges towards the ends of the bone, osteoclasts start to break down the new spongy bone to form the **medullary cavity** in the centre of the bone, where the bone marrow will be located. Primary ossification therefore proceeds inwards from the external surface to the centre of the bone.

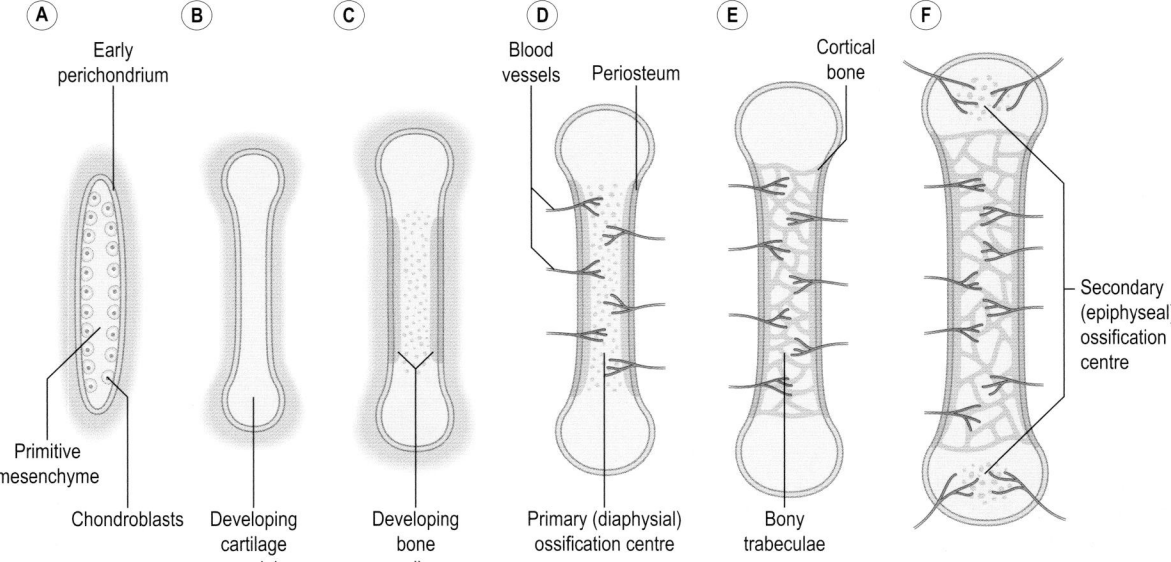

Fig. 9.5 **Endochondral ossification.**

Primary ossification forms the diaphysis or shaft of the long bones, composed of an outer core of compact bone, lined with spongy bone surrounding a medullary cavity which is filled with red bone marrow. **Secondary ossification centres** form the epiphyses at the ends of the long bones and these usually develop at around the time of birth. The formation of bone in the secondary ossification centres is much the same as for that in the primary ossification centres. However, there is one difference in that spongy bone remains in the interior of the epiphyses. Secondary ossification also proceeds in an outward direction from the centre of the epiphysis towards the outer surface of the bone.

The still-growing bone has two regions composed of hyaline cartilage: the first is the cap of **articular cartilage** that covers the epiphyses at both ends of the bone, and the second is the **epiphyseal growth plate** located between the epiphysis and the diaphysis, which is responsible for the growth in length of the bones during childhood. The articular cartilage cap at the end of the bone is retained throughout life and helps to reduce the friction between the articulating bones.

Intramembranous ossification

The second process by which bone is formed is **intramembranous ossification**, where bone forms directly in the condensed mesenchymal cells without first going through a cartilage step (Fig. 9.6). This type of ossification tends to be found in the flat bones of the skull, the lower jaw, and the scapula of the pectoral girdle. At the site of future bone the mesenchymal cells condense as for endochondral ossification, but they differentiate into osteogenic cells rather than chondroblasts. The osteoblasts cluster together forming a centre of ossification and secrete the organic bone matrix around themselves. Once surrounded, the osteoblasts become osteocytes located in lacunae and they extend fine cytoplasmic processes into canaliculi in all directions.

Calcium and other mineral salts are deposited in the matrix within a few days and this hardens and calcifies forming **bony spicules**. The matrix develops into spongy bone with **trabeculae** (small pieces of bone) separated by spaces. The connective tissue associated with the blood vessels in the trabeculae differentiates into red bone marrow that fills the spaces. On the outside of the bone the mesenchyme condenses and develops into the periosteum. Finally, the most superficial layers of spongy bone are remodelled into compact bone with spongy bone remaining in the centre.

BONE GROWTH

During childhood the bones grow both in thickness and in length. The bones continue to grow in length until about 25 years of age, although they may still increase in thickness after this time.

Bone growth in length

Bone growth in length, especially the long bones, is by the addition of new bone on the diaphyseal side of the epiphyseal growth plates. The epiphyseal growth plate is composed of hyaline cartilage and separates the epiphyses from the diaphysis of the growing bones. It can be divided into four zones (Fig. 9.7).

- Zone 1 is the zone of **resting cartilage**. It is closest to the epiphysis and is made up of small, scattered chondrocytes that have a low rate of proliferation. These cells do not have a function in the growth of the bone; their role is to anchor the epiphyseal growth plate to the bone of the epiphysis and to provide the supplies for the developing cartilage cells and to store the necessary materials (lipids, glycogen, proteoglycan aggregates) for growth.
- Zone 2 is the zone of **proliferating cartilage**. The chondrocytes are slightly larger and are stacked like

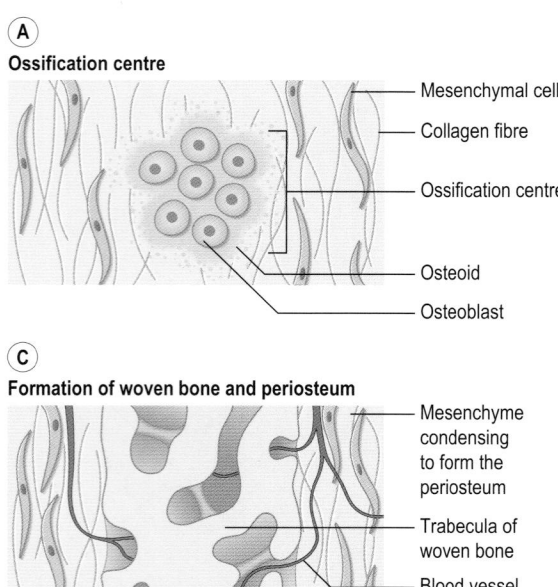

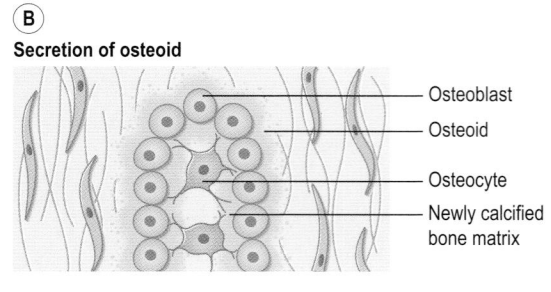

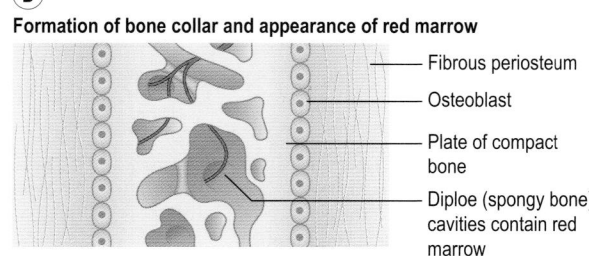

Fig. 9.6 Intramembranous ossification.

coins. The chondrocytes are dividing and replacing the ones that are dying at the diaphyseal side of the epiphyseal growth plate. These chondrocytes produce the necessary matrix and are responsible for longitudinal growth of the bone via active cell division.

- Zone 3 is the zone of **hypertrophic cartilage**. This zone can be further subdivided into maturation, degeneration, and provisional calcification zones. The chondrocytes increase in size, still in their columns, and they accumulate calcium within their mitochondria; this causes them to deteriorate, and ultimately leads to their cell death. Upon their death, calcium is released from matrix vesicles, impregnating the matrix with calcium salt. The calcification of the matrix is necessary for invasion of metaphyseal blood vessels, destruction of cartilage cells, and the formation of bone along the walls of the calcified cartilage matrix. No active growth occurs in this layer; columns of cells extending toward the metaphysis are at various stages of maturation. This is the weakest portion of the physis and is commonly a site of fracture or alteration (e.g. widening, as in rickets).
- Zone 4 is the zone of **calcified cartilage**. This layer is only a few cells thick and is composed of mainly dead or dying chondrocytes, because they have become surrounded by a calcified matrix. The calcified matrix is removed by the action of osteoclasts and invaded by osteoblasts. The osteoblasts lay down new bone matrix and therefore result in the diaphyseal border being firmly attached to the epiphyseal growth plate. It is only by the action of the epiphyseal growth plate that the diaphysis can increase in length. Cartilage is replaced by bone at the diaphyseal end of the growth plate and new

chondrocytes are added to the epiphyseal growth plate to maintain its size. Thus the thickness of the epiphyseal growth plate is maintained.

Between the ages of 18 and 25 the epiphyseal growth plates begin to close. The main stimulus for growth by the epiphyseal growth plate is **growth hormone (GH)**, which is secreted by the pituitary gland and promotes growth during childhood and adolescence. Growth hormone acts on the liver and other tissues to stimulate production of **insulin-like growth factor 1 (IGF-1)**, which is responsible for the growth-promoting effects of growth hormone and also reflects the amount produced. The amount of hGH, and so IGF-1, declines with age.

When the levels of GH and IGF-1 begin to decline the chondrocytes in zone 2 stop dividing and so the thickness of the epiphyseal growth plate gets thinner as bone gradually replaces the cartilage. Eventually only the epiphyseal line remains as a bony feature on the bones, indicating that the bones have stopped growing. The last bone to finish growing is the clavicle. On X-rays of children and young adults, the epiphyseal growth plates are visible as a radiolucent area between the bone of the epiphysis and the diaphysis, as cartilage is radiolucent. If a fracture damages the epiphyseal growth plate while it is still open, then the fractured bone may be shorter than normal. This is because the epiphyseal growth plate is an avascular structure and damage to it accelerates the closure of the plate and so growth of the bone is reduced. If the rate of bone formation is reduced then the affected bone will be shorter and may cause misalignment of joint surfaces, and in severe cases shorter stature (Clinical Box 9.4).

Growth in bone thickness

Bone can increase in thickness by **appositional growth**. The periosteal cells at the bone surface differentiate into osteo-

Resting (quiescent) zone	Zone 1
Growth (proliferation) zone Cartilage cells undergo mitosis	Zone 2
Hypertrophic zone Older cartilage cells enlarge	Zone 3
Calcification zone Matrix becomes calcified; cartilage cells die; matrix begins deteriorating	Zone 4
Ossification (osteogenic) zone New bone formation is occurring	Zone 5

Fig. 9.7 **Bone growth in length.** Redrawn with permission from Young B, Heath JW 2006 Wheater's functional histology, 5th edn. Edinburgh, Churchill Livingstone.

Clinical box 9.4	Achondroplasia (without cartilage formation)

Achondroplasia is the commonest cause of short stature, with an average adult height of about 1.2 m (4 ft) for affected men and women, and it occurs in around 1 : 22 000 live births. Achondroplasia is an autosomal dominant disorder, but approximately 75% of cases represent new dominant mutations. The gene for achondroplasia has recently been found. Achondroplasia is due to a change in the **fibroblast growth factor** receptor 3 gene, with most of the mutations occurring at the same position. The diagnosis of achondroplasia is based on a number of very specific features that can be seen in X-rays.

During fetal development and childhood, the majority of the bones have a cartilage precursor that becomes ossified and forms bone (endochondral ossification, see above). In individuals with achondroplasia, something goes wrong during this process, especially in the long bones of the upper and lower limbs. The rate at which cartilage cells in the growth plates of the long bones turn into bone is slow, leading to short bones and reduced height.

Children affected with achondroplasia frequently have delayed motor milestones, otitis media, and bowing of the knees. Most individuals with achondroplasia are of normal intelligence and lead independent and productive lives.

blasts and components secrete collagen fibres and other organic forming the bone matrix. The osteoblasts become surrounded by the matrix and develop into osteocytes. This forms bone ridges along the bone on either side of a periosteal blood vessel. As more bone matrix is produced the ridges grow and create a groove for the blood vessel. The ridges eventually fuse together and form a tunnel for the blood vessel. The former periosteum now becomes endosteum that lines the tunnel.

Bone deposition continues from the osteoblasts in the endosteum forming concentric lamellae that proceed towards the centre of the tunnel. Once the tunnel is filled in with bone it is a new osteon. As an osteon is forming, osteoblasts under the periosteum deposit a new circumferential lamella, which further increases the thickness of the bone. This process continues as new periosteal blood vessels become enclosed.

As new bone is being added on the outer surface of the bone, the bone lining the medullary cavity is being destroyed by osteoclasts in the endosteum. Therefore, the medullary cavity gets larger as the bone increases in diameter.

Factors affecting bone growth

Adequate dietary intake of minerals and vitamins is essential to maintain the growth of bone, as well as sufficient levels of several hormones.

Calcium and phosphorus are needed in considerable quantities during bone growth. Fluoride, magnesium, iron and manganese are required in smaller amounts. Vitamin C is required for the synthesis of the collagen – which is the main bone protein – and is also needed for the differentiation of osteoblasts into osteocytes. The vitamins K and B_{12} are required for protein synthesis, and vitamin A stimulates the activity of osteoblasts.

IGFs are the most important hormones during childhood to stimulate growth of the bones. IGFs are produced by the bone tissue itself and also by the liver. They act by promoting cell division and synthesis of new bone proteins at the epiphyseal growth plate and periosteum. The production of IGF is stimulated by **hGH** produced by the anterior pituitary. The thyroid hormones T_3 and T_4 and insulin are also required for normal bone growth.

At puberty the ovaries and testes secrete sex steroids. Initially the sex steroids cause a sudden growth spurt and the oestrogens in the female start to cause changes in the female skeleton, such as a wider pelvis. The sex steroids, especially oestrogens, contribute to the shutting down of the epiphyseal growth plate. Females have more circulating oestrogens than males, who have higher androgens; therefore, the lengthwise growth of bones stops earlier in females than males.

Bone remodelling

In normal life there is constant bone remodelling, where the resorption of bone by osteoclasts matches the formation of new bone by the osteoblast cells. Osteoclasts attach to the surface of old bone that is about to be resorbed. The ruffled border of the osteoclast faces the bone surface; they seal themselves onto the bone surface when activated. They secrete enzymes such as **collagenases** and **lysosomal**

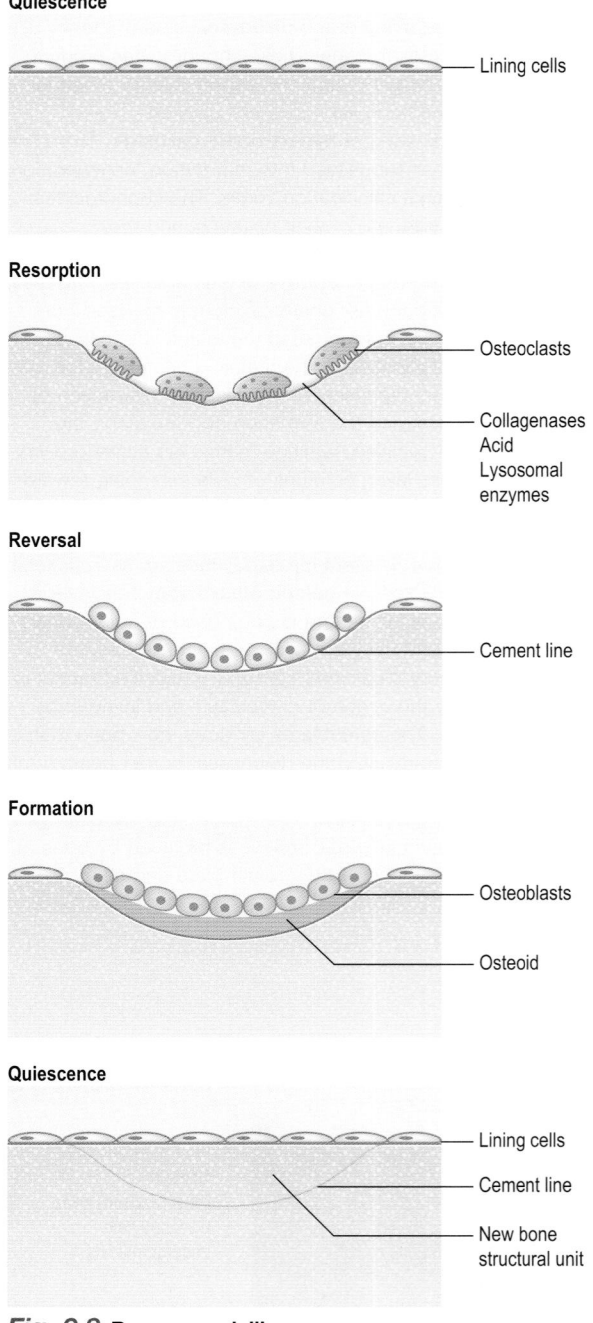

Fig. 9.8 **Bone remodelling.**

enzymes that attack the organic portion of the bone under the leak-proof seal beneath their ruffled border. They also secrete acid to dissolve the inorganic salts of the bone matrix. Both bone proteins and minerals – mainly calcium salts – enter the osteoclasts and pass through to be excreted into the extracellular space (Fig. 9.8). The next step is that osteoblasts migrate into the hollowed out space prepared by the osteoclasts. They synthesise **type 1 collagen**, **osteocalcin** (also known as **bone Gla protein**), and the other organic components of bone such as proteoglycans and growth factors. The osteoblasts also control the mineralisation of the bone. The osteoid matrix is gradually coated in calcium salts and hardens. As the osteoblasts become embedded in the mineralising matrix, they slow down their production of matrix protein and become osteocytes. The bone is now in a resting phase of the remodelling cycle.

This cycle is the same for both compact cortical bone and the trabecular network of the internal spongy bone. This constant remodelling means that old bone is removed before it can deteriorate, and also redistributes the bone matrix along lines of mechanical stress. Uncoupling bone resorption from bone formation leads to the bone conditions with a loss or increase in the body's bone mass, as seen in osteoporosis, osteomalacia or Paget's disease (Clinical Box 9.5).

The whole process of bone remodelling takes between 160 and 200 days from when the osteoclasts begin to remove the old bone and when the osteoblasts have become embedded in the mineralised bone matrix. The final stage of bone healing after a fracture occurs by the same process as happens in bone remodelling (see below).

BONE'S ROLE IN CALCIUM HOMEOSTASIS

The main calcium store for the body is the bone, with 99% of the total body calcium stored in the skeleton; serum calcium represents less than 1% of the body's total calcium. The serum calcium level is extremely important for many vital bodily functions, such as blood clotting, nerve cell activity, and many other cellular activities. The concentration of calcium ions in the blood plasma is therefore very closely regulated to be maintained within 8.5 mg/100 mL and 10.5 mg/100 mL, as even small changes outside of this narrow window can be fatal, by heart or respiratory arrest due to either calcium concentrations that are too high or low respectively. The level of calcium in the blood must therefore be very tightly regulated by controlling the rate of calcium resorption from bone into the blood, and calcium deposition into the bones. There are two major hormones and one minor hormone that control calcium homeostasis.

Parathyroid hormone

Parathyroid hormone (PTH) is an 84-amino acid peptide which is secreted by the four parathyroid glands, which are located on the back of the thyroid gland in the neck. PTH is the most important regulatory hormone of calcium concentration in the bone and blood and is linked to several negative feedback systems that adjust blood calcium ion concentration. A fall in blood calcium ions is detected by the PTH receptors, and PTH synthesis is increased and is released into the blood. PTH affects the activity of osteoclasts, which increase the resorption of bone, thus resulting in the release of calcium from the bone into the blood. PTH also acts on the kidneys to increase calcium reabsorption, phosphate excretion and 1,25-dihydroxyvitamin D synthesis. Normally 95% of the calcium filtered by the kidney is reabsorbed, PTH actually decreases calcium reabsorption from the proximal tubule but increases the reabsorption from the distal nephron. There is also decreased phosphate reabsorption from the proximal tubule, which results in its increased excretion.

Vitamin D

1,25-dihydroxyvitamin D (dihydroxycholecalciferol) is the second factor that controls serum calcium levels. Vitamin D is derived from two sources: the diet (D_3) or by synthesis in the skin (D_2). This is then converted to **25-dihydroxyvitamin D** in the liver, which is then converted to the active 1,25-dihydroxyvitamin D in the kidneys. 1,25-dihydroxyvitamin D is a very potent stimulator of intestinal calcium and phosphate absorption, and is also a stimulator of bone resorption, although only at high concentrations. At normal physiological levels 1,25-dihydroxyvitamin D is necessary for proper bone mineralisation, and the lack of vitamin D either due to dietary deficiencies or lack of sunlight exposure leads to osteomalacia (Clinical Box 9.6).

The principal role of 1,25-dihydroxyvitamin D is the increased mineralisation of the bone matrix, a part of this is due to the raised plasma Ca^{2+} levels from the action of 1,25-dihydroxyvitamin D on the gut. 1,25-dihydroxyvitamin D can

---

Clinical box 9.5   Paget's disease (osteitis deformans)

In **Paget's disease** there is accelerated bone turnover, which is indicated by an increased osteoclast-mediated bone resorption. The osteoclasts seen in Paget's disease patients are numerous and large, with up to 100 nuclei in them. The alkaline phosphatase levels are very high as well indicating increased osteoblast activity. The increase in bone turnover leads to thicker but softer bones and is frequently associated with fractures.

Paradoxically there is also **bone thickening**, but the new bone is new woven bone as there is no remodelling to stronger compact and trabecular bone. This thickening of the bone may trap nerves, resulting in severe bone pain. Untreated, the disease progresses and the legs may bow, the spine develops a curvature and the skull may increase in size with the person's hat size going up several sizes. If there is severe skull enlargement there can be problems with the patient's vision and hearing as the nerves become trapped. Treatment includes the administration of drugs that reduce bone turnover, such as bisphosphonates and analgesics.

Clinical box 9.6   Osteomalacia

Osteomalacia is a softening of the bones and the childhood variety of this condition is **rickets**. There is no loss in the mass of the bones, but the ratio of matrix to mineral changes so that there is more bone matrix and less bone mineral than in the normal bones. It can produce similar symptoms to osteoporosis. It is due to the inadequate mineralisation of newly formed bone matrix. Rickets is only seen before the epiphyseal growth plate has closed, and causes a bowing of the legs as the bones are softer and bend. This may be due to a lack of dietary calcium or to a lack of activated vitamin D, which is needed for the absorption of calcium from the gut. In children, the bones are soft anyway because they are growing, so the deformities produced by osteomalacia may be severe, with curvature of the spine and bowed legs. In children the epiphyseal growth plate is widened and may be cup or trumpet shaped, and the line of ossification is less distinct. In adults, because the bones have stopped growing, the deformities are less severe, and the symptoms are more like osteoporosis. On an X-ray of an adult with osteomalacia, there may be pseudofractures visible on regions of bones that have muscle attachments. These radiolucent lines on the bones are called 'Looser's zones or lines'.

also stimulate the proliferation and activity of the osteoblasts, which are producing the new bone matrix.

Calcitonin

Calcitonin also contributes to controlling the blood plasma concentration of calcium. It is released from the parafollicular cells of the thyroid gland and can directly inhibit osteoclast activity. Therefore, calcitonin leads to less calcium resorption from the bones and more calcium is incorporated into the bone tissue. Under normal physiological conditions calcitonin has only minor effects, which are the opposite of PTH.

Other factors affecting bone mass

Oestrogen

Oestrogen increases the activity of osteoblasts and decreases the activity of the osteoclasts that remove the bone. It therefore has a protective effect in women and the loss of oestrogen at the menopause removes this protective effect and there is a rapid loss of bone mass in the 5 years around the time of the menopause (Clinical box 9.7).

Exercise

As bone is continually being formed and broken down it has the ability to alter its strength in response to **mechanical stress**. More new bone is deposited along the lines of stress, and calcitonin production is increased to inhibit bone resorption. With no mechanical stress, bone does not undergo normal remodelling and bone resorption outweighs bone formation. The main mechanical stress that bone encounters is from the contraction of skeletal muscles and the pull of gravity. If a person is bedridden or has a fractured bone that is placed in a cast, the strength of the unstressed bones reduces. Astronauts who live in a low gravity environment for even a short length of time lose bone mass dramatically – as much as 1% a week. The bone of athletes on the other hand, whose bones are continually under repetitive stress, become thicker. Any weight-bearing activity helps to maintain bone mass and this is especially vital just prior to the closure of the epiphyseal growth plate, as it helps to build up bone mass prior to the inevitable loss with age. Even in the elderly, weight-bearing activities can help to slow the loss of bone mass.

Diet and bone mass

A calcium intake of between 800 mg and 1500 mg per day is considered to be adequate for most adults; children and teenagers require higher levels of calcium in their diet as their bones are actively growing. However, the amount of calcium required to be taken in from dietary sources must be considered alongside those of the other dietary components that affect absorption of calcium from the gut, and also those factors that influence calcium losses.

Calcium is lost from the body in urine, gut secretions and sweat. To avoid a net loss of calcium from the bones the calcium absorbed from food in the gut must balance the losses. Otherwise, the body will take calcium from bone to maintain the required level of calcium in the blood. The body contains about 1 kg of calcium in the bones. Even a small excess in the loss of calcium compared with absorption of

---

Clinical box 9.7 **Osteoporosis**

Osteoporosis literally means porous bones, and there is a generalised loss of bone mass making the bones more insubstantial and brittle. In both men and women, bones reach their maximum density in early adulthood. By the age of 20 years, 90–95% of the peak bone mass has being attained and from around 40 years of age there is a gradual loss of bone mass. However, in women, the loss of oestrogen at the menopause means that the protection the hormone provides in preventing osteoclast activity is now removed, and bone loss is increased. As women's skeletons tend to be lighter to begin with a relatively small loss of bone mass can have severe implications on the health of their bones. There is a loss in the bone mass but the ratio of bone matrix to mineral is unchanged.

The condition is usually diagnosed from the X-ray appearance of the bones where they appear more radiolucent and less dense than normal. However, normal X-rays are relatively insensitive to the loss of bone mass and as much as 50% of the bone mass has to be lost for it to be clearly seen on an X-ray. In most cases of osteoporosis the loss of bone is not evenly distributed; trabecular bone has a higher rate of bone remodelling and so bones that contain a large trabecular bone framework are particularly at risk. The loss of bone mass is greatest in the trabecular bone with a reduction of between 2% and 3% per year, and in the cortical bone the loss averages 1–2% per year. This includes the vertebral body and the neck of the femur.

The loss of bone mass has no clinical effect unless a fracture occurs. Fractures of the vertebral bodies create a loss in the anterior height of the vertebrae, leading to kyphosis (excessive posterior curvature) of the back. Fracture of the neck of the femur increases with age until by the age of 75 it is the most common type of fracture, due to the osteoporosis seen in the elderly.

Genetic, hormonal, nutritional and activity factors all play a role in the development of osteoporosis. Excessive glucocorticoid activity, either naturally from an adrenal tumour or from artificial sources such as the prolonged use of corticosteroids, also lead to the loss of bone mass and osteoporosis. Excessive alcohol, caffeine and smoking can also lead to the loss of bone mass and brittle bone.

To prevent osteoporosis, children and especially young girls should be encouraged to maintain an adequate dietary intake of calcium, and to exercise, both of which will build up the strength of the bones. Throughout life adequate dietary calcium and exercise should be continued, not to prevent bone loss but to minimise the rate of loss. In women the use of hormone replacement therapy has been shown to slow down the development of osteoporosis in postmenopausal women.

Apart from hormone replacement therapy another treatment available for osteoporosis is the class of drugs known as the bisphosphonates. These are pyrophosphate analogues that bind to the hydroxyapatite crystals of the bone matrix and so inhibit bone breakdown. They also inhibit osteoclast attachment to the bone matrix, as well as stimulating osteoblasts to inhibit osteoclast formation.

---

just 30 mg per day, will at the end of the year result in a 1% loss of calcium from the bones.

The typical diet of North Americans and Europeans contains four dietary components with equal importance that lead to a net calcium loss: high sodium, high protein, low potassium and low bicarbonate intakes.

- Increasing the sodium intake from 1000 mg to 4000 mg per day causes an additional 52 mg of calcium loss per day. Increasing the protein intake from 40 g to 100 g per day will cause an additional calcium loss of 66 mg per day.

- Decreasing the potassium intake from 8000 mg to 2000 mg per day will increase calcium losses by 31 mg per day.
- Finally, decreasing the bicarbonate intake from 100 mmol to 20 mmol per day will increase calcium losses by 32 mg per day.

In children, adolescents and younger adults, calcium absorption is more efficient and adapts better to increased losses with better production of 1,25-dihydroxyvitamin D. Older individuals of both sexes show a decline in calcium absorption of about 30–40% less at 80 years than at 30 years, and so they are affected more by these dietary factors.

The best foods for increasing calcium absorption without effecting calcium loss are the green leafy vegetables such as kale and spring greens. Surprisingly, all dairy foods increase calcium loss as well as providing calcium. Foods such as meat, fish and eggs, which are low in calcium but which also drive high calcium losses should be eaten in moderation, while low-calcium foods which reduce losses, such as peppers, bananas and oranges, provide a modest boost.

The Asian diet is not without problems for calcium absorption as well. Phytic acid is found in high quantities in *chapatti* flour and combines with calcium in the gut to make it unabsorbable. This diet may be deficient in calcium to begin with and osteomalacia and the juvenile form of this disease, rickets, may be the result.

The pH of the blood also plays a significant factor in osteoblast and osteoclast activity. As the blood pH drops, the balance is shifted in favour of osteoclasts and therefore bone density declines. The pH of the blood decreases with age, as the kidney efficiency declines, and it is also more sensitive to the balance between acid and bicarbonate from the diet. Consuming alkaline foods, which are typically high in potassium relative to protein, will increase the pH of the blood, thereby shifting the balance in favour of the osteoblasts. However, a low protein diet causes a decline in the production of growth hormones and even of bone proteins such as collagen. It is therefore very important to maintain adequate protein intakes while eating plenty of alkaline foods such as fruits and vegetables to balance the acid from the protein. It should be noted that proteins that come from vegetable sources (other than grains and some nuts) are usually alkaline, whereas proteins from animal sources are usually acidic.

BONE HEALING

A **fracture** is any break in the bone; the process of bone healing is an ordered progression of steps. Bone is about the only tissue in the body that when it heals it is stronger than before the fracture. Usually scar tissue is weaker than the original, but with bone the healing process leads to new bone tissue which is as strong if not stronger than the old bone that broke.

The first step in the repair process is the formation of a **fracture haematoma**. There are numerous blood vessels throughout the bone. As a result of the fracture the blood vessels that cross the fracture line are damaged and blood leaks out into the fracture site. A blood clot forms 6–8 hours after the fracture. The blood supply to the bone cells that lie on either side of the fracture is disrupted, and they begin to die. The dead cells induce macrophages and osteoclasts to start removing the dead bone and other cells from the fracture site and these cause a localised swelling and inflammation. The haematoma serves as a focus for the healing process.

The next step in the healing process is to re-establish the blood supply to the fracture area, so that new cells can begin to heal the fracture. Blood capillaries grow into the haematoma. It is during this stage that the presence of nicotine in the system can inhibit this capillary ingrowth, and for smokers there is an increased length of fracture healing compared with non-smokers. This stage may last several weeks.

The next step is the formation of a **fibrocartilaginous callus**, the new blood vessels that grow into the haematoma begin to organise it into a granulation tissue, called initially a **procallus**. Fibroblasts from the periosteum, and osteogenic progenitor cells from the periosteum, endosteum and the red bone marrow start to invade the procallus. Collagen is produced by the fibroblasts, which become chondroblasts, and these connect the two ends of the fracture together. The osteogenic progenitor cells enter the bordering regions of healthy bone on the edges of the dead bone, ready to start making new bone matrix. As more chondroblasts form they begin to make fibrocartilage which replaces the procallus. This stage lasts about 3 weeks. The procallus and the fibrocartilaginous callus that replace it are very soft in the first 4–6 weeks of fracture healing, so there is need for adequate support and bracing until the callus begins to ossify.

The next step in the healing process is the formation of the **bony callus**. The osteogenic progenitor cells that invaded the procallus and migrated to the borders of the dead/healthy bone region form into osteoblasts and begin to secrete bone matrix. They form spongy bone trabeculae which at this stage are not arranged in an ordered way and so the new bone is called **woven bone**. The trabeculae join the living bone tissue on either side of the fracture. Depending on the size of the bone and the severity of the injury, it may take up to 3 months for the whole of the fibrocartilaginous callus to be transformed into bone of adequate strength.

The final step in the healing process is bone remodelling. The woven bone lattice is re-arranged into the normal cortical and spongy bone arrangement. The woven bone is removed gradually by the action of the osteoclasts and replaced by other osteoblasts. Sometimes the repair is so good that the fracture line is undetectable even on an X-ray.

JOINTS

Joints occur at the joins between two or more bones and can be classified according to the type of connecting material into three types:

- Fibrous joints
- Cartilaginous joints
- Synovial joints.

They can also be classified according to the amount of movement that is possible at the joint:

- Synarthroses – fixed, unmovable joints
- Amphiarthroses – where some movement is possible
- Diarthroses – which are freely movable.

Synarthroses are mainly found in the limbs and amphiarthroses predominate in the axial skeleton.

FIBROUS JOINTS

Fibrous joints are connected via fibrous tissue, with no cavity between them. These are **synarthroses**, as there is usually very little movement at the joint because the bones are held together very closely via fibrous tissue crossing the joint. There are four types of fibrous joint:

■ Suture
■ Syndesmosis
■ Gomphosis
■ Schindylesis.

Suture

A type of fibrous joint called a **suture** is found between the bones of the skull where dense connective tissue is found between the closely interlocked bones. At birth the bones of the skull vault are separated via broad fibrous bands of tissue called **fontanelles**. These allow an easier passage of the baby's head through the birth canal (pelvic outlet) during labour, by letting the skull mould, with the parietal bones over-riding each other. This makes the baby's head temporarily smaller and a few days after birth the head returns to its normal shape. The fontanelles are also vital *after* birth as they also allow the brain to grow.

The anterior fontanelle is the largest and generally closes by 18–24 months after birth. While it is open it can be used to help in the diagnosis of raised intracranial pressure. As the fontanelle is composed of fibrous tissue rather than bone it can be gently palpated; a fontanelle that is dome-shaped and does not depress when gently pressed indicates a raised intracranial pressure.

The fontanelles remain open until at least 18 months after birth; however, the sutures are still separated by fibrous tissue. The sutures can still be seen on the adult skull, as most never fully close. A suture which does close completely, with bone forming between the bones in the suture, is that between the left and right frontal bones. This is then called a **synostosis** (see Clinical box 9.8). Other synostoses may form in old age.

Syndesmosis

Another type of fibrous joint is a **syndesmosis**. These are formed by either a bundle or sheet of fibrous tissue between the bones. The bundles are **ligaments** while the sheets are called **interosseous membranes**. Syndesmoses are found in the lower legs between the distal tibia and fibula, forming the **distal tibiofibular joints**. These joints have a short ligament between the bones so they are very rigid. Another syndesmosis is found in each lower arm between the radius and ulna, forming the **radioulnar interosseous joints**. These bones are connected by an interosseous membrane so these joints do allow a little movement between the bones and so functionally are **amphiarthroses**.

Gomphosis

Each tooth is connected to the bone of the upper or lower jaw via a fibrous joint called a **gomphosis**. The dense fibrous

connective tissue between the tooth and its socket in the alveolar bone is called the **periodontal ligament**. In most healthy cases there should be no or only very limited movement between the elements of the joint; only in dental gum disease does the gomphosis become weakened and the tooth loosen in its socket.

Schindylesis

The last type of fibrous joint is the **schindylesis**; this is an articulation where a thin plate of bone is received into a cleft or fissure formed by the separation of two laminae in another bone. An example of a schindylesis is the articulation of the rostrum of the sphenoid and perpendicular plate of the ethmoid with the vomer, or in the reception of the latter in the fissure between the maxillae and between the palatine bones.

CARTILAGINOUS JOINTS

Cartilaginous joints are generally classified as amphiarthroses in that they allow slight movement. In this class of joints, the bones are connected via cartilaginous connecting material and there is no synovial cavity between the bones. There are two types of cartilaginous joints:

■ Primary
■ Secondary.

Primary cartilaginous joints called **synchondroses**, where the joint is bridged by hyaline cartilage, tend to be temporary and are associated with the growth of the bones (especially the long bones). The epiphyseal growth plates are examples of a primary cartilaginous joint. They are temporary in that the epiphyseal growth plate will close and become bone when bone growth stops. There is little or no movement possible at these growth plates although the hyaline cartilage that joins the two parts of the bone can slip and cause problems such as slipped upper femoral epiphysis (SUFE). A persistent synchondrosis is the joint between the first rib and the manubrium of the sternum, which usually remains cartilaginous throughout life but may ossify in later life.

The secondary type of cartilaginous joint is the **symphysis**; these are permanent joints that are designed for strength, resilience and limited mobility. The ends of the bone are covered by hyaline cartilage, with fibrocartilage connecting the bones together. An example of this type of joint is the pubic symphysis, where the two coxal bones of the pelvis are joined at the front; other examples are the anterior intervertebral joints between the vertebrae, and the manubriosternal and xiphisternal joints, which join the manubrium (superior) and xiphoid process (inferior) to the body of the sternum. All symphyses are located in the midline of the body.

SYNOVIAL JOINTS

Synovial joints are the largest and most important class of joints. They are all **diarthroses** in that they allow free movement of the joint. Most of the joints in the body are of this type and all the limb joints are synovial.

The normal synovial joint is highly effective at allowing low friction movement between the articular surfaces of the opposing bones. To achieve this low friction the articular cartilage is elastic, and the joint is filled with fluid, which is kept in place by a relatively impervious layer of calcified cartilage and bone. Load-induced compression of the articular cartilage forces the interstitial fluid to flow laterally within the tissues through adjacent cartilage, which assists in protecting the cartilage from mechanical injury.

Synovial joint structure

Synovial joints all have the same characteristic features (Fig. 9.9). These are:

- **Articular cartilage** covering the ends of the bones
- An **articular capsule** consisting of a **fibrous capsule** surrounding the joint and a **synovial membrane** lining the cavity
- A **joint cavity** filled with **synovial fluid**.

The joint is usually reinforced by ligaments, external and/or internal. Besides these features, which are present in all these joints, several other structures can be found in some synovial joints such as articular discs (menisci), labrum, ligaments and fat pads.

Articular cartilage

The ends of the bones are covered by a layer of **articular cartilage**. This is hyaline cartilage, except for a few cases where they are covered by fibrocartilage. Hyaline cartilage provides the joint with a very smooth and slippery surface, which helps to reduce the friction between the articulating bones and helps to absorb shock through its content of water and extracellular matrix proteoglycans. Loss and damage of the articular cartilage can lead to osteoarthritis (Clinical box 9.9).

Clinical box 9.9   Osteoarthritis

Osteoarthritis is a degenerative condition which primarily affects the articular cartilage. It is often known as wear and tear arthritis as this is the leading cause of the condition. It mainly affects the main weight-bearing joints of the body such as the hip and knee, although for unknown reasons the ankle is often spared.

It is characterised by the loss of articular cartilage from the joint surface of the bone, leading to bone being exposed. As the articular cartilage reduces the friction at the joint and also acts as a shock absorber, these properties are reduced in affected joints and bone rubs on bone, leading to reduced joint movement and pain. On an X-ray you can see a loss of joint space as the articular cartilage is lost from the ends of the bones: as cartilage is radiolucent, and does not show up on the X-ray, most of the gap seen between the adjacent bones is the articular cartilage.

The bone tries to compensate for the loss of the articular cartilage by producing new bone, leading to the growth of bony spurs (**osteophytes**) at the joint margins, which may reduce the movement at the joint even further. They can grow quite extensive, and may eventually break off, leading to loose bodies in the synovial fluid that may cause the joint to seize up completely. The production of osteophytes also leads to the presence of calcium pyrophosphate crystals in the synovial fluid; this is known as pseudo-gout. In the knee these calcium phosphate crystals may become embedded in the menisci and lead to their calcification, which is visible in X-rays as a white line in the middle of the joint.

As the articular cartilage is lost over the articular surface and bone is exposed, the underlying bone responds by making new bone subchondrally. This leads to a thickening of the bone or **bone sclerosis**, immediately under the remaining articular cartilage of the joint. However, the new bone produced is disorganised and weaker than normal bone, and may not withstand the normal stresses, leading to trabecular fractures. These are small fractures in the underlying bone, due to the new compression forces on the bone from being exposed to the synovial fluid directly, which can cause subchondral **cysts** to form. These may be the result of a group of trabecular fractures collapsing to form a cavity in the bone.

The end point of untreated osteoarthritis is that the head region of the bone may collapse completely and the complete loss of the articular cartilage may lead to **arthrodesis** of the joint. This is the fusion of the bone on each side of the joint, which leads to the complete loss of function of that joint with the joint becoming immovable.

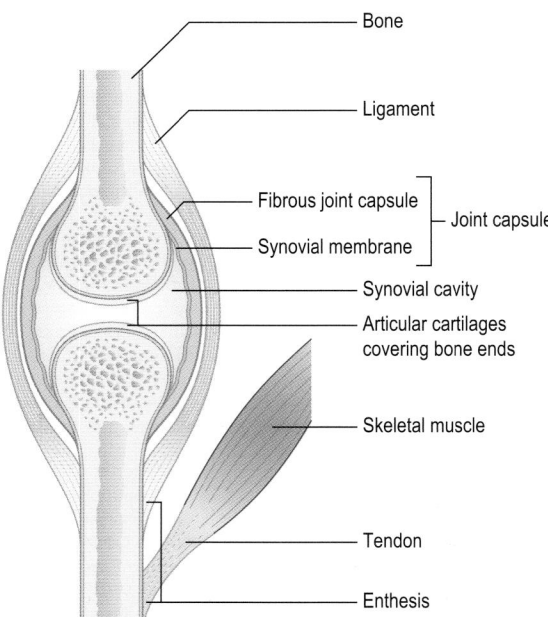

Fig. 9.9 **Structure of a synovial joint.**

Labels: Bone; Ligament; Fibrous joint capsule; Synovial membrane; Joint capsule; Synovial cavity; Articular cartilages covering bone ends; Skeletal muscle; Tendon; Enthesis

Articular capsule

The **articular** or **joint capsule** is a sleeve-like structure that surrounds and encloses the synovial cavity; it also acts to join the articulating bones together. It is composed of two layers.

1. There is an outer **fibrous capsule**, which is composed of dense irregular connective tissue attached to the periosteum of the articulating bones. The fibrous capsule allows considerable movement while still maintaining great tensile strength. These features give synovial joints a great degree of movement with stability. Often there are fibres arranged into parallel bundles incorporated into the fibrous capsule. These are **ligaments** and often have individual names. Ligaments give added strength to the joint and help to prevent dislocations of the articulating bones.
2. The inner layer of the articular capsule is the **synovial membrane**. This is composed of areolar connective tissue with elastic fibres. These allow the capsule to stretch during movement and to return to the resting position after the movement has stopped.

In many joints, the synovial membrane has accumulations of adipose tissue, which are called **articular fat pads**. The knee has several of these fat pads.

The synovium

The **synovium** is the inner lining layer of the joint cavities. It is composed of a layer of specialised cells, between one to three cells thick, called **synoviocytes** and a **subintima** (Fig. 9.10). The synoviocytes line the inner surface of the synovium, which is composed of at least two types of synoviocytes, designated type A and type B, and is sometimes called the **intima**.

Type A synoviocytes are derived from the bone marrow macrophage lineage. These synoviocytes mediate cytokine release in response to small immune complexes. There are also dendritic cells, which are antigen-processing cells that are involved in the generation of an immune response.

Type B synoviocytes are of the fibroblast-like mesenchymal cell lineage. These synoviocytes keep the surface intact, smooth and non-adherent. The type B synoviocytes synthesise large amounts of the proteoglycan, hyaluronic acid, which then passes into the synovial fluid (see below). The synovium is permeable to water, small molecules and small proteins, but not to hyaluronic acid. This allows the synovium to trap the synovial fluid within the cavity.

The synoviocytes lie in a matrix of collagen fibrils and proteoglycans which is not separated from the subintima by a basement membrane so is one continuous layer. The subintima is made from loose connective tissue and contains a dense network of fenestrated capillaries, which allow the diffusion of nutrients and metabolic waste between the synovium and the blood. Lymphatic capillaries remove large molecules from the synovium. The synovium contains nerve endings that produce pain, particularly during inflammation (Clinical box 9.10). Tendon sheaths and bursae are also lined with similar synovium (see below).

The synovial fluid

The **synovial fluid** is present in relatively small quantities in normal synovial joints, even the largest joints such as the knee and the hip may only have a few millilitres of fluid. Normal synovial spaces contain only a microscopic film of fluid (about 50 µm thick) at subatmospheric pressure. In the healthy joint, the synovial fluid should be clear and a very pale straw colour, or colourless; it is a relatively acellular liquid and has high viscosity. Synovial fluid is formed by the ultrafiltration of the blood into which hyaluronic acid is secreted. Hyaluronic acid is a long-chain glycosaminoglycan (see Ch. 2) with a molecular mass of about 1 million. Normal synovial fluid contains 3–4 mg/mL hyaluronic acid. The

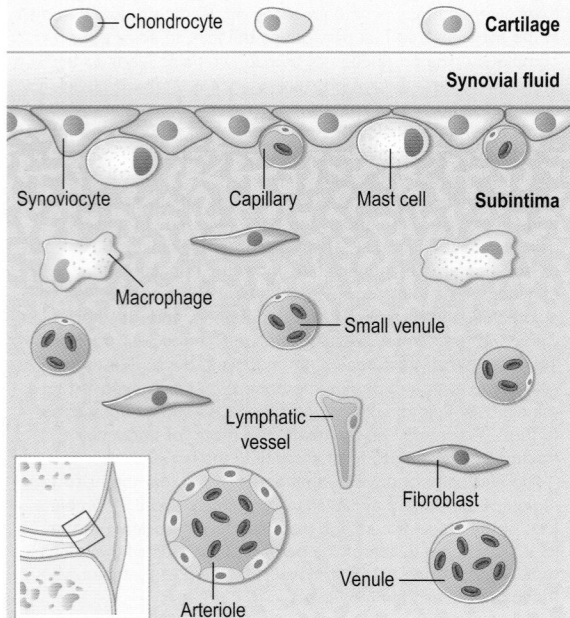

Fig. 9.10 **Structure of the synovium.**

Clinical box 9.10 **Rheumatoid arthritis**

Rheumatoid arthritis is the classic inflammatory arthropathy (joint disease). The synovium undergoes characteristic changes histologically, although these are not specific for the disease. Eventually the changes in the synovium may lead to the destruction of the articular cartilage and result in the destruction of the joint.

In the early stages of rheumatoid arthritis, the synovium becomes swollen with excess fluid, thickened and hyperplastic with the synovial cells multiplying to such an extent that the synovium develops villi. In the later stages of the disease, the inflamed synovium develops a layer of inflamed fibrous tissue known as **pannus**. In the pannus new blood vessels form and allow more pannus formation. The pannus may spread over and even invade the articular cartilage, depriving the cartilage of its nutrients and leading to the death of the cartilage, and erosion of the bone underneath.

The synovial fluid often appears cloudy owing to the increased number of white blood cells, mainly neutrophils, which it now contains. It tends to have a lower viscosity than normal synovial fluid because of the biochemical breakdown of hyaluronic acid.

Unlike osteoarthritis, rheumatoid arthritis often involves periarticular structures as well as the joints, with any structure that has a synovial membrane affected; this includes tendon sheaths and bursae.

hyaluronic acid gives the synovial fluid its high viscosity so it acts as a lubricant for the movement of the articular cartilage against each other. Not only does the synovial fluid have lubricant abilities but it also allows the exchange of metabolites between the plasma and the surrounding synovial membrane and articular cartilage. The half-life of hyaluronan in the joint cavity is about 24 hours. It eventually seeps out by a process of 'reptate diffusion', which can be considered as molecular 'snaking' through the tissue surface.

Lubricin, also known as proteoglycan 4, is a specialised glycoprotein which plays an important role in lubricating synovial joints at the boundary interface between opposing articular cartilage surfaces. The hyaluronic acid as well as helping to lubricate the joint also helps to maintain the thickness of the lubricating fluid film.

Water is able to enter the joint very quickly during inflammation, but once it mixes with the hyaluronan it cannot leave as quickly, and so a joint may swell within a few hours but the inflammation may take several days to reduce. The synovial fluid also provides a cushion for the synovial lining by filling the crevices, which the synovial tissue cannot reach. The synovial lining cannot fill the space between the cartilage surfaces perfectly in all positions. If it did the joint would be like a vacuum pack and the synovium would probably be caught between the articular cartilages and damaged. If the joints are stretched suddenly, even the fluid does not fill all the space and the lining may jump into the vacuum formed, which is how people 'click' their finger joints. Clicking one's joints does not lead to osteoarthritis or damage to the joint – it is just a habit in some people.

Accessory ligaments

Many of the synovial joints have accessory ligaments, which are also called **extracapsular** and **intracapsular** ligaments, depending on whether they lie outside or inside the articular capsule. Examples of the extracapsular ligaments are the medial and lateral collateral ligaments of the knee. The intracapsular ligaments lie within the articular capsule but are excluded from the synovial cavity by folds in the synovial membrane. Examples of this type of accessory ligament are the anterior and posterior cruciate ligaments of the knee.

Articular discs

In some joints there are pads of fibrocartilage inside the synovial cavity, which are attached to the fibrous outer capsule and lie between the articular surfaces. These pads are called **articular discs** or **menisci**. The knee joint has lateral and medial menisci; they modify the shape of the articular surfaces of the bones so that they fit together better. They also direct the synovial fluid to the areas of greatest friction, thus giving added stability to joints and protecting the joint from damage during heavy work.

Blood and nerve supply to the joint

The nerves that supply the joint are the same that supply the skeletal muscles around the joint. The nerve endings are distributed around the articular capsule and associated ligaments. Some of the nerve endings convey pain from the joint to the brain. Others convey the degree of stretch that the joint is undergoing (see below).

The arteries around the synovial joint send out many branches that supply the ligaments and articular capsule with

oxygen and nutrients. The veins remove the waste products of metabolism from the joints. However, because cartilage lacks a blood supply, the articular cartilage gets its nutrients from the synovial fluid and not directly from the blood supply of the joints.

Types of synovial joints

There are six subtypes of the synovial joint, although they all have a similar underlying structure.

- Planar joints
- Hinge joints
- Pivot joints
- Condyloid joints
- Saddle joints
- Ball and socket joints.

The different types of synovial joints are named after the shape of the bones, or the type of movement that is performed at the joint (Fig. 9.11). Movement can occur in a variety of axes.

- Non-axial: gliding movement only in a single plane
- Uniaxial/monoaxial: in a single axis
- Biaxial: in two axes
- Multiaxial: in many axes.

Planar or gliding synovial joints

The **planar** or **gliding joints** are non-axial joints which have the form of two flat plates which slide against each other. The articulating surfaces of these joints are usually flat or only slightly curved; there is only a limited range of movement possible at these joints. They allow a side-to-side, back and forth movement. Examples of planar joints are the intercarpal and intertarsal joints in the hands and feet (see Anatomy box 9.5 below) and between the vertebrae.

Hinge joint

The **hinge joint** consists of a convex part of one bone which fits into the concave part of another to allow uniaxial movement, as in a door hinge. Examples include the humeroulnar joint of the elbow (see Anatomy box 9.3) and the interphalangeal joints of the fingers and toes. The knee is also considered to be a hinge joint although it is a far more complex joint, and also has condylar and planar joint elements (see below). The movement possible at a hinge joint is a simple opening and closing movement – **flexion** and **extension** (Information box 9.1).

Pivot joints

The **pivot joint** allows uniaxial movement and in this type of joint there is usually a peg of bone that fits into another bone

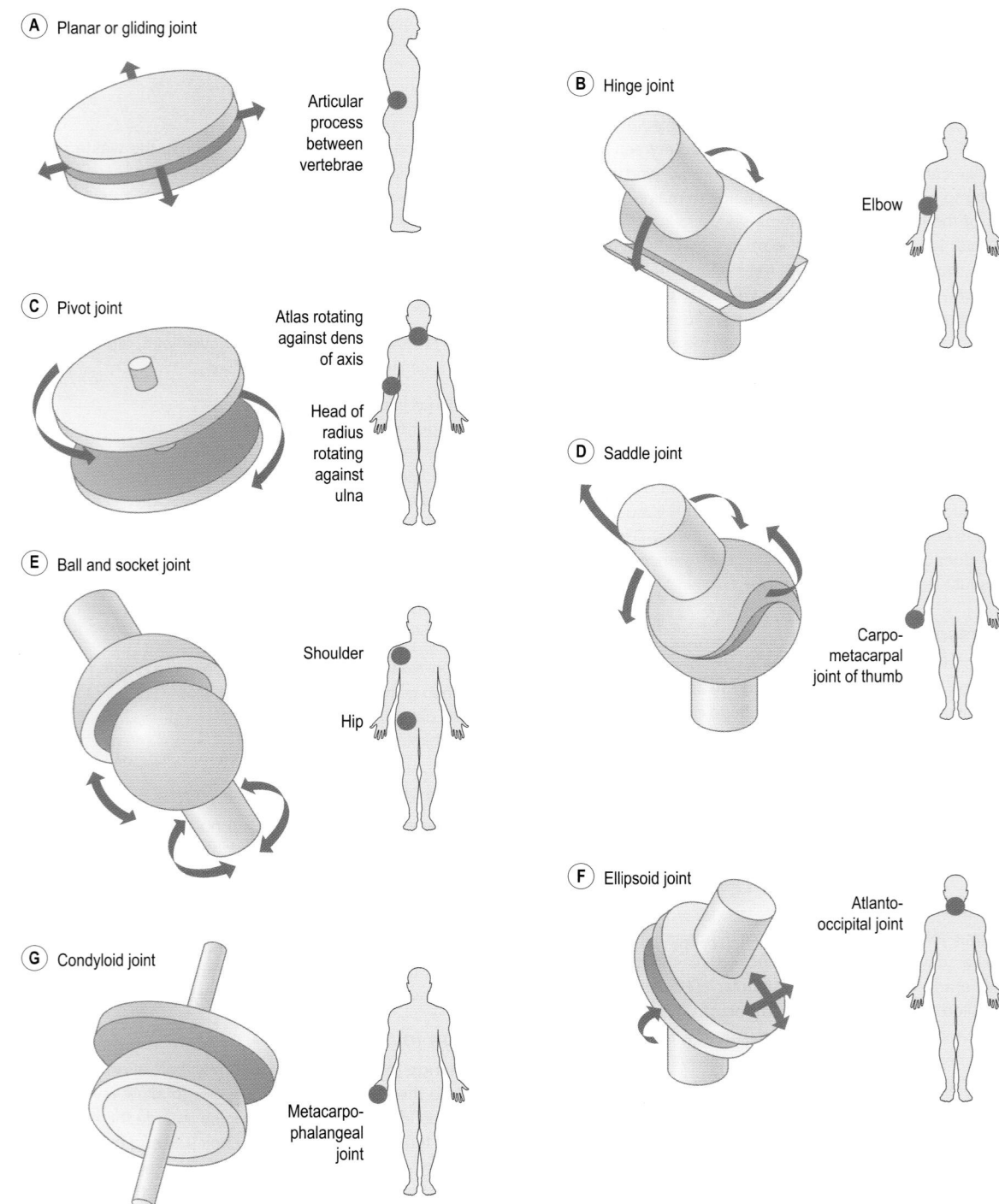

Fig. 9.11 **Types of synovial joint.**

Information box 9.1   Movements at joints

The different movements at the joints have specific names (Fig. 9.12). These are particularly useful in describing the available movement during a clinical examination.

- **Flexion** – decreasing the angle of the joint. For example, moving the head forwards at the neck or raising the arm above the head.
- **Extension** – increasing the angle of the joint. For example, moving the arm behind the body line.
- **Dorsiflexion** – upward movement of the foot, lifting the toes towards the front of the leg.
- **Plantar flexion** – lowering the toes away from the ankle (pointing the toes).
- **Abduction** – away from the midline of the body. For example, raising the arm to the side or spreading of the fingers.
- **Adduction** – towards the midline of the body. For example moving the arm towards the body or closing the fingers.
- **Circumduction** – this is a combination of extension, flexion, abduction and adduction which allows a limb to draw a cone in space in a sort of stirring motion.

Special movements at particular joints

- **Supination and pronation** – this refers to a rotation of the hand involving the radius and ulna. Supination rotates the palm upwards and pronation rotates the arm to face the palm downwards.
- **Inversion and eversion** – this turns the sole of the foot. Inversion turns the sole inwards, facing the other leg, and eversion turns it outwards.
- **Protraction and retraction** – these movements move the body part forwards and backwards in the transverse plane. Jutting out the jaw is protraction and holding the shoulders back is an example of retraction.
- **Elevation and depression** – this is moving the body part upwards (elevation) or downwards (depression) in the frontal plane. An example of this is chewing where the lower jaw (mandible) is alternately elevated and depressed.

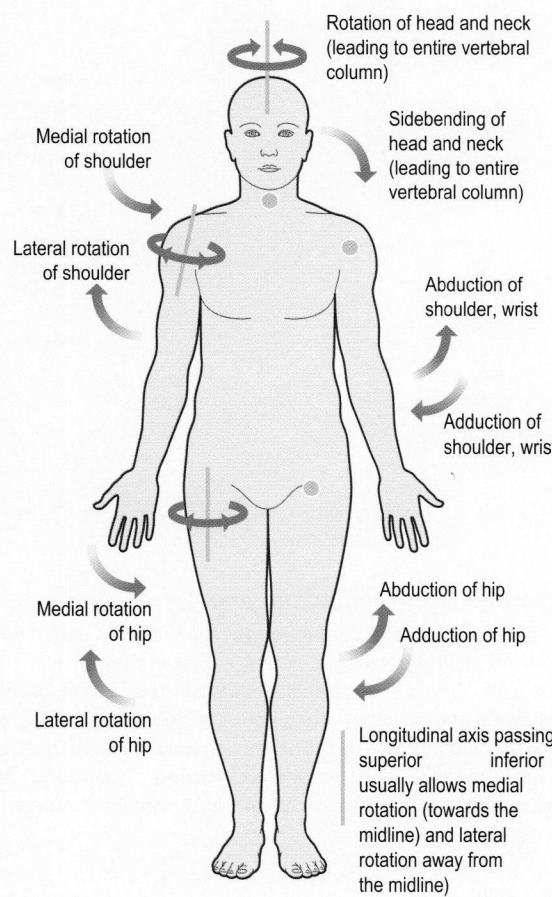

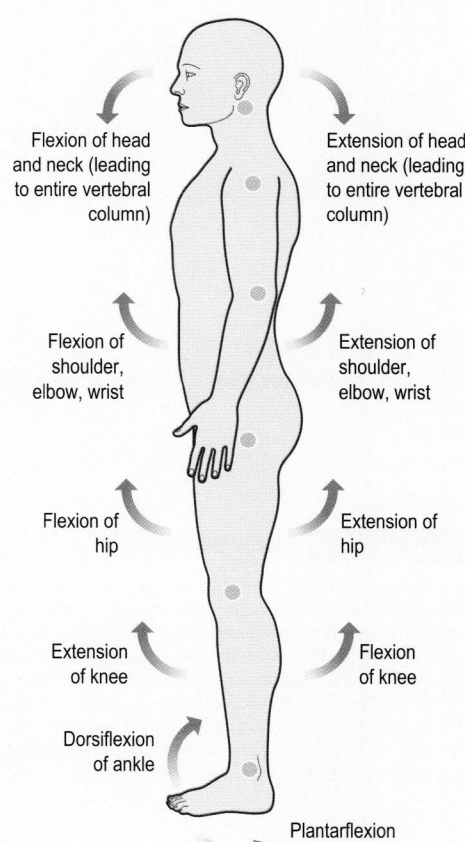

Fig. 9.12 **Anatomical movements.**

A **Anatomy box 9.3**   **A simple hinge joint: the elbow**

The elbow is possibly the most important joint of the upper limb as it brings the hands towards the head and the body. The elbow flexors are the 'hand to mouth' muscles producing movements which are vital in everyday life, such as in eating, washing and dressing.

The elbow extensors allow the upper limb to form a firm brace that can be used to push objects away from the body. People who have lost the use of their lower limbs rely on the elbow extensors to lift their body so that they can use crutches and to rise from a chair. The elbow is a hinge joint, but the forearm can rotate so that the lower end of the radius rotates around the ulna, carrying the hand with it (pronation or supination).

The elbow joint is a complex of three joints functionally, with all three joints within the same synovial cavity (Fig. AB3). The three joints are the:

- Humeroradial
- Humeroulnar
- Superior (proximal) radioulnar.

The humeroradial and humeroulnar joints allow flexion and extension of the elbow. The superior (proximal) radioulnar joint allows the pronation and supination of the forearm and hand.

The hinge joint between the humerus and ulna has bony surfaces that are interlocked in such a way as to constrain the flexion and extension movements of the elbow, preventing hyperextension and flexion of the joint. The flexion of the joint is not restricted by the ligaments that surround the elbow joint, but extension is limited by the contact of the olecranon process of the ulna with the floor of the olecranon fossa of the humerus. Adduction and abduction on the other hand are limited by the ligaments that surround the joint.

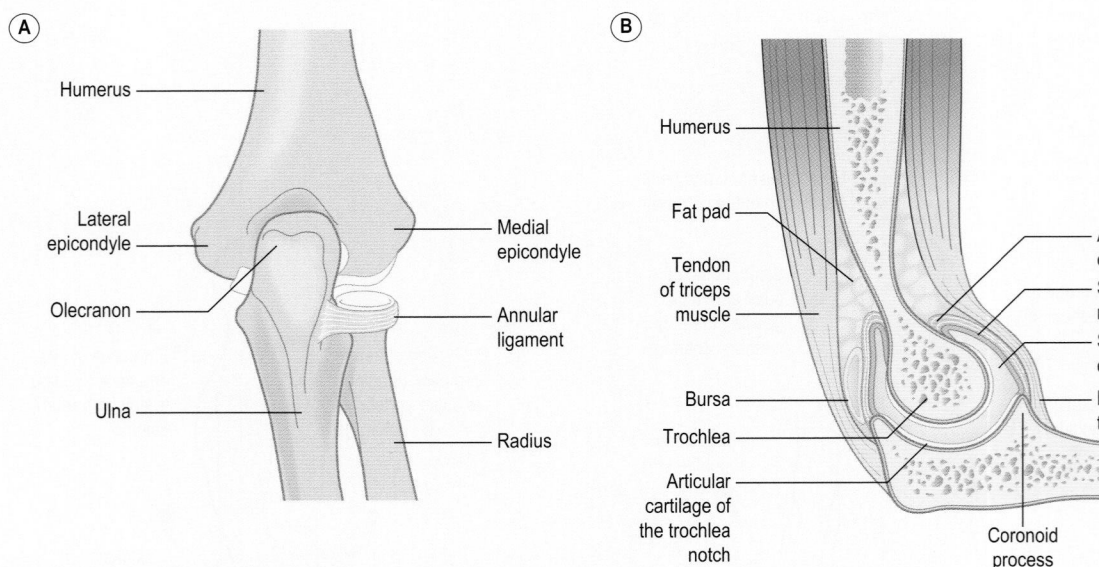

Fig. AB3 **The elbow joint.** (A) External view. (B) Cross-sectional view.

Clinical box 9.12   **Elbow dislocation**

The elbow may dislocate posteriorly in children who fall on their hands with their elbows flexed. The distal end of the humerus is driven through the weak anterior part of the elbow joint's fibrous capsule as the radius and ulna are displaced posteriorly. There is often an associated fracture of the head of the radius, coronoid process or olecranon processes of the ulna. Because of the posterior displacement of the radius and ulna, the ulnar nerve may be stretched or torn and results in numbness of the little finger and weakness in flexion and adduction of the wrist.

or ligament. An example of this type of joint is the atlantoaxial joint (between the C_1 (atlas) and C_2 (axis) vertebrae) in the neck. The movement is a rotational movement, thus the atlantoaxial joint allows one to say 'no' by turning the head from side to side. Another pivot joint is the superior (proximal) radioulnar joint, where the head of the radius fits into the annular ligament of the ulna. This joint allows one to **pronate** and **supinate** the forearm and hand.

Condyloid or ellipsoidal joints

Condyloid or ellipsoidal joints allow biaxial movement; the metacarpophalangeal joints are examples of this type of joint. One of the articular surfaces has a convex oval shape while the other has a concave depression into which the convex surface fits. The movements possible at these types of joints are **extension**, **flexion**, **abduction and adduction;** a mixture of all these movements producing **circumduction**.

Saddle joints

Saddle joints can be considered a modified condyloid joint; they allow multiaxial movement, compared with the biaxial movement of the condyloid joint, so the movement is freer. In the saddle joint, one bone is the rider and the other bone the saddle – one example is the carpometacarpal joint of the thumb. At these types of joints a slightly larger range of movement is possible than at the condylar joints (see Anatomy box 9.5).

A Anatomy box 9.4   Muscles of flexion and extension, the brachial artery and cubital fossa

Muscles of flexion and extension

There are two muscles that bring about extension of the forearm, the large **triceps brachii** and the much smaller **anconeus**, which are both contained in the posterior compartment. The three flexors are all in the anterior compartment. The two main flexors are the **biceps brachii** and **brachialis**, which insert into the radius and ulna, respectively. The **brachioradialis** is only really effective when the forearm is partially flexed as it originates on the distal humerus and inserts into the distal radius (Fig. AB4).

The biceps brachii muscle is also the main supinator and this action prevents it being an effective flexor of the pronated forearm. The **supinator** and **pronator quadratus** muscles are roughly equal in strength but the great size of the biceps brachii relative to the **pronator teres** muscle enables a person to supinate the forearm with much greater force than he or she can pronate the forearm. This fact, in combination with the preponderance of right-handed people, has meant that screws are constructed so that they can be tightened by supination of the right forearm.

The brachial artery

The **brachial artery** is a continuation of the axillary artery and begins at the lower border of teres major. The brachial artery descends through the arm in the flexor compartment of the arm. The **profunda brachii** artery is given off from the brachial artery soon after its origin. It descends deep through the arm following the spiral groove on the posterior side of the humerus, along with the radial nerve, and thus may be damaged by a mid-shaft fracture of the humerus.

The brachial pulse may be palpated by pressing the artery from the medial aspect against the humerus. The brachial artery passes anterior to the elbow joint; it then bifurcates in the cubital fossa into the **radial** and **ulnar** arteries. However, in some individuals, the bifurcation occurs higher up in the arm.

The cubital fossa

The triangular area in front of and slightly distal to the elbow is the **cubital fossa**, or antecubital fossa. The fossa is bounded proximally by an imaginary line joining the two humeral epicondyles and distally by the pronator teres muscle on the ulnar side and the brachioradialis on the radial side. The floor of the fossa is formed by the brachialis and supinator muscles. The roof of the fossa is formed by the deep fascia and the bicipital aponeurosis.

The cubital fossa usually contains the terminal part of the brachial artery before it divides into the ulnar and radial arteries. The brachial artery lies between the biceps tendon, which has to be pushed aside to feel the brachial pulse, and the median nerve. Accompanying the arteries are the deep veins so the brachial vein or veins are located in the fossa. The tendon of biceps brachii and the median nerve all pass through the fossa. Superficial to the fossa are the superficial veins, such as the median cubital vein, which makes the fossa a good site for injections into the superficial veins.

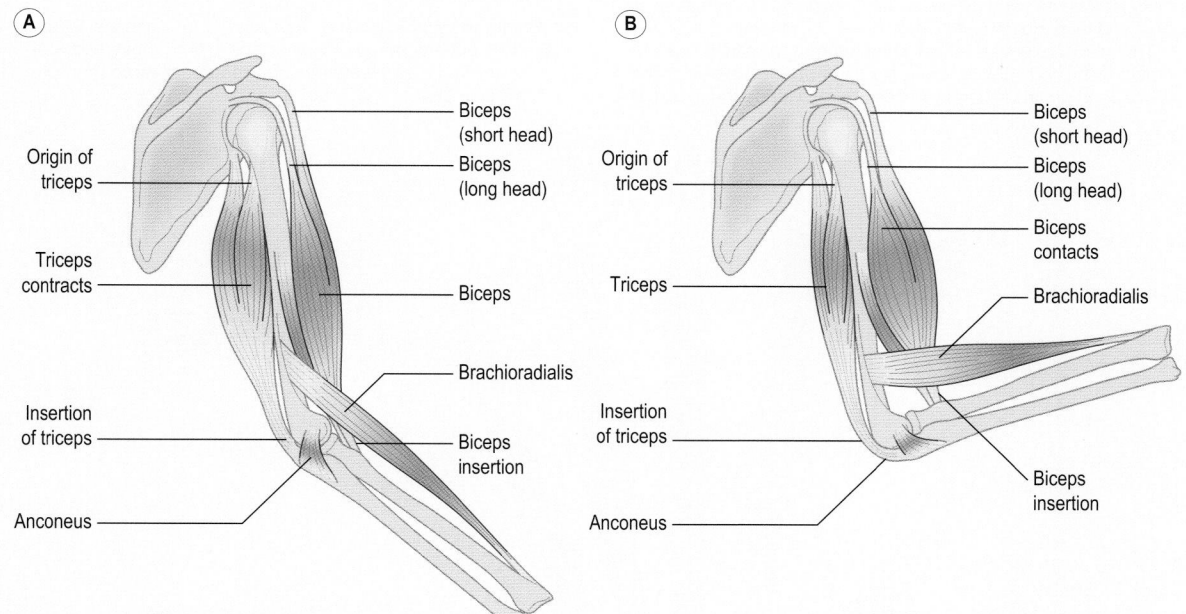

A

- Origin of triceps
- Biceps (short head)
- Biceps (long head)
- Triceps contracts
- Biceps
- Brachioradialis
- Insertion of triceps
- Biceps insertion
- Anconeus

B

- Origin of triceps
- Biceps (short head)
- Biceps (long head)
- Biceps contacts
- Triceps
- Brachioradialis
- Insertion of triceps
- Biceps insertion
- Anconeus

Fig. AB4 **Extensor and flexor muscles of the elbow.**

Clinical box 9.13   Tennis elbow

Pain around the lateral epicondyle of the humerus may be due to **tennis elbow**, also known as **lateral epicondylitis**. It is an overuse injury, causing inflammation of the common extensor tendon insertion. The main muscle that is affected is the extensor carpi radialis brevis, although the other extensor muscles may also be involved. The clinical signs of tennis elbow are a localised tenderness over the epicondyle and pain on resisted extension of the wrist or middle finger. A similar condition can occur over the medial epicondyle called golfer's elbow and is an inflammation of the flexor tendons. Both of these conditions can occur in individuals who do not play tennis or golf and are caused by repetitive wrist activity.

Anatomy box 9.5 **A pivot joint – the wrist joint**

The joint of the wrist is vital to ensure the manual dexterity which is essential for both work and leisure activities.

The distal radioulnar joint forms a **pivot type synovial joint**. The rounded head of the ulna articulates with the ulnar notch on the medial side of the radius, so that during pronation and supination of the forearm, the head of the ulna rotates within the ulnar notch of the radius.

The eight carpal bones are arranged in two rows, the **scaphoid** and **lunate** bones articulate with the radius with the **pisiform** and **triquetrum** bones situated more medial to the lunate bone. The four distal bones (the **hamate**, **capitate**, **trapezoid, and trapezium**) articulate with the metacarpals of the fingers (Fig. AB5).

Two sets of movements are possible at the wrist joint, caused by radial and ulnar deviation, respectively:

- Flexion/extension
- Abduction and adduction.

Flexion-extension takes place about a mediolateral axis through the lunate and, due to the mobility of the carpal bones, also about the mediolateral axis of the capitate bone. Muscles passing anterior to these axes will act as flexors, while the muscles that pass posterior to these axes will act as the extensors.

The flexors of the wrist are the:

- Flexor carpi radialis
- Palmaris longus
- Flexor carpi ulnaris.

These muscles all have a common point of origin on the medial epicondyle of the humerus. The tendons of these three muscles can be seen on the anterior surface of the wrist when the hand is made into a fist and the wrist is flexed.

The palmaris longus is the central tendon, with flexor carpi radialis lying next to it on the radial (thumb) side. The tendon of flexor carpi ulnaris is harder to see but runs along the ulnar (little finger) side of the wrist. It is estimated that in 13% of the population, palmaris longus is missing, and the absence of the muscle has no significant effect on the flexion of the wrist.

Palmaris longus is composed of a very short body of muscle with a long tendon, and many believe that it is gradually being lost from the population. It is a weak wrist flexor and its main action is to tense the palmar aponeurosis. As it is missing in a significant percentage of people and they can function normally without it, it is a prime candidate for surgical removal for use as a tendon for the repair of damaged ligaments or tendons elsewhere in the body, such as for anterior cruciate knee ligament replacement.

The extensor muscles of the wrist are the:

- Extensor carpi radialis longus
- Extensor carpi radialis brevis
- Extensor carpi ulnaris.

The common point of origin for these muscles is the lateral epicondyle of the humerus. Abduction and adduction occurs about the anteroposterior axis through the head of the capitate, the largest and centrally positioned carpal bone of the wrist region.

The abductors of the wrist are:

- Flexor carpi radialis
- Extensor carpi radialis longus
- Extensor carpi radialis brevis
- Abductor pollicis longus.

The adductors of the wrist are:

- Flexor carpi ulnaris
- Extensor carpi ulnaris.

As all the muscles of the wrist except for palmaris longus have two actions across the wrist joint, pure movements at the wrist require simultaneous contraction of more than one of the muscles.

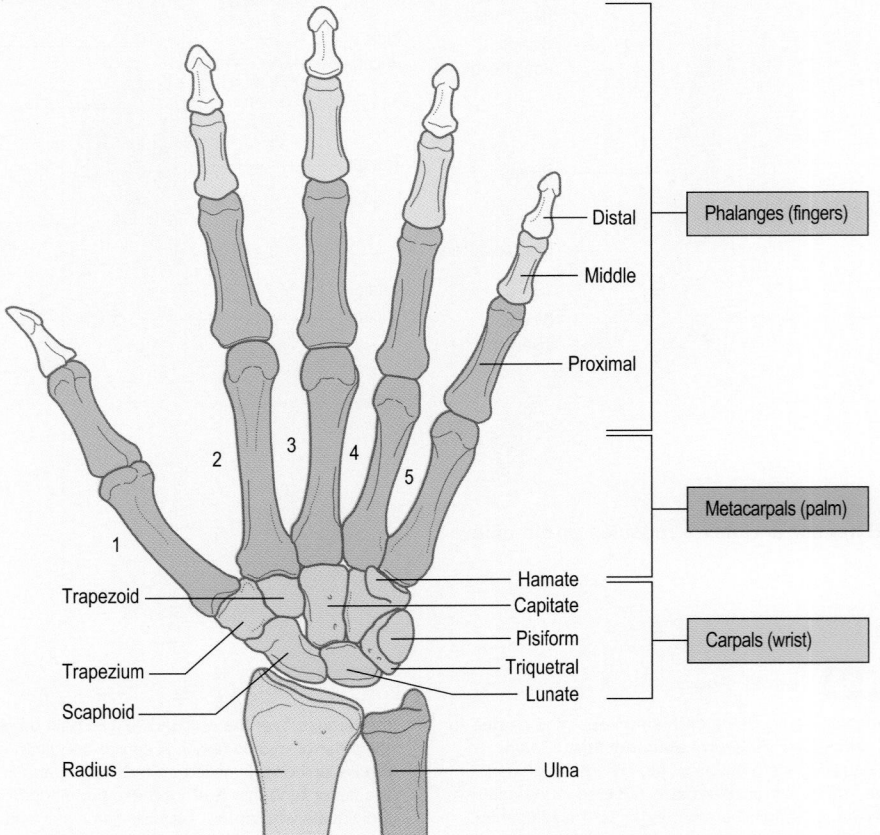

Fig. AB5 **Bones of the hand.**

Colles' and Smith's fractures

Colles' fractures are very common, and distal wrist injuries such as these account for 17% of fractures treated in the emergency department. A Colles' fracture occurs when a person falls onto their outstretched hand in the pronated position. The fracture site is usually 2–3 cm up the radius and the fragment is displaced proximally, causing a shortening of the radius. The fragment is also usually displaced dorsally giving the broken wrist the resemblance to a dinner-fork.

Smith's fracture is a reverse Colles' fracture and is caused by falling backwards onto the palm of an outstretched hand, which leads to pronation of the upper extremity while the hand is fixed to the ground.

Ball and socket joints

The most versatile type of synovial joint is the **ball and socket joint**. There are only four ball and socket joints in the body, the two shoulder (glenohumeral) joints and the two hip (femoral-acetabular) joints (see Anatomy box 9.6). These joints allow multiaxial movement and have the greatest range of movement among the joints, allowing extension, flexion, abduction, adduction, medial and lateral rotation and circumduction.

Ⓐ Anatomy box 9.6 **Ball and socket joints: the shoulder**

Both the shoulder and the hip joints are ball and socket joints. However, there are significant differences between these joints which relate to their flexibility and the load bearing capacity of the different joints.

Shoulder joint
The shoulder joint itself is the joint between the head of the **humerus** and the **glenoid cavity** of the scapula: the **glenohumeral joint**. This is the most mobile joint in the body (Fig. AB6); the joint is so mobile because it is held away from the trunk via the **pectoral girdle**, which itself is largely suspended from the trunk via muscles rather than through joints.

The **clavicle** (collar bone) and the **scapula** (shoulder blade) form the **pectoral girdle**, which links the upper limb and the trunk. There is a large range of movements possible for the scapula and a large part of the overall mobility of the shoulder is due to the mobility of the scapula. This is in contrast to the lower limb where the pelvis (the equivalent of the pectoral girdle) is firmly fixed to the axial skeleton, and so sacrifices mobility for increased stability and better load bearing capacity.

The head of the humerus lies in a rather flat **glenoid fossa**, and so its movements are not constrained by bony boundaries. The humeral head is four times larger than the glenoid cavity; this allows the head of the humerus a great range of movement around the glenoid cavity. The glenoid fossa is deepened a little by a ring of fibrocartilage called the **glenoid labrum**, and this does give the joint a small degree of stability. The joint capsule for the glenohumeral joint is also

rather 'baggy', especially inferiorly, which allows the arm to be raised above the head. As well as being lax and loose, the articular capsule of the shoulder is also relatively weak, giving the glenohumeral joint plenty of 'give' before the extent of the joint capsule is reached and movement restricted.

The **coracohumeral ligament**, which extends from the coracoid process of the scapula to the humerus, is the only strong ligament around the glenohumeral joint and this serves mainly to support the weight of the arm. There are three **glenohumeral ligaments**, the superior, middle and inferior, which are only simple thickenings of the joint capsule. This means that the ligaments of the glenohumeral joint are relatively weak, and the muscles around the joint – the four **rotator cuff muscles** and their tendons – are the main stabilisers for the joint. These muscles are:

- Supraspinatus
- Infraspinatus
- Teres minor
- Subscapularis.

All four originate on the scapula and insert close to the humeral head onto either the greater or lesser tubercles of the humerus. Their main role is to stabilise the head of the humerus in the glenoid fossa, and to work with the other larger muscles such as the deltoid to act on the shoulder, mainly to rotate the humerus and to help in the abduction of the humerus. Another stronger stabiliser is the **intracapsular tendon of biceps** (long head) which runs through the joint capsule and helps to stabilise the shoulder joint as well as moving the shoulder.

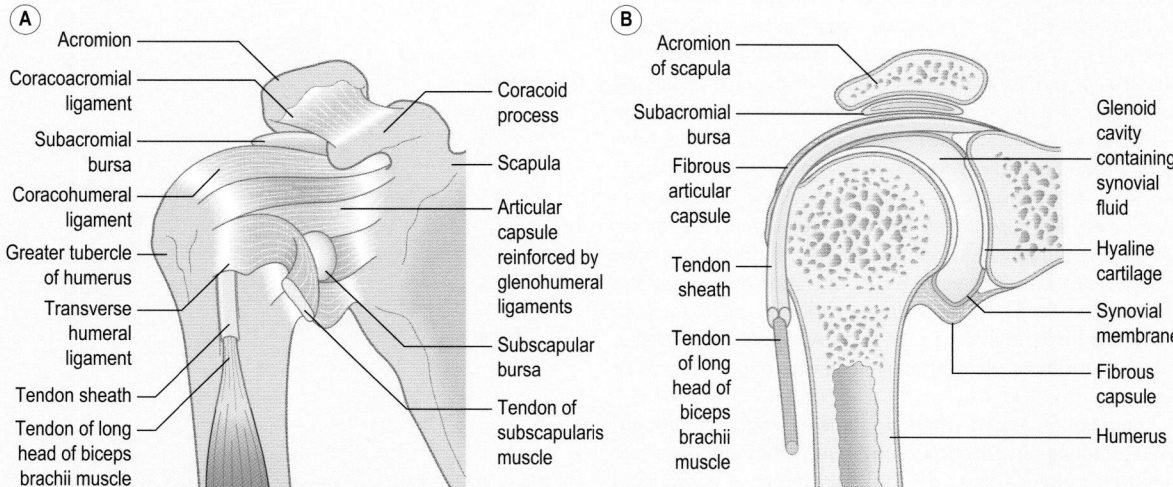

Fig. AB6 **The shoulder joint.** (A) External view. (B) Cross-sectional view.

Clinical box 9.15   **Shoulder dislocations**

As a consequence of the freedom of movement of the glenohumeral joint, it is likely to be dislocated by either a direct or indirect injury. Because of the positions of the reinforcing elements and the position of the acromion and coracoid processes of the scapula, most dislocations are downwards (inferior) and forwards (anterior).

Two types of movement commonly produce dislocation of the shoulder:

- Excessive extension and lateral rotation of the humerus can drive the head of the humerus inferoanteriorly, which may tear the inferior part of the glenoid labrum as it is forced out of the joint. This is known as Bankart's lesion.
- A hard blow to the humerus when the glenohumeral joint is fully abducted tilts the head of the humerus inferiorly onto the weaker part of the joint capsule. This may result in tearing the capsule and dislocates the shoulder so that the head of the humerus now lies inferior and anterior to the glenoid cavity.

After dislocation the strong flexor and abductor muscles around the joint pull the head of the humerus into a subcoracoid position. The patient is unable to use the arm and commonly will support it with the other hand.

Two consequences of a shoulder dislocation are clinically relevant:

- The axillary nerve may be damaged by the displaced humeral head. This denervates the deltoid muscle and gives cutaneous denervation to a small area of skin covering the central part of the deltoid. Testing for the loss of sensation over the deltoid muscle is a sign of axillary nerve damage. If the axillary nerve is damaged then the deltoid muscle may waste and the rounded profile of the shoulder will be lost.
- The glenoid labrum may be torn. This forms a weak spot so that in the future the shoulder is easier to dislocate again and requires less force to do so.

Almost all the muscles that move the shoulder are innervated by the branches of the **brachial plexus** so damage to the brachial plexus, which can occur when the limb is pulled hard or by a severe blow to the top of the shoulder, can cause weakness and/or paralysis to the whole upper arm.

Ligaments and tendons

Ligaments attach bone to bone (or cartilage) and are variable in how elastic they are. **Tendons**, which are made of very strong dense regular connective tissue, attach muscles to bone and so they tend to be inelastic in order to transmit the muscles' power to the bones. The joint capsule is usually composed of a network of independently moving ligaments and tendons associated with sheets of coarse fibrous connective tissue called **fascia**. Some joints, such as the sacroiliac joint, are surrounded almost exclusively by ligaments while others are surrounded by tendons, such as the rotator cuff muscle tendons around the shoulder. Tendons can pass through joint cavities, such as in the shoulder where the tendon of the long head of the biceps muscle enters the joint cavity and helps to stabilise the joint. **Aponeuroses** are flat, sheet-like tendons which attach muscles to bones or to other muscles.

The point on a bone where a ligament, tendon or aponeurosis attaches is called an **enthesis**. The entheses are important because they are the main target in a group of inflammatory disorders known collectively as the **seronegative spondyloarthropathies** (Clinical box 9.17).

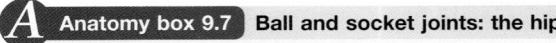

Anatomy box 9.7   **Ball and socket joints: the hip**

The hip joint, where the **head of the femur** articulates with the **acetabulum** of the pelvis, is a strong weight-bearing joint but it has much less flexibility than the shoulder. Like the shoulder, the hip joint is another ball and socket synovial joint, but the acetabulum into which the head of the femur fits is already deep and is deepened even further by the presence of a ring of fibrocartilage, the **acetabular labrum** (Fig. AB7).

The joint has a strong fibrous **joint capsule** that is attached to the acetabular margin and to the pelvis and anterior femur. Inferiorly the capsule extends some way down the medial border of the femur; this gives the capsule enough slack to allow abduction of the hip joint. The fibres of the capsule form three strong ligaments that help to

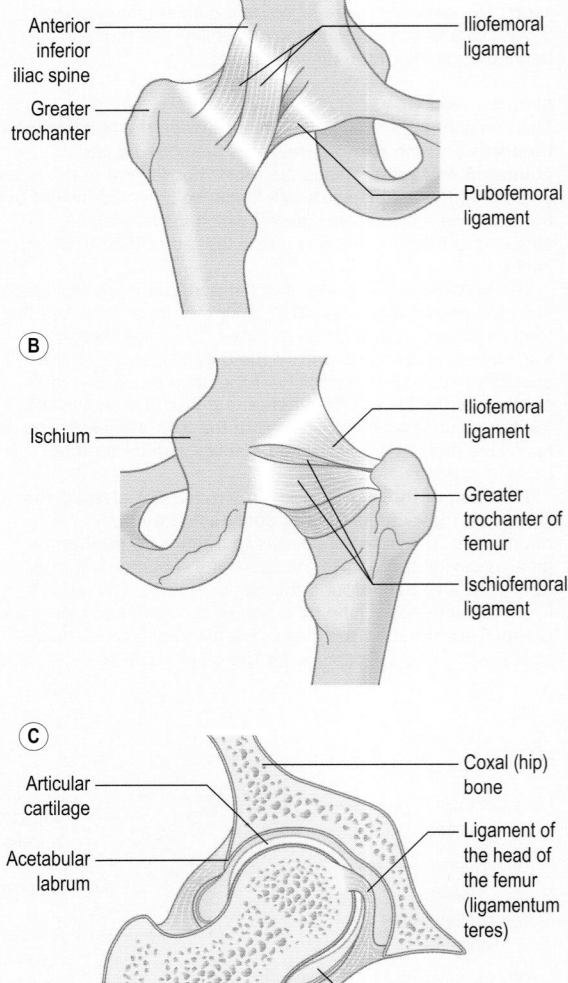

Fig. AB7 **The hip joint.** (A) Anterior external view. (B) Posterior external view. (C) Cross-sectional view.

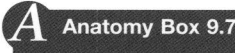

Anatomy Box 9.7 **Ball and socket joints: the hip—cont'd**

stabilise the joint. The **iliofemoral ligament** strengthens the front of the joint capsule, and the **pubofemoral** and **ischiofemoral ligaments** reinforce the back of the joint capsule.

The large muscles and tendons which cross the joint increase the stability of the joint but this is insignificant compared with the stability produced by the deep acetabulum and strong ligaments.

Clinical box 9.16 **Hip fractures**

Due to its stability, dislocations of the hip joint are rare, but **fractures of the femoral neck** are fairly common, especially in elderly women or any person with **osteoporosis**. The head and neck of the femur are mainly supplied with blood from the gluteal and obturator arteries (branches of the internal iliac artery). Following a fracture of the femoral neck, if the gluteal artery is damaged **avascular necrosis** of the femoral head may occur as the obturator artery is not sufficient to maintain the bone of the head of the femur. Avascular necrosis of the femoral head may occur in children spontaneously and is called **Perthes' disease**.

The nerve supply to the hip joint is via branches of the femoral, obturator, sciatic and gluteal nerves. Some of these nerves also give off branches that supply the knee joint as well as the hip. Therefore, pain originating in the hip may be referred to the knee.

Clinical box 9.17 **Seronegative spondyloarthropathies**

Diseases that fall into this class of inflammatory conditions (which are associated with the human leucocyte antigen (HLA)-B27 class I allotype) are **ankylosing spondylitis**, **psoriatic arthritis** and **reactive arthritis**. Typically, there is inflammation in the synovium and bony entheses. The synovium in these conditions may be difficult to distinguish from rheumatoid arthritis microscopically but the synovium does not develop extensive pannus formation and consequently there is less invasion of the bone and articular cartilage than in rheumatoid arthritis.

The enthesis becomes infiltrated by non-specific granulation tissue. In more severe forms of the disease, enthesopathy is followed by calcification and ossification of the enthesis, thus reducing the movement possible at the joints affected. Because there are many entheses around the spine, due to the large number of joints and muscle/tendon insertions, the spine is often affected by such conditions.

The characteristic history is of insidious onset of low back pain associated with marked stiffness lasting for an hour or more after waking in the morning. The pain and stiffness is usually relieved by exercise and begins again when resting.

Bursae and tendon sheaths

Bursae and **tendon sheaths** are flattened sacs made of fibrous material containing synovial fluid. The synovial lining of these structures is similar to that found within the joints, with a slippery non-adherent surface that allows movement between the planes of the tissues. The sacs lie under and around structures in the joint to reduce friction.

Clinical box 9.18 **Inflammation of the bursae**

Diseases that affect the synovial joints usually also affect all types of synovial cavity, which include bursae and tendon sheaths. The overuse of muscles or tendons in regions where bursae are found, as well as continuous external compression or trauma, can cause **bursitis** (inflammation of the bursae). The symptoms of bursitis include swelling, pain and often a loss of muscular strength and range of motion in the joint. Repeated cumulative trauma may eventually lead to the formation of calcium deposits and to degeneration of the internal lining of the bursa.

Bursitis of the shoulder is often seen in athletes who participate in sports that require repetitive throwing and swinging motions and who use the shoulder joint throughout its entire range of motion, such as in swimming, gymnastics, and tennis to name a few.

The knee joint contains a number of bursae, and bursitis of the prepatellar bursa is colloquially known as 'housemaid's knee'. Tendon sheaths are elongated bursae which surround the tendon where it could be subjected to friction. The synovial tendon sheaths line the tendons only where they pass through narrow passages or **retinacula** such as in the palm of the hand, the wrist and around the ankles. Elsewhere the tendon lies in a bed of loose fibrous tissue.

Clinical box 9.19 **Ganglion**

If there is a small hole in the tendon sheath specifically, the synovial fluid may leak out and expand the tough fibrous outer connective tissue layer. Water and small molecules are able to diffuse away leaving the hyaluronan behind. This forms a very thick hyaluronan-rich fluid sac called a ganglion. These often form at the wrist where there are many long tendon sheaths passing over the wrist into the hand. A ganglion can be excised if it causes pain by pressing on nerves.

Bursae are located at sites where the muscle or fascia may experience shearing forces due to being close to the surface or being embedded in the subcutaneous tissues. For example, in the shoulder there is a bursa which lies between the outside of the joint capsule and the overlying ligament (Clinical Box 9.18). Many bursae form during development but new or adventitious bursae can occur at sites of occupational friction. Bursae are located predominantly between bony prominences, muscles or tendons, and their main function is to provide cushioning and support in areas where repetitive motion occurs.

SKELETAL MUSCLE

Skeletal muscle is the most abundant of the three types of muscle found in the body. Its main function is to provide the force for locomotion; to do this it converts chemical energy to mechanical energy. Skeletal muscle is under the voluntary control of the nervous system. Besides its role in locomotion, it has other functions as well, such as acting as a reservoir for 80% of the body's water and as a pool for the storage of intracellular ions such as potassium. Its conversion of chemical energy to mechanical work generates heat and contributes to the maintenance of the body's temperature.

A   **Anatomy box 9.8**   **A complex joint: the knee**

Perhaps the most complex joint in the body is the **knee joint**. It is partly a hinge joint, allowing flexion and extension, but it also has **condylar joint** characteristics, which adds rotational movements to the list of movements possible at the knee. Standing in the anatomical position the knee is in extension in a stable configuration.

The knee is a compromise between mobility and stability. It is most stable when fully extended as it 'locks', making the lower limb a solid column and well adapted for weight-bearing. However, for locomotion the knee must unlock, and for this to happen the **popliteus muscle** contracts, causing the femur to rotate laterally so that flexion of the knee can occur. The knee joint is one of the most frequently used joints and as a result one of the most frequently injured joints.

The knee joint is surrounded by strong muscles and by ligaments that are arranged both inside and outside the fibrous joint capsule, which help to maintain the stability of the knee joint when it is straightened.

The knee is composed of articulations between three bones:

- Femur
- Tibia
- Patella.

The knee consists of three joints that are combined together (Fig. AB8). At the centre of the knee is the **femoropatellar joint**, a plane joint between the patella and the distal femur. The patella is a sesamoid bone that is held at the front of the knee between the tendon of the quadriceps muscle and the **patellar ligament**. The other two joints are between the medial and lateral condyles of the femur and tibia, the **tibiofemoral joints**. Unusually the joint cavity is only covered by the capsule on the lateral and posterior sides. On the anterior surface the joint is covered by ligaments.

The menisci and the ligaments of the knee joint

The condyles of the femur and tibia do not fit very closely so to help with the stability of the joint there are two semicircular rings of fibrocartilage called the **menisci**. The **lateral and medial menisci** help to pack the joint so that the femur and tibia fit together better. They also help to distribute the load and direct the synovial fluid to the most stressed part of the joint.

The medial meniscus is partly attached to the **medial (tibial) collateral ligament**. This ligament is a broad band that partly blends with the joint capsule and so is partly attached to the medial meniscus. Often when one is injured the other is also damaged due to this connection. The lateral meniscus is completely separate from the lateral collateral ligament. The **lateral (fibular) collateral ligament** is a rope-like structure that is also separated from the joint capsule. These collateral ligaments prevent the knee joint from opening medially and laterally. They help to supply stability when the knee moves from side to side or when you make sharp twisting movements. Other ligaments outside the joint capsule are the **oblique and arcuate popliteal ligaments**, which reinforce the posterior of the knee. The front of the knee is stabilised in the middle by the patellar ligament and by the **lateral and medial patellar retinacula** ligaments, which extend from the quadriceps femoris muscle to the articular capsule on either side of the knee.

Inside the joint are two more ligaments that prevent the tibia from moving too far forwards or backwards on the femur. These are the cruciate ligaments, as they cross each other. The **anterior cruciate ligament** originates near the back of the femur and runs downwards to attach to the anterior of the tibia, while the **posterior cruciate ligament** runs from the anterior of the femur to the posterior of the tibia. On the tibia they attach to the tibial spines while on the femur they attach to the intercondylar notch.

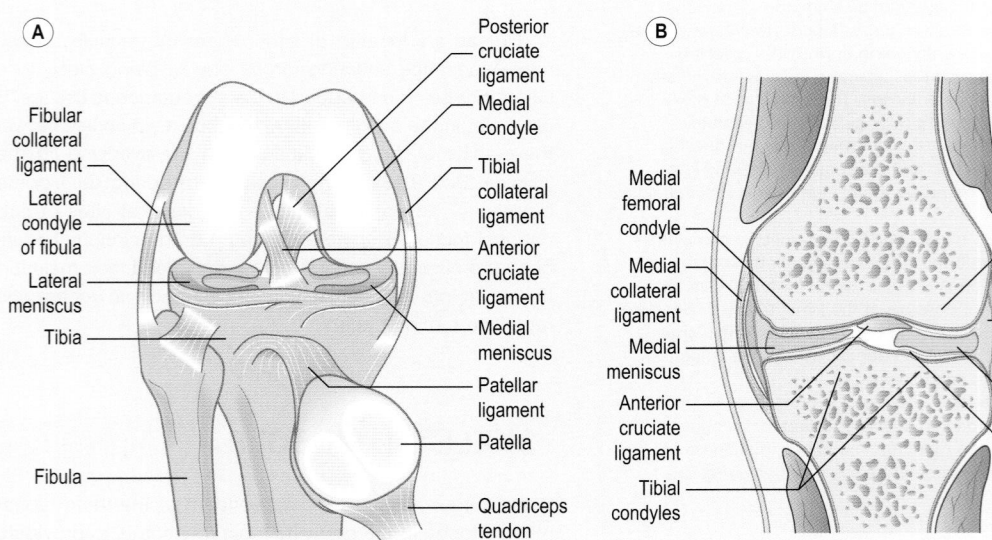

Fig. AB8 **The knee joint.** (A) External view. (B) Cross-sectional view.

Anterior cruciate injuries

The anterior cruciate ligament is easily injured and accounts for 70% of cruciate ligament injuries. This high proportion of injuries is in part due to the close association it has with the medial meniscus, so that damage to the medial meniscus can cause tears not only in the medial collateral ligament but also in the anterior cruciate. Likewise damage to the anterior cruciate can lead to damage to the medial meniscus and collateral ligament. This is often called the 'triad' of knee injuries.

The popliteal fossa
The **popliteal fossa** is a diamond-shaped fossa located at the back of the knee joint. Its boundaries are the hamstring muscles superiorly and the two heads of the gastrocnemius muscle inferiorly. The fossa is important as all the important blood vessels and nerves from the thigh pass through the popliteal fossa to reach the leg.

The **popliteal artery** is a continuation of the femoral artery; it runs immediately next to the posterior surface of the femur and is thus the deepest structure in the fossa. It can be vulnerable to a fracture of the supracondylar femur when the pull of the gastrocnemius on the distal fragments can cause the artery to be severed by the sharp bone. The **popliteal pulse** can be difficult to locate because of its deep location and because of the overlying leg fascia. It is felt by pressing from behind against the back of the femur, but to feel the pulse the leg muscles must be relaxed and the knee flexed, which helps to relax the popliteal fascia.

At the lower border of the popliteal fossa the popliteal artery bifurcates to give rise to the **posterior tibial artery**, which travels down through the posterior compartment of the leg, and the **anterior tibial artery**, which descends in the anterior compartment of the leg. The posterior tibial artery usually gives off the **fibular artery**, which runs close to the fibula in the posterior compartment of the leg.

The **sciatic nerve** usually divides into the **tibial and common fibular nerves** at the upper border of the popliteal fossa. The tibial nerve descends vertically down the leg, while the common fibular passes laterally around the neck of the fibula. Both nerves are vulnerable to trauma in the fossa. The **sural nerve**, the sensory branch of the sciatic nerve in the posterior calf, is composed from nerve fibres from both the tibial and the fibular nerves. As the common fibular nerve winds round the neck of the fibula it is vulnerable to damage from strikes to the lateral leg. Unfortunately, the neck of the fibula is the right height for impacts from car bumpers and damage to the common fibular nerve causes foot drop.

THE SKELETAL MUSCLE FIBRE

Each muscle is composed of a collection of muscle fibres, which are bound together by connective tissue (Fig. 9.13). Each fibre within the muscle is itself formed by the fusion of many myogenic cells into a single multinucleated cell. Individual muscle fibres can measure up to 10 cm in length with a diameter ranging from 10 µm to 100 µm. In the mature muscle fibre the nuclei are arranged around the periphery of the fibre, as the fibre is packed with contractile proteins, but during development or repair after damage the nuclei of the newly added myogenic cells appear in the centre of the muscle fibre.

Each muscle fibre contains many **myofibrils**. These long rod-like structures run the entire length of the cell and contain the contractile proteins. Each fibre contains between hundreds and thousands of myofibrils depending on its size. The myofibrils take up more than 80% of the cell volume, with the **sarcoplasm** (muscle cell cytoplasm), mitochondria and the other cellular components packed in between. The sarcoplasm contains relatively high levels of glycogen and the red, oxygen-carrying molecule, **myoglobin**.

Duchenne muscular dystrophy

Duchenne muscular dystrophy (DMD) is a genetic disorder caused by a defect in the muscle protein **dystrophin**. Dystrophin is an accessory muscle protein that helps to reinforce the muscle fibres' plasma membrane and in its absence the plasma membrane can be damaged more easily, leading to muscle fibre degeneration and even muscle fibre death. This results in a loss of muscle bulk and replacement with fibrous scar tissue in affected individuals. The gene for dystrophin is located on the X chromosome and so is commonly found in males. The gene is very long (nearly 2.5×10^6 base pairs) and mutations in the gene are relatively common. DMD has an occurrence of 1 in 3500 male births and is therefore one of the most common genetic disorders. DMD presents with progressive muscle weakness, which results in affected individuals being wheelchair-bound by puberty and dying, usually in their early to mid twenties, from respiratory and cardiac failure.

The contractile proteins

As in all types of muscle, the contractile proteins of skeletal muscle are **actin** and **myosin**, plus a number of accessory muscle proteins (See Ch. 2, Table 2.9). Actin and myosin form the **thin** and **thick** filaments, respectively, which are arranged in a very ordered lattice arrangement (Fig. 9.14), giving skeletal muscle its other name of 'striated muscle'. The interactions between the thick and thin filaments form the basis of muscle contraction by the binding of myosin and actin in the presence of calcium and ATP (adenosine triphosphate).

The thin and thick filaments are attached at regular intervals to accessory proteins, which are visible as lines that divide the myofibril into its functional unit, the **sarcomere**. The actin filaments insert into the **Z line**, while the myosin filaments insert into the **M li**ne (Fig. 9.14A). Each sarcomere extends from one Z line to the next and is composed of alternating light and dark bands. These are formed depending on the overlap between the thin and thick filaments. The length of the thick filaments is shown by the **A band**, whose length remains constant even during muscle contraction. The light band called the **H zone** is the region that contains just myosin filaments whereas the light **I band** is where there are only actin filaments.

Thin filaments
The thin filaments are made from actin plus two regulatory proteins, troponin and tropomyosin.

Long strands of actin, **F-actin** (fibrous actin), form by the polymerisation of the **G-actin** (globular actin) subunits. Two F-actin strands coil around each other forming the thin filaments. The thin filaments are attached to the Z-line and extend into the sarcomere, partly overlapping with the myosin chains that extend from the M-line. In a muscle fibre there are approximately twice as many actin filaments as myosin filaments, leading to an array where each myosin filament is associated with six actin filaments, and each actin filament with three myosin filaments (Figs 9.14 and 9.15).

Two other proteins, **tropomyosin** and **troponin**, are associated with the actin filament. Tropomyosin is a filamentous protein that lies in the groove of the coiled F-actin filaments. It strengthens and stiffens the F-actin, and at rest, in the

Muscle
(organ)

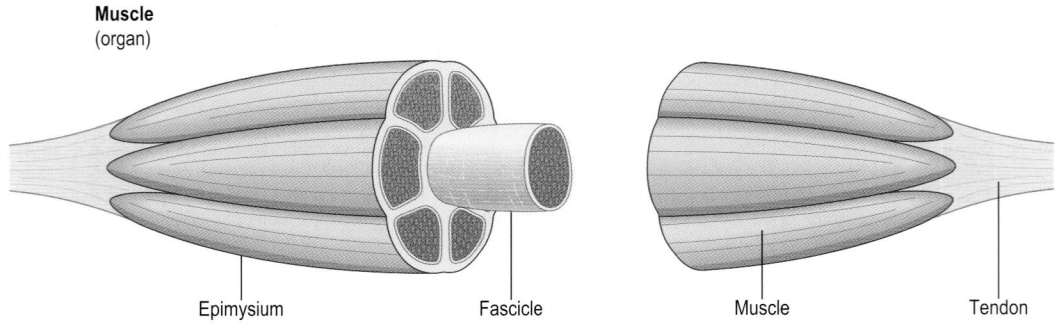

Epimysium   Fascicle   Muscle   Tendon

Fascicle
(a portion of the muscle)

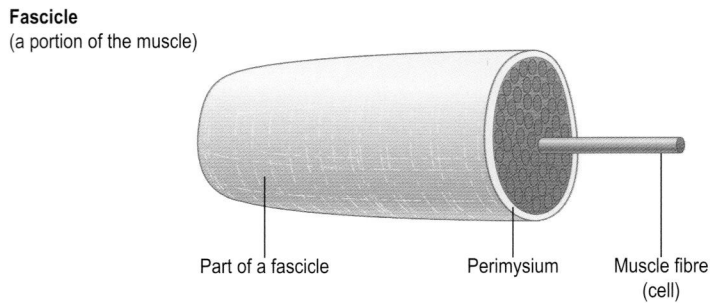

Part of a fascicle   Perimysium   Muscle fibre
(cell)

Muscle fibre
(cell)

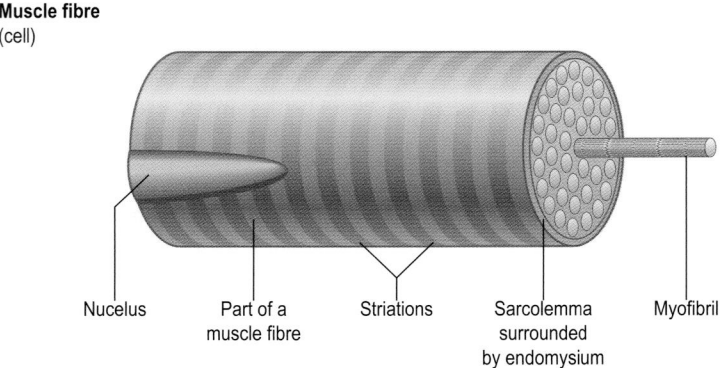

Nucelus   Part of a   Striations   Sarcolemma   Myofibril
muscle fibre   surrounded
by endomysium

Myofibril or fibril
(complex organelle composed of bundles of myofilaments))

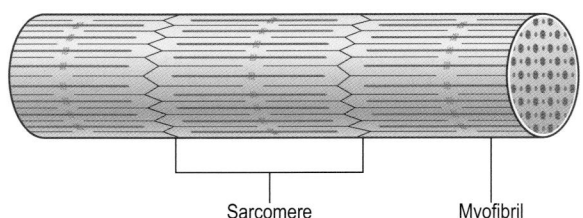

Sarcomere   Myofibril

Fig. 9.13 **Macroscopic structure of skeletal muscle.**

absence of Ca^{2+}, covers the myosin-binding site on the actin filament. Troponin consists of three proteins:

- Troponin T which binds to tropomyosin
- Troponin C which binds calcium
- Troponin I which is an inhibitory subunit.

During muscle contraction, interactions between calcium, the troponins and tropomyosin control the interactions between actin and myosin.

Thick filaments

The thick filaments are made up mainly of myosin. Myosin is a multimeric elongated protein with two globular heads and is made up of two heavy and four light chains. The two heavy chains form an extended alpha helix, while at each end of the two heavy chains a light chain binds to form a globular domain sometimes called the head region. A flexible hinge region near the globular head divides the protein into **light meromyosin** (LMM, helical region) and **heavy meromyosin**

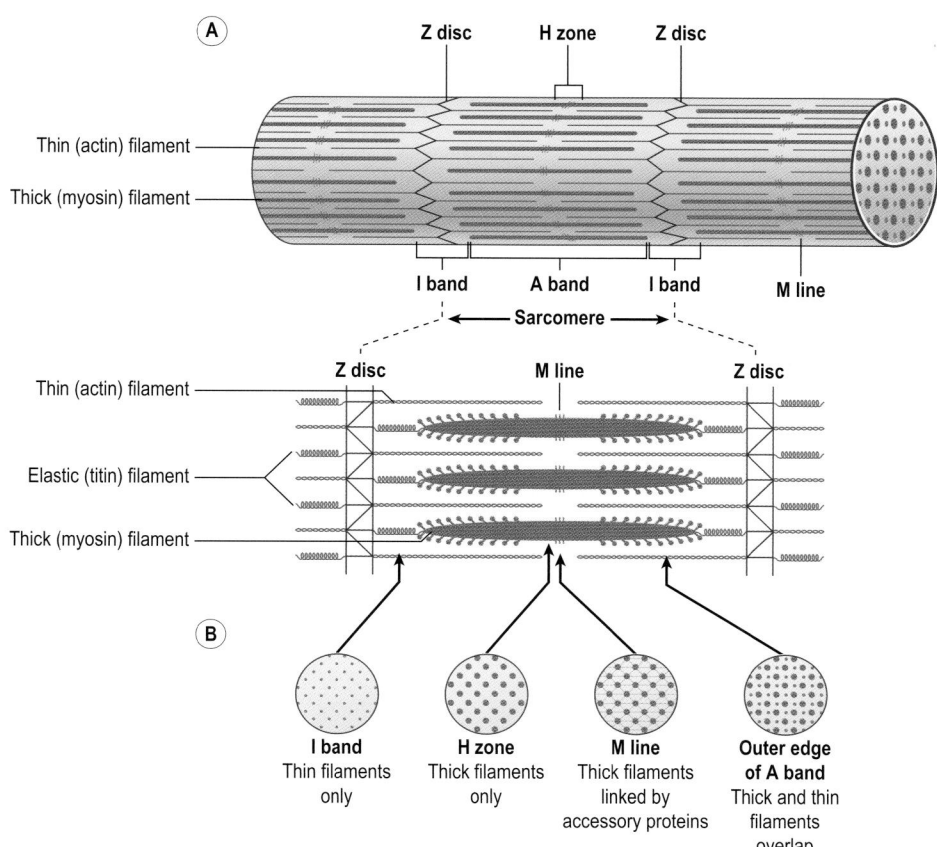

Fig. 9.14 The sarcomere. (A) Longitudinal view showing A and I bands, M and Z lines and H zone. (B) Cross-sectional view showing geometrical arrangement of thick and thin filaments.

(HMM, the short helical region and the globular domains). The thick filaments of muscle are formed by the self-association of LMM helices, with up to 400 myosin molecules in each thick filament. The thick filaments extend outward from the M line towards the Z line of each myofibril, with the globular heads protruding from the bundles of myosin molecules. A second hinge region is between the short helical and globular regions of the HMM.

Each of the globular domains contains a calcium-dependent ATPase. Binding of ATP to ATPase reduces the affinity of binding between actin and myosin, and hydrolysis of ATP by ATPase provides the energy required to shorten the muscle.

The sliding filament model of muscle contraction

During muscle contraction it can be seen that while each sarcomere shortens, the length of the separate thin and thick filaments does not change. This is because during contraction the thin and thick filaments slide along one another with increasing degrees of overlap.

1. At rest, when the muscle is at its maximum length, there is only a small amount of overlap between the thin and thick filaments, as shown by the wide H zone and I band (Fig. 9.15A).
2. As the muscle shortens the H zone gradually disappears as the ends of the thin filaments get closer. The I band

also narrows as the ends of the thick filaments get closer to the Z lines (Fig. 9.15B).
3. At maximum contraction the thin filaments from the opposing ends of the sarcomere overlap where the H zone was and the thick filaments reach the Z bands, thus abolishing the I band. The A band is the same length as at rest with the thick filaments now filling the space between the two Z lines (Fig. 9.15C).

The method by which the muscle shortens is due to a cycle of making and breaking of **cross-bridges** between the thick and thin filaments. At each cycle the energy from the hydrolysis of ATP causes the myosin head region to move backwards (towards the tail region) pulling the thin filament along the thick filament (see below).

THE CONTRACTILE PROCESS

Muscle contraction is triggered by the activity in the motor neuron supplying the muscle. The process by which the electrical signal produces contraction is called **excitation-contraction coupling**.

Excitation-contraction coupling

Intracellular calcium release

The **sarcolemma** (muscle fibre plasma membrane) has invaginations that penetrate deep into the muscle fibre, called **T tubules** (transverse tubules). These occur at the Z

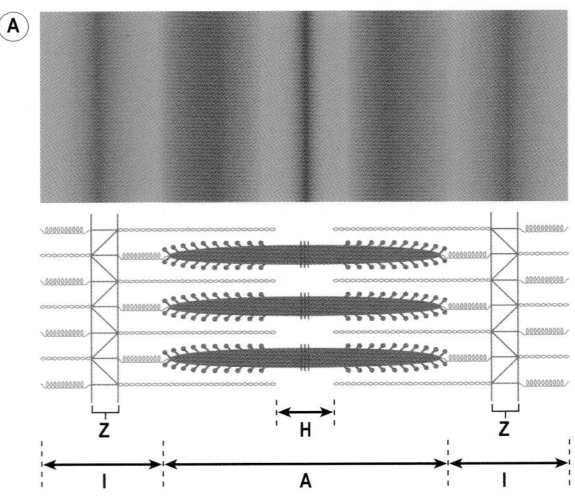

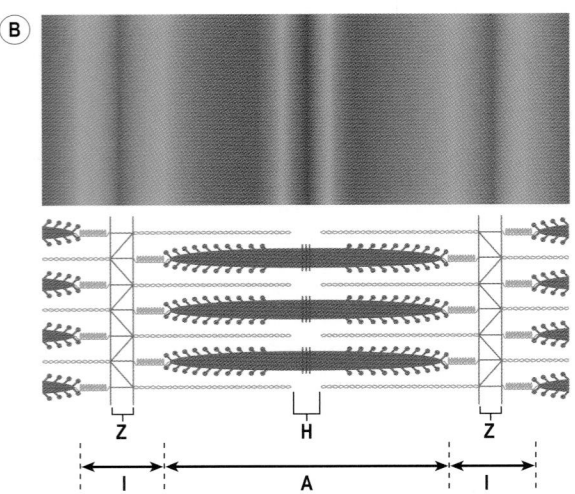

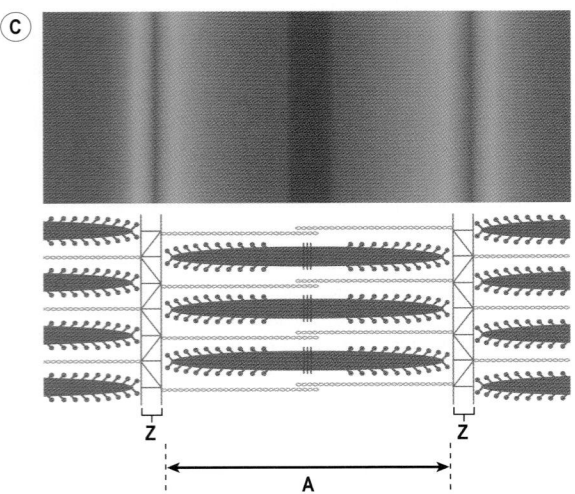

***Fig. 9.15* Sliding filament model of muscle contraction:** (A) at rest, (B) during contraction and (C) fully contracted.

lines where, along with the terminal cisternae of the **sarcoplasmic reticulum** (SR, the endoplasmic reticulum of the muscle), they form a structure called a triad where the T tubules and the SR are linked by structures called **endfeet**. The SR stores high concentrations of calcium whereas free

calcium levels in the sarcoplasm at rest are very low (about 10^{-8} M).

When the sarcolemma is depolarised by the motor neuron at the neuromuscular junction, the electrical impulses are propagated across the surface of the muscle and deep into the T tubules by the activation of voltage-dependent sodium channels. The T tubule system allows the simultaneous contraction of all the muscle fibres in the muscle, thereby avoiding damage to the muscle from parts of the muscle contracting while other parts are inactive.

In the T tubules (transverse tubules) modified L-type calcium channels transmit the signal to the endfeet, which are a specialised type of calcium channel with a very high conductance called **ryanodine-sensitive calcium channels**. These channels open rapidly to allow the efflux of large amounts of calcium from the SR into the sarcoplasm, reaching 10^{-5} M.

Cross-bridge formation and muscle contraction

Prior to contraction, the binding of ATP to the myosin ATPase and its subsequent hydrolysis to ADP and P_i move the myosin head to point forwards along the axis of the myosin filament in a high energy conformation. ADP and P_i remain bound to the myosin head and this complex has a high affinity for the binding site on the actin filaments. However, this is inhibited by tropomyosin which blocks the binding site.

When Ca^{2+} is released from the SR it binds to troponin C, which undergoes a conformational change allowing the myosin binding sites to become available. The myosin heads now bind to the thin filaments forming **cross-bridges**. This binding triggers a conformation change in the myosin head, releasing the stored energy, which moves the head region backwards, pulling the thin filament about 10 nm along the thick filament. This also releases the ADP and P_i from the ATPase.

The myosin ATPase now binds ATP, which causes the release of the cross-bridge, followed by hydrolysis of the ATP and movement of the myosin head back to the forward-pointing position. This high-energy conformation is then ready to reattach to the thin filament and repeat the stroke 10 nm further along.

This cycle of cross-bridge formation, movement and release is repeated over and over again by all the myosin heads until the Ca^{2+} is removed or ATP is depleted. Because, at any given time, about half of the cross-bridges will be attached, this prevents the filaments sliding apart.

Calcium removal and muscle relaxation

During a muscle contraction the muscle will typically shorten by about 30%, which requires many cross-bridge cycles. The contraction is terminated by the removal of Ca^{2+} from the sarcoplasm by the action of Ca^{2+}-ATPase pumps present on the SR membrane which actively transport Ca^{2+} back into the SR. As the Ca^{2+} levels drop in the sarcoplasm of the muscle fibre, the troponin–tropomyosin complex once again covers the myosin-binding sites on the actin filament, and so the cross-bridges detach. In the SR the Ca^{2+} is sequestered by a calcium-binding protein called **calsequestrin**. This allows the concentration of Ca^{2+} to be 10 000 times greater than in the cytosol.

During contraction the actin and myosin filaments slide past each other and so the sarcomere reduces in length. During relaxation the sarcomere returns to its resting length. The sarcomere may decrease by as much as 70% during muscle contraction, although typically muscles contract by about 30%. If another depolarisation occurs before all the Ca^{2+} is removed then contraction is sustained and is strengthened until, at high frequencies of stimulation, a maximum sustained contraction occurs, called **tetanus** (see below).

Muscles cannot actively lengthen and in order to return to their resting length they must be actively stretched, either by their antagonist, e.g. a relaxed flexor muscle is stretched by the contraction of its extensor and vice versa, or by the effects of gravity or other forces acting on the muscle.

Muscle length and tension

The optimal overlap between the actin and myosin filaments is at a sarcomere length of 2.0–2.4 μm, and at this length the muscle fibre is able to develop its maximum tension. If the muscle fibre is stretched so that overlap between the actin and myosin is reduced, fewer myosin cross-bridges are able to make contact with the actin filament, and thus the muscle cannot generate the same degree of tension. At 170% of its optimal length there is no overlap between the actin and myosin, and the muscle will not generate any tension. If the sarcomere length becomes shorter the tension that can be generated by the muscle again is reduced. This is because the myosin filaments are compressed and crumple against the Z line, and consequently, fewer myosin heads are able to make contact with the actin filament. The resting length of muscle is held very close to the optimal length by the firm attachments of the skeletal muscle to the bones via their tendons.

Clinical box 9.22	Malignant hyperthermia (hyperpyrexia)

Malignant hyperthermia is a rare genetic defect which is caused by a defect in the control of calcium release from sarcoplasmic reticulum (SR). It is only manifested when the susceptible individual is given halothane anaesthesia or a muscle relaxant. Muscle spasms result due to excessive calcium release that triggers massive cross-bridge cycling and ATP consumption, and a rapid rise of body temperature, due to the heat generated by the regeneration of large quantities of ATP. Metabolism can become anaerobic, resulting in the generation of lactic acid with subsequent metabolic acidosis. Depletion of ATP leads to the release of high levels of K^+ from muscle, causing hyperkalaemia with a risk of cardiac arrhythmias. As well as supportive treatment, the drug dantrolene, which inhibits the ryanodine-sensitive Ca^{2+} channels in the membranes of the SR, is used to prevent further Ca^{2+} release.

MUSCLE METABOLISM

Muscle goes from times where it is virtually inactive and using only small amounts of ATP, to contracting continually, where ATP is being used at a rapid rate. The ATP stored in muscle is only enough to power contraction for a few seconds, so additional ATP must be continually synthesised if contraction of the muscle is to continue without fatigue.

Muscle has three sources of ATP synthesis:

- Creatine phosphate
- Anaerobic cellular respiration
- Aerobic cellular respiration.

The first of these is unique to muscle fibres, while all cells utilise the other two sources of ATP and are considered elsewhere (see Ch. 2).

Creatine phosphate

When the muscle is relaxed and at rest, excess ATP is being produced and some of this excess ATP is diverted to the synthesis of **creatine phosphate**. This is an energy-rich molecule produced by the enzyme creatine kinase. The enzyme catalyses the transfer of one high energy phosphate group from ATP to creatine, forming creatine phosphate and ADP. In the sarcoplasm of the muscle fibre, creatine phosphate is three to six times more abundant than ATP. As contraction of the muscle begins, the ADP levels begin to rise and creatine kinase catalyses the return of the high-energy phosphate group from creatine phosphate back to ADP, forming ATP. The creatine phosphate and ATP stores in muscle can fuel muscle contractions for about 15 seconds, which is sufficient for short bursts of activity.

Creatine supplementation

Creatine is a small amino acid-like molecule, which the body can synthesise, as well as it being derived from the diet. Adults need to synthesise and ingest around 2 g of creatine daily to replace the loss of creatine as its breakdown product **creatinine**, which is expelled in the urine. During intense exercise improved performance has been shown in subjects who had taken creatine supplements of up to 15 g per day for 28 days prior to the exercise. The subjects also gained muscle mass and were able to lift greater weights. However, such a large intake of creatine causes the body's own production of creatine to stop, and no long-term studies have been done to check whether after cessation of supplementation, the body's own synthesis of creatine is restored to normal levels again.

Muscle fatigue

After a prolonged period of muscle contraction the muscle becomes fatigued. However, this is not due to a lack of ATP in the muscle, as the levels of ATP in fatigued muscle are often not much lower than in resting muscle. The depletion of creatine phosphate may trigger muscle fatigue as may insufficient oxygen, depletion of glycogen and other nutrients, the build up of lactic acid and ADP, and the failure of the action potential in the motor neuron to release sufficient acetylcholine (ACh). Certain muscle fibres are more resistant to fatigue such as the type 1 slow fibres, while the type 2b fast glycolytic fibres are the easiest to fatigue.

TYPES OF MUSCLE FIBRES

Muscle fibres can be divided on the basis of their morphology and physiochemical characteristics into one of two main groups which have different functions.

■ **Type 1 muscle fibres** are slow in their speed of contraction and have high resistance to fatigue. The metabolism of type 1 fibres is oxidative and they have an increased concentration of myoglobin, which gives them their red appearance and an increased capacity to hold oxygen. The type 1 fibres tend to have more mitochondria and generally a larger capillary blood supply than type 2 fibres.

■ **Type 2 muscle fibres** use glycogen as their energy source and an anaerobic metabolism. The fibres contract at a faster rate and have a lower resistance to fatigue. Type 2 fibres may be further subdivided into **type 2a** and **type 2b** fibres. Type 2a have a mixed metabolism, that is oxidative and glycolytic, and therefore have a mixed phenotype with some features of a type 1 fibre.

During development the pattern of fibre types is established before innervation, but in the adult, fibre types are maintained by the innervation to that fibre, although circulating hormones such as thyroid hormone can also influence the fibre types in muscle. All the muscle fibres supplied by a single neuron are of the same histological type. The proportions of different fibre types within a muscle can vary because of exercise or inactivity.

The distribution of type 1 and type 2 fibres depends on their function, so that more type 1 fibres are located in the deeper muscles and are involved in the maintenance of posture, while the type 2 fibres are located more superficially and are mainly associated with movement.

THE CONNECTIVE TISSUE OF MUSCLE

Surrounding each muscle is the **fascia** (bandage); it lies deep to the skin and is a sheet of fibrous connective tissue.
Several layers of the fascia can be identified.

■ The **superficial fascia** separates the muscles from the skin. It allows a route for nerves and blood vessels to both enter and exit the muscle, and therefore it is composed of a loose areolar connective tissue. There is also a layer of adipose tissue, which helps to protect the underlying muscle from everyday traumas, as well as acting as an insulator that prevents too much loss of the heat generated by the muscles.

■ The **deep fascia** is composed of dense irregular connective tissue. It separates functionally similar muscles together. The nerves and blood vessels travel between the sheets of the deep fascia.

Around each individual muscle is the **epimysium**. The **perimysium** separates the muscle fibres into **fascicles** of around 10–100 muscle fibres. Finally, around each individual muscle fibre is the **endomysium**. Both the epimysium and the perimysium are made up of dense, irregular connective tissue, while the endomysium is composed of an areolar connective tissue.

The deep fascia, epimysium, perimysium and the endomysium are continuous with and contribute collagen fibres to the tendons (see above). The tendons are dense regular connective tissue cords and bands that connect muscle to the bone's periosteum. The tendon that attaches the muscle to the stationary part of the body is known as the **origin**, while the tendon that connects the muscle to the more mobile part of the body is known as the **insertion**. These terms are not precise as in some cases the muscle will act over several joints and both ends of the muscle are therefore mobile, but usually the distal end of the muscle has the 'insertion' tendon attachment.

MUSCLE GROWTH AND REPAIR

Skeletal muscle is able to repair itself by the activation of a population of resident muscle precursors that lie under the basal lamina of the muscle fibres, called **satellite cells**. These satellite cells remain quiescent until the muscle fibre is damaged, when they become activated to re-enter the cell cycle. They initially undergo symmetrical division (producing two identical daughter cells) like any stem cell population and then a proportion will undergo asymmetric division and one of the daughter cells will drop out of division and will fuse with the damaged muscle fibres and differentiate. The muscle contractile proteins of the differentiated cell will span the damaged region, repairing the defect.

The activated satellite cells that do not differentiate and help repair the damaged region will become quiescent again and remain dormant until needed. In this way, there is always a population of repair cells available to the muscle, although with age the ability of the satellite cells to re-enter the cell cycle declines and thus repair in the elderly is reduced. This may have to do with the number of cell divisions that the satellite cells have had to undergo in a lifetime, reducing their ability to replicate. This has implications for muscle diseases such as muscular dystrophy as the satellite cells are constantly having to repair damaged muscle. It is thought that one of the reasons for the reduced lifespan of these patients is that their satellite cells reach their maximum number of divisions earlier in life than in normal individuals and are thus unable to repair the muscle after the early to mid twenties (see Clinical box 9.21).

After growth has stopped no new muscle fibres are formed and any increase in muscle bulk is due to the incorporation of more myogenic cells into pre-existing fibres **(hyperplasia)**. This also means that if a muscle fibre is extensively damaged, the satellite cells cannot repair the damage, and the fibre is lost and replaced by fibrocollagenous scar tissue.

Recently, evidence has emerged of a circulating population of stem cells derived from bone marrow, which can also contribute to the repair of muscle. However, satellite cells still make up the majority of the repair cells in muscle and are responsible for replacing cells lost in the day-to-day microtrauma that muscle has to withstand. The newly identified stem cells form only a very small proportion of the muscle repair mechanism and are only activated after extensive muscle fibre damage.

THE NEUROMUSCULAR JUNCTION AND MUSCLE INNERVATION

Skeletal muscle is under voluntary control and the axons of the motor neurons extend to the muscles and form synapses at the neuromuscular junctions. The neuromuscular junction is located at the centre of the muscle fibre rather than at the ends. As muscle fibres can be up to 10 cm in length, the neuromuscular junction is located near the midpoint and the action potential is then propagated towards both ends of the fibre. This allows a near simultaneous activation and contraction of the fibre.

At the neuromuscular junction the motor neuron axon branches into a number of endings (Fig. 9.16). Each of the axon branches ends with an elongated terminal bouton, which contains thousands of synaptic vesicles loaded with the neurotransmitter **acetylcholine** (ACh). The sarcolemma of the muscle fibre under these endings is thrown into ruffles or 'junctional folds'.

Neurotransmitter release

An action potential in the motor neuron causes the exocytosis of several hundred vesicles into the synaptic cleft. Each synaptic vesicle contains approximately 10^4 ACh molecules so the simultaneous release of so many vesicles results in large amounts of ACh being released (Information box 9.3).

---

i Information box 9.3   Botulinum toxin

There are several plant substances and drugs that selectively block the neuromuscular junction. The toxin produced by *Clostridium botulinum* (botulinum toxin) prevents the exocytosis of ACh from the synaptic vesicles. Therefore, no ACh is released and the muscle does not contract. The bacteria can be found in improperly canned foods, and the toxin is one of the most lethal chemicals known, causing death by paralysis of diaphragm.

Recently, however, the toxin has been marketed as Botox. In the clinic, Botox injections into the muscle can help patients with strabismus, blepharospasm or cerebral palsy, by relaxing the muscles. Its other uses have been cosmetic, with injections into the facial muscles reducing the appearance of fine lines and wrinkles, by again relaxing the muscles attached to the skin of the face. The long-term risks of Botox injections have not been assessed.

Acetylcholine receptors

Following release ACh diffuses across the synaptic cleft to the ruffled sarcolemma of the muscle fibre where ACh receptors (AChRs) are located (see Fig. 9.16). There are 30–40 million AChRs embedded into the muscle fibre membrane at each synapse and the postsynaptic membrane is thickened with cytoskeletal proteins that hold the receptors in place. All of the AChRs on skeletal muscle are nicotinic acetylcholine receptors (nAChR). These are ligand-gated ion channels that open an integral ion channel permeable to Na^+ and K^+ in response to the binding of two molecules of ACh. This leads to depolarisation of the sarcolemma, which is propagated across the muscle fibre and into the inside of the muscle fibre by the T tubules.

Neuromuscular blockade

Several drugs produce muscle paralysis by affecting AChRs. They are used during surgery to produce relaxation of skeletal muscle. Much surgery requires the separation of muscle layers, and this requires these layers to be relaxed. The use of muscle relaxants requires the patient to be artificially ventilated via an endotracheal tube (intubation), which also cannot be inserted without relaxation of the muscles of the larynx.

The two types of muscle relaxant are:

- Non-depolarising drugs such as **tubocurarine** and its safer synthetic alternatives are competitive antagonists of nAChRs. These drugs bind to AChRs but do not cause depolarisation. They are fairly long-lasting (up to 60 min) and can be reversed by drugs, such as neostigmine, which increase the local concentration of ACh.
- Depolarising drugs such as **succinylcholine** are ACh agonists. They bind to AChRs and cause a long-lasting depolarisation of the muscle which, after disorganised initial contractions called fasciculations, produces a flaccid paralysis possibly due to AChR desensitisation.

Succinylcholine is normally rapidly metabolised by circulating cholinesterases and so is short acting. It is usually used only to provide relaxation during intubation. However, about 1 in 3000 patients have a type of plasma cholinesterase which does not metabolise succinylcholine so the neuromuscular blockade lasts several hours during which the patient must be continually ventilated.

Breakdown of acetylcholine

ACh is broken down in the synaptic cleft by cholinesterase enzymes concentrated on the basement membrane, which hydrolyses approximately 30% of the released ACh before it

---

i Information box 9.4   Curare

Curare is derived from a South American plant, and is used by the local Indians to tip their arrows and darts. It causes muscle paralysis, by binding to the AChR and blocking normal activation of the receptor. Curare-like drugs, such as cisatracurium, are often used as muscle relaxants before surgery. **Neostigmine** (an anticholinesterase) is used as an antidote for curare poisoning and terminates its effect after surgery. Neostigmine is usually administered with atropine to block the muscarinic effects of increasing the amount of circulating ACh.

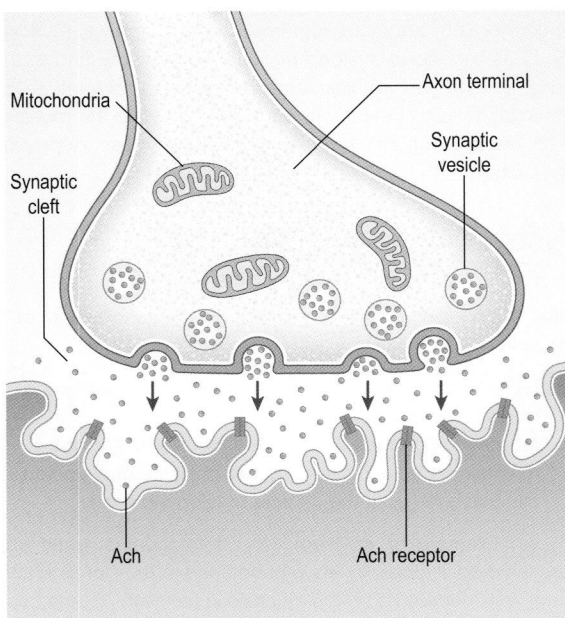

Fig. 9.16 **The neuromuscular junction.**

The ACh receptors (AChRs) on skeletal muscle normally turnover with a half-life of 10 days, with new receptors constantly being made and incorporated into the postsynaptic junctional folds, and the old receptors removed and degraded by lysosomes.

In **myasthenia gravis** the immune system makes antibodies to the AChR. The antigen–antibody complex has a half-life of only 2 days, leading to a progressive loss of AChRs. Certain muscles are affected more than others; those innervated by the cranial nerves, for example, are affected more than the somatic muscles of the body. For this reason myasthenia gravis clinically is characterised by muscle weakness of the muscles in the face and this is especially noticeable in the muscles around the eyes and mouth. The limb muscles are usually less affected but in severe cases these will be weakened as well. In the most severe cases, the muscles of swallowing and respiration are affected and this can be life-threatening.

Treatment for myasthenia gravis involves the administration of an anticholinesterase drug such as **neostigmine**. This prevents the breakdown of ACh as it is released from the motor axon and allows it to bind to the remaining AChRs, thus improving the contractile power of the muscles.

The antibodies that are produced originate in the thymus gland which in affected individuals is hyperplastic, and in 10% of cases there is a lymphoid tumour in the thymus gland. The removal of the thymus may therefore be beneficial in individuals with severe symptoms that are not controlled by the usual drug regimen.

reaches the postsynaptic membrane of the muscle fibre. However, as ACh is released in such large quantities, with up to 10 times more ACh being produced than is needed, muscle contraction is usually assured. For muscle contraction to fail, 90% of the receptors must be blocked (Clinical box 9.23).

ACh is broken down into acetic acid and choline. The choline is taken back into the synapse by the action of a specific Na^+-dependent choline transporter. This is a rate-limiting step for the synthesis of ACh and this transporter can be blocked by the drug, **hemicholinium**. This results in a depletion of ACh in the synapse and a reduction in ACh release. Another drug, **vesamicol**, prevents the transport of synthesised ACh into vesicles.

Motor units

Each muscle is innervated by at least one motor neuron which branches to supply a number of muscle fibres within the muscle. The motor neuron and all the muscle fibres it supplies are called a **motor unit**. The average number of fibres in a motor unit is about 150 but the number varies according to the degree of fine movement or force required from that muscle. The number of fibres innervated by a single neuron varies enormously, from hundreds in large, weight-bearing muscles such as those around the hip to as few as four in the tiny ocular muscles which control eye movements.

The fibres innervated by a single motor unit are distributed through a muscle so activation of a single motor unit causes a weak contraction of the whole muscle. As more motor units are activated, fibres throughout the muscle are activated until maximum tension is reached with the activation of all the motor units supplying a given muscle.

Development of sustained tension

A single action potential in a motor neuron will cause a small twitch in a muscle, and repeated low frequency stimulation will produce a series of twitches which match the frequency of stimulation.

When a skeletal muscle is stimulated at 20–30 times a second, it is only partly able to relax between the stimuli. This results in a sustained but wavering contraction called **unfused tetanus**. Stimulating the muscle at 80–100 times a second results in no relaxation between repeated stimuli and a **fused tetanus** occurs with a sustained constant tension.

In both unfused and fused tetanus the level of Ca^{2+} builds up inside the muscle and the peak tension that can be generated is 5–10 times greater than for a single contraction.

Muscle tone

In skeletal muscle, a muscle is never totally inactive; a few motor units are always being activated to produce a sustained contraction of their muscle fibres. The proportion of the motor units that are active is only very small and so the muscle is relaxed but has 'tone'. The motor units that are active constantly shift so that fatigue does not set in. Muscle tone keeps the muscle firm but is not strong enough to cause movement. For example, when standing the muscles of the leg and back help to maintain an upright posture but are mainly relaxed with only a few motor units active to stop us from falling down.

Sensory innervation of muscle

Apart from the motor neuron innervation of muscle there is also sensory innervation of skeletal muscle. Sensory nerves convey information about muscle length and tension in order to coordinate muscle contraction. The main sensory organ in muscle, the muscle spindles, which are embedded between the contractile fibres, are up to 1 cm in length and can vary in number from a dozen to several hundred in different muscles. They are more numerous in the antigravity muscles such as the muscles along the vertebral column and in the legs, and in the intrinsic muscles of the hand. All these muscles tend to have more type 1 fibres while the muscles rich in type 2 fibres tend to have fewer muscle spindles (see Ch. 8).

ISOTONIC VERSUS ISOMETRIC CONTRACTION

Not all muscle contraction results in the shortening of a muscle:

- **Isotonic** contractions result in muscle shortening and move the body and external objects
- **Isometric** contractions stabilise joints and are vital in maintaining posture; they do not produce movement but still use energy as the muscle tension increases.

An example of an isometric contraction is when you are holding a book in an outstretched arm. Considerable tension is generated by the muscles in the arm – as the book drags the arm down, the shoulder and arm muscles must compensate by contracting. Therefore, the stretching and contraction of the muscle in opposite directions keeps the arm level.

Isotonic contractions can be subdivided into concentric and eccentric contractions:

- **Concentric contractions** cause a muscle to shorten and produce a movement that reduces the angle at a joint (flexion). Picking up a book from a table is a result of a concentric contraction of the biceps brachii muscle in the front of the upper arm.
- **Eccentric contractions** are where a muscle contracts but the length of the muscle gets longer. As you lower the book gradually to the table the biceps brachii still contracts to prevent the book from dropping, yet the actual length of the muscle increases.

Repeated eccentric contractions produce more damage to the muscle fibres as it is thought that the myosin heads are pulled off the actin filaments by the stretching of the muscle that takes place. In most daily activities there is a mixture of isotonic and isometric contractions.

MUSCLE NOMENCLATURE

Muscle shape

The arrangement of the fascicles in each muscle can vary and is used to describe the shape of the muscle (Fig. 9.17).

The deltoid muscle is a **pennate** muscle which has its fascicles arranged in a feather-like arrangement. Pennate muscles may be uni-, bi-, or multi-pennate muscles, examples of each being the extensor digitorum longus, rectus femoris and the deltoid, respectively.

The biceps brachii muscle is an example of a **fusiform** muscle, which is spindle shaped, with tapered ends and a fatter belly. The biceps brachii is also a **bicipital** muscle that has two heads which are separate proximally, but which at the distal end merge into one tendon. A **quadrate** muscle has four equal sides; an example is the pronator quadratus muscle.

When the muscle fibres surround an opening, and contraction of the muscle causes a constriction of the opening, these are called **circular** or **sphincter** muscles, such as the orbicularis oculi and oris muscles in the face.

Muscle names

Muscles are named according to several factors, including their **location** and **function**. Some are named according to the bones they are attached to. For example:

- The cricothyroid muscle in the neck attaches to the cricoid cartilage inferiorly, and to the thyroid cartilage superiorly.
- The abductor digiti minimi abducts the little finger.

Muscle names may also be derived from their **position** (for example the flexor digitorum superficialis is the superficial flexor of the digits) or **length** or **size** (the extensor pollicis longus and extensor pollicis brevis are the long and short extensor muscles of the thumb, respectively).

Some muscles are named according to the **shape** and **direction** of their fascicles. For example, the deltoid muscle is roughly triangular (deltoid means triangle) whereas the rectus abdominus has its fascicles running straight (rectus) with respect to the midline.

These simple rules will help remind you about where and what each muscle does.

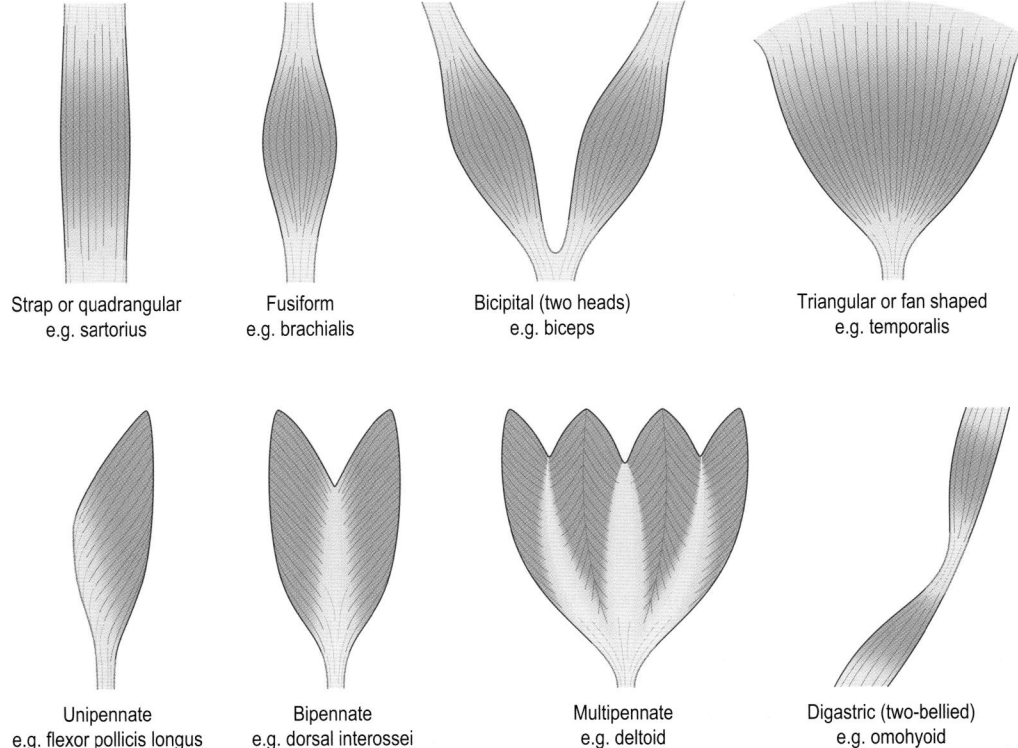

Strap or quadrangular
e.g. sartorius

Fusiform
e.g. brachialis

Bicipital (two heads)
e.g. biceps

Triangular or fan shaped
e.g. temporalis

Unipennate
e.g. flexor pollicis longus

Bipennate
e.g. dorsal interossei

Multipennate
e.g. deltoid

Digastric (two-bellied)
e.g. omohyoid

Fig. 9.17 **Muscle shapes.**

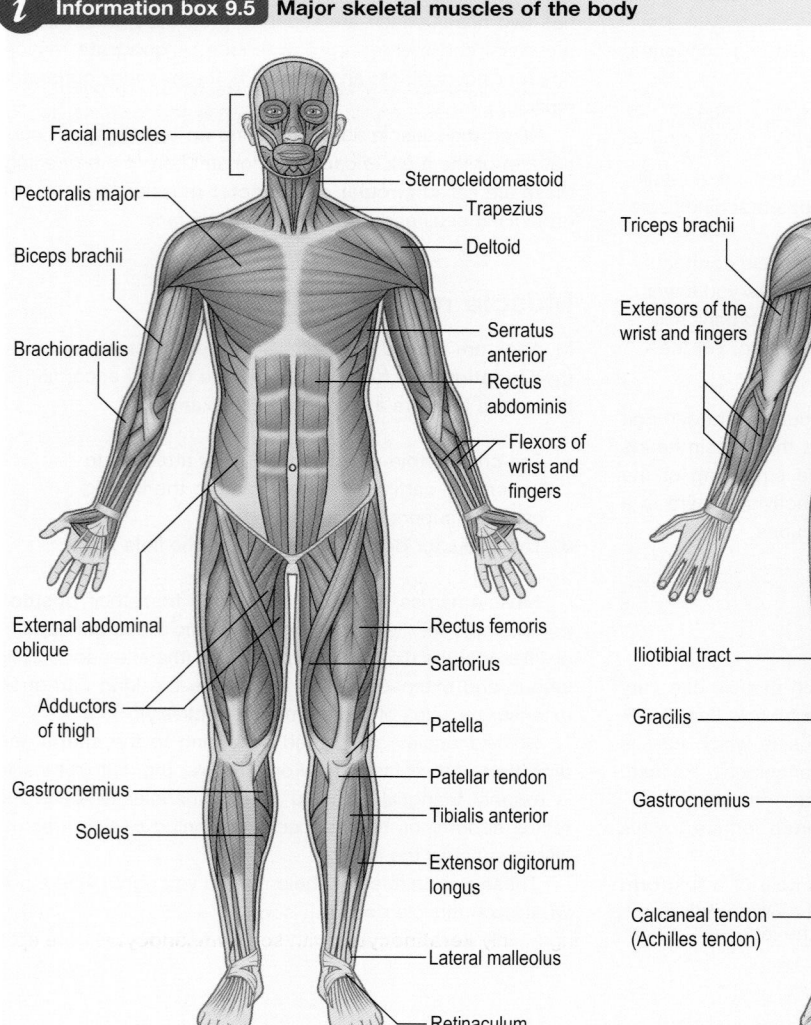

Facial muscles
Pectoralis major
Biceps brachii
Brachioradialis
Sternocleidomastoid
Trapezius
Deltoid
Serratus anterior
Rectus abdominis
Flexors of wrist and fingers
External abdominal oblique
Adductors of thigh
Gastrocnemius
Soleus
Rectus femoris
Sartorius
Patella
Patellar tendon
Tibialis anterior
Extensor digitorum longus
Lateral malleolus
Retinaculum

Fig. 9.18 **Superficial muscles of the body: anterior view.**

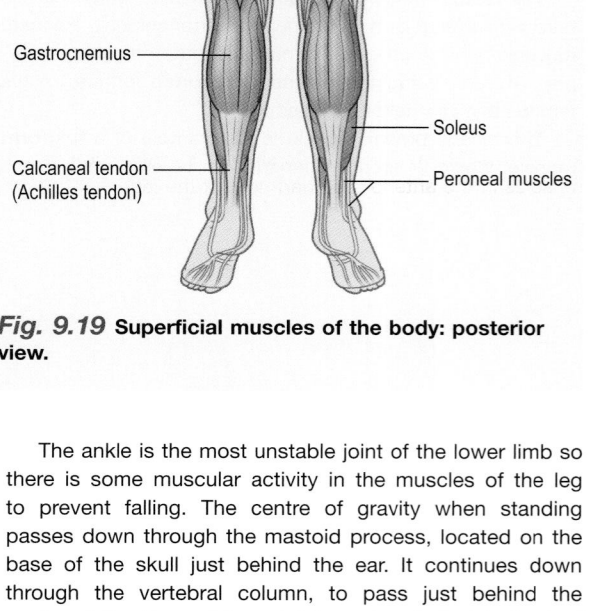

Triceps brachii
Extensors of the wrist and fingers
Iliotibial tract
Gracilis
Gastrocnemius
Calcaneal tendon (Achilles tendon)
Sternocleidomastoid
Trapezius
Deltoid
Latissimus dorsi
External abdominal oblique
Gluteus maximus
Adductor
Hamstrings
Soleus
Peroneal muscles

Fig. 9.19 **Superficial muscles of the body: posterior view.**

POSTURE AND LOCOMOTION

Posture refers to the arrangement of the limbs, trunk and head in relation to the centre of gravity. It is controlled by reflexes which enable the body position to remain stable, especially during movement which moves the centre of gravity. Postural reflexes which automatically adjust the body position in response to sensory input are organised by the brainstem (see Ch. 8). The main muscles involved in posture are the axial trunk extensors and the proximal limb muscles.

STANDING

When standing normally the feet are slightly apart and laterally rotated with the toes pointing outwards. Because of the arrangement of the joints in the lower limb, they tend to be in their most stable position when standing, with the hip and knee extended. This means that when standing there is little muscular activity needed to maintain the upright position.

The ankle is the most unstable joint of the lower limb so there is some muscular activity in the muscles of the leg to prevent falling. The centre of gravity when standing passes down through the mastoid process, located on the base of the skull just behind the ear. It continues down through the vertebral column, to pass just behind the centre of the hip and knee joints and ends just in front of the ankle joint.

WALKING

Movement involves the coordinated activity of the central nervous system at different hierarchical levels which involve parts of the cortex, basal ganglia, cerebellum, brainstem nuclei and spinal cord pathways and circuits (see Ch. 8). The basic patterns of muscle activity needed for locomotion are provided by spinal cord networks called central pattern generators which are subsequently modified by sensory input.

Walking is a complex process that requires coordination of the two legs; it also requires transfer of the body's weight from both legs to one leg. A basic understanding of locomotion is important as changes in the gait of an individual are indicative of joint, muscle and nervous system disorders.

When walking on a level surface the walking cycle can be divided into swing and stance phases; these phases look at the movements of a single leg as you walk.

- The **stance phase** begins with heel-strike and ends with toe-off; it is the longer portion of the walking cycle and accounts for 60% of the cycle.
- The **swing phase** is the smaller part of the walking cycle, only taking up 40% of the time; it begins with toe-off and ends when the heel makes contact with the ground.

Stance phase

At **heel-strike** the foot is dorsiflexed and usually inverted (for terms related to gait see Information box 9.1), and as the body weight is transferred to that leg the foot comes into full contact with the ground. At **toe-off** the foot is plantar-flexed and slightly everted.

If the triceps surae (gostrocnemius and soleus) is paralysed or the calcaneus tendon is ruptured, toe-off is less effective, the gluteus maximus and hamstrings can lift the leg off the ground by extending the thigh at the hip joint but the movement is not as efficient.

Swing phase

During the swing phase the toes are prevented from dragging on the ground by the simultaneous flexion of the hip and knee joints. The foot is also dorsiflexed by the action of the muscles in the anterior compartment of the leg.

During normal walking the quadriceps and gluteus maximus contribute little but become more active when walking up and down hills or when climbing stairs.

Stabilisation

Stabilisation is very important when walking, especially as you go from a double support to a single support. When the weight is transferred to one lower limb there is a tendency for the unsupported pelvis to drop, this is prevented by the contraction of the hip abductors, the gluteus medius and minimus, on the supporting side to pull the pelvis level. Weak hip abductors, dislocation of the femoral head or fracture of the greater trochanter all lead to the pelvis dropping to the unsupported side. This is known as **Trendelenburg's sign**.

The invertors and evertors of the foot are the main stabilisers of the foot, with movements adjusting to the ground constantly.

Gait analysis

Gait analysis can be used for both normal and abnormal gaits. Markers are applied to anatomical landmarks such as the bony landmarks on the pelvis, knee and ankles. As the patient walks along a walkway they are videoed from several angles and strain gauges in the floor measure the forces applied by the feet. This allows the movement of each joint to be analysed. Specific conditions can be diagnosed and possible treatments suggested.

Clinical box 9.24 Gait defects

Disorders of gait can be caused by both mechanical and neurological problems. Mechanical causes include osteoarthritis, muscle strains and blisters, while neurological problems include deficits in perception and damage to nerves.

A commonly seen abnormal gait is seen in Parkinson's disease, with short shuffling steps and rigidity in the knee and hip extensors.

SKIN, HAIR AND NAILS

Skin covers the whole body with a surface area (adult) of between 1.5 m^2 and 2 m^2. As well as providing a flexible, waterproof protective surface it is also involved in regulating body temperature (see Ch. 11) and providing sensory input about the external world (Ch. 8).

STRUCTURE OF SKIN

The skin is composed of three layers (Fig. 9.20):

- Epidermis, the most superficial layer of the skin, formed mainly of keratinocytes.
- Dermis, the middle layer containing large quantities of connective tissue and the dermal capillaries which provide nutrients to the skin.
- Subcutaneous layer, the deepest layer, formed from loose connective tissue and fat cells (adipose tissue).

Epidermis

The **epidermis** is a stratified squamous epithelium containing mainly **keratinocytes** with some **melanocytes**. The epidermis sits on a basement membrane composed mainly of type IV and VII collagens. Defects in these collagens results in skin fragility.

The epidermis is composed of four to five layers which represent different stages in the maturation of **keratin**, a fibrous protein which is secreted by the keratinocytes. The surface layers of the epidermis consist of toughened dead cells which are continually being shed. They are replaced from below by new cells produced at the base of the epidermis, the entire epidermis being replaced about every 40 days.

- **Stratum basale** (basal layer) is the layer closest to the basement membrane and contains the youngest keratinocytes which are rapidly dividing from stem cells. These columnar keratinocytes are anchored to the basement membrane by **hemidesmosomes**.
- **Stratum spinosum** (spiny layer) consists of several layers of polyhedral keratinocytes linked by **desmosomes**. These cells contain bundles of **prekeratin** which form **tonofilaments** which confer strength and distribute stress horizontally. The 'spines' are artefacts of tissue fixation but the name remains.
- **Stratum granulosum** (granular layer) consists of three to five layers of flattened keratinocytes. These cells have thickened membranes and, as well as tonofilaments, contain two types of granule: **keratohyalin granules** (see below) and **lamellar granules** containing waterproofing glycolipids which are secreted into the extracellular space. This waterproofing slows water loss

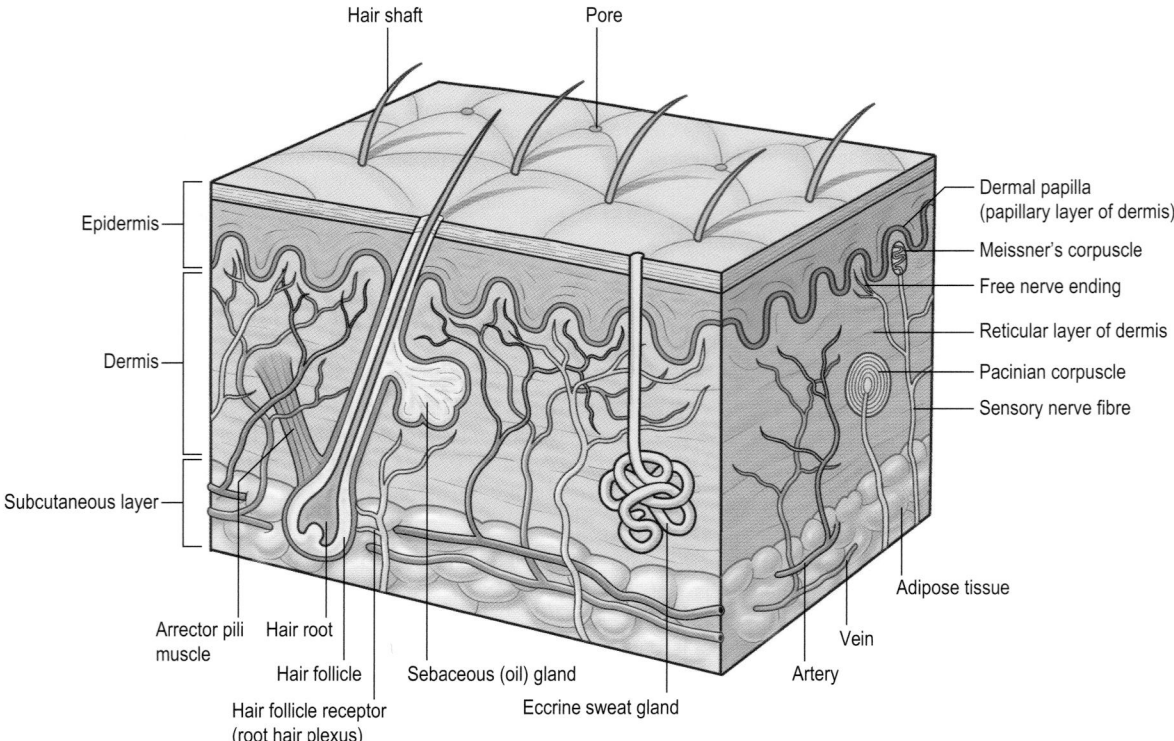

Fig. 9.20 **Structure of skin.**

across the skin. Above this layer the cells are dead as they are too far away from the dermis to receive adequate nutrition.

■ **Stratum lucidum** (clear layer) is only present in thick skin (palms, fingertips and soles of the feet) and consists of a few layers of dead keratinocytes with the keratin fibrils formed from the association of keratohyalin and tonofilaments.

■ **Stratum corneum** (horny layer) is the thickest layer, 20–30 cells thick, and consists of dead cells called **corneocytes** filled with keratin fibrils. Their thick membranes and their waterproof coating produce a strong impermeable layer which protects the body from damage and dehydration. Cells from this layer are continually being shed, and can been seen as skin flakes and dandruff.

Melanocytes

Melanocytes are found in the stratum basale where they synthesise **melanins**, which give the skin its characteristic colour (Information box 9.6). Melanin accumulates in melanocytes as membrane-bound melanosomes which move along the arm like processes of the melanocytes, where they are then taken up by the nearby keratinocytes. The melanin granules take up position above the keratinocyte nucleus. As melanins absorb ultraviolet radiation by scavenging for free radicals, they protect the skin from the damaging effects of exposure to sunlight (Clinical box 9.25).

The epidermis also contains **Langerhans' cells (epidermal dendritic cells)**, a type of macrophage, mainly in the stratum spinosum. They not only ingest foreign material but also activate the immune system as they present antigens to lymphocytes. **Merkel's cells** are found in the stratum basale and consist of sensory receptors which respond to touch (see Ch. 8).

𝒊 Information box 9.6 **Skin colour**

The relative number of melanocytes is the same in all humans; therefore an individual's skin colouration is dependent on the kind and amount of melanin that is made. Melanin is manufactured from tyrosine and is produced in two forms:

■ Eumelanin – this is the most common and gives the skin a brown-black colour.
■ Phaeomelanin – this gives a yellow-red colouration, seen particularly in red-haired individuals.

Skin colour depends on the type and quantity of melanin present in the skin. Darker-skinned individuals produce more of the darker form of melanin and it is retained for longer. It is thought that the lighter skin of individuals living at more northerly or southerly latitudes, where the incident radiation is less, has evolved in response to the need to produce sufficient vitamin D in the skin.

Melanin production is stimulated by exposure to the sun to give a 'tan'; however, this also increases cross-linking of collagen fibres in the skin which produces wrinkles and there is an increased risk of skin cancer. The low rates of skin cancer in dark-skinned individuals, especially in countries with a high incident solar radiation, shows how effective melanin is as a sun shield.

Albinos, who lack all melanin, are at grave risk of skin cancer unless they avoid going in the sun and use high strength sun creams.

Dermis

The dermis consists of connective tissue containing cells such as fibroblasts and macrophages in a matrix of collagen and elastin. The dermis has large numbers of capillaries, nerve endings and lymphatics.

While there are many types of benign tumours of the skin, exposure to UV radiation, especially in light-skinned individuals, is one of the major causes of malignant skin cancer. This is thought to be due to the inhibition of the tumour suppressor gene, p53.

There are three main types:

● **Malignant melanoma** – this tumour, derived from melanocytes, is the most dangerous with 5-year survival rates for the severe forms being less than 40%. Treatment involves surgical removal of the cancer plus a wide surrounding region with subsequent chemotherapy.
● **Basal cell carcinoma** – this tumour is derived from basal keratinocytes, and it is the most common type of skin cancer and the least dangerous. Also known as rodent ulcers, these cancers are slow growing and can usually be cured by simple excision.
● **Squamous cell carcinoma** – this tumour is derived from mature differentiated keratinocytes, and these tumours can metastasise to local lymph nodes.

Public awareness campaigns aim to encourage the use of powerful sunscreens, limiting sun exposure times and periodic examination of any new lesions as a way of preventing and limiting skin cancer.

The dermis consists of two layers:

■ Papillary layer – this thin uppermost layer has numerous raised projections which interdigitate with the epidermis. These either contain loops of capillaries or sensory nerve endings.
■ Reticular layer – this layer contains bundles of collagen fibres which give strength and flexibility to the skin. This layer contains the sweat and sebaceous glands and the hair follicles.

Damage to the dermis can occur when the skin is burnt (Clinical box 9.26). Different types of burn affect different layers.

Sweat glands

Sweat glands, which are found over most of the body, secrete water with varying amounts of sodium chloride and other metabolic compounds.

There are two types of sweat glands:

■ **Eccrine glands** – these are found everywhere on the body except mucous membranes, and they secrete a watery hypotonic fluid which produces cooling of the skin as it evaporates. This varies from a minimum of 0.5 L/day to a maximum of 2 L/hour. This is a major mechanism in the control of body temperature, although it is much less effective when the external humidity is high. The fluid is slightly acidic (pH 4–6), which reduces fungal growth and also lubricates the skin surface. The glands consist of a simple secretory coil in the epidermis with a duct that opens onto the skin surface with a pore.
■ **Apocrine glands** are found mainly in the axillae (armpits) and anogenital area. Their secretions are more viscous as they contain more fats and proteins than eccrine secretions and are not secreted onto the skin but into hair follicles. Although the secretions are initially odourless, bacteria on the skin break them down to give a musky smell which is the basis of body odour. They

Acute trauma such as digging the garden with a spade can cause shearing forces between the epidermis and the dermis of the hands, producing a blister. The separation between the epidermal and dermal layers of the skin is filled with fluid that leaks from the capillaries in the dermis.

Burns

When the skin is burnt this can lead to large losses of fluids and electrolytes which, if sufficiently extensive, can be life-threatening, so initial treatment is concentrated on maintaining fluid balance. If the patient survives this, then the major problem is infection due to the loss of the protective barrier. The extent of burns (in adults) is estimated by the **rule of nines** which divides the body into 11 regions (Table 9.1), each of which represents 9% of the surface area (total 99%) plus the perineum (1%).

Burns are classified according to the thickness of the burnt layer.

● **First-degree burns** only involve damage to the epidermis. There is swelling, pain and localised redness, but the epidermis heals in 2–3 days without specialist treatment. Unless severe, sunburn is usually a first-degree burn.
● **Second-degree burns** involve the epidermis and the upper dermis. They produce blistering but if infection is avoided there are enough remaining live cells to produce regeneration within about 4 weeks.
● **Third-degree burns** involve the destruction of the entire epidermis and dermis and so are called **full-thickness burns**. These burns are not painful as the nerve endings are also destroyed but due to the complete loss of tissue they can only regenerate round the edge, which is very slow, so treatment usually involves skin grafting. New techniques involving growing the patient's own epidermal cells in culture to provide unlimited sheets of tissue with no rejection problems may eliminate many of the problems associated with traditional methods.

Table 9.1	**Rule of nines**	
Area		**%**
Head and neck		9
Anterior upper trunk		9
Posterior upper trunk		9
Anterior lower trunk		9
Posterior lower trunk		9
Anterior arms		9
Posterior arms		9
Anterior leg (×2)		18
Posterior leg (×2)		18
Perineum		1
Total		100

only become active after puberty and there are suggestions that they may be involved in sexual signalling.

Sebaceous glands

These glands secrete an oily substance called **sebum** usually into the hair follicles or occasionally onto the skin. This softens the hair and skin and helps to reduce water loss from the skin surface. Sebum is also strongly bactericidal. They are especially numerous on the face and scalp. They are activated by androgens and become particularly active during puberty when they may cause acne (Clinical box 9.27).

Subcutaneous layer

This layer, which is also called the **hypodermis**, consists of areolar connective tissue and adipose tissue. As well as providing an energy store, the fat layer also acts as a shock absorber and insulator. The hypodermis allows the skin to slide over the underlying structures, reducing the severity of trauma.

HAIR

Structure of hair

Although humans are relatively hairless compared with most other mammals, most of the body is covered with hairs of some kind. Hair consists of the hair shaft, which is the external hair, and the root, which lies in the dermis and epidermis.

The hair shaft consists of three concentric rings of keratinocytes, which contain hard keratin:

- Medulla – an inner core of large cells
- Cortex – several layers of flattened cells
- Cuticle – a single layer of overlapping highly keratinised cells.

Structure of hair follicle

In the dermis the **hair follicle** is where the hair shaft is produced. The developing shaft is surrounded by the **root sheath** which consists of two layers: the **inner** and **outer** root sheath. At the base of the follicle is the **hair bulb**. This consists of a loop of capillaries which project into a dermal papilla, which is covered by a single layer of cells from the stratum basale. Growth signals from the papilla reach a group of stem cells situated just above the hair bulb, called the **hair matrix**, and cause the cells to divide. This pushes the older cells upwards towards the skin surface. Just as in the different layers of the epidermis, the cells become more keratinised until they die and form the hair shaft.

Hair growth is not continuous, otherwise all our hair would keep growing until it broke. There are three phases of hair growth:

- **Anagen** – the active growth phase.
- **Catagen** – the resting phase during which no growth occurs, the hair bulb partially atrophies and the hair shaft is released from the matrix with a short club root.
- **Telogen** – during this phase the hair is shed and a new hair shaft develops at the matrix. The old hair is either pushed out by new hair or it falls out.

Most (80–90%) of the scalp hair is in anagen and about 10–20% in catagen. Fewer than 1% of scalp hair is in telogen, with the loss of about 90 hairs per day.

Hair growth is usually out of phase so there is no detectable reduction in hair volume, but a number of factors, such as stress, fever, surgery and childbirth, can cause synchronisation during anagen and so large numbers of hairs are lost at the same time leading to hair thinning (Clinical box 9.28). A common cause of hair thinning in women is iron-deficiency anaemia and this is reversed after treatment of the anaemia. However, other types of hair loss may be permanent. Women may also have excessive hairiness due to high levels of androgen hormones (Clinical box 9.28).

Each hair follicle is connected to a smooth muscle called the **arrector pili**, which can pull the hair into a more vertical position in response to cold or fear. In humans this gives the skin a dimpled appearance known as 'goose bumps' but in more hairy mammals this can either increase heat retention by trapping more air between the hairs or give the impression that the animal is larger (and possibly fiercer).

Types of hair

There are three types of hair, of different length and thickness:

- **Lanugo** are fine, long hairs which are produced in utero and are shed before birth, hence they are usually only seen in premature babies.
- **Vellus** hairs are the short, fine hairs which cover most of the body, particularly in women and children.
- **Terminal** hairs are the thicker, longer hairs which cover the scalp and eyebrows. They grow in the axillae and pubic regions of both sexes after puberty and also form the beard and chest hairs in males.

The rate of hair growth is dependent on many factors including nutritional and hormonal status and normally is about 0.4 mm per day. But the length of hairs in the different areas of the body is dependent on the length of time the hair follicles are in their active phase. Scalp hair is in the anagen phase for between 3 and 7 years but for eyebrow hair this is less than 4 months.

The hair shaft which projects from the skin varies in its cross-section. Straight hair is round while wavy hair is oval and curly hair is flattened. Hair colour is dependent on melanocytes in the hair follicle, which transfer melanins to the cortex of the growing hair. Grey or white hair is due to reduced quantities of melanin being produced.

NAILS

Nails are derived from the epidermis and consist of hardened keratin which forms the hard **nail plate**. Nails grow from the proximal end, which consists of a **nail matrix** that produces the keratinocytes. These become heavily keratinised as they emerge to form the nail plate. The area of the nail matrix can be seen as a white crescent called the **lunula**, at the base of the nail. Under the nail plate lies the nail bed, which is pink due to the presence of dermal capillaries. Skin lies over the nail plate on each side, forming the **lateral nail folds**, and over part of the matrix, the **cuticle**.

Finger nails grow faster than toe nails; it takes 6 months to replace a finger nail and 12 months for a toe nail. However, there are many disease processes which can affect nail growth and distinctive patterns in nail growth can reflect previous medical history. **Beau's lines** are ridges in the nail caused by a temporary halt in nail growth. **Finger clubbing**, which is a change in the angle of the nail bed, is an important clinical sign associated with a number of respiratory, cardiovascular and other diseases.

10

Endocrine and reproductive systems

Alan Longstaff

INTRODUCTION

Most of the 10^{15} cells of which an adult human is made are linked by networks of signalling molecules. These coordinate the activities of cells so that the physiology of the individual is appropriate for current needs. The networks consist of thousands of secreted and cell surface molecules and their respective receptors located on target cells.

The first signalling molecules to be discovered were called **hormones**. They are released from **endocrine glands** directly into the bloodstream. This transports them to widely distributed **target cells**, which have specific hormone receptors. The signalling network that includes endocrine glands, hormones and their target cells is referred to as the **endocrine system**, and its study is called **endocrinology**.

The functions of hormones are:

- Regulating fuel metabolism by optimising the availability and utilisation of energy substrates to the prevailing physiological state, e.g. feeding or fasting, exercise, pregnancy, etc. (see Ch. 3)
- Controlling sexual development and reproductive cycles, and influencing sexual behaviour
- Organising the growth and maturation that takes a baby to adulthood
- Modulating behaviour over the long term.

The classic hormone-secreting endocrine organs are the hypothalamus, the pituitary, thyroid, parathyroid and adrenal

---

Information box 10.1   Non-endocrine signalling molecules

Many signalling molecules are not the province of endocrinology because they are not produced by specific glands, or they are secreted into the extracellular space rather than blood (**paracrine** not endocrine secretion), so operate over short distances, or they are not secreted at all but instead are cell surface molecules. These include:

- **Cell adhesion molecules** – usually transmembrane glycoprotein molecules that interact with each other and with the extracellular matrix. They allow cells to recognise and interact with their immediate neighbours, e.g. cadherins and integrins.
- **Growth factors** – proteins concerned with cell division, differentiation, growth and maturation, e.g. erythropoietin, which stimulates red cell production. Many growth factors are liberated into the extracellular space. Disordered growth factor function is implicated in some cancers.
- **Cytokines** – about 200 small proteins that act as intercellular mediators to coordinate the functions of cells in the immune system (Ch. 6), e.g. interleukins and interferons. These are usually liberated into the blood. Many act on the cells which secrete them; this is **autocrine** secretion.
- **Neurotransmitters and neuromodulators** – signalling molecules that underpin information processing in the nervous system (Ch. 8), e.g. glutamate and endorphins. These are secreted into the synaptic cleft, part of the extracellular space. This **neurocrine** signalling is highly local – the distances involved are of the order of tens to hundreds of micrometres – and occurs by diffusion on a millisecond to second timescale.

glands, gonads (testes and ovaries) and pancreatic islet cells (endocrine pancreas). However, not all hormones are produced by the classic endocrine glands. These include atrial natriuretic peptides produced by the heart (Chs 11 and 14), and peptides released by the gut that help to control gut function and appetite (Chs 15 and 16).

GENERAL PRINCIPLES OF ENDOCRINOLOGY

ENDOCRINE SIGNALLING

Diffusion is too slow to transport molecules over the large distances needed for communication between cells that are separated by more than a few millimetres. The circulatory system, however, can transport hormones rapidly over large distances. Given an adult resting cardiac output of 5 L/min and a blood volume of 5 L, the **average** transit time for circulating blood is 1 minute. This defines the timescale for target cells to recognise secreted hormones.

PROPERTIES OF ENDOCRINE SYSTEMS

Chemistry of hormones

Hormones can be classified by their chemistry into three major groups (Table 10.1). With the exception of the steroids, which are lipid soluble, and thyroid hormones for which there is a specific membrane transporter, hormones are recognised by cell surface receptors. By contrast, the steroid and thyroid hormones, which cross the cell membrane, interact with nuclear receptors (see also Ch. 4).

Amino acid derivatives

Adrenaline and **noradrenaline** (epinephrine, norepinephrine) are synthesised by the adrenal medulla (Ch. 4) from the amino acid, tyrosine. These catecholamine hormones are water soluble and circulate free in the blood or weakly bound to albumin. They have short half-lives and activate G-protein-coupled receptors.

Thyroid hormones are produced from iodinated tyrosine moieties in a large precursor molecule, **thyroglobulin**. Two mature molecules are released from thyroglobulin, differing only in their number of iodide residues; **thyroxine** (T_4) has four and **triiodothyronine** (T_3) has three. Barely soluble in water, the hormones are transported in blood bound to plasma proteins. They have long half-lives, with a timescale of days. Thyroid hormones are transported across cell membranes by a specific transport system and bind to nuclear receptors that belong to the steroid receptor superfamily.

Steroid hormones

Steroid hormones are secreted by the adrenal cortex, gonads and placenta. They are derived from cholesterol and contain the **cyclopentanoperhydrophenanthrene** ring structure. A general scheme for steroid metabolism (Fig. 10.1) shows that steroids can be classified by the number of carbon atoms in them. The numbering of the carbon atoms in the ring is used in steroid nomenclature to specify the location of substituents. Steroids are non-polar, so they are sparingly water soluble and transported in blood bound to plasma proteins. They are, however, highly lipid soluble, so that they diffuse readily through plasma membranes to interact with steroid receptors either in the nucleus or the cytoplasm (see also Ch. 4).

Steroid hormone receptors have extremely high affinities for their ligands, with equilibrium dissociation constants of order 10^{-10} M. Consequently steroids are effective even at the very low free (i.e. unbound) concentrations at which they are present in the plasma.

Table 10.1	The chemical nature of some key hormones (closely related peptides/ proteins are grouped together)
Chemical class	**Hormone**
Amino acid derivative	Adrenaline (epinephrine) Thyroid hormones (T_3, T_4)
Steroid	Oestrogens (e.g. oestradiol) Androgens (e.g. testosterone) Progesterone Cortisol Aldosterone
Peptides	Thyrotropin-releasing hormone (TRH) Gonadotropin-releasing hormone (GnRH) Vasopressin Oxytocin (OT) Vasoactive intestinal peptide (VIP) Glucagon Adrenocorticotropic hormone (ACTH) Somatostatin
Proteins	Insulin Insulin-like growth factors (IGFs) Growth hormone (GH) Prolactin (PRL) Placental lactogen (PL) Parathyroid hormone (PTH)
Glycoproteins	Thyroid-stimulating hormone (TSH) Follicle-stimulating hormone (FSH) Luteinising hormone (LH) Chorionic gonadotropin (CG)

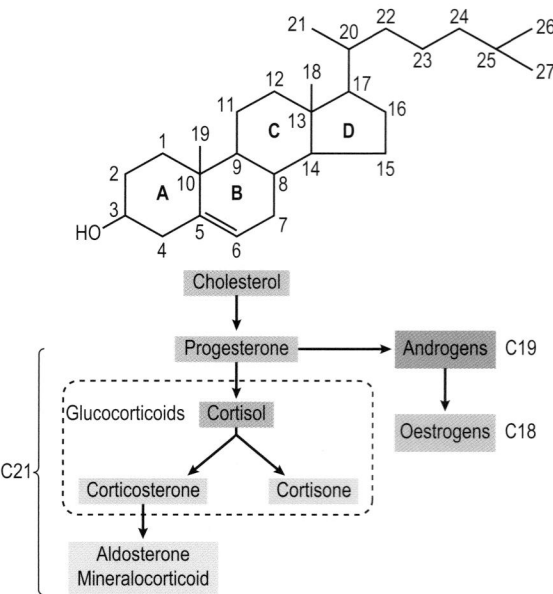

Fig. 10.1 Outline of steroid synthesis from cholesterol. Note the nomenclature of the steroid nucleus rings and carbon atoms.

Protein hormones

Proteins hormones include:

- **Peptides**: which consist of a single subunit, are relatively small and may have a modest number of amino acid residues (e.g. thyrotropin-releasing hormone has only three amino acid residues).
- **Peptide multimers**: which are larger and consist of peptide subunits linked by disulfide bonds (e.g. insulin).
- **Glycoproteins**: which are large glycosylated proteins (e.g. gonadotropins).

After their synthesis on polyribosomes, protein hormones are handled in the same way as any other secreted protein (Ch. 2). Cleavage of the signal peptide from the N-terminal end of the inactive **preprohormone** generates either a hormone or a **prohormone**, which may be biologically inactive. Prohormones are subject to further proteolytic cleavage to generate the mature hormone and this usually occurs in the Golgi apparatus or the secretory vesicles. Some prohormones contain the sequences for several hormones. Protein hormones are secreted by exocytosis in a calcium-dependent fashion, are water soluble, do not generally bind plasma proteins and have short half-lives (minutes). Many peptide and protein hormones are small enough to cross the renal filtration barrier to appear in the urine.

Three superfamilies of cell surface receptor (G-protein-coupled receptors, tyrosine receptor kinases and guanylyl cyclase receptors; Ch. 4) are responsible for mediating the effects of protein hormones. This not only reflects the great variety of this group of hormones but also shows the diversity of intracellular signalling mechanisms that can be activated by them.

Patterns of hormone secretion

Hormone secretion varies with time (Fig. 10.2). The secretion can be periodic, ranging from 2 hourly to 24 hourly. Secretion that varies regularly over 24 hours is termed **circadian**. This periodicity is usually driven by the brain. A circadian clock in the suprachiasmatic nucleus of the hypothalamus, for example, generates an intrinsic rhythm that is entrained by environmental cues, such as light, to have a period of 24 hours. Circadian release is quite marked for growth hormone and cortisol. If the period for hormone release is shorter than 1 day the secretion is described as **ultradian** or **pulsatile**. Protein hormones of the anterior pituitary gland are released in a pulsatile fashion, with periods of between 90 and 120 minutes. Pulsatile release can be crucial for hormone function, e.g. female rhesus monkeys fail to ovulate when the pulsatile release of gonadotropins is replaced by continuous delivery. Many hormones are secreted in response to specific physiological stimuli. This **episodic release** is seen, for example, with insulin, which is stimulated by the rise in plasma glucose concentration that occurs after eating (see also Ch. 3).

The secretion of a given hormone may be driven by several superimposed rhythms with different frequencies. For example, growth hormone secretion from the anterior pituitary is both circadian and ultradian. In addition, stimulus-evoked secretion is often superimposed on periodic releasing. Growth hormone release is triggered both by a fall in blood glucose concentration and by exercise.

Measurements of hormone concentration must take account of the variations in hormone release. Multiple frequent samples are needed to reliably measure ultradian and circadian hormones, not only to assess whether their concentrations are within the normal range, but because these rhythms are often disturbed in disease. Fasting, resting values are generally used because they exclude most of the variation due to physiological stimuli.

Feedback regulation of hormone secretion

Endocrine systems are controlled by feedback mechanisms, the most fundamental being negative feedback, in which a system maintains its status quo in the face of influences that tend to perturb it (Ch. 1). This basic control is then modified by additional signals, generally produced by the nervous system, in response to physiological state (e.g. sleeping and waking, feeding and fasting, exercise, pregnancy), psychological stresses (e.g. anxiety, depression) and pathological stresses (e.g. trauma, myocardial infarction).

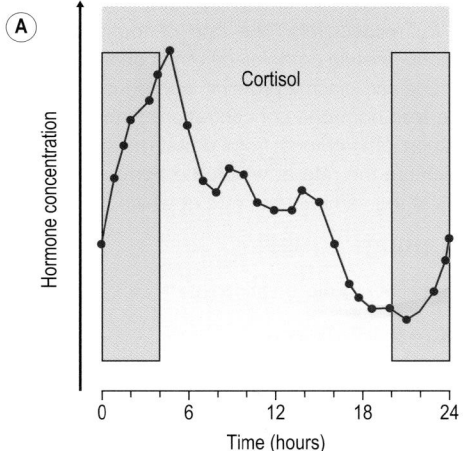
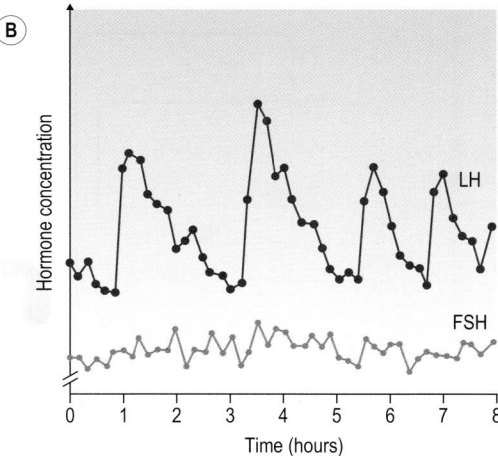

Fig. 10.2 Temporal patterns in plasma hormone concentrations. (A) Circadian variations in cortisol concentrations. Redrawn from DeGroot LJ et al 1979 Endocrinology, vol 3, Grune & Stratton, New York. (B) Ultradian variation in luteinising hormone (LH) and follicle-stimulating hormone (FSH). Redrawn from Naftolin F et al 1973 Journal of Clinical Endocrinology and Metabolism 36:285.

Closed loop negative feedback

Secretion of most hormones is under **closed loop negative feedback** control. The controlled variable can be the basal plasma concentration of a hormone, when negative feedback is accomplished by the hormone acting to inhibit its own release. An endocrine system can also regulate the blood concentration of a variable such as glucose.

It is easy to imagine how the speed of a car is better regulated by provision of both accelerator and brake than with accelerator alone. Similarly, many physiological variables are regulated by two feedback loops with antagonistic actions. For example, a rise in blood glucose concentration triggers the release of insulin by the endocrine pancreas, stimulating the transport of glucose into a variety of cell types, reducing blood glucose concentration to basal levels. Another feedback loop (actually one of several) operates in the opposite direction. A fall in blood sugar triggers glucagon secretion, which stimulates glycogenolysis (Ch. 3), causing the release of glucose into the circulation, which restores basal glucose concentration.

Negative feedback maintains a steady state but this is often not appropriate. For example, in response to stress, the nervous system stimulates the release of a number of hormones (adrenaline, glucagon, cortisol, growth hormone) to act in concert to raise blood glucose concentrations (see Fig. 10.3). Stress, however, also activates sympathetic nerves to the endocrine pancreas, which inhibit the secretion of insulin (and enhance glucagon secretion). This overrides the normal feedback control by the pancreas, allowing a sustained rise in blood glucose.

Open loop negative feedback

Open loop negative feedback allows hormone levels to rise in response to a physiological stimulus, but is self-limiting. For example, infant suckling stimulates the secretion of **oxytocin**, a peptide hormone secreted by the posterior pituitary gland, which stimulates smooth muscle contraction in the breast, and thereby triggers milk ejection. This is self-limiting, because eventually the infant becomes sated, stops suckling, and oxytocin secretion is curtailed.

Positive feedback

Positive feedback (Ch. 1) is relatively unusual in normal endocrinology because it causes a system to flip dramatically between two stable states that may be very different. One example is childbirth. In the Ferguson reflex that operates during labour, stretching of the cervix triggers the reflex secretion of oxytocin during the first stage. This causes the smooth muscle of the uterus to contract, so further stretching and dilating the cervix in a self-reinforcing manner. This positive feedback eventually causes the woman to make the transition from pregnant to non-pregnant state. Birth terminates the feedback.

Role of plasma proteins in hormone transport

The catecholamine and peptide hormones are water soluble and circulate either freely or weakly bound to albumin. Hydrophobic hormones, such as thyroid hormones and steroids, which are barely soluble, are carried in the blood stream, bound to a variety of plasma proteins (carrier proteins). The kinetics of hormone binding to plasma proteins follows the law of mass action, which says that the rate of a chemical reaction is directly proportional to the concentration of each of the reactants. By studying these kinetics it is possible to calculate the effect plasma proteins have on the concentration of free hormone in the blood and hence deduce what functions plasma proteins might have.

Kinetics of hormone binding to plasma proteins

Hormone binding to plasma protein is generally of low affinity but high capacity (Ch. 2). Hence most of the hormone released into the blood becomes bound, keeping the free hormone concentration low. Only the free hormone is available to bind to the high affinity receptor sites on target cells, but as it does so, the hormone dissociates from the binding proteins to maintain the free hormone concentration. It is possible to quantify the free hormone concentration because hormone (H) binding to plasma proteins (P) obeys the law of mass action:

$$H + P \underset{k_d}{\overset{k_a}{\rightleftharpoons}} HP$$

The association and dissociation rate constants are k_a and k_d, respectively. The rate of formation of the bound hormone–protein complex depends on the concentrations of hormone and plasma proteins, and is just k_a [H][P], where [H] is the **free** hormone concentration. Similarly the rate of dissociation of hormone from protein is given by k_d [HP]. At equilibrium the rate at which the hormone–protein complex forms is the same as the rate at which it dissociates:

$$k_a [H][P] = k_b [HP]$$

The equilibrium dissociation rate $K_D = k_d / k_a$ so:

$$K_D = [H][P]/[HP]$$

from which,

$$[H] = K_D [HP]/[P]$$

It is worth noting that the above derivation is based on exactly the same principles that apply to substrate binding to enzymes (Ch. 2) and the binding of drugs to receptors (Ch. 4).

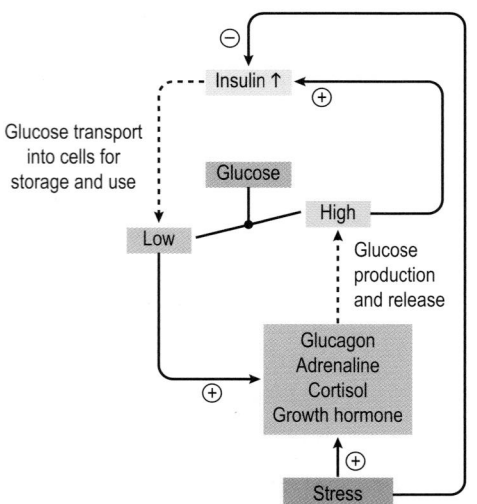

Fig. 10.3 **Modulation of glucose homeostasis in stress.**

At the capillary/target cell interface, more detailed modelling of hormone binding to plasma proteins shows that free hormone concentration is not constant across a capillary but is, not surprisingly, lower in the layer of blood close to the vessel walls as a result of uptake by tissues. This favours dissociation of hormone from the binding proteins in this layer, making more hormone available. In addition, a higher concentration of bound hormone results in a greater flux of hormone liberated from bound to free form. In other words, protein binding **favours** hormone delivery to tissues.

Endocrine status correlates better with free than with bound hormone concentration, because it is only free hormone that is available to receptors both for target organ effects and feedback control. It is therefore more useful to measure free hormone than total hormone concentration. This can be difficult, but in some cases (e.g. steroids) free hormone in the blood equilibrates with saliva, in which it can be assayed.

Measuring hormone concentrations

A mainstay in the evaluation of endocrine status is the measurement of hormone concentrations. This can reveal if the quantity and rhythm of hormone secretion are within the normal range or disturbed by disease. Hormone measurements can be taken from 24-hour urine samples or saliva, but more usually from plasma. Because plasma hormone

levels are generally low, immunological techniques, which are very sensitive and highly specific, are almost invariably used for measuring hormone concentrations.

Concentrations of hormones with a long half-life (e.g. T_3 and T_4) vary little over time, so that basal measurements are useful. Concentrations of hormones such as oestrogens and progesterone vary according to the timing of the menstrual cycle, so measuring these at appropriate times can provide information about reproductive health and fertility. The time of day for taking samples is important when assessing hormones secreted in a circadian fashion. For hormones released on an ultradian basis, a time series of samples needs to be taken. It is usual to take fasting, resting values for hormones that are secreted in response to physiological stimuli such as eating or exercise.

 Information box 10.3 **Immunological techniques for measuring hormone concentrations**

Immunological methods for measuring hormone concentrations rely on specific anti-hormone antibodies (usually monoclonal) raised in animals. In the case of non-peptide hormones they are first covalently bound to a protein carrier molecule; the resulting conjugate is immunogenic.

The most common methods are immunometric assays and immunoassays. Immunometric assays are more sensitive and more readily automated than immunoassays, and therefore more widely used.

Immunometric (sandwich) assays

- This method uses two antibodies that bind to different epitopes on the hormone.
  - One antibody is adsorbed onto the surface of a multi-well plate. This serves to anchor the unknown amount of hormone present in the samples added to the wells. The antibody must be present in large excess to ensure all the hormone is captured.
  - The second **reporter antibody** is now added and the amount of this antibody that binds is in direct proportion to the amount of anchored hormone. The reporter antibody is so called because it bears an easily measured marker such as a fluorescent tag or an enzyme.
- When the marker is an enzyme the assay is called an **enzyme-linked immunosorbent assay** (**ELISA**) (see also Ch. 6).

Immunoassay (IA)

The principle of **immunoassay** is that an unknown amount of hormone and a known amount of labelled hormone compete for a limited number of binding sites on anti-hormone antibodies.

- Known amounts of labelled hormone and antibody are added to samples containing an unknown hormone concentration. The label may be a radioactive tracer (**radioimmunoassay**, **RIA**), a fluorescent molecule or some other marker.
- The lower the unknown concentration of hormone in the samples, the greater the amount of labelled hormone that binds the antibody.
- A variety of methods are then used to separate antibody-bound and free hormone and the ratio of bound to free labelled hormone (B/F) is measured.
- The B/F ratio is a measure of the competition between labelled and non-labelled hormone and the unknown hormone concentration is found by comparison with a standard curve prepared from a range of known concentrations of unlabelled hormone.

 Information box 10.2 **Function of hormone binding by plasma proteins**

Several functions for plasma protein binding of hormones have been proposed:

- To enable poorly water-soluble hormones to be transported in sufficient concentration in the bloodstream.
- To act as a store that attenuates rapid changes in hormone concentration due to altered secretion or peripheral demand (the amount of bound hormone can correspond to several days' worth of secretion). Moreover, the plasma proteins can be far from saturated, so increases in secretion will be 'mopped up' rather than contributing to a rise in free hormone. Therefore, changes in hormone secretion cannot effect **short-term** homeostatic regulation. What purpose does this buffering of rapid fluctuations in concentration serve? It has been suggested that it avoids changes in target cell sensitivity due to receptor down- or up-regulation (see below), or that it ensures an even distribution of hormone to tissues.
- To increase hormone half-life: this can be affected in at least two ways. First, small molecules of free hormone may be rapidly eliminated in the liver or kidneys. Plasma proteins are too big to cross the renal filtration barrier, so bound hormone is not lost in the urine. Second, bound hormone may be less readily metabolised. The rate of hormone elimination, and therefore the half life, can vary from minutes (e.g. insulin) to hours (e.g. steroids) to days (e.g. thyroid hormone).
- To increase hormone delivery: binding proteins may increase delivery of hormone to target tissues (see kinetic argument above).

Remarkably, genetic abnormalities resulting in the loss of specific binding proteins need not cause pathological defects. For example, in thyroxine-binding globulin deficiency, although total T_3 and T_4 are low, free hormone concentrations and TSH are the same as in normal subjects.

Stimulation and suppression tests

Sometimes measuring basal concentrations of hormones cannot provide sufficient information about the operation of an endocrine system. To examine whether endocrine systems have properly functioning feedback systems, or can respond appropriately to stimuli, hormone concentrations are measured after stimulation or suppression tests. Stimulation tests are used to confirm deficient hormone secretion. For example, the ability of the pituitary gland to secrete growth hormone can be tested by intravenous injection of arginine or growth-hormone-releasing hormone (GHRH). Suppression tests are used to confirm hormone excess. Thus, the injection of low doses of the synthetic steroid dexamethasone into a normal individual acts by negative feedback to suppress cortisol secretion. In patients with Cushing's disease, who over-produce cortisol, this suppression is not seen.

Action of hormones

At the target cells, hormones act on a variety of receptors through a range of signal transduction mechanisms (see Ch. 4).

Receptors

Hormone receptors are either located in the cell surface, or within the cell, usually the nucleus, of target cells. The specificity of hormone action arises from the fact that generally a hormone only acts on a subset of cells in the body. For example, most of the physiological effects of insulin can be accounted for by its actions on the liver, skeletal muscle and fat (Ch. 3), since these are the cell types that express insulin receptors on their surface.

Biochemistry of hormone action

Hormone receptors act through several transduction mechanisms (Table 10.2). The steroid receptor superfamily of receptors are **transcription factors**. They are nuclear receptors which bind to specific sequences of DNA and when activated by hormone modify (usually increasing) the transcription of specific genes. Hence steroid and thyroid hormones act at the level of the genome. This can produce profound changes over long periods of time (e.g. cell differentiation and proliferation that accompanies puberty) and these actions can be viewed as an extension of the developmental programme that begins with the first mitotic division of the zygote.

Cell surface receptors act through **second messenger systems**. In essence, these operate by switching on or off the functions of specific target proteins by altering their phosphorylation state (see Ch. 4). The target proteins include enzymes, ion channels, transporters, and receptors and can provide a basis for interactions between hormones. However, second messenger systems can also act at the level of the genome. For example, one of the targets of cAMP is a transcription factor called **cAMP response element binding protein (CREB)**. cAMP stimulates the phosphorylation of CREB via protein kinase A, and phosphorylated CREB binds to the promoter region of genes bearing **cAMP response elements (CREs)**, activating transcription. Given that there

Table 10.2	Receptor and transduction mechanisms for some key hormones	
Transduction mechanism	**Receptor**	**Hormone**
Activates adenylate cyclase (increases cAMP)	β-Adrenergic V2	Adrenaline Vasopressin ACTH Glucagon PTH Calcitonin TSH FSH LH CG
Inhibits adenylate cyclase (decreases cAMP)	α_2-Adrenergic	Adrenaline Somatostatin
Stimulates PLC (Ca^{2+} mobilisation)	α_1-Adrenergic OT V1 AT1	Adrenaline Oxytocin Vasopressin GnRH Angiotensin
Modulates gene transcription: steroid (nuclear) receptor superfamily	ER AR PR GR MR T3R D3R RAR/RXR	Oestrogens Androgens Progesterone Cortisol Aldosterone T_3 Calcitriol Retinoic acid
Activates tyrosine kinases	RTK (intrinsic tyrosine kinase activity) Class I cytokine (couples to soluble tyrosine kinases)	Insulin IGFs GH PRL
Activates serine/threonine kinases	ActRIIA/betaglycan TGF-β receptors	Inhibin Müllerian inhibiting factor

PLC, Phospholipase C; ER, oestrogen receptor; AR, androgen receptor; PR, progesterone receptor; GR, glucocorticoid receptor; MR, aldosterone receptor; T3R, thyroid hormone receptor; D3R, calcitriol receptor; RAR/RXR, retinoic acid receptors (vitamin A); IGF, insulin-like growth factor; TGF, transforming growth factor; for other abbreviations see Table 10.1. No receptor is shown for protein hormones having a single receptor subtype that takes the name of its hormone.

are so many intracellular mechanisms that can be influenced by a given hormone it is not surprising that their physiological effects can be so various and include:

- Stimulating cell division, differentiation and growth
- Regulation of pathways involved in intermediary metabolism
- Modification of all modes of secretion, including exocrine secretion
- Control of smooth muscle contraction and influence on the contractile properties of skeletal and cardiac muscle
- Regulation of ion transport.

Hormone action can be terminated by converting the hormone to an inactive metabolite, or by processes operating at receptors or further downstream, which are usually triggered by prolonged agonist exposure, for example:

- G-protein-coupled receptors undergo desensitisation.
- Both tyrosine kinase receptors and G-protein-coupled receptors can be internalised. The receptor may be recycled back to the membrane or effectively down-regulated by lysosomal degradation.
- Second messenger systems have in-built termination mechanisms such as the intrinsic GTPase of G proteins, phosphodiesterases to degrade cyclic nucleotides, transport mechanisms to remove Ca^{2+} from the cytoplasm, and phosphatases to flip target proteins back into inactive conformations.
- In the case of intracellular receptors, the stimulated transcription and protein synthesis ceases when the hormone dissociates, but any pre-existing mRNA protein molecules continue to be active until they are enzymically degraded. Hence reversal of the effect of steroid and thyroid hormone action is slow, and is clinically relevant.

Up- and down-regulation of receptors

Increasing the number of a particular receptor is known as **up-regulation**, and decreasing the number, **down-regulation**. These processes occur in response to exposure to their own hormone or to others, which may be normal physiological responses regulating the sensitivity of target cells to hormones. For example, **prolactin** induces the expression of its own receptors, while **oestradiol** induces the expression of progesterone receptors (see below).

Changes in receptor number can occur in disease. For example, insulin resistance is a prominent feature in the metabolic syndrome, obesity and type II diabetes, all characterised by high plasma insulin *and* glucose concentrations. In insulin resistance, insulin receptors are down-regulated so that there is a reduced ability to transport glucose into cells (see Ch. 3). Receptor up-regulation can account for **synergism** in which two hormones acting together produce a much greater physiological response than either hormone acting individually.

Permissive action of hormones

Some hormones have a **permissive action** in that they must be present for other hormones to exert their effects. Permissive actions are seen particularly between steroid and thyroid hormones themselves, or between either of these and other hormones. In the first case it is due to the need for both hormones to activate some members of the steroid receptor superfamily of receptors, and in the second it is because the steroid or thyroid hormones increase the transcription of genes coding for proteins that are part of the signalling cascade for the other hormones, e.g. receptors, protein kinases or their substrates.

Hormone metabolism and excretion

After exerting their actions, hormones are inactivated by further metabolic processes: conjugation, proteolysis and hydrolysis. The metabolites are excreted in the urine, so that measurement of urinary hormone metabolites can be used for diagnosis (e.g. urinary vanillylmandelic acid (VMA) in phaeochromocytoma, urinary human chorionic gonadotropin (hCG) in pregnancy).

Adrenal catecholamines

Circulating adrenaline and noradrenaline are metabolised mainly in the liver by methylation and oxidative deamination, catalysed by **catechol-*O*-methyltransferase** and **monoamine oxidase**, respectively.

Thyroid hormones

Peripheral tissues deiodinate thyroid hormones to produce inactive metabolites. These hormones can also be conjugated in the liver to form glucuronides and sulphates, which enter the bile and then the intestine for elimination.

Steroid hormones

Adrenal and gonadal steroids are conjugated in the liver, and the resulting steroid glucuronides and sulphates are inactive and much more water soluble than the parent steroids, so they are excreted in the urine. Binding of steroids to plasma proteins can increase their half-life; aldosterone, which does not have a specific transport protein, has a shorter half-life than the steroids, which do.

Protein hormones

Two processes are responsible for inactivating protein hormones:

- Receptor-mediated endocytosis in which the bound protein is internalised and degraded
- Proteolysis by enzymes.

NEUROENDOCRINOLOGY

Many endocrine systems are regulated by the hypothalamus and pituitary gland. The study of these systems, summarised in Figure 10.4, is called **neuroendocrinology**. Among other effects, destruction of the pituitary results in the atrophy of three endocrine glands: gonads, adrenal and thyroid. The functional links between hypothalamus and pituitary, and the glands they support, are known as **hypothalamic–pituitary axes**.

HYPOTHALAMUS

The hypothalamus is discussed in detail in Chapter 8. It lies at the base of the brain, and is part of the forebrain. As well as being a critical component of neuroendocrine systems, it regulates many functions, such as sleep/wakefulness, core temperature homeostasis, feeding and drinking.

PITUITARY GLAND

The pituitary gland lies in a cavity of the sphenoid bone, the **pituitary fossa**, also known as the **sella turcica**, so named

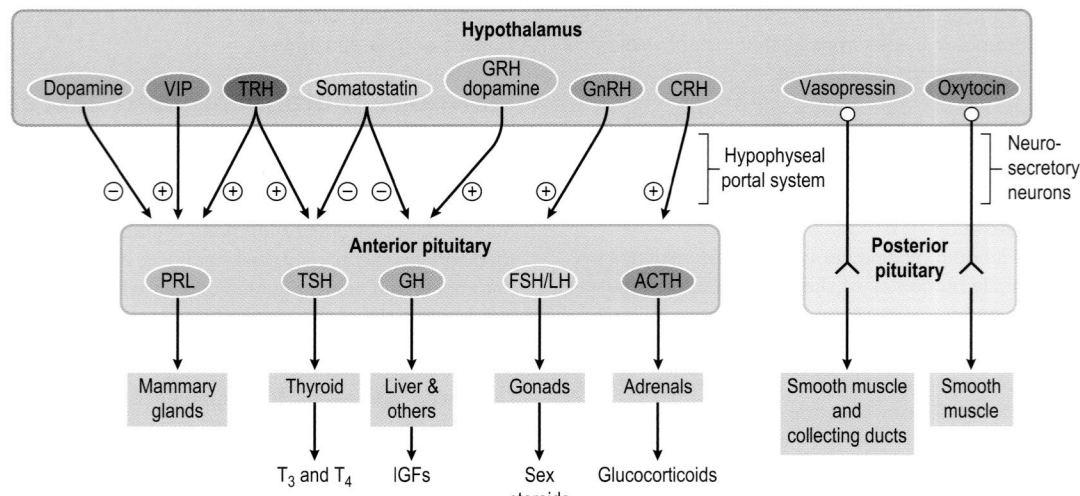

Fig. 10.4 **Endocrine relations of the hypothalamus and pituitary gland.** Hypophysiotropic hormones: VIP, vasoactive intestinal peptide; TRH, thyrotropin-releasing hormone; GRH, growth hormone-releasing hormone; GnRH, gonadotropin-releasing hormone; CRH, corticotropin-releasing hormone. Anterior pituitary hormones: PRL, prolactin; TSH, thyroid-stimulating hormone; GH, growth hormone; FSH, follicle-stimulating hormone; LH, luteinising hormone; ACTH, adrenocorticotropic hormone.

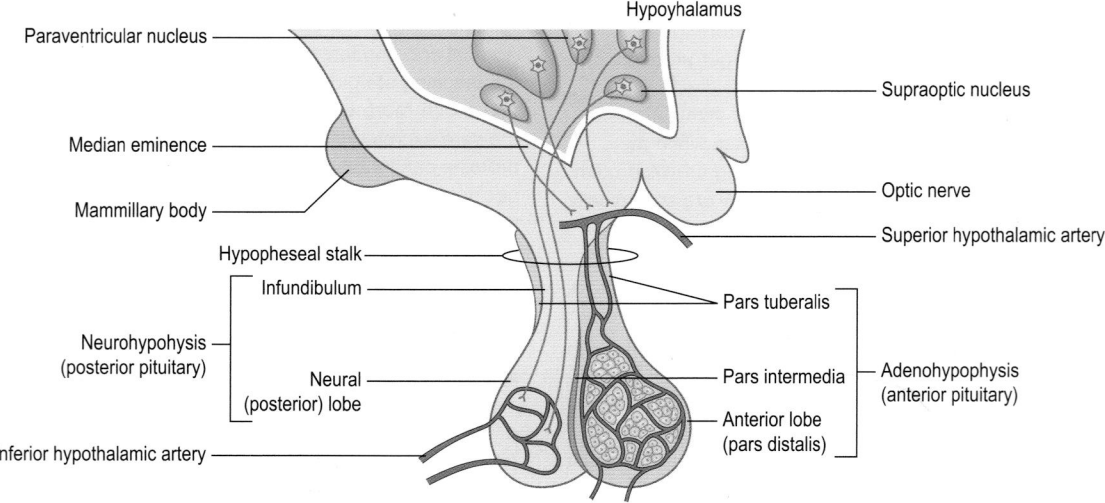

Fig. 10.5 **Anatomy of the human pituitary gland and its vasculature.**

because it resembles a Turkish saddle. It is connected to the hypothalamus by the **pituitary stalk** (**infundibulum**). The pituitary gland is encapsulated by dura mater. The **sellar diaphragm** is placed superiorly, and is the part of the dura that is pierced by the pituitary stalk. Communication between the hypothalamus and pituitary via the pituitary stalk is both neural and humoral.

Functional anatomy of the pituitary gland

The adult human pituitary has two principal parts: posterior and anterior.

Posterior pituitary

The **posterior pituitary** (**neurohypophysis**) (Fig. 10.5) consists of the core of the pituitary stalk, the **infundibular stalk**, which is an extension of the **median eminence**, and the **posterior** (**neural**) **lobe**. Large (**magnocellular**) neuroendocrine cells located in the bilaterally paired **supraoptic** and **paraventricular** nuclei of the hypothalamus send their axons through the median eminence and infundibulum to terminate in the posterior lobe. The terminals have large secretory vesicles which release the peptide hormones oxytocin and vasopressin (also called anti-diuretic hormone (ADH)) into fenestrated capillaries. The axons of these neuroendocrine cells do not contain ribosomes; the peptide hormones are synthesised in their cell bodies and move by axonal transport into the terminals. Hence, the posterior pituitary is the site of hormone secretion but *not* of synthesis.

Anterior pituitary

The **anterior pituitary** (**adenohypophysis**) is largely the **anterior lobe** (**pars distalis**), plus a thin collar of cells on the outside of the pituitary stalk termed the **pars tuberalis**. The anterior lobe contains several populations of polygonal-shaped secretory cells. The blood supply of the anterior pituitary, the **hypothalamic–pituitary portal system**, is remarkable. The superior hypophyseal arteries form a primary capillary bed in the median eminence. This drains into long portal vessels which run through the pituitary stalk, giving rise to a secondary capillary bed in the anterior lobe. Small (**parvocellular**) neuroendocrine cells in several hypothalamic nuclei send axons to the median eminence where they secrete **hypophysiotropic hormones**. These are conveyed by the hypothalamic–pituitary portal system into the anterior lobe to regulate its secretion. Cells in the anterior pituitary are specialised to synthesise and secrete particular hormones, and can be distinguished by differences in histological staining.

Hypophysiotropic and anterior pituitary hormones

Hypophysiotropic hormones produced by the hypothalamus control five separate endocrine axes by either stimulating or inhibiting the synthesis and secretion of hormones by the anterior pituitary. All bar one are peptides. The exception is dopamine, which is a catecholamine (see Ch. 4). Anterior pituitary hormones in turn regulate the synthesis and release of hormones from a variety of other, more peripheral target organs (see Fig. 10.4). The five hypothalamic–pituitary axes are:

- Hypothalamic–pituitary–gonadal axis: **gonadotropin-releasing hormone** (**GnRH**) from the anterior pituitary regulates the synthesis and release of **follicle-stimulating hormone** (**FSH**) and **luteinising hormone** (**LH**). Together, FSH and LH are termed **gonadotropins**. FSH and LH act on the gonads to regulate the secretion of **testosterone** in males, and **oestrogens** and **progesterone in** females.
- Growth hormone axis: **GHRH** stimulates the synthesis and release of **growth hormone** by the anterior pituitary. Growth hormone has a tropic effect on the liver, which produces **insulin-like growth factor** (**IGF**), but it also has a direct action on tissues, such as bone and muscle, to stimulate growth. **Somatostatin** inhibits the synthesis of growth hormone.
- Prolactin axis: **prolactin**, secreted by the anterior pituitary gland, has a direct endocrine action on breast tissue, stimulating lactation (milk production). This hormone is mainly under inhibitory control by dopamine from the hypothalamus.
- Hypothalamic–pituitary–thyroid axis: **thyrotropin-releasing hormone** (**TRH**) stimulates the synthesis and release of **thyroid-stimulating hormone** (**TSH**) by the anterior pituitary gland. TSH stimulates its target organ, the thyroid gland, to produce the thyroid hormones **thyroxine** (T_4) and **triiodothyronine** (T_3). **Somatostatin**, secreted by the pancreas, inhibits TSH secretion.
- Hypothalamic–pituitary–adrenal axis: **corticotropin-releasing hormone** (**CRH**) and **vasopressin** stimulate the biosynthesis and release of **adrenocorticotropic hormone** (**ACTH**), which targets the adrenal cortex to secrete the glucocorticoid **cortisol**.

Posterior pituitary hormones

The hormones of the posterior pituitary gland are oxytocin and vasopressin. The paraventricular and supra-optic nuclei of the hypothalamus synthesise and package these hormones, which are then carried by the axons of the neurosecretory neurons to the posterior pituitary (Fig. 10.4). The hormones are secreted into the circulation by the posterior pituitary. Oxytocin and vasopressin are both peptides.

- Oxytocin acts on the smooth muscle of the uterus to maintain labour (parturition), and the lactating breast to eject milk.
- Vasopressin acts on vascular smooth muscle (Ch. 11), and on renal collecting tubules where it functions to promote water reabsorption and so is critical for water homeostasis (Ch. 14).

Disorders of hypothalamic–pituitary axes

Defects in endocrine systems controlled by the hypothalamus and pituitary are classified by the locus of the fault:

- **Primary** endocrine disorders are when the problem occurs in the target organ, such as gonads, adrenal or thyroid gland.
- Se**condary** endocrine disorders result from a defect of the pituitary.
- **Tertiary** disorders are due to defects in the hypothalamus.

Disorders of hypothalamic–pituitary axes may be selective or multiple and result in excess or deficiency of hormone production (Table 10.3). Excess pituitary hormone secretion can be due to enhanced hypophysiotropic hormone

Table 10.3	Common endocrine disorders of the pituitary	
Hormone	**Deficiency (–)/ Excess (+)**	**Disorder**
PRL	–	None
	+	Infertility and galactorrhoea in both sexes
TSH	–	Hypothyroidism: child, cretinism; adult, myxoedema
	+	Hyperthyroidism: Graves' disease
GH	–	Child, dwarfism
	+	Child, gigantism; adult, acromegaly
FSH/LH	–	Hypogonadism: infertility in both sexes
	+	None
ACTH	–	Addison's disease
	+	Cushing's disease
Vasopressin	–	Diabetes insipidus
	+	Hypertension
Oxytocin	–	None reported
	+	None reported
All hormones	–	Panhypopituitarism (empty sella syndrome)

secretion (tertiary) or to pituitary tumours. Prolactin-secreting microadenomas are the commonest pituitary tumour. Pituitary hormones can also be secreted by tumours outside the pituitary (e.g. some bronchial carcinomas produce prolactin). This is termed **ectopic secretion**. Selective deficiencies are typically genetic or due to autoimmune disease. For example, one type of dwarfism is caused by a defect in expression of growth hormone receptor.

Multiple loss of anterior pituitary hormones (**panhypopituitarism**) occurs as a result of any agent that destroys the pituitary, including tumours, infections, trauma, infarction, radiation, and the condition reflects the combined loss of secretion by gonads, adrenals and thyroid, and of growth hormone.

FEMALE REPRODUCTIVE ENDOCRINOLOGY

Female reproductive biology is orchestrated by a hormonal dialogue between the ovaries and the brain. The outcome of this is a cyclical output of gonadotropins and gonadal steroids – the menstrual cycle – which ensures that ovulation occurs at a time when the female reproductive tract is in the optimal state to receive and nurture a conceptus. Once pregnancy is established it is the conceptus that becomes the major hormonal influence.

FEMALE REPRODUCTIVE TRACT

The female reproductive tract consists of the paired, intra-abdominal ovaries and oviducts (fallopian tubes), together with the uterus and vagina.

Ovaries

Anatomy

Each ovary is surrounded by a fibrous **tunica albuginea**, and covered by a specialised mesothelium, which is analogous to membranes covering other organs, such as peritoneum. It is anchored medially to the uterus by the **ovarian ligament**, and laterally to the pelvic wall by the **suspensory ligament**, through which run ovarian vessels and nerves (Fig. 10.6). In a woman of child-bearing age the ovary has an outer **cortex** containing ovarian follicles (most primordial, but a few at various stages of development) and an inner **medulla** consisting of connective tissue and blood vessels. The ovarian arteries emerge from the aorta, and a pampiniform plexus of veins drains into the uterine plexus.

Functional microanatomy

At 5 weeks after conception, primordial **sex cells** migrate from the yolk sac (see below) into the undifferentiated gonad. In the female fetus, the **oogonia** (sex cells) undergo repeated mitotic division until mid-gestation to produce some seven million **primary oocytes**. Each becomes surrounded by a single layer of epithelial cells derived from the cortex of the developing ovary to form **primordial follicles**.

Within each follicle, the primary oocyte commences its first meiotic division (Fig 10.7), but this is arrested in prophase I until it is capable of responding to LH and subsequent ovulation (see Chs 2 and 5). All but 400 000 primordial follicles undergo apoptosis by puberty. It has been assumed that women are born with all the primary oocytes they are ever going to have. For reasons that are poorly understood, an increasing proportion of oocytes become defective after 30 years, accounting for the decline in fertility seen in women after 30 years of age. One possible explanation, based on work in mice, is that germline stem cells continue to divide in adults, constantly renewing the population of primary oocytes. It remains to be seen whether this is also the case in women, but if so it means that the reproductive decline in older women may be due to a fall in the quality of germline stem cells with age. Confirming this could have significant consequences for fertility treatment.

Uterus

Functional anatomy

The uterus is a hollow organ consisting of an upper **body**, and a lower **cervix** which projects into the vagina. A pair of

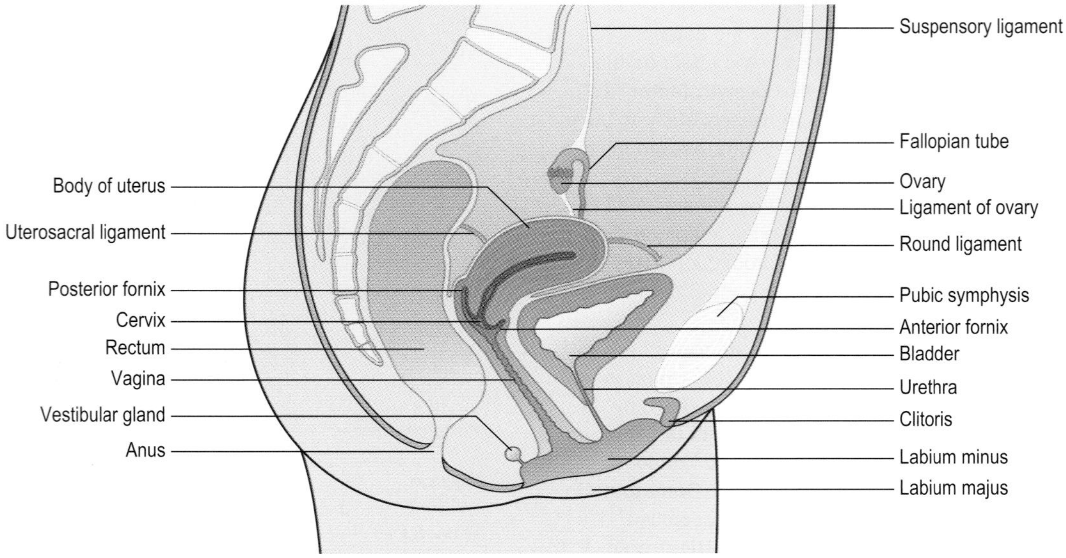
Suspensory ligament
Fallopian tube
Ovary
Ligament of ovary
Round ligament
Pubic symphysis
Anterior fornix
Bladder
Urethra
Clitoris
Labium minus
Labium majus
Body of uterus
Uterosacral ligament
Posterior fornix
Cervix
Rectum
Vagina
Vestibular gland
Anus

Fig. 10.6 **Midsagittal section through the adult female pelvis.**

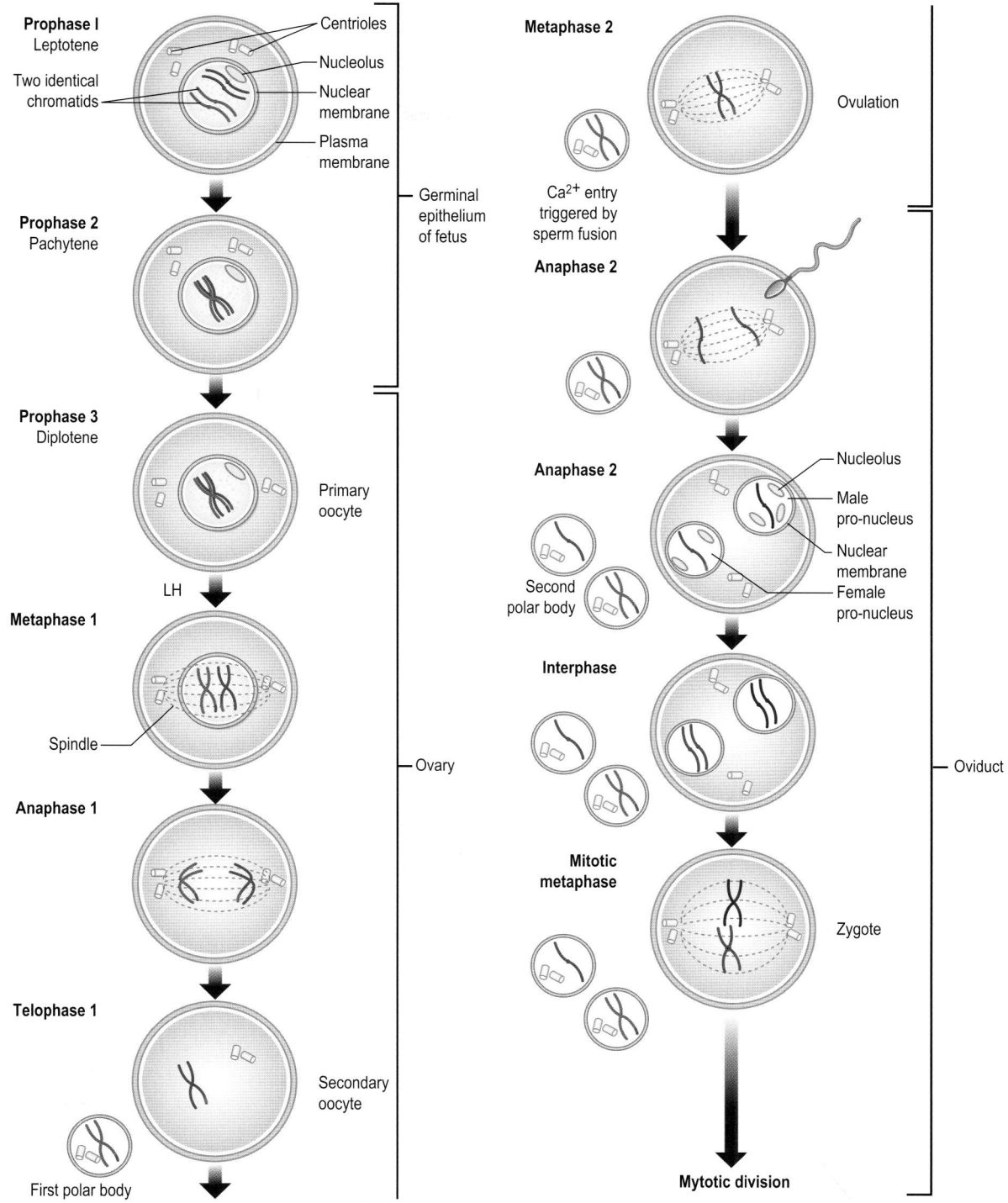

Fig. 10.7 **Cell divisions in the oocyte.**

oviducts (**fallopian/uterine tubes**), largely made of smooth muscle, arise from the superior part of the body of the uterus and terminate with trumpet-shaped fimbriated ends close to (but not attached to) the ovaries. At ovulation, an oocyte (surrounded by a cluster of follicle cells) is released from a ruptured follicle into the peritoneum and is swept by the fimbria into the fallopian tube, down which it is transported by ciliary action and smooth muscle peristaltic contractions. Spermatozoa enter the oviducts from the uterine end. Fertilisation normally occurs in the oviduct.

The bulk of the uterus is made of smooth muscle, the **myometrium**. The cavity of the uterus is lined by the **endometrium**. This is a secretory epithelium consisting of two layers: a deep **basal layer**, which is unresponsive to steroid hormones, overlain by a **functional layer**, which regenerates from the basal layer and is hormone responsive. The functional layer consists of low columnar epithelium over a stroma. The epithelium invaginates to form simple glands (Fig. 10.8). The functional layer is regenerated and lost with each menstrual cycle.

The cervical canal is filled with mucus secreted by the cervical endometrium. Cervical mucus is generally viscous, the glycoproteins in the mucus being arranged in a tight mesh that it is difficult for motile bacteria (or sperm) to penetrate, forming a barrier to ascending infection. At ovulation, the influence of oestrogens increases the water content of the cervical mucus so that the glycoproteins rearrange into widely separated parallel strands that the spermatozoa can swim between.

Gross anatomy

The uterus is supported by the pelvic floor and several pairs of ligaments that run in a side-to-side peritoneal fold, termed the **broad ligament**, which projects from the pelvic floor. The oviduct forms the upper edge of the broad ligament, which effectively divides the female pelvis into anterior and posterior parts containing bladder and rectum, respectively. The uterus is normally anteverted (the long axis of the uterus is at about 90 ° to the long axis of the vagina) and anteflexed (the body curves downward). Retroversion or retroflexion can cause problems during pregnancy and delivery. The non-gravid (non-pregnant) uterus is about 8–10 cm in length, but the fundus, the top of the body of the uterus, is palpable abdominally during pregnancy after about 14 weeks' gestation. Fundal height can be used as an approximate assessment of gestational age.

The **uterine arteries** are branches of the internal iliac arteries. They ascend one each side of the uterus and join up with the ovarian arteries. Branches of the uterine artery in the myometrium are highly tortuous **helicine arteries**. The **spiral arteries** which grow into the functional layer of the endometrium are also tightly coiled. The uterine venous plexus is continuous with plexuses of the ovary and vagina, emptying into uterine veins which drain into the internal iliac veins. The uterus has visceral sensory afferents and an autonomic nerve supply.

Vagina

The **vagina** is a distensible fibromuscular tube lined by stratified squamous epithelium that readily tolerates the friction of coitus. The ducts of a pair of **vestibular glands** open near the vaginal entrance. Secretion from the glands contributes to vaginal lubrication during sexual excitement. Oestrogen-stimulated vaginal mucosa secretes glycogen, which is anaerobically metabolised to lactate by resident bacteria. The low pH reduces the risk of infection (e.g. by *Candida*, the yeast which causes 'thrush') but is hostile to sperm. The vagina of young and prepubertal girls and post-menopausal women is alkaline because oestrogen levels are low.

OVERVIEW OF EVENTS IN THE OVARIAN AND MENSTRUAL CYCLES

A sequence of events in the ovary (the **ovarian cycle**), coupled to a sequence of events in the endometrium (the **menstrual cycle**) ensure that ovulation coincides with the optimal state of the reproductive tract for fertilisation and implantation. The cycles are synchronised and last approximately 28 days; the first day of the menstrual bleed is counted as day 1 of the cycle, with ovulation occurring on about day 14. The duration of the cycles in women is variable.

In the first half of the ovarian cycle, the **follicular phase**, under the influence of gonadotropins from the pituitary gland several ovarian follicles grow, but one comes to dominate and eventually ovulates. During this phase the follicle secretes oestrogens. The follicular phase corresponds to the **proliferative phase** of the menstrual cycle because the functional layer of the endometrium regenerates and proliferates under the influence of oestradiol. Ovulation is followed by the second half of the ovarian cycle, the **luteal phase**, so called because the follicle becomes a **corpus luteum**, which produces progesterone as well as oestrogens. The luteal phase corresponds to the **secretory** phase of the menstrual cycle because the endometrium develops simple glands and becomes secretory at this time.

If pregnancy does not happen, the corpus luteum degenerates and the functional layer of the endometrium that was sustained by its steroid output is shed during menstruation. There is, therefore, a sudden fall in the levels of oestradiol and progesterone and menstrual flow occurs over an average of 3–5 days during which period 6–50 mL blood is lost.

Hypothalamic–pituitary–ovarian axis

The events in the ovarian and menstrual cycles are orchestrated by an endocrine dialogue between brain and ovary (Fig. 10.9). Neuroendocrine cells with their cell bodies in the **arcuate nucleus** of the hypothalamus secrete **GnRH** (also referred to as **luteinising hormone releasing hormone**, **LHRH**) into fenestrated capillaries in the median eminence. From here GnRH is transported by the

---

> **Clinical box 10.2** | **Tubal occlusion**
>
> Ascending bacterial infections from the vagina and uterus to the oviducts can cause scarring, with occlusion of the tubes. Tubal occlusion is associated with increased risk of:
>
> - Infertility
> - Ectopic pregnancy.
>
> Tubal occlusion prevents normal entry and descent of the oocyte down the tube, preventing fertilisation by spermatozoa, which normally takes place in the oviducts. This is a common cause of infertility. Should fertilisation take place, but the fertilised ovum cannot proceed down the occluded tube to the uterus, implantation takes place in the tube, when an ectopic (tubal) pregnancy ensues.

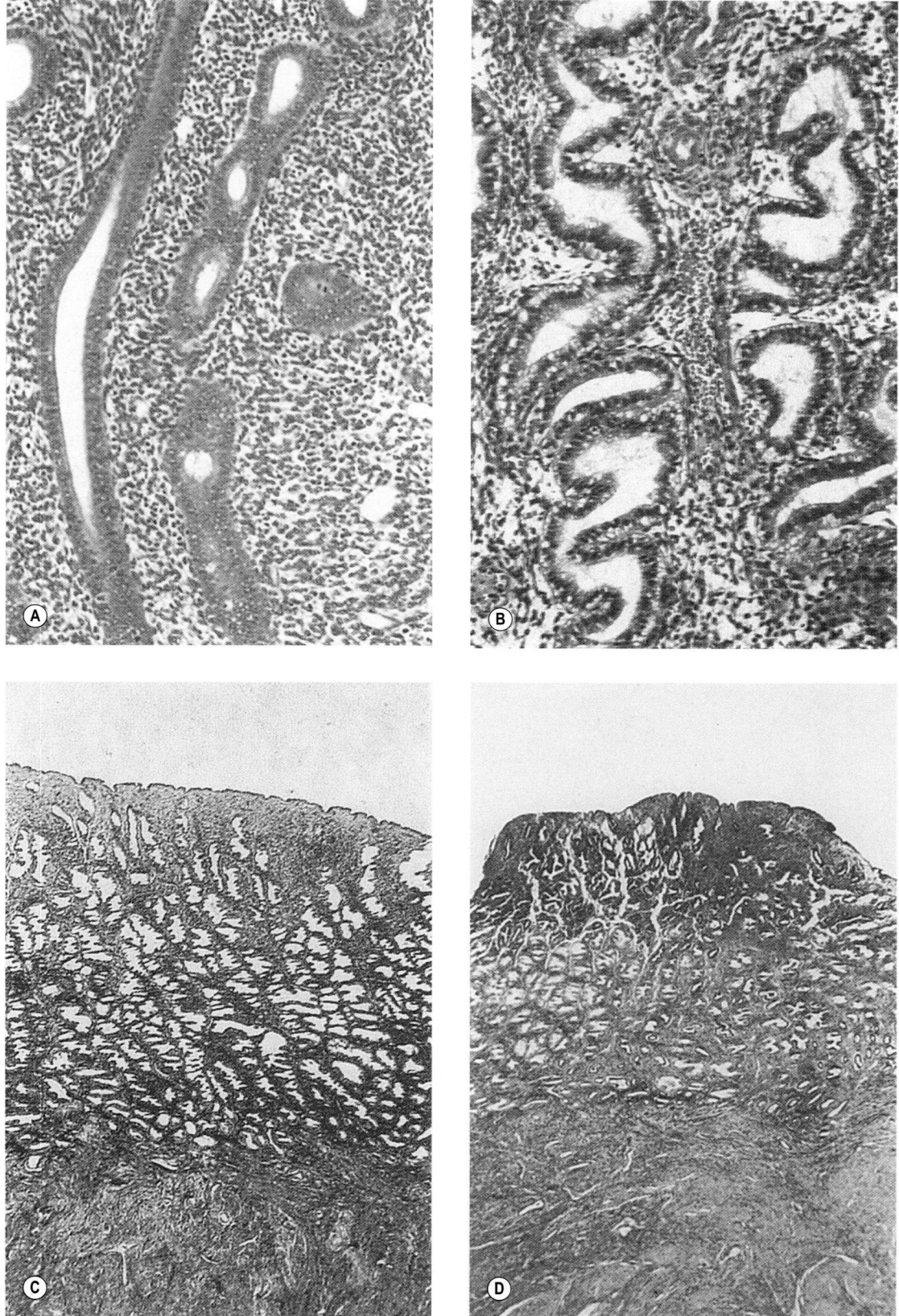

Fig. 10.8 **Endometrial histology during the menstrual cycle** (×8): (A) proliferative phase; (B) early secretory phase; (C) late secretory phase; (D) menstruation. Reproduced with permission from Young B, Lowe JS, Stevens A, Heath JW 2006 Wheater's functional histology, 5th edn. Churchill Livingstone, Edinburgh.

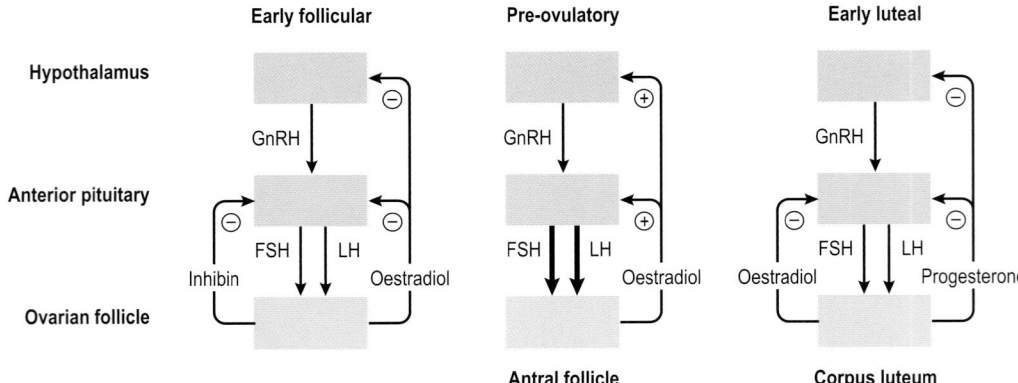

Fig. 10.9 **Feedback mechanisms in the hypothalamic–pituitary–ovarian axis during the menstrual cycle.** GnRH, gonadotropin-releasing hormone; FSH, follicle-stimulating hormone; LH, luteinising hormone.

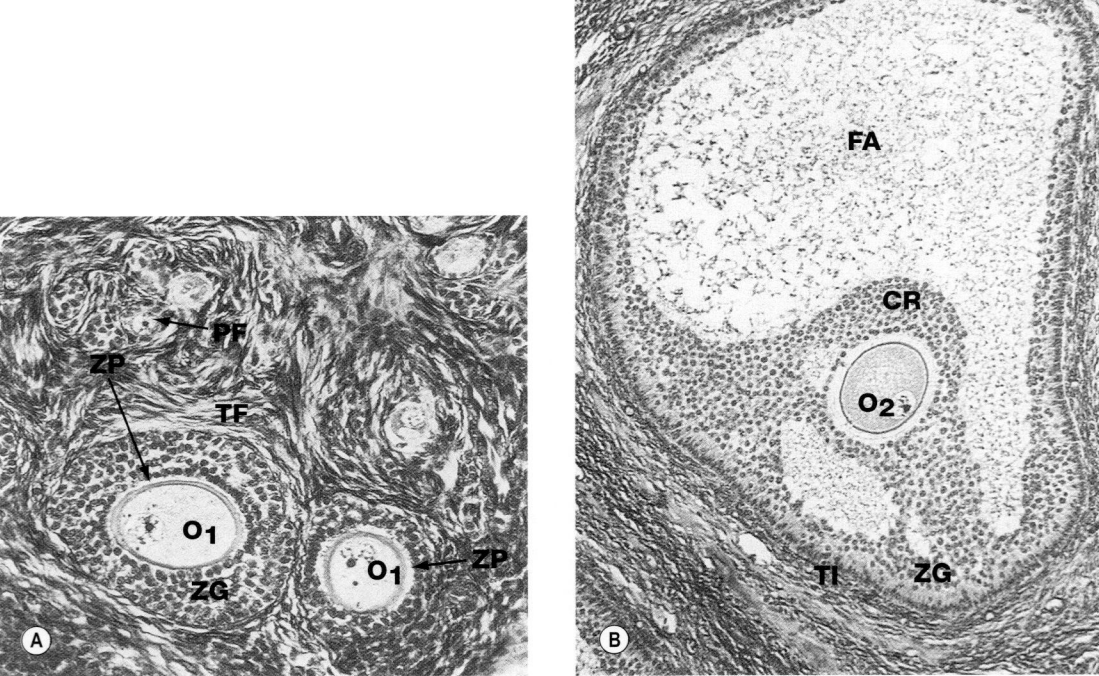

Fig. 10.10 **Follicular development.** (A) Primordial and primary follicles in the ovarian cortex. (B) Antral follicle. TA, tunica albuginea; O_1, primary oocyte; PF, primordial follicle; TF, thecal cells; ZG, granulosa cells; ZP, zona pellucida; CR, corona radiata (cumulus oophorus), FA follicular antrum; O_2, secondary oocyte; TI, theca interna. Reproduced with permission from Young B, Lowe JS, Stevens A, Heath JW 2006 Wheater's functional histology, 5th edn. Churchill Livingstone, Edinburgh.

hypothalamic–pituitary portal system to the anterior pituitary where it stimulates the secretion of two **gonadotropins** from a specific population of cells in the anterior pituitary called **gonadotrops**. The gonadotropins **FSH** and **LH**, both large glycoproteins, are secreted into the systemic circulation. Their target is the ovarian follicle. (Although named for their functions in females, the gonadotropins have homologous roles in males.)

Follicle development

A few primordial follicles (Fig. 10.10) about 30 μm across start growing each day **independently** of hormones, so there is always a continuous trickle of developing **primary follicles** from fetal life to the menopause. Each primary follicle consists of a **primary oocyte**, which secretes a thin layer of mucoproteins, the **zona pellucida**. This is surrounded by a single layer of follicle cells. A primary follicle grows to become a 200 μm diameter **pre-antral follicle** in which the follicle cells differentiate into two cell types; adjacent to the oocyte are **granulosa cells** and outside these are **theca interna cells**. The oocyte increases its RNA and protein synthesis at this time, growing from 20μm to 100 μm. The amino acids, nucleotides and nutrients the oocyte needs for this are supplied via gap junctions with granulosa cells.

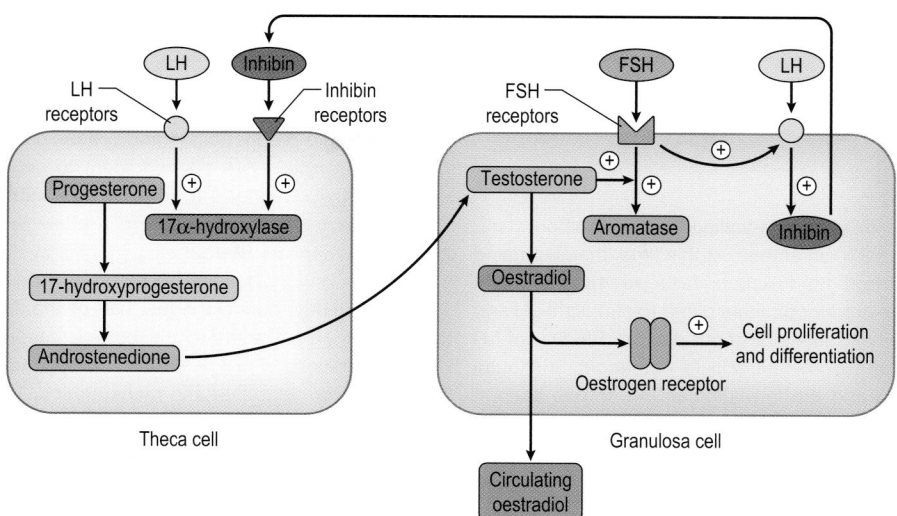

Fig. 10.11 **Ovarian steroid biosynthesis in the late follicular phase.** FSH, follicle-stimulating hormone; LH, luteinising hormone.

Pre-antral follicles acquire gonadotropin receptors and continue to grow in a hormone-dependent manner for about 2 months to become **antral** (**secondary, Graafian**) follicles, provided they are exposed to adequate concentrations of FSH and LH. If follicles are not exposed to gonadotropins at this time, for example in prepubescent girls, they undergo apoptosis. In women of reproductive age, 6–12 antral follicles embark on a rapid hormone-dependent growth phase towards the end of each luteal phase, one of which is destined to ovulate in the next cycle.

In an antral follicle, steroid metabolism is shared between thecal and granulosa cells (Fig. 10.11). LH acts on thecal cells to induce the expression of 17α-hydroxylase, an enzyme which catalyses the synthesis of androgens from progesterone and its metabolites. The androgens diffuse into the granulosa cells where they are converted to oestradiol by aromatase, an enzyme activated by FSH. Granulosa cells are the only FSH-responsive cells in a woman's body.

At the beginning of a cycle FSH concentrations are raised somewhat. (Figure 10.12 shows the pattern of hormone secretion and related events during a single ovarian and menstrual cycle.) The antral follicles vary in their maturity with one, the **dominant follicle**, requiring little additional FSH to progress to ovulation. The dominant follicle effectively has the greatest sensitivity to FSH. It rapidly produces high levels of aromatase and hence synthesises most oestradiol. Rarely there are two dominant follicles and if all goes well the result is **dizygotic** (non-identical) **twins**.

Two molecules exert negative feedback to reduce the blood concentrations of FSH (see Fig. 10.9), suppressing further development of follicles that are still FSH dependent. Oestradiol and **inhibin**, a peptide heterodimer, both produced by granulosa cells, act on the anterior pituitary to dampen the output of FSH. Follicles for which there is not enough FSH to progress undergo apoptosis.

By day 7 the dominant follicle (now termed a **preovulatory** follicle) is about 1 cm in diameter and several events complete its development.

■ Granulosa cells acquire oestrogen receptors. Oestradiol now acts as an autocrine, stimulating its own receptors to bring about granulosa cell proliferation (i.e. further

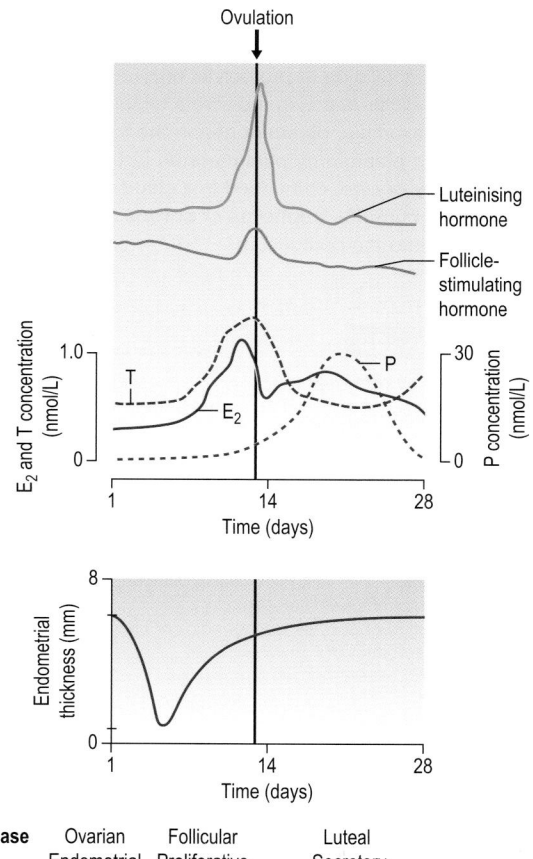

Fig. 10.12 **Hormone concentrations during a single ovarian and menstrual cycle.**

follicle growth) and ever greater oestradiol output. This positive feedback is responsible for the surge of circulating oestradiol in the late follicular phase (about day 11–15).

■ To match the oestradiol production in the granulosa cells, inhibin acts as a paracrine signal on thecal cells to stimulate synthesis of the precursor androgens.

■ FSH induces the expression of LH receptors and these are able to stimulate aromatase activity and inhibin synthesis. Hence the follicle is now responsive to LH but loses its dependence on FSH.

Ovulation

By mid-cycle the follicle is thin-walled, filled with about 6 mL of fluid, and about 2.5 cm across. At this time, the ever-rising oestradiol output from the follicle drives a **positive** feedback response from the anterior pituitary gland to stimulate LH and FSH secretion, which peaks at about day 14. Binding of LH to receptors on the dominant follicle (for about 36 hours) leads to ovulation and the formation of the corpus luteum. The large pulse of LH triggers several events.

■ Resumption of meiosis. The primary oocyte, which has a diploid karyotype, is held arrested in prophase I of meiosis by an **oocyte maturation inhibitor** secreted by granulosa cells. LH causes meiosis to resume and continue as far as metaphase II, when meiosis is again arrested (see Fig. 10.7). This process generates a secondary oocyte, which is haploid and contains most of the cytoplasm, and a **first polar body**.
■ Ovulation. Rupture of the follicle is caused by LH-mediated activation of proteolytic enzymes which digest the intercellular matrix in a discrete region of the follicle wall. For example, **plasminogen** in the follicular fluid is cleaved to **plasmin** by **plasminogen activator**. The secondary oocyte, embedded in a cloud of granulosa cells (the **cumulus oophorus** or **corona radiata**) is expelled into the peritoneum.

Clinical box 10.3

Premature ovarian failure
Premature ovarian failure (POF, premature menopause) is a cause of infertility, defined as ovarian failure in women before the age of 40, and has an estimated overall incidence of 1%. There is a persistently high gonadotropin concentration, indicating that concentrations of ovarian oestrogens are no longer sufficient to exert negative feedback on the pituitary and hypothalamus. The causes are:

● **Idiopathic** (i.e. of unknown cause), although it may be due to an autoimmune disorder
● Destruction of oocytes during radio- or chemotherapy, or oophorectomy
● A genetic basis – ovarian dysgenesis.

Pathology
Normal recruitment of primordial follicles into the pool of primary follicles is irreversible, and triggered by a mechanism intrinsic to the ovary. The overall rate of recruitment may be influenced by circulating factors. Any activated follicles not selected for further growth undergo apoptosis. POF may be due to a faster initiation of primordial follicles, which are therefore depleted earlier than normal.

Animal model
Female mice lacking the specific gene (*foxo3a*) that codes for a transcription factor for folliculogenesis have POF. Early FOXO3A expression suppresses follicular activation and so is a candidate component for the ovarian mechanism controlling recruitment. The *foxo3a* product is expressed in the ovaries of human newborn and adult ovaries, and defects in a related molecule are associated with POF in women. Study of the roles played by these transcription factors could lead to the development of therapeutic agents that delay follicular activation in women at risk of POF.

Corpus luteum

After ovulation the follicle becomes a corpus luteum. The LH stimulates the granulosa cells to express low-density lipoprotein (LDL) receptors. These take up cholesterol, which is converted to pregnenolone and progesterone faster than the 17α-hydroxylase can convert them to androgens and then oestrogens. Hence the release of oestrogens falls and progesterone release rises from virtually zero to peak in the mid-luteal phase. Steroid biosynthesis by the corpus luteum depends on LH, but the LH surge is over by day 16 or so. Consequently, during the last half of the luteal phase, if no pregnancy has resulted, the corpus luteum regresses and concentrations of progesterone and oestradiol fall, leading to endometrial cell death and menstruation. The fall in circulating progesterone and oestradiol releases FSH secretion from intense negative feedback inhibition, allowing the next menstrual cycle to begin (see Fig. 10.12).

Site of steroid feedback

For most of the menstrual cycle oestradiol concentrations are low and exert a negative feedback effect on gonadotropin output. However, the high level of oestradiol in the late follicular phase triggers a positive feedback surge of LH and FSH which peaks at day 14. The LH surge is brief because the positive feedback is turned off by progesterone, the concentration of which rises 6 hours after ovulation.

Steroids exert their feedback effects by acting on both the hypothalamus and anterior pituitary. Just before ovulation the high oestradiol concentration acts in the arcuate nucleus to cause GnRH release to occur in high frequency, low amplitude, pulses. This pattern allows upregulation of GnRH receptors on the anterior pituitary gonadotropes, which become exquisitely sensitive to the releasing hormone. Consequently there is a rapid rise in LH and FSH secretion. The oestradiol induces the expression of progesterone receptors in the arcuate nucleus. Rising progesterone concentrations after ovulation act on these to switch the secretion of GnRH into a low frequency, high amplitude, pattern of release. This down-regulates GnRH receptors in the anterior pituitary so that gonadotropin secretion plummets in the luteal phase.

However, in humans the anterior pituitary is able to generate a normal pattern of gonadotropin output even if exposed to pulses of GnRH of **constant** frequency and amplitude. Evidence for this comes from women with **Kallmann's syndrome**, who have a deficiency in GnRH secretion caused by

---

Clinical box 10.4 | Clinical uses of GnRH

Hypothalamic hypogonadotropic hypogonadism in both sexes can be treated with GnRH. The hormone is delivered intravenously as discrete 5 μg pulses every 90 minutes via a portable, battery-powered, programmable pump. The effectiveness of the treatment is assayed in women by measuring plasma oestradiol concentrations and determining the diameter of follicles by ultrasound scan, and in men by plasma testosterone concentrations and sperm counts.

Continuous (i.e. non-pulsatile) delivery of GnRH causes cessation of gonadotropin secretion, probably by down-regulating GnRH receptors in the anterior pituitary. This is exploited by giving long-acting **GnRH agonists** in conditions in which suppression of the hypothalamic–pituitary–gonadal axis to reduce sex steroid concentrations is desirable, e.g. prostatic cancer, polycystic ovary syndrome, endometriosis, precocious puberty or uterine fibroids.

Clinical box 10.5 Polycystic ovary syndrome

Polycystic ovary syndrome (**PCOS**) results from a defect in the hypothalamic–pituitary–ovarian axis. This is a relatively common form of secondary hypogonadism where there is a permanent cycle of positive feedback between oestrogens and LH release. High levels of LH stimulate stromal cells in the ovary to produce large amounts of androgens (particularly androstenedione) that are aromatised peripherally to oestrogens (oestrone). The high oestrogen concentration drives positive feedback LH secretion.

The causes of PCOS are unclear, but may be associated with peripheral insulin resistance leading to secondary hyperinsulinism. The increased circulating insulin and IGF stimulates ovarian androgen secretion. The androgens:

- Inhibit follicle development, resulting in anovulation and amenorrhea
- Cause **hirsutism**, with a male pattern of hair distribution.

Clinical box 10.6 Hormonal contraception and abortion

The effects of sex steroids on the hypothalamic–pituitary–ovarian axis are exploited in the use of hormones to prevent pregnancy – contraception. However, many endogenous steroids are inactive orally because of substantial first-pass metabolism by the liver; consequently a number of synthetic oestrogenic and progestagenic molecules are used for contraception.

Synthetic oestrogens (e.g. ethinylestradiol, mestranol) inhibit FSH release by negative feedback, suppressing follicular development. Synthetic progesterone-like compounds, progestins (e.g. norethisterone, desogestrel), block the oestrogen-mediated positive feedback surge in LH release, preventing ovulation, and in addition render cervical mucus sperm hostile. Endometrial development in response to synthetic hormones is scanty and not favourable for implantation of a fertilised ovum.

Mifepristone is a progesterone (and glucocorticoid) receptor antagonist which blocks hormonal support of the endometrium. It is an effective abortifacient for early pregnancy, sometimes used in conjunction with prostaglandin E1, which stimulates contraction of uterine smooth muscle.

the failure of GnRH neurons to migrate properly during development. These women do not release gonadotropins, do not experience a natural puberty and are infertile, a state of affairs termed **hypothalamic hypogonadotropic hypogonadism**. However, they can have normal menstrual cycles induced, exhibiting both negative and positive feedback, if given constant size GnRH pulses. The implication is that the number of GnRH receptors on anterior pituitary cells (and hence their sensitivity to GnRH) can be regulated directly by steroids.

Roles of oestradiol and progesterone

During the menstrual cycle oestradiol and progesterone, the major ovarian steroids, prepare the female reproductive tract for possible fertilisation and implantation. One function of oestradiol is to induce the expression of progesterone receptors in target tissues. In other words, sensitivity to progesterone produced by the corpus luteum is **primed** by prior exposure to the oestrogen secreted during the follicular phase of the menstrual cycle.

Tubal epithelium

Oestradiol stimulates the proliferation of highly ciliated columnar epithelium lining the fallopian tubes and the secretion of a sugar-rich fluid. The secretion presumably supplies nutrients to the egg cell mass during its sojourn in the tube. Progesterone reduces the number of cilia and secretion in the fallopian tubes.

Endometrium

During the follicular phase of the ovarian cycle (see below), oestradiol stimulates hyperplasia and hypertrophy of both columnar epithelium and stroma cells in the functional layer of the endometrium. Stromal cells secrete osmotically active mucopolysaccharides into the stroma, which becomes oedematous. Endometrial glands elongate and spiral arteries grow into the functional layer from the basal layer.

Progesterone and oestradiol operate together in the secretory phase of the menstrual cycle (see below) to stimulate further growth and to activate secretion from the endometrial glands. The glandular secretion supplies the embryo with sugars and amino acids. As ovarian steroid concentrations fall at the end of the secretory phase (see below) of the menstrual cycle, prostaglandin $F_{2\alpha}$ ($PGF_{2\alpha}$) liberated from cell membranes causes the spiral arteries go into vasospasm, the functional layer becomes ischaemic, dies, and is sloughed off as the menstrual flow. $PGF_{2\alpha}$ also triggers the release of lysosomal proteolytic enzymes which digest the endometrium and destroy blood clotting factors. Consequently, menstrual flow does not coagulate.

Smooth muscle

Oestradiol up-regulates receptors for prostaglandins and oxytocin. Spontaneous and stimulated activity of smooth muscle of the fallopian tubes and myometrium is increased. By contrast, progesterone produces relaxation of smooth muscle both in the reproductive tract and elsewhere, reducing the sensitivity of smooth muscle to oxytocin by receptor down-regulation.

Cervix

Under the influence of oestradiol in the late follicular phase (see below), cervical mucus becomes more plentiful, more alkaline and less viscous. In this state sperm are much more able to swim through it. Progesterone reduces mucus volume and increases its viscosity, making it hostile to sperm.

PUBERTY IN GIRLS

Puberty is the period during which the hypothalamic–pituitary–gonadal axis matures to its adult state. It is heralded by the adolescent growth spurt (**adrenarche**) and its progress assessed by the development of **secondary sexual characteristics** such as the growth of pubic hair and breasts. Puberty ends with the **menarche**, the first menstrual period. The mean age of the menarche in the developed world is 12.5 years and the median length of puberty about 4 years, but these averages mask large individual variation.

Adrenarche and secondary sexual characteristics

During adrenarche a rise in androgen secretion from the adrenal cortex drives the adolescent growth spurt and the growth of pubic and axillary hair. Oestradiol, at first derived from the aromatisation of adrenal androgens and later from the ovaries, not only stimulates the growth of long bones by enhancing the secretion of growth hormone, but also promotes the closure of the epiphyseal plates. Hence the sex steroids both stimulate but eventually bring to an end the adolescent growth spurt.

Hair growth is stimulated by dihydrotestosterone (DHT) formed locally from testosterone by 5α-reductase. During puberty androgens transform fine, less pigmented, **vellus hair** which covers the body and face (except the palms of the hands, soles of the feet, and back of the ears), into coarser pigmented **androgenic terminal hair**. It is termed **androgenic hair** because its growth is stimulated by androgens (unlike terminal head hair). Hair in the pubic region is most sensitive to androgens and hence transforms first. Quantitative differences in circulating testosterone lead to the characteristic patterns of male and female body and facial hair distribution. Enhanced androgenic activity in women (such as increased androgen secretion, reduced SHBG (sex hormone-binding globulin) and hence a higher free androgen concentration, or increased 5α-reductase activity in target tissues) can result in hirsutism and virilisation.

Breast development begins about 1.5 years after the start of the growth spurt. Branching and growth of the lobuloalveolar ducts is stimulated by oestrogens and progesterone from the ovaries. For these steroids to be effective corticosteroids, prolactin, growth hormone and IGF-1 must also be present. Oestradiol stimulates cell division, and increases the transcription of actin and myosin genes in smooth muscle of the uterus. Oestrogens are also responsible for the female pattern of fat deposition, including that in the breasts.

Triggers for puberty

During childhood, plasma gonadotropin concentrations (and consequently steroid concentrations) are low. This probably results from tonic GABAergic inhibition on the hypothalamic neurons that secrete GnRH. The arrival of puberty is marked by high amplitude pulses of LH and FSH, firstly during sleep and subsequently throughout the day. The rise in gonadotropin output is unrelated to ovarian steroids because it is seen in girls with gonadal dysgenesis. Hence, it is clearly **triggered** by some central mechanism rather than a change in responsiveness to steroid hormones. It could be due to a reduction of GABAergic inhibition on GnRH secretion. A secondary effect seems to be an up-regulation of GnRH receptors on gonadotropes, which consequently become more sensitive to the releasing hormone.

What triggers the brain to switch on GnRH release is uncertain but it is clearly some sort of metabolic signal which is related to body fat because lean girls start puberty later. Leptin is a candidate molecule, but whether it is the primary trigger or has a permissive role is not known. Menarche occurs when a girl's body mass exceeds about 47 kg, so overweight girls have their first period earlier than their lighter peers. The fall in the age of menarche recorded in Europe over the past 130 years is attributed largely to better nutrition. Dancers, athletes and anorexics become anovulatory and cease menstruating if their body mass falls too low.

MENOPAUSE

Menopause is the permanent age-related cessation of menstrual cycles. The median age of the menopause in the developed world is 51.5 years (range 45–55 years). The menopause is preceded by irregular cycles that have a shorter follicular phase and may be anovulatory. It is generally assumed to be due to primary ovarian failure, but apparently normal oocytes are found in post-menopausal ovaries, so changes in central control of GnRH release may also play a part. Whatever the exact cause, the concentrations of oestradiol and progesterone fall and the loss of negative feedback results in a rise in the concentrations of the gonadotropins, FSH and LH. The rise in FSH is greatest, because of the loss of inhibin secretion from follicles. Gonadotropins isolated from the urine of post-menopausal women can be used to induce ovulation in women with secondary hypogonadism. Sex steroids continue to be produced in post-menopausal women at a low level, principally by the adrenal glands. Oestrogens (mainly oestrone) are derived from aromatisation of androgens by fat cells in small amounts.

MALE REPRODUCTIVE ENDOCRINOLOGY

MALE REPRODUCTIVE TRACT

The male gonads, the **testes**, are paired organs situated outside the abdominal cavity. Each **testis** consists of several hundred highly convoluted **seminiferous** tubules, 30–70 m in length and 0.3 mm across, connected at both ends to the **rete testis**, a tubular anastomosing network. From the rete testis, **efferent ductules** merge into a single highly coiled tube, the **epididymis**, which drains into the **vas deferens** (Fig. 10.13). The vas deferens passes through the inguinal canal into the abdominal cavity to reach the **prostate gland**. Here, the vas deferens converges with the duct of a **seminal vesicle** to become an **ejaculatory duct**. The two ejaculatory ducts enter the prostatic urethra. The ducts of the two **bulbourethral glands** join the urethra where it enters the penis. The mucous secretion of the bulbourethral glands lubricates the urethra.

Testis

Gross anatomy of the testis and its relations

In the fetus, an evagination of the peritoneal cavity, the **processus vaginalis**, precedes the descent of the testis from its abdominal, retroperitoneal position, through the inguinal canal into the scrotum. Hence the testis, encapsulated in a connective tissue **tunica albuginea**, becomes ensheathed in a double layered **tunica vaginalis**, derived from the visceral and parietal peritoneum (Fig. 10.14).

After the testis descends (normally before birth) the processus vaginalis is obliterated; should it remain patent abdominal contents can herniate through the inguinal canal into the scrotum (**indirect inguinal hernia**). Excess secretion of serous fluid into the cavity of the tunica vaginalis causes **hydrocele**, which is usually asymptomatic. Failure of the testes to descend (**cryptorchidism**) is problematic because undescended (ectopic) testes tend to undergo malignant change.

As the testis and epididymis descend through the **inguinal canal** they become covered successively with **internal spermatic fascia**, **cremaster muscle** and **external spermatic fascia**, derived from the transversalis fascia, internal oblique and external oblique aponeurosis, respectively; the

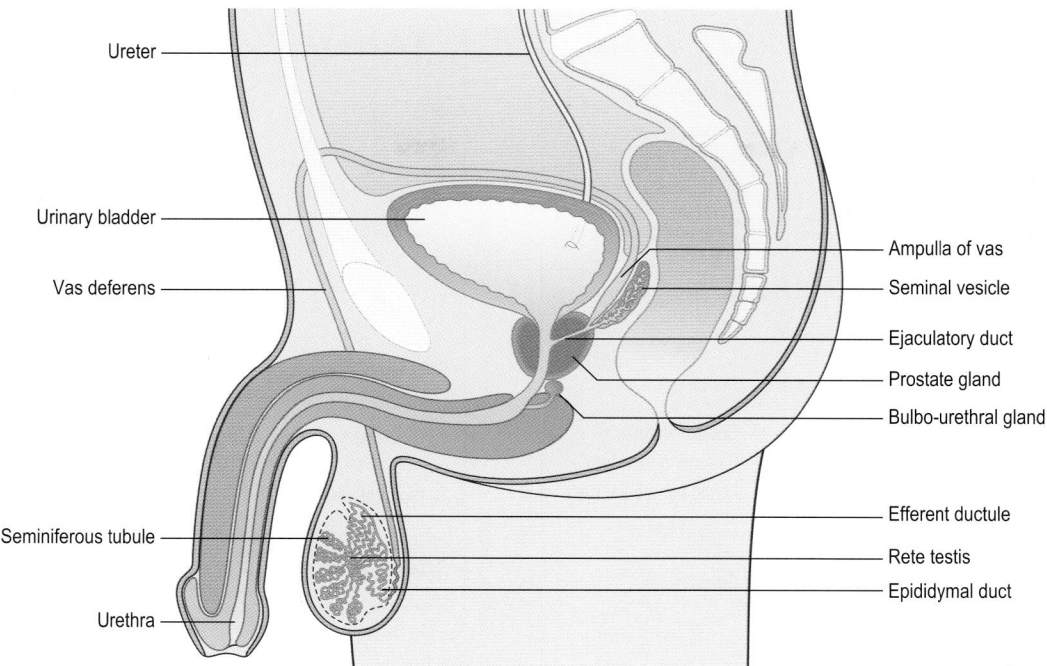

Fig. 10.13 **Midsagittal section through the male pelvis.**

Labels (figure 10.13):
Ureter
Urinary bladder
Vas deferens
Seminiferous tubule
Urethra
Ampulla of vas
Seminal vesicle
Ejaculatory duct
Prostate gland
Bulbo-urethral gland
Efferent ductule
Rete testis
Epididymal duct

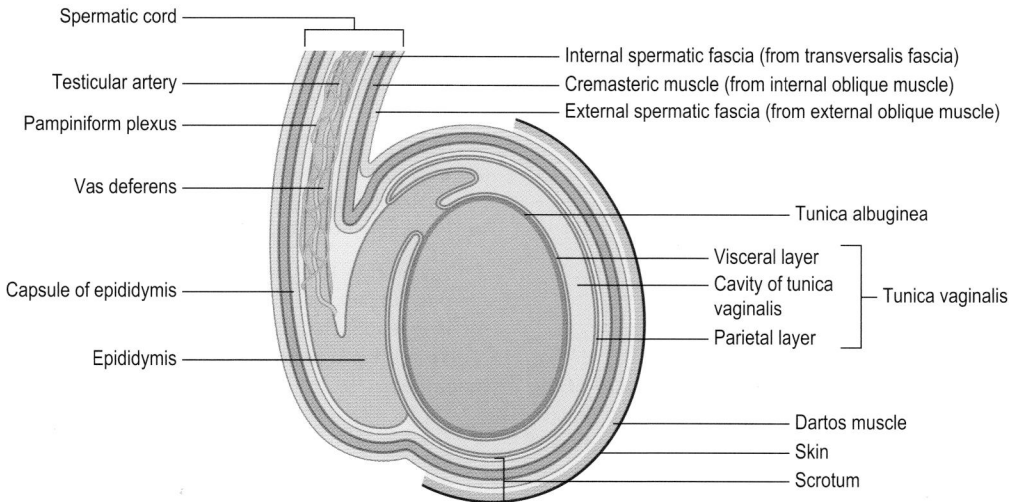

Fig. 10.14 **Coverings of the testis and spermatic cord.**

Labels (figure 10.14):
Spermatic cord
Testicular artery
Pampiniform plexus
Vas deferens
Capsule of epididymis
Epididymis
Internal spermatic fascia (from transversalis fascia)
Cremasteric muscle (from internal oblique muscle)
External spermatic fascia (from external oblique muscle)
Tunica albuginea
Visceral layer
Cavity of tunica vaginalis
Parietal layer
Tunica vaginalis
Dartos muscle
Skin
Scrotum

associated blood vessels, nerves and the vas deferens are similarly invested to form the **spermatic cord**. Reflex contraction of the cremaster, and of the **dartos** (smooth) **muscle** in the scrotum, in response to touch, cold or during exercise, serve to retract the testis against the abdominal wall.

The **testicular arteries** come from the aorta. A plexus of veins (**pampiniform plexus**) surrounding the arteries in the spermatic cord are drained by the testicular veins which enter the inferior vena cava (left side) or renal vein (right side). Blood returning in the venous plexus cools incoming arterial blood. Their extra-abdominal position, plus the heat exchange mechanism, keep the temperature of the testes at about 3°C below core temperature, optimal for sperm production. If the testis rotates about the spermatic cord, the testicular artery can occlude to cause testicular ischaemia. This sequence of events is termed **testicular torsion**. The pampiniform plexus veins contain valves. When these become incompetent the veins become varicose, which leads to the development of a **varicocele**.

Cellular physiology of the testis

The seminiferous tubule epithelium (Fig. 10.15) is bounded by a basement membrane that is surrounded by a thin coat of myoid **peritubular cells**. Resting on the basement membrane are **Sertoli cells** that are coupled together by tight junctions to form a **blood–testis barrier**. Sandwiched between the basement membrane and the Sertoli cell gap junctions are spermatogonia. These cells divide and differentiate into

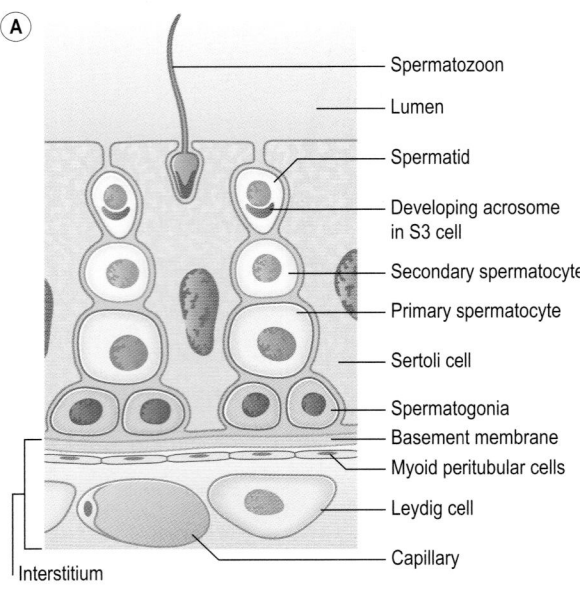

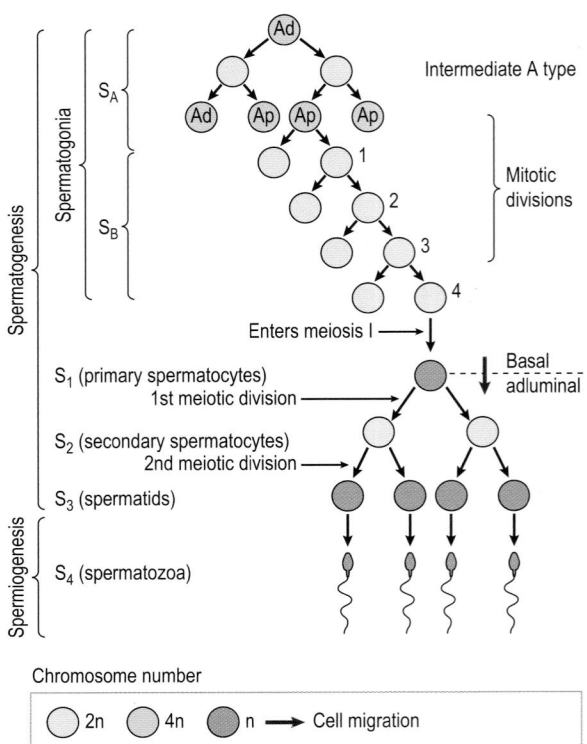

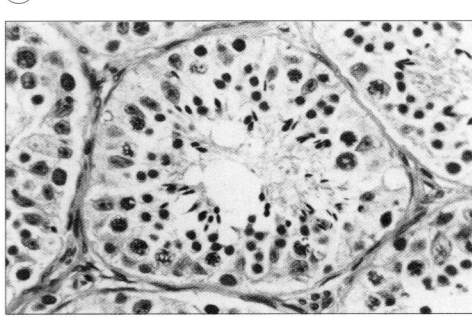

Fig. 10.15 Seminiferous tubule, transverse section: (A) cytoarchitecture; (B) micrograph (×640). Reproduced with permission from Young B, Lowe JS, Stevens A, Heath JW 2006 Wheater's functional histology, 5th edn. Churchill Livingstone, Edinburgh.

Fig. 10.16 Spermatogenesis. Cell types: Ad, dark-type A spermatogonia (dormant stem cells); Ap, pale-type A spermatogonia (clonal expansion of each Ap cell yields 16 type B spermatogonia (S$_B$) by four successive mitotic divisions, and eventually 64 sperms).

spermatozoa. Spermatogonia are on the blood side of the blood–testis barrier in the **basal compartment** of the testis. Nestling between adjacent Sertoli cells on the testis side of the blood–testis barrier, in the **adluminal compartment**, are spermatocytes and spermatids, cells derived from spermatogonia, that are busy differentiating into sperm. These cells express cell surface antigens that would be recognised as foreign by the immune system, because sperm are not made during the time when the fetal immune system learns to distinguish self from non-self. This explains why they are effectively isolated from circulating immune system cells on the testis side of the blood–testis barrier. The integrity of the blood–testis barrier requires androgens synthesised by Leydig cells (see below) and so it is not formed until puberty. Sertoli cells, stimulated by FSH, have numerous functions other than forming the blood–testis barrier, including:

- Synthesis of anti-Müllerian hormone
- Releasing chemical signals that control sperm formation and nutrients for the sperm progenitor cells
- Producing **testicular fluid**, the transport medium for sperm
- Aromatisation of testosterone to oestradiol

- Manufacture of sex-hormone binding globulin, which acts to maintain high concentrations of testosterone and oestradiol locally in the testis and seminal fluid
- Production of inhibin.

Located in the interstitial compartment between seminiferous tubules are **Leydig cells** which synthesise androgens in response to chorionic gonadotropin in utero and LH. There are three periods during which Leydig cells produce androgens:

- 8–24 weeks' gestation for differentiation of internal and external genitals
- 8–12 weeks' post-natally, which may be the time when brain sexual differentiation occurs
- From puberty onwards, with a gradual decline after about 50 years.

Steroid biosynthesis in the testis

As in the ovarian follicle the synthesis of steroids is shared between two major cell types. Leydig cells are homologous to theca interna cells, whereas Sertoli cells are homologous to the granulosa cells. Spermatogenesis requires testosterone but some testicular functions need oestrogens; for example, fluid reabsorption in the epididymis.

Spermatogenesis

Spermatogenesis begins at puberty, in response to rising concentrations of testosterone and FSH, and is thereafter continuous. The production of mature spermatozoa from a spermatogonium takes about 64 days (Fig. 10.16). About two million spermatogonia enter the spermatogenesis cycle each day, with neighbouring cells dividing in synchrony.

At 5 weeks' post-conception, primordial **gametes (sex cells)** migrate from the yolk sac into the undifferentiated gonad. The testis develops between 6 and 12 weeks' gestation, during which time the sex cells divide to become **type Ad spermatogonia**. These are diploid stem cells that retain the ability to divide throughout life, giving rise to spermatozoa (sperm). Spermatogenesis takes place in the seminiferous tubules of the testes in four stages.

1. Spermatogonial stage (cell multiplication): stem cells undergo two mitotic divisions and multiply to generate:
   - Another type **Ad spermatogonium** that does not progress to spermatogonia, but maintains the stem cell number
   - Three **type Ap spermatogonia**, each of which undergoes four successive mitotic divisions to form a clone of 16 **type B spermatogonia (S_B)** that enter the next stage of spermatogenesis.
2. Spermatocyte stage (growth): each S_B cell enters prophase of meiosis I, at which stage they arrest for 20 days, becoming **primary spermatocytes (S_1)**. These cells migrate between adjacent Sertoli cells so that they come to lie on the adluminal side of the blood–testis barrier. The clonal expansion of a single Ap cell generates 64 sperm, because each primary spermatocyte gives rise to four sperm by meiosis
3. Maturation: completion of meiosis I produces **secondary spermatocytes (S_2)** and reduction division of meiosis II then generates haploid **spermatids (S_3)**. Cytokinesis is incomplete in these cells, which consequently remain connected via narrow bridges of cytoplasm.
4. Differentiation of spermatids into mature **spermatozoa (S_4) (spermiogenesis)** now occurs. This involves:
   - The Golgi apparatus forming a lysosome-like organelle called the **acrosome** which is filled with the hydrolytic enzyme, **hyaluronidase** and which enables the sperm to gain access to the ovum

- Formation of the flagellum (sperm tail) from microtubules
- Division of mitochondria and their assembly around the proximal part of the flagellum
- Loss of cytoplasm.

HYPOTHALAMIC–PITUITARY–TESTICULAR AXIS

GnRH released from neuro-secretory cells in the arcuate nucleus of the hypothalamus stimulate the release of FSH and LH from the anterior pituitary (Fig. 10.17).

- LH receptors in Leydig cells stimulate testosterone biosynthesis and secretion. Loss-of-function mutations of LH receptors prevents testosterone secretion and causes a total failure of spermatogenesis.
- Sertoli cells are the only cells to express FSH receptors in the male. FSH enhances spermatogenesis via its actions on Sertoli cells; however, loss-of-function mutations on FSH receptor genes, although resulting in low sperm counts, does not cause infertility.
- Inhibin produced by Sertoli cells in response to the gonadotropin exerts negative feedback inhibition on FSH release from pituitary gonadotropes.
- Testosterone from Leydig cells exerts negative feedback inhibition on LH release from pituitary gonadotropes.

Actions of androgens

Testosterone mainly originates in the testes, but some is secreted by the adrenal glands. Only about 2% of circulating testosterone is free (unbound). The remainder is bound to either plasma protein (about 50%) or **sex-hormone-binding globulin (SHBG)**.

At many target tissues testosterone is converted to **dihydrotestosterone (DHT)** by the enzyme 5α-reductase. DHT has a higher affinity for androgen receptors than testosterone and so is the more potent androgen. Hence much of the effect of testosterone on spermatogenesis, gonadotropin

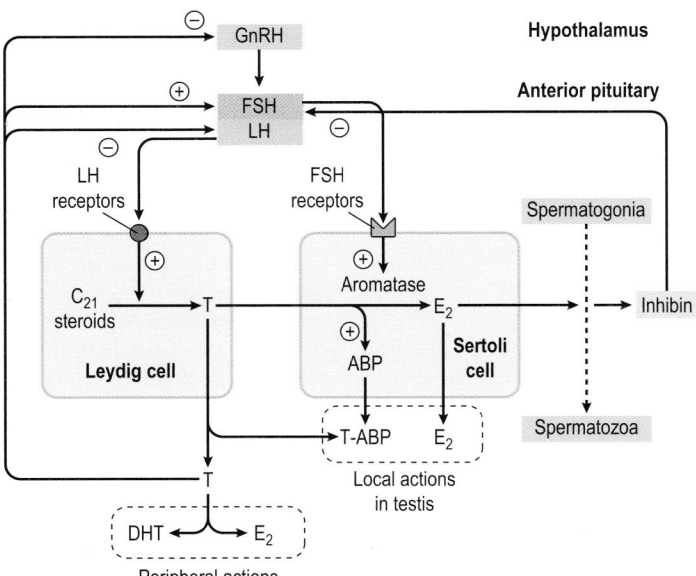

Fig. 10.17 **Regulation of testicular function by the hypothalamic–pituitary–gonadal axis.** ABP, androgen binding protein; DHT, dihydrotestosterone; E_2, oestradiol; T, testosterone.

regulation, sexual differentiation of the male reproductive system in utero, and the development of male secondary sexual characteristics at puberty are mediated by dihydrotestosterone.

Testosterone also affects behaviour in both men and women by acting on the hypothalamus. These behavioural effects may require testosterone to be aromatised to oestradiol first, which then binds to oestrogen receptors located in the neurons that synapse with GnRH-secreting neurons of the arcuate nucleus.

Sex-hormone-binding globulin

SHBG is a glycoprotein with a single steroid-binding site that has a higher affinity for testosterone than oestradiol. Synthesis of SHBG by the liver is reduced by androgens so its concentration in men is half that in women.

Sertoli cells also secrete SHBG into testicular fluid – when it is often referred to as **androgen-binding protein** (**ABP**). Unlike the liver, expression of the *shbg* gene in Sertoli cells is enhanced by androgens. In the testis, SHBG serves to maintain the high concentration of androgens in Sertoli cells and the testicular fluid needed for spermatogenesis.

PUBERTY IN BOYS

In boys, puberty starts about a year later than in girls. It is assessed by the growth of pubic hair, testes and penis. As in girls, it is preceded by adrenarche, but as testosterone secretion from the testis is added to that from the adrenals, its plasma concentration rises to become 10- to 20-fold higher in boys than girls.

Male secondary sexual characteristics

At puberty, androgens:

- Enhance long bone growth by stimulating growth hormone secretion, but promote closure of the epiphyses (these actions require that testosterone is converted to oestradiol)
- Enhance growth of the larynx
- Stimulate muscle protein synthesis
- Enhance synthesis of erythropoietin, consequently haematocrit is greater in men than women
- Activate growth and development of internal and external genitals
- Stimulate secretion by seminal vesicles, prostate and bulbourethral glands
- Generate male pattern hair growth by transforming vellus hair to terminal hair
- Stimulate secretion of sebaceous glands.

Most of the above effects are mediated by dihydrotestosterone. Unlike terminal androgenic hair, which is stimulated by DHT, the same steroid gradually reduces the thickness of head hair, and so is responsible for **male pattern baldness**.

Gonadotropin secretion

As in girls, it is thought that hypothalamic neurons responsible for triggering pulsatile GnRH release are inhibited in childhood by central GABAergic input. Puberty may be triggered

by relaxation of this inhibition, and secondary rise in sensitivity of the anterior pituitary to the releasing hormone.

SPERM TRANSPORT

Mature spermatozoa are transported from the seminiferous tubules through the male reproductive organs, and are prepared for fertilisation of an ovum during this process (see below).

Testis

Spermatozoa (sperm) in the seminiferous tubules are propelled by the pressure of seminiferous tubule fluid, and activity of a thin layer of myoid peritubular cells that surround the seminiferous tubules, into the epididymis. Here, sperm are concentrated about 100-fold by fluid absorption, facilitated by oestrogens, and sufficient numbers are stored for one ejaculate (equivalent to about a day's production). Sperm are metabolically inactive in the epididymis because of the lack of energy substrates and oxygen, and are non-motile. Sperm take about 12 days to transit the epididymis, during which time proteins secreted by its columnar epithelium confer on them the ability to fertilise an ovum (**capacitation**, see below). However, a number of **decapacitation factors** suppress capacitation. Consequently, sperm are only capable of fertilisation after spending about 4 hours in the female reproductive tract.

From the epididymis, the sperm enter the vasa deferens, which eventually carry the sperm to the urethra. The vas deferens has both circular and longitudinal smooth muscle and peristalsis propels sperm and tubule fluid along its length.

Seminal vesicles

The **seminal vesicles** are glands that form by evagination of the wall of the ampulla of the vas deferens. Seminal vesicles secrete seminal fluid (about 60% of the volume of the semen), which is rich in energy substrates such as fructose (which sperm metabolise anaerobically) and citrate. It is slightly alkaline, and contains phosphate and bicarbonate buffers to neutralise the acid pH of the vagina, thus improving sperm motility and survival.

Seminal fluid contains enzymes which cause ejaculated semen to clot, and has a high potassium concentration that inhibits sperm motility. The clotting of semen after ejaculation limits gravitational losses. Prostaglandins in seminal vesicle secretion are thought to stimulate contraction of the smooth muscle of the female reproductive tract, thereby helping uptake of clotted semen into the cervix, and subsequent sperm transport by stimulating contraction of smooth muscle in the fallopian tubes.

As the clot subsequently dissolves, potassium concentration and viscosity falls so that sperm become motile. The fall in pH, as buffer capacity is overwhelmed by hydrogen ions in the vaginal secretions, activates **acid phosphatase** (a prostatic secretion, see below), making more energy substrates available.

Prostate

The **prostate** is an exocrine gland surrounding the root of the male urethra. Prostatic secretions contain proteases that digest semen clots, citrate and **acid phosphatase**. Acid phosphatase cleaves phosphorylcholine and phosphocreatine in seminal vesicle secretion to provide energy substrates. Prostatic acid phosphatase secretion is elevated in prostate cancers and correlates with tumour progression. The prostate also produces a merocrine secretion of **prostasomes**, submicron lipid bilayer-enclosed organelles containing **tissue factor** that triggers the clotting cascade. Prostasomes bind to sperm to facilitate motility, and contain proteins that suppress immune cells or inhibit complement so as to limit immune attack by the female on the sperm.

Prostate-specific antigen (PSA) is a glycoprotein specific to the prostate. PSA liquefies semen, enabling sperm to 'swim' more easily. PSA is also thought to dissolve cervical mucus to facilitate entry. PSA levels are increased in prostatic cancers. Although not very reliable, serum PSA is used as a screening test for prostate cancer. It is a useful marker for tumour progression and for monitoring response to treatment.

Sperm count

Sperm counts are performed during investigation of infertility (see below), when the number, morphology and motility of the spermatozoa are examined. Sperm counts are normally of order 10^8 /mL semen. Sperm counts below 20×10^6/mL or lower than 60% sperm with normal morphology or motility are associated with male infertility.

Endocrine determinants of libido

Libido or sex drive is the motivation to engage in sexual activity. Although numerous factors influence libido in humans, it seems to be enhanced by testosterone in both men and women. In men the frequency of orgasms correlates with plasma DHT concentration; low testosterone concentration or castration is associated with diminished libido that can be restored by testosterone replacement. However, testosterone supplements in men with normal plasma testosterone concentrations do not enhance libido; testosterone is not an aphrodisiac! Treatment with the anti-androgen **cyproterone acetate** lowers libido.

A controlled study of ovariectomised women given either long-acting androgen plus oestrogen, or oestrogen alone, or no treatment, showed a substantial rise in sexual desire, sexual arousal and frequency of sexual fantasies in the group that had received the androgen plus oestrogen than in the other two groups. In addition, there was a significant correlation between these measures of libido and plasma testosterone, but not plasma oestradiol. This is evidence that testosterone is a hormonal determinant of libido in women.

There is a modest tendency for women not using oral contraceptives to have sex more often around the time of ovulation (which correlates with peak plasma testosterone concentration in women) and just before menstruation, but less during the mid-luteal phase of the cycle. However, this cyclic variation can be explained by differences in when men initiated sex. It is suggested that this arises from alterations in the women's sexual attractiveness, rather than changes in her libido. One possibility is that high progesterone concentrations during the mid-luteal phase exert an anti-oestrogenic effect, reducing the secretion of a vaginal **pheromone** that normally acts as an olfactory sexual attractant for men. Oral contraceptives which suppress endogenous progesterone production, abolishes the mid-luteal dip in coital frequency.

PREGNANCY

In humans, a normal pregnancy begins with fertilisation of a mature ovum by a spermatozoon in the fallopian tube, and ends with the delivery of a healthy baby. From fertilisation to delivery, the period of embryonic development and fetal growth is referred to as **gestation**.

For a successful pregnancy several key conditions must be met. The conceptus must subvert the maternal immune system so that it is not rejected. Initially, the female reproductive tract must provide the proper environment for fertilisation and implantation to occur. Subsequently, the placenta becomes an endocrine gland producing a variety of hormones which maintain the uterus in a fit state to nurture the developing fetus, and alters maternal biochemistry to meet the needs of the fetus. The placenta must allow an adequate supply of nutrients from mother to conceptus. Major changes to maternal physiology are required to facilitate this and for the woman to accommodate the growing uterus and its contents.

FERTILISATION

Of the $\sim 10^8$ sperm ejaculated into the posterior fornix of the vagina only 1% make it through the cervical mucus, and just a few hundred reach the oocyte in the ampulla of the fallopian tube. The remainder drain out of the vagina, are killed by its acidity, or are phagocytosed by leucocytes in the uterine cavity. The journey is facilitated by prostaglandin-triggered contractions of uterine and tubal smooth muscle, and undulating wave-like motions of the sperm tail which gives a forward velocity of about 1 mm/min. Sperm appear in the fallopian tube in as little as 5 minutes and may remain viable in situ for up to 72 hours. Since the ovum is only viable typically for 6–24 hours, the time window for fertilisation is quite narrow; normally coitus must occur no earlier than 3 days before ovulation and no later than 1 day after.

To become capable of fertilisation, and to penetrate the cumulus oophorus and the zona pellucida (see above), the sperm are prepared by two processes:

- Capacitation
- Acrosome reaction.

CAPACITATION

Capacitation is the loss of surface glycoprotein from the sperm, caused by proteolytic enzymes secreted from the uterine endometrium. This process takes about 4 hours, and enables the sperm to fertilise the ovum.

ACROSOME REACTION

Sperm have to get through the cumulus oophorus and zona pellucida to reach the oocyte. Enzymes liberated from many sperm are needed to breech these barriers. On arrival in the vicinity of the ovum, progesterone secreted by the cumulus oophorus activates Ca^{2+} influx through the outer plasma membrane of the sperm head so that it fuses with the

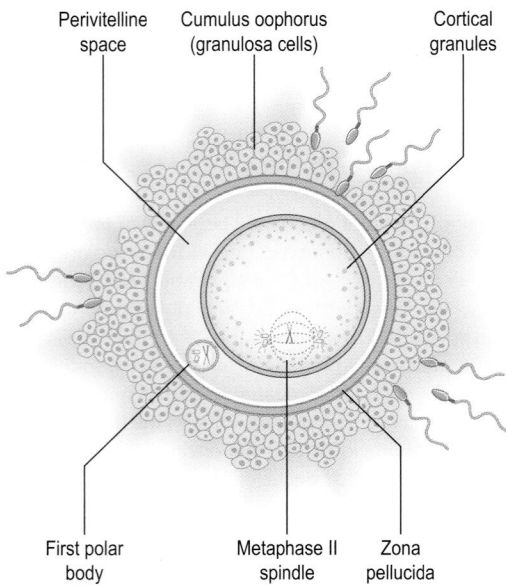

Fig. 10.18 **Secondary oocyte immediately before sperm fusion.**

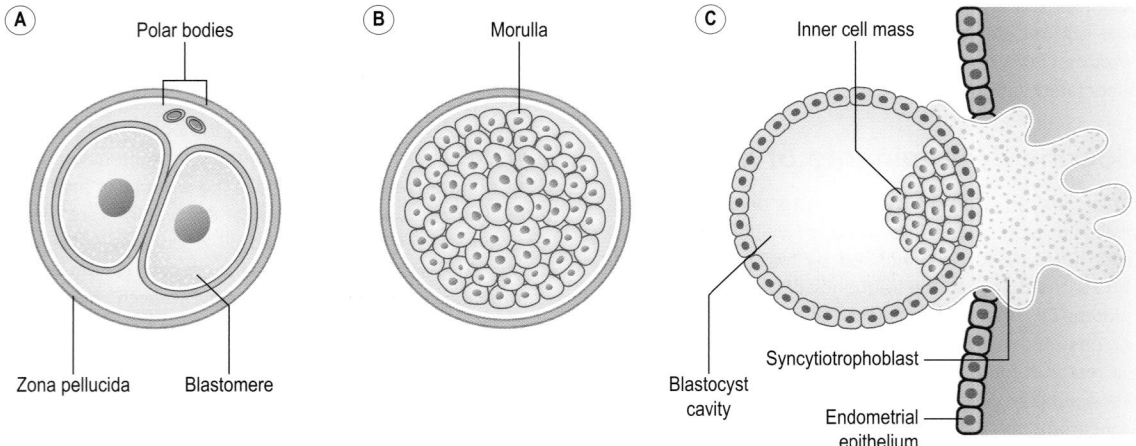

Fig. 10.19 Early development of the pre-embryo: (A) two-cell stage, 2 days; (B) morula, day 4; (C) implanting blastula, day 7.

acrosome membrane beneath. This is the **acrosome reaction** and permits the release of enzymes from the acrosome. **Hyaluronidase** digests the intercellular matrix between the cumulus oophorus cells. This allows sperm access to the zona pellucida which contains a specific glycoprotein to which they bind. Here a trypsin-like enzyme from the acrosome, **acrosin**, digests a path through the zona pellucida and large thrashes of the tail drive sperms into the **perivitelline space** (Fig. 10.18). For sperms, fertilisation is a race. The first to fuse with the plasma membrane of the ovum, the vitelline membrane, is the winner.

ZYGOTE FORMATION

About 2–3 hours after a sperm fuses, the oocyte reactivates metaphase II of meiosis. This proceeds to telophase II in which unequal cytokinesis gives rise to an ovum containing a **female pronucleus** and a second polar body (see Fig. 10.7). During this time the sperm nucleus has entered the ovum to become the **male pronucleus**. Fusion of the two

haploid pronuclei and DNA replication gives rise to a single diploid nucleus and a **zygote** ready to embark on its first mitotic division (Fig. 10.19A).

INFERTILITY (SUBFERTILITY)

Most couples (84%) having regular sexual intercourse (two to three times a week) without contraception will conceive within 1 year, and half of the remainder will conceive within 2 years, resulting in 92% of couples conceiving overall. Infertility is generally regarded as the inability of a couple to achieve a pregnancy after 12 months of unprotected intercourse. In about one-third of cases, infertility can be attributed to the male, about one-third to the female, 15% to a combination of both, while about 19% remain unexplained after both partners have been through all the standard tests (**idiopathic infertility**).

Primary infertility refers to cases where the woman has never conceived and **secondary infertility** to cases where a pregnancy has been achieved in the past, but the couple has not managed a pregnancy following unprotected intercourse for at least 1 year. An age-related decline in fertility is seen in both women and men after about 35 years and contributes to secondary infertility in couples who delay having second and subsequent babies. Infertility in both sexes is commonly associated with lifestyle (smoking, excessive alcohol, obesity or anorexia) and with concurrent disease, e.g. diabetes mellitus and hypertension.

Disorders of the hypothalamic–pituitary–gonadal axis make up only a small proportion of the known causes of infertility in both sexes. For example, failure to ovulate occurs in only 5% of women and most of these cases are secondary hypogonadism, particularly due to PCOS. Over-secretion of prolactin, most commonly caused by pituitary tumour, results in infertility in both sexes by suppressing GnRH secretion and responsiveness. By far the commonest cause of female infertility is occlusion of the fallopian tubes by whatever cause, e.g. pelvic inflammatory disease following infection (e.g. sexually transmitted disease), endometriosis or following an ectopic pregnancy. About 10% of infertile men produce anti-sperm antibodies, presumably as a result of a breakdown in the blood–testis barrier, due mostly to infection or injury.

A significant number of women are infertile because they produce antibodies against their partner's sperm and these are secreted into the cervical mucus. Most sperm spend up to 12 hours sequestered in cervical mucus before embarking on their journey up the fallopian tube, and infertility in which the woman's cervical mucus is hostile to her partner's sperm for any reason, accounts for many of the cases of infertility that cannot be attributed to the male or female alone.

EMBRYONIC AND FETAL DEVELOPMENT

The development of the conceptus is traditionally divided into three stages:

1. Until implantation the conceptus is a **pre-embryo**
2. After implantation those cell layers destined to become the baby are termed an **embryo** until 8 weeks' gestation
3. After 8 weeks the developing baby is termed a **fetus**, while the remainder of the conceptus is the placenta and fetal membranes.

Clinical box 10.7   Treatments for infertility

Ideally, treatment of any condition is aimed at prevention or treating the cause. For example, avoiding sexually transmitted infection reduces the risk of infertility in both men and women. Many causes of infertility are, however, untreatable, so that many therapeutic interventions are empirical.

Assisted reproduction techniques (ART)
If the gonads are incapable of producing gametes (spermatozoa or oocytes), then gamete donation becomes necessary: sperm donation, **artificial insemination by donor (AID)** or egg donation. When sperm and oocytes are present, albeit defective, then a variety of rapidly developing artificial reproduction techniques are available for treatment of infertility. For ART to be effective, sperm capable of fertilisation, healthy oocytes and a physiologically normal and receptive uterus are necessary.

Ovulation induction
This is appropriate when secondary hypogonadism prevents the proper development of an ovarian follicle (e.g. PCOS or hypogonadotropic hypogonadism). Two pharmacological therapies are in common use:

- **Clomifene citrate**, a partial agonist at oestrogen receptors, blocks negative feedback inhibition of gonadotropin release by endogenous oestradiol. This allows gonadotropin concentrations to rise to stimulate follicular growth and ovulation.
- **Human menopausal gonadotropins** are given to stimulate the development of ovarian follicles. A single dose of hCG is then given – mimicking the normal mid-cycle LH surge – after at least one follicle has reached a diameter of 17 mm and endometrial thickness is a minimum of 8 mm.

Ovulation occurs after 36–48 hours. Rarely, ovarian hyperstimulation occurs (**ovarian hyperstimulation syndrome**) in which an excessive number of ovarian follicles develop Ovarian stimulation has to be closely monitored by assaying blood oestradiol concentrations and ultrasound scanning of the ovaries. The chance of pregnancy is 15–25% per treatment cycle. This is about the same probability as occurs with unprotected sexual intercourse between a fertile couple at around the time of ovulation.

In vitro fertilisation
In vitro fertilisation (IVF) techniques are used when the cause of infertility is likely to be the inability of spermatozoa to fertilise the ovum in the fallopian tube, which may include defects in sperm motility or oligospermia, cervical anti-sperm antibodies or tubal occlusion, among others.

A gonadotropin analogue is administered to inhibit the normal release of FSH and LH. By breaking the normal pituitary control over follicle development, an average of 10–12 dominant follicles can be generated. Ovulation is then induced using gonadotropins. Usually, 2 days after ovulation induction the IVF procedure is performed as follows:

1. **Egg retrieval**: mature and apparently healthy oocytes are harvested by means of a fine needle inserted into each follicle, via an endoscope under ultrasound guidance.
2. **Sperm preparation**: sperm (fresh or frozen, from husband/ partner or donor) are prepared for fertilisation by removing inactive sperm and semen, and capacitation triggered by exposure to oestrogen.
3. **Fertilisation**: each oocyte is placed in a Petri dish with the prepared sperm that have been treated so that they capacitate. Fertilisation is confirmed microscopically by the presence of 2 pronuclei. Incubation is continued until a six to eight cell pre-embryo develops. These are usually referred to as 'embryos' in the context of ART.
4. **Embryo transfer**: several of the morphologically 'best' embryos are then either transferred directly to the uterus, or sometimes intravaginally. In the UK and some other countries, the number of embryos transferred is regulated to a maximum of **2**, to reduce the risk of multiple pregnancies. In cases where there is a risk of genetic abnormality a single cell can be removed for **pre-implantation diagnosis**. The woman's menstrual cycle is artificially regulated by endocrine manipulation so that embryo transfer is performed at a time when the uterine endometrium is receptive for implantation.

The pregnancy rate with IVF in the UK is 10–28% per treatment session and depends heavily on the age of the woman. Surplus oocytes or embryos can be frozen for use in further cycles or donated to women unable to produce their own.

Gamete intra-fallopian transfer
When there is a male cause of infertility, such as low sperm count or (rarely) a defective acrosome reaction, or if the woman produces cervical anti-sperm antibodies, **gamete intra-fallopian transfer (GIFT)** can come to the rescue. It requires a patent fallopian tube. In this procedure oocytes are retrieved as in IVF, mixed with sperm and endoscopically transferred to the fallopian ampulla. The success rate with GIFT is reported to be somewhat higher than for IVF. In a variation on this theme, in **intra-cytoplasmic sperm injection (ICSI)**, a single sperm (or even a spermatid) is injected into the cytoplasm of a harvested oocyte before it is placed into the fallopian tube.

Pre-embryo development

The pre-embryo takes 3 days to travel down the fallopian tube and remains for a further 2–3 days in the uterine cavity before implantation. During this time, the early pre-embryo undergoes **cleavage** (repeated mitotic divisions) to produce a solid ball of 16 cells, a **morula** (Fig. 10.19B). Cleavage is an unusual form of cell division because it is not accompanied by cell growth. The morula is no bigger than the original zygote and remains entrapped within the zona pellucida.

By the 64-cell stage, the pre-embryo has become a hollow fluid-filled sphere with a single layer of cells, a **blastocyst** (Fig. 10.19C). These cells secrete enzymes that digest the zona pellucida. At this stage, the blastocyst is suspended in and nourished by uterine secretions.

Oviduct transport

During the late proliferative phase of the menstrual cycle, oestrogens up-regulate sympathetic activation of α-adrenoceptors, which stimulates peristalsis of oviduct smooth muscle. This facilitates the movement of sperm to reach the ampulla, but curtails movement of the pre-embryo in the reverse direction towards the uterus. In the secretory phase, progesterone up-regulates β-adrenoceptors, which relax tubal smooth muscle, enabling migration of the pre-embryo to the uterus.

Decidual reaction

Once the pre-embryo arrives in the uterine cavity it attaches itself to the endometrium. This, together with the high concentrations of progesterone and oestrogens present in the late luteal phase, triggers a **decidual reaction** at the implantation site which transforms the functional layer of the endometrium into the **decidua** (so called because it becomes part of the placenta that will be shed at delivery). There is an ingrowth of capillaries, an increase in capillary permeability causing endometrial oedema and morphological alterations to the epithelial cells. Stromal cells enlarge, change from spindle shape to rounded, and become **decidual cells**, which:

- Develop enlarged nucleoli and extensive endoplasmic reticulum with numerous polysomes, all testament to massively increased protein synthesis
- Synthesise glycogen and store it in granules
- Develop large numbers of lysosomes
- Acquire lipid droplets
- Secrete a number of proteins that control implantation, including prolactin.

One function of the decidual reaction is to limit the invasiveness of the blastocyst during implantation.

Implantation

At implantation, the blastocyst consists of an outer shell of flattened cells, the **trophoblast**, which is destined to become part of the placenta and outer fetal membranes (chorion), and an **inner cell mass** that develops into the embryo, extra-embryonic mesoderm, yolk sac and inner fetal membranes (amnion). The blastocyst becomes embedded in the endometrium, usually in the upper portion of the posterior wall of the body of the uterus. How the site of implantation is determined is not known but if the mechanism is thwarted then:

- Implantation can occur too low down so that the placenta straddles the cervix. This is **placenta praevia**, for which elective caesarean section before labour starts is indicated
- Implantation can occur outside the uterus. This is termed **ectopic pregnancy** (Information box 10.5).

The trophoblast differentiates into two layers, an inner **cytotrophoblast** and an outer **syncytiotrophoblast**, in which individual cells have merged to produce a single multinucleate cell (see Fig. 10.19C). The syncytiotrophoblast is phagocytic. It invades the endometrium, engulfing decidual cells, capillary endothelial cells, endometrial glands and subepithelial connective tissue. By 12–14 days the blastocyst is completely embedded within the endometrium and the epithelium grows back over it. For the first month the conceptus is nourished by phagocytosis of the endometrium.

Human chorionic gonadotropin

The syncytiotrophoblast produces **hCG**, a glycoprotein with high homology to LH. It binds to LH receptors on the corpus luteum, which consequently continues its steroid output. This maintains the endometrium.

Chorionic gonadotropin is detectable in maternal blood 7 days after fertilisation, its concentration rises steeply to peak between 8 and 10 weeks and is in mid-decline by 15–16 weeks. Because hCG has a half-life of 30 hours, substantial concentrations accrue even from the small secretory capacity of the conceptus. A modest hCG output occurs throughout pregnancy. Pregnancy becomes independent of the corpus luteum when placental output of steroid hormones is sufficient to support the endometrium, from about 7–9 weeks. Before this time, ovariectomy results in abortion.

All modern pregnancy tests are immunological and rely on binding of antibodies to the β subunit of hCG in blood or urine.

ⓘ Information box 10.5 Ectopic pregnancy

The majority of ectopic pregnancies (about 95%) occur in the oviduct (tubal pregnancy), but they also occur in the ovary, peritoneum and cervix. When implantation occurs in the oviduct, blastocyst invasiveness is very high because the decidual reaction of tubal endometrium is weak. Consequently, in over half of all tubal pregnancies the fallopian tube ruptures and haemorrhages. This is a surgical emergency. In the remaining cases, the embryo dies and the conceptus is absorbed.

Although any functional or anatomical impediment to the transport of the conceptus down the oviduct increases the risk of a tubal pregnancy, the commonest cause is pelvic inflammatory disease. This usually results from ascending infection. Both *Neisseria gonorrhoeae* and *Chlamydia trachomatis* preferentially infect fallopian tubes and infection may be asymptomatic. Infection and inflammation damage the ciliated epithelium, thus compromising conceptus transport, and produce scar tissue that can lead to tubal occlusion.

One explanation for the mistaken association of intrauterine contraceptive devices (IUCDs) with ectopic pregnancy is that IUCDs are more effective in preventing intrauterine pregnancy than ectopic pregnancy, so implantation is more likely to occur in an ectopic location.

Formation of the embryonic membranes

As implantation is occurring the inner cell mass of the blastocyst differentiates into two cell blocks: a dorsal **epiblast** and a ventral **hypoblast** (Fig. 10.20A).

- Hypoblast cells give rise to a layer of **extraembryonic mesoderm**, which surrounds a **primary yolk sac**. This is filled with an energy substrate-rich fluid generated by the phagocytic activities of the trophoblast.
- At the same time (~day 8 after fertilisation) a primordial amniotic cavity forms in the epiblast. Dorsal epiblast cells form the **amnion**.

Where epiblast and hypoblast cells are in contact, the **embryonic disc** forms. Here, epiblast cells become a single layer of columnar **ectoderm**, whereas hypoblast cells differentiate into a single layer of cuboidal **endoderm**.

The primary yolk sac shrinks to form the **secondary yolk sac** as the **chorionic cavity (extraembryonic coelom)** opens up in the extraembryonic **mesoderm** (Fig. 10.20B). The **chorion**, which surrounds the chorionic cavity, consists of an outer layer of trophoblast and an inner layer of mesoderm. Proliferating endodermal cells on the ventral surface of the embryonic disc migrate to enclose the secondary yolk sac. An outgrowth of the yolk sac, the allantois, grows through the connecting stalk of extraembryonic mesoderm to contribute to the formation of the umbilical cord.

Amnion

The amniotic cavity enlarges to enclose the embryo entirely. The amnion is the innermost fetal membrane, forming the outer layer of the umbilical cord and the fetal surface of the placenta. Amniotic fluid is derived from maternal blood and fetal lungs. Later, the fetus swallows amniotic fluid and urinates into it. (Defecation in utero is a sign of fetal distress.) Fetal ventilatory movements cause amniotic fluid to be inspired and expired. Amniotic fluid volume at term is 0.5–1 L and serves as a buoyant cushion to dampen acceleration of embryonic motion caused by mother's movements, while allowing the embryo to move about.

Chorion and decidua

The chorion is the outermost fetal membrane and forms the fetal part of the placenta. The maternal contribution to the placenta is the **decidua basalis**, which lies between the conceptus and myometrium. Initially the non-placental part of the chorion is covered by the **decidua capsularis**, the part of the endometrium overlying the implanted conceptus (Fig. 10.21). The endometrium lining the remainder of the uterus is the **decidua parietalis**. By the third month the capsularis and parietalis have been pushed together by the expanding conceptus, and these two layers eventually undergo atrophy. The fetus is then surrounded by the fetal membranes, chorion and amnion.

Yolk sac

The cells of the yolk sac secrete nutrient-rich fluid to sustain the embryonic disc until the placenta begins to function. These cells have three fates:

- To form part of the gut
- To give rise to the earliest **haemopoietic** (blood-forming) stem cells
- To generate the primordial germ cells which migrate to seed the undifferentiated gonads.

Gastrulation

By the end of the second week after fertilisation, the embryonic disc has elongated and broadened anteriorly, but still consists of two layers, ectoderm and endoderm. The ectoderm has become two to four cells thick. A raised groove, the **primitive streak**, appears in the midline of the posterior end of the dorsal (ectodermal) face of the disc, oriented along the long axis of the embryo (Fig. 10.22). On about day 16, surface ectodermal cells migrate medially, penetrating the primitive streak to insinuate themselves between the ectoderm and endoderm by migrating laterally between these layers. The result of this process, **gastrulation**, is a three-layered structure: an outer ectoderm and inner endoderm with mesoderm sandwiched in between. Each of these is destined to differentiate into particular structures (Table 10.4).

> **ℹ Information box 10.7** **Neural tube defects**
>
> Failure of embryonic neural tube closure leads to **neural tube defects** (malformations of the brain and spinal cord) of varying severity. The precise aetiology is unknown, but may be due to the defective expression of a gene or genes, as yet unidentified. Clinically, women with folic acid deficiency are at higher risk of having babies with neural tube defects.
>
> **Pathogenesis**
> - Failure of the embryonic neural tube to close anteriorly causes **anencephaly**, in which the fetus lacks large components of forebrain and cranium. This condition is invariably lethal.
> - Defects in closure of the posterior end of the embryonic neural tube, corresponding to the lumbosacral spinal cord, result in **spina bifida**.
>   - Most severe is **meningomyelocele**, in which part of the spinal cord, cauda equina and meninges herniate through a defect in the vertebral column and overlying tissues.
>   - More commonly, spina bifida defects are restricted to bone and/or meninges.
>   - Spina bifida is associated with hydrocephalus.
>
> **Screening and diagnosis**
> α-Fetoprotein (AFP) is excreted from the fetal circulation via the urine into the maternal amniotic fluid. AFP can also leak from the open fetal neural tube into amniotic fluid. Consequently, maternal circulating AFP increases above normal, at about 15–20 weeks gestation. Together with accurate, ultrasound dating of gestational age, maternal serum AFP is used as a screening test for neural tube defects, and amniotic AFP concentrations are used for diagnosis.

> **ℹ Information box 10.6** **Amniocentesis**
>
> Amniotic fluid can be sampled via a needle pushed through the abdominal wall into the uterus (under ultrasound guidance to avoid damage to fetus or placenta) to obtain fetal cells. The genetic make-up of these cells can be analysed for the presence of abnormality, e.g. trisomy 21, in diagnosis of Down's syndrome. Several measurements of amniotic fluid provide information about the metabolic state of the fetus, e.g. lecithin/sphingomyelin ratio to measure fetal lung surfactant (Ch. 13).

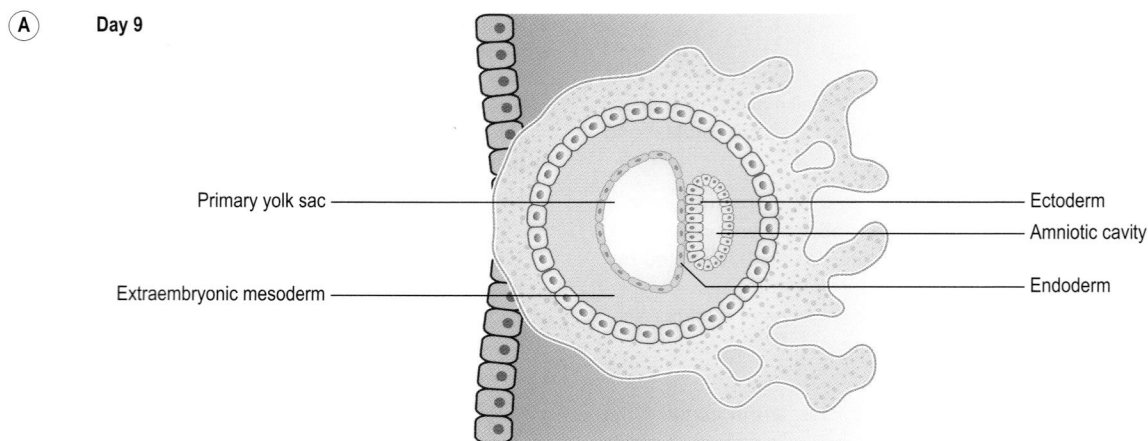

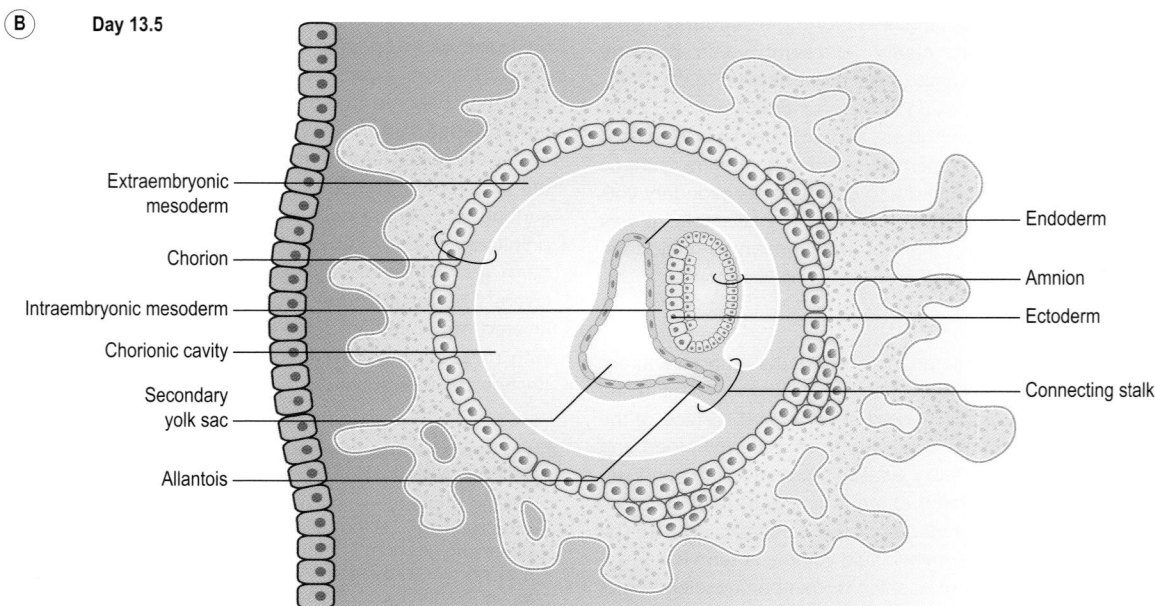

Fig. 10.20 **Implanted conceptus:** (A) day 9; (B) day 13.5.

Table 10.4	**Fate of cells in the germ layers**		
Ectoderm		**Mesoderm**	**Endoderm**
Nervous system		Cartilage and bone	Anterior pituitary
Posterior pituitary		Connective tissues	Thyroid
Retina		Skeletal muscle	Parathyroid
Adrenal medulla		Cardiac muscle	Thymus
Smooth muscle of iris		Smooth muscle*	Pancreas
Skin		Blood vessels	Liver
Epithelia of:		Urogenital system†	Epithelium of:
■ Eye		Adrenal cortex	■ Gut§
■ Nose		Teeth‡	■ Airways
■ Mouth			■ Urogenital system
■ Parotid glands			
■ Ears			
■ Anal canal			
■ Distal urethra			
■ Penis			
■ Vulva			

*Except of the iris.
†Except the epithelium.
‡Except the enamel.
§Including all glands except the parotids.

Uterine contents at 28 days

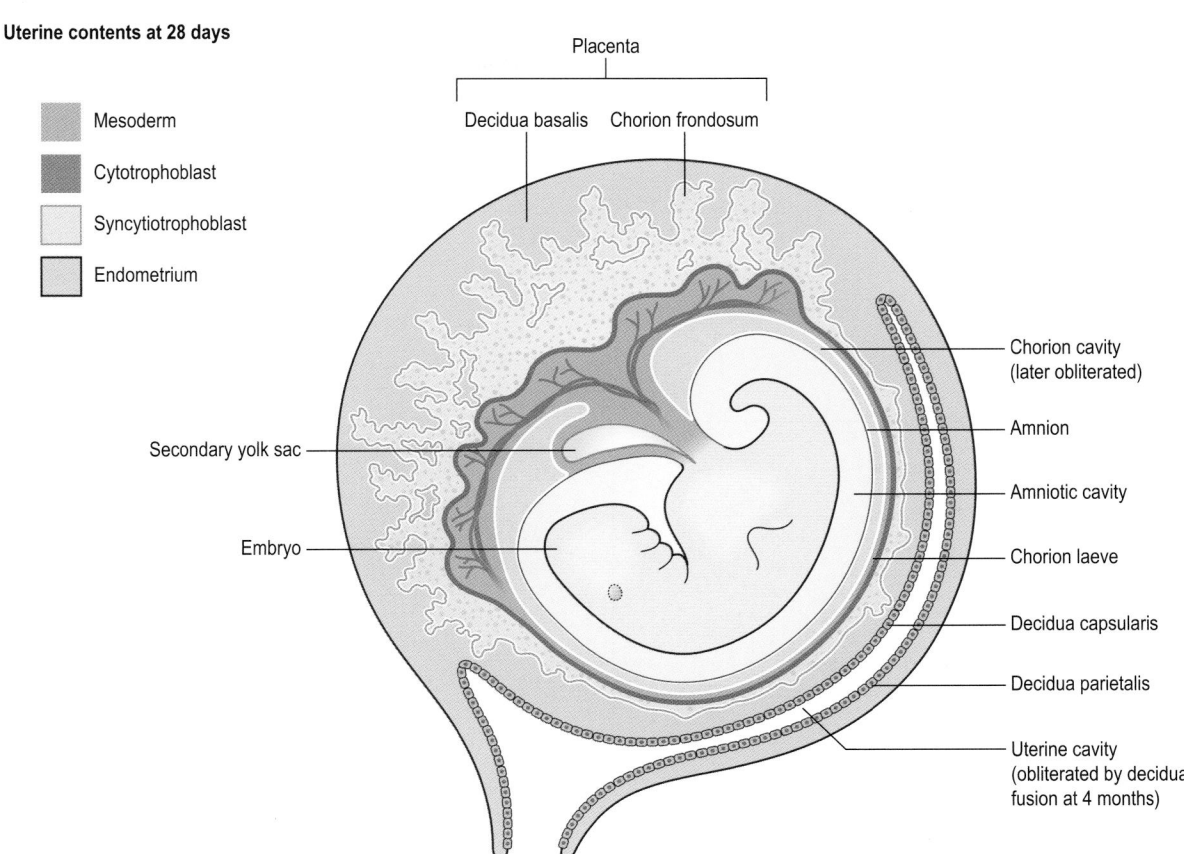

Fig. 10.21 **Uterine contents at 28 days showing the origin of the fetal membranes.**

An elongated central core of mesoderm just anterior to the primitive streak becomes the **notochord**, the first axial support for the embryo.

Neural tube formation

In parallel with gastrulation, the first steps in organisation of the nervous system are taking place, known as **neurulation** (Fig. 10.23). In response to chemical signals from the notochord, the ectoderm thickens to become the **neural plate**. This develops a midline groove that deepens, and the neural folds at the margins grow over it to form the **neural tube**, the primordial central nervous system. Neural tube formation starts in the middle at about day 23 and spreads both anteriorly and posteriorly, being complete by about day 28. Cells at the dorsal border of the neural tube migrate laterally as the **neural crest**, which gives rise to much of the peripheral nervous system.

Endoderm differentiation

While the neural tube is forming, the embryonic disc both folds laterally to form a cylinder and curls up from its rostral and caudal ends to give rise to the **head fold** and **tail fold**. The endoderm folds inwards along its length to fuse at the midline (Fig. 10.24), enclosing part of the yolk sac as a tube, the **primitive gut**, destined to become the **epithelial lining** of the gastrointestinal tract (except mouth and anal canal) and other structures.

From the anterior end of the primitive gut, the **foregut** or **pharyngeal endoderm**, various evaginations become

the respiratory tract, thyroid, parathyroid glands and thymus. The **midgut** gives rise to the liver, pancreas, and trigone of the bladder. The adrenal medulla, urinary bladder (except the trigone) and reproductive tract epithelium develop from the **hindgut**.

Mesoderm differentiation

At the same time as neurulation, the mesoderm differentiates mediolaterally into paraxial, intermediate and lateral parts.

■ The **paraxial mesoderm** becomes split by a series of transverse grooves to form prismatic blocks, **somites**, adjacent to the neural tube. This is **metameric segmentation** and establishes the ground plan for the axial skeleton and associated skeletal muscle, and for segmentation of the nervous system. Somite formation starts at about day 20, proceeds in the rostrocaudal (head to tail) direction, and is complete by the end of the fourth week. There are 40 pairs of somites: 5 that give rise to the cranium form in the region of the hindbrain; 8 cervical, 12 thoracic; 5 lumbar; 5 sacral; 5 coccygeal. Each somite has three regions:
  ■ **Sclerotome** cells migrate to invest the neural tube and notochord and go on to form the vertebrae and ribs.
  ■ **Myotome** cells give rise to the bulk of the skeletal muscles.
  ■ **Dermatome** cells on the dorsal surface of the somite form the dermis of the dorsal surface of the body.

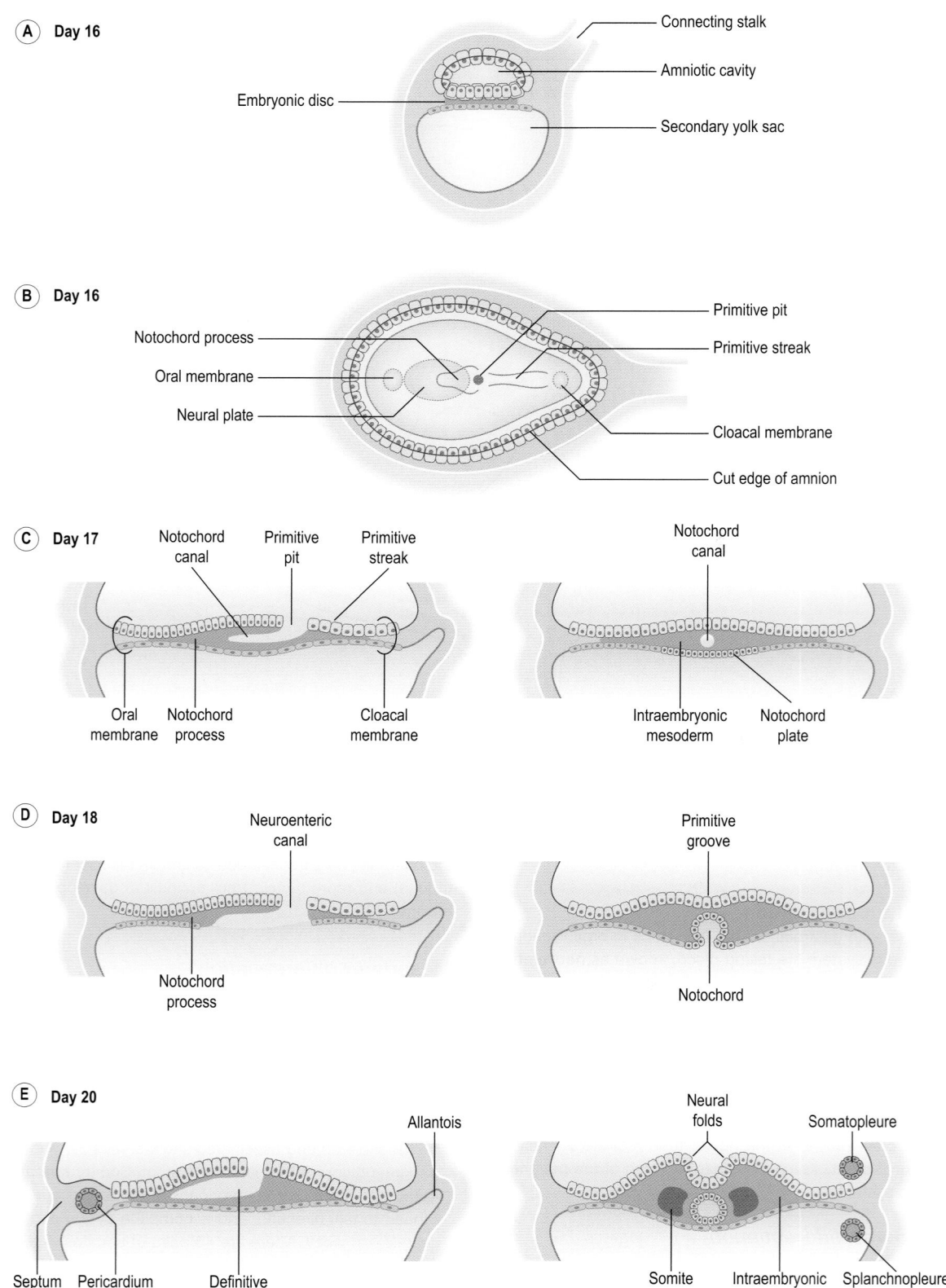

***Fig. 10.22* Early embryonic development.** (A) Day 16: dorsal aspect; (B) day 16: longitudinal section. (C) Day 17: longitudinal section (*left side*) and transverse section (*right side*). (D) Day 18: longitudinal section (*left side*) and transverse section (*right side*). (E) Day 20: longitudinal section (*left side*) and transverse section (*right side*).

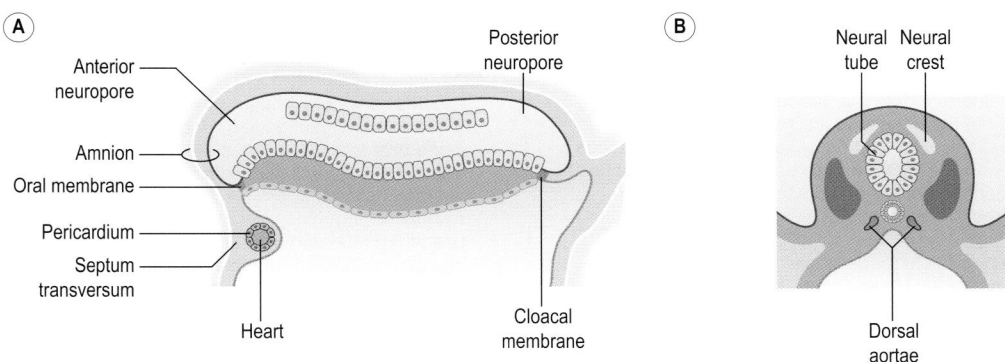

Fig. 10.23 Formation of the neural tube: (A) longitudinal section; (B) transverse section.

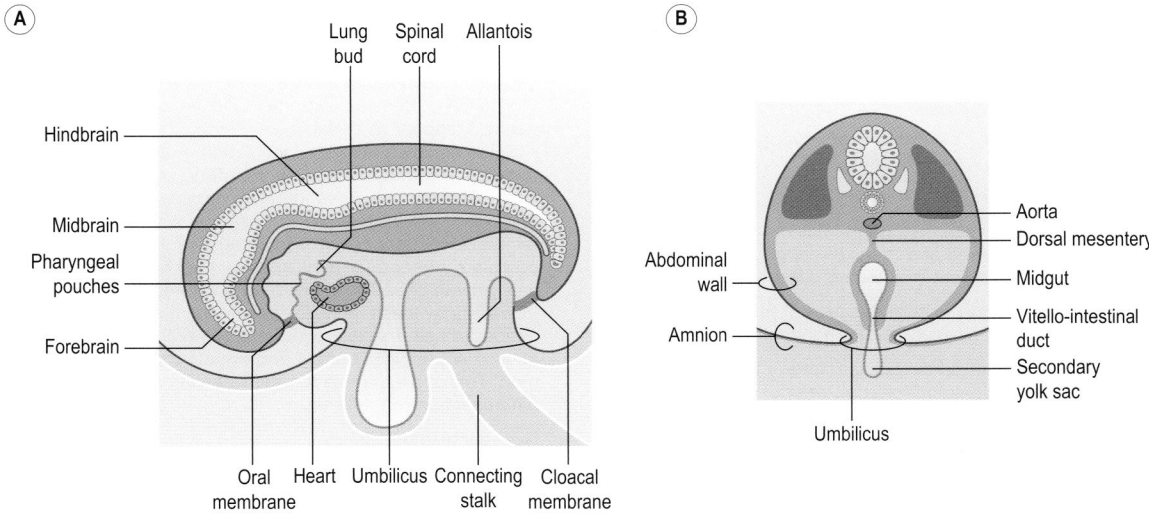

Fig. 10.24 Human embryo at day 28 (crown–rump length 5 mm): (A) longitudinal section; (B) transverse section.

- **Intermediate mesoderm** forms the gonads (but the gamete-forming cells are derived from yolk sac), the Müllerian and Wolffian ducts, kidneys, ureters, trigone of the urinary bladder and adrenal cortex.
- The **lateral mesoderm** forms two sheets, somatic and splanchnic mesoderm, lying dorsally and ventrally, respectively. The gap between these sheets becomes the **coelom**, the ventral body cavity.
- The **somatic mesoderm** becomes:
  - Limb buds that produce limb bones and some limb muscles
  - (Parietal) serosal lining of thorax and abdomen
  - Dermis (skin) of the ventral surface of the body.
- The **splanchnic mesoderm** generates connective tissues (including bone and cartilage), the entire cardiovascular and lymphatic systems, haemopoietic stem cells, smooth muscle and (visceral) serosal coverings of thorax and abdomen.

Sex determination

Sex chromosomes

The normal karyotype for female and male are 46XX and 46XY, respectively. In females, in the late blastocyst stage of embryonic development one of the X chromosomes in each somatic cell is inactivated and appears as a **Barr body** in the cell nucleus. The choice of which X chromosome is inactivated appears to be random.

Testis-determining factor

Before 6 weeks, the gonads of the human embryo have the potential to become either testes or ovaries. The signal which switches on testis development is the **testis-determining factor**, a DNA binding protein encoded by the *TDF* gene, located in the **sex-determining (SRY) region** on the short arm of the Y chromosome. Exactly how testis-determining factor operates is not known but it is thought to allow the binding of transcription factors to promoters of autosomal genes necessary for testis differentiation. In the absence of a *TDF* gene the undifferentiated gonads become ovaries.

Congenital hypogonadism

Sex cells which go on to form oocytes (egg cells) do not inactivate X chromosomes. While initiation of normal gonadal development occurs when **mesenchymal** cells have one Y (testis) or one X (ovary), its completion requires exactly one X (testis) or XX (ovary) in the sex cells. Consequently a failure of proper gonad development (**gonadal dysgenesis**) occurs

Information box 10.8 **Klinefelter's syndrome**

- Most common cause of primary hypogonadism in males.
- Usually due to a defect in meiosis (maternal non-disjunction) that results in an ovum with two XX chromosomes. Fertilisation of such an ovum produces a zygote with a 47, XXY karyotype. Sometimes meiotic non-disjunction of spermatocytes is responsible.
- One of the X chromosomes is inactivated in somatic cells.
- At puberty, afflicted individuals have:
  - High levels of LH and SHBG, because Leydig cells produce low amounts of testosterone
  - High levels of FSH, because their seminiferous tubules become fibrotic and so fail to produce sperm (**azoospermia**) or secrete inhibin.
- Abnormally high oestradiol/testosterone ratio causes varying degrees of feminisation, including:
  - Gynaecomastia (inappropriate breast growth)
  - Female pattern of hair growth.

 Information box 10.9 **Turner's syndrome**

- Is the commonest cause of primary hypogonadism in females.
- Karyotype 45, XO.
- Gonads fail to develop: although Müllerian duct structures are formed and the external genitals are female, patients do not experience puberty.
- Patients are of short stature because of the lack of oestradiol to enhance growth hormone release.
- Patients may suffer cardiovascular and/or autoimmune disorders for reasons that are not clear.

in 47, XXY males (Klinefelter's syndrome) and 45, XO females (Turner's syndrome). These are both examples of primary hypogonadism.

Sexual differentiation

By about 5 weeks after conception, the embryonic **Wolffian** (**mesonephric**) and Müllerian (**paramesonephric**) ducts have the potential to develop into either male or female urogenital tracts (Fig. 10.25).

Wolffian and Müllerian ducts

In males, by 8 weeks, the hCG secreted by the placenta stimulates the production of testosterone by Leydig cells in the embryonic gonad. The testes develop and testosterone acts in a paracrine fashion to cause differentiation of the Wolffian duct into a number of male urogenital tract components (Table 10.5). Simultaneously, Sertoli cells of the testis release **anti-Müllerian hormone** (**AMH**), a paracrine growth hormone which triggers apoptosis of the cells in the Müllerian duct, which are consequently reabsorbed.

In females, the Wolffian ducts regress in the absence of testosterone, and the lack of AMH preserves the Müllerian ducts, which differentiate into components of the female urogenital tract. The ovaries play no part in sexual differentiation. In the absence of gonads, female internal and external genitalia develop. Defects in Müllerian duct development are

 Information box 10.10 **Disorders of sexual differentiation**

Pseudohermaphroditism occurs when errors of sexual differentiation result in individuals with testes acquiring some characteristics of the female phenotype (i.e. genital tract, external genitalia and/or secondary sexual characteristics that are female-like) or individuals with ovaries having male phenotypic characteristics. Male pseudohermaphroditism includes androgen insensitivity syndrome and 5α-reductase deficiency. In females, pseudohermaphroditism most commonly arises as a result of errors in steroid metabolism, e.g. congenital adrenal hyperplasia.

Androgen insensitivity syndrome
Loss-of-function mutations in the androgen receptor gene (located on the X chromosome) in individuals with a 46,XY karyotype and (undescended) testes is known as the **androgen insensitivity syndrome** (**AIS**). The loss of androgen responsiveness varies in severity. Without any functional androgen receptors, the Wolffian ducts regress, but so do the Müllerian ducts because of the presence of AMH. Consequently, there are no internal genitalia except a short blind-ending vagina because the lower third of the vagina is not derived from the Müllerian ducts. The external genitalia appear to be female.

Since negative feedback regulation of androgens cannot take place without androgen receptors, androgen concentrations are very high from puberty onwards. The androgens are aromatised to oestrogens, which produce female secondary sexual characteristics. Hence adults with complete AIS appear female, except for having little body hair, growth of which depends on skin androgen receptors. Interestingly, these individuals have female gender identity, gender role and sexual orientation: they think of themselves as women, act like women and are sexually attracted to men. This implies a role for androgens in sexual differentiation of the brain.

5α-reductase deficiency
A deficiency of 5α-reductase reduces the conversion of testosterone to DHT, resulting in male pseudohermaphroditism. Internal genitalia develop normally because this relies directly on testosterone, but the external genitalia may be incompletely masculinised as to be mistaken for female at birth. At puberty, masculinisation may take place if there is some residual enzyme activity, because of the huge increase in testosterone concentration, accounting for the 'penis at 12' syndrome.

relatively common and result in abnormalities such as bicornate uterus.

External genitalia

The structures which become the embryonic external genitalia are bipotential. A female phenotype develops in the absence of *any* sex steroids, whereas a male phenotype requires testosterone secretion from the embryonic testis. Testosterone is not directly responsible for the differentiation of male external genitalia, but acts as a prohormone. It is converted to **DHT** by **5 α-reductase** locally. Differentiation occurs between 9 and 12 weeks. Exposure of female fetuses to androgens during this time masculinises the external genitalia, and, conversely, a lack of androgens causes incomplete masculinisation of male external genitalia. A common consequence is **hypospadias**, in which the urethra opens onto the ventral surface of the penis.

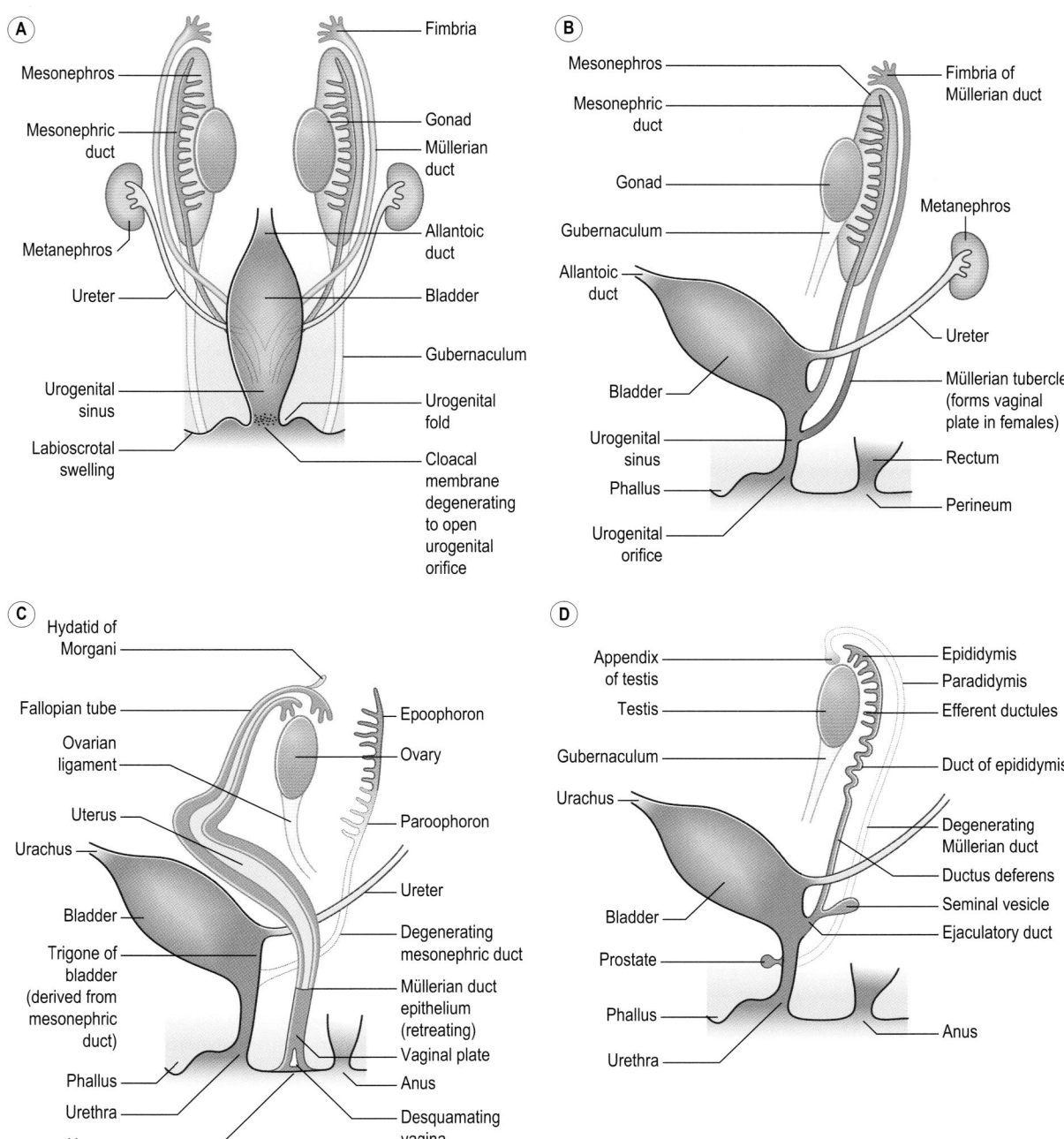

Fig. 10.25 Sexual differentiation of the internal genitalia. Undifferentiated human embryo (week 7): (A) frontal aspect; (B) lateral aspect. Differentiated state (week 12), lateral aspect; (C) female; (D) male.

Table 10.5	Fates of the Müllerian and Wolffian ducts and related structures	
Müllerian duct	**Wolffian duct**	
Appendix of testis (in males)	Efferent ductules	
Fallopian tubes	Epididymis	
Uterus	Vas deferens	
Upper vagina	Ejaculatory duct	
	Part of bladder and urethra in both sexes	

Sexual differentiation of the brain

The human brain is sexually dimorphic: there are significant anatomical and cognitive differences between the brains of women and men. Much of human sexuality is undoubtedly culturally determined, but there is circumstantial evidence to show that early exposure to androgens is, at least in part, responsible for male brain differentiation. In the absence of androgens or their receptors female brain differentiation occurs.

There are two peaks in gonadotropin (FSH and LH) secretion in early life, one in the fetus at about 20 weeks and another in the neonate at 2–3 months. The gonadotropins stimulate testosterone production in males, but the ovaries remain quiescent at these times. In males, the fetal gonadotropin and testosterone surge (no negative feedback operates in the fetus) coincides with completion of internal and external genitalia differentiation. However, the absence of either oestrogen or androgen receptors in the fetal brain at this time rules out pre-natal hormonal brain sexual differentiation in humans. The function of the neonatal testosterone surge is uncertain, but it may be the time when the male brain becomes sexually differentiated by hormone exposure.

> ### ⓘ Information box 10.11 Homosexuality
>
> Hundreds of mammal and bird species, including non-human primates, exhibit homosexual behaviour though usually it is not exclusive. The physiological basis for homosexuality is unknown. Human male homosexuality has been studied more thoroughly than lesbianism.
>
> A genetic predisposition for male homosexuality has been suggested. There is a higher concordance rate for male homosexuality in monozygotic than in dizygotic twins. A study of 200 men has shown that those who were homosexual had more homosexual relatives in their maternal lineage. Moreover, maternal relatives of homosexual men (mothers and aunts) produce more offspring than those of heterosexuals. The implication is that X-linked genes predispose to homosexuality, while boosting the reproductive fitness of women. (However, to date no genetic markers on the X chromosome linked to male homosexuality have been unambiguously demonstrated.) It also provides one explanation for the apparent paradox that genes for homosexuality have not been selected against. Other explanations for alleles linked to homosexuality surviving in the population include:
>
> - Kin selection; gay men spend more time with their nieces and nephews and hence promote their own gene survival vicariously.
> - Promotion of social cohesion: this requires that natural selection can act at the group as well as the individual level, a controversial claim.
> - Heterozygote fitness: this pre-supposes that individuals homozygous for a homosexual allele are homosexual but heterozygotes are heterosexual and that this confers superior fitness compared with males lacking the homosexual allele altogether. For example, heterozygotes may be more attractive to women (sexual selection) or produce sperm with a competitive advantage.
>
> There is a positive correlation between the probability that a man is homosexual and the number of older brothers he has. One hypothesis suggests that this is due to in utero exposure to antibodies produced by the maternal immune system to the H–Y antigen. This is a membrane protein expressed early in embryonic development, but only in males. H–Y antigen is found in brain cells and implicated in male brain differentiation. The more male pregnancies a woman has, the higher her H–Y antibody titre is likely to be, and the greater the chance that these will bind H–Y antigen in her male fetus to affect brain differentiation.
>
> An hypothesis that homosexuality is due to altered brain sexual differentiation is based on the finding that three brain structures differ in size between men and women (third interstitial nucleus of the anterior hypothalamus, suprachiasmatic nucleus and anterior commissure), and are the same size in male homosexuals as in women. It has been proposed that inadequate early (neonatal) exposure to androgens accounts for both the anatomical findings and the sexual orientation of male homosexuals.

Fetal development

At the end of week 8, all the organ systems have been laid down in the embryo. Although more differentiation continues during the fetal stage, much of the remainder of pregnancy is taken up by growth. At this stage of gestation, the embryo has a **crown–rump length** (measured from the top of the head to the buttocks) of ~3 cm. Table 10.6 shows the developmental progress of the fetus.

Fetal endocrinology

By 12 weeks, the fetal **hypothalamus** and **anterior pituitary gland** can synthesise all their hormones, although the portal circulation between them is not functional until 18 weeks. At this time, levels of anterior pituitary hormones are high because of the immaturity of negative feedback systems. Fetal growth, however, is stimulated by prolactin rather than growth hormone.

The fetal **thyroid gland** is stimulated by hCG rather than TSH from the fetal anterior pituitary or placenta, but does not become capable of secreting sufficient hormones for brain development until after 10 weeks. Until this time maternal thyroid hormones cross the placenta to provide fetal needs.

The fetal **endocrine pancreas** is competent from 15 weeks, but fetal blood glucose is regulated by the mother and placental transport. If the mother has diabetes, her high blood glucose concentration will increase fetal blood concentration, stimulating insulin secretion from the fetal pancreas. Since insulin is a growth-promoting hormone for the fetus, babies born to diabetic women often have a significantly higher birth weight than normal.

The fetal **adrenal cortex** has two zones:

- The outer **definitive zone** is the precursor to the zona glomerulosa, and a middle transitional zone that becomes the zona fasciculata, which produces cortisol, and zona reticularis, which produces precursors of sex hormones in the adult. The zona fasciculata produces cortisol from about 30 weeks. Cortisol stimulates the production of surfactant in the fetal lungs. Infants born before surfactant production is adequate suffer from **neonatal respiratory distress syndrome** (**NRDS**) (see Ch. 13).
- The inner **fetal zone**, which comprises 80% of the adrenal cortex at this stage, makes mostly dehydroepiandrosterone sulphate (DHEAS, a testosterone precursor), which is transported to the placenta where it is desulphated and aromatised to oestrogens. Fetal zone steroidogenesis starts at 7 weeks and the zone regresses in the early post-natal period.

Although the fetal **parathyroid glands** are functional from 15 weeks, the high fetal blood calcium concentration, produced by placental parathyroid hormone-related peptide (PTHrP)-mediated mobilisation of maternal Ca^{2+}, inhibits fetal PTH output.

Placenta

The **placenta** originates from both the conceptus (trophoblast) and the mother (the uterine endometrium). Its functions include respiratory gas exchange, transport of nutrients to, and metabolic waste products from, the conceptus, the pro-

Table 10.6	Developmental progress of the fetus	
Gestational age/weeks	**Crown–rump length (mm)**	**Developmental landmarks**
8	30	All organ systems laid down Pentadactyl limb plan complete Basic brain structure present (neural tube closed at 4 weeks) Optic cup has retina and lens Cartilaginous otic capsule (inner ear) in place Synchronous neuron firing established Weak spontaneous contraction of skeletal muscle Blood circulation established (from week 4) Liver production of blood cells Ossification commences
12	90	Rudimentary cerebellum Cervical and lumbar enlargements of spinal cord Cochlea developed Differentiation of epidermis and dermis Sexual differentiation of internal genitalia Notochord degenerating, rapid bone ossification Fusion of palate Endodermal-derived glands formed Smooth muscle layers of gut forming Bile secretion commences Blood cell formation starts in bone marrow
16	140	Rapid development of cerebellum Blinking Sucking Fully differentiated kidneys
20	190	Quickening (fetal movements felt by mother) Lanugo covers skin, sebaceous glands active Fetal position adopted due to lack of space
30	280	Primary gyri present in cerebral cortex Myelination of spinal cord starts Bone marrow becomes sole site of haemopoiesis Surfactant production starts (inadequate for normal ventilation) Ossification of distal limb bones starts Descent of testis complete High growth rate
40	360–400	Maximum density of synapses in cerebral cortex Subcutaneous fat deposited, no lanugo Surfactant production sufficient for normal ventilation High growth rate

duction of hormones that both sustain the conceptus and produce adaptive changes to maternal physiology. Alcohol and some prescribed drugs readily cross the placental barrier, and drug metabolism may be altered during pregnancy; this must be allowed for when prescribing during pregnancy (see Ch. 4).

Development of the placenta

The proliferating trophoblast develops a layer of **extra-embryonic mesoderm** on its inner surface to become the **chorion**, one of the fetal membranes. **Chorionic villi** project into **maternal lacunae**, spaces in the surrounding decidua, which have been eroded by the phagocytic activity of the trophoblast and are filled with circulating maternal blood (Fig. 10.26). Blood enters the maternal lacunae from spiral arteries that are highly convoluted and dilated so that pressure drops to 2–2.5 kPa. Angiogenesis occurs in the mesodermal cores of the chorionic villi and the newly formed vessels grow into the embryo as the two umbilical arteries and umbilical vein.

Early on, the embryonic capillaries are separated from the maternal circulation by a 10 μm syncytiotrophoblast layer, but towards the end of pregnancy this has shrunk to only 1–2 μm. Thus the placental barrier, formed by the syncytiotro-phoblast and embryonic capillary endothelium, gets smaller as fetal size and metabolic demands increase – facilitating oxygen diffusion.

Placental transport

Blood gases, water, urea and non-polar molecules such as cholesterol, steroids and fatty acids are transported from the maternal circulation across the placenta by passive diffusion. Transport of O_2 across the placenta is much less efficient than in the lung. This, plus a high O_2 consumption by the fetus, contributes to a steep O_2 gradient between maternal and fetal blood; maternal arterial and fetal umbilical venous pO_2 are ~12 and 5 kPa, respectively. The fetus is adapted to the resulting low oxygen diffusion rate in that it has **fetal haemoglobin** (Ch. 12) – which has a greater affinity for oxygen than the adult molecule – and high blood flow rates.

Specific transporters exist for ions, hexoses (glucose is the major energy substrate of the fetus), amino acids and water-soluble vitamins. Several large molecules are transported by receptor-mediated endocytosis (e.g. low-density lipoprotein (LDL), IgG). Towards term, the placental barrier can become leaky and allow fetal red blood cells to enter the maternal circulation. This may provoke an immune response

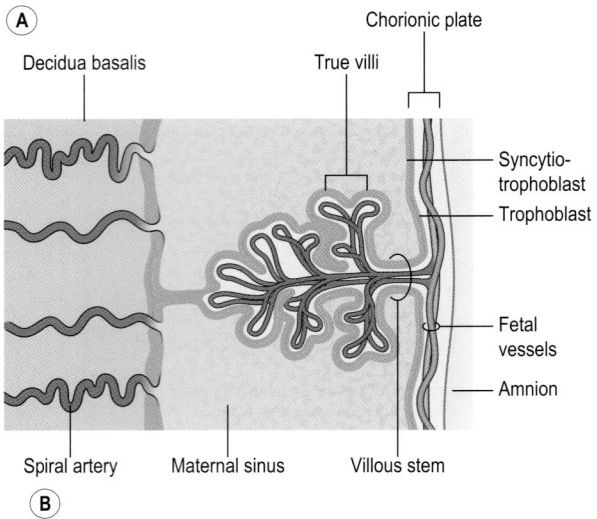

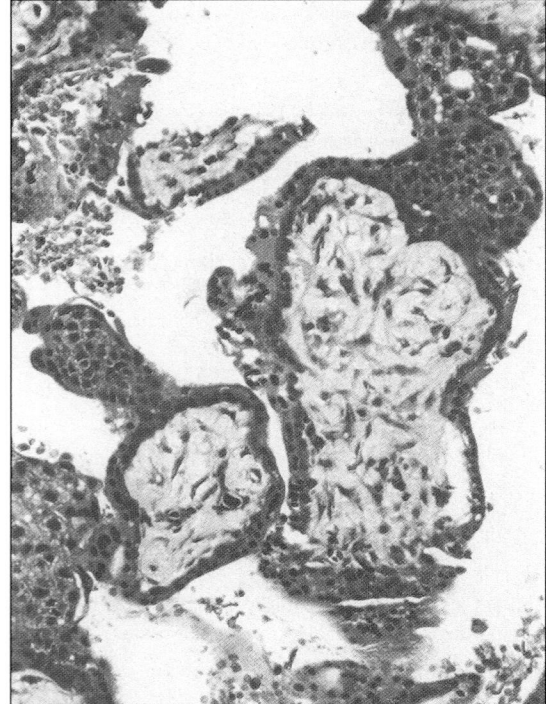

Fig. 10.26 Structure of the early placenta: (A) a chorionic villus; (B) histological section (×150) Reproduced with permission from Young B, Heath JW 2006 Wheater's functional histology, 5th edn. Churchill Livingstone, Edinburgh.

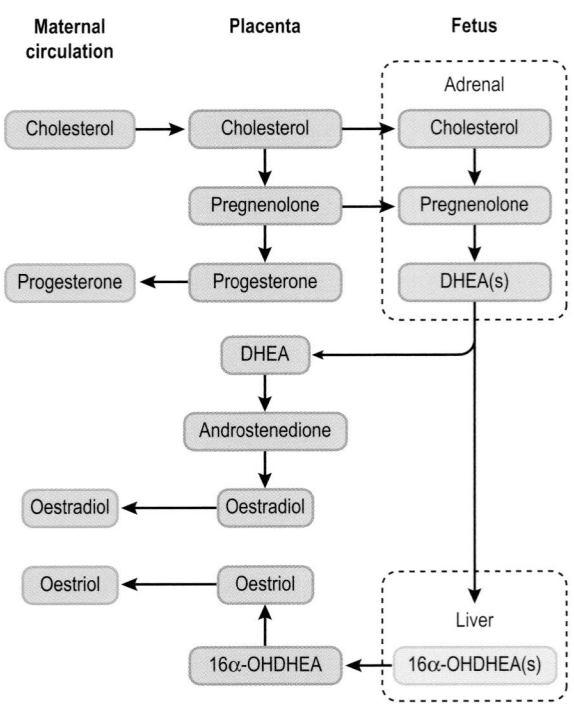

Fig. 10.27 **Steroid biosynthesis by the fetoplacental unit.** OHDHEA, hydroxydehydroepiandrosterone; DHEA(S), dehydroepiandrosterone sulphate.

against fetal antigens by the mother, for example in rhesus incompatibility and neonatal jaundice (see Ch. 12).

Immunoprotection of the conceptus

Because trophoblast cells are derived from the conceptus they contain paternal major histocompatibility complex (MHC) genes (Ch. 5) and might be allergenic to the mother. However, the expression of most MHC genes is switched off in the trophoblast. An exception is the human leucocyte antigen gene, *HLA-G* (which codes for an MHC class Ib molecule), expression of which allows the placenta to fend off attack from natural killer cells (see Ch. 6). In addition,

progesterone, among other placental products, and prolactin from the anterior pituitary, suppress maternal immune responses against the conceptus.

Spontaneous abortion

It is estimated that 30–40% of pregnancies are spontaneously aborted before 20 weeks' gestation because the conceptus does not implant or form a proper placenta. Whether this represents a failure of these processes per se, an underlying pathophysiology (such as an immune attack by the mother on the conceptus), loss of endocrine support, or is a consequence of genetic abnormalities in the conceptus, is not clear.

Hormone biosynthesis by the fetoplacental unit

Secretion of steroids by the corpus luteum falls after 8 weeks despite continuing hCG stimulation. By this stage the placenta becomes an endocrine organ, secreting the oestrogens and progesterone needed to maintain the pregnancy. In fact progesterone and oestrogen production now becomes a cooperative activity between fetus and placenta (Fig. 10.27), which together are referred to as the **fetoplacental unit**. The process is controlled solely by substrate availability, there being no negative feedback on steroidogenesis by the fetoplacental unit. The syncytiotrophoblast is unable to synthesise cholesterol but uses maternal LDL taken up by receptor-mediated endocytosis. From cholesterol the placenta produces pregnenolone. Some of this acts as a precursor for placental progesterone whereas some is exported to the fetus. The placenta lacks the P450c17 enzyme needed to cleave the C20,21 side chain to produce C19 androgens, but the fetal adrenal glands and liver synthesise and release androgens. The fetal androgens are delivered back to the placenta where they are aromatised to oestrogens.

Two mechanisms protect the fetus from the effects of the high concentrations of steroid hormones in pregnancy:

- Fetal androgens are sulphated and have low androgenicity. Without this, female fetuses would be masculinised. Furthermore, the placenta has a **sulphatase** which cleaves the sulphate moiety from the androgens so that maternal oestrogens are unopposed and have full biological activity.
- The fetal yolk sac and subsequently liver secrete **AFP** into the fetal circulation where it binds oestrogens.

Normally AFP is excreted by the fetal kidneys into amniotic fluid, but high levels are associated with open neural tube defects, such as spina bifida, and low levels with trisomy 21 (Down's syndrome). Because maternal blood AFP concentration increases with the number of fetuses and rises appreciably during the second trimester, peaking at 30 weeks, care is needed if it is to be used as a marker for abnormalities.

ENDOCRINE SUPPORT OF PREGNANCY

Hormones supporting pregnancy are provided by both the mother and the fetus.

Steroid hormones

Oestradiol acting on oestrogen receptors in the myometrium increases expression of genes for proteins that promote contractility, e.g. actin and myosin, gap junction proteins, oxytocin receptors and prostaglandin receptors. In addition, oestradiol increases fetoplacental steroid biosynthesis by stimulating placental uptake of LDL, and activating the placental enzyme P450scc to convert cholesterol to pregnenolone (see above). Since pregnenolone is a precursor for oestradiol, the oestrogen is locked into a positive feedback cycle that promotes its own synthesis. Pregnenolone is also the substrate for progesterone synthesis, and progesterone promotes relaxation of smooth muscle, opposing the actions of oestradiol. This is crucial for maintenance of pregnancy.

The major placental oestrogen quantitatively is **oestriol**, but it contributes little to maintaining the uterine contents directly because of a very high rate of conjugation and low potency as an oestrogen receptor activator. Oestriol functions to raise uterine blood flow by stimulating endothelial cells to produce nitric oxide (NO), a potent vasodilator.

Placental protein hormones

The placental syncytiotrophoblast synthesises several protein hormones that are homologues of anterior pituitary hormones (Table 10.7). **Human placental lactogen (hPL)** is structurally related to growth hormone and prolactin, having some functions of both. hPL alters maternal metabolism to make glucose more readily available to the fetus. By antagonising the actions of insulin, glucose transport into maternal cells is decreased, raising the blood glucose concentration in the mother (the **diabetogenic effect** of pregnancy, see Ch. 3). In addition, hPL increases proteolysis and lipolysis, providing more amino acids for the fetus and non-esterified fatty acids for the mother, respectively. Fetal growth is not promoted by

Table 10.7	Placental protein hormones and their homologues	
Placental hormone	**Anterior pituitary homologue**
Chorionic gonadotropin (CG)	LH
Placental lactogen (hPL)	PRL/GH
Chorionic thyrotropin (CT)	TSH
CRH	CRH
ACTH	ACTH
PTHrP	PTH
Relaxin	

PTHrP, parathyroid hormone-related peptide; for the rest of the abbreviations see Table 10.1.

GH, but by hPL, which stimulates production of IGFs (mostly IGF-II). hPL becomes detectable in maternal blood by 3 weeks after fertilisation and rises with placental growth.

MATERNAL ADAPTATIONS TO PREGNANCY

The growth of the fetus and placenta increases metabolic demand on the mother, which is met mainly by hormone-driven physiological adaptations. The gain in maternal weight during pregnancy averages about 12.5 kg, of which about half is uterus, conceptus and breast, and about 3 kg is fat reserves in preparation for lactation (see Ch. 16).

Circulatory adaptations

For a singleton pregnancy, the maternal plasma volume increases about 40% between 6 and 32 weeks' gestation by activation of the renin–angiotensin–aldosterone system. This occurs because the rapidly growing size of the uteroplacental vascular bed acts as an arteriovenous anastomosis, lowering total peripheral resistance (TPR, Ch. 11). This is augmented in three ways:

- Inhibition of vascular smooth muscle tone by progesterone
- Oestrogen activation of nitric oxide synthase in endothelial cells, increasing their NO production
- Release by placental endothelial cells of large amounts of prostacyclin, a potent vasodilator.

Reduced TPR lowers the pressure in renal afferent arterioles, triggering the release of renin. Blood volume increases because aldosterone stimulates sodium and hence water reabsorption by the kidney. The capacity of the renin–angiotensin–aldosterone system to respond in this way is augmented by the stimulation of renin synthesis by the renal tubules, and angiotensinogen synthesis in the liver by oestrogens. Healthy pregnant women maintain normal arterial blood pressure in the face of higher angiotensin II concentrations because of the efficacy of the mechanisms, listed above, that favour vasodilation.

Although plasma osmolality falls during pregnancy, there is no corresponding reduction in vasopressin secretion by the posterior pituitary gland. It is thought that the set point of the osmoreceptors falls, hence the ability to excrete a water load decreases in pregnancy and this contributes to the rise in total body water. Progesterone, hPL and prolactin stimulate erythropoiesis, but the rise in red cell mass is not enough to offset the rise in plasma volume, so red cell count, haematocrit and the haemoglobin level are all reduced. This is the **physiological anaemia of pregnancy**.

The fall in TPR leads to a rise in cardiac output, which drives increased blood flow to uterus, breasts and skin. The increase in skin blood flow allows more heat loss in the face of the rise in metabolic rate. Pressure of the gravid uterus on the vena cava can restrict venous drainage from the legs, damaging the valves in the veins and resulting in varicose veins.

Respiratory adaptations

Progesterone triggers an increase in maternal core temperature, raising metabolic rate, by effects on the hypothalamus. Oxygen consumption rises about 15% during pregnancy to meet the added metabolic demands of the growing pregnancy, and this is facilitated by the increased oxygen carrying capacity of blood. Progesterone also increases the sensitivity of central chemoreceptors to CO_2, increasing pulmonary ventilation by 40% by raising tidal volume but not ventilation

rate (see Ch. 13). This large response is needed to overcome a reduction in the rate of gas exchange in the lungs caused by changes in the alveolus brought about by oestrogens. The functional residual capacity is decreased by displacement of abdominal contents into the thorax, but tidal volume increases by using more of the inspiratory reserve volume.

Gastrointestinal changes

Energy intake needs to increase by only 1200 kJ/day by the end of pregnancy to satisfy the additional demands. Gastrointestinal tone and motility are reduced due to relaxation of smooth muscle by progesterone, the effects of which include:

- Increased transit time for food
- Gastro-oesophageal reflux leading to heartburn
- Constipation.

The nausea and vomiting that sometimes occurs in the first trimester of pregnancy is caused by the rising levels of ovarian steroids.

 Information box 10.12   **Pregnancy-induced hypertension, pre-eclampsia and eclampsia**

Pregnancy-induced hypertension
Hypertension is a common complication of pregnancy. **Pregnancy-induced hypertension (PIH, gestational hypertension)** is a rise in blood pressure in a previously normotensive woman, usually during the second half of pregnancy, occurring in about 10% of normal pregnancies. PIH probably results from modest perturbations in blood pressure control wrought by the changing hormone status of the pregnant woman and is usually benign.

Pre-eclampsia
Pre-eclampsia is a disorder of pregnancy characterised by hypertension, proteinuria and oedema. It affects 2–8% of pregnancies and it can occur from week 20. It is most common in first pregnancies, especially in woman who have had little exposure to sperm (perhaps because they are sexually inexperienced or use barrier methods of contraception) or when a woman who has had previous pregnancies has conceived by a new partner. In late pregnancy, pre-eclampsia can progress to **eclampsia** in which the underlying pathology affects the brain, resulting in seizures and possibly coma.

Pathology of pre-eclampsia
Defective placental implantation has been implicated. It is clearly a disease of the trophoblast since it is seen in **hydatidiform mole**, a condition in which the conceptus lacks an embryo, and it almost invariably resolves on delivery of the placenta. There is evidence from examining placentas from normal and pre-eclamptic pregnancies to show that, owing to failure to express the appropriate **cell-adhesion molecules**, the invasiveness of trophoblasts is defective in pre-eclampsia. The trophoblast fails to invade and remodel the maternal endometrial spiral arteries, which is necessary for the dilation of spiral arteries to accommodate the increased blood flow required by the growing placenta. This leads to poor placental perfusion, and the placenta becomes ischaemic and is poorly developed. Hypoxia, due to poor perfusion, leads to up-regulation of inflammatory mediators secreted by the fetoplacental unit. These products damage the placental and maternal vascular endothelium, leading to endothelial dysfunction. Why the trophoblast is compromised in pre-eclampsia is unclear, but a defect in the immune suppression that prevents the mother from rejecting the fetus has been suggested. Evidence for the immunological nature of the pathology includes:

- The trophoblast does not invade the endometrium so deeply and its cells suffer widespread apoptosis, just as if it were under immune attack.
- Placental vessel pathology closely resembles that in arteries of transplant organs during rejection; there is an acute atherosclerosis, triggered by reactive oxygen species, with platelet aggregation, thrombosis and infarction, contributing to placental ischaemia.

Changes in the endothelial cells of both placental and maternal vasculature increase vascular resistance:

- They produce less prostacyclin.
- Their receptors for angiotensin II become more sensitive to the peptide.
- They secrete more endothelin I, a potent and long-lasting vasoconstrictor.

Increased vascular resistance in the placenta further reduces blood flow (adding to placental ischaemia) and in the mother it results in **hypertension**. Renal arteriolar vasoconstriction stimulates fluid retention and **oedema**, and causes glomerular damage and **proteinuria**.

In severe pre-eclampsia damage to maternal vessels produces a low-grade disseminated intravascular coagulation, low platelet count (thrombocytopenia) and haemorrhages. The brain, kidneys and liver are particularly prone to injury. When brain involvement is sufficiently bad as to precipitate seizures, pre-eclampsia has become **eclampsia**, a life-threatening condition seen in 0.05% of deliveries. The fetus does not escape the effects of pre-eclampsia but may suffer **intrauterine growth retardation (IGR)** in which, because of placental ischaemia, blood supply to the fetus is compromised so that fetal growth is delayed. The infant is born with a low birthweight (small for dates), and in severe cases, may suffer brain damage.

Rationale for treatment of pre-eclampsia and eclampsia
Unless prompt delivery of the infant is a viable option, pre-eclampsia may not be easy to manage. Unfortunately many antihypertensive drugs and diuretics lower placental perfusion and further compromise fetal survival. Labetalol, a combined α- and β-blocker, is useful because it lowers blood pressure without reducing cardiac output. In severe pre-eclampsia, intravenous magnesium sulphate is given, because it reduces the risk of seizures by blocking N-methyl-D-aspartate (NMDA) receptors. Eclampsia is treated with anticonvulsants such as diazepam.

Brain adaptations

Many pregnant women report an increased sense of calm and well-being, and there are reduced neuroendocrine responses to stress in pregnancy. This may be the result of increased GABAergic inhibition caused by the direct action of a progesterone metabolite on $GABA_A$ receptors.

Neuroendocrine adaptations

The maternal pituitary increases in size by 30–50% during pregnancy, largely due to increased synthesis of prolactin by the anterior pituitary gland, and also because of increased ACTH and oxytocin production.

- Prolactin is required, together with oestradiol and progesterone, for breast development (because it does not cross the placenta, *maternal* prolactin has no effect on the fetus.)
- The increased secretion of ACTH stimulates the synthesis and release of cortisol from the adrenal cortex. The rise in free cortisol concentration that results is modest, because oestrogens stimulate a twofold rise in plasma **cortisol-binding protein** concentration, and the effects of cortisol are moderated by progesterone, which is a competitive inhibitor at glucocorticoid receptors. The rise in cortisol down-regulates insulin receptors, reducing glucose uptake by maternal tissues. This makes more glucose available to the fetus and contributes to the diabetogenic effect of pregnancy. Cortisol is probably responsible for the **abdominal striae** (stretch marks) of pregnancy because it inhibits fibroblast collagen synthesis. The rise in ACTH concentration causes **pigmentation** of some areas of skin, including chloasma (increased pigmentation of the face, in the 'mask' area), the areolae and nipples.
- Oxytocin synthesis occurs in the posterior pituitary during pregnancy and the hormone is stored because release is somewhat inhibited until after birth by mechanisms that all depend on progesterone or oestradiol. Oxytocin stimulates uterine contractions during labour and milk ejection during lactation.

Changes in thyroid status

The thyroid gland increases in size during pregnancy, and total T_4 and T_3 can double. This is not caused by placental TSH (or maternal TSH, which is held low by negative feedback) but by hCG, which has very high homology with TSH. However, the free concentrations of T_4 and T_3 do not rise much in pregnancy because oestrogens stimulate the synthesis of **thyroxine-binding globulin (TBG)**. Maternal bound T_4 acts as a reservoir to supply the fetus with thyroid hormone (see above).

Changes in calcium handling

PTHrP increases placental calcium transport from mother to fetus. The fall in maternal blood Ca^{2+} stimulates PTH output. PTH increases maternal:

- Gut Ca^{2+} absorption
- Renal reabsorption of Ca^{2+}
- Mobilisation of Ca^{2+} from bone.

These mechanisms ensure that the fetus is well supplied with calcium. When maternal dietary intake of calcium is inadequate, mobilisation of the ion from bone predominates

 Information box 10.13 **Assessing gestational age**

Human pregnancy is regarded in the UK as lasting 40 weeks, or 280 days from the first day of the last menstrual period (**gestational age**), 2 weeks longer than **fertilisation age**, which assumes that conception occurs on day 14 of the menstrual cycle, and is an approximate estimation. A study of over 400 000 pregnant women showed that the peak number of deliveries (the **mode** of the gestational age distribution) was at 283 days after the first day of the last menstrual period. A more accurate estimation of gestational age may be important because, with the assumed 280 days of gestation, a significant number of women may be spuriously regarded as late for dates, and unnecessary interventions such as induction of labour and caesarean sections may be performed. Some ante-natal screening and diagnostic tests require an accurate assessment of gestational age.

Gestational age can be assessed clinically by measuring fundal height, which is an inaccurate but convenient method. A more accurate assessment of gestational age is by **ultrasound scanning**, measuring the biparietal diameter of the fetal skull (to a resolution of 1 mm).

and may contribute to the increased risk of dental caries in the third trimester.

PARTURITION – LABOUR

Parturition is the process of giving birth to an infant. This normally occurs when the fetus has reached maturation, and involves **labour**, the process in which the fetus is expelled from the uterus. Although not fully understood, it is thought that labour is initiated by hormonal changes in the **fetus**.

Initiation of labour

Towards the end of pregnancy the synthesis of oestrogens from DHEAS accelerates, and the rise in oestrogens increases the excitability of the myometrium, which consequently engages in weak, irregular, painless **Braxton Hicks contractions** with increasing frequency. The initiation of labour is probably a result of the accumulated effect of several processes that eventually overcomes the inhibitory effects of progesterone on the myometrium. One model for triggering parturition in humans (Fig. 10.28) is that cortisol from the fetal adrenal gland provokes a positive feedback rise in CRH from the placenta which:

- Stimulates adrenal DHEAS synthesis, accelerating placental oestrogen production
- Stimulates prostaglandin synthesis by the myometrium.

Both oestrogens and prostaglandins increase myometrial contractility, and prostaglandins produce **cervical ripening**, a softening of the cervix that is a pre-requisite for cervical dilation.

Maintaining labour

Once labour has been triggered, it is maintained by positive feedback release of oxytocin from the posterior pituitary gland. This is mediated by a neural **Ferguson reflex** which is activated by stretch receptors in the cervix in response to the pressure of the fetal head (see above). Oxytocin stimulates uterine contractions. The stress of labour may help to

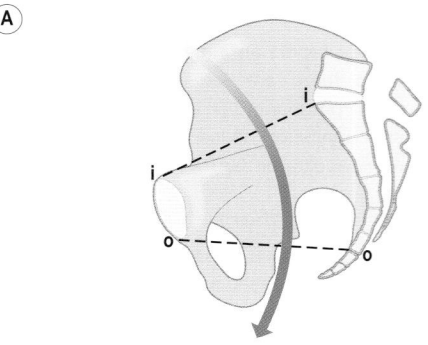

ℹ Information box 10.14   Premature labour

Premature labour, if not halted, leads to childbirth before 37 weeks' of gestation (**preterm birth or premature birth**). Infants born prematurely are at greater risk of death in the first year of life, and have a higher risk of a variety of disabilities, such as cerebral palsy, and of chronic respiratory and cardiovascular disease in later life. The shorter the gestation period the greater the risk of severe complications. In a prospective cohort study published in 2008 no infant born at 22 weeks' gestation survived. This marks the limit of extrauterine viability for the fetus with current technology.

The causes of premature labour are unknown, though several risk factors have been identified, including a history of premature labour, maternal age (under 18 or greater than 35), concurrent disease (diabetes, pre-eclampsia) and abnormalities of the uterus. Therapeutic interventions for postponing premature labour include:

- β$_2$-agonists, which cause relaxation of uterine smooth muscle
- Prostaglandin synthesis inhibitors, such as aspirin or ibuprofen
- Oxytocin receptor antagonists (see below).

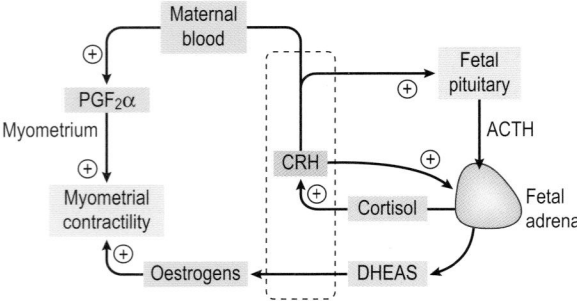

Fig. 10.28 A model for hormonal triggering of parturition. The contribution of the fetal membranes has been omitted for simplicity. PGF, prostaglandin F; CRH, corticotropin-releasing hormone; ACTH, adrenocorticotropic hormone; DHEAS, dehydroepiandrosterone sulphate.

Fig. 10.29 Dimensions of the bony pelvis: (A) midsagittal view showing the location and orientation of the pelvic inlet (i–i) and outlet (o–o); (B) anteroposterior (AP), oblique and transverse diameters of the bony pelvis.

	Diameter (cm)		
	AP	Oblique	Transverse
Inlet	11	12	13
Mid cavity	12	12	12
Outlet	13	12	11

reinforce contractions via increased sympathetic activity to the uterus and elevated concentrations of circulating catecholamines. While α-adrenoceptors stimulate contraction of uterine smooth muscle, this is tempered by β-adrenoceptor-mediated relaxation. The anxiety, pain and sometimes fear experienced by women in labour activates noradrenaline release and adrenoreceptor activation. This preferentially stimulates contractions of the lower uterine segment, leading to uncoordinated uterine contractions that are ineffective for expelling the fetus, and prolonging labour (**dystocia**, see below).

Progress of normal labour

During normal labour the fetus is propelled through the **birth canal**, formed by the fully dilated cervix and vagina, by powerful and regular uterine contractions. The fetal head negotiates the widest diameter offered by the **true pelvis** (Fig. 10.29) at each part of its journey. This journey is tortuous because the diameter of the bony pelvis varies throughout its cavity. Labour lasts for an average of 14 hours in first-time mothers (**primiparous** women) and 7.5 hours in **multiparous** women.

Uterine contractions

Initially in labour, regular contractions lasting 10–30 seconds commence in pacemaker cells in the upper part of the uterus and spread downwards. These occur at intervals of 15–30 minutes at the beginning and their frequency and amplitude goes up as labour progresses. Physiological smooth muscle contractions are not usually painful. Contractions during labour become so because uterine muscle becomes hypoxic. This is because during the contraction the pressure in the myometrium exceeds the pressure in the branches of the uterine arteries supplying the muscle, resulting in periodic ischaemia. Contractions shorten the upper uterine segment (the smooth muscle fibres do not return to their initial length at the end of a contraction) so that the lower segment thins and the cervix thins and dilates. The overall effect is to pull first the lower segment and then the cervix over the fetal head.

Once the cervix is dilated sufficiently to allow passage of the fetal head, the fetus is generally delivered within 50 minutes in primiparous women and 20–30 minutes in multiparous women. At this stage, uterine contractions occur every 2–3 minutes and each lasts about 1 minute. Because the pressure developed in the myometrium during contractions can exceed the local mean arterial pressure, maternal blood supply to the placenta is severely reduced. This leads to intermittent fetal hypoxia. Healthy fetuses are well adapted to this, providing labour is not too prolonged. Expulsive efforts are helped by engaging abdominal muscles during contractions, but are not necessary.

Bony anatomy of the birth canal

Prior to or during early labour the fetal head **engages**, i.e. it enters the **pelvic inlet** (defined by the brim of the maternal bony pelvis). This is facilitated by rupture of the fetal membranes, which allows amniotic fluid in front of the fetal head to escape from the vagina.

In most cases the **occipitofrontal diameter**, which is 12 cm across in a 3 kg fetus (Fig. 10.30A), is oriented along the **transverse diameter** of the pelvic inlet, which is 13 cm across. This is termed the **occipitotransverse** position. Because the long axis of the lumbar vertebral column is inclined at 135 ° to the pelvic inlet, one parietal eminence is lower than the other. This asymmetry causes reaction forces of the pelvic floor between contractions to rotate the fetal head as it negotiates the **mid-cavity** of the pelvis, which is 12 cm across in all directions. In 95% of **vertex** (head first) deliveries, the end result is that the occiput of the fetal skull

comes to lie anteriorly, the **occipto-anterior position** (Fig. 10.30B). This allows the occipitofrontal diameter of the fetal head to negotiate the largest (13 cm) **anteroposterior diameter** of the **pelvic outlet**.

During delivery, because the anterior wall of the pelvis is shorter than the posterior wall, the fetal head extends as it passes through the vagina. As the head is born the shoulders engage with the transverse diameter of the pelvic inlet and they rotate as they descend, just as the head did, because one shoulder (usually the anterior) leads. The shoulders negotiate the anteroposterior diameter of the pelvic outlet, and the head rotates to take up its usual alignment with the shoulders. After delivery of the anterior shoulder, the rest of the infant slips out easily.

Transition to extrauterine life

Stimulated by hypoxia and cold, the infant takes its first breath, normally within 1 minute of delivery. This requires considerable effort since it must overcome the high surface tension forces (Ch. 13) in closed alveoli. The infant's cardiovascular system flips from fetal to neonatal state (Ch. 11).

Expulsion of the afterbirth

Within 15–20 minutes of delivery under natural conditions, the placenta and fetal membranes detach from the uterine wall and are expelled as the **afterbirth** by continuing powerful uterine contractions. Umbilical vessels constrict in response to cold, damage and high levels of circulating catecholamines. Catecholamines also constrict uterine blood vessels so that maternal blood loss is generally only 200–300 mL. Loss in excess of 500 mL is regarded as **postpartum haemorrhage**. The routine intramuscular injection of oxytocin analogues immediately after delivery has reduced the risk of this potentially fatal condition. A thin layer of decidua remains and this is shed over the next few days leaving just the basal layer of endometrium.

Post-partum maternal endocrine adaptation

With the loss of the placenta, maternal concentrations of steroid and protein hormones fall at a rate determined by

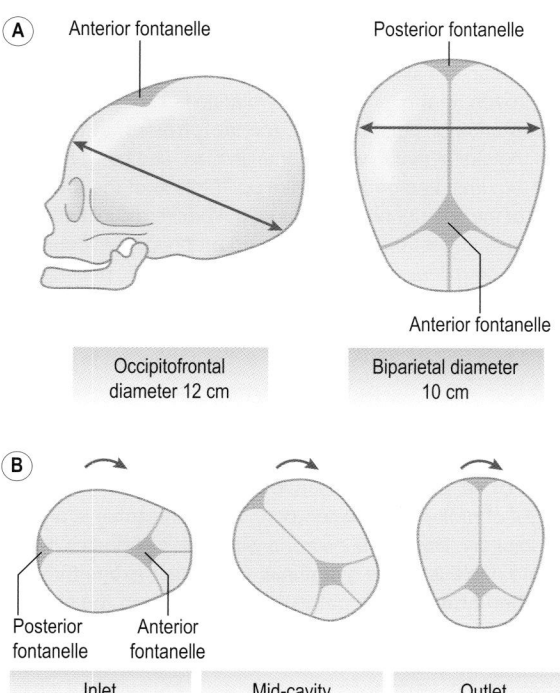

Fig. 10.30 **Fetal head during parturition**: (A) dimensions of the head that engage the largest diameters of the bony pelvis during a normal labour (vertex presentation, occipito-anterior position); (B) rotation of the fetal head during its passage through the bony pelvis (right occipito-anterior position).

> **ℹ Information box 10.15** **Dysfunctional labour**
>
> **Dysfunctional labour (dystocia)** is abnormal or difficult and prolonged labour. Uterine failure (uncoordinated uterine contractions) is rarely a primary cause of dysfunctional labour, but usually confounds other causes and contributes to prolonged labour. The commonest cause of dystocia is **cephalopelvic disproportion (CPD)** in which the fetal head and pelvic diameters are too similar.
>
> - **Relative CPD** will allow normal delivery if the fetal position is correct and the mechanics of labour work properly.
> - **Absolute CPD** rules out the possibility of vaginal delivery, but is rare in the developed world. CPD may be due to a large fetus (for example, in women with uncontrolled diabetes), constitutionally small pelvis, deformed pelvis due to rickets, trauma or congenital abnormalities, or fetal hydrocephalus.
>
> Dystocia also occurs if the mechanics of labour results in **malpositions** (e.g. occipitoposterior position caused by rotation of the head in the wrong direction as it moves through the mid-cavity), or **malpresentations**, in which the wrong part of the head (face, brow) or some other part of the fetus (e.g. buttocks) is first into the pelvis.

Feelings of anxiety and depression are very common in women for a few days after giving birth and are also experienced by some women just before menstruation. These are termed the **post-partum syndrome** (**PPS**) and **pre-menstrual syndrome** (**PMS**), respectively. What they have in common is a considerable fall in progesterone concentration. Hence it has been suggested that PPS and PMS may be the result of progesterone withdrawal. In the brain, progesterone is converted to a metabolite which acts on GABA$_A$ receptors to increase GABAergic inhibition. However, although all women get post-partum progesterone withdrawal, only about 10–15% experience PPS. Studies of PPS pregnancy hormone levels have not generally found a correlation in differences in progesterone concentration between women with and without PPS. Uncommonly, PPS involves psychosis or obsessive compulsive disorder, the underlying biology of which is not understood.

Hyperprolactinaemia is the overproduction of prolactin, and may be physiological, e.g. during pregnancy and lactation. Pathological causes include:

- Prolactin-secreting tumours, which account for over 70% of all anterior pituitary tumours (commonly a microadenoma)
- Lesions of the hypothalamus or pituitary stalk
- Dopamine (D$_2$) receptor antagonist drugs, which interfere with dopaminergic inhibition of prolactin secretion, e.g. metoclopramide, phenothiazines.

Hyperprolactinaemia causes infertility in both sexes by suppressing:

- The secretion of GnRH
- The gonadotrope response to GnRH
- The response of the gonads to LH.

their individual half-lives, restoring the pre-pregnancy endocrine state by about 72 hours. There is, however, a great fall in circulating progesterone. Progesterone is converted to a metabolite which acts on GABA$_A$ receptors to increase GABAergic inhibition (see above). A sudden fall in GABAergic inhibition may be the reason that some women experience temporary anxiety and/or depression.

Breasts and lactation

The breast consists of the mammary gland, plus adipose tissue in women. Apart from secreting milk in post-partum women, the female breast is a sexual signal and erogenous zone, and hence a determinant of sexual behaviour in both sexes.

Anatomy of the breast

The **mammary gland** of the breast consist of many **lobules**. Each lobule resembles a bunch of grapes, with branched tubules, the **lobuloalveolar ducts**, from which numerous **alveoli** evaginate. In lactating women, each alveolus consists of a single layer of secretory epithelium surrounded by capillaries and a network of myoepithelial cells. Several lobules drain into a single lactiferous duct that opens at the **nipple**. This structure constitutes a lobe. Each breast has 15–20 lobes, plus associated adipose tissue, separated by fibrous septa. The mammary glands are rudimentary in the non-pregnant state and develop during pregnancy, stimulated by oestrogens, progesterone, prolactin, human placental lactogen, growth hormone and insulin.

The breast is supported by connective tissue suspensory ligaments attached to the skin, especially of the upper part of the breast, and deep fascia. The nipple is surrounded by the **areola**, an area of skin containing modified sebaceous (Montgomery's) glands that have an oily secretion that lubricates the nipple during suckling. The ducts of these glands open in tubercles (Montgomery's tubercles) on the areolar surface. The areola becomes pigmented and darkens in early pregnancy (usually first pregnancy) in response to increased ACTH; the pigmentation is permanent. There is no subcutaneous fat underlying the areola and nipple. The base of the nipple has circularly arranged smooth muscle fibres, contraction of which causes the nipple to become erect. This is produced by mechanical stimulation generally and particularly by suckling, sexual excitement and cold.

The male breast consists of a mammary gland in a rudimentary state, although the nipple is erectile. In healthy men with a normal body mass index, it does not serve as a fat store.

Prolactin

Prolactin (**PRL**), along with oestrogens and progesterone, stimulates development and growth of the female breasts during puberty and pregnancy. In the post-partum period, prolactin is responsible for milk secretion, by activating the transcription of genes responsible for milk proteins and enzymes involved in lactose synthesis.

Prolactin is a single chain peptide that shares homologies with growth hormone and hPL. Prolactin is secreted by specialised anterior pituitary cells, the **lactotropes**, at baseline rates that are higher in women than in men, and has a half-life of 20 minutes. Lactotropes make up 15–25% of the total cell count of the anterior pituitary gland, but proliferate in response to the rise in oestrogen levels during pregnancy, accounting for the doubling of the size of the anterior pituitary in pregnancy.

Prolactin acts at tyrosine kinase receptors, which also have some affinity for GH. This class of receptors phosphorylate signal molecules, which migrate to the nucleus, where they activate transduction of specific genes.

Control of prolactin secretion

Control of prolactin secretion by the hypothalamus is primarily inhibitory. Dopamine neurons with their cell bodies in the arcuate nucleus of the hypothalamus project axons through the **tuberoinfundibular pathway** to terminate in the median eminence. Dopamine is released into the hypothalamic–pituitary portal system and carried to the anterior pituitary. Lactotropes have dopamine D$_2$ receptors, activation of which inhibits prolactin release.

Like other anterior pituitary hormones, prolactin release is pulsatile. It is also circadian, increasing during sleep. A number of factors raise prolactin concentrations including arousal, breastfeeding, breast stimulation (in women but not men), exercise, and stressors such as fear and trauma.

Oestradiol stimulates the proliferation and hypertrophy of lactotrophs and their synthesis of prolactin mRNA, accounting for the rise in prolactin secretion at puberty in girls and during pregnancy.

Treatment of hypoprolactinaemia with a D_2 receptor agonist (e.g. bromocriptine) is usually effective. Surgery may be required for pituitary tumours.

Lactation

Lactation is the production of milk, an apocrine secretion. Milk secretion depends on high concentrations of prolactin. Lactation does not occur during pregnancy because the high levels of oestrogens and progesterone render the alveolar cells resistant to prolactin. Lactation is **initiated** by:

- The rise in cortisol at parturition, which induces the enzymes needed for milk synthesis
- The dramatic fall in sex steroid concentrations at birth, which causes a 20-fold up-regulation of prolactin receptors (oestrogens or D_2 receptor antagonists can be used to inhibit lactation).

Maintenance of lactation requires prolactin. Suckling triggers prolactin secretion by a neuroendocrine reflex pathway that runs in the anterolateral columns and median forebrain bundle to inhibit dopamine secretion. The high, steady concentration of prolactin falls after 8 weeks to non-pregnant baseline levels punctuated by episodic surges that coincide with suckling. Each surge is responsible for secreting the milk that will be baby's next meal. Suckling at frequent intervals (2 hours) usually produces sufficient circulating prolactin to suppress ovulation, but this is an unreliable form of contraception. In the absence of suckling, milk secretion stops within days and the alveoli involute.

Milk ejection reflex

Milk ejection is stimulated by **oxytocin**. Suckling triggers a second neuroendocrine reflex, the **milk ejection (milk let-down) reflex**, which releases oxytocin from the posterior pituitary gland. Oxytocin stimulates contraction of the myoepithelial cells around the alveoli, ejecting milk into the ductal system of the mammary glands. It is not necessary for the infant to get a good seal around the areola or suck hard to get a feed, milk is squirted at some pressure (1–2 kPa) from the breast. The reflex can be conditioned by the sight or sound of the baby. **Catecholamines** inhibit oxytocin neurons, so that stress can prevent milk ejection, even when the breasts are full. Lactating women may eject milk during sexual intercourse when mechanical force on the cervix stimulates oxytocin release, just as it does during parturition.

Breast pheromone

Infants seek and find the nipple at least partly on the basis of smell. Immediately after birth babies are attracted to the smell of amniotic fluid, subsequently pre-feeding behaviour is triggered by the odour of unwashed breast. Hence human breasts seem to secrete a pheromone, whether in the milk, as reported in rabbits, or from the Montgomery's glands or elsewhere is not known.

Milk composition

The composition of human milk is shown in Table 10.8. A woman feeding a single infant makes about 800 mL of milk per day, with an energy content of 27 kJ/L.

Table 10.8	Composition of mature human breast milk*	
Substance	**Concentration**
Carbohydrate	70 g/L
Lactose	55 g/L
Oligosaccharides	15 g/L
Protein	10 g/L
Fat	40 g/L
Na^+	6 mmol/L
K^+	13 mmol/L
Cl^-	13 mmol/L
Ca^{2+}	5×10^{-3} mmol/L
Vitamins	
Fat-soluble:	
A	670 µg/L
D	0.5 µg/L
E	2300 µg/L
K	2 µg/L
Water-soluble:	
B_6	90 000 µg/L
B_{12}	1 µg/L
Biotin	4 µg/L
Vitamin C	40 000 µg/L
Folate	85 µg/L
Niacin	1500 µg/L
Pantothenic acid	1800 µg/L
Riboflavin	350 µg/L
Thiamine	210 µg/L
Trace elements	
Iron	300 µg/L
Iodine	100 µg/L
Zinc	1200 µg/L

*Large variations are associated with these data because milk composition varies with nutritional status, parity, period of lactation, and during each individual feed.

Carbohydrate

Lactose is the major carbohydrate energy substrate in milk. For people in parts of the world where milk continues to be drunk after weaning, the enzymes needed for lactose catabolism continue to be produced. Inhabitants of countries where milk is not part of the normal diet (large parts of Asia) lose the ability to induce these enzymes in response to a lactose challenge after weaning and become **lactose intolerant**. When they consume milk they suffer osmotic diarrhoea. The oligosaccharides have bactericidal activity.

Proteins

Many milk proteins are highly glycosylated and hence resistant to proteolysis. In addition, milk contains anti-protease activity. Hence rather than being digested, a large number of milk proteins remain intact in the infant in whom they exert specific biological activities. These include:

- **Immunoglobulins**: largely IgA but some IgM and IgG, which confer passive immunity
- **Lactoferrin** and **lysozyme**: which are bactericidal
- **Cytokines**: which boost immune responses by attracting neutrophils and lymphocytes into the milk, activate macrophages and T cells, and enhance IgA production
- **Casein**: which is hydrolysed to peptides with a number of actions including: preventing attachment of *Helicobacter pylori* to the infant's gastric mucosa; opioid agonist activity which increases pain threshold and elevates mood

- **Growth factors** and **glycoprotein hormones** (e.g. prolactin): which are absorbed from the gut to exert physiological effects in the baby
- **Digestive enzymes** such as **amylase** and bile-salt-dependent **lipase**: which compensate for the very low activities of salivary amylase and pancreatic lipase in infants at 4–6 months, when milk is beginning to be supplemented with other foods.

Fat

Although the carbohydrate and protein content of milk is fairly constant the fat content and composition depend on the mother's diet. Long-chain polyunsaturated fatty acids such as arachidonic acid, docosahexaenoic acid (DHA) and eicosapentaenoic acid, supplied by a maternal diet rich in animal fats (particularly oily fish), are crucial for neonatal brain development and are secreted into the milk even at the expense of depleting maternal reserves.

Vitamins and minerals

If maternal intake of specific vitamins is low then so is the vitamin content of the mother's milk. Vitamin supplements (particularly of water-soluble vitamins) raise vitamin concentrations in milk. The vitamin D content of breast milk is extremely low and is not much increased by giving massive doses to the mother. For this reason, babies should be allowed to sunbathe regularly for brief periods.

The milk concentrations of some minerals (e.g. iron and fluoride) seem to be independent of maternal nutrition, but others (notably iodine) depend on the mother's intake. The high bioavailability of iron in human milk means breastfeeding can supply a baby's total iron requirements until he or she is about 6 months old. This is a major factor in determining the appropriate time to introduce a baby to solid foods.

Colostrum

For the first few days, a mother produces about 100 mL/day of **colostrum**, a watery fluid, rich in the immunoprotective proteins, phospholipids and cholesterol, but poor in lactose and triacylglycerols. Hence newborn babies invariably lose weight in the first week. From about day 7 transitional milk is produced and the transition to mature milk occurs normally by 14–21 days. This slow start to mature milk secretion probably reflects an immaturity in the infant's ability to use nutrients, because milk produced by women who deliver prematurely differs from that produced after a full-term pregnancy in that the transition to mature milk is much slower. Hence preterm infants are particularly well protected immunologically by their mother's milk.

ℹ Information box 10.17   **Long-term benefits of breastfeeding**

Human milk is not only beneficial in infancy. The incidence of Crohn's disease and diabetes mellitus is lower in adults who were breastfed as infants. Preterm infants have been shown to have significantly better cognitive development at age 8 years when fed human milk rather than formula milk. This has also been reported for full-term babies. Moreover, breastfeeding reduces the incidence of breast cancer in the mother.

Oxytocin and reproductive behaviour

The presence of oxytocinergic neurons in the hypothalamus (e.g. paraventricular nucleus and nucleus of the anterior commissure) that project to limbic structures, medulla and spinal cord, shows that oxytocin is a neurotransmitter likely to be involved in more than parturition and milk ejection. Animal studies implicate oxytocin in several aspects of reproductive behaviour.

Pair bonding

Studies of monogamous **voles** shows that pair bonding appears to be facilitated by oxytocin. In **humans**, sexual intercourse causes firing of oxytocinergic neurons in both women and men. Oxytocin release becomes classically conditioned by repeatedly having intercourse with the same partner, so that eventually seeing them is sufficient to evoke release. Furthermore the neurotransmitter actions of oxytocin increase libido in women, and is predicted to do so in men. This closes a positive feedback loop which motivates a couple to stay together (**pair bonding**).

Over time, the reinforcing properties of sexual pleasure become associated with other characteristics of the partner that become secondary reinforcers. Brain imaging studies show that brain areas (e.g. anterior cingulate cortex) that are active when a woman is shown photographs of her lover (but not platonic male friends) are those that respond to oxytocin. It is currently argued that sexual and romantic love can be thought of as addictive behaviour towards a specific individual, organised by oxytocin.

Maternal behaviour

There is evidence from animal experiments (rats) to show that oxytocin may be involved in triggering maternal behaviour after parturition. At parturition, there is a dramatic fall in progesterone concentration whereas oestradiol levels remain high. Oestradiol triggers maternal behaviour (pup retrieval, licking), probably by upregulating oxytocin receptors in limbic structures. Several studies show that increasing brain oxytocin enhances maternal behaviour, while oxytocin antagonists and lesions of the paraventricular nucleus reduce it. The hypothesis is that, initially, the episodic surges of oxytocin generated by suckling trigger maternal behaviour – via the oestradiol-mediated increase in oxytocin sensitivity in the limbic system – and over time the surges come to be associated with the smell of the pups so that eventually the smell is sufficient to maintain maternal behaviour.

Imaging studies reveal that women shown pictures of their own children (but not those of their friends) engage brain areas that overlap extensively with those implicated in romantic love and oxytocin neurotransmission.

Paternal behaviour

Almost nothing is known about parenting behaviour in men, but interestingly new fathers have lower blood **testosterone** and **cortisol** concentrations and higher **oestradiol** concentrations than age-matched controls.

GROWTH

Growth can be defined as an increase in height or mass and reflects increases in cell number and cell size. Growth is also accompanied by cell differentiation and tissue remodelling in which apoptosis (programmed cell death) often plays a part (see Ch. 2). Final size and body stature depends in complex ways on genetic, environmental and nutritional factors which give rise to large variations between ethnic groups. For example, Eskimos have a short, stocky build whereas Somalis are tall and lean. These are adaptations to the climate in which certain peoples have lived for hundreds of generations.

Although a number of hormones influence growth rate, pre-eminent among them after birth is growth hormone and its downstream effectors, the IGFs.

CHARACTERISTICS OF GROWTH

Throughout life, growth does not occur evenly. Measurements of height and weight in different populations at various ages are taken to construct growth curves.

Growth curves

Humans grow most rapidly in utero, and by 1 year of age a child has reached almost half of their adult height. From approximately 1 to 10 (girls) or 12 (boys) years, children gain height at a constant rate that is the same for both sexes, at the end of which they are about 85% of their adult height. Subsequently there is a rapid acceleration in growth rate (the **adolescent growth spurt**) which lasts longer in adolescent boys than girls (Fig. 10.31) that completes normal growth. Because the growth spurt is triggered by the secretion of androgens from the adrenal glands, it is sometimes referred to as the **adrenarche**.

ENDOCRINE DETERMINANTS OF GROWTH

Many hormones contribute to growth at different times. During the prenatal period, prolactin and human placental lactogen are key players, along with a variety of growth factors such as insulin and the IGFs that are important throughout life. Growth hormone is responsible for spurring much post-natal growth, with thyroid hormone having a crucial permissive role. The adolescent growth spurt is driven by the added contribution of sex hormones at puberty, which, paradoxically, also impose a limit on the growth of long bones.

Characteristics of growth hormone

Growth hormone (**GH**, **somatotropin**) is actually a mixture of two single-chain proteins generated by alternative splicing of mRNA from a single gene. The larger form has 191 amino acids and accounts for 90% of growth hormone. Growth hormone is very similar to prolactin and hPL; there is some overlap between the activities of these molecules and all bind to members of the tyrosine kinase receptor superfamily. Because growth hormone is highly species-specific, only the human hormone can be used as replacement treatment for growth hormone deficiency.

About half of the growth hormone in blood is bound to a plasma protein that is identical to the extracellular domain of the growth hormone receptor. It is generated by proteolytic cleavage of native receptor in the plasma membrane. This protein binding serves to keep growth hormone in the vascular compartment (free growth hormone crosses capillary endothelium) and prolongs its half-life to 20 minutes. Most growth hormone is destroyed following glomerular filtration by receptor-mediated endocytosis into renal tubular cells.

Growth hormone secretion

One-third of all cells in the anterior pituitary are growth-hormone-secreting **somatotropes** and 10-fold more growth hormone is produced than any other pituitary hormone. Growth hormone secretion is pulsatile, with a period of about 3 hours, and the pulse amplitude is increased by deep non-rapid eye movement sleep (NREM, see Ch. 8). This circadian release is not light entrained and hence this phase shifts in people who work at night. Superimposed on these rhythms are brief episodes of growth hormone secretion evoked by

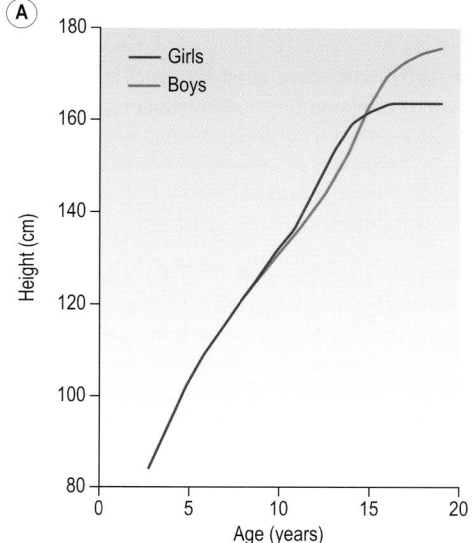
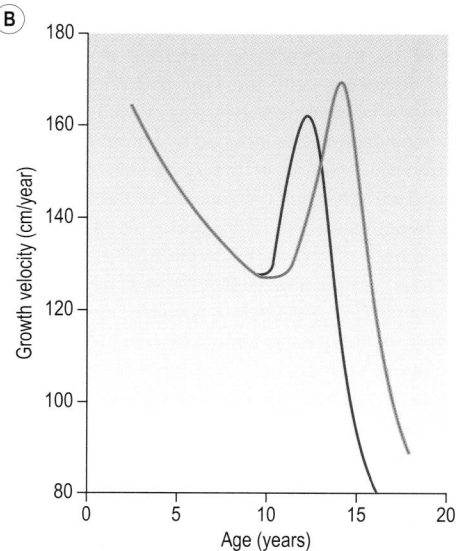

Fig. 10.31 **Non-linear growth from infant to adult**: (A) growth curves; (B) rate of change of growth; note the high growth velocity in the infant and during the growth spurt at puberty.

Table 10.9	Factors influencing the secretion of growth hormone	
Stimulates secretion	**Inhibits secretion**	
Energy substrates		
Decreased plasma glucose	Increased plasma glucose	
Increased plasma amino acids (arginine, leucine)		
Hormones		
Growth-hormone-releasing hormone	Somatostatin	
Thyrotropin-releasing hormone		
Vasopressin		
Dopamine		
	Insulin-like growth factors Hypothyroidism	
Physiological states		
Exercise		
Deep non-rapid eye movement sleep		
Puberty		
Stress	Emotional deprivation in childhood	

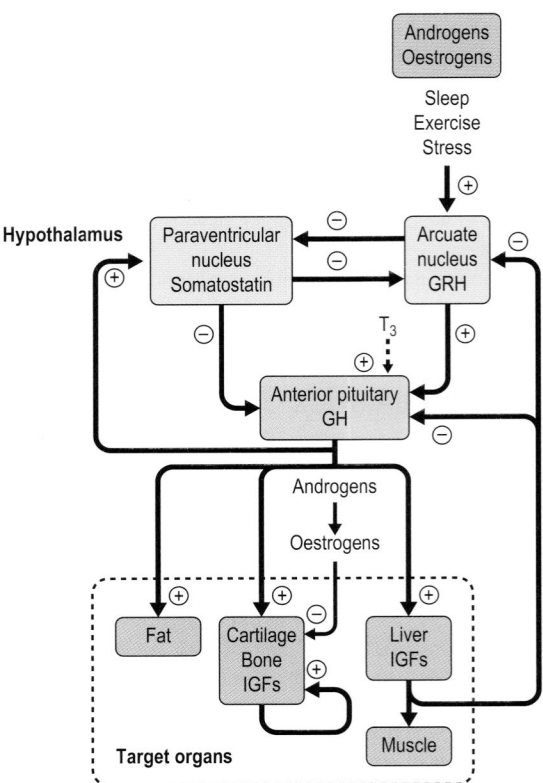

Fig. 10.32 Control of growth hormone (GH) secretion. Note the autocrine actions of insulin-like growth factors (IGFs) on some target tissues, particularly cartilage and bone. Circulating IGFs from the liver are responsible for negative feedback on GH secretion. GRH, growth-hormone-releasing hormone.

stressors, principally hypoglycaemia and exercise, but also trauma or psychogenic stress (although long-term emotional deprivation in children results in reduced GH release). A rise in the blood concentration of some amino acids, e.g. arginine and leucine, also provokes growth hormone secretion. Intravenous arginine can be used to test the ability of the pituitary to make and release growth hormone, as a safer alternative to insulin-induced hypoglycaemia (Table 10.9).

Growth hormone secretion falls fivefold after puberty, by the age of 20 years, and is one of the factors that leads to the loss of lean body mass and rise in fat stores usually seen from middle age in individuals leading sedentary lives.

Hypothalamic–pituitary control of growth hormone secretion

Two hypothalamic neuropeptides control growth hormone secretion. **Growth hormone releasing hormone (GRH)** is manufactured by neurosecretory neurons in the arcuate nucleus and stimulates both the synthesis and secretion of growth hormone by somatotropes (Fig. 10.32). Inhibition of growth hormone secretion is induced by somatostatin, which is synthesised by neurons in the paraventricular nucleus. Both GRH and somatostatin gain access to the anterior pituitary via the hypothalamic–pituitary portal blood.

Pulsatile output of growth hormone occurs because the arcuate nucleus and paraventricular nucleus have reciprocal inhibitory connections with each other and together act as a central pattern generator: bursts of GRH secretion alternating with bursts of somatostatin secretion. Growth hormone secretion is also regulated by negative feedback. IGF-I from the liver suppresses growth hormone synthesis and secretion by:

■ Down-regulating GRH receptors on somatotropes
■ Inhibiting GRH secretion by the arcuate nucleus cells.

Growth hormone exerts short loop control by stimulating the secretion of somatostatin but inhibiting that of GRH.

Growth hormone and sex hormones
Oestrogens promote growth hormone secretion by stimulating GRH release. This is the drive for the adolescent growth spurt. At first, the oestrogens are derived by aromatisation of adrenal androgens in both sexes (adrenarche). Subsequently they are produced by the ovaries in girls, or by hypothalamic aromatisation of testicular androgens in boys.

Growth hormone and thyroid hormones
Thyroid hormones are necessary for proper growth. Untreated hypothyroidism in children causes stunted growth. This is largely because T_3 is needed for somatotropes to respond to GRH. Hence a lack of thyroid hormone results in growth hormone deficiency.

Biochemical effects of growth hormone
Growth hormone stimulates growth and has other metabolic actions. It stimulates cell division in chondrocytes, osteoblasts, connective tissue, muscle, liver and fat cells, and activates transcription of specific genes within all these cells. Growth hormone also affects signal transduction by insulin receptors, reducing sensitivity to insulin (see below).

Endocrine control of long bone growth
Growth-hormone-mediated division of chondrocytes in the epiphyseal plates of long bones is responsible for growth of the shaft of long bones, which is one of the determinants for

height. Proliferation of osteoblast precursors in the periosteum surrounding the shaft causes the thickening of long bones.

The increase in sex steroids during puberty has two effects. First, both androgens and oestrogens stimulate the secretion of growth hormone. However, they subsequently act locally on the epiphyseal plates to inhibit growth-hormone-stimulated chondrocyte mitosis. Hence, while on the one hand enhancing growth, sex steroids eventually terminate long bone growth. Importantly, the influence of androgens on bone growth requires that they are aromatised to oestrogens. It is oestrogens that bring about the acceleration of growth at puberty and closure of the epiphyses *in both sexes*. This explains why people with AIS have an adolescent growth spurt and are of normal stature. It also means that girls with hypogonadism, who do not experience a growth spurt and are of short stature, can have their growth enhanced by treatment with oestrogens.

Insulin-like growth factors

The growth effects of growth hormone are not direct but mediated by two **IGFs** (**somatomedins**). Growth-hormone-evoked IGF secretion requires the presence of insulin. It occurs:

- In growth-hormone-responsive tissues (e.g. epiphyses); this paracrine release is responsible for growth and some metabolic effects, such as opposing the action of insulin
- From the liver into the circulation, from where they exert negative feedback inhibition on growth hormone release from the pituitary.

Both **IGF-I**, the predominant peptide in adults, and **IGF-II**, the chief peptide in the fetus, have a high homology with pro-insulin and bind to **type I IGF receptors** that belong to the same family of protein tyrosine kinases as insulin receptors. In the fetus the stimulus for IGF-II production is not growth hormone but prolactin and human placental lactogen.

IGFs are transported in the blood bound to **insulin-like growth factor-binding proteins** (**IGFBPs**), which confines them to the vascular compartment, or sequesters them in the extracellular matrix of connective tissues, and gives them a long half-life (~15 hours). IGFs are inactivated in the liver.

Metabolic actions of growth hormone

Protein synthesis

Growth hormone is a protein anabolic hormone. It promotes the transport of amino acids and net protein synthesis in muscle and connective tissue cells. Hence growth hormone generates a positive nitrogen balance and reduces urea production.

Fat mobilisation

Growth hormone mobilises neutral fats from adipose cells by activating **hormone-sensitive lipase**. This raises the concentration of free fatty acids (FFAs) and increases their uptake and oxidation.

Glucose metabolism

Many of the effects of growth hormone on glucose metabolism arise as a consequence of elevated FFAs which (see Ch. 3):

- Inhibit glucose uptake into muscle and fat
- Stimulate gluconeogenesis and hence glucose release from the liver.

Also, growth hormone inhibits signal transduction by insulin receptors to produce **insulin resistance**, a reduction in sensitivity to insulin. Clearly the overall effect is to increase blood glucose concentration, the **diabetogenic effect** of growth hormone. Excess growth hormone secretion over time may lead to diabetes mellitus, as insulin response to high blood glucose concentrations falls.

Growth hormone in starvation and stress

In hypoglycaemia, growth hormone secretion is stimulated (above) but insulin secretion falls. Growth hormone cannot evoke IGF secretion *without* insulin; hence, in **starvation** (defined as fasting for longer than 24 hours) IGF production is inhibited – even though growth hormone levels are high – because insulin concentrations are low. This is adaptive because it means that in lean times, metabolic resources are not squandered on growth. The effect of growth hormone on fat cells is direct (adipocytes lack IGF receptors), so in starvation the blood concentration of FFAs is raised, and consequently so is blood glucose (see above), and these energy substrates can be harnessed for immediate energy needs. In **stress**, growth hormone secretion is elevated but insulin secretion is inhibited by sympathetic activity on the endocrine pancreas, similar to the pattern seen in starvation.

Not surprisingly long-term **under-nutrition** in children, like that seen in developing countries, stunts growth. Growth is also suppressed in protein-poor diets, even when energy intake is adequate, because growth hormone secretion is suboptimal when blood amino acid concentrations are low.

Disorders of growth

Growth in childhood can be compromised by a wide variety of factors including: lack of growth hormone function, hypothyroidism, congenital adrenal hyperplasia, diabetes mellitus and vitamin D deficiency. Emotional deprivation in childhood is associated with low growth, probably by lowering growth hormone output.

THYROID GLAND

The thyroid gland is the source of two hormones derived by the iodination of tyrosine residues. The iodine for the synthesis of thyroid hormones is supplied in the diet. Thyroid hormones increase basal metabolic rate and enhance the actions of catecholamines.

Anatomy

Gross anatomy

The thyroid gland is a saddle-shaped structure that straddles the trachea, just below the larynx.

Gross anatomy

The thyroid gland has right and left lateral lobes, both being attached to a central isthmus. It lies closely attached to and in front of the upper trachea and thyroid cartilage, so that it moves on swallowing. It has a copious blood supply. The **superior thyroid artery** on each side supplies the upper half

Information box 10.18 | **Growth hormone deficiency – dwarfism**

A lack of growth hormone after closure of the epiphyses has no effect on growth, but may be a cause of a syndrome in adults characterised by hypoglycaemia, increased body fat/lean ratio and muscle weakness.

Pituitary dwarfism is due to deficits in growth hormone secretion during childhood. It may be associated with lack of other anterior pituitary hormones, such as gonadotropins and therefore hypogonadism. Pituitary dwarfs are normal at birth and grow rapidly in the first few months. By about 1 year growth rate drops and, if untreated, their final height is about 1.2 m. Pituitary dwarfs have disproportionately small maxillary and mandibular bones, short limbs and juvenile distribution of body fat. Their metabolic disturbances are quite predictable from the known effects of growth hormone and include fasting hypoglycaemia, low blood insulin concentrations, with increased insulin sensitivity.

Apart from accidents that result in panhypopituitarism, pituitary dwarfism can arise from genetic defects in the synthesis or secretion of growth hormone, or IGFs, or low target cell responsiveness. Autosomal recessive growth hormone deficiency results from lack of, or loss-of-function mutations on, the growth hormone gene. **Laron dwarfs** have a genetic defect in the expression of growth hormone receptors. These individuals have high circulating concentrations of growth hormone, but no IGFs. **African pygmies** have a blunted rise in IGF-I at puberty (IGF-II concentrations are normal) probably because of a loss of functional mutation of the growth hormone receptor gene.

Deficient growth hormone production can be assayed by measuring:

- Growth hormone release during deep NREM
- Growth hormone secretion in response to intravenous arginine
- Response to L-dopa (which mimics the physiological release of growth hormone by dopamine)
- The response to insulin-induced hypoglycaemia (but this carries a risk of hypoglycaemic seizures, coma and death).

Treatment of growth hormone deficiency is by replacement with **human growth hormone (hGH)** synthesised using recombinant DNA biotechnology. Laron dwarfs will not, of course, respond to growth hormone replacement.

Information box 10.19 | **Growth hormone excess**

Gigantism

An excess of growth hormone in childhood results in **gigantism** in which an individual grows to be exceptionally tall. It is associated with glucose intolerance, high circulating insulin levels and cardiac hypertrophy (since growth hormone stimulates the growth of viscera).

Acromegaly

If growth hormone excess continues, or does not occur until after closure of the epiphyses, the consequence is **acromegaly** (acro, extremity; megaly, enlargement). Growth can only occur as a result of stimulating osteoblasts in the periosteum, consequently there is no increase in height, but there is a characteristic thickening of cranium, maxilla, mandible, and the bones of the feet and hands. Growth hormone also stimulates chondrocytes at the costochondral junctions of the ribs, so the thorax enlarges. Growth hormone excess is usually due to growth-hormone-secreting pituitary tumours.

of the gland, usually emerging from the external carotid artery just superior to its origin. The **inferior thyroid artery** is a branch of the **thyrocervical trunk**, itself a branch of the first part of the subclavian artery. The inferior thyroid artery also supplies the four parathyroid glands embedded in the posterior aspect of the thyroid gland. A venous plexus on the surface of the thyroid drains via the thyroid veins into the internal jugular and brachiocephalic veins.

The thyroid has sympathetic and parasympathetic nerve supply from the cervical ganglia and vagus nerve, respectively. Sympathetic activity increases blood flow and probably hormone secretion also, while parasympathetic activity has the reverse effects. The **recurrent laryngeal nerve** is a branch of the vagus that ascends deep to the common carotid artery, in a groove between the trachea and oesophagus, to supply all the laryngeal muscles except the cricothyroid. Swelling of the thyroid or thyroidectomy may damage this nerve, paralysing the vocal cord on the damaged side and reducing the voice to a whisper.

Microanatomy

The thyroid consists of numerous roughly spherical **follicles** 50–500 μm across (Fig. 10.33). Each consists of a single layer of secretory epithelium that is cuboidal normally, but columnar in highly stimulated, or squamous in quiescent, glands. Occupying the lumen of the follicle is **colloid**, consisting of the high relative molecular mass (660 kD) glycoprotein **thyroglobulin (TG)**, with a large number of tyrosyl residues. Iodination of some of these tyrosyl residues in situ is the starting point for the synthesis of the thyroid hormones. In the stroma outside the follicles are **parafollicular (C)** cells that make calcitonin, and blood vessels.

Thyroid hormones

There are two **thyroid hormones**, **triiodothyronine (T_3)** and **thyroxine (T_4)** that differ chemically only in the number of iodide residues they possess. The thyroid gland also produces calcitonin, concerned with endocrine control of calcium homeostasis.

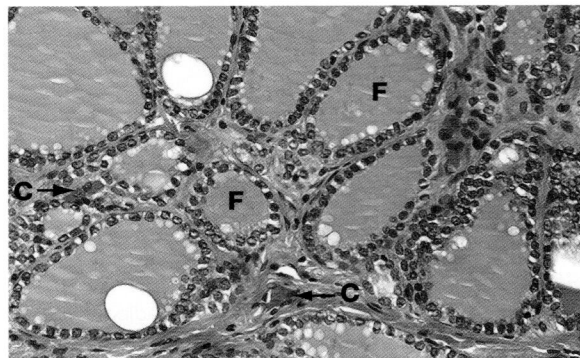

Fig. 10.33 Histology of the thyroid gland (×150). F, follicles containing thyroglobulin; C, capillaries with highly eosinophilic (*pink-stained*) red blood cells. Reproduced with permission from Young B, Heath JW 2006 Wheater's functional histology, 5th edn. Churchill Livingstone, Edinburgh.

Biochemistry

About 90% of thyroid hormone is T_4. Thyroxine has a lower affinity for thyroid hormone receptors than T_3, and is regarded as a **prohormone**. T_4 is converted to T_3 by thyroid hormone-responsive cells in target tissues, so most of the biological effects of thyroid hormones are due to T_3.

Iodide trapping

Circulating iodide is taken into follicular cells by an **iodide pump** (an iodide-Na^+ symport) in the basolateral membrane (Fig. 10.34). The thyroid uptake of iodide (~75 μg/day) is regulated by the amount of thyroid hormone synthesised. The cation pump normally responsible for maintaining the sodium gradient in cells (Na^+/K^+-ATPase) provides the energy for the iodide uptake against a large concentration gradient (iodide concentration may be as much as 250-fold higher in follicular cells than in blood). The iodide diffuses out of the follicular cell through its apical membrane via a carrier-mediated transporter, **pendrin**.

Thyroid hormone synthesis

Within the follicle lumen the iodide is used to iodinate tyrosine residues in thyroglobulin (TG), a process termed **organification**. Only 10% of the 132 tyrosyl residues in each TG

dimer are accessible for iodination. Two transmembrane enzymes in the apical border of the follicular cells are required for the iodination. **Thyroid oxidase** generates hydrogen peroxide (H_2O_2). This is a substrate for **thyroid peroxidase (TPO)** which catalyses the oxidation of the iodide to a reactive intermediate, a necessary step for tyrosyl iodination, also catalysed by TPO. The initial result is TG with monoiodotyrosyl (MIT) and diiodotyrosyl (DIT) residues. Normally, more DIT residues are synthesised than MIT, but when dietary iodide is scarce the ratio is reversed. The TPO subsequently catalyses **coupling reactions** in which ether linkages are made between two close DITs (or one DIT and one MIT) moieties to yield a T_4 (or a T_3) substituent. Only 20% of DIT and MIT residues take part in coupling (those near the ends of the TG molecules), the remainder serve as an iodide store that can be recycled for thyroid hormone synthesis (see below).

---

i Information box 10.20   Thyroid imaging

The thyroid gland can be imaged by ultrasound or by radionuclide scanning after administration of I^{125}. The maximum uptake of I^{125} by the thyroid (after 18–24 hours) is a measure of thyroid function; it is high and low in hyper- and hypothyroidism, respectively. However, it can also be low in thyroid hormone overdose (often deliberate in individuals attempting to lose weight), excessive iodide ingestion (e.g. seaweed in Japanese cuisine, radio-opaque dyes) or ectopic thyroid hormone production.

---

i Information box 10.21   Wolff–Chaikoff block

The Wolff–Chaikoff block, or effect, is the inhibition of iodide organification and thyroid hormone synthesis by high doses of iodine. In most cases, the effect is transient, and the normal thyroid escapes from this block after about two weeks. In susceptible individuals, however, the effect can result in iodine myxoedema (see below). Iodide administration therefore has a place in the short-term treatment of hyperthyroidism, for example during preparation for thyroid surgery. The thyroid gland is highly sensitive to radioactive isotopes of iodine because of its selective uptake and concentration of iodine, which carries a high risk of thyroid cancer. It is possible to exploit the Wolff–Chaikoff effect to block the uptake of radioactive iodine (e.g. in the event of a nuclear accident) by giving large doses of non-radioactive iodide prophylactically to people at risk of exposure to radioactive iodine, thereby reducing the risk of subsequent thyroid cancer.

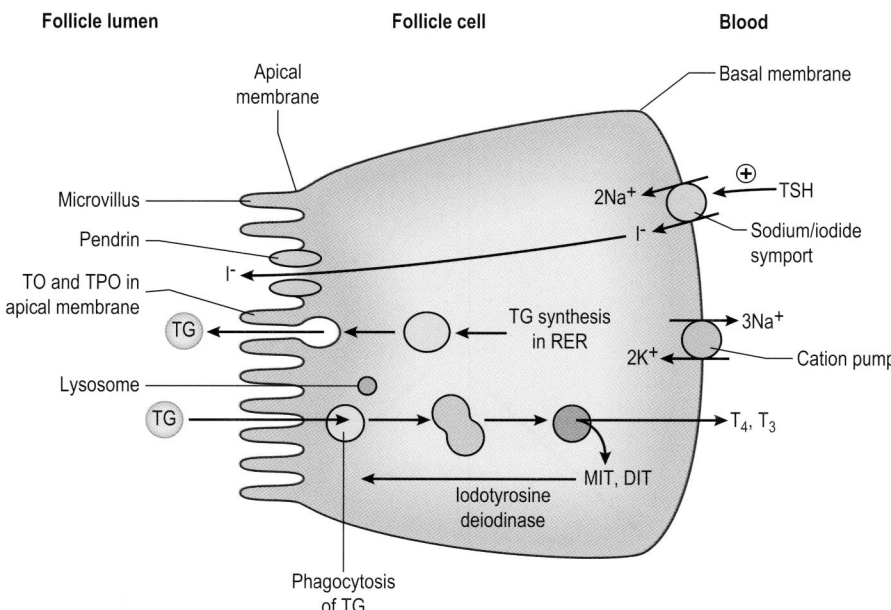

Fig. 10.34 Outline of thyroid hormone synthesis by follicle cells: TO, thyroid oxidase, and TPO, thyroid peroxidase, are responsible for iodination of tyrosyl residues in TG (thyroglobulin) and coupling reactions. MIT, monoiodotyrosyl; DIT, diiodotyrosyl; RER, rough endoplasmic reticulum; TSH, thyroid stimulating hormone.

Storage of thyroid hormone

Thyroglobulin is synthesised by follicular cells and secreted into the follicular lumen. This protein, which comprises about 30% of the mass of the thyroid gland, acts as an extracellular store of thyroid hormone sufficient for 2–3 months. About 90% of the body's entire iodide pool is in the thyroglobulin DIT and MIT residues that do not undergo coupling.

Secretion of thyroid hormone

Thyroglobulin is taken into follicular cells by endocytosis and packaged into lyso-endosomes where it is degraded into peptides, free amino acids, T_4, T_3, DIT and MIT (see Fig. 10.34). Of these, only the T_4 and T_3 are secreted into the circulation. The DIT and MIT residues are deiodinated by microsomal tyrosine deiodinases and the liberated iodide is recycled for the iodination of thyroglobulin. This recycling is important because it provides twice as much iodide for hormone synthesis as the iodide pump. Genetic deficiency of microsomal deiodinases, characterised by the abnormal urinary excretion of DIT and MIT, causes the same effects as dietary iodide deficiency.

Transport of thyroid hormone

Three plasma proteins bind thyroid hormones. **Thyroxine-binding globulin (TGB)**, **transthyretin (TTR, thyroxine-binding prealbumin)** and albumin. Of these TGB is quantitatively the most important because, despite being present in only small amounts, it has a high affinity for the hormones. An equilibrium is established between the various bound forms, which leaves only 0.04% of T_4 and 0.4% of T_3 free. Because T_3 is bound with lower affinity than T_4 it diffuses more rapidly from capillaries into cells, and hence exerts its effects more quickly; it also has a shorter half-life – 1 day, compared with 6 days for T_4. Bound thyroid hormone is a substantial reservoir (it represents about 3 days turnover) which can buffer short-lived reductions in secretion. Because the plasma proteins are nowhere near saturated, even big temporary increases in thyroid hormone secretion will have no effect on free concentrations.

Thyroxine-binding globulin levels are increased by oestrogens, and hence are raised in pregnancy and in women taking oestrogen-containing oral contraceptives. By contrast, androgens and glucocorticoids decrease TBG concentrations.

Thyroid hormone metabolism

Thyroxine is deiodinated by three enzymes (Fig. 10.35):

- **Type I deiodinase (DI)**: this is mainly found in liver and kidney, and can remove an iodide from either the outer (phenolic) ring of T_4 to give the more active T_3, or catalyse inner (tyrosyl) ring deiodination to yield the inactive **reverse triiodothyronine (rT$_3$)**. This enzyme is responsible for generating most circulating T_3.
- **Type II deiodinase (DII)**: this catalyses outer ring deiodination, and is present in many target tissues (including brain and pituitary) and is responsible for supplying local demand for T_3. DII activity is regulated by hormones; it is expressed more highly when blood T_4 concentrations are low.
- **Type III deiodinase (DIII)**: this is also found in target tissues and catalyses inner ring deiodination to give rT$_3$.

The relative activities of the DII and DIII enzymes clearly determine how much free T_4 ends up as active hormone (T_3) in tissues. If DII activity falls, T_3 concentration drops. This is seen during starvation and debilitating illness and may be a way in which metabolic rate is decreased in these states to conserve energy substrates.

T_3 and rT$_3$ are successively deiodinated to diiodothyronine, monoiodothyronine and finally thyronine. All of these metabolites are inactive and excreted in urine.

Hypothalamic–pituitary–thyroid axis

Neurons in the anterior hypothalamus produce **TRH**, which is released into the hypothalamic–pituitary–portal system. TRH evokes the synthesis of **TSH** by **thyrotropes** in the anterior pituitary, by increasing its transcription and post-translational processing. TRH also increases the secretion of TSH. TSH, a glycoprotein that resembles the gonadotropins, stimulates the growth of the thyroid gland and its synthesis of thyroid hormones, probably by increasing the activities of

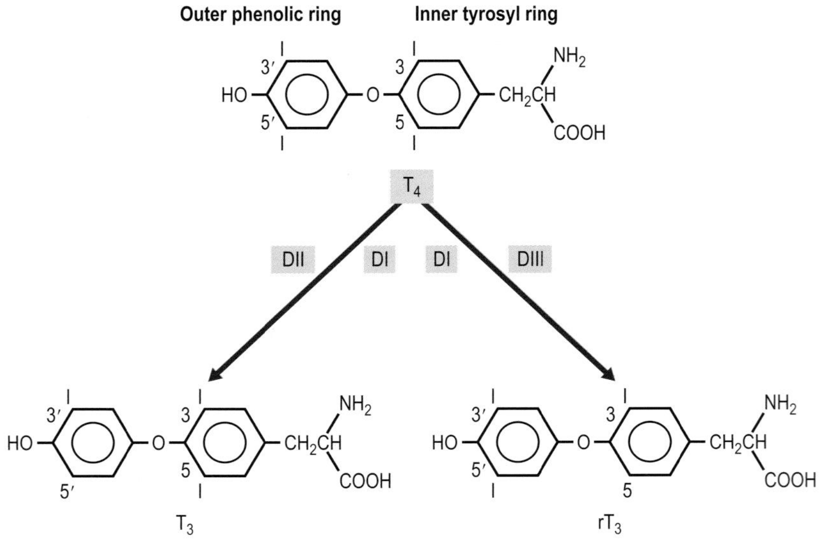

Fig. 10.35 **Deiodination of thyroxine (T$_4$).** DI, type I deiodinase; DII, type II deiodinase; DIII, type III deiodinase.

the iodide pump and thyroid peroxidase secretion. The hypothalamic–pituitary–thyroid axis is activated by cold exposure and suppressed by stress.

Control of thyroid hormone secretion

Negative feedback operates at the level of the anterior pituitary and hypothalamus. At the anterior pituitary, circulating T_4 is deiodinated by DII in the thyrotropes and the T_3 released decreases TSH synthesis and secretion. The TSH response to intravenous injection of TRH can be used to distinguish between:

- Primary (thyroid) hyperthyroidism
- Secondary (anterior pituitary) hyperthyroidism
- Tertiary (hypothalamic) hypothyroidism.

If the defect lies in the thyroid gland, baseline TSH levels are high because of the lack of feedback, and TRH evokes a robust and rapid secretion of TSH. This response is completely lacking in the case of secondary hypothyroidism. In hypothalamic hypothyroidism, TSH is released in response to TRH but the secretory response in blunted and slower than that seen in primary hypothyroidism. The great majority of disorders of the hypothalamic–pituitary–thyroid axis are primary, i.e. they are due to dysfunction of the thyroid gland.

Actions of thyroid hormones

Thyroid hormone receptors

Thyroid hormones are transported across the plasma membrane by several organic anion and amino acid transporters. **Thyroid hormone receptors** (**THRs**) are members of the steroid receptor superfamily (Ch. 4), and have a much higher affinity for T_3 than T_4. Unlike most other nuclear receptors they bind their cognate response elements (**thyroid hormone response elements**, **TREs**) in gene promoters in the *absence* of ligand. THRs bind either as monomers, homodimers or heterodimers (usually with **retinoid X receptors**), and act as transcription factors, altering the expression of specific genes (see Ch. 5).

 Information box 10.22   **Goitre**

A **goitre** is an enlarged thyroid gland. Goitre may be **diffuse**, where the swelling is uniform throughout the gland, or **nodular** where the swelling is patchy. When it occurs in the presence of low or normal thyroid hormone levels it is said to be **non-toxic goitre**. **Toxic goitre** is found in conjunction with elevated thyroid hormone levels and is typically seen in patients with Graves' disease (see below).

Worldwide, diffuse non-toxic goitre is usually caused by dietary iodide insufficient for normal thyroid hormone production giving rise to borderline hypothyroidism. This leads to excessive TSH production, stimulating thyroid enlargement. **Endemic goitre** is common in mountainous areas (northern India, Central Africa, Chile, Peru, the Alps in Europe, and parts of Indonesia). People with goitre may be hypothyroid or euthyroid. Women living in 'endemic goitre' regions are at high risk of giving birth to infants with cretinism. The simple expedient of making iodised table salt cheaply available to these women solves this problem, as recommended by the World Health Organization.

Ingestion of substances which inhibit iodide trapping (**goitrogens**) also cause diffuse non-toxic goitres. These include anions such as thiocyanate, which are present in large amounts in some vegetables (e.g. cassava and cabbage), and certain drugs, e.g. sulphonylureas and lithium.

Two genes (**THRA** and **THRB**) encode thyroid hormone receptors and alternative splicing of each gene product gives rise to four THR isoforms. Three isoforms ($TR\alpha_1$, $TR\beta_1$ and $TR\beta_2$) bind T_3, but $TR\alpha_2$ does not. The $TR\beta_2$ isoform is highly expressed in the brain and anterior pituitary and mediates the negative feedback effects of T_3. Mutations which silence the *THRB* gene cause **thyroid hormone resistance**. Affected individuals have very high T_4, T_3 and TSH concentrations, and goitre, because of the lack of feedback. Tissues expressing the $TR\alpha_1$ receptor isoform (e.g. heart, bone) are over-stimulated, resulting in a chimera for hyperthyroidism (partial hyperthyroidism).

Selective gene knockout experiments in mice show that loss of the $TR\alpha_2$ isoform is lethal, so it appears to be a critical transcription factor. Loss of any one of the isoforms that bind T_3 produces only modest symptoms of hypothyroidism, but combined absence of all produces more severe hypothyroidism, so these THRs appear to have overlapping functions. However, the symptoms are mild compared with those of animals with normal receptors but no thyroid hormone. It is thought that the normal role of THRs is to silence genes and T_3 binding suppresses their expression. So this form of hypothyroidism is a failure to release genes from the brake imposed by THR binding, and is worst when there are receptors but no hormone.

Effects on sympathetic transmission

Thyroid hormones enhance the effect of catecholamines at least in part by upregulating β-adrenoceptors. This is responsible for many of the metabolic and physiological effects of thyroid hormones.

Regulation of basal metabolic rate

Thyroid hormones raise the basal metabolic rate (BMR) in all tissues except adult brain, testis and spleen. This can be measured by an increase in oxygen consumption and results in a rise in heat production, the **calorigenic effect** of thyroid hormones (see Ch. 16). This action of thyroid hormones is important in long-term adaptation to cold. Since the metabolic actions of thyroid hormones responsible for the rise in BMR have latencies of several hours, these hormones cannot help adjust to brief periods of cold exposure. Cold exposure in adult humans does not cause a rise in TSH output. However in many cells the rise in cAMP that accompanies the sympathetic activity induced by cold stress activates DII deiodinase and hence enhances the conversion of T_4 to T_3.

Biochemistry of BMR regulation by thyroid hormones

Broadly speaking the increase in BMR occurs in the following ways:

- Thyroid hormones frequently activate both anabolic and catabolic metabolic processes so as to produce futile cycling.
- Thyroid hormones increase the number and activity of Na^+/K^+-ATPase molecules. Every time ATP is split in metabolic reactions, or in driving the cation pump, some heat is produced.
- By upregulating the activity of **uncoupling proteins** (**UCPs**, **thermogenins**) thyroid hormones uncouple oxidative phosphorylation so that the proton flux through the inner mitochondrial membrane is used to generate heat rather than synthesise ATP. This method of heat

ⓘ **Information box 10.23**   **Hyperthyroidism**

Hyperthyroidism is overactivity of the thyroid gland. Many of the consequences of exposure to excess thyroid hormone – **thyrotoxicosis** – are related to the physiological effects of the hormones.

Graves' disease
The commonest form of hyperthyroidism is **Graves' disease**, an autoimmune disorder in which naïve T helper lymphocytes (Th2 cells) are inappropriately primed to recognise TSH receptors on thyroid follicle cells. The activated Th2 cells stimulate cognate B lymphocytes to produce antibodies to the TSH receptors. These are termed **thyroid-stimulating immunoglobulins** because in effect they act as agonists of the TSH receptor and the consequence is unregulated thyroid hormone production. The high thyroid hormone concentration clamps TSH at low levels by intense negative feedback.

Thyroid eye disease in Graves' disease (ophthalmopathy)
Retro-orbital connective tissues suffer autoimmune attack by activated Th2 cells because they express TSH receptors:

- Fibroblasts secrete glycosaminoglycans, generating oedema, which pushes the eyes forward (**proptosis**) and may produce visual impairment by compression of the optic nerve.
- Cytokines from activated lymphocytes stimulate abnormal growth of the extraocular eye muscles causing disturbance to gaze and vision.
- Overactivity of sympathetic transmission (an effect of elevated thyroid hormone levels) retracts the eyelids; inability to cover the eyes results in conjunctival oedema and corneal damage, with scarring.

Total thyroidectomy and treatment with radioactive iodine (I^{131}) are the most effective treatments for ophthalmopathy because they remove the source of self-antigens. Less drastic management includes corticosteroids to suppress the autoimmune inflammatory response.

Neonatal Graves' disease
Graves' disease can occur in neonates due to placental transfer of thyroid-stimulating immunoglobulins from an afflicted mother. The disorder resolves over 4–12 weeks as the infant clears the offending antibodies.

Management of hyperthyroidism
- Anti-thyroid drugs inhibit thyroid peroxidase, blocking iodide organification and coupling reactions. The main ones are the thioamides (carbimazole or its metabolite methimazole, and propylthiouracil). Because of the long half-life of T_4, it can take 3–4 weeks for clinical improvement.
- **Iodides** (e.g. potassium iodide) at high concentrations suppress organification and thyroid hormone synthesis via the Wolff–Chaikoff effect. Because iodide administration produces improvement within 2–7 days, it is used (along with β-blockers which antagonise the Th-mediated increase in β-adrenoceptors, and other measures) in **thyrotoxic crisis** (or **'thyroid storm'**), a rare but rapid, life-threatening, worsening of hyperthyroidism that is usually triggered by stress.
- **Iodine radioisotope**: I^{131} is rapidly absorbed by the gut and concentrated in the thyroid by iodide trapping. It decays by emitting electrons (β⁻ particles), and has a **biological** half-life of 5 days. The electrons have sufficient energy to penetrate 0.4–2.0 mm and kill large numbers of thyroid cells. Because I^{131} crosses the placenta and is secreted into milk it is not used in pregnant or lactating women. Early fears that the radiation would lead to increased incidence of leukaemias or thyroid cancers have not been borne out. It restores normal thyroid hormone levels in most patients, but hyperthyroidism often reoccurs.
- **Subtotal thyroidectomy**: care must be taken not to remove all the parathyroid glands and to avoid damaging the recurrent laryngeal nerve.

production is **called non-shivering thermogenesis**. In humans most non-shivering thermogenesis is carried out by **brown fat** (its colour coming from its huge numbers of mitochondria), and is most important in infants, since relatively little brown fat is seen in human adults. Brown fat thermogenesis is stimulated by sympathetic activity because noradrenaline (norepinephrine) induces the expression of an uncoupling protein.

Physiology of BMR regulation by thyroid hormones

The increase in oxygen consumption driven by thyroid hormones must be matched by a rise in oxygen supply if it is to be maintained. This is brought about either directly, by the potentiation of sympathetic transmission wrought by thyroid hormones, or indirectly by a rise in cardiac output which occurs because there is:

- Increased metabolism in cells causing opening of vascular beds and hence a fall in peripheral resistance
- A rise in force and rate of cardiac contraction due to enhanced sympathetic activity (although in part the inotropic effect is due to thyroid-hormone-mediated changes in myosin and calcium ATPase gene transcription)
- The net result is increased stroke volume, and increased systolic but decreased diastolic pressure, i.e. larger pulse pressure.

In addition, thyroid hormones potentiate oxygen-carrying capacity, raising red cell number by stimulating erythropoietin production, and increase resting ventilation rate.

Thyroid handling in pregnancy

Oestrogens increase the synthesis of TBG so that during pregnancy a woman can have a total blood T_4 concentration that is twice normal. The free thyroid hormone concentrations, however, are little changed. This phenomenon is described as being **hyperthyroxinaemic** (high T_4) but **euthyroid** (i.e. her thyroid function is normal). The increase in thyroid hormone binding in pregnancy probably ensures an adequate hormone reservoir for fetal requirements.

Thyroid hormones are critical for brain development (particularly synapse formation and myelination) in the first trimester of pregnancy. Towards the end of pregnancy they become important for growth. Because the fetal thyroid gland is non-functional for the first 10 weeks, the fetal thyroid hormone requirements are provided by the mother during early pregnancy. Maternal T_4 is deiodinated by DII in the placenta to deliver T_3 to the fetus. As the fetal thyroid comes on-stream the placenta switches its deiodinase to the DIII type. Maternal T_4 is now converted to rT_3 which the fetus uses as the iodide source for making its own thyroid hormones. Clearly if a woman is hypothyroxinaemic (low total T_4 concentration) her fetus risks hypothyroidism. The rise in TBG that makes women physiologically hyperthyroxinaemic during pregnancy has presumably evolved as providing a safety margin against such a catastrophe.

ADRENAL CORTICOSTEROIDS

Adrenal hormones

The adrenal glands are crucial for life. Their principal secretions are **adrenaline** (epinephrine), and three functional classes of steroid (see Table 10.10):

Information box 10.24   Hypothyroidism

Underactivity of the thyroid gland is hypothyroidism, also known as **myxoedema**. The clinical features are related to the physiological action of thyroid hormones; for example the neurological symptoms illustrate that thyroid hormones are needed for adult brain function. Treatment is usually by life-long replacement therapy with synthetic thyroxine (e.g. levothyroxine).

Hashimoto's thyroiditis

The most common cause of hypothyroidism in the Western world is **Hashimoto's thyroiditis**, an autoimmune disorder in which antibodies against thyroid peroxidase are produced. Initially the disease may present as hyperthyroidism because destruction of the thyroid parenchyma causes a transient release of stored hormone. With continuing lymphocyte infiltration and autoimmune attack, thyroid function drops and TSH concentrations rise. Other endocrine autoimmune disorders sometimes accompany Hashimoto's thyroiditis.

Hypothyroidism and fertility

Hypothyroid women frequently have anovulatory sterility, possibly because noradrenergic neurons are involved in driving the positive feedback surge in GnRH release in response to high oestradiol concentrations, and thyroid hormones are needed for proper catecholamine neurotransmission. Conception rate is low and miscarriage rate is high. However, administration of thyroid hormones to anovulatory euthyroid women has no influence on their infertility.

Information box 10.25   Cretinism

Inadequate thyroid hormone during fetal development results in congenital hypothyroidism. If untreated, severe hypothyroidism results in **cretinism**, characterised in infants by signs of **neurological cretinism** (mental retardation, deafness, pyramidal tract signs, muscle weakness), growth failure, and myxoedema due to the accumulation of glycosaminoglycans. Dietary iodine deficiency in the mother is the most common reason. All newborn infants in the UK and other developed nations are screened for primary hypothyroidism. A small amount of blood, obtained by heel prick, is assayed for T_4. If the infant is hypothyroxinaemic (i.e. low T_4 concentration) a diagnosis of primary hypothyroidism is then confirmed by a concomitant high blood TSH concentration. Cretinism is preventable by administering T_4, preferably starting within the first two weeks of birth.

- **Mineralocorticoids** regulate extracellular sodium concentrations and hence extracellular fluid volume. By far the most important is **aldosterone**.
- **Glucocorticoids**, so called because their metabolic effects raise blood glucose concentration. The major glucocorticoid in humans is **cortisol**.
- **Sex steroids**; i.e. androgens and oestrogens.

Together mineralocorticoids and glucocorticoids are also known as **corticosteroids**. Adrenaline and cortisol are important in adaptation to stress. It is just about possible to survive without these hormones, provided the living is easy, but a lack of aldosterone is fatal within days.

Adrenal gland anatomy

Gross anatomy

The adrenal (suprarenal) glands lie above the kidneys, encapsulated by the renal fascia and embedded in perinephric fat.

Table 10.10	Relative potencies of endogenous and synthetic corticosteroids*	
Steroid	**Glucocorticoid activity**	**Mineralocorticoid activity**
Cortisol	1.0	1.0
Corticosterone	0.3	15
Aldosterone	0.3	3000
Deoxycorticosterone	0.2	100
Cortisone	0.7	1.0
Prednisolone	4	0.8
Dexamethasone	25	<0.01

*From: Porterfield SP 2001 Endocrine Physiology, 2nd edn. Mosby, Edinburgh.

Each adrenal gland has an outer **cortex**, which produces steroids, and an inner **medulla**, which secretes adrenaline and noradrenaline.

Three adrenal arteries, from the aorta, inferior phrenic, and renal arteries, anastomose to form a subcapsular plexus. This gives rise to fenestrated sinusoids that pass radially into the gland, draining into a single medullary vein. Arterioles emerge directly from the adrenal arteries to supply the medulla. Hence the medulla gets a dual blood supply. Medullary venules drain into the medullary vein, which leaves the hilus of the gland, entering the inferior vena cava (right side) or left renal vein.

The medulla receives a large number of myelinated pre-ganglionic cholinergic sympathetic fibres from the coeliac ganglion. Medullary chromaffin cells are in effect postganglionic sympathetic neuroendocrine cells.

Corticosteroid synthesis and the functional microanatomy of the adrenal cortex

The synthesis of all steroid hormones begins with cholesterol, which is converted to corticosteroids in the adrenal cortex, and sex hormones in the gonads (See Fig. 10.1).

Beneath the adrenal capsule, three layers can be distinguished in the adult adrenal cortex (Fig. 10.36). The superficial **zona glomerulosa** is the only layer that has the 18-hydroxylase needed to synthesise the mineralocorticoid aldosterone from corticosterone. Angiotensin II stimulates both the growth of the zona glomerulosa and the synthesis of aldosterone from corticosterone. Because it lacks 17α-hydroxylase/17,20-lyase (CYP17) the zona glomerulosa is unable to make either cortisol, androgens or oestrogens.

The middle and inner layers, **zona fasciculata** and **zona reticularis**, respectively, both have the CYP17 enzyme and hence can manufacture cortisol and the sex steroids (see Fig. 10.37).

Mineralocorticoid: aldosterone

Aldosterone is the main mineralocorticoid that promotes the reuptake of sodium and hence water by the kidneys, and thereby maintains extracellular sodium concentration (Ch. 14); it is also involved in the long-term regulation of blood volume and blood pressure (Ch. 11).

Control of aldosterone secretion

Aldosterone secretion is controlled by the **renin–angiotensin–aldosterone system** (see Ch. 14). Briefly, three signals activate the release of renin from the juxtaglomerular apparatus of the kidney:

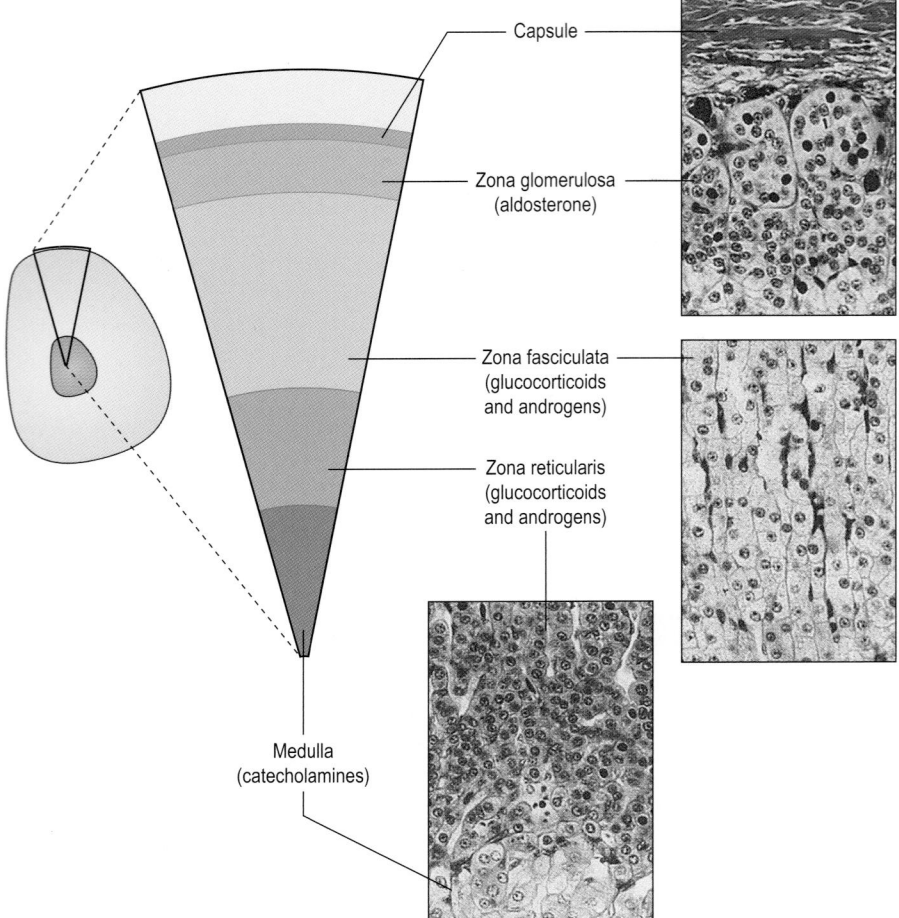

Capsule

Zona glomerulosa
(aldosterone)

Zona fasciculata
(glucocorticoids
and androgens)

Zona reticularis
(glucocorticoids
and androgens)

Medulla
(catecholamines)

Fig. 10.36 **Structure of the adrenal glands.** Images reproduced with permission from Young B, Lowe JS, Stevens A, Heath JW 2006 Wheater's functional histology, 5th edn. Edinburgh, Churchill Livingstone.

- A drop in perfusion pressure in the renal afferent arterioles
- Activation of sympathetic nerve supply to afferent and efferent arterioles in the kidney
- A decrease in the flux of NaCl past the macula densa.

Renin, a proteolytic enzyme cleaves a plasma protein **angiotensinogen** to generate a decapeptide **angiotensin I**. This is further cleaved by **angiotensin converting enzyme (ACE)**, located in pulmonary endothelial cells, to an eight amino acid peptide **angiotensin II (AII)**, by a single pass through the lungs. Angiotensin II is a powerful vasoconstrictor and it stimulates the release of aldosterone from the zona glomerulosa. Aldosterone acts on the distal convoluted tubules and collecting ducts of the kidneys to increase the reuptake of Na^+, in exchange for H^+ and K^+ (Ch 14). Chloride ions and water follow. Thus the renin–angiotensin–aldosterone system is a negative feedback system (one of several) which defends extracellular fluid volume (see Ch. 6).

Transport of aldosterone

Aldosterone binds with a low affinity to aldosterone-binding globulin, corticosteroid-binding-globulin (CBG) and albumin, so that only about 60% of the steroid is bound, i.e. almost half of the circulating aldosterone is free. Consequently it has a short half-life of 20 minutes.

Mineralocorticoid receptors for aldosterone

Aldosterone diffuses readily across plasma membranes to enter the cytoplasm where it binds to **mineralocorticoid receptors (MRs)** that belong to the steroid receptor superfamily. The hormone–receptor complex translocates to the nucleus, where it binds to specific sequences of DNA in control regions of specific genes that are subject to regulation by aldosterone. Mineralocorticoid receptors are found mostly in the kidneys and the brain.

MRs have equal affinity for aldosterone and cortisol so cannot distinguish between them. Since free cortisol concentration in the blood is 100-fold higher than aldosterone, how is it that MR responses reflect the concentration of aldosterone rather than cortisol? The reason is that co-localised with mineralocorticoid receptors is **11β-hydroxysteroid dehydrogenase II (HSD II)**. This enzyme converts cortisol to **cortisone**, which has a low affinity for MRs and is released into the blood. Therefore, MR responses reflect the concentration of aldosterone rather than cortisol.

Apart from the adrenals, the kidneys are the major source of cortisone. Patients with genetic defects in HSD II suffer from symptoms of mineralocorticoid excess. Cortisol is regenerated from circulating cortisone by a similar enzyme (HSD I) in the liver.

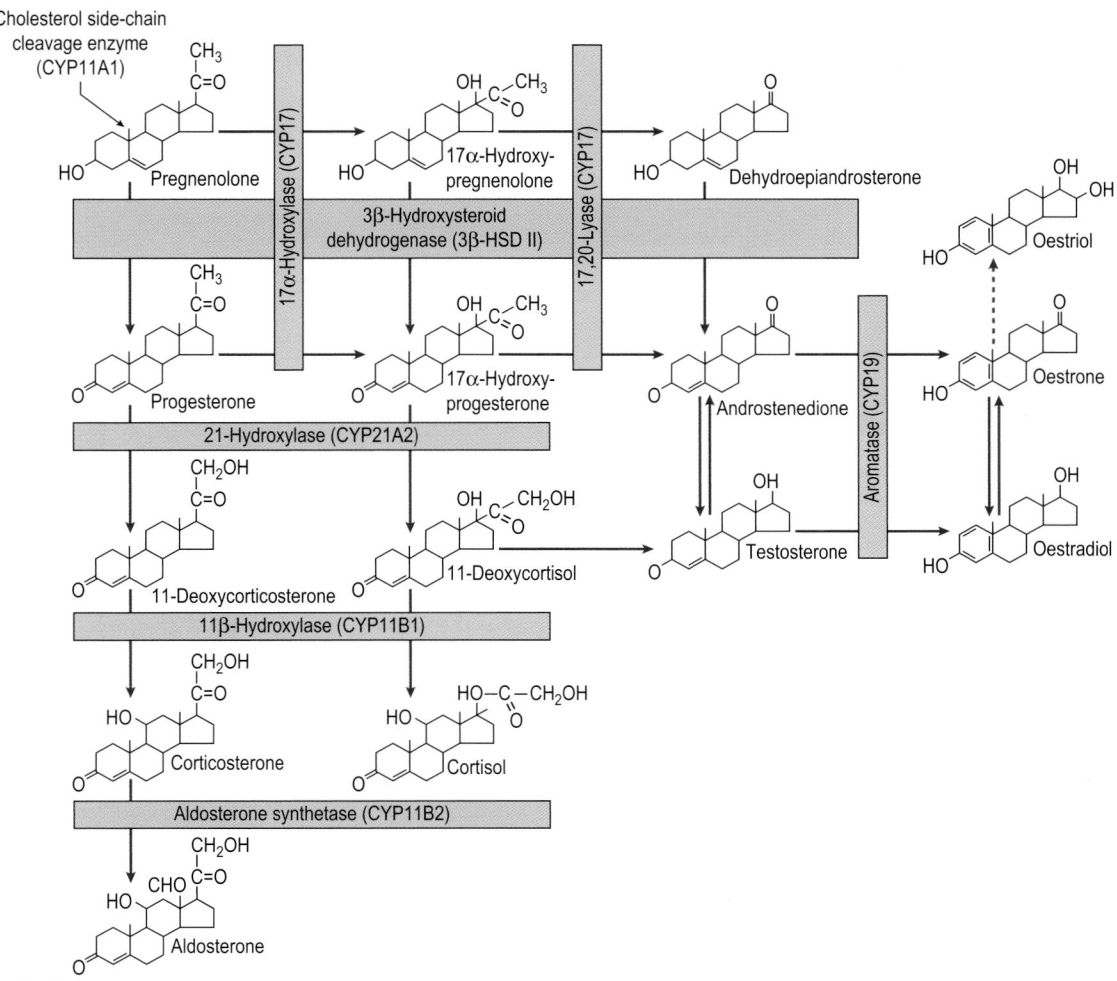

Fig. 10.37 Steroid metabolism.

Information box 10.26   Hyperaldosteronism

Primary hyperaldosteronism – Conn's syndrome
Conn's syndrome is the consequence of excessive
aldosterone output from the adrenal cortex, usually the result
of an aldosterone-secreting tumour or of adrenal hyperplasia.
It is characterised by:

- Excessive renal tubule Na⁺ reabsorption leading to
  hypertension and hence low plasma renin concentration
- Loss of K⁺ and H⁺.

Although extracellular fluid volume expands, oedema is
uncommon because the hypervolaemia stimulates atrial
natriuretic hormone secretion from the heart and this brings
about natriuresis.

Deoxycorticosterone excess
Types II and V congenital adrenal hyperplasia (CAH, see Table
10.11) result in excess production of deoxycorticosterone.
Because this steroid has mineralocorticoid activity, CAH
effectively resembles primary hyperaldosteronism. However,
the hypertension caused by the sodium retention in these
disorders actually suppresses aldosterone secretion.

- Type II CAH, arising from **11β-hydroxylase (CYP11B1)**
  deficiency, causes the signs and symptoms of
  mineralocorticoid excess by blocking the synthesis of
  cortisol and corticosterone from their 11-deoxy derivatives.
  In the absence of cortisol the unrestrained ACTH release

drives excessive synthesis of the corticosteroids
upstream of the missing enzyme. This includes
11-deoxycorticosterone (DOC), which has
mineralocorticoid activity. Females with this disorder
will be masculinised by the resulting excess androgen
production.

- Type V CAH, due to the lack of **17α-hydroxylase (CYP17)**,
  shunts steroid metabolism away from androgen synthesis
  and towards deoxycorticosterone production.

Secondary hyperaldosteronism
The majority of cases of secondary hyperaldosteronism are of
renal origin. There are two forms, depending on whether
hypertension is present.

- With hypertension: renovascular disease (atherosclerosis or
  fibromuscular hyperplasia) produces renin and hence
  aldosterone secretion that is inappropriately high and this
  results in hypertension.
- Without hypertension, as a result of:
  - Renal diseases in which sodium reabsorption is com-
    promised (sodium-wasting nephropathy, renal tubular
    acidosis)
  - Loss-of-function mutations of the mineralocorticoid
    receptor gene
  - Bulimia, in which vomiting and laxative misuse depletes
    extracellular fluid volume via the gastrointestinal tract.

Glucocorticoids

Glucocorticoids, such as cortisol, raise blood glucose concentrations by a variety of mechanisms. They also have powerful effects on the immune system that can be qualitatively (as well as quantitatively) different, depending on whether they are present at physiological or supra-physiological concentrations. These effects are frequently exploited clinically. Cortisol analogues are a mainstay in the management of a great variety of conditions in which the suppression of immune function or inflammatory responses is likely to be beneficial, such as allergies, autoimmune disorders, infections and organ transplants.

Hypothalamic–pituitary–adrenal axis

The **hypothalamic–pituitary–adrenal axis** regulates the production of glucocorticoids from the adrenal cortex.

ACTH secretion

A distinct population of neurons in the **paraventricular nucleus (PVN)** of the hypothalamus releases corticotropin-releasing hormone (**CRH**) into the hypothalamic–pituitary portal capillaries. CRH has two effects on corticotropes of the anterior pituitary gland:

- It switches on the synthesis of **ACTH**, by activating the transcription of **prepro-opiomelanocortin (POMC)**, the 31 kDa preprohormone for ACTH. POMC is then cleaved by trypsin-like endopeptidases to generate ACTH.
- It stimulates ACTH secretion.

A second population of neurons in the PVN releases **arginine vasopressin (AVP)** which finds its way to the corticotropes via the hypothalamic–pituitary portal system. The stimulation of ACTH secretion by CRH is greatly amplified by the co-release of AVP.

Cortisol secretion

ACTH stimulates hypertrophy of cells in the zona fasciculata and zona reticularis and their synthesis and secretion of cortisol.

Transport and inactivation of cortisol

About 75% of circulating cortisol is bound to CBG and 15% is bound to albumin. Cortisol has a half-life of 70 minutes and is inactivated mainly by conjugation with glucuronide or sulphate in the liver and then excreted by the kidneys.

Modulation of the hypothalamic–pituitary–adrenal axis

The output of the hypothalamic–pituitary–adrenal axis is regulated in several ways (Fig. 10.38). Glucocorticoid secretion is subject to negative feedback control, is both ultradian and circadian, and is activated by stress.

Negative feedback

Negative feedback by cortisol is brought about by binding to glucocorticoid receptors in the pituitary and hypothalamus. At both levels the feedback has two components. At first there is suppression of release of either ACTH or CRH, possibly by activating the transcription of potassium channel genes, in effect rendering their respective cells less excitable. This is followed by a fall in ACTH or CRH synthesis, brought

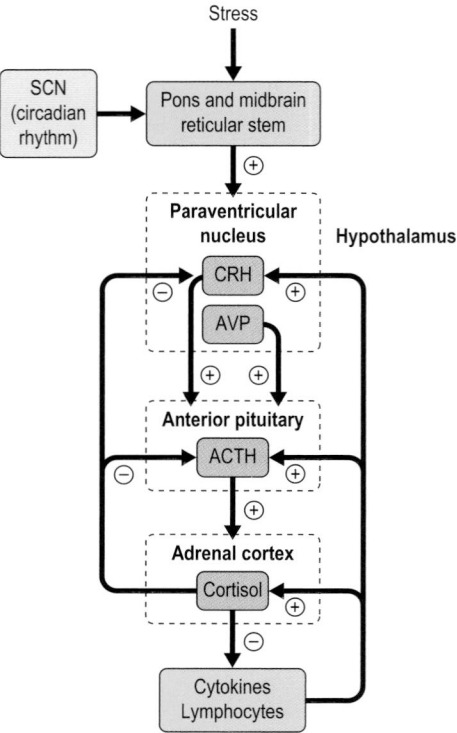

Fig. 10.38 Control of the hypothalamic–pituitary–adrenal axis. AVP, arginine vasopressin; SCN, suprachiasmatic nucleus; ACTH, adrenocorticotropic hormone; CRH, corticotropin-releasing hormone.

about by decreases in transcription of the genes for POMC and CRH.

Many synthetic glucocorticoids (e.g. **dexamethasone**) have negative feedback effects. This has clinical implications.

- In the **dexamethasone suppression test** the administration of dexamethasone (usually at night) can help tease out the nature of excessive cortisol secretion. In a normal hypothalamic–pituitary–adrenal axis, dexamethasone produces a marked reduction in blood cortisol concentration. By contrast, the steroid concentration stays high if there is an autonomous cortisol-secreting or ACTH-secreting tumour.
- Chronic exposure to high levels of cortisol, as a result of disease or long-term therapeutic administration of cortisol analogues, causes a functional atrophy of the hypothalamic–pituitary–adrenal axis which can last for several months after the end of exposure. For this reason it is important to wean patients gradually from corticosteroids.

Ultradian and circadian release

Like other anterior pituitary hormones, ACTH release is pulsatile, but the frequency is higher – about three pulses per hour. There is also a pronounced circadian rhythm; concentrations of ACTH and cortisol rising during sleep to peak just before waking and falling to their lowest levels in the evening. The alterations in secretion are due to changes in pulse amplitude rather than frequency.

The circadian rhythm for ACTH secretion is driven by hypothalamic CRH release, and happens because the sensitivity of the paraventricular neurons to cortisol varies during

Information box 10.27 Congenital adrenal hyperplasias

Any enzyme deficiency that results in reduced cortisol synthesis (see Fig. 10.37) will increase ACTH secretion and produce adrenal hyperplasia. Several inborn errors of metabolism, caused by recessive mutations in autosomal genes for steroid metabolism, result in a decrease in cortisol production by the adrenal cortex. This lifts the normal negative feedback on ACTH release from the anterior pituitary. The rise in circulating ACTH stimulates the growth of the adrenal cortex. These disorders are termed **congenital adrenal hyperplasias (CAHs)**.

There are several types of CAH (Table 10.11), the signs and symptoms of which depend on which enzyme is defective, how much the enzyme activity is reduced and the sex. All CAHs are characterised by high blood concentrations of ACTH but low concentrations of cortisol. The commonest is type I, caused by deficiency of the CYP21 enzyme responsible for hydroxylation of the methyl group on C21 of progesterone and 17α-hydroxyprogesterone. It is estimated that 1% of humans overall have mild type I CAH, though the incidence is higher in some ethnic groups (e.g. Hispanics). The most severe is type VI in which the absence of cholesterol side-chain cleavage enzyme results in the failure of the synthesis of all adrenocortical and gonadal steroids. Three types of CAH are causes of primary adrenal insufficiency (II, IV and VI) and two result in mineralocorticoid excess (III and V, see Information box 10.26, Primary hyperaldosteronism).

CAH also results in disorders of sexual differentiation.

- In types I–III there is secretion of large amounts of androgens which causes **virilisation** of female external genitals, including enlargement of the clitoris and some degree of fusion of the genital folds. The virilisation continues into adulthood with the development of male secondary sexual characteristics (**adrenogenital syndrome**).
- In types IV–VI there is a failure of androgen synthesis and incomplete or failed masculinisation of external genitals in affected males resulting, for example, in hypospadias. Female pseudohermaphroditism also occurs with these types.

Occasionally, the inappropriate presence or absence of androgens in CAH coincides with development of the internal genitalia, and these will then also be abnormal.

Table 10.11 Congenital adrenal hyperplasias

CAH Type	Missing enzyme*	Effect on steroid biosynthesis	Clinical profile	Effects on sexual differentiation
I	P450c21, CYP21A2 (21-hydroxylase)	↓ cortisol →↑ ACTH → ↑ androgens	Signs and symptoms of androgen excess, but not of mineralocorticoid deficiency, wide spectrum of severity	XY: Virilisation XX: Virilisation with enlarged clitoris and partial labioscrotal fusion
II	P450c21, CYP21A2 (21-hydroxylase)	↓ cortisol →↑ ACTH → ↑ androgens ↓aldosterone	Salt-losing version of type I; ↓ Na⁺→↑ renin, ↑ K⁺, Addison's disease, premature adrenarche	XY: Virilisation XX: Ambiguous external genitals
III	P450c11, CYP11B1 (11β-hydroxylase)	↑ 11-deoxycorticosterone, ↑ 11-deoxycortisol, ↓ cortisol →↑ ACTH → ↑ androgens	Hypertension	XY: Virilisation XX: Wide range of virilisation (mild to severe)
IV	3β-Hydroxysteroid dehydrogenase	↓ cortisol →↑ ACTH ↓ androgens, ↓ oestrogens, ↓ aldosterone	↓ Na⁺→↑ renin, ↑ K⁺, Addison's disease	XY: Incomplete masculinisation (hypospadias) XX: Mild clitoral enlargement
V	P450c17, CYP17 (17α-hydroxylase)	↑ 11-deoxycorticosterone, ↑ corticosterone, ↓ aldosterone (because of hypertension)	↑ Na⁺ (but ↓ renin), ↓ K⁺, ↓ H⁺ (hypokalemic alkalosis), hypertension	XY: Juvenile female or ambiguous external genitals XX: Juvenile female external genitals, delayed puberty
VI	P450scc, CYP11A (cholesterol side chain cleavage)	Loss of all adrenal and gonadal steroids	Addisonian crisis, hypogonadism	XY: Juvenile female external genitals, no Wolffian duct structures (no androgens), no Müllerian duct structures (because testis produces AMH) XX: Juvenile female external genitals, delay or failure of puberty

*See also Fig. 10.37.
AMH, anti-Müllerian hormone; ACTH, adrenocorticotropic hormone.

the day; in effect the set point changes. However, cortisol concentrations are precisely controlled by negative feedback at all times; the set point alters with time, but it does not disappear.

Although the nocturnal ACTH peak is not related to any specific stage of sleep, it is at least in part entrained by sleep–wake transitions because it is rescheduled over a period of days in people who go on night shifts. It is also entrained by light since the rhythm is abolished by constant exposure to light or dark, by blindness and unconsciousness. **Jet lag**, the disruption to sleep–wake patterns caused by flying across several time zones, is in part attributable to the disruption in circadian output of cortisol caused by the phase lag between sleep–wake and light–dark cycles.

Stress

Stress is the major activator of the hypothalamic–pituitary–adrenal axis. Virtually any stressor is effective: hypoxia, dehydration, hypoglycaemia, starvation, infection, trauma, anaesthesia, surgery, psychological stresses, anxiety and depression. Indeed, blood ACTH and cortisol concentrations are used as markers of stress in clinical and experimental studies. Moderate stress activates the hypothalamic–pituitary–adrenal axis by raising the set point for negative feedback, but severe stress overrides feedback so that high Rates of ACTH secretion are maintained even in the face of the maximum output of cortisol. Not surprisingly, high levels of chronic stress produces significant enlargement of the adrenal glands. Stress also flattens the pituitary circadian output, although the pulsatile nature of the release is unaffected.

Neural substrates for stress

Generally, stress affects the hypothalamic–pituitary–adrenal axis via extensive neural connections to the PVN from many parts of the brain. Neurons using a variety of neurotransmitters excite the PVN to drive neuroendocrine stress responses, including noradrenaline, acetylcholine, serotonin and angiotensin II. For example, the rise in osmolality contingent on dehydration activates osmoreceptors which project to the PVN via neurons that are sensitive to angiotensin II. These neurons stimulate the release of AVP as part of the usual homeostatic mechanism to restore blood osmolality and volume, *and* the release of CRH as a stress response to dehydration. Interestingly the enkephalins and endorphins, released during intense exercise, are inhibitory on the PVN and therefore dampen stress responses.

Neuroendocrine-immune system cross-talk

Not all neuroendocrine responses to stress are initiated by the brain. **Cytokines**, released by immune cells in response to trauma or infection or any other stress that stimulates the immune system, activates the hypothalamic–pituitary–adrenal axis (Fig. 10.38). In particular, macrophages release **interleukin (IL)-1** and T helper cells release **IL-2** and **IL-6**, all of which stimulate release of CRH and ACTH and hence promote the secretion of cortisol from the adrenal glands. However, negative feedback mechanisms operate, holding the immune system in check:

- ACTH dampens macrophage activation.
- Glucocorticoids reduce the number of circulating lymphocytes by sequestering them in the spleen.
- Glucocorticoids suppress the production of cytokines, especially those (e.g. IL-2) produced by Th1 cells responsible for local inflammatory responses.

These actions limit unrestrained immune system action and excessive inflammatory responses.

Actions of glucocorticoids

Glucocorticoid receptors

Glucocorticoids are lipophilic and diffuse readily across plasma membranes of cells. In the cytoplasm they bind to **glucocorticoid receptors** (**GRs**), which are members of the steroid superfamily of nuclear receptors. Having bound glucocorticoid, the receptors translocate to the nucleus where they act as transcription factors, binding to glucocorticoid responsive elements in control regions of specific genes.

Glucocorticoids also bind with lower affinity to mineralocorticoid receptors and so have weak but significant mineralocorticoid activity, promoting sodium reabsorption but loss of potassium.

Actions on glucose metabolism

Glucocorticoids raise blood glucose concentrations by:

- Inhibiting the insulin-dependent transport of glucose into muscle and fat cells, thus reducing glucose utilisation by these tissues

- Increasing gluconeogenesis (Ch. 3) and consequently glucose release by the liver.

The glucocorticoid-evoked rise in blood glucose concentration allows more glucose to be taken up by tissues that do not have insulin-dependent glucose transporters, e.g. brain. In the liver, because glucocorticoids stimulate glycogenesis, much of the new glucose is subsequently stored there as glycogen. Hence, glucocorticoids control the distribution of glucose to tissues, making more available to critical organs such as the brain.

Gluconeogenesis is in part promoted by provision of more substrates by other actions of glucocorticoids:

- An increased rate of lipolysis in adipose tissue, providing glycerol and free fatty acids
- Stimulation of protein breakdown, releasing amino acids into the circulation.

How are glucocorticoids adaptive in stress?

Patients with adrenal insufficiency due to lack of pituitary ACTH secretion have low constant baseline output of glucocorticoids. Even relatively innocuous stress can prove lethal to these people, demonstrating that glucocorticoids are important for adapting to stress. Although the exact mechanisms for this are unclear there are several possibilities.

- **Metabolic**: glucocorticoids turn long-term energy substrates, fats and proteins into short-term, readily available energy sources, free fatty acids (FFAs), glycogen and glucose. Moreover, the glucose is not squandered but reserved for the brain, while the FFAs are the preferred fuel for the heart. This harnessing, but economic use, of energy substrates may contribute to stress tolerance.
- **Permissive effects on actions of catecholamines**: the enhancement of the actions of adrenaline and noradrenaline by glucocorticoids enables other adaptive stress responses to occur. For example, glucocorticoids increase α-adrenoceptor sensitivity, potentiating sympathetic vasoconstriction.
- **Effects on the immune system**: the physiological effects of glucocorticoids are immunosuppressive in vivo and include reduction in the number of circulating lymphocytes and inhibited production of some cytokines. These actions are thought to be adaptive. Moreover, although some cytokines stimulate the hypothalamic–pituitary–adrenal axis, negative feedback loops act to dampen immune system action (see above). This is clearly adaptive in the acute stress of injury and infection. However, chronic exposure to high levels of glucocorticoids, either physiologically released in response to long-term stress, or the highly potent synthetic glucocorticoids used clinically, can be maladaptive. For example:
  - Prolonged exposure to high concentrations of glucocorticoids kills cells in the hippocampus and may lead to learning deficits.
  - Immune suppression, seen in chronic and/or intense stress, has been shown to increase the risk of a variety of viral, bacterial and parasitic infections.

Additional actions of glucocorticoids
Connective tissues

Glucocorticoids decrease the synthesis of collagen by fibroblasts. By decreasing calcium absorption by the intestine and reabsorption in the kidney, glucocorticoids reduce blood ionised calcium (Ca^{2+}) concentration. This causes increased secretion of PTH, which mobilises Ca^{2+} from bone by increasing demineralisation.

In the long term, therapeutic oral administration of glucocorticoids leads to osteoporosis. This can be offset to some extent by co-administration of vitamin D to patients on long-term glucocorticoids. Vitamin D acts on the kidneys to promote calcium reabsorption and maintain blood calcium concentration.

Red blood cell formation
Glucocorticoids stimulate erythropoietin production and therefore red cell formation, raising the red cell count and haematocrit.

Gastrointestinal effects
Glucocorticoids stimulate:

- Growth of gastrointestinal mucosa
- Gastrointestinal motility
- Gastric acid and enzyme production.

Nervous system
Apart from their actions in regulating the hypothalamic–pituitary–adrenal axis, glucocorticoids have central nervous system (CNS) effects which increase appetite, enhance vasopressin secretion, and influence sleep and mood in complex and poorly understood ways.

 Information box 10.28   **Adrenocortical insufficiency**

Primary adrenocortical insufficiency – Addison's disease
Failure of the adrenal cortex to secrete aldosterone and cortisol is most commonly due to autoimmune disorder or tuberculosis. Other autoimmune disorders (e.g. type 1 diabetes mellitus, Hashimoto's thyroiditis, Graves' disease, vitiligo) are commonly seen in patients with autoimmune Addison's disease. The signs and symptoms are predictable from the actions of the missing hormones (Table 10.12). Pigmentation of the skin, due to the excess ACTH secretion from the anterior pituitary released from its glucocorticoid negative feedback, is often the first manifestation and distinguishes it from secondary adrenocortical insufficiency.

Secondary adrenocortical insufficiency
Loss of ACTH secretion from the anterior pituitary, either because of hypopituitarism or because of atrophy of corticotropes induced by long-term glucocorticoid treatment,

results in a failure of the zona fasciculata and zona reticularis to secrete glucocorticoids and androgens. However, the output of aldosterone by the zona glomerulosa is normal. **Secondary adrenal insufficiency** is easily distinguished from primary:

- There is no pigmentation.
- ACTH concentrations are low.
- ACTH injection will stimulate cortisol secretion. (Note that in very long-standing cases of secondary adrenocortical insufficiency, the response will be slow, so that at least a 3-day test will be needed).
- No effects attributable to lack of aldosterone are seen.
- Other evidence of pituitary failure (hypogonadism, hypothyroidism) except when the insufficiency follows withdrawal of long-term glucocorticoid therapy.

Table 10.12   **Clinical features of primary adrenal insufficiency (Addison's disease)**

Loss of aldosterone	Loss of cortisol
Na+ loss: hyponatraemia, hypovolaemic shock, raised plasma renin	Reduced gluconeogenesis, increased glucose transport and utilisation by muscle and fat: hypoglycaemia
Impaired excretion of K+ and H+: hyperkalaemia, metabolic acidosis	Loss of enhanced catecholamine actions: postural hypotension, hypotension
	Loss of appetite stimulation and gastrointestinal tropoic effects: anorexia, weakness, fatigue, nausea, vomiting
	Increased adrenocorticotropic hormone (ACTH) from loss of negative feedback: hyperpigmentation
	Decreased secretion of adrenal androgens: loss of pubic and axillary hair in women

---

 Information box 10.29   **Effect of excess glucocorticoids: Cushing's syndrome**

Long-term therapeutic use of pharmacological doses of synthetic glucocorticoids is the commonest cause of **Cushing's syndrome**. The condition could also be secondary to an ACTH-secreting adenoma of the pituitary or ectopic ACTH sources (e.g. small cell carcinoma of the lung). Primary Cushing's disease is uncommon and usually due to an adrenal tumour. Major features of Cushing's syndrome are:

- Skin pigmentation, which is infrequent in the secondary syndrome, but is seen, particularly, in the case of ectopic ACTH-secreting tumours. It is not seen in the primary disease since here ACTH concentrations are low
- Hyperglycaemia – which results because of the **diabetogenic effect** of glucocorticoids. i.e. they raise blood glucose concentration

- Increased appetite, with truncal obesity adding to insulin resistance
- Increased proteolysis – which reduces muscle mass, with weakness and wasting, especially of the proximal limb muscles
- Enhanced actions of catecholamines resulting in hypertension
- Bone demineralisation and hence osteoporosis, which often leads to pathological fractures
- Decreased collagen synthesis, which increases wound healing time and is the cause of abdominal striae
- Immune suppression, which increases the risks of infection
- Increased erythropoietin production which increases red cell number.

ENDOCRINE CONTROL OF ENERGY METABOLISM

Normal cellular metabolism requires an adequate supply of glucose (see Ch. 3). Blood glucose concentrations fluctuate depending on when and what an individual last ate, their recent exercise history and how stressed they are. In health it is tightly controlled by hormones within a range of 3.5–8.0 mmol/L. Several hormones are concerned with the regulation of glucose homeostasis, including insulin and glucagon, secreted by the endocrine pancreas, together with adrenaline and cortisol from the adrenal gland. In controlling the rate of energy metabolism, thyroid hormones are the major endocrine players in the rate of glucose utilisation, by actions on mitochondria which set the BMR (see Ch. 16).

ENDOCRINE PANCREAS

The endocrine pancreas produces two hormones that are directly responsible for controlling blood glucose concentration and glucose utilisation:

- **Insulin**, released in response to a rise in blood glucose concentration that accompanies feeding, enhances glucose use by liver, fat and muscle, and lowers blood glucose. Insulin is essential for maintaining normal blood glucose concentration.
- **Glucagon**, produced during the post-absorptive and fasting states when blood glucose concentrations fall, raises blood glucose. In normal subjects, several other hormones with similar actions on blood glucose, for example adrenaline and cortisol, can raise blood glucose in the absence of glucagon.

Insulin, being the major regulator of intermediary metabolism, is vital to life. Failure of the endocrine pancreas to secrete insulin, or of target cells to respond to it, results in diabetes mellitus. This is the most common endocrine disorder in the Western world and its treatment uses at least 5% of total healthcare costs. Diabetes is also an important risk factor for ischaemic heart disease and cerebrovascular disease, which themselves take a huge toll in both morbidity and mortality. Furthermore, the most prevalent form, type 2 diabetes, is shown by epidemiological evidence to be essentially a disorder of modern Western lifestyle, and consequently the number of people with diabetes looks set to rise to epidemic proportions during this century.

BLOOD GLUCOSE

Normal values

Normally blood glucose concentrations fluctuate around an average value of 5 mmol/L (for glucose concentrations in mg/dL multiply the value in mmol/L by 18.) Glucose concentration is homeostatically quite tightly regulated by a number of hormones including insulin, glucagon, adrenaline, cortisol and growth hormone. Only one hormone, insulin, decreases blood glucose concentrations, all others increase it.

On feeding, blood glucose concentrations rise and this stimulates insulin release from the endocrine pancreas. Insulin reduces blood glucose by increasing its uptake and utilisation by skeletal muscle and fat, and by inhibiting its production (gluconeogenesis and glycogenolysis) in the liver. In diabetes mellitus, there is either insufficient insulin secre-

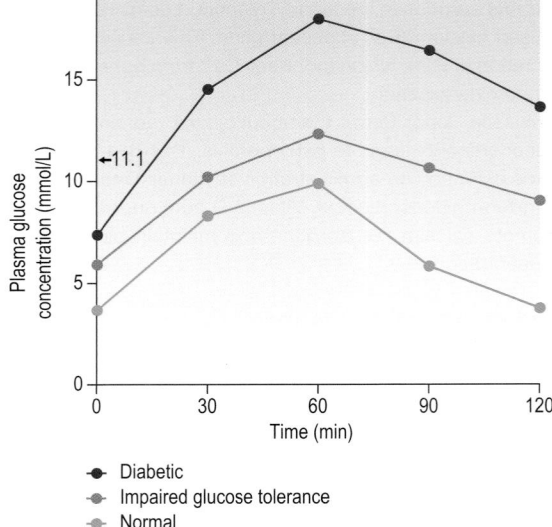

Fig. 10.39 Typical oral glucose tolerance curves. After fasting, the first venous blood sample is taken at time $t = 0$ and the patient drinks a solution containing 75 g glucose; blood samples are then taken at 30-minute intervals.

tion, or cellular response to insulin, and consequently blood glucose concentrations are excessive (**hyperglycaemia**).

Hyperglycaemia

The homeostatic regulation of blood glucose is assessed by an **oral glucose tolerance test** (**OGTT**, Fig. 10.39). Blood glucose concentrations are measured after a 10-hour fast, and then 30, 60, 90 and 120 minutes after ingesting 75 g of glucose. Currently, a fasting blood glucose in excess of 7.0 mmol/L is regarded as diagnostic of diabetes mellitus on the basis that this is consistent with a blood glucose concentration 11.1 mmol/L two hours into an OGTT, a value that lies at the threshold for **microvascular damage**. Consequently a random sample of blood (i.e. non-fasting) with a glucose concentration > 11.1 mmol/L is also a diagnostic criterion for diabetes if it is associated with the cardinal symptoms of diabetes, polyuria, polydipsia and unexplained weight loss.

Individuals with a fasting glucose between 6.1 mmol/L and 7.0 mmol/L and a glucose concentration between 7.8 mmol/L and 11.1 mmol/L 2 hours after a 75 g glucose load have **impaired glucose tolerance** and are at increased risk of developing diabetes.

Hypoglycaemia

An abnormally low blood glucose, **hypoglycaemia**, is defined as blood glucose concentration <2.8 mmol/L. Physiologically it may occur with prolonged starvation or exercise. It also occurs after excessive alcohol consumption (Ch. 3), and commonly results from insulin excess in people with diabetes who are experiencing difficulties in controlling their disease.

Pancreatic islets

The endocrine pancreas consists of about one million clusters of cells, **pancreatic islets** (**islets of Langerhans**) 50–500 µm across, scattered throughout the exocrine pancreas, but making up only 1–2% of its total mass (Fig. 10.40).

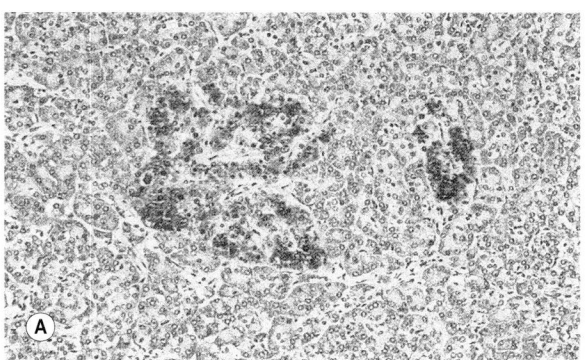
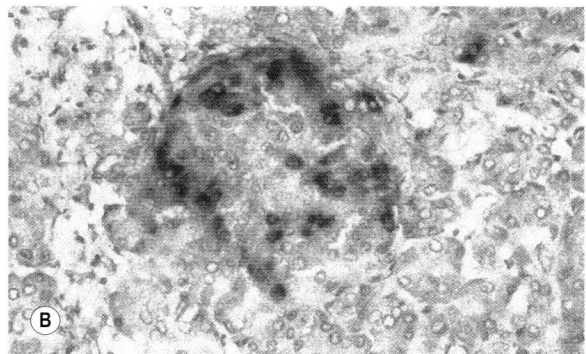

Fig. 10.40 **Islets of Langerhans:** (A) stained for insulin; (B) stained for glucagon. Note the peripheral location of the glucagon-staining cells. Reproduced with permission from Young B, Lowe JS, Stevens A, Heath JW 2006 Wheater's functional histology, 5th edn. Churchill Livingstone, Edinburgh.

Functional microanatomy of the islets

The pancreatic islets contain three populations of cells:

- A (α) cells secrete glucagon and glucagon-like peptides (GLPs).
- B (β) cells release insulin and C peptide.
- D (δ) cells secrete somatostatin.

The islets consist of a central medulla in which B cells are clustered, surrounded by a cortex containing the other cell types. B cells make up about three-quarters of the total number of islet cells. Gap junctions couple A cells to each other, B cells to each other, and A cells to B cells. These relationships may account for the synchronised secretion seen from these cells. Arterioles supplying the islets enter the medulla and break up into an anastomosing network of sinusoids that drain into more peripheral venules. This arrangement delivers insulin released from the central B cells to the cortical A and D cells, on which it acts as a paracrine. For example, insulin inhibits glucagon secretion from A cells. The venous drainage of the islets carries their secretions into the portal vein. The islets are supplied by both divisions of the autonomic nervous system.

Insulin

Synthesis and structure

Insulin is produced from a precursor, **proinsulin**, that is packaged into secretory granules by the Golgi apparatus, and has about 8% the biological activity of insulin itself. Inside the granule, proinsulin is cleaved by proteases (at least four, all Ca^{2+}-dependent) to produce insulin and **C** (**connecting**) **peptide** (Fig. 10.41). **Insulin** is a dipeptide with its A and B chains linked by two disulphide bonds.

C-peptide has no known biological activity, but it is co-released in equimolar proportions with insulin, so it is a marker for **endogenous** insulin production in diabetic patients being treated with exogenous human insulin. Conversely, an absence of C-peptide in severe, recurrent hypoglycaemia with raised insulin concentration indicates overtreatment with exogenous insulin (or insulin misuse).

Secretion of insulin

Insulin secretion is Ca^{2+}-dependent and is evoked principally by the rise in blood glucose after eating. The biochemistry of insulin secretion in response to glucose is well understood.

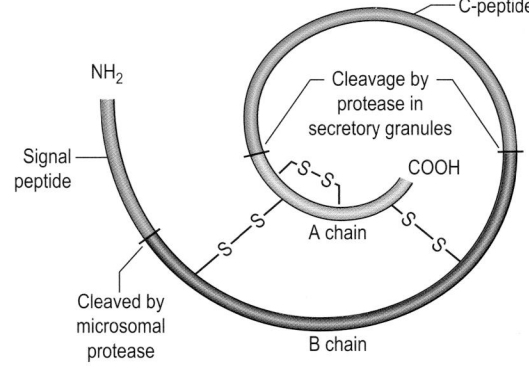

Fig. 10.41 **Molecular components of preproinsulin.** The signal peptide is cleaved as the nascent protein is secreted into the endoplasmic reticulum. Note that equimolar quantities of insulin and C-peptide are generated in the secretory granules.

Glucose enters B cells in proportion to its concentration in the blood because the GLUT2 transporter responsible for B cell glucose uptake has a high capacity and is hard to saturate (see Ch. 3). Glucose oxidation raises the ATP/ADP ratio inside the B cell which closes an ATP-sensitive potassium channel. The fall in K^+ influx depolarises the cell, opening calcium channels. Calcium entry then activates the secretory machinery.

Some amino acids liberated after a protein-rich meal, principally arginine, lysine and leucine (Table 10.13), also evoke insulin secretion, but only when glucose concentration is normal. This facilitates storage of dietary amino acids as proteins rather than their being used for gluconeogenesis. This is because insulin shifts glucose metabolism towards glycolysis and away from gluconeogenesis (Ch. 3). Insulin secretion is also stimulated by *high* concentrations of fatty acids and ketones, and this acts as a negative feedback mechanism to curtail their production because insulin inhibits lipolysis and β-oxidation.

B cells are innervated by both branches of the autonomic nervous system. Insulin secretion is stimulated by parasympathetic activity (e.g. when eating) but inhibited by sympathetic activity. The rise in blood glucose that is seen during stress is in large measure due to the sympathetic suppression of insulin release. Insulin secretion, triggered by eating a mixed meal, has two phases.

Table 10.13	Physiological stimuli affecting insulin release	
Stimulates insulin secretion		**Inhibits insulin secretion**
Increased plasma:		Decreased plasma:
Glucose		Glucose
Amino acids		Amino acids
Fatty acids		Fatty acids
Ketones		
Parasympathetic stimulation		Sympathetic stimulation
Adrenaline (β-adrenoceptors)		Adrenaline (α-adrenoceptors)
Glucose stimulated insulotropic peptide (GIP)		Somatostatin
Glucagon-like peptide (GLP)		Leptin
Gastrin		
Cholecystokinin (CCK)		
Secretin		

Table 10.14	Major biochemical actions of insulin		
Process	**Tissue**		
	Liver	**Skeletal muscle**	**Adipose tissue**
Glucose transport	(GLUT2) ↑ by activating glucokinase	↑ GLUT4	↑ GLUT 4
Glycolysis	↑	↑	↑
Gluconeogenesis	↓		
Glycogenesis	↑	↑	
Glycogenolysis	↓	↓	
Fatty acid biosynthesis	↑		
Lipogenesis	↑		↑
Lipolysis	↓		↓
β-Oxidation	↓		↓
Amino acid uptake		↑	
Protein synthesis		↑	
Proteolysis		↓	

- A **fast phase** is seen almost immediately and occurs before glucose levels rise in the portal circulation. It is brought about, in response to eating, by activation of the parasympathetic supply to the B cells. It lasts only a few minutes because it relies on the release of preformed insulin.
- A **slow phase** is triggered by hormones **glucose-stimulated insulotropic peptide (GIP)** and **GLPs**, secreted by the gut, and by the rise in concentrations of glucose, amino acids and fatty acids that enter the circulation via the portal vein. The slow phase of insulin secretion begins after about 10 minutes, rises over a period of about 1 hour, and is sustained by de novo insulin synthesis.

Insulin receptors

Receptors for insulin are members of the **tyrosine kinase** superfamily (Ch. 4). Hormone-binding triggers autophosphorylation of its tyrosine kinase domains. Once this has taken place the receptor can activate a number of intracellular signalling cascades by way of tyrosine phosphorylation of insulin receptor substrates, even in the absence of any further insulin. The effects of insulin are complex and not well understood at the molecular level. Apart from modulating the activities of a large number of enzymes via phosphorylation, insulin is known to regulate the expression of at least 150 genes.

Actions of insulin

Insulin regulates carbohydrate, fat and protein metabolism primarily by actions on skeletal muscle, adipose tissue and the liver (Table 10.14). This has been discussed in Chapter 3.

Insulin-dependent glucose transport

A major action of insulin is in determining the rate at which glucose is utilised, by regulating glucose transport, the rate limiting step in most cells. The facilitated diffusion of glucose into cells is controlled by four distinct transporters (Ch. 3). Only one of these, the GLUT4 transporter, expressed on skeletal and cardiac muscle and on fat cells, is insulin dependent. Insulin causes the GLUT4 transporters in the cytoplasm to be inserted into the plasma membrane and so become functional. About 80% of insulin-dependent glucose uptake is mediated by skeletal muscle.

Actions in the liver

Glucose transport

As transport of glucose into hepatocytes is via the high capacity GLUT2 transporter, it is not rate-limiting until glucose concentrations are abnormally high. Hence insulin increases the uptake of glucose into the liver by stimulating glucokinase, which phosphorylates glucose. Raising the rate at

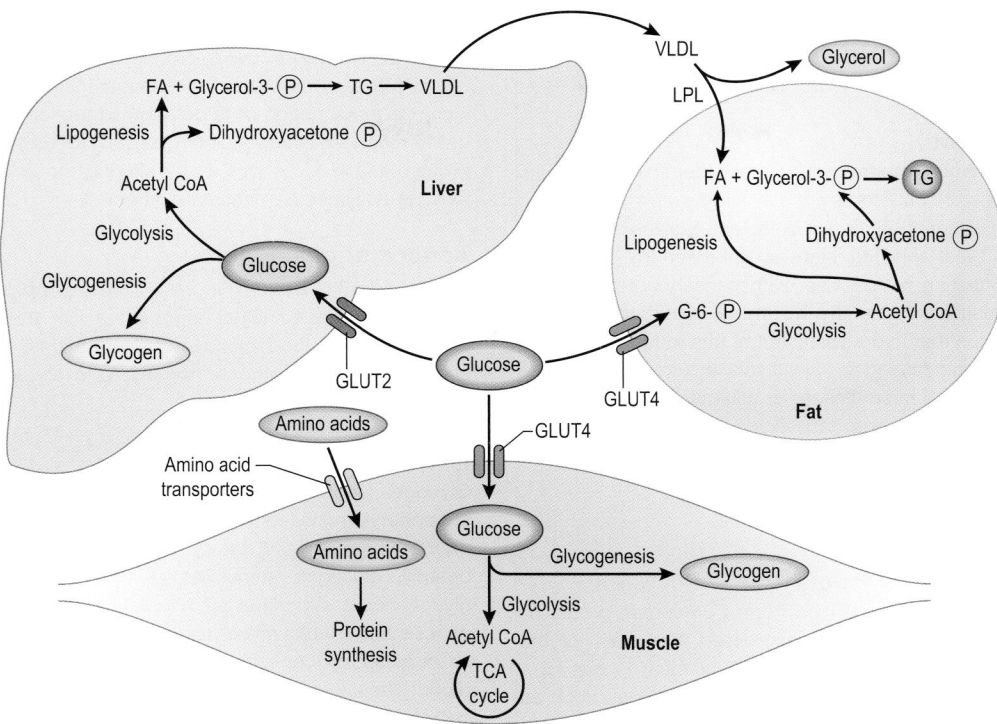

Fig. 10.42 Metabolism in the fed state dominated by the actions of insulin. FA, fatty acids; LPL, lipoprotein lipase; TG, triacylglycerol; VLDL, very-low-density lipoprotein.

which glucose is phosphorylated in this way increases the glucose concentration gradient across the cell membrane.

Glucose metabolism

Insulin increases glycolysis and glycogenesis while inhibiting gluconeogenesis and glycogenolysis (Fig. 10.42). The overall effect is that when blood glucose levels are high it is taken up by the liver and either used to provide acetyl CoA for fatty acid synthesis or is stored as glycogen. In contrast, when glucose – and consequently insulin – concentrations are low, glucose derived from gluconeogenesis and glycogenolysis is released from the liver.

Fatty acid biosynthesis

In humans, the principal site for fatty acid biosynthesis is the liver. Several enzymes involved in this are stimulated by insulin, including **acetyl CoA carboxylase**, which catalyses the first step in fatty acid biosynthesis, the carboxylation of acetyl CoA to malonyl CoA (see Ch. 3). Glycerol is phosphorylated by liver glycerol kinase to glycerol-3-phosphate (G-3-P), which is then esterified with fatty acids to produce triacylglycerols. These are packaged with cholesterol and apolipoproteins for release into the circulation as very-low-density lipoproteins (VLDLs). The triacylglycerols in VLDLs are hydrolysed by lipoprotein lipase in peripheral tissues to provide fatty acids, and are used as a fuel for muscle and for lipogenesis by fat cells.

Actions in muscle

Glucose transport

Glucose is transported into muscle by the insulin-dependent GLUT4 transporter. Insulin stimulates muscle glycogenesis. In resting muscle, when glucose and insulin levels are high, glucose is stored as glycogen. This is the rationale for using a high carbohydrate diet by athletes: to maximise muscle glycogen stores so as to increase endurance.

For reasons that are unclear, exercising muscle, even in trained athletes, cannot get more than about 70% of its energy needs from oxidation of fats. During exercise, the release of adrenaline stimulates glycogenolysis in muscle, providing it with an endogenous source of glucose. (Muscle cannot release glucose into the circulation because, unlike liver, it lacks glucose-6-phosphatase, see Ch. 3.) Also, adrenaline increases both glycogenolysis and gluconeogenesis in the liver, which consequently delivers more glucose to the blood. However, sympathetic activity during exercise completely shuts down insulin secretion. In working muscle, glucose transport via GLUT4 is stimulated in the absence of insulin. The decreased oxygen concentration in working muscle causes translocation of GLUT4 transporters into the plasma membrane.

During exercise or fasting, when insulin concentration is low, glucose entry into non-working muscle is at a low rate. The basal metabolic requirements of resting muscle are met largely by fatty acids.

Amino acids

Insulin stimulates the transport of amino acids, particularly the branched chain amino acids (leucine, isoleucine, valine) into muscle, where they are incorporated into proteins. Protein synthesis is enhanced by insulin in several ways, e.g. by promoting the phosphorylation of initiation factors that allow ribosomes to bind mRNA. Insulin also limits protein breakdown, though how is not well understood.

When insulin concentration is low, enhanced muscle proteolysis, together with extensive amino acid transamination reactions, provides the gluconeogenic amino acids, particularly alanine. This forms part of the glucose–alanine cycle, which mirrors the Cori cycle (Ch. 3), and allows muscle to sustain glycolysis without de novo glucose synthesis (see Fig. 10.43).

Actions in fat

Glucose transport into fat cells is insulin dependent (see Fig. 10.42 and Ch. 3). Fat stores are only laid down when glucose and insulin concentrations are sufficient. For many individuals in the West this fed state is unbroken by significant periods of fasting or exercise, with consequent obesity. In addition, insulin inhibits the **hormone-sensitive lipase** in adipose tissue that hydrolyses neutral fats to fatty acids and glycerol. During fasting insulin levels are low, so glucose transport into adipose tissue is minimal and lipolysis is increased, which releases fatty acids into the circulation to provide fuel for skeletal and cardiac muscle.

Glucagon

Glucagon structure

Glucagon is a peptide cleaved from a precursor, proglucagon. The proglucagon gene, expressed in A cells of the pancreatic islets, intestine and hypothalamus, is one of a superfamily of genes that code for gut hormones such as secretin, vasoactive intestinal peptide (VIP), GIP, GLPs and GHRH.

Secretion and metabolism of glucagon

Glucagon is packaged into secretory granules by the Golgi apparatus and secreted by exocytosis like other peptide hormones. It circulates without being protein-bound and has a half-life of 5 minutes. It is degraded by peptidases in the liver, kidney and plasma. The key stimuli for glucagon release are:

- Fall in blood glucose concentration
- Rise in concentrations of amino acids, mainly alanine and arginine
- Sympathetic stimulation of β-adrenoceptors on A cells
- Gut hormones, e.g. gastrin, cholecystokinin.

Glucagon secretion is inhibited in paracrine fashion by insulin, and by circulating glucose and free fatty acids. Glucagon synthesis is inhibited at blood glucose concentration of 11.1 mmol/L. The inhibition is lifted as glucose levels falls, reaching to nil at 2.8 mmol/L. Hence glucagon secretion is minimal after a carbohydrate-rich meal, but increases gradually as glucose concentration falls. How the A cells monitor blood glucose and produce a proportionate secretory response is not known. One possibility is that inhibition of glucagon secretion by glucose is brought about indirectly by the paracrine action of insulin secreted in response to the rise in glucose concentration. The direction of blood flow in the islets is consistent with this idea.

Stress is an important stimulus for glucagon release. This is mediated by β-adrenoceptor stimulation brought about by activation of the sympathetic fibres to the A cells and by circulating adrenaline. The stimulation of glucagon secretion by amino acids and gut hormones probably has two roles. It primes the liver to synthesise glucose from amino acids when these are plentiful and it ensures that some glucagon is released after a meal, counteracting the hypoglycaemic actions of insulin.

Glucagon receptors

Glucagon receptors are G-protein-coupled receptors that use cAMP as their second messenger. Glucagon is able to increase transcription of target genes by phosphorylation of cAMP response element binding protein (CREB) mediated by protein kinase A, as well as by altering the activity of pre-existing enzymes by phosphorylation.

Actions of glucagon

The actions of glucagon (Fig. 10.43) are the opposite to those of insulin, and its principal target is the liver. Its major effect is to increase blood glucose concentrations, an action it shares with several other hormones, for example adrenaline, cortisol and growth hormone.

Liver

Glycogen phosphorylase and glycogen synthase are both phosphorylated in response to glucagon, but while the phosphorylase is activated, the synthase is de-activated. Consequently, glucagon stimulates glycogenolysis but inhibits glycogenesis. Glucagon also rapidly stimulates gluconeogenesis and inhibits glycolysis in the liver (see Ch. 3). Clearly, as increased gluconeogenesis and reduced glycolysis cause blood glucose levels to rise, this dampens further glucagon secretion; this is negative feedback at work.

Glucagon stimulates the hepatic uptake of precursors for gluconeogenesis, such as alanine, glutamate, pyruvate and lactate. The amino groups from the amino acids are converted to urea so that glucagon increases urinary nitrogen excretion. Glucagon increases the β-oxidation of fatty acids in the liver by causing the phosphorylation and inactivation of acetyl CoA carboxylase. Consequently, with acetyl CoA not being used for fatty acid biosynthesis, its concentration builds up, but because β-oxidation depletes NAD it is not much oxidised by the tricarboxylic acid (TCA) cycle. This has two effects. First, glycolysis is inhibited. Second, acetyl CoA is metabolised to ketones (for this reason glucagon is described as ketogenic). The **ketone bodies β-hydroxybutyrate** and **acetoacetate** are formed by the condensation of two molecules of acetyl CoA. Ketones can serve as metabolic fuels, particularly for the brain.

Fat

Hormone-sensitive lipase in adipocytes is stimulated by glucagon so that free fatty acids and glycerol are released from adipose tissue. This lipolysis is limited by virtue of the inhibitory effect that fatty acids have on glucagon secretion.

Somatostatin

Somatostatin is a short peptide, secreted by D cells of the pancreatic islets, with several roles. It acts as a neurotransmitter in the cerebral cortex and as a hypophysiotropic hormone that inhibits growth hormone release. Although it has been suggested that somatostatin has a paracrine role in the islets, inhibiting insulin and glucagon release, the direction of blood flow in the microcirculation means that somatostatin does not reach B cells. It may have an endocrine role instead, exerting negative feedback on gut hormone secretion.

As for insulin, somatostatin secretion is stimulated by increases in blood glucose, amino acid and fatty acid concentrations, plus gastrointestinal hormones such as gastrin, secretin and cholecystokinin.

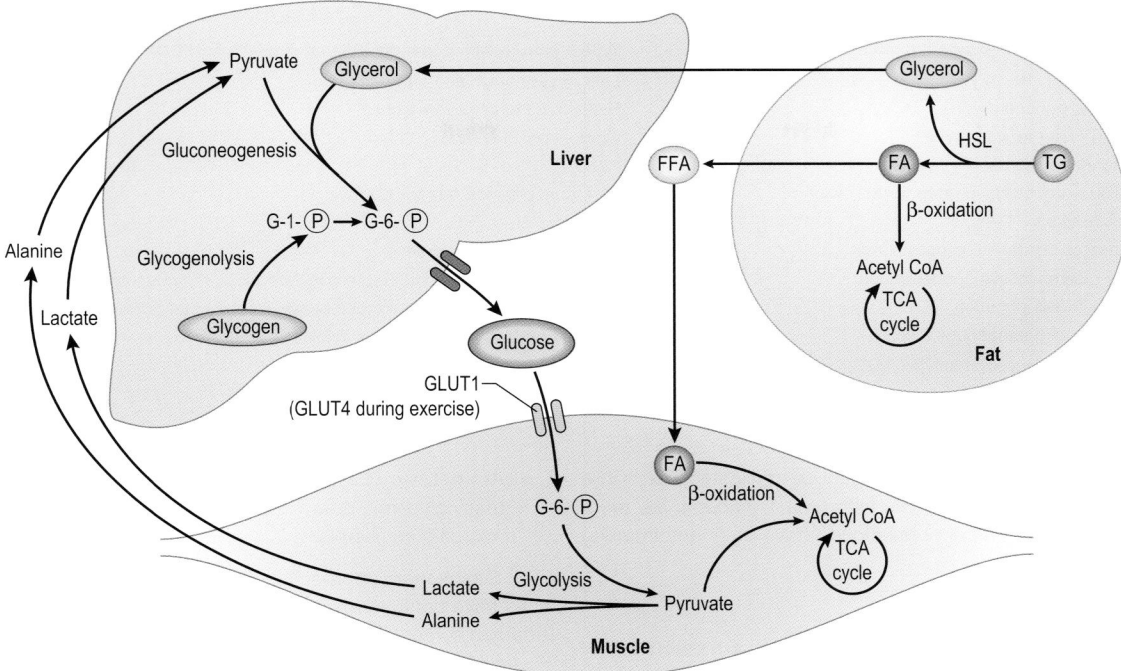

Fig. 10.43 **Metabolism in the fasting (post-absorptive) state, dominated by the actions of glucagon.** FA, fatty acids; FFA, free fatty acids; HSA, hormone-sensitive lipase; TG, triacylglycerol.

Actions of somatostatin

Somatostatin probably serves to ensure that gut function matches the ingested nutrient load, optimising absorption, by:

- Inhibiting the release of gastrin, secretin and cholecystokinin, hence curtailing their effects (see Chs 15 and 16)
- Inhibiting the transport of glucose, amino acids and fatty acids across intestinal epithelia.

Effects of feeding and fasting on pancreatic hormones

Immediately after a meal, in the **fed** (**post-prandial, absorptive**) state, insulin is secreted while glucagon release is inhibited (see Fig. 10.42; Chs 3 and 16). This favours the storage of metabolic fuels. In contrast, the **fasting** (**post-absorptive**) state is dominated by the secretion of glucagon, while insulin release is minimal (Fig. 10.43). Metabolism now is directed to maintaining blood glucose concentrations by increased hepatic breakdown of glycogen and gluconeogenesis. In this state, at rest 80% of glucose uptake is insulin-independent of which fully half is into the brain. Muscle and fat are the main tissues responsible for the remaining 20% of uptake that is insulin dependent.

As the period without food gets longer, at first the contribution of gluconeogenesis to maintaining glucose concentration becomes increasingly important as liver glycogen stores fall. This is augmented by gluconeogenic precursors from muscle, lactate (via the Cori cycle) and the gluconeogenic amino acids alanine and glutamate, derived from increased proteolysis. In addition, lipolysis increases, providing glycerol for gluconeogenesis and fatty acids as metabolic fuels for muscle (Ch. 3).

In prolonged fasting (>24 hours), hypoglycaemia stimulates maximal glucagon output and the release of growth hormone. This favours the use of free fatty acids as the dominant energy source (Chs 3 and 16; growth hormone activates hormone-sensitive lipase in adipocytes), and stimulates gluconeogenesis, while sparing proteins from being broken down to provide gluconeogenic amino acids. Because growth hormone inhibits glucose transport into tissues and because oxaloacetate concentration is depleted by gluconeogenesis, glucose oxidation in the TCA cycle is reduced. The result is that acetyl CoA concentration rises and this leads to ketone production.

Diabetes mellitus

Classification

Diabetes mellitus is a group of metabolic disorders characterised by hyperglycaemia, which causes long-term problems. It afflicts 2% of the population in the West and its incidence is rising. There are two major forms, type 1 and type 2, the principal features of which are summarised in Table 10.15. The major endocrine distinction between the two is that in type 1 there is an absolute deficiency of insulin, whereas in type 2 there is insulin resistance and a relative deficiency of insulin secretion as the disease progresses.

Epidemiology and etiology

Type 1 diabetes

Type 1 diabetes is an autoimmune disorder. Autoantibodies to islet cells, histological evidence that B cells are subject to immune attack, and infiltration of the islets by mononuclear cells, all testify to the nature of the disease. There is an association with specific MHC alleles (the HLA DR3 and DR4 loci increase the risk, while the DR2 locus reduces the risk) but in some cases the autoimmune attack is triggered by environmental factors such as viral infection (mumps, rubella

Table 10.15	Main features of type 1 and type 2 diabetes
Type 1 (insulin-dependent diabetes mellitus, IDDM)	**Type 2 (non-insulin-dependent diabetes mellitus, NIDDM)**
Early onset (10–14 years)	Late onset (fourth and fifth decades)
Patients generally lean	Patients generally overweight
Rapid onset (days to weeks)	Gradual onset (years)
Autoantibodies usually present	
30–50% concordance rate for MZ twins	90% concordance rate for MZ twins
HLA markers	No markers
Seasonal incidence, viruses?	Poor diet/lack of exercise
Low plasma insulin concentration	Insulin resistance (plasma insulin concentrations may be low, normal or high)
Ketoacidosis common	Ketoacidosis unusual (non-ketotic hyperosmolar state possible)
Always need exogenous insulin	Most do not require exogenous insulin

HLA, human leucocyte antigen; MZ, monozygotic.

and cytomegalovirus are among those implicated), exposure to toxins, or stress. Patients with type 1 diabetes are more likely than the general population to have other autoimmune disorders.

Type 2 diabetes

Type 2 diabetes is a heterogeneous set of metabolic disorders associated with over-consumption of a diet rich in fats and high glycaemic index carbohydrates (those which produce a rapid and large rise in blood glucose concentration after ingestion), obesity and lack of exercise. The epidemiological evidence is unassailable. The prevalence of type 2 diabetes is extremely low in developing, rural societies, increasing with urban lifestyle and greater average wealth, and its incidence rises in people migrating from the developing to developed world. Recent studies predict that one-third of all North Americans born in 2000 will develop diabetes and this is likely to be reflected across the developed world.

One-third of obese people develop type 2 diabetes. The risk of diabetes, severity of the insulin resistance, and risk of cardiovascular disease are all positively correlated with the amount of **abdominal visceral fat**, which can be estimated crudely by the waist–hip circumference ratio (**central obesity**). Abdominal fat deposition seems to be enhanced by psychosocial stress and elevated cortisol levels. Over 85% of individuals with type 2 diabetes are obese and successful weight loss, better diet and exercise will improve or even ameliorate the disorder.

Type 2 diabetes has an inherited component:

■ Concordance rates for type 2 diabetes and its precursor state, impaired glucose tolerance, are consistently higher in monozygotic than dizygotic twins.
■ Sibling reoccurrence rates are somewhat higher than the prevalence in the normal population.
■ There are correlations between some common single-nucleotide polymorphisms and the risk of developing type 2 diabetes.

A number of rare monogenic mutations have been characterised at the molecular level.

Type 2 diabetes may occur in conjunction with inter-related metabolic disorders in the **metabolic syndrome**. This is defined as being a combination of:

■ At least one of: type 2 diabetes, impaired glucose tolerance, insulin resistance

plus

■ At least two of: hypertension, obesity, elevated blood triacylglycerols or low high-density lipoproteins (HDLs), microalbuminaemia.

Evolutionary approaches to the genetics of type 2 diabetes have concentrated on the notion of **thrifty genes**. Early human hunter–gatherers would have faced prolonged periods when food was in short supply. These famines would selectively favour the survival of individuals who could most efficiently store energy substrates and use them sparingly when times were hard. Essentially this means evolutionary pressure is to maximise the amount of adipose tissue (since fat is the most efficient way to store energy) and to preserve glucose for use by the brain by having peripheral tissues that are resistant to insulin. In the modern developed world, with unrestricted access to food and sedentary lifestyles, thrifty genes are maladaptive and contribute to the two linked epidemics: obesity and type 2 diabetes.

A variation on the thrifty genes hypothesis is the notion of a **thrifty phenotype**. This postulates that fetal malnutrition results in altered gene expression for enzymes whose activities are linked to energy stores. The altered pattern of gene expression favours economical use of energy substrates in utero and in post-natal life, leading to obesity and type 2 diabetes. This idea is supported by the clear correlation between low birthweight and later diabetes in many populations investigated. The correlation is also seen in identical twins discordant for type 2 diabetes, showing that it is epigenetic (see Ch. 5) modification in response to the in utero environment, rather than just genotype that is important.

Several candidates for thrifty genes have been proposed. One that is currently receiving a great deal of attention is the gene encoding leptin. **Leptin** is a hormone secreted by adipose tissue that inhibits food intake by acting as a satiety signal in the brain and accelerating energy metabolism. Lack of leptin leads to obesity and insulin resistance in both rodents and humans. The amount of leptin secreted is normally proportional to the amount of adipose tissue. Hence leptin is a signal encoding the size of the fat store. Except in the rare instances in which obesity is a consequence of a defective leptin gene, obesity is associated with elevated leptin concentrations. During starvation blood leptin concentrations fall, stimulating hunger and reducing metabolic rate. Interestingly, in women whose body mass is so low that they become amenorrhoeic (e.g. some dancers and athletes), leptin replacement restores normal menstrual cycles. Hence, leptin may be a link ensuring that reproduction is only possible for women who are well nourished.

Biochemistry

Type 1

Most patients with type 1 diabetes present with a classic triad of symptoms:

- Polyuria and polydipsia
- Weight loss
- Blurred vision.

The principal sign in type 1 diabetes is fasting hyperglycaemia (see above for diagnostic criteria). When blood glucose exceeds about 11.1 mmol/L the glucose transporters in the renal tubules become saturated and excess glucose is renally excreted (**glucosuria**). This causes an osmotic diuresis (**polyuria**) which results in dehydration, thirst and hence excessive drinking (**polydipsia**). The weight loss occurs because with the low insulin/glucagon ratio lipolysis increases, as does proteolysis to provide amino acids for gluconeogenesis. Excessive eating (**polyphagia**) may also result because satiety neurons in the hypothalamus that monitor blood glucose concentrations rely on insulin-dependent GLUT4 glucose transporters. Blurred vision is due to osmotically driven changes to the shape of the lens.

The low insulin/glucagon ratio causes **dyslipidaemia** by:

- Increasing the activity of hormone-sensitive lipase, increasing lipolysis by fat cells, so raising blood free fatty acid concentration
- Decreasing lipoprotein lipase activity, which limits the uptake of fatty acids from VLDLs so that circulating VLDL levels rise
- Reducing the recruitment of LDL receptors into plasma membranes of hepatocytes and cells of peripheral tissues so that blood LDL and cholesterol concentrations rise.

The increase in lipolysis and β-oxidation of fatty acids leads to a rise in concentration of acetyl CoA, but crucially this cannot be effectively oxidised by the TCA cycle by muscle or fat because the inability to transport glucose into these tissues, due to insulin lack, depletes their oxaloacetate levels (Fig. 10.44). Consequently, much of the acetyl CoA condenses to form ketones. This can give rise to **ketoacidosis**.

Glucagon and diabetes

The clinical picture of type 1 diabetes is due not simply to insulin lack but also to an excess of glucagon. While hyperglycaemia might be thought to lower glucagon levels, this does not happen appropriately in individuals with impaired glucose tolerance and diabetes. This is partly because the lack of insulin means that other stimuli for glucagon-release remain. Because, normally, insulin stimulates amino acid transport into cells, in diabetes blood amino acid concentrations – a potent stimulant of glucagon secretion – are elevated. Hence, much of the biochemistry of diabetes can be understood as being due to glucagon turning the liver into a net producer of glucose. Since this is usually a response seen in fasting, but neither glucose nor fatty acids can be used efficiently as metabolic fuels, type 1 diabetes may be regarded as a disorder in which a patient starves in the midst of plenty.

There is considerable evidence that abnormal A cell function is needed to account for the full expression of diabetes.

Information box 10.30 **Diabetic ketoacidosis**

Pathophysiology

Diabetic ketoacidosis occurs in untreated or poorly controlled type 1 diabetes:

- Excessive ketone formation (**ketogenesis**) in the liver by condensation of acetyl CoA causes a rise in blood ketone concentration (**ketonaemia**) and a fall in blood pH – metabolic acidosis. Stimulation of central chemoreceptors in the medulla oblongata by the acidosis causes hyperventilation (**Kussmaul's respiration**).
- The concentration of ketones in the blood may exceed the transport maximum for ketone reuptake by renal tubule cells so that ketones are excreted in the urine (**ketonuria**), enhancing the osmotic diuresis brought about by glucose excretion. The diuresis results in dehydration and electrolyte loss.
- The central problem, hyperglycaemia, is aggravated by the release of stress hormones, adrenaline, cortisol and growth hormone, as well as increased secretion of glucagon, all of which tend to increase blood glucose concentration.

Treatment rationale

- Fluid replacement should take first priority since the major risks are circulatory failure due to hypovolaemic and cardiogenic shock. Fluid replacement in hypovolaemic shock will lower blood glucose concentration by shutting down the secretion of the stress hormones.
- Insulin increases potassium uptake into cells, so when insulin is lacking, potassium is released into the circulation, particularly from skeletal muscle. Renal excretion of potassium is enhanced in diabetes because of the diuresis. Consequently, patients with ketoacidosis are usually potassium depleted and this must be corrected by suitable intravenous fluid replacement. Without this, insulin administration will provoke potassium uptake and hypokalaemia, the cardiac effects of which are dangerous.

The evidence for this is that individuals with type 1 diabetes whose glucagon secretion is suppressed with somatostatin, have blood glucose concentrations only slightly above normal, have much reduced hyperglycaemia and hyperketonaemia following acute withdrawal of insulin, and show much better diabetic control with long-term suppression. Hence in diabetes, the failure of hypoglycaemia to stimulate glucagon secretion increases the risk of severe hypoglycaemia in individuals with poor therapeutic management.

Type 2

Patients with type 2 diabetes may present with the classic triad of symptoms, but rapid onset, ketonuria and ketoacidosis are rare. This is because there is usually sufficient reserve of insulin secretion in type 2 diabetes to inhibit lipolysis. This limits the availability of free fatty acids from adipose tissue to act as precursors for hepatic ketogenesis. An unambiguous differential diagnosis can be made on biochemical grounds because type 1 is characterised by:

- Presence of autoantibodies
- Absence of C peptide.

C peptide is present in type 2 diabetes because this is generally due to a reduced ability to **respond** to insulin, rather than a lack of the hormone; insulin concentrations are commonly normal.

An early and invariable defect in type 2 diabetes is **insulin resistance** in which, despite the presence of insulin, uptake

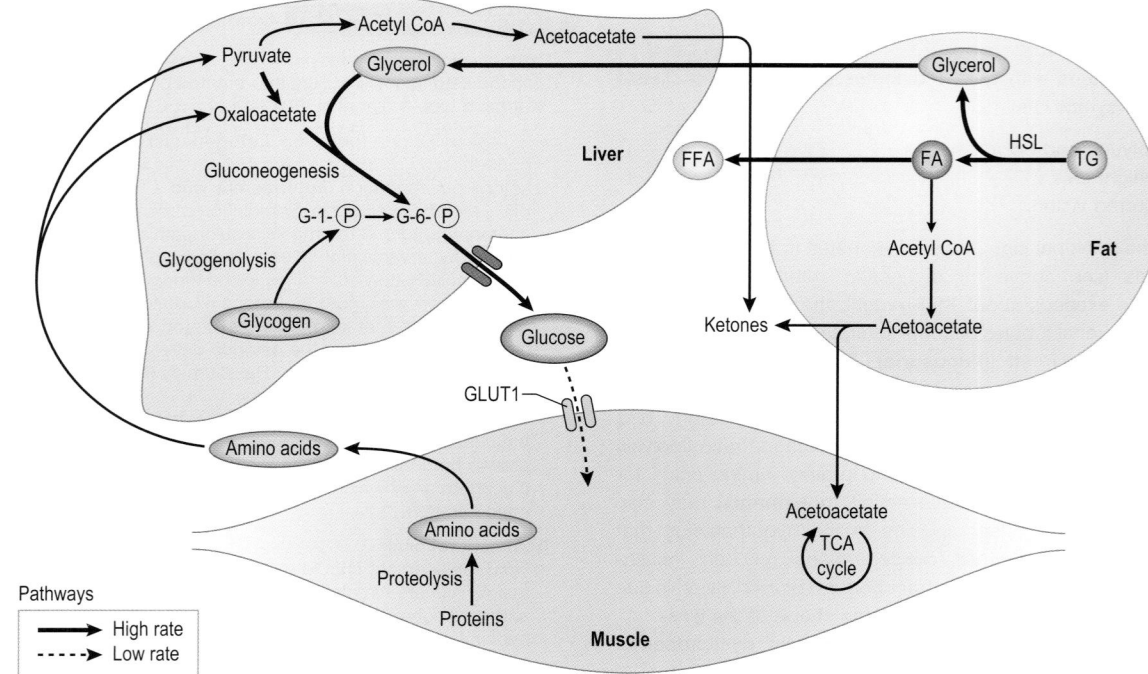

Fig. 10.44 **Dominant metabolic pathways in type 1 diabetes mellitus.** FA, fatty acids; FFA, free fatty acids; HSL, hormone-sensitive lipase; TG, triacylglycerol.

of glucose by muscle and fat is decreased. It is also seen in many obese people in whom a mild hyperglycaemia occurs in the face of an inappropriately high insulin concentration (**hyperinsulinaemia**). A number of mechanisms have been postulated to account for it (see Ch. 3). Any successful theory must account for the link between hyperglycaemia and raised concentrations of free fatty acids in the blood because this results in insulin resistance in animal studies and in humans who have a diet high in fat and high glycaemic index carbohydrates, take insufficient exercise, are typically obese, and who consequently have excessive blood concentrations of glucose and free fatty acids. The hunt for the biochemical links between nutrient excess and insulin resistance is a topic of ongoing research. A widely accepted model is that elevated blood glucose or free fatty acid concentration overactivates a biochemical pathway, dampening insulin receptor signalling and impairing the incorporation of the insulin-dependent GLUT4 glucose transporter into the plasma membrane of skeletal muscle and fat cells (see Information box 10.31).

Although early on in type 2 diabetes insulin resistance is usually accompanied by normal or even elevated insulin levels, later in the disease the B cell secretory response to glucose gradually fails, with the fast phase of insulin secretion being the first to be lost. The number of B cells in islets fall and those that remain may be misshapen. Hence in those with longer-standing or more severe disease, insulin concentrations are low.

Normally, biochemical mechanisms operate to ensure that B cell mass (the net result of mitotic division of existing B cells, production of new B cells from stem cells, B cell growth and B cell apoptosis) produces sufficient insulin to match changes in metabolic load and insulin sensitivity. These regulate B cell mass throughout life, but the effect is particularly dramatic during pregnancy, when B cell numbers can double under stimulation by prolactin and human pla-

cental lactogen, and in obese, non-diabetic, individuals who have an increased B cell mass in their islets to compensate for the high-energy substrate intake and insulin resistance.

Long-term consequences of diabetes

Pathophysiology

Persistent hyperglycaemia gives rise to pathophysiological changes seen in long-standing diabetes. These include:

■ **Macrovascular** disease (ischaemic heart disease, cerebrovascular disease and peripheral vascular disease) in which atherosclerosis is the key player, is a common consequence of long-standing type 2 diabetes. In up to 20% of patients with type 2 diabetes, vascular disease produces **renal stenosis**, and so hypertension, by activating the renin–angiotensin–aldosterone system. The hypertension adds to the vascular damage. Free radicals produced in mitochondria as a result of hyperglycaemia are partly responsible for the accelerated development of atherosclerosis, and hence the macrovascular disease.

■ **Microvascular** disorders, characterised by vasoconstriction, increased capillary permeability, proliferation of extracellular matrix and capillary occlusion, is more usually seen in type I than type 2 diabetes. Microvascular damage contributes to nephropathy, retinopathy and neuropathy.

■ **Diabetic nephropathy** is the most common reason for end-stage renal failure worldwide. The glomerular filtration barrier opens, there is renal arteriolar vasodilation and increased glomerular pressure which raises glomerular filtration rate. **Angiotensin-converting enzyme (ACE) inhibitors** have produced major reductions in morbidity and mortality associated with diabetic nephropathy not only by their antihypertensive action but because they dilate renal **efferent arterioles**,

Information box 10.31   Biochemistry of insulin resistance

Hexosamine synthesis pathway

About 3% of glucose entering glycolysis is diverted into the **hexosamine synthesis pathway** (**HSP**). Entry into the HSP is catalysed by the conversion of fructose-6-phosphate and glutamine into glucosamine-6-phosphate (GlcN-6-P) and glutamate by the rate-limiting enzyme **glutamine–fructose-6-phosphate transaminase** (**GFAT**). After a few further steps the hexosamine sugar **UDP-*N*-acetylglucosamine** (**UDP-GlcNAc**) is formed. This is the substrate for the enzyme **O-GlcNAc transferase** (**OGT**) which catalyses the transfer of GlcNAc to serine and threonine residues of numerous proteins. The serine and threonine residues are usually sites for the phosphorylation of the proteins and their glycosylation acts as another level of regulation of protein function. Many of the proteins glycosylated in this way are involved in signalling by the insulin receptor.

Stimulating the HSP

Excessive blood concentrations of glucose and free fatty acids stimulate the hexosamine biosynthetic pathway, thereby elevating concentrations of **O-GlcNAc**. High levels of glucose are thought to do this by generating a high number of superoxide anions in mitochondria as it is catabolised. These reactive oxygen species inhibit **glyceraldehyde-3-phosphate dehydrogenase** (**GAPDH**), essentially blocking glycolysis, so that concentrations of substrates upstream of the GAPDH reaction rise, including fructose-6-phosphate. This increases the flux into the hexosamine pathway. Free fatty acids may exert their effects by a similar inhibition of glycolysis or by increasing the transcription of GFAT.

In the light of the above, it is interesting to speculate that insulin resistance may have evolved to protect cells from free radical damage produced by nutrient overload. If so, the Western lifestyle is testing this adaptation to its limits.

Effects downstream of the HSP (Fig. 10.45)

One of the actions of insulin is to recruit the enzyme **OGT** to the plasma membrane of the target cell, where it catalyses the transfer of O-GlcNAc to proteins involved in insulin signalling, attenuating insulin responses. (This is thought to be a normal negative feedback control mechanism.) However, with O-GlcNAc concentrations raised by higher flux through the HSP, insulin responses are excessively suppressed. Over-expression of OGT in mice causes insulin resistance and dyslipidaemia. A key protein glycosylated in this fashion, and hence inhibited, is **insulin receptor substrate-2**. Normally activated by the insulin receptor, IRS-2 stimulates **phosphatidylinositol-3-OH kinase** (**PI(3)K**). This enzyme converts phosphatidylinositol 4,5-bisphosphate into the second messenger phosphatidylinositol 3,4,5-trisphosphate, which in turn activates a number of proteins. A major player among these is **Akt** (**protein kinase B**, there is no sensible expansion of Akt) the actions of which include:

- Stimulating lipogenesis and glycogen synthesis
- Inhibiting gluconeogenesis
- Recruiting the GLUT4 glucose transporter into the plasma membrane.

Glycosylation of IRS-2 curtails the entire signalling cascade and could account for insulin resistance by reducing the incorporation of GLUT4 into plasma membranes. Mice genetically engineered to lack Akt have insulin resistance.

Normally B cell growth and survival is promoted by Akt. In type 2 diabetes B cell mass falls because of increased apoptosis. This appears to result from inhibition of the signalling cascade between IRS-2 and Akt. Hence events triggered by the HSP that lead to insulin resistance also result in the decline in B cell numbers seen in type 2 diabetes.

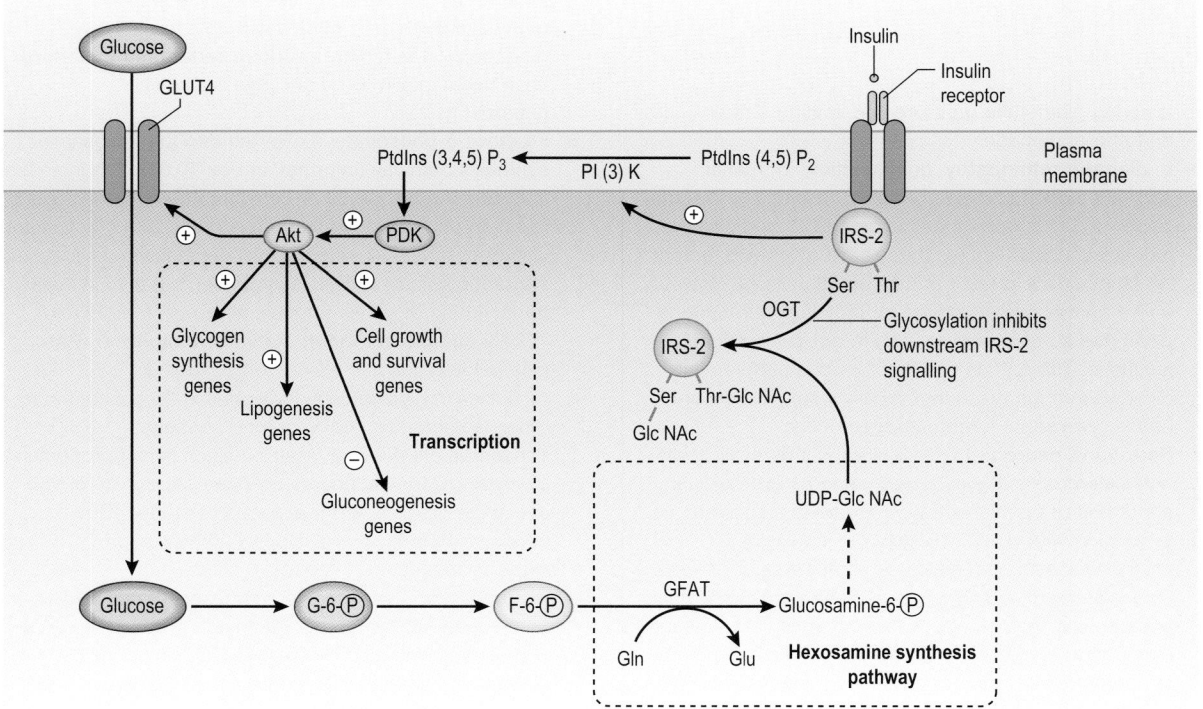

***Fig. 10.45* Effect of the hexosamine synthesis pathway on aspects of insulin signalling.** Akt, protein kinase B; GFAT, glutamine–fructose-6-phosphate transaminase; GLUT4, insulin-dependent glucose transporter; IRS-2, insulin receptor substrate-2; OGT, *O*-GlcNAc transferase; PDK, phosphatidylinositol-dependent kinase; PI(3)K, phosphatidylinositol-3-OH kinase; PtdIns (4,5)P_2, phosphatidylinositol 4,5-bisphosphate; PtdIns (3,4,5)P_3, phosphatidylinositol 3,4,5-trisphosphate; UDP-GlcNAc, UDP-*N*-acetylglucosamine.

Information box 10.31 Biochemistry of insulin resistance—cont'd

Fat cell signalling

Controversy exists as to whether increased *O*-GlcNAc is required for insulin resistance in all insulin-sensitive cells. Currently it is well established for fat cells, but there are conflicting results about whether it operates in skeletal muscle cells. However, fat cells release a number of **adipokines**, which regulate insulin sensitivity in other cell types, such as skeletal muscle, under physiological conditions.

At least two adipokines, leptin and **adiponectin**, increase insulin sensitivity. Population studies show that individuals with high concentrations of adiponectin are less likely to develop type 2 diabetes than those with low concentrations. Treatment with thiazolidinedione, the antidiabetic agent, which reduces insulin resistance, increases adiponectin concentrations.

Several adipokines are also cytokines, that is they are also released by immune cells such as macrophages. These include tumour necrosis factor-α (TNF-α) and interleukin-6 (IL-6). Both TNF-α and IL-6 are potent inhibitors of adiponectin expression in human fat cells, and they also inhibit the signal transduction pathways of both leptin and insulin. Hence these agents reduce insulin sensitivity. Insulin resistance in muscle cells may partly rely on inhibition of adiponectin release from fat cells, or by inhibition of the actions of leptin and/or insulin by TNF-α and IL-6 liberated from fat cells and macrophages.

The release of cytokines by both adipose cells and macrophages is intriguing because it suggests links between the response to infection and metabolic regulation. One possibility is that the ability to survive not just starvation, but also infection, is improved by peripheral insulin resistance, which by maintaining blood glucose concentration ensures an adequate glucose supply to the brain.

Information box 10.32 **Hyperosmolar non-ketotic syndrome (HONK)**

- Occurs in some patients with type 2 diabetes
- Shares some of the characteristics of ketoacidosis
- It is characterised by extreme hyperglycaemia and osmotic diuresis severe enough to cause dehydration and hypernatraemia
- The plasma osmolality is >340 mOsmol/L because of the high glucose and sodium concentrations
- Acidosis is sometimes seen but usually reflects other pathology; mild ketosis may occur if the patient has felt too ill to eat properly
- Onset of HONK may be insidious, with polyuria and polydipsia over the previous weeks. The most serious sequelae are hypovolaemic and cardiogenic shock so it is managed by fluid replacement.

lowering glomerular pressure and limiting further endothelial damage.

- In **diabetic retinopathy**, tight junctions of retinal capillaries open and leak proteins, resulting in **macular oedema**. Later, capillaries become occluded and the retinal ischaemia causes the release of growth factors, which stimulate growth of new blood vessels. However, unlike normal retinal capillaries, they lack surrounding **pericytes** so cannot autoregulate or develop tight junctions. The outcome is that blood is preferentially diverted through these intrinsically weak vessels and hence **pre-retinal haemorrhages** occur.
- **Peripheral neuropathy**, in which focal demyelination and loss of distal axons is seen, occurs eventually in about half of people with type 1, and in a smaller proportion with type 2, diabetes. It is usually a progressive symmetrical sensorimotor disorder in which sensation mediated by large diameter fibres is preferentially lost. However, loss of small fibre function is not uncommon and may manifest as loss of pain or temperature sensation or autonomic deficits (e.g. erectile dysfunction, sweating, disordered gastrointestinal motility).

Biochemistry

Most of the unpleasant consequences of chronic hyperglycaemia can now be understood in terms of increased flux through four biochemical pathways. Free radicals (reactive oxygen species, such as the superoxide anion, $O_2^{•-}$) produced in mitochondria as a result of hyperglycaemia inhibit the glycolytic enzyme **glyceraldehyde-3-phosphate dehydrogenase (GAPDH)** and thereby divert upstream glycolysis intermediates into alternative pathways (Fig. 10.46).

- Glucose itself is siphoned off into the **polyol pathway** which results in the elevated production of **sorbitol** in tissues expressing **aldose reductase**. Schwann cells, neurons, blood vessels and lenses of the eyes are among those expressing this enzyme. The conversion of glucose to sorbitol depletes these cells of the NADPH needed to regenerate reduced **glutathione**, a potent intracellular antioxidant. Hence activation of the polyol pathway leaves cells more vulnerable to oxidative damage by free radicals. **Aldose-reductase inhibitors** have been shown to be effective in diabetic neuropathy.
- Fructose-6-phosphate is diverted into the hexosamine synthesis pathway (Information box 10.31). The increase in *O*-GlcNAc glycosylation of a large number of proteins (including transcription factors) is responsible for a great variety of metabolic effects, including insulin resistance and apoptosis of B cells (see above), but also increased transcription of genes for several growth factors (e.g. TGF-β) and **plasminogen activator inhibitor 1 (PAI-1)** (see below).
- Increases in glyceraldehyde-3-phosphate concentration drives a rise in dihydroxyacetone phosphate concentration, the end result of which is inappropriate synthesis of the second messenger diacylglycerol and activation of the β and δ isoforms of protein kinase C. This increases the expression of numerous proteins, with consequences:
  - Endothelin – vasoconstriction (exacerbated by PKC-mediated reduction of nitric oxide synthase and hence a reduction in the vasodilator nitric oxide)
  - Vascular endothelial growth factor – increased capillary permeability
  - TGF-β – increased production of collagen and fibronectin, capillary occlusion
  - PAI-1 – decreased fibrinolysis and hence vascular occlusion
  - NF-κB transcription factor – increased expression of numerous pro-inflammatory proteins

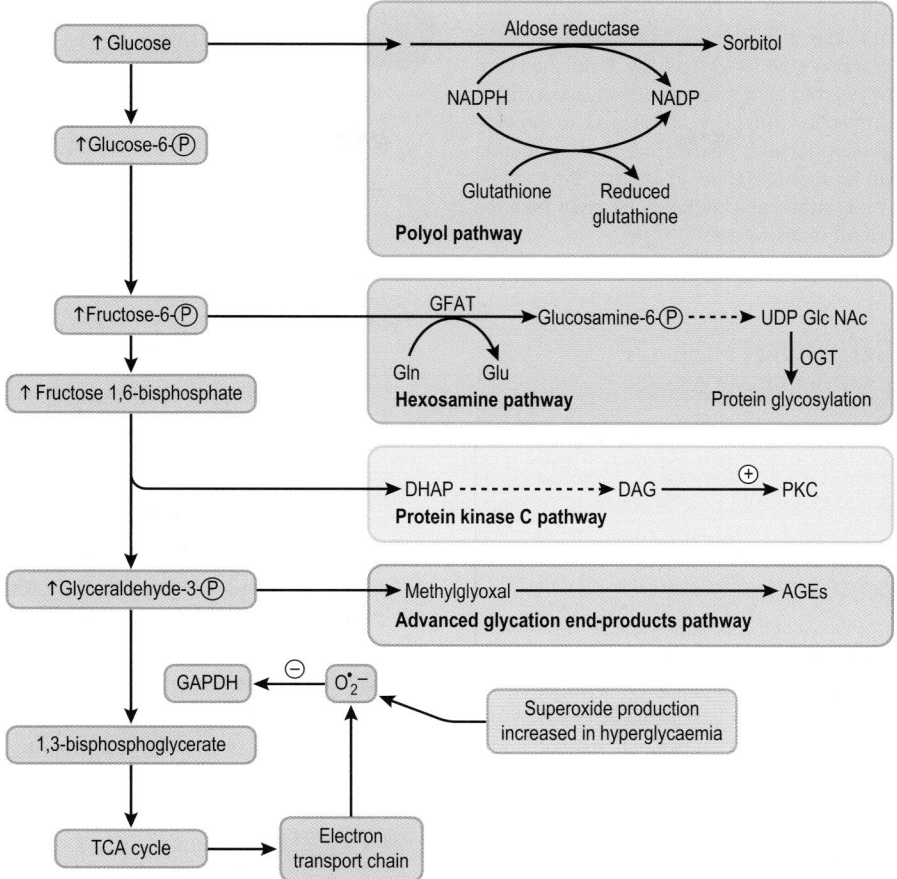

Fig. 10.46 Biochemical pathways implicated in the pathology of long-standing diabetes mellitus. DAG, diacylglycerol; DHAP, dihydroxyacetone phosphate; GADPH, glyceraldehyde-3-phosphate dehydrogenase; GFAT, glutamine–fructose-6-phosphate transaminase; TCA, tricarboxylic acid.

■ Elevated glyceraldehyde-3-phosphate levels also generate **advanced glycation products (AGEs)** inside cells and extracellularly. Extracellular AGEs produce abnormalities in matrix proteins such as collagen and laminin, one consequence of which is to reduce the elasticity of large vessels. The altered matrix proteins disrupt interactions between cells and the extracellular matrix. One consequence of this is failure of neurite outgrowth by neurons. Extracellular AGEs bind to AGE receptors on the surface of endothelial cells, mesangial cells of the kidney, and macrophages. This results in the expression of numerous cytokines and growth factors incriminated in microvascular pathology. AGE inhibitors (e.g. aminoguanidine) partly prevent microvascular changes that occur in diabetic nephropathy, retinopathy and neuropathy.

Hormone responses to stress

The metabolic response to stress (e.g. exercise, trauma, major surgery, infection, see Ch. 16) resembles that in prolonged fasting except that as well as glucagon, catecholamines released by sympathetic activity, cortisol provided by activation of the hypothalamic–pituitary–adrenal axis and more growth hormone are added to the cocktail. All have actions antagonistic to insulin and are synergistic, so that glucagon, adrenaline and cortisol together raise blood glucose much more and for longer than their individual actions would suggest. This is reinforced by the sympathetic block to the secretion of insulin, and by the sympathetic stimulation of glucagon release, which occurs in stress.

Adrenaline

Adrenaline (epinephrine) stimulates glycogenolysis and gluconeogenesis via β-adrenoceptors. This helps to maintain blood glucose concentration. This is important because, apart from ketones, glucose is the only metabolic fuel the brain can use. Adrenaline is also a potent stimulator of lipolysis by activating hormone-sensitive lipase in adipocytes. Indeed the mobilisation of fatty acids by adrenaline is quantitatively more important than its effects on hepatic glucose output, which is one reason that regular, sustained, moderately intense exercise is an effective way of losing weight (Ch. 16).

Cortisol

Increased cortisol secretion is important because it:

■ Inhibits the uptake of glucose into muscle and fat, hence sparing glucose for the brain
■ Stimulates gluconeogenesis by inducing transcription of the same genes as glucagon
■ Has a permissive role in the actions of catecholamines.

In intense stress there is an increase in insulin-independent glucose transport into muscle brought about by the actions of cytokines such as TNF-α and IL-1. TNF also enhances glycogenolysis in muscle, which enables muscle to utilise its own glucose stores more readily. Cytokines (e.g. IL-6) stimulate lipolysis but also muscle proteolysis; in other words, in stress, muscle protein is harnessed to provide substrates for gluconeogenesis, despite the protein-sparing attempts of growth hormone. Hence, in intense stress there is a loss of lean body mass and negative nitrogen balance as well as a loss of fat reserves (see Ch. 16).

ENDOCRINE CONTROL OF CALCIUM HOMEOSTASIS

ROLES OF CALCIUM

Free ionised calcium (Ca^{2+}) in the cytosol is required by all cells for cell division, regulation of the activities of many enzymes and as an intracellular signalling molecule involved in transducing the actions of many hormones, cytokines and growth factors. Ca^{2+} also acts as a signal for:

- Excitation–secretion coupling in neurons (i.e. neurotransmitter release), endocrine, paracrine and exocrine secretion and in degranulation of immune system cells (e.g. mast cells)
- Excitation–contraction coupling in skeletal, cardiac and smooth muscle

Other roles in normal physiology include:

- Providing a Ca^{2+} concentration gradient across the plasma membranes of excitable cells (neurons, all types of muscle and some endocrine cells such as insulin-secreting B cells) to maintain an appropriate threshold for excitability
- Acting as a cofactor for several proteases in the blood clotting cascade
- Its inclusion in the mineral **calcium hydroxyapatite** ($Ca_{10}[PO_4]_6[OH]_2$), which provides bone with stiffness and compressive strength.

CALCIUM HOMEOSTASIS

Calcium regulatory hormones

Calcium has a crucial role in biochemistry and physiology and the extracellular fluid concentration of Ca^{2+} is normally regulated to quite high precision by two hormones with opposing actions. The several actions of parathyroid hormone all raise blood Ca^{2+} while those of **calcitonin** reduce them. In addition, **vitamin D₃** is a precursor for its metabolite, **calcitriol**, which can be thought of as a hormone secreted by the kidney with similar actions to parathyroid hormone.

Hypocalcaemia and hypercalcaemia

Normal blood calcium concentration ranges between 2.2 mmol/L and 2.5 mmol/L, but only 50% of this is free Ca^{2+}, the rest is bound either to plasma proteins such as albumin or to citrate, lactate and phosphate. Only the free ionised calcium is directly regulated by hormones and available for active participation in physiological processes. The ratio of free to bound calcium is determined by blood pH. Increased hydrogen ion concentration ($[H^+]$) reduces calcium binding

---

_i_ Information box 10.33 **Bone resorption and hypercalcaemia**

Long-term reduction in mechanical forces applied to bone results in increased bone resorption. This occurs:

- In the sedentary elderly (contributing to osteoporosis in this group)
- With immobility due to prolonged illness
- In the low gravitational forces experienced by astronauts; indeed it is one of the serious physiological constraints to long manned space flights.

The release of calcium from resorbing bone can result in hypercalcaemia, for example in Paget's disease when bone resorption is greatly increased. Hypercalcaemia can also occur with hyperparathyroidism and cancers.

Clinical consequences of hypercalcaemia include:

- Raising the combined concentrations of calcium and phosphate in any body fluid compartment beyond the **solubility product** for calcium phosphate allows this mineral to precipitate out. When this occurs in the extracellular compartment the result can be calcification of soft tissues with a consequent reduction in function (e.g. renal calcification may lead to renal failure). When there is increased renal **excretion** of calcium this can result in calculi (stones) in the renal pelvis (Ch. 14)
- Osmotic diuresis and thirst due to renal excretion of calcium
- Stimulation of gastrin secretion resulting in elevated gastric acid release and eventually peptic ulceration
- Decreasing neuron excitability, causing constipation via effects on the enteric nervous system, and a plethora of CNS symptoms–predominantly depression and cognitive impairment.

---

while decreased $[H^+]$ raises calcium binding. Hence in acidosis free $[Ca^{2+}]$ is elevated, while in alkalosis free $[Ca^{2+}]$ falls. A blood $[Ca^{2+}]$ of below 2.2 mmol/L is defined as **hypocalcaemi**a, whereas concentrations above 2.5 mmol/L are termed **hypercalcaemia**. Both of these are problematic, even in the short term, because of effects on muscle and neuron excitability.

Calcium distribution and fluxes

Average required daily dietary intake of calcium is about 25 mmol (1 g), of which 5 mmol reaches the blood after intestinal absorption (7.5 mmol) and excretion (2.5 mmol) are accounted for (Fig. 10.47). The net uptake of calcium from food is therefore inefficient; most dietary calcium (20 mmol each day) is excreted in the faeces. The calcium uptake is enough to replace the calcium loss of 5 mmol per day in the urine, which is the net difference between the amount filtered through the glomerulus and the amount reabsorbed by the renal tubules. Bone is a massive repository of 25 mol (1 kg) of calcium, a tiny fraction of which, 10 mmol per day, is exchanged with that in the blood by bone resorption matched by an equal amount of bone mineralisation. Many of these fluxes can be altered by one or more hormones so as to maintain blood calcium concentration, which takes first priority.

Intracellular calcium

Although the free cytosolic $[Ca^{2+}]$ is five orders of magnitude lower than the free $[Ca^{2+}]$ in extracellular fluid, cells contain large calcium pools in organelles (e.g. endoplasmic reticu-

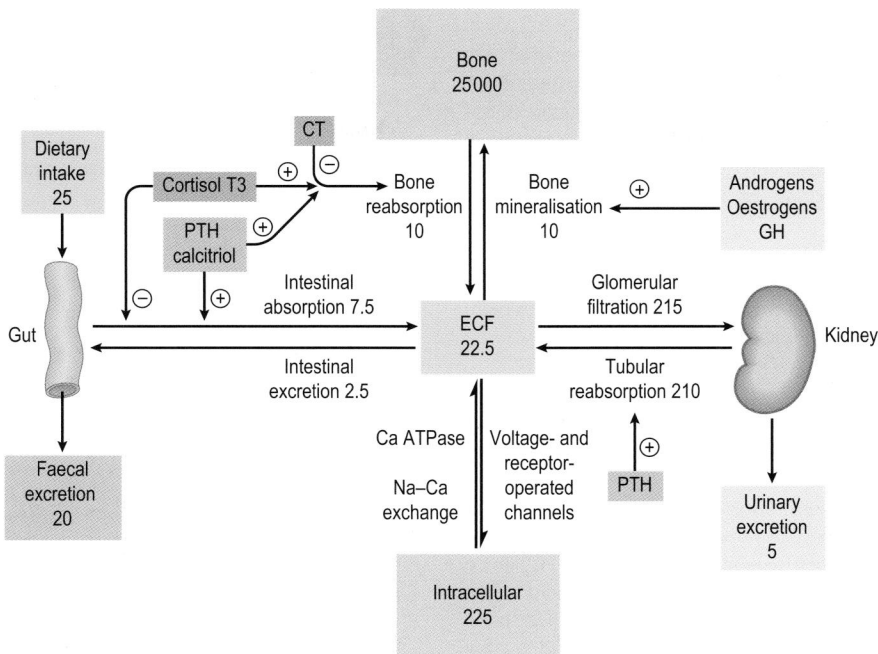

Fig. 10.47 **Endocrine regulation of calcium fluxes and distribution.** Fluxes are the quantities of calcium shifting per unit of time (mmol/day). Calcium amounts are in mmol.

lum), so there is 10-fold more calcium sequestered inside cells (225 mmol) than in extracellular fluid (22.5 mmol).

Free $[Ca^{2+}]$ in the cytosol is tightly regulated because of the involvement of calcium in so many biochemical processes within cells. The resting cytosolic $[Ca^{2+}]$ is maintained at about 100 mmol/L by protein buffering within the cytosol and by a variety of transporters which pump calcium into internal stores, such as endoplasmic reticulum, or sarcoplasmic reticulum, or which actively transport calcium out of cells. Calcium signals – transient increases in free cytosolic $[Ca^{2+}]$ generated in cells by excitation, hormones, etc. – are produced by either calcium influx into cells through voltage- or receptor-operated channels or the liberation of calcium from intracellular stores by second messengers such as inositol trisphosphate (see Chs 2 and 3).

CONTROL OF BLOOD CALCIUM AND PHOSPHATE CONCENTRATIONS

Serum calcium is mainly regulated by two hormones with opposing actions. The several actions of parathyroid hormone (secreted by the parathyroid glands) all raise blood Ca^{2+} while those of **calcitonin** (secreted by the thyroid gland) reduce it.

In addition, **vitamin D₃** is a precursor for its metabolite, **calcitriol**, which is a hormone secreted by the kidney, has similar actions to parathyroid hormone, and is also found in many target organs. Adrenal and gonadal steroids (in particular testosterone and oestrogen) and growth hormone also have regulatory effects on calcium homeostasis.

Parathyroid hormone

Parathyroid glands

Most people have four parathyroid glands, each a flattened ellipsoid 6 mm long, attached to the posterior surface of the lateral lobes of the thyroid gland or embedded within it. The glands have a rich blood supply from the inferior thyroid arteries and contain cords of **chief cells** that secrete parathyroid hormone (parathormone; **PTH**) and small clusters of larger **oxyphil cells** with no known function.

Synthesis, storage, release and metabolism

PTH is a single peptide molecule with 84 amino acids, but all the biological activity resides in the N-terminal 34 amino acids. Close to basal levels of secretion of PTH occurs in bursts 1–3 times per hour at a blood $[Ca^{2+}]$ of approximately 2.5 mmol/L. There is also a circadian rhythm which appears to be an intrinsic property of chief cells, with a peak at midnight and nadir just before midday. PTH secretion rises about fourfold in an almost linear fashion in response to a fall in blood $[Ca^{2+}]$ from 2.6 mmol/L to 2.1 mmol/L. The Ca^{2+} sensor in the chief cell plasma membrane is a G-protein-coupled receptor structurally related to the glutamate metabotropic receptors and coupled to phospholipase C (Ch. 3). Activation of the calcium receptor by Ca^{2+} (or less potently by Mg^{2+}) reduces PTH secretion. Increases in blood phosphate concentration stimulate PTH secretion indirectly by ionic bonding to calcium, which reduces blood free $[Ca^{2+}]$.

Parathyroid cells store only sufficient PTH to sustain the maximum secretion rate for about 90 minutes; the hormone is synthesised and degraded to match secretory demand. When $[Ca^{2+}]$ is high, proteolytic enzymes within the secretory granules are stimulated and as much as 90% of stored hormone is degraded to inactive fragments that are co-released along with the small remaining quantity of intact PTH.

PTH has a circulating half-life of only 2–4 minutes, being rapidly hydrolysed by proteases in the liver and kidneys. PTH fragments are small enough to cross the renal filtration barrier and be excreted in the urine.

Actions of PTH

PTH acts through G-protein-coupled receptors that are coupled to the cyclic AMP second messenger system. Both short-term effects due to protein A kinase-mediated phosphorylation of target proteins and longer-term alterations in gene expression, via regulation of cAMP response elements, are seen. All the actions of PTH raise blood calcium concentration.

Bone

PTH increases osteoclastic bone resorption, and calcium and hence phosphate mobilisation (Ch. 9).

Kidney

PTH activates the synthesis of vitamin D_3 (1,25-$(OH)_2D_3$) from vitamin D. Vitamin D_3 is a precursor of **calcitriol**, which has a similar action to PTH.

About 90% of calcium reabsorption occurs in the proximal convoluted tubule. The remaining reabsorption by the thick ascending loop of Henle is increased by PTH. Hence PTH increases the **fractional** reabsorption of calcium, but because the overall effect of PTH is to raise blood $[Ca^{2+}]$, the hormone increases the amount of calcium filtered by the kidney and increases renal calcium excretion. The details of hormone-sensitive calcium reabsorption are summarised in Figure 10.48.

PTH reduces the transport maximum for phosphate reabsorption by the proximal convoluted tubule, increasing phosphate excretion. This is achieved by translocation of the sodium–phosphate cotransporter in the luminal membrane of the tubule cells into intracellular vesicles. This is so powerful an effect that even though PTH mobilises phosphate from bone and raises its absorption by the gut, blood phosphate concentrations fall.

> ### ⓘ Information box 10.34 — Disorders of the parathyroid gland
>
> **Hypoparathyroidism**
>
> Lack of PTH leads to low blood calcium concentration in conjunction with high blood phosphate concentration. The low $[Ca^{2+}]$ increases neuromuscular excitability causing:
>
> - **Paraesthesia** (tingling sensation in lips, fingers and toes)
> - **Tetany** – sustained, abnormal and repetitive muscle contractions (muscle cramps).
>
> **Trousseau's sign**: Even when calcium concentrations are not low enough to cause frank tetany, thumb adduction, triggered in the hand by occluding the arterial blood supply to the arm with a sphygmomanometer cuff for 3 minutes, is taken as diagnostic of hypocalcaemic tetany. The hypoxia inhibits the cation pump in muscle and neuron plasma membrane, so that the extracellular potassium ion concentration rises causing depolarisation (Ch. 10). This is sufficient stimulus, together with the increased excitability, to generate skeletal muscle tetany.
>
> A reduced excitability is found in **cardiac muscle** at the calcium concentrations encountered in hypoparathyroidism, and this can precipitate first-degree heart block (Ch. 3).
>
> **Pseudohypoparathyroidism**
>
> - Failure to respond to exogenous PTH is caused by defects in the cyclic AMP second messenger system recruited by the PTH receptor, despite a lower serum calcium concentration.
> - About half of the cases arise from mutations in the α subunit of the G_s G protein, and patients have resistance to other hormones that act through cyclic AMP.
>
> **Hyperparathyroidism**
>
> - Excess PTH activity causes increased blood calcium concentration, usually accompanied by a reduced blood phosphate concentration
> - **Primary hyperparathyroidism** is most commonly caused by excess PTH secretion by parathyroid gland adenomas.
> - **Secondary hyperparathyroidism** generally results from vitamin D deficiency and renal failure (see Clinical box 10.9).

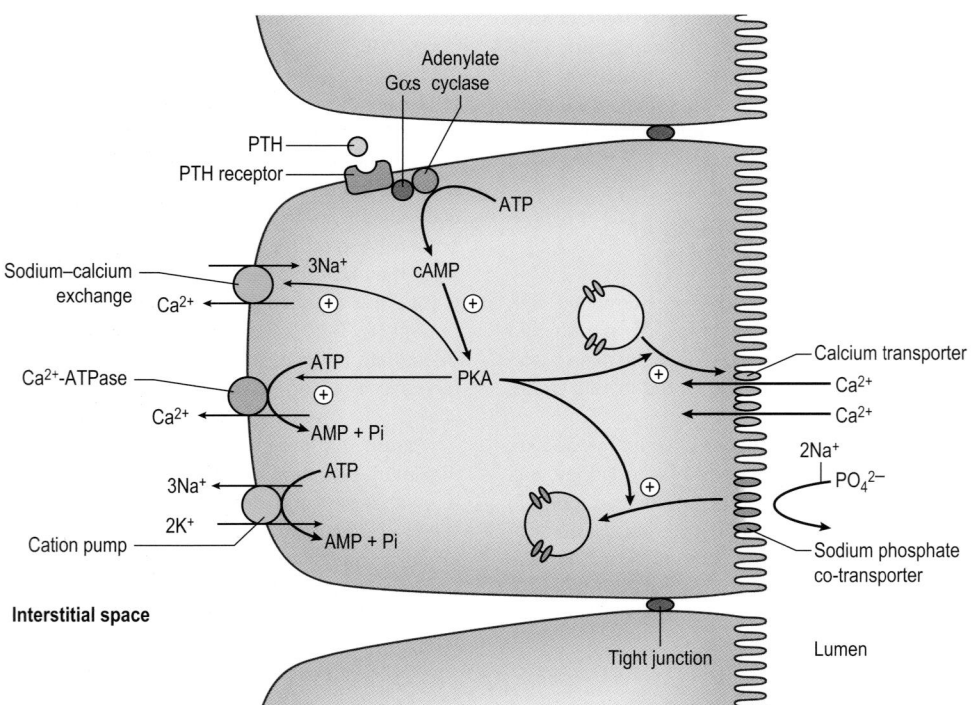

Fig. 10.48 Effects of parathyroid hormone (PTH) on calcium and phosphate ion (Pi) transport across renal tubular epithelium. NB: Phosphate and calcium are reabsorbed in the proximal and distal tubules, respectively.

Gastrointestinal tract

PTH increases the absorption of calcium and phosphate by the gut indirectly by stimulating the transcription of 1α-hydroxylase in the kidney. This enzyme catalyses the synthesis of calcitriol, the direct agent for absorption.

Calcitonin

The actions of **calcitonin** (**thyrocalcitonin**) are antagonistic to PTH and tend to lower blood calcium concentration.

Synthesis and metabolism

Calcitonin is produced by **parafollicular** (C) cells which lie singly or in clusters scattered among the thyroid follicles. The biochemistry of C cells has some similarities to A cells of the pancreatic islets and to chromaffin cells, such as those of the adrenal medulla, in that they can take up and decarboxylate amines. This could account for the frequent association of the malignancy seen in these three types of cells.

Calcitonin is a peptide of 32 amino acid residues coded by a gene, the transcript of which is subject to alternative splicing in other tissues to generate **calcitonin gene-related peptide** (**CGRP**). This molecule is a neuropeptide with potent vasodilator and positive cardiac inotropic effects.

Calcitonin has a half-life of about 5 minutes; it is subject to proteolysis and cleared from the blood mainly by renal excretion.

Secretion

Parafollicular cells express the same metabotropic receptors for Ca^{2+} as the chief cells of the parathyroid glands and respond over the same range of blood calcium concentrations, but in the opposite direction to PTH; calcitonin secretion increases as $[Ca^{2+}]$ rises. Calcitonin secretion is also increased by the release of the gut hormones, gastrin, cholecystokinin, and secretin, which are liberated after a meal. This may:

- Limit the rise in blood $[Ca^{2+}]$ in response to a high load of ingested calcium
- Favour bone mineralisation when blood $[Ca^{2+}]$ rises after eating.

Actions of calcitonin

The G-protein-coupled receptors for calcitonin share a high homology with those for PTH and are coupled to G_s proteins and the cyclic AMP second messenger system. The major effect of calcitonin is to lower blood calcium and phosphate levels by inhibiting the activity of osteoclasts (Ch. 9). The hormone probably has no effects on any other type of bone cell.

In the kidney, calcitonin can increase the excretion of calcium and phosphate by curtailing their reabsorption by the proximal convoluted tubules, but in humans this is too small and transient an effect to be of physiological importance.

Role of calcitonin in calcium regulation

In humans, calcitonin is probably not important in calcium regulation in the short term. No obvious perturbation of calcium homeostasis or disease state is seen in its absence or when it is produced in excess. However, its inhibition of osteoclastic activity may act as a protective agent against excessive bone resorption in the long term.

Clinical uses of calcitonin

The inhibition of osteoclast activity is exploited in the treatment of osteoporosis and in Paget's disease, a disorder of unknown aetiology that causes localised increases in bone turnover (see Ch. 9). Calcitonin has an analgesic effect which reduces the pain of these disorders and does produce modest increases in bone density, but without effect on the incidence of bone fractures. Unfortunately with long-term use, the salmon calcitonin which is most commonly used generates antibodies in about 20% patients, who become resistant to its effects.

Calcitriol

A metabolite of vitamin D_3, **calcitriol** (**1, 25-dihydroxycholecalciferol**) has PTH-like effects on bone and mediates the effects of PTH on the absorption of calcium and phosphate by the gut.

Synthesis and transport

Vitamin D_3 (**cholecalciferol**), a steroid in which the B ring has been opened up, comes either from the diet or is synthesised in the skin by the action of near-ultraviolet radiation in sunlight on **7-dehydrocholesterol** (see Fig. 10.49). It is hydroxylated first in the 25 position by the liver and then again in the 1 position ($1,25-(OH)2D_3$) in the proximal convoluted tubule cells of the kidney to give calcitriol.

Calcitriol may be thought of as a hormone because it is synthesised from a precursor and can be made endogenously (vitamin D_3) by the joint actions of two organs and released directly into the circulation. Calcitriol is not very soluble in water and 99% circulates bound to **transcalciferin** giving it a half-life of about 15 hours.

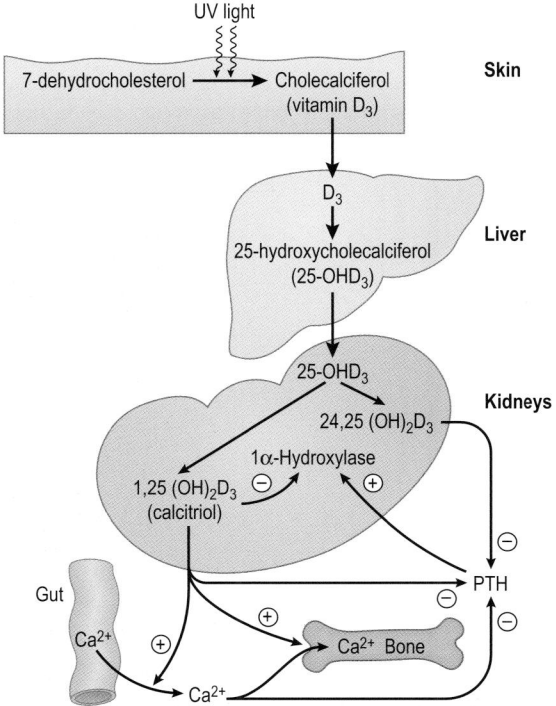

Fig. 10.49 Synthesis and actions of calcitriol.

One of the first consequences of glomerular impairment in chronic renal failure is a reduction in phosphate clearance and consequent **hyperphosphataemia**. The excess phosphate causes the solubility product for calcium phosphate to be exceeded so extracellular calcium concentration falls as calcium phosphate is precipitated out of solution. The fall in calcium levels stimulates PTH secretion, so these individuals have hypocalcaemia in the face of secondary hyperparathyroidism. Patients with chronic renal failure often cannot produce sufficient calcitriol from vitamin D_3 to suppress this PTH secretion because of reduced expression of renal 1α-hydroxylase (see Fig. 10.49). Moreover, the diminished calcitriol impairs gut absorption of calcium (and phosphate), which exacerbates the hypocalcaemia. The excess PTH secretion stimulates bone resorption, aggravating the hyperphosphataemia. In summary, in chronic renal failure there is hyperphosphataemia, hypocalcaemia, low calcitriol but high PTH concentrations and bone demineralisation. This unpleasant combination is called **renal osteodystrophy**. Calcium supplements may help, but calcitriol is problematic because it increases phosphate as well as calcium reabsorption.

Actions of calcitriol

The major effect of calcitriol is to increase the calcium and phosphate concentrations of extracellular fluid by acting on intestine, bone and kidney. It acts via members of the steroid receptor superfamily of nuclear receptors.

Intestine

Calcitriol increases the active transport of calcium and phosphate across epithelial cells of the small intestine, possibly by stimulating the transcription of Ca^{2+}-ATPase and a specific high affinity cytosolic binding protein termed **calbindin**. Upregulating the Ca^{2+}-ATPase effectively increases the calcium permeability of the brush border while calbindin may shuttle calcium to Na^+–Ca^{2+} antiports in the basolateral membrane. How calcitriol enhances phosphate absorption is not certain.

Bone

Calcitriol has direct PTH-like effects, increasing the activity of osteoclasts to promote bone resorption (Ch. 9) but its principal effect is to mobilise sufficient calcium and phosphate concentrations in bone fluid to favour mineralisation. A deficiency of vitamin D_3 in the diet, coupled with a lack of exposure to sunlight, results in inadequate calcitriol synthesis. This impairs gut calcium and phosphate absorption and hence proper bone mineralisation. In children this manifests as **rickets** and in adults as **osteomalacia** (see Ch. 9).

Kidney

Calcitriol increases the expression of calbindin in cells of the distal nephron and so increases calcium reabsorption. This may not be of much importance in humans.

Regulation of calcitriol

The hydroxylation of 25-hydroxycholecalciferol by 1α-hydroxylase in the kidney to give calcitriol is a key regulated step. It is stimulated by PTH (which is thus acting as a tropic hormone) and by low concentrations of phosphate. 1α-hydroxylase is inhibited by calcitriol, which therefore is exerting negative feedback on its own synthesis. In addition, calcitriol inhibits the secretion of PTH from the parathyroid glands. Because there is some unavoidable urinary excretion of calcium, even a moderate period of fasting will result in hypocalcaemia. Initially this raises PTH secretion, which stimulates calcitriol production to increase the efficiency of gut calcium absorption, after about 24 hours.

Adrenal and gonadal steroid effects on calcium metabolism

Adrenal and gonadal steroids increase osteoblast activity, enabling calcium uptake into bone, while inhibiting osteoclast-mediated bone resorption. They also decrease renal calcium and phosphate excretion, and decrease intestinal calcium excretion, the overall effect being to conserve calcium.

Growth hormone effects on calcium metabolism

The effect of growth hormone on bone is mediated through the action of IGF, which increases osteoblast activity. This is an anabolic effect, promoting skeletal growth.

11

The cardiovascular system

Patricia Revest

INTRODUCTION

BASIC FUNCTIONS OF THE CARDIOVASCULAR SYSTEM

The main role of the cardiovascular system is to supply the appropriate levels of metabolic substrates to the different tissues of the body and to remove the waste products from those tissues. Oxygen and nutrients, such as glucose, fatty acids and amino acids, must be provided to the approximately 100 trillion (100×10^{12}) cells of the body in amounts which vary according to the current metabolic demands. The waste products of the cellular processes, such as carbon dioxide and urea, must also be removed. Thus the cardiovascular system is not static but adapts constantly according to what the whole body is doing. The system must continu-

Table 11.1	Deaths by cause (UK 2006)	
Cause of death	**Number of deaths**	**Per cent**
Coronary heart disease (CHD)	94 381	16.5
Stroke	55 098	9.6
Other cardiovascular deaths	48 288	8.5
Lung cancer	34 183	6.0
Colorectal cancer	15 965	2.8
Breast cancer	12 323	2.2
Other cancer	95 330	16.7
Respiratory disease	77 729	13.6
Injuries and poisoning	20 465	3.6
All other causes	117 272	20.5
Total	571 034	100.0

Sources: Office for National Statistics England and Wales; General Register Office, Scotland; General Register Office, Northern Ireland.

ally monitor and adjust its function in order to balance the demands of different tissues over a wide range of conditions.

Other functions of the cardiovascular system include:

- Transport of signalling molecules, such as hormones, in the blood from source to target
- Movement of immune cells around the body
- Regulation of body water
- Maintenance of the correct internal temperature.

The roles of the cardiovascular system are so diverse that any impairment of cardiovascular function can have severe consequences. Cardiovascular disease accounts for a high proportion of deaths, the largest proportion of which are due to coronary heart disease (CHD) (Table 11.1).

BASIC STRUCTURE OF THE CARDIOVASCULAR SYSTEM

As is obvious from its name, the cardiovascular system consists of two major components: the heart and the blood vessels or vasculature (Fig. 11.1).

The heart

The pumping action of the heart provides the energy which propels the blood around the body in two separate circuits. The heart contracts about 70 times in every minute; in a lifetime of 75 years, this is almost three billion (3×10^9) beats, hopefully without stopping. At each beat, blood returning from the tissues is pumped into the lungs, where it gains oxygen and loses carbon dioxide. Simultaneously, oxygenated blood, which has just returned from the lungs, is pumped into the aorta, from where it is distributed around the body. The separation of these two circulations, the **pulmonary** and the **systemic**, ensures that there is no mixing of oxygenated and deoxygenated blood, thus facilitating an efficient transfer of oxygen from the lungs to the tissues. It also allows the two independent circulations to function at different pressures. The **systemic circulation** requires high pressures in order to propel the blood to the most distant capillaries, whereas the **pulmonary system** works at much lower pressures, required by the delicate nature of the thin-walled tissues of the lungs.

The blood vessels

The blood vessels, which total about 100 000 km in length, consist of a closed system of tubular structures which can be divided into three major groups.

Arteries and arterioles

The arteries act as the conduits for the distribution of blood to the various parts of the body. There are two types of artery – **elastic** and **muscular** – and they have different roles in smoothing out the fluctuations of blood pressure produced by the heart's pumping action and in the distribution of blood to the organs. The smallest arteries, called **arterioles**, have a major role in the control of blood flow to specific areas and in the maintenance of central (arterial) blood pressure.

Capillaries

Capillaries are the smallest blood vessels and it is at the level of the capillaries that virtually all the exchanges between the blood and the tissues occur. In parts of the body there are different types of capillary which have diverse permeability characteristics. For example, in the brain, only blood gases and water can move freely across the specialised capillaries (the blood–brain barrier; see Ch. 8), whereas in the liver the spaces between the capillary endothelial cells are so large that even red blood cells can move in and out of the circulation.

Veins and venules

The venules and veins drain blood from the capillaries and return it to the heart. These thin-walled vessels are highly distensible so their capacity can vary and they can contain up to 70% of the total blood volume. They are not involved in tissue exchange but are important in the control of blood pressure as changes in the muscular tone of veins can change the central blood volume, a key determinant of blood pressure. This is particularly important in situations of fluid loss, such as haemorrhage, when constriction of the veins can increase the volume of blood returning to the heart. Veins from the legs move blood against gravity, and so they have valves to ensure that blood flow is unidirectional.

Lymphatic system

Although the blood vessels return most of the blood to the heart during the circulation of blood around the body, a certain amount of fluid and protein is lost into the interstitial fluid. If this accumulates then the tissues become distended and oedematous. The lymphatic system consists of a series of blind-ended tubes which arise in the tissues as lymphatic capillaries. These capillaries remove the excess fluid and protein, termed **lymph**, from the extracellular spaces and they form a network of vessels that merge as they lead towards the thorax, where they empty into the venous circulation. The lymphatic system also has a major role in the immune system as the lymphatic vessels contain clusters of lymph nodes where cells of the immune system are located (see Ch. 6).

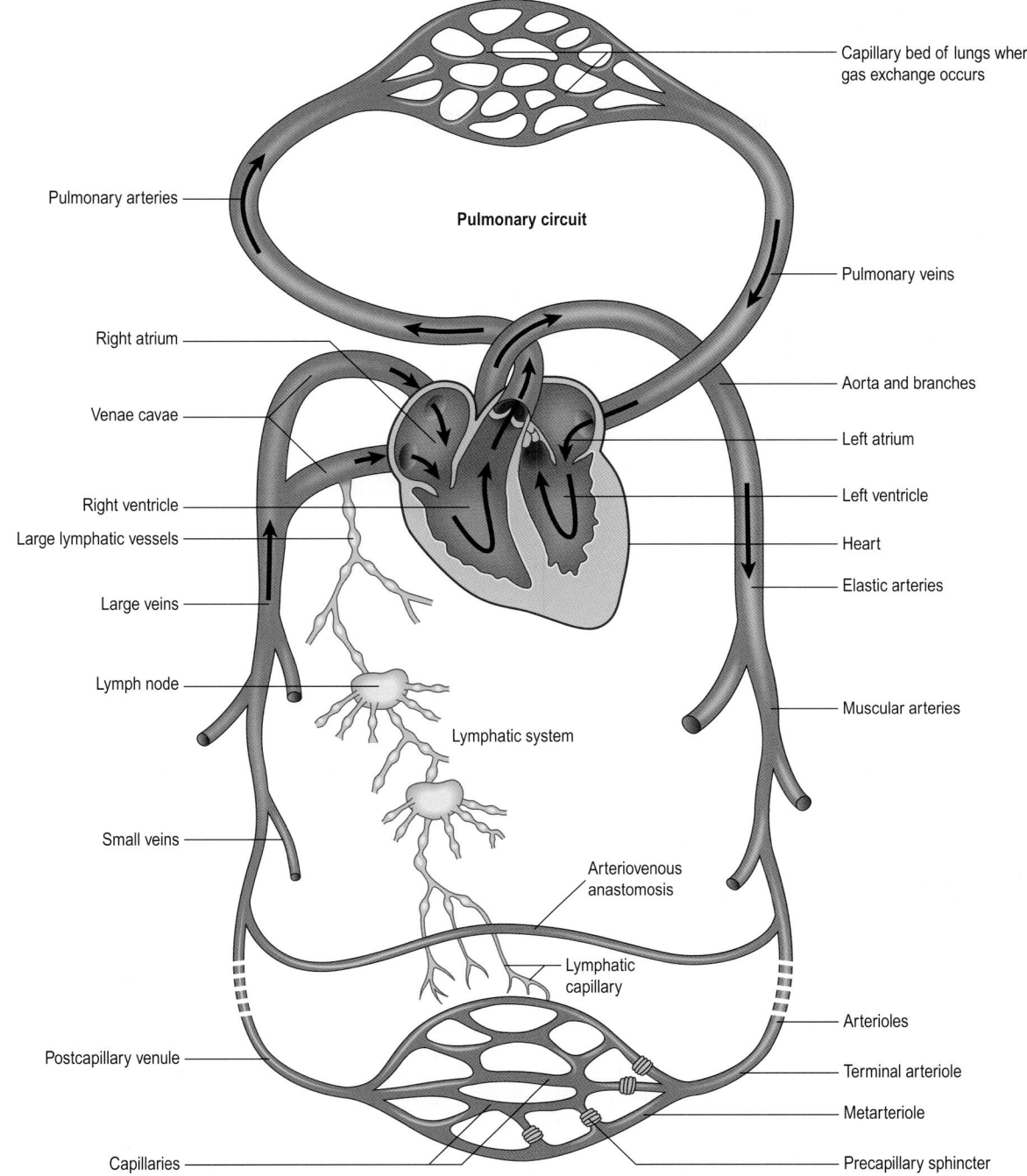

Capillary bed of lungs where gas exchange occurs

Pulmonary arteries

Pulmonary circuit

Pulmonary veins

Right atrium

Aorta and branches

Venae cavae

Left atrium

Right ventricle

Left ventricle

Large lymphatic vessels

Heart

Large veins

Elastic arteries

Lymph node

Lymphatic system

Muscular arteries

Small veins

Arteriovenous anastomosis

Lymphatic capillary

Arterioles

Postcapillary venule

Terminal arteriole

Metarteriole

Capillaries

Precapillary sphincter

Fig. 11.1 **Overview of the systemic and pulmonary circulations.** Oxygenated blood is shown in *pink*, deoxygenated in *blue* and the lymphatic system is *green*. Redrawn, with permission from Marieb EN 2004 Human anatomy and physiology, 6th edn. Pearson Benjamin Cummings, San Francisco.

ANATOMY OF THE CARDIOVASCULAR SYSTEM

GROSS ANATOMY

The heart

The heart is a double pump working in tandem, consisting of four chambers, two atria and two ventricles (Fig. 11.2). Blood returning from the body, via the great veins, drains into the **right atrium** from where it flows into the **right ventricle**. Blood from the right ventricle leaves by the pulmonary trunk and travels to the lungs from where it drains into the **left atrium** and **left ventricle**. Blood from the left ventricle then travels via the **aorta** to all parts of the body.

In adults, the heart is about the size of a clenched fist and weighs between 250 g and 350 g. It is located in the centre of the thorax, in the medial mediastinum, between the lungs and above the diaphragm. The heart itself consists of three layers of tissue:

- A thin **epicardium**
- A thick **myocardium** composed largely of cardiac muscle fibres tethered to spiral bundles of connective tissue
- A thin **endocardium**, which is made up of connective tissue layers and a layer of endothelium which lines the internal structures of the heart and is continuous with the endothelial lining of the blood vessels.

These layers, particularly the myocardium, are richly supplied with blood from the coronary vessels.

The pericardium

The heart is surrounded by the pericardial sac, which has two layers: a layer of fibrous tissue (**fibrous pericardium**) and a double layer of serous membranes (**serous epicardium**) (Table 11.2). The serous epicardium is divided into two layers: a parietal layer which is fused to the fibrous pericardium, and a visceral layer that covers the heart itself and the large blood vessels leaving the heart. The space between the two layers of epicardium is known as the **pericardial cavity** and this

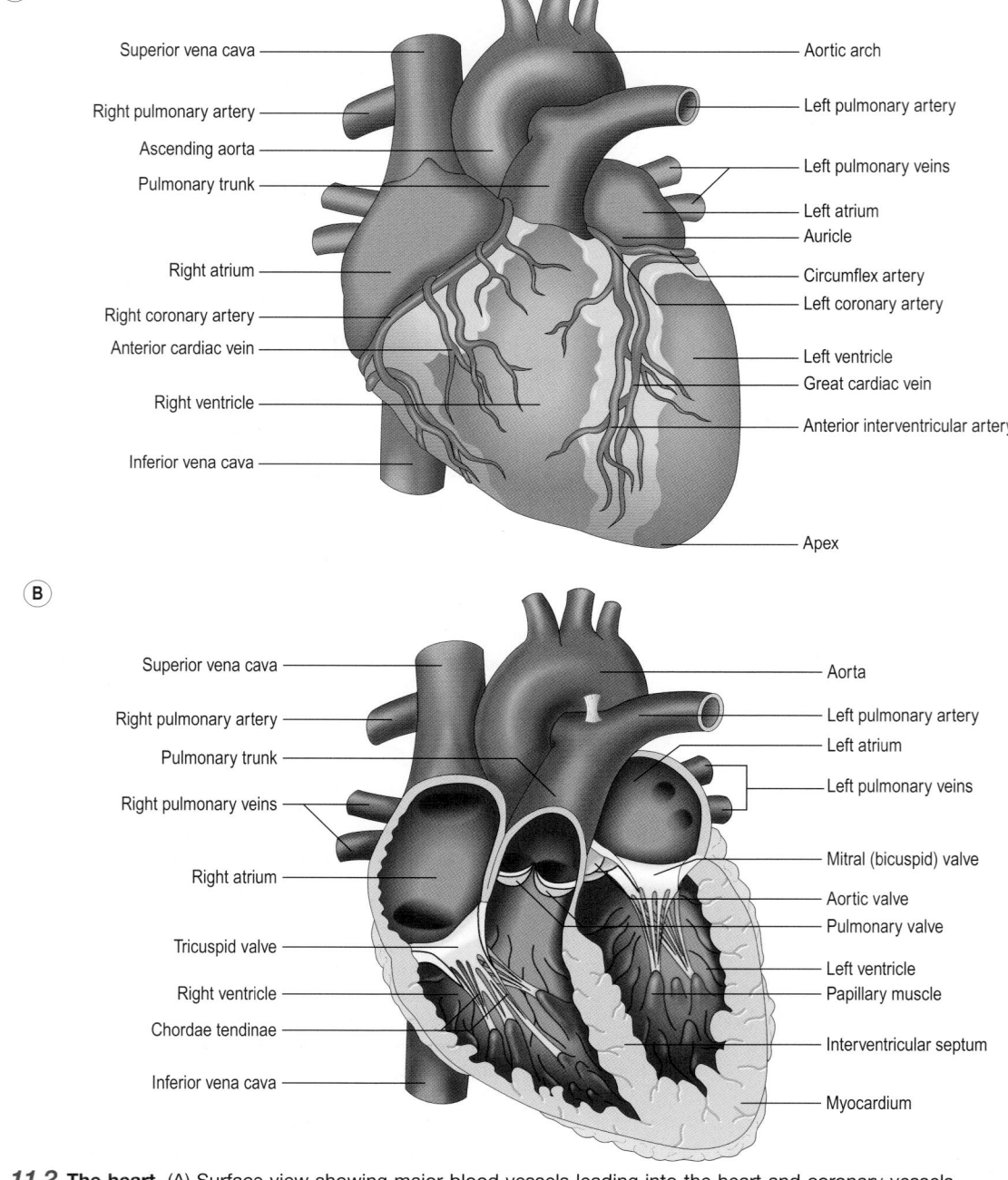

Fig. 11.2 **The heart.** (A) Surface view showing major blood vessels leading into the heart and coronary vessels. (B) Frontal section showing the heart chambers and valves. Redrawn, with permission from Marieb EN 2004 Human anatomy and physiology, 6th edn. Pearson Benjamin Cummings, San Francisco.

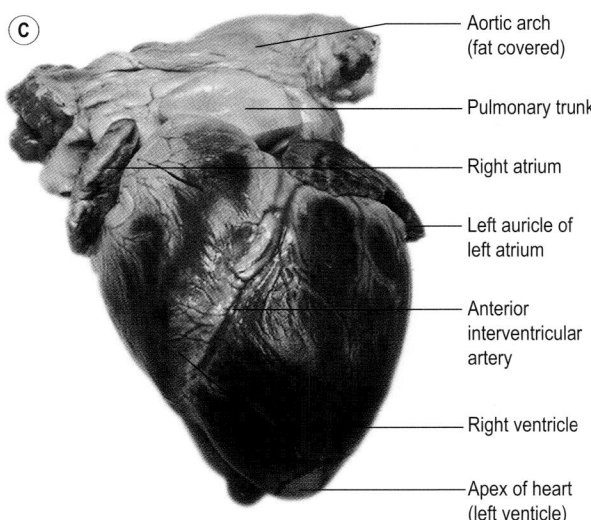

Aortic arch
(fat covered)

Pulmonary trunk

Right atrium

Left auricle of
left atrium

Anterior
interventricular
artery

Right ventricle

Apex of heart
(left venticle)

Fig. 11.2, cont'd (C) External appearance of a human heart. Adapted from Marieb EN 2004 Human anatomy and physiology, 6th edn. Pearson Benjamin Cummings, San Francisco.

Table 11.2	Tissue layers of the heart from the external surface of the heart working inwards
Fibrous pericardium	
Parietal pericardium	
Pericardial fluid	
Visceral pericardium (epicardium)	
Cardiac muscle (myocardium)	
Connective tissue and endothelium (endocardium)	

Clinical box 11.1   Pericarditis

Pericarditis or inflammation of the pericardium leads initially to a reduction in the amount of pericardial fluid. This allows the heart to rub against the pericardial sac, causing chest pain and a characteristic rustling sound known as **pericardial friction rub**. In later stages there is overproduction of fluid, called a **pericardial effusion**, which accumulates around the heart, eventually reducing the ability of the heart to expand and contract, a condition known as **cardiac tamponade**.

contains the **pericardial fluid**. This fluid and the slippery surfaces of the serous membranes ensure that the heart moves in a relatively frictionless space (Clinical box 11.1).

The atria and the ventricles

The atria are the initial collecting chambers for blood entering the heart. They are thin walled and only contract slightly to propel blood into the ventricles. The ventricles make up the major bulk of the heart mass with the right ventricle being prominent on the anterior surface and the left ventricle making up most of the posterior aspect. The thick-walled ventricles generate the force required to propel the blood round the two vascular circuits, with the left ventricle having a thicker myocardium because it generates a much higher pressure than the right ventricle.

The heart valves

Heart valves ensure that the flow of blood through the heart is unidirectional. They are not vascularised, which means that they are occasionally prone to infection, and also that they are not very immunogenic, so they can be replaced by synthetic prostheses.

Situated between the atria and the ventricles are the two **atrioventricular (AV) valves** (Fig. 11.3A): the **mitral (bicuspid) valve** on the left and the **tricuspid valve** on the right. These are opened by blood flowing from the atria into the ventricles and are closed when the ventricles contract and pressure in the ventricles exceeds the atrial pressure. The **chordae tendineae** are thin cords which run between the cusps of the AV valves to the papillary muscles which emerge from the wall of the ventricles. These prevent the valves inverting when they are closed and the pressure in the ventricles rises. As the heart contracts the papillary muscles contract in order to keep the chordae tendineae taut.

At the base of the aorta and the pulmonary trunk are the **aortic** and **pulmonary semilunar valves**, which are flattened against the artery walls when blood flows out of the ventricle (Fig. 11.3B). They prevent back flow of blood into the heart from the elastic arteries, forming three cup-like structures which occlude the vessels when the pressure in the arteries exceeds that in the ventricles. The closing of all these valves produces distinctive sounds, which can be heard with a stethoscope (see below).

The heart skeleton

In order to do work all muscle contraction requires a fulcrum, a fixed point about which contraction can occur. This is provided by the rigid heart skeleton which consists of the connective tissue of the myocardium, attached to rings of dense connective tissue situated round the base of the aorta, the pulmonary trunk and around the junction between the atria and ventricles (the **annulus fibrosus**). The valves and heart muscle are all attached to these rings (see Fig. 11.3). The annulus fibrosus also has the effect of separating the atria and ventricles electrically (see below).

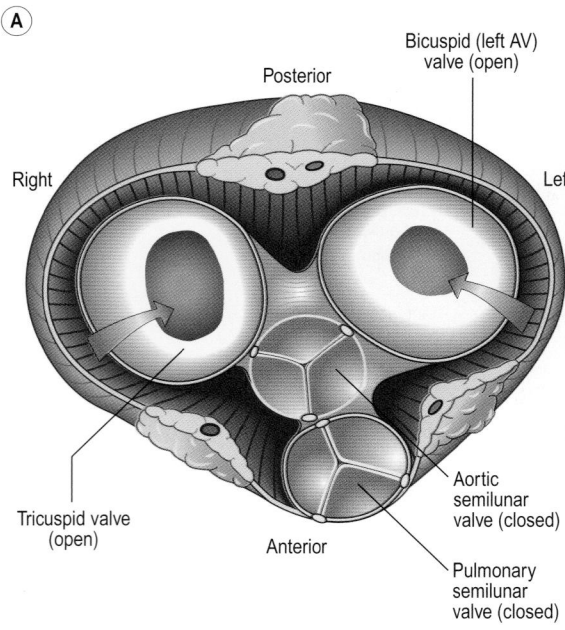

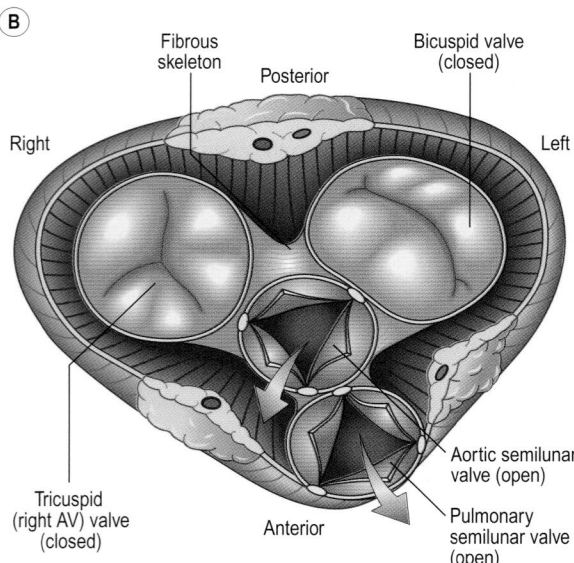

Fig. 11.3 **Transverse section of the heart showing the atrioventricular (AV) (mitral and tricuspid) and semilunar (aortic and pulmonary) valves.** Superior view with the atria and vessels removed. *Arrows* indicate direction of blood flow. (A) When the heart is filling with blood the AV valves are open and the semilunar valves are closed. (B) When blood is leaving the heart the semilunar valves are open and the AV valves are closed. Redrawn, with permission, from Martini FH and Nath JL 2009 Fundamentals of anatomy and physiology, 8th edn. Pearson Benjamin Cummings, San Francisco.

Systemic arterial circulation

Blood leaving the heart via the **aorta** is directed into a number of parallel circuits which supply different parts of the body (Fig. 11.4). Each separate circuit receives its own supply of well-oxygenated blood at relatively high pressure. The division of blood flow into separate circuits allows the flow in each of the branches to be regulated separately in response

to the demands of the organs supplied and the ultimate requirement to maintain blood flow at sufficient pressure to the most critically important organs of the body – the brain and the heart.

After emerging from the heart, the aorta, which is about 2–3 cm in diameter, forms the aortic arch (Fig. 11.5A). Branching off from the ascending limb of the **aortic arch** are the **coronary arteries**, which provide the blood supply to the heart muscle. The top of the aortic arch gives off three major branches:

- Brachiocephalic artery
- Left common carotid artery
- Left subclavian artery.

The **brachiocephalic artery** divides into the **right common carotid artery** and the **right subclavian artery**. Between them, the subclavian and the carotid arteries supply blood to the head, neck, arms and part of the wall of the thorax.

The **descending** or **thoracic aorta** runs down the back of the thorax (corresponding to vertebrae T5–T12), where pairs of small arterial branches supply tissues in the chest, the bronchi, pericardium, intercostal muscles, superior diaphragm and oesophagus, and passes through the diaphragm at the level of T12. Below this the **abdominal aorta**, as it is now known, descends to the level of L4 where it divides into the **left** and **right common iliac arteries**. These are the vessels which supply the pelvic organs (bladder, rectum and reproductive organs, excluding gonads) and the lower limbs. The abdominal organs are supplied by branches of the abdominal aorta. After giving off the paired **phrenic arteries**, which supply blood to the inferior diaphragm, the abdominal aorta gives off a major branch, the **coeliac trunk**, which divides into the **common hepatic, splenic** and **left gastric arteries**. These arteries supply the stomach, duodenum, pancreas, liver and spleen.

Just below the paired **suprarenal arteries**, which supply the adrenal glands, the **superior mesenteric artery** supplies the small and large intestines and part of the colon. Two subsequent pairs of branches are the arteries that supply the kidneys – the **renal arteries** – and the **gonadal arteries** (ovarian arteries in females and testicular arteries in males). The last major branch of the aorta, before it divides into the left and right **common iliac arteries** to supply the lower limbs, is the **inferior mesenteric artery** – which provides blood to the lower parts of the intestinal tract, the colon and rectum.

Although the liver receives some blood directly via the hepatic artery, a large proportion of its supply comes from the veins draining the digestive organs, which all supply a common vessel – the **hepatic portal vein**. Blood laden with absorbed nutrients is then supplied directly to the liver, where they are taken up rapidly, and it also allows the liver to detoxify potentially harmful chemical substances that are not normally present in the body, **xenobiotics**, which have been absorbed along with the nutrients. The blood supply to the digestive tract and the liver is in series, rather than parallel – an arrangement called a **portal system**. The kidney also has an internal portal system whereby blood is supplied directly to the kidney glomerular capillaries via the renal arteries. The efferent arterioles then supply the peritubular capillaries. In portal systems the blood supplied to the second capillary bed is at a much lower pressure and oxygen saturation than normal. This has important consequences when blood pressure is low.

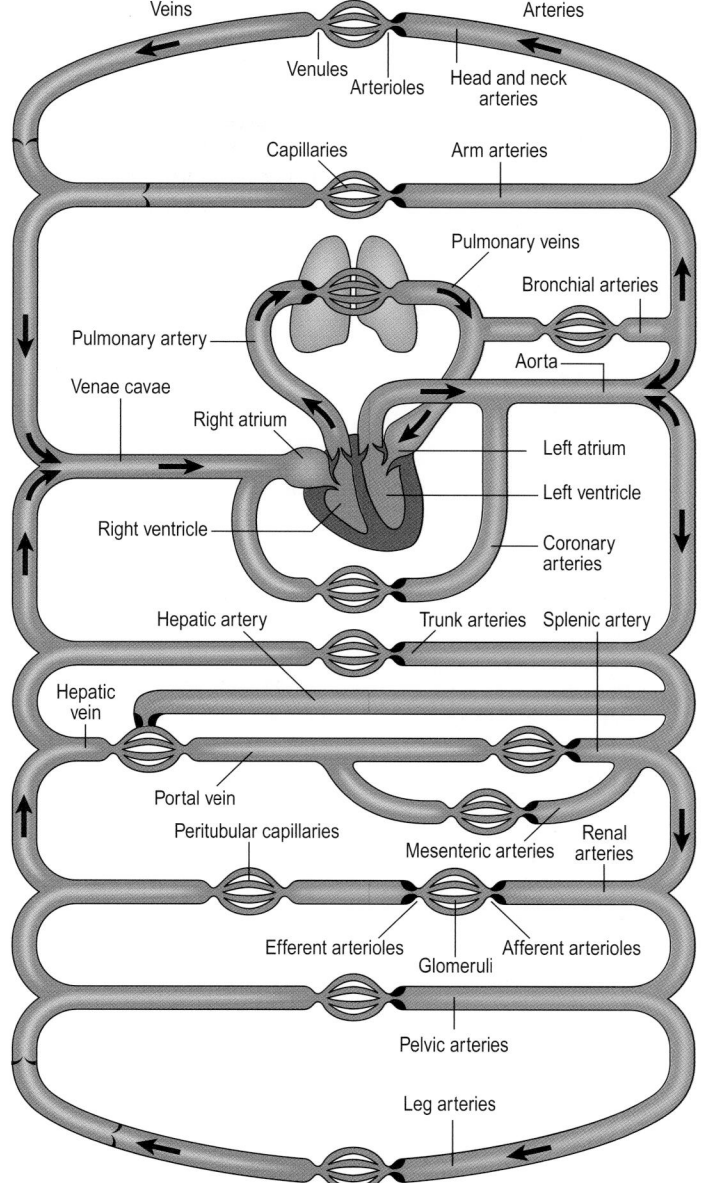

Fig. 11.4 **Circulatory routes in the body.** The diameter of the arterioles at the beginning of the capillary bed controls blood flow through the capillaries, and hence regulates blood flow. Redrawn, with permission, from Berne RM and Levy MN 2001 Cardiovascular physiology, 8th edn. Mosby, St Louis.

Coronary circulation

The coronary arteries provide blood to the myocardium, and branch from the aorta immediately behind the cusps of the aortic valve. The large arteries run over the surface of the heart and small arteries dive into the cardiac muscle (see Fig. 11.2B).

The **right coronary artery** supplies blood mainly to the right ventricle, part of the interventricular septum, and both atria, whereas the **left coronary artery**, which soon divides into two branches, the **circumflex artery** and the **anterior interventricular** (**anterior descending**) **artery**, supplies both atria, the rest of the interventricular septum and most of the left ventricle. There are extensive anastomoses between the left and right supplies. For example, the circumflex artery passes behind the heart to link to the right coronary artery, and individual variations are common. However, these anas-

tomoses are not large enough to allow sufficient blood flow to compensate if one of the major arteries becomes blocked (see below).

Systemic venous circulation

Many veins run parallel to the arteries, which in general run deep inside tissues where they are protected from superficial injuries. These veins often share the names of the arteries; for example, the **femoral veins** – which drain the legs – follow the route of the femoral arteries. However, there are also superficial veins which run just below the skin and can be easily observed. Their names do not correspond to the names of arteries, for example the **great saphenous vein**, which drains the leg. Veins are commonly interconnected by linking vessels, called **anastomoses**, providing alternative

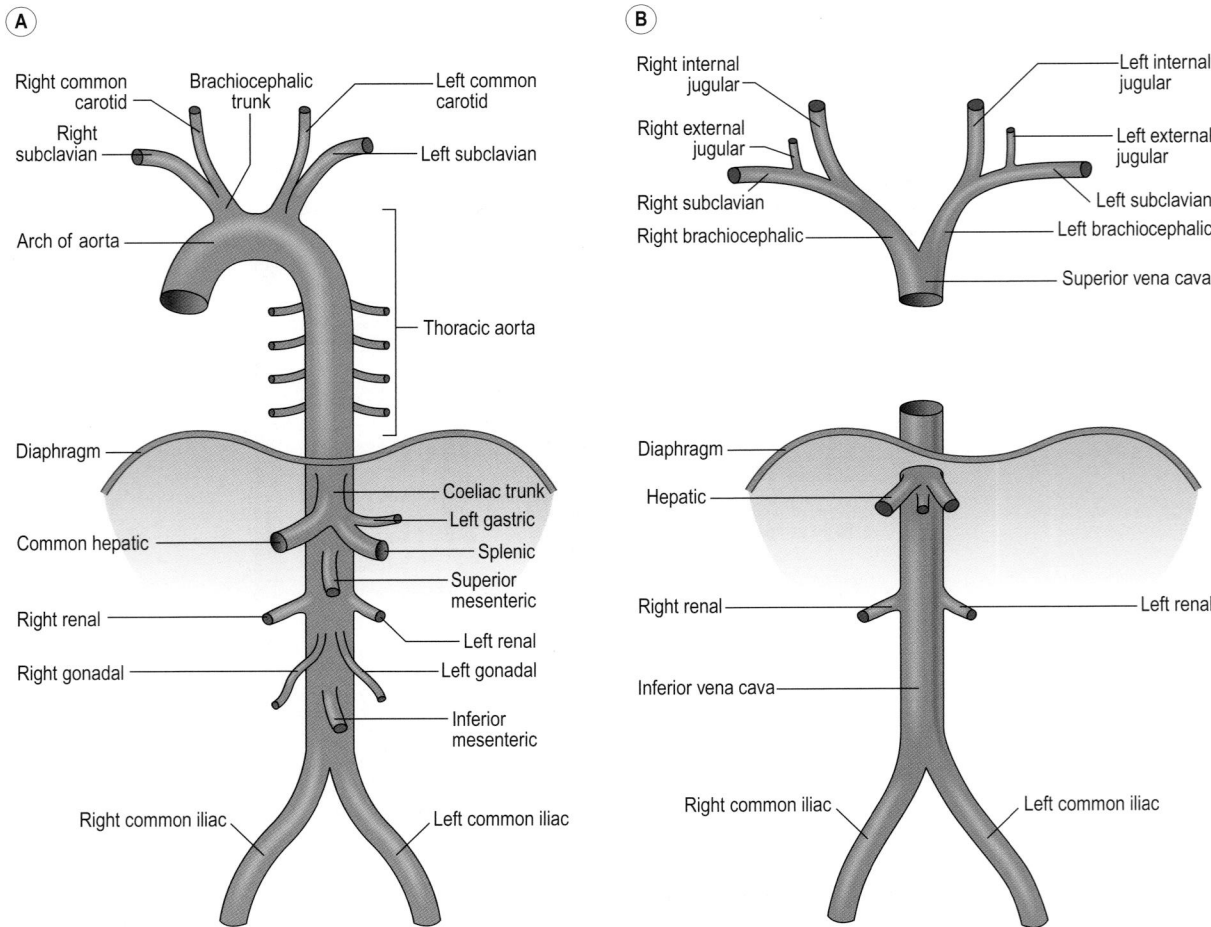

Fig. 11.5 **(A) Major branches of the aorta. (B) Major tributaries of the superior and inferior venae cavae.**

routes back to the heart in the event that these low pressure superficial vessels are occluded by external pressure.

All the systemic arteries originate from the aorta, but the veins do not all converge into a single vein entering the heart. There are three separate routes by which blood returns to the heart (Fig. 11.5B):

■ The **coronary capillaries** converge to form the cardiac veins, most of which join to form a large vessel called the **coronary sinus**. This then drains directly into the right atrium, although the small coronary veins of the right ventricle and the **thebesian veins**, which run through the myocardium, open directly in the heart chambers.

■ The veins draining the brain empty into the dural sinuses, the enlarged vessels in the dura mater (Ch. 8), before going mainly into the **internal jugular veins**. These merge with the **subclavian veins** coming from the arms to form the **brachiocephalic veins**. The two brachiocephalic veins then join to form the **superior vena cava**, which drains into the right atrium.

■ The veins which drain the parts of the body originally supplied by the abdominal aorta all merge into the **inferior vena cava**, which empties into the right atrium.

The legs are drained by the **common iliac veins** that merge to form the start of the inferior vena cava. This is then joined by two major sets of veins, first the **renal veins**, which

drain the kidneys, and then the **hepatic veins**. Much of the blood supplied to the intestinal organs goes to the liver via the **hepatic portal vein**, which in turn drains into the hepatic veins.

The veins of the legs and the arms have valves which prevent the back flow of blood due to gravity. These are particular effective during rhythmical muscular activity when the squeezing of the veins, due to muscle shortening, forces blood towards the heart. Under conditions where the pressure in the veins is raised the valves may become leaky (**incompetent**). When this occurs in the superficial veins of the leg this leads to bulging, unsightly, **varicose veins**.

Much of the thorax drains via the **azygos system**, which, after collecting blood from much of the region supplied by the branches of the thoracic aorta, empties via the **azygos vein** into the superior vena cava.

Pulmonary circulation

Blood leaves the right ventricle via the pulmonary trunk, which immediately divides into the **left** and **right pulmonary arteries**. These then divide in turn into the three right and two left **lobar arteries** which supply blood for each lobe. The pulmonary capillaries form a dense network surrounding the alveoli, where gases can diffuse rapidly across the thin capillary endothelial and alveolar cells (see Ch. 13). The capillaries from each lung converge to form venules which further

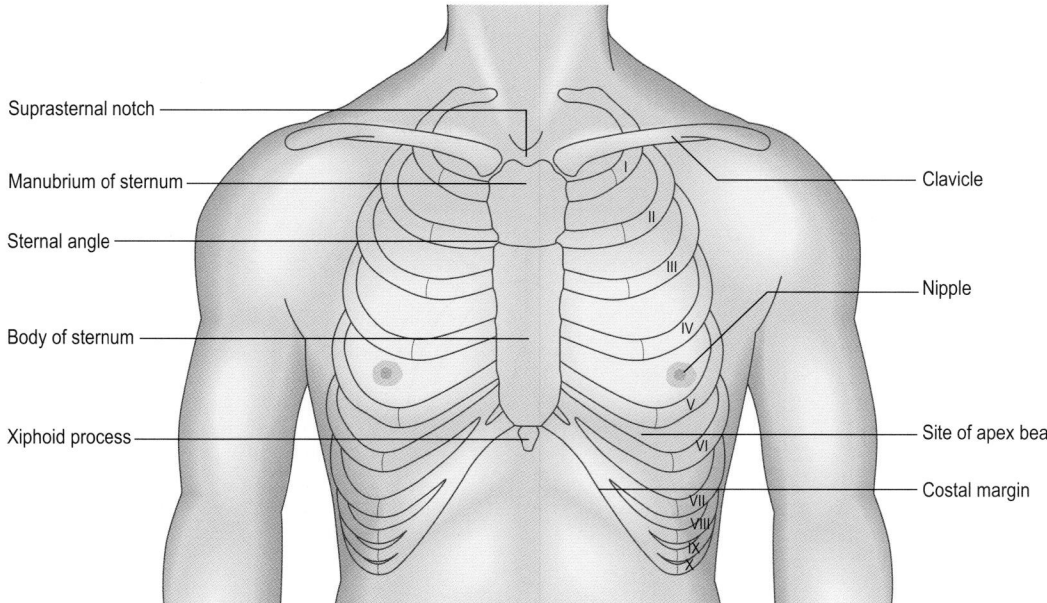

Fig. 11.6 Surface anatomy of the chest (male).

converge to form a pair of pulmonary veins. The four **pulmonary veins** then enter the left atrium on the posterior aspect of the heart.

SURFACE ANATOMY

Surface anatomy of the heart

An understanding of the surface anatomy of the chest and upper back is useful during the clinical examination to locate the position of the heart. It is also important to be able to recognise surface landmarks when listening to heart sounds and when attaching electrodes to produce an electrocardiogram (ECG).

Location of the sternum and ribs

The first landmarks which should be identified are the **clavicles** (collar bones) and the **sternum** (breast bone) (Fig. 11.6). The sternum has two parts. The upper end of the body of the sternum is attached at a slight angle to the **manubrium**. The curved upper end of the manubrium and the medial ends of the clavicles form a recess called the **suprasternal notch**. In the depths of the notch the firm cartilage of the trachea can be felt.

The manubrium and body of the sternum are joined at the **manubriosternal joint**. The **sternal angle** (angle of Louis) is the angle made by this joint. The sternal angle can be used to find the medial end of the costal (rib) cartilage of the second rib and further laterally the rib itself. All ribs may be counted from this point by moving an examining finger systematically down the chest wall from one rib to another, noting the soft **intercostal space** between them. Ribs are numbered according to the vertebra to which they are attached posteriorly. The true ribs (1–7) attach directly to the sternum. The false ribs are either attached to costal cartilage (8–10) or do not attach anteriorly (11 and 12). Intercostal spaces are named after the rib above. At the lower end of the sternal body is a tongue of cartilage called the **xiphoid process**. The costal margin is formed by the **costal carti-**

lages of the seventh to tenth ribs. It forms the lower border of the thorax. Posteriorly, the eleventh and twelfth ribs are usually separate from the costal margin.

The anatomical term for the armpit is the axilla or **axillary fossa**. The upper part of the lateral chest wall lies in the space between the axillary folds, which come into prominence when the upper limb is raised above the head. The chest is marked by three imaginary vertical lines which are used for orientation:

- Passing through the centre of the manubrium and the sternum is the **mid-sternal line**.
- Passing through the mid-point of the clavicle is the **mid-clavicular line**.
- Passing midway between the axillary folds is the mid-axillary **line**.

Location the apex of the heart

The beat of the heart can be felt through the chest wall at the apex of the heart, which is the tip of the left ventricle. In a normal individual, the apex can be felt by placing the fingers over the left anterior chest wall. It is usually found in the fifth intercostal space, left to the mid-clavicular line (Fig. 11.7), but by moving the fingers along the intercostal spaces the maximum pulsation can be located. The position of this and the nature of the beat can give important information about heart function.

Auscultation of the heart

The opening and closing of the valves of the heart (**heart sounds**) can be heard on **auscultation** using a stethoscope at specific positions the anterior surface of the chest (Fig. 11.7). The positions do not correspond to the exact positions of the valves but are at a slight distance, where each heart sound can be heard more distinctly than the others. Because of the way that the pulmonary artery and aorta wrap around one another as they leave the heart the aortic area is found, not on the left, but on the right side of the sternum with the pulmonary area on the left. The mitral area is at the apex of

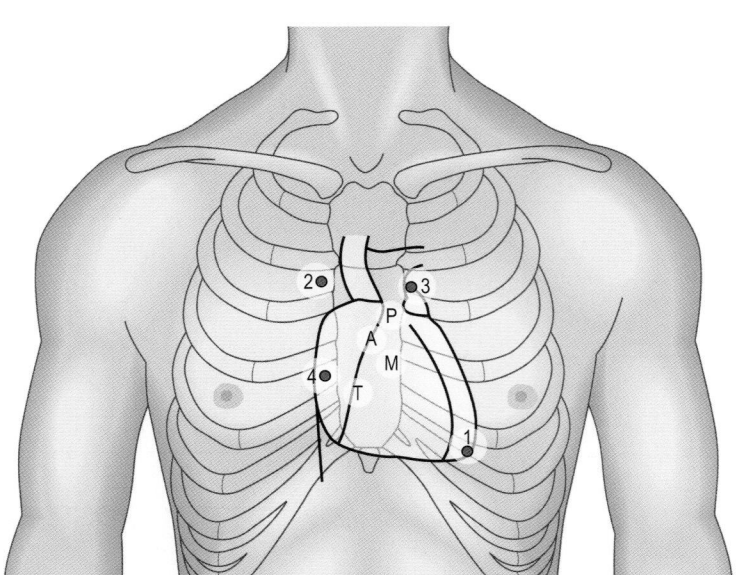

Fig. 11.7 Surface anatomy of the chest. The letters A (aortic), P (pulmonary), T (tricuspid) and M (mitral), also known as bicuspid) indicate the surface positions corresponding to the heart valves within the chest. The opening and closing of the four heart valves can be heard best at the areas marked 2 (aortic), 3 (pulmonary), 4 (tricuspid) and 1 (mitral). The numbers indicate the positions where particular heart sounds and added sounds (including flow murmurs) may be heard best (see text for details). Murmurs can be heard in more than one position.

the heart. When the valves are diseased, the blood flow through them may be increased or turbulent and this manifests as murmurs on auscultation. Murmurs, like heart sounds, are *not* best heard over the surface of the chest corresponding to the position of the valves, but at the positions where the blood meets an obstruction while going through a valve, setting up the disturbance in blood flow.

On auscultation:

- Normally, the first and second heart sound are best heard over the left fifth intercostal space, left to mid-clavicular line (where the apex beat can be palpated, see above and Fig. 11.7, number 1).
- Mitral valve sounds are best heard in an area over the left fifth intercostal space, left to mid-clavicular line and the left lower sternal border, but may radiate to the left mid axillary line (mitral regurgitation) (Fig. 11.7, near number 1).
- Aortic valve sounds are best heard at the right second intercostal space and the right upper sternal border (Fig. 11.7, number 2).
- Pulmonary valve sounds are best heard in an area over the left second intercostal space and the left upper sternal border (Fig. 11.7, number 3).
- Tricuspid valve sounds are best heard over an area over the right fourth intercostal space and the right mid-sternal border (Fig. 11.7, number 4).

Electrode placement

In order to measure the electrical activity of the heart (see below) electrodes need to be positioned in a standard way so that different records can be compared. The exact positions depend on being able to locate numbered intercostal spaces and the vertical lines (see above) which divide the chest (see Table 11.4 below).

Pulses

When the blood leaves the heart it produces pulsations in the arteries that can be felt through the skin at various points on the body (by palpation). The examination of these pulses not only gives information about the heart function, such as rate, rhythm and strength, but can also inform about the condition of the circulation. If blood flow is impaired by disease then pulses distal to the blockage are reduced or even eliminated.

Peripheral arterial pulses

The pulse which is most commonly palpated is the **radial pulse** in the wrist; it is routinely used to measure heart rate. However, many other pulses can be felt (Fig. 11.8). The most commonly used are:

- **Carotid pulse**; very useful for monitoring heart rate in shock where more peripheral pulses may be unobtainable or very weak.
- **Brachial pulse**; the sounds produced by turbulent blood flow in the brachial artery are commonly used to assess blood pressure.
- **Femoral, popliteal, posterior tibial and dorsalis pedis pulses**; these are all palpated in order to assess the blood flow to the lower limbs, which may be impaired due to atherosclerosis and/or thrombosis.

Jugular venous pulse

There are no valves between the internal jugular veins draining the head and the right atrium, so normally blood flows downwards into the heart by the force of gravity. The internal jugular vein is not visible in a normal subject sitting upright. The top of the venous column normally lies about 4 cm above the manubriosternal angle so can be seen only if the person

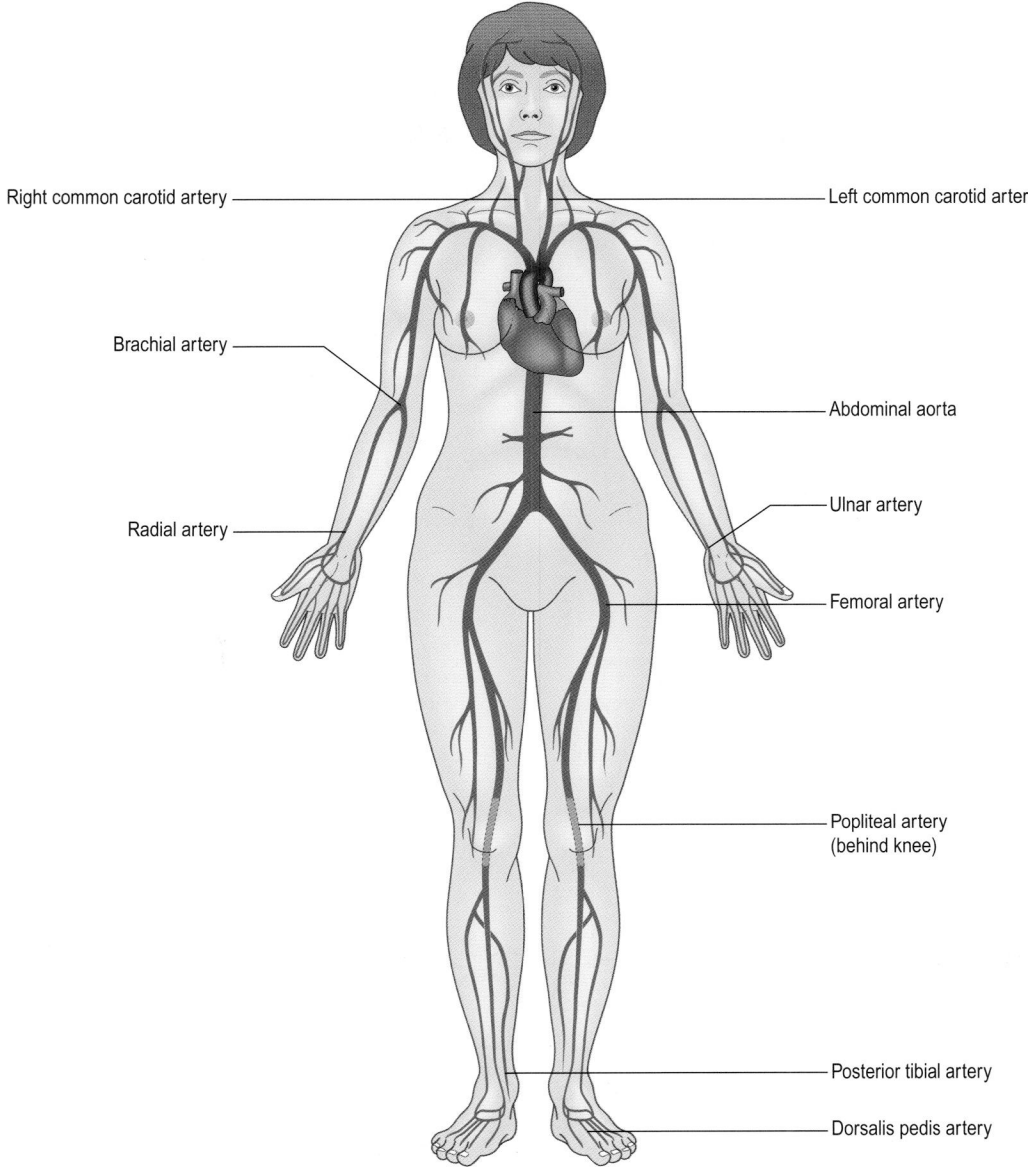

Right common carotid artery

Left common carotid artery

Brachial artery

Abdominal aorta

Radial artery

Ulnar artery

Femoral artery

Popliteal artery
(behind knee)

Posterior tibial artery

Dorsalis pedis artery

Fig. 11.8 Common arterial pulse points.

is lying down in a more prone position. However, if the pressure in the right atrium is raised above normal then blood will accumulate in the veins leading into the heart, and the level of the column of blood in the internal jugular vein will rise. In severe cases, if the patient is sitting upright, this can be observed as pulsations in the neck.

CARDIAC MUSCLE FUNCTION

CARDIAC MYOCYTES

The myocardium is made up of cardiac muscle cells (**myocytes**) which are striated, like skeletal muscle, but in a less organised manner (Fig. 11.9). The cells are small and branched, forming a dense network with a rich capillary supply and connected by an arrangement of their membranes called an **intercalated disc**. This provides both structural support, via desmosomes, and electrical connections

through large numbers of gap junctions, which are formed from pore-forming transmembrane proteins called **connexins** (see Ch. 2). These allow currents to pass from cell to cell and in this way the muscle can act in a coordinated manner, as a functional syncytium. The myocytes contain large numbers of mitochondria in order to provide the ATP required to power the contractile machinery. This consists of a similar arrangement as in skeletal muscle: thin actin and thick myosin filaments with **sarcomeres** showing M lines, Z discs and the A, H and I bands (see Fig. 11.9).

Heart muscle is almost exclusively dependent on aerobic respiration and thus requires a constant supply of oxygen by the dense capillary network; however it can switch readily between fuel molecules and can use glucose, fatty acids and even the lactic acid produced by the anaerobic respiration of other tissues. Cardiac muscle has **T tubules** and **sarcoplasmic reticulum** (SR), similar to that in skeletal muscle (see Ch. 9). However, compared with skeletal muscle, the T tubules are wider and less common and the SR is less well

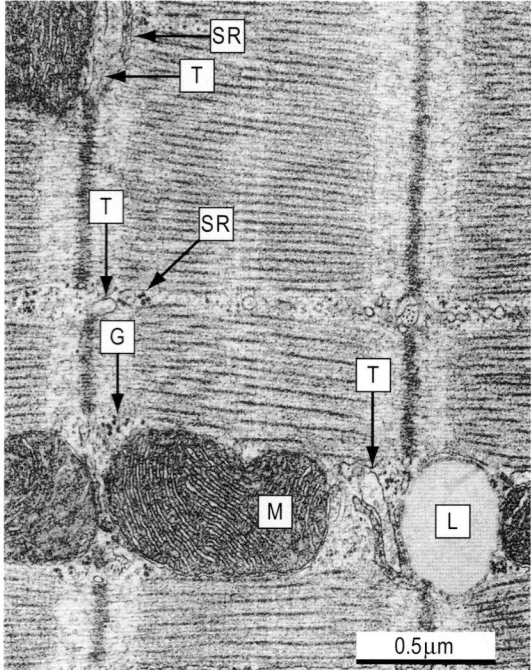

Fig. 11.9 **Electron micrograph of cardiac myocytes** (×38 000). G: glycogen granules; L: lipid droplet; M: mitochondrion; SR: sarcoplasmic reticulum; T: T tubules. From Young B, Lowe J, Stevens A et al 2006 Wheaters functional histology, 5th edn. Churchill Livingstone, Edinburgh.

developed. The ends of the SR form terminal cisternae which are closely opposed to the T tubules, although they do not make direct contact (Fig. 11.10). The combination of T tubule and terminal cisternae form diads; the triads seen in skeletal muscle are only found occasionally.

CARDIAC EXCITATION AND CONTRACTION

Cardiac contraction is brought about by a rise in the Ca^{2+} concentration inside the myocytes. The contraction of the atrial and ventricular myocytes is triggered by action potentials which run across the surface of the myocytes and down the T tubules. These are mediated by voltage-dependent sodium channels (see Ch. 8) which allow sodium influx to produce depolarisation (Fig. 11.11). These channels are opened when the plasma membrane is depolarised from its normal resting membrane potential, which in ventricular myocytes is about −90 mV, to the threshold potential of −65 mV. This depolarization triggers calcium entry into the cytoplasm in two ways:

- In the plasma membrane, particularly in the T tubules, there are voltage-sensitive calcium channels, of a type sensitive to a group of drugs called dihydropyridines, known as **L-type calcium channels** (see Ch. 3). These channels open at a slower rate than the sodium channels and produce the sustained depolarisation known as the **plateau phase** of the action potential.

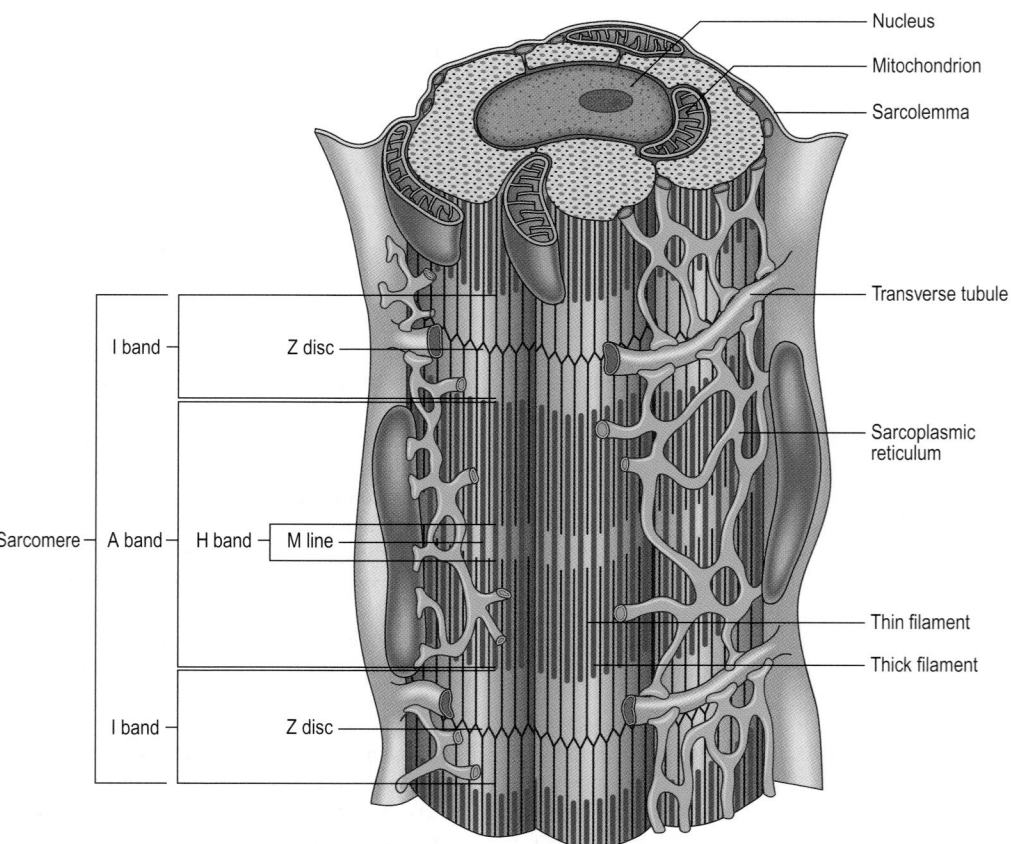

Fig. 11.10 Cardiac muscle showing arrangement of transverse tubules, sarcoplasmic reticulum and the divisions of the sarcomeres.

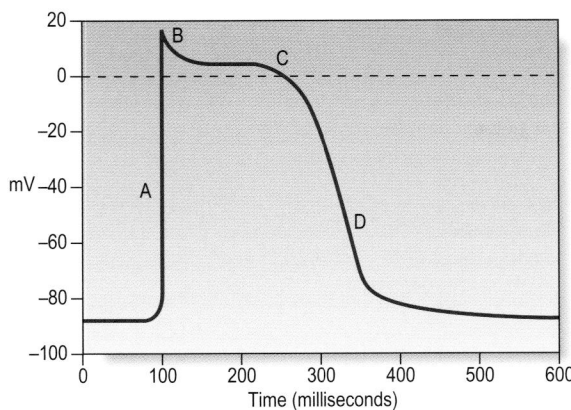

Fig. 11.11 **Action potential in cardiac ventricular myocytes.** A: Na^+ influx (fast inward); B: K^+ efflux (transient); C: Ca^{2+} influx (slow inward); D: K^+ efflux (delayed rectifier).

- Some of the calcium which enters through the L-type calcium channels binds to receptors on the SR known as **ryanodine receptors**, which, in turn, release calcium from the SR, a process known as **calcium-induced calcium release**. This process provides about 80% of the calcium required for muscle contraction.

The calcium inside the myocyte interacts with troponin C in a similar manner to skeletal muscle to cause muscle contraction.

Relaxation

The repolarisation of the action potential is brought about by the opening of **potassium channels** which allow potassium efflux to return the membrane potential to its resting level. As in skeletal muscle, the sodium channels inactivate when they close and remain inactivated until the resting membrane potential is restored. The myocyte cannot be re-excited until after this refractory period. The long action potential of cardiac muscle and the refractory period ensure that, unlike skeletal muscle, the muscle cannot be excited again before it has fully relaxed, ensuring that each heart beat is separate from the previous one and the heart has time to refill with blood before it contracts again. Relaxation of the muscle is caused by the removal of calcium from the cytoplasm by two types of **calcium transporter**:

- **Calcium-ATPase** pumps on the SR and plasma membrane return about 80% of the calcium into the SR and remove a small amount from the cell.
- **Na^+/Ca^{2+} cotransporters** on the plasma membrane remove excess calcium in exchange for sodium, which itself is then removed by the Na^+/K^+-ATPase.

Changes in the contractility of cardiac muscle are known as **ionotropic effects**. Many drugs which affect the contractility of cardiac muscle do so by mechanisms which change intracellular calcium levels, either by increasing calcium influx or reducing calcium removal (see below). A number of endocrine and renal disorders produce changes in the plasma concentrations of potassium and calcium which have profound effects on the cardiac action potential (Information box 11.1).

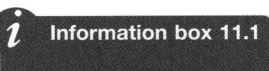

Information box 11.1 **Cardiac excitation is sensitive to levels of potassium and calcium**

Hypokalaemia
Changes in the plasma potassium concentration alter the resting membrane potential of cardiac myocytes, which can change their excitability. Normal potassium levels are 3.5–5.0 mM but if levels fall below 5 mM then the myocytes will become hyperpolarised. This means that myocytes must be stimulated more to reach threshold and cardiac excitation is reduced. Many diuretics used to treat heart failure and hypertension can cause **hypokalaemia** as Na^+ is exchanged for K^+ and H^+ in the distal tubules. This can be reduced by the addition of potassium-sparing diuretics such as amiloride and triamterene.

Hyperkalaemia
Potassium levels can rise if renal excretion is impaired, usually due to renal failure or drugs which interfere with renal excretion of potassium. If the potassium concentration rises above 5.5 mM (**hyperkalaemia**) at first the cardiac excitation increases as the membrane potential of the myocytes gets closer to threshold. This can produce arrhythmias and may lead to ventricular fibrillation. However, if potassium levels increase further, then **heart block** may occur as the voltage-dependent sodium channels become inactivated. The inactivation of these types of channels is dependent on the membrane potential. At normal resting potentials about 50% of the channels are in the inactivated state. This percentage increases rapidly with depolarisation, so that if the membrane potential is maintained near to threshold then all the sodium channels are in the inactivated state and so are non-excitable. Levels of potassium above 7 mM can cause complete heart block, which is a medical emergency.

Hypocalcaemia
About 20–25% of the calcium required for cardiac contraction comes from extracellular calcium, so a reduction in plasma calcium (**hypocalcaemia**) to below the normal levels of about 1.8 mM causes a reduction in cardiac contraction. It also reduces the size of the intracellular calcium stores. Very low levels of calcium can destabilise membranes in excitable tissues and make them hyper-excitable although it is doubtful if these extreme levels could be attained in vivo.

Hypercalcaemia
Extreme **hypercalcaemia** causes arrhythmias and cardiac arrest because of an increase in intracellular calcium. This occurs in systole with the heart in full contraction.

THE ORIGIN OF THE HEART BEAT

The coordinated contraction of the heart is due to an **action potential** being initiated in one region of the heart from where it is conducted through a specialised conducting system, via specific routes, to the rest of the heart. As the action potential travels through the heart muscles, it triggers the different areas of the heart to contract in a sequence that ensures the efficient pumping of blood.

All cardiac myocytes exhibit a property known as **auto-rhythmicity**, that is they can spontaneously fire action potentials in a regular pattern, without the need for nervous inputs; because of this cardiac contraction is said to be **myogenic**. The most important place where this occurs is at the **sinoatrial node** (SA node), a small area of tissue located in the posterior wall of the right atrium. This is called the **cardiac pacemaker** and is normally responsible for the initial depolarisation and subsequent contraction of the whole heart because its intrinsic rate of firing is higher than that of other

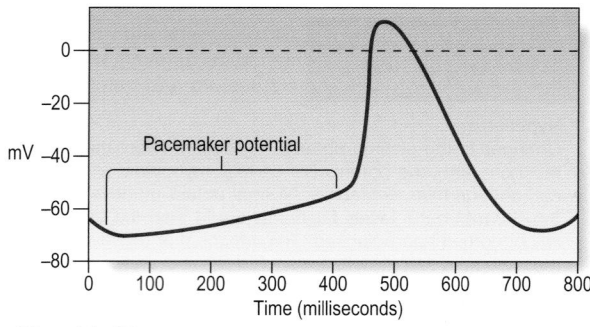

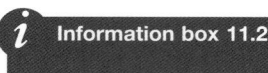

Fig. 11.12 Pacemaker potentials in the SA node. Sinoatrial nodal cells show an unstable resting membrane potential due to a combination of slow inward sodium and calcium currents.

Table 11.3	Conduction pathways in the heart	
Pathway	Duration/sec	Conduction velocity m/sec
Sinoatrial node to atrioventricular node	0.04	1
Atrioventricular node to bundle of His	0.11	0.05
Bundle of His to Purkinje fibres	0.01	4
Purkinje fibres to ventricular myocytes	0.05	0.7

> ### Information box 11.2 | Cooling the heart slows it down
>
> The pacemaker cells are sensitive to temperature and the heart rate will be increased when there is an increase in body temperature, for example during a fever. The heart rate will also be reduced when the heart is cooled. This can be exploited during open heart surgery, where cooling the heart can slow it down.

areas of the heart. In these myocytes the resting membrane potential of −60 mV, which is less polarised than normal ventricular myocytes, is unstable; that is, it tends to drift towards the threshold for firing an action potential (which in these cells is about −40 mV).

This **pacemaker potential** (Fig. 11.12) is due to the action of different populations of ion channels in these cells. The SA node myocytes have sodium and calcium channels that allow slow, inward, background currents to gradually depolarise the cells. At the same time the background potassium current reduces, increasing the net depolarisation until the threshold is reached. These cells do not have voltage-dependent sodium channels so the depolarisation phase of their action potentials is solely due to an influx of calcium, giving the action potential a very different shape than that seen in neurons (Fig 11.11).

The slope of the pacemaker potential determines the rate of firing of the SA node cells, a pattern known as **sinus rhythm**, which is the normal rhythm of the heart. A steeper slope increases the rate and a shallower one reduces it (see Information box 11.2). In the absence of any nervous or hormonal input, the SA node fires about 100 times per minute; however, the normal resting heart rate is slower, at about 70 beats per minute. This is due to the influence of the autonomic nervous system, which reduces the resting rate. Changes in the heart rate are known as **chronotropic effects** (Greek: *khronos*, time) and many drugs which affect the heart rate do so by changing the slope of the pacemaker potential.

THE ELECTRICAL CONDUCTION SYSTEM OF THE HEART

From the SA node the electrical depolarisation spreads from myocyte to myocyte, through gap junctions, across both atria. As in nerve cells, the depolarisation spreads faster through larger cells. Conduction towards the **atrioventricular (AV) node** and the ventricles is fastest through the three **internodal tracts** of larger atrial myocytes (Fig. 11.13).

The AV node is located in the **interatrial septum** which divides the two atria, just above the tricuspid valve. Here the muscle fibres, called **transitional myocytes**, are smaller with fewer gap junctions. Thus, the spread of electrical activity is slowed for about 0.1 s (Table 11.3). This AV delay allows the atria to complete their contraction before ventricular contraction starts. The depolarisation then spreads down the AV bundle. This is the only conduction pathway available between the atria and the ventricles, as the annulus fibrosus acts as an electrical insulator between them. The **AV bundle**, also called the **bundle of His** then splits into two, the **left** and **right bundle branches**, which travel down the **interventricular septum** and finally onto the **Purkinje fibres**. These are large diameter muscle cells which distribute the excitation over the walls of the ventricles to all the ventricular myocytes. The contraction of the interventricular septum gives a rigid fulcrum about which the ventricles can contract. As the apex of the heart contracts, blood is pushed upwards towards the arteries leading out of the heart.

Other regions of the heart also have pacemaker potentials, but under normal conditions the SA node predominates because it has the fastest intrinsic rhythm. Their activity can been seen when there are defects in the conduction pathways. The AV node has an intrinsic rhythm of about 50 beats/min while the Purkinje fibres depolarise at about 30 beats/min.

THE ELECTROCARDIOGRAM

The coordinated electrical activity of the cardiac cells can be detected on the surface of the body using **electrocardiography**. This technique is extremely useful because it is easy and relatively cheap to carry out, and in the hands of an experienced practitioner it can be used to detect a wide range of cardiac pathologies.

Recording an ECG

The **electrocardiogram** (**ECG**) is performed by attaching surface electrodes to the skin at specific sites on the body where signals of about 1 mV can be detected. The standard clinical ECG uses 12 sets of recordings (confusingly called leads). Three of the electrodes, called the **limb leads**, are traditionally attached to the left and right arms and the left leg, forming a triangle with the heart at its centre, although these days they are more usually attached to points on the

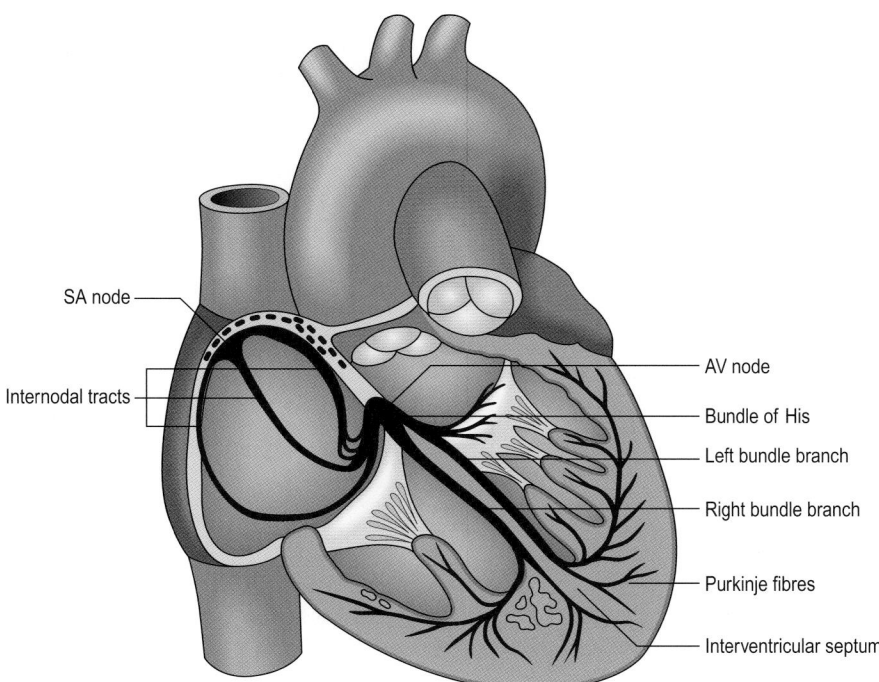

Fig. 11.13 **Conduction pathways of the heart.** Normally, excitation spreads from the sinoatrial (SA) node via internodal pathways to the atrioventricular (AV) node, from where it travels down the interventricular septum and across both ventricles.

Table 11.4	Placement of the chest leads
Chest lead	**Position**
V_1	Fourth intercostal space, just right of the sternum
V_2	Fourth intercostal space, just left of the sternum
V_3	In between V_2 and V_4
V_4	Fifth intercostal space, mid-clavicular line
V_5	Anterior axillary line, level with V_4
V_6	Mid-axillary line, level with V_4 and V_5

Table 11.5	The 12-lead ECG	
Lead	**Positive electrode**	**Negative or reference electrode**
Bipolar leads		
I	Left arm	Right arm
II	Left leg	Right arm
III	Left leg	Left arm
Augmented bipolar leads		
aVR	Right arm	Zero (left arm + left leg)
aVL	Left arm	Zero (right arm + left leg)
aVF	Left leg	Zero (left arm + right arm)
Unipolar leads		
V_1–V_6	See Fig. 11.14	Zero (all three limb leads)

thorax. Another six electrodes, called the **chest or precordial leads**, are placed at specific positions on the chest (Table 11.4 and Fig. 11.14).

The 12 recordings obtained are combined into three groups (Table 11.5):

- The **standard bipolar limb leads**, called leads I, II and III, record the potential difference between two of the limb leads. The most commonly seen recordings are those from **lead II**. This records the difference between the left leg (+) and the right arm (−). Because this follows the main direction of electrical conduction from the SA node to the apex of the heart, this lead shows the main features of the ECG particularly clearly.
- Using the same limb leads, but recording from each one with respect to zero, are the **augmented bipolar limb leads,** aVL, aVR and aVF. The zero potential is estimated by attaching together the other two limb leads.
- The chest leads are **unipolar leads** which are recorded with reference to zero, estimated from connecting together the three limb leads.

The way in which the different arrangements of the electrodes 'look' at the heart can be shown on a diagram known as **Einthoven's triangle** (Fig. 11.15). This represents the positions of the three limb leads with the heart at its centre.

- The leads I–III are represented as looking at the electrical activity of the heart, parallel to each of the sides of the triangle.
- The augmented limb leads, aVR, aVL and aVF, are equivalent to looking at the heart from each of the points of the triangle.
- The chest leads allow an even closer look at the heart from the six positions around the chest wall. Because the zero reference point is equivalent to a point behind the heart this records signals in an anterior to posterior direction.

The normal ECG

The electrical activity of the heart shown by the ECG can be related to the different phases of contraction and relaxation of the heart muscle. Looking at a typical recording from lead

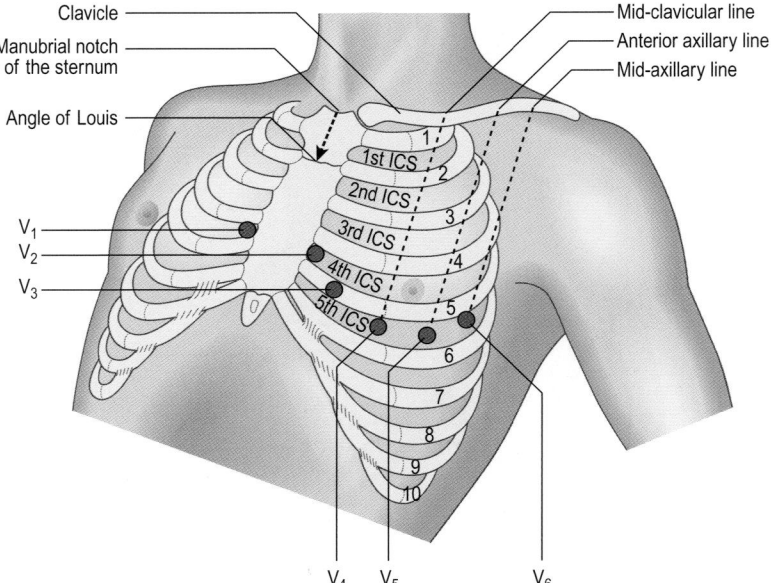

Fig. 11.14 Positions of the chest leads. ICS; intercostal space; ribs numbered 1–10. Redrawn with permission from Kumar P, Clark M 2006 Clinical medicine, 6th edn. Elsevier, Edinburgh.

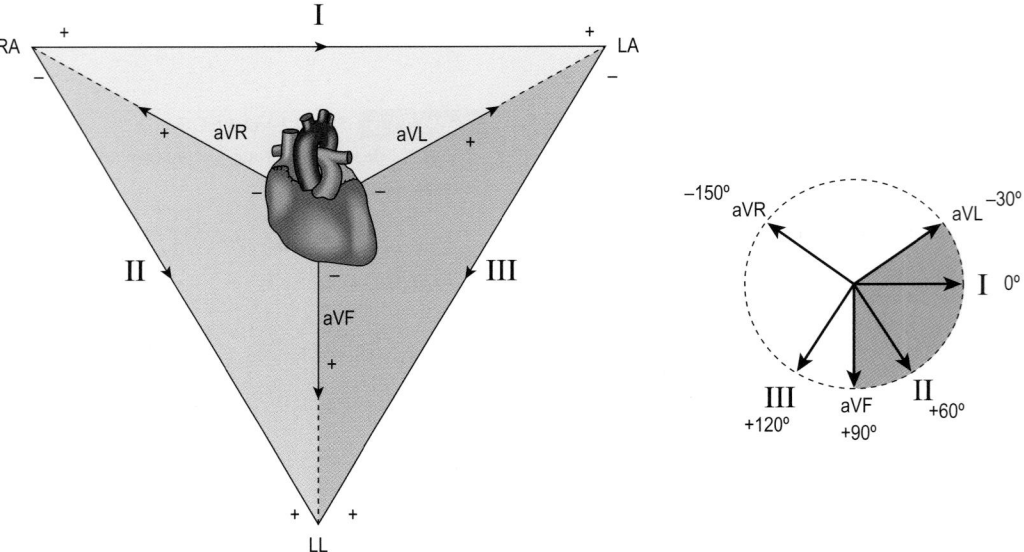

Fig. 11.15 Einthoven's triangle. The six recordings from the different combinations of the limb leads record the signals from the heart from different directions. LA, left arm; RA, right arm; LL, left leg. The normal range for the electrical axis of the heart is between –30° and +90°.

II (Fig. 11.16) the different deflections from the baseline are labelled as follows:

■ The **P wave** is produced by the depolarisation of the atria, giving a positive deflection as the wave of depolarisation moves towards the positive electrode.
■ The **QRS complex** shows the depolarisation of the ventricles, which also masks the repolarisation of the atria. This is a complex signal in that it comprises:
  ■ Q: the depolarisation of the interventricular septum from left to right
  ■ R: the depolarisation of the main mass of the ventricles

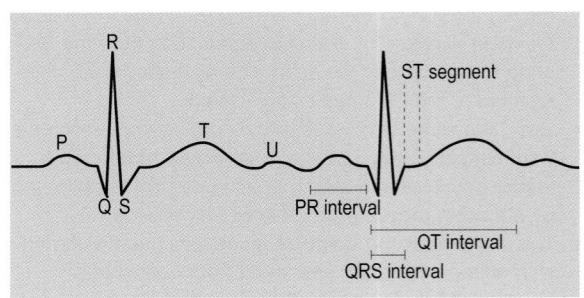

Fig. 11.16 Typical normal electrocardiogram as recorded from lead II. The duration of each beat (RR interval) is approximately 0.8 s.

Table 11.6	Directions of waves of the ECG	
Type of signal	**Direction of movement**	**Deflection of ECG**
Depolarisation	Towards electrode	Positive
Repolarisation	Towards electrode	Negative
Depolarisation	Away from electrode	Negative
Repolarisation	Away from electrode	Positive

Table 11.7	Timing of the normal ECG	
	Duration (sec)	**Corresponds to**
P wave	0.11	Atrial depolarisation
PR interval	0.12–0.20	Atrial depolarisation, atrioventricular conduction, spread through bundle of His, bundle branches to Purkinje fibres
QRS interval	0.06–0.10	Ventricular depolarisation
QT interval	Varies with heart rate (see note below)	Ventricular depolarisation and repolarisation

Note: the QT interval is usually expressed as QTc which equals QT divided by the square root of the RR interval (QTc = QT/√RR). However, as a rough guide the normal QT interval should be less than half the RR interval.

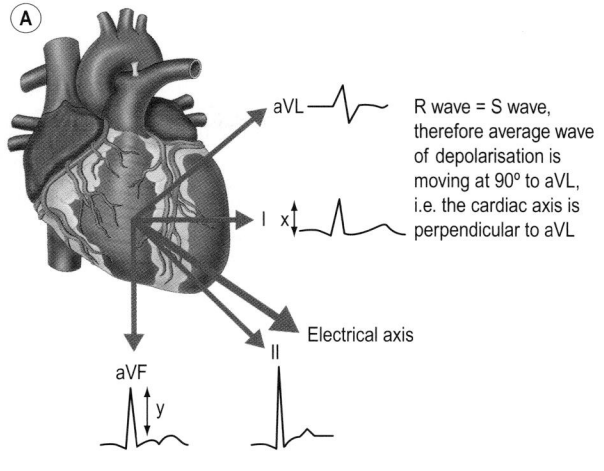
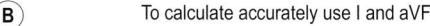

(Greatest R wave= axis is close to direction of II)

To calculate accurately use I and aVF

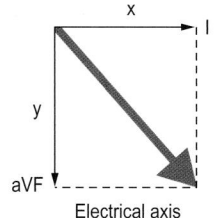

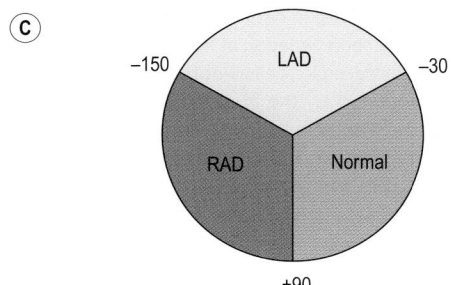

Fig. 11.17 Calculating the electrical axis of the heart. (A) Calculation of the electrical axis by inspection; (B) x and y represent the heights of the QRS complex in leads 1 and aVF, respectively; (C) normal axis – LAD, left axis deviation; RAD, right axis deviation.

- S: the depolarisation of the area of the heart near the base. The waves are tall because of the large muscle mass and the rapidity of depolarisation.
- The **T wave** shows ventricular repolarisation and is spread out because, although the muscle mass is large, its contraction rate is relatively slow. This is a positive wave because, although it is produced by a repolarisation, it is moving away from lead II as the wave of repolarisation of the heart moves from the apex of the heart towards the base (Table 11.6).
- The **U wave** which follows the T wave is often unseen. This small wave is of uncertain origin but may be due to the repolarisation of the Purkinje fibres.

In the normal ECG, the **ST segment** is **isoelectric**: that is it has a zero potential. However, in certain conditions this is not the case. After a myocardial infarction, where heart muscle is damaged due to the interruption of normal blood flow, the ST segment can appear raised or lowered because of changes in the baseline.

There is a slight delay in the spread of excitation at the AV node which allows the atria to complete their contraction before the ventricular depolarisation. The **PR interval** corresponds to the time taken for the excitation to spread across the atria, through the AV node and down the bundle of His (Table 11.7). If there is damage to this pathway then changes are seen in the length of the interval and, in extreme cases, the transmission may be blocked entirely.

The electrical axis of the heart

The maximum current generated by the ECG, which corresponds to the main depolarisation of the ventricle, is called the **electrical axis** of the heart. This can be calculated from the different vectors of the ECG (Fig. 11.17) and gives information about the size and position of the contracting heart muscle. The axis is normally close to lead II although it may be anywhere between −30 and + 90° (see Fig. 11.15 and Clinical box 11.2). The electrical axis can be estimated by plotting the size of the height of the QRS complex (with respect to the isoelectric ST interval) from leads I and aVF on a diagram that represents the directions of the two leads (Fig. 11.17B) and calculating the resultant vector as shown in the diagram.

Cardiac arrhythmias

By obtaining a detailed understanding of the shape, size and timing of the ECG components it is possible to diagnose a wide range of complaints, especially irregular rhythms (**arrhythmias**) (Fig. 11.18).

A normal type of arrhythmia is called **sinus arrhythmia**, which is the change in the heart rate due to inspiration and expiration. During expiration there is a reduction in the heart rate (**sinus bradycardia**), followed by an increase (**sinus tachycardia**) during inspiration (Fig. 11.18B and C). These variations are particularly noticeable in children and young adults and are due to phasic changes in the nervous input to the SA node from the vagus nerve.

Another commonly seen variation in heart rate is the presence of occasional extra beats called **ectopics** or extrasystoles, which are produced by the aberrant firing of a group of cells, often in the ventricle, prior to the SA node. This produces an ECG with an extra QRS complex. Subsequently, when the SA node fires the myocytes are in the refractory phase so they do not depolarise. There is then a longer gap before the heart beats again, the compensatory pause. The following beat may be felt by the patient as a larger beat, due to a longer filling time. Ectopic beats may also occur in the atria. Many of them are harmless but under certain conditions they can precipitate more serious arrhythmias. Other kinds of arrhythmias are seen when the normal conduction pathways through the heart are damaged:

- **First-degree AV block** occurs when conduction through the AV node takes longer than normal. This extends the PR interval, slowing the heart rate.
- **Second-degree AV block** occurs when not all of the P waves are transmitted to the ventricles; this is shown by the fact that not all P waves have a corresponding QRS complex. This may occur in regular patterns, for example with the ventricle being excited by every second P wave, called 2 : 1 type.
- **Third-degree (complete) AV block** occurs when the atria and ventricles are completely separated and beat independently. In this case the atria will beat at a much faster rhythm than the ventricles, which will beat at the rate of the fastest pacemaker in the ventricles, usually about 30 beats/min (bpm).

If delays occur in the transmission of excitation through the intraventricular septum (**bundle branch block**), this causes specific changes in the ECG traces in certain leads. Some abnormal rhythms result from conditions where cells are excited by recurring circles of depolarisation, where ventricular cells are re-excited the moment they emerge from the refractory period, a phenomenon known as **re-entry**. This may lead to extremely rapid rates of ventricular contraction, known as **ventricular tachycardia**, where the heart may beat at over 200 bpm (Fig. 11.18E). **Atrial fibrillation** occurs when the same re-entry occurs in the atria. This leads to an ECG where there are no regular P waves, the atrial contractions appear as an irregular baseline, upon which are superimposed normal but irregular QRS complexes (Fig. 11.18F). This condition is quite common in the elderly.

The most dangerous form of arrhythmia is **ventricular fibrillation**, which occurs when the heart is subjected to poor blood flow, producing myocardial ischaemia. The ECG shows no regularity, indicating that ventricular contraction is not coordinated (Fig. 11.18G). In this condition there is virtually no pumping of blood from the heart, and unless this is corrected immediately it leads to death. Treatment involves **electrical defibrillation**. An electric shock of initially 200 J is transmitted via two paddles placed on the chest wall across the heart. The high voltage which passes through the heart muscles has the effect of putting all the myocytes into the refractory period simultaneously. In many cases, the first cells to fire will be the pacemaker cells, which can then re-establish an organised heart beat.

Anti-arrhythmic drugs

A wide range of drugs are able to influence the rate and rhythm of the heart and many of these are used to treat arrhythmias. Many of them act by either blocking the ion channels which are opened during the cardiac action potential or by affecting the receptors which control the heart rate and force of contraction.

There are several methods of classifying anti-arrhythmic drugs; the most well known is the **Vaughan–Williams classification** (Table 11.8), which classifies the drugs according to their effect on the cardiac action potential. However, there are a number of other drugs, not included in this classification, which have effects on other targets, such as **digoxin**, which slows the heart rate by its effects on the activity in the vagus nerve, and **atropine** and **adenosine**, which act on muscarinic (M_2) acetylcholine receptors and adenosine (A_1) receptors in the heart muscle.

A more recent approach to the classification of anti-arrhythmic drugs is called the **Sicilian Gambit**, which organises drugs according to the potency of their action on the ion channels, ion pumps and receptors and their clinical effects.

THE CARDIAC CYCLE

The sequential excitation of the cardiac myocytes results in an organised sequence of muscle contraction, leading to the pumping of blood through the heart. The sequence of events which make up each heart beat is called the **cardiac cycle** and is summarised in Figure 11.19. The different phases of the cardiac cycle can be related to the changes in pressure which occur in different parts of the heart. These changes in

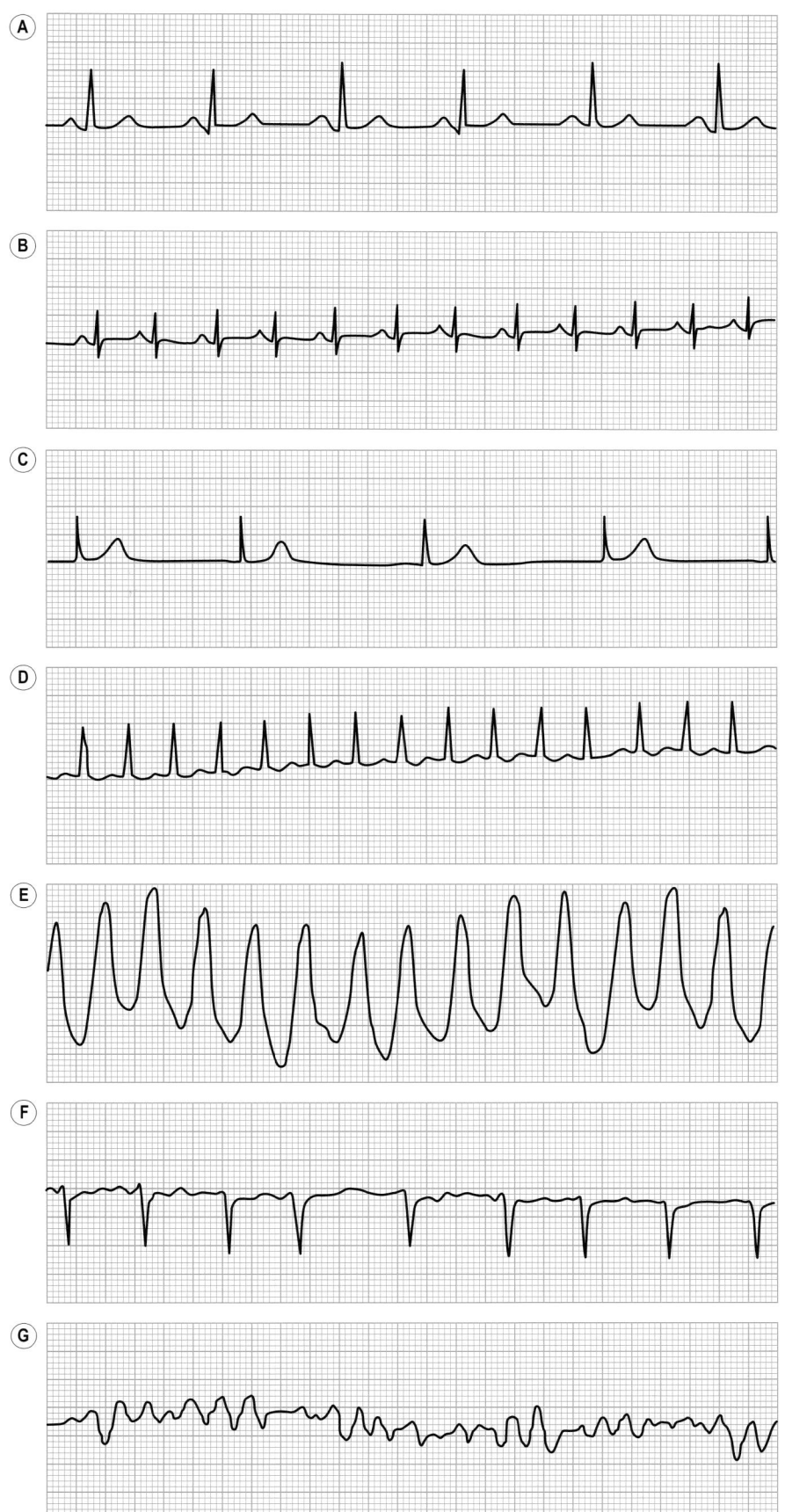

Fig. 11.18 **Different types of heart rhythm.** (A) normal sinus rhythm; (B) sinus tachycardia; (C) sinus bradycardia; (D) supraventricular tachycardia; (E) ventricular tachycardia; (F) atrial fibrillation; and (G) ventricular fibrillation. Redrawn, with permission from Marieb EN 2004 Human anatomy and physiology, 6th edn. Pearson Benjamin Cummings, San Francisco.

Table 11.8	Vaughan–Williams classification of anti-arrhythmic drugs		
Class	Type of drug	Action	Examples
Ia	Na$^+$ (open) channel blocker	Lengthens action potential	Quinidine, disopyramide
Ib	Na$^+$ (inactivated) channel blocker	Shortens action potential	Lidocaine, mexiletine
Ic	Na$^+$ (open) channel blocker	Slows upstroke and conduction speed	Flecainide
II	β-adrenoceptor antagonist	Acts on sinoatrial node to block increases in the slope of the pacemaker potential	Propranolol, atenolol
III	K$^+$ channel blocker	Prolongs the action potential by slowing repolarisation	Amiodarone
IV	Ca^{2+} channel blocker	Reduces conduction predominantly at the atrioventricular node	Verapamil, diltiazem

pressure determine the opening and closing of the heart valves and the flow of blood through the heart.

The amount of blood pumped at each heart beat is called the **stroke volume** (**SV**), which is about 70 mL in an 'average' person at rest, and the amount of blood pumped per minute in called the **cardiac output** (**CO**). Given that an average resting heart rate is about 70 bpm, this gives an average cardiac output at rest of about 5 L/min. However, cardiac output varies widely between individuals, dependent on their energy demands.

The period of contraction of the heart muscle is called **systole** and the period of relaxation is called **diastole**. The atria and the ventricles contract and relax at different phases of the cardiac cycle so there are separate phases of atrial systole and diastole and ventricular systole and diastole. However, when the terms are used on their own they usually refer to the ventricles.

ATRIAL SYSTOLE

Atrial systole is the first phase of the cardiac cycle which occurs just after the P wave of the ECG. Before this the blood returning to the heart has been entering the atria and passively flowing into the ventricles. The atria then contract and blood is forced into the ventricles. However, at rest, most of the blood enters the ventricles by passive filling and the atrial contraction only increases the amount of blood in the ventricles by about 15–20%. This is why patients with atrial fibrillation, and thus no regular atrial systole, have a reasonable cardiac output.

VENTRICULAR SYSTOLE

The contraction of the ventricles commences immediately after the QRS complex of the ECG and the first thing that occurs is that the increase in pressure in the ventricle causes the AV (mitral and tricuspid) valves to close. The closure of the AV valves ensures that blood cannot move back into the atria. The closure of the AV valves produces the **first heart sound** (**S1**), mainly caused by the movement of blood in the ventricles and the vibration of the ventricular walls (Fig. 11.19 trace B). The sound is best heard near the apex of the heart and is sometimes described as a 'lubb' sound.

The first part of ventricular systole occurs without a change in the volume of the ventricle, as the semilunar valves (aortic and pulmonary) are still shut. This is because the pressures in the aorta and the pulmonary trunk are higher than in the ventricles. This phase is called **isovolumetric contraction** (IVC), during which time the pressure in the ventricles rises rapidly. When the pressure in the ventricles exceeds the pressures in the large arteries, the semilunar

valves open and blood starts to flow out of the ventricles. During this **ventricular ejection phase** the volume of the ventricles is reduced and blood is forced into the arteries where the pressure starts to rise.

The ventricular contraction starts at the apex and spreads towards the base. This means that blood is forced upwards towards the openings of the semilunar valves. During this period the atria relax and start to fill with blood. The AV valves are still closed and the atrial pressure starts to rise.

VENTRICULAR DIASTOLE

When the T wave of the ECG occurs, signalling ventricular depolarisation, the ventricles start to relax. As the pressure in the ventricles falls below that in the aorta and pulmonary trunk, the back pressure of blood in the arteries closes the semilunar valves ensuring that blood cannot flow back into the heart. Closure of the semilunar valves produces the **second heart sound** (**S2**). The second heart sound is shorter, but quieter than the first, is described as 'dubb' and is best heard towards the base of the heart. Because the pulmonary and systemic circulations operate at different pressures this does not always occur simultaneously, and so the second heart sound is frequently heard as two split sounds.

The closure of the aortic valve results in a slight increase in the pressure in the aorta as blood rebounds from the closed valves. This is seen as a small dip on the pressure trace measured in the aorta, which coincides with aortic valve closure, followed by a rise and then gradual decline in aortic blood pressure. This complex blip in the pressure trace is called the **dicrotic notch** (Fig. 11.19C, *red line*). This initial phase of ventricular relaxation occurs without any change in ventricular volume and is known as **isovolumetric relaxation** (IVR). During this time the atria have continued to fill with blood and when the pressure in the atria exceeds that in the ventricles the AV valves open and the blood flows rapidly into the ventricles. This produces rapid ventricular filling with an increase in volume.

The ventricular volume at the end of atrial systole, after ventricular filling, is called the **end-diastolic volume** (EDV) and is typically about 120 mL. However, not all of this blood is expelled and the volume of blood remaining in the ventricle at the end of ventricular systole, called the **ESV**, is typically about 40–50 mL. Thus the stroke volume is the difference between EDV and ESV, which at rest is around 70 mL. If the heart muscle is weakened in a way which prevents full contraction, then the stroke volume will fall and hence cardiac output will be reduced. Drugs that increase the force of contraction help to maintain cardiac output by increasing the stroke volume.

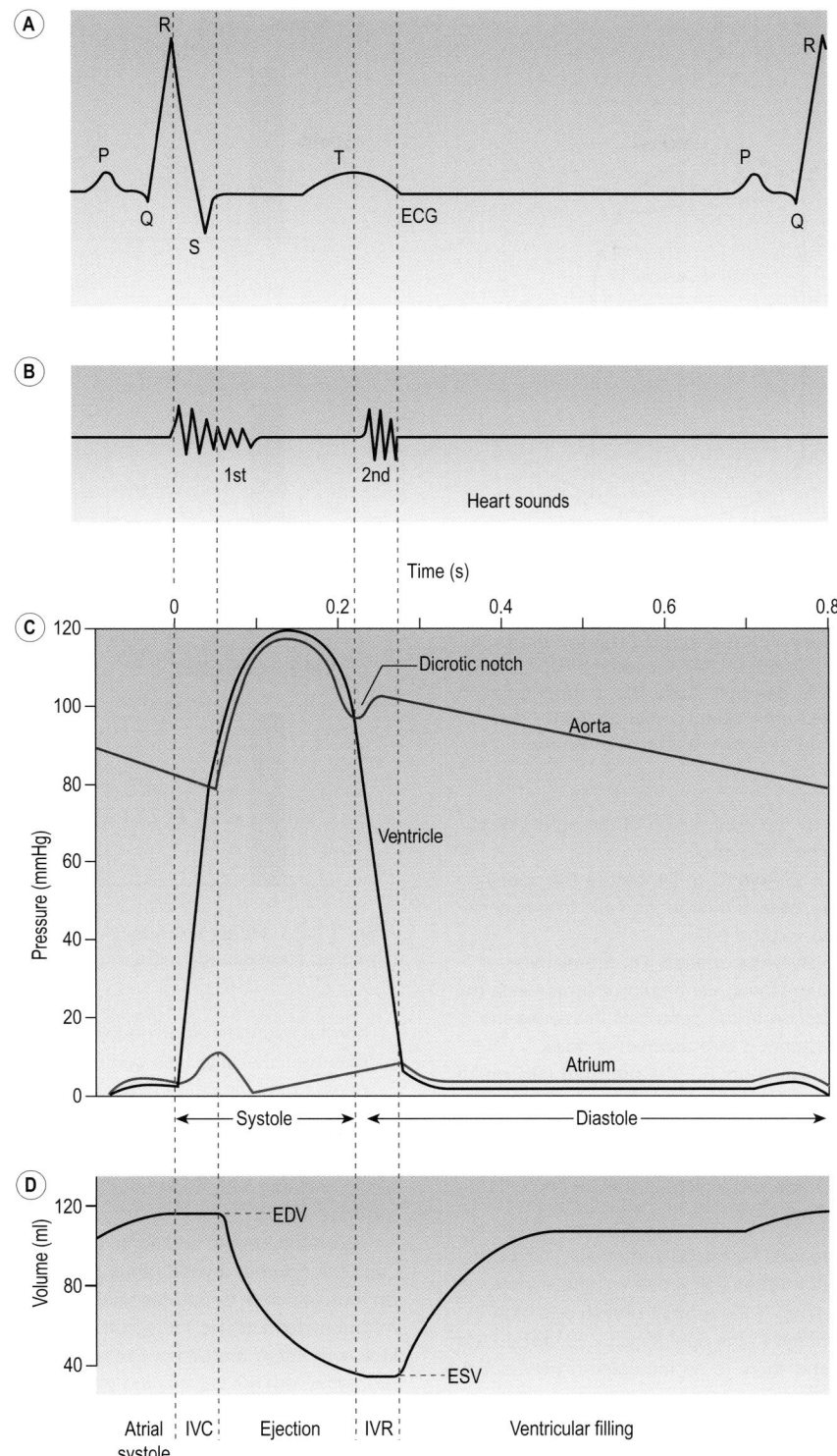

Fig. 11.19 **The cardiac cycle showing:** (A) electrocardiogram (ECG); (B) heart sounds; (C) left ventricular pressure (*black line*), aortic pressure (*red line*), left atrial pressure (*blue line*); and (D) left ventricular volume. Redrawn with permission from Marieb EN 2004 Human anatomy and physiology, 6th edn. Pearson Benjamin Cummings, San Francisco.

THE PRESSURE–VOLUME LOOP

Another way of looking at the changes in pressure and volume in the left ventricle during the cardiac cycle is the **pressure–volume loop** (Fig. 11.20). Similar changes occur in the right ventricle but at much lower pressures.

- At A, the mitral valve opens and the ventricle starts to fill passively from its ESV of about 40 mL.
- The ventricular volume increases but the pressure falls slightly as the ventricles relax and distend.
- At the end of diastole there is a small rise in both ventricular pressure and volume, due to active

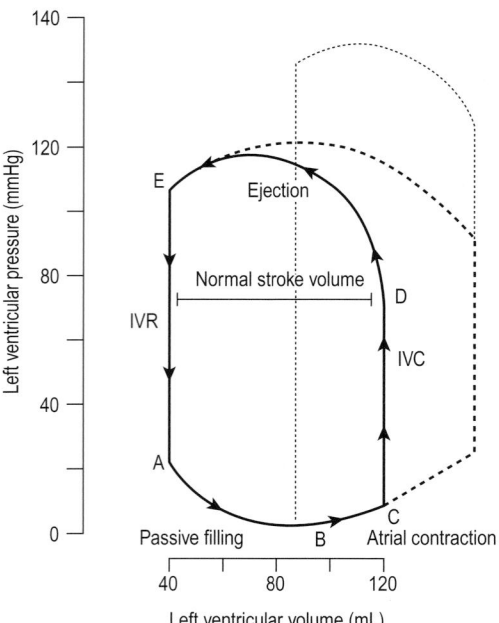

Fig. 11.20 **Pressure–volume loop of the left ventricle.**
IVC, isovolumetric contraction; IVR, isovolumetric relaxation.
For description of A–E, see text. *Solid line*, normal function;
dashed line, increased end-diastolic volume (EDV); *dotted
line*, increased EDV and increased arterial pressure.

ventricular filling by the contraction of the atrium (B to
C). The EDV reaches 120 mL.

- The first period of systole (C to D), before the opening
  of the aortic valve, shows a large increase in pressure
  with no change in volume IVC.
- Once the aortic valve has opened (D), the ejection of
  blood shows a decrease in ventricular volume while the
  continuing contraction of the ventricles increases the
  pressure slightly before it falls as ejection falls.
- Once the aortic valve shuts (E), the pressure falls rapidly
  in the ventricle with no change in volume (IVR) and the
  loop is closed (E to A).
- The stroke volume is shown by the distance between
  the segments CD and EA, which, in this example, is
  approximately 80 mL.

If the EDV is increased by raised ventricular filling due to
increased venous return, then the stroke volume is increased
(Fig. 11.20, *dashed line*). If the arterial pressure is high then
the whole curve is shifted to the right (Fig. 11.20, *dotted line*).
The ESV is raised and there is an increase in EDV but the
stroke volume is reduced.

HEART SOUNDS AND MURMURS

On auscultation of the heart, besides the two main heart
sounds (S1 and S2), two additional sounds may be heard in
normal individuals during diastole (Fig. 11.21):

- The **third heart sound (S3)** is due to rapid ventricular
  filling and can be heard at the apex of the heart as the
  AV valves open. It is a normal sound in young people
  and children but can indicate heart failure or volume
  overload in older subjects.
- The **fourth heart sound (S4)** occurs during atrial systole
  and is due to the rapid ventricular filling. This is a

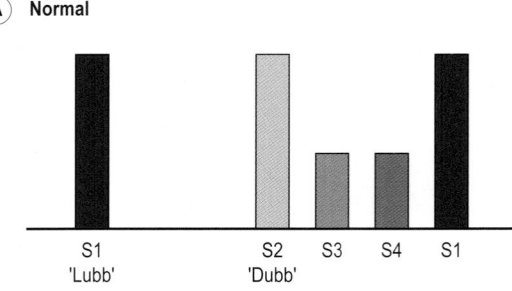

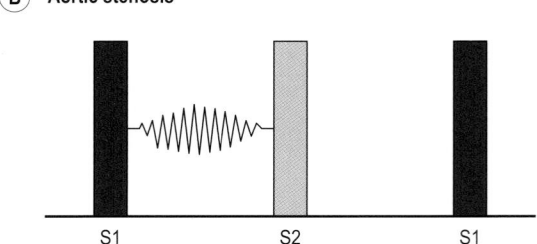

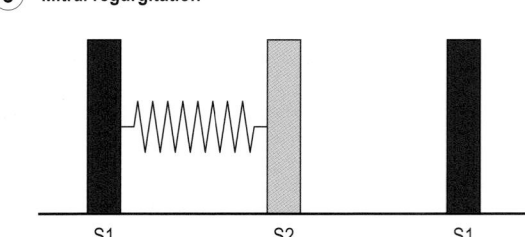

Fig. 11.21 **Heart sounds.** (A) normal heart sounds;
(B) aortic stenosis; (C) mitral regurgitation.

normal sound in elderly subjects whose heart muscle
may be stiffer and less compliant, but in younger
people may indicate increased ventricular stiffness.

Completely smooth flowing blood is silent, but when
blood flow is turbulent then sounds are produced due to the
blood colliding with heart structures, which then vibrate and
produce sound.

As stated above, additional sounds, known as **murmurs**,
can occur due to a wide range of causes and many of them
do not indicate a pathological condition. These innocent
murmurs tend to be fairly soft and occur in early systole.
However, there are distinctive sounds that are indicative of
problems with the valves, and the type, intensity and position
of these sounds can be used to help with diagnosis (see
Clinical box 11.3).

FACTORS AFFECTING CARDIAC OUTPUT

The cardiac output (CO) is determined by the stroke volume
(SV) and the heart rate (HR):

$$CO = SV \times HR$$

Although heart rate is predominantly affected by nervous
input (see below), a number of factors can change stroke
volume and thus affect cardiac output.

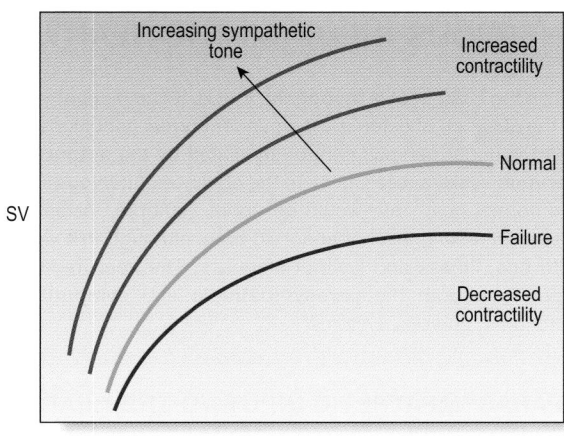

Fig. 11.22 Starling's curves. SV, stroke volume; EDP, end-diastolic pressure.

Clinical box 11.3 | **Damaged valves produce murmurs**

There are two major categories of valve damage:

● **Stenosis**, in which the valve is narrowed
● **Incompetence**, in which the valve does not close properly.

If the aortic valve is narrowed, it is **stenotic**, and blood flowing through it will cause an extra sound called an **ejection (mid-systolic) murmur** between S1 and S2 during the ventricular ejection phase (Fig. 11.21B).

Another distinctive sound is produced when the AV valves fail to close properly. **Incompetent** AV valves allow blood to flow back into the atria during ventricular systole and this regurgitation of blood produces a long murmur that lasts the whole length of systole, called a **pan-systolic murmur** (Fig. 11.21C).

PRELOAD AND STARLING'S LAW

When heart muscle is stretched, just like skeletal muscle, the increase in length can lead to an increase in tension up to a limit, after which the tension falls (Ch. 9). In an individual at rest, heart muscle cells are usually shorter than their optimal length so if they are stretched this can increase the force they can generate. **Starling's law** of the heart states that the energy released during contraction depends on the initial fibre length. The amount of stretch of the heart muscle depends on the **EDV**. This can be affected by two factors:

■ The inherent compliance of the muscle. As we age, the heart muscle becomes stiffer and less compliant and therefore it becomes more difficult for the heart to stretch.
■ The **end-diastolic pressure** (**EDP**) or **preload**. This is the filling pressure of the heart and is determined by the pressure in the great veins, the **central venous pressure** (**CVP**). If EDP is plotted against stroke volume the resulting curve, known as **Starling's curve** (Fig. 11.22), shows that stroke volume increases with increase in EDP until the muscle is overstretched and the stroke volume starts to fall.

One of the major consequences of Starling's Law is that the output of the left ventricle matches the output of the right ventricle. For example, if there is an increase in the stroke volume of the left side of the heart, this increases the filling pressure of the right side, which increases the right EDV and hence increases the right stroke volume.

CONTRACTILITY

The ability of myocytes to contract varies with their length but can also vary due to changes in intracellular biochemistry. This change in the force for a constant length is known as **contractility** and can be changed by factors that alter the calcium handling inside the cell.

Compounds which affect contractility are known as **ionotropes**:

■ **Positive ionotropes** increase contractility. They include compounds that stimulate the receptors present on cardiac muscle. Increased plasma calcium levels, which may be due to increased temperature and a range of drugs that increase intracellular calcium, also increase contractility.
■ **Negative ionotropes** include drugs that block cardiac receptors and calcium-channel blockers. Conditions such as hypoxia also have similar effects.

Changes in contractility affect Starling's curve; positive ionotropes move the curve upwards (Fig. 11.22 *blue lines*) and negative ionotropes move the curve downwards (*red lines*).

AFTERLOAD

If the pressure in the aorta is increased, the flow of blood out of the heart is reduced. This **afterload** increases the **ESV** and hence reduces stroke volume. If the ESV is increased the blood remaining in the heart will increase the EDV of the next beat and Starling's law means that the stroke volume of the following beat will be increased. This means that, up to a certain limit, the heart can maintain cardiac output despite increase in aortic pressure. However, if the afterload becomes too great, the heart muscle becomes overstretched and the force generated will start to fall.

Besides Starling's law, another mechanism related to the size of the heart affects the force generated during contraction. **Laplace's law** states that the pressure (*P*) inside a sphere increases with the wall tension (*T*) and decreases with radius (*r*).

$$P = 2T/r$$

In the heart this means that as the EDV increases (increasing *r*) the efficiency of the heart decreases. This fall in efficiency with increasing size works against the Starling mechanism but does not become dominant until the heart becomes grossly enlarged. When this happens, not only does the force generated start to fall because the myocytes have been overstretched, reducing the number of cross-bridges, but also Laplace's law means that the force generated is reduced.

Ventricular hypertrophy

When the afterload to the heart is chronically increased, such as in hypertension (high blood pressure), the ventricular muscle responds like any other muscle when trained and grows thicker (hypertrophy):

- Constant increased wall stress causes the cardiac muscle to thicken in order to maintain contraction.
- The increased muscle mass increases the oxygen demand of the heart.
- The thickened wall has increased stiffness, which leads to higher ventricular pressures.

If this occurs in the left ventricle, due to systemic hypertension, the higher ventricular pressures are transmitted to the left atrium and pulmonary veins, resulting in **pulmonary oedema** (see under Microcirculation below). If this occurs in the right ventricle, the result is systemic oedema.

HEART FAILURE

Heart failure occurs when the heart is unable to maintain the necessary cardiac output despite normal venous pressures. This may be due to well-identified causes such as a chronic increase in afterload due to hypertension, or a reduction in contractility due to ischaemic heart disease. It can also occur due to a failure of the myocytes to generate sufficient force. Starling's curve is shifted downwards (Fig. 11.22 *red line*) with a lower stroke volume for all values of EDV.

Blood tends to accumulate in the venous circulation, causing a rise in **CVP**. Because there are no valves between the internal jugular vein and the right atrium, pressures in the internal jugular vein reflect the atrial pressures. This means that if there is any accumulation of blood in the right atrium and vena cava this can back-up in the internal jugular vein, and the **jugular venous pressure (JVP)** will be raised, reflecting the high right atrial pressure. In patients with heart failure, the CVP is raised and the column of blood in the internal jugular vein can be observed when the patient is sitting upright as a pulsation in the vein in the neck. Drugs used to treat heart failure have a variety of actions and work in a number of different ways (Information box 11.3).

> ℹ️ **Information box 11.3** | **Drug treatments for heart failure**

Compounds that increase the contractility of the heart muscle will shift Starling's curve upwards and increase stroke volume (see Fig. 11.22). For example **digoxin**, which is extracted from the foxglove (*Digitalis* sp.), inhibits the Na^+/K^+-ATPase of the plasma membrane. The increase in intracellular sodium concentration leads to an increase in intracellular calcium, because of reversal of the Na^+/Ca^{2+} exchange pump. The raised intracellular Ca^{2+} is pumped into the sarcoplasmic reticulum, from where it can be released during excitation–contraction coupling, thus enhancing muscle contraction.

Many of the other drugs used to treat heart failure act by reducing the preload and afterload in some way.

1. Reduction in preload: many patients have an increased blood volume, which is a normal response, initiated by the kidney, to a reduced perfusion pressure. This volume overload can be reduced by the use of **diuretics**, which increase water loss in the kidney and hence reduce blood volume. This reduces venous return and hence reduces preload.
2. Reduction in afterload: a mechanism which lowers afterload is through a reduction in the total peripheral resistance – by reducing the resistance to blood flow from the heart. This is achieved by widening blood vessels using a variety of drugs that reduce vasoconstriction.

NERVOUS INPUT TO THE HEART

While the heart beat is **myogenic**, that is, it can be generated in the absence of external input, under normal conditions the heart is under nervous control, mediated by the **autonomic nervous system** (see Ch. 4). In the absence of nervous input the normal heart rate would be about 100 bpm, instead of the usual resting level of about 70 bpm, although this varies with age, fitness and level of alertness. The heart receives input from both the **parasympathetic** and **sympathetic** autonomic nervous systems.

PARASYMPATHETIC INPUT TO THE HEART

The parasympathetic supply via the **vagus nerve** provides input to the sinoatrial (SA) and atrioventricular (AV) nodes.

- The SA node is supplied by the right vagus nerve and reduces the firing rate of the pacemaker cells.
- The AV node is innervated by the left vagus, which slows conduction through the node.

The preganglionic fibres terminate within the heart muscle and synapse onto postganglionic fibres, which release **acetylcholine** on to M_2 muscarinic acetylcholine receptors (mAChR). Activation of these G-protein-coupled receptors leads to slowing of the heart by causing a reduction in the slope of the pacemaker potentials as well as a slight hyperpolarisation in the nodal cells (Fig. 11.23C). The reduction in the slope of the pacemaker is caused by the decrease in cyclic adenosine monophosphate (cAMP) mediated via a G protein. The reduction in cAMP reduces activation of the ion channels which contribute to the depolarisation of the pacemaker potential. The reduction in the initial resting membrane potential is due to the opening of G-protein-sensitive K^+ channels in the myocytes, which shift the potential to a value close to the potassium equilibrium potential.

No parasympathetic nerves supply the ventricular heart muscle, so the parasympathetic nervous system has no effect on the force of contraction.

SYMPATHETIC INPUT TO THE HEART

The sympathetic nerves, which originate from the spinal cord segments T1–T5, innervate both the nodal tissue and the heart muscle. The preganglionic fibres synapse in the **stellate** and **cervical ganglia**, close to the spinal cord, and the long postganglionic neurons travel in the **cardiac nerves** to the heart. The sympathetic nerve terminals release **noradrenaline** (norepinephrine) onto β_1-adrenoceptors, which are found on the plasma membranes of the cardiac muscle. These receptors are linked via a G protein to increases in cAMP within the cells. Noradrenaline and the other catecholamine, **adrenaline** (epinephrine), which is released into the blood stream, have a number of chronotropic (change in rate) and ionotropic (change in force) effects on the myocytes.

- The heart rate is increased by increasing the slope of the pacemaker potential (Fig. 11.23B). An increase in the inward sodium and calcium currents depolarises the cells faster and they reach threshold quicker.
- The action potential of the myocytes is shortened by an increase in the potassium current responsible for repolarisation.

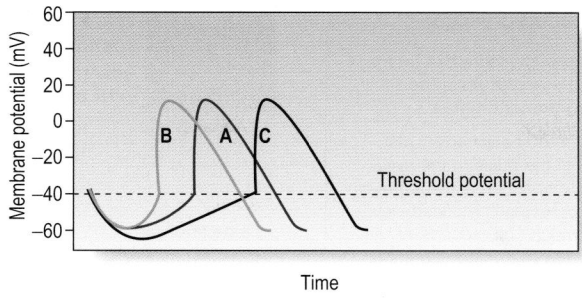

Fig. 11.23 **Autonomic effects on the heart.** (A) control; (B) sympathetic stimulation; (C) parasympathetic stimulation.

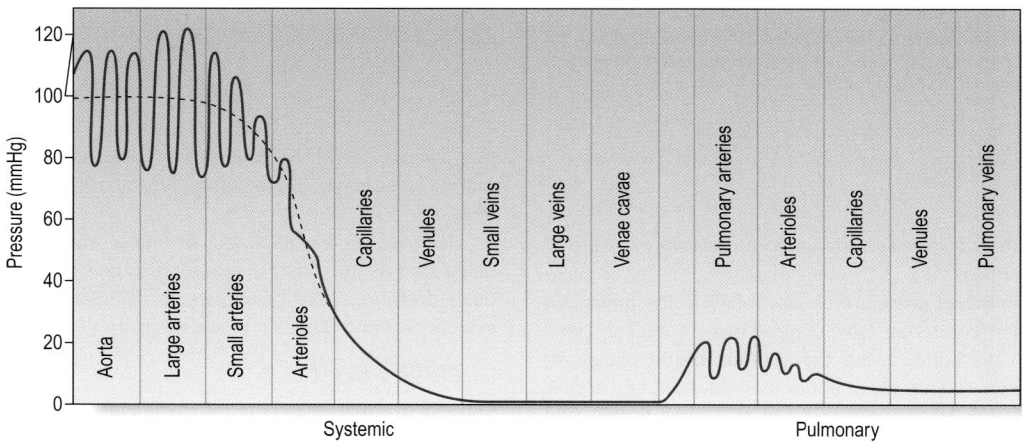

Fig. 11.24 **Pressure changes in the systemic and pulmonary circulations.** Most of the resistance to flow in the systemic system occurs at the arterioles. Pressures in the pulmonary system are much lower.

ⓘ Information box 11.4 β-Blockers

Antagonists of β₁-adrenoceptors, called **β-blockers**, are an important group of drugs which are widely used to treat a number of cardiovascular diseases, especially high blood pressure (**hypertension**). These drugs have a range of effects, some of which are not understood, but some of their actions are due to a blockade of the β₁-adrenoceptors on heart muscle causing a reduction in heart rate and contractility. However, there are also β₁ receptors in other tissues, which are also affected, and other types of adrenoceptors (α₁, α₂ and β₂) may be affected by β-blockers that are less selective for the β₁ subtype, producing unwanted side effects. Examples of β₁ ('cardioselective')-adrenoceptor antagonists are atenolol and metoprolol.

- Relaxation is faster due to a more rapid sequestration of the intracellular calcium in the sarcoplasmic reticulum.
- The conduction through the AV node is faster.
- There is an increase in the calcium current during the plateau phase, which increases the intracellular calcium concentration and hence increases the force of contraction.

All these effects are mediated intracellularly by the increased levels of cAMP. These include:

- Direct effects of cAMP on ion channels
- Via activation of intracellular regulatory enzymes, such as protein kinase A, which acts via phosphorylation of ion channels, and by increasing the activity of the Ca^{2+}-ATPase pump on the sarcoplasmic reticulum.

ADRENAL MEDULLA

The autonomic nervous system also controls the release of catecholamines, predominantly adrenaline but also some noradrenaline, from the **adrenal medulla**. Anatomically, the adrenal medulla receives input from sympathetic preganglionic neurons, and the cells of the adrenal medulla act as postganglionic cells in releasing adrenaline. However, this adrenaline is released not directly onto the target tissue but into the blood and thus is classified as a hormone.

Adrenaline acts on the β₁-adrenoceptors of heart muscle in the same way as the does noradrenaline released from nerves. Its release is thought to be a particularly important component of the increase in cardiac contractility seen in exercise. Adrenaline has other effects on both the vasculature, increasing the blood supply to working muscle, and the liver, increasing the supply of glucose to fuel muscle contraction (see below).

MECHANICS OF BLOOD FLOW

The rate at which blood flows through the closed system of the cardiovascular system is determined by two main parameters: the **pressure** and the **resistance**. Blood flows from high pressure to low pressure. The pressure in the different parts of the systemic vasculature falls from an average of approximately 100 mmHg in the aorta to about 25 mmHg in the capillaries, to almost zero in the venae cavae (Fig. 11.24). The same rule applies in the pulmonary circulation except that the pressures are much lower, going from a maximum

Accurate direct measurements of arterial pressure can be made using a cannula inserted in an artery. However, it can be measured indirectly by using a **sphygmomanometer**.

- An inflatable cuff is placed over the brachial artery just above the elbow and inflated until the pulse in the radial artery can no longer be felt. A stethoscope is placed over the brachial artery and the cuff pressure is reduced slowly until a tapping sound is heard, which corresponds to systolic pressure. The sounds are due to blood spurting through the artery at each beat and vibrating the artery walls. This first happens when the cuff pressure is just below the peak arterial blood pressure – the systolic pressure.
- The cuff pressure is reduced further until these sounds become muffled and then disappear. This corresponds to the diastolic pressure and occurs when the cuff no longer compresses the artery and the blood flow is smooth and silent.

Table 11.9   Velocity of blood flow and cross-sectional area in the vasculature. Approximate values for a resting human with a CO = 5 L/min

Type of vessel	Total cross-sectional area (cm²)	Velocity of blood flow (cm/s)	Relative velocity
Aorta	5	17	1
Large arteries	9	9.3	0.6
Small arteries	40	2.1	0.13
Capillaries	3000	0.03	0.002
Small veins	100	0.8	0.050
Large veins	30	2.8	0.17
Vena cava	7	12	0.7

of 25 mmHg in pulmonary arteries to a capillary pressure of about 10 mmHg.

The term **blood pressure** usually refers to the pressures in the systemic arteries (see Clinical box 11.4). The peak pressure in the aorta, called the **systolic blood pressure**, reaches about 120 mmHg at about the mid-point of the ventricular ejection phase (see Fig. 11.19C, *red trace*). The lowest pressure in the aorta, the **diastolic pressure**, occurs just before the opening of the aortic valve and is about 80 mmHg. These values are averages, which vary with many physiological and pathological factors.

DARCY'S LAW AND MEAN ARTERIAL BLOOD PRESSURE

The relationship between pressure and resistance in a fluid is illustrated by **Darcy's law**:

$$Q = \Delta P / R$$

where, between two points, Q = flow rate, ΔP = pressure difference and R = resistance. This is the fluid equivalent of Ohm's law. In terms of blood flowing through the vasculature the components of this equation are as follows:

ΔP = **pressure difference between the aorta and the great veins**
   = **mean arterial blood pressure (MABP) – CVP**

In practice, because normal CVP is nearly zero:

$$\Delta P = MABP$$

and

R = **total resistance to flow in the vasculature (total resistance in all the vessels – arteries, capillaries and veins – some of which are arranged in series and some in parallel)**
   = **total peripheral resistance (TPR).**

Using these terms, **Darcy's law** can be re-stated for **cardiac output**:

$$CO = MABP / TPR$$

The MABP is not just the simple average of the systolic and diastolic blood pressures, because at rest diastole is longer than systole, so MABP should be the area under the curve of the pressure wave in the aorta (Fig. 11.19C, *red trace*) over time.

However, as a reasonable estimate, the MABP can be calculated as the diastolic blood pressure (P_d) plus one-third pulse pressure. Pulse pressure is the difference between the systolic (P_s) and diastolic blood pressure (P_d):

$$MABP = P_d + (P_s - P_d)/3$$

Thus for average values of P_s (110 mmHg) and P_d (80 mmHg), which give a pulse pressure of 30 mmHg:

$$MABP = 80 + 30/3 = 90 \text{ mmHg}$$

which can also be expressed as:

$$MABP = 2/3(P_d) + 1/3(P_s)$$

VELOCITY OF BLOOD FLOW

Cardiac output is about 5 L/min at rest. As this flows through the different parts of the vasculature the velocity of the blood changes. The velocity (v) of that flow in different vessels is inversely proportional to the total cross-sectional area of the vessels (A).

$$v \propto 1/A$$

Thus for a give cardiac output:

$$v = CO/A$$

If the whole flow were through a single tube and if that tube were to become narrower, then the velocity would increase. However, if the total flow is divided into flows through a number of tubes then the velocity depends on the sum of their cross-sectional areas. If the total area is increased then the velocity will decrease and vice versa. In the vasculature this is demonstrated by flow through the aorta (a single vessel) followed by flow through a number of arteries, then through many capillaries, then into fewer veins and then to the two vena cavae. As the aorta divides into arteries and millions of capillaries, the cross-sectional area increases, with corresponding falls in blood velocity, which reaches a minimum in the capillaries. As blood travels back towards the heart the cross-sectional area becomes smaller again and the velocity increases. The functional consequence of this is that the low velocity in the capillaries allows time for the blood to exchange substances across the capillary walls (Table 11.9).

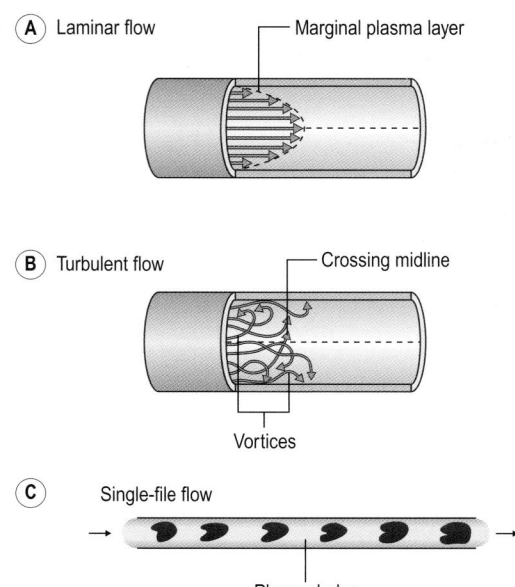

Fig. 11.25 **Types of blood flow.** (A) Profile of laminar flow with marginal plasma layer. (B) Turbulent flow showing eddies. (C) Bolus flow in capillaries.

TYPES OF BLOOD FLOW

Many of the theoretical laws which determine the flow of fluid in tubes do not strictly apply to blood flow in vivo:

- Blood is not a Newtonian fluid. That is, it is not a homogeneous fluid like water but a suspension. This means that certain properties relating to shear stress and shear rate do not apply.
- Blood flow is not steady; because of the heart pumping it is pulsatile.
- Blood vessels are not rigid, straight and uniform.

Despite these caveats, useful conclusions can be drawn from laws that have been shown to govern flow under more standard conditions. Two main types of flow occur in tubes: laminar and turbulent (Fig. 11.25).

- **Laminar flow** is smooth, with parallel streams of fluid moving along the tubes.
- **Turbulent flow** has eddies and swirls, with fluid moving in irregular patterns.

Reynolds' numbers

Whether flow is laminar or turbulent is determined by **Reynolds' number (Re)**. This ratio is determined by the velocity (v), the diameter of the tube (D), and the density (ρ, rho) and viscosity (η, eta) of the fluid.

$$\mathbf{Re = (v \times D \times \rho)/\eta}$$

In straight, uniform rigid tubes with steady flow, at low values of Re (that is, below 2000), flow is laminar. However above this critical value of Re, laminar flow breaks down and turbulence appears. In most blood vessels these high values of Re are not reached, even though in blood vessels the critical value of Re is actually lower because the flow is pulsatile and the vessels are neither straight nor uniform. However, at branch points and regions which are narrowed due to

disease, turbulence can arise at values of Re much lower than 2000.

Laminar flow

During laminar flow of a fluid in a tube, the fluid moves at different rates depending on its position with respect to the walls (Fig. 11.25A). The fluid closest to the walls is motionless due to forces between the wall and the fluid, called the **no-slip condition**. The layers (or laminae) closer to the centre of the tube move at faster and faster rates, reaching a maximum in the centre of the tube. This gives a velocity profile which is parabolic. Each layer slides past the slower layer and the shear stress between the layers has two important consequences in a suspension such as blood:

- The cells are displaced towards the centre; this leaves no cells in the layer next to the wall, the **marginal plasma layer**, which aids blood flow. Thus red cells tend to accumulate in the centre of vessels where the velocity is greatest. This effect is known as **axial streaming** and means that red cells transit the circulation faster than plasma.
- The red cells, which are flattened discs, tend to orient themselves along the long axis of the vessel.

Another consequence is that when smaller vessels branch off from a larger vessel they receive their blood from the layers nearer the wall which have fewer red cells. This is called **plasma skimming** and means that the blood in these vessels is plasma rich, which reduces its viscosity (see below).

Turbulent flow

Turbulent flow occurs at high values of Re (Fig. 11.25B). The blood no longer moves solely along the axis of the vessel and mixing of blood from the different laminae occurs. During turbulent flow some energy is dissipated as heat, so a greater pressure is required to move a fluid during turbulent flow. This increases the workload of the heart. During the ejection phase of ventricular systole, the peak velocity which is reached in the aorta is sufficient to exceed the critical Re value and turbulence is produced. This is sometimes sufficient to produce a murmur, known as an **innocent systolic ejection murmur**.

In severe anaemia, two factors may contribute to the production of cardiac murmurs. The reduced viscosity of the blood and the increased cardiac output both serve to increase the value of Re and produce turbulent flow.

Turbulent flow also occurs normally in the ventricles, where it serves to mix the blood from the pulmonary veins, thus ensuring that the blood leaving the heart is evenly oxygenated.

Bolus flow

Red blood cells are about 8 μm in diameter, which is larger than the capillaries (5–6 μm diameter) through which they travel. This means that red cells have to deform and pass in single file (Clinical box 11.5). Between each individual red cell there will be a bolus of plasma which is obliged to travel at the speed of the red cell, hence the name **bolus flow** (Fig. 11.25C).

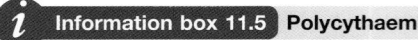
POISEUILLE'S LAW AND RESISTANCE TO FLOW

During laminar flow the presence of the no-slip condition means that any resistance to flow is because of the properties of the fluid itself and not the friction between the walls of the tube and the fluid. Poiseuille discovered that the resistance (R) to steady laminar flow in a Newtonian fluid depends on the viscosity of the fluid (η), the length of the tube (L) and the internal radius of the tube (r):

$$R = 8\eta L/\pi r^4$$

Thus one of the greatest determinants of the resistance is the radius of the vessel. A small change in radius produces a large change in resistance to flow; reducing the radius by half will increase the resistance 16-fold (2^4). Combining this equation with Darcy's law ($Q = \Delta P/R$, see above) gives the equation known as **Poiseuille's law**.

$$Q = \Delta P\pi r^4/8\eta L$$

This law relates to flow along a *single* tube. However, when the flow is divided between a number of tubes in series, such as in the transition from arteries to capillaries, then the total resistance is the sum of the different resistances. In the whole vasculature this then means that:

$$TPR = R_{arteries} + R_{arterioles} + R_{capillaries} + R_{venules} + R_{veins}$$

But if the tubes are connected in parallel then their resistances are combined in a different way because the total flow (Q_t) is equal to the sum of the flows through the different vessels (Q_1, Q_2, Q_3...)

$$Q_t = Q_1 + Q_2 + Q_3 + ...$$

Hence for a pressure difference (ΔP) across the parallel tubes:

$$Q_t/\Delta P = Q_1/\Delta P + Q_2/\Delta P + Q_3/\Delta P + ...$$

Because $Q_t/\Delta P = 1/R_t$ (from Darcy's law):

$$1/R_t = 1/R_1 + 1/R_2 + 1/R_3 + ...$$

The actual resistance per unit length is lowest in the aorta and highest in the capillaries. However, when the pressure in the different parts of the vasculature are measured, the greatest change is seen at the arterioles and very small arteries. This is because of the large number of parallel circuits in the capillaries, and the fact the capillaries are short. This is evident when one examines total resistance change according to the number of parallel elements.

In a system with three elements, each with an identical resistance R, the total resistance R_t is equal to $1/3R$.

$$1/R_t = 1/R + 1/R + 1/R = 3/R$$

where $R_t = R/3$. Similarly, in a system with five elements, $R_t = R/5$ and the total resistance is reduced. A major con-

sequence of these relationships is that small changes in diameter can change the resistance to flow in a specific vessel without having a major effect on the total resistance. In this way blood flow to specific areas can be controlled without major effects on the blood pressure.

BLOOD VISCOSITY

This is a measure of the internal friction within a fluid. In plasma, the presence of plasma proteins makes its viscosity slightly greater than water. However, the viscosity of whole blood (**relative viscosity**) is about four times that of water and is mainly determined by the volume of packed red cells per unit volume of blood (**PCV**), i.e. the **haematocrit**. This is normally about 0.42–0.53 in men and 0.36–0.45 in women (see Information box 11.5).

When blood is moving quickly, the central laminae move faster than the layers closer to the wall (see Fig 11.25A). The relative velocity of these adjacent layers is called the **shear rate** and at high levels of shear the apparent viscosity of the blood is reduced (**shear thinning**). This is partly due to the axial streaming, and is also due to the fact that at low velocities red cells tend to aggregate, forming stacks of cells known as **rouleaux**. The tendency of red cells to aggregate depends on the levels of plasma proteins, particularly fibrinogen. When fibrinogen levels are high, such as in inflammation or infection, the increased rouleaux formation is measured as an increase in the **erythrocyte sedimentation rate** (**ESR**) (see Ch. 12).

The apparent viscosity of blood is dependent on the size of the vessel. The **Fahraeus–Lindqvist effect** is the observation that in tubes with diameter smaller that 1 mm, the apparent viscosity decreases with the decreasing size of the tube. This has the effect that in small vessels such as arterioles the relative viscosity is only 2.5, and in capillaries the blood viscosity is almost as low as plasma, which has a relative viscosity of 1.2 at normal blood temperature. The resultant fall in viscosity means that the pressure needed to perfuse the microcirculation is also reduced. This effect is due partly to axial streaming and partly to the fact that in very small vessels the red cells assume a single file, which also lowers the viscosity.

ARTERIES

The function of arteries is to carry blood at high pressure from the heart to the tissues. To do this they need to be strong. Like all blood vessels, except capillaries, they consist of the following three layers (Fig. 11.26):

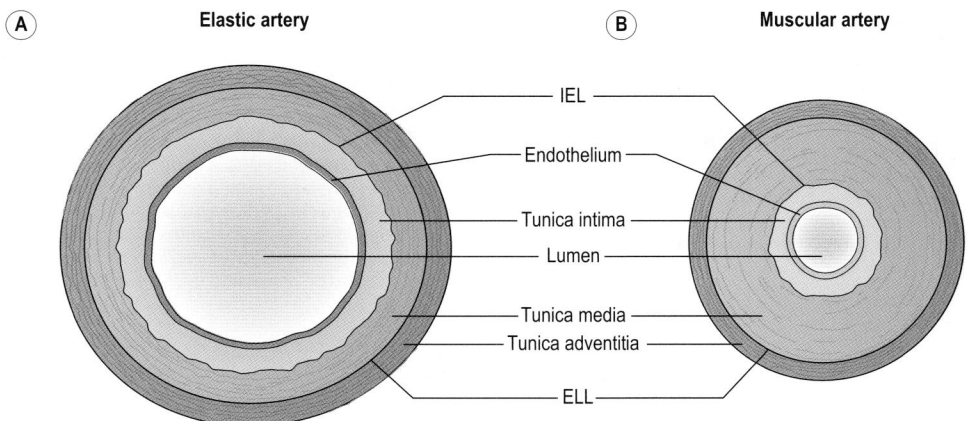

Elastic artery   Muscular artery

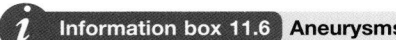

Fig. 11.26 **Structure of (A) elastic and (B) muscular arteries.** EEL, external elastic lamina; IEL, internal elastic lamina.

■ **Tunica intima**: lining the lumen, this is the innermost layer and consists of a thin layer of endothelial cells that are in direct contact with the blood and surrounded by a thin layer of connective tissue. **Tight junctions** between endothelial cells prevent the diffusion of large molecules and cellular components out of the blood. Endothelial cells secrete many substances which affect vasoconstriction and vascular permeability. They also have an important role in both blood clotting (see Ch. 12) and the growth of new blood vessels.

■ **Tunica media**: this middle layer is made up of circular and spiral layers of smooth muscle cells (see below). It also contains large amounts of elastin and collagen which provide the vessel with strength and elasticity. The smooth muscle is innervated by sympathetic nerves that control the contraction of the smooth muscle and hence the diameter of the blood vessel.

■ **Tunica adventitia** (or tunica externa): this outermost layer consists of connective tissue, mainly collagen and some elastin, and contains nerves, fat cells and fibroblasts. In large vessels this layer contains small blood vessels called **vasa vasorum**, which provide nutrients for the outer regions of the vessel wall.

On both sides of the tunica media are the **internal** and **external elastic lamina**, which form the innermost and outermost sheets of the elastic tissue surrounding the tunica media. There are two main types of arteries:

■ elastic or conducting arteries
■ muscular or distributing arteries.

The two types of artery differ mainly in the proportion of elastic tissue and smooth muscle in their walls.

ELASTIC ARTERIES

The large vessels (1–2 cm diameter) that leave the heart, the aorta and the pulmonary arteries and their major branches, are all **elastic arteries**. The tunica media of these arteries contains large fenestrated sheets of elastin which allow the vessels to stretch under pressure. The relatively thin adven-

> ### *i* Information box 11.6 Aneurysms
>
> Sometimes the wall of an artery becomes locally weakened, leading to a permanent dilation called an **aneurysm**. These are defined by their shape and location. The most common aneurysms occur in the aorta, although they may also occur in the cerebral vessels forming the **circle of Willis** and in other organs. Bleeding may occur in between the layers of the artery or into extravascular space. The weakening can be caused by a number of different causes, including atherosclerosis, degenerative conditions of either elastin or collagen, such as **cystic medial necrosis** or **Marfan's syndrome**, infections of the arterial wall, such as syphilis and tuberculosis, and inflammatory diseases such as **giant cell arteritis**.

titia is mainly made of collagen, which prevents overstretching and tears (Information box 11.6).

The high elasticity of the arterial walls allows the intermittent pumping action of the heart to be converted into a steady flow at a constant pressure. The resistance to flow in the vasculature is greatest in the capillaries, which limit the blood flow (at a given pressure). If the arteries were completely rigid the pressure in them would rise and fall as it does in the left ventricle, from about 120 mmHg at the peak of systole to about 9 mmHg at the end of diastole. There would be a certain amount of blood flow into the capillaries during systole, but this would cease when the pressure dropped (see Information box 11.7).

A constant flow into the capillaries is maintained because, as the blood is ejected from the heart into the elastic arteries, the arteries expand under the pressure. A large proportion of the stroke volume (70–80% at rest) and the energy of ejection is thus stored in the stretched arteries, and as the ejection pressure drops the arteries recoil maintaining pressure and the flow of blood towards the periphery. The maintenance of arterial pressure during diastole is patently evident as the aortic pressure does not fall below 80 mmHg.

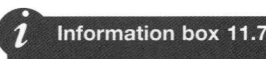

Information box 11.7 | **Compliance of arteries changes with age**

The compliance or stretchiness of arteries decreases with increasing age. This is the result of **arteriosclerosis**, a generalised stiffening of the arterial wall mainly due to hypertrophy of the smooth muscle in the tunica media and tunica intima. Calcification stiffens the wall further. The loss of compliance leads to an increase in pulse pressure as the elastic arteries fail to stretch during systole.

Clinical box 11.6 | **Blood loss can be reduced in muscular arteries**

When traumatic injury to a limb occurs it is possible for the blood loss to be almost completely inhibited by the contraction of the muscular artery, which can prevent a fatal haemorrhage. During the Falklands War, a number of potentially fatal casualties survived, despite not being treated immediately. This was thought to be partly because of the contractile mechanism reducing blood loss, and also because of the activation of clotting mechanisms, as well as intense peripheral vasoconstriction stimulated by the extreme cold.

MUSCULAR ARTERIES

The medium to small arteries (1 mm–1 cm diameter) like the cerebral, brachial and popliteal arteries are called **muscular arteries** because the proportion of smooth muscle in their walls is higher and their tunica media is much thicker than in elastic arteries. Their large diameter, in comparison to the arterioles and capillaries, makes them act as low resistance distributing arteries, carrying blood quickly to the extremities. The thick wall ensures that these vessels do not collapse easily under external compression, and the high proportion of smooth muscle allows ready contraction or relaxation. In response to increased energy demands, vessels supplying active skeletal muscle can dilate, while at the same time blood flow to non-essential organs can be reduced by contraction (Clinical box 11.6).

ARTERIOSCLEROSIS AND ATHEROSCLEROSIS

Arteriosclerosis is the generic name for a group of diseases where there is thickening of the arterial wall, which then loses elasticity. **Sclerosis** means hardening, hence the name often given to these diseases 'hardening of the arteries'. The commonest and most serious of these is **atherosclerosis**, a disease of the large- and medium-sized arteries that involves the development of fatty **plaques** within the walls of the arteries.

Evolution of atherosclerotic plaques

The first visible stage in the formation of atheromatous plaques is the development of **fatty streaks**, which are seen as yellow streaks running along the aorta and other arteries. There is a suggestion that the early formation of fatty streaks is a relatively normal process, as they are seen in most individuals at 1 year of age, and by the age of 10 about 10% of the aorta may show streaks. However, in underdeveloped

countries these streaks show no further development, in contrast with developed countries, where streaks continue to form and develop into plaques by about age 30. The development of atheromatous plaques has three main stages:

1. Endothelial damage
2. Uptake of modified **low-density lipoprotein** (**LDL**) particles, adhesion and infiltration of macrophages
3. Smooth muscle proliferation and formation of a fibrous cap.

Endothelial damage

The event that is thought to precipitate the development of plaques is damage to endothelial cells, changing their function without actual observable damage. A number of factors have been proposed that promote plaque formation:

- Shear stress is higher at arterial branch points, which also tend to be regions of atheroma formation. Hypertension increases shear stress.
- Toxic damage by exposure to chemicals, for example those present in cigarette smoke.
- Exposure to abnormally high levels of lipids, such as in familial hypercholesterolaemia, in diabetes mellitus, and in people consuming a high-fat diet.
- Viral or bacterial infection. One study found that 79% of patients undergoing surgery for removal of plaques from the coronary arteries (coronary atherectomy) tested positive for *Chlamydia pneumoniae*.

Uptake of modified LDL particles, adhesion and infiltration of macrophages

Damaged endothelium loses its ability to restrict the movement of circulating lipoproteins into the subendothelial layers. Lipoproteins are categorised into five major classes depending on their source, size, lipid constituents and associated apoproteins (Table 11.10). Lipoproteins are acted on by

Table 11.10	Types of lipoprotein	
Type	**Main constituents**	**Notes**
Chylomicrons	Triacylglycerols (90%)	Carry dietary lipids from the intestine to the peripheral tissues from where their remnants go to the liver
VLDL (very-low-density lipoprotein)	Triacylglycerols (50%)	Produced in the liver from endogenous lipids which are carried to peripheral tissues
IDL (intermediate-density lipoprotein)	Cholesterol (30%)	Produced from VLDL remnants, these are then converted to LDL
LDL (low-density lipoprotein)	Cholesterol (50%)	Produced from IDL, carries cholesterol from the liver to peripheral tissues
HDL (high-density lipoprotein)	Phospholipid (30%), cholesterol (30%)	Transport cholesterol from peripheral tissues to the liver

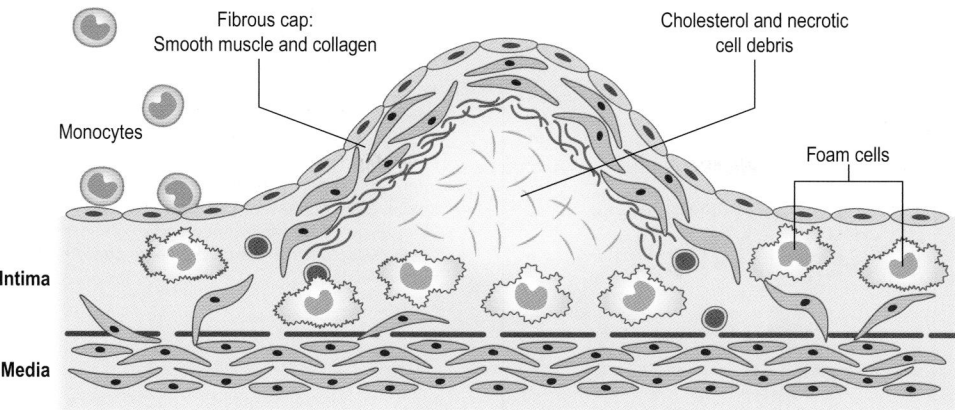

Fig. 11.27 An atheromatous plaque. Calcification of the fibrous cap increases the possibility of rupture. Exposure of the collagen stimulates the formation of a thrombus.

lipoprotein lipases, which remove fatty acids, gradually reducing the size of the lipoproteins and proportionally increasing the amount of cholesterol, phospholipid and protein.

LDL, when found in the subendothelial space, can be modified by both oxidation and glycation. **Oxidation** is facilitated by the presence of reactive oxygen species, such as those produced by smoking, and **glycation** is facilitated by the presence of high glucose levels, such as encountered in diabetes mellitus. Oxidised LDL stimulates the overlying endothelial cells to express inflammatory mediators, including adhesion molecules for monocytes, which are precursors of phagocytic macrophages. The bound monocytes cross the endothelium and are transformed into macrophages by factors released by other macrophages, attracted by the modified LDL.

Under normal conditions, macrophages ingest LDL using the LDL-receptor-mediated endocytosis. The LDL receptor recognises the apolipoprotein B-100, which is only present in lipoproteins VLDL, IDL and LDL. The levels of LDL are controlled by a negative feedback mechanism, by which internal accumulation of LDL downregulates the LDL receptor numbers, reducing further LDL uptake. However, modified LDL is not recognised by the LDL receptor, but is taken into phagocytic macrophages via a scavenger receptor. The important point about the scavenger receptor is that it is not subject to negative feedback and so modified LDL uptake is not limited. Hence, large amounts of modified LDL are taken up by the subendothelial macrophages, where it accumulates in large droplets known as **foam cells**. Dead foam cells allow lipids to accumulate in droplets in the region below the endothelium.

This accumulation of foam cells and lipid causes a raised area known as a fatty streak. The endothelial surface does not appear damaged but the area is raised and protrudes into the lumen.

Smooth muscle proliferation and formation of fibrous cap

The development of the fatty streak into a mature plaque is caused by growth factors released by the damaged endothelial cells and macrophages. These growth factors cause the proliferation of smooth muscle cells in the intima (**myointimal cells**), and the deposition of collagen. The internal elastic

lamina is broken down and pressure on the media causes muscle atrophy and an increase in collagen. Some smooth muscle cells become foam cells by taking up modified LDL.

As the plaque increases in size it bulges into the lumen of the artery (Fig. 11.27). This can reduce blood flow and cause symptoms such as **angina** (chest pain – if the blockage occurs in the coronary arteries) or **claudication** (leg cramp, which is caused by reduced blood flow to the limbs). Reduced blood flow in the renal arteries can produce an increase in blood volume and hypertension, partly due to the reduced glomerular filtration and partly by triggering the renin–angiotensin pathway.

The collagen forms a fibrous cap over the plaque, but this is fragile and easily ruptured. Its fragility is increased by calcification of the plaque, which makes the artery rigid. Rupture of the cap exposes blood to collagen, which triggers the formation of a thrombus (see Ch. 12). This can increase the volume of the plaque and reduce blood flow by narrowing the vessel lumen (Fig. 11.28). Blockage of the vessel leads

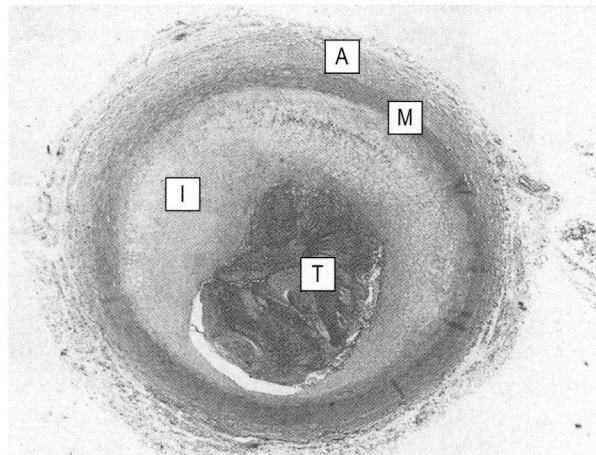

Fig. 11.28 Transverse section of a coronary artery. The tunica intima (I) has been thickened by atheroma. A thrombus (T) has blocked the lumen of the vessel. The tunica media (M) and tunica adventitia (A) are normal. Redrawn with permission from Stevens A, Lowe JS 2005 Human histology, 3rd edn. Elsevier, Edinburgh.

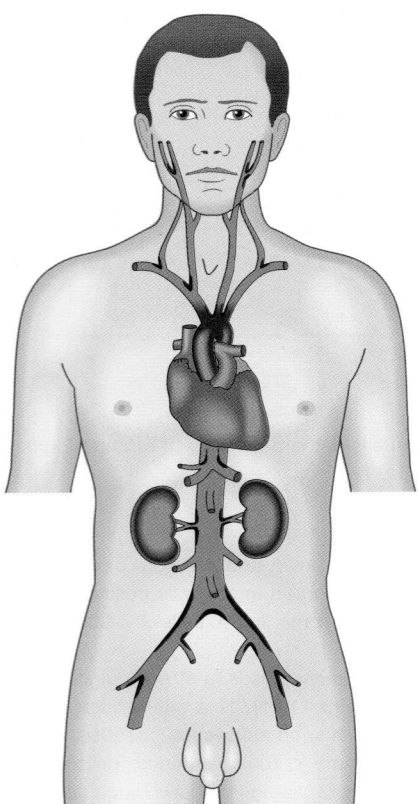

Fig. 11.29 **Common sites of atheroma formation**, shown in *blue*.

to tissue death (infarction) when either the vessel is completely occluded by the thrombus, or if parts of the thrombus break off (**embolise**) and lodge in smaller, distal arteries. Rupture of the plaque can also result in haemorrhage and aneurysm because it weakens the wall of the artery.

Plaques do not form uniformly in all arteries but are prone to develop at points where arteries branch, where blood flow may be turbulent and the endothelium is under more shear stress (Fig. 11.29). However, in advanced atherosclerosis, plaques may be extensive.

Risk factors for atherosclerosis

The known risk factors for the development of atherosclerosis can be divided into factors that are unmodifiable and factors that can be altered or even eliminated through treatment or by changes in lifestyle.

Unmodifiable risk factors

Risk factors for atherosclerosis that cannot be modified by changes in lifestyle or by treatment are:

- **Age**: the risk of developing atheroma increases with age, although if this were due simply to the inevitable accumulation of LDL over time, a very low fat intake could reduce the risk.
- **Gender**: men are more at risk than women, although risk for women increases after the menopause and the coexistence of diabetes removes the premenopausal benefit. It was thought that reduction in oestrogen after

---

Familial hypercholesterolaemia is an inherited autosomal dominant condition which is associated with high levels of early heart disease. Mutations of the gene for the LDL receptor (chromosome 2) cause a reduction in the number of LDL receptors. This increases the levels of circulating LDL (and intermediate density lipoprotein – IDL), which is thought to increase the amount of LDL that infiltrates the artery walls. Homozygotes for the mutation often die in childhood and heterozygotes have elevated plasma cholesterol (often twice the normal level).

the menopause was causative but studies of oestrogen replacement have not shown a benefit, and some studies have shown an increased risk.
- **Family history**: a positive family history for coronary heart disease (CHD) is a strong risk factor for atherosclerosis, even after the exclusion of genetically inherited diseases such as **familial hypercholesterolaemia** (See Clinical box 11.7). It is thought that many different genes may contribute to an increased susceptibility for the formation of atheroma.

Modifiable risk factors

Many of the following modifiable risk factors can be reduced and some even eliminated:

- **Lipids**: risk is increased with increasing levels of LDL and serum cholesterol and reduced with increasing levels of HDL. Risk can be lowered by reducing dietary fats, particularly saturated fat.
- **Smoking**: one of the most effective measures to reduce risk is to stop smoking. Smoking increases LDL and reduces HDL, as well as increasing the amounts of reactive oxygen species which can damage the endothelium. Nicotine is also toxic to endothelium.
- **Hypertension** is a risk factor, especially when associated with raised cholesterol.
- **Diabetes** increases risk, both by causing increased glycation due to raised blood glucose and by causing dyslipidaemia. **Insulin resistance** also increases risk.
- **Obesity**, particularly central obesity, where large amounts of fat are stored around the abdominal organs, is a risk factor independent of raised blood sugar and lipids.
- **Lack of exercise**: regular physical activity favourably alters the LDL: HDL balance, lowers blood pressure, reduces insulin resistance and improves general cardiac function. Thus a sedentary lifestyle lacking in physical exercise could be a risk factor for atherosclerosis.
- **Increased plasma homocysteine**: high levels are found in some patients with atherosclerosis, although it is not yet clear if this is a consequence of the disease or a cause.
- **Increased fibrinogen** levels accelerate plaque development.
- **Infection** with *Chlamydia pneumoniae*: atherosclerosis is considered to be an inflammatory condition and various infectious agents have been isolated from plaques and identified as possible risk factors. Antibiotic therapy has, so far, not shown any benefit.

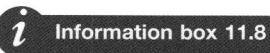

Information box 11.8   Universal treatment for risk factors using a super pill

Many patients do not know they have atherosclerosis before they have a serious episode of CHD. As a preventive measure, it has been suggested that large numbers of people, without obvious heart disease, should take statins to reduce their risk of developing atherosclerosis. A further development of this idea suggests that a 'super pill' or polypill, which would also contain low-dose aspirin, low doses of three drugs to reduce blood pressure, and folic acid to reduce homocysteine levels, would produce a very significant reduction in mortality from atherosclerosis-associated conditions. The proposers of this idea, Professors Law and Wald from Barts and the London School of Medicine and Dentistry, claim that if this pill were taken by all patients with known cardiovascular disease and all suitable individuals over 55 then cardiovascular disease could be reduced by 80%.

Treatment of atherosclerosis

As many of the risk factors for atherosclerosis are modifiable by changes in lifestyle, increasing effort is being made to try to prevent the development of atherosclerosis and subsequent heart disease. Government initiatives include increased taxation and public information campaigns aimed at helping reduce smoking, and encouragement to take more exercise and eat healthily (the five portions of fruit or vegetables per day, as well as reducing dietary fat and sugar intake). Exercise is being encouraged, especially in the young, because obesity is increasingly recognised as a potential major problem for the next generation.

If the risk to a particular patient is high and in people in whom lifestyle changes are either not sufficient or not adhered to, there are a number of drugs that can be used to lower the risk of developing CHD (see also Information box 11.8). The point at which drug therapy should be started can be calculated using charts that take into account risk factors such as blood lipids and blood pressure, as well as sex, age, smoking or diabetes. These charts calculate the per cent risk of having a CHD event within 10 years.

Much recent drug treatment has concentrated on reducing plasma lipids. **Statins**, such as simvastatin, are a group of drugs which inhibit the enzyme HMG CoA in the pathway for cholesterol synthesis. This leads to a reduction in cholesterol in cells, which triggers an increase in the numbers of LDL receptors on the cell surface, increasing LDL uptake. This further leads to a reduction in plasma cholesterol levels. Other therapeutic and preventive measures can be used to reduce blood pressure (see below) and to treat diabetes.

Non-atheromatous arteriosclerosis

Arteriolosclerosis

Narrowing of small arteries and arterioles may be the result of thickening caused by the accumulation of plasma proteins and lipids in the intima, media and basement membrane. The thickening has a glassy appearance and is also called **hyaline arteriosclerosis**.

This type of arterial disease is a prominent feature of systemic hypertension. The inability of the vessels to dilate, and the reduction in lumen size, cause ischaemia down-stream of the affected areas. The upstream increase in pressure further contributes to the hypertension and increases the risk of developing atherosclerosis.

Mönckeberg's sclerosis

Mönckeberg's sclerosis is also known as **medial calcific sclerosis**. It is an uncommon idiopathic condition of the elderly, where medium-sized arteries develop areas of calcification, visible on radiographs. This results in rigid vessels but is of limited consequence as there is no narrowing of the lumen.

VASCULAR SMOOTH MUSCLE AND THE CONTROL OF BLOOD FLOW

The blood flow in a particular region of tissue (called a vascular bed) is controlled by the constriction and relaxation of the small arteries (100–500 µm diameter) and arterioles (<100 µm diameter) supplying the bed. These are known as the **resistance vessels**. The contraction and relaxation of the smooth muscle in the walls of these vessels controls the diameter of the lumen and hence controls the resistance to flow (see above).

VASCULAR SMOOTH MUSCLE

Structure of vascular myocytes

The smooth muscle cells of the tunica media, also called **vascular myocytes**, are spindle-shaped cells, up to about 60 µm in length (Fig. 11.30). They have a single central nucleus and no visible striations (see also Ch. 2, Table 2.28). They contain the contractile proteins actin and myosin, which, like skeletal and cardiac muscle, shorten using ATP in response to increased intracellular calcium. However, in smooth muscle the process is controlled by different mechanisms.

The actin and myosin are arranged in bundles lying along the long axis of the cell, with the thick myosin filaments surrounded by thin actin filaments. The filaments are longer than in cardiac muscle, which allows a higher degree of shortening. The ends of the actin filaments are anchored to structures called **dense bodies** on the inner face of the plasma membrane. These dense bodies are themselves linked to intermediate filaments that make up the cell cytoskeleton. At the cell membrane they are attached to integrins within the cell membrane (see Ch. 2). When contraction occurs, the overlap between the actin and myosin increases and the dense bodies and bands are pulled together so the entire cell shortens and thickens.

The sarcoplasmic reticulum is not as extensive as in other muscle types, being less than 6% of the cell volume. It is less developed in the smooth muscle of resistance vessels than it is in larger vessels. Therefore most of the calcium required for contraction enters the cell from the extracellular fluid. This is not a problem because smooth muscle cells have small invaginations called **caveolae** on their surface, which gives them a high surface area to volume ratio compared with other muscle types, and thus giving them a large surface area across which calcium can be moved. Because

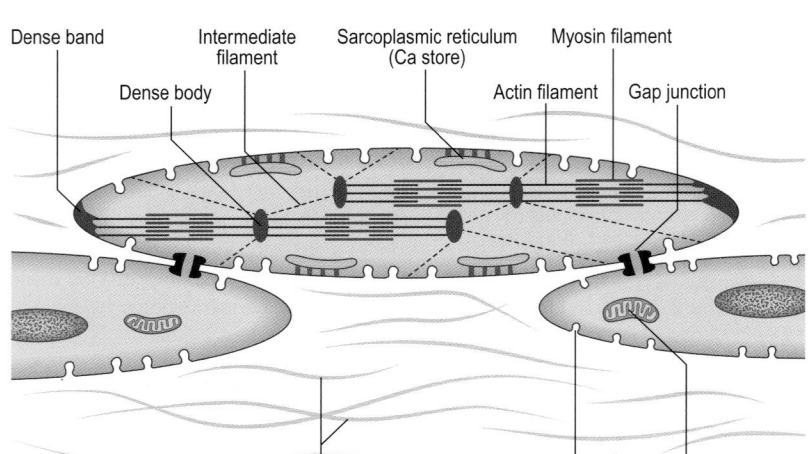

Fig. 11.30 **Structure of a vascular myocyte showing dense bodies and intermediate filaments.**

of their reliance on extracellular calcium, resistance vessels are particularly sensitive to drugs that block this influx (see below). In places the sarcoplasmic reticulum is closely associated with the cell membrane, which may allow for interactions between influx of calcium from external sources and the release of calcium from the sarcoplasmic reticulum, known as **calcium-induced calcium release**.

Like cardiac muscle cells, individual smooth muscle cells are linked via gap junctions to neighbouring smooth muscle cells. Although this electrical connection is not as extensive as it is in cardiac myocytes, it does allow some spread of excitation between cells.

Innervation of vascular smooth muscle

In arteries and arterioles, smooth muscle is innervated by nerve fibres in the adventitia and the outer tunica media. They do not have highly structured terminals like the neuromuscular junctions of skeletal muscle (see Ch. 9); instead they have long strings of up to 1000 swellings along the ends of their axons. These **varicosities** have vesicles containing neurotransmitters, which are released close to the surface of the smooth muscle cells. A single smooth muscle cell may receive neurotransmitter from multiple varicosities.

EXCITATION–CONTRACTION COUPLING IN SMOOTH MUSCLE

Unlike skeletal and cardiac muscle contraction, smooth muscle contraction does not rely on the interaction between calcium and troponin C, which is absent in smooth muscle; it is the **phosphorylation of myosin** which triggers muscle contraction in smooth muscle. This phosphorylation is dependent on the levels of calcium in the cell and occurs by a cascade of interactions:

1. Calcium entering the cytoplasm from the different sources (external calcium or calcium released from stores) binds to four binding sites on the calcium-binding protein **calmodulin**.
2. Calcium-bonded calmodulin activates **myosin light-chain kinase (MLCK)**.

3. MLCK phosphorylates the light chains of the myosin heads which form cross-bridges with the actin filaments.
4. Myosin head cycling pulls the actin filaments along the myosin chain, shortening the muscle.

Smooth muscle contracts slowly but is capable of maintaining contraction for long periods of time without the consumption of large amounts of ATP, and uses only 1/300 of the ATP required by skeletal and cardiac muscle. This is due to both the low rate of cycling of the cross-bridges (about a 1/10 of that of skeletal muscle) and the existence of a 'latch state' in which the myosin heads remain attached to the actin filaments, maintaining muscle tension without consuming ATP. This is very important as most arteries and arterioles are maintained at a low continual level of contraction. This **basal tone** allows these vessels to be either dilated or constricted when appropriately stimulated, enabling dynamic control of blood flow into vascular beds. Without basal tone, blood flow could only decrease.

Contraction is stimulated by circulating hormones, e.g. adrenaline (and noradrenaline) from the adrenal medulla, and neurotransmitters, e.g. noradrenaline, ATP and neuropeptide Y released from sympathetic nerve endings. It occurs in two phases (Fig. 11.31).

1. Electromechanical coupling
   - **Activation of MLCK and phosphorylation of myosin**: this accounts for the first minute of contraction, during which calcium levels inside the cell rise from the resting level of 0.1 μM to about 0.6 μm.
   - **Inhibition of myosin light-chain phosphatase (MLCP)**: sustained calcium levels activate a kinase, **rhoA**, inhibiting the enzyme MLCP, which would normally, in the absence of calcium, dephosphorylate MLCK and cause relaxation. This inhibition of MLCP thus maintains contraction, even though intracellular calcium levels are falling. Vasoconstriction and vasodilation occur through the activation of a variety of receptors. Many of these activate common pathways, cause changes in levels of intracellular second messengers and result in increases or decreases in intracellular calcium.
   - Some of these changes are dependent on alterations in the membrane potential, including firing action

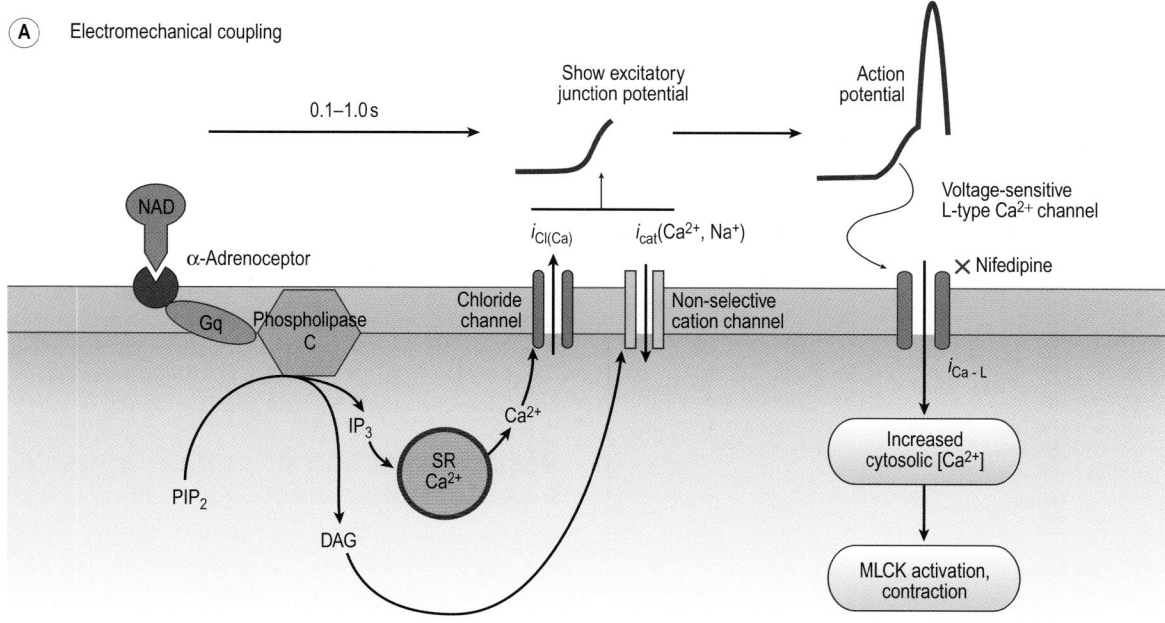

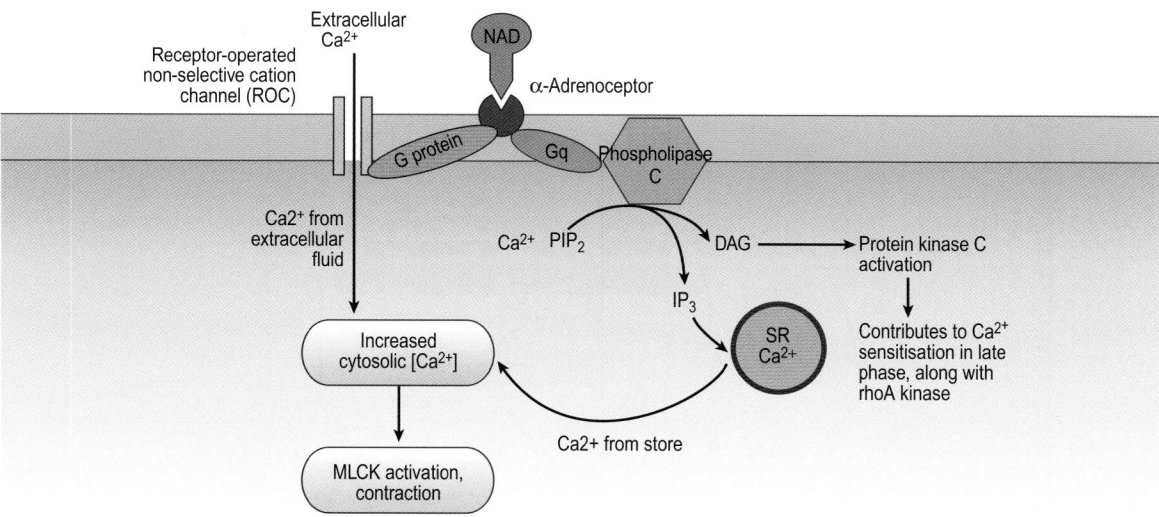

Fig. 11.31 **The pathways involved in the two phases of contraction in smooth muscle cells.** NAD, noradrenaline; IP_3, inositol trisphosphate; DAG, diacylglycerol; MLCK, myosin light chain kinase; MLCP, myosin light chain phosphatase; MLC, myosin light chains; PIP_2, phosphatidylinositol 4,5-bisphosphate; SR, sarcoplasmic reticulum. Not all the intermediate steps are shown. Redrawn with permission from Levick JR 2003 An introduction to cardiovascular physiology, 4th edn. Arnold, London.

potentials, which trigger the opening of **voltage-sensitive calcium channels (VSCCs),** mainly L-type calcium channels.

2. Pharmacomechanical coupling

Some receptors do not require changes in membrane potential and produce calcium influx through voltage-independent channels, called **receptor-operated non-selective cation channels (ROCs).** This mechanism occurs particularly in large arteries which do not fire action potentials. The diffusion gradient for calcium entry is very steep. Calcium levels outside the cell are about 1.5–2 mM, while resting levels of intracellular calcium are about 0.1 µM. So calcium tends to

diffuse into the cell continually, as well as entering when the cell is depolarised. Calcium that enters the cytoplasm is removed by three main mechanisms:

- Ca^{2+}**-ATPase** present on the sarcoplasmic reticulum returns some of the calcium to the stores.
- Ca^{2+}-ATPase present on the plasma membrane pumps calcium out of the cell into the extracellular space.
- **Sodium/calcium cotransport** exchanges intracellular calcium for extracellular sodium. This is driven by the large sodium gradient across the cell membrane. The sodium is then removed from the cell by Na^+/K^+-ATPase.

Table 11.11	Some important endogenous vasoconstrictors and vasodilators
Vasoconstrictors	**Receptors activated***
Noradrenaline (adrenaline)	α-Adrenergic
Endothelin	ET_A
Angiotensin II	AT1
Vasopressin	V_1
Thromboxane A_2	TP
Vasodilators	
Adrenaline (noradrenaline)	β_2-adrenergic
Adenosine	A_2
Bradykinin	Bradykinin$_1$ and bradykinin$_2$
Prostacyclin	IP
Nitric oxide	Guanylate cyclase

*All the receptors shown here are types of G-protein-coupled receptors (GPLR) except for guanylate cyclase, which is an intracellular enzyme.

Many different compounds can cause vasoconstriction and vasodilation, and some compounds have contrasting effects in different vascular beds, for example adrenaline and noradrenaline. This is entirely dependent on the receptor population of a particular smooth muscle (see Table 11.11). While adrenaline and noradrenaline act on both α- and β-receptor types, noradrenaline, which is released from sympathetic nerves, has a higher specificity for α-adrenoceptors, while adrenaline, which is the main catecholamine released from the adrenal medulla into the blood, is more active on β-adrenoceptors. Despite adrenaline secretion from the adrenal gland, at rest plasma levels of adrenaline are lower than those of noradrenaline due to the diffusion into the blood of noradrenaline released from sympathetic nerve terminals into the blood.

Vasoconstriction of smooth muscle by catecholamines

Noradrenaline and **adrenaline** act on α-adrenoceptors to constrict vascular smooth muscle (Fig. 11.32). They do this

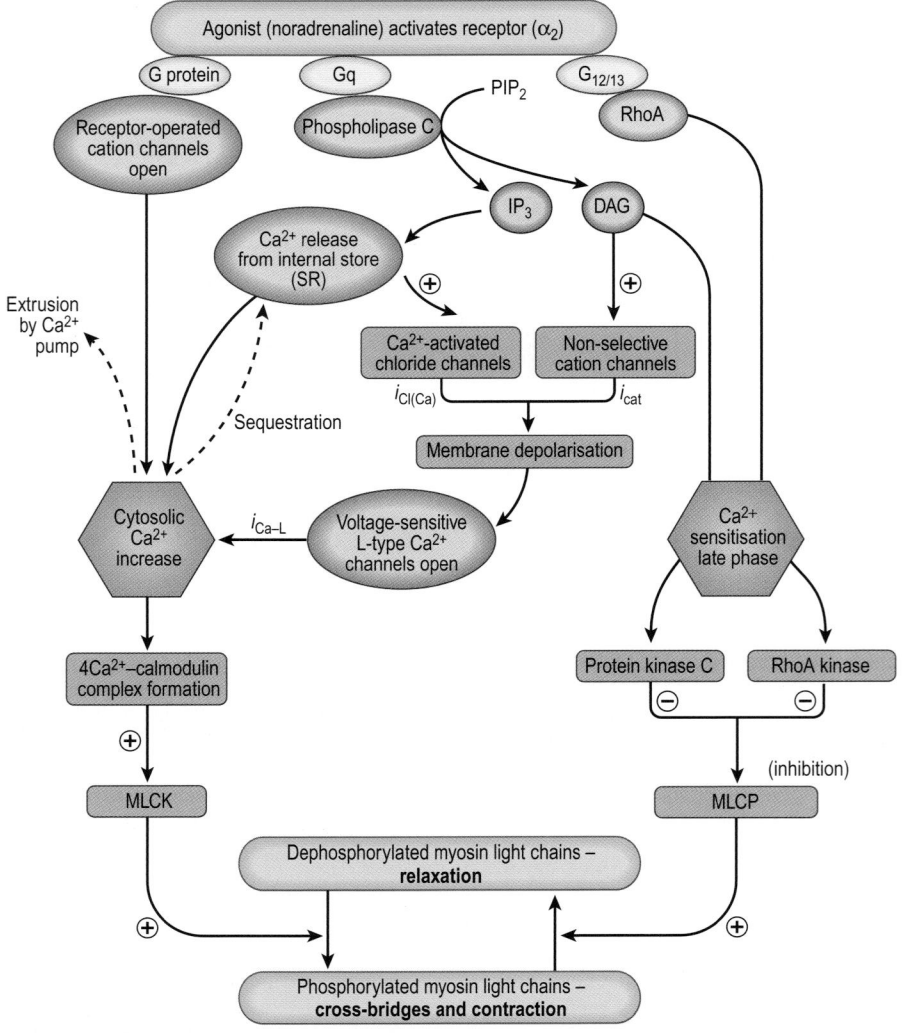

***Fig. 11.32* Vasoconstriction of smooth muscle by catecholamines.** G_q, G protein type q; PIP_2, phosphatidylinositol bisphosphate; IP_3, inositol trisphosphate; DAG, diacylglycerol; MLCK, myosin light chain kinase; MLCP, myosin light chain phosphatase. Redrawn with permission from Levick JR 2003 An introduction to cardiovascular physiology, 4th edn. Arnold, London.

by both electromechanical and pharmacomechanical coupling:

- They bind to α-adrenergic receptors, which are a type of **G-protein-coupled receptor**.
- α-Adrenergic receptors are linked via the G protein, G_q, to the enzyme phospholipase C, which generates the second messengers **inositol trisphosphate (IP$_3$)** and **diacylglycerol (DAG)** from the membrane lipid PIP_2 (phosphatidylinositol 4,5-bisphosphate) (see Ch. 2).
- IP_3 releases calcium from intracellular sarcoplasmic reticulum and, as well as increasing intracellular calcium, it also opens **calcium-activated chloride channels** in the plasma membrane.
- The efflux of chloride from the cell through the channels produces a slowly developing depolarisation.
- The depolarisation causes voltage-sensitive calcium channels (VSCCs) to open.
- In cells with sufficient numbers of VSCCs, there is a positive feedback effect and an action potential occurs, opening any remaining VSCCs. This causes a sharp rise in intracellular calcium.

Larger vessels do not have as many VSCCs as arterioles and small arteries and do not fire action potentials. In small arteries, catecholamines also open ROCs, although the mechanism is not clear. Some evidence suggests that these channels may be opened directly by a G protein. The DAG that is generated at the same time as IP_3 activates **protein kinase C**. This enzyme, which is also calcium-dependent, can inhibit MLCP, thus increasing the sensitivity to calcium (Fig. 11.32).

A group of drugs called **calcium-channel blockers** are used therapeutically to prevent the entry of calcium into cells through L-type calcium channels. They are also sometimes referred to as calcium antagonists, which is not correct as they do not block the effects of calcium (see Ch. 3 for a definition of antagonist). Calcium-channel blockers are used mainly for their cardiovascular effects, especially their effects on heart rate, blood pressure and vasoconstriction, and are

used to treat hypertension, angina and cardiac arrhythmias (see Information box 11.9). They do not affect other calcium-dependent processes, such as neurotransmitter release, as these are mediated by other types of calcium channel and these drugs are also relatively selective for L-type channels.

Vasodilation of smooth muscle by catecholamines

Most arterioles are constricted by noradrenaline and adrenaline acting on α-adrenergic receptors. However, in some tissues, particularly the liver, skeletal muscle and cardiac muscle, adrenaline causes vasodilation (Fig. 11.33). This is mediated by a different group of G-protein-linked receptors, β$_2$-adrenergic receptors, which, through activation of the G protein G_s cause an increase in intracellular cAMP. This

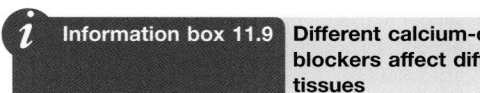

Information box 11.9   Different calcium-channel blockers affect different tissues

Usefully from a clinical point of view, the L-type calcium channels are not all exactly the same, with different isoforms being present in different tissues. The different types of calcium channel blockers have different effects in different tissues. There are three main classes of calcium-channel blockers:

- Phenylalkylamines, e.g. verapamil (cardioselective): verapamil acts mainly on the heart, reducing myocardium oxygen consumption by slowing electrical conduction through the heart.
- Dihydropyridines, e.g. nifedipine (vascular selective): nifedipine acts predominantly as a vasodilator. Acting on coronary arteries it increases coronary blood flow, and acting on peripheral vessels it reduces peripheral resistance in arterioles. The potent vasodilatory effects can, however, produce significant side effects: hypotension, headache and peripheral oedema.
- Benzothiazepines, e.g: diltiazem (intermediate).

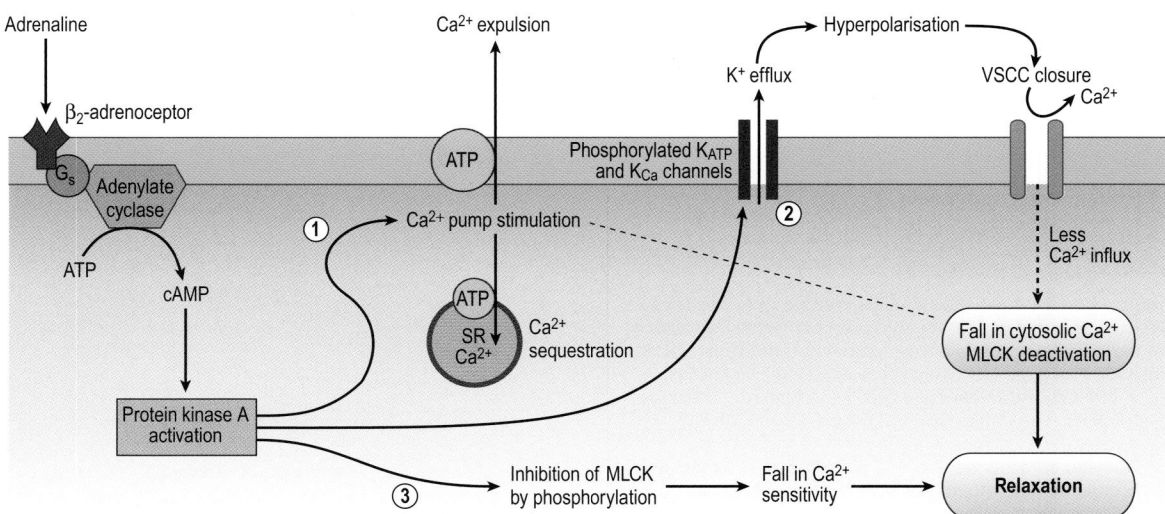

Fig. 11.33 Vasodilation of smooth muscle by adrenaline. G_s, G protein type s; cAMP, cyclic adenosine monophosphate; VSCC, voltage-sensitive calcium channel; MLCK, myosin light chain kinase; MLC, myosin light chains. Redrawn with permission from Levick JR 2003 An introduction to cardiovascular physiology, 4th edn. Arnold, London.

second messenger activates **protein kinase A (PKA)**, which has multiple actions, all of which lead to relaxation of smooth muscle and vasodilation:

- Calcium levels in the cytoplasm are reduced as the Ca^{2+}-ATPase is stimulated by PKA. This results in more calcium being pumped into the sarcoplasmic reticulum and out across the plasma membrane.
- PKA also phosphorylates K^+ channels in the plasma membrane. This opens the channels causing hyperpolarisation, which prevents the opening of VSCC.
- PKA also phosphorylates myosin light-chain kinase, inactivating it. This decreases the sensitivity to calcium.

Vasodilation of smooth muscle by nitric oxide

A different mechanism which does not involve cAMP underlies the vasodilatory action of **nitric oxide (NO)**. NO is a small molecule, produced in endothelial cells, which due to its small size and high solubility can diffuse freely across cell membranes. It is a free radical (it has an unpaired electron; see Ch. 2) and because of this it is highly reactive. It therefore has a short half-life, limiting its actions in both time and space.

- NO is synthesised in endothelial cells by the enzyme **nitric oxide synthase (NOS)** (see Information box 11.10) from the amino acid L-arginine, stimulated by increased calcium in the endothelial cell. This can be caused by a number of factors including shear stress on the endothelium (see below).
- NO diffuses across the plasma membrane into the tunica media, where it diffuses into the smooth muscle cells, activating the cytoplasmic enzyme guanylate cyclase.
- Guanylate cyclase produces the second messenger cyclic guanosine monophosphate (cGMP).
- cGMP activates protein kinase G (PKG).

It is thought that PKG causes relaxation in similar ways to PKA (see above).

FACTORS THAT CONTROL FLOW IN BLOOD VESSELS

The resistance vessels form two groups which reflect the factors controlling them:

> **ℹ Information box 11.10 Excess NO synthesis can produce severe hypotension**
>
> Nitric oxide synthase (NOS) exists in more than one form. Normal amounts of NO are produced continually by a form of the enzyme which is always present: **constitutive NOS (cNOS)**. However, NO can also be produced by another form of NOS, **inducible NOS (iNOS)**, induced by bacterial endotoxins. The transcription of large amounts of iNOS is stimulated by cytokines, such as TNF-α, released by monocytes in response to these endotoxins. The resulting high unregulated amounts of NO cause widespread vasodilation with associated hypotension. Current research into treatment for this potentially fatal hypotension includes the use of specific iNOS inhibitors in an attempt to block the excess NO production.

- **Extrinsic factors** control the small arteries and arterioles with relatively thick walls which form the first-order or proximal resistance vessels. These have a dense nerve supply and are mainly controlled by nervous input from the central nervous system and circulating hormones.
- **Intrinsic factors** control the smaller **terminal arterioles** (10–40 μm diameter). These have less smooth muscle and are poorly innervated. They are controlled predominantly by local factors.

This dual control ensures that while local needs can be met as much as possible with blood flow matched to tissue demand through the opening and closing of the terminal arterioles, these local needs can be overridden by central (extrinsic) control mechanisms that balance the demands of different organs under a range of conditions. For example, arterial blood pressure can be maintained by central regulation of total peripheral resistance. This is important in physiologically demanding situations, such as exercise. However, it is particularly critical in pathological conditions, such as haemorrhage, where individual tissues may be shut down in order to preserve central blood pressure even if this causes damage to the tissue.

Intrinsic factors

Stretch and autoregulation of blood flow

Over quite a wide range, changes in arterial blood pressure do not affect the blood flow through most vascular beds (except in the pulmonary circulation) (Fig. 11.34). In response to increased perfusion pressure, the flow initially increases but then falls back. This is due to, first, stretching of the vessel, which reduces resistance, thus increasing blood flow, followed by vasoconstriction of the vessel, which increases resistance and reduces blood flow. Known as the **myogenic response**, this is thought to be due to the activation of mechano-sensitive ion channels in the myocyte plasma membrane. These allow the myocytes to depolarise, increasing the influx of calcium through voltage-sensitive calcium

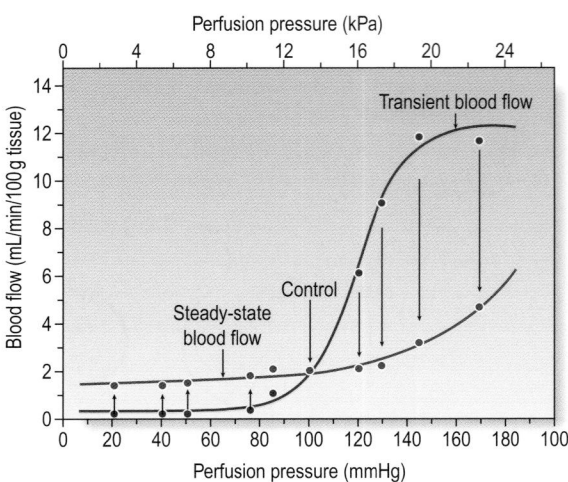

Fig. 11.34 Autoregulation of blood flow. When the perfusion pressure is changed there is a transient change in flow but this rapidly reverts to the steady-state. Redrawn with permission from Levick JR 2003 An introduction to cardiovascular physiology, 4th edn. Arnold, London.

channels and hence increasing contraction. This contraction is self-limiting due to two mechanisms:

- Calcium-activated efflux of potassium through the K^+_{Ca} channels in the smooth muscle limits the depolarisation and hence the constriction.
- Under normal conditions, the main stimulus for NO production in the endothelial cells lining the blood vessels is the shear stress exerted by blood as it passes through the vessel. Increased pressure in the vessel further increases shear stress and thus NO production. Increased NO opposes the myogenic response, balancing vasoconstriction with vasodilation. It has been shown that inhibiting this basal NO production causes hypertension, underlining the importance of NO in the control of normal blood pressure.

At very low pressures, however, this **autoregulation** is not able to maintain flow, and in severe hypotension, blood flow can be significantly reduced (see below).

Metabolic activity and local vasodilation

Autoregulation does not mean that blood flow always remains constant. In response to increases in metabolic rate the 'set point' around which autoregulation occurs can be reset at a higher value in order to match tissue requirements. When local metabolism increases, a number of factors are released into the extracellular fluid and act on the arterioles to cause vasodilation. Different **metabolic vasodilators** seem to affect some tissues more than others, but the actions generally include:

- Increases in CO_2 (hypercapnia)
- Reduction in O_2 (hypoxia)
- Increases in H^+ (particularly increases in lactic acid)
- Increased phosphate ions (from the breakdown of ATP and creatinine phosphate)
- Increased osmolarity
- Increased K^+ (as a result of increased action potential frequency in nerves and muscles)
- Increases in extracellular adenosine (a byproduct of ATP metabolism).

All of these factors act on smooth muscle by a variety of mechanisms, including receptor activation, hyperpolarisation and stimulation of ion transport, all of which result in the relaxation of the arterioles and increased blood flow. This is called **metabolic hyperaemia**, also known as active or functional hyperaemia (Fig. 11.35A). Importantly, pulmonary arterioles do not dilate in response to hypoxia; they constrict. This diverts blood away from areas of the lung that are hypoxic, and under normal conditions ensures that regions of the lung that are not ventilated are not perfused (see Ch. 13).

If metabolic activity is sustained then the increase in blood flow is maintained, but when the metabolic activity decreases, blood flow returns to its previous rate. This is because of two effects:

- The metabolic vasodilators are no longer being produced.
- Those that are produced are washed out by the increased flow.

With the removal of the vasodilators, the vasoconstriction produced by stretch (see earlier) reduces blood flow to previous levels. Reduced levels of metabolic vasodilators may

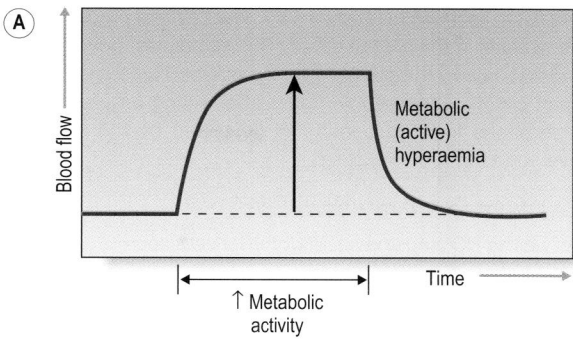

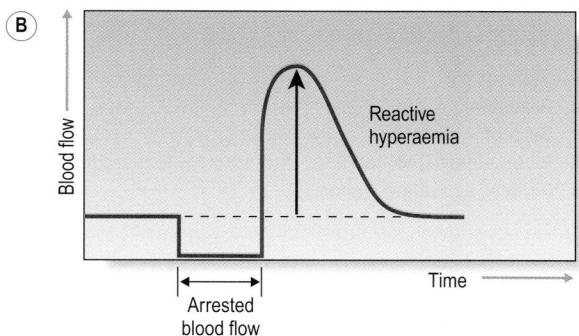

Fig. 11.35 **(A) Metabolic and (B) reactive hyperaemia.**

> ### Information box 11.11   Pressure sores
>
> If external pressure prevents blood flow for long enough then tissue damage occurs. In individuals who are unable to move about sufficiently (or at all in the case of unconscious or paralysed patients), the impairment of blood flow can lead to local tissue damage and pressure sores (bed sores) can develop.

also play a role in autoregulation as the transient increased flow that occurs when pressure increases washes out local vasodilators. However, in situations where both flow and pressure are reduced, the metabolites accumulate and vasodilation occurs.

External pressure applied to an artery can compress the vessel and impair flow. This occurs normally during the cardiac cycle when the contraction of the myocardium during systole compresses the coronary arteries (see below). However, flow is only transiently interrupted and blood flows during diastole. If blood flow is stopped for long periods of time, the tissue becomes ischaemic and damage may occur (see Information box 11.11). When the pressure is relieved the blood flow to the tissue is increased above normal for a period of time. This is called **reactive hyperaemia** (Fig. 11.35B). An example can be seen in the skin of the buttocks after sitting for a long period of time. The reddening that occurs on standing is a reflection of the increased blood flow. The hyperaemia occurs because of the accumulation of metabolic vasodilators in the tissue when blood flow is low. Although wash-out starts to occur the moment that the pressure is removed, initially the vasodilation is high. Normally, the tissue ischaemia produces substances that produce pain sensations in the area affected. This stimulates movement in order to relieve the pressure on the affected area and can be seen clearly when people fidget after sitting on uncomfortable chairs for long periods of time, and by the fact that everyone turns during sleep.

Local vasoactive chemicals

As well as NO (see above), endothelial cells secrete a number of substances which can act on vascular smooth muscle. Apart from NO the most important of these is a vasoconstrictor peptide called **endothelin**. In contrast to NO, this has a long lasting effect which may have a role in maintaining the basal tone of blood vessels. However, raised levels of endothelin have been observed in some cardiovascular diseases. Other local hormones include:

- Histamine
- Bradykinin
- Serotonin (5-HT)
- Eicosanoids (prostanoids, thromboxanes, leukotrienes)
- Platelet activating factor.

These substances are produced by a variety of cells present in the blood and tissues, and are mainly involved in the control of bleeding and in the response to infection and inflammation (see Ch. 6).

Extrinsic factors

In order to exercise a coordinated control of blood flow to the tissues, local factors can be overridden by nervous input to the first-order arterioles. Circulating hormones produced by other organs, including the brain, can also control blood flow, although their effects are most important in the long-term control of blood pressure rather than in mediating short-term control of blood flow.

Nervous input to blood vessels

Most of the nerves supplying blood vessels are sympathetic nerve fibres that release noradrenaline (with co-release of ATP and neuropeptide Y). Noradrenaline causes vasoconstriction in all vascular beds through its action on α-adrenoceptors. While some tissues also have high numbers of β₂-adrenoceptors, noradrenaline has little effect on them, so α-mediated vasoconstriction predominates.

The pathway which controls the firing of these sympathetic nerves originates in the brainstem, in the **nucleus tractus solitarius (nTS)** in the medulla (Fig. 11.36). The nTS receives sensory input about the blood pressure and blood volume, from the heart and carotid sinus, which, along with information from the cortex and hypothalamus, determines their firing. These projections synapse in the **rostral ventrolateral medulla** from which nerves project to the preganglionic

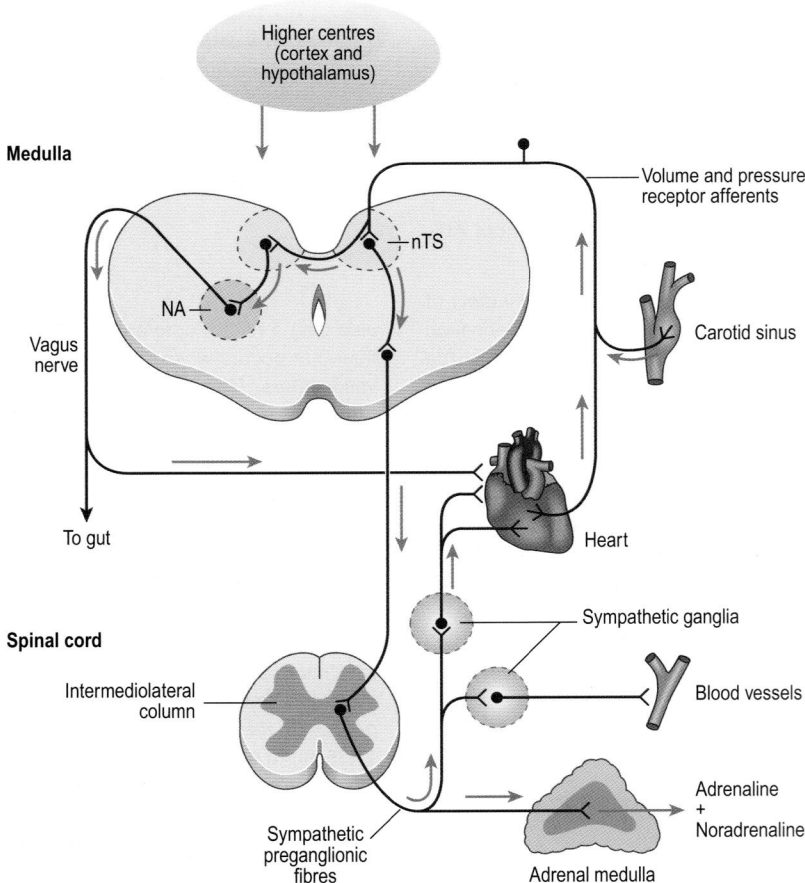

Fig. 11.36 Sympathetic innervation of the heart, blood vessels and adrenal medulla. *Dotted arrows* show sensory feedback from the heart and carotid sinus.

neurons in the spinal cord. These synapse on sympathetic ganglia from which postganglionic neurons project to the blood vessels (and the heart). These pathways have a tonic firing rate which contributes to the resting tone of the vessels. In this way reduction in the basal firing rate can cause vasodilation in tissues that only have α-adrenoceptors.

Uniquely, blood vessels in the sweat glands are innervated by sympathetic fibres which release acetylcholine. These cause vasodilation and an increase in the production of sweat. In a small number of tissues, there are also vasodilator parasympathetic nerve fibres which release acetylcholine and another **non-adrenergic, non-cholinergic (NANC)** transmitter, which is thought to be predominantly the neuropeptide **vasoactive intestinal peptide (VIP)**. Other NANC transmitters include neuropeptide P and NO.

Hormones that affect blood flow

Four hormones mainly affect blood flow:

- Adrenaline
- Vasopressin (also called antidiuretic hormone – ADH)
- Angiotensin II
- Atrial natriuretic peptide (ANP).

Adrenaline has potent effects throughout the body:
- The **main** effect of adrenaline is to increase heart rate and contractility, and so cardiac output increases.
- Adrenaline released by sympathetic stimulation of the adrenal medulla also acts directly on adrenergic receptors on smooth muscle. Depending on which receptors are present it can produce vasoconstriction or vasodilation. When there is widespread activation of the sympathetic system, the **fight and flight response**, adrenaline will allow blood flow to skeletal muscle to increase, while vasoconstriction will occur in many other tissues, mediated by both noradrenaline and adrenaline. This has the effect of maintaining total peripheral resistance (TPR) at normal levels.
- Circulating adrenaline affects liver metabolism, switching on the breakdown of glycogen to glucose (glycogenolysis) and stimulating new glucose production (gluconeogenesis). Adrenaline also activates β-adrenoceptors in adipose tissue to stimulate fat mobilisation through lipolysis. These effects on metabolism provide the energy needed by heart and skeletal muscle during periods of higher activity.

Unlike adrenaline, the hormones vasopressin, angiotensin II and ANP all have effects on blood volume (described below), through actions on the kidney (see also Ch. 14) as well as on vascular tone. The effects of **vasopressin** on blood flow are seen if blood volume becomes very low, as in severe haemorrhage. High concentrations of vasopressin acting on V_1 receptors cause generalised vasoconstriction in all tissues, except the coronary and cerebral vessels. In the latter tissues, vasopressin stimulates the release of NO, resulting in vasodilation. This has the effect of maintaining perfusion to the heart and the brain. **Angiotensin II** is more powerful than adrenaline in producing vasoconstriction, which it does by a variety of mechanisms:

- Acting directly on smooth muscle to activate contraction via AT_1 receptors
- Acting presynaptically, to enhance the release of noradrenaline
- Acting centrally, to promote increased sympathetic vasoconstrictor activity.

ANP is a vasodilator, acting by increasing cGMP levels in smooth muscle in a similar manner to NO.

MICROCIRCULATION

The purpose of the heart and large blood vessels is to transport blood quickly around the body and supply all the tissues with nutrients. While the luminal surfaces of the large blood vessels are maintained by the direct diffusion of nutrients from the blood, all other tissues receive what they need by diffusion from the **exchange vessels** – which are:

- The smallest **arterioles**
- The capillaries
- The small post-capillary **venules**

However, by far the majority of material is transferred across capillaries.

VESSELS OF THE MICROCIRCULATION

Capillaries are very small (5–10 μm diameter) and between 0.3 mm and 1 mm long (Fig. 11.37). They are very thin, consisting solely of endothelial cells and a basement membrane. Capillaries are extremely numerous, so the diffusion distance between most cells and their nearest capillary is very small (maximum 40–80 μm). Some tissues, such as cartilage, do not contain capillaries but rely on diffusion from nearby tissues. The lung, in contrast, is served by capillaries that have a surface area of 3500 cm^2/g of lung tissue.

Most capillary beds start with a tuft of capillaries that are branches of the **terminal arterioles**. The flow into the tissue is controlled by the vasoconstriction of the small and terminal arterioles. Capillaries drain into **postcapillary venules**, which have **pericytes** in their walls. These cells vary in number in the venules in different tissues and, while some of them are contractile, their role is not clear. From these blood drains into the **venules**, which contain smooth muscle.

Metarterioles and AV shunts

Some tissues, such as the mesentery, have **metarterioles** (10–20 μm diameter) branching off from the terminal arteriole.

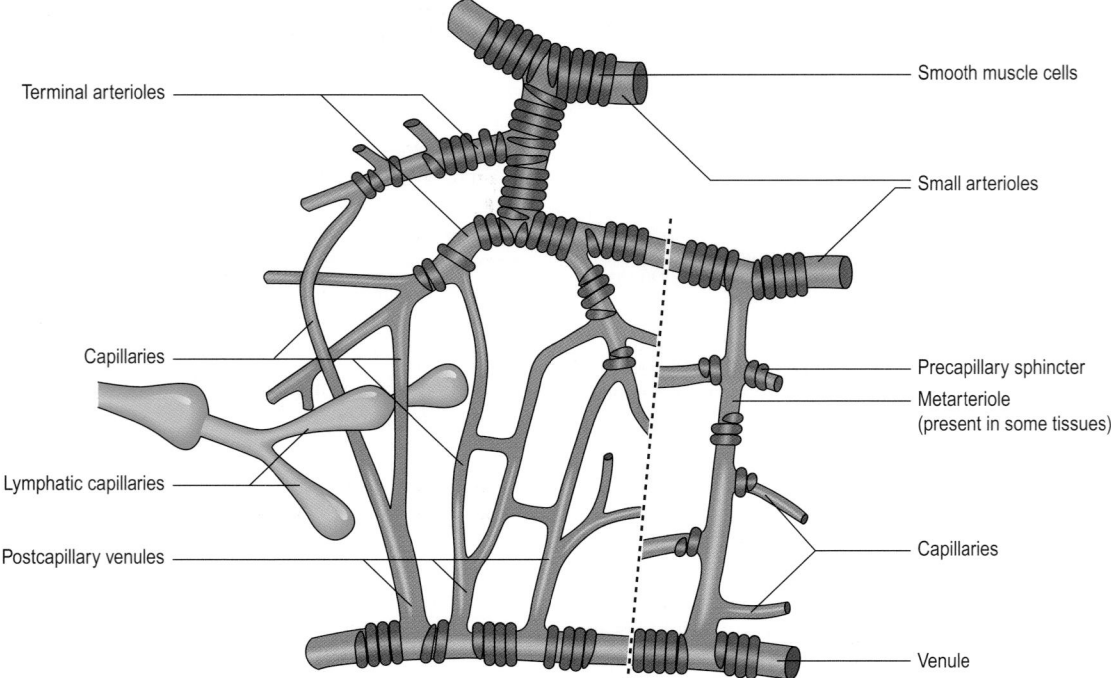

Fig. 11.37 **Anatomy of the microcirculation.** Redrawn with permission from Aaronson PI, Ward JPT 1999 The cardiovascular system at a glance. Blackwell Science, Oxford.

These vessels are similar to capillaries but are larger and have a single layer of discontinuous smooth muscle. Metarterioles directly connect arterioles to venules and can serve as bypass channels for blood. True capillaries branch from the metarterioles with rings of smooth muscle, **precapillary sphincters**, controlling whether blood flows from the metarteriole directly into the venules or through the capillaries. In other tissues, blood flow through the capillary bed can be bypassed by the presence of **arteriovenous anastomoses** or **AV shunts**. These are short, highly muscular vessels which can shunt blood from the arterioles to either venules or venous plexuses. They are mainly found in the skin of the extremities and are involved in temperature regulation (see below).

TRANSPORT MECHANISMS ACROSS THE ENDOTHELIUM

Diffusion of solutes

Diffusion is the main mechanism by which substances move from the blood to the extracellular fluid or vice versa. **Fick's law of free diffusion** describes how the rate of diffusion (J_s) is dependent on a number of variables (see also Ch. 2).

$$J_s = -DA\, \Delta c / \Delta x$$

where Δc is the concentration difference and Δx is the distance of diffusion and together they make up the concentration gradient. A is the surface area over which diffusion occurs and D is the diffusion coefficient. The minus sign indicates that diffusion occurs down a concentration gradient. The diffusion coefficient, D, depends on the temperature, the viscosity of the solvent and the size of the solute. Generally, small solutes diffuse more quickly than

larger ones so D is inversely proportional to the molecular weight.

Free diffusion describes how a solute moves through a large volume of the solvent (which in plasma is water). However, if the diffusion has to occur across a membrane the situation becomes more complex. Some solutes can only move through pores of a given size in the membrane, thus reducing the surface area (A) available for diffusion. The distance of diffusion, Δx, may be longer because the pore does not take the shortest route across the membrane. There may be frictional drag between the pore and the solute, which impedes its progress if the solute is larger than the pore size. All these factors can be included in a revised version of Fick's law:

$$J_s = -PA\, \Delta c$$

where P is the permeability of the membrane to the solute.

The permeability of the membrane is extremely important in determining the ability of a given solute to pass from the blood into the tissue. In the kidney, for example, the permeability must be high in order for solutes to pass from blood into the urine to be excreted. However, in the brain, it is equally important that the neurons be protected from fluctuations in blood chemistry, which could adversely affect brain function, so permeability across the blood–brain barrier is low.

The diffusion of a given solute depends on its chemistry and the availability of different pathways across the membrane, that is, a solute can use different types of pore so that the effective surface area for diffusion varies. Models of diffusion of a wide range of solutes across the endothelium postulate the existence of two groups of pores in the membrane of differing size and frequency.

Diffusion of lipid-soluble compounds

If a compound is lipid soluble, it can diffuse freely across the endothelial cell membranes without the need for pores. This is the case for both **oxygen** (O_2) and **carbon dioxide** (CO_2), which can therefore diffuse across the whole surface area of the capillary.

The degree to which a solute is lipid soluble can be measured using the oil:water partition coefficient. This measures how easily solutes dissolve in water and an organic solvent (usually ether). Oxygen has an oil:water partition coefficient of 5 and carbon dioxide a value of 1.6, which makes them both very permeable. Free lipids (not bound to membrane proteins) such as **cholesterol** can diffuse freely across capillaries, as can anaesthetic drugs. The potency of **inhalation anaesthetics**, such as halothane and nitrous oxide, are closely correlated with their lipid solubility.

Diffusion of lipid-insoluble molecules

Small lipid-insoluble molecules include **water**, ions and small hydrophilic molecules such as urea, glucose and some amino acids. Although water is about 300 times less permeable than oxygen, water flows relatively freely across capillaries, both through water-selective channels, **aquaporins**, present in the cell membranes and through gaps between adjacent endothelial cells – the **paracellular pathway**. These gaps, and the connective tissue surrounding the capillaries, forming the equivalent of **small pores** of about 4 nm wide, also allow the passage of ions, urea and glucose. They are relatively sparse and cover only about 0.03% of the total capillary area. They allow the passage of molecules of molecular weight (MW) <10 000. The gaps are not present in 'tight' barriers, such as the blood–brain barrier, which relies more on specific transport mechanisms. Glucose, which has a molecular weight 10 times that of water, is 0.6 times as permeable.

Larger lipid-insoluble molecules, such as **albumin** (MW 69 000), do not pass through the interendothelial clefts, but can only pass through large gaps between endothelial cells. In most capillaries these types of gaps do not exist, which is why albumin is largely restricted to the blood plasma. In some disease states, however, the permeability of the capillary increases enough to allow proteins and other blood components to move into the extracellular space (see below).

Despite albumin being largely restricted to the blood plasma, there is a small but measurable permeability (0.000 1 relative to water). Additionally, in order for protein-bound molecules, such as thyroxine and the hormones testosterone and oestradiol, to move into the tissues it has been suggested that there are very few **large pores** (4000 times fewer than small pores) with a radius of 20–30 nm. Unlike the small pores, which are represented by the inter-endothelial clefts, the physical identity of the large pores is still under discussion. It has been suggested that transient trans-endothelial channels form from fused vesicles across the endothelium.

Other transport mechanisms across endothelium

Apart from diffusion, there are two other mechanisms that allow the movement of lipid-insoluble molecules across the endothelium:

- **Pinocytosis**: this is a form of bulk transport where small areas of membrane containing water and solutes are endocytosed on one face of the endothelium. These vesicles are then moved across the endothelium, where they release their contents by exocytosis. This type of endocytosis/exocytosis is also used to transport specific molecules across the blood–brain barrier, using **receptor-mediated endocytosis** (see Ch. 2) as a means of trapping specific molecules, for example, transferrin which is used to transport iron in endocytotic vesicles.
- **Specific transport mechanisms**: glucose moves into the brain by facilitated diffusion using a series of **glucose transporters** (**GLUT**). The transport is kept moving in the right direction because the concentration gradient for glucose drops progressively from blood to endothelial cell to brain extracellular fluid (ECF) to neuron, and each type of glucose transporter in the chain has a higher affinity for glucose.

Limiting factors for exchange across endothelium

The rate of blood flow in a capillary has important effects on the exchange of solutes across a capillary. For substances with a high permeability, the equilibration of concentrations across the capillary occurs so rapidly that before the blood has reached the end of the capillary, no more exchange occurs. This is called **flow-limited diffusion** because if the flow rate is raised, the amount of a solute transferred per unit time is increased, as it continues to equilibrate further down the capillary. This occurs in the lung, where O_2 and CO_2 are exchanged very rapidly across the alveoli. If the permeability of the solute is much lower, equilibration does not occur before the end of the capillary. The amount of a solute delivered to a particular tissue can be increased by reducing the rate of blood flow, allowing the solute more time to diffuse into the tissues (**diffusion-limited diffusion**).

TYPES OF CAPILLARIES

Three main types of capillaries are present in different tissues. They have different permeability characteristics which determine the types of solute diffusing across them and the rate at which this occurs.

Continuous capillaries

The most common type of capillary is the **continuous capillary** (Fig. 11.38). The endothelial cells form a continuous layer around the lumen and the endothelial cells are linked to each other by **tight junctions** (see Information box 11.13). However, in most tissues the tight junctions are not completely continuous and allow the passage of small molecules (see above). The entire capillary is surrounded by the basement membrane, which contains collagen and other proteins. Continuous capillaries are found in a wide range of tissues, such as skin, muscle and fat.

Fenestrated capillaries

Fenestrated capillaries contain pores (20–100 nm diameter) within a circular structure that looks somewhat like a cartwheel. Between the spokes there are the fenestrae (windows) which are usually covered by a thin membrane. These fenestrae have a much higher permeability than continuous capillaries and fenestrated capillaries are found in tissues where there is either substantial filtration and/or absorption, such as the kidney tubules and the intestinal mucosa, or in endocrine glands that are actively secreting compounds into the blood. In the kidney glomerulus, where the primary filtrate which goes to produce urine is filtered from blood, the membrane is absent, allowing even greater passage of solutes. (Note that the barrier to filtration of solutes in the kidney glomerulus is not the capillary but the basement membrane see Ch. 14).

Discontinuous or sinusoidal capillaries

In a small number of capillaries, called **discontinuous** or **sinusoidal capillaries**, there are gaps between the endothelial cells and the basal lamina which allow any of the components of blood, including blood cells, to move freely between the tissue and the vasculature. These only occur in organs such as the liver, spleen and bone marrow, which process blood cells in some way. In order to prevent blood leaking from these organs into the body cavities, these organs are all encapsulated. The **spleen** is covered by a fibrous capsule, the **liver** by the visceral peritoneum and the **bone marrow**, which is found in spongy bone, is covered by compact bone.

> *i* **Information box 11.13** | **The blood–brain barrier causes problems in drug development**
>
> In the brain, continuous capillaries form the **blood–brain barrier** (see Ch. 8). In these capillaries, the tight junctions between the endothelial cells are complex and have a high electrical resistance which indicates a low permeability. In order to protect the brain from toxic substances in the blood and fluctuations in blood chemistry, the blood–brain barrier prevents the entry of most solutes into the brain. This is particular important in the case of solutes such as K^+ and catecholamines, which could affect neuronal firing patterns. The blood–brain barrier is also extremely impermeable to many lipophilic molecules.
>
> This poses a considerable problem for the development of drugs for central nervous system disorders. Not only must these drugs be designed so as to be active but they must also have a structure which allows them to penetrate the blood–brain barrier. Some drugs can be transported across the blood–brain barrier using existing transporters; the drug used to treat Parkinson's disease, levodopa, crosses the blood–brain barrier using the endogenous dopamine transporter. Research on transiently opening the blood–brain barrier continues, but at present the approach is used only for the administration of drugs requiring limited use for life-threatening conditions.

> *i* **Information box 11.14** | **Removal of the spleen following trauma**
>
> The capsule of the spleen is relatively fragile and may be ruptured by trauma to the abdomen. In such circumstances it is usually necessary for it to be removed (splenectomy) in order to prevent fatal haemorrhage. In adults, the spleen is not an essential organ, but its removal may leave patients at increased risk of infection.

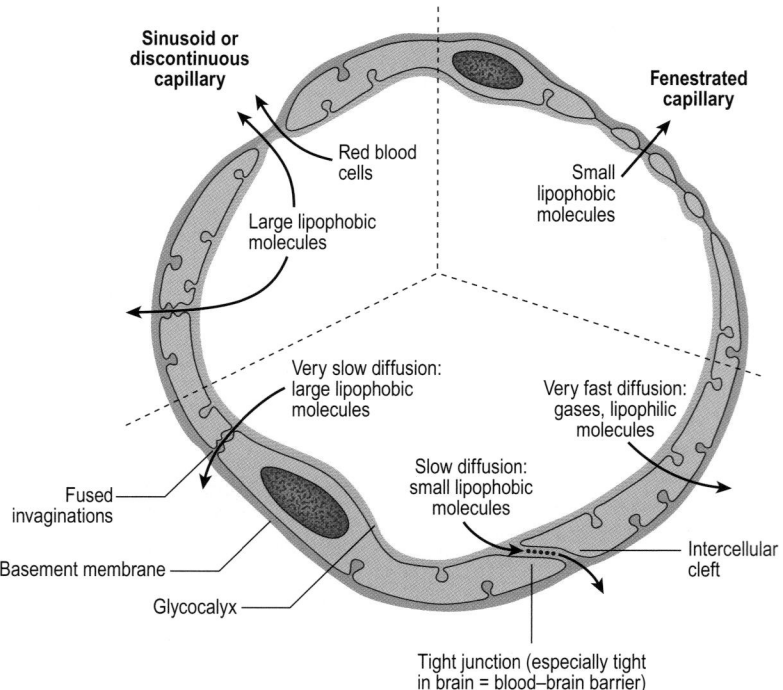

Fig. 11.38 Types of capillary. Redrawn with permission from Aaronson PI, Ward JPT 1999 The cardiovascular system at a glance. Blackwell Science, Oxford.

FLUID MOVEMENTS BETWEEN THE VASCULAR AND EXTRAVASCULAR COMPARTMENTS

Due to its small size and the presence of sufficient pores and aquaporins, water moves freely between the blood and the extracellular fluid (see above). There are two forces which cause water to move across capillaries:

- **Hydrostatic pressure**: water moves from a region of high pressure to a region of lower pressure. Interstitial hydrostatic pressures are very low (and may even be negative) so the normal blood pressure in the capillaries tends to force water from the capillaries into the tissues.
- **Oncotic pressure**: water moves by osmosis from areas of low solute concentration to areas of high solute concentration. In blood, the effective osmotic pressure is largely produced by the plasma proteins. These large proteins are called **colloids** so the osmotic pressure of blood is known as the **colloid osmotic pressure** or **oncotic pressure**. As the extracellular fluid contains much less protein than the blood, this colloid osmotic pressure tends to draw fluid into the capillaries.

The balance of these two opposing forces will determine whether fluid moves in or out of the capillary. They were first described by Ernest Starling in 1896 and are often called **Starling forces**.

Starling forces

The hydrostatic and oncotic forces acting across the capillary can be described using a few simple terms (Fig. 11.39A):

1. **Hydrostatic pressure of blood, P_c**: this is the change in pressure through the circulation which drives blood flow, blood pressure falling along the whole length of the circulation (Fig. 11.39). The hydrostatic pressure (P_c) of the blood in a well-perfused capillary is about 32 mmHg at the arteriolar end, falling with distance along the capillary to about 17 mmHg at the venous end for a 1 mm long capillary. These values change depending on the degree of vasoconstriction, which reduces the arteriolar pressure (and hence the venous pressure).

2. **Hydrostatic pressure of interstitial fluid, P_i**: although hard to measure, in many tissues the interstitial fluid (P_i) is probably maintained at a pressure slightly below atmospheric pressure, at about –3 mmHg. This negative pressure is thought to be caused by the suction of fluid from the extracellular spaces by the lymphatic system (see below). In encapsulated organs such as the liver the pressure may be slightly positive.

3. **Oncotic pressure of plasma, π_c**: most of the osmotic pressure of the plasma (about 6000 mmHg) is produced by the electrolytes and other small molecules present in the blood. As these are also present in the ECF, they do not produce osmotic movements of water. However, the plasma also contains large plasma proteins (60–80 g/L) at much higher concentrations than in the ECF. It is this difference which produces the effective difference in osmotic potential between the blood and the ECF, the **colloid osmotic potential**, which is normally about 27 mmHg.

4. **Oncotic pressure of ECF, π_i**: the ECF normally contains low levels of protein (about 20–30 g/L) and has an average oncotic pressure of about 8 mmHg (see below, inflammation).

Filtration pressure

The net force across the capillary is the net filtration pressure. It can be calculated as follows:

Net filtration pressure (FP) = net hydrostatic pressure – net oncotic pressure

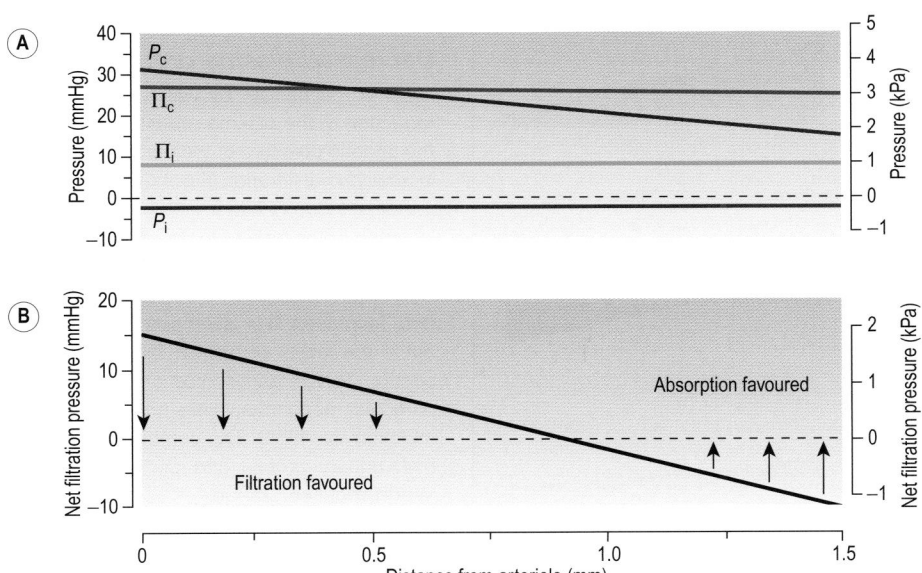

Fig. 11.39 **Starling forces and filtration pressure.** (A) Starling forces along a capillary; (B) net filtration pressure along a capillary. For explanation of abbreviations see text. P_c: *purple line*, P_i: *red line*; π_c, *blue line*; π_i, *green line*.

Therefore:

$$FP = (P_c - P_i) - (\pi_c - \pi_i)$$

The net filtration pressure at each end of the capillary can be calculated as follows:

At the arteriolar end:

$$FP = (32 + 3) - (27 - 8) = 16 \text{ mmHg}$$

At the venous end

$$FP = (17 + 3) - (27 - 8) = 1 \text{ mmHg}$$

The results of these pressure differences means that at the arteriolar end of the capillary filtration is high and water moves out of the capillary, and at the venous end filtration is reduced almost to nothing, with net filtration being reduced gradually along the length of the capillary (see Fig. 11.39B). This description is a simplification, assumes a well-perfused capillary and does not take into account factors such as the degree of arteriolar constriction, which may reduce the hydrostatic pressure at the arteriolar end and hence at the venous end. It is suggested that when vasoconstriction occurs, pressures fall sufficiently for absorption to occur at the venous end (Fig. 11.40B). However, this absorption is transient because there is both a change in concentration of plasma proteins along the capillary as water is drawn into the ECF and a reduction in the interstitial hydrostatic pressure due to the removal of water by absorption. However, if the arteriole alternates between periods of constriction and relaxation then over time large amounts of fluid can be reabsorbed.

Under normal conditions, a state of equilibrium exists between the amount of water leaving and entering the circulation. Calculations of the mean pressures for the entire capillary circulation show a slight excess of filtration over absorption of only 0.3 mmHg. Only a very small percentage of the total plasma water is filtered and reabsorbed in this way but, given the large volumes which pass through the

capillary circulation each day, any imbalance between the ECF and the plasma can produce large movements of fluid over time. Only about 0.2–0.3% of plasma is filtered by most tissues, but with a total fluid movement of 4000 L per day this leads to the net filtration of 12 L per day. More than 80% of this is returned to the circulation by reabsorption, and the remainder is removed by the lymphatic system and returned to the circulation by that route.

In the kidney glomerulus, the net filtration is much higher, about 20% of the plasma is filtered. This could lead to the loss of 800 L, rather more than the total volume of the body. However, more that 99% of the fluid is returned to the circulation by reabsorption in the tubules and the remaining 1% is returned by the lymphatics. In the lungs, the low capillary hydrostatic pressure (10 mmHg) would suggest that net absorption should occur in lung tissue. However, the reverse is true as lymph forms in the lungs. This is because lung tissue fluid contains more plasma protein and therefore the oncotic pressure of the interstitial fluid is much higher (16–20 mmHg), favouring net filtration.

Oedema

Oedema occurs when net filtration exceeds lymphatic drainage. This can occur in a number of conditions by four different mechanisms:

- Increased capillary pressure
- Decreased plasma proteins
- Reduction in lymphatic drainage
- Increased capillary permeability.

Increased capillary pressure

Filtration in capillary beds is not increased by an increase in systemic arterial pressure. If the arterial pressure is raised, as in hypertension, there is no significant increase in the arteriolar capillary pressure, due to autoregulation (see Fig. 11.34). In contrast, raised venous pressure changes the pressure gradient across the capillary bed to favour filtration (*red area*) over absorption (*green area*) This is shown in Figure 11.41B, where an increase in venous pressure reduces the slope of the line P_{net} (*dotted line*).

Decreased plasma proteins

Another mechanism by which oedema occurs is if there is reduction in the plasma protein concentration. This reduces the oncotic pressure of the blood, reducing reabsorption and increasing net filtration (Fig. 11.41C). This reduction in plasma proteins is due to either a reduction in their production or an increase in their excretion by the kidney.

Increased loss of protein in urine due to damage to the renal glomerulus occurs in a number of kidney diseases. At first, increased liver synthesis maintains the protein levels, but if the levels of protein fall below 25 g/L then oedema occurs. This is generalised oedema, but often the face, in particular, appears swollen in the morning due to fluid accumulation overnight. The combination of low plasma protein, high urinary protein and oedema is known as **nephrotic syndrome** (see Ch. 14).

Reduction in lymphatic drainage

If the amount of fluid in the tissues increases, this can initially be removed by an increased rate of lymph flow. It has been estimated that lymph flow can increase 10 to 50-fold, also

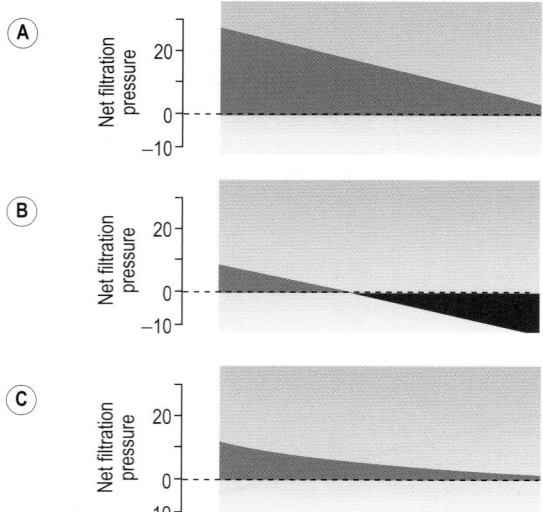

Fig. 11.40 **Changes in pressure across the capillary**: (A) well-perfused capillary; (B) vasoconstriction – early transient; and (C) vasoconstriction – later steady-state. Blue shows net filtration and red net absorption.

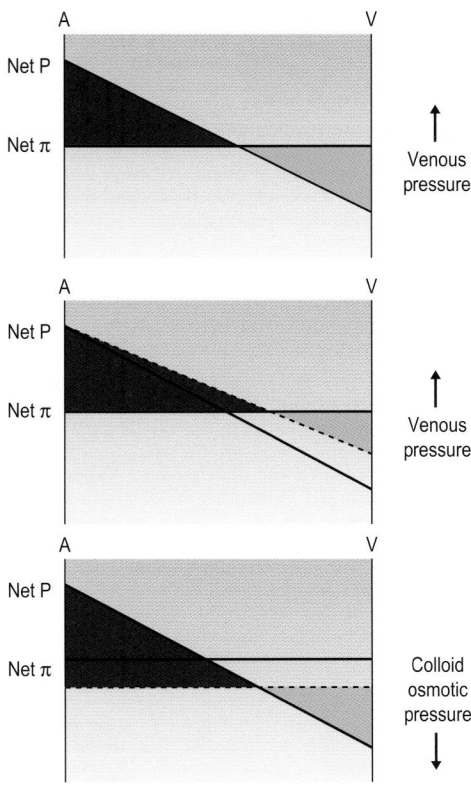

Fig. 11.41 Effect of pressure on filtration rate.
(A) Normal pressure. (B) Increased net filtration due to raised venous pressure (*dotted line*). (C) reduced osmotic pressure (*dotted line*). Normal pressures are shown by the *black lines*. Net filtration is filtration (*red area*) minus absorption (*green area*).

carrying away proteins in the extracellular fluid, which themselves could increase filtration. This increase in lymph drainage is the equivalent of an increase of about 7 mmHg on normal filtration pressure. However, if the rate of fluid production exceeds the capacity of the lymphatic system, then fluid accumulates.

If lymphatic drainage is impaired, both fluid and protein accumulate in the tissues. This produces a sometimes dramatic and painful swelling in the affected area. Lymph nodes can be obstructed by tumours, or may be damaged following radiotherapy, which stimulates fibrosis. Removal of lymph nodes during surgery for breast cancer will also limit drainage. Lymph node removal was more common when radical mastectomy (removal of the entire breast and underlying tissue) was the standard treatment for breast cancer.

Inflammation and increased capillary permeability

The classic symptoms of inflammation are **rubor** (redness), **calor** (heat), **dolor** (pain) and **tumor** (swelling). Inflammation is caused by the local release of a wide range of inflammatory mediators in response to a pathogen or injury (see Ch. 6). They stimulate a cascade of events that includes local vasodilation (which leads to the redness and heat) followed by local slowing of blood flow (stasis) and a local increase in

Information box 11.15 Heart failure leads to oedema

In heart failure, the inability of the heart to maintain cardiac output leads to an accumulation of blood in the venous circulation. This increases the pressure in the venous circulation.

If the heart failure only affects the left side of the heart, the pulmonary venous pressure will be raised. When the pulmonary venous pressure exceeds 20 mmHg, fluid accumulates in the lung, increasing the diffusion distance for blood gases and reducing pulmonary compliance. One of the common symptoms of heart failure is breathlessness (**dyspnoea**) which is made worse by lying down (**orthopnoea**). Patients may experience **paroxysmal nocturnal dyspnoea**; that is, they are woken up by severe breathlessness. Lying down leads to reabsorption of fluid from the extremities, which raises blood volume and increases venous pressure. Many patients with this condition have to sleep with the upper part of their body upright so that more fluid remains in the lower extremities. Pulmonary oedema can be seen on X-rays as a butterfly-shaped shadow (see Ch. 13, Fig. 13.8).

In patients with right-side heart failure, the increase in venous pressure occurs in the systemic veins, and so oedema occurs in the periphery. This is most obviously seen as swelling in the ankles and feet, which gets worse during the day. In heart failure, the arterial pressure is usually low, which reduces filtration in the kidney and hence leads to accumulation of salt and water. This raises blood volume, making things worse. In addition, reduced perfusion of the kidney activates the renin–angiotensin–aldosterone system, leading to further retention of salt and water. A common treatment in heart failure is to give diuretics, which increase fluid loss, thus reducing the blood volume and hence lowering preload.

Information box 11.16 Cirrhosis of the liver can cause oedema

In **cirrhosis** of the liver, which is most frequently caused by excess alcohol intake or by a viral infection (**hepatitis**), there is fibrosis and loss of normal function. This reduces the ability of liver cells to produce plasma proteins and results in a generalised oedema. In this condition, oedema is also often seen as **ascites**, a large accumulation of fluid in the abdominal cavity. The fibrosis in the liver raises the pressure in the hepatic portal vein, which drains blood from the intestine. This leads to an increased venous capillary pressure in the intestinal capillaries, resulting in increased filtration of fluid into the abdominal cavity. This is further exacerbated by the reduced plasma oncotic pressure, allowing large amounts of fluid to accumulate.

capillary permeability. The increase in capillary permeability is caused by endothelial cells loosening their tight junctions and contracting their actin–myosin cytoskeleton in order to allow neutrophils from the blood to access the infected or injured tissue. However, it also allows protein to leak into the surrounding tissue. This increases the interstitial oncotic pressure and produces movement of fluid out of the capillary, leading to local swelling. The protein-rich fluid is called an **exudate**, in contrast with protein-poor fluid, which is called a **transudate**.

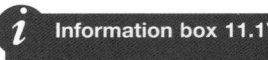

Information box 11.17 **Infection with nematode worms can block lymph drainage**

Oedema is a serious problem in tropical and subtropical countries due to infections with the nematode worms responsible for **filariasis**, *Wuchereria bancrofti* and *Brugia malayi*. These parasites, whose larvae are transmitted through the bite of affected mosquitoes, grow in the lymphatics and the lymph nodes, where they eventually impede the flow of lymph. This results in sometimes huge oedematous swellings of the dependent tissues. The skin also changes, becoming thick and rough which, along with the swelling, is often referred to as **elephantiasis**.

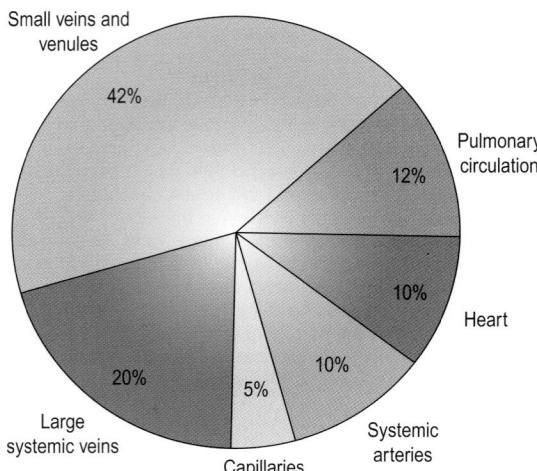

Fig. 11.42 Distribution of blood in the different parts of the circulation at rest.

VEINS

The venules and veins, which drain blood from the capillary beds and return it to the heart, have a three-layered structure similar to arterioles and arteries except that the walls are thinner and much more compliant. The lumen of a vein is larger, relative to its diameter, than that of other large blood vessels, and veins are much more numerous; this combination results in a large cross-sectional area and a low resistance to flow. The venous system is a low-pressure system, with pressures falling from about 17 mmHg at the venous end of the capillary bed to 0 mmHg in the venae cavae. Because of this, veins are easily compressed if the pressure in the surrounding tissue is raised slightly. The muscular tunica media is much thinner than in arteries and the elastic tunica adventitia is the thickest layer, often several times thicker than the media. With their high stretchability, venules and veins act as reservoirs, or capacitance vessels, containing about two-thirds of the circulating blood volume (Fig. 11.42). Stretching is limited, however, by the presence of collagen in the adventitia, which prevents too much pooling of blood, particularly in the veins of the legs.

Most medium-sized veins, particularly in the limbs, have valves which permit flow only in the direction of the heart. These **semilunar valves** are formed from the tunica intima

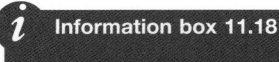

Information box 11.18 **Varicose veins are caused by incompetent valves**

Varicose veins occur when the veins become distended and the valves, which can no longer meet in the middle, cannot stop the backflow of blood. Although varicose veins are often inherited, they may also be caused by conditions that reduce venous return, such as:

- Prolonged standing without moving, where blood pools in the veins of the legs
- Pregnancy, where the enlarged uterus presses on the veins in the groin, reducing venous return
- Obesity, where the enlarged abdomen has the same effect.

Varicosities occur more often in the **superficial veins**, which are not well supported by surrounding tissues. The saphenous veins of the legs are the most commonly affected. Other sites can be affected when venous pressure is raised. For example, in the anal veins, where straining during bowel movements can produce **haemorrhoids**, and in the oesophageal veins, where **oesophageal varices** can develop due to high pressure in the hepatic portal vein, often due to liver damage.

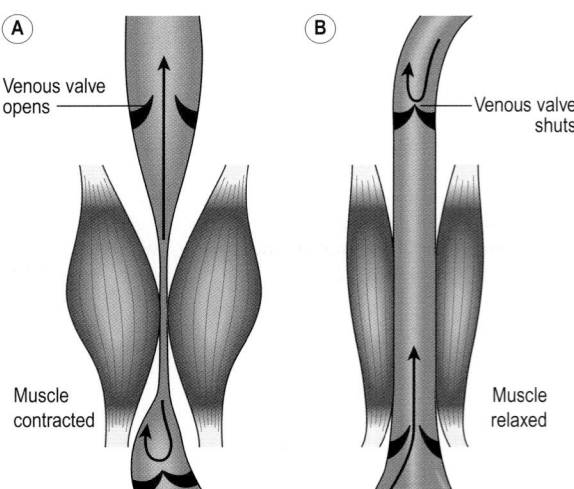

Fig. 11.43 Skeletal muscle pump: when the muscle contracts blood is pushed towards the heart, and when the muscle is relaxed the vein refills from below.

and prevent blood from flowing backwards. This is particularly important in the legs, where gravity opposes the flow of blood upward towards the heart (see Information box 11.18).

Venous return from the deep veins in the limbs is aided by the action of the **skeletal muscle pump**. When the skeletal muscle surrounding the veins contracts, it shortens and thickens, putting pressure on the veins (Fig. 11.43A). This squeezes the blood in the veins, and, because backflow is prevented by the valves, the blood has to move towards the heart. When the skeletal muscle relaxes the pressure on the veins drops and they refill from the venules and the superficial veins (Fig. 11.43B). The blood which was pushed towards the heart cannot flow back down because of the valves. In this way blood is pumped towards the heart, lowering the venous pressure in the legs.

Blood flow in the large **thoracic veins** is affected by respiration. During inspiration, the pressure in the thoracic cavity falls, expanding the thoracic veins. At the same time, as the diaphragm descends, the intra-abdominal pressure rises, compressing the veins and aiding flow towards the thorax. During expiration the reverse occurs. This **respiratory pump** affects the venous return to the two sides of the heart differently. Inspiration increases right ventricular filling, but the capacity of the lung vasculature is increased at the same time, which reduces left ventricular filling. The situation is reversed during expiration and the output of the two ventricles averages the same over time.

VENOCONSTRICTION

Veins are well supplied with sympathetic vasoconstrictor nerves that control the diameter of the veins, thereby also regulating the volume of the blood reservoirs. This controls the filling pressure of the heart and has a major influence on cardiac output. Unlike arteries, veins have very little basal tone and do not show the myogenic response to stretch.

The skin contains a large reservoir of blood which can be added to the central blood volume when needed. In **haemorrhagic hypotension** the profound venoconstriction diverts blood from the skin, producing a characteristic pallor. In exercise, the conflicting demands of increasing cardiac output and temperature regulation lead to an initial venoconstriction, which diverts blood to the working muscle, followed by a venodilation when the core temperature rises. Veins in the gastrointestinal tract, the liver and the spleen contain about 20% of the total blood volume. During exercise and hypotension they also contract to help maintain central venous pressure (CVP).

Some vasoactive compounds have different effects on veins and arteries. **Glyceryl trinitrate** and **isosorbide mononitrate** are more effective on veins than arteries. When given for the treatment of angina, they act to reduce the filling pressure of the heart and hence cardiac work, whereas **sodium nitroprusside** acts on both arteries and veins, reducing both preload and afterload.

VENOUS RETURN AND CARDIAC OUTPUT

Stroke volume is dependent on the end-diastolic pressure (EDP) in the ventricle. The right atrial pressure, which is equivalent to the CVP, is almost equal to the ventricular EDP because the atrioventricular valve between the atria and ventricle offers no significant resistance. Given that cardiac output is directly dependent on stroke volume, and assuming no changes in heart rate and contractility, Starling's curve (see Fig. 11.22) can be redrawn with cardiac output as a function of CVP. This is described as a cardiac output curve, also called the **cardiac function curve**.

The **vascular function curve** represents the venous return, which equates to cardiac output to the CVP. At high atrial pressures the pressure gradient driving flow back to the heart is reduced and venous return is low. If atrial pressure reaches 7 mmHg, which is the **mean circulatory pressure (MCP)**, venous return falls to zero. MCP is determined by blood volume and is the pressure that would be reached at equilibrium if all circulation stopped. As atrial pressure falls, venous return increases until it reaches a plateau. If these two curves are plotted on the same axes (Fig. 11.44) they intersect at a point (A) where cardiac output equals venous

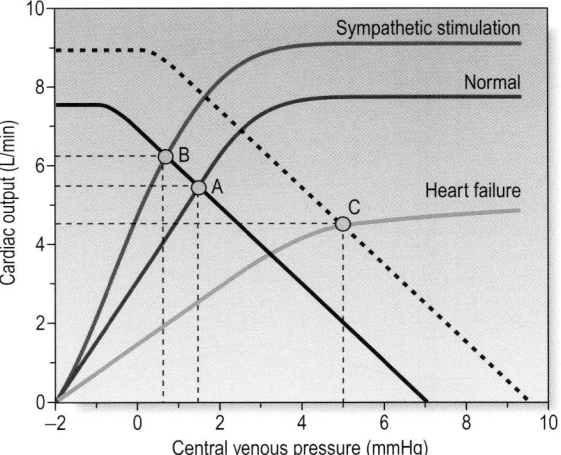

Fig. 11.44 **Cardiac and vascular function curves.** Cardiac function curves; normal (*black*); increased volume (*dashed*). Vascular function curves; normal (*red*); sympathetic stimulation (*blue*); heart failure (*green*).

return, at a value of about 5 L/min at a CVP of about 1.5 mmHg, which is the normal steady state.

The utility of this analysis can be seen when considering changes in cardiovascular function as a result of sympathetic stimulation. The cardiac function curve becomes steeper and has a higher plateau as heart rate and contractility increase. The point of intersection with the vascular function curve moves up and to the right. The new steady state (B) has a raised cardiac output with very little change in CVP.

In heart failure, the cardiac function curve is depressed because of the reduced contractility of the heart, but the vascular function curve is shifted by an increase in blood volume due to salt and water retention (**hypervolaemia**). In this example, a new steady state is reached (C) where cardiac output is maintained at a value approaching normal, but at a raised CVP. To reduce CVP, either the vascular function curve can be shifted back leftwards by the use of diuretics, or the cardiac function curve could be raised by the use of drugs, such as **digoxin**, which increase cardiac contractility. Reducing the total peripheral resistance (TPR) using vasodilators has complex effects on both the cardiac and vascular function curves (not shown in Fig. 11.44). Decreasing TPR increases cardiac output by reducing afterload. This shifts the cardiac function curve in a similar manner to digoxin. The vascular function curve also changes without changing the MCP, but with a steeper slope. This has the effect of increasing cardiac output without reducing CVP from its elevated level.

VENOUS THROMBOEMBOLISM

A **thrombus** is a solid mass formed in the circulation from the constituents of blood. There are two main types:

- In the arterial circulation, thrombi usually form in association with atheromatous plaques, or they come from the left side of the heart following myocardial infarction, or they form on damaged or infected heart valves. These **white thrombi** are formed when platelets adhere to damaged endothelium, and they contain large quantities of platelets.

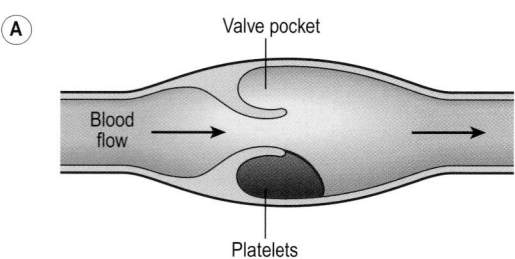

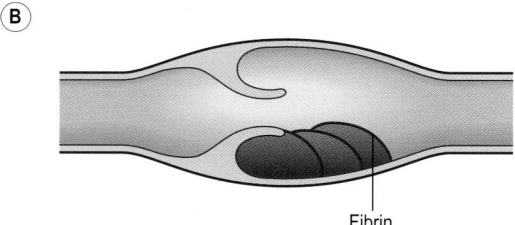

Fig. 11.45 Evolution of venous thrombosis. (A) Platelets aggregate behind the valve pocket. (B) Fibrin and red blood cells stabilise the clot. Subsequent layers of platelets form a distinctive coral-like structure.

- **Venous thrombi** are formed in apparently normal vessels as a consequence of **Virchow's triad**:
  - Reduced blood flow leading to stasis
  - Hypercoagulability
  - Vascular damage.

About 20% of cases of venous **thrombosis** are the results of inherited conditions, such as a deficiency in clotting factor V. About 40% of venous thrombi are acquired, and the remainder are idiopathic.

Deep vein thrombosis

Venous thrombi are found mainly in the deep veins of the legs, especially in the calf venous sinuses, and are formed largely from red cells and fibrin, hence the name **red thrombus**. These thrombi are particularly liable to embolise (see below). Thrombi often form behind the open flaps of venous valves where the initial event is platelet adhesion (Fig. 11.45A). The thrombus forms in layers and is seen in section as alternating bands of platelets and red cells with fibrin. The bands are called **lines of Zahn** (Fig. 11.45B).

If a vessel becomes completely occluded with thrombus, the column of blood heartwards of the blockage up to the next venous junction becomes static and prone to clotting. At this junction point, a new thrombus forms and the process repeats, propagating the thrombus along the vessel. The leg with deep vein thrombosis (DVT) is painful and swollen and feels warm to the touch. If there is complete occlusion then there will be severe oedema which, if unresolved, can lead to gangrene.

DVT often occurs after periods of immobility (see Information box 11.19), such as bedrest following surgery or illness. Because of this, it is common practice to provide all patients with pressure stockings to reduce venous pooling in the legs and to mobilise patients as soon as possible following surgery. Daily injections of long-acting heparin are also given to reduce the coagulability. An increase in the viscosity of the

---

> **ℹ Information box 11.19** | **DVT and long-haul air travel**
>
> It is thought that DVT can also be caused by the long periods of immobility that occur during long-haul air travel. Airlines are being asked to provide more leg room and to encourage passengers to move about regularly during flights. The dehydration that often occurs may also increase the risk, so drinking plenty of water or soft drinks is advisable. Alcohol intake should be limited as it can also lead to dehydration. The use of pressure stockings and low-dose aspirin may also help to reduce the risk.

blood, either because of an increase in blood components, such as red cells in polycythaemia, or because of reduction in plasma volume by dehydration, can increase the risk of DVT and subsequent embolism. Other factors known to increase the risk of DVT are oral contraceptives and hormone replacement therapy, certain tumours, nephrotic syndrome and diabetes mellitus. There is a strong correlation between cigarette smoking and the risk of DVT and other vascular diseases.

Pulmonary embolism

Embolism occurs when part of a thrombus breaks off and travels through the circulation to lodge in a distal vessel. The most common sites of embolism occur in the pulmonary circulation following DVT. A portion of the thrombus breaks off within the deep veins of the legs and travels through the great veins and the right side of the heart to lodge in the pulmonary circulation. The embolus blocks the blood flow in the pulmonary vessel and so reduces oxygenation. This produces breathlessness if it occurs in a small vessel, but blockage of a large vessel can prove fatal.

Other emboli

Not all emboli are caused by thrombi. The term embolus applies to anything that blocks an artery, and emboli can be produced by:

- **Air**: possibly introduced during surgery, transfusion or dialysis
- **Nitrogen**: the 'bends', produced after spending too long at high atmospheric pressure (divers or tunnellers) without sufficient time for decompression
- **Fat**: commonly following trauma
- **Bone marrow**: especially in the elderly after external cardiac massage with fracture of the breast bone
- **Debris**: from atheromatous plaques
- **Cells**: from metastasising tumours.

CONTROL OF BLOOD PRESSURE

In order to maintain perfusion of vascular beds, arterial blood pressure must not be allowed to fluctuate too much. However, this does not mean that blood pressure (or more strictly speaking mean arterial blood pressure, MABP) remains constant at all times. For example, during exercise, both systolic and diastolic blood pressures change significantly in order to

Table 11.12	Sensory pathways of the baroreceptors	
	Aortic arch baroreceptors	**Carotid sinus baroreceptors**
Afferent fibres	Aortic nerve Vagus (tenth cranial)	Carotid sinus nerve Glossopharyngeal (ninth cranial)
Cell bodies	Petrous ganglion	Nodose ganglion
Terminals	Nucleus tractus solitarius	Nucleus tractus solitarius

increase cardiac output and supply working muscles with more oxygen.

Blood pressure also varies within and between individuals and changes with age. The average blood pressure in a population also seems to depend on ethnicity. A large number of factors have been identified which contribute to increases in blood pressure and which may lead to hypertension (see below).

Mean arterial pressure is determined by cardiac output and TPR, and blood pressure is regulated, in the short term, by reflexes that serve to control the MABP around a **set point** that can be altered both centrally and peripherally. These reflexes also control TPR, the venous return, and the heart rate and contractility. They are:

- Baroreceptor reflex
- Chemoreceptor reflexes
- Cardiopulmonary reflexes.

THE BARORECEPTOR REFLEX

The **baroreceptor reflex** is a reflex arc consisting of sensory elements (**baroreceptors**) that supply information about the blood pressure to areas in the brainstem which control sympathetic and parasympathetic nervous system output to the heart and blood vessels to return the pressure to its set point.

Baroreceptors and their responses

Baroreceptors are mechanosensitive sensory nerve endings found in the adventitia of the elastic arteries in the **aortic arch** (transverse arch) and the **carotid sinus** (a region at the base of the internal carotid artery) (Fig. 11.46). They respond to the stretching of the arteries by firing action potentials. The baroreceptor neurons are bipolar, with long afferent fibres leading from the arteries to cell bodies located in the petrous and nodose ganglia and with their axons terminating in the nTS (Table 11.12).

Baroreceptors have two types of response: static and dynamic (Fig. 11.47). Many baroreceptors fire action potentials continuously at normal blood pressure (S1). It has been shown that when blood pressure is increased (and not allowed to be reflexly adjusted) they have an initial burst of firing (D1) followed by a sustained higher firing rate (S2), intermediate between the burst rate and the initial base rate. The rate of the initial burst indicates the rate of change of blood pressure (**dynamic response**) and the new sustained rate reflects the new higher blood pressure (**static response**). A similar effect occurs when the pressure is reduced, initially falling silent (D2), and then resuming at a new lower rate (S1).

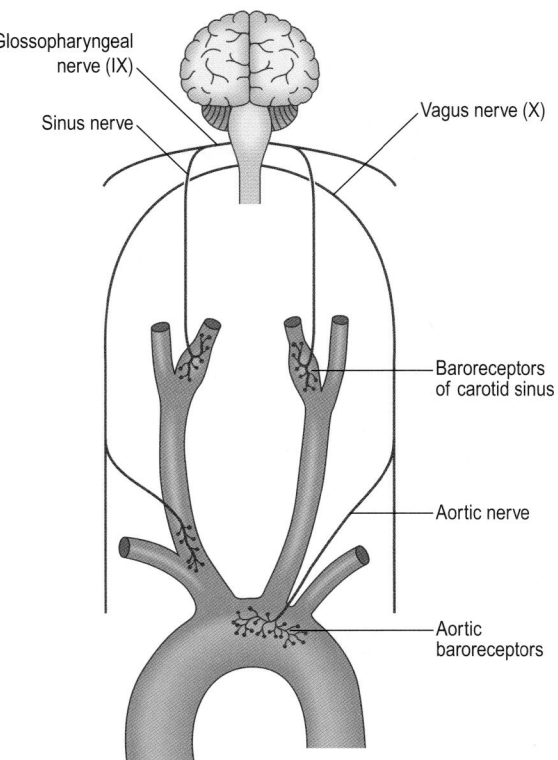

Fig. 11.46 **Arterial baroreceptors.** Afferent sensory fibres from the aortic and carotid baroreceptors have their cell bodies in the petrous and nodose ganglia and synapse in the nucleus tractus solitarius.

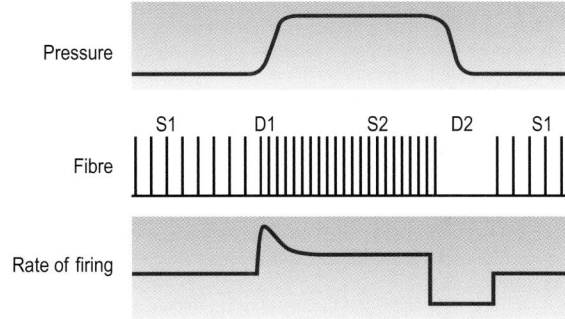

Fig. 11.47 Dynamic (D) and static (S) responses of baroreceptors.

There are two types of baroreceptors in the aortic arch and carotid sinus:

- **A fibres** are activated at low pressures (30–90 mmHg) and reach their maximum firing rate at about 150 mmHg (Fig. 11.48 *red line*). Therefore, they are active at normal blood diastolic pressures and fire bursts of action potentials at each systole. Their large myelinated fibres have a high firing rate and are extremely sensitive to changes in pressure between about 80 mmHg and 140 mmHg.
- **C fibres** are only activated at higher pressures (70–140 mmHg). They have a lower firing rate than A fibres and are less sensitive, but they can still signal changes in pressure above 200 mmHg (Fig. 11.48 *black line*). They are more numerous than A fibres and are small unmyelinated fibres.

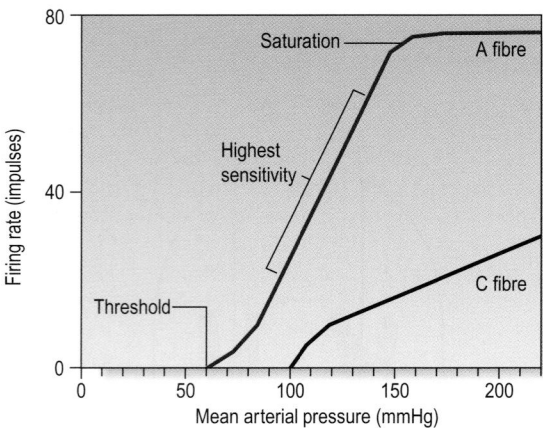

Fig. 11.48 **Different types of baroreceptor signal different ranges of blood pressure.** A fibres: *red line*; C fibres: *black line*. Redrawn with permission from Levick JR 2003 An introduction to cardiovascular physiology, 4th edn. Arnold, London.

Clinical box 11.8	Baroreceptor stimulation to treat resistant hypertension

Normally the baroreceptor reflex keeps the blood pressure within the normal range, with an average blood pressure of 120 mmHg systolic and 80 mmHg diastolic. However, there are many people with abnormally raised blood pressure (hypertension, see below).

Whilst many patients with hypertension can be successfully treated using a combination of lifestyle changes and drugs, there are a significant proportion who still have an abnormally high blood pressure despite taking a number of different medicines. This is known as **resistant hypertension** and carries a high risk of developing cardiovascular disease.

A recent study has introduced a novel treatment for resistant hypertension using a pacemaker-like device which electrically stimulates the baroreceptors in an effort to reduce blood pressure. The device consists of a pulse generator, which is implanted in the chest, and electrodes which are attached to the carotid sinus to electrically stimulate the baroreceptors. The rationale behind the treatment is that stimulation of the baroreceptors will result in signals being conveyed to the brain which will trigger the autonomic nervous system reflexes to reduce blood pressure, such as vasodilation, a reduction in heart rate and the production of hormones which lower blood pressure.

In recent trials around the world using this device, a relatively small group of patients, all of whom had a systolic blood pressure of over 160 mmHg, showed reductions in their systolic and diastolic blood pressures and in their heart rate. Their average systolic blood pressure after 3 months' treatment had been reduced by about 20 mmHg and there were still significant reductions after 12 months. There were no significant safety issues despite the necessity of surgery to implant the devices. This was only a small study, and following these positive results a much larger trial with 300 patients is being undertaken.

Because individual baroreceptor fibres have different thresholds over a wide range of pressures, more and more baroreceptors start firing, and the firing rate of each fibre increases with pressure. This gives a wide range of possible responses and great sensitivity.

Effects of baroreceptor activity

In response to an increase in blood pressure, the rate of firing from the baroreceptors increases. The response from the nTS is an increase in the rate of firing of the vagus nerve supplying the heart and a decrease in the activity of the sympathetic nerves supplying the heart and vasculature. This leads to:

- A rapid decrease in the heart rate and a reduction in cardiac contractility, reducing cardiac output
- Reduction in sympathetic vasoconstrictor activity which produces vasodilation, reducing TPR
- Reduction in both cardiac output and TPR, which reduces the MABP

In response to a fall in blood pressure, the opposite effects are stimulated:

- A decrease in vagal activity and an increase in sympathetic nervous system output, which increases the heart rate and contractility
- Widespread vasoconstriction, especially of the veins draining the gastrointestinal tract and the liver, forcing blood into the central veins, thus increasing venous return to the heart, which causes an increase in stroke volume due to Starling's law.

These responses of the baroreceptor reflex to low pressure are particularly important in maintaining blood pressure in acute hypotension. Severe vasoconstriction also leads to increases in blood volume, which again may be important in maintaining blood pressure in acute hypotension. Net filtration in the capillaries is dependent on the balance between the pressures at both ends of the capillaries. If arterioles are severely constricted then the downstream pressure falls (at least in the short term). This fall in hydrostatic pressure reduces net filtration and hence more water is retained in the blood. Furthermore, increased sympathetic activity in the nerves supplying the kidney increases renin secretion and hence increases blood volume via the renin–angiotensin–aldosterone system (see Ch. 14).

Resetting of the baroreceptor reflex

The set point of the baroreceptor reflex can be altered by both central and peripheral mechanisms. During exercise the blood pressure is still controlled, but the set point is raised. This allows cardiac output to increase to meet demands. A sustained increase in pressure in the periphery causes the baroreceptors to reset to the new higher pressure. This is thought to be important in hypertension, where a slight increase in blood pressure (possibly caused by increased blood volume or high vasoconstrictor tone) could produce a shift in the set point; if this continued, the set point could gradually move upwards.

CHEMORECEPTOR REFLEXES

Lying adjacent to the aorta and the carotid sinus are chemoreceptors called the **aortic** and **carotid bodies**. These arterial chemoreceptors consist of groups of cells richly supplied with blood and have sensory nerve endings that respond to low levels of oxygen and high levels of carbon dioxide and hydrogen ions in the blood. Under normal conditions, they are primarily involved in the control of breathing (see Ch. 13) but they have important effects on the cardiovascular system during severe hypotension. At very low pressures the baroreceptors are mostly below their threshold for activation so little information is being carried to the central nervous system.

However, as hypotension produces hypoxia due to reduced perfusion of the chemoreceptors and metabolic acidosis develops, the chemoreceptors are strongly stimulated. This leads to sympathetic vasoconstriction, which helps to maintain central blood pressure.

CARDIOPULMONARY REFLEXES

Cardiopulmonary receptors are a diverse group of receptors which have vagal afferent fibres and are situated in the heart and at the junctions with the great veins and pulmonary arteries.

Veno-atrial mechanoreceptors, found in the atria and the great veins, respond to stretch and monitor venous volume and pressure. Activation of these large myelinated afferents produces reflex tachycardia by sympathetic stimulation of the cardiac pacemaker. This is called the **Bainbridge reflex** and may possibly serve to move blood rapidly from the venous circulation into the systemic circulation during exercise. This reflex also causes an increase in urine flow by a decrease in renal sympathetic activity, which reduces renin secretion. Other mechanoreceptors are present in the atria and ventricles (mainly the left). These numerous, small non-myelinated afferents form a network of fibres that fire during atrial filling and ventricular systole, respectively, and produce bradycardia and vasodilation, respectively.

In the walls of the heart there are chemosensitive unmyelinated vagal and sympathetic fibres which respond to substances released by ischaemic heart muscle, such as bradykinin and prostaglandins. The sympathetic fibres are responsible for signalling the pain associated with myocardial infarction and angina.

OTHER FACTORS WHICH AFFECT BLOOD PRESSURE

There are two other types of input which affect the cardiovascular system. First, there are receptors in muscle which help to initiate the changes in heart rate, contractility and blood pressure that occur during exercise (see below). Cardiovascular reflexes can also be activated by pain, temperature and alerting stimuli, such as sudden noises.

CENTRAL REGULATION OF CARDIOVASCULAR REFLEXES

The afferent nerves from the baroreceptors and other cardiovascular receptors terminate in the medulla in the nTS. Neurons in the nTS integrate the signals from the different inputs and send outputs to:

- Other areas of the **medulla**, which control autonomic output
- The **hypothalamus**, which receives inputs from the cerebral cortex
- The **cerebellum**, which coordinates muscular activity.

The hypothalamus and cerebellum, in turn, feedback to the medulla. In the medulla, the **nucleus ambiguous** and the **dorsal motor nucleus** contain the cell bodies of the parasympathetic vagal preganglionic neurons which, when activated, slow the heart. Inputs to the ventrolateral medulla also control efferent neurons which mediate the activity of sympathetic preganglionic neurons on the spinal cord.

In the hypothalamus there is a group of neurons called the **depressor area**, which, when activated, produces a fall in blood pressure due to an activation of vagal afferents and an inhibition of sympathetic activity. There is also another area of the hypothalamus that seems to be responsible for the 'flight and fight' alerting response. This response increases heart rate, raises blood pressure and produces changes in blood flow, preparing for action. This defence area has inputs from the limbic system and the frontal cortex. The cerebral cortex can activate cardiovascular responses in the absence of input from the periphery, which suggests a 'central command' role.

LONG-TERM CONTROL OF BLOOD PRESSURE

The reflexes initiated by baroreceptors and other cardiovascular reflexes are all short-term mechanisms to control blood pressure. The long-term control of blood pressure is thought to be due to the long-term control of blood volume by a combination of mechanisms that involves both the endocrine and renal systems (see also Ch. 14).

Hormones that control blood volume

In normal human beings, the daily fluid intake is about 2300 mL, ingested as food and drink, with an extra 200 mL produced by metabolic activity. This is balanced by losses which total about 1000 mL from sweat, faeces, skin and lungs, and urine production is about 1500 mL. In very hot climates, the water losses are much greater, and even though urine production would fall, a minimum of 500 mL of urine continues to be produced per day in order to excrete urea and creatinine. Because water intake can vary enormously, there are mechanisms which control blood volume and osmolarity very closely. A number of hormones interact to control blood volume:

- Vasopressin
- Angiotensin II
- Aldosterone
- Atrial natriuretic peptide (ANP).

Vasopressin

Vasopressin is released from the **supraoptic** and **paraventricular** nuclei of the hypothalamus in response to a rise in osmolarity of the blood sensed by **osmoreceptors** in the hypothalamus. The same receptors also stimulate thirst and so can increase voluntary water intake. Vasopressin has its main effect in the kidney where it promotes water retention, thus restoring blood volume and restoring normal osmolarity. It acts through a series of reactions:

1. Binds to V_2 receptors in the cells of the collecting duct
2. This stimulates an increase in intracellular cAMP
3. cAMP promotes the fusion of intracellular vesicles with the luminal membrane.

These vesicles contain aquaporins, which increase the water permeability of the duct. Water moves from the urine into the kidney medulla concentrating the urine.

Vasopressin is also released in response to low blood volume. This release can be extremely high, and with a large reduction in blood volume, it can occur even if plasma osmolarity is low.

Angiotensin II

Angiotensin II is a potent vasoconstrictor, but also promotes the release of aldosterone, which promotes retention of salt and water in the kidney. Angiotensin II is formed via a cascade which starts with the release of **renin** from the **juxtaglomerular cells** in the kidney glomerulus. There are three different stimuli for this release:

- A fall in the perfusion pressure in the arterioles supplying the kidney
- Stimulation of β_1-adrenoceptors on juxtaglomerular cells by circulating adrenaline or sympathetic nerve stimulation
- a reduction in sodium concentration in the distal tubule.

Renin is a proteolytic enzyme that activates **angiotensinogen** to produce **angiotensin I**. Angiotensin I is cleaved by the enzyme **angiotensin converting enzyme** (**ACE**) to produce the active form, **angiotensin II**. ACE is found on the surface of endothelial cells, particularly in the lung where, because of the large surface area of endothelium, most of the conversion takes place.

Aldosterone

Aldosterone is a steroid hormone that enhances Na^+ reabsorption and K^+ secretion from the kidney. It acts on nuclear receptors in cells in the distal tubules to increase the synthesis of Na^+/K^+-ATPases present on the abluminal side of these cells. These cells enable the transport of more sodium into the renal medulla. As well as being stimulated by angiotensin II, aldosterone release can be stimulated by reduced blood volume, reduced plasma sodium and other stimuli, such as trauma and stress.

Atrial natriuretic peptide

ANP and a closely related substance called **brain natriuretic peptide** (**BNP**) are released by specialised atrial myocytes in response to stretch caused by increased pressure, indicating a high blood volume and possible volume overload. The effects of ANP are the opposite to those of the other hormones described above in that it increases salt and water excretion by the kidney. It acts to:

- Increase the glomerular filtration rate by relaxing the afferent arterioles supplying the glomerulus, while constricting the efferent arterioles, thus increasing the pressure in the capsule
- Reduce sodium reabsorption in the tubules and hence reduce water reabsorption
- Inhibit the release of a number of vasoconstrictors, including angiotensin II, aldosterone and endothelin.

In heart failure, levels of ANP, and especially BNP, are raised significantly and may play a role in offsetting the increase in fluid volume. These peptides have a short half-life in plasma and there is interest in the possible therapeutic benefits of inhibiting their breakdown and thus extending their action.

HYPERTENSION

Hypertension is chronically raised blood pressure. It is a very common disorder that leads to an increased risk of strokes and heart disease, as well as causing damage to the kidneys and the retina. Unfortunately, on its own, it is symptomless;

Table 11.13	**Main types of hypertension**
Type	**Per cent of hypertensive patients**
Essential hypertension	95
Secondary hypertension	
Renal parenchymal	2–4
Renovascular	1
Phaeochromocytoma	0.2
Coarctation of the aorta	0.1
Primary hyperaldosteronism	0.1
Cushing's syndrome	0.1

Table 11.14	**Classification of blood pressure**		
Classification	**Systolic blood pressure (mmHg)**		**Diastolic blood pressure (mmHg)**
Normal	<120	and	<80
Prehypertension (borderline or mild)	120–139	or	80–89
Hypertension stage I (moderate)	140–159	or	90–99
Hypertension stage II (severe)	≥160	or	≥100

Joint National Committee on Prevention, Detection, Evaluation and Treatment of High Blood Pressure. US Department of Health (JNC 7; 2003).

this means that, unless it is diagnosed as part of a routine medical check-up or as incidental to another condition, it may not be detected until damage has already been produced.

In **primary** or **essential hypertension** there is no obvious underlying cause, although many risk factors may be present. In about 5% of cases, the hypertension has an identifiable cause and this is known as **secondary hypertension** (Table 11.13).

Hypertension could be defined as a level of blood pressure that produces an increase in mortality and morbidity but, because blood pressure is normally distributed across a wide range of values, for practical purposes hypertension is classified as **systolic** and **diastolic** blood pressures above certain values. The actual definition of hypertension and the decision whether to treat or not is controversial. Different criteria set the level at which hypertension is deemed to be present and these vary from 160/95 mmHg to 140/90 mmHg (Table 11.14).

Treatment should not be started on the basis of a single measurement, which could be raised due to anxiety about having blood pressure measured (**white coat hypertension**). Furthermore the decision to treat depends on a number of factors, which include blood pressure and other cardiovascular risk factors present.

Risk factors for essential hypertension

Essential hypertension is strongly associated with a family history of the condition. Many genes are thought to predispose an individual to develop high blood pressure, particularly in the presence of other risk factors, such as:

- Low birth weight
- African ancestry
- Low socio-economic and educational background
- Increasing age
- Male sex (although both systolic and diastolic blood pressures increase in women after the menopause).

A number of environmental factors have been shown to be correlated with a higher incidence of hypertension. The major ones are:

- High salt diet
- Obesity (especially central obesity where fat is deposited largely in the abdominal cavity)
- Excessive alcohol intake (>6 units/day)
- Stress and anxiety.

Other factors have been suggested as contributing to hypertension and are certainly risk factors for heart disease:

- Smoking
- Dietary cholesterol/saturated fat
- Diabetes mellitus (and impaired glucose tolerance).

Causes of essential hypertension

Epidemiological research into the causes for essential hypertension has led to a number of theories on why the condition develops.

- **Response to increased sympathetic drive**: some theories suggest that while most patients with established hypertension show normal cardiac output but with a raised peripheral resistance, the initial problem is a raised cardiac output due increased sympathetic drive. The increase in peripheral resistance then develops as a compensatory mechanism in order to maintain capillary perfusion pressures at the normal (low) levels.
- **Stress hypothesis**: high levels of stress produce sympathetic stimulation, leading to increased cardiac output and peripheral vasoconstriction. If this is sustained, the resulting hypertrophy of the smooth muscle of the resistance vessels (the small arteries and arterioles) will reduce the diameter of the lumen, thus increasing resistance to flow even when the sympathetic stimulation ceases.
- **High salt intake**: Given the relationship between blood volume and blood pressure, there has been a lot of interest in the relationship between salt, water retention and hypertension. A high salt diet has been shown to exacerbate hypertension in some patients and a reduced salt intake has been shown to be efficacious.
- **Effect of renin**: most patients with hypertension do not have raised renin levels, although reduction in the activity of the renin–angiotensin system or reduction in blood volume both have beneficial effects on blood pressure.
- **Multifactorial**: this hypothesis suggests that, as the long-term regulation of blood pressure involves a combination of different neural and hormonal influences, then hypertension only occurs in genetically susceptible individuals when more than one mechanism for controlling blood pressure is faulty.

Causes of secondary hypertension

Renovascular hypertension

Renovascular hypertension is caused by stenosis of one or both renal arteries. This produces increased renin release and an increase in angiotensin II and aldosterone, which together produce vasoconstriction and increase blood volume.

Renal parenchymal hypertension

Renal parenchymal hypertension results from damage to the nephrons of the kidney, reducing their ability to excrete normal amounts of salt and water, leading to an increase in blood volume and cardiac output.

Endocrine hypertension

Endocrine hypertension is mostly due to tumours that secrete excessive and unregulated amounts of hormones (see Ch. 10). Many of these hormones are involved in the normal regulation of salt and water, blood volume and blood pressure.

- A **phaeochromocytoma** is a tumour of the phaeochromocytes (or **chromaffin cells**). These are the **catecholamine**-secreting cells of the adrenal medulla that secrete adrenaline and noradrenaline, although chromaffin cells can also be found throughout the sympathetic nervous system. Most of the tumours occur in the adrenal medulla, but about 10% of phaeochromocytomas are extramedullary.
- **Primary hyperaldosteronism** (**Conn's syndrome**) is usually caused by an aldosterone-secreting tumour.
- **Cushing's syndrome** is an excess of adrenocortical hormones, such as cortisol. In Cushing's disease, this is due to an excess of adrenocorticotropic hormone (ACTH) from a tumour, most often in the pituitary gland. Another common cause is the long-term use of exogenous corticosteroids.
- **Congenital adrenal hyperplasia** is an inherited condition where an enzyme deficiency (21-hydroxylase) reduces cortisol synthesis, and most patients with this condition develop hypotension. However, some patients have a deficiency of 11β-hydroxylase, an enzyme further along the synthetic pathway, and have elevated levels of the precursor to cortisol, **deoxycortisol** (**DOC**). DOC has significant mineralocorticoid activity and high levels of DOC cause salt and water retention, causing hypertension.

Drug-induced hypertension

Oral contraceptives can increase blood pressure because oestrogens increase the synthesis of the precursor to angiotensin II, angiotensinogen. The progestogen-only pill does not have this effect, but is also a less-effective contraceptive. **Monoamine oxidase inhibitors**, used to treat depression and parkinsonism, have a side effect known as the 'cheese reaction', where tyramine-containing foods such as some cheeses, red wine, and yeast products such as Marmite, produce acute hypertension by actions that mimic sympathetic stimulation. Because of these interactions clinical use of these drugs is in decline.

Cardiovascular hypertension

Coarctation of the aorta is a rare congenital malformation which narrows the aorta. It causes hypertension by reducing renal blood flow and hence stimulating the renin–angiotensin system. Additionally, raised pressures in the aorta proximal to the narrowing stimulate hyperplasia of the tunica media, which reduces both compliance and the sensitivity of the baroreceptor reflex.

Pregnancy-induced hypertension

Hypertension diagnosed in the first half of pregnancy is usually due to pre-existing hypertension. If hypertension develops in the latter half of pregnancy this normally reverts after delivery. **Pre-eclampsia** consists of hypertension and proteinuria. It is thought to be caused by an immunological reaction which disturbs placental function (see Ch. 10). It can lead to **eclampsia**, which includes severe hypertension among many other potentially life-threatening symptoms. Eclampsia remains the main cause of maternal death in the developed world.

Malignant hypertension

Hypertension usually develops slowly. However, in rare cases blood pressure rises rapidly and causes rapid damage to the walls of blood vessels. This is known as **malignant hypertension** and requires immediate treatment.

Treatments for hypertension

Assessment of patients with hypertension must first exclude possible secondary causes before a diagnosis of essential hypertension can be made. Once diagnosed, it is important to assess the severity of the condition before recommending appropriate management.

In patients with mild or prehypertension, primary treatment often consists of advice on reducing of risk factors related to lifestyle:

- Weight loss
- Reduced salt intake
- Healthy diet (low fat, reduced saturated and total fat, plentiful fruit and vegetables)
- Reduced alcohol consumption
- Increased aerobic exercise.

If the changes in lifestyle are not sufficient to reduce the blood pressure, or if hypertension is more severe, then drug therapy should be considered. The risk of developing cardiovascular disease can be assessed in the light of a patient's other risk factors.

The drugs of choice will depend on the severity of the hypertension, the risk factors present, and the evidence of organ damage, such as retinopathy, nephropathy, etc. (Table 11.15), and the patient's clinical history. Some of the drugs can be used in combination (e.g. diuretics and β-blockers) while others should not be used in patients with particular associated conditions (e.g. β-blockers should be avoided in patients with a history of asthma or bronchospasm).

Resistant hypertension

Hypertension that is resistant to normal medication needs further investigation. The principal causes of resistant hypertension are:

- Improper measurement of blood pressure
- Excess sodium intake
- Inadequate diuretic therapy
- Medication
  - Inadequate dose
  - Drug actions and interactions (e.g. non-steroidal anti-inflammatory drugs, illicit drugs, sympathomimetics, oral contraceptives)
  - Over-the-counter drugs and herbal supplements
- Excess alcohol intake
- Identifiable causes of hypertension (secondary hypertension).

Drugs that may be used to treat resistant hypertension include centrally acting drugs such as **moxonidine** and vasodilators such as **hydralazine** and **minoxidil**.

NORMAL ALTERATIONS IN BLOOD PRESSURE AND FLOW

ORTHOSTASIS

When going from sitting or lying to standing upright (literally **orthostasis**), stroke volume decreases and heart rate increases. Cardiac output falls by about 20%, but TPR increases, increasing MABP by about 10 mmHg. When the normal physiological response fails to do this sufficiently **orthostatic hypotension** or **postural hypotension** occurs.

On moving from supine (Fig. 11.49A) to the vertical position, about 500 mL of blood is shifted from the central compartment into the veins in the legs. This increases pressures below the heart and decreases pressures above the heart. In

Table 11.15	Drugs used to treat hypertension	
Class of antihypertensive drug	Example	Mode of action
Thiazide diuretics	Bendrofluazide	Initial reduction in blood volume by increasing sodium (and water) excretion. Later fall in TPR by unknown mechanism/s
β-Blockers	Atenolol	Initial reduction in heart rate and contractility, and inhibition of renin release. Sustained reduction in blood pressure by unknown mechanism/s.
Calcium-channel blockers	Nifedipine	Block entry of calcium into vascular smooth muscle, reducing TPR. May also affect entry of calcium into cardiac myocytes
ACE inhibitors	Captopril	Block production of angiotensin II and breakdown of bradykinin. Leads to reduced vasoconstriction and hence reduces TPR
Angiotensin II antagonists	Losartan	Block of angiotensin II receptors for patients who cannot tolerate ACE inhibitors
α-Blockers	Prazosin	Inhibition of α-adrenoceptors on vascular smooth muscle to reduce TPR

ACE, angiotensin-converting enzyme; TPR, total peripheral resistance.

the feet, pressures are increased by about 90 mmHg in both veins and arteries (Fig. 11.49B). This results in an arterial pressure in the foot of about 185 mmHg and a venous pressure of about 95 mmHg. Flow is maintained because the arteriovenous difference is the same, but the increase in venous pressure stretches the veins, increasing their capacity, and unless adjustments are made, the increase in capillary hydrostatic pressure leads to excess filtration and oedema.

The fall in blood pressure in the upper part of the body on standing immediately activates the baroreceptor reflex causing an increase in heart rate and vasoconstriction. In the feet, with the compensatory vasoconstriction and autoregulation, this leads to a reduction in the capillary pressure at the arteriolar end, but the increase in venous capillary pressure still results in an increased net filtration (Fig. 11.49C). In the absence of other measures to reduce pressures in the feet, the increased filtration can lead to a loss of central blood volume and a reduction in cerebral perfusion, followed by loss of consciousness (fainting).

The action of the skeletal muscle pump reduces pressures in the feet, and hence the formation of oedema. During muscle contraction, pressures are reduced in the veins and arteries by compression (Fig. 11.49D). During relaxation, the movement of blood in the veins (and lymphatics), supported by the one-way valves, reduces the weight of the blood in the veins. This lowers the mean capillary pressure to a level that normally reverses the net filtration and allows fluid to be removed from the tissue by the lymphatics (Fig. 11.49E).

Fainting

Baroreceptor reflexes act rapidly to counteract the fall in upper body blood pressure that happens on standing up, but in individuals with impaired autonomic reflexes, or in conditions where there is a high degree of peripheral vasodilation (such as during hot weather or after a long hot bath), the transient reduction in blood flow to the head may be sufficient to cause brief dizziness. In severe cases, this may

---

_i_ **Information box 11.20** | **Fainting due to prolonged standing**

Prolonged standing still can result in a faint. This used to be seen occasionally among soldiers on guard duty in Horse Guards Parade in London, who were not allowed to move for long periods. It was realised that fainting was not a weakness, but an inevitable physiological response. Once this was explained, the guards were allowed to walk occasionally in order to activate the skeletal muscle pump. Another type of faint, **psychogenic fainting**, is caused by psychological stress, such as at the sight of blood. Mediated by a marked increase in vagal activity from stimulation of chemoreceptors in the left ventricle as a result of a brief stop in breathing (**apnoea**), the heart rate slows (bradycardia) and blood vessels dilate, causing the blood pressure to fall, hence the alternative name, **vasovagal syncope**. It has been suggested that this is the human equivalent of the 'playing dead' response of some animals when faced with extreme danger.

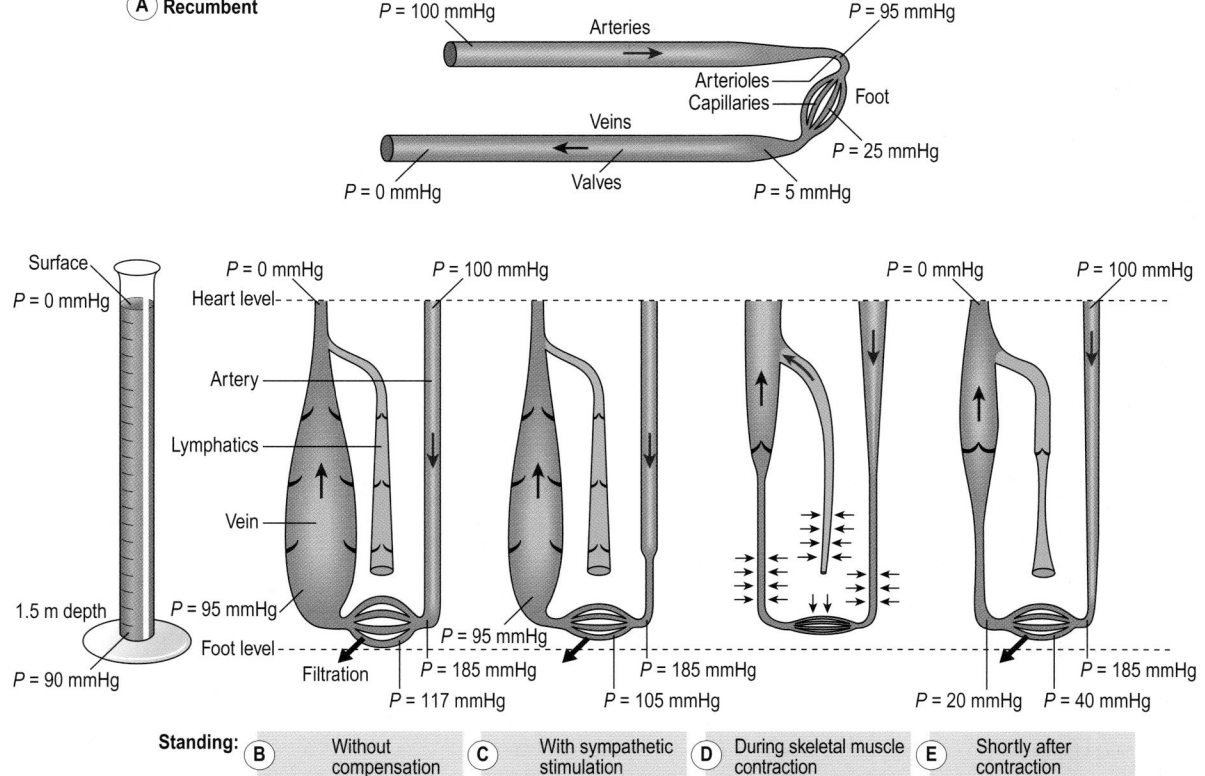

Fig. 11.49 **Effect of orthostasis on vascular pressures in the feet.** Redrawn with permission from Mohrman DE 1991 Cardiovascular physiology, 3rd edn. McGraw-Hill, New York.

cause the person to faint. Fainting, or **syncope**, occurs when the pressure in the cerebral arteries drops below 40 mmHg (equivalent to a MABP at heart level of about 70 mmHg).

Whatever the cause of the faint, an individual who has fainted should be left lying down (as long as they are in a safe location) because the supine position aids cardiac filling and helps to increase cardiac output and blood flow to the head.

EXERCISE

Most of the preceding descriptions of cardiovascular function have been concerned with the heart and vasculature at rest. However, while not everyone can run a marathon or a sprint race, the increased demands of any level of activity over and above sleeping require cardiovascular adjustments.

Changes in cardiac output

In exercise, cardiac output increases in proportion to the increase in oxygen consumption. Cardiac output increases from about 5–6 L/min at rest to 20 L/min at maximal exercise levels, in the young, to more than 30 L/min in trained athletes. This occurs through increase in heart rate and stroke volume.

Heart rate increases about threefold to a maximum value that can be calculated roughly as 220 minus age in years (beats/min). Increases in **stroke volume** depend more on the posture. The increases are small in supine exercise (10–20%), but in upright exercise can increase significantly. Trained athletes have a much larger increase in stroke volume than ordinary subjects and achieve their maximal level of cardiac output at lower heart rates. This is because they have more efficient hearts with enlarged ventricular cavities, which give a larger end-diastolic volume. There are limits to the ability of an individual to increase exercise:

- **Diffusion of oxygen into the lung capillaries**: with a high cardiac output the transit time in the lung is not long enough to fully saturate the blood. Therefore, at very high work rates, the oxygen concentration of blood starts to fall.
- **Rate of cardiac filling during diastole**: as the heart rate increases, the length of diastole is reduced more than systole. Because most ventricular filling occurs during diastole, if diastole becomes very short, the end-diastolic volume is reduced. If the heart rate increases further the filling time is reduced even more, resulting in a decrease in cardiac output, rather than an increase. In rhythmic exercise, however, the skeletal muscle pump aids venous return, as does the respiratory pump.

Changes in patterns of blood flow and blood pressure

During exercise, blood flow changes in many different vascular beds (Table 11.16). The only organ to which blood flow remains constant is the brain. Blood flow to the exercising muscle increases largely through **metabolic hyperaemia**, thought to be due to increased osmolarity and acidity. This not only increases flow rates through capillaries that are open at rest but also opens unperfused capillaries in order to support the increased metabolism. In addition to the increased blood flow to the muscle:

- Capillary recruitment reduces the diffusion distance for nutrients and wastes
- Increased oxygen and glucose consumption in the working muscle reduces their concentration in the tissues. This aids their transfer by increasing the diffusion gradient
- Increased temperature, carbon dioxide and acidity in the working muscle shift the oxygen dissociation curve to the right, increasing the ability of haemoglobin to unload oxygen at low partial pressures.

Tissue perfusion during exercise varies according to the tissue involved and the type and extent of exercise, but normal physiological events act to maintain blood pressure. Factors that act to lower TPR, and hence also blood pressure, are:

- Increased blood flow to muscle tissue and local vasodilation, due to metabolic hyperaemia as described above
- Increased blood flow to the heart and local vasodilation as oxygen consumption by cardiac muscle increases with the greater force and frequency of heart contraction
- Increased skin vasodilation as core temperature rises in order to lose heat.

These factors are balanced by factors that increase blood pressure:

- Skin vasoconstriction in the early stages of exercise
- Increased cardiac output
- Vasoconstriction in the splanchnic (visceral) circulation, kidneys and non-working muscle tissue.

Of course, as cardiac output increases, the tissue with the largest increase in blood flow is the lungs, which receive the entire increase in blood flow. During exercise, perfusion pressure increases and with the increased ventilation more of the lung tissue is perfused, leading to a fall in resistance.

Table 11.16	Changes in blood flow to different organs during exercise		
Blood flow (mL/min)	**At rest**	**Strenuous exercise**	**Change**
Brain	750	750	None
Heart	250	750	Threefold increase
Muscle	1250	12 500	10-fold increase
Skin	500	2000	Fourfold increase
Kidney	1100	550	Halved
Abdominal organs	1400	700	Halved
Other	600	400	Reduced by one-third
Total	5850	17 650	Threefold increase

Differences in static and dynamic exercise

Changes in blood pressure are not the same during static and dynamic exercise. During **dynamic exercise**, such as running or rowing, while blood flow through working muscles may be impeded during contraction, the action of the muscle pump ensures rapid flow during relaxation so there is no sustained impediment to flow. During dynamic exercise, the systolic blood pressure increases due to the increased cardiac output but diastolic pressures remain constant and even decrease at high levels of exercise, leading to only a slight elevation of MABP.

However, the situation is very different during **static exercise** such as weightlifting, when the contraction of the working muscle is sustained. The long contraction impairs blood flow and also induces a reflex known as the **exercise pressor reflex**. This reflex is stimulated by receptors in muscle that respond to various stimuli associated with exercise, including raised K^+ concentration. The reflex produces an increase in heart rate, contractility and peripheral vasoconstriction. This produces an increase in both systolic and diastolic blood pressures, with a concomitant increase in MABP. The increase in MABP is thought to be a way of increasing blood flow in under-perfused muscle. This is not a problem for fit, weightlifting athletes. However, the same reflex is triggered in the lifting needed to carry a suitcase, resulting in the same rapid and large increase in MABP; this is the reason why such weight-bearing activity should be avoided in patients with ischaemic heart disease.

HAEMORRHAGE AND SHOCK

When tissues are under-perfused, and if this under-perfusion is maintained, cells become **hypoxic** (starved of oxygen) and eventually die. Some tissues are much more resistant than others to the effects of hypoxia. For example, skin can be deprived of blood flow for many hours whereas brain and cardiac tissue, with their high metabolic rates, start to be damaged after only a few minutes. This is called **shock** and has many different causes.

Medically, shock is not the withdrawn mental state that often follows psychological trauma, but is a condition that occurs when **cardiac output** is not sufficient to maintain adequate tissue **perfusion**.

There are many different causes for the lack of perfusion but they can be grouped into a small number of categories:

- Hypovolaemic
- Cardiogenic
- Neurogenic
- Anaphylactic
- Vasodilatory.

TYPES OF SHOCK

Hypovolaemic shock

Hypovolaemic shock results from a reduction in the plasma or blood volume. This is most commonly caused by haemorrhage, but can also be caused by the loss of plasma alone. **Haemorrhage** is most obvious when there are open wounds on the skin and blood is lost directly from damaged blood vessels. The most dangerous ruptures occur in arteries, where the blood loss is pulsatile and the higher pressure causes a higher flow rate. The blood appears bright red due to the oxygenated haemoglobin. Blood loss from veins is usually slower for the same-sized vessel because of the lower pressures in the venous circulation. However, significant haemorrhage can also occur without the external appearance of blood, for example in a closed fracture of the femur, where large amounts of blood can be lost internally.

The loss of 10% of blood volume (about 500 mL), which is the amount removed during blood donation, does not usually produce any of the symptoms of shock and is well tolerated by healthy individuals. Only a highly trained athlete might notice a drop in performance at this loss in oxygen-carrying capacity. A 10% loss is normally restored fairly rapidly.

The loss of 20–30% of blood volume over a short period of time produces **shock**, which if treated rapidly enough should not cause serious long-term problems. Blood pressure may not fall very much, due to the many compensatory mechanisms that are triggered (see below), and the patient will show the signs and symptoms of shock (see below). Even this degree of blood loss can be dangerous, however, if not treated quickly or in elderly or already ill individuals.

The loss of 30–40% of blood volume (up to 2 L), or the equivalent in fluid, such as ascites fluid, for example, can cause severe shock which may be irreversible (see below). Whereas haemorrhage causes the loss of whole blood, circulating blood volume can be reduced by the loss of plasma alone. For example:

- Skin burns increase capillary permeability and result in plasma loss
- Intestinal obstruction reduces plasma volume, because the swollen intestine will collapse the veins, causing an increase in capillary filtration into the abdominal cavity.

Dehydration also reduces circulating blood volume. This can be due to diarrhoea and/or vomiting and may occur in several conditions:

- In **cholera**, the massive loss of water from the diarrhoea and vomiting causes a severe shock which is the cause of death. If body fluid levels can be maintained then mortality is massively reduced. Oral rehydration therapy is a cheap and easy remedy for cholera and infant diarrhoea (see Ch. 2, Clinical box 2.12). Oral rehydration therapy consists of salt (sodium chloride) plus some potassium, citrate and sometimes bicarbonate, plus glucose.
- In some types of **renal disease**, where large amounts of water are lost via the kidneys
- In **Addison's disease**, where the destruction of the adrenal cortex results in a reduction in aldosterone (see Ch. 10).

Cardiogenic shock

Cardiogenic (**cardiac**) **shock** occurs when the pumping ability of the heart is impaired. This may occur subsequent to a myocardial infarction or in severe heart failure when the ability of the heart to pump is impaired. It can also occur if there is a build up of fluid in the pericardium due to pericardial effusion. Because the pericardium has a limited extensibility, if the volume and rate of effusion production are large enough, the pressure within the pericardium rises and the expansion of the heart during filling is impaired, causing a fall in cardiac output. The fluid may be a transudate, an exudate (produced by local infection) or can be the result of a haemorrhage.

Cardiac shock almost always occurs in severe myocardial infarction if more than 40% of the left ventricle is affected. The condition is self-perpetuating, because the low cardiac output produces a reduced blood flow in the coronary arteries, depriving the heart of oxygen still further, thus producing a vicious circle of low output and low power.

Neurogenic shock

Neurogenic shock occurs when there is a loss of the normal basal tone in blood vessels throughout the body, leading to a massive vasodilation. Venodilation is particularly important because it leads to large volumes of blood pooling in the venous system, which reduces venous return and thus reduces cardiac output.

Neurogenic shock can be caused by general anaesthetics which, if they produce a sufficiently deep sedation, depresses the vasoconstrictor activity of the brain stem. Inhibition of the autonomic sympathetic outflow by spinal anaesthesia can also produce vasodilation. A common cause of neurogenic shock is damage to the brainstem.

Anaphylactic shock

Anaphylactic shock is a large drop in blood pressure due to an immune reaction. This is a type I hypersensitivity reaction, which is an allergic response that triggers a rapid response to an allergen. Previous exposure to the allergen leads to the generation of IgE antibodies which bind to F_c receptors on mast cells. On subsequent exposure the allergen binds to the IgE antibodies on mast cells, triggering the release of **histamine** and other inflammatory mediators.

The type of response varies from relatively mild reactions to pollens, as in hay fever, to the life-threatening reactions sometimes seen on exposure to peanuts or bee stings. The inflammatory mediators cause massive vasodilation, reducing blood pressure, and bronchoconstriction, which impairs breathing. Rapid treatment with adrenaline (epinephrine) is necessary to produce vasoconstriction and bronchodilation, with antihistamine and hydrocortisone to block the further effects of histamine and to reduce the inflammatory response.

Anaphylactic shock can also occur in response to drugs, most often with antibiotics, and in particular penicillin and cephalosporin. This is the 'classic' type I reaction occurring after previous exposure to the drug, usually in patients who already have a history of allergic reactions. A type of shock that is very similar to anaphylactic shock (**anaphylactoid shock**) may also occur in response to novel agents, such as the contrast dyes used in angiography. This does not require prior exposure to the antigen, but is treated in the same way. Anaphylactoid shock is only occasionally fatal.

Vasodilatory shock (septic shock)

Unlike the other causes of shock, which all produce widespread vasoconstriction, **vasodilatory shock** (**septic shock**) produces hypotension due to a failure of vascular smooth muscle to constrict and with the stimulation of arterial vasodilation. Usually it is caused by an extensive systemic bacterial infection, but may also follow long-lasting shock from any cause. It can also be caused by poisoning by carbon monoxide or nitrogen and a number of other chemicals, such as cyanide and the oral anti-diabetic drug, metformin.

Despite raised levels of catecholamines and activation of the renin–angiotensin system, the smooth muscle fails to contract. While different initial mechanisms may trigger vasodilatory shock there seem to be a number of common pathways which cause the vasodilation:

- Opening of ATP-sensitive potassium channels by decreases in ATP. The resulting efflux of potassium hyperpolarises the cell, preventing the opening of voltage-dependent calcium channels and hence reducing the amount of calcium that is required for muscle contraction.
- Increased synthesis of nitric oxide by cytokine-induced activation of inducible nitric oxide synthase. Levels of cytokines are increased by endotoxins, released by bacteria. The nitric oxide has two effects:
  - Increases cGMP levels, producing vasodilation
  - Opens membrane potassium channels (normally opened by calcium) which hyperpolarise the cell (see above).
- Reduction in vasopressin levels. While vasopressin levels in early shock are raised markedly, producing vasoconstriction and water retention, after a prolonged period of shock vasopressin levels fall. There is evidence that this may be due to depletion of vasopressin stores in the pituitary.

SIGNS AND SYMPTOMS OF SHOCK

Many of the signs and symptoms of hypovolaemic shock are common to all types of shock (Fig. 11.50), although there are some that are specific to particular types of shock, e.g. warm skin in septic shock. Most of the signs are due to the compensatory responses of the cardiovascular reflexes which normally control blood flow and maintain blood pressure. In severe shock, however, there are other reflexes which are activated only at very low pressures.

The first response to shock is an activation of the **baroreceptor**, **reflex** by a fall in blood pressure. which produces an increase in heart rate (**tachycardia**) and, except in the case of vasodilatory shock, peripheral vasoconstriction and venoconstriction. Because of the combination of raised heart rate and peripheral vasoconstriction, the pulse is weak (thready). Initially, this has the effect of maintaining mean blood pressure, and the perfusion of the heart and brain, even though pulse pressure is reduced. During mild shock there may be no reduction in blood pressure because of these compensatory responses, so arterial blood pressure is not a good indicator of the extent of any blood loss. There are a wide range of other systemic effects and consequences of the shock:

- There is a generalised activation of the sympathetic nervous system, which leads to an increase in liver glycolysis, increasing blood glucose levels.
- The increase in anaerobic metabolism produces more lactic acid, which uncouples glycolysis leading to

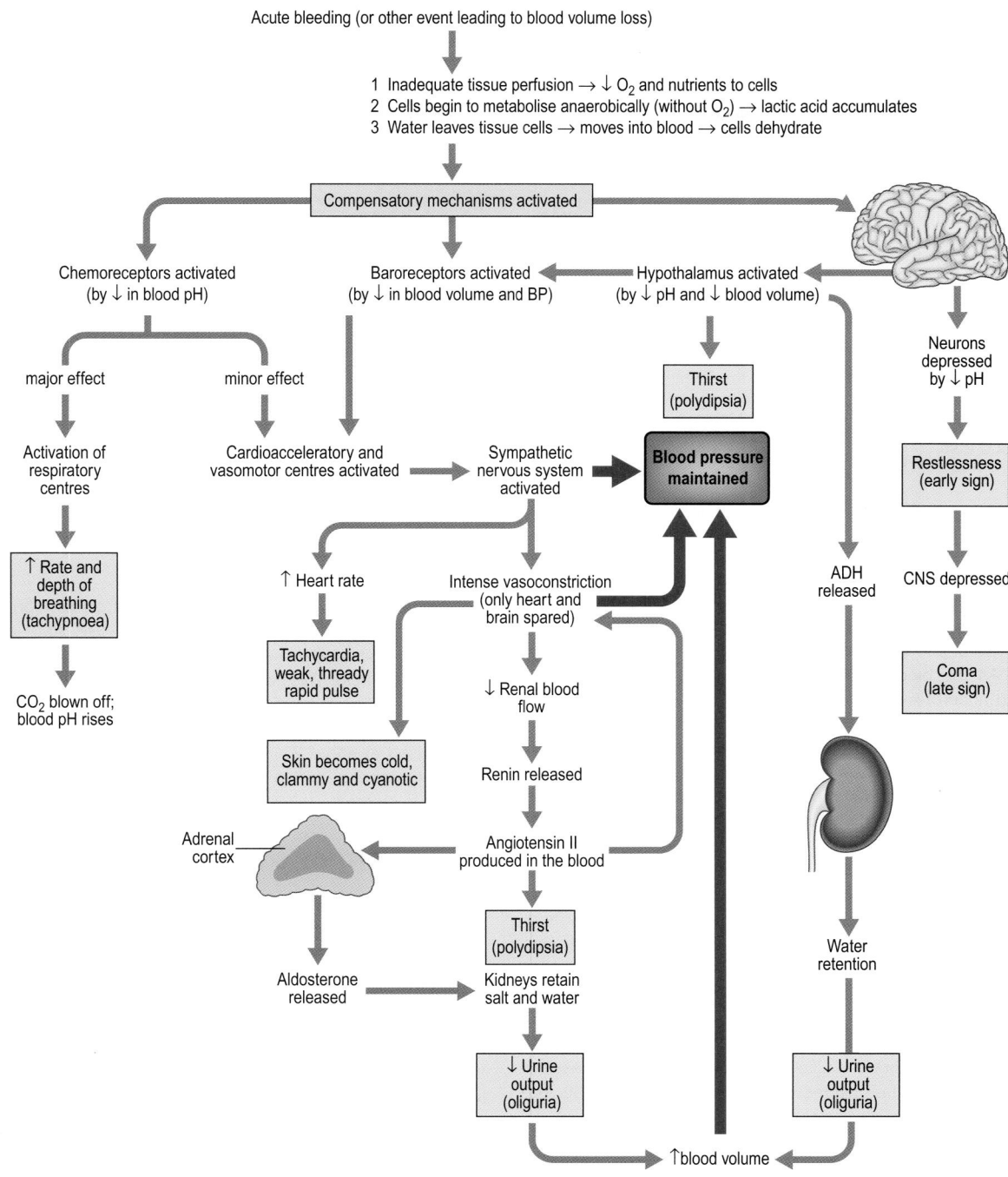

Acute bleeding (or other event leading to blood volume loss)

1 Inadequate tissue perfusion $\rightarrow \downarrow O_2$ and nutrients to cells
2 Cells begin to metabolise anaerobically (without O_2) $\rightarrow$ lactic acid accumulates
3 Water leaves tissue cells $\rightarrow$ moves into blood $\rightarrow$ cells dehydrate

Compensatory mechanisms activated

Chemoreceptors activated
(by $\downarrow$ in blood pH)

Baroreceptors activated
(by $\downarrow$ in blood volume and BP)

Hypothalamus activated
(by $\downarrow$ pH and $\downarrow$ blood volume)

major effect   minor effect

Activation of
respiratory
centres

Cardioacceleratory and
vasomotor centres activated

Sympathetic
nervous system
activated

Thirst
(polydipsia)

Blood pressure
maintained

Neurons
depressed
by $\downarrow$ pH

Restlessness
(early sign)

$\uparrow$ Rate and
depth of
breathing
(tachypnoea)

$\uparrow$ Heart rate

Intense vasoconstriction
(only heart and
brain spared)

ADH
released

CNS depressed

Tachycardia,
weak, thready
rapid pulse

$\downarrow$ Renal blood
flow

Coma
(late sign)

CO_2 blown off;
blood pH rises

Skin becomes cold,
clammy and cyanotic

Renin released

Adrenal
cortex

Angiotensin II
produced in the blood

Thirst
(polydipsia)

Aldosterone
released

Kidneys retain
salt and water

Water
retention

$\downarrow$ Urine
output
(oliguria)

$\downarrow$ Urine
output
(oliguria)

$\uparrow$blood volume

Fig. 11.50 **Signs and symptoms of hypovolaemic shock.** ADH, antidiuretic hormone (vasopressin). Redrawn with permission from Marieb EN 2004 Human anatomy and physiology, 6th edn. Pearson Benjamin Cummings, San Francisco.

reduced myocardial function, and causes a fall in the blood pH.

■ The low blood pH activates medullary chemoreceptors to increase the rate and depth of breathing (**tachypnoea**).

■ In the brain, neuronal activity is depressed by the fall in pH. An early sign of this is restlessness but as shock progresses the patient becomes comatose.

■ The sympathetic activation causes an increase in sweating, but as the skin is poorly perfused, due to the vasoconstriction, the skin surface is cool and so the sweat does not evaporate, resulting in the patient

feeling cold and clammy. This will not be seen in vasodilatory shock because of the lack of vasoconstriction in this particular form of shock.

■ In patients with light skin colour the peripheral vasoconstriction will be evident in the skin, which will show a **pallor**, and lips, which may appear **cyanotic**.

■ There is an increased reabsorption of fluid from the interstitial fluid in response to **hypovolaemia**, which may add 500 mL of fluid to the vascular compartment.

■ The fall in blood volume results in a decrease of the usual inhibition of vasopressin release, acting through the baroreceptors, allowing **vasopressin** to increase**,** which reduces water loss from the kidney, leading to decreased urine output (**oliguria**).

- The reduction in renal perfusion will trigger activation of the **renin–angiotensin–aldosterone system**, which will produce further vasoconstriction, as well as salt and water retention.
- The production of angiotensin II through the renin–angiotensin activation also stimulates thirst (**polydipsia**) by acting on receptors in the brain.

In the long term, the reduced fluid loss from the kidney and increased water intake will restore fluid balance. The liver will replace the plasma proteins (mainly albumin), which will increase the colloid osmotic pressure of blood. The hypoxia in the kidney will have stimulated the release of erythropoietin, which will act on precursor cells in the bone marrow to stimulate the production of new red blood cells to replace blood loss.

IRREVERSIBLE (DECOMPENSATED) SHOCK

If the degree of shock is large and is not treated rapidly then blood pressure can no longer be maintained by compensatory responses. This is called **decompensated shock** and is a type of positive feedback.

As the blood pressure falls, so does tissue perfusion, and anaerobic metabolism increases. At a MABP between 50 mmHg and 70 mmHg, the perfusion of the heart and brain fall significantly. The reduction in perfusion of the myocardium reduces the contractility of the heart, which reduces cardiac output, further reducing perfusion that can no longer be compensated for. There is evidence that this kind of shock releases a substance from pancreatic lysosomes, a **myocardial depressant factor**, which causes direct myocardial depression by an unknown mechanism.

There is almost no perfusion of the kidney and liver and the lack of peripheral perfusion leads to **vascular stasis**. This produces the release of local vasodilators and an increase in endothelial permeability with the subsequent loss of fluid and proteins into the interstitial fluid. The static blood agglutinates in the capillaries causing blockage. The reduction in blood flow to the brain leads to depression of neurons in the vasomotor areas of the brain, reducing the sympathetic discharge and so reducing the vasoconstriction and tachycardia. When blood pressure falls to below 50 mmHg, there is a 'last ditch' attempt by the brain, mediated by ischaemic brainstem neurons, to increase arterial blood pressure by an intense sympathetic vasoconstriction, called the **central nervous system ischaemic response**.

Organ damage in shock

In severe shock, the liver and kidney eventually deteriorate so that, even if the patient recovers, there may be significant tissue damage. Because both the kidney tubules and the liver receive their blood supply via portal systems, the blood pressure and oxygen saturation are already compromised and, during shock, can fall to extremely low levels. Damage tends to be less at the arteriolar end of the capillary bed. In contrast, in the liver, the centres of the liver lobules, which are the last to receive blood, suffer the most damage.

Inflammatory damage to lung tissue can cause the development of **adult respiratory distress syndrome** (**ARDS**), which can lead to acute respiratory failure and death (see Ch. 13). Due to its association with shock, this condition is also known as **shocked lung syndrome**.

Cellular damage in shock

Cellular damage in shock is due to a failure of the supply of ATP, which leads to a reduction in ATPase activity:

- Failure of the plasma membrane Na^+/K^+-ATPase, one of the largest consumers of ATP in the cell, leads to an increase in intracellular Na^+.
- A reduction in Na^+/Ca^{2+} exchange also reduces Ca^{2+}-ATPase activity, leading to an increase in intracellular Ca^{2+}, which then saturates the regulatory proteins and disrupts mitochondrial function.
- Lysosomes release proteases into the cytoplasm, which destroy intracellular proteins.
- The increase in intracellular cations leads to an influx of Cl^- and, by osmosis, an increase in cell water. This causes swelling of the cell and eventually cell death by lysis.

In severe shock, the reserves of ATP and creatine phosphate are depleted. ATP is metabolised to ADP, AMP and finally adenosine, which enters the blood where it is converted to uric acid. This cannot be used to resynthesise ATP, so adenosine has to be synthesised from nitrogenous bases, sugars and phosphate (see Ch. 2). However, this can only be synthesised at about 2% per hour, which means that once these high-energy phosphate stores are depleted they are difficult to restore.

TREATMENT OF SHOCK

The initial treatment of shock is based on restoring haemodynamic control by correcting the circulating blood volume. Further treatment then aims to restore tissue perfusion to all organs, and to achieve a correct fluid balance. Although the major problem in shock is tissue hypoxia, oxygen therapy does not always have a significant effect as, due to the shape of the oxygen/haemoglobin saturation curve, in many cases the oxygenation of blood in the lungs is already high and it is the delivery of oxygen to the tissues that is reduced.

Fluid replacement

The fluid chosen depends partly on the type of shock. For example, in hypovolaemic shock, if the shock is haemorrhagic, the most appropriate treatment is usually the transfusion of red cells and fluid. However, rapid correction of circulating blood volume by immediate transfusion of an electrolyte solution or a plasma substitute (see Information box 11.21) is essential – even before there has been time to source and test the appropriate blood (see Ch. 12). If the loss is solely of plasma (e.g. in burns), plasma is the most appropriate fluid; if the loss is due to dehydration, an electrolyte solution is used.

Drug treatment

There are two ways in which drugs can be used to treat shock, either by increasing **cardiac contraction** or by chang-

Information box 11.21   Replacement fluids

Crystalloid solutions

- Electrolyte solutions contain water and salts (e.g NaCl) in concentrations that are iso-osmolar with blood. These may also contain sugars such as dextrose and glucose, and lactate. They are called crystalloid because they are true solutions and pass freely across semi-permeable barriers, e.g. capillary endothelium. Normal saline solution contains 0.9% sodium chloride, which provides 154 mmol/L of both sodium and chloride ions, giving a total of about 300 mOsmol.
- A disadvantage of saline solutions is that they move freely from the vasculature into the interstitial fluid: so to increase blood volume by 1 L, 3 L of saline must be transfused. Care must be taken not to administer too much fluid because overload can lead to pulmonary oedema and heart failure. However, dextrose solutions also increase intracellular volume as dextrose is taken into cells and water follows osmotically.

Colloid solutions

- These are not true solutions; they are suspensions of particles. They include blood and plasma and a variety of synthetic preparations. Synthetic colloids are suspensions of high molecular-weight compounds, e.g. dextrans (40–70 kDa), derivatives of gelatine (30–35 kDa) and albumin.
- Because the particles are too large to pass through the capillary endothelial layer, the colloid osmotic pressure increases and fluid remains within the vasculature, which increases circulating volume rapidly.
- In **vasodilatory shock** or in **advanced shock**, endothelial permeability is increased. Thus the colloids can leak out of the vasculature, increasing the interstitial fluid volume and interstitial oncotic pressure. This leads to **oedema**, which is particularly dangerous if it occurs in the lungs because it reduces gas exchange.

ing **peripheral resistance** by altering vasoconstriction. In most types of shock the aim is to increase cardiac output and organ perfusion, particularly of the kidneys and the liver. In vasodilatory shock, vasoconstriction is useful in reducing the hypotension but carries the risk of reducing organ perfusion.

Drug treatments require careful balancing of the advantages and disadvantages of each type of drug, and their effects must be closely monitored and dosages adjusted continually to maximise their benefit.

Problems which can arise are:

- Increasing the force and rate of cardiac contraction increases cardiac output, but these drugs also increase the oxygen demand of the heart, which can exacerbate myocardial ischaemia.
- Vasodilation increases perfusion, but it also reduces blood pressure.
- Vasoconstriction in some vascular beds, while reducing perfusion in those organs, can increase perfusion in others.

Many of the drugs used are agonists that act on adrenoceptors, called **sympathomimetics**.

- **Adrenaline** (epinephrine) at low doses acts predominantly on β-receptors to increase the force and rate of cardiac contraction (via β_1-receptors) and decrease peripheral resistance (via β_2-receptors on skeletal and heart muscle vasculature), but at higher doses acts on α-receptors to produce vasoconstriction.

- **Noradrenaline** (norepinephrine) acts mainly on α-receptors causing vasoconstriction.
- **Dopamine** also acts on α- and β-receptors as well as at dopaminergic D_1 and D_2 receptors. D_1 receptors are postsynaptic and produce vasodilation. D_2 receptors are presynaptic and inhibit noradrenaline release. At low doses, dopamine produces vasodilation, particularly in the renal, coronary and cerebral circulations. Some patients benefit from vasodilation because of the reduction in afterload, which is particularly important in patients with heart failure. At high doses, vasoconstriction predominates as dopamine is converted to adrenaline. Analogues of dopamine, dopexamine and dobutamine, have similar effects with varying potencies at the different receptors.

THE CIRCULATION IN SPECIFIC ORGANS

CORONARY CIRCULATION

The heart pumps continuously, hardly without a pause from before birth to death. It is able to do this only because it is supplied with sufficient oxygen and nutrients (mainly fatty acids). The coronary circulation has the shortest transit time – of only 6–8 seconds – and has a very high density of capillaries, approximately one per myocyte, which are all perfused continuously. This means that the diffusion distance is small. There are high levels of oxygen extraction (65–75%), compared with the average for the whole body (25%), and during exercise, extraction rates rise to 90%. These levels are necessary because the rate of oxygen consumption is 20 times higher in cardiac muscle than in the skeletal muscle at rest.

The major factor controlling coronary blood flow is **metabolic hyperaemia**, which causes blood flow to increase linearly with oxygen consumption, with adenosine being the main metabolic vasodilator. Basal tone in the arterioles is maintained by sympathetic vasoconstrictor nerves releasing noradrenaline onto α-adrenoceptors. During exercise, however, the circulating adrenaline acts on β_2-adrenoceptors to produce vasodilation that reinforces the metabolic vasodilation.

The small coronary blood vessels run through the cardiac muscle. Because muscle shortens (and fattens) when it contracts, this produces a mechanical restriction to flow during systole. This leads to blood flow in the coronary vessels being extremely pulsatile, with blood flow in the coronary artery being stopped and even reversed during systole (Fig. 11.51). In addition, because the openings of the coronary arteries lie behind the cusps of the aortic valve, they are covered during systole and only after the closure of the aortic valve can the recoil of the aorta push blood into them. As a result, over 80% of coronary blood flow occurs during diastole, when the relaxation of the muscle reduces the external pressure on the arteries.

Ischaemic heart disease

If blood flow to the heart through the coronary vessels is reduced or the oxygenation of the blood is insufficient, then the heart muscle will be damaged. **Ischaemic heart disease**

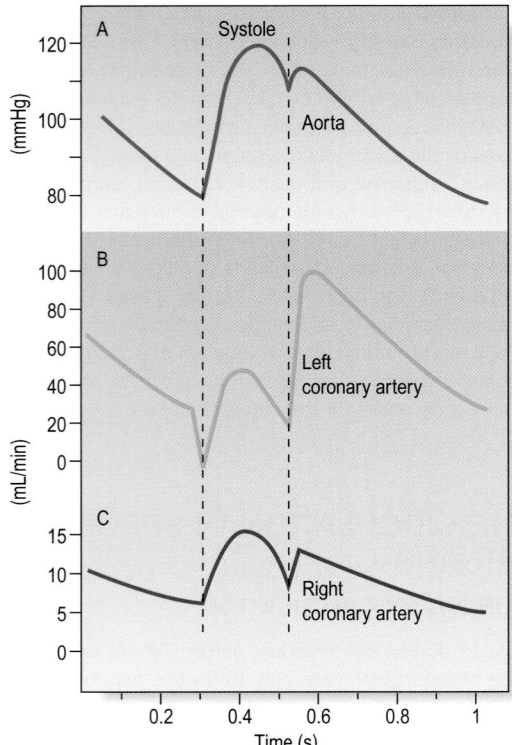

Fig. 11.51 Blood flow in the coronary arteries during the cardiac cycle. Pressure in the aorta (*A*); flow in the coronary arteries (*B*, *C*).

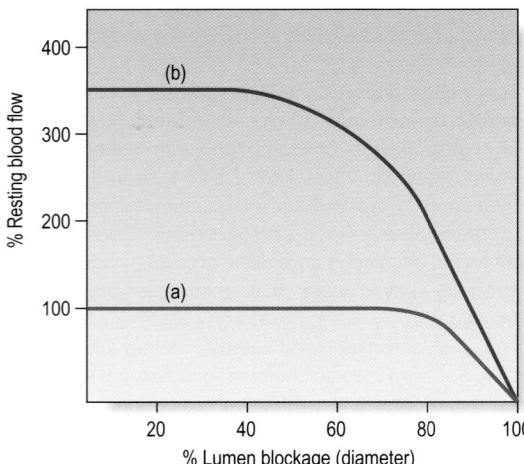

Fig. 11.52 Blood flow is reduced by decreasing lumen diameter: (a) resting blood flow and (b) maximal blood flow.

is a major cause of death in the Western world. Over two-thirds of deaths from **coronary artery disease** occur outside hospitals, with few prior symptoms and often no warning. The two most common manifestations of ischaemic heart disease are **angina** and **myocardial infarction**.

The major factor in the development of ischaemic heart disease is the narrowing of the coronary arteries by the formation of atheroma. At rest, the blood flow is only impaired if the artery diameter is reduced by more that 80% (Fig. 11.52

line (a)). However, at higher rates of blood flow the effect of reduced diameter is increased (Fig. 11.52 line (b)). If the ischaemia develops slowly then this encourages the development of anastomoses between the blood vessels, but these are relatively narrow vessels.

Angina

If the blood flow to the heart muscle does not provide an adequate supply of oxygen for its requirements, the muscle becomes ischaemic and pain occurs. This substernal, central chest pain, which is often described as 'crushing', and which may radiate to the arms, neck or jaw, is due to **angina** (**angina pectoris**) and may be caused by a number of factors.

Stable angina

Stable angina can be evoked by intense sympathetic stimulation, which causes vasoconstriction. While this can occur in response to severe stress or severe cold, it is usually caused by a narrowing of a coronary artery due to atheroma. Although the atheroma may not impair flow significantly at rest, it can prevent the increase in flow required during exercise (**exertional angina**).

Exertional angina occurs consistently on exercise and subsides after 3–10 minutes of rest. This type of angina can be investigated using ECGs. While many patients with angina may have a normal resting ECG, when the heart rate is raised, such as in an exercise stress test, they show a depression of the ST segment. The narrowing of the arteries can be observed using **coronary angiography** or **Doppler ultrasonography** (Information box 11.22).

Variant angina

Variant angina, also known as **Prinzmetal's angina**, is a rare condition in which vasospasm of the coronary arteries occurs at rest, often in the early hours of the morning. It is thought to be caused by an exaggerated response to vasoconstrictors such as adrenaline and 5-hydroxytryptamine.

Unstable angina

Unstable angina is a medical emergency because there is a high risk of a subsequent myocardial infarction. It occurs as a result of the transient blockage of a coronary artery by a thrombus that has formed at the site of an atheromatous plaque. There is anginal pain at rest and the ECG shows ST segment depression or elevation. Patients should be admitted to a coronary care unit for pharmacological therapy and possible cardiac catheterisation.

Treatment of angina

An important part of the treatment of angina involves reduction of the risk factors for atherosclerosis and treatment of underlying hypertension, diabetes and hyperlipidaemia. Drug treatment is useful as follows:

- Enteric-coated aspirin can be used prophylactically in patients with stable angina to reduce platelet aggregation and reduce the risk of thrombi forming on atherosclerotic plaques.
- Angina attacks are rapidly relieved by drugs such as glyceryl trinitrate, isosorbide dinitrate and isosorbide mononitrate. These act by releasing NO, which then causes vasodilation of both arteries and veins. This sequentially reduces venous return, preload, peripheral

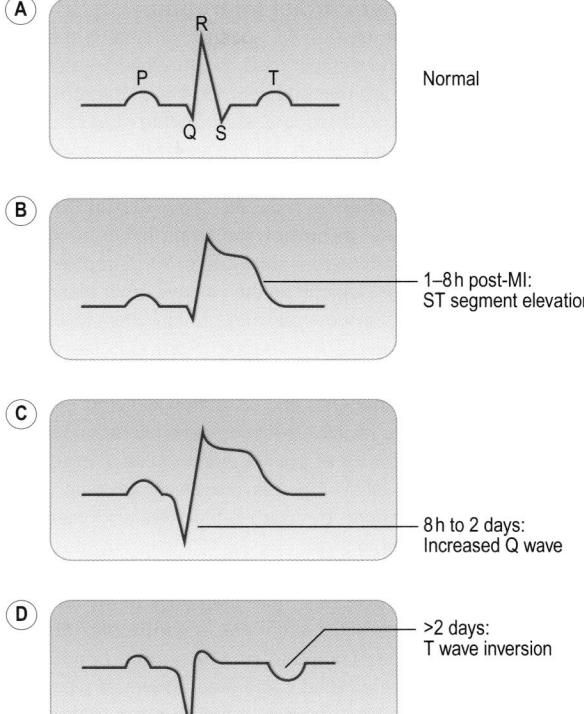

Fig. 11.54 Evolution of typical changes in the ECG following myocardial infarction (MI).

Information box 11.22

i **Information box 11.22** | **Coronary angiography and Doppler ultrasonography**

Coronary angiography involves the injection of a radiocontrast dye into the left and right coronary arteries. X-ray images are taken from various angles in order to observe fully any narrowings. This information may be useful in assessing the degree to which vessels may be narrowed (Fig. 11.53), but it cannot determine the degree of physiological impairment. Dye can also be injected into the left ventricle in order to assess ventricular function. There is, however, a low but significant risk associated with this procedure.

A non-invasive alternative, now in more common use, is **Doppler ultrasonography**. This measures the direction and speed of blood flow and has more commonly been used to evaluate the degree of impairment in patients with heart failure. However, improvements in resolution and processing mean that it can now also be used to evaluate blood flow in the coronary vessels.

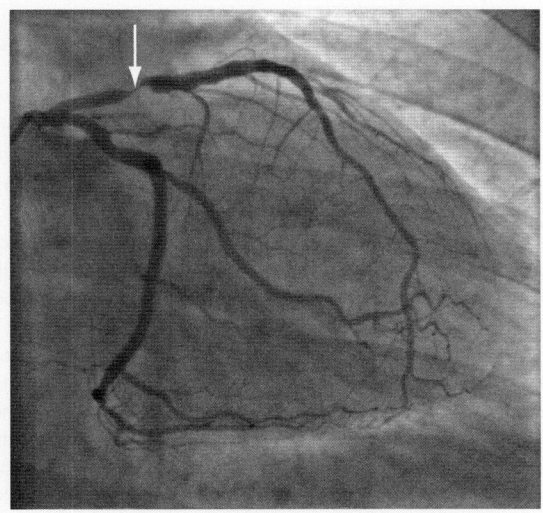

Fig. 11.53 **Coronary angiogram from a patient with stable angina.** There is severe stenosis of the left main stem (*arrow*). From Haslett C, Chilvers E, Boon N et al (eds) 2002 Davidson's principles and practice of medicine, 19th edn. Churchill Livingstone, Edinburgh.

resistance and, subsequently, afterload. Their effect on coronary arteries will not increase flow through stenosed vessels, because the obstruction is fixed, but will increase blood flow through other arteries, which may increase collateral circulation.

■ **β-Blockers** can be used to relieve angina and prevent ischaemic attacks by decreasing the heart rate and myocardial contractility, thus reducing the myocardial oxygen demand.

■ **Calcium-channel blockers** can be used instead of β-blockers and are useful in variant angina.

Surgical intervention may be recommended in particular cases to open up the coronary vessels. The main procedures used are:

■ **Percutaneous transluminal coronary angioplasty (PTCA):** which involves dilating the artery with a balloon catheter.

■ **Stents**: these are thin wire mesh structures that act as a permanent lining to keep the artery open. Stenting may be used in combination with PTCA.

■ **Coronary artery bypass grafting (CABG):** this is an operation in which the diseased artery is replaced with a short piece of vessel, such as a piece of the great saphenous vein in the leg, or a piece of the internal mammary artery.

Myocardial infarction

Myocardial infarction occurs when there is persistent blockage of a coronary artery, leading to the death of heart muscle by necrosis. This medical emergency is extremely grave as the risk of dying due to **ventricular fibrillation** is very high, particular for the few hours following the onset of symptoms. The typical chest pain at rest (more commonly reported in men) is described as constricting around the chest, radiating to the arms, neck and jaw. It may be accompanied with anxiety, sweating, nausea and vomiting. The pulse may be increased or decreased, and blood pressure may be normal or reduced. If the systolic pressure is less than 90 mmHg, this may indicate cardiogenic shock.

Within a few hours of the onset of symptoms the ECG shows **ST segment elevation** and in the following days there is a series of ECG changes (Fig. 11.54). There is elevation in the plasma of a number of enzymes released from dying cells. A peak in **creatine kinase** is followed by a rise in **aspartate transaminase** and then **lactate dehydrogenase** (see Ch. 2). The muscle proteins **troponin T** and **troponin I**, both indicators of myocardial necrosis, are also detected in plasma.

Treatment for myocardial infarction

The immediate treatment for MI consists of limiting the size of the thrombosis and reducing cell death. While areas at the centre of the infarct will become necrotic 15–30 minutes after the blockage occurs, there are surrounding areas, called **stunned myocardium**, which will recover if their blood flow is restored early enough.

Platelet aggregation is reduced using aspirin and the clot can be dissolved (**thrombolysis**) using either streptokinase or tissue plasminogen activator (tPA). Streptokinase binds to plasminogen, which can then cleave other plasminogen molecules to produce plasmin, which then lyses the fibrin clot. Streptokinase is extracted from cultures of the streptococcal bacteria and cannot be given more than once within a year as it antigenic and its action blocked by antibodies that develop rapidly following administration. tPA is an endogenous activator of plasminogen which is produced using recombinant DNA. Opiates are given for pain relief. Cardiac work is reduced by using β-blockers and vasodilators such as ACE inhibitors.

The major risk following myocardial infarction is **cardiac failure**, which often occurs if more than 20% of the left ventricle is affected. The other major risk is **ventricular fibrillation**, caused by the disruption of the normal conduction pathways during the cardiac cycle (see above). If pieces of the thrombus break off, they may travel to other organs and cause embolism (or stroke in the case of the brain). Following the initial cell death, the dead tissue is invaded by neutrophils, and there is breakdown of the old tissue and its replacement with scar tissue. During this process the tissue becomes very soft and prone to rupture. This is very often fatal and accounts for about 10% of deaths following myocardial infarction.

SKELETAL MUSCLE CIRCULATION

The two types of skeletal muscle have very different blood flow rates.

- **Tonic muscles**, also known as **red** (due to their high numbers of mitochondria) or **slow postural** muscles, have moderate flow rates of about 15 mL/min per 100 g tissue.
- **Phasic** (**white, fast twitch**) **muscles** have a low flow rate when resting (3–5 mL), but at maximal exercise this can rise to more than 60 mL/min per 100 g and can consume 80–90% of the total cardiac output. This rise is mainly as a result of **metabolic vasodilation** due to increases in extracellular K^+ and osmolarity.

A major mechanism which allows this increase in blood flow is the opening of a large number of capillaries that are not perfused at rest. This **capillary recruitment** effectively increases the capillary density and reduces the diffusion distance. Oxygen extraction increases from 25% to 90% in intense exercise. Even so, there is often a build up of lactic acid due to a degree of anaerobic metabolism, so after the exercise ends blood flow is still increased (**post-exercise hyperaemia**) until the oxygen debt is repaid. The increase in the number of perfused vessels can be seen clearly by the increase in volume of exercising muscle.

CUTANEOUS CIRCULATION

The skin not only provides a protective covering and a sensitive surface but also is the main means by which humans regulate body temperature. The cutaneous circulation is unusual in that there are two routes by which blood can pass from the arterial to the venous side:

- Via **arterioles** that supply the capillaries which provide the blood supply to the dermis. Changes in these arterioles are responsible for autoregulation and reactive hyperaemia
- Through relatively large coiled **arteriovenous anastamoses** (**AVAs**) directly into the **venous plexus**. The venous plexi are wide vessels running under the dermal papillae that can accommodate a high rate of blood flow. These are found mainly in the skin of the extremities. The smooth muscle walls of the AVAs are not sensitive to local metabolism, but are almost completely under sympathetic nervous control.

Temperature regulation

Heat can be lost from the skin by **radiation**, **convection**, **conduction** and **evaporation**, but all of these processes only occur if warm blood is brought close to the surface of the skin. The resting naked human is thermoneutral at 27–28 °C, that is, able to maintain a core temperature of 37 °C without using heat gaining or heat losing mechanisms. At this temperature the blood flow is about 10–12 mL/min per 100 g tissue. Under the dermis are layers of subcutaneous fat that insulate the body and prevent heat loss.

Changes in core temperature are monitored by receptors in the hypothalamus. In the cold, the AVAs are closed, the arterioles are constricted and only small amounts of blood pass through the capillary bed – less than 10 times than at thermoneutral. When the core temperature rises, the arterioles dilate and the AVAs open up (Fig. 11.55). This allows a high flow rate in the venous plexi, which have a large surface area and act like radiators in order to lose heat. Flow rates of up to 200 mL/min per 100 g tissue allow heat loss across the skin. However, the amount of heat lost depends on the ambient temperature, which determines the temperature gradient, and the humidity, which determines the degree to

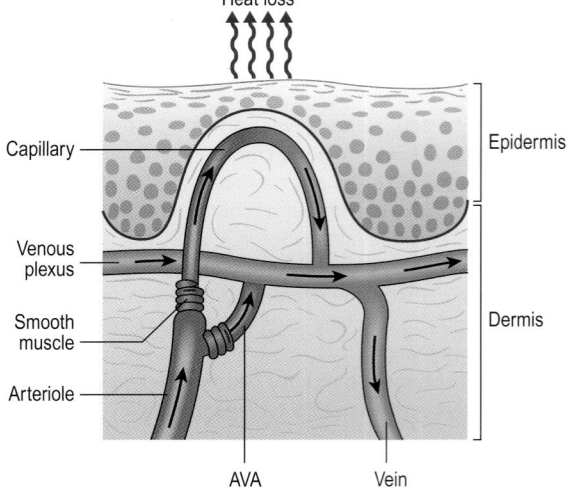

***Fig. 11.55* The cutaneous circulation.** Blood can flow either through the capillary loops or via the arteriovenous anastomoses (AVAs) into the venous plexus. The diameter of the AVAs is controlled by sympathetic vasomotor discharge.

which sweat evaporates. The latent heat of evaporation of water is very high, so sweating is a very efficient way of losing heat, but if the humidity is high then water does not evaporate. This is why a hot humid day feels much hotter than a dry day at the same temperature.

CEREBRAL CIRCULATION

Due to the high metabolic rate of brain tissue, especially the grey matter, the brain receives 15% of the cardiac output at rest, even though it comprises only 2% of body weight. The grey matter is very sensitive to hypoxia and, at normal body temperatures, damage can occur within 5 minutes of an interruption to the supply. The blood supply to the brain is maintained at a nearly constant flow rate, despite variations in blood pressure from about 60 mmHg to 160 mmHg. This is due to the **myogenic response** and **autoregulation**, with very little control by extrinsic nervous input.

The cerebral vessels are sensitive to levels of carbon dioxide. **Hypercapnia** (increased carbon dioxide) causes vasodilation, which helps to improve blood flow in asphyxia. **Hypocapnia** causes vasoconstriction. This can be seen during hyperventilation, when the excessive breathing lowers the concentration of CO_2 and so brain blood flow is reduced. This leads to a feeling of dizziness and can produce fainting.

Blood flow to different brain regions varies with metabolic activity. Brain imaging shows that different areas of the brain are more metabolically active during certain tasks. For example, limb movements can be seen to increase blood flow in the motor and sensory areas of the brain. This hyperaemia is caused by local increases in the K^+ concentration around active neurons.

The capillaries of the brain are continuous capillaries which have particularly tight junctions (See Information box 11.13).

PULMONARY CIRCULATION

The pulmonary capillary bed is very large, so the overall resistance to flow is small compared with the systemic circulation. This enables the pulmonary circulation to function at much lower pressures (about 10 mmHg), which do not stress the delicate alveolar tissue. While damage to the alveoli by high pressures rarely occurs in humans, the high arterial pressures that occur in racehorses during racing can lead to pulmonary haemorrhages, seen as blood blowing out of the nostrils.

Capillary perfusion is controlled by oxygen levels. Pulmonary arterioles respond to hypoxia in the *opposite* way to systemic arterioles, that is, they constrict. This is extremely important, because it ensures that only regions of the lung with sufficient ventilation, which therefore contain oxygen, are perfused (see Ch. 13). At rest, only part of the lung is ventilated at each breath, so only those regions receive blood and the unventilated regions are not perfused. During deep breathing more of the lung is ventilated and so more of the lung is then perfused (see Information box 11.23).

DEVELOPMENT OF THE HEART

Congenital abnormalities of the heart occur in about 6–8 live births/1000 and are thought to arise very early in embryonic

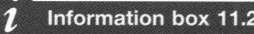

Information box 11.23 | **Hypoxic lung disease can lead to heart failure**

The constriction of pulmonary arterioles in response to hypoxia can cause severe problems. Lung diseases that reduce ventilation and cause hypoxia, such as **chronic obstructive pulmonary disease** (**COPD**), can produce heart failure due to the constrictor response of pulmonary capillaries.

The constriction of the pulmonary arterioles causes an increase in the resistance to flow in the pulmonary arteries. The increased pulmonary artery pressure causes the right side of the heart to pump harder to compensate. Increased pumping causes the right side of the heart to hypertrophy and become dilated due to the back pressure of blood, a condition known as **cor pulmonale**. The mechanical efficiency of the right ventricle is thus reduced and, if the condition persists, eventually the right side of the heart fails. Two common symptoms result:

- Raised jugular venous pressure, which can be observed as pulsation of the jugular vein when the patient is sitting upright.
- Peripheral oedema, which is particularly noticeable as swelling of the ankles, worse at the end of the day.

development (about 5–8 weeks). Knowledge of how the heart develops gives an understanding of the processes which produce the different defects.

FORMATION OF THE EARLY HEART

In the very early embryo, the exchange of gases and nutrients occurs by diffusion. However, the increasing size of the embryo soon requires that substances are moved more quickly than can occur by diffusive processes. At about day 17 after fertilisation, **mesenchymal cells** start to form two **endothelial tubes**, and by day 22 these have partially fused. This **heart tube** has an inner layer which becomes the **endocardium** and an outer muscular layer which eventually becomes the **myocardium**.

At the same time as the development of the embryonic heart, clumps of mesodermal cells, called **blood islands**, form vascular tubes which grow towards each other and the heart, forming a basic vascular system. By 23 days the primitive heart tube starts to beat, producing a circulation of blood in an embryo which is less than 5 mm long. The rudimentary heart develops bulges, which go on to form the heart chambers (Fig. 11.56A). Blood flows into the heart in the same direction from the two vessels that become the great veins, into the (in order):

- **Sinus venosus** (which becomes part of the right atrium and coronary sinus, as well as the sinoatrial node)
- **Atrium** (separated from the ventricle by the AV canal)
- **Ventricle** (forms the left ventricle)
- **Bulbus cordis** and **truncus arteriosus** (which form the right ventricle, the aorta and the pulmonary artery).

As the heart enlarges it then bends, forming a loop which brings the atria above the ventricles (Fig. 11.56B). At this point, there is no division of the heart into left and right, nor are there any valvular structures.

FETAL PULMONARY CIRCULATION

In the fetus, there is very little blood flow through the pulmonary circulation. The fetus makes respiratory movements in

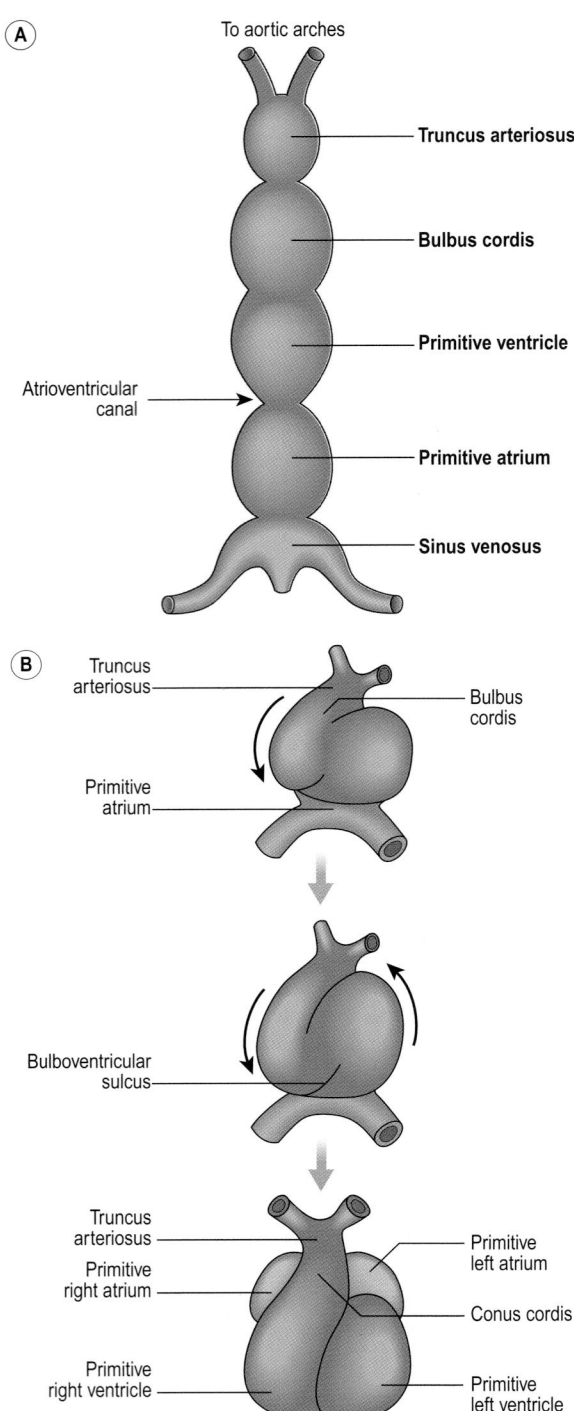

Ⓐ

To aortic arches

Truncus arteriosus

Bulbus cordis

Primitive ventricle

Atrioventricular canal

Primitive atrium

Sinus venosus

Ⓑ

Truncus arteriosus

Bulbus cordis

Primitive atrium

Bulboventricular sulcus

Truncus arteriosus

Primitive right atrium

Primitive right ventricle

Primitive left atrium

Conus cordis

Primitive left ventricle

Fig. 11.56 **Early fetal heart development.** (A) straight heart tube (22 days). (B) Formation of the heart loop. Redrawn, with permission, from LS Lilly (ed) 2003 Pathophysiology of heart disease, 3rd edn. Lippincott, Williams & Wilkins, Baltimore.

FORMATION OF THE HEART CHAMBERS

The septa that divide the two atria and ventricles into the four-chambered heart, and the valves that control the direction of blood flow through the heart, develop during the fourth and fifth weeks. The division between the atria and the ventricles grows inwards to become the **endocardial cushions**, which divide the AV canal into left and right and give rise to the **tricuspid** and **bicuspid (mitral) valves**.

The **interatrial septum** forms in two steps that produce a wall of tissue, the **septum secundum**, between the two atria, which is perforated by an opening called the **foramen ovale**. This opening is covered by a flap of tissue, the **septum primum**, on the left side of the hole. The septum primum works like a one-way valve, allowing blood entering the right side of the heart to cross into the left atrium, but not vice versa. At birth, this opening normally closes (see below) preventing mixing of blood between left and right sides of the heart. However, in the fetus it enables oxygenated blood entering the heart from the inferior vena cava to pass from the right atrium directly into the left atrium and be pumped around the rest of the body.

At about week 5, a pair of inward-growing ridges in the bulbus cordis and the truncus arteriosus, called the **bulbar ridges**, fuse and spiral to form the **aortic septum**, which divides this part of the heart tube into two arteries: the **aorta** and the **pulmonary artery**. At the same time, tissue around the openings of the arteries forms the **aortic and pulmonary valves**. The **interventricular septum** grows from the apex of the heart towards the atria but does not fuse with the endocardial cushions, which grow inwards from the AV canal until week 7, when fusion normally occurs and division of the heart chambers is thus completed. At the top of the pulmonary trunk, where the left and right pulmonary arteries branch, there is a vessel called the **ductus arteriosus**, which joins the pulmonary arterial circulation to the aorta. This is situated at a point just after the three branches that supply the head and upper limbs, at the top of the thoracic aorta. This means that in the fetus there are two routes by which blood entering the right side of the heart can bypass the lungs.

THE FETAL CIRCULATION BEFORE AND AFTER BIRTH

Fetal circulation before birth

The fetus has a different circulatory pattern to the newborn. During gestation, the fetus receives oxygen and nutrients through the placenta, via the **umbilical vein** (Fig. 11.57A). Remember that, although the umbilical vein carries oxygenated blood, it is travelling towards the fetal heart. Waste products, including carbon dioxide, leave the fetus by the **umbilical arteries** which are branches of the **iliac arteries** supplying the lower limbs.

The highly oxygenated blood in the umbilical vein (80% saturated) is divided roughly equally between the liver and the **ductus venosus**, which bypasses the liver and joins the **inferior vena cava**, where it is mixed with oxygen-depleted blood from the lower body of the fetus, giving an oxygen saturation of about 67% when it enters the right atrium. Blood can also enter the right atrium from the **superior vena cava**; however, this blood is oxygen poor, having passed around the head, coronary circulation, upper limbs or lungs,

utero but the lungs are not inflated and do not receive oxygen until after birth. Blood vessels in the lung constrict in hypoxia (see Ch. 13) so pulmonary pressures are higher than those in the systemic circulation, preventing much of the blood flow in the fetal lung. However, the heart develops in a way that ensures that the adult pattern of dual circulation can be immediately activated once the lungs are inflated.

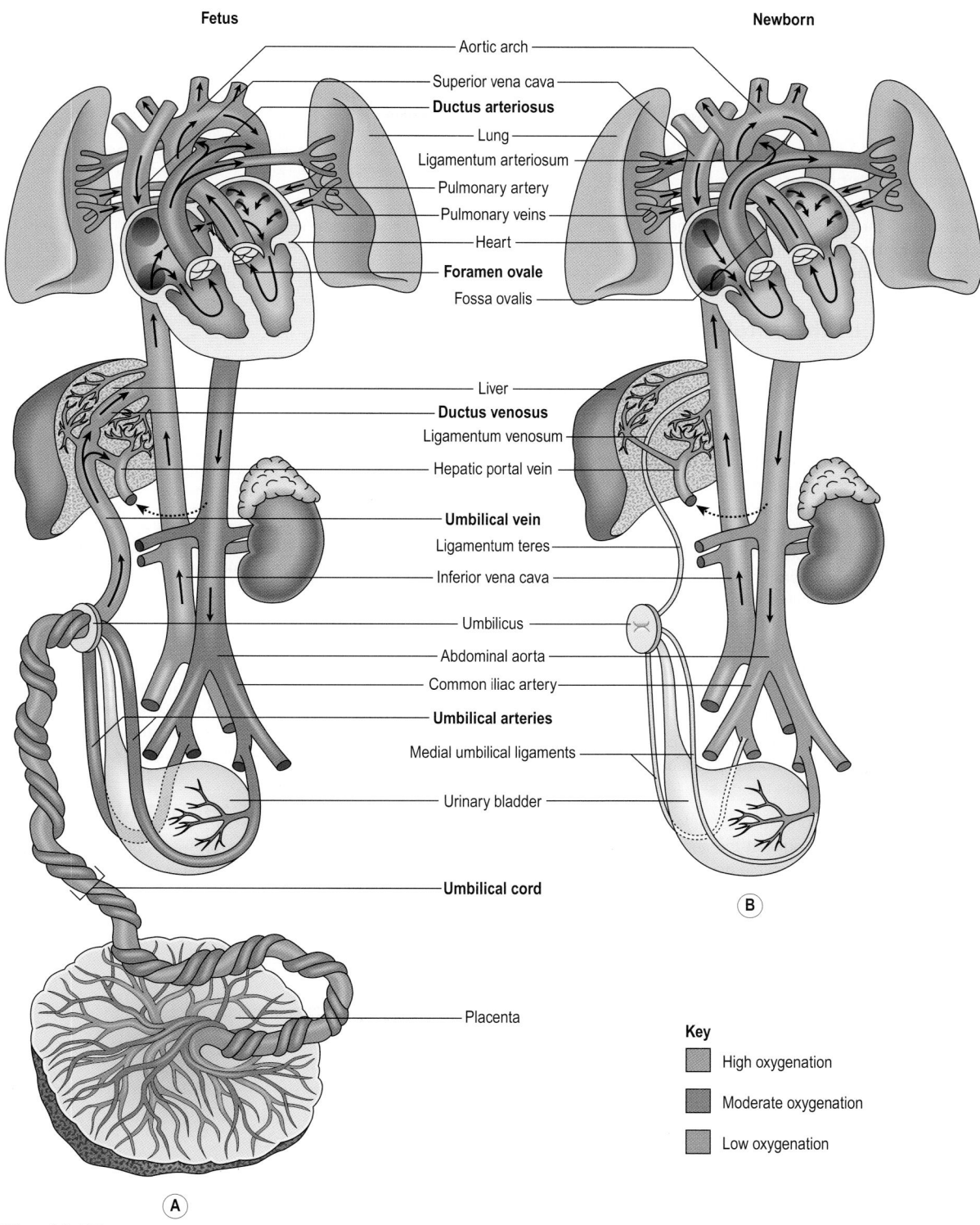

Fetus

Newborn

- Aortic arch
- Superior vena cava
- **Ductus arteriosus**
- Lung
- Ligamentum arteriosum
- Pulmonary artery
- Pulmonary veins
- Heart
- **Foramen ovale**
- Fossa ovalis

- Liver
- **Ductus venosus**
- Ligamentum venosum
- Hepatic portal vein

- **Umbilical vein**
- Ligamentum teres
- Inferior vena cava

- Umbilicus
- Abdominal aorta
- Common iliac artery
- **Umbilical arteries**
- Medial umbilical ligaments
- Urinary bladder

- **Umbilical cord**

(B)

- Placenta

Key

High oxygenation

Moderate oxygenation

Low oxygenation

(A)

Fig. 11.57 **Comparison of fetal and newborn circulation.** (A) Fetal circulation before birth. The ductus venosus allows blood to bypass the liver. The ductus arteriosus and foramen ovale allow blood to bypass the lungs. (B) After birth these close allowing the blood flow to develop the normal adult pattern. Redrawn with permission from Marieb EN 2004 Human anatomy and physiology, 6th edn. Pearson Benjamin Cummings, San Francisco.

which have all reduced the oxygen content to about 35% saturated.

These two streams of blood do not mix completely in the right atrium. The more oxygenated blood from the inferior vena cava mainly passes through the foramen ovale into the left atrium. This blood is then pumped out of the left ventricle

into the cerebral arteries, coronary arteries and the upper limbs. Blood entering via the superior vena cava mainly flows into the right ventricle from where it is pumped into the pulmonary trunk. A small fraction (about 12%) flows through the lungs (which also consume oxygen) but most passes through the ductus arteriosus into the aorta. This blood then supplies the viscera and lower limbs. Below the descending aorta some of the blood returns to the placenta via the umbilical arteries, while the rest supplies the lower limbs. The relatively high oxygen demand of the liver is met by blood supplied directly by the portal sinus from the umbilical vein.

Due to the low resistance of the large vessels of the placenta, which produces a low pressure in the aorta and the high pressure in the pulmonary arteries, the relative blood pressures in the left and right sides of the heart are the reverse of those in the adult. Right-side pressures are higher in the fetus, which maintains the patency of the foramen ovale.

Changes in the fetal circulation at birth

At birth the fetal circulation must switch rapidly to a different pattern (Fig. 11.57B). With the baby's first breaths, the lungs inflate, which stretches the capillaries, and the rise in oxygen levels in the lungs causes the blood vessels to dilate. This immediately causes the pulmonary vascular pressures to fall, which aids blood flow through the lungs. In addition, blood flow in the umbilical cord is stopped, either by clamping the cord or by the natural constriction which occurs in response to stretch, a fall in temperature or a rise in the oxygen content of the blood in the umbilical vein. This approximately doubles the systemic vascular resistance, which increases the pressures in the aorta, left ventricle and left atrium, reversing the pressure gradient between the right and left atria.

Closure of fetal shunts

At the same time as the reversal of the pressure gradient, the three shunts through the ductus venosus, the foramen ovale and the ductus arteriosus are closed.

- Due to the higher pressure in the left atrium, the septum primum is pressed against the septum secundum, covering the foramen ovale and preventing the right-to-left atrial shunt. Within a few months to years this valve is permanently closed by the fusion of the two septa, but even if this fusion does not occur, as long as the left atrial pressure remains higher than that in the right atrium the valve will remain closed.
- Initially, the higher pressure in the aorta causes a reversal of blood flow through the ductus arteriosus. However, within a few hours of birth the muscular walls of the ductus constrict, and within 1–8 days this is sufficient to prevent backward blood flow (see Clinical box 11.9). This closure is caused by the rise in oxygen tension. During gestation, the relatively low oxygen levels in the fetus stimulate the production of high levels of prostaglandin E_1 (PGE_1), which relaxes the smooth muscle walls of the ductus arteriosus. After birth, when oxygen levels rise, the levels of PGE_1 fall, which allows vasoconstriction. During the following months, this closure becomes permanent with the growth of fibrous tissue.

Development of the ventricles

In the fetus, more blood is pumped out of the right ventricle than the left ventricle. Only one-third of the total blood entering the heart passes through the left ventricle, so the right ventricle is more developed than the left. After birth, with the separation of the two sides of the heart, the cardiac

---

Clinical box 11.9 **Patent ductus arteriosus**

In some babies, especially those born prematurely, the ductus arteriosus fails to close (remains patent), leaving a shunt between the pulmonary trunk and the aorta (**patent ductus arteriosus**). Immediately after birth, the pressure in the pulmonary trunk is only slightly higher than in the aorta so any failure in the closure of the ductus arteriosus does not produce a large left–right shunt. However, as the muscular wall of the left ventricle develops, the mean pressures in the systemic system rise gradually from about 70–80 mmHg at birth to 90–100 mmHg at the age of 6. This increases the backflow of blood through the patent duct and the raised pressure tends to increase the diameter of the ductus, making the situation worse. In an older child, up to two-thirds of the blood leaving the left ventricle flows into the pulmonary circulation. Compensation by the left ventricles increases cardiac output, which can reach up to seven times normal resting levels. This massively reduces the reserve for exercise and causes hypertrophy of the left side of the heart, which can lead to left ventricular failure and pulmonary oedema.

In the newborn with this condition there are no abnormal heart sounds, due to the low flow rate through the patent ductus. However, as the flow increases a type of continual murmur, known as a **machinery murmur**, is heard in the pulmonary area, which is louder during systole. A few hours after birth the ductus venosus also constricts. This increases pressure in the hepatic portal vein to about 10 mmHg, which increases flow through the sinuses of the liver. This very rarely fails to occur and the stimulus for closure is unknown.

---

outputs of the two sides become equal and, due to the higher pressures in the left side of the heart and the reduction in the right side pressures, the walls of the left thicken, while those of the right become relatively thinner.

CONGENITAL HEART ABNORMALITIES

Congenital heart abnormalities are rare and may be due to either genetic or environmental causes. Known environmental causes include:

- Rubella infection
- Systemic lupus erythematosus
- Alcohol misuse.

Known genetic causes include:

- Trisomy 21 (Down's syndrome – an additional chromosome 21)
- Marfan's syndrome (a connective tissue disorder)
- Turner's syndrome (loss of an X chromosome in females).

Congenital heart abnormalities often do not produce any deleterious effects before birth, while the left and right ventricles pump in parallel. However, after birth, when the switch to two separate serial circulations occurs and babies must oxygenate their own blood, their effects become apparent.

Many of these defects cause blood to be shunted between the pulmonary and systemic circulations. Shunts can occur from either left-to-right or right-to-left. Abnormalities are often categorised as **cyanotic** or **acyanotic**, depending on whether or not the patient shows cyanosis, a blue-purple colouration of the skin and mucous membranes. Cyanosis is due to a high level of deoxygenated haemoglobin in the blood (at least 40 g/L) produced by a low level of oxygen saturation in the blood. Left-to-right shunts do not cause cyanosis, but right-to-left shunts allow blood to bypass the lungs, reducing its oxygenation. Many defects cause turbulent blood flow with accompanying murmurs that can aid diagnosis.

Ventricular and atrial septal defects

The most common congenital defect is a **ventricular septal defect (VSD)**, in which a hole in the interventricular septum allows blood to flow between the ventricles. In the fetus, the blood is shunted from right to left and, if the hole is large, the left ventricle is overloaded and left heart failure develops. After birth, the shunt will reverse as left ventricular pressure rises and the large quantities of blood entering the right ventricle will cause pulmonary hypertension.

Atrial septal defects (ASD) occur most commonly in the region of the foramen ovale, or at the endocardial cushions, by a failure of the developing septum primum and secundum. Both of these types of ASD lead to an open hole between the atria, which allows shunting. In contrast, in cases where the valve covering the foramen ovale fails to fuse with the interatrial septum, called a **patent foramen ovale**, blood does not flow from the left atrium to the right because the higher left side pressure pushes the valve against the septum. The effects of this are not evident unless there is an increase in right atrial pressure, for example in pulmonary hypertension.

Both pulmonary hypertension and right heart failure allow the pressure in the right side of the heart to rise, which leads to right-to-left shunting in patients with septal defects. Deoxygenated blood bypasses the lungs and enters directly into the systemic circulation, producing cyanosis. The resulting pulmonary hypertension due to the reversal of the left-to-right shunt is known as **Eisenmenger's syndrome**, which manifests with cyanosis and other symptoms of hypoxaemia such as **finger clubbing** and **reticulosis** (a skin lesion).

Narrowing of the aorta or heart valves

Coarctation (narrowing) of the aorta most commonly occurs in the region of the aorta immediately below the point where the ductus arteriosus joins the aorta. It is usually due to tissue which forms the ductus extending into the aorta. When the ductus arteriosus constricts after birth, the area of aortic tissue also constricts, leading to a narrowing of the aorta and an increase in the load on the left ventricle, which can produce heart failure. The femoral pulses are weak and delayed due to the narrowing of the aorta impeding the pressure wave.

Congenital stenosis of the aortic or pulmonary valves produces raised ventricular pressure, leading to ventricular hypertrophy, low cardiac output and heart failure.

Complex developmental defects

Two complicated defects that produce cyanotic ('blue babies') lesions are **Fallot's tetralogy** and **transposition of the great arteries**.

Fallot's tetralogy

Fallot's tetralogy is a complicated defect, which consists of four simultaneous problems:

- A ventricular septal defect
- An overriding aorta: a misalignment of the aorta which then receives blood from both ventricles
- Stenosis of the pulmonary trunk (below the pulmonary valve)
- Right ventricular hypertrophy (caused by the stenosis)

The condition is thought to arise from a single defect in the position of the developing interventricular septum, which is displaced anteriorly. Due to the pulmonary stenosis there is a high right ventricular pressure which shunts blood to the left ventricle, bypassing the lungs. This leads to hypoxaemia and cyanosis.

Children with this condition often feel dizzy on exertion because the reduction in total peripheral resistance increases the proportion of blood flowing through the shunt. These dizzy spells can be alleviated by squatting, which increases the TPR by reducing blood flow in the femoral arteries. Early treatment may involve reduction of the pulmonary stenosis to improve pulmonary blood flow, prior to later surgical repair.

Transposition of the great arteries

Transposition of the great arteries occurs when the developing aortic and pulmonary arteries do not spiral correctly and the output of the left and right ventricles is reversed, going into the pulmonary trunk and aorta, respectively. Patients with this condition can only survive if there is a shunt, either an atrial or ventricular septal defect, or a patent ductus arteriosus. The shunt allows blood entering the right ventricle from the periphery to pass through the shunt into the left ventricle, from where it can enter the pulmonary circulation. Similarly, blood draining from the pulmonary veins can pass through the shunt and enter the aorta.

The only permanent treatment for this condition is surgical switching, although administration of PGE_1 to maintain the patency of the ductus arteriosus, or the insertion of a balloon catheter between the atria, can maintain the circulation prior to surgery.

12

Haematology

Drew Provan and Adrian C Newland

THE HAEMOPOIETIC SYSTEM

BLOOD AND ITS CONSTITUENTS

Blood is one of the body's largest tissues, comprising a mixture of cells within a fluid (plasma). Blood permeates all organs and tissues, and maintains homeostasis and body temperature, carries oxygen, acts as a buffering system, and has many other functions. Definitions and explanations of many of the terms that are used throughout the chapter are given in Table 12.1.

Blood plasma

Plasma makes up about 60% of our blood volume and is a complex mixture of water (90%) absorbed from the gut, proteins (8%), molecules such as glucose, and a variety of other dissolved chemicals.

Blood cells

The average adult has around 24×10^{12} red cells (making up a third of the total number of cells in the body), which live for around 120 days with a daily death rate of 2×10^{11} cells. This equates to the breakdown of 400×10^{12} haemoglobin molecules *per second* (Information box 12.1).

Red cells (erythrocytes)

Red cells are biconcave disc-shaped cells that lack a nucleus, since this is extruded while the cell is maturing in the bone

Information box 12.1   **Key features of blood**

A 70 kg man will have approximately:

- 5 L of blood:
  - 60% as plasma
  - 40% as cells – referred to as the packed cell volume (PCV).

The main blood cell types and their quantities are:

- Red blood cells: $4.5–6.5 \times 10^{12}$/L ($3.9–5.8 \times 10^{12}$/L females)
- White blood cells: $4–11 \times 10^{9}$/L
- Platelets: $150–400 \times 10^{9}$/L.

marrow (Fig. 12.1). The reason red cells have no nucleus is not known. Perhaps the cells are consequently more pliable and can travel through small blood vessels more easily. This cannot be the complete answer, however, since birds have red cells that contain nuclei. The diameter of a red cell is around 6.7–7.7 μm. The principal function of red cells is to carry oxygen and carbon dioxide round the body. The biconcave shape provides an increased surface area compared with a sphere, making gas exchange faster, and is maintained by a complex cytoskeletal system.

White blood cells (leucocytes)

There are several types of white blood cell (Fig. 12.1), but those most numerous in peripheral blood are neutrophils and lymphocytes. Other cell types found in blood, but in smaller numbers, are eosinophils, monocytes and basophils. Some

Table 12.1	Terms used in haematology
Term	**Explanation**
-aemia	Of the blood
Anisocytosis	Red cells of different sizes
APTT	Activated partial thromboplastin test
Bite cell	Irregular red cells with indentations that look like bites
Blast	Primitive blood cell
-cyte	Cell
ESR	Erythrocyte sedimentation rate
Haemoglobinuria	Red urine due to presence of haemoglobin from lysed red cells
Hyperplasia	Abnormal cellular increase
Hypochromic	Red cells with reduced haemoglobin
Leucopenia	Reduced white cell numbers
Macrocytic	Red cells that are larger than normal
MCH	Mean (red) cell haemoglobin in picograms (pg)
MCHC	Mean cell haemoglobin concentration in %
MCV	Mean cell volume in femtolitres (fL)
Megaloblast	Red cell precursor (blast) in bone marrow that is abnormally large (megalo)
Microcytic	Red cells that are smaller than normal
Normocytic	Red cells of a normal size
-osis	Too much
Pencil cells	Elongated red cells
-penia	Not enough
-philia	Affinity for
Poikilocytes	Red cells with abnormal shape
Polychromasia	Red cells showing a bluish tinge because they contain little haemoglobin
PT	Prothrombin time
Reticulocytes	Young red cells containing ribosomal remnants that can only be seen with reticulum stains – an increase in reticulocytes in blood is an indicator of increased red cell production
Spherocytes	Small red cells with no central pallor
Target cells	Red cells which appear pale but have a central dark area making them look like targets due to an increased surface membrane to volume ratio
Thrombocytopenia	Reduced platelet numbers
TT	Thrombin time

cells engulf foreign particles – they are phagocytic – for example neutrophils, eosinophils and monocytes/macrophages, while others are non-phagocytic, such as lymphocytes. White cells that have granules visible in their cytoplasm (neutrophils, eosinophils and basophils) are often referred to as granulocytes. White cells are an important part of the immune system, whose role is to protect the body from invading pathogens.

Neutrophils

Neutrophils are the commonest white cell found in peripheral blood (50–70% total white cells) with a lifespan of around 8–10 hours. Characteristically, the nucleus has two to five lobes. The cytoplasm has granules that contain proteolytic enzymes used to break down ingested material, such as pathogenic bacteria. The function of neutrophils is primary defence against bacteria and fungi. This defence is non-specific as neutrophils do not recognise specific antigens in the same way as other cells of the immune system, such as lymphocytes.

Neutrophils are attracted to sites of infection by chemo-attractant chemicals to which they are very sensitive. Chemo-attractant molecules include bacterial cell wall proteins and endothelial cell molecules, such as leukotrienes. The cells have receptors for a variety of adhesion molecules, such as fibronectin and complement, and migrate towards the site of infection.

Killing of ingested bacteria within neutrophils involves a variety of mechanisms including oxygen-dependent pathways. The various neutrophil granules contain several different proteins that fulfil the different functions of adhesion and bacterial killing; their release (neutrophil degranulation) is stimulated by leukotrienes and chemoattractants. The azurophilic granules contain enzymes that kill bacteria, such as lysozyme and myeloperoxidase, and others that facilitate the process, such as by increasing membrane permeability. The killing mechanism involves superoxide (O_2^-), hydrogen peroxide (H_2O_2) and other oxygen species, generated from O_2 and NADPH:

$$2O_2 + NADPH \rightarrow 2O_2^- + NADP^+ + H^+$$

Most of the O_2^- is converted into H_2O_2, which reacts with myeloperoxidase and halides in the neutrophils producing a series of toxic chemicals that are thought to kill the ingested microorganisms. A recent study in mice has suggested that the proteins cathepsin G and elastase are more important in this respect. Further, lactoferrin within the neutrophils binds iron, essential for bacterial growth, which therefore has a bacteriostatic effect.

Monocytes and macrophages

Monocytes are larger than neutrophils and make up around 5% of our circulating white cells. The nucleus is characteristically kidney shaped (indented) and there are usually vacuoles within the cytoplasm. Monocytes contain granules that store acid hydrolases and myeloperoxidase. Monocytes and macrophages can ingest pathogenic material, degrade it and present peptides or peptide fragments to T lymphocytes. Because of this function, monocytes and macrophages are called **antigen-presenting cells**, since they present antigen to these T cells. Monocytes circulate for about 10 hours in the blood before they mature into tissue macrophages. Their main role is to kill intracellular microorganisms, such as *Listeria*, mycobacteria and some fungi.

Eosinophils

Eosinophils make up 1–6% of the total white cells in a healthy individual and have a striking orange appearance due to the cytoplasm that takes up eosin dye when blood films are stained. Eosinophils circulate in the peripheral blood for 4–5 hours and then make their way to the tissues, where their main function is to provide defence against helminth (worm) parasitic infestations. Certain cytokines stimulate the increased production of these cells (**eosinophilia**).

Basophils

These dark-staining cells are present in peripheral blood in very small numbers (up 0.2% total white cell count). Basophils possess granules that contain a variety of mediators of inflammation including histamine, leukotrienes and proteases. After migrating to the tissues, basophils become

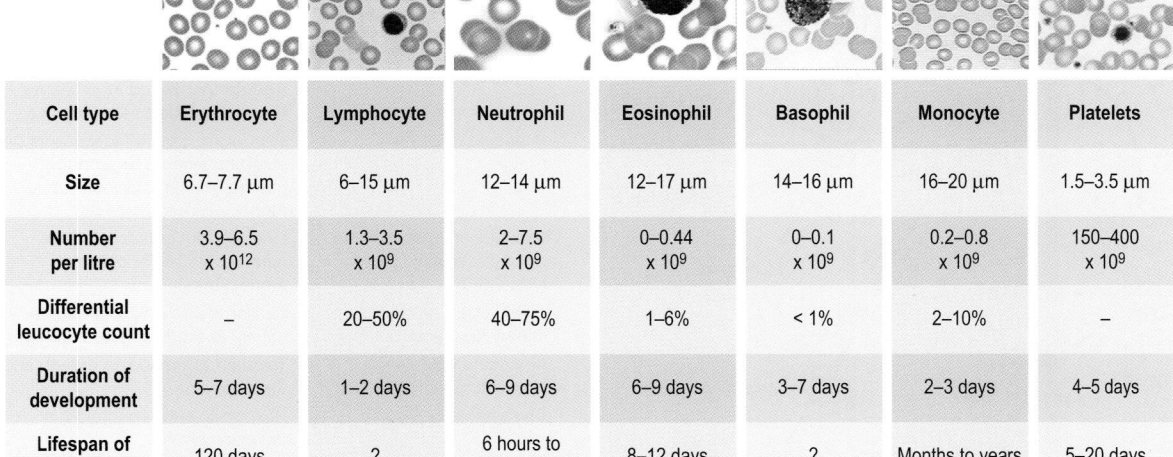

Cell type	Erythrocyte	Lymphocyte	Neutrophil	Eosinophil	Basophil	Monocyte	Platelets
Size	6.7–7.7 μm	6–15 μm	12–14 μm	12–17 μm	14–16 μm	16–20 μm	1.5–3.5 μm
Number per litre	3.9–6.5 x 10^{12}	1.3–3.5 x 10^{9}	2–7.5 x 10^{9}	0–0.44 x 10^{9}	0–0.1 x 10^{9}	0.2–0.8 x 10^{9}	150–400 x 10^{9}
Differential leucocyte count	–	20–50%	40–75%	1–6%	< 1%	2–10%	–
Duration of development	5–7 days	1–2 days	6–9 days	6–9 days	3–7 days	2–3 days	4–5 days
Lifespan of mature cell	120 days	?	6 hours to a few days	8–12 days	?	Months to years	5–20 days

Fig. 12.1 **Blood cells.** Redrawn with permission from Young B, Lowe JS, Stevens A et al 2006 Wheater's functional histology: a text and colour atlas, 5th edn. Churchill Livingstone, Edinburgh.

mast cells. Both basophils and mast cells possess receptors for the Fc portion of IgE, and after activation by IgE the cells degranulate, spilling their granule contents into the peripheral blood.

Lymphocytes

Most lymphocytes are small cells, roughly the same size as a red cell, with a round nucleus and very little cytoplasm. Lymphocytes make up 20–40% of all white blood cells. Their lifespan is much longer than the other white cells. Some may live for many years and act as 'memory' cells. There are two main types of lymphocyte, indistinguishable microscopically, called **B and T lymphocytes**. Functionally these have very different roles. Other types of lymphocyte, including **natural killer (NK) cells** have also been identified and these take part in antibody-dependent cellular cytotoxicity reactions.

Platelets

These small cells (Fig. 12.1) are actually fragments of **megakaryocytes** that bud off in the bone marrow before entering the peripheral blood, and are non-nucleated. Megakaryocyte nuclei are large polyploid structures with chromosome contents between diploid (2N) to 64N, where N is a single set of chromosomes. Such polyploid status is achieved through a process termed nuclear endoduplication, where there is successive doubling of the chromosome content in the absence of cell division. A single megakaryocyte can generate around 3000 platelets, of which 20–30% are pooled in the spleen. In health, the peripheral blood platelet count is 150–400 × 10^{9}/L but this fluctuates, for example following heavy exercise, 'stress', and throughout the menstrual cycle.

The main role of platelets is to plug a small hole in the blood vessel wall (primary haemostasis): when blood vessels are damaged the platelets form a primary plug, which stops or slows down bleeding, while the clotting cascade generates fibrin to seal off the damaged area. In health, platelets live for 10–12 days. Platelets have no nucleus but contain two types of granule: **dense bodies** and **α granules**. Dense bodies contain adenosine diphosphate (ADP), adenosine tri-

phosphate (ATP), 5-hydroxytryptamine (5-HT), calcium and pyrophosphate. The α granules contain platelet factor (PF) 4, β thrombospondin, platelet-derived growth factor (PDGF), von Willebrand's factor (vWF), fibrinogen, factor V and fibronectin. The contents of these granules are integral components of the platelet's biological activities, and are required for normal platelet function.

Stem cells and their role in haemopoiesis

Haemopoiesis is the production of new red cells, white cells and platelets, all of which have specialised functions throughout the body. The renewal of blood cells relies on the **stem cells**. Stem cells represent the most primitive form of blood cell that is capable of multiplying and they can generate cells of any lineage, e.g. red cell, granulocyte, lymphocyte and other cell types. Once a stem cell has begun to differentiate as it matures, it will no longer be able to produce new stem cells. There is a delicate balance in the bone marrow between stem cell multiplication (i.e. renewal) and differentiation. This is necessary because if there are insufficient numbers of stem cells, the number of mature cells falls. The mechanisms controlling stem cell renewal and differentiation are poorly understood but probably involve the **bone marrow stroma** and cytokines or other hormones interacting with stem cells. The stroma is the supporting network or matrix and is capable of passing signals to stem cells, as well as controlling various replicative pathways and differentiation events.

Stem cells are multipotent

There appear to be several types of stem cell, some more primitive (multipotent, or pluripotent) than others. A multipotent cell can differentiate into any cell type since the cell has not become committed to any specific lineage (Fig. 12.2).

There is a major difficulty in agreeing what constitutes a stem cell when looking at bone marrow in a stained preparation, since these are indistinct cells and look rather unremarkable, resembling small lymphocytes. Stem cells can,

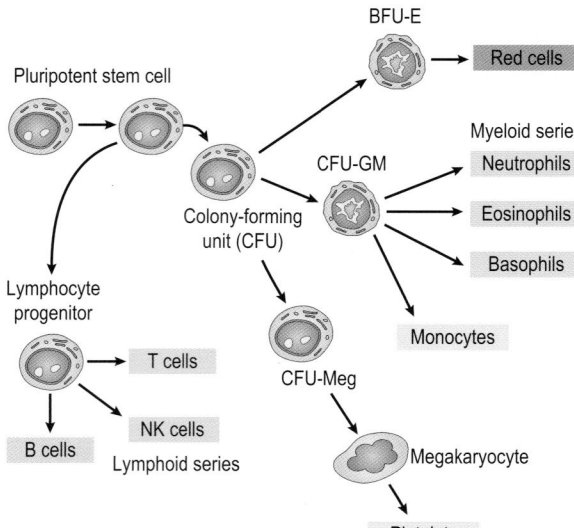

Fig. 12.2 **Growth factors act on stem cells and early progenitor cells to stimulate haemopoiesis.** BFU-E, erythroid burst-forming unit; CFU, colony-forming unit; GM, granulocyte macrophage; Meg, megakaryocyte; NK, natural killer.

however, be detected using monoclonal antibodies against specific cell membrane proteins such as CD34 (stem cell antigen) and CD38 (an activation marker). Stem cells are typically CD34 positive and CD38 negative.

BLOOD CELL PRODUCTION AND THE BONE MARROW MICROENVIRONMENT

Stem cells derive from mesenchymal tissue in the yolk sac, forming **blood islands** of stem cells at about 6 weeks of gestation, migrating initially to the fetal liver, then the spleen. By 6–7 months of development the stem cells migrate to the bone marrow, which is the principal site of haemopoiesis in children and adults. In haematological diseases haemopoiesis may take place at other sites, including the spleen and liver. This is termed **extramedullary haemopoiesis**.

Regulation of haemopoiesis

The bone marrow stroma

The marrow stroma provides the ideal environment for growth and development of stem cells. The stroma comprises blood vessels and specific supporting cell types including fat cells, fibroblasts, endothelial cells, macrophages and sinusoids. The stromal cells maintain the delicate cellular balance of the bone marrow by secreting a variety of hormones and other molecules such as collagen, fibronectin, thrombospondin and glycosaminoglycans, in addition to growth factors, or **cytokines**.

Growth factors

■ Coordination of the various growth factors is controlled by hormone production and their interaction with specific receptors on the developing cells (Table 12.2). Hormones or growth factors that play a major role in the

Table 12.2	Growth factors and their function
Growth factor	**Function**
Stem cell factor (SCF)	In the fetus: helps haemopoietic cells move from the yolk sac to liver and then bone marrow
	After birth: needed at all stages for normal blood cell production
Interleukin 3 (IL-3)	With other growth factors acts on early progenitors to produce mature red cells, granulocytes, monocytes and platelets
Granulocyte macrophage colony-stimulating factor (GM-CSF)	Like IL-3 but acts to produce neutrophils, eosinophils and monocytes
Granulocyte colony-stimulating factor (G-CSF)	Similar to GM-CSF but directed mainly at producing neutrophils
Monocyte colony-stimulating factor (M-CSF)	Targeted at monocyte growth and development
Erythropoietin (Epo)	Responsible for erythroid cell development
Thrombopoietin (Tpo)	Responsible for megakaryocytic development

Clinical box 12.1 | **Therapeutic use of growth factors**

Advances in molecular biology have meant that many growth factor genes have been cloned and sequenced, enabling the synthetic production of these molecules for therapeutic use. Because of the concern of inducing leukaemia if growth factors that act early in haemopoiesis are given, there is more emphasis on the clinical use of growth factors that act late and are lineage specific. Important clinical growth factors in use are:

● G-CSF – for treatment of patients with neutropenia
● Epo – used especially to treat anaemia associated with renal disease. rEpo is manufactured by inserting the relevant DNA sequence into a host cell, such as a bacterium, leading to a 'recombinant' rDNA that codes for the protein.

growth and differentiation of myeloid and erythroid cells are called **colony-stimulating factors** (**CSFs**), and those that are responsible for lymphocyte development are **lymphokines**. They are all glycoproteins.

Some growth factors act on more than one lineage; others act only on a single pathway, or at a particular state of haemopoiesis, stimulated by the acquisition of specific receptors on the cell surface. Usually more than one growth factor is involved in each stage of maturation (Fig. 12.3).

Haemopoietic receptors

The various growth factor receptors are distinct from other types of cell surface receptors, but, individually, are similar in structure and span the plasma membrane. Once receptors are bound by a growth factor they are activated, forming a dimeric complex with another receptor unit. These complexes can activate tyrosine kinase, which signals the start of cell division.

■ Chromosome 5 carries many of the receptor genes in a small area on the long arm and deletions in this region are associated with the development of acute leukaemia.

Growth factors are also synthesised for therapeutic use (Clinical box 12.1).

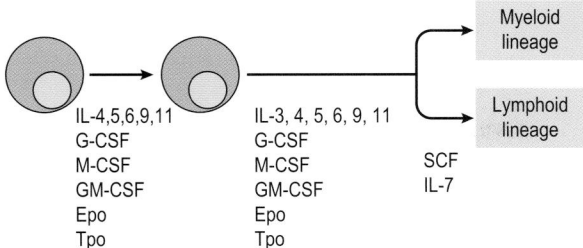

Fig. 12.3 Many growth factors are required in concert to drive differentiation of stem cells. IL, interleukin; G-CSF, granulocyte colony-stimulating factor; M-CSF, monocyte colony-stimulating factor; GM-CSF, granulocyte macrophage-colony stimulating factor; Epo, erythropoietin; Tpo, thrombopoietin; SCF, stem cell factor.

> ### *i* Information box 12.2 — Disordered erythropoiesis occurs in severe anaemia
>
> Severe anaemia stimulates rapid red cell production in one or two days. The stress produced by anaemia results in red blood cells that:
>
> - Are macrocytic (due to skipped cell division)
> - Possess the i (fetal) red cell surface antigen instead of the I (adult) antigen (due to insufficient time to go through the biochemical process needed for the change)
> - Have inclusion bodies (debris that is normally produced but accumulates due to the rapid processing of the cell from marrow to blood). Many inclusion bodies are removed as cells pass through the spleen by a process known as 'pitting' in which small parts of the cell are removed.

RED CELLS

The main function of red cells is delivery of oxygen from the lungs to the tissues. The bone marrow produces approximately 10^{10} cells per hour in order to maintain a steady state, but must be able to adapt rapidly to maintain oxygen delivery in situations where blood is lost.

The production of red cells from stem cells is driven by various transcription factors that further influence the expression of growth factors and adhesion molecules necessary for cell differentiation.

TRANSCRIPTION FACTORS IN ERYTHROPOIESIS

Tal-1/SCL

This factor is thought to be important at very early stages of erythropoiesis, at the multipotent or myeloid-erythroid stem cell level. Studies in mice have shown that disrupting the gene for this factor results in uterine death with no blood production, whereas an overexpression leads to increased erythroid differentiation.

Rbtn2/LMO2

This protein, rhombotin 2, seems to form a complex with Tal-1/SCL and is of similar importance, as mice lacking the gene also cannot produce blood and die in utero.

GATA-2

Laboratory animals, such as zebrafish, provide the opportunity for much molecular research. GATA-2 expression in this animal is associated with areas of haemopoiesis. Also found on multipotent stem cells, increased expression of GATA-2 leads to proliferation of these cells, and a reduction results in a loss of haemopoiesis.

GATA-1

While GATA-1 is found in association with multipotent progenitors and several blood cell lineages, its absence leads to a failure of erythroid cell production with cells not developing beyond the primitive proerythroblast. The interaction between GATA proteins and another transcription factor, **PU.1**, appears to influence whether uncommitted stem cells commit to either the erythroid or myeloid lineages; overexpression of PU.1 leads to cells developing down the myeloid lineage.

GROWTH FACTORS IN ERYTHROPOIESIS

Committed erythroid cell production begins with the primitive **erythroid burst-forming unit (BFU-E)**. With a combination of growth factors the erythroid progenitors divide to form **erythroid colony-forming units (CFU-E)** that subsequently develop sequentially into **proerythroblasts** (the earliest recognisable erythroid cell), **erythroblasts**, **normoblasts** and **reticulocytes**, where the nucleus is then extruded to form the mature red cell over about five days. Erythropoiesis may speed up in certain clinical conditions (Information box 12.2).

The most important of the growth factors is **erythropoietin or Epo**, which appears to be essential for the differentiation of the CFU-E progenitors. Other growth factors involved in erythropoiesis include SF (Steel factor) – 'Steel mutant' mice are very anaemic – interleukin (IL)-3, GM-CSF, insulin and activin.

Erythropoietin controls the red cell mass

The rate of production of red cells is governed by erythropoietin, a glycosylated protein of 165 amino acids produced by the kidney (90%), and to a lesser extent by the liver. Glycosylation is a *post-translational modification* and adds sugar molecules to the protein, which helps prolong its half-life.

The body has no stores of erythropoietin and its regulation is at the gene transcription (i.e. mRNA) level. This means that when Epo is needed the DNA must be transcribed into mRNA, which is then translated into protein. The **hypoxia-inducible factor-1 (HIF-1)** has two subunits, α and β. The α form interacts with oxygen sensors to activate Epo transcription. It is seen only in hypoxic (low oxygen) situations; when oxygen levels reach a high level a molecule hydroxylates HIF-1α, which then binds to **von Hippel–Lindau (VHL) protein**, activating a ligase complex that destroys HIF-1α so that Epo transcription is rapidly stopped.

The kidney responds to reduced oxygen tension with production of erythropoietin by the interstitial peritubular cells, resulting in a higher rate of red cell production by stimulating proliferation of BFU-E and CFU-E. As the number of red cells increases, so does the oxygen delivery to the

Information box 12.3 **Secondary polycythaemia**

Secondary polycythaemia results from an increased production of erythropoietin, leading to increased red cell production. It can be due to a number of causes:

Cause	Reasons	Explanation
Decreased oxygen concentration	High altitude	Low ambient oxygen concentration
	Sleep apnoea (stopping breathing while asleep)	Hypoventilation of the lung alveoli
	High levels of carboxyhaemoglobin from carbon monoxide exposure	Exposure to smoking or exhaust fumes
Impaired blood perfusion of the kidneys	Blocked or thickened renal arteries	
	Renal failure	
	Renal transplantation	
Increased stimulation of Epo	Tumours secreting Epo	
	Chuvash polycythaemia	Mutation in VHL gene, preventing Epo production from being switched off
	Blood doping	Self-administration of rEpo by athletes resulting in an increase in red cells, and thus the oxygen carrying capacity

tissues and erythropoietin production falls (Fig. 12.4). It is believed that erythropoiesis is controlled by the kidneys because the kidney represents the only organ in which oxygen consumption parallels blood flow.

Epo production involves a negative feedback loop

As the number of red cells increases, and the red cell mass rises, oxygen is delivered more easily to tissues. The kidney senses this increase in oxygen delivery and erythropoietin levels drop. Where oxygen levels are low (**hypoxia**), erythropoietin levels rise, and red cell production increases, until oxygenation returns to normal. In effect, this is a simple feedback loop (Fig. 12.5). An abnormal increased production of erythropoietin leads to the clinical condition of polycythaemia (Information box 12.3).

STROMAL MOLECULES IN ERYTHROPOIESIS

In addition to haemopoietic cells the bone marrow stroma contains endothelial cells, fibroblasts, macrophages and associated stromal proteins. The stroma appears to have several functions that are essential for cell differentiation and facilitating release of cells from the marrow.

- Adhesion proteins, such as **fibronectin**, bind to the **very late antigen** (**VLA**) on erythroid cells; as the cell differentiates into a reticulocyte the adhesion is lost. Interaction between VLA on erythroid cells and the **vascular adhesion molecule** (**VAM-1**) is also thought to be important.
- **Macrophage deoxyribonuclease II** may be instrumental in the ability for red cells to lose their nuclei.
- Cells must pass through small endothelial pores in order to enter the blood and need to be flexible. Only mature cells have that flexibility.

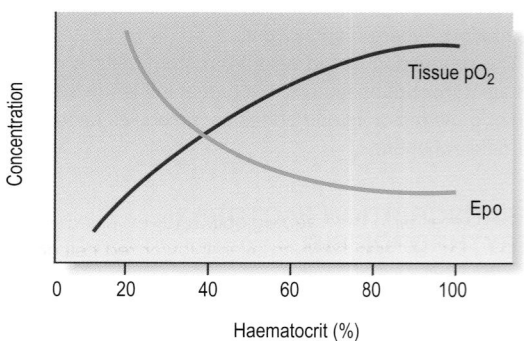

Fig. 12.4 **Erythropoietin (Epo) levels are driven by tissue oxygenation, in an inverse relationship.** Redrawn with permission from Provan A, Gribben J 2005 Molecular Haematology, 2nd edn. Blackwell, Oxford.

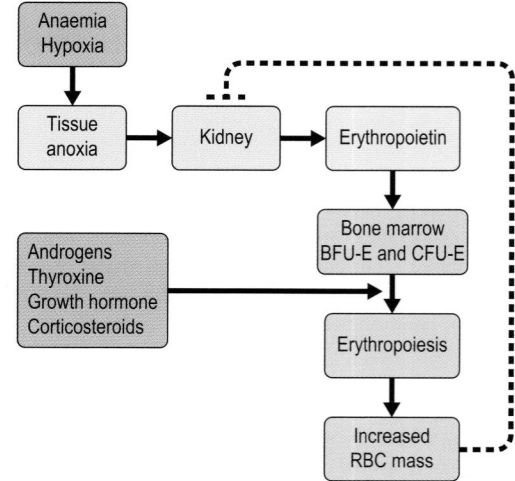

Fig. 12.5 **Oxygen levels are sensed by the kidney, which then modulates Epo production in combination with other hormones.** BFU-E, erythroid burst-forming unit; CFU-E, erythroid colony-forming unit; RBC, red blood cell.

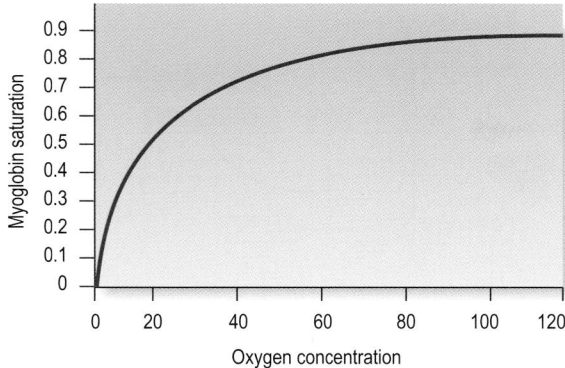

Fig. 12.6 **Myoglobin saturation curve.**

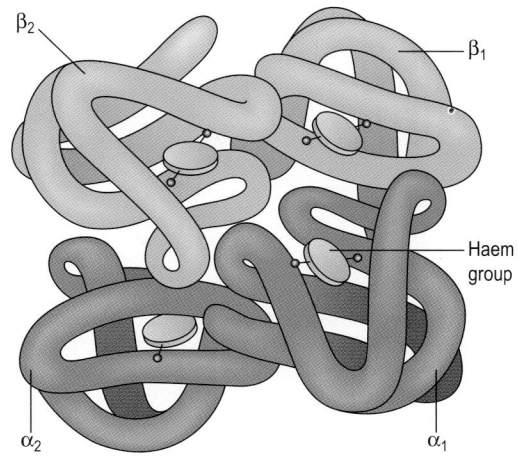

Fig. 12.7 **A haemoglobin molecule is made up of two α and two β globin chains and four haem groups.**

Other hormones that influence haemoglobin production

Although erythropoietin is the main hormone controlling red cell production, other hormones such as corticosteroids, androgens, growth hormone and thyroxine also play a role.

Red cell production during life

- Babies are born with very high red cell counts and high haemoglobin levels, since fetal haemoglobin binds oxygen very tightly, shifting the **oxygen dissociation curve** to the left. This is a normal physiological adaptation.
- Soon after birth the haemoglobin and red cell count drop and children have an overall lower red cell count and haemoglobin level than adults.
- After puberty, under the hormonal control of the androgen testosterone, males have higher haemoglobin levels than females.
- Finally, elderly people have lower haemoglobin levels than their younger counterparts, but males retain a higher level in comparison with elderly females.

TRANSPORT OF OXYGEN BY HAEMOGLOBIN

At rest an adult uses around 0.25 L of oxygen per minute. Oxygen consumption and carbon dioxide production increase dramatically with exercise. In general, oxygen is not particularly soluble in water and requires a carrier molecule to transport it from the lungs to the tissues. Respiratory pigments serve this purpose, and in humans take the form of **haemoglobin** and **myoglobin**. In both of these molecules oxygen molecules are bound to Fe^{2+} within the haem moiety.

- **Myoglobin** is found predominantly in muscle and is made up of a single globin protein chain with an associated haem group, which has an iron core (Fe^{2+}). Oxygen binds to myoglobin and easily saturates the molecule, resulting in a hyperbolic curve (Fig. 12.6).
- **Haemoglobin**, by comparison, is a tetramer (2α-like + 2β-like globins) each subunit of which has an associated haem group (Fig. 12.7).

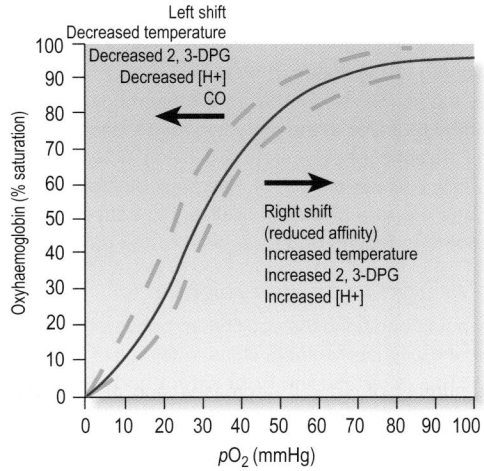

Fig. 12.8 **The oxygen dissociation curve.** 2,3-DPG, 2,3-diphosphoglycerate. Adapted from Baynes WJ, Dominiczak M 2004 Medical biochemistry, 2nd edn. Mosby, Edinburgh.

The oxygen dissociation curve

Binding of oxygen to the first haem is quite difficult, but as each haem takes up an oxygen molecule, the binding of subsequent oxygen molecules becomes easier, resulting in a sigmoid-shaped curve, which flattens out when haemoglobin becomes saturated with oxygen (Fig. 12.8). At the steepest part of the curve a small change in oxygen tension (pO_2 concentration) results in rapid release or uptake of oxygen (reflected in the large change in haemoglobin oxygen saturation). This ensures rapid delivery to the tissues where oxygen tensions are lower.

When blood returns to the lungs, carbon dioxide will diffuse out into the alveoli to be breathed out. Blood pCO_2 will be reduced, and pH will increase (becoming more alkali) – due to a decrease in blood carbonic acid. The curve will shift to the left and, at any given alveolar pO_2, the amount of oxygen that binds to haemoglobin will increase.

At the capillaries, carbon dioxide diffuses in from the tissues – the curve shifts to the right as the blood becomes more acidic and oxygen will be displaced from haemoglobin, delivering oxygen to the tissues.

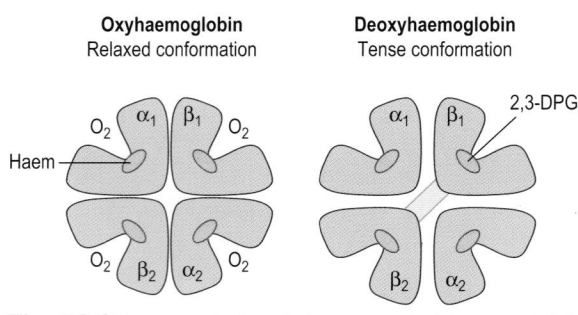

Oxyhaemoglobin
Relaxed conformation

Deoxyhaemoglobin
Tense conformation

Fig. 12.9 Oxygenated and deoxygenated haemoglobin molecules. 2,3-DPG, 2,3-diphosphoglycerate. Redrawn with permission from Hoffbrand AV, Perit JE 1993 Essential haematology, 3rd edn. Blackwells, Oxford.

In order to function as an oxygen carrier, haemoglobin needs a high affinity for oxygen in the lungs and a low affinity for oxygen in the tissues. Haemoglobin exists in two principal tertiary forms: **relaxed** (R), with high oxygen affinity, and **tense** (T) in the absence of oxygen, with a low affinity for oxygen (Fig. 12.9). Induced by lower levels of oxygen in the tissue, oxygen is released from the haemoglobin molecule. The α and β chains in the molecule rotate, allowing the entry of the 2,3-diphosphoglycerate (2,3-DPG) molecule. This then produces a lower affinity of haemoglobin for oxygen and increases the rate of oxygen delivery in active tissues. This is reflected in Figure 12.8 by a 'shift to the right'.

Role of acid in oxygen release

Under acid conditions the equilibrium between deoxyhaemoglobin and oxyhaemoglobin shifts in favour of deoxyhaemoglobin. This is termed the **Bohr Effect** and is very useful in physiological terms, since oxygen will dissociate from haemoglobin when muscle tissue is acidic. The acidity occurs during exercise when carbohydrates are metabolised to lactic acid in an anaerobic reaction. This is shown by the oxygen dissociation curve shifting to the right under the influence of H^+ ions.

At any pO_2 level the oxygen saturation of blood is much lower in a right shifted curve, reflecting the move of oxygen into the tissues. Typically the partial pressure of oxygen in body cells is about 40 mmHg, when the haemoglobin saturation will be around 70%. At this same partial pressure, when the curve is shifted to the right, the haemoglobin saturation reduces to around 60% as oxygen is released.

Role of 2,3-DPG in oxygen release from haemoglobin

2,3-Diphosphoglycerate (2,3-DPG) is a by-product of glycolysis and present in red cells at the same concentration as haemoglobin. The binding of more 2,3-DPG to haemoglobin promotes the release of oxygen to the tissues.

Levels of 2,3-DPG rise during exercise, altitude and anaemia, shifting the oxygen dissociation curve to the right, ensuring that oxygen is off-loaded more easily.

TRANSPORT OF CARBON DIOXIDE

Carbon dioxide is taken from the tissues where it is produced, and eventually ends up in the lungs where it is breathed out. CO_2 carriage is more complex than oxygen transport. Figure 12.10 illustrates this.

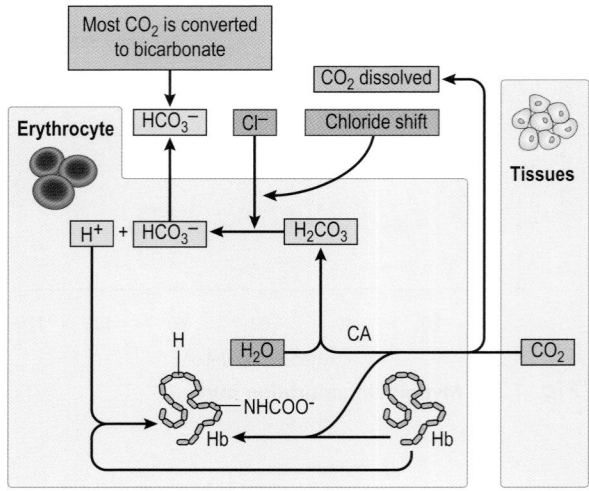

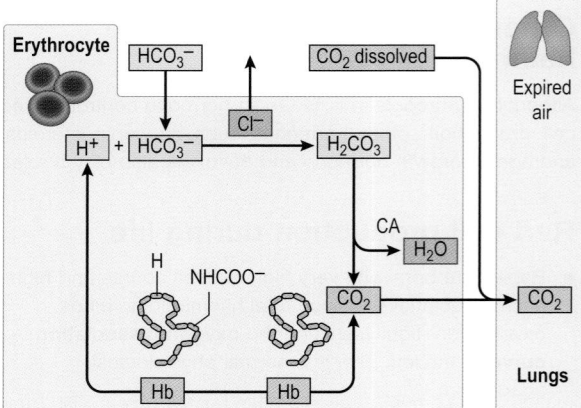

Fig. 12.10 The role of red cells in CO₂ transport. Most of the CO_2 produced in tissues is converted to HCO_3^- for transport to the lungs: approximately 20% of the total amount is transported bound to haemoglobin as carbamino groups, and small amounts are transported as dissolved gas in plasma. CA, carbonic anhydrase. Redrawn from Baynes WJ, Dominiczak M 2005 Medical biochemistry, 2nd edn. Mosby, Edinburgh.

- In the tissues, CO_2 is produced from catabolic reactions and enters the red cell where the enzyme carbonic anhydrase converts it to **carbonic acid** (H_2CO_3). The release of oxygen from oxyhaemoglobin buffers the acidic carbonic acid by taking up H^+ ions and releasing bicarbonate HCO_3^-, which diffuses back into the plasma and is carried in the venous circulation back to the lungs. The movement of HCO_3^- into the plasma is counterbalanced by the movement of chloride ions (Cl^-) into the red cell (**chloride shift**). This exchange maintains electroneutrality.

- About 10% of CO_2 is transported as **carbamino haemoglobin**, where it is covalently linked to the N-terminal valine residues of the haemoglobin subunits:

$$CO_2 + HbN \rightarrow HbNH \cdot COO^- + H^+$$

Thus further H^+ ions are available, in addition to those released from carbonic acid. Not all are taken up by haemoglobin and thus venous blood plasma is more acidic (reflected by the higher pCO_2 and lower pO_2) than arterial blood.

On arrival at the lungs, the reduced haemoglobin is oxygenated and this results in release of H^+ ions. For HCO_3^- to move back into the red cell, the negatively charged chloride ion must take its place, and the H^+ ions react with HCO_3^- to produce H_2CO_3 again. Here the carbonic anhydrase catalyses the reverse reaction, releasing H_2O and CO_2 gas, which then diffuses out of the capillaries to be expired through the lungs.

THE RED CELL MEMBRANE

Like most cell membranes of higher organisms, the red cell membrane is a lipid bilayer made up of phospholipids, cholesterol and glycolipids. The protein compartment contains about 10–15 major proteins and many minor proteins, including band 3 protein (anion exchange channel) and glycophorins.

The cell membrane and cytoskeleton are responsible for maintaining the disc shape of the red blood cell, but at the same time must allow great flexibility in order to allow the red cells to travel through blood vessels that are much narrower than the red cell diameter.

Spectrin

This is the major structural protein. It is 100 nm long, is highly pliable, and comprises two subunits, α and β. Each subunit is made up of tandem repeats (106 amino acid repeats). The subunits are aligned side by side and form heterodimers, cross-linked at their tail ends by **actin** filaments. The membrane cytoskeleton is linked to integral proteins in the lipid bilayer by **ankyrin** and **protein 4.1**. Ankyrin binds to β spectrin near a self-association site and links it to the cytoplasmic portion of band 3. This meshwork of proteins, which underlies the plasma membrane, restricts the lateral mobility of the integral proteins.

We know that these are important molecules since mice lacking spectrin or ankyrin have gross haemolysis (increased red cell breakdown). In humans, diseases such as **hereditary spherocytosis** and **hereditary elliptocytosis** are caused by defects in the red cell membrane (see the section on inherited anaemias).

HAEMOGLOBIN

Haemoglobin molecules each comprise four polypeptides, two α-like and two β-like globin molecules, in addition to a haem group, which is synthesised in the mitochondria.

The main adult haemoglobin is **HbA**, which comprises two α globin and two β globin polypeptide chains ($\alpha_2\beta_2$). Other important haemoglobins found in adults are **HbA$_2$** ($\alpha_2\delta_2$) and **HbF** ($\alpha_2\gamma_2$).

Coordinating haemoglobin production throughout life

Different types of globin molecule are produced at varying stages of human development. After conception the human embryo produces three types of early Hb called haemoglobins **Gower 1**, **Gower 2** and **Portland** (Table 12.3). The structure of these molecules follows the same rules as all Hb molecules, namely two α-like globin molecules linked to two β-like globin molecules to produce the familiar tetrameric structure.

The genes for all globins related to α globin are found on chromosome 16, the β-like globins are found on chromo-

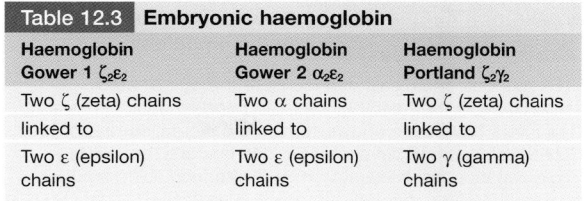

Table 12.3	Embryonic haemoglobin	
Haemoglobin Gower 1 $\zeta_2\epsilon_2$	**Haemoglobin Gower 2 $\alpha_2\epsilon_2$**	**Haemoglobin Portland $\zeta_2\gamma_2$**
Two ζ (zeta) chains linked to	Two α chains linked to	Two ζ (zeta) chains linked to
Two ϵ (epsilon) chains	Two ϵ (epsilon) chains	Two γ (gamma) chains

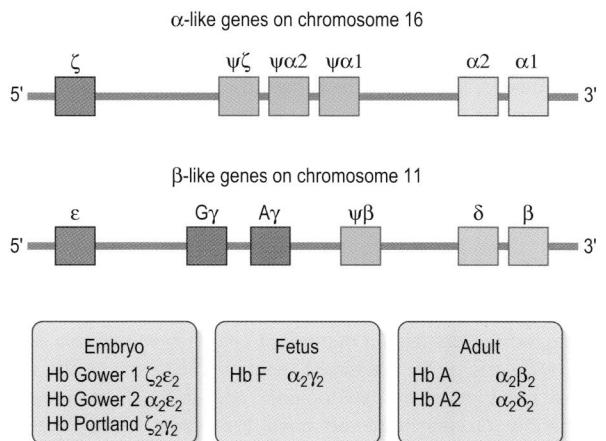

Fig. 12.11 **Arrangement of globin-producing genes on chromosomes and haemoglobins formed during human development.** Adapted with permission from Kumar P, Clark M 2002 Clinical medicine. WB Saunders, Edinburgh.

some 11, and the order of the different genes on each of the chromosomes reflects the order in which different haemoglobin molecules are produced during embryonic development.

Figure 12.11 illustrates the arrangement of α-like globin genes on chromosome 16 and the β-like globin genes on chromosome 11. Three pseudogenes Ψ (psi) are also present on chromosome 16 and one pseudogene on chromosome 11.

- From left to right, ζ (zeta) is the first α-like globin to be produced in the embryo by the ζ gene. After ζ expression stops, α is switched on (so-called $\zeta \rightarrow \alpha$ switch), resulting in the production of a α globin chains.
- On chromosome 11 the arrangement of β-like globins follows the order (from left to right) ϵ (epsilon) $\rightarrow \gamma$ (gamma) $\rightarrow \delta$ (delta) $\rightarrow \beta$, which mirrors the β-like globin chains produced during development. There are two γ genes, Gγ and Aγ, differing only by one amino acid, guanine and alanine, respectively, at position 136.

As the embryo develops into a fetus, production of ζ stops and α is produced instead. α-Globin combines with γ chains and produces $\alpha_2\gamma_2$, which is also called **fetal haemoglobin or HbF**. Both G and A forms are produced. HbF is the main haemoglobin type in the fetus leading up to birth.

After birth, γ chain production drops and both δ and β chains are produced. The main adult Hb is **HbA** ($\alpha_2\beta_2$) although a small amount of **HbA$_2$** ($\alpha_2\delta_2$) and **HbF** ($\alpha_2\gamma_2$) is produced.

The mechanisms underlying the switch are, at least in part, physiological. We know that HbF ($\alpha_2\gamma_2$) binds oxygen much more tightly than adult Hb (oxygen dissociation curve shifts to the left). This ensures adequate oxygen delivery to the developing fetus, which has to extract its oxygen from the mother's circulation. After birth the lungs expand, the oxygen is derived from the air the baby breathes and β chains are produced instead of γ, leading to an increase in adult Hb ($\alpha_2\beta_2$).

RED CELL ENZYMES ARE REQUIRED TO MAINTAIN RED CELL COMPONENTS

The red cell contains a number of enzymes whose role is to provide energy for metabolic reactions. In addition, the red cell must maintain haemoglobin and red cell membrane integrity. Oxygen transport does not require energy but, in order to survive for around 120 days, the red cell membrane requires regular maintenance and this relies on energy.

The following maintenance processes require energy:

- Red cell membrane integrity
- Red cell enzymes and haemoglobin sulphydryl groups must be maintained in reduced form
- Red cell shape (biconcave disc)
- Haem iron must be kept in reduced (Fe^{2+}) form
- K^+ and Ca^{2+} gradients.

If there is insufficient energy the red cell cannot maintain these functions, ionic gradients fail and the red cell adopts a spherical shape (**spherocyte**). These abnormal cells are quickly removed by the spleen and by other reticuloendothelial (phagocytic) cells. In addition, during a normal day, about 2% of the total body haemoglobin becomes oxidised to form **methaemoglobin**. The latter cannot combine with oxygen and is functionally useless, requiring energy to re-reduce it to its functional form. Abnormally increased methaemoglobin compromises tissue oxygenation (Information box 12.4).

Glucose is the main source of red cell energy

Glucose is metabolised mainly via the glycolytic pathway (see Ch. 3), which uses glucose in a series of steps that do not require oxygen (**anaerobic**).

One mole of glucose generates 2 moles of ATP, with lactate and pyruvate as the end-products of the pathway. NADH, required to maintain Hb in the reduced ferrous form, is produced in the glycolytic pathway. About 10% of the glucose is metabolised in the **pentose phosphate pathway** (also called the **hexose monophosphate shunt**) and results in the generation of NADPH, a cofactor required to maintain glutathione on the red cell membrane in its reduced form.

Since red cells lack a nucleus there is no capacity for further gene transcription. Instead the red cell must maintain its cell membrane and haemoglobin molecules using only the mRNA and enzymes it already contains. The red cell probably has enough mRNA to manufacture enzymes for a few days after losing its nucleus and leaving the bone marrow, but for most of its life it will rely on the preformed red cell enzymes for all these housekeeping functions.

MAINTENANCE AND RECYCLING OF RED CELLS

Fate of old red cells

Normal red cells live for around 120 days, showing signs of age towards the end of this time:

- Become more rigid
- Glycolysis slows down
- ATP levels fall
- Membrane lipid levels reduce
- Cell gradually desiccates
- Haemoglobin cross-links to spectrin
- Antibodies are produced against neoantigens (new antigens) that have been revealed by ageing.

The markers of senescence are poorly understood but it is likely that increasing red cell rigidity, caused by a reduction in normal red cell enzyme function, marks red cells for destruction by the reticuloendothelial system. Old red cells are phagocytosed and digested by macrophages found throughout the reticuloendothelial system, and particularly within the spleen.

Recycling of red cell components

At the end of their life, red cells are broken down (around 1% each day) and most constituents are used in the production of new red cells (Fig. 12.12).

- Free haemoglobin is released into plasma and binds avidly to **haptoglobin** (**Hp**), an 85 kDa α2 glycoprotein present in plasma. The HpHb complex is rapidly cleared by the liver. Excess haemoglobin can result in its excretion in the urine (Information box 12.5).
- Iron from the haem group is released and recycled via plasma **transferrin**, which passes the recycled iron to developing red cells in the marrow (these cells expressing transferrin receptors).
- The haem porphyrin ring is broken down and generates unconjugated **bilirubin**, which is transported bound to albumin. After processing by liver hepatocytes, bilirubin becomes conjugated and excreted as **urobilinogen** in urine and through the gut.

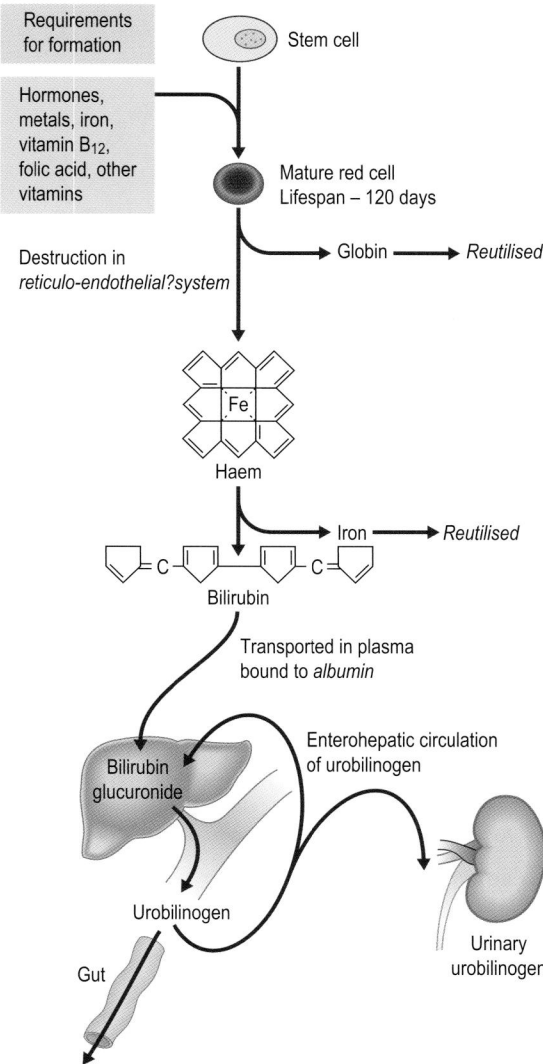

Fig. 12.12 Steps in the production and breakdown of red blood cells. Redrawn with permission from Kumar P, Clark M 2005 Clinical medicine, 6th edn. Elsevier Saunders, Edinburgh.

Table 12.4	Clinical indications of anaemia	
Signs more likely		**Signs less likely**
Severe anaemia		Mild anaemia
Elderly		Younger patients
Sudden drop in haemoglobin concentration		Gradual drop in haemoglobin
Other pathologies e.g. cardiorespiratory disease		Absence of other diseases

Table 12.5	Symptoms and signs of anaemia	
Symptoms of anaemia		**Signs**
Tiredness		Pallor, e.g. seen by looking at palmar creases, nail bed, conjunctivae (all generally unreliable in the assessment of anaemia)
Fainting		Rapid heart beat (**tachycardia**)
Shortness of breath		Bounding pulse
Worsening of heart-related pain (**angina**) or pain in limbs (**claudication**)		Systolic flow murmur
Rapid heart beat (**palpitations**)		Cardiac failure
		Retinal haemorrhages

ANAEMIAS

General features of anaemia

The term **anaemia** implies a reduction in red cell haemoglobin concentration, in comparison with that found in a population of similar age and sex (Table 12.4). Anaemia is not a diagnosis in itself as there is always an underlying cause.

Mostly the signs and symptoms of anaemia simply reflect a reduction in haemoglobin concentration, and hence delivery of O_2 to the tissues. These may be minimal or even absent, especially if the anaemia is mild and the individual is physically fit.

Anaemia in an adult male is defined as having a haemoglobin level of less than 13.5 g/dL and in a female of less than 11.5 g/dL. Anaemia is the commonest blood disorder worldwide, affecting some 30% of the world population.

Signs and symptoms may be general, and found in all types of anaemia, or specific and limited to specific causes of anaemia. The signs and symptoms of anaemia may reflect the fact that less oxygen is being delivered to tissues, or may be the result of the compensatory mechanisms that try to restore oxygen delivery towards normal (Table 12.5).

Physiological adaptations to anaemia

The body is equipped with a variety of mechanisms that are able to offset the effects of a reduced haemoglobin level and these explain, in part, why individuals with reduced haemoglobin may have very few symptoms. As discussed earlier, 2,3-DPG binding to β globin shifts the oxygen dissociation curve to the right, making haemoglobin offload oxygen to tissues more easily. With increased 2,3-DPG, oxygen delivery may increase by 40%.

Tissues and perfusion

The total blood volume in anaemia is generally much the same as normal, but blood may be diverted from less vital tissues, such as the skin and kidney, to more vital organs such as the heart, brain and muscle in an attempt to increase the flow of oxygen to sites which need it for energy production.

Cardiovascular system

As the haemoglobin drops to below 7–8 g/dL, the output of blood from the heart is increased, with an increase in heart rate and stroke volume. This is usually well tolerated, unless the individual has coexisting cardiovascular disease, such as coronary heart disease, in which case **angina** (heart pain) may develop or worsen.

Classification of anaemia

(1) Using the mean cell volume (MCV)

As with most diseases, anaemias may be:

- **Acute** (sudden) or **chronic** (of long standing)
- Inherited or acquired
- Primary or secondary.

Table 12.6	Causes of different forms of anaemia according to red cell volume	
Small red cells		
MCV <76 fL		
Microcytic	Iron deficiency Thalassaemia	
Normal sized red cells		
MCV normal		
Normocytic	Acute blood loss Anaemia of chronic disease e.g. infections, malignancy, connective tissue diseases Renal failure Hypothyroidism Bone marrow infiltration with leukaemia, or other cancers	
Large red cells		
MCV >96 fL		
Macrocytic	Megaloblastic marrow	Vitamin B$_{12}$ or folate deficiency
	Normoblastic marrow	Alcohol
		Myelodysplasia

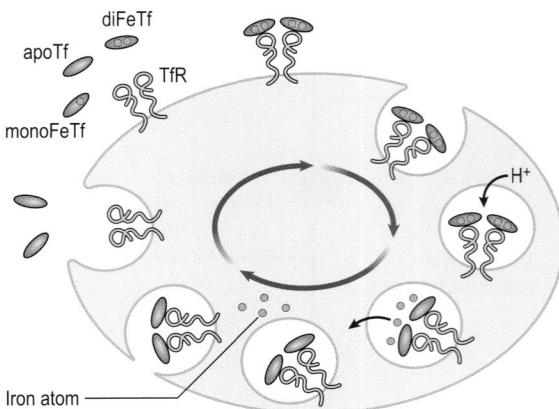

Fig. 12.13 **Schematic representation of cellular iron uptake.** Tf, transferrin; TfR, transferrin receptor; monoFeTf, transferrin bound to 1 iron atom; diFeTf, transferrin bound to 2 iron atoms; apoTf, transferrin lacking bound iron.

Classification of anaemias on the basis of the red cell size is also useful and helps the clinician to select investigations that are likely to determine the underlying cause (Table 12.6).

The MCV in anaemia may be **normocytic**, **microcytic** or **macrocytic** and will be associated with differing conditions. For example:

- Normocytic anaemia is associated with **renal failure**
- Microcytic anaemia is associated with **iron deficiency**
- Macrocytic anaemia is associated with **vitamin B$_{12}$ deficiency**

(2) Acquired or inherited

There are many reasons for developing anaemia. These can be due to acquired or inherited conditions. While some are discussed in some detail (shown in bold in the Table 12.7), the reader is advised to consult a specialist haematological text for more information about other causes.

Acquired anaemias due to deficiencies

Iron deficiency

Iron is one of the commonest elements on the earth but, despite this, iron deficiency is the commonest cause of anaemia worldwide. Iron is a key component of haemoglobin and without iron there is a defective synthesis of haemoglobin, resulting in red cells that are both microcytic and **hypochromic**.

Iron metabolism

Iron plays a major role in many metabolic processes, but carriage of oxygen by haemoglobin, where it is the core component, is the most important.

The average adult contains 3–5 g of iron, of which two-thirds is in the oxygen-carrying molecule haemoglobin. A normal Western diet provides about 15 mg of iron daily, of which only 5–10% is absorbed (~1 mg), principally in the proximal end of the small intestine where the acidic conditions help its absorption in the ferrous form. The body can increase its iron absorption if there is increased demand, e.g. in pregnancy, lactation, growth spurts, and iron deficiency. Table 12.8 lists the average daily iron requirements.

Once absorbed from the bowel, iron is transported across the mucosal cell to the blood, where it is carried by the protein **transferrin** to developing red cells in the bone marrow.

Our bodies have two main types of iron store:

- **Ferritin**, a readily accessible source of iron, and
- **Haemosiderin**, an insoluble form of storage iron found mainly in macrophages.

Iron loss

Only around 1 mg of iron a day is lost from the body in urine, faeces, sweat, and cells shed from the skin and gastrointestinal tract. Menstrual losses of an additional 20 mg a month and the increased requirements of pregnancy (500–1000 mg) contribute to the higher incidence of iron deficiency in women of reproductive age. Humans have no specific mechanism for eliminating iron from the body other than the passive mechanisms listed above. In the adult male 90% of cycling iron is that released from old recycled red blood cells.

Iron is transported by **transferrin** to developing red blood cells where it is reused. Some 20 mg iron is recycled daily for erythropoiesis, and several milligrams are required to replenish the haem and non-haem iron of cycling tissue cells. Figure 12.13 illustrates the uptake of iron by the cells. The transferrin receptor (TfR) expressed on the cell surface binds transferrin (Tf) when bound to two iron atoms. The Tf-TfR complex is internalised, iron dissociates, moves into cytosol, and Tf-TfR recycles to plasma and dissociates. Unbound transferrin, measured as the **total iron binding capacity (TIBC)** in plasma will be increased when iron levels are low.

Iron homeostasis: regulation of ferritin and transferrin receptor levels

Iron balance relies on two proteins that readily take up iron:

- **Transferrin**, responsible for iron transport and the recycling of iron
- **Ferritin**, a protein that safeguards iron entry into the body, and maintains surplus iron in a safe and readily

Table 12.7   Causes of acquired and inherited forms of anaemia

Acquired anaemia		Inherited anaemia	
Deficiencies	Iron Vitamin B$_{12}$ Folate	Red cell membrane defects	e.g. Hereditary spherocytosis
Blood loss	Acute or chronic	Red cell enzyme defects	e.g. Glucose-6-phosphate dehydrogenase deficiency
Anaemia of chronic disease	Chronic infections, chronic inflammatory diseases, renal failure and malignancies	Globin abnormalities	e.g. Sickle cell anaemia Thalassaemia
Haemolysis	Immune (auto-immune e.g. autoimmune haemolytic anaemia (AIHA); allo-immune, e.g. haemolytic disease of the newborn (HDN)) Non-immune (red cell fragmentation syndromes)	Other rare inherited disorders	e.g. Fanconi anaemia
Marrow infiltration	E.g. leukaemia, lymphoma, cancers radiation, fibrosis	Other disorders (inherited or acquired)	e.g. Sideroblastic anaemia
Aplastic anaemia	E.g. red cell aplasia, cytotoxic therapy		

Table 12.8   Average daily iron requirement

Daily dietary iron requirements	mg/24 hours
Male	1
Adolescence	2–3
Female (menstruating)	2–3
Pregnancy	3–4
Infancy	1

Clinical box 12.2   Diagnosis of iron deficiency anaemia

The concentration of ferritin in plasma is a good indicator of iron stores, and low levels are only seen in deficiency. Normally the levels are about 40–200 ng/mL and virtually everyone with levels below 15 ng/mL is iron deficient although deficiency might be suspected at any level below normal. This test shows high sensitivity, but specificity is not so good if a 15 ng/mL level is used as a cut-off point.

Measurement of soluble transferrin receptor concentration has both high sensitivity and specificity for identifying iron deficiency.

Diagnostic test sensitivity and specificity

A test that has high sensitivity (is very good at detecting a disease that is present) and high specificity (is very good at detecting when a disease is not present) will have few false positives or false negatives, and so a negative result (soluble transferrin receptor concentration normal) is a very good pointer to the disease (iron deficiency) not being the cause of the anaemia.

accessible form. Ferritin is one of the substances that can be measured in order to make a diagnosis of iron deficiency anaemia (Clinical box 12.2).

When iron is in short supply transferrin receptor levels are upregulated, encouraging more iron to be taken up by the cells and incorporated into haemoglobin molecules, and ferritin levels fall. Conversely, when iron is abundant, ferritin levels rise with a concomitant fall in transferrin receptor concentration. Thus there appears to be close coordination of expression of the genes encoding ferritin, transferrin receptor and the haem biosynthetic enzymes.

Recent studies of the iron regulatory proteins, **IRP**, have provided an insight into the mechanisms of this coordinated response.

- Ferritin messenger RNA (mRNA) has a 5′ untranslated region (5′UTR) which contains a stem-loop structure, termed the **iron responsive element (IRE)**. The IRE is recognised by **IRP-1**, a soluble polypeptide which has a similar amino acid sequence to the TCA (citric acid) cycle enzyme, aconitase. In the absence of iron, IRP-1 represses ferritin mRNA translation and blocks the attachment of initiation factors for translation.
  - The active site of IRP-1 is an [4Fe-4S] cluster; when cytoplasmic iron levels are high the cluster is complete. In this form IRP-1 cannot bind to mRNA, and thus the ferritin message is translated and more ferritin produced.
  - However, if cytoplasmic iron levels are low, IRP-1 will bind mRNA, resulting in prevention of translation of the ferritin message. Ferritin is therefore reduced.

- IRP-1 also controls the expression of the **transferrin receptor (TfR)** gene, located on chromosome 3 close to the gene encoding transferrin. The 3′UTR region of the TfR gene contains five potential stem-loop structures that are very similar to the ferritin IRE. These conserved regions of the TfR mRNA bind the same protein as the IRE of ferritin, with resulting stabilisation of the message and increased levels of TfR in iron deficient states.

Causes of iron deficiency

Diet alone is seldom the sole cause for iron deficiency anaemia in developed countries except when it prevents an adequate response to a physiological challenge, e.g. pregnancy. Table 12.9 lists various causes.

Laboratory findings in iron deficiency

A full blood count and blood film is used to investigate the anaemia, but abnormalities typical of iron deficiency can also be seen in other disorders, such as the globin chain disorder, thalassaemia. Measurements of iron binding proteins can help confirm the diagnosis: Table 12.10 lists typical features and Figure 12.14 shows a blood film from a patient with iron deficiency.

Megaloblastic anaemia

In **megaloblastic anaemia** there is an impairment of DNA synthesis, but not RNA synthesis, and the **megaloblastic** cells are characteristically large because they are unable to divide by mitosis. The nucleus also has an immature appearance.

Although we are primarily concerned in this chapter with blood cells, megaloblastic changes will affect *all* actively dividing cells, including those of the gut lining. Megaloblastic red cells in the bone marrow will give rise to **macrocytic** red cells in the peripheral blood.

The terms 'megaloblastic' and 'macrocytic' are often used as though they mean the same thing; however, 'macrocytic' simply implies that the red cells are larger than normal (the MCV is >96 fL). There are other instances where the red cells are macrocytic, while the marrow cells are completely normal: for example, chronic alcohol ingestion may give rise to a raised MCV, but in these cases the cells in the marrow are normal.

Why are vitamins B₁₂ and folate important?

All actively dividing cells require DNA synthesis in order to undergo mitosis. The metabolic pathways involved in replication of DNA are complex, and involve both **vitamin B₁₂** and **folate** within the same pathway: hence a deficiency of these substances results in the same clinical picture.

Vitamin B₁₂ (cobalamin, Cbl)

The **cobalamins** are compounds that have three main components:

- A corrin nucleus (a porphyrin-like structure around a cobalt atom)
- A nucleotide
- A β group linked to cobalt. The β group may be cyanide (in cyanocobalamin), hydroxyl (hydroxocobalamin), methyl (methylcobalamin) or ado (adenosylcobalamin).

Table 12.9	**Causes of iron deficiency**
Causes of iron deficiency	
Blood loss	Heavy periods are the most likely cause in young females
Gastrointestinal	Bleeding peptic ulcer
	Inflammatory bowel disease
	Carcinoma of stomach, colon or rectum
	Abnormal blood vessels in gut (angiodysplasia)
	Malabsorption, e.g. coeliac disease
Dietary	Vegans
	Elderly
Infection	Hookworm infestation is commonest worldwide cause
Normal	Physiological demands e.g. growth spurts in children
	Pregnancy

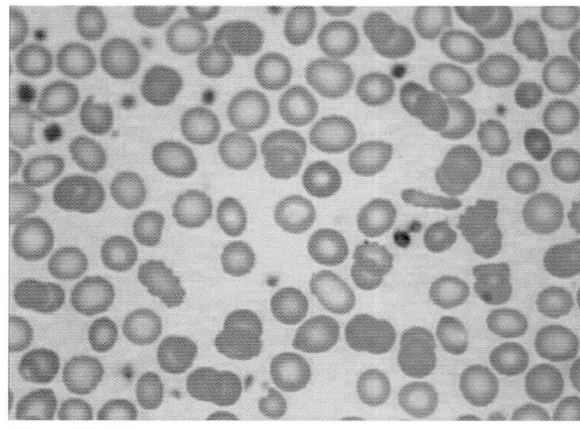

Fig. 12.14 Typical blood film in chronic iron deficiency anaemia: note the pale red cells with pencil (elongated) cells seen in this patient.

Table 12.10	**Laboratory findings in iron deficiency**	
Source	**Finding**	**Explanation**
Blood count	Low Hb concentration	Insufficient precursor iron
	Low red cell indices, MCV and MCH	
Blood film	Microcytic hypochromic red cells	A reduced rate of haemoglobin synthesis due to lack of precursors results in more cell division time as red cells develop until they reach the critical haemoglobin concentration – resulting in smaller cells
		Lower levels of haemoglobin in the cells make them appear pale
	Pencil cells	Unbalanced surface membrane to cytoplasmic volume due to reduced haemoglobin
	Target cells	Decreased cytoplasmic volume due to reduced haemoglobin
Biochemical	Low serum ferritin. Normal levels do not exclude iron deficiency as ferritin is an acute phase protein that may be raised for other reasons	Low iron represses ferritin production
	Low serum iron	Reduced iron availability
	Increased serum total iron-binding capacity (TIBC)	More free transferrin available to bind to iron

Vitamin B_{12} is only manufactured by microorganisms and is ingested through eating meat and dairy products from animals contaminated with these bacteria. Vegans therefore need to take supplements to avoid a deficiency in this vitamin. The average Western diet provides about 5 μg per day and the total liver store is about 2–5 mg, which is sufficient for about 3–4 years in the absence of vitamin B_{12}.

1. In the *stomach*, **Cbl** is released from non-specific binding proteins due to the acid environment.
2. Cbl then binds to pepsin-resistant **R protein**.
3. In the *duodenum*, trypsin digests the R protein and vitamin B_{12} is then bound to **intrinsic factor (IF)**, which is produced by gastric parietal cells.
4. Once it reaches the terminal *ileum*, the **cobalamin-IF** complex binds to a receptor, named '**cubulin**' after the **CUB domains** that make up most of the protein. A CUB domain is a highly conserved sequence consisting of 110 amino acid residues and found in many regulatory proteins, but in a particularly high concentration in this protein.
5. Cbl dissociates from IF and the Cbl is transported by **transcobalamin II (TC II)**, which carries the B_{12} into the *portal circulation*.
6. TC II binds to specific receptors on the cell surface and is internalised. Then Cbl is released and the transport protein is degraded by cellular enzymes. Within the liver cell, Cbl acts as a coenzyme in the complex pathway leading to DNA synthesis.

Tetrahydrofolate (THR) is the biologically active form of folate. Its role is to acquire and donate carbon atoms to biosynthetic pathways that make thymidine nucleotides and methionine, an essential amino acid.

■ Folate, in the form of **5-methyl-tetrahydrofolate (5-methyl-THF)** transfers a carbon atom through action of the **methyl-transferase** enzyme to Cbl, and then on to **homocysteine** to form the amino acid, **methionine** and then **S-adenosyl methionine**.
■ **S-adenosyl-methionine** is needed to donate a methyl group to maintain the protein, **myelin**.
■ Free THF is then used to transfer a single carbon atom through a series of folate coenzymes to **deoxyuridine monophosphate (dUMP)**, thus producing **thymidylate (TMP)**, required for nucleotide synthesis.
■ TMP formation also involves the transfer of two hydrogen ions, producing **dihydrofolate (DHF)** which must be reduced to THF by **dihydrofolate reductase (DHFR)**. THF can then enter the metabolic cycle again.

There are two main consequences of a B_{12} deficiency:

1. A lack of S-adenosyl-methionine methylation is associated with demyelination of nerves and peripheral neuropathy.
2. A block in the production of THF means that 5-methyl-THF accumulates, and folate coenzymes needed for nucleotide biosynthesis are limited (the **methyl trap hypothesis**). This produces a pseudo-folate deficiency, with an anaemia that resembles that seen in true folate deficiency. In B_{12} deficiency, treatment with folate will, therefore, correct the anaemia, but not the neuropathy.

Figure 12.15 shows a simplified DNA synthesis pathway, illustrating the role of vitamin B_{12} and folate in this process.

Causes of vitamin B_{12} deficiency

Reduced absorption, rather than dietary deficiency, is the commonest cause of vitamin B_{12} deficiency in the UK. The most severe cases, resulting in a condition known as **pernicious anaemia**, are due to an autoimmune condition in which the lining of the gut atrophies. This results in a loss of

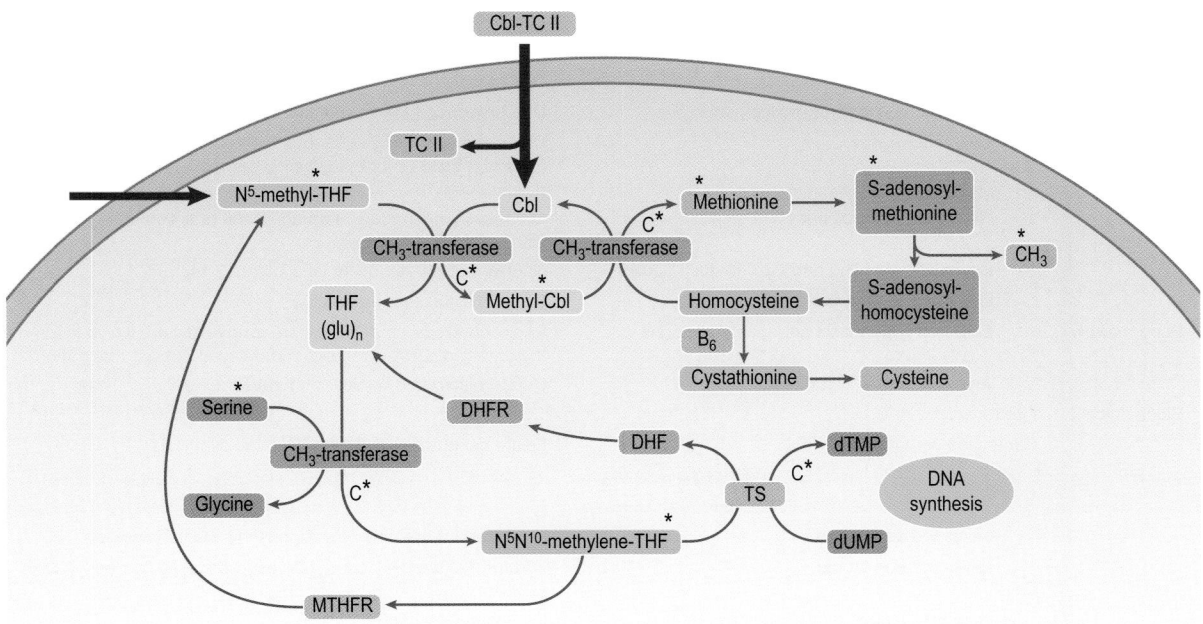

***Fig. 12.15* Cobalamin-folate metabolism.** *Indicates the carbon atoms that are transported through a series of biochemical reactions. TC II, transcobalamin II; Cbl, cobalamin; THF, tetrahydrofolate; DHF, dihydrofolate; DHFR, dihydrofolate reductase; MTHFR, methylene tetrahydrofolate reductase; TS, thymidylate synthase; dUMP, deoxyuridine monophosphate; dTMP, deoxythymidine monophosphate. Redrawn with permission from Israel LG, Israel ED 1998 Mechanisms in hematology, 3rd edn. Core Health Sciences, Canada.

the intrinsic factor production, required for absorption of B_{12} (see Ch. 16).

Vitamin B_{12} deficiency also can occur after total or partial gastrectomy, and may also be seen in association with other bowel diseases or dietary deficiency.

Folate

The other key player in DNA synthesis is **folate**, derived from folic acid. Folate comprises three components:

- Pteridine component
- Para-aminobenzoic acid component
- An L-glutamine residue

Folates are found in green vegetables, and are easily destroyed by cooking (see Ch. 16). The average requirement in adults is 100 µg per day (diet provides about 250 µg daily) and the liver can store 8–20 mg. Compared to Cbl, the body stores of folate are therefore quite small, and will only last about 4 months if supply stops.

Folate is absorbed in the upper small intestine, and the dietary form is predominantly polyglutamates. The polyglutamic form has a side chain of multiple glutamic acids joined in peptide linkages and this side chain must be cleaved before absorption can occur. The monoglutamate form is therefore most easily absorbed and can enter cells either by diffusion or by being taken up by specific folate-binding proteins. This form is employed therapeutically.

Causes of folate deficiency

The most common cause of folate deficiency is nutritional, due to poor diet and/or alcoholism. Table 12.11 lists these and other causes.

Table 12.11	Causes of folate deficiency
Causes of folate deficiency	
Poor nutrition	Seen in poverty, old age, alcoholics
Increased requirements for folate, or excessive loss	Pregnancy (rapid growth of fetus), malignancy (increased cell turnover), chronic red cell haemolysis (increased red cell production)
Malabsorption	Coeliac disease, Crohn's disease and other malabsorptive states
Drugs	Phenytoin, barbiturates, valproate (anti-epileptics), oral contraceptives
Antifolate drugs	Methotrexate (cytotoxic drug), trimethoprim (antibiotic), pentamidine (antiprotozoal drug)

Laboratory findings in B_{12} and folate deficiency

Clinically B_{12} and folate deficiencies present with a macrocytic, megaloblastic anaemia, which may be mild or severe (Hb < 6.0 g/dL) but only B_{12} deficiency produces neurological changes. Table 12.12 lists typical features of these diseases.

Acquired anaemias due to blood loss

Acute blood loss

When large volumes of blood are lost from the body in a short space of time there are general features of volume depletion:

Table 12.12	Laboratory findings in B_{12} and folate deficiency		
Source	**B_{12} deficiency**	**Folate deficiency**	**Explanation**
Blood count	Reduced haemoglobin, often severe		Ineffective erythropoiesis
	Raised MCV (often severe)		Due to cells being unable to divide efficiently
	Leucopenia and thrombocytopenia		Due to reduced DNA synthesis
Blood film	Oval macrocytes		DNA synthesis is impaired, but not RNA synthesis and so there is a build up of cytoplasmic components in a slowly dividing cell
	'Tear drop' poikilocytes		Often seen when there is an abnormal proliferation of cells within the bone marrow
	Basophilic stippling and Howell–Jolly bodies		Nuclear activity remnants (see Table 12.14)
	Hypersegmented neutrophils		Disordered nuclear maturation
Bone marrow	Erythroid hyperplasia and giant neutrophil precursors		Poor conversion of deoxyuridate to thymidylate, which leads to slowing of DNA synthesis and delayed nuclear maturation
	Atypical nuclear chromatin		Due to disordered nuclear maturation
Biochemical	Reduced serum B_{12}		
	Increased serum folate		Folate cannot be used for nucleotide synthesis
		Reduced serum folate	
		Reduced red cell folate	
	Increased serum iron		Increased iron turnover in response to megaloblastosis
	Increased iron stores		Iron from effete cells cannot be used because of block in DNA synthesis
	Increased lactate dehydrogenase (LDH)		Increased cell death
Immunological	Gastric parietal cell antibodies		Autoimmune condition leading to reduced intrinsic factor production
	Intrinsic factor antibodies		Autoimmune condition blocking Cbl attachment to intrinsic factor, or the attachment of the complex to receptors in the ileum

- Increased heart beats (**tachycardia**)
- Low blood pressure.

The haemoglobin concentration will be normal for several hours following the bleed; in fact a full blood count taken immediately after the bleed will be normal because red cells and plasma are lost together. Anaemia only develops once the blood volume has been restored through the movement of fluid from the extravascular to the intravascular space. The MCV remains normal and so this anaemia may be described as **normocytic**.

Chronic blood loss

In the developed world this is the most common cause of iron deficiency anaemia. Examples might be unrecognised loss from a bleeding gastric ulcer, or heavy menstruation.

Acquired anaemias due to chronic disease

Anaemia of chronic disease (ACD)

This is very common in medical practice and generally reflects the presence of other underlying disease, such as chronic infection (e.g. tuberculosis, osteomyelitis), chronic inflammation (e.g. rheumatoid arthritis, systemic lupus erythematosus (SLE)) or malignancy. By definition the anaemia is normocytic.

Mechanism of ACD

Why should the presence of a chronic disorder induce anaemia? Previously called **reticuloendothelial block**, since there is abundant iron in the bone marrow macrophages, the iron is not, however, passed to developing red cells.

The molecular and cellular mechanisms are still poorly understood, but appear to be multifactorial.

- In chronic renal failure the erythropoietic drive does not seem to be able to release iron from the reticuloendothelial system at the expected rate, which could be due to a depressed response to erythropoietin.
- In other cases the problem may be due to disruption of iron metabolism in the developing red cells. Key molecules involved in iron uptake are the transferrin receptor, ferritin and the red cell enzyme, 5-aminolaevulinic acid synthase. These are controlled, post transcription, by iron regulatory proteins that bind to mRNA when intracellular iron is low and it is possible that cytokines (inflammatory mediators), such as tumour necrosis factor (TNF)-α, could interfere with this process.
- Inflammatory cytokines also upregulate ferritin synthesis, diverting iron into storage, rather than release.

Diagnosis of ACD

Diagnosis may be difficult because of the varying causes but generally there is a mild normocytic anaemia often associated with increases in acute phase proteins, such as ferritin and **C-reactive protein** (**CRP**) and an increased **erythrocyte sedimentation rate** (**ESR**), due to inflammatory changes in plasma proteins.

If the process is longstanding, the picture may resemble iron deficiency, but the patient will *not* respond to iron therapy.

Anaemias due to haemolysis

Haemolytic anaemias are disorders in which the red cells are destroyed faster than normal; i.e. they have a reduced lifespan. Anaemia occurs because the bone marrow cannot produce sufficient new red cells to keep pace with the rate of destruction. Instead of 120 days, red cells may live for as little as 20 days. Consequently, in haemolytic anaemias, red cell breakdown will be increased and red cell production will be increased as a response to the anaemia. If the bone marrow can increase erythropoiesis sufficiently the patient may not even be anaemic.

Haemolytic anaemias may be acquired (and due to immune or non-immune processes) or inherited. Whatever the cause of the red cell breakdown there are metabolic consequences that are reflected in the clinical and laboratory picture. Figure 12.16 illustrates these.

Acquired autoimmune haemolytic anaemia (AIHA)

These anaemias are characterised by:

- Autoantibodies (i.e. antibodies directed against the individual's own antigens)

or

- Complement, which attaches to red cells and either causes destruction via macrophages in the reticuloendothelial system within the spleen (mainly IgG coated red cells), or the liver (mainly complement coated red cells), resulting in an extravascular breakdown of red cells.

Red cells become coated with antibody, most often IgG. These antibodies react with Fc receptors on the macrophages leading to phagocytosis of the red cells. If the phagocytosis is incomplete the remaining portion of the red cell continues to circulate as a spherocyte (note that phagocytosis is usually complete if complement is involved) (Fig. 12.17).

The autoantibodies are of various types: 'warm', in which haemolysis occurs at normal body temperature; 'cold', in which haemolysis occurs at low temperatures, and the condition may be idiopathic (of unknown cause) or associated with other diseases. Some anaemias appear to be drug induced, leading to complement-induced haemolysis.

Most of the red cell breakdown takes place in the spleen causing it to enlargen from the debris (**splenomegaly**). Removal of the spleen (**splenectomy**) can resolve the anaemia.

Laboratory findings in AIHA

Examination of a blood film shows features typical of haemolytic anaemia: spherocytes and polychromatic red cells (Fig. 12.18). Table 12.13 details other features associated with AIHA.

Other acquired anaemias

Anaemia can also be caused by a variety of other mechanisms that interfere with either red cell production or the normal life span of the red cell:

Non-immune haemolytic anaemias

- **Paroxysmal nocturnal haemoglobinuria** (**PNH**) is a rare defect of red cells that makes cells vulnerable to

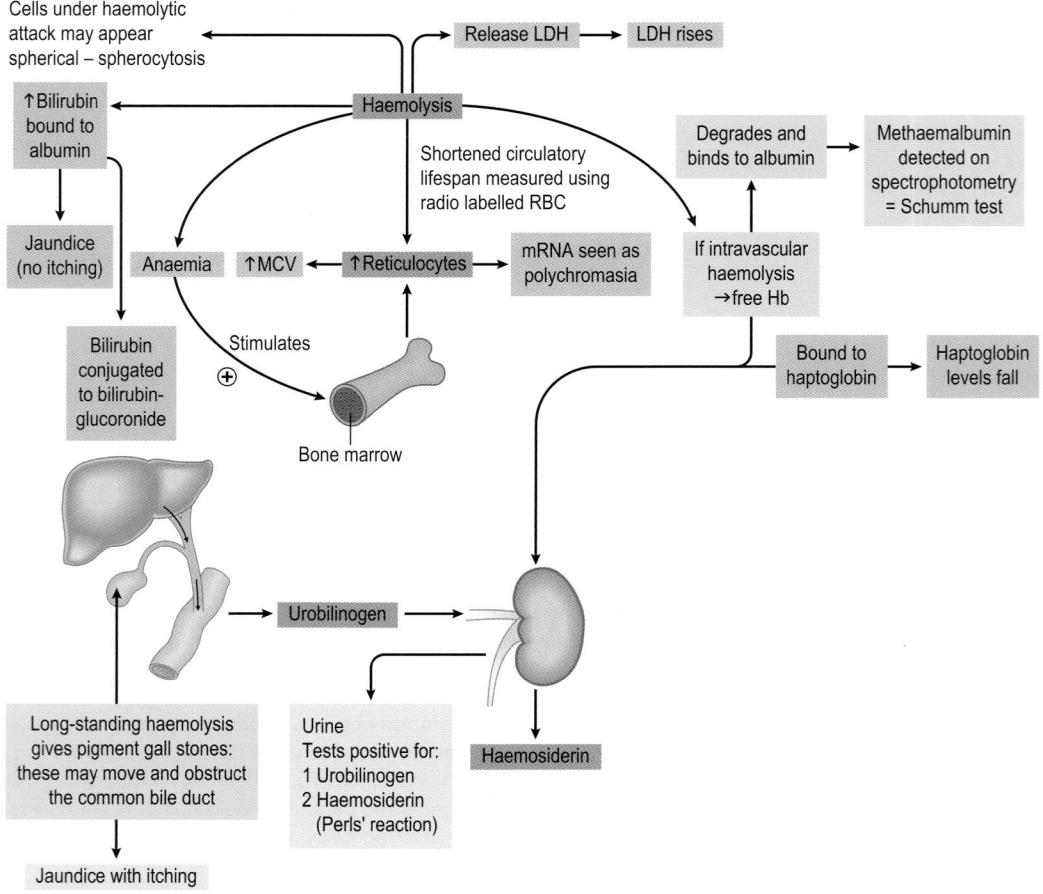

Fig. 12.16 **Metabolic effects of increased red cell breakdown.** LDH, lactate dehydrogenase; MCV, mean cell volume; RBC, red blood cell.

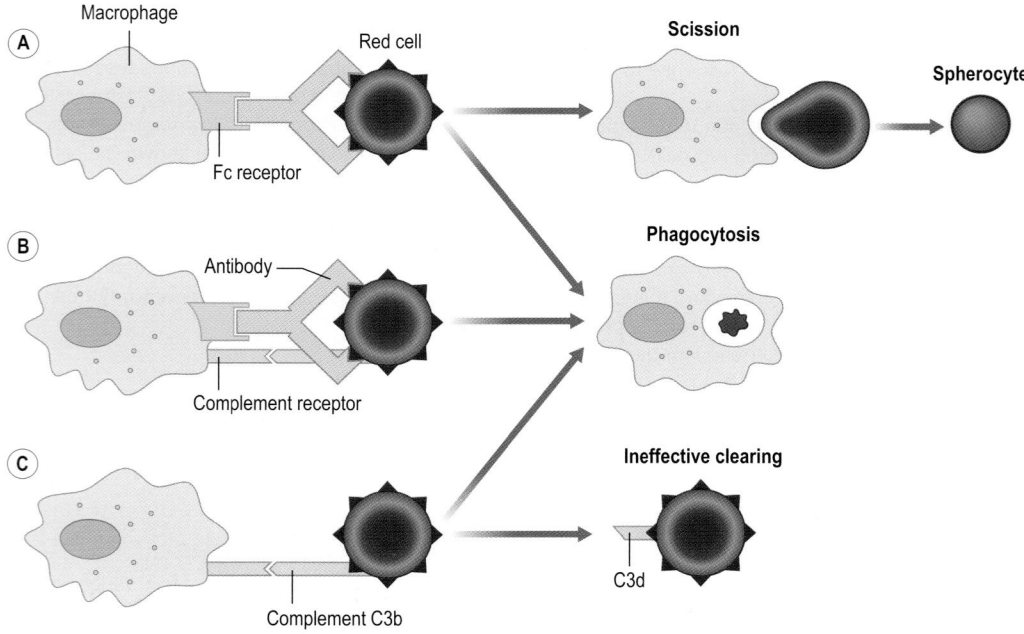

Fig. 12.17 **Extravascular haemolysis is due to interaction of antibody-coated cells with cells in the reticuloendothelial system, predominantly in the spleen.** (A) Spherocytes result from partial phagocytosis. (B) Complete phagocytosis may occur and this is enhanced if there is complement as well as antibody on the cell surface. (C) Cells coated with complement only are ineffectively removed and circulate with C3d or C3b on their surface. Redrawn with permission from Kumar P, Clark M 2005 Clinical medicine, 6th edn. Churchill Livingstone, Edinburgh.

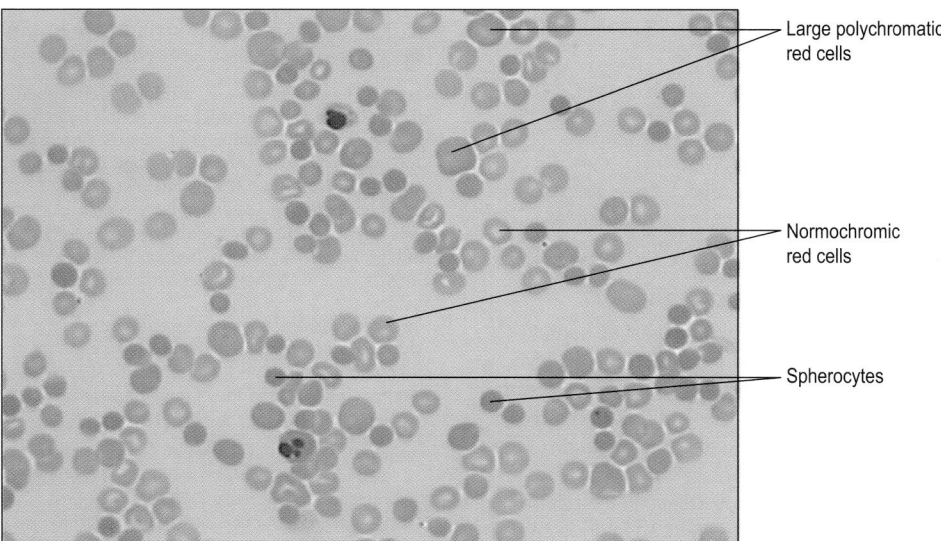

Large polychromatic
red cells

Normochromic
red cells

Spherocytes

Fig. 12.18 **Blood film from patient with autoimmune haemolytic anaemia.** Note the presence of spherocytes and polychromatic cells.

Table 12.13	Laboratory findings in AIHA	
Source	**Finding**	**Explanation**
Blood count	Reduced haemoglobin	Destruction of red cells
	Increased reticulocytes	Response of bone marrow to haemolysis
Blood film	Spherocytes	Due to a partial loss of the red cell membrane, possibly during partial phagocytosis stimulated by antibodies on the cell surface
	Polychromatic cells	Young red cells or reticulocytes produced in response to the haemolysis
Biochemical	Increased lactate dehydrogenase (LDH)	Released from red cells as a result of the haemolysis
	Decreased haptoglobin (Hp)	Haptoglobin binds free haemoglobin and the Hp–Hb complex is removed by the reticuloendothelial system
Other	Positive direct antiglobulin test (DAT)	Detection of red cells coated with antibody or complement

destruction by **activated complement**. The breakdown of red cells reveals itself in dark-coloured urine (**haemoglobinuria**), particularly evident in the morning when urine is more concentrated, although it was originally thought to be due to red cell breakdown at night due to increased acidosis – hence nocturnal and paroxysmal (intermittent). PNH is caused by a mutation in the **pig-A** (phosphatidyl inositol glycan complementation group A) gene, which makes a protein that anchors complement-protective proteins to the red cell surface.

Mechanical red cell fragmentation
This can occur in several conditions:

- Artificial heart valves – damaged valves can shear the red cells
- **Microangiopathic haemolytic anaemia (MAHA)** – in some conditions the micro-environment that the red cells encounter may produce fragmentation
- **March haemoglobinuria** – caused by traumatic exercise (such as prolonged marching in a military exercise)
- Heat – burns where red cells are exposed to heat over 47 °C will result in the cells being fragmented
- **Malaria** – parasite-infected red cells are fragmented.

Marrow infiltration
When the marrow is taken over by clonal expansion of a particular cell, such as can occur in leukaemia, normal red cell precursors are squeezed out.

Marrow failure
Aplastic anaemia – is caused by a failure of the *pluripotent stem cells*. This failure can affect all blood cell precursors, or just one line, as in **red cell aplasia**. It can be caused by a variety of drugs, but is often the intentional consequence of the therapeutic use of certain cytotoxic drugs.

Rare inherited anaemias
Fanconi's anaemia is an autosomal recessive disease that results in skeletal, skin and organ abnormalities, as well as an aplastic anaemia. Several genes on different chromosomes are involved in making a complex essential for DNA repair. Individuals with this condition have cells that are hypersensitive to genotoxic agents, such as mitomycin. Cells are seen to have increased chromosome breaks.

Inherited anaemias

Hereditary anaemias are virtually all haemolytic in nature and may be classified by the pathological process causing decreased red cell lifespan. These can be separated into three major groups of disorders affecting:

- Red cell membrane
- Red cell enzymes
- Haemoglobin molecule.

Clinical and laboratory findings reflect those seen in the acquired haemolytic disorders but may be more severe and can be associated with some specific findings.

Red cell membrane disorders

The red cell membrane is a typical lipid bilayer containing integral membrane proteins. These externally carried glycoproteins are responsible for the various blood group systems. Internally these integral proteins are bound to a protein cytoskeleton, which is responsible for the maintenance of the shape and flexibility of the red cell.

The principal cytoskeletal proteins identified are **spectrin**, **ankyrin**, **actin** and **protein 4.1**, of which spectrin is by far the most abundant. **Hereditary spherocytosis** and **hereditary elliptocytosis** represent a group of disorders in which there are deficiencies or dysfunction of these skeletal proteins.

Hereditary spherocytosis

Spectrin deficiency is the most common cause of hereditary spherocytosis and leads to instability in the red cell cytoskeleton, producing spherocytes. Different point mutations result in different forms of the disease:

- Mutations of α spectrin result in a recessive condition.
- Mutations of β spectrin are seen in families that show an autosomal dominant inheritance.

The reason for the difference in inheritance manifestation is because α spectrin synthesis normally occurs in excess, unlike β spectrin synthesis, with unwanted chains being degraded. Individuals who are heterozygotes will therefore normally produce enough α spectrin to balance the normal β spectrin production.

The laboratory findings are similar to other haemolytic anaemias with many of the red cells showing the characteristic spherical or elliptical shape. Often the MCV will be increased, because of the high prevalence of larger reticulocytes. The MCHC may also be increased because spherical cells can hold more haemoglobin than disc-shaped normal red cells. The increased haemoglobin breakdown will result in increased serum bilirubin in plasma, urobilinogen in urine and stercobilinogen in faeces. Special tests help to confirm the diagnosis (Clinical box 12.3).

Red cell enzyme disorders

Although haemolytic anaemia can be the result of defects in any of the red cell enzymes, only three disorders are common: **glucose-6-phosphate dehydrogenase (G6PD) deficiency**, **pyruvate kinase (PK) deficiency**, and **pyrimidine 5′ nucleotidase deficiency**.

Glucose-6-phosphate dehydrogenase deficiency

G6PD deficiency is the commonest red cell enzyme defect leading to haemolytic anaemia. The enzyme plays an important role as part of the pentose phosphate pathway (hexose monophosphate shunt) reducing NADP to NADPH (see also Ch. 3).

Clinical box 12.3	Diagnosis of hereditary spherocytosis

Osmotic fragility is the test used to detect spherocytosis. The degree of red cell lysis (rupture) caused by incubating red cells in sodium chloride solutions of various strengths is measured. Curves are drawn for normal and test samples and the mean corpuscular fragility (MCF) is calculated (Fig. 12.19). This is the saline concentration at which 50% lysis occurs. Normal red cells remain intact until the saline concentration reaches 50% and lysis increases as the solution becomes more hypotonic. Spherocytes, with their lower surface area to volume ratio, lyse more readily.

In normal subjects the curve is steep and symmetrical, whereas in spherocytic anaemias the span and shape of the curve is altered and, characteristically, in hereditary spherocytosis, a long tail of highly fragile cells will be seen.

Radioactive studies may also be helpful:

- Red cell lifespan – this can be determined by labelling the patient's red cells with radioactive chromium and measuring loss of radioactivity over time.
- Red cell destruction sites – this will often be combined with the former, the body being scanned for hot spots of radioactivity where cells are being destroyed.

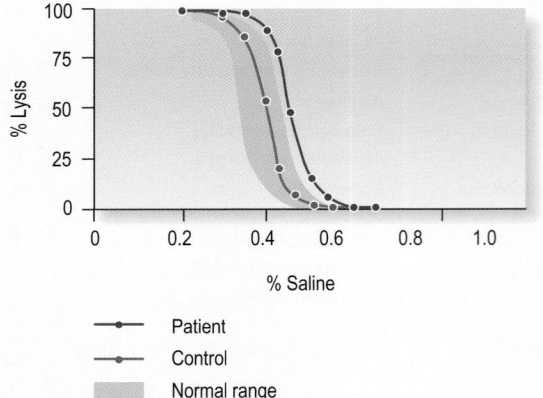

Patient
Control
Normal range

Fig. 12.19 Osmotic fragility test. The patient's red cells are more prone to rupture (lysis) than the control red cells at the same saline concentration because the patient's red cells are spherical rather than disc-shaped.

NADPH maintains glutathione in its reduced form, protecting the red cell from oxidative damage by detoxifying hydrogen peroxide produced by bacteria and certain drugs. G6PD is the only source of NADPH in red cells and a fully functioning biochemical pathway is needed to keep the red cell intact.

Oxidative damage leading to a haemolytic crisis may be caused by various factors:

- Drugs such as analgesics, antimalarials (primaquine) and antibiotics
- Ingestion of fava beans
- Sepsis.

G6PD deficiency is inherited in an X-linked recessive manner, so males are affected more frequently than females, although females who are heterozygous may still show features of the disorder. The condition is commonest in the tropics but has become increasingly common in northern Europe, the UK, and North and South America.

The disease is extremely variable both in terms of its phenotype and genotype, with several hundred variants already described. Many of the mutations are point mutations in the 18 kilobase structural gene for G6PD found at Xq28. Three major forms of G6PD deficiency exist:

- G6PD A
- G6PD A−
- G6PD Mediterranean.

The last variant is the most severe form and associated with acute haemolytic crises. Patients may have a mild anaemia or are asymptomatic until they experience an oxidative 'stress' that results in an acute attack.

In addition to the typical findings associated with haemolytic anaemia the red cells often show particular characteristics:

- **Heinz bodies** are seen with particular stains where haemoglobin has been rendered unstable due to oxidant damage.
- **Bite cells** are thought to result from the processing of cells through the spleen and removal of Heinz bodies.

Haemoglobin disorders

These may be due to structural abnormalities of the haemoglobin molecule, e.g. **sickle haemoglobin**, or due to defective and imbalanced globin chain production, e.g. **thalassaemia**.

Sickle cell disease

Sickle cell disease results from a single base change in the β globin gene, resulting in a change of amino acid number 6 glu→val due to the point mutation GAG→GTG. The resultant haemoglobin produced by the β^S gene is referred to as **HbS**.

Red blood cells containing the sickle haemoglobin elongate under conditions of reduced oxygenation, and form characteristic sickle shaped cells. These do not flow well through small vessels, and are more adherent than normal RBCs to vascular endothelium, leading to vascular occlusion and **sickle cell crises**. Sickling is initially reversible but red cells become progressively more rigid due to membrane defects. Sickled red cells have reduced lifespan and result in chronic haemolysis.

The sickle gene is widespread throughout Africa, Middle East, the parts of India and the Mediterranean. In the African Caribbean population of the UK the gene is found in 10% of individuals. Screening programmes offer early diagnosis of this and other inherited disorders of haemoglobin (Clinical box 12.4). Despite the deleterious nature of the sickle gene it has remained at high frequency because heterozygous carriers have increased resistance to malaria.

Sickle cell disease is generally due to homozygous HbSS ($\alpha_2\beta^S_2$), but may also be due to interactions with other abnormal haemoglobins, such as:

- **HbC** (resulting in HbSC, $\alpha_2\beta^S\beta^C$)
- **β thalassaemia** (resulting in HbSβ⁺ thalassaemia, $\alpha_2\beta^S\beta^+$thal or β° thal)
- **HbD** (resulting in HbSD, $\alpha_2\beta^S\beta^D$).

All of these produce significant symptoms but SS and Sβ° are the most severe. The parents of individuals with HbSS sickle cell disease are both carriers of the β^S gene, i.e. they usually both have **sickle cell trait**.

Clinical box 12.4   Screening for the sickle gene

The identification of individuals who carry the sickle gene, and other inherited abnormal haemoglobins, is important in order to reduce morbidity and mortality. Screening tests are undertaken on adults at risk who may experience problems under anaesthesia, and for genetic counselling.

Infants with sickle cell disease are normally healthy at birth because of the high levels of fetal haemoglobin. The early recognition of affected infants is important in order to make plans for their care. Use of prophylactic penicillin and comprehensive care has reduced the mortality among children with sickle cell disease in their first 5 years from approximately 25% to less than 3%.

Elevated fetal haemoglobin levels are beneficial

Adult Hb comprises **HbA** ($\alpha_2\beta_2$), which makes up the majority of Hb, along with **HbA₂** ($\alpha_2\delta_2$). Sickle cell disease is not detected at the time of birth since the main haemoglobin in early life is **HbF** ($\alpha_2\gamma_2$), which does not contain the β chain. When γ chain production diminishes and β globin production increases, sickle cell disease becomes apparent and is normally diagnosed before the age of 2 years.

Precipitants of sickle cell disease

Sickle cell disease is highly variable. Many patients have few symptoms, since HbS has reduced O_2 affinity and oxygen is given up more easily, although they are often severely anaemic. The anaemia is chronic, however, and patients are generally well adapted until an episode of decompensation occurs, resulting in a sickle cell crisis and an accompanying severe haemolytic anaemia (Fig. 12.20).

Precipitants include:

- Infection
- Dehydration
- Cold
- Hypoxia
- Acidosis.

Laboratory findings in sickle cell disease

Table 12.14 summarises the laboratory findings associated with sickle cell disease.

Specialist tests are also available to confirm the presence of haemoglobin S.

- Sickle test screen – the presence of HbS produces a turbid appearance when blood is left in a dilute solution of potassium dihydrophosphate. This test will not discriminate between sickle cell trait and homozygous disease and will not detect other abnormal haemoglobins.
- Haemoglobin electrophoresis (Information box 12.6) – confirmation of a homozygous state requires haemoglobin electrophoresis, which will show 80–95% sickle Hb ($\alpha_2\beta^S_2$) with no normal HbA ($\alpha_2\beta_2$). Fetal haemoglobin ($\alpha_2\gamma_2$) may be elevated to about 15% (range 5–15%). The parents will have features of sickle cell trait.

The thalassaemias

This group of disorders arises as a result of diminished or absent production of one or more globin chains. The net result is unbalanced globin chain production. Globin chains

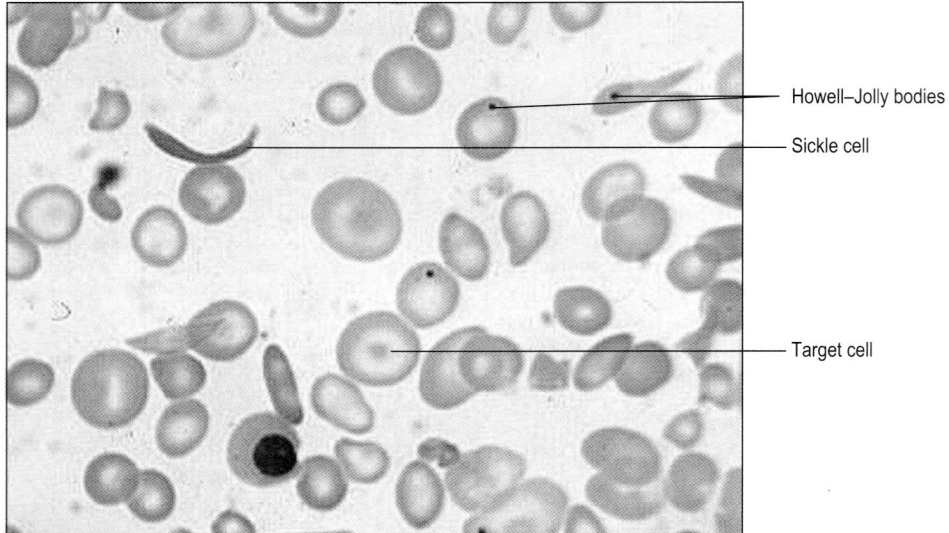

Howell–Jolly bodies

Sickle cell

Target cell

Fig. 12.20 **Blood film of sickle cell crisis.** The blood film shows several sickle cells as well as a nucleated red cell, target cells and cells with inclusion bodies (Howell–Jolly body).

Table 12.14	Laboratory findings in sickle cell disease	
Source	**Finding**	**Explanation**
Blood count	Low haemoglobin (6–9 g/dL)	Destruction of sickled red cells
	High reticulocytes (20–39%)	Increased bone marrow production of red cells
Blood film	Sickle cells	Haemoglobin S aggregates and distorts cell shape
	Target cells	Decreased cytoplasmic volume due to reduced haemoglobin
	Basophilic stippling and Howell–Jolly bodies	Evidence of nuclear remnant from cells undergoing rapid erythropoiesis
	Polychromatic cells and nucleated red cells	Immature red cells released from the bone marrow to compensate for the acute anaemia

in excess precipitate within red cells, leading to chronic haemolysis.

Thalassaemias occur at high frequency in parts of Africa, the Mediterranean, Middle East, India and Asia, and are found mostly in areas where malaria is endemic. Like the sickle gene, inheritance of thalassaemia probably offers some protection against malaria.

Thalassaemia is further classified after the gene affected, e.g. in α thalassaemia, the α globin gene is altered in such a way that either α globin synthesis is reduced (α^+) or abolished (α°) from red blood cells. The severity varies and depends on the type of mutation or deletion of the α globin or β globin gene. The consequence of impaired production of globin chains leads to red cells being microcytic and hypochromatic.

α Thalassaemia

α Thalassaemia is generally caused by large deletions within the α globin complex (compared with β thalassaemia, which is usually due to point mutations). There are two α globin genes on each chromosome 16, making a total of four α globin genes per cell (the normal person is designated αα/αα). Like sickle cell anaemia, patients can have:

- Mild α thalassaemia where one (α–/αα **silent α thalassaemia**) or two (α–/α– **α thalassaemia trait**) α globin genes are affected; severe α thalassaemia if three (α–/–– **Haemoglobin H disease**) or four (––/–– **Haemoglobin Barts hydrops fetalis**) of the genes are affected.

- In its mild form those with α thalassaemia have no symptoms and no treatment is required.
- Patients with HbH disease may have some features of red cell haemolysis, but treatment is not normally required. Up to 40% of the haemoglobin is HbH (β_4) and the remainder HbA, HbA_2 and HbF.
- When all four α globin genes are affected no functioning α globin genes remain. The γ chains form tetramers (γ_4) which bind oxygen very tightly, resulting in poor tissue oxygenation – the oxygen dissociation curve is shifted to the left. Most of the haemoglobin is Hb Barts (γ_4) with small amounts of HbH (β_4). Inheritance of this severe condition usually results in a stillbirth at 34–40 weeks gestation, or the baby dies soon after birth. Haemoglobin Barts hydrops fetalis is a common cause of stillbirth in Southeast Asia.

β Thalassaemia

Most **β thalassaemias** are due to single point mutations in the β globin gene and are not as deleterious as α thalassaemia (Clinical box 12.5).

- Normally there are two copies of the β globin gene per cell, one inherited from each parent. An abnormality in one β globin gene results in the asymptomatic **β thalassaemia trait** (the patient has increased HbA_2 ($\alpha_2\delta_2$)).
- If both β globin genes are affected the patient has **β thalassaemia major** and most of the haemoglobin will be HbF ($\alpha_2\gamma_2$).

Information box 12.6 Haemoglobin electrophoresis

Haemoglobin electrophoresis is an electrical method for separating molecules on the basis of overall electrical charge. Electrophoresis allows the separation of different haemoglobins providing they have differing charges (if different types of Hb have the same charge these will move together on the gel and cannot be distinguished).
Electrophoretic methods in current use are:

- Cellulose acetate (at pH 8.6)
- Citrate agar (at pH 6.0)
- Isoelectric focusing (IEF)
- High-performance liquid chromatography (HPLC).

Some haemoglobin variants travel together through one type of gel and must be separated using another type of electrophoresis. There is no single electrophoretic method that allows each different type of haemoglobin molecule to be identified – usually two techniques are required to be absolutely certain that the haemoglobins have been fully separated.

Cellulose acetate electrophoresis
This is a common test which, although fairly old, is still used (Fig. 12.21). Different haemoglobins that have the same net charge will run together on the gel, e.g. HbS will run in the same band as HbD (hence cannot be distinguished using this method). Similarly HbG, and HbC will run with HbE. In order to separate these bands the electrophoresis needs to be repeated using an acid pH (citrate agar).

Citrate agar
This is very similar to cellulose acetate but uses a pH gradient to separate different haemoglobins. HbD and HbG cannot be distinguished from HbA with this method but HbS will be distinguished from HbD.

Isoelectric focusing (IEF)
IEF is a high resolution method for separating different Hb molecules and the basic principle of the test relies on the fact that all proteins and amino acids have a pH at which their net charge is zero (**isoelectric point**). At this pH there is

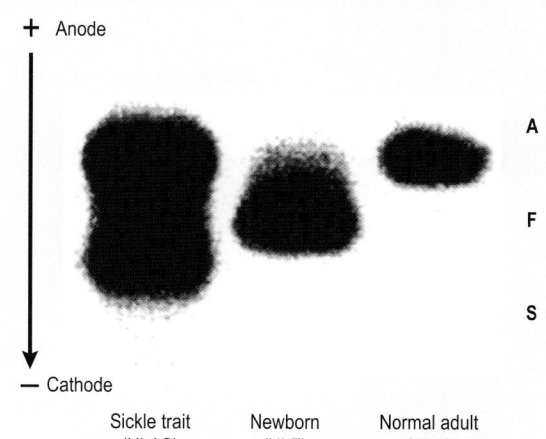

Fig. 12.21 Cellulose acetate haemoglobin electrophoresis of blood from a patient with sickle cell trait (Hb AS), a newborn baby (Hb F) and a normal adult (HbA).

no net movement in the presence of an externally applied electric field. The Hb molecules are subjected to a pH gradient. This method has the advantage of high resolution but is more expensive than standard electrophoresis.

High-performance liquid chromatography (HPLC)
HPLC is used for analysis of haemoglobin molecules. Haemoglobins are passed through a matrix column and eluted from the column at varying times, and their absorbance measured. Detection of standard haemoglobin variants is simple and the technique has the added advantage that novel haemoglobin variants can be detected. HPLC can separate proteins that cannot be resolved using other techniques.

Clinical box 12.5 Thalassaemia

Infants with this disease fail to thrive once HbF has declined and suffer severe anaemia needing lifelong blood transfusion (every 4–6 weeks) to suppress ineffective erythropoiesis and stimulate normal growth and development in childhood. They will suffer from an enlarged liver and spleen (due to production and destruction of red cells by these organs) and iron overload (leading to heart failure, endocrine dysfunction and chronic hepatitis) and are likely to need injections of desferrioxamine to chelate the excess iron.

- Microcytic hypochromic cells (because of the severe imbalance of globin chain synthesis).
- Increased reticulocytes, polychromasia and nucleated red cells (due to the bone marrow response to the severe anaemia).
- Poikilocytosis, especially in β thalassaemia, seen because the excess α chains precipitate, distorting the cells and damaging the cell membrane, leading to intravascular haemolysis.

- To date more than 150 mutations have been identified. These may result in reduced β globin synthesis (β⁺) or absent β globin production (β°).

Laboratory findings in the thalassaemias
The findings depend on the severity of the disease.

- α Thalassaemia shows limited changes in red cell indices. In contrast, individuals with β thalassaemia have a significantly reduced MCV and increased red cell count.
- In the more severe disease (HbH disease, or β thalassaemia major) anaemia can be severe (Hb 3–9 g/dL) and the blood film shows changes that reflect this:

ONCOGENESIS AND DISORDERS OF BLOOD CELL PRODUCTION

In health, the bone marrow regulates the number of cells in the peripheral blood to match requirements. Our bodies make sufficient red cells to transport oxygen to our tissues. White cell numbers are maintained to provide defence against infection and platelet numbers are adequate for normal primary haemostasis. However, the bone marrow may malfunction and produce excess numbers of cells (**myeloproliferative diseases**), or the bone marrow may produce cells that are functionally defective, a large proportion of which are destroyed within the marrow, leading to low numbers in the circulation (**myelodysplastic syndromes**). Finally, in extreme cases the marrow may produce excess numbers of malignant cells that spill out into the peripheral blood whilst within the marrow they suppress the production of normal cells (**leukaemias**).

NORMAL BLOOD PRODUCTION RELIES ON COORDINATED GENE EXPRESSION

Normal cell division and differentiation are complex processes, controlled by many regulatory genes and proteins. When these processes go wrong we see disordered growth of bone marrow cells. Why these events occur is poorly understood but we have learned a great deal by studying animal leukaemia models, in addition to examining haematological malignancies in humans.

ONCOGENESIS

The search for oncogenes in human blood disease

When **oncogenes** (cancer genes) were found in animals, researchers turned their attention to human cancers to look for similar associations. The research has been fairly rewarding in the case of solid tumours (lung, breast, colon and others) but undoubtedly the most significant advances have been made in blood disorders. Some leukaemias, such as **chronic myeloid leukaemia** (**CML**), have been intensively studied and CML is arguably the paradigm of human haemopoietic malignancy. Through the efforts of many clinicians and scientists we know much about this disease at the molecular level. This molecular knowledge has been used to full advantage, and we now have treatment aimed at specifically deactivating molecular targets implicated in the disease.

Oncogenes and tumour suppressor genes

Neoplasia is a process whereby uncontrolled growth occurs, and results from a loss of the normal process governing coordinated cellular growth. Two major classes of gene have been implicated, namely **oncogenes** and **tumour suppressor genes**.

Oncogenes

Oncogenes appear to cause malignancy through their direct effects. This group of genes includes growth factors, growth factor receptors and DNA binding proteins. Such genes are part of our normal genetic makeup and serve useful purposes, although, as **proto-oncogenes**, by definition they have the potential to become oncogenes. Once altered, through mutation or other processes, such as chromosomal translocation or viral activation, they become oncogenes, which have detrimental effects on cell growth and differentiation. Human cancers often involve the activation of one or more oncogene along with a loss of tumour suppressor gene(s).

Mutations

Point mutations induced by mutagens, such as UV light and ionising radiation, can lead to the production of oncogenes from their normal counterparts.

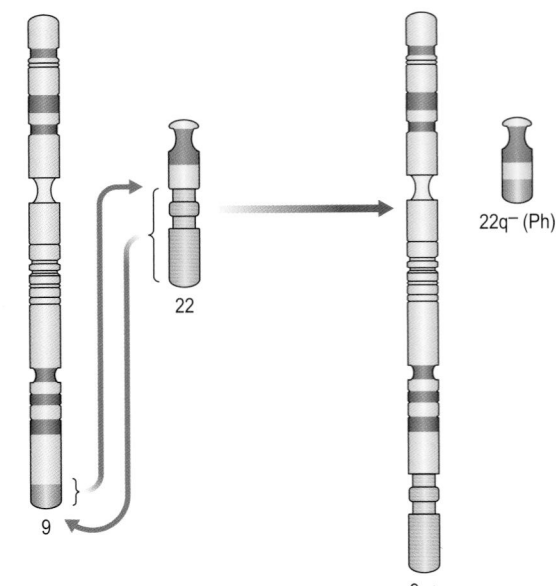

Fig. 12.22 The Philadelphia chromosome (Ph). The long arm (q) of chromosome 22 has been shortened by the reciprocal translocation with chromosome 9. Redrawn with permission from Kumar P, Clark M 2005 Clinical medicine, 6th edn. Elsevier Saunders, Edinburgh.

Chromosome translocations

Translocation of DNA from one chromosome to another, or within the same chromosome, can result in novel fusion genes. The best studied example is the **Philadelphia chromosome** (Fig. 12.22) (t(9;22)) in which **ABL** from chromosome 9 becomes fused to **BCR** on chromosome 22. The resulting *BCR-ABL* fusion gene, through its gene product (BCR-ABL protein), gives rise directly to the typical phenotype seen in chronic myeloid leukaemia (CML). This disease occurs because *BCR-ABL* is a tyrosine kinase and its action results in uncontrolled growth of haemopoietic cells.

Viral activation

Viral genes may become incorporated into the host chromosomes, directly stimulating adjacent genes. In addition, viruses may pick up pieces of host DNA and transduce these into the next host, inducing cancer by this mechanism. Animal experiments have shown that the **Rous sarcoma virus** (**RSV**) in chickens may pick up the **ras oncogene** from one host and transmit it into another host, inducing **sarcoma** (a cancer of the mesoderm – bone, cartilage, muscle) in the new host.

Tumour suppressor genes

Tumour suppressor genes are implicated in a variety of malignant disorders, including myelodysplasia (MDS), leukaemia and lymphomas (Information box 12.7).

Tumour suppressor genes are able to result in malignancy through *loss or inactivation* (compare this with oncogenes, which induce malignancy through their activity). It seems that, under normal circumstances, tumour suppressor genes suppress uncontrolled cell growth, or at least they are key players in the regulation of cell growth. Uncontrolled cell growth will result if the suppressive effect is lost. Many tumour suppressor genes have now been identified that are associated with diseases such as **familial retinoblastoma** (cancer of the eye in children), **Wilm's tumour** (a kidney cancer in children) and **familial adenomatous polyposis** (leading to colon cancer).

THE LYMPHOID SYSTEM

The lymphoid system is found throughout the body (Clinical box 12.6) and acts to protect the body from foreign antigens. Specialised tissues have different functions and neoplastic transformations within the tissues lead to a variety of associated diseases.

Primary lymphoid tissues

In the bone marrow, primitive cells (**stem cells**) are stimulated by **cytokines** to mature into blood cells that enter the peripheral circulation. Lymphocytes are programmed in primary lymphoid tissue:

- **Pre-B lymphocytes** mature to form **B cells** in the bone marrow, which then circulate within the secondary lymphoid tissues.
- **T lymphocytes** are attracted to the **thymus** gland by chemotactic factors. Self-antigens enter through the capsule that surrounds the gland and come into contact with lymphocytes, where thymus epithelial cells promote the different steps of T cell differentiation and maturation. This is done through direct contact, allowing presentation of antigens (presentation of the **major histocompatibility complex**) enabling the recognition of 'self', and through hormonal influence, producing **helper T cells** and **cytotoxic T cells**.

Secondary lymphoid tissues

Lymph nodes are collections of cells, surrounded by a capsule, that are placed in areas of the body through which body fluid drains. Macrophages that line the sinuses beneath the capsule collect antigens present within fluid. Within the nodes lie the cortex, composed of follicles, and in the centre is the medulla. Different areas of the nodes have different functions:

- **B cells** proliferate in the follicles in response to antigen sensitisation.
- **T cells** differentiate and proliferate in the inter-follicular region, also in response to antigens.
- **Plasma cells** are present in the medulla and positioned close to the sinuses to facilitate delivery of immunoglobulins to react with foreign antigens.
- **Mucosa-associated lymphoid tissue** (**MALT**) is found along mucosal surfaces to protect antigen entry through this route. **Tonsils** are an example of MALT tissue. They are similar to lymph nodes but are filled mainly with B cells. Their position in the nasopharynx means they are suited to detect antigens within breathed-in air.

MYELOPROLIFERATIVE DISEASES

This is a diverse group of conditions with one feature in common: they are all **clonal** proliferations that may eventually (after several years) transform into acute leukaemia. The clinical and laboratory features reflect the predominant cell type in each.

The myeloproliferative diseases

- **Polycythaemia rubra vera** (proliferation of red cells)
- **Essential thrombocythaemia** (proliferation of platelets)
- **Myelofibrosis** (proliferation of myeloid cells)
- **Chronic myeloid leukaemia** (proliferation of leukaemic myeloid cells)

Polycythaemia

Polycythaemia is an increase in haemoglobin concentration, packed cell volume (PCV) and red cell count. Depending on whether there is a real increase in the red cell mass (RCM) or a reduction in plasma volume, polycythaemias fall into two major groups:

- Absolute erythrocytosis (true increase in red cell mass)
- Relative erythrocytosis (RCM normal but plasma volume reduced).

The three main groups (Fig. 12.23) are:

- **Primary proliferative polycythaemia** (PPP; also called polycythaemia rubra vera, PRV)
- **Secondary polycythaemia** – due to an increase in erythropoietin which may be physiological and appropriate, or produced inappropriately by a variety of tumours
- **Relative polycythaemia**, which is also called **apparent polycythaemia** – due to a reduced plasma volume making the red cell count relatively higher than normal.

Polycythaemia rubra vera

In **PRV** there is an absolute erythrocytosis (a true elevation of the red cell mass) often accompanied by an increase in

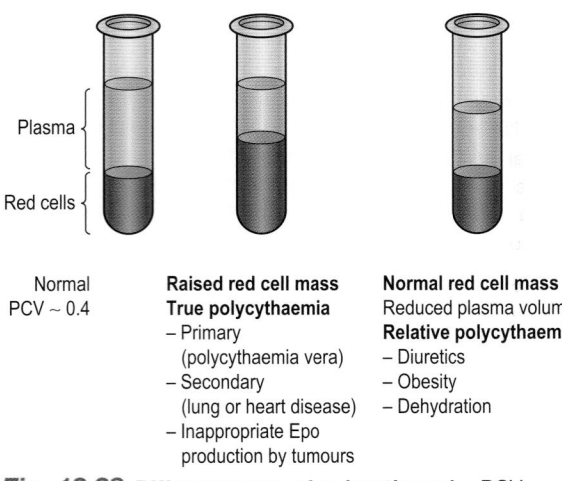

Normal
PCV ~ 0.4

Raised red cell mass
True polycythaemia
 – Primary
   (polycythaemia vera)
 – Secondary
   (lung or heart disease)
 – Inappropriate Epo
   production by tumours

Normal red cell mass
Reduced plasma volume
Relative polycythaemia
 – Diuretics
 – Obesity
 – Dehydration

Fig. 12.23 **Different types of polycythaemia.** PCV, packed cell volume.

granulocytes and platelets. The underlying cause is unknown but is likely to be due to acquired genetic changes in the stem cell leading to disturbance of the normal cellular growth pattern.

Cell culture studies have shown that the red cell precursors are more sensitive than normal to a variety of growth factors, including **Epo** and **thrombopoietin (Tpo)**. Precursor red cells are usually critically dependent on Epo. Cellular proliferation is believed to be driven through protein phosphorylation, and the tumour suppressor gene, SHP-1, appears to be a suitable candidate influencing this process; SHP-1 interacts with a variety of growth factor receptors including that of Epo.

The disease is generally found in older people with non-specific and variable symptoms, often resulting in PRV being unrecognised. Once diagnosed it is often treated by:

■ Venesection – removal of a unit of blood at regular intervals to relieve symptoms
■ Chemotherapy (hydroxyurea) – to control thrombocytosis and risk of vascular complications
■ Allopurinol – to block uric acid production.

Essential thrombocythaemia

Essential thrombocythaemia is a malignant clonal disorder affecting the bone marrow megakaryocytes. These increase in number and produce excess platelets. As with PRV, this disorder is commoner from middle age onwards. Thrombosis and haemorrhage may occur; the former occurs because there are excess platelets, and haemorrhage may result from interference in platelet function.

Myelofibrosis

Myelofibrosis is an uncommon myeloproliferative disease in which there is megakaryocyte hyperplasia in the bone marrow, with intense bone marrow fibrosis. Extramedullary haemopoiesis (production of blood at unusual sites) in the spleen, liver and at other sites is common.

MYELODYSPLASTIC SYNDROMES (MDS)

The **myelodysplastic syndromes** comprise clonal stem cell disorders characterised by abnormal blood cell develop-

ment. There is a highly proliferative bone marrow but with peripheral blood cytopenia. This is caused by the cells within the bone marrow being destroyed before being released into the circulation. Although the bone marrow is trying to produce adequate numbers of cells, these are largely defective. This leads to anaemia, with reduced white cell and platelet counts.

Some forms of MDS have a tendency to transform into acute leukaemia, and MDS was previously termed **preleukaemia**. However, many patients never develop leukaemia so this term has been abandoned. MDS is probably the commonest haematological neoplasm, with an incidence of about 1 : 10 000, and is primarily a disease of the elderly.

Overall, 5q– (a deletion in the long arm of chromosome 5) is the commonest cytogenetic finding in MDS and constitutes a separate clinical syndrome, usually affecting elderly females, and carries a good prognosis. Mutations of p53 have also been found and are associated with a poor prognosis and increased tendency to progress to acute leukaemia.

LEUKAEMIAS

Leukaemia literally means 'white blood', so-called because of the enormous numbers of white cells in the peripheral blood in patients with leukaemia at diagnosis. Classically, the leukaemias are divided into **acute** and **chronic** forms:

■ **Acute leukaemia** tends to present more dramatically, and must be treated early or death will occur within a short period of time.
■ In general, **chronic leukaemia** is more indolent (slow growing) and in some cases may not require therapy for years.

In both acute and chronic leukaemias there is progressive accumulation of abnormal white blood cells in the bone marrow or other organs, which spill out into the peripheral blood. There is progressive bone marrow failure with a reduction in the other normal cell types. Patients therefore tend to also have a reduced number of red cells (producing anaemia) and megakaryocytes (leading to low platelets and bleeding).

Acute leukaemia is uncommon and may occur at any age. There is a peak in early childhood and a progressive increase with age. The overall incidence is 4/100 000 per year. Leukaemias are categorised into either **childhood** (<15 years) or **adult** disease.

The acute leukaemias

Childhood and adult acute leukaemias differ in their frequencies, with **acute myeloid leukaemia (AML)** primarily a disease of adults and **acute lymphoblastic leukaemia (ALL)** affecting mainly children. Their response to treatment is also quite different; for example, children with ALL would be expected to be cured if treated, whilst adults with ALL do badly. The reasons for these age-related differences are complex and not fully understood. The acute nature of the disease is experienced through:

■ Tiredness, shortness of breath and anaemia – due to reduced red cells
■ Increased susceptibility to infection – due to reduced white cells

Table 12.15 Causes of acute leukaemia

Implicated agent	Mechanism	Examples
Ionising radiation	Induces genetic damage to haemopoietic progenitor cells. The peak incidence is 7–8 years after exposure	X-ray workers
		Post-atomic bomb survivors
		Irradiation used as part of therapy for Hodgkin's disease, non-Hodgkin's lymphoma, and other cancers
Chemical agents	DNA damage	Benzene and its derivatives
		Alkylating agents (anti-cancer drugs)
Genetic factors	Unstable chromosomes	Down's syndrome (trisomy 21)
		Fanconi's anaemia
Viruses	Some may integrate their DNA into the host and influence (e.g. upregulate) regulatory genes	Evidence exists for the role of viruses in causing leukaemia in animals but less so for humans. One human disease for which a virus has been shown to be causative is acute T cell leukaemia/lymphoma (ATLL), which is induced by the virus HTLV-1

■ Bruising or bleeding – due to reduction in platelets
■ Bone pain in children – accumulation of leukaemic cells in long bones
■ Respiratory and neurological symptoms – due to large numbers of white cells in the peripheral blood causing hyperviscosity and sludging of the blood.

Incidence and causes

As with many malignancies the underlying causes are not fully elucidated. However, there are environmental and genetic factors that predispose to the development of acute leukaemia; these are shown in the Table 12.15.

Laboratory findings

While it may be clear from the blood film that the patient has an acute leukaemia, differentiation between the myeloid and lymphoid forms are likely to need specialist tests.

Examination of the bone marrow will usually show an increased cellularity with most of the cells being abnormal blast cells. The blood film reflects the contents of the marrow with reduced numbers of normal red cells, white cells and platelets (because there is limited room in the marrow for the normal lineages), and immature white cells (leukaemic blast cells). Specialist tests are used to provide a formal diagnosis (Clinical box 12.7).

Chronic leukaemias

Chronic myeloid leukaemia (CML) and chronic lymphocytic leukaemia (CLL) have very little in common, apart from the fact that they are chronic in nature. Both may be discovered by chance.

Chronic myeloid leukaemia

CML is an uncommon clonal stem cell disorder making up 15% of all leukaemias. Presentation is more common in adults between the ages of 40 and 60 years. CML is characterised by a high white cell count, of granulocytic lineage, and the presence of the Philadelphia chromosome (Ph). There are two different forms of the resulting BCR-ABL mutation, depending on where the join to the 3′ end of BCR is placed. One type, seen in about 30% of patients, is associated with a more rapid progression of disease. The mutation leads to transcription of proteins with high tyrosine kinase activity. Tyrosine kinases are important in cell growth and

Table 12.16 Clinical features of chronic leukaemia

Chronic myeloid leukaemia	Chronic lymphocytic leukaemia
Non-specific – tiredness, fatigue and weight loss	
Abdominal discomfort – due to enlarged spleen and/or liver	
Progressive anaemia – due to marrow infiltration	
Gout – due to increased cell turnover producing high levels of uric acid	
Mild fever, night sweats – due to hypermetabolism	Enlarged lymph nodes – due to clonal B cell production
	Petechiae – pin point blood spots in the skin – due to reduced platelets
	Increased infection rate – due to reduced immunoglobulin

differentiation. CML was the first human malignancy shown to be associated with a specific chromosome translocation.

CML has three main phases: chronic phase, which lasts about 5 years before progressing to an accelerated phase, with increased numbers of blast cells, and finally blast crisis. The crisis resembles an acute leukaemia; there may be features of acute myeloid leukaemia in 80% of cases and lymphoid in 20%. Frequently there is evidence of other cytogenic abnormalities, such as another Ph-positive clone, trisomy 8, 9, 19 or 21, loss of one chromosome 17, or deletion of the Y chromosome.

Chronic lymphocytic leukaemia (CLL)

CLL is the commonest adult leukaemia in Western societies with a peak incidence in patients aged between 60 and 80 years of age, and a male to female ratio of 2:1. CLL is a slow-growing disorder characterised by progressive accumulation of neoplastic cells in the bone marrow, spleen, liver and lymph nodes. In some cases there is bone marrow failure with marked reduction in the normal cell lines. Both disease and treatment complications are causes of death. Table 12.16 summarises the clinical features of CLL (and CML).

The cause is largely unknown and most cases of CLL are of B cell lineage, their maturation arrested. Although the cells look like mature lymphocytes, examination of cell surface antigens reveal some differences and the cells have very low levels of surface immunoglobulin. Cytogenic abnormalities are also common: about 50% have a deletion of 13q, and other deletions or trisomy may be seen.

Clinical box 12.7   **Diagnosis of acute leukaemia**

Cytochemistry

Blood films are stained with different stains to detect specific proteins, carbohydrates and lipids that are characteristic of certain cell lineages (Fig. 12.24).

Immunophenotyping using flow cytometry

This technique has improved the diagnosis of leukaemia and other haematological disorders. It uses a panel of powerful monoclonal antibodies (MAbs) to determine the presence or absence of specific antigens on the surface (or inside) leukaemic cells. The MAbs are very sensitive and specific and will only bind to one target antigen. We now know the pattern of expression of antigens on the cells of most leukaemias, making it relatively easy to determine whether blast cells are lymphoid or myeloid.

Leukaemic cells are incubated with a variety of MAbs after which they are passed through a fluorescence activated cell sorter (FACS) machine. The FACS plots forward and side scatter and provides a guide to positivity or negativity for the antigens tested (Fig. 12.25).

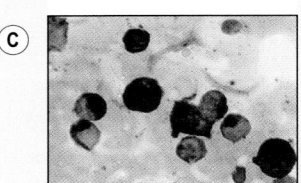

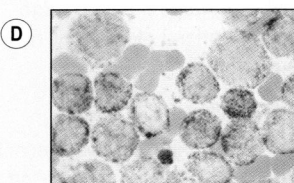

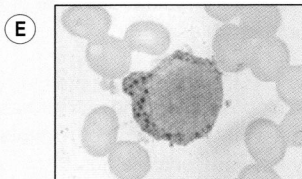

Fig. 12.24 **Cytochemical staining for acute leukaemia helps to distinguish between different forms of leukaemia.** (A) AML blast with Auer rod (top left) (May–Grunwald–Giemsa stain). (B) ALL blasts (May–Grunwald–Giemsa stain). (C) AML blasts: Sudan black stains lipids black. Lipids are rarely seen in lymphocytes. (D) ALL blasts: acid phosphatase positive staining in T cell subsets in ALL. (E) ALL blasts: Periodic acid–Schiff (PAS) stains glycogen red in ALL blasts. Glycogen is not present in normal lymphocytes.

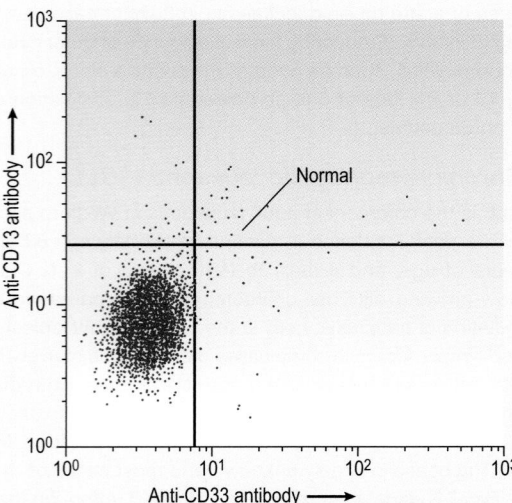

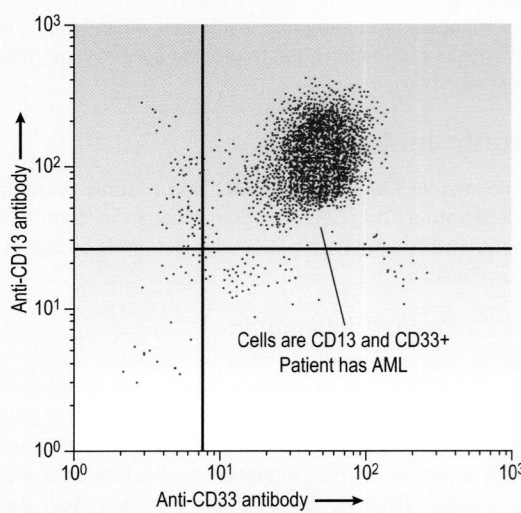

Fig. 12.25 **Flow cytometry using different monoclonal antibodies to cell surface molecules can distinguish between normal (*left*) and acute myeloid leukaemia (AML) (*right*).**

Table 12.17	Laboratory findings in chronic leukaemia	
Chronic myeloid leukaemia	**Chronic lymphocytic leukaemia**
White count very high, up to >100 × 10⁹/L, reduced haemoglobin	
Mainly granulocytic with full range of precursors (Fig. 12.26A)	Mainly mature looking lymphocytes with 'smear' cells. These are produced when the blood film is made (Fig. 12.26C)
Bone marrow hypercellular – mostly granulocytes (Fig. 12.26B)	Bone marrow has increased number of small lymphocytes

An overexpression of **BCL2** is seen in the disease. This proto-oncogene is a suppressor of **apoptosis** (programmed cell death) and thus the affected cells have a longer lifespan.

Research has shown that somatic mutation of the variable regions of the immunoglobulin heavy chain genes (IgH V region genes) predicts a favourable outcome, whereas patients in whom the IgH V genes are not mutated fare less well. The reason for the influence of IgH V gene mutational status on survival is that B CLL lymphocytes, in which the IgH V genes are mutated, have passed through the lymph node germinal centres and are by definition more competent. By contrast, those with unmutated IgH V genes are pre-germinal.

Laboratory findings

In chronic leukaemia the white cell count is very high, typically greater than 100 × 10⁹/L, and the types reflect the disease (Table 12.17). In myeloid leukaemia the full range of precursors are seen in the blood, and the bone marrow is hypercellular (Fig. 12.26A, B), whereas in lymphoid leukaemia the cells appear mature but are often accompanied by 'smear' cells, produced when the blood film is made (Fig. 12.26C).

LYMPHOMAS

Lymphomas are malignancies affecting lymphoid tissue, i.e. lymphocytes, and comprise the **non-Hodgkin's lymphomas (NHLs)** and **Hodgkin's disease**.

Non-Hodgkin's lymphoma (NHL)

In **NHL** there is a clonal expansion of lymphoid cells, mostly of B cell origin. Several different mechanisms are thought to be involved.

Chromosome translocations

Different chromosomal translocations and molecular rearrangements influence the pathology and disease prognosis.

- t(14;18) involves an apoptotic inhibitor oncogene, bcl-2, leading to its overexpression, and is particularly associated with **follicular lymphoma**.
- t(11;14) leads to overexpression of the cell cycle regulator, bcl-1, associated with **mantle cell lymphoma**.
- t(8;14) leads to movement of the c-myc proto-oncogene and results in its deregulation, leading to cell

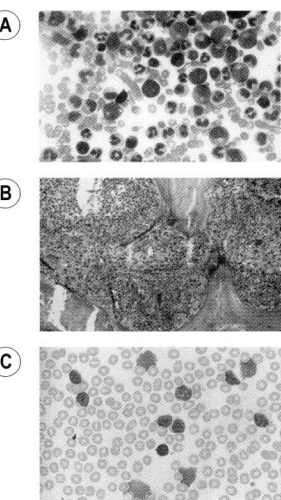

Fig. 12.26 **Chronic leukaemia.** (A) CML blood film: note the large numbers of granulocytic cells, in particular neutrophils, at all stages of development. (B) CML bone marrow trephine biopsy showing a packed marrow with granulocytic cells similar to those are found in the peripheral blood. (C) CLL blood film showing numerous mature-looking lymphocytes, with 'smear' cells.

proliferation, associated with **Burkitt and human immunodeficiency virus (HIV)-infection associated lymphomas**.
- t(2;5) links two genes (NPM) and (ALK1) and produces a new protein which is found in associated **anaplastic large cell lymphomas**.
- t(11;18) links an apoptosis inhibitor gene with the MALT1 gene and produces a protein that is associated with **MALT lymphomas**.

Viral infection

Viral infection can lead to chronic antigenic stimulation and dysregulation of cytokines, resulting in B or T cell proliferation. Several viruses are implicated and their geographical locations may influence the prevalence of different disease expression:

- Epstein–Barr virus (EBV)
- Human T cell leukaemia virus type 1 (HTLV-1)
- Hepatitis C virus (HCV)
- Kaposi's sarcoma-associated herpes virus (KSHV).

Other implicated factors

- Environmental: chemicals (organic solvents, pesticides, hair dye, etc) or radiation exposure.
- Immunodeficiencies: congenital (severe combined immunodeficiency disease); acquired (acquired immune deficiency syndrome (AIDS)); induced (immunosuppressive therapy).
- Chronic inflammation of MALT tissues.
- Helicobacter pylori infection.

Hodgkin's disease

Hodgkin's disease is less common and potentially curable. There are two incidence peaks: one in young adults, and the second in older individuals. The cause is unknown but **EBV infection** may have a role. The annual incidence is 2–3 per

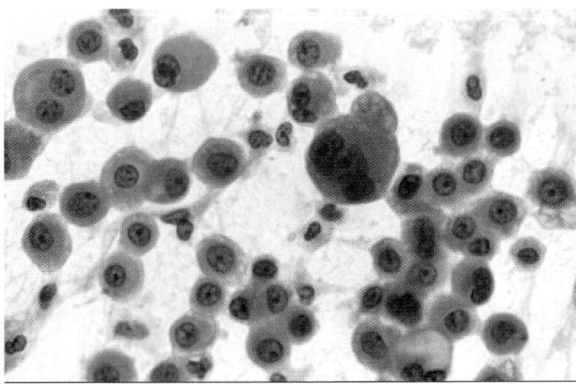

Fig. 12.27 **Reed–Sternberg cells in Hodgkin's disease.** These cells appear as abnormal giant and often multinucleated cells.

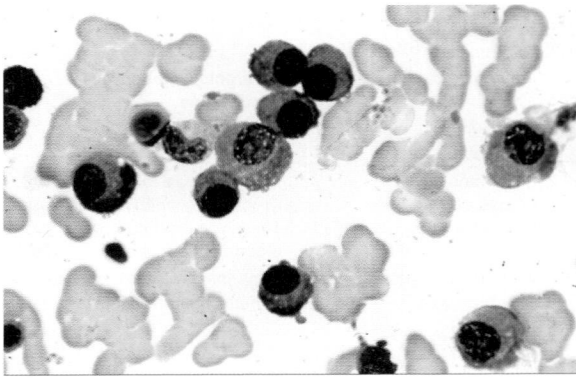

Fig. 12.28 **Plasma cells showing characteristic features:** an eccentric nucleus; very dark blue cytoplasm; a paler region close to the nucleus (perinuclear halo).

100 000. **Reed–Sternberg cells** (Fig. 12.27) are characteristically seen when lymph nodes are biopsied. These cells are B lymphocytes that originate in the lymph node germinal centre but have lost the ability to produce antibodies.

PLASMA CELL DISORDERS

Plasma cells are terminally differentiated B cells (cannot divide any further) whose main role is the production of antibody. Plasma cell diseases include:

- Monoclonal gammopathy of undetermined significance
- Multiple myeloma
- Plasmacytoma
- Plasma cell leukaemia.

Multiple myeloma

Myeloma has an incidence of 4 per 100 000 individuals, with 2500 new cases in the UK each year. The incidence increases with age and most patients are over 60 years of age; the disease is rare in individuals under the age of 40 years. For reasons not understood, myeloma is commoner in black Americans. Genetic associations and environmental chemical exposure have both been linked to development of the disease.

The malignant **plasma cells** accumulate in the bone marrow and suppress normal cell production. Most myelomas produce large quantities of **monoclonal immunoglobulin** (i.e. antibody molecules that are identical, as opposed to the normal polyclonal pattern seen in health).

Clinical feature of multiple myeloma

About 60% of patients have bone disease. Bones are destroyed due to activation of osteoclasts by cytokines such as TNF-α and IL-1α, produced by the neoplastic cells. The osteoclasts also make and secrete IL-6, which is a growth factor for plasma cells.

Almost 30% of patients experience renal failure. Damage to the kidneys may be by direct injury to the tubules by proteins, amyloidosis (deposition of insoluble protein in the tissues) or plasmacytoma interference (soft tissue mass of plasma cells).

In addition, the patients also experience anaemia (multifactorial), infection (due to defective humoral and cellular immunity) and neurological problems (from hyperviscosity,

Table 12.18	Laboratory features of multiple myeloma	
Source	**Finding**	**Explanation**
Blood count	Reduced haemoglobin	Plasma cell proliferation interferes with normal cell production
Blood film	Plasma cells	Overproduction of malignant cells
Other	Very high erythrocyte sedimentation rate (ESR)	See Information box 12.8
Biochemistry	Abnormal urea and electrolytes	If renal impairment or renal failure is present
	Raised serum calcium	Excess calcium from bone destruction
	Monoclonal globulin in electrophoresis	Malignant plasma cells produce a single gamma globulin
	Bence Jones protein in urine	Free light chains from the excess abnormal globulin

producing headaches and hazy vision, or from spinal cord compression).

Laboratory features of multiple myeloma

While patients might have experienced symptoms of anaemia and bone pain these may be dismissed as something common in the older patient, which is the key target group for this disease. A blood film may well reveal the presence of characteristic plasma cells (Fig. 12.28). Table 12.18 lists other typical findings.

HAEMOSTASIS AND THROMBOSIS

NORMAL HAEMOSTATIC MECHANISMS

The haemostatic system is designed to ensure that there is no major leakage of blood following injury and consists of a complex system of proteins and enzymes. In health, any local bleeding is arrested by an interaction between platelets and blood vessel endothelial cells, followed by a cascade of coagulation factors. Any defect in these may result in bleeding or thrombosis.

The erythrocyte sedimentation rate (ESR)

This is a laboratory test undertaken by placing anticoagulated blood in a narrow vertical tube. Red cells fall through the plasma under gravity, dropping only a few millimetres in an hour under normal conditions (Fig. 12.29).

A non-specific test with high rates (high ESR) being associated with acute and chronic inflammation (including infections and cancer), autoimmune diseases and multiple myeloma (due to the changes in plasma proteins), anaemia (due to the reduction in red cell content), sickle cell disease (due to the shape of the red cells). It is particularly useful in the diagnosis of **temporal arteritis** (chronic inflammation of the large arteries of the head) and **polymyalgia rheumatica** (shoulder and pelvic joint stiffness).

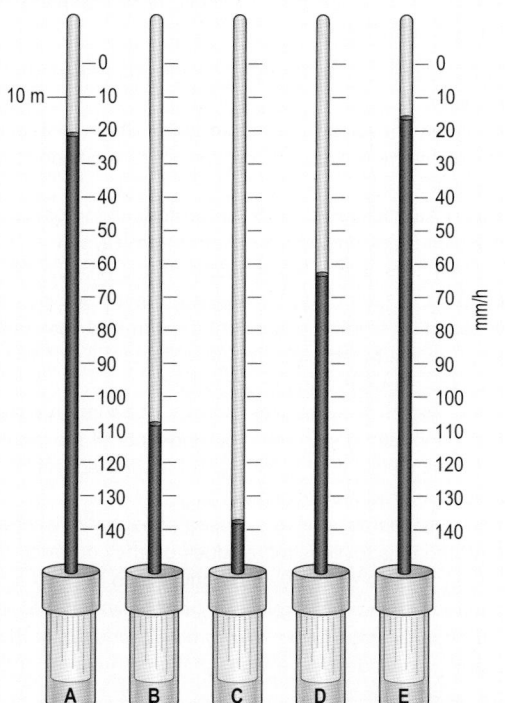

Fig. 12.29 **Erythrocyte sedimentation rate (ESR):** the rate at which red cells precipitate (in a Westergren tube) in mm/h. The rate increases in inflammatory diseases. Blood samples A and E show normal ESR, B, C and D show greatly increased ESR; each division is 10 mm.

The role of the endothelium and platelets in the maintenance of haemostasis

Endothelial cells line all blood vessels and these play a central role in preventing unwanted thrombosis. The endothelium provides an effective barrier between the thrombogenic subendothelial cells and the blood coagulation factors. Agents produced by endothelium include:

- **Thrombomodulin** (protein involved in thrombin control)
- **Heparan sulphate** (a naturally occurring heparin that leads to inhibition of thrombin)
- Enzymes that degrade platelet-derived molecules, such as ADP, the latter encouraging platelets to aggregate.
- **Prostacyclin** and **nitric oxide** (**NO**), which are potent inhibitors of platelet aggregation, discouraging platelets from sticking to the vessel wall.

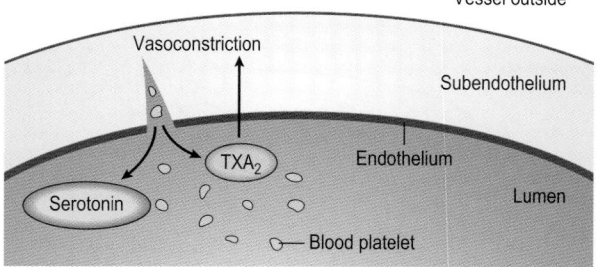

Fig. 12.30 **Early involvement of platelets and blood vessel subendothelium.** Platelets are attracted to subendothelial material when the endothelial layer is breached, plugging the gap and stimulated to release substances that enhance vasoconstriction in order to further reduce blood loss from the vessel. TXA$_2$, thromboxane A$_2$.

When tissue damage occurs, the subendothelium is exposed to blood cells, including platelets. Figure 12.30 illustrates the components involved.

1. Prostacyclin concentration is lower in the subendothelium than in the endothelium.
2. Lower levels of prostacyclin, along with collagen and other subendothelial molecules, attract platelets causing them to stick, producing a platelet plug.
3. **Thromboxane A$_2$** and **serotonin** are released from the activated platelets. These are vasoconstrictors, serving to reduce the vessel lumen and thus also blood flow and loss.

For minor breaches in vessel integrity these events may be sufficient for repair, but in severe breaches, or high flow, more is needed.

Platelets do not have a nucleus and so have limited ability to provide energy for their necessary functions. Glycogen stores and mitochondria within platelets provide energy through **microtubules** to change their shape, facilitating aggregation, and allowing release of substances from **dense** and **α granules** present within the platelet cytoplasm.

1. Platelets adhere to the connective tissue through a glycoprotein receptor (**GpIb-Ix**) in combination with von Willebrand's factor (**vWF**).
2. More platelets adhere to the site, binding to each other through the **GPIIa-IIIb** platelet receptor in combination with the plasma protein, **fibrinogen**.
3. Platelets are discouraged from extending along the vessel wall by the high concentration of **prostacyclin** in the intact endothelium.
4. At this point, although platelets have changed shape and aggregated together, this action is reversible and platelets can return to normal and be released back into the circulation.
5. Once granule release takes place the aggregation becomes irreversible.

Amongst other substances, **ADP**, **thrombin** and **thromboxane A$_2$** are released. These serve to recruit even more platelets to the site and thrombin acts to change fibrinogen into fibrin, thereby helping to stabilise the platelet plug. **Platelet factor 4** and the structurally related **β-thromboglobulin** promote clotting by neutralising heparin and heparin-like substances.

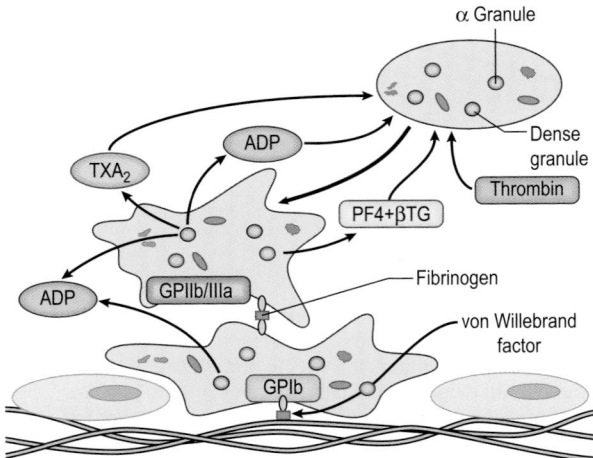

Fig. 12.31 Platelet–vessel–wall interactions.

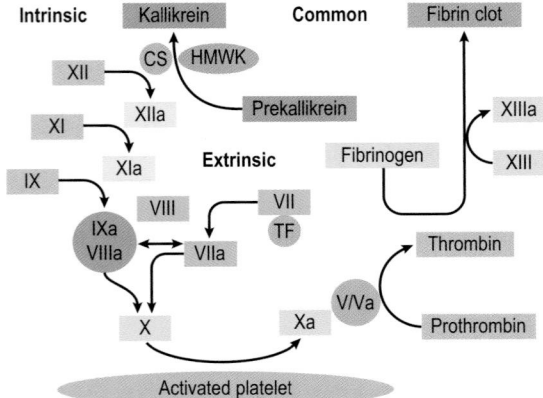

Fig. 12.32 The coagulation cascade. Clotting factors are indicated with roman numerals and their active forms by the 'a'. For example, VIII is inactive factor VIII, and VIIIa is the active form. TF, tissue factor; CS, contact surface; HMWK, high-molecular-weight kininogen.

Platelet factors are also an integral part of the coagulation cascade that is subsequently stimulated by the release of tissue factor and thrombin. Fig. 12.31 illustrates the initial involvement of platelets in the maintenance of haemostasis.

Coagulation cascade

This comprises two main components:

- **Coagulation** – production of the blood clot, in order to arrest bleeding.
- **Fibrinolysis** – to dissolve the clot once it has served its purpose.

Most of the clotting factors are present in the circulation as inactive proteins called **zymogens**, probably a safety feature to prevent unwanted blood clotting. These inactive proteins require activation, usually by other clotting factors, to an active form in order to take part in a coagulation reaction.

Figure 12.32 shows the entire coagulation cascade, which comprises **intrinsic** and **extrinsic** pathways. Both of these

terms are somewhat dated, and we no longer view the cascade in this manner. Nonetheless, it does help explain some of the tests used to detect coagulation cascade abnormalities. The cascade is normally triggered by local damage, which brings coagulation factors into contact with negatively charged phospholipid surfaces and non-endothelial surfaces.

The intrinsic pathway

Prekallikrein, high-molecular-weight kininogen (HMWK), calcium ions, phospholipids from platelets and clotting factors XII, XI, IX, VIII and X are required for this pathway, which is initiated on exposure to a negatively charged non-endothelial surface, such as collagen, finally resulting in the production of factor Xa.

1. Contact phase components convert prekallikrein to kallikrein.
2. Kallikrein activates factor XII to factor XIIa, which also stimulates more kallikrein production to maintain the cascade.
3. Factor XIIa activates factor XI to produce factor XIa and releases bradykinin (a vasodilator) from HMWK.
4. Calcium ions and factor XIa activate the proenzyme factor IX to factor IXa, the serine protease activity being released by binding of calcium to vitamin K-dependent γ-carboxyglutamate (gla) residues (factors II, VII and X are also gla-containing proenzymes).
5. Active factor IX hydrolyses factor X at an internal arg-ile bond and, along with other components of the tenase complex (calcium ions, VIIIa and IXa, and activated platelets) produces activated Xa.
6. Activated platelets have exposed phosphatidylserine and phosphatidylinositol residues on their surface.
7. Factor VIII is a cofactor, and activated to VIIIa by small amounts of thrombin, released from activated platelets, although the high levels of thrombin produced in the clotting cascade cleave VIIIa, limiting the extent of the coagulation cascade.

The extrinsic pathway

The cascade is initiated by tissue factor (TF), also known as factor III, which is present on the blood vessel endothelial cells and also involves factor VII.

1. Factor VII is activated by thrombin to factor VIIa, and also further activated by factor Xa from the intrinsic pathway.
2. Factor VIIa and its cofactor, TF, is involved in the activation of factor X to Xa, in the same way as factor IXa.

The common pathway

The two pathways converge with the production of factor Xa. Production of a clot further involves factors II, I and XIII.

1. Factor Xa cleaves prothrombin (factor II) at two sites to form a two-chain active thrombin molecule (factor IIa), each chain being held by a single disulphide bond on the surface of activated platelets within a prothrombinase complex.
2. The prothrombinase complex is similar to the tenase complex and involves the phospholipids on activated platelets, calcium, prothrombin, factor Xa and factor Va as a cofactor.

3. Factor V is activated to factor Va by small amounts of thrombin, like factor VIII.
4. Thrombin reinforces the clotting cascade by further activating factor XI, VIII and V and also converts fibrinogen (factor I) to form the fibrin clot.
5. Fibrinogen is composed of three pairs of polypeptides, linked with disulphide bonds. The polypeptides have residues that have a high negative charge, making fibrinogen soluble in plasma. Activation with thrombin releases the polypeptides for monomers that spontaneously aggregate to form a weak fibrin mesh.
6. Thrombin also activates factor XIII to form factor XIIIa (transglutaminase) which cross-links the fibrin with covalent bonds between glutamine and lysine residues to consolidate the clot.

Natural anticoagulants are required to maintain the balance

In addition to the possession of a highly effective coagulation mechanism there needs to be an anticoagulant system in place to maintain the homeostatic balance. The body has several molecules that serve this purpose:

- **Thrombomodulin**, a glycoprotein present on endothelial cells that combines with thrombin.
  - The thrombomodulin-thrombin compound activates **protein C** to protein Ca.
  - Protein Ca and its cofactor, **protein S**, degrade factors Va and VIIIa.
- **Antithrombin** combines with its substrates, which include factor Xa and thrombin, to limit action of the coagulation pathways.
- **Heparin cofactor II** inhibits thrombin.

Both antithrombin and heparin cofactor II are stimulated by **heparin**, which is used clinically as an anticoagulant.

The fibrinolytic system

After a blood clot has served its purpose it requires breaking down in order to restore normal flow in the blood vessel. The fibrinolytic system is responsible for this activity and, much the same as the coagulation cascade, consists of a series of coordinated enzyme reactions.

The key player in the whole process is **plasmin**. The zymogen (inactive proenzyme) **plasminogen** must first be converted, through activators, to plasmin, whose main role is to break down fibrin molecules, in addition to coagulation factors V and VII. This leads to the release of **fibrin degradation products** (FDPs).

The largest fragment produced by fibrin degradation is **fragment X**, generated by plasmin cleavage of the terminal α and β chains of the fibrin molecule. Fragment X is then cleaved by plasmin to form two fragments Y and DXD. Finally, through further enzyme cleavage, **D-dimers** are produced (D-D). D-dimers represent in vivo lysis of fibrin rather than fibrinogen. This is important clinically since laboratories used to measure FDPs for the diagnosis of disorders such as **disseminated intravascular coagulation** (DIC), but FDPs cannot distinguish between fibrin and fibrinogen degradation. The newer D-dimer assay is now used as a measure of in vivo fibrinolysis since D-dimers represent only fibrin degradation.

Clinical box 12.8 **Clot-busting drugs**

The understanding of the physiology of clot breakdown has led to the development of drugs serving the same purpose. These are useful where thrombosis has occurred within a vessel, causing life-threatening consequences. One example of this is in **myocardial infarction**. In this situation a thrombus occludes one or more of the coronary arteries, compromising blood flow to the heart muscle.

Streptokinase is an example of an agent that can be administered in the acute situation in order to break down the clot and restore blood flow.

- Streptokinase is isolated from β-haemolytic streptococci, and is a polypeptide that binds to plasminogen, which then undergoes a change in conformation.
- The active site of plasminogen is exposed and the molecule then resembles plasmin (although it is not plasmin, since no cleavage of plasminogen has occurred; however, functionally it acts as though it *is* plasmin).

Streptokinase is used therapeutically, but has several disadvantages:

- Its half-life is very short.
- The streptokinase–plasminogen complexes degrade fibrin *and* fibrinogen, which is undesirable (increases bleeding).
- Streptokinase is very antigenic and can cause severe allergic reactions. This occurs because streptokinase is derived from bacteria to which most individuals have been exposed.

Human tissue plasminogen activator (**tPA**) was shown to have advantages over streptokinase:

- Not antigenic
- 1% lower mortality at 12 months
- *but* – more patients were likely to have an early stroke after treatment with tPA, compared with streptokinase.

Clinical consequences of fibrin degradation products

Apart from FDPs being used as indicators of continuing thrombosis/haemostasis, they have major functional consequences for haemostasis itself, contributing to the ongoing intravascular coagulation that is seen in **disseminated intravascular coagulation** (DIC).

Fibrin breakdown products possess antithrombin activity, and they interfere with normal polymerisation of fibrin monomers. The larger of the fragments, X and Y, are the most inhibitory. These fragments also coat platelets and interfere with normal platelet function, thereby worsening the haemorrhagic tendency.

Plasminogen activators: tissue and urinary plasminogen activator (tPA and uPA)

Tissue plasminogen activator (**tPA**) is a glycoprotein produced by endothelial cells. tPA is found in blood and most body fluids. The binding of tPA to fibrin leads to cleavage of plasminogen, producing plasmin. Excess tPA in the blood is rapidly cleared by the liver. Synthetic tPA is used therapeutically to treat patients who may be experiencing a heart attack (Clinical box 12.8).

Urinary plasminogen activator (**uPA**) is made by the renal tubules and collecting ducts. The molecule has many similarities to tPA but its primary role is not clear; it appears to be involved in cell differentiation but may also be involved in the breakdown of fibrin clots deposited in the excretory ducts.

Fibrinolysis inhibitors

- Fibrinolysis inhibitors are required in vivo to prevent prolonged or unwanted degradation of fibrinogen. Several natural inhibitors have now been described, including **plasminogen activator inhibitor** 1 and 2 (PAI-1, PAI-2), α_2-antiplasmin, adhesion molecules and thrombin-activated fibrinolysis inhibitor.
- Free tPA and uPA are rapidly inhibited by PAI of which PAI-1 is the most important. PAI-1 is made by endothelial cells of blood vessels and is also found in platelet α granules. Increased levels of PAI-1 predispose individuals to thrombosis and are one cause of thrombophilia.
- Free circulating plasmin is inhibited by α_2-**antiplasmin**.
- Thrombin binds to and releases G protein protease activated receptors (PARs) that signal release of interleukins (IL-1 and IL-6) to increase the secretion of intercellular adhesion molecule-1 (ICAM-1) and vascular cell adhesion molecule-1 (VCAM-1) – increasing platelet activation and leucocyte adhesion.
- Thrombin activates **thrombin-activated fibrinolysis inhibitor** (**TAFI**), which impairs plasminogen activation, and therefore also fibrinolysis.

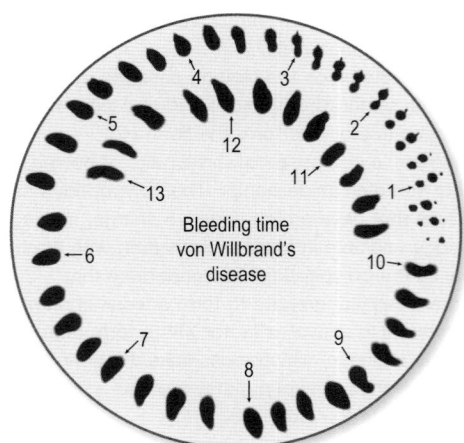

Fig. 12.33 **Bleeding time record in a patient with von Willebrand's disease.** It took more than 13 minutes for this patient to stop bleeding.

Assessment of the coagulation system

Over the years a number of tests have been developed that help to determine which component of the haemostatic mechanism is functioning incorrectly.

Full blood count and film

A full blood count will detect any abnormalities in platelet number. A high platelet count will not necessarily mean that there is no danger from bleeding. A blood film is useful to confirm the automated platelet count and also allows the morphology of the platelets to be assessed – some inherited platelet disorders are associated with large platelets.

The bleeding time

This crude test is useful for assessing the in vivo function of the platelets, since platelets are responsible for providing the first line of defence in bleeding. By inflicting controlled depth incisions into the skin using a template bleeding time device, bleeding is induced (Fig. 12.33). Platelets plug up the defect in the blood vessels and the bleeding will stop, usually within 9 minutes. If platelet function is defective, or if the platelet number is low, bleeding will occur for much longer. Platelet function may also be abnormal due to inherited disorders or drug ingestion (e.g. aspirin).

Coagulation tests

These are used to determine the function of the intrinsic and extrinsic components of the coagulation system. Blood is taken from the patient and placed into tubes containing sodium citrate. The normal functioning of the coagulation cascade requires calcium. Citrate binds calcium, and blood taken into citrate is therefore anticoagulated and will not form a clot until further calcium is added (Fig. 12.34).

The principal tests in current use are:

- **Prothrombin time** (**PT**) – used to assess the extrinsic pathway (Fig. 12.34A). Calcium is added to plasma to replace that removed by citrate anticoagulant and brain

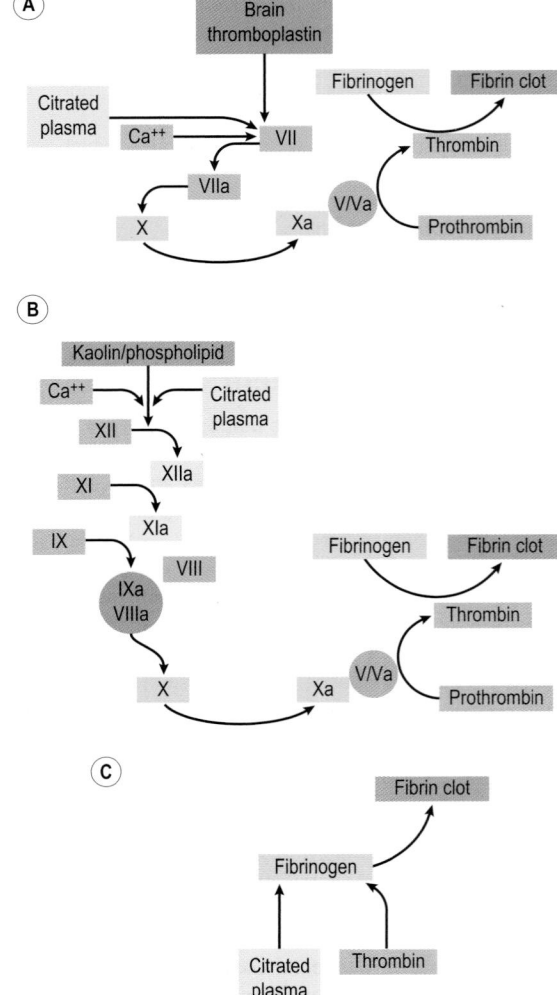

Fig. 12.34 **(A)** Principle of the prothrombin test. **(B)** Principle of the activated partial thromboplastin time (APTT). **(C)** Principle of the thrombin time.

thromboplastin is added to substitute for tissue factor. Clotting normally takes 12–15 seconds and the test time is compared with a standard normal control in a ratio – the **international normalised ratio** (**INR**). The test is used to assess liver function and monitor warfarin therapy.

- **Activated partial thromboplastin time** (**APTT**) – used to assess the intrinsic pathway (Fig. 12.34B). Calcium is added to plasma to replace that removed by citrate anticoagulant, then kaolin and phospholipids are added to substitute for contact factor. Clotting normally takes 25–36 seconds. The test is used to check for factor deficiencies and monitor heparin therapy.
- **Thrombin clotting time** (**TCT**) – used to assess the common pathway (Fig. 12.34C). Calcium is added to plasma to replace that removed by citrate anticoagulant, then thrombin is added to substitute for the products of the intrinsic and extrinsic pathways and to assess the conversion of fibrinogen to fibrin. The test is used to check for **disseminated intravascular coagulation** (**DIC**) but will also be prolonged in the presence of **heparin**.
- **Correction tests** – if the clotting time is prolonged. The patient's plasma is mixed 50:50 with normal plasma containing all clotting factors. If *correction* occurs, this implies that the patient's sample has a **factor deficiency**. If addition of normal plasma *fails to correct* the prolongation, this would tend to indicate that a **clotting factor inhibitor** is present. The inhibitor interferes with the normal clotting pathway.
- **Coagulation factor assays** to determine the actual deficiency.

COAGULATION FACTOR DISORDERS

Coagulation factor disorders may be inherited or acquired.

Inherited disorders

Inherited disorders include:

- Haemophilia A (factor VIII deficiency)
- Haemophilia B (factor IX deficiency)
- von Willebrand's disease (vWD)
- Inherited platelet disorders.

Haemophilia A
Haemophilia A is an inherited X-linked disorder where mutations within the factor VIII gene lead to defective function of the factor VIII-C molecule in the coagulation cascade, although about a third of diagnoses are new mutations. A large number of different genetic mutations have been described in this gene which has 26 exons and 25 introns at 28q on the X chromosome, leading to different manifestations of what is, nevertheless, a significant bleeding diathesis. About 40% of diagnoses are due to a major inversion of part of the tip of the long arm of the X chromosome, one break point of which is situated within intron 22 of the gene.

As a key protein in the intrinsic pathway, deficiency of factor VIII leads to prolongation of the APTT coagulation screening test, whereas the PT test is normal. Haemophilia A affects 1 in 5000 males and the disease is classified according to the factor VIII level.

Males, who only have one X chromosome, are the main sufferers of this condition, with females generally only having one of their X chromosomes affected. Such females are referred to as **carriers**, and their male children will have a 50% chance of having haemophilia. Female children of the union of a male haemophiliac with a female carrier will also have a 50% chance of having haemophilia.

Haemophilia B (Christmas disease)
Haemophilia B is an inherited X-linked disorder, where mutations within the factor IX gene leads to defective function of the factor IX molecule in the coagulation cascade. Like haemophilia A, about a third are new mutations. While most mutations are point mutations, at various sites, a variety of other mutations have been described. The original factor IX deficient subject, Mr Christmas, was a severely deficient patient whose mutation was cys-206-ser.

Like haemophilia A, a deficiency in factor IX leads to an abnormal APTT with a normal PT. Haemophilia B however is not as common, affecting about 1 in 30 000 males. The pattern of disease in males, with female carriers, is identical to that in patients with haemophilia A.

Clinical and diagnostic features of haemophilia
Patients with very low factor levels, who experience repeated and painful bleeds into their joints and muscles, are given factor replacement. Originally the factors were produced from plasma pooled from a large number of individuals. This led to a large number of haemophiliac patients also being infected with HIV in the 1970s and 1980s. Since 1998, children have only received recombinant factors. Porcine factor replacement is also used.

Typically, in severe disease, factor levels are less than 1% of normal levels. The APTT screening test is prolonged, but the bleeding time is normal (because primary platelet plug formation is not affected).

Von Willebrand's disease
Von Willebrand's disease (vWD) is an autosomal dominant inherited disorder associated (although some forms are recessive), with a deficiency in circulating vWF. The *vWF* gene is found on chromosome 12 and a variety of quantitative and qualitative defects have been described that result in reduced expression of vWF. vWF is a large glycoprotein, released, in response to stimuli, from platelet storage granules and endothelial cells. vWF has two major roles:

- Mediating platelet adhesion to sites of vascular injury (see Fig. 12.31)
- Binding and stabilising factor VIII.

vWD is the most common inherited bleeding disorder. Clinically it affects about 125 per million people and leads to a mild bleeding disorder affecting males and females equally. Bleeding is typically seen in mucocutaneous tissues (skin and mucous membranes) because of the high capillary density; these tissues particularly depend on the efficient formation of platelet plug to stop bleeding.

Because of its links to factor VIII, low levels of vWF, like haemophilia A, also result in a prolonged APTT test and reduced factor VIII clotting activity. Unlike haemophilia A, patients have a prolonged bleeding time because of a failure in platelet–vessel wall interaction.

Inherited platelet disorders

The best known of these are:

- Glanzmann's thrombasthenia
  - Autosomal recessive inheritance
  - Abnormality in platelet Gp IIb–IIIa interaction (see Fig. 12.31) preventing platelet aggregation.
- Bernard Soulier syndrome
  - Autosomal recessive inheritance
  - Reduced complex of GpIb, factor IX, and factor V, which serves as a receptor for vWF, leading to lack of platelet plug formation (see Fig. 12.31).

Acquired disorders

A range of acquired platelet and clotting factor disorders have been described that are often associated with other diseases. For example, **acquired haemophilia** is the result of stimulation and production of an autoantibody that reduces factor VIII levels (factor VIII inhibitor).

THE THROMBOCYTOPENIAS

Thrombocytopenia, a reduction in platelet count, may be caused by:

- Impaired production
- Increased destruction
- Altered distribution.

Patients with thrombocytopenia are likely to have the following clinical features:

- Pin-point skin haemorrhagic spots (**petechiae**) that result from capillary bleeds (Fig. 12.35). These red spots do not 'blanch' when pressed.
- Bruising and mucous membrane bleeding resulting in **epistaxis** (blood from nose), **melaena** (blood in faeces) and **menorrhagia** (heavy periods).

Thrombocytopenia caused by impaired platelet production

This can be drug induced, or the result of a bone marrow failure. For example, cytotoxic drugs that are myelosuppressive will inhibit megakaryocyte stem cells, and hence may cause thrombocytopenia.

Aplastic anaemia is an uncommon disorder with an incidence of 2–5 per million population per year. When the bone

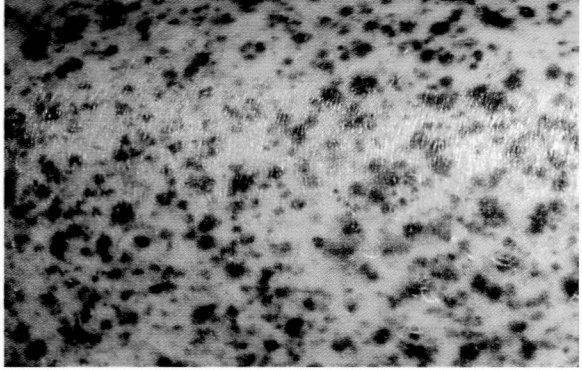

Fig. 12.35 **Skin with petechial haemorrhages.**

marrow is examined there are hardly any cells present and this is reflected in a lack of all the mature cells in the blood. The cells, when seen, appear morphologically normal. The lack of platelets in this condition results in problems with primary haemostasis.

Thrombocytopenia caused by increased platelet destruction

These may be immunological or non-immunological in origin.

Non-immune causes of thrombocytopenia

Disseminated intravascular coagulation (DIC)

Disseminated intravascular coagulation (**DIC**) is characterised by excessive activation of the coagulation cascade and may be triggered by the release of tissue thromboplastins that contain a high concentration of phospholipids following trauma, surgery, mismatched blood transfusion and a variety of other triggers, such as premature separation of the placenta (**abruptio placenta**). Unrecognised and untreated it can lead to uncontrolled bleeding as all the clotting factors are used up, and may result in death.

Thrombocytopenia due to an altered distribution, or dilution

In health, **the spleen** may pool up to one third of the total platelet mass, but in disease states this may rise to 90%. If the spleen is removed there is a large rise in the platelet count. Platelets can pool in the spleen in conditions such as liver cirrhosis and this leads to a relative thrombocytopenia.

Massive transfusion, when a patient's total blood volume is replaced over a short time period, may lead to thrombocytopenia. The degree is largely related to the amount of blood transfused, but the mechanism is *not* purely dilutional since there appears to be an element of platelet consumption as well.

Immune causes of thrombocytopenia

The more important immune-mediated causes of thrombocytopenia are:

- Neonatal alloimmune thrombocytopenia (NAIT)
- Post-transfusion purpura (PTP)
- Idiopathic thrombocytopenic purpura (ITP)
- Drug-induced thrombocytopenia
- Heparin-induced thrombocytopenia (HIT).

Platelet antigens can be platelet specific, or shared with other cells. Important shared antigens include human leucocyte antigen (HLA) class I and ABH (blood group A and B) antigens. Platelet-specific antigens fall into five well-defined human platelet antigen (HPA) groups: HPA-1, HPA-2, HPA-3, HPA-4 and HPA-5, each of which has an 'a' and a 'b' allele. Because some platelet glycoproteins carry antigenic sites that play a major role in platelet function, platelet alloantibodies may not only cause thrombocytopenia but also affect primary haemostasis.

Idiopathic thrombocytopenic purpura (ITP)

In **idiopathic thrombocytopenic purpura** (**ITP**), platelets are coated with anti-platelet autoantibodies and removed prematurely by the reticuloendothelial system, leading to a reduced peripheral blood platelet count. It is thought to be due to an inappropriate response to an environmental trigger. The cause, however, is unknown and the clinical course is variable and unpredictable. ITP has an incidence of around 60 new cases per million population per year.

- Childhood ITP generally leads to an illness that is seasonal, typically follows a trivial viral infection or vaccination, and in most cases is transient, requiring no treatment. There is spontaneous recovery in 80% of cases.
- In most cases of adult ITP the platelet glycoprotein (Gp) antigen targets are GpIIb/IIIa and GpIb/IX.

Heparin-induced thrombocytopenia (HIT)

Thrombocytopenia in patients treated with heparin is fairly common, but in most cases has no serious consequences. HIT is caused by the production of antibodies against heparin–PF4 complexes. In some patients an immune response is induced, leading to platelet activation and thrombin generation, and rarely can result in large thromboses or massive bleeding due to the consumption of platelets and clotting factors.

THE THROMBOPHILIAS

Thrombophilias are conditions associated with excessive clotting. The coagulation system is a delicately balanced series of coagulation and fibrinolytic events and a defect or deficiency in one of the natural anticoagulants (e.g. **protein C or S**) will swing the balance towards thrombosis. There are two principal types of hypercoagulable state:

- Inherited – where the patient has a specific defect in one of the natural anticoagulant mechanisms.
- Acquired thrombophilia – which represents a heterogeneous group of disorders associated with an increased risk of thromboembolism.

Thromboembolism is responsible for nearly 50% of all adult deaths in the UK and thrombophilia plays an important role. Inherited thrombophilias should be considered in all patients under 40–50 years of age who experience a venous thrombosis.

The inherited thrombophilias

Table 12.19 summarises the prevalence and incidence of thrombotic events among individuals with an inherited thrombophilia.

Protein C deficiency

Protein C is a vitamin K-dependent glycoprotein that acts as one of the major regulatory inhibitory proteins of the coagulation system. Protein C is activated to form activated protein C on endothelial surfaces by the **thrombin thrombomodulin complex**. Protein C acts as an anticoagulant by degrading activated factor V (Va) and VIII (VIIIa).

Protein C deficiency is inherited as an autosomal dominant disorder. Affected heterozygotes have protein C levels of around 50%. Some 75% of affected individuals have venous thromboembolism in young adulthood.

Protein S deficiency

Protein S was isolated and characterised in Seattle (hence protein S). It is a non-enzymatic cofactor of activated protein

Table 12.19	Inherited thrombophilias		
Inherited disorders	**% in population**	**% with thrombosis**	
APCR: factor V Leiden mutation	3–8 of Caucasians	20–25	
Prothrombin G20210A	2–3 of Caucasians	4–8	
Antithrombin deficiency	1 in 2000–5000	1–1.8	
Protein C deficiency	1 in 300	2.5–5.0	
Protein S deficiency	Unknown	2.8–5.0	
Hyperhomocysteinaemia	11	13.1–26.7	

C. Like protein C, protein S is a vitamin K-dependent protein and is synthesised by the liver endothelial cells and it is also found in α granules of platelets. Inherited protein S deficiency is autosomal dominant.

Activated protein C resistance

Dahlback and others described APCR in 1993 as a mechanism for recurrent thrombosis. They described patients whose plasma exhibited a poor response to activated protein C in an APTT assay. A mutation in the factor V gene (**factor V Leiden**) was identified as the major cause. Factor V Leiden is a point mutation at the site at which activated protein C cleaves factor Va; this mutation makes the Va molecule biochemically resistant to inactivation by activated protein C.

Factor V Leiden deficiency has been demonstrated in more than 20% of thrombotic patients and has a prevalence of around 5% in the general population. APCR therefore may represent the commonest cause of inherited thrombophilia. Patients who co-inherit protein C deficiency are at an even greater risk of thrombosis.

The acquired thrombophilias

A large number of conditions are associated with thrombotic events, but the most important are shown in the following list, in order of the risk involved:

- Femoral and tibial fractures
- Hip, knee, gynaecological or prostate surgery
- Adenocarcinoma
- Chronically elevated factor VIII
- Oral contraceptives
- Pregnancy
- Hormone replacement
- Homocysteinaemia due to vitamin deficiency
- Anti-phospholipid syndrome

Anti-phospholipid syndrome

Anti-phospholipid syndrome (**APS**) is the most common acquired thrombotic disease and is associated with antibodies in the form of **lupus anticoagulant** or **anticardiolipin antibody**.

The mechanisms producing the thrombotic events are not clear. The 'two-hit' hypothesis refers to the coexistence of an anti-phospholipid antibody with vascular endothelial damage.

Lupus anticoagulant

This is due to an antiphospholipid antibody (IgG or IgM or both) but is often recognised because it prolongs the phospholipid-dependent APTT clotting assay. Although seen in about 25% of patients with **SLE**, a generalised autoimmune condition, the term is a misnomer since it occurs frequently in patients with no evidence of SLE and is seen in association with other autoimmune disease, drugs, infections, malignancy and in many otherwise normal individuals.

Anti-cardiolipin antibody

Discovered in the 1980s, these antibodies to combinations of phospholipids and serum proteins, such as β_2-glycoprotein I or prothrombin, have been associated with thrombotic events of the APS.

BLOOD GROUPS AND TRANSFUSION MEDICINE

DEFINITION OF A BLOOD GROUP

In its widest sense this can just mean an observation of characteristics in blood that differ between individuals. When we refer to a **blood group**, it is usually used in a much more restricted sense.

Three characteristics define a blood group: a variation (or **polymorphism**) detected in the blood; the variation is seen in a protein, glycoprotein or glycolipid on a blood cell surface membrane (usually a red cell); which are also antigens (can produce antibodies that bind to the antigen).

BLOOD GROUP ANTIGENS

Blood group antigens are generally found only on the red cell, but some are also found throughout the body. The antigens are usually made by the red cells but some are adsorbed on to the red cell from plasma.

Antigens are generally:

- Proteins, produced by blood group genes
- Carbohydrates on glycoproteins or glycolipids. The blood group genes produce glycosyltransferase enzymes that produce the different antigenic variants.

It is not known why there are different blood groups, but those that have reached a significant frequency in the population have probably provided individuals with a selective advantage. Some blood groups are associated with resistance to parasitic infections (Duffy blood group). It has been suggested that the exploitation by microorganisms allowing them to invade red cells occurs through receptors on glycoproteins and glycolipids. Polymorphisms may simply be chance mutations that have had a selective advantage because the parasite cannot interact with the altered receptor. The selective factors may no longer exist but the polymorphisms will remain until other selective factors interact with them.

ANTIBODY PRODUCTION

Antibodies are produced by B lymphocytes when an antigenic structure is recognised as foreign (i.e. non-self) by the immune system – for example by transfusion of blood cells with different red cell antigens on their surface. Usually macrophages, dendritic cells or other antigen-presenting cells 'process' the antigen, which generally involves digesting it into smaller subunits and presenting it to a T cell. The T cells, in turn, instruct the B cells to make antibodies against the antigenic substance.

BLOOD GROUP SYSTEMS IN TRANSFUSION MEDICINE

Knowledge of blood groups is of key importance in providing safe blood and blood products for transfusion, as well as minimising the risk of diseases such as haemolytic disease of the newborn. It is the interaction between an antigen and its antibody, and the effect of that interaction on the red cells that defines whether a blood group system is seen as being clinically important.

There are 26 different blood group systems, controlled by single, or related clusters of genes, and about 270 blood group antigens have been authenticated. The most important blood group systems in transfusion medicine are **ABO** and **Rhesus**, although others may also produce clinically important antibodies.

The ABO system

The genes for ABO are inherited in a Mendelian manner, giving rise to a variety of different types (**phenotypes**). Blood group 'O' is so called because it lacks both A and B (more like 'zero').

ABO antigens

The ABO system is sugar, rather than protein, based. **H substance** is the precursor of the A and B antigens and whether a person produces A or B antigens is dependent on which enzyme he or she inherits.

The **FUT 1 (H/h)** and **FUT 2 (Se/se)** genes on chromosome 19 give rise to the enzyme **H-fucosyltransferase** which leads to the production of the H antigen. Most people have the H antigen on their red cells.

People without H are rare and this is the result of various genetic changes in the FUT 1 gene. The earliest description was of a group of people without H from India – they were said to have the **'Bombay' type**. Other genetic changes that result in no H antigen (h) have been described since.

The FUT genes act in different tissues:

- FUT 1 is active in tissues of endodermal and mesodermal origin.
- FUT 2 is active in tissues of ectodermal origin and produces the soluble H antigen found in secretions, such as urine and saliva, of those 80% of people who have inherited the Se form of the gene, referred to as being 'secretors'.

A and B genes are found on chromosome 9 and code for two different **glucosyltransferases**. The action of the enzymes produced by A and B genes on the H antigen (**H substance**) dictates which blood groups are produced.

- If there is *no* active enzyme, the H antigen is modified and is described as the O allele (**blood group O**).
- Action of α1,3-*N*-acetyl-D-galactosaminyltransferase on the H antigen modifies it to the A antigen, producing the A allele (**blood group A**).
- Action of α1,3-*N*-D-galactosyltransferase on the H antigen modifies it to the B antigen, producing the B allele (**blood group B**).
- Inheritance of both enzymes from their parents will result in red cells that express both antigens (**blood group AB**).

ABO blood groups can be determined by mixing the red cells with serum containing antibodies to A and B. For example, anti-A antibody will agglutinate A cells, but not B cells or O cells. Figure 12.36 illustrates this.

The antigens we *detect* on the red cells determine the **phenotype** of the individual. Antigens A and B are each recognised by agglutination with the respective antibody, but the O antigen is defined by a lack of agglutination with anti-A and anti-B, and so is not detected in the presence of cells carrying the A or B antigens.

- An individual who is blood group O must have inherited the 'O' allele from both parents, and will have an OO **genotype**.
- An individual who is blood group A, must have blood that agglutinates with anti-A, and therefore must have inherited the 'A' allele from one parent, but we are unable to tell from the agglutination test whether he will also have inherited an 'A' allele (genotype AA) or an 'O' allele (genotype AO) from the other parent. Table 12.20 illustrates the possible genotypes of people with each blood group.
- As we inherit half our genes from one parent, and half from the other, sometimes our red cells have a different phenotype from our parents. For example, a father with genotype AO (phenotype A) and a mother with genotype BO (phenotype B) can produce children who are

phenotype A (genotype AO), phenotype B (genotype BO), phenotype AB (genotype AB) or phenotype O (genotype OO).
- Sometimes the genotypes that a person must have can be inferred from knowledge of the blood groups of their true parents. For example, a mother and father who are both blood group O (phenotype O, genotype OO) can only produce children with a phenotype O (genotype OO).
- The frequency of different blood groups differs between populations.
  - In comparison with the UK, blood group O is more common in America (particularly south and central), and in some parts of Africa.
  - Blood group A is quite prevalent in Europe, particularly Scandinavia.
  - Higher levels of blood group B are found in central Asia, and across Europe the frequency declines from east to west.
- Knowledge of these different distributions has implications for planning of blood stocks for transfusion in a multiracial community.

Changes in blood groups

Many rare variants of ABO groups have been described but do not change within an individual.

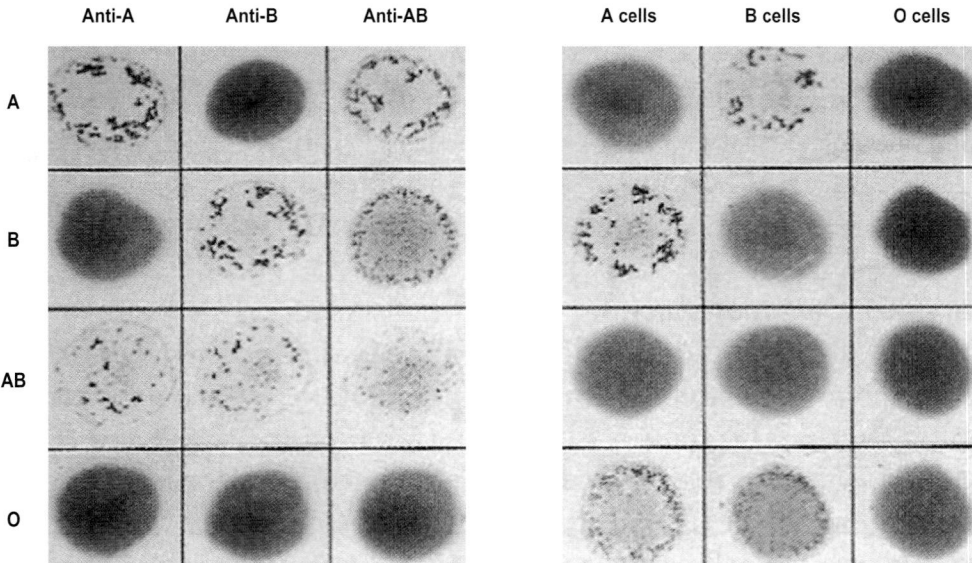

***Fig. 12.36* Blood grouping on a glass tile.** The agglutination (clumping) of red cells in response to their antibody is clearly shown on the tile and illustrates the potential seriousness of this reaction occurring within a person. In the left half is shown the interaction between red cells from a person of blood group A, B, AB and O (shown down the left side of the tile) and serum containing the anti-A, anti-B, and anti-AB antibodies. In the right half is shown the interaction between serum or plasma from a person of the various blood groups, with group A, group B and group O red cells. (The terms 'serum' and 'plasma' are sometimes used interchangeably, but strictly 'serum' is used when blood is placed in a glass tube without anticoagulants and clots, the clotting factors within the plasma having been used up.)

Table 12.20	ABO blood group phenotypes, antigens, defining antibodies and blood group genotypes			
ABO blood group (phenotype)	Frequency in UK Caucasians (%)	Antigens on red cells	Agglutinated by	Genotypes
O	44	O	None	OO
A	45	A	Anti-A	AO or AA
B	8	B	Anti-B	BO or BB
AB	3	AB	Anti-A and Anti-B	AB

Table 12.21	Rh haplotypes and relative population frequencies			
CDE (Fisher–Race)	Rh-Hr (Wiener)	UK Caucasian	Black African	South-East Asian
CDe	R¹	0.42	0.06	0.73
cDE	R²	0.14	0.12	0.19
CDE	Rᶻ	<0.01	<0.01	<0.01
cDe	Rᵒ	0.03	0.59	0.03
Cde	r′	0.01	0.03	0.02
cdE	r″	0.01	<0.01	<0.01
cde	r	0.39	0.20	0.02
CdE	rʸ	<0.01	<0.01	<0.01

Table 12.22	Antibodies found in people of different ABO blood groups	
ABO group		Antibodies in serum
O		Anti-A, B
A		Anti-B
B		Anti-A
AB		None

- Loss of A activity – apparent changes in ABO blood group are sometimes observed in patients with leukaemia, with patients who are group A losing ability to agglutinate with anti-A. Lower expression of the antigen is usually associated with a reduction in A- or B-glucosyltransferase.
- **Acquired B** – a weak B antigen develops on group A cells and is associated with digestive tract disease. The phenomenon is likely to be due to a bacterial deacetylation of *N*-acetylgalactosamine

The Rhesus system

The **Rhesus (Rh) blood group** system is more complex than ABO and is the second most important blood group system in terms of blood transfusion practice because of its high immunogenicity. In all there are around 50 Rh antigens but only five are common, namely D, C, c, E and e. We use the term **Rh positive** for individuals who are Rhesus (D) positive, which is the case in 83% of Caucasians and higher for Africans and Asians, and **Rh negative** for those individuals who do not have the D antigen.

Inheritance of the Rh genes puzzled scientists for many years and it was originally proposed (the **Fisher–Race theory**) that there were possibly either three closely linked genes (C, D and E) or multiple alleles of a single gene (**Wiener's Rh-Hr theory**). In 1986 Tippett proposed a new model, and subsequent molecular analysis in the 1990s has shown this to be more accurate. There appear to be at least two Rh genes, **RHD** expressing D, and **RHCE** expressing C or c, and E or e, both found close to each other on chromosome 1.

Some eight different **haplotypes** have been defined consisting of a 'C or c', 'D or no-D' and 'E or e' components. (A haplotype is the configuration of the genes on one chromosome.) Note that the d antigen has not been found; we now know that 'd' represents deletion (not mutation) of *D*. Anti-d therefore cannot exist. Haplotypes are shown in the Table 12.21 in Fisher–Race and Wiener nomenclature, with their relative population frequencies. In the Fisher–Race system **D** is used for Rh positive and **d** for **no-D**, or Rh negative. In the Weiner system the presence of D is indicated by **R**, and no-D by **r**.

Examination of Rh-family genes has helped in the understanding of human evolution. Like humans, chimpanzees and gorillas have the two Rh genes, RHD and RHCE, whereas other primates have only one, suggesting that the gene duplication happened in the common ancestor some 8–11 million years ago.

The ancestral Rh haplotype is thought to be **cDe**, the other haplotypes developing from a point mutation, gene conversion or deletion, each followed by rarer recombination events, reflecting the rarer haplotypes. Note that this particular haplotype is very common in black African communities (about 60%) compared with less than about 3% in non-African populations – supporting the 'Out of Africa' origin of modern human populations.

The presence or absence of the D antigen, D+ or D–, is what is normally referred to as Rhesus positive or (Rh+) or Rhesus negative (Rh–). The frequency of D+ is close to 100% in the Far East, with about 95% of black Africans also being D+. The frequency is lowest among Europeans and in white North Americans is at a minimum of 82%.

Production of antibodies to blood group antigens

Antibodies can be 'natural', not needing exposure to non-self blood group molecules through transfusion or pregnancy, or 'immune' where such exposure is required. Both types of antibody are encountered in transfusion medicine.

ABO blood group system antibodies

Anti-A and anti-B antibodies are almost always present in the serum of people lacking these antigens, other than newborn infants. We know from animal work that bacterial proteins resembling A and B molecules present in food result in the production of anti-A and anti-B. Chickens, which normally develop anti-B within a few months after hatching, fail to produce anti-B if kept in a sterile environment. Because these antibodies arise naturally they are called 'naturally occurring' antibodies. The antibody molecules are IgM in contrast with 'immune' antibodies, which are usually IgG.

These ABO antibodies are generally detected from around 3 months of age and appear to be the result of immunisation by A and B antigens present in the environment. People of blood group O don't have *both* antibodies: it is thought likely that people of blood group O develop an antibody (anti-A,B) that recognises a structure common to both A and B antigens. Table 12.22 lists these naturally occurring antibodies.

Rh blood group antibodies

In contrast with the ABO blood group system, immune reactions, produced as a result of exposure to a foreign antigen through blood transfusion or pregnancy, may lead to the production of **immune IgG antibodies**. Antibodies produced against Rh system antigens are an important example of IgG antibody development. IgG antibodies react best in the warm.

Rh(D) is the most important of the Rh antigens since it is extremely immunogenic. This means that very few Rh(D) positive cells are required to induce anti-D formation if given to an Rh(D) negative individual. Development of antibodies

Haemolytic disease of the newborn

HDN describes a situation in which there is incompatibility between the mother and the fetus, and leads to a destruction of the newborn infant's red cells. Several blood group antigens are implicated in severe HDN: in North America and Europe the disease is most commonly due to Rh(D), but in South America, Africa and Asia, ABO incompatibility is an important cause.

Any person who is Rh(D) negative and exposed to Rh(D) positive red cells, for example, will most likely make anti-D. Such exposure may occur through:

- Transfusion
- Pregnancy (by leakage from the fetal circulation)
  - During birth delivery
  - Amniocentesis and other obstetric investigations
  - Termination of pregnancy.

In HDN, the exposed mother's immune system will generate IgG antibodies against the D antigen that they do not possess. Since IgG can cross the placenta, the mother's IgG anti-D will attack fetal Rh(D) positive red cells, causing haemolysis within the fetus.

With severe haemolysis there can be:

- Significant anaemia
- Significant rise in fetal bilirubin levels – the baby appears jaundiced
- Irreversible brain damage (**kernicterus**) due to unconjugated bilirubin being deposited in the basal ganglia
- Massive oedema (**hydrops fetalis**) due to abnormal transport of water
- Perinatal death.

Of women who develop this antibody, about 20% lose their infants in their first affected pregnancy and this rate increases further in subsequent pregnancies. For this reason, exposure to Rh(D) positive blood through blood transfusion in women who may become pregnant is avoided wherever possible.

Rhesus HDN is not common today, however, due to the introduction in 1967 of **anti-D prophylaxis** programmes (Fig. 12.37):

- Pregnant women are checked during pregnancy for the presence of anti-D (and other antibodies) and, if detected, are measured serially in order to check whether the antibody levels are rising.
- To prevent Rhesus HDN, pregnant women who are Rh(D) negative are now given anti-D injections during pregnancy at 28 and 34 weeks, to mop up any fetal cells that might enter the circulation. This prevents the immune system from forming antibodies and thus protects the fetus.
- Rh(D) negative women who subsequently deliver a Rh(D) positive child are given a further injection within 72 hours of the birth.

This programme has been very successful: before its introduction there were around 1.6 perinatal deaths per 1000 births; this had dropped to around 1 death per 10 000 births by 1986.

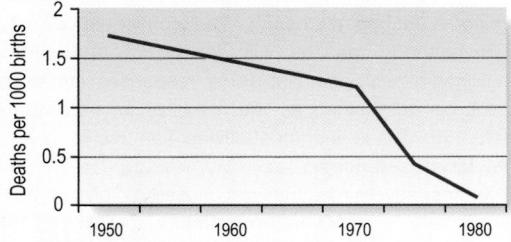

Fig. 12.37 **Fall in perinatal death rate following introduction of anti-D prophylaxis.** Perinatal death rates fell between 1950 and 1970 because of better medical care but the introduction of the policy for anti-D immunoglobulin prophylaxis (100 µg) within 72 hours of birth led to a dramatic fall in the death rate.

can result in serious reactions to blood transfusion and anti-D is the principal cause of **haemolytic disease of the newborn** (**HDN**) (Clinical box 12.9).

Other blood group systems

There are too many to discuss in detail but a few will be mentioned that are particularly important in transfusion and neonatal medicine:

- Kell
- Duffy
- I/i
- HPA (a non-red cell system).

Kell

Like Rhesus, **Kell** is highly immunogenic. **Anti-K** is generally caused through blood transfusion and may also arise in pregnancy. Anti-K is common because the K gene is only present in about 9% of Caucasians, and is even rarer in the black and East Asian populations. Its production may result in subsequent transfusion reactions.

A woman who is herself Kell negative, carrying a fetus which is Kell positive, may develop IgG anti-K antibodies. IgG is the only immunoglobulin that can cross the placenta and anti-K may lead to haemolytic disease of the newborn, much as in Rh incompatibility. All women of child-bearing age are now given Kell negative blood in order to reduce the incidence of Kell associated HDN.

Duffy

There are two main antigens in the **Duffy** (**Fy**) system, namely **Fya** and **Fyb**.

Individuals may have either: Fy(a+b–) or Fy(a–b+), or both: Fy(a+b+). A GATA-1 transcription factor binding site upstream of the Duffy gene has produced a mutation that prevents expression of the Duffy glycoprotein on red cells. This mutation, **Fy(a–b–)**, is extremely common in the black population due to natural selection because of **malaria** exposure. Individuals with this phenotype are refractory to the malarial parasite *Plasmodium falciparum*, and resistant to *Plasmodium vivax* infection, which requires an interaction between the parasite and the Duffy glycoprotein to invade red cells.

Antibodies to the Fy antigens may arise through transfusion or pregnancy. They can lead to:

- Delayed transfusion reactions, i.e. haemolysis occurring several days after an incompatible red cell transfusion
- HDN.

I/i

These are interesting since different antigens are present at different stages of development.

- **i** is found on cord blood (taken from the placental cord at birth) or the red cells of neonates (I is absent)
- Adult red cells have mainly **I** with little i.

Antibodies against I are naturally occurring IgM antibodies that react best in the cold. IgM anti-I may be found in diseases such as **cold haemagglutinin disease** characterised by cold-induced haemolysis. Pneumonia caused by *Mycoplasma pneumoniae* may give rise to antibodies with anti-I specificity.

| Clinical box 12.10 | Neonatal alloimmune thrombocytopenic purpura |

In **NAITP**, the mother and fetus are incompatible in terms of their platelet antigens.

- The mother lacks the platelet antigen present in the fetus and makes an IgG antibody against it.
- The IgG crosses the placenta and destroys the fetal platelets causing marked thrombocytopenias.
- The fetus may bleed in utero (e.g. intracerebral), but more commonly the disorder is diagnosed after birth.
- The antigen most commonly implicated is **HPA-1a**.
- NAITP affects 1 in 2000 live births and makes up 20% of neonatal thrombocytopenias.

| Clinical box 12.11 | Avoiding transmission of variant Creutzfeldt–Jakob disease (vCJD) through blood transfusion |

In the UK the blood transfusion service has introduced a number of measures in order to protect individuals from possible transmission of vCJD. These include:

- Withdrawal and recall of any blood components, plasma derivatives or tissues obtained from any individual who later develops vCJD (December 1997).
- Import of plasma from the US for fractionation to manufacture plasma derivatives (October 1999).
- Leucodepletion (removal of white cells) of all blood components (Autumn 1999).
- Importation of clinical fresh frozen plasma from the US for patients born on or after 1 January 1996 (introduced in Spring 2004).
- Deferral of donors who have received a blood transfusion in the UK since 1980 (announced March 2004, implemented April 2004).

Platelet antigens

Blood cells such as platelets and neutrophils have antigens specific for these cell types. Platelet antigens include **human platelet antigen** (HPA)-1, HPA-2, HPA-3, HPA-4 and HPA-5; in addition, each can have an a or b allele. These are relevant to disorders such as **neonatal alloimmune thrombocytopenic purpura** (**NAITP**; see Clinical box 12.10).

BLOOD TRANSFUSION

Whereas blood transfusion is normally considered to be a transfusion of red cells, and originally that meant whole anticoagulated blood, today donated blood is processed to produce the separate different components that might be required for medical or surgical purposes, for example: red cells, white cells, platelets, fresh frozen plasma, heat-treated plasma, and other more specialised fractionations of whole blood.

Blood has never been an unlimited resource and blood transfusion can no longer be considered as a safe process. The aims of good transfusion medicine should always be to limit unnecessary exposure to blood products and there is good evidence to show that much of the blood transfusion that has been considered normal in the past – for example to raise the haemoglobin to normal in a patient who is anaemic after a surgical operation, in order to increase the oxygen carrying capacity of the blood – is ineffective in the latter terms and therefore unnecessary and risky to the patient.

Guidelines for safe transfusion

Sometimes blood transfusion is indicated, and great care must be employed to reduce the associated risk, not only in *what* is transfused, but *how* the process of blood provision is managed in order to ensure that the blood is of the highest quality (Clinical box 12.11).

Management of the blood transfusion process

A survey of UK blood transfusion in 1993 identified an incidence of blood being transfused to the wrong patient for 1 in 30 000 units of blood. Over 18 months there were 111 incidences of **incompatible transfusion** and 12 of these patients died as a result. The deaths were as a result of errors in:

- Collection or labelling of the sample for blood grouping
- Laboratory error
- Failure of final pre-transfusion checks.

In the UK these incidences are monitored by the Serious Hazards of Transfusion (SHOT) initiative.

Transfusion reactions

Transfusion reactions may be:

- **Haemolytic** – due to an antigen-antibody reaction as a result of an incompatible transfusion, resulting in severe or fatal intravascular haemolysis.
- **Non-haemolytic** – due to damaged blood products that release high levels of cytokines, leading to fever and rigor. Usually benign.
- **Allergic** reactions (IgE mediated) – leading to rashes and itching. Benign.
- **Anaphylactic** reactions (IgA mediated) in certain patients. Potentially, but rarely, fatal.
- Transfusion of antileucocyte antibodies – leading to **transfusion-related acute lung injury** (**TRALI**). Can be fatal.
- Due to **volume overload** – leading to acute pulmonary oedema. Outcome depends on the other conditions.
- Transfer of **bacteria** – leading to endotoxaemia (as a result of free bacterial toxins) and septicaemia. Potentially fatal.

Haemolytic transfusion reactions are the most important of these. The transfusion of an antigen into someone who does not possess that antigen results in the recognition of that antigen, either by production of an antibody against it, or by reaction between an already pre-existing antibody (ABO antibodies, or immune antibodies stimulated as part of a previous antigen exposure). The consequences of the antigen–antibody reaction will depend on the particular immunogenic response, but some responses are extreme and will be determined as the result of an **incompatible transfusion**. These incompatibilities can result in shock, kidney failure and death.

The most severe reactions are caused by IgM antibodies, such as seen in **ABO incompatibility**, particularly when group A, or group AB blood cell antigens are transfused into group O recipients. For example:

- If blood of group A is transfused to a group O person then the anti-A in the group O plasma will react with the transfused A cells – an antigen–antibody reaction.

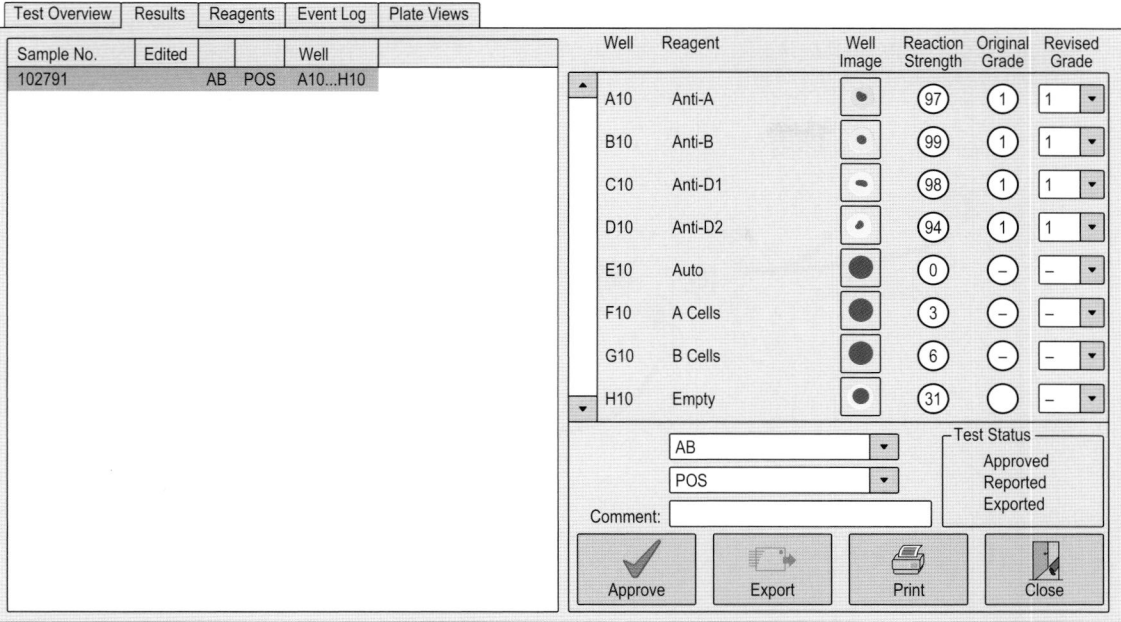

Fig. 12.38 **Automated blood group typing.** A computer generated output from an automated blood grouping instrument of a patient who is blood group AB Rh(D) positive, showing images of the reaction and the automated interpretation of the results.

- The antigen-antibody reaction also activates **complement**, which rapidly ruptures the incompatible cells (**haemolysis**), resulting in haemoglobin being released into the plasma (**haemoglobinaemia**).
- Ruptured cell membrane debris activates the coagulation pathway within blood vessels (**disseminated intravascular coagulation – DIC**).
- DIC can lead to **renal failure** and **death**.

Group O blood, if transfused into a group A, B or AB patient, does not normally produce a reaction because the blood is transfused as red cells, without the plasma that would normally contain the anti-A and anti-B found in group O plasma, and the recipient antibodies do not react against the O antigen. Hence group O blood has been referred to as being **universal donor** blood. In contrast, plasma from a group O individual, which *will* contain the anti-A and anti-B antibodies, would not be given to a group A or B individual. Use of the 'universal donor' term (and **universal recipient** for someone of blood group AB, who can theoretically receive red cells from any ABO group donor) is discouraged as this only really applies to red cells and hence transfusion practice now recommends the use of ABO identical components.

IgG antibody–antigen reactions that might be seen in incompatible blood group Rh, Kell, Duffy, Kidd and Ss (MNSs blood group) transfusions, in particular, where the relevant antibody has previously been stimulated, produce a milder, but still clinically significant reaction.

Tests used in transfusion medicine

Blood grouping

For transfusion purposes we are normally only concerned with:

- **ABO blood group** – because of the danger of incompatibility to the patient

- **Rh(D) blood group** – particularly in women because of the danger of subsequent HDN.

Other blood groups may become important to consider if a person develops an antibody to a particular antigen, since it is then important not to expose someone to that antigen again to avoid transfusion reactions.

Before automation, blood grouping was carried out using glass tiles and polyclonal antisera derived from human blood (see Fig. 12.36). A whole panel of antisera was required, each one recognising different blood group antigens. This type of grouping technique was carried out by placing drops of red cells of unknown group (e.g. the patient) onto the tile, after which one drop of antiserum was added. The red cells and antiserum were mixed on the tile and agglutination (clumping of red cells) noted. Agglutination occurs when there is a positive reaction.

Nowadays a number of automated blood grouping machines are available that can perform blood group typing on large numbers of samples efficiently and safely. The results are read by computer (Fig. 12.38) and stored within blood group databases. Accuracy is provided through rigorous operating procedures and use of bar codes for computerised verification.

The antibody screen

Antibody screening exposes the patient's plasma to pools of red cells which contain *all* the common blood group antigens in all the important blood group systems. Use of cells from blood group O ensures that the naturally occurring ABO antibodies are not picked up. Thus agglutination will indicate the *presence of an immune antibody*. Once the particular antibody has been defined using a series of different antigen pools, compatible blood, without the antigen, can be provided.

While antibodies, such as those IgM antibodies found in the ABO blood group system can easily be detected by

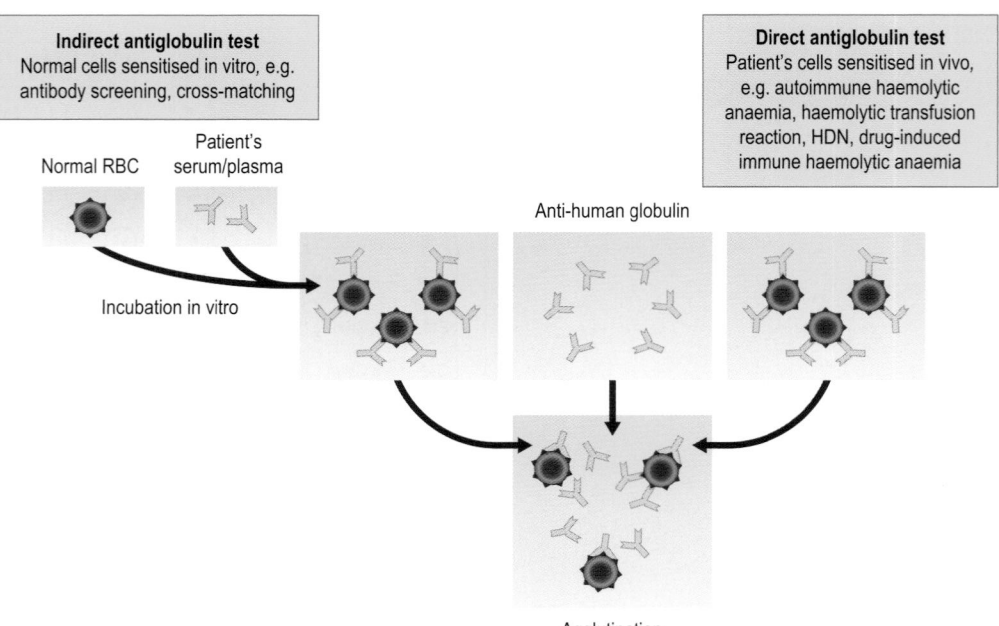

Fig. 12.39 **Principles of the antiglobulin test.** HDN, haemolytic disease of the newborn. Redrawn with permission from Kumar P, Clark M 2005 Clinical medicine, 6th edn. Elsevier Saunders, Edinburgh.

simple mixing of serum and red cells at room temperature, another strategy has been developed to detect the smaller IgG antibodies, such as those seen after immunisation in the Rhesus system. This is known as the **antiglobulin test**.

The antiglobulin test

This test was devised by Coombs in 1945 and until recently was known as the **Coombs test** but has now been renamed the **antiglobulin test** (Fig. 12.39). Coombs recognised that red cells can be coated with antibody but fail to show agglutination in the test tube (in vitro). The reason for this is because the antibody molecules are too small to link the red cells and cause agglutination. This occurs mainly with IgG molecules.

Coombs' strategy was to generate another antibody that would bind to any human antibody already present on the red cells, bound to its respective antigen, and agglutinate these. This test is called the **direct antiglobulin test** (**DAT**) since it detects antibody *bound* to the surface of the red cells. The **indirect antiglobulin test** (**IAT**) detects the presence of antibody in the patient's serum (i.e. free unbound antibody). In other words it detects immune antibodies in the patient that have been stimulated by exposure to a foreign antigen. This is the basis of the **antibody screen**.

The cross-match (compatibility test)

The **cross-match** is designed to ensure that any blood transfused into a recipient is compatible with the recipient and will not cause a transfusion reaction. Transfusion reactions occur when there is a blood group antibody in the recipient's serum which reacts with the transfused red cells. In order to detect this, red cells from the donated blood (intended for transfusion) are mixed with some of the recipient's serum.

- Agglutination indicates a positive reaction
- No agglutination indicates a negative reaction.

Only when there is a negative reaction between the two can the blood be issued and transfused into the recipient. Because ABO antibodies are potentially always present it is usually *only ABO compatibility* that is being tested. Only where the antibody screen indicates that immune antibodies are present do we need to cross-match for other blood group antigens. Antibodies that will usually result in clinically important transfusion reactions include those from the Rh, Kell, Duffy, Kidd and Ss (MNSs) blood groups.

While cross-matching implies the physical mixing of the patient's serum and the red cells to be transfused, in the UK an 'electronic' cross-match is often performed. Provided the antibody screen is negative at the time then the patient can simply be transfused with ABO compatible red cells – and generally, for the good reasons referred to above, Rh(D) compatible cells as well. Electronic cross-matching can only be used where the systems of information technology and labelling are safe and robust.

NON-RED CELL TRANSFUSION

A variety of other components of blood are used for administration to patients in certain circumstances.

Platelet transfusion

Platelet transfusion is indicated to prevent or treat haemorrhage that may be the result of thrombocytopenia or platelet function defects. Platelets are expected to be at a very low level ($<10 \times 10^9$/L) before platelet transfusion is needed. Prophylactic transfusion may also be recommended at such low levels in conjunction with bone marrow failure, to provide surgical cover, or to treat medical emergencies, such as DIC or immune thrombocytopenias.

White cell transfusion

Transfusion of white cells in the form of **bone marrow** or **stem cells** is undertaken for bone marrow transplant to treat conditions such as leukaemia. White cell engraftment occurs after bone marrow ablation, where a patient's marrow is destroyed (along with its cancer cells) and replaced with that from a compatible donor.

Frozen plasma and plasma concentrate transfusion

Fresh frozen plasma (**FFP**) and concentrates such as **cryoprecipitate** may be transfused. Indications for **FFP** administration include **DIC**, if there is active bleeding. It is never indicated to reverse **warfarin anticoagulant therapy**, unless bleeding is very severe. A **pathogen-reduced plasma** (**PRP**), sourced from counties with a low incidence of bovine spongiform encephalopathy (BSE), is recommended for all children born after 1995.

Cryoprecipitate is the cryoglobulin fraction of fresh frozen plasma and is particularly rich in FVIII, vWF, FX111, fibronectin and fibrinogen. It is usually used in conditions where fibrinogen levels are low (**hypofibrinogenaemia**).

13

The respiratory system

Gavin Donaldson

INTRODUCTION

The primary function of the respiratory system is to move air into the lungs to supply oxygen for the metabolic processes of the body, while removing sufficient carbon dioxide to maintain the acid–base balance of the blood. It involves actively drawing air in (**inspiration**) through the nose, mouth and trachea into the lungs, and expulsion (**expiration**). In the lungs, oxygen and carbon dioxide move across the barrier between air and blood, made up of lung tissue (alveolar wall) and capillaries, by simple diffusion. The rate of diffusion depends on the lung surface area, alveolar wall thickness and partial pressure difference (i.e. concentration gradient of oxygen and carbon dioxide). This process is called **gaseous exchange**. In general, respiratory diseases interfere with the efficient operation of this process.

The lungs also carry out other functions apart from gaseous exchange:

- Expulsion of air from the lungs to produce sound and speech (phonation)
- Conversion of angiotensin I to angiotensin II in the regulation of blood pressure and volume
- Local production of surfactant (a phospholipid) to lower surface tension in the alveolar cells
- Act as a reservoir of blood
- Filtration of small blood clots from the blood to prevent them entering the systemic circulation
- Synthesis of arachidonic acid metabolites, the eicosanoids that play an important part in the body's defence mechanisms in inflammation and homeostasis
- Inactivation of noradrenaline, bradykinin, 5-hydroxytryptamine (5-HT) to prevent constriction of the airways
- Secretion of immunoglobulin (mainly IgA) into bronchial mucus in response to allergic challenges
- Maintenance of acid–base balance – by excretion of carbon dioxide.

EPIDEMIOLOGY OF RESPIRATORY DISEASE AND ITS SOCIAL IMPACT

Respiratory disease is an important cause of mortality and morbidity at all ages. In 1999, chronic obstructive pulmonary disease (COPD) was the fifth leading cause of death globally (4.8% of total deaths), and acute lower respiratory infections were the second most common cause of death in Africa (10.3% of total). Worldwide, the prevalence of lung cancer and asthma has been rising. Tuberculosis is also increasing in incidence and prevalence, particularly related to the compromised immune systems in individuals with human immunodeficiency virus/acquired immune deficiency syndrome.

In the UK, asthma is a common chronic disease in children, but mortality from asthma is confined to those aged over 45 with only a small proportion occurring in children (2 per million aged 0–4 years). In adults, chronic obstructive lung diseases are important causes of sickness absence from work, reduced quality of life, disability and hospital admissions (Table 13.1).

Acute upper respiratory tract infections (common colds) occur frequently, with two to four episodes per year in adults and six to eight episodes per year in children. These infections are costly in terms of absenteeism from school and work, and the purchase of 'over-the-counter drugs'. The inflammatory processes and symptomatic deterioration triggered by upper respiratory tract infections account for a substantial number of hospital admissions and mortality at all ages.

SMOKING AND RESPIRATORY DISEASE

Much of adult respiratory disease is tobacco related (Fig. 13.1). Cigarette consumption became well established during the first world war, but did not become popular among women until the second world war. The Tobacco Advisory Council in the UK estimated that in 1948, 65% of men and 41% of women smoked manufactured cigarettes, and that by 1996, these figures had fallen to 29% and 28%, respectively. This decrease has been in all age groups except those aged 20–24, where there has been a steady increase since 1988. However, as a consequence of people smoking in the 1940 and 1950s, deaths attributed to COPD, which is overwhelmingly caused by smoking, are currently rising to such an extent that this disease has recently risen to being the fourth leading cause of mortality worldwide.

CLASSIFICATION OF COMMON RESPIRATORY DISEASES

The classification of respiratory diseases is difficult as patients may have one or a combination of diseases or conditions. A useful way of thinking about respiratory diseases is to consider them to be of two main types: obstructive and restrictive. Also both types can be chronic or acute in onset (Information box 13.1).

- **Obstructive pulmonary disease**, where the overall volume of the lungs available for gas exchange is unchanged, but there is *obstruction* to the flow of gases along the airways. Obstructive pulmonary disease has many possible causes.
- **Restrictive pulmonary disease** is less common than obstructive disease. The available lung volume for gaseous exchange is reduced, or *restricted*, but there is no obstruction to airflow.

Clinical box 13.1	Chronic obstructive pulmonary disease (COPD)

COPD is a chronic respiratory disease which has the symptoms of:

- Productive cough
- Wheeze
- Shortness of breath, especially on exertion.

The airways become obstructed with forced expiratory volume in 1 second (FEV_1) <70% of predicted and FEV_1/forced vital capacity (FVC) ratio <0.7. This obstruction is not relieved by bronchodilators.

COPD gets progressively worse and usually occurs in smokers, although a few cases (5%) occur in non-smokers. While most patients with COPD are smokers and severity is related to the number of cigarettes smoked, the susceptibility of individual smokers varies widely. About 50% of smokers do not develop any significant deficit and only 15% will get clinically significant COPD.

Table 13.1	Emergency hospital admissions for respiratory diseases in England during the financial year 1999/2000	
		No. of admissions
Chronic obstructive pulmonary disease, excluding asthma, in patients aged 65 years and over		75 600
Asthma in children		28 500
Lower respiratory infections, pneumonia and acute bronchitis		97 000
Pneumonia in patients aged 65 years and over		47 200
Acute bronchitis in children		21 800
Total		182 800

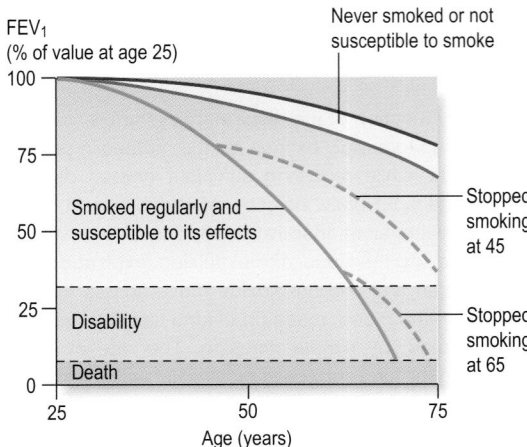

Fig. 13.1 **Influence of smoking on airflow limitation.** FEV_1, the forced expiratory volume in 1 second, is a sensitive indicator of lung function and reductions in FEV_1 can indicate respiratory disease.

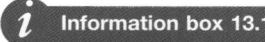

Information box 13.1 **Classification of lung diseases**

Chronic lung diseases

- **COPD**: a chronic, slowly progressive disease characterised by a fixed airflow obstruction that cannot be reversed by bronchodilator therapy. Commonly associated with smoking.
- **Asthma**: a pulmonary disease characterised by reversible airway obstruction, airway inflammation, and bronchospasm to a variety of stimuli.
- **Emphysema**: destruction of the alveolar walls leading to enlarged air spaces.
- **Atelectasis**: collapsed areas of lung with no gas exchange.
- **Bronchiectasis**: irreversible dilation of the bronchial walls.
- **Pulmonary fibrosis** (idiopathic, occupational, etc.).

Acute lung diseases

- **Acute bronchitis**: acute inflammation of the trachea and bronchi. It is usually self-limiting.
- **Pleurisy**: inflammation of the pleura.
- **Pneumonia**: acute inflammation of lung substance, usually bacterial.
- **Pneumothorax**: free air between the visceral and parietal pleurae.
- **Pulmonary embolism**: obstruction of blood flow in a section of the lung which prevents perfusion and gas exchange.
- **Adult respiratory distress syndrome (ARDS)**: an inflammatory response which causes non-cardiogenic pulmonary oedema leading to hypoxaemia and respiratory failure.
- **Pulmonary fibrosis**: lung scarring and cyst formation arising from inflammation of the airways.

OBSTRUCTIVE PULMONARY DISEASE

Obstructive pulmonary disease is due to narrowing of the airways that conduct air into and out of the lungs. This may be caused by:

- Inflammation of the lining of the airways, particularly of the smaller airways, when the lining swells and causes blockage
- Mucus plugs obstructing the lumen of the airways, which occurs in acute or chronic infections when there is excessive mucus secretion
- Constriction of the smooth muscles in the walls of the airways, causing airway narrowing. The commonest example is asthma
- Loss of elasticity in the airways, usually caused by chronic infection. The elasticity of the airways is normally instrumental in keeping the airways open, so that stiffness would lead to obstruction when the airway collapses (particularly on expiration).

Common examples of obstructive pulmonary disease are asthma, COPD, chronic bronchitis and emphysema.

RESTRICTIVE PULMONARY DISEASE

Restrictive pulmonary diseases are due to reduced total lung capacity (TLC), but airflow and airway resistance are normal. Restriction may be caused by:

- Intrinsic lung disease, when lung tissue (parenchyma) is destroyed, which reduces lung volume. In acute situations, the air spaces become filled with inflammatory exudates and debris. Chronic inflammation with scarring and fibrosis (interstitial fibrosis) destroys air spaces, thereby reducing lung volume. Large parts of the lung parenchyma cannot function for gaseous exchange.
- Extrinsic disorders of the muscles of respiration, the chest walls, connective tissue, pleura or the nerve supply that impair movement during inspiration. The inability of the chest to expand for whatever reason mechanically restricts ventilation, and respiratory failure ensues.

Examples of restrictive pulmonary disease are pneumothorax, pulmonary embolism, adult respiratory distress syndrome (ARDS) and pulmonary fibrosis.

ANATOMY OF THE RESPIRATORY SYSTEM

The respiratory system consists of the **upper respiratory tract** (Fig. 13.2), which is concerned mainly with **conduction** of gases from the air to and from the lungs, and the **lower respiratory tract**, which is partly concerned with conduction and mainly with **gaseous exchange**. The upper airway or the upper respiratory tract is made up of the:

- Nasal cavity
- Pharynx
- Larynx.

The lower respiratory tract consists of:

- Conducting airways
- Respiratory airways.

The **conducting airways** are made up of the trachea, main bronchi and those bronchioles which make up branches 1–16 of the **tracheobronchial tree** (see below and Fig. 13.5). They are lined with specialised ciliated pseudostratified columnar (or columnar) epithelial cells, macrophages, goblet cells, Clara cells and glands, with cartilage and smooth muscle in the walls. This part of the respiratory tract is not concerned with gaseous exchange (non-respiratory). These air passages have the function of:

- Protecting the lower airways by removing dust particles, atmospheric pollutants and other debris from the airways
- Humidifying and warming inspired air.

The **respiratory airways**, where gaseous exchange takes place, consist of the smaller bronchioles which are branches 16–23 of the tracheobronchial tree and the alveoli.

The alveoli:

- Are where the alveolar walls form the thinnest possible barrier between the air and the blood
- Consist of type I (squamous epithelium) and type II (cuboidal) alveolar cells (also called pneumocytes)
- Contain macrophages, lymphocytes and granulocytes.

Gaseous exchange of oxygen and carbon dioxide, or respiration, takes place at the interface between the alveoli and the pulmonary circulation (see Fig. 13.7 below). This interface is known as the **alveolar–capillary barrier**. The **pulmonary circulation** and the **pulmonary lymphatics** provide the blood supply and fluid drainage of the lungs,

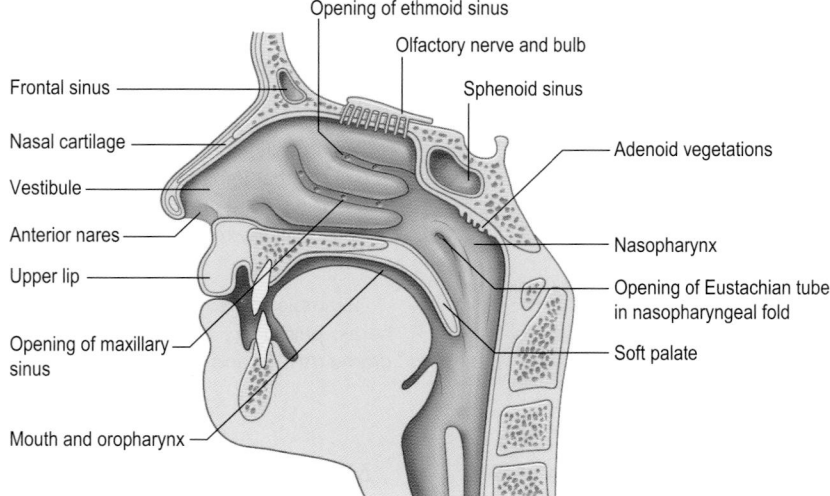

Fig. 13.2 **Upper respiratory tract.**

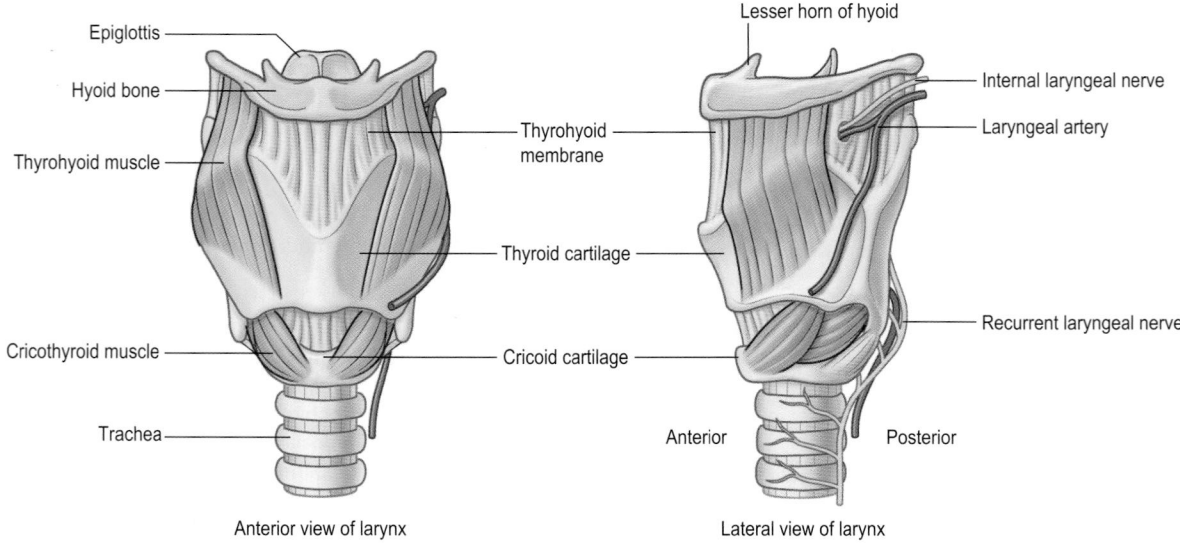

Fig. 13.3 **Views of the larynx.**

respectively. The alveoli have a very extensive blood supply and extracellular fluid is drained from the alveoli by the lymphatics.

ANATOMY OF THE UPPER AIRWAYS

Nasal cavity

Air drawn into the lungs via the **nasal cavity** (Fig. 13.2) passes highly vascular nasal mucous membranes, which, with the exception of the nasal entrance, are covered by ciliated columnar epithelium. These nasal membranes moisten the entering air, remove large particles of dust and can warm it sufficiently to raise the temperature of the air inspired from 6 °C to 30 °C. Inhaled air is then fully humidified and warmed to body temperature (37 °C) as it travels through the trachea. Expired air is always below body temperature because it gives up heat when it leaves the nasal passages. This **counter-current exchange system** prevents excessive heat loss from the body core.

Pharynx

The **pharynx** is divided by the soft palate into an upper **nasopharyngeal** and a lower **oropharyngeal** region. The area contains lymphoid structures such as the **adenoids** and **tonsils**. The airway can be opened during anaesthesia or emergency resuscitation by tilting the head backwards at the atlanto-occipital joint (between C1 and skull). The airway can also be opened by protruding the jaw to lift the tongue forward. A partial blockage of the airways by the tongue during sleep leads to turbulence in airflow which is heard as snoring.

Larynx

The **larynx** (Fig. 13.3) consists of a number of articulated cartilages, vocal cords, muscles and ligaments, which keep the airway open during breathing and closed during swallowing. It can remain closed and withstand the highest pressures generated by the thorax (90 cmH$_2$O) prior to sudden release during **coughing**. It is innervated by the laryngeal nerve.

Trachea

The **trachea** begins at the lower border of the cricoid cartilage of the larynx, at the level of the sixth cervical vertebra. It has a mean diameter of 1.8 cm and a length of 11 cm. It is supported by C-shaped cartilaginous rings to prevent kinking during head and neck movement. It can, however, be compressed by moderate external pressure of between 50 cmH$_2$O and 70 cmH$_2$O or by internal pressure from a haematoma (blood clot) following surgery or accident.

GROSS ANATOMY OF THE LUNGS

The two lungs (Fig. 13.4) are divided into lobes:

- The **right lung** is divided into three lobes: upper, middle and lower.
- The **left lung** has only two lobes: upper and lower.

Invaginations of the **pleurae** (see below) separate the lobes of the lungs. The upper and lower lobes are separated by an **oblique fissure**, the right middle lobe being further demarcated by the **horizontal fissure**. Each lobe is further divided into **bronchopulmonary segments**, which in turn are divided into pyramidal lobules with their apices towards the **bronchiole** (see below) that supplies them. Divisions of the bronchioles eventually end in the blind, balloon-like **alveoli**. The bronchopulmonary segments are separated by fibrous septa, which are extensions of the pleura.

The tracheobronchial tree

The trachea divides into two bronchi. The right **bronchus** is wider than the left and makes a smaller angle with the trachea. The right bronchus is therefore more likely to receive inhaled foreign bodies. After the trachea has divided into two main bronchi, it continues to subdivide (Fig. 13.5) into four lobar bronchi, 16 segmental bronchi, and thereafter into small bronchi, **terminal bronchioles**, **respiratory bronchioles** and **alveolar ducts**. Eventually, 23 generations of division result in about 8 million **alveolar sacs**. These sacs are the last blind generation of air passages and, from each, about 17 **alveoli** arise. These alveoli account for about half of the 250–300 million alveoli, and the other half arise directly from the alveolar ducts. They have a total surface area of about 75 m^2 (adult male).

The trachea, bronchi and bronchioles are tubular structures that are designed for conducting air. Their walls consist of an outer fibrous layer with supporting pieces of **cartilage**, and **bronchial smooth muscle**. The bronchial smooth muscle is arranged in clockwise and anticlockwise helical bands and there is a matrix of elastic tissue supporting the muscles. The lumen of the airways decreases in size with progressive numbers of divisions in the tracheobronchial tree:

- As the airways get smaller, the supporting cartilage, which maintains the rigidity of the walls so that the larger airways remain patent during expiration, gradually disappears so that the proportion of muscle increases.
- The walls of the bronchioles consist of smooth muscle, collagen and reticular fibres for support. There is *no* cartilage in bronchiolar walls. Bronchial smooth muscle occupies as much as 20% of the walls of the smallest bronchioles.
- With further divisions, the bronchiolar muscle layer becomes progressively thinner.
- The airways are lined with **epithelium** containing ciliated and goblet cells (see below), with a **submucosa** containing mucus-secreting cells. These cells function to ensure that inhaled air is adequately humidified and irritants or foreign bodies are removed from the airways.

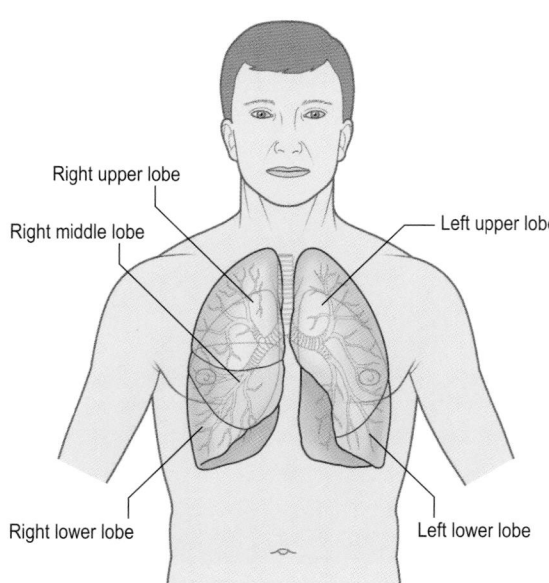

Fig. 13.4 **Gross structure of the lungs**, showing the lobes and fissures.

Right upper lobe
Right middle lobe
Right lower lobe
Left upper lobe
Left lower lobe

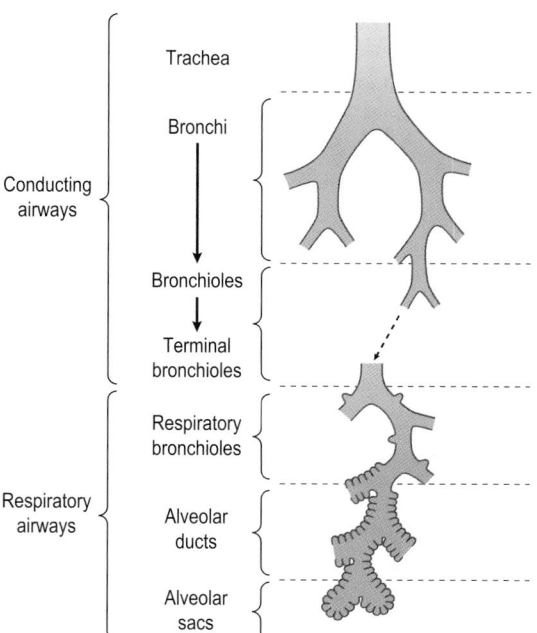

Fig. 13.5 **The tracheobronchial tree.** There are about 23 orders of branching from the trachea to the alveoli. Only the smallest respiratory bronchioles and the alveoli are involved in gas exchange. (Based on Weibel 1963.)

Trachea
Bronchi
Conducting airways
Bronchioles
Terminal bronchioles
Respiratory bronchioles
Respiratory airways
Alveolar ducts
Alveolar sacs

- The lining of the tracheobronchial tree also contain **endocrine cells** – the Kulchitzky or APUD (amine precursor uptake and decarboxylation) cells containing 5-HT. These cells are capable of secreting hormones that have an effect on smooth muscle.
- As the bronchioles become smaller, the epithelium becomes progressively thinner until it is only one cell thick, containing mostly ciliated cells, very few goblet cells and non-ciliated Clara cells (see below).

From the trachea, as far down as the smallest bronchioles, the functions of these air passages are solely conduction and humidification, but beyond this point there is a gradual transition to the function of gas exchange and so the covering of smooth muscle stops.

Breath sounds

Breath sounds are caused by movement of air through the trachea, bronchi and alveoli. They can be heard using the diaphragm of a stethoscope (use a bell in patients with lots of hair on their chest) and can be used to diagnose a number of respiratory conditions. Normal breath sounds are:

- Vesicular, i.e. inspiratory breath sounds are longer than expiratory sounds (which are very brief) with no distinct gap between the end of inspiration and the beginning of expiration
- Loudest over the upper lobes anteriorly.

Breath sounds may be loud in a thin healthy subject, or soft in patients with emphysema, or have a prolonged expiratory phase when the airways are narrowed, as in asthma.

> ### Information box 13.2 Abnormal breath sounds
>
> - **Bronchial breathing**: inspiration and expiration are of equal length, with a short gap in between. These sounds mimic the sound heard over the trachea or between the scapulae at the level of the fourth thoracic vertebra where the trachea bifurcates. Bronchial breathing is heard over areas of consolidation (pneumonia), collapse, bronchiectasis or fibrosis because of narrowing of the airways.
> - **Reduced or absent breath sounds**: when there is severe narrowing of the airway (severe asthma), extensive lung damage (e.g. emphysema) over a pleural effusion, a pneumothorax or when there is no air going in to that part of the lung because of an obstruction such as a neoplasm.
> - **Expiratory wheezes**: heard in airways obstruction, e.g. asthma and chronic bronchitis/chronic obstructive pulmonary disease (COPD). The wheezes may vary in tone and sound high pitched when there is narrowing of numerous small airways, or harsh and monophonic in obstruction of a single large airway, e.g. bronchial cancer. Wheezes are not always heard in airways obstruction, e.g. in asthma when the airflow is very restricted.
> - **Crackles**: brief crackling sounds, fine or coarse, which may be caused by the opening of previously closed airways. Early inspiratory crackles are heard when there is diffuse airflow limitation, as in COPD, and late inspiratory crackles occur in pulmonary oedema, fibrosis and bronchiectasis.
> - **Pleural rub**: heard as a creaking or rubbing, and sometimes palpable, occurs with inflammation, often accompanied by pain.
> - **Stridor** is an inspiratory wheeze which is audible without a stethoscope. It is louder over the larynx and indicates an upper airway obstruction. This may be life-threatening, especially in children, where the epiglottis can compromise the airway.

Vocal resonance

The sound of spoken words (e.g. 99) is heard as an indistinct resonance. Intensity reflects the conductivity of the lung substance; for example, when there is consolidation the sounds are heard much more clearly.

Specialised tracheobronchial cells

The tracheobronchial tree is lined by cells that have a protective function. Their defensive actions remove dust and other noxious particles, and destroy invading bacteria.

Cilia and macrophages

From the nose to the bronchioles, the respiratory tract is lined by ciliated columnar epithelium cells. Where these border the tract, they each have several hundred cilia 1–5 μm long and 0.3 μm wide. The cilia beat synchronously about 20 times per minute with a rapid forward movement followed by a slower return movement. They sweep particles and mucus towards the main bronchi and trachea, where they are finally expelled from the airway by coughing.

The lower respiratory tract also contains macrophages. Smaller particles (<10 μm diameter) which may reach the alveoli are phagocytosed by macrophages and eventually eliminated via the trachea (by coughing) and the gastrointestinal tract (i.e. swallowed). Alveolar macrophages vary from 15 μm to 30 μm in diameter and there are an estimated 16 macrophages per alveolus in the human lungs. Macrophages also immobilise and destroy bacteria.

Goblet cells and the mucociliary escalator

Goblet cells are found predominately in the epithelium from the nose to the bronchi. They are columnar, tapering towards the base. Their function is the secretion of mucus, a sticky, gelatinous substance. Mucus is relatively impermeable to water, forming a layer, like a gelatinous 'blanket', around the cilia of the epithelial cells. Under normal circumstances, the tips of the cilia extend into the mucus layer. Movement of the cilia then sweeps the mucus upwards. This process is called the mucociliary 'escalator' (Fig. 13.6). Along with the cilia, mucus is part of airways defence. Inhaled particles, macrophages, cell debris and bacteria are trapped in the sticky mucus to be swept away on the **mucociliary escalator**. The mucociliary escalator can be slowed by inhaled or general anaesthetics, airborne pollution, bacterial or viral infection and tobacco smoke. Cigarette smoking not only

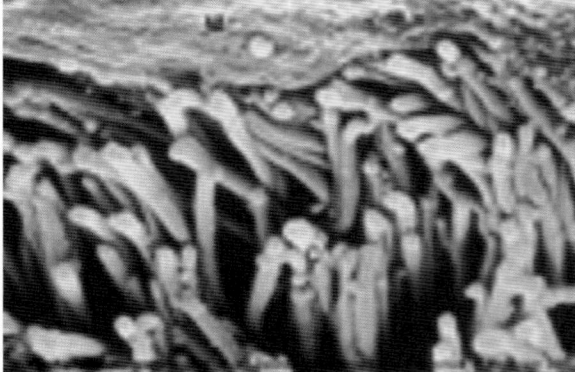

Fig. 13.6 **The mucociliary escalator.** Scanning electron micrograph of the respiratory epithelium showing large numbers of cilia overlaid by a mucus 'raft'.

contributes to recurrent bronchial infection by slowing down mucociliary transport, but also allows more prolonged contact with carcinogens.

Cilia may be slowed by genetic diseases that predispose to ciliary dyskinesia (as is the 'immotile cilia' syndrome); these diseases invariably result in chronic infections of the nose, sinuses and lower airways. Increase in mucus viscosity, for example by diseases such as cystic fibrosis, will also results in more frequent and often chronic infection of the airway.

Clara cells

Clara cells are found mainly in the distal conducting airways, the terminal bronchioles and alveolar ducts. They are not ciliated, they possess large quantities of smooth endoplasmic reticulum and have a protruding apical cap that contains dense granules. These granules contain secretory protein that produces a form of surfactant which covers the surface of the bronchiolar and alveolar ducts to prevent their col-

---

Clinical box 13.2 | **Cystic fibrosis**

Cystic fibrosis is an inherited disease which affects all exocrine glands. It is relatively common in Caucasians, affecting 1 in 2500 live births in the UK. Its major effects are on the respiratory system and the gastrointestinal tract. It is caused by mutations in an autosomal recessive gene located on chromosome 7. The gene codes for a cAMP-regulated chloride (Cl^-) transporter called the cystic fibrosis transmembrane regulator (CFTR). There are more than 300 different mutations which affect the *CFTR* gene, although the commonest is the deletion of a single amino acid, phenylalamine at position 508 (ΔF508). Defects in Cl^- transport lead to the production of sticky mucus that obstructs the small airways and leads to chronic infections. Long-term changes in the bronchi result in chronic hypoxia, pulmonary hypertension and eventual right heart failure.

Cystic fibrosis can be diagnosed using a sweat test as cystic fibrosis patients produce sweat containing high Cl^- concentration. This can then be confirmed by genetic testing. The prognosis for cystic fibrosis patients is improving due to early diagnosis and treatment, with a current median survival of 31 years.

---

lapse. Clara cells also contain enzyme systems that detoxify inhaled noxious pollutants. This function is not yet well understood. There is evidence to suggest that the number of Clara cells are decreased after prolonged tobacco smoke inhalation.

The alveoli

Alveoli are minute balloon-like structures at the end of the terminal bronchioles and alveolar ducts (Fig. 13.7A). Extremely thin layers of tissue form known as **alveolar septa**, the walls between neighbouring alveoli. Each alveolus contains an **alveolar space**. Clusters of alveoli open into spaces, **alveolar sacs**, giving the appearance of tiny bunches of grapes. A few alveoli open directly into terminal bronchioles. The walls of some alveoli have holes, the **pores of Kohn**, that allow communication between adjoining alveoli or alveolar sacs.

The alveoli are the principle sites for **gaseous exchange**, where inspired gases enter the blood in the pulmonary circulation from the alveolar space and expired gases leave the pulmonary circulation to enter the alveolar space. The gap between the alveolar space and the pulmonary circulation, known as the **gas–blood barrier** (or the **alveolar–capillary barrier**), has to be extremely thin to allow rapid gaseous exchange.

The alveoli are regular polyhedrons between 70 μm and 300 μm in diameter. They are smaller in the more dependent (lower) parts of the lungs because they are generally less well inflated. At maximal inflation, as when taking the deepest possible breath in, these lower alveoli become larger so that the vertical gradient in size disappears.

The gas–blood barrier

The thinnest possible membrane between the alveolar spaces and pulmonary capillaries, the **gas–blood barrier**, facilitates rapid and efficient **gaseous exchange** (Fig. 13.7B). Gases such as oxygen have to diffuse across the gas–blood barrier to reach the blood. Carbon dioxide travels in the opposite direction.

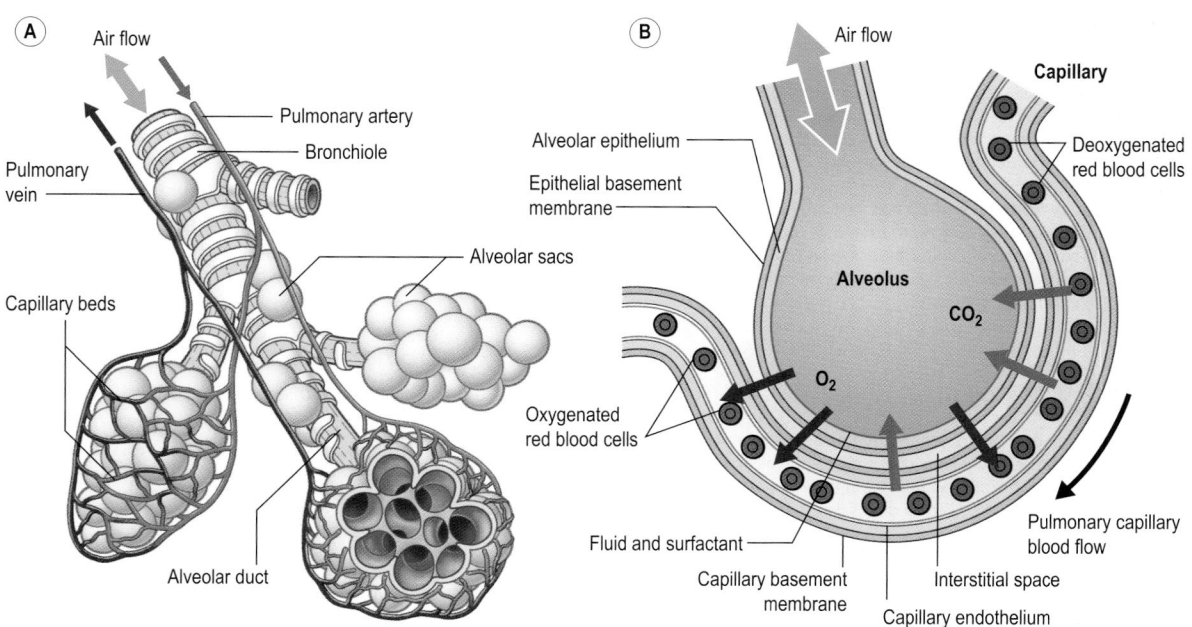

Fig. 13.7 (A) **Lung alveolar tissue** and (B) **Its blood supply**.

The gas–blood barrier is only 0.5 µm wide, and consists of:

■ Alveolar epithelium (type I and type II alveolar cells – see below)
■ Fused membrane of the alveolar epithelial cells and capillary endothelium
■ Vascular epithelium of the pulmonary capillaries (the capillary endothelial cells).

The total surface area of the gas–blood barrier is estimated to be 70–100 m² in the adult man. Gaseous exchange takes place by diffusion, when there is a gradient in pressures across the gas–blood barrier.

Cell types at the alveolar level

Gaseous exchange takes place at the alveoli, where oxygen is taken into the bloodstream, and carbon dioxide off-loaded into the alveolar gases.

Capillary endothelial cells

Very thin-walled alveolar capillaries, lined with **capillary endothelial cells**, form a dense network in the alveolar walls. This gives a large surface area that facilitates rapid gaseous exchange between the pulmonary circulation and the alveoli. Each capillary endothelial cell has a thickness of only 0.1 µm except in its nuclear region, where it is wider to accommodate the nucleus. The cells abut loosely against each other and the junctions between cells are about 5 nm wide. These junctions permit the passage of large molecules, and macrophages can also pass easily through them. This is unlike the walls of most systemic capillaries, which do not allow migration of large molecules or cells.

Type I alveolar cells

The epithelial lining of alveoli consist mainly of **type I alveolar cells** (also known as **type I pneumocytes**). These are large, flat, squamous cells with few organelles and thin cytoplasm. They cover about 93% of alveolar surface area. Their primary

---

Clinical box 13.3 **Small airway diseases**

● **Emphysema**: is due to the breakdown of the alveolar membranes giving rise to large spaces called emphysematous bullae, common in chronic obstructive pulmonary disease (COPD).
● **Bronchiectasis**: results from inflammatory destruction of bronchi leading to irreversible bronchial dilation. Clinically characterised by a chronic cough with production of large amounts of purulent sputum. Common in COPD and emphysema.
● **Pulmonary fibrosis**: see Clinical box 13.4 of tissue.
● **Occupational lung diseases**: may develop as the result of prolonged exposure to dust particles and fumes at work. Coal miners' pneumoconiosis, asbestosis and silicosis are probably the best known.

Clinical box 13.4 **Pulmonary fibrosis**

Pulmonary fibrosis is characterised by the development of stiff lungs caused by the thickening of the alveolar walls with the proliferation of fibroblasts and the laying down of abnormal levels of collagen. Severe fibrosis could result in ipsilateral deviation of the trachea (and mediastinum).

It is caused by many different factors among which are dust and/or gas inhalation, infection, drug side effects and sarcoidosis. Two occupational causes are inhalation of coal dust or asbestos fibres.

---

purpose is air–blood gas exchange. The junctions between these cells are narrow (1 nm). This tightness is necessary for preventing the escape of fluid into the alveoli. Flooding the alveoli (alveolar oedema, see below) with fluid would prevent effective gaseous exchange by increasing the diffusion distance for gases.

Type II alveolar cells

Type II alveolar cells (**type II pneumocytes**) are domed cuboidal cells in the alveolar epithelium containing lamellar bodies that secrete **surfactant**. They cover only ~5% of the alveolar surface area. Pulmonary surfactant forms a thin film covering the whole alveolar surface. The film consists of:

■ A basal layer mostly made up of protein
■ A surface layer of a phospholipid, dipalmitoyl lecithin.

Surfactant is continuously synthesised and secreted by type II alveolar cells. It reduces alveolar surface tension throughout the lungs, in order to:

■ Prevent the basically spherical alveoli from collapsing during expiration
■ Decrease the effort needed to expand the alveoli at the next inspiration (increase **pulmonary compliance**).

Macrophages

Alveoli also contain **macrophages**, which enter the alveolar lumen to phagocytose dust particles and bacteria. Macrophages are part of the pulmonary defence mechanism.

Collateral ventilation

As well as the main air pathways from the trachea through the bronchi and into the alveoli, other pathways link the different regions of the lungs and allow collateral ventilation. The pathways include the pores of Kohn and accessory bronchiolo–alveolar communications. These allow communication between adjacent alveoli, which equalises pressure and provides collateral ventilation. When small airways are blocked, these alternative pathways provide a means for maximising the use of all available alveoli.

The pleura

The outer surface of the lungs is covered by a membrane – the **visceral pleura**. This is separated by a thin fluid film from the **parietal pleura** which covers the thoracic walls and upper surface of the diaphragm. The pleural layers can only be separated by considerable force but can slide easily over each other (like two wet microscope slides). The space between the two layers is called the **pleural cavity** and contains a few millilitres of fluid that acts as a lubricant.

Pleurisy and other pleural conditions

Pleurisy is an inflammation of the pleura, which gives rise to sharp pain on inspiration. The inflammation and roughing of the pleura may be associated with a pleural rub (a creaking sound) at the lung bases, best heard posteriorly. The pain and rub disappear when the pleurae become separated by fluid.

Pleural effusion occurs when fluid fills the space between the visceral and parietal pleurae. It is more common at the lung bases, i.e. is dependent on posture. The chest wall over the effusion is dull to percussion, sometimes 'stony dull'.

Breath sounds at the site of effusion are reduced or absent, and if heard are vesicular. **Empyema** is a collection of pus and occurs when a pleural effusion becomes infected.

A **pneumothorax** is the entrance of air into the pleural space which then prevents the lung from expanding. With a large pneumothorax, the trachea (and mediastinum) may be deviated contralaterally. The side of the chest containing the pneumothorax is resonant to percussion (see Clinical box 13.5). Breath sounds are reduced or absent.

Pulmonary lymphatics

The channels providing lymphatic drainage in the lungs lie in the interstitial spaces between the alveolar cells and the endothelial cells of the alveolar capillaries. These lymphatic

channels drain into a network of lymph nodes that follow the tracheobronchial tree towards the hilum. In the normal, healthy state, pulmonary lymphatic drainage is highly efficient.

The alveolar surfaces are continually moistened by a net filtration of fluid. Any Excess fluid is removed by the lymphatics. Under normal physiological conditions, these channels can hold up to 500 mL of fluid. Fluid will leak into the interstitial spaces giving rise to **pulmonary oedema** if excessive fluid filtration beyond the capacity of the pulmonary lymphatic channels occurs.

When pulmonary oedema is present, the pulmonary lymphatic channels become engorged, as do the hilar lymph glands. This will appear as a butterfly shadow on a chest radiograph (Fig. 13.8). As the left heart pressure increases, thickening of the interlobular septa may be visible as linear shadows on a chest X-ray, known as Kerley B lines. These are more easily seen at the costophrenic angles, but may disappear as the hydrostatic pressure increases further, leading to alveolar oedema.

Pulmonary oedema

The alveoli are the primary units for gaseous exchange in the lungs. They therefore have to be kept relatively 'dry' in order to facilitate rapid and efficient gaseous exchange. The normal balance between capillary hydrostatic pressure/interstitial hydrostatic pressure and capillary oncotic pressure/interstitial oncotic pressure has the overall effect of maintaining a net filtration of fluid to continually moisten the alveolar surface. Excessive accumulation of fluid in the pulmonary interstitial spaces (interstitial oedema) or alveoli (alveolar flooding) leads to pulmonary oedema. Pulmonary oedema may be produced by excess filtration from the pulmonary capillaries or normal filtration with impaired drainage of fluid:

Clinical box 13.5 **Pneumothorax**

There are three types of pneumothorax:

- **Spontaneous**: this occurs without an obvious cause in a patient without an underlying respiratory disease. It typically occurs in tall thin young men and maybe caused by the rupture of a localised defect. It often occurs without exertion but can be associated with the pressure changes due to diving or high-altitude flying.
- **Traumatic**: this occurs when air enters through a wound, usually a knife wound. It can also be caused by rib fractures.
- **Tension**: this occurs when air can enter the pleural space through a defect that acts like a one-way valve. Air moves into the space during inspiration but is trapped during expiration. The rise in pressure in the pleural space can displace the mediastinum affecting the central vessels and reducing cardiac performance. High pressures can result in cardiac tamponade – where the pumping of the heart is impaired.

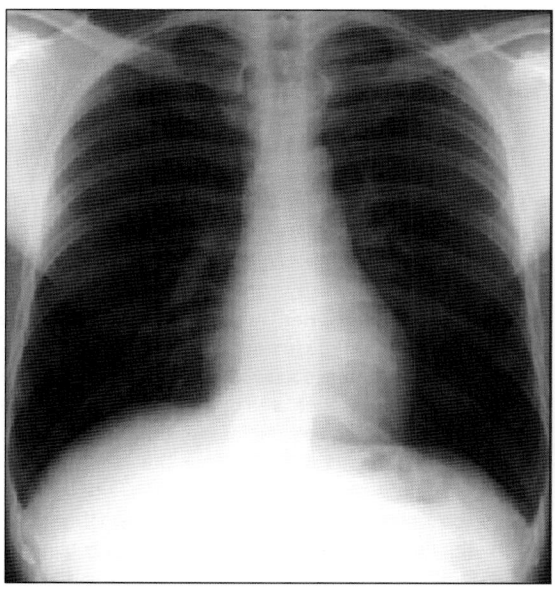
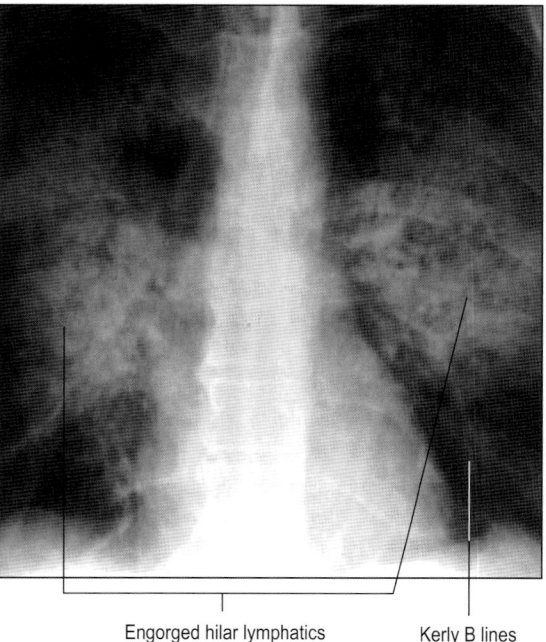

Engorged hilar lymphatics
and glands   Kerly B lines

Fig. 13.8 **Appearance of the normal lung (left) and the lung in pulmonary oedema (right).** The shadowing in oedema typically has a 'butterfly' shape.

- Increased capillary hydrostatic pressure
- Decreased oncotic pressure across the capillary membrane (rare)
- Increased capillary permeability (to both fluid and protein)
- Impaired lymphatic drainage.

In the blood surrounding the alveoli, the oncotic pressure of the plasma proteins (25 mmHg) normally exceeds the hydrostatic capillary blood pressure (10 mmHg) in the pulmonary circulation. However, there is a high protein concentration in the lungs, about 70% that of the plasma, which gives an oncotic pressure in the lungs of about 18 mmHg.

Thus, in conditions such as heart failure where there is even a small rise in left atrial pressures to 20 mmHg or above, there is an increase in pulmonary venous pressure, so net filtration exceeds the capabilities of the lymphatic drainage, and consequently pulmonary oedema occurs. Alveolar oedema occurs when the pulmonary venous pressure exceeds 30 mmHg.

ANATOMY OF THE PULMONARY CIRCULATION

In order to ensure maximum efficiency in oxygen transfer between the alveoli and the blood, the pulmonary circulation is at very low pressure with very thin-walled vessels. The pressure in the alveoli being close to atmospheric pressure, the pressure in the gaseous compartment of the lungs (the alveoli) is greater than the pressure in the blood compartment, so that the lungs are in effect surrounded by negative pressure.

The lungs have two sources of blood supply (Fig. 13.9) delivered by two separate sets of blood vessels:

- **Deoxygenated blood** from the systemic circulation is carried to the lungs by the pulmonary artery from the right ventricle. After successive divisions that follow the bronchi and bronchioles, the pulmonary artery ends as thin-walled pulmonary capillaries in the alveolar walls to form the alveolar–capillary complexes, where gaseous exchange takes place (see Fig. 13.7). Oxygenated blood is collected via the pulmonary venous circulation into the pulmonary veins, which empty into the left atrium for onward distribution.
- **Oxygenated blood** from the descending aorta supplies the bronchial circulation, carrying nutrients to the lungs via the bronchial arteries. Bronchial veins drain deoxygenated blood from the lung parenchyma, bronchial tree, pleura and nerves. Most of this blood is returned to the right side of the heart via the superior vena cava. Blood from the deeper lung parenchyma drains into the pulmonary vein, and is therefore returned to the left side of the heart.

Although the two sets of circulation through the lungs are considered to be separate, there are overlaps where there are communications between the pulmonary and bronchial vascular systems (right-to-left shunt, see below). In total, these pulmonary blood vessels contain about 24% of the body's total blood volume (about 1.2 L of a total blood volume of about 5 L). Their capacity is variable and decreases during expiration, thus affecting inflow into the left atrium and beat-to-beat output of the left ventricle.

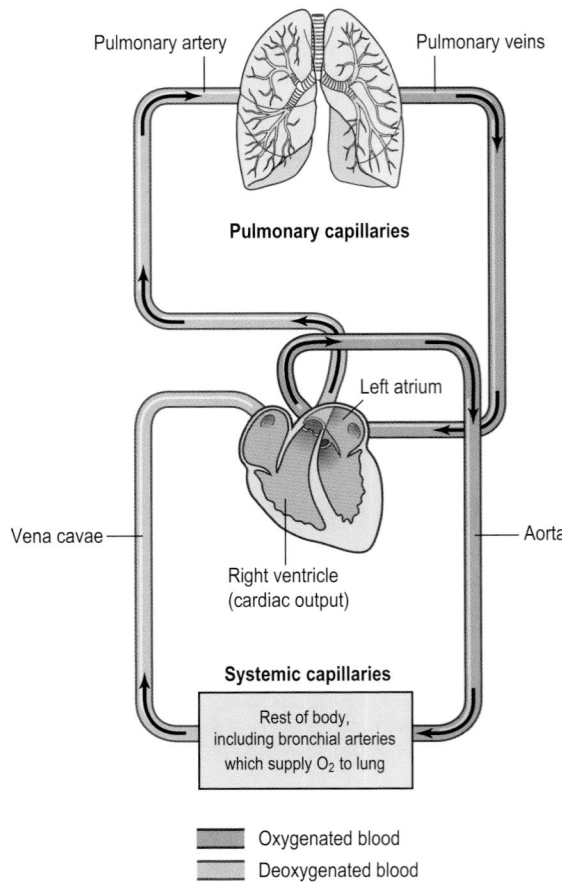

Fig. 13.9 **Anatomy of the pulmonary circulation.** The alveoli have two supplies of blood, from the pulmonary artery and from the aorta.

Arteries

The main **pulmonary artery** divides into two arteries, one for each lung. Their resistance is about one-sixth of the resistance of systemic arteries that have the same blood flow. Structurally, the pulmonary artery is primarily elastic, with the muscular media layer of the arterial wall about half the thickness of equivalent systemic arteries. Maximum muscularity occurs in vessels about 200–100 μm diameter, but muscular tissue is lost as the vessels narrow from 100 μm to 30 μm.

Pulmonary capillaries arise abruptly from the larger vessels; each is about 8 μm in length and diameter (see Fig. 13.7). They form a dense network or sheet around the alveoli, with an estimated surface area of 30–50 m^2. A capillary is not confined to one alveolus but passes from one alveolus to another, and blood traverses a number of alveolar septa before it reaches a venule.

The **bronchial arteries** enter each lung and their branches follow the larger bronchi and bronchioles. They supply arterial blood to bronchial smooth muscle as far as the respiratory bronchioles, the intrapulmonary nerves, nerve ganglia, pleura, interstitial lung substance, lymphoid tissue and vasa vasorum of the pulmonary artery. **Vasa vasorum** are the blood vessels that supply the walls of large blood vessels such as the aorta.

Veins

Blood from the pulmonary capillaries drains into the pulmonary vein and thence into the left atrium. Blood from the bronchial arteries can either drain back to the heart via the true **bronchial veins** into the right atrium or via the **pulmonary vein** into the left atrium. Blood from the systemic circulation can therefore reach the pulmonary circulation by way of the bronchial vascular system. There are also connections (**anastomoses** or **shunts**) between these two circulatory systems at the capillary level. As the bronchial arteries are carrying oxygenated blood at systemic pressures and the drainage is via the low-pressure pulmonary venous system, the bronchial circulation becomes an arteriovenous shunt.

Right-to-left (arteriovenous) shunts

Shunting of blood refers to the phenomenon whereby deoxygenated blood from the right side of the heart bypasses the ventilated areas of the lungs and enters the systemic circulation without effectively taking up oxygen and off-loading carbon dioxide. This lowers the partial pressure of oxygen in the arterial blood due to mixing of blood from various sources:

- Oxygen-depleted blood from the bronchial circulation entering the pulmonary vein and thus the left ventricle
- Congenital abnormalities of the heart where there is addition of deoxygenated blood from the right side directly to the left, e.g. atrial septal defects, Fallot's tetralogy, patent ductus arteriosus
- Vascular anomalies such as pulmonary arteriovenous fistulas (direct connection between an artery and a vein)
- Coronary venous drainage directly into the left ventricle (Thebesian veins)
- Blood flow through diseased or damaged areas of the lungs that are poorly or not ventilated, where gaseous exchange is inefficient.

Pulmonary blood flow

Blood flow through the pulmonary artery is usually taken to be equal to cardiac output even though 1–2% of blood pumped out of the right ventricle bypasses the lungs via shunts. This relationship is the basis of direct (invasive) and numerous indirect (non-invasive) methods for estimating cardiac output using the **Fick equation** (See Clinical box 13.6). Table 13.2 lists the commonly used respiratory symbols and abbreviations.

The normal value for pulmonary blood flow or cardiac output in the average man at rest is 5 L/min or, when expressed as the cardiac index, 3.0 L/min/m^2 body surface area. Output from the right ventricle is not distributed equally to the two lungs: about 45% of deoxygenated blood passes through the left lung and 55% through the right. The time for blood to pass through the lungs from pulmonary artery to left atrium is about 5 seconds. Gaseous exchange at the alveolar–capillary complex takes about 0.75 seconds. Although this falls to 0.3 seconds during strenuous exercise, the blood is **fully saturated** in that time because **haemoglobin** has such a high affinity for oxygen.

Volume of blood in lungs

There is an estimated 100 mL of blood in the pulmonary capillaries. The pulmonary blood volume can vary under dif-

Clinical box 13.6	Determining pulmonary blood flow or cardiac output

- Blood is sampled from the aorta and pulmonary artery using catheters inserted into the heart.
- The concentration of oxygen (O_2) or carbon dioxide (CO_2) is measured in the respective arterial (a) and mixed venous (v) blood.

The **Fick principle** states that the rate at which oxygen is taken up from the atmosphere (O_2 consumption) is equal to the flow of blood passing through the lungs and the increase in oxygen concentration of blood passing through the lungs. Thus:

$$CO = \frac{O_2 \text{ consumption}}{a - v \ O_2 \text{ concentration difference}}$$

or

$$CO = \frac{CO_2 \text{ production}}{v - a \ CO_2 \text{ concentration difference}}$$

- Normal O_2 consumption is 250 mL/min, the arterial O_2 concentration 190 mL/L blood and the venous O_2 concentration 140 mL/L blood
- Normal CO_2 production is 200 mL/min, the venous O_2 concentration 520 mL/L blood and the arterial O_2 concentration 480 mL/L blood

Using either O_2 consumption or CO_2 consumption should give the same answer.

$$CO = (250 \text{ mL/min})/(190 - 140 \text{ mL/L blood})$$
$$= (250 \text{ mL/min})/50 \text{ mL/L}$$

or

$$CO = (200 \text{ mL/min})/(520 - 480 \text{ mL/L blood})$$
$$= (200 \text{ mL/min})/(40 \text{ mL/L})$$

Both of which give a pulmonary blood flow or cardiac output = 5 L/min.

ferent conditions and therefore acts a reservoir. This reservoir of blood is important in ensuring that the left side of the heart is filled during diastole. This ability of the lungs to store blood means that it can buffer minor irregularities in the output of the two ventricles.

Pulmonary arterial and venous pressure

Pulmonary arterial pressure is much lower than systemic arterial pressure, at about 25/8 mmHg (mean 11–15 mmHg) compared with 120/80 mmHg in the aorta. The pulmonary arterial walls are about half as thick as corresponding vessels in the systemic circulation. Pressures can be measured directly by inserting a catheter through a large leg vein via the left side of the heart, through the chambers into the pulmonary artery. Pressures inside the pulmonary artery are the same as in the right ventricle.

There are no valves between the left atrium and the pulmonary vein, so pressures in the left atrium are equivalent to those in the pulmonary vein and left atrial pressure may be taken as a measure of **pulmonary venous pressure**. Left atrial pressures are measured by inserting a catheter into the heart via an artery (normally the femoral artery). The mean left atrial pressure, equivalent to the pulmonary venous pressure, varies from 0 mmHg to 5 mmHg. This suggests that the pressure drop across the lungs is about 12 mmHg.

Table 13.2	**Respiratory abbreviations**	
Symbol	**Definition**	**Examples**
p	Partial gas pressure	p_aCO_2, arterial CO_2 pressure
V	Gas volume	V_T, tidal volume
$\dot{V}$	Gas volume per unit time (flow)	$\dot{V}$, volume of expired air/min
F	Fractional gas concentration	F_iO_2, fractional concentration of O_2 in inspired gas
D	Diffusing capacity	DO_2, diffusing capacity of O_2 (e.g. 50 mL O_2/min/mmHg)
Q	Volume of blood	Q_c, volume of blood in pulmonary capillaries
$\dot{Q}$	Volume flow of blood per unit time	$\dot{Q}$, blood flow through pulmonary capillaries/min
C	Concentration of gas in blood	C_aO_2, mL O_2 in 100 mL arterial blood
S	% saturation of haemoglobin with O_2	S_vO_2, saturation of haemoglobin with O_2 in mixed venous blood
Gas symbols		
A	Alveolar gas	
B	Barometric	
D	Dead space gas	
E	Expired gas	
I	Inspired gas	
L	Lung	
T	Tidal gas	
Blood symbols		
a	Arterial blood	
v	Venous blood	
c	Capillary blood	

A dash (–) above any symbol indicates a mean value ($\bar{p}_cO_2$, mixed venous pO_2).
A dot (.) above any symbol indicates a time derivative.

Pulmonary blood vessels

The pulmonary blood vessels are supplied by sympathetic vasoconstrictor fibres. Little is known about regulation of pulmonary vessel diameter, but there must be a certain level of resting tone since, during exercise, pulmonary resistances must decrease to accommodate a sixfold increase in pulmonary blood flow. Pulmonary blood vessels, unlike vessels in the systemic circulation, are constricted by hypoxia or acidosis. The response to hypoxia is non-linear and partly dependent on the carbon dioxide levels. **Hypoxic vasoconstriction** is very important as a means of diverting blood flow away from lung regions where the oxygen tension is low, to regions where oxygen is available to be taken up by haemoglobin. Chronic hypoxia, as seen in COPD, will lead to pulmonary hypertension and the development of right heart failure (**cor pulmonale**).

Variations in pulmonary blood flow

Pulmonary blood flow varies during normal breathing. Intrathoracic pressure falls during **inspiration**, so that blood flows more readily through the veins. There is increased filling of the right ventricle and so increased right ventricular output. Pulmonary arterial pressure rises and pulmonary blood vessels engorge. However, pulmonary venous outflow falls, possibly because of the expansion in capillary volume, and there is a reduction in left ventricular filling and a slight fall in left systemic pressure.

During **expiration** the increased volume of blood in the lungs is expelled through the pulmonary veins with the result that the left ventricular output increases, causing a rise in systemic blood pressure. Simultaneously the higher intrathoracic pressure reduces the return of blood to the right ventricle and the mean pulmonary artery pressure falls.

Clinical box 13.7	**Clinical conditions associated with defects in the pulmonary circulation**

Cor pulmonale is a condition in which there is right heart (ventricular) failure resulting from raised blood pressure in either the pulmonary arteries or the pulmonary veins – pulmonary hypertension. Right heart failure is caused by a primary disorder of the respiratory system, or may be secondary to some other cardiopulmonary disease.

Chronic cor pulmonale is associated with right ventricular hypertrophy. Common causes include:

- Chronic obstructive pulmonary disease (COPD)
- Pulmonary fibrosis from whatever cause
- Cystic fibrosis
- Primary pulmonary hypertension
- Chronic thromboembolic pulmonary disease
- Obstructive sleep apnoea.

Right ventricular dilatation occurs in acute cor pulmonale. Acute cor pulmonale is reversible, and may occur with massive pulmonary embolism. Symptoms of cor pulmonale are mainly associated with right ventricular failure and the underlying lung disease. Physical signs are those of pulmonary hypertension and right ventricular failure, together with the underlying lung condition.

Pulmonary oedema occurs in left ventricular failure from whatever cause. Symptoms include:

- Shortness of breath (dyspnoea) on exertion
- Orthopnoea – dyspnoea when lying flat
- Paroxysmal nocturnal dyspnoea – acute shortness of breath while asleep, causing patient to wake from sleep.

The presence of bilateral fine, basal crackles on auscultation of the chest is the cardinal physical sign of pulmonary oedema.

Effect of gravity on pulmonary blood flow

Gravity has an effect on pulmonary blood flow. In the upright posture, the contents of the thorax are like a semi-liquid column. Due to gravity, the hydrostatic pressure in the lower part of the column would be higher than the upper part. The negative pressure in the lower parts of the lungs is therefore less 'negative' than that in the top parts.

This higher pressure has the effect of increasing blood flow through the lower parts of the lungs by opening up the capillaries that are collapsed as the result of negative pressure. As a result, the lower parts of the lungs are better perfused than the upper parts, and these have been described as three 'zones' (see below, Uneven perfusion, Fig. 13.24). At rest, and in the upright position, the upper zone capillary bed is closed, but it may open up during exercise due to increased oxygen demand.

SURFACE ANATOMY OF THE RESPIRATORY SYSTEM

The surface anatomy of the respiratory system gives an indication of the underlying structures, and it is essential to know these surface markings when performing clinical examinations or procedures.

Larynx and trachea

The larynx is made up of the prominent thyroid cartilage (thyroid prominence: Adam's apple) and the cricoid cartilage just beneath it, and is palpable in the anterior part of the neck. Its complex structure reflects the variety of muscles attached to it. The vocal cords lie within the larynx behind the thyroid cartilage. The first of the cartilaginous rings of the trachea can be felt in the midline in the depths of the suprasternal notch. The trachea ends just right of the midline at the level of the sternal angle (see below).

Surface markings of the thorax

Anterior surface of the chest

The **clavicles** (collar bones) and the **sternum** (breastbone) form the single bony articulation (joint) between the upper limb and the thorax. The sternum is in two parts and can be felt throughout its entire length at the bottom of a furrow, the sternal furrow, situated between the pectoralis major muscles. The upper end of the body of the sternum is attached at a slight angle to the **manubrium**. The curved upper end of the

---

---

manubrium and the medial ends of the clavicles form a recess called the **suprasternal notch**, where the cartilage of the trachea may be felt. The sternocleidomastoid muscles appear as oblique cords narrowing and deepening the notch. The **xyphoid process (xiphisternum)** is a tongue of cartilage at the lower end of the sternal body (Fig. 13.10).

The manubrium and body of the sternum are joined by the manubriosternal joint The **sternal angle** (angle of Louis) is the angle made by this joint. The sternal angle can be seen and felt and is used to mark the medial end of the costal (rib) cartilage of the second rib and further laterally the rib itself. All ribs may be counted from this point systematically down the chest wall from one rib to another, with the soft intercostal spaces between them. Ribs are numbered according to the vertebra to which they are attached posteriorly. **Intercostal spaces** are named after the rib above. The lower border of the pectoralis major at its attachment corresponds to the fifth rib. The vertical line that passes through the mid-point of the clavicle is the midclavicular line.

The costal margin is formed by the costal cartilages of the seventh to tenth ribs marking the lower border of the thorax. Posteriorly, the eleventh and twelfth ribs are usually separate from the costal margin. The twelfth rib is small and is more difficult to feel because it is buried in bulky muscles.

Lateral surface of the chest

The anatomical term for the armpit is the axilla or axillary fossa. The upper part of the lateral chest wall lies in the space between the **axillary folds**, which come into prominence when the upper limb is raised above the head. The anterior fold is formed by the lower border of a large muscle, the pectoralis major. The posterior fold is formed by the tendon of the latissimus dorsi muscle as it passes round the lower border of the teres major muscle. The vertical line midway between the axillary folds is the midaxillary line.

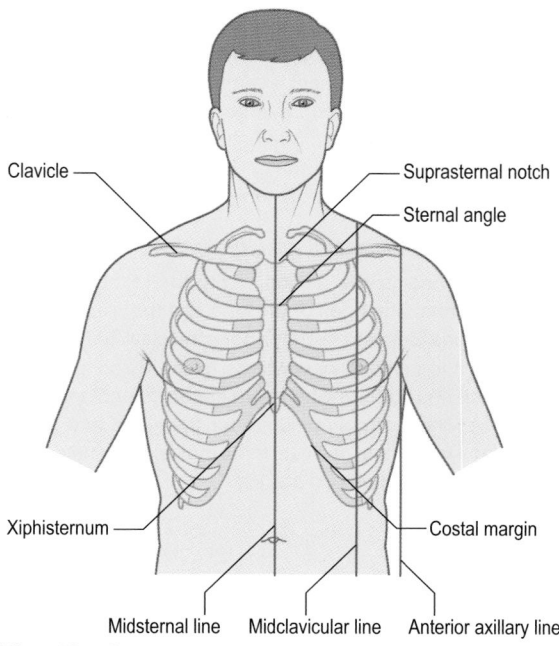

Clavicle — Suprasternal notch — Sternal angle

Xiphisternum — Costal margin

Midsternal line   Midclavicular line   Anterior axillary line

Fig. 13.10 **Surface anatomy of the anterior chest (male).**

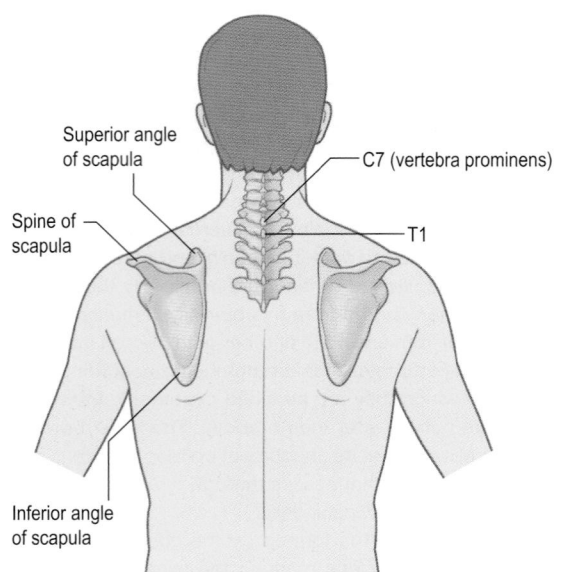

Fig. 13.11 **Surface markings of the posterior chest wall.**

Posterior surface of the chest

The spinous processes of the 12 thoracic vertebrae are visible as plate-like knobs and can be felt, providing attachments for large muscles. The first palpable (and visible) spinous process is that of the seventh cervical vertebra (C7, vertebra prominens). The spinous processes of the first thoracic vertebrae is inferior (caudal) to the vertebra prominens. The spinous process of each thoracic vertebra lies immediately posterior to the body of the one below.

The scapula is a prominent landmark on the posterior wall of the chest, shaped to form a large surface for attachment of the powerful muscles that move the upper limb in relation to the thorax (Fig. 13.11). It has a lower point (apex) and a spine that projects from its posterior surface.

The lungs and pleural cavity

The lungs lie inside the pleural cavity and almost entirely beneath the ribs. The apex of the lung and the pleural cavity which surround it extend slightly above the clavicles by about 3 cm. They then extend downwards to the diaphragm, and between the ribs and the diaphragm as the costodiaphragmatic recess. The surface markings for the lungs and pleura are similar except that the lungs do not extend below the vertebral level of T10 (Fig. 13.12).

MECHANICS OF BREATHING

Ventilation (movement of air into and out of the lungs) is produced by changes in the size of the thoracic cavity. When

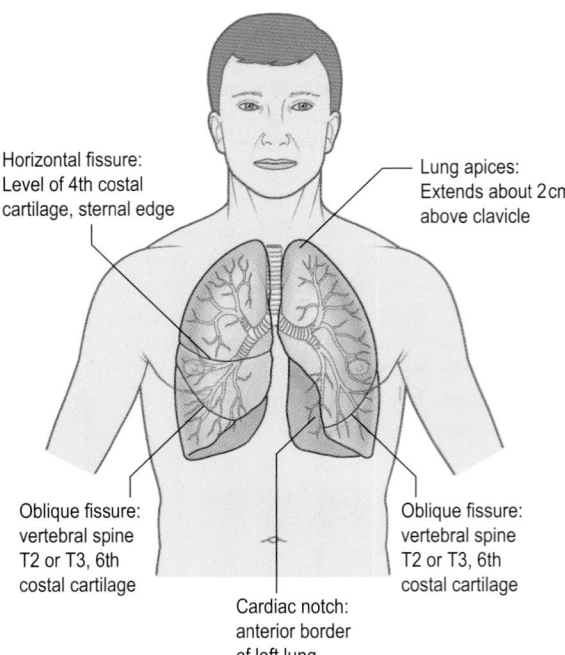

Fig. 13.12 **Surface markings of the lungs.**

the cavity enlarges during inspiration, air flows into the lungs because at that instant the pressure in the atmosphere is greater than that in the lungs.

THE DIAPHRAGM AND OTHER MUSCLES USED IN BREATHING

The **diaphragm** is the main muscle of respiration. It is a dome-shaped sheet of skeletal muscle separating the thoracic and abdominal cavities and consisting of muscle fibres and a central tendinous portion. The fibres run upwards from their origin at the inner part of the thoracic cage and then arch towards the midline.

During normal, **quiet respiration**, the diaphragm contracts and moves downwards in inspiration and the diaphragmatic parietal pleura descends. This movement pulls down the visceral pleura so that the airways and alveoli expand and air is sucked in. The diaphragm relaxes in expiration and the recoil of the elastic tissues in the lung expels air from the alveoli and airways. Movement of the **ribcage** also contributes to respiration by increasing the diameter of the chest, thereby increasing the thoracic volume and making the negative pressure in the lungs more 'negative', allowing air to be sucked in. The joints between the posterior ends of the ribs and the transverse processes of the vertebrae enable the lower ribs to swivel upwards and outwards to increase the lateral diameter of the chest, while the anterior ends of the ribs move up and out to increase the anteroposterior diameter. The diaphragmatic movement contributes about 75% and movement of the ribcage contributes 25% to the increase in thoracic volume.

During **forced respiration**, when there is increased demand for oxygen, as in exercise or disease, **accessory muscles of respiration** come into play. These are muscles that are not primarily involved in respiration, but enlarge the ribcage in any way possible during inspiration to increase the amount of air, and therefore oxygen, breathed in (Fig. 13.13).

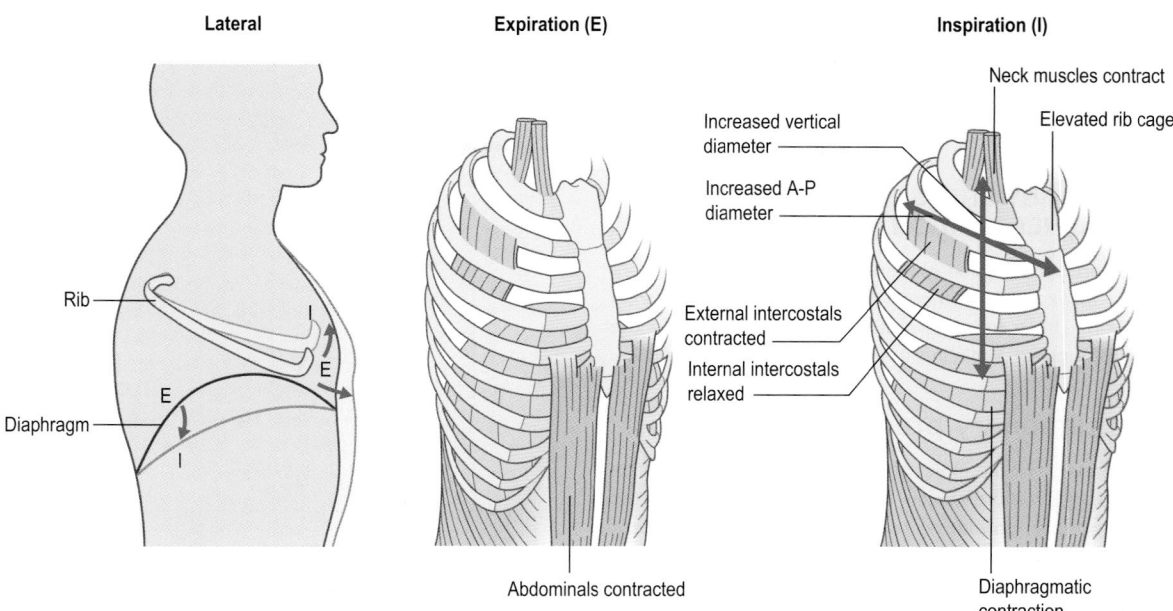

Lateral   Expiration (E)   Inspiration (I)

Neck muscles contract

Increased vertical
diameter

Elevated rib cage

Increased A-P
diameter

External intercostals
contracted

Internal intercostals
relaxed

Rib

Diaphragm

Abdominals contracted

Diaphragmatic
contraction

Fig. 13.13 **Chest and rib movements contribute to chest expansion.** The accessory muscles assist in increasing chest capacity in forced respiration. A-P, anteroposterior.

Clinical box 13.10   **Accessory muscles of respiration in respiratory distress**

The use of accessory muscles of respiration is a sign of respiratory distress or failure. Breathing becomes laboured and the accessory muscles of respiration may be seen clearly in the neck and abdomen. Intercostal recession occurs because of the external intercostal muscles contracting to move the ribcage up and outwards. This is accompanied by tachypnoea and dyspnoea, and sometimes cyanosis is present.

The external intercostal muscles move the ribcage upwards and outwards to increase the lateral and anteroposterior diameter of the thorax. The neck muscles pull the ribcage upwards; the sternocleidomastoids will elevate the sternum while the scalenus major and minor muscles will elevate both the first two ribs and the sternum. The oblique, transversus and rectus abdominis muscles will pull the ribcage downwards. By fixing the shoulder girdle, the pectoralis major and latissimus dorsi muscles will pull the ribcage outwards.

These muscles can be seen hard at work in patients with respiratory distress (Clinical box 13.10) as in acute asthma, and in athletes at the end of a hard race. Contraction of the abdominal muscles also increases intra-abdominal pressure and pulls the ribcage downwards and medially in forced expiration.

Inspiration

The diaphragm is the main muscle of **inspiration**. It has a motor nerve supply from cervical segments C3–C5 via the left and right phrenic nerves. The sensory supply is also through the phrenic nerve centrally and branches of the intercostal nerves peripherally. When stimulated, the diaphragm moves downwards, increasing the size of the thoracic cavity. This has the effect of making the negative intrapulmonary

pressure more negative, and thus drawing air into the lungs. In **eupnoea** (normal breathing) the diaphragm may move by 1.5 cm, and in deep breathing it may show as much as a 7 cm excursion.

In spinal cord injuries, only breaks above C3–C4 will affect the phrenic nerve and result in apnoea (absence of breathing) and death. If the phrenic nerve is severed by accident but the spinal cord remains intact, ventilation can be adequately accomplished by contraction of the external intercostal muscles. The intercostal muscles are innervated by motor neurons from vertebrae T1–T12. The muscles move the chest wall upwards and outwards.

The position of the diaphragm varies with body posture. In an upright posture, the abdominal contents sink under gravity as does the diaphragm. The diaphragm also flattens out, increasing its cross-sectional area. Thus, in the upright posture, the diaphragmatic movement required to achieve expansion of the thoracic cavity is smaller than that required to achieve the same expansion in the supine posture, when the diaphragm is more dome-shaped. This explains why patients with respiratory diseases, particularly those involving respiratory muscle fatigue, prefer an upright posture.

Expiration

In quiet breathing, **expiration** is usually passive and results from the elastic recoil of the lungs and chest wall, and the inward pull of surface tension in the pleural space.

1. Muscles of the diaphragm and intercostals relax.
2. Thoracic and intrapulmonary volumes decrease.
3. Intrapulmonary pressures increases to about 1 mmHg above atmospheric pressure.

Forced expiration during maximal ventilation or against an obstruction is an active process: the abdominal muscles contract and increase intra-abdominal pressure. This movement forces the diaphragm upward and depresses the lower ribs, so decreasing the volume of the thoracic cavity and expelling air. Lung emptying can be enhanced by contraction of the internal intercostal muscles. This displaces the ribs down and back, again decreasing the volume of the thorax and expelling air from the lungs.

PULMONARY PRESSURE CHANGES DURING VENTILATION

The diaphragm, muscles of respiration and chest wall work together to expand the thorax and inflate the lungs during inspiration. These muscles reduce their effort, causing the thorax to contract, deflating the lungs during expiration.

Intrapulmonary pressure

With expansion of the chest and the accompanying inflation of the lung, pressure within the alveoli of the lungs, the **intrapulmonary pressure**, falls to about 3 mmHg below the atmospheric pressure. As the lungs fill, this gradient decreases, and by the end of inspiration the intrapulmonary pressure equals atmospheric pressure. During expiration, intrapulmonary pressures become positive relative to atmospheric (+3 mmHg) but return to atmospheric pressure once expiration is complete.

Intrapleural pressure

Intrapleural pressure refers to pressures within the pleural space, i.e. between the visceral and parietal pleural layers. These are normally subatmospheric (−4 mmHg) because of the elastic recoil of the lungs continually trying to separate the two layers. During normal breathing and movement of the diaphragm and ribcage, intrapleural pressures will fall or rise by about 5 mmHg relative to this subatmospheric pressure. A deep inspiration can drop the intrapleural pressures by as much as 30 mmHg below atmospheric. Intrapleural pressures can be measured by inserting the tip of a needle connected to a manometer into the pleural cavity. Less invasively, changes in intrapleural pressure can be measured by a balloon catheter in the oesophagus at the level of the mediastinum.

Maximal respiratory pressures

Maximal respiratory pressures are used to measure the strength of inspiratory and expiratory muscles. Muscle weakness will restrict maximal inspiration, whereas stiff lungs will stretch less for the same muscular effort. In disease conditions such as multiple sclerosis, poliomyelitis or spinal injuries, these pressures may be used to monitor the effectiveness of interventions to strengthen the respiratory muscles. The maximal expiratory pressures (PE_{max}) that can be developed are 150–200 cmH$_2$O at high lung volume, while maximal (negative) inspiratory pressure (PI_{max}) is 100 cmH$_2$O at low lung volumes.

PULMONARY VENTILATION

Pulmonary ventilation is the process for moving gases in and out of the lungs. In the healthy state, the amount of gas (or air) that can be accommodated will depend of the size of the lungs and thorax, which is related to the age, sex, height and ethnicity of the individual. This is referred to as **lung**

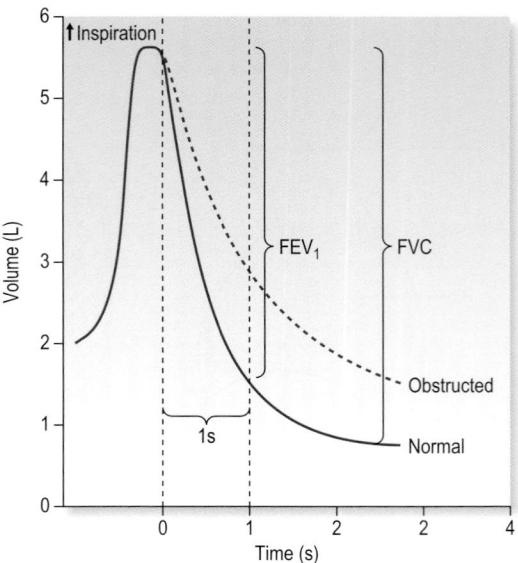

Fig. 13.14 Lung volumes as measured using a spirometer. Subjects breathe out as fast as possible from maximum inspiration. The volume expelled relates to lung capacity. The volume expelled in the first second (FEV$_1$) is used expressed as a percentage of the total forced expiratory capacity (FVC); this normally should be >80%.

capacity. The amount of gas (or air) that can be moved with respiration is known as **lung volume**, and will depend on inspiratory and expiratory effort. Pulmonary disease will affect both lung capacity and the volume of gases that the lungs can move in and out of the alveoli. Pulmonary ventilation is defined as the amount of gas moved in or out of the lungs per minute.

Lung volumes and capacities

The changes in the volume of the lungs during breathing can be measured with a spirometer. There are various types of spirometer but a modern version is a rolling seal spirometer. Figure 13.14 shows the lung capacities and lung volumes recorded on a spirometer.

Lung capacities are made up from two or more 'volumes' (Fig. 13.15):

- **Total lung capacity** (TLC): the maximum amount of gas the lungs can accommodate. TLC is the sum of four 'volumes'.
  - **Tidal volume** (TV): the amount of air inspired and expired at each breath at any level of activity. During normal, quiet breathing this is about 0.5 L, but TV can increase to 1 L or more during exercise and with training.
  - **Expiratory reserve volume** (ERV): the amount of gas that could be expelled with maximum expiratory effort at the end of normal, quiet expiration – about 1.5 L.
  - **Residual volume** (RV): the volume of air that still remains in the lungs – about 1.0 L.
  - **Inspiratory reserve volume** (IRV): the amount of air that can be breathed in with a maximum inspiration from the end of a normal inspiration – about 3.0 L.

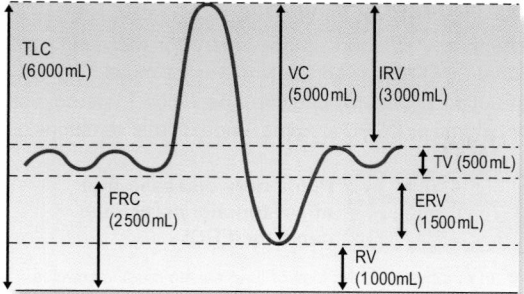

Fig. 13.15 **Lung volumes** can be considered as having various components. The figure shows lung volumes measured with a spirometer during quiet breathing with one maximum breath. Volumes shown are for an average-sized healthy young man. RV, residual volume; ERV, expiratory reserve volume; IRV, inspiratory reserve volume; TLC, total lung capacity; FRC, functional respiratory capacity; TV, tidal volume; VC, vital capacity.

■ **Forced vital capacity (FVC)** or **vital capacity (VC)** is the maximum possible breath that can be taken, typically 5 L. FVC (VC) is made up of three 'volumes':

VC = TV + ERV + IRV

■ **Functional residual capacity (FRC)**: the volume of air left in the lungs at the end of normal quiet expiration when all respiratory muscles are relaxed. For a healthy, resting, recumbent young man (1.7 m^2 body surface) breathing at sea level, an average FRC would be 2.5 L.

FRC = RV + ERV

■ VC + RV = TLC, which is about 6 L.

Total lung capacity (TLC) is equal to VC plus RV, which is about 6 L:

TLC = VC + RV

RV cannot be determined by the use of a simple spirometer, nor therefore can FRC because it is given as the sum of RV + ERV; other means have to be used (see Clinical box 13.11).

Dead space

Dead space is the volume of the respiratory tract not involved in gas exchange. The **anatomical dead space** lies between the mouth/nose entrance and the respiratory bronchioles where the tissue walls are too thick and blood vessels too few to allow diffusion of gases into the blood. Some air may also enter parts of the lungs where gaseous exchange is not fully efficient because these parts of the lungs are either relatively poorly perfused or relatively overventilated. The total volume of air not involved in oxygenation of blood is termed the **physiological dead space** and encompasses this and the anatomical dead space. In healthy people, the physiological dead space is identical to the anatomical dead space.

At rest, typically the respiratory rate (RR) is 12–15 breaths per minute and the tidal volume (TV) 500 mL. Therefore:

Pulmonary ventilation = RR × TV
$$= 12 \times 500$$
$$= 6 \text{ L/min.}$$

However, not all of the breath can take part in gaseous exchange. About 150 mL of each breath fills the so-called

---

Clinical box 13.11 **Measurement of residual volume or functional residual capacity**

This open-circuit method is based on the fact that air contains a fixed concentration (about 80%) of nitrogen (N_2) that is neither absorbed nor produced by the body. So, by washing all the N_2 out of the lungs and measuring its volume, the volume of air that was in the lungs can be estimated. That is:

Volume of gas in the lung (V) × concentration of N_2 in the lung = Volume of gas exhaled × concentration of N_2 in gas exhaled

● To wash the N_2 from the lungs, the subject breathes O_2 (N_2-free) gas and breathes out through a turbine volume–flow meter for a few minutes. Normally 2 minutes are required in healthy adults but longer (7 minutes) may be necessary for people with asthma or emphysema.
● The expired gas is collected and its N_2 concentration measured and its volume determined.

Example: If 40 L of expired gas was collected and it contained 5% nitrogen, then:

$$V \times 80/100 = 40 \times 5/100$$

$$V = 40 \times 0.05/0.80$$
$$= 2.5 \text{ L}$$

If this test is begun precisely at the moment of complete and maximal expiration, then **RV** is measured, while if it is begun at the end of a normal expiration, **FRC** is measured.

Clinical box 13.12 **Measurement of physiological dead space**

● Ask a volunteer to breathe into a Douglas bag and measure the volume of air collected while counting the number of breathes exhaled into the bag. Calculate the tidal volume (TV).
● Measure the CO_2 concentration in the bag ($F_E CO_2$).
● Ask the volunteer to make a rapid and deep expiration into a Haldane tube (a tube about 1 m long and 2.5 cm diameter with a sample tap near the mouthpiece). Sample air with a syringe at the end of the expiration but before the volunteer removes their mouth, to prevent contamination by room air. Measure the CO_2 concentration of the sample gas ($F_A CO_2$).

DS = TV × ($F_A CO_2 - F_E CO_2$)/($F_A CO_2$) (Bohr equation)

The underlying assumptions are that:

● The Haldane tube sample contains the last air to be expelled from the lungs and can be taken to be alveolar air
● Exhaled tidal volume is diluted by the air in the physiological dead space (DS), thus:

(TV − DS) × %CO_2 in alveolar air = TV × %CO_2 in expired air

● Air in the dead space has 0% CO_2.

---

anatomical dead space (DS). The volume of air that participates in gas exchange because it is in contact with perfused alveoli is termed the alveolar ventilation, and is less than pulmonary ventilation. Using the figures above:

Alveolar ventilation = RR × (TV − DS)
$$= 12 \times (500 - 150)$$
$$= 4.2 \text{ L/min.}$$

In disease the physiological dead space will increase with pulmonary embolism, emphysema, artificial ventilation and hyperventilation.

Functional residual capacity

Functional residual capacity refers to the volume of air left in the lungs at the very end of normal expiration. At this stage, all the muscles of respiration are at rest, and the intrapulmonary pressure equals atmospheric pressure (see above). The importance of FRC is that it corresponds to the point where the outward elastic recoil forces of the chest wall are balanced by the inward elastic recoil of the lungs. This balance is changed in a number of respiratory diseases (Clinical box 13.13).

Measuring rates of airflow

In many respiratory diseases it is important to be able to measure the degree to which airflow is limited. Two measures of this are the forced expiratory volume (FEV_1) and peak expiratory flow rate (PEFR)). A more sophisticated measure is flow rates against volume: flow–volume loops. This test can identify the site of airways obstruction (see below).

Forced expiratory volume

A type of spirometer known as a vitalograph can be used to measure FEV_1, which is the amount of air that can be forcibly expelled from a maximal breath in 1 second. Vitalographs can also measure the FVC. FEV_1 and FVC are related to height, age and sex, from which they can be predicted (Fig. 13.16). Their value will also vary with ethnicity and patterns of activity. Swimmers, divers and brass musical instrument players typically have larger than expected FEV_1 and FVC.

Peak expiratory flow rate

Although not as good as spirometry for measuring airflow limitation **PEFR** is a convenient way of measuring airways obstruction as patients can use a peak flow meter to monitor their asthma or COPD at home. Wide diurnal variations occur

---

Clinical box 13.13   **Pulmonary diseases that affect functional residual capacity (FRC)**

- In emphysema, the loss of lung elastic recoil increases FRC so that the thorax is overinflated. This gives rise to the barrel chest of obstructive airways disease. Expanding already overexpanded lungs also makes breathing in harder work.
- Conversely, a low FRC occurs in restrictive lung disorders. The increased lung stiffness in pulmonary oedema, interstitial fibrosis and other restrictive disorders decreases FRC.
- Space occupying intra-abdominal masses also reduce FRC, for example pregnancy, ascites and hepatosplenomegaly.
- Kyphoscoliosis, with deformity of the thoracic cage, leads to a decrease in lung volumes because a stiff, non-compliant chest wall restricts lung expansion.

Clinical signs of hyperinflation of the chest
The anteroposterior diameter of the thorax increases as the chest is continually overinflated giving rise to the following characteristics:

- The 'barrel' shaped chest
- Relatively horizontal ribs
- Protruding abdomen
- Hyper-resonance on percussion.

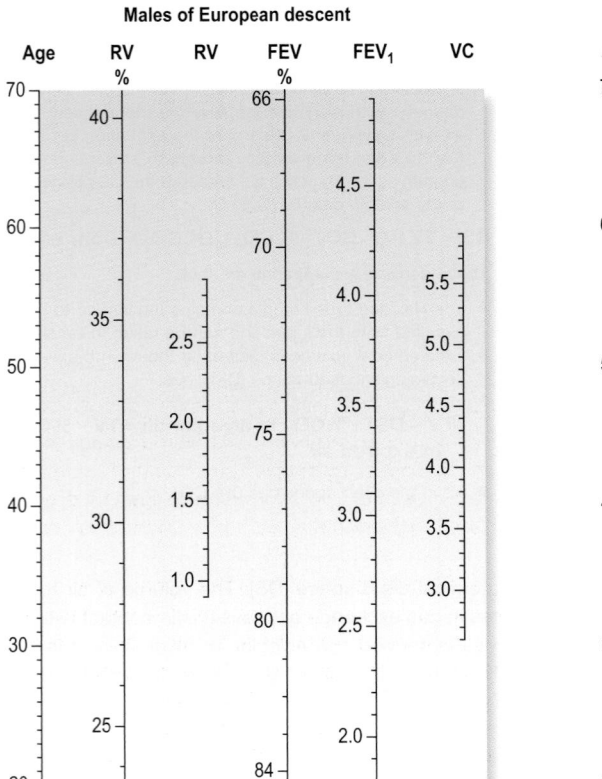
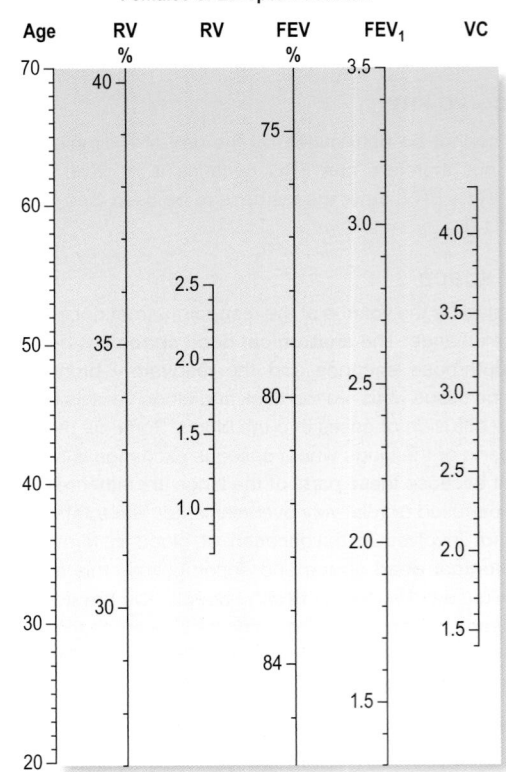

Fig. 13.16 **Nomogram showing predicted airflow values for different ages.** FEV, forced expiratory volume; RV, residual volume; VC, vital capacity. Percentages are related to the total forced expiratory volume; FEV_1, volume expelled in the first second.

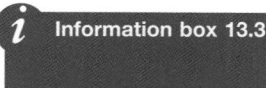

Clinical box 13.14 Measurement of forced expiratory volume (FEV)

- The patient should be upright (FEV$_1$ will be greater in the upright posture), a nose clip should be worn (but is not absolutely essential), a sterile mouthpiece should be used with the lips sealed firmly around it, and the patient verbally encouraged by the operator (because measurement is effort dependent) to fully empty their lungs.
- The patient is asked to make a maximal inspiration followed by a single, forced and long expiration.
- Patients with severe airflow limitation may have a prolonged forced expiratory time so any test should not be prematurely terminated. With a vitalograph-type spirometer the recording takes about 5 seconds in healthy people.

Reductions in FEV$_1$ and forced vital capacity (FVC) can be used to distinguish between diseases (Fig. 13.17). Expression of FEV$_1$ as a percentage of the predicted FEV$_1$ is a good measure of airflow limitation and is used clinically in comparisons of disease severity between patients. In healthy people it is normally greater than 75%. The FEV$_1$/FVC ratio (or FEV$_1$ expressed as a percentage of FVC) is a useful measure of airway obstruction:

- In patients with an obstructive lung disease (asthma, COPD, emphysema) the ratio is less than 75%. Asthmatic patients with air trapping will have reduced FEV$_1$ and FVC, but FEV$_1$ as a percentage of FVC would also be reduced.
- With a restrictive lung disease, i.e. interstitial lung disease, respiratory muscle weakness and thoracic cage deformities such as kyphoscoliosis (kyphosis: dorsal curvature; scoliosis: side-to-side curvature of the spine), both FEV$_1$ and FVC are reduced but the FEV$_1$/FVC ratio is normal (FEV$_1$ as a percentage of FVC is normal).

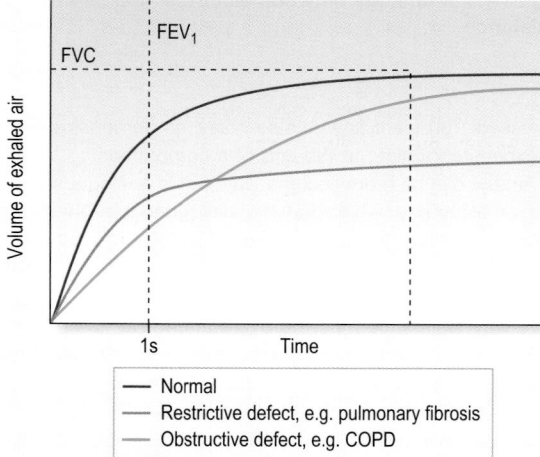

Fig. 13.17 Changes in the forced expiratory volume in 1 second (FEV$_1$) and the forced expiratory capacity (FVC) in obstructive and restrictive pulmonary disease. COPD, chronic obstructive pulmonary disease.

in PEFR, with the highest readings in the evening and the lowest in the early hours of the morning. PEFR is less dependent on effort than the FEV$_1$ but only measures expiratory flow rate. The unit used is L /min or L /s.

Reversibility of airflow limitation

Measurements of FEV$_1$ and PEFR made before and after inhalation of a bronchodilator (e.g. the β-adrenoceptor agonist salbutamol) can be used to distinguish between asthma and chronic obstructive lung disease.

Information box 13.3 Measuring airflow limitation in chronic obstructive pulmonary disease (COPD)

Patients with COPD, as in asthma, experience periods of acute deterioration in symptoms and increased airway inflammation, with respiratory viruses being an important trigger. Exacerbations are an important cause of mortality, morbidity, excess winter hospital admissions and impairment of quality of life.

The best guide to the severity and progression of COPD is the change in forced expiratory volume (FEV$_1$) over time. FEV$_1$ normally declines after the age of 30, but this decline is accelerated in COPD.

- 90% of patients with COPD aged <60 with an FEV$_1$ >50% of predicted will survive for 3 years.
- 80% of patients with COPD aged >60 with an FEV$_1$ >50% of predicted will survive for 3 years.
- 75% of patients with COPD aged >60 with an FEV$_1$ 40–49% of predicted will survive for 3 years.

There is evidence that acute exacerbations of COPD lead to an increased rate of FEV$_1$ decline. No drug treatment has yet been shown to affect the rate of FEV$_1$ decline.

Clinical box 13.15 Measuring peak expiratory flow rate (PEFR)

To measure PEFR, subjects are asked to breath in fully and blow out forcefully into a peak flow meter, sometimes called a Wright flow meter after its inventor. The exhaled air pushes a plastic pointer along a graduated scale. The device should be held horizontally, and certainly not pointed downwards, and the best of three readings taken. The meter is cheap and simple and can be used by patients at home to monitor disease progression and treatment response in, for example, asthma. The maximum flow usually occurs during the first 2 ms of the exhalation.

- In asthma, the airways constriction is reversible so that the FEV$_1$ and PEFR would be restored to normal after salbutamol.
- In COPD, the airways constriction is irreversible, or nearly irreversible. There would be <15%, or <200 mL/s, improvement in FEV$_1$ and PEFR after salbutamol.

WORK OF BREATHING

Breathing costs energy. About half of the work done during a respiratory cycle is dissipated during inspiration (as heat) to overcome resistance to airflow. The remaining energy is stored as potential energy in the elastic structures of the lungs and chest wall, and this stored energy is the driving force for normal expiration. The amount of work done is given by the area within the **flow–volume loop** that describes pressure and volume changes during inspiration and expiration (Fig. 13.18).

Flow–volume loops measure the velocity of air flowing through the airways in relation to the volume of air moved during inspiration or expiration. The measurements therefore reflect both the condition of the conducting airways and lung capacity. Analysis of flow–volume loops gives a better idea of where airflow limitation occurs in the lungs. Different pulmonary diseases give different flow–volume loops, so that an experienced chest physician is able to make a diagnosis from the shape of the loop.

In normal individuals, at rest, the work performed by the muscles of respiration is small at between 2% and 5% of the

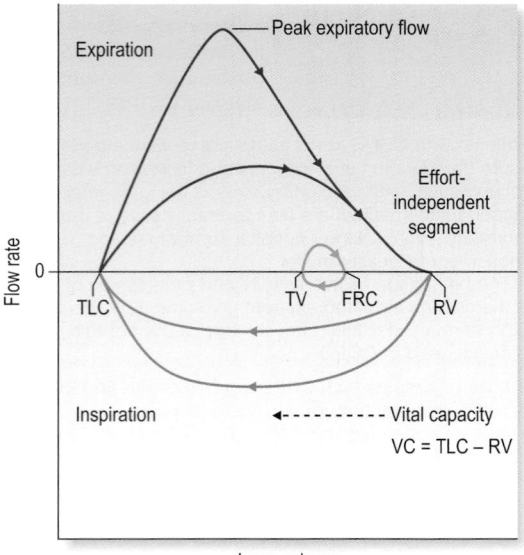

Fig. 13.18 Normal flow–volume loop for increasing inspirations. Both meet in a common effort-independent segment. A normal tidal volume (TV) breath is shown. TLC, total lung capacity; FRC, functional respiratory capacity; RV, residual volume.

resting oxygen consumption, but with maximal hyperventilation, the work of breathing is at about 30% of the resting oxygen consumption. The work of breathing increases disproportionately with increasing airflow because:

- As the speed of airflow increases, the air moves in whirls in the airway, rather than in parallel with the walls of the airway, creating 'turbulent flow' (see below)
- The resistance to airflow increases with turbulent flow, requiring the driving pressure for moving the air along to increase by the power of 2, thus increasing the work involved.

The work of breathing can also become much greater when the elastic properties of the lung/chest wall or airway resistance to airflow increases. The elastic load will increase with lung 'stiffness', as in pulmonary interstitial fibrosis, while the flow resistance will be increased with obstructive lung diseases. If the workload becomes too great, respiratory fatigue will develop. When respiratory fatigue develops, the muscles of respiration cannot ventilate the lungs sufficiently to satisfy oxygen requirements. Under these circumstances, patients often require mechanical ventilation unless pharmacological measures can rapidly and dramatically reduce their work of breathing.

Airway resistance

Airway resistance is the result of frictional forces opposing the flow of air. Under normal conditions, air flowing through the conducting airways is streamlined, known as **laminar flow**. There is very little resistance to laminar airflow. Air at the centre of the tube moves faster than air near the walls of the tube. This is analogous to blood flow (see also Ch. 11).

Where the airways branch or become narrower, or when ventilation increases, the air flows in eddies and whirls rather than parallel to the walls of the tubes. The smooth laminar flow changes to **turbulent flow** and airway resistance is

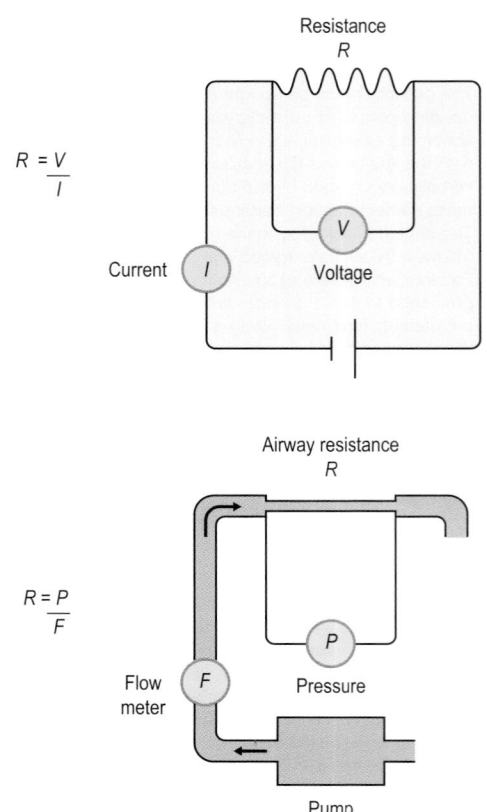

Fig. 13.19 Analogy between electrical and airway resistance.

increased. Turbulent flow is also noisy, as demonstrated by an exhausted athlete at the end of a competition.

Airflow can be modelled in a way that is analogous to the flow of electricity, which can be described by Ohm's law where $R = V/I$ (V = voltage, I = current and R = resistance). In this model $R = P/F$ where resistance to flow (R) is equal to pressure (P) divided by flow (F) (Fig. 13.19).

Airway resistance must be overcome for air to flow. It is analogous to electrical resistance to the flow of electrical current. Greatest resistance is found close to the walls of the airways and least in the centre of the airways. The resistance for laminar airflow (without turbulence) is described by **Poiseuille's equation**:

$$\text{Resistance} = \frac{8 \times \text{length} \times \text{viscosity of gas}}{\pi \times (\text{radius})^4}$$

This equation indicates that resistance increases dramatically as the airways narrow, although in practice, most of the resistance to airflow in lungs is offered by the large airways, trachea and bronchi of more than 2 mm diameter (80–90%) rather than by the smaller airways. This is counter-intuitive because, usually, the narrower the tube the greater the resistance. However, the resistance arises because there are many more smaller airways in parallel so the effective cross-sectional area is much larger at lower points in the tracheobronchial tree (see Fig. 13.5). In the trachea, which has a diameter of about 20 mm, the cross-sectional area is 3 cm². At generation 23 of the airways, which are 0.4 mm in diameter, the cross-sectional area is much greater at 4×10^5 cm² because there are so many of them (3×10^8). If this was not the case it would be virtually impossible to ventilate the alveoli.

Airway resistance can be increased by **bronchospasm** (constriction) in smaller, muscular airways, as in asthma, or by airway narrowing with **increased mucus production**, as in COPD. Airway resistance can also be increased by pressure due to:

■ Structures outside the conducting airways, such as tumours, mediastinal masses or hilar lymph nodes
■ Laryngeal spasm
■ Blockage of the airways with gastric contents or blood
■ The tongue falling backwards due to relaxation of the genioglossus muscle during anaesthesia
■ Aspirated objects, such as peanuts and pretzels.

Asthma

In asthma the airways are obstructed, increasing resistance and reducing airflow. This obstruction has a number of causes including:

■ Constriction of airway smooth muscle, in response to a wide range of stimuli which is usually reversible with bronchodilators
■ Inflammation of the bronchi that causes oedema and mucus plugging. Eosinophils and lymphocytes infiltrate the airways and the epithelium is damaged.

These factors cause pathophysiological changes that lead to airway obstruction and non-uniform ventilation. The triad of **bronchoconstriction**, **inflammation** and **secretion** is useful to bear in mind when considering the principles for appropriate treatment.

Bronchoconstriction

Typically, all asthma patients with active disease have hyper-responsive (hyper-reactive) airways. Bronchomotor tone is mainly under control of the parasympathetic system. The constriction is mediated by efferents from the vagus to ganglia in the walls of the small bronchi, from which short postganglionic fibres lead to nerve endings which release acetylcholine to act on muscarinic receptors in the bronchial smooth muscle, causing bronchoconstriction. Many different triggers can cause bronchospasm. Stimulants include:

■ Noxious substances such as cigarette smoke, atmospheric pollution, some occupational sensitizers and chemicals, particles (including nebulised water), cold air and exercise
■ Histamine, released from mast cells, which affects the parasympathetic system and has a direct action on airway smooth muscle
■ Non-adrenergic non-cholinergic fibres that pass to bronchial smooth muscle can also cause constriction by releasing vasoactive intestinal polypeptide.
■ Some classes of drugs, such as non-steroidal anti-inflammatory drugs (notably aspirin) and β-adrenoceptor blocking drugs.

Inflammation and secretion

Many **inflammatory mediators** are found in the airway secretions of patients with asthma, causing mucus secretion, bronchoconstriction and gaps in the capillary endothelium. Leakage of protein into the interstitium leads to submucosal oedema, which narrows the lumen, increasing airway resistance, and contributes to bronchial hyper-responsiveness. Inflammatory mediators are released from mast cells, neutrophils and eosinophils.

Clinical box 13.16	Conditions leading to loss of lung tissue

Atelectasis is a failure of the lungs to expand. This is most commonly caused, whether acutely by foreign bodies or chronically by tumours, when complete obstruction of the airways prevents air inflating the alveoli. Air in this distal region is absorbed and the alveoli collapse. Secretions then accumulate and may become infected. If the lung remains collapsed, irreversible fibrosis occurs. Atelectasis may also be caused when compression, for example due to pleural effusion or pneumothorax, opposes inflation.

Bronchiectasis is the condition of permanently dilated bronchi with chronic infection. It is most commonly caused by severe respiratory infection (often in childhood) leading to permanently dilated bronchi, although it can also be caused by congenital abnormalities of the cilia which reduce the removal of mucus from the lungs.

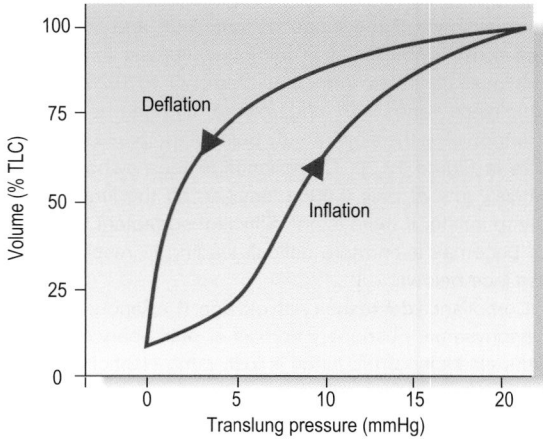

Fig. 13.20 **Pressure–volume relationship in the lung.**

Mast cells are activated by the attachment of the Fc portion of immunoglobulin IgE and other complement fractions. This leads to a rise in intracellular calcium ions as calcium channels open, and the release of range of mediators, primarily **histamine**, that is stored within granules inside the mast cells. Activation of mast cells will also lead to synthesis of arachidonic acid derivatives such as the leukotriene C4 that cause a slow but sustained contraction of bronchial smooth muscle (see Ch. 6).

Lung inflation and deflation

The force required for inflation and deflation of the lung depends on the stiffness of the lung, the compliance and the effect of liquid on the surface of the alveoli which produces surface tension.

Pressure–volume relationship

During inflation and deflation the pressure around the lung changes with lung volume (Fig. 13.20). During inspiration, there is only a small volume change until a pressure of more than 5–6 mmHg is reached. Subsequent expansion is non-linear until complete expansion is reached at about 15 mmHg. During deflation, the curve is displaced to the left, so that the pressure at any volume is less on expiration than inspiration. This phenomenon, known as **hysteresis**, is attributed to the presence of surface tension at the interface of air and fluid lining the alveolar walls and the effect of surfactant.

Compliance

Compliance is a measure of how easily the lungs can be distended. The elastic properties of the lungs tend to pull them away from the thoracic walls, giving rise to a negative intrapleural pressure (Fig. 13.21). The strength of this elastic force is related to lung volume, so that more inflated lungs that are more stretched give rise to more negative intrapleural pressure. Lung **compliance** is the measure of the relationship between the inflating pressure and lung volume.

Compliance is defined as the ratio of the change in volume to the change in intrapleural pressure, i.e.:

$$\text{Compliance} = \frac{\Delta V}{\Delta P}$$

The changes in lung volume are measure by spirometry. The change in inflating pressure is the difference between atmospheric pressure and intrapleural pressure, measured by an oesophageal balloon. The compliance of the lungs is therefore lower if the lungs become stiff and less elastic, because ΔV is smaller, as in pulmonary fibrosis. In the healthy adult male it varies from 0.09 L/cmH$_2$O to 0.26 L/cmH$_2$O. Compliance varies with lung volume, and can be estimated by determining the slope at any point of the pressure–volume curve in Figure 13.20. Compliance in the newborn child is relatively low at only 0.005 L/cmH$_2$O, so the lungs are not easy to inflate. If there is not sufficient surfactant, then inflation becomes even more difficult leading to respiratory distress (see below).

Compliance decreases with old age. It is seriously reduced in emphysema, pulmonary fibrosis or pulmonary congestion as the elasticity of the lungs is lost. Lung elasticity can also be lost if the pleurae stiffen, for example in chronic emphysema because of the fibrous covering of the pleurae, in chest deformity (kyphoscoliosis) or if the skin tightens around the chest because of scars, for example from severe burns. A sustained external pressure is also sufficient to prevent expansion of the lungs, such as crushing in crowds or when buried under rubble or snow.

Surface tension

Alveoli are nearly spherical structures, rather like tiny, interconnecting bubbles. The alveolar surfaces are covered with a thin film of fluid, and surface tension at the air–water interface produces forces that act to reduce the area of the interface. For example, in a soap bubble blown at the end of a tube, the surface contracts as much as it can, forming a sphere and thus minimising the surface area for a given volume. This surface tension generates a pressure inside the bubble that can be predicted using **Laplace's equation**:

$$P = 2 \times \text{surface tension/radius}$$

The surface tension in the alveolus is inversely proportional to its radius. At a constant surface tension, smaller alveoli would generate a greater pressure and might be expected to collapse into larger alveoli. Surfactant, however, differentially reduces surface tension more at lower volumes than higher volumes, stabilising the alveoli and preventing collapse.

Experiments on foam generated from fluid extracted from alveoli show it to exert a very low surface tension. Surfactant reduces the surface tension of the thin liquid film covering the whole alveolar surface, where gaseous exchange takes place. This makes the lungs easier to inflate during inspiration, thus increasing compliance and reducing the effort needed for expansion.

Flow-related airway collapse

Air may be trapped behind a collapsed conducting airway during **expiration**. Airways beyond generation 11 in the tracheobronchial tree have no cartilage and hence no structural rigidity and rely on the elastic recoil of the surrounding tissue to prevent collapse.

When making a forced, rapid expiration, intrathoracic pressure must be raised well above atmospheric to generate the required flow rate. As air flows from the alveoli to the mouth, the pressure in the airway will drop due to airway resistance. Thus, at some point along the airway the forces maintaining airway patency matches the intrathoracic pressure, and the pressure across the airway wall (the transmural pressure) is zero (Fig. 13.21). Further downstream, i.e. towards the mouth in expiration, the transmural pressure gradient is reversed and the airway collapses. This collapse is temporary, because the occlusion of the airway will increase the pressure behind it (i.e. upstream), raising the intra-airway pressure to open the airway again and restore airflow. This flow-related collapse during a forced expiration accounts for the brassy sound which is occasionally heard. A similar mechanism narrows large airways during coughing to increase the velocity and the scouring action by the rapidly moving exhaled air on the airway walls.

The 'collapse point' moves backwards (upstream), towards the smaller airways as the elastic recoil of the lungs is reduced with decreasing lung volume. Flow-related collapse in small air passages is common in certain diseases where there is loss of recoil pressure, particularly asthma and emphysema. Airway collapse over time can lead to hyperinflation of the chest because inhaled air is not as fully expired and is thus trapped within the lungs.

Closing capacity and posture

In the upright posture, the airways in the dependent, lowest, parts of the lungs are compressed and narrowed by the weight of the overlying tissues. In these regions, expiration will reduce the volume of air in an airway to a point where the airway closes. The lung volume at which this occurs is known as the **closing capacity**. In young adults, the closing capacity is less than FRC, but it becomes equal to FRC at an approximate age of 44 years in the supine posture and at 66 years in the upright posture. When the closing capacity exceeds the FRC, it begins to compromise gaseous exchange.

PRINCIPLES OF GAS EXCHANGE

DIFFUSION

The movement of gases, principally oxygen and carbon dioxide, across the alveolar–capillary barrier takes place by simple diffusion. The rate of diffusion is related to the concentration gradient of the gases in solution on either side of the blood/gas membrane. The gases flow down a gradient, from a higher to a lower concentration. The fundamental law governing this situation is **Fick's equation**.

$$\text{Rate of diffusion } \frac{dn}{dt} = D \times A \times \frac{dc}{dx}$$

where dn/dt is the rate of linear diffusion (quantity n, time t), D is the diffusion coefficient (cm^2/s), A is the surface area,

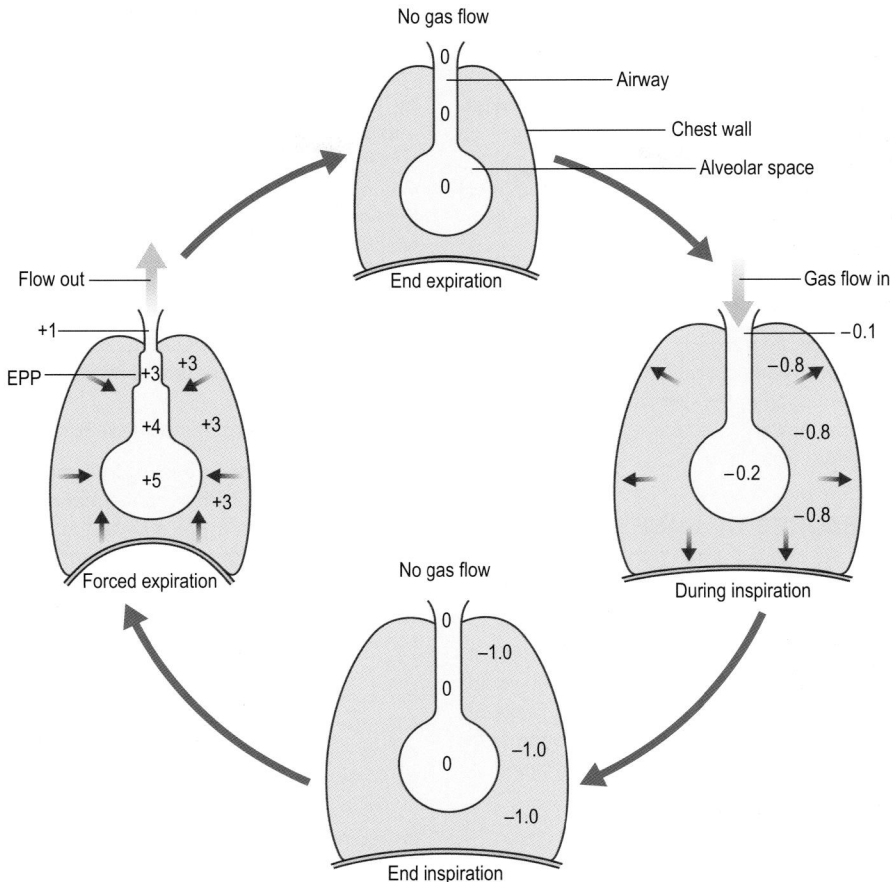

Fig. 13.21 **Pressure changes in the chest and lung during inspiration and forced expiration.** The pleural pressure around the airways is usually negative (less than atmospheric). During inspiration the chest wall expands and there is a greater negative pleural pressure, drawing air into the airways. At forced expiration, the pleural pressure may become positive, forcing air out. The equal pressure point (EPP) is where airway pressure equals pleural pressure.

dc is the difference in gas partial pressures and dx is the thickness.

The diffusion coefficient, or diffusion constant (D), is defined as the volume of gas (in mL) which diffuses through 1 cm^2/min under a pressure of 1 mmHg. This is related to the size and shape of the gas molecules, so that D is proportional to the gas solubility (S) but inversely proportional to the square root of the molecular weight of the gas (MW), i.e.:

$$D(\propto)S/\sqrt{MW}$$

The efficiency of pulmonary diffusion will also depend on the thickness of the alveolar–capillary membrane barrier (dx), which is only about 0.5 μm and may be as little as 0.2 μm in places. It comprises the alveolar epithelium (~0.2 μm), a very thin tissue space with a common basement membrane and the capillary endothelium (~0.2 μm) (see Fig. 13.7B). Once across this barrier, oxygen needs to enter a red blood cell. The red blood cells are similar in size to pulmonary capillaries, have to deform to squeeze through and so are in intimate contact with the capillary endothelium.

Pulmonary diffusion capacity

Pulmonary diffusion capacity is the ability of the lungs to transfer a gas, usually oxygen (O_2), or carbon dioxide (CO_2), across the alveolar–capillary membrane. The diffusing capacity for both oxygen (D_LO_2) and carbon dioxide (D_LCO_2) is difficult to measure, and therefore not often used clinically. The **single breath carbon monoxide (CO) diffusion test** is the more usual test of pulmonary diffusion capacity. Interpretation of D_LCO needs to be in the context of other clinical and physiological findings.

Values for oxygen diffusion capacity at rest vary between 15 mL/min/mmHg and 35 mL/min/mmHg. The average is about 20 mL/min/mmHg. Diffusion capacity is increased in exercise, to values of 65 mL/min/mmHg or more, presumably due to dilatation of the capillaries and opening up of the closed capillary bed in the lung apex. In disease, diffusion capacity is reduced. Thickening of the alveolar–capillary interface can occur in scleroderma, asbestosis, pulmonary fibrosis, pulmonary oedema and sarcoidosis. Reduction of the area of the alveolar–capillary interface may occur through emphysema or surgery.

Measuring lung diffusion capacity – single breath CO testing (D_LCO)

CO is used in testing pulmonary diffusion capacity. It is a non-reactive gas which binds to haemoglobin with such a high affinity that virtually all of the CO will reach the alveolar space. A single breath from a volume of gas containing a known small quantity of carbon monoxide is inspired. The breath is held for 10 seconds, then rapidly and forcibly expired (as in measuring FVC). The expired gas is analysed to determine the amount of CO that was absorbed during the breath, from which the CO diffusing capacity (D_LCO) is calculated. Major types of lung disease causing decreased D_LCO include:

- Destruction of the lung parenchyma with a reduction in the surface area of the alveolar–capillary interface resulting in a reduction in gas transfer (particularly emphysema and possibly cystic fibrosis)
- Interstitial lung disease with thickening of the alveolar–capillary membrane causing a reduction in gas transfer, e.g. fibrosing alveolitis, asbestosis
- Pulmonary vascular disease particularly with vascular occlusion and a reduction in the pressure gradient across the alveolar–capillary interface, e.g. pulmonary embolism, pulmonary hypertension.

PARTIAL PRESSURES OF GASES IN AIR

Air is a mixture of oxygen (20.93%), carbon dioxide (0.03%), argon (0.93%), nitrogen (78.09%) and a number of other trace gases, but for all practical purposes, air can be thought to consist of 21% oxygen and 79% nitrogen (Table 13.3). If this mixture was enclosed in a sealed container, then it would exert a pressure as the molecules collided into the walls of the container. The total pressure exerted would be the sum of the separate pressures exerted by each of the gases. A

Clinical box 13.17 — Measuring oxygen diffusing capacity (D_LO_2)

The effectiveness of oxygen transfer in the lungs depends on D_LO_2. This is measured as the amount of O_2 taken up by pulmonary capillary blood from the alveoli per minute, per unit of average O_2 pressure gradient between alveolar gas and pulmonary capillary blood. Quantification of the diffusing capacity of the lung for oxygen can be achieved by dividing the rate of oxygen transfer by the pressure gradient across the alveolar–capillary interface ($p_A - p_C$).

The amount of O_2 transferred from alveoli to pulmonary capillaries per minute

$$p_A - p_C$$

Obviously, the rate of transfer is equal to the oxygen consumption, which is easy to measure. The mean alveolar pO_2 (p_AO_2) is also relatively easy to measure using spirometry. The difficulty lies in measuring capillary pO_2 (p_CO_2) as direct measurements are not possible. Nor can arterial pO_2 be used as an approximation because it contains deoxygenated blood from the bronchial circulation, anterior cardiac and Thebesian veins that empty into the left side of the heart (the so-called physiological right-to-left shunt). Thus, there are uncertainties with estimates of capillary pO_2. Similar calculations using CO_2 can measure D_LCO_2.

partial pressure is therefore the pressure one of these gases would exert if it occupied the same total volume alone. If the container was not pressurised, then the total pressure exerted by the gas mixture inside the container would equal the outside barometric pressure.

The concept of partial pressures also applies to liquids. Gas molecules will enter a liquid until the partial pressure in the liquid matches that in the surrounding air. The speed at which equilibrium is achieved depends on solubility and chemical binding. Gas volumes are typically stated to be dry or moist, and at:

- **STP**: standard temperature (20 °C) and pressure
- **BTP**: body temperature, normally taken as 37 °C, and partial pressure
- **ATP**: atmospheric temperature and pressure.

The **partial pressure of a dry gas** can be calculated by multiplying its fractional concentration by the barometric pressure. Barometric pressure is the atmospheric pressure exerted by the weight of a column of air on the surface of a unit area at sea level, which is around 760 mmHg. For example, in air, oxygen has a concentration of 21% (a fractional concentration of 0.21). Its partial pressure at a barometric pressure of 760 mmHg is 0.21×760 or 160 mmHg. If the barometer pressure was to fall from 760 mmHg to 400 mmHg while ascending to an altitude of 4800 m (16 000 ft), the partial pressure of oxygen would fall proportionally to 84 mmHg.

When liquids vaporise they also contribute to the total pressure. But the vapours of liquids, for example water, exert partial pressures at different temperatures. **Water vapour** complicates the situation as its pressure is independent of barometric pressure, but dependent on temperature. So the partial pressure of gaseous components of humidified air must be reduced so that the total will equal barometric pressure *less* water vapour pressure.

The vapour pressure of fully saturated air at 37 °C is 47 mmHg. In moist air at normal body temperature, oxygen has a partial pressure of $0.21 \times (760 - 47)$ or about 150 mmHg. Expired air is normally fully saturated with water at 37 °C. Inspired air may not be fully saturated and the pressure it exerts will be less than at full saturation. The saturation of inhaled air depends on humidity, which is in turn dependent on climatic conditions. Expired air also contains more carbon dioxide and less oxygen, the levels of which depend on alveolar ventilation.

PARTIAL PRESSURES OF GASES IN ALVEOLI AND BLOOD

In human respiration, the partial pressures of O_2 and CO_2 are of particular importance. Partial pressures in alveoli (p_A), know as **alveolar tension**, would obviously affect the

Table 13.3 Partial pressures of the various constituents of air under various conditions

	Dry gas (%)	Partial pressure of dry gas, at sea level (mmHg)	Partial pressure of dry gas, at 4800 m (16 000 ft) (mmHg)	Partial pressure at sea level (mmHg), moist air at 37 °C	Partial pressure of at 4800 m (16 000 ft) (mmHg) moist air at 37 °C
Oxygen	21	160	84	150	74
Carbon dioxide	0	0	0	0	0
Nitrogen	79	600	316	563	279
Water vapour	0	0	0	47	47
Total	100	760	400	760	400

efficiency of gaseous exchange. There is a reciprocal relationship between p_AO_2 and p_ACO_2 so that CO_2 retention in the alveoli reduces p_AO_2 and less O_2 enters the blood. Arterial p_aO_2 is reduced, which in turn affects the oxygen-carrying capacity of the blood (see below). Normally, the alveolar–arterial oxygen difference ($p_{A-a}O_2$) is small, but increases with disease. Clinically, this can be influenced by the administration of O_2 or administering air under pressure (i.e. effectively increasing the barometric pressure).

CARRIAGE OF OXYGEN BY THE BLOOD

One of the functions of the circulation is to deliver O_2 to the tissues to sustain metabolism, and tissue demand for O_2 will vary according to consumption. For example, O_2 consumption will increase many times during exercise. Large amounts of gaseous O_2 would have to be carried around the body, which has evolved an ingenious way for doing this efficiently, while minimising the effort needed by the heart. O_2 can be carried by blood in two ways:

- Dissolved in the plasma
- Combined with haemoglobin in the red blood cells.

The amount of O_2 dissolved in the plasma is quite small (0.3 mL per 100 mL of arterial blood and 0.13 mL per 100 mL of venous blood). So most oxygen is transported and stored by oxygenated **respiratory pigments**. Almost all of the O_2 is carried by **haemoglobin** in red blood cells, or combined with **myoglobin** in muscle. These two molecules have different functions. Haemoglobin is the main transporter of oxygen to all tissues, whereas myoglobin carries the oxygen reserve for tissues that have variable demand for oxygen (see Ch. 11).

RESPIRATORY PIGMENTS

Haemoglobin and myoglobin both consist of protein chains, the **globin** portion, and a haem group which contains ferrous **iron**. The O_2 molecule combines with an iron molecule in the **haem** part of haemoglobin and myoglobin. Haemoglobin (Hb) and myoglobin (Mb) are structurally different, so that they can fulfil their different functions. Haemoglobin is made up of four subunits each containing one globin chain and one haem group; myoglobin consists of single globin and haem molecules. Haemoglobin therefore has the capacity to carry four molecules of O_2 whereas myoglobin can only carry one molecule of O_2. The presence of haemoglobin greatly increases the O_2-carrying capacity of the blood (see Ch. 12).

Oxygen dissociation curve

A distinction should be made between the O_2 content of the blood and O_2 saturation:

- O_2 **content** refers to the amount of O_2 carried by 1 L of blood
- O_2 **saturation** (S) is the percentage of O_2-carrying sites on the haemoglobin molecule occupied by O_2

Under normal physiological conditions, arterial O_2 saturation, S_aO_2, would be around 100%. The amount of oxygen that is

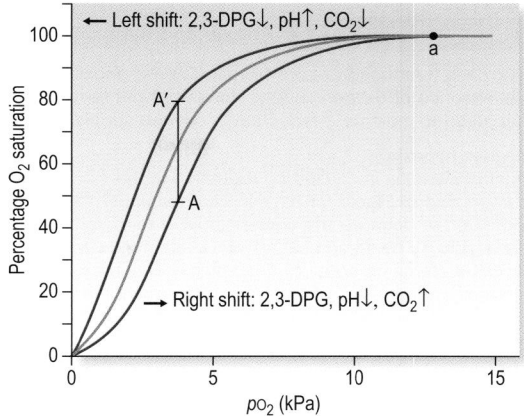

Fig. 13.22 Oxygen saturation curve, with the Bohr effect and effect of 2,3-diphosphoglycerate (2,3-DPG). In the tissues, where there is increased 2,3-DPG (a product of energy metabolism), CO_2 and [H⁺] (i.e. pH is lower), the shift of the curve means that less O_2 can be carried by haemoglobin at the same pO_2 (A′ to A) and so O_2 is released to the tissues.

available for haemoglobin to take up to the point where it is fully saturated depends on the partial pressure of oxygen, pO_2. This relationship is described by the O_2 dissociation curve, which has a sigmoidal or S shape (Fig. 13.22). This relationship ensures that small reductions in p_aO_2 will not affect the O_2 content of the blood. Both haemoglobin and myoglobin saturates with O_2 below the p_AO_2 normally found in alveoli.

Haemoglobin

As discussed above, haemoglobin consists of four subunits of haem and globin. The alteration in the structure in one subunit by binding with O_2 alters the structure of the other subunits, changing their affinity for haemoglobin. Full saturation is not reached until the alveolar p_AO_2 exceeds 100 mmHg. This greatly increases the efficiency of haemoglobin as the main O_2 transporter in the blood. O_2 uptake by haemoglobin is extremely rapid, and O_2 off-loading to tissues is even faster. A number of factors can favour unloading of O_2 from haemoglobin including:

- Hydrogen ions
- Temperature
- 2,3-Diphosphoglycerate (2,3-DPG).

Hydrogen ions (H⁺) reduce haemoglobin affinity for O_2 by altering the haemoglobin structure so that it binds less easily with O_2. This is known as the **Bohr effect**. When tissue pH is reduced (i.e. a rise in H⁺), as for example with the accumulation of lactic acid in exercising muscle or the accumulation of CO_2 from metabolic processes in solution, O_2 dissociates more rapidly from haemoglobin so that the O_2 is unloaded to the tissues needing it (Fig. 13.22). Heat also reduces haemoglobin affinity for O_2. Working tissues generate heat so that more O_2 is given up to it at any pO_2. The haemoglobin affinity for O_2 is reduced by increasing the concentration of 2,3-DPG in the red cells, thus releasing O_2 more easily. 2,3-DPG is produced in response to hypoxia, as in anaemia and high altitude. 2,3-DPG is low in transfused blood.

Information box 13.4　Anoxia and hypoxia

Hypoxia is a reduced level of oxygen supply; anoxia is a total absence of oxygen supply. However, both terms are often used to indicate a reduction in oxygen supply.

Anaemic hypoxia

Anaemic hypoxia is caused by reduction in the haemoglobin available for oxygen carriage either through blood loss or because the haemoglobin is rendered unavailable by being combined with a substance with which it forms a stable compound. Examples of the latter are chlorates and nitrates, which convert haemoglobin to methaemoglobin, or carbon monoxide, which forms carboxyhaemoglobin.

Stagnant anoxia

Stagnant anoxia arises due to slowing of the circulation. This may occur locally due to cold-induced vasoconstriction or obstruction to the venous outflow, or because of cardiac failure.

In stagnant anoxia, arterial oxygen saturation is normal but circulation is slowed and blood dwells too long in the capillaries. Thus the arteriovenous oxygen difference ($p_{a-v}O_2$) is increased and much of the oxygen is delivered at a reduced tension.

Clinical box 13.18　Cyanosis

Cyanosis is the bluish discoloration that occurs because of high levels of deoxygenated haemoglobin.

- Central cyanosis occurs when there is more than 50 g/L of deoxyhaemoglobin present. It is seen in the buccal mucosa, lips and tongue and may indicate hypoxia.
- Peripheral cyanosis is seen in the fingers and earlobes and may indicate reduced blood flow.

In anaemia when haemoglobin levels are low, cyanosis may not be apparent even if the patient is hypoxic.

Myoglobin

Myoglobin is found in muscles, particularly those involved in slow repetitive contractions, e.g. leg muscles or heart muscle of large mammals. Myoglobin has a single protein chain, contains one iron per molecule and its oxygen dissociation curve is a simple rectangular hyperbola. It can easily take up oxygen from haemoglobin at low oxygen pressures and is 95% saturated at a pO_2 of 40 mmHg. It will rapidly release oxygen under hypoxic conditions. Myoglobin acts as an oxygen reserve when the oxygen demands of muscles increase as muscular contraction increases the muscles' cross-sectional area, thus compressing local blood vessels and sharply reducing the flow of blood to the muscle.

CARRIAGE OF CARBON DIOXIDE BY THE BLOOD

CO_2 is the end-product of tissue metabolism, and has to be transported from the tissues to the lungs. CO_2 also has a role in the maintenance of normal acid–base balance, so that disturbance of CO_2 concentrations is the basis for respiratory acidosis or alkalosis (see below and Ch. 1). It diffuses across cell membranes more easily than O_2, and can be carried in the blood in three ways:

 Information box 13.5　Key points in the formation of bicarbonate (HCO_3^-)

- The speed of this reaction is sufficiently fast for the rapid uptake of CO_2 when blood traverses the tissue capillaries. The concentration of bicarbonate in the red blood cells exceeds that of the plasma, so that most of it will pass back into the plasma. Plasma carries about two-thirds and the red cells one-third of the bicarbonate.
- The formation of bicarbonate increases the osmotic gradient into the red cells so that the cells increase in size by taking up water. This increases the packed cell volume (**haematocrit**) of the blood by 3%.
- The hydrogen ions (H^+) are 'mopped up' by the histidine residues of the α and β amino acid chains of haemoglobin (see Ch. 12). Haemoglobin therefore has a central role in transporting both O_2 and CO_2, by virtue of its ability to bind with both O_2 and H^+.
- Electrical neutrality is maintained by the movement of negatively charged chloride ions into the red cells (Na^+ and K^+ cannot easily pass through the red cell membrane). This so-called **chloride shift** means that venous blood contains about 2% less chloride than arterial plasma.
- The whole process is reversed in the lungs, with chloride leaving the red cells; bicarbonate enters to be converted by carbonic anhydrase to CO_2 and then diffuses into the alveolar air.

- In solution in red cells and plasma
- Combined with the protein subunits of haemoglobin and with other plasma proteins
- As sodium bicarbonate in the plasma.

About 3 mL of CO_2 per 100 mL of blood is dissolved in the blood at a pCO_2 of 40 mmHg. A further 0.1–0.2 mL CO_2 per 100 mL blood will be in the form of carbonic acid, which is formed when CO_2 is dissolved in water:

$$CO_2 + H_2O \rightleftharpoons H_2CO_3$$

Carbon dioxide can form neutral carbamino compounds with the amino acid subunits of haemoglobin and to a lesser extent with other plasma proteins. Carbon dioxide reacts with the amine (NH_2) groups of the protein. When deoxygenated, blood carries about 4 mL of CO_2 as carbamino per 100 mL of blood. The remaining carbon dioxide (45 mL per 100 mL deoxygenated blood) is carried in the blood as hydrogen and bicarbonate ions (HCO_3^-). These are formed rapidly within the red blood cells by the enzyme **carbonic anhydrase** (CA), which catalyses the rapid formation of carbonic acid. Carbonic acid then dissociates into H^+ and HCO_3^-:

$$CO_2 + H_2O \rightleftharpoons H_2CO_3 \rightleftharpoons H^+ + HCO_3^-$$

Carbonic anhydrase is a zinc-containing enzyme that can be inhibited by cyanide and the enzyme acetazolamide. Much use has been made of acetazolamide in experimental investigations into the role of carbonic anhydrase in other organs – gastric mucosa, pancreas and renal tubular cells – but it also acts as diuretic and is used in treatment of raised intraocular pressure (glaucoma) and altitude sickness.

CARBON DIOXIDE DISSOCIATION CURVE

At a given pCO_2, the degree of oxygen saturation will influence the CO_2-carrying capacity of the blood. In the lungs, as haemoglobin becomes fully saturated, CO_2 is displaced and

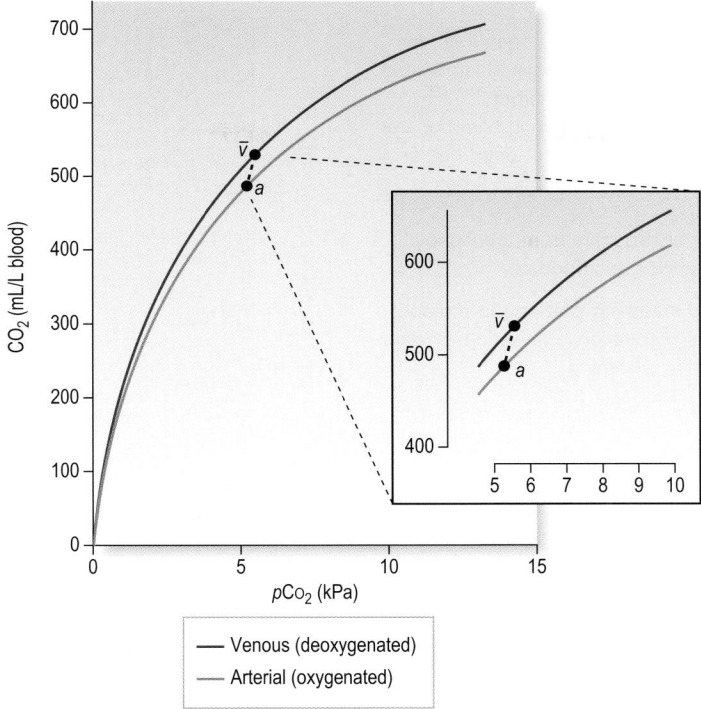

Fig. 13.23 **The carbon dioxide dissociation curve.** The ability of deoxygenated blood to carry more CO_2 than oxygenated blood is called Haldane's effect. The enlarged part of the curve shows how this effect 'steepens' the true physiological curve and enables deoxygenated blood in the tissues to pick up in excess of 50 mL more CO_2 per litre than it would if it remained oxygenated.

therefore excreted, whereas in the tissues, the off-loading of O_2 from haemoglobin enables it to increase its affinity for CO_2 (Fig. 13.23).

Haemoglobin reacts more readily with CO_2 to form carbamino compounds as it off-loads O_2, increasing the CO_2-carrying capacity of blood. The opposite occurs as haemoglobin becomes oxygenated, with a decrease in CO_2-carrying capacity. This is known as **Haldane's effect**, and mirrors the Bohr effect for O_2. The overall relationship between carbon dioxide content and pCO_2 is curvilinear, but over the physiological range, i.e. between the extremes of arterial and venous blood (40 mmHg and 46 mmHg, respectively) it is essentially linear. The relationship is quite steep: approximately 0.7 mL CO_2 per 100 mL blood is unloaded for 1 mmHg drop in pCO_2. This ability to load or unload CO_2 with minimal change in pCO_2 helps to minimise the change in pH between arterial and venous blood.

DISTURBANCES OF ACID–BASE BALANCE

The physiology of renal and metabolic acid–base control is discussed elsewhere (Ch. 1) but it is intimately linked to respiratory acid–base control. Respiration is in part under regulation by the hydrogen ion concentration of the cerebral spinal fluid in the brain (c.f. control of breathing below). This feedback system will cause hyperventilation to lower plasma pH or hypoventilation to increase plasma pH. Thus, in patients with metabolic disorders, ventilation can be used to quickly compensate for disturbances in acid–base balance. Conversely, chronic respiratory disease will lead to disturbance in the balance that can only be slowly compensated for by excretion or retention of hydrogen ions in the urine,

although most hydrogen ions are buffered in the urine by bicarbonate or phosphate, or converted to ammonia.

Hydrogen ion concentrations ([H^+]) in the blood are normally very low at about 40 nmoles/L, i.e. 10^{-7} L, expressed by the term **pH**, which is the log 1/[H^+]. Water has a pH of 7 and is regarded as neutral. An increase in the hydrogen ion concentration in the blood, and thus lowering the pH to below 7, is described as **acidaemia** or **acidosis**, while a reduction (rise in pH) is described as **alkalaemia** or **alkalosis**. There are four classes of acid–base disorder depending on whether it causes acidaemia or alkalaemia, and whether the problem is caused by the respiratory system or a metabolic problem.

The four classes of acid–base disorder

Respiratory acidosis

■ Is caused by retention of carbon dioxide: the blood p_aCO_2 rise and pH falls.
■ Is associated with impaired efficiency of gaseous exchange. Common causes include type II respiratory failure in COPD and respiratory depression from drugs or paralysis of respiratory muscles (see below).

Respiratory alkalosis

■ p_aCO_2 falls and pH rises.
■ Causes are overbreathing (hyperventilation), blowing off excessive CO_2, due to hysteria, aspirin poisoning, cerebral diseases such as viral infection (encephalitis) or head injuries.

Metabolic acidosis

- Caused by excessive production of hydrogen ions, for example in diabetic ketosis or with increased lactic acid production following shock or cardiac surgery.
- Can also occur with the loss of fluid rich in bicarbonate from the small intestines, e.g. because of diarrhoea or loss of intestinal contents through aspiration tubes or fistulae.
- Less common is loss of bicarbonate from the kidney due to a defect in reabsorbing bicarbonate.

There are characteristic breathing patterns in metabolic acidosis called Kussmaul's respiration, consisting of deep sighing, with rapid but regular breathing.

Metabolic alkalosis

- Caused by excessive intake of bicarbonate in the treatment of peptic ulceration, or by loss of acidic fluids by vomiting gastric contents.
- Respiratory compensation is often slight, and it is rare to encounter a p_aCO_2 above 6.5 kPa (50 mmHg) even with severe alkalosis.

MATCHING LUNG VENTILATION TO LUNG PERFUSION

Ventilation is the movement of air in and out of the lungs. Specifically, alveolar ventilation refers to the movement of air in and out of the alveoli. The rate at which oxygen exchange can take place at the alveolus then depends on the blood flow through the alveolar tissues, called **perfusion**. The efficiency of gas exchange thus concerns both ventilation and perfusion.

VENTILATION–PERFUSION RATIO

In the healthy resting adult about 4 L of air ventilate the alveoli (V_A) and 5 L of blood pass through the lungs (Q) each minute. Hence, the mean ventilation–perfusion ratio (V_A/Q) is 4/5 or 0.8.

Uneven perfusion

In health, efficient exchange of gases between alveolar air and the blood would occur if alveolar ventilation matched the alveolar perfusion. However, blood flow through different parts of the lungs is uneven. In the upright position, blood flow is maximal at the lung bases, decreasing linearly to the apices. There is a 7–10-fold increase in perfusion at the bases relative to the apex of the lungs. This can be explained by the differences in hydrostatic pressure within the blood vessels in different parts, or zones, in the lungs (Fig. 13.24).

Zone 1 is at the top of the lungs where blood flow is poor, because the mean pulmonary artery pressure of 11–15 mmHg is barely sufficient to propel blood the 15 cm to the lung apices in an upright individual. Should pulmonary arterial pressure (p_a) fall below alveolar pressure (p_A), the capillaries would collapse and no blood flow would be possible. In this case, despite normal alveolar ventilation, there is no perfusion and gaseous exchange cannot take place. This zone then becomes an alveolar dead space. This phenomenon

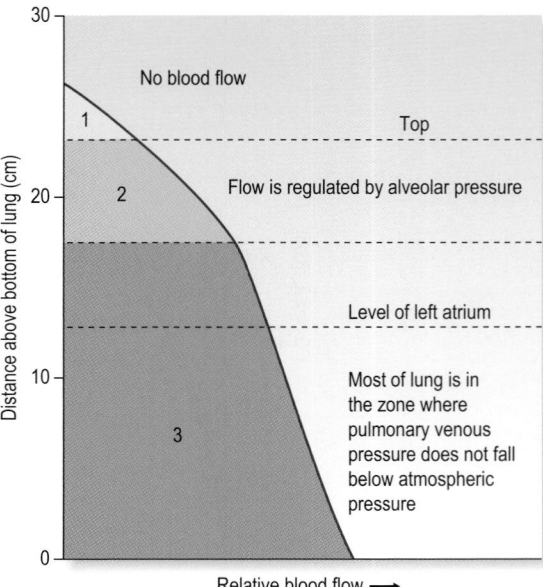

Fig. 13.24 Uneven distribution of blood flow in the lungs results in regional differences in gas exchange down the normal lung. Three zones can be identified. Zone 1 is where alveolar pressure exceeds capillary pressure and so no blood flow occurs. This will be very small and at the apices of the lung in normal healthy people. In zone 2, gas exchange will vary with the balance of alveolar pressure and capillary pressure. The latter increases in systole, forcing open more capillaries. In zone 3, the hydrostatic pressure in the column of blood above the heart is sufficient to keep the alveolar capillaries open.

occurs when pulmonary arterial pressure falls, for example due to blood loss. Perfusion is then dependent on the difference between p_a and p_A.

The effect of hydrostatic pressure increases pulmonary arterial pressure lower down in the upright lungs, in zone 2, where it exceeds alveolar pressure. Pulmonary venous pressure (p_v), however, is still below alveolar pressure. Pulmonary venous pressure only affects perfusion when it exceeds alveolar pressure, and this occurs in zone 3, the lung bases. Gravity, together with hydrostatic pressure, further raises arterial pressure, but venous pressure also rises due to gravity. Blood flow here is determined by the difference between arterial and venous pressure. The perfusion pressure is equivalent to the pulmonary artery pressure, and there is a hydrostatic pressure of about 15 cm of blood due to gravity.

Uneven ventilation

The distribution of inspired air is also not uniform, with a 1.5–3-fold greater ventilation of the base in healthy individuals. This occurs because there are regional differences in **airway resistance** and **compliance** that influence the alveolar filling time in each region. The situation is further complicated by the time constants for alveolar filling being affected by the rate, duration and frequency of inspiration. Other factors affecting ventilation involve airway closure, the right bronchus being at less of an angle to the trachea than the left, and the conformation of the chest and diaphragm.

Clinical box 13.19   Pulmonary embolism

Pulmonary embolism is a condition in which blood clots migrate into the pulmonary arterial system, blocking the circulation and preventing deoxygenated blood from passing through the ventilated parts of the lungs. These areas of lung are ventilated, but not perfused, creating a **dead space** where gaseous exchange cannot take place. Many emboli originate from deep vein thrombi in the legs or pelvis and most of these lodge in the large or intermediate pulmonary arteries. Fat emboli can be released from fractured bones and usually end up in the smaller pulmonary vessels. Once lodged in the lung, the thrombi start to lyse but massive emboli can cause rapid death.

In order to prevent pulmonary emboli in patients undergoing surgery, deep vein thromboses are avoided by rapid mobilisation after the operation, the use of elastic pressure stockings to prevent vascular stasis and the prophylactic use of anticoagulants.

Ventilation–perfusion mismatch

Ideally, the amount of ventilation (V_A) to a given area of lung should be matched with the amount of blood perfusing (Q) that area for the efficient exchange of oxygen and carbon dioxide. The ventilation–perfusion ratio is commonly used to describe their mismatch. Because of the variations in perfusion and ventilation, the V_A/Q ratio varies from 3.3 at the apex of the lungs to 0.6 in the base. The effect of V_A/Q mismatch on gaseous exchange can be minimised. Localised hypoxia in underventilated areas of the lungs causes local vasoconstriction, so that blood is diverted to better ventilated areas. The importance of V_A/Q matching is illustrated by an often quoted example of one lung being ventilated but not perfused while the other is perfused but not ventilated. If this absurd situation arose suddenly, the individual would soon die from asphyxia. Clinical conditions leading to uneven ventilation include:

- Asthma
- COPD
- Emphysema
- Pneumothorax
- Pulmonary fibrosis.

Uneven blood flow may arise from:

- Anatomical shunts (right to left): blood flow through an area of lung with no ventilation due to airway obstruction or collapse
- Regional destruction of vascular beds by emphysema
- Pulmonary embolism or tumour preventing blood flow to an area of the lung
- Increased pulmonary vascular resistance due to heart failure.

CONTROL OF BREATHING

The requirement for O_2 by the human body varies widely, being low during sleep and at rest, and rising during exercise. At the same time, CO_2 output also varies. Yet, despite these variations, the partial pressures of arterial O_2 and CO_2 are kept within narrow limits. Breathing control for effective gas exchange in the lungs to maintain a normal p_aO_2 and p_aCO_2 is regulated by the nervous system.

Receptors (sensors) collect information, which is relayed to the respiratory centres:
- Chemoreceptors:
  Central: in ventral surface of medulla
  Peripheral: in carotid bodies and aortic arch

- Lung receptors:
  Pulmonary stretch receptors
  Cough or lung irritant receptors
  J-receptors

- Other receptors:
  Nasal and upper airway receptors
  Muscle stretch receptors
  Joint proprioceptors
  Arterial baroreceptors

Afferent

Central respiratory centres control automatic breathing
Brain stem:
- Medulla: inspiratory and expiratory areas
- Pons: apneustic and pneumotaxic areas

Cortical control of voluntary breathing can override respiratory centre control

Efferent

Effectors are the respiratory muscles:
- Diaphragm (main muscle of respiration)
- Intercostal muscles
- Abdominal muscles
- Accessory muscles

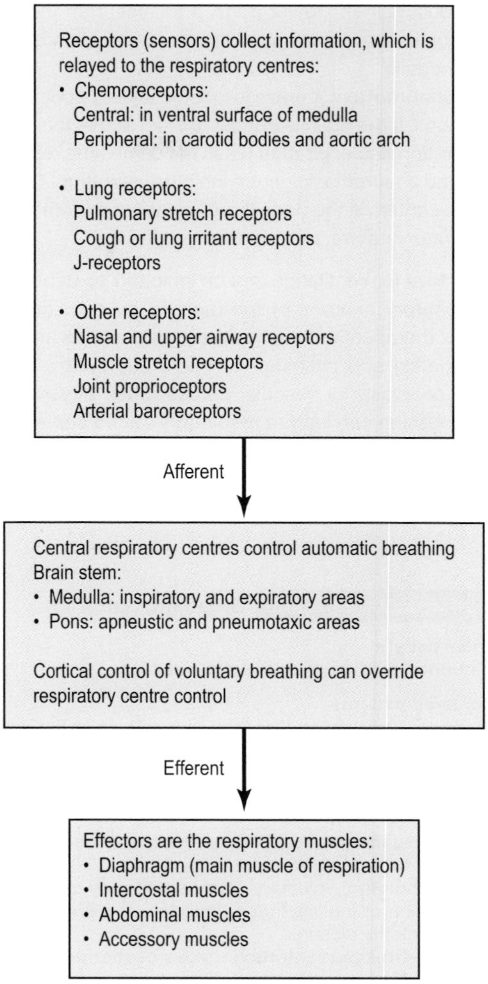

Fig. 13.25 **The component parts in the control of breathing.**

Respiration is controlled by the nervous system, and like all neural systems the process has:

- An afferent pathway, where receptors or sensors collect information to be relayed to
- A central control in the brainstem
- An efferent, or effector pathway to the muscles of respiration.

The reflex control of breathing can, however, be overridden by higher, cortical centres when voluntary respiration becomes necessary (Fig. 13.25).

THE RESPIRATORY CENTRE

The **respiratory centre** is a collection of neurons situated in the **medulla** of the brainstem which control the **pattern of breathing**. This **primary centre** consists of a collection of separately arranged neurons that are capable of altering their firing threshold so that activity oscillates between them during inspiration and expiration. The neurons responsible for inspiration are in the dorsal medulla, and those for expiration are in the ventral medulla. The **primary centre** is under the influence of two centres in the pons:

- The **apneustic centre** (apneusis = prolonged inspiration or gasping inspiration) is located at the level of the area vestibularis in the lower pons. Impulses from the apneustic centre may stimulate the inspiration areas of the medulla.

■ The **pneumotaxic centre** is located in the upper part of the pons. If the brain is transected just above this centre, inspiration and expiration takes the same time, suggesting that the pneumotaxic centre inhibits inspiration. Cells in these centres in the pons therefore affect rhythm in the respiratory centre, but are not essential.

The drive for ventilation can be inhibited by depression of the respiratory neurons of the medulla by hypoxia, a wide variety of therapeutic drugs (opiates, barbiturates and anaesthetic agents) and inhibition of blood supply (by pressure, trauma, neoplasm or vascular catastrophe). Severe respiratory depression can lead to respiratory failure and eventually death. There is a wide range of different breathing patterns that are produced under different conditions (Information box 13.6).

ⓘ Information box 13.6 ▎Breathing patterns

Normal pattern
■ **Eupnoea**: normal spontaneous breathing.

Disordered patterns
■ **Apnoea**: absence or cessation of breathing in the resting expiratory position.
■ **Apneusis**: respiration ceases in the inspiratory position, because of sustained contraction of the inspiratory muscles.
■ **Biot's respiration**: sequences of uniformly deep gasps, apnoea, then deep gasps.
■ **Breath-holding**: voluntary apnoea, either by continuous contraction of the inspiratory muscles, or relaxation against glottis closure.
■ **Cheyne–Stokes respiration**: cycles of alternating hyperventilation and apnoea. Typically, over a period of 1 minute, a 10–20 second episode of apnoea or hypopnoea is observed followed by respirations of increasing depth and frequency. The cycle then repeats itself. However, despite periods of apnoea, significant hypoxia rarely occurs.
■ **Dyspnoea**: is a sensation of discomfort during the act of breathing. It applies to both severe exercise and to the dyspnoea of respiratory failure or cardiac failure. Dyspnoea is also common during acute hypoxia at high altitude. It can be evoked by breathing high CO_2 concentrations.
■ **Hyperpnoea**: ventilation above normal level.
■ **Hyperventilation**: increase in alveolar ventilation relative to metabolic demands.
■ **Hypopnoea**: ventilation below normal level.
■ **Hypoventilation**: ventilation less than required by metabolic demands.
■ **Kussmaul's respiration**: deep, sighing regular hyperventilation.
■ **Orthopnea**: dyspnoea experienced only in the recumbent position, usually supine, and relieved by sitting or standing. It often occurs in patients with left ventricular insufficiency.
■ **Paroxysmal nocturnal dyspnoea**: orthopnea at night, due to accumulation of fluid in the lungs (pulmonary oedema) when the patient lies flat while sleeping, the patient wakening with dyspnoea.
■ **Panting**: breathing pattern both very rapid and shallow. In some conditions, this pattern is adopted to dissipate heat (thermal panting).
■ **Periodic breathing**: abnormal breathing pattern, with a series of cycles separated by pauses.
■ **Tachypnoea**: increased rate of breathing (also hyperpnoea).

RESPIRATORY RECEPTORS

The neurons in the respiratory centre also respond to many afferent impulses arising from a wide variety of respiratory receptors. These receptors control ventilation by increasing or decreasing the volume of air breathed in or out, whereas the medullary centres control the patterns of respiration.

Respiratory chemoreceptors

There are two groups of chemoreceptors:

■ Central chemoreceptors respond to changes in the pH of cerebrospinal fluid (CSF)
■ Peripheral chemoreceptors respond to changes in the O_2 and CO_2 content in the blood.

Central chemoreceptors

The central chemoreceptors lie just below the anterolateral surfaces of the medulla, close to the origins of the glossopharyngeal (IX) and vagus nerves (X), but are anatomically separate from the medullary respiratory centre. They respond to changes in the pH of the surrounding CSF. A rising pH (lowering the hydrogen ion – H^+ – concentration) inhibits ventilation, whereas lowering the pH (rising H^+ concentration) stimulates it. The composition of the CSF is determined by partly by blood flow and metabolic processes.

The **blood–brain barrier** separates the CSF from the blood. Hydrogen ions cannot pass through the blood–brain barrier, but CO_2 diffuses through it easily. CO_2 crossing the blood–brain barrier combines with water to form carbonic acid, which is then ionised to release H^+. CSF is relatively poorly buffered, so that CSF H^+ concentration is proportional to arterial p_aCO_2.

Through this mechanism, a rise in arterial p_aCO_2 (**hypercapnia**) would thus cause a rise in brain extracellular H^+ (fall in pH, acidosis), and increased ventilation. This central response to an increase in p_aCO_2 is relatively slow when compared to the response by peripheral chemoreceptors (see below). There is also considerable variation between people in the ventilatory response to CO_2. However, p_aCO_2 is the most important factor in the regulation of ventilation and 80% of the stimulus to ventilation originates in the medullary chemoreceptors.

Peripheral chemoreceptors

Peripheral chemoreceptors are located in:

■ The carotid bodies, found above or near the bifurcation of the common carotid artery on either side of the neck
■ The aortic bodies in the aortic arch.

Clinical box 13.20 ▎Sleep apnoea

Obstructive sleep apnoea occurs when airflow through the nose or mouth is obstructed. This results in a reduction in arterial oxygen and an increase in carbon dioxide which often wakes the patient up, often with a loud gasp. This repeatedly disrupts the sleep pattern and leads to problems in the daytime, with a loss of concentration and a tendency to fall asleep during the day. The patient often snores which also disrupts the sleep of partners.

It is caused by the collapse of the flexible nasopharyngeal region of the upper airway. This is partially due to a naturally narrow airway plus the effects of gravity and the muscle relaxation which occurs during sleep. Obesity, alcohol and sedating drugs make the problem worse.

The carotid and aortic bodies are surrounded by sinusoidal capillaries which allow the cells within them to be bathed directly by blood. Specialised cells called glomus cells in the small carotid bodies respond to hypoxia by releasing dopamine onto afferent nerves of the carotid sinus nerve which run to the glossopharyngeal nerve and thence to the medullary respiratory centres. Afferents from the aortic body run via the aortic nerve to the vagus.

The peripheral chemoreceptors respond rapidly, within 1–3 seconds, to falls in p_aO_2 (hypoxia) and pH, or rises in p_aCO_2 (hypercapnia), to increase ventilation. Experiments show that gas mixtures containing little O_2 will stimulate ventilation only if the nerves to these chemoreceptors are intact, suggesting that peripheral chemoreceptors respond to an O_2 deficit, whereas the central chemoreceptors do not.

The carotid bodies are extremely well perfused (2000 mL/min per 100 g tissue), although in absolute terms the blood flow through them is small (40 µL/min). Likewise, their O_2 consumption on a relative scale is high (9 mL/min per 100 g). They undergo hypertrophy during chronic hypoxia such as in COPD or during acclimatisation to high altitude.

Lung receptors

Pulmonary stretch receptors

Pulmonary stretch receptors lie close to or in the smooth muscle of the bronchi and trachea. Whether they also exist in bronchiolar smooth muscle is less clear. The receptors are localised chiefly at the points of bronchial branching, where the smooth muscle is thickest. Drugs that increase bronchial tone increase stretch receptor discharge. Stretch receptors can also be found at the lower end of the trachea and the main bronchi.

The afferent fibres from pulmonary stretch receptors run in the vagus nerve in large myelinated fibres to send impulses to the respiratory centre. Inflating the lungs stimulates these receptors. Thus, during normal breathing, vagal impulse activity from stretch receptors increases with the onset of inspiration, dying down as expiration begins. Stimulation of the stretch receptors by maximally inflating the lungs in humans inhibits inspiration, thereby limiting tidal volume, and also slows respiratory rate. This so-called **Hering–Breuer lung inflation reflex** (first described in 1868) is important in situations in which an increased depth and rate of breathing is needed, such as during exercise. Although it is thought that this reflex is inactive in adult human beings until the tidal volume exceeds 1 L, the reflex produces an increase in respiratory frequency by shortening the time for inspiration. Thus the need to increase ventilation is satisfied. There is an added benefit in that the energy expenditure involved in breathing is minimised since deep breathing requires more energy than more frequent smaller volume breaths. There is evidence to suggest that this reflex is more important in infants.

Cough or lung-irritant receptors

Cough is a common symptom in a range of respiratory diseases and can be a useful diagnostic tool. It is a sudden explosive expiratory manoeuvre that tends to clear material such as sputum from the airways. It also helps protect the lungs against aspiration. Coughing is caused by the stimulation of receptors by foreign bodies and sputum in the bronchi or trachea. Histological studies show that there are receptors throughout the airways from the trachea to the bronchioles which respond to foreign bodies in the bronchi or trachea, and reflexively cause coughing.

Myelinated afferent fibres from the cough or lung-irritant receptors run in the vagus to the respiratory centre in the central nervous system. The receptors also respond to irritants, such as sulphur dioxide, but stimulation of these receptors in the intrapulmonary bronchi and the bronchioles does not cause coughing; hence these are named **lung-irritant receptors**. Stimulation of these receptors causes hyperpnoea (deep inhalation) and reflex bronchial or laryngeal constriction. Coughing occurs when an expiratory effort against a closed glottis is suddenly released.

The nose and upper airways contain receptors that respond to chemical and mechanical stimulation in a similar way to the lung-irritant receptors. Reflex responses include sneezing, coughing and bronchoconstriction. These reflexes need to be abolished with local anaesthetics when passing an endotracheal or nasogastric tube.

Haemoptysis

Haemoptysis occurs when there is bleeding from the airways. This can vary from streaks of blood in the sputum to massive bleeding. Bleeding usually arises from the bronchial circulation rather than the pulmonary circulation, unless trauma or erosion by a granulomatous or calcified lymph node or a tumour has damaged a major pulmonary vessel. Haemoptysis is a symptom complained of by the patient, and needs to be distinguished from haematemesis (bringing up blood from the stomach). It is a serious symptom and must always be investigated.

Clinical box 13.21   CO₂ levels and oxygen therapy

The responsiveness of the respiratory centre and the central and peripheral chemoreceptors to variation in p_aO_2 and p_aCO_2 underpin the principles of oxygen therapy, particularly for patients with chronic obstructive pulmonary disease (COPD) and chronically elevated p_aCO_2 who may need long-term O_2 therapy.

In chronic lung diseases, such as COPD, CO_2 retention occurs so that p_aCO_2 is chronically elevated. The central chemoreceptors adapt to this chronic state of hypercapnia, becoming unresponsive to the elevated p_aCO_2, so that the main drive for maintaining ventilation comes from the peripheral chemoreceptors, which respond to hypoxia.

Patients with chronic CO_2 retention who go into type II respiratory failure (see later) risk respiratory arrest if given high-partial pressure O_2 therapy, which removes the main respiratory drive (low p_aO_2).

Clinical box 13.22   Different types of cough

Different types of cough are characteristic of different conditions. Conditions such as pneumonia and chronic obstructive pulmonary disease (COPD) cause a productive cough. The cough may be intermittent or persistent, or may be worse in the morning or at night. Coughing can also be stimulated by non-respiratory causes such as gastro-oesophageal reflux or treatment with angiotensin-converting enzyme inhibitors. A productive cough (i.e. one with sputum) should not be suppressed as the mucus needs to be cleared. Mucolytics reduce the viscosity of the mucus, aiding clearance. Anti-tussives, such as codeine, suppress coughing by acting centrally. Expectorants are also intended to reduce the viscosity of the mucus and increase the fluid in the respiratory tract although their effectiveness is disputed.

J-receptors

The **J-receptors** (juxtacapillary receptors) lie in the alveolar walls, close to the capillaries. Impulses from these receptors travel along slowly conducting nerve fibres in the vagus nerve when the receptors are stimulated by the presence of interstitial fluid in the alveoli and by histamine and other inflammatory mediators. They may be the cause of the dyspnoea and the rapid, shallow breathing in left ventricular failure and interstitial pulmonary disease.

Other receptors

Receptors located in parts of the body other than the respiratory system can also respond to the need for more oxygen. Stimulation of these receptors leads to increased inspiration.

Muscle stretch receptors

Muscle stretch receptors are located in the **muscle spindles** of the diaphragm and the intercostal muscles. The intercostal muscles contain numerous muscle spindles whereas the diaphragm (the main respiratory muscle) is sparsely supplied. The spindles are richly innervated and lie in parallel with the muscle fibres. As the muscle is stretched so too are the spindles, leading to an increased rate of discharge of their action potential. The rate of increase is dependent on the rate of muscle movement; thus they can signal both instantaneous length and the velocity of stretch. These receptors reflexively control the strength of muscle contraction to increase the depth of breathing. They may give rise to dyspnoea when large breathing efforts are required, for example in airways obstruction or when breathing through a narrow tube.

Joint proprioceptors

The costovertebral joints contain mechanoreceptors that are sensitive to rib displacement. These **joint proprioceptors** are the thought to be the main site of impulses giving rise to the conscious sensation of lung distension since this sensation is still present when the vagus is severed and input from the pulmonary and intercostal stretch receptors is lost. These joint proprioceptors are involved in the sensation of dyspnoea arising from absence of chest movement during, e.g. breath-holding (see below). Impulses from the movement of the limbs may signal increased breathing during early stages of exercise.

Baroreceptors

A rise in blood pressure detected by the carotid or aortic sinus **baroreceptors** tends to depress respiration, causing hypoventilation or apnoea. The reverse occurs when blood pressure falls, leading to hyperventilation. The afferents run in the carotid sinus nerve or glossopharyngeal nerve.

HIGHER CENTRE CONTROL OF BREATHING

Breathing is voluntary to some extent, and within limits, cortical activity can over-ride reflex control of ventilation. Voluntary hyperventilation (deep, rapid breathing) can blow off CO_2 to halve p_aCO_2, causing a rise in pH. The resultant alkalosis effectively leads to hypocalcaemia, which may cause tetany with muscle spasm in the hand and foot (car-

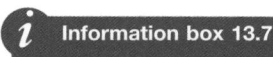

Information box 13.7 | **Common respiratory reflexes**

- **Gasping**: application of cold water to the skin during a cold shower will cause gasping followed by hyperventilation.
- **Sneezing**: this is the sudden expiratory blast through the nose produced by irritation of the nasal mucosa and stimulation of the nasal branches of the maxillary nerve, which is the second division of the trigeminal nerve (cranial nerve V). Droplets may spread to 5 m, making this a significant mode of spread for many respiratory infections.
- **Hiccups**: this term refers to the repetitive spasmodic contraction of the diaphragm and external intercostal muscles during which the glottis closes suddenly and further entrance of air into the chest is prevented, thus producing the characteristic sound and sensation.

popedal spasm). Hypoventilation or breath-holding is more difficult because the duration of breath-holding is restricted by either p_aCO_2 or p_aO_2 (see later). Breathing patterns can also be altered by emotions such as fear or anger.

ENERGY PRODUCTION AND OXYGEN CONSUMPTION

The primary function of respiration is to supply oxygen for the combustion of foodstuffs and to remove carbon dioxide. This is described by the **respiratory quotient** (RQ), which is the ratio of the CO_2 production to the O_2 consumption. The RQ is affected by:

- Changes in acid–base balance from whatever cause
- Hyperventilation
- The type of food consumed (metabolic fuels).

RESPIRATORY QUOTIENT AS AN INDICATION OF METABOLIC FUEL

If only carbohydrates are metabolised, e.g. glucose ($C_6H_{12}O_6$), the volume of CO_2 produced is equal to the volume of O_2 used, and the RQ is equal to 1.

$$C_6H_{12}O_6 + 6O_2 \rightleftharpoons 6CO_2 + 6H_2O$$

Thus

$$RQ = \frac{6CO_2}{6O_2} = 1$$

The metabolism of fatty acids alone gives an RQ of about 0.7. For example, stearic acid is converted in a two-stage process:

$$C_{17}H_{35}COOH + 8O_2 \rightleftharpoons 3C_6H_{12}O_6$$

$$C_6H_{12}O_6 + 6O_2 \rightleftharpoons 6CO_2 + 6H_2O$$

Overall, the reaction is

$$C_{17}H_{35}COOH + 26O_2 \rightleftharpoons 18CO_2 + 18H_2O$$

Thus $RQ = 18/26 \approx 0.7$

The RQ for protein depends on the precise amino acid composition of the protein but RQ for the average protein is about 0.8. RQ can to used to calculate energy consumption in humans using indirect calorimetry (see below). This has i   Information box 13.8   **Respiratory quotient (RQ) changes with diet and ventilation**

- A person eating a mixed Western diet containing carbohydrates, fats and proteins will have an overall or average RQ of 0.85.
- A highly physically active person on a predominately carbohydrate diet will have a higher RQ, closer to 1.
- A diabetic patient will have a low RQ due to the increased utilisation of fats and decreased metabolism of carbohydrates.

RQ can be affected by changes in pulmonary ventilation that are unrelated to food metabolism:

- Hyperventilation (voluntary hyperpnoea) will wash out excessive quantities of CO_2 from the body and RQ will rise above 1.
- RQ will rise in acidosis and will fall in alkalosis from metabolic causes, because of the raised and lowered CO_2 excretion produced by respiratory compensation.
- RQ will rise in severe exercise as lactic acid is produced and ventilation is overstimulated.

clinical significance, as energy consumption increases or decreases in diseases such as hyperthyroidism.

METHODS FOR ESTIMATING ENERGY CONSUMPTION

Energy consumption in healthy human beings varies according to nutritional status and physical activity (see Ch. 16). This can be measured as the **basal metabolic rate (BMR)** plus the energy needed in fuel metabolism, to combat cold and for physical activity. It may be altered by disease processes, for example thyroid disease, when energy consumption could be increased or decreased by the effects of disordered hormone activity.

Basal metabolic rate

BMR refers to the minimum energy used by the body to maintain the essential activities of the brain, heart and lungs. BMR is commonly expressed as a fraction of the body's surface area. A person of average height 1.7 m and weight 70 kg has a surface area of 1.8 m^2. Before the discovery of immunoassays for thyroid hormones, BMR was the standard test for the diagnosis of hypo- and hyperthyroidism. There are two methods of measuring BMR:

- **Direct calorimetry** – which is based on the principle that energy expended by the body is eventually lost as heat
- **Indirect calorimetry** – which is based on the principle that energy consumption depends on oxygen consumption, which can be easily measured.

For a man the average BMR is about 46 W/m^2 and for women 42 W/m^2. The lower figure of women is probably due to their greater fat content and lower muscle mass. In newborn babies, for whom the surface area is not known, BMR is given by the oxygen consumption as 4.8 mL/min/kg. On the day after birth, it averages 6.6 mL/min/kg and then is about 7.0–7.2 mL/min/kg for the next 18 months. After that, BMR falls gradually with age.

Table 13.4	Oxygen consumption at different levels of activity	
Exercise	**Oxygen consumption (mL/min)**
Rest	200
Brisk walking (5 km/h)	1000
Running (12 km/h)	3000
Severe exercise	4000
Elite rowers, for a brief period*	6600

*Source: Clark et al (1983) J Appl Physiol 55:440.

CHALLENGES TO NORMAL RESPIRATION

EXERCISE

During exercise, both ventilation and oxygen consumption increase linearly with work load (Table 13.4). The severity of exercise is a subjective sensation which appears related more to the oxygen consumption than the work done.

The mechanism by which ventilation during exercise is controlled is unclear. Arterial blood gases are substantially unchanged by exercise up to an O_2 consumption of 3 L/min at sea level, and so cannot easily explain the increased ventilation. This is not to say that chemoreceptors cannot feed into the respiratory control system, as administering pure O_2 during exercise will depress ventilation. Factors thought to play a role in regulating ventilation during exercise include:

- Feedback from joint proprioceptors
- The anticipation of exercise
- Increased venous return and cardiac output
- Rising core temperature
- Increased sensitivity of the peripheral chemoreceptors to oscillations in arterial pH and pCO_2.

In severe exercise, ventilation may be further increased by lactic acid from muscles lowering blood pH and the release of potassium ions from exercising muscles. This increased ventilation may actually lower p_aCO_2 as CO_2 is blown off. During heavy exercise, ventilation cannot supply sufficient O_2. The difference is made up by anaerobic metabolism, which produces lactic acid. The point when anaerobic metabolism starts is called the aerobic threshold. The threshold can be raised by physical training; available evidence (mercifully!) suggests no difference in the benefit of continuous or intermittent training at the threshold.

The phenomenon of a **second wind** during exercise, which can be marked in untrained individuals, occurs when the initial dyspnoea and raised p_aCO_2 disappears. It coincides with increased body temperature and onset of sweating.

ALTITUDE

As a person ascends a mountain or in an aircraft, barometric pressure falls but the fractional concentration of oxygen and the saturated vapour pressure of the air remains constant (see Table 13.3). Thus, the inspired pO_2 falls according to.

$$\text{Inspired } pO_2 = 0.21 \times (\text{barometric pressure} - 47)\,\text{mmHg}$$
$$= 74\,\text{mmHg}$$

Physiological responses to high altitude

Sudden exposure to high altitude, as in ascent in a balloon or unpressurised aircraft, leads to acute, severe hypoxia and loss of consciousness. O_2 must therefore be provided in unpressurised aircraft for passengers above 3700 m (12 000 ft), which will provide protection from unconsciousness up to 12 000 m. Pilots are required to use oxygen above 3000 m to ensure safety.

During more gradual exposure to high altitude, as when climbing a mountain, the peripheral chemoreceptors are the first to respond to hypoxia, leading to hyperventilation. As CO_2 is washed out, p_aCO_2 is lowered, and consequently the pH of the blood and CSF rises (alkalosis). This hypocapnia places a brake on the ventilation response to the hypoxia, so that hyperventilation is less than would otherwise occur if p_aCO_2 remained normal.

In a few hours, active transport of bicarbonate out of the CSF brings the pH of CSF under control, but the kidneys take longer to excrete the bicarbonate and bring arterial pH under control. It should be remembered that haemoglobin without O_2 is also more alkaline and this adds to the alkalosis. Increased bicarbonate excretion leads to diuresis. Dehydration may occur. Water and electrolyte imbalance such as potassium deficiency and sodium retention could accompany mountain sickness (see below). In the longer term, hypoxia causes an increase in pulmonary vasoconstriction and may lead to pulmonary oedema. Hypocapnia, from hyperventilation, decreases cerebral blood flow giving rise to symptoms of cerebral dysfunction. Cerebral oedema may also occur, although the pathophysiology is not clear.

To compensate for the low alveolar pO_2, the body attempts to increase the blood O_2-carrying capacity by increasing red cell volume. Renal erythropoietin secretion increases so that haemoglobin concentrations rise from an average of 141 g/L to 196 g/L after 4 weeks (polycythaemia) (see also Ch. 12). At altitude, the accompanying increase in blood viscosity increases resistance to blood flow which may be offset by a general vasodilatation.

Acclimatisation to altitude

Over time, a series of integrated physiological adaptations takes place in people living at high altitudes to restore tissue oxygenation to normal levels: acclimatisation. This process includes:

- Hyperventilation
- Correction of persistent alkalosis
- Polycythaemia
- Increased cardiac output
- Increased tolerance for physical exercise.

Mountain sickness

The unacclimatised mountaineer becomes aware of breathlessness at about 2000 m (6600 ft) and may experience the symptoms of **mountain sickness** (headache, nausea, loss of appetite, difficulty in sleeping and performing exercise). At 5500 m, feelings of unreality, amnesia and dizziness become apparent. Disturbances to sleep arise from sleep apnoea, the commonest form of which is Cheyne–Stokes breathing, during which periodic apnoea occurs between periods of increasing tidal volume. Some people are more susceptible than others to the effects of high altitude, and symptoms vary among individuals. The clinical manifestations and severity of mountain sickness are therefore a spectrum of conditions.

BREATH-HOLDING

When a breath is held, p_aCO_2 and p_ACO_2 rise to a remarkably constant **breaking point**, when the respiratory chemoreceptors triggers respiratory stimulation, at which point the next breath has to be taken. Hyperventilation prior to breath-holding will reduce the p_aCO_2 but not increase p_aO_2 and extends the breath-holding time, thus demonstrating the dominance of the CO_2 drive to ventilation. Mental determination can be another important factor in determining the breaking point, as can re-breathing into a bag, which overcomes the discomfort due to the absence of rhythmic chest movements.

Prolonging the held breath

The duration of apnoea in a breath-hold can be increased by **hyperventilation** which 'blows-off' CO_2 and lowers p_aCO_2. Thus there is a longer period before the p_aCO_2 rises sufficiently to trigger the central chemoreceptors, when the so-called CO_2 breaking point is reached and the person must take another breath. Hyperventilation prior to breath-hold diving carries the risk of fainting underwater since dangerous levels of hypoxia will be reached before the CO_2 drive forces breathing. There are unconfirmed reports of this occurring in synchronised swimmers so that less emphasis should be placed on the length of time of set underwater routines during competitions.

DIVING

The simplest method of diving is **breath-hold diving** (also known as 'free' diving), when the diver does not use any artificial aids to breathing, such as the self-contained underwater breathing apparatus (SCUBA) or specialised deep diving equipment, but simply holds his or her breath. After breathing air, breath-holding times are normally limited to 60–75 seconds. In people who practise breath-holding, such as synchronised swimmers or sponge divers, longer times can be achieved. It is unclear whether this is due to training or to an inherited ability, which, as it increases the success rate, effectively selects people for these activities.

Effects of pressure in free diving

The pressure exerted by water increases rapidly as greater depths are reached. During a breath-hold dive, lung volumes decrease as the external pressure rises according to Boyle's law. At a depth of 50 m a starting lung volume of 6.0 L would be reduced to 1.0 L. Lung volume cannot be reduced below residual volume, so that further increases in water pressure during descent may lead to undesired effects. Conversely, lung volume will increase during ascent.

At a depth of only 1.6 m the increase in pressure will exceed 100 mmHg. At this point, the inspiratory muscles cannot overcome the external water pressure, so that, for some people, it becomes impossible to breath in. This has important significance for diving while breathing air through a rigid hose, a snorkel. The length of the snorkel should therefore be limited for use near the surface (34 cm).

Effects of pressure during ascent

At a depth equivalent to 2 atm the partial pressures of O_2 and CO_2 in the lungs will be doubled even though the percentage concentration remains unchanged. It is therefore possible that the tension of CO_2 in the lungs will be higher than that of the blood, which is incompressible. CO_2 will therefore pass in the reverse direction to normal. Oxygen will continue to enter the blood and maintain an adequate O_2 tension due to the affinity of haemoglobin for O_2 (the diver does not feel a lack of O_2). This constitutes a danger when returning to the surface, as on ascent the partial pressure of O_2 in the lungs may fall below that of the blood. Consequently, O_2 will leave the blood and pass into the lungs. This will lead to acute anoxia and may lead to unconsciousness. Another risk exists during escape from submarines. Air must be breathed out during ascent as the gases in the chest expand, otherwise lung rupture is almost certain.

Effects of pressure in deep diving

At greater depths using underwater breathing apparatus (aqua-lung or SCUBA) the air is supplied at the environmental pressure so that the normal pressure differential between the lungs and outside the chest wall is maintained. The risks of acute anoxia and lung rupture are, however, still present.

At very great depths, helium oxygen mixtures are used (98% helium, 2% oxygen) but supplied at the environmental pressure. Only 1–2% O_2 is required because of the high partial pressures. At depth, nitrogen is replaced by helium because of three properties of nitrogen:

- It is an anaesthetic and at 30 atm can cause full surgical anaesthesia.
- It has increased solubility in tissues, which is a problem during decompression, when gas bubbles may be produced, variously known as the 'bends' or 'chokes'.
- Its density increases at pressure which hinders breathing.
- Nitrogen narcosis ('narks', raptures of the deep) may occur if breathing compressed air during deep diving (40 m), when loss of consciousness and drowning is preceded by euphoria.

Helium is not without problems. It increases voice pitch, making it squeaky, and so communication becomes difficult. Helium under pressure is a good conductor of heat and can cause hypothermia unless the diver's environment is heated. Slow decompression is also required to prevent the bends.

DIVER'S REFLEX

The diver's reflex is a response to hypoxia when oxygenated blood is directed from the heart to the brain. Observations in diving mammals, such as seals, show that during a dive, primary bradycardia (vagal in origin) and vasoconstriction to the skin, muscle, gastrointestinal tract and kidneys effectively 'shut down' the peripheral circulation, ensuring adequate O_2 to the heart, lungs and brain. However, ventilation drive is **suppressed**. This is contrary to the normal response to hypoxia, when hyperventilation occurs in response to the low p_aO_2 and raised p_aCO_2, with an associated secondary tachy-

cardia. This reflex is triggered by submersion in cold water, and may in part explain survival in cases of near drowning in man (see below).

DROWNING

Most drowning victims eventually inhale water into the lungs, either before or after losing consciousness. In some cases, drowning will occur without inhalation when entry of cold water into the upper airways causes laryngeal spasm, closing the glottis, and produces apnoea thus preventing the water from entering into the lungs. In fresh water, most of the water entering the lungs will move into the circulation causing haemodilution. Sea water is hypertonic with three times the osmolarity of blood and so will remain in the lungs and tend to draw fluid from the circulation to cause haemoconcentration. Both conditions lead to heart failure, which can complicate efforts to resuscitate victims of drowning. It is also usual for drowning people to swallow large quantities of water and then regurgitate or vomit, further complicating the drowning with acid aspiration.

There are remarkable accounts of survival of children for as long as 40 minutes in cold water. It is clear that reduction in cerebral metabolism by cooling is protective, but very rapid cooling (>1 °C/min) would be required to lower metabolism before the anoxia caused brain cell death. Cooling by simple immersion would be too slow. Other factors which could better explain the survival of these children include reflex apnoea, reflex closure of the glottis or the diver's reflex.

HIGH OXYGEN LEVELS

The body most commonly has to deal with low oxygen levels. Prolonged exposure to high oxygen concentrations can cause disease because of oxygen toxicity. Exposure to oxygen at partial pressure in excess of 2 atm can occur during deep sea dives or during hyperbaric oxygen therapy.

Neurological oxygen toxicity

The central nervous system, especially the brain, responds adversely to too much O_2 and seizures are common. High levels of O_2 lead to the generation of damaging free radicals (see Chs 2 and 16).

Cellular oxygen toxicity

The use of inspired oxygen during mechanical ventilation is part of the routine care for treating critically ill or injured patients. However, there is some question as to the level of inspired oxygen that creates a toxic effect to the lungs and reduces their ability to produce surfactant.

Continuous exposure to high concentrations of oxygen can damage the lungs. This has to be taken seriously when giving continuous oxygen therapy: the lowest concentrations of oxygen for adequate arterial oxygenation should be used. Newborn babies can develop retrolental fibrosis leading to blindness if the incubator pO_2 is too high.

CARBON MONOXIDE POISONING

CO has a very high affinity for haemoglobin, about 250 times that of O_2. So it easily displaces O_2 to form HbCO and effectively reduces the amount of haemoglobin available for gas transport.

Low levels of HbCO (less than 2%) are normal, but smokers have 5–10% HbCO and significant amounts of HbCO are found in the blood of fetuses whose mothers smoke. Acute levels below 20% are usually asymptomatic in individuals with no cardiorespiratory disease but levels above 60% may lead to coma. However, lower chronic exposure can lead to headaches and nausea and may lead to permanent neurological damage.

Treatment of CO poisoning is by 100% O_2 in order to displace the CO, although in some centres patients are treated with 100% O_2 in a high pressure chamber (hyperbaric oxygen) in order to displace the CO even faster.

RESPIRATORY FAILURE

Respiratory failure is when alveolar ventilation in not sufficient to maintain normal arterial blood gases. It is defined practically as:

- $p_aO_2 < 8$ kPa (60 mmHg)

  or

- $p_aCO_2 > 7$ kPa (55 mmHg)

  although the extreme limits of survival are:

- $p_aO_2 < 2.7$ kPa (20 mmHg)

  and

- $p_aCO_2 > 11$ kPa (83 mmHg).

CAUSES OF RESPIRATORY FAILURE

Respiratory failure occurs when either pulmonary gas exchange or the respiratory muscles fail, or both. Disturbances in ventilation and perfusion in pulmonary disease lead to V_A/Q imbalance, so that the balance of p_aO_2 and p_aCO_2 becomes disrupted, with the ensuing disturbance in acid–base balance. There are two types of respiratory failure:

- **Type I** where p_aO_2 is low (hypoxaemia), and p_aCO_2 is normal or low
- **Type II** where p_aO_2 is low, and p_aCO_2 is high (hypercapnia).

Although type I and type II respiratory failure have distinct blood gas patterns, physiologically they represent a continuum. For example, mild to moderate right-to-left shunts could give rise to a type I respiratory failure where, although the p_aO_2 is low, the p_aCO_2 is maintained as normal or low through compensation by hyperventilation. However, as the lung disease progresses and larger areas of lung damage give rise to more severe right-to-left shunting, the central respiratory drive (hyperventilation) can no longer compensate for the rise in p_aCO_2 and hypercapnia ensues, giving rise to type II respiratory failure.

Type I respiratory failure

Type I respiratory failure occurs in **restrictive lung disease**, when there is a significant, and sometimes sudden, reduction in lung volume leading to acute hypoxaemia. This could be the result of right-to-left shunts, when unventilated parts of the lungs are perfused so that gaseous exchange does not take place effectively. Alternately, there is severe ventilation–perfusion (V_A/Q) mismatch. Clinical conditions leading to type I respiratory failure include those in which lung tissue is damaged or reduced, as in:

- Pneumonia
- Pulmonary oedema
- Adult respiratory distress syndrome (ARDS)
- Pneumothorax
- Fibrosing alveolitis (more chronic respiratory failure).

Type II respiratory failure

Type II respiratory failure occurs mainly with obstructive lung disease. Although lung volume is unchanged, airflow is reduced so that alveolar ventilation is reduced. The alveoli fail to adequately oxygenate the blood and excrete sufficient CO_2. The commonest cause is COPD. Other causes include asthma, chest wall deformity, respiratory muscle weakness and depression of the respiratory centre. p_aO_2 is depressed, giving rise to hypoxia, while CO_2 accumulates leading to hypercapnia.

Reactive hyperventilation to hypercapnia, similar to adaptation to high altitude, blows off CO_2 while increasing O_2. But whereas the body puts up with mild alkalosis at altitude, the respiratory centre becomes less sensitive to hypercapnia in type II respiratory failure.

Asthma

Airways obstruction in asthma results from intermittent, reversible constriction of airways due to smooth muscle spasm, and mucosal inflammation. Excess mucus secretion leads to further narrowing of the airways, increasing airway resistance. Voluntary respiratory effort has to increase in order to expel air against increasing resistance and small airways collapse before tidal volume is expelled. The FRC increases, leaving over-expanded lungs (hyperinflation), which make inspiration more and more difficult.

These changes lead to varying degrees of airway obstruction and to ventilation that is uneven and patchy. Continued blood flow to some hypoventilated areas (right-to-left shunt) causes V_A/Q imbalance, resulting in arterial hypoxaemia. Early in an attack, a patient typically compensates by hyperventilating the unobstructed areas of the lung, resulting in a decrease in p_aCO_2 (type I respiratory failure). As the attack progresses, the capacity for hyperventilation is impaired by the increased FRC, more extensive airway narrowing and muscle fatigue. Hypoxaemia worsens, and p_aCO_2 begins to rise (hypercapnia), leading to respiratory acidosis. At this point, the patient is in type II respiratory failure.

COPD

Chronic, persistent irreversible airways obstruction, increased inflammation and mucus secretion are present in COPD. The vast majority of cases are caused by cigarette smoking and severe atmospheric pollution. Other currently proposed risk factors include poor nutrition in utero, α_1-antitrypsin deficiency and pre-existing bronchial hyper-responsiveness.

Small airways collapse easily due to destruction of pulmonary elastic tissue causing further obstruction. As with asthma, the FRC increases, giving rise to the 'barrel chest' of COPD. Furthermore, the effort required to ventilate the alveoli against increasing resistance gives rise to dyspnoea on exertion, where even speech becomes difficult in severe cases. As for asthma, airways obstruction causes inadequate ventilation. Destruction of alveolar walls lead to the formation of larger air sacs (emphysema, see below) that are inefficient for gaseous exchange. The varying combinations of airway disease and pulmonary emphysema lead to hypoxia of respiratory origin (hypoxic hypoxia) and hypercapnia, and thus chronic, type II respiratory failure of varying severity.

Emphysema

Emphysema is an enlargement of the alveolar sacs by the destruction of the alveolar walls. Large spaces called bullae form, which reduce the surface area for gas exchange. The bullae can also rupture to cause a pneumothorax. The main cause of the enlargement is the destruction of elastin fibres in the lung tissue by the unusual activity of the enzyme neutrophil elastase.

Emphysema occurs in about 20–30% of heavy smokers. A few patients with emphysema are deficient in α_1-antitrypsin, which inhibits the elastase. However, it is not known why some smokers with normal levels of α_1-antitrypsin develop the disease and others do not. There are different types of emphysema, according to the anatomical distribution of the damage.

Clinical effects of respiratory failure

Hypoxia interferes with aerobic metabolism, so that cellular function is disrupted. Effects on the brain give rise to confusion and drowsiness, progressing to coma and death in severe cases. To compensate for the reduced p_aO_2, renal tubular cells increase erythropoietin production so that polycythaemia results to increase the O_2-carrying capacity of the blood. Pulmonary vasoconstriction to divert blood from poorly ventilated parts of the lungs leads to pulmonary hypertension and, eventually, cor pulmonale (see above).

Hypercapnia adds to the effects of hypoxia on the brain and also causes respiratory acidosis as the result of

inadequate CO_2 excretion. In chronic respiratory failure (e.g. COPD), the respiratory centre becomes desensitised to hypocapnia, so that the central ventilatory drive from the elevated p_aCO_2 no longer operates. Renal retention of bicarbonate can, to some extent, compensate for the respiratory acidosis, but this takes time. The combination of hypoxia and acidosis could be fatal.

LUNG DEFENCES AGAINST INFECTION

The seasonality of respiratory disease is important in understanding the pathology of infective respiratory disease. The inhalation of particles and airborne microbes is an unavoidable consequence of inhaling approximately 10 000 L of air per a day, and infections of the upper respiratory tract can lead to infections of the lower respiratory tract with viruses and bacteria. Elaborate systems have evolved to defend the lungs but when activated these processes can also damage the lungs. The nasopharyngeal airways trap particles >10 µm diameter and is relatively effective in filtering particles >5 µm diameter. The nasopharynx also absorbs soluble and reactive gases such as sulphur dioxide.

THE UPPER AIRWAYS

The nose and upper airways have two major defences against infection:

- The physical barrier of a continuously moving layer of mucus that lines the airway
- A local immune response involving phagocytic polymorphonuclear leucocytes and other leucocytes such as natural killer cells.

Airway cooling in winter is likely to compromise both these mechanisms of respiratory defence and predispose to respiratory infection by slowing the mucociliary escalator and the phagocytic activity of macrophages. Others factors may be of importance, such as staying indoors in cold weather as the greater proximity to other people allows the spread of infections. Cross-infection explains the peak in general practitioner consultations and hospital admission of children with asthma, which has been exacerbated by infections when they return to school after the summer vacation.

CONDUCTING AIRWAYS

Mucins and ciliary action

Particulates larger than 2 µm diameter become trapped in the viscous 5 µm thick mucus blanket that covers the airway epithelial cells. This mucus is formed from mucins, a group of glycosylated proteins. Mucins are synthesised by goblet cells in the surface epithelium and mucous cells in the submucosal layers. A sublayer of water underlies the mucous layer and provides less resistance to the movement of cilia. The cilia are just long enough to catch the base of the viscous mucus layer and propel it forward (see Fig. 13.6). Each ciliated epithelial cell has about 200 cilia that beat at 12–14/s. Microbes can be cleared from the trachea within 30 min and from the distal airways with a half-time of hours. Cigarette smoking, bacterial or viral infection, anaesthetics and cold

---

Clinical box 13.23 **Other causes of respiratory failure**

- **Acute neurological disorders**: traumatic injury to the brain and spinal cord or strokes may result in total or partial loss of respiratory muscle function.
- **Guillain–Barré syndrome**: this is an acute, multifocal disease that demyelinates peripheral nerves. In about 50% of cases it follows a viral infection. Muscle weakness and paralysis commonly begin in the lower extremities and progress upwards to include the respiratory muscles. Maximum weakness develops within 2–4 weeks. Most patients recovery fully.
- **Chronic muscle disease**: examples are Duchenne's muscular dystrophy, which is an X-linked recessive disorder caused by mutations of the gene for the protein dystrophin, and myotonic dystrophy, which is characterised by delayed muscular relaxation and muscle weakness.
- **Paralytic poliomyelitis**: before the use of poliovirus vaccines, poliomyelitis was the most frequent neuromuscular disorder to result in respiratory failure, although only a minority of infected persons developed paralysis.

exposure can slow cilia or destroy airway epithelium, delaying clearance, and increase the likelihood of recurrent infection.

Other factors

The airways also secrete a number of factors that inhibit bacteria or limit the damage they cause. Lactoferrin is released by epithelial cells and by binding iron limits the growth of bacteria since a supply of iron is essential for the production of the bacteria's transport proteins. Lysozyme is secreted (10–20 mg/day) and catalyses the hydrolysis of bonds between bacterial cells walls. The anti-proteases (α_1-antitrypsin and α_2-macroglobulin) secretory leukoprotease inhibitor inhibit the enzymes chymotrypsin, trypsin and elastase.

INNATE IMMUNITY

With innate immunity, carbohydrates in the microbial cell wall identify the organism as harmful and it is destroyed by a system involving macrophages, natural killer cells, complement factors and defensins (see Ch. 6).

Destroying the invading organism

Pulmonary macrophages normally lie within the alveoli and airways and are derived mainly from monocytes that enter the lung from the circulation. There are four aspects to the microbicidal action of macrophages:

■ Recognition
■ Migration
■ Ingestion and
■ Secretion of mediators.

Macrophages recognise the microbe using surfaces receptors to specific carbohydrates, e.g. lipopolysaccharide (LPS), which is commonly found on Gram-negative bacteria, or mannose that is found in yeasts, mycobacteria and *Pneumocystis carinii*. Macrophages also have receptors for the third component of **complement**. Complement is present in bronchial fluid and when activated generates C3b, an opsonin that promotes receptor-mediated phagocytosis. The microbes are killed once recognised and engulfed, but killing is not fully activated until certain signals are received. These activation stimuli can be produced by the macrophages themselves, such as the release of interferon (IFN)-α and IFN-β, induced by LPS, or the release of granulocyte-macrophage colony-stimulating factor or IFN-γ by natural killer cells.

Defensins

Oxidative and non-oxidative processes are use to kill the phagocytosed microbes, but macrophages are not as effective as monocytes or neutrophils, as they are deficient in myeloperoxidase, an essential part of the MPO–hydrogen peroxide–halide system. The non-oxidative mechanisms involve **defensins** that fill many Gram-positive organisms (*Staphylococcus aureus*) and Gram-negative species (*Escherichia coli*, *Klebsiella pneumoniae*) and fungi, and inactivate certain viruses.

Surfactant proteins

Also under the umbrella of innate immunity are type 2 alveolar cells that secrete **surfactant proteins** A and D which enhance the phagocytosis and agglutination of Gram-positive bacteria.

INFLAMMATORY RESPONSES

Macrophages are capable of dealing with low levels of bacterial infection and minimally virulent organisms. However, when the lungs are infected with numerous bacteria or virulent encapsulated organisms such as *Pseudomonas aeruginosa* or *Streptococcus pneumoniae*, the recruitment of polymorphonuclear neutrophils for containment and clearance is essential. Simply, the process is:

1. Bacteria or their products stimulate macrophage production of cytokines (tumour necrosis factor (TNF)-α, interleukin (IL)-1, IL-8, leukotriene B4) or cause the production of complement activations products C5a and C3a. These molecules act as chemoattractants or stimulate production of further cytokine production by epithelial cells or fibroblasts.
2. The chemoattractants induce the migration of neutrophils from the capillaries into the alveolar space.
3. The neutrophils phagocytose the bacteria and kill them with a 'respiratory burst' of reactive oxygen metabolites such as hydrogen peroxide, hydroxyl radicals and singlet oxygen.
4. These reactive oxygen molecules are derived from the reduction of oxygen by an NADPH (nicotinamide adenosine dinucleotide phosphate (reduced form)) oxidase present in the phagocyte cytoplasm or from the synthesis of nitric oxide. Besides damaging the invading microbe, they are also toxic to the host cells.

Neutrophils also release the enzyme elastase, which produces a number of side effects: excessive mucus secretion, epithelial cell damage and a significant slowing of the beat frequency of the ciliated epithelium.

DEVELOPMENT OF THE LUNGS AND CHANGES IN THE NEWBORN

EARLY LUNG DEVELOPMENT

Embryonic phase

The earliest, embryonic, phase of lung development occurs at 4 weeks with the formation of the **lung bud** or **respiratory diverticulum**, an outgrowth on the ventral surface on the wall of the foregut just below the primordial pharynx (Fig. 13.26). This then divides into two buds which will eventually make up the two main bronchi. The right bud is slightly larger and is more vertically orientated, a relationship which persists in the adult. By the end of week 8 these main bronchial buds have further divided to produce the segmental bronchi, which will form the lobes, two on the left and three on the right. These buds continue to divide to form the bronchioles. By 24 weeks there are about 17 orders of branching, with the remaining seven orders developing after birth. The lung buds are closely associated with the visceral pleura which covers the lobes and each lung is covered with the parietal pleura, which encloses the pleural cavity.

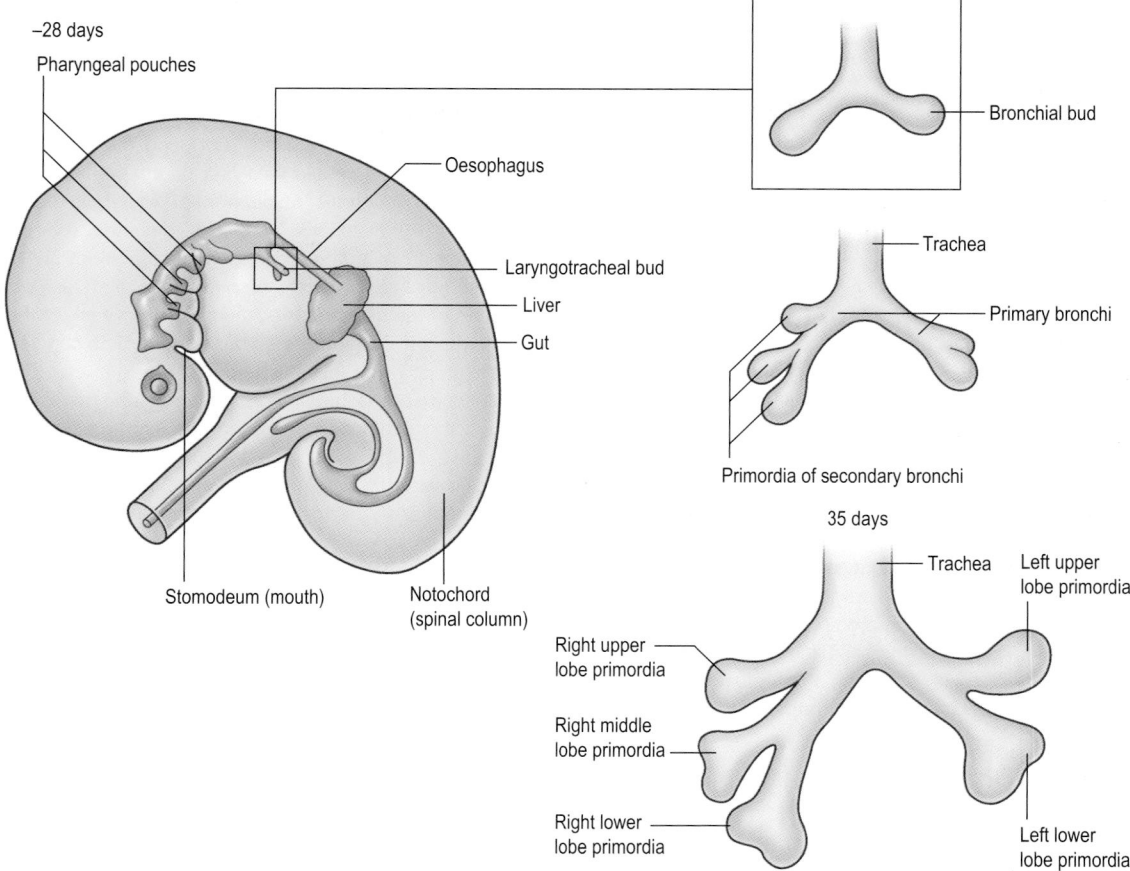

Fig. 13.26 Early lung development. The lung bud develops at 4 weeks as an outgrowth of the embryonic foregut (the laryngotracheal bud). The whole of the epithelium lining the entire respiratory tract is, therefore, derived from endoderm. This bud forms two subsections, with the smaller bud on the left, initiating the asymmetry of the bronchi at this early stage. By 8 weeks the right and left segmental bronchi have formed and the pleura cover the lungs.

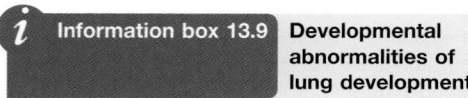

Information box 13.9 **Developmental abnormalities of lung development**

When it first forms, the lung bud is connected directly to the foregut, but a band of tissue forms between the nascent trachea and oesophagus called the **tracheoesophageal ridge**, which separates them. In some cases this ridge does not develop correctly, producing a range of abnormalities. The most common of these (>85% of cases) occurs when the trachea remains connected to the lower part of the oesophagus, giving a connecting passage, a **fistula**, between them. The upper part of the oesophagus has a blind end called oesophageal **atresia**. Other rarer abnormalities can lead to different combinations of atresia and fistulas.

STAGES IN LUNG MATURATION

Once the basic structure has been laid down the lung develops and matures in four phases which span a long period from 6 weeks post-conception to 8 years after birth. The four phases are:

- Pseudoglandular phase
- Canalicular phase
- Terminal saccular phase
- Alveolar phase.

Pseudoglandular phase (6–16 weeks in utero)

During the **pseudoglandular phase**, so called because the lung tissue resembles an exocrine gland, the lung consists of the terminal bronchi which are surrounded by connective tissue which contain capillaries. However, there are no respiratory bronchioles so there is no possibility of survival for fetuses born during this period. Towards the end of the pseudoglandular phase, the lumen of the bronchi starts to enlarge and the epithelia become thinner.

Canalicular phase (16–24 weeks in utero)

In the **canalicular phase**, the terminal bronchioles divided to form respiratory bronchioles which themselves divide to form alveolar ducts and the capillaries. At the end of the canalicular phase these can support some respiration, because the ends of some of these ducts have developed into **terminal saccules** (primordial alveoli with thin walls which are highly vascularised). However, fetuses born before 24 weeks may not survive due to the immaturity of other systems as well as poor respiratory function.

Saccular phase (24 weeks in utero to birth)

The **saccular period** is where the number of terminal saccules increases and the epithelium covering them thins to form the **blood–air barrier**. The epithelium differentiates into mainly type I alveolar cells (type I pneumocytes) although there are also type II alveolar cells (type II pneumocytes), which secrete surfactant. The capillary and lymphatic network develops around the terminal saccules, providing a short diffusion distance for dissolved gases.

The increases in surface area provided by the thinning of the epithelium and the increase in surfactant production, especially after week 30, mean that fetuses born in this period have much higher survival rates.

Alveolar phase (32 weeks – 8 years)

The **alveolar phase** overlaps with the saccular phase as it depends on the definition of an alveolus. After 36 weeks the walls of the alveoli are so thin that the capillaries bulge into the alveoli. Most fully mature alveoli do not appear until after birth and form from the division of the terminal saccules which become the alveolar ducts. New alveoli arise by the formation of septa across the enlarging immature alveoli and the development of new capillaries. While there is a large increase in their number soon after birth, alveoli continue to be produced in large numbers for about 3 years and this process is complete by about 8 years of age.

Breathing movements with aspiration of amniotic fluid occur for several months before birth. These stimulate lung development and may help to condition the respiratory muscles. Lung growth is also inhibited by lack of space and inadequate amniotic fluid (**oligohydramnios**).

RESPIRATORY SYSTEM CHANGES AT NORMAL DELIVERY

At birth, passage through the pelvis expels much of the amniotic fluid contained within the lungs (although this does not occur with caesarean sections), the baby takes its first breath and the placental circulation ceases. Before the first breath, the alveoli are not inflated and their small size means that the surface tension is high, and pressures in the order of 30 cmH_2O are needed to inflate an excised lung of a full-term baby. This presents little difficult as the baby can develop pressures of 90 cmH_2O during the first respiratory effort. Most babies take their first breath within 20 seconds of delivery. Rhythmic respiration of about 30 per minute (range 14–60) is reached within 90 seconds. Average tidal volume is 17 mL, with a crying vital capacity of 56–110 mL. The stimulants to initiate respiration at birth are probably cooling of the skin and mechanical. The release of the compression caused by passage through the birth canal will also passively draw air into the lungs.

Inflation of the lungs and reduction of the hypoxic pulmonary vasoconstriction following the first breath causes a decrease in the resistance to pulmonary circulation. This coupled with the rise in the systemic circulation causes the right atrial pressure to fall below the left atrial pressure and results in closure of the foramen ovale, which is then followed by closure of the ductus arteriosus (see Ch. 11). The pulmonary capillaries and the relatively large lymphatic vessels in the fetal lung allow remaining fluid to be reabsorbed rapidly from the lungs. In stillborn infants this does not occur, so their lungs are filled with fluid, not air.

RESPIRATORY DISTRESS SYNDROME OF THE NEWBORN

Respiratory distress syndrome of the newborn (RDS) is usually caused by a deficiency in surfactant and often occurs in premature infants. The lungs contain a protein-rich fluid which has a glassy, membranous appearance. With low surfactant levels, lung compliance is decreased, and the work of inflating the stiff lungs is increased. In newborn infants, the ribs are more easily deformed (compliant) than the lungs, so breathing results in deep sternal retractions but poor air entry. Rapid, laboured, grunting respirations will usually develop immediately or within a few hours after delivery.

Surfactant production can be increased by the administration of corticosteroids, which stimulate lung development and surfactant production, although this is of little use in an emergency delivery. However, the administration of exogenous surfactant can also aid breathing and reduce the severity of RDS.

Newborn infants have a lower p_aO_2 than adults, 50–70 mmHg compared with 100 mmHg in adults. At these levels the fetal haemoglobin is almost fully saturated due to the higher affinity for O_2 of fetal haemoglobin. While most cases of RDS in the neonate are due to prematurity there are rare cases because of other causes, including congenital absence of a component of surfactant.

The renal system

Malcolm Segal

INTRODUCTION

The kidney is an essential organ for life and plays a central role in homeostasis. Homeostasis, originally defined by the great French physiologist Claude Bernard, refers to the stability and maintenance of the internal environment of the body; the so called 'milieu intérieur' (see Ch. 1). Key renal functions may be deduced from what happens when the kidneys cease to function or fail.

FUNCTIONS OF THE KIDNEY

The functions of the kidneys may be summarised as:

- Homeostasis – consisting of filtration, when the blood is filtered to remove waste products of metabolism and toxic substances but retains essential nutrients, which is followed by reabsorption and secretion of water and essential electrolytes, to maintain acid–base balance, water (fluid) and electrolyte balance, and a normal blood pressure. Urine is produced in the process.
- Hormone secretion – independent of the endocrine system, the kidneys secrete erythropoietin to stimulate red cell production, renin as part of the blood pressure control mechanism, and the active form of vitamin D.

   Therefore, the kidney:

- Controls the volume, osmolarity and acid–base balance of the plasma and extracellular fluid
- Controls the level of electrolytes in blood and extracellular fluid (ECF)
- Recovers all the small molecules filtered by the nephron, such as sugars and amino acids
- Excretes nitrogenous waste and 'fixed' acid from protein metabolism, mainly urea, uric acid and creatinine

- Excretes a variety of toxic metabolites and excess electrolytes and water
- Maintains red cell production by the secretion of the hormone, erythropoietin
- Produces the active form of vitamin D and hence maintains calcium balance
- Controls blood pressure over the long term.

URINE VOLUME AND COMPOSITION

In a healthy person the kidneys form about 1.5–2 L of urine every 24 hours, which is equivalent to 1 mL/min entering the bladder. Urine composition differs from plasma:

- First, the levels of urinary nitrogenous waste products, mostly in the form of urea and ammonia, are much higher, whereas protein, glucose and amino acids are all very much lower.
- Second, although in any given 24 hours the total amount of any urinary constituent, such as salts (NaCl, KCl, $NaHCO_3$) and urea, are excreted at a fairly constant rate, the volume of water in which they are contained can vary widely, so that the amount of solute excreted is independent of the volume of urine.

   Normally, urine is a slightly acidic, pale yellow fluid, with a pH of about 6. However, when large volumes of water are ingested, it can rapidly change to an almost colourless fluid, the excreted volume matching the intake and the osmolarity falling to a minimum of 50 mOsm. In contrast, if sweating is increased by hard exercise or if the water intake is restricted, the volume of urine will fall and a dark concentrated fluid is produced with an osmolarity which can rise to 1400 mOsm. Plasma has a constant osmolarity of just less than 300 mOsm (285 mOsm).

Osmolarity measures the concentration of 'particles' that are capable of exerting osmotic pressure, so that the osmolarity of a solution reflects the number of 'particles' in a given volume of fluid that can exert an osmotic pressure across a membrane. The kidneys are vital in keeping the osmolarity of blood and the ECF constant. The kidneys are therefore a key element in the control of electrolytes and acid–base balance in the body. Sodium as NaCl and $NaHCO_3$ is conserved, whereas potassium is eliminated and 'fixed' acid is excreted in the form of ammonia and phosphate ions in the urine.

Table 14.1	Water balance and factors which disturb the balance		
Sources for the input of water	**Litres**	**Sources of output**	**Litres**
Water content in food	1.0	Urine osmotic load	0.7
Food metabolism	0.5	Urine from choice drinking	0.8
Drinking minimum	0.5	Lungs and airways	0.4
Drinking by choice	1.0	Skin insensible loss	1.0
		Faeces	0.1
Total	3.0	Total	3.0

Factors disturbing balance	Composition and route
Hyperventilation/fever	Loss of pure H_2O – diffusion through skin
Sweating	H_2O + Na^+, Cl^- – sweat glands and ducts
Air conditioning (dry air)	0.5–1 L per day pure H_2O – diffusion into lungs
Diarrhoea – cholera	20 L in 48 h Na^+, Cl^-, HCO_3^-, K^+– small bowel/colon
Lactation – milk	Isotonic salts – milk secretion, breasts

BALANCE OF FLUID INTAKE AND LOSS

In a healthy human being, the daily intake of water roughly equals loss in the steady state. The principal source of water is drinking water and other fluids and in food (oral), and most of the loss is in urine, via the kidneys. Some water is lost as 'insensible loss', via respiration, skin, sweating and faeces. Table 14.1 shows the approximate balance of the total intake and loss of water by the body over 24 hours and the electrolyte balance, and the factors that can disturb this balance.

RENAL FAILURE

In a person whose kidneys are beginning to fail, there is at first no detectable sign or symptom of damage, since human beings have a massive overcapacity in renal function. Few changes are seen until three-quarters of the normal renal function is lost. An early sign of renal failure is a rising blood urea concentration. Figure 14.1 shows blood urea concentration plotted against creatinine clearance, which measures the glomerular filtration rate (GFR) by all the nephrons (see later). In healthy individuals, the GFR is a very large volume of fluid – 125 mL/min in the young male (equivalent to 180 L per 24 h). For a normal person on a mixed diet the level of plasma urea is about 5 mM and it does not begin to change until the GFR has fallen by about 75%.

However, this response does depend on the diet – a high protein intake of a meat eater would cause the plasma urea to rise more rapidly in renal disease, whereas a vegetarian

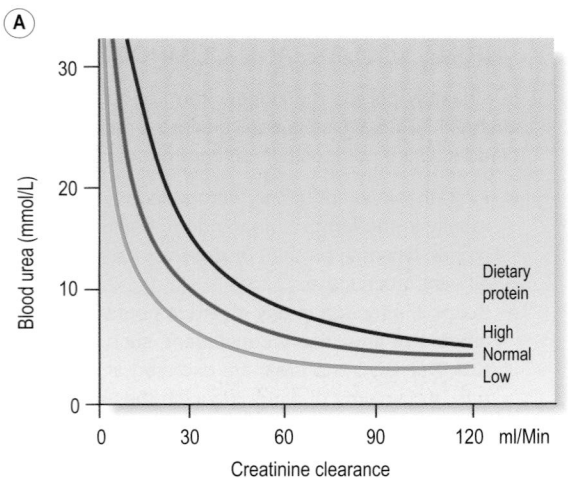
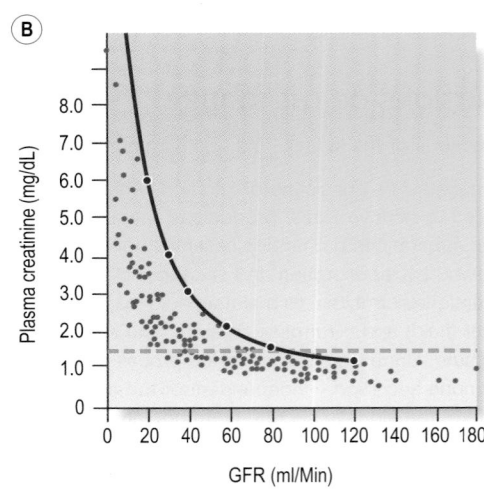

Fig. 14.1 **(A) The relationship between blood urea concentration and creatinine clearance showing the effect of high, normal and low protein intakes. (B) Relationship between true glomerular filtration rate (GFR) (as measured by inulin clearance) and plasma creatinine concentration in 171 patients with glomerular disease.** The *open circles* joined by the *solid red line* represent the relationship that would exist if creatinine were excreted solely by glomerular filtration; the *dotted line* represents the upper limit of 'normal' for plasma creatinine concentration of 1.4 mg/dL. In the patients (*dark dots*), variations in GFR between 129 and 60 mL/min were often associated with a plasma creatinine concentration that remained within the normal range due to increased creatinine excretion, which becomes saturated at a plasma concentration above 1.5–2 mg/dL; as a result, plasma creatinine concentration rises as expected with further reductions in GFR. Redrawn with permission from Richards P, Truniger B 1983 Understanding water electrolytes and acid base balance. William Heinemann, London.

The consequences of renal failure are related to kidney functions other than fluid balance and excretion, which include:

- Hypertension – the kidneys secrete the enzyme renin in response to impaired renal perfusion. Renin activates angiotensin-converting enzyme (ACE) to convert angiotensin I to angiotensin II, which is a powerful systemic vasoconstrictor and stimulates aldosterone secretion to promote sodium and water retention (see below and Ch. 4). Chronic disruption of the renin-angiotensin-aldosterone system in renal failure leads to hypertension. Pharmacological treatment with ACE inhibitors is used in the management of hypertension (see below). Before the advent of effective hypotensive drugs, nephrectomy was performed to prevent renal hypertension.
- Anaemia – renal interstitial cells secrete erythropoietin, which stimulates red cell production (see Ch. 12). Destruction of renal tissue in chronic renal failure results in erythropoietin deficiency.
- Vitamin D deficiency – the distal convoluted tubules secrete the enzyme 1α-hydroxylase. Naturally occurring vitamin D needs to be hydroxylated to an active metabolite in the liver, then further converted by 1α-hydroxylase to produce the metabolically active 1,25-dihydroxychlolecalciferol (vitamin D_3). Chronic renal failure thus leads to disorders of bone (renal osteodystrophy), calcium metabolism and secondary hyperparathyroidism (see Chs 10 and 16).
- Hypoproteinaemia – the persistent and chronic urinary protein loss in chronic renal failure leads to hypoproteinaemia, which can lead to impaired protein binding with consequent adverse reactions from therapeutic agents (see Ch. 4), wasting and malnutrition (see Ch. 16).
- Other metabolic complications – e.g. defective excretion of urate leads to gout; defective insulin excretion may lead to hypoglycaemia in insulin-dependent diabetics.
- Other endocrine disorders – these may arise owing to defective protein binding of hormones consequent to hypoproteinaemia (e.g. thyroid hormone), or impairment of hormone action and excretion (e.g. hyperprolactinaemia leading to gynaecomastia in men, growth retardation secondary to complex defects of growth hormone secretion and action in uraemic children).
- Neurological complications – severe, persistent uraemia depresses cerebral function and may lead to convulsions (see also Ch. 3).

diet would delay this rise until an even greater loss of renal function had occurred. Often, prior to the rise in plasma urea, the blood pressure begins to increase to high levels at rest (hypertension) and this can be an early warning sign of renal problems.

In addition to the raised blood urea (uraemia), the level of creatinine also increases. Creatinine is a product of muscle metabolism and is normally formed at a fixed rate related to the muscle mass. The plasma level is normally constant at about 0.06–0.12 mM and only becomes raised in renal failure. Creatinine is mostly filtered and can also be used as an index of GFR.

Another sign of renal failure is cloudy and frothy urine caused by protein and cells appearing in the urine. In time, in response to the protein loss, there is peripheral oedema, an elevation of plasma potassium from its normal value of 4 mM and a fall in plasma pH (raised H^+, i.e. acidosis). These two latter changes lead to cardiac arrhythmias and finally to death.

ANATOMY OF THE KIDNEY

GROSS STRUCTURE

The adult kidneys are two 'bean'-shaped structures weighing about 150 g each, lying on either side of the vertebral column (at about the level of T12–L3) in the midline, but outside the peritoneum in the abdominal cavity (retroperitoneal). The concave aspect of each kidney faces medially (towards the vertebral column). Here, the hilum (an opening in the medial aspect of the kidney) allows passage of the renal artery and vein, nerve supply and ureters (Fig. 14.2).

The kidney consists of two layers, an outer cortex and an inner medulla (see Fig. 14.2), contained in a thick inelastic capsule. The thickness of the capsule is necessary to withstand the high tissue pressure of 10 mmHg generated within the tissue ECF by the filtration process.

The renal cortex lies under the capsule, and contains the renal corpuscles and tubules (apart from the 'hairpin' loop of Henle), blood vessels and the cortical collecting ducts (see below). The renal filtration processes take place in the cortex. The renal medulla, which is deep to the cortex, is made up of 10–20 pyramids containing the numerous loops of Henle, collecting ducts and blood vessels.

Renal pyramids

In longitudinal section, the kidney is divided into a number of conical structures, the renal pyramids (see Fig. 14.2). The gross structure also reflects the highly organised microstructure with linear feature, the medullary rays, arranged into the inner and outer stripes. These are related to the capillary networks and to the straight tubular elements of the loop of Henle, the vasa recta and the collecting ducts (see below). The tip of each pyramid forms a papilla which is enclosed in a funnel-shaped extension of the renal pelvis, the calyx. It is these structures which collect the urine draining from the collecting ducts and merge together to form the renal pelvis. Urine in the renal pelvis is then carried by peristaltic waves down the ureter and into the bladder.

THE NEPHRON

The fundamental unit of the kidney is the nephron, of which there are some 1.5 million in each kidney. Each nephron consists of the renal corpuscle, where the primary urine is first formed, and the renal tubule, a highly coiled tube where this primary urine is modified. A simplified overall structure of the nephron is shown in Fig. 14.3.

The renal corpuscle

The renal corpuscle, the filter in the kidney sited in the cortex, consists of the glomerulus, which is a knot of capillaries, surrounded by the Bowman's capsule where fluid is forced out of the plasma into Bowman's space to form the glomerular filtrate. Bowman's capsule, also known as the glomerular capsule, elongates to become the renal tubule.

The renal tubule

The renal tubule is the reabsorptive part of the renal system. It is a highly convoluted structure, varying in size throughout its length, consisting of:

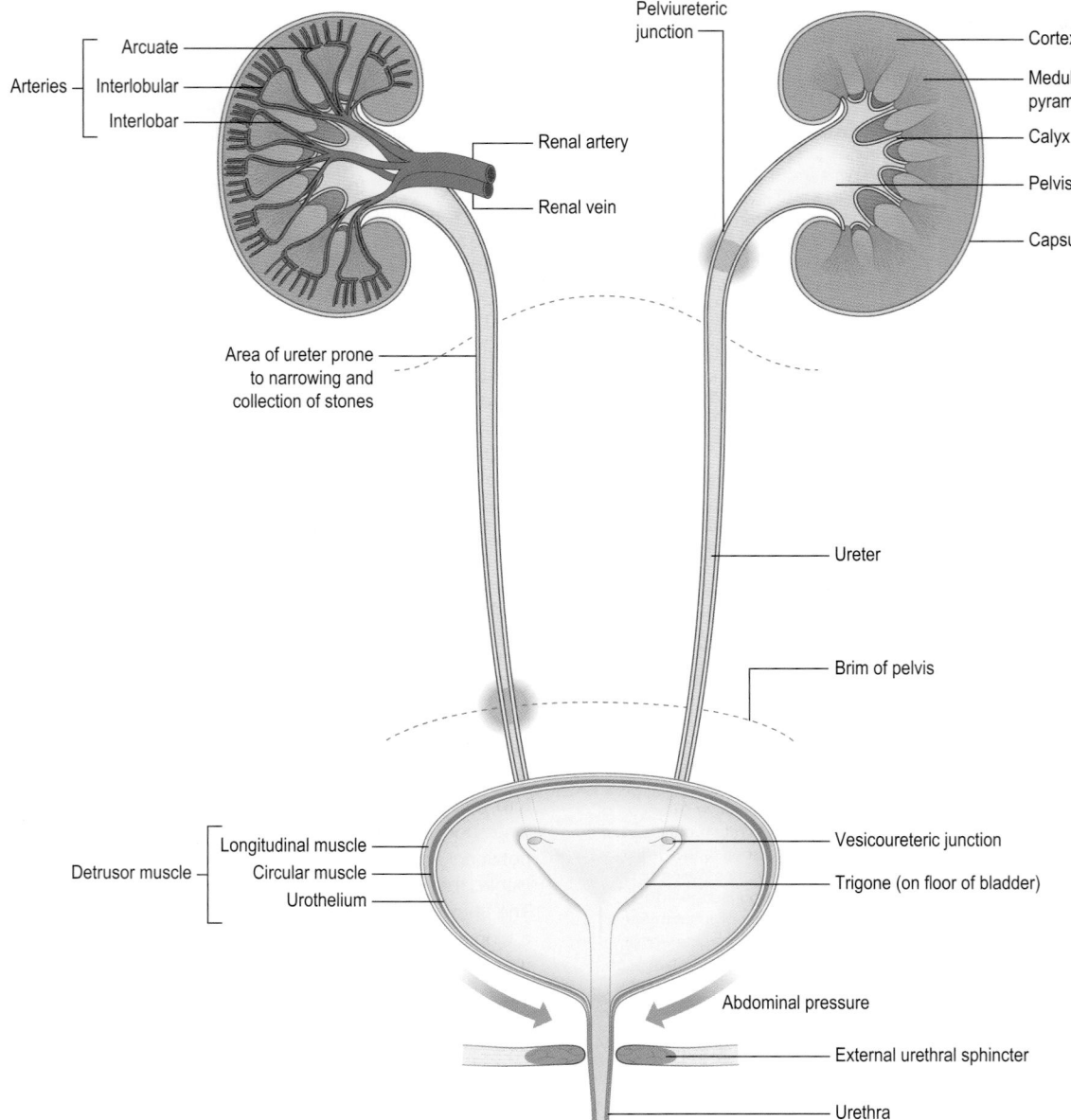

Fig. 14.2 The major components of the urinary tract and bladder. Note the pelviureteric junction, the brim of the pelvis and the vesicoureteric junction, which are sites where renal stones can lodge and impede urine flow, so causing back pressure and renal damage.

- Proximal convoluted tubule
- Loop of Henle
- Distal convoluted tubule
- Collecting ducts.

Although originating in the renal cortex, the renal tubule descends into the medulla as the hairpin loop of Henle (see below), which doubles back so that the distal convoluted tubule returns to the cortex ending next to the glomerulus of the same nephron.

Proximal convoluted tubule (PCT)

The fluid formed by the glomerular capillaries flows from Bowman's space along the nephron into the highly coiled structure of the PCT. In the PCT the cells have fine microvilli on the luminal side (urine side). Each cell is joined to the others around it, close to the luminal boundary, by an occlud-

ing band of tight junctions. The base of each cell (blood side) is inwardly convoluted in many folds which interdigitate with the cells around it. These structures enormously expand the surface of the cell for exchange processes. The cells are also filled with mitochondria, which are always present in cells that are metabolically active and use energy generated from glucose and oxygen.

Loop of Henle

After the PCT, the nephron then descends from the cortex towards the medulla via the hairpin loop of Henle. There are three types of loop:

- Loops from juxtaglomerular nephrons which are very long and extend all the way down to the renal pyramids (medulla).

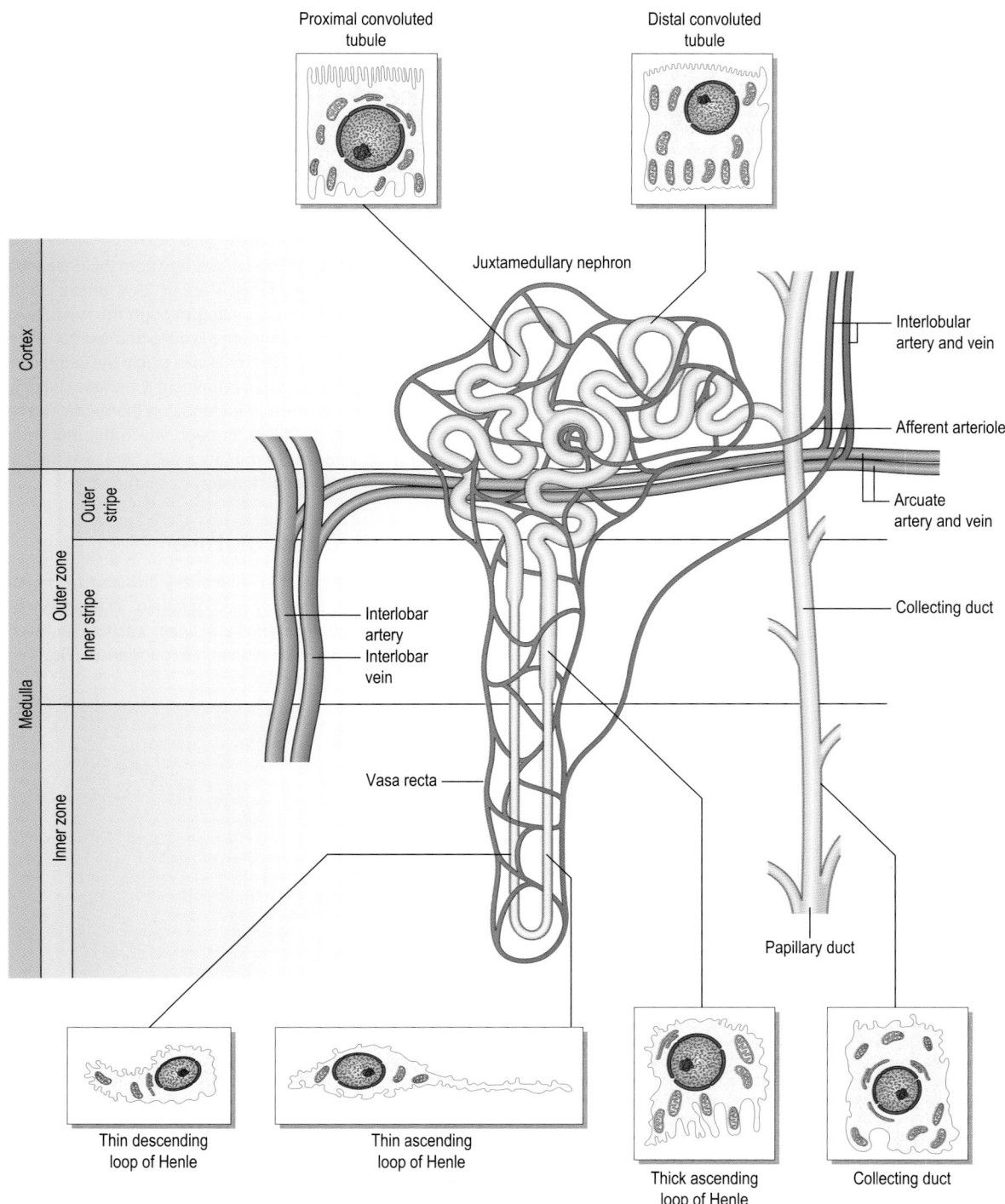

Proximal convoluted tubule

Distal convoluted tubule

Juxtamedullary nephron

Cortex

Outer stripe

Outer zone

Inner stripe

Medulla

Inner zone

Interlobar artery

Interlobar vein

Vasa recta

Interlobular artery and vein

Afferent arteriole

Arcuate artery and vein

Collecting duct

Papillary duct

Thin descending loop of Henle

Thin ascending loop of Henle

Thick ascending loop of Henle

Collecting duct

Fig. 14.3 **Structure of the nephron.** Primary urine formed within the glomerulus is modified during its passage along the kidney tubules before entering the collecting duct from where it goes to the bladder for excretion. The zones of the kidney are shown on the left hand side with the major blood vessels that supply the kidney. The nephron shown is the juxtaglomerular nephron, consisting of the proximal convoluted tubule (PCT), which dips deep into the medulla as the thin descending loop of Henle then bends acutely as the thin ascending loop of Henle and then becomes the thick ascending loop. The thick ascending loop of Henle emerges into the cortex to form the distal convoluted tubule (DCT). The DCTs merge to form the collecting duct which again descends into the medulla and forms the urine. The changing morphology of the tubule walls reflects the differences in permeability and function. The macula densa, a densely packed group of specialised cells lining the DCT, is at the top of the thick ascending loop of Henle, a key site for the control of sodium balance. Some nephrons only penetrate into the outer medulla, the cortical nephrons. It is thought the nephrons with the longest loops of Henle are responsible for forming the most concentrated urine.

- Loops from cortical nephrons which are short and only reach the cortex/medulla border. About 80% of nephrons have short loops.
- A few intermediate loops between the above types.

The functional reasons for the differences in the length of the loops are not fully understood but desert animals that produce a highly concentrated urine have the highest proportion of the long loops. The loop of Henle consists of several cell types; the bulk of this structure is the thin descending and thin ascending loops. The cells of this region are sparse in number, and are narrow with few infoldings on either face and few mitochondria. The loop of Henle is amazingly long, the length being about 1000 times the diameter, and if Fig. 14.3 was drawn to scale, it would be as high as a 20-storey building! After the thin ascending loop, the next section undergoes a major change in structure becoming the thick ascending loop. The cells in this section are thick, complex and rich both in mitochondria and cellular inclusions which reflects their active transport functions.

Distal convoluted tubule

Fluid now leaves the loop of Henle and enters the DCT, which is in the renal cortex. Here, 10–15% of ions and fluid of the filtrate are recovered. Tubules from five to six nephrons then merge to form the larger collecting duct, which re-enters the renal medulla. Up to this point the fluid recovery is a fixed proportion of that which has been filtered, and is said to be constitutive.

Collecting ducts (CD)

The CDs are derived from a different embryological origin than the rest of the nephron, and are divided into a cortical section (CCD) and a medullary section (MCD). In these ducts the fluid recovery can be varied either to produce a dilute or a concentrated urine under the influence of the antidiuretic hormone (ADH), also called vasopressin (see below).

RENAL VASCULATURE

Each kidney is supplied by a large artery from the descending aorta and together they receive about 20% of the cardiac output (1.2 L/min). After circulating through the medulla and cortex, blood from renal capillaries is collected in renal venules and leaves the kidney via the renal vein to join the inferior vena cava. The kidneys also have a prominent lymphatic drainage.

The renal arteries enter the kidney on the medial surface of each kidney via the hilum, through which the renal artery enters and the veins and lymphatics exit; here also the renal nerves enter and leave the kidney.

Renal microvasculature

On entering the kidney, the renal artery divides to form interlobar vessels, which supply each pyramid. These then subdivide to form arcuate arteries and finally interlobular arteries supplying the grape-like glomerular capillaries (Fig. 14.4), where the renal filtrate is formed.

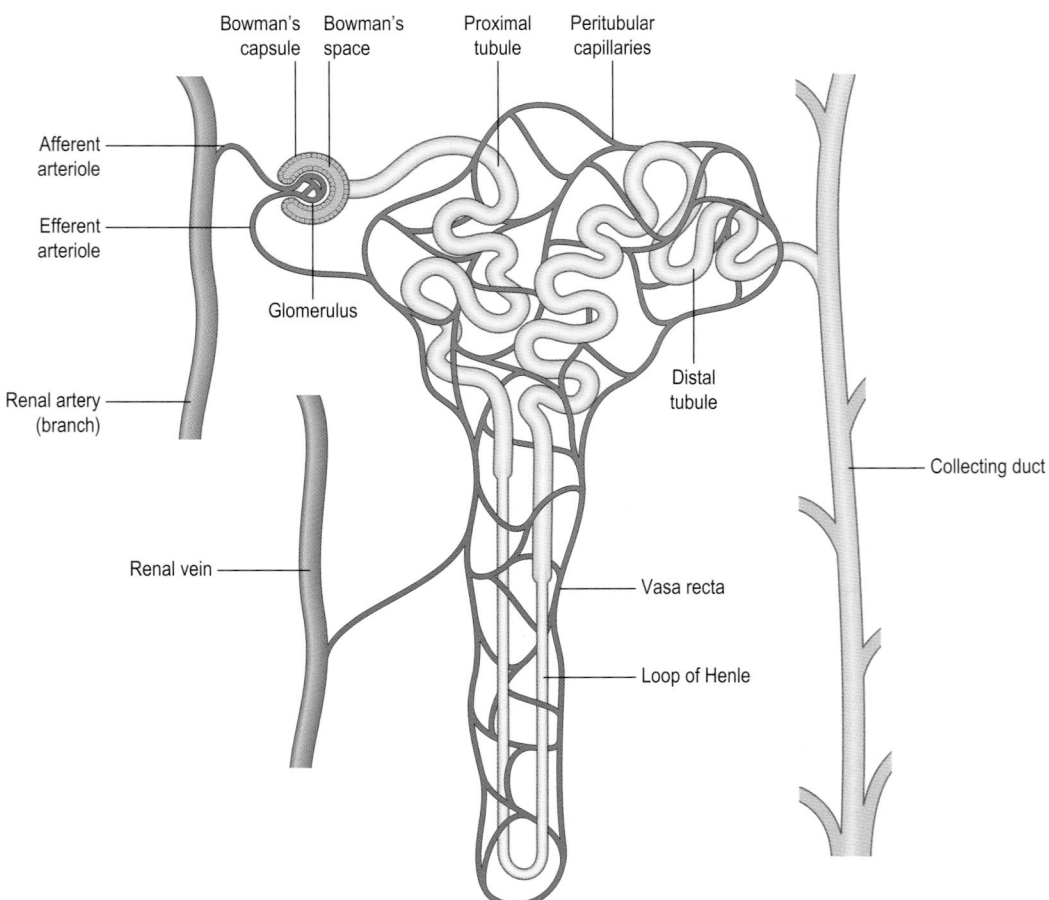

***Fig. 14.4* Renal vasculature.** The blood supply originates from the renal artery (*red*) and leaves via the renal vein (*blue*). Blood passes through two capillary beds, the glomerular capillaries followed by the vasa recta.

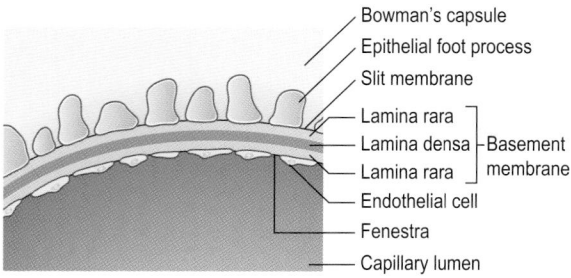

Fig. 14.5 **Glomerular capillary wall.** The structure of the glomerular capillary wall, which is the filtration pathway. By Cuppage from Sullivan and Grantham 1982.

The arterial supply enters the start of the nephron at the blind-ended dilation, the Bowman's capsule, and divides into a knot of capillaries, the glomerulus. The glomerular capillaries are unusual in that they have an arteriole at the start of the capillary bed, the afferent arteriole, and a second arteriole, the efferent arteriole, at the end of the glomerulus, where the capillaries combine to emerge from Bowman's capsule.

Peritubular capillaries

The glomerular capillaries reunite into an efferent arteriole which then divides again to form a second capillary bed becoming either the peritubular capillaries, which envelop both the proximal and distal convoluted tubules, or descend as looped capillaries into the medulla of the kidney as the vasa recta around the loop of Henle (see Fig. 14.4).

Blood flowing through the glomerular capillaries is under high pressure, whereas the tubular capillaries and vasa recta are under low pressure.

Glomerular filtration barrier

Filtration of the blood entering the glomerulus at the afferent arteriole relies on the permeability of the glomerular capillary walls that make up the filtration bed, which is characterised by (Fig. 14.5):

- Fenestrations (holes) in the layer of endothelial cells lining the capillary walls.
- Podocytes (foot processes), which are finger-like projections of the capillary epithelium that interdigitate and enclose and strengthen the vessels, so enabling them to withstand the large filtration pressures which are needed to form the urinary filtrate.
- A basement membrane consisting of a fibrillar network of matrix proteins, rather like an irregular fishing net, but with holes of a fairly consistent size. Each of these 'holes' has negative charges on the surface of the matrix, so molecules with a similar charge would be repelled by these charges. In health, this prevents negatively charged molecules from being filtered out of the blood (see below). Matrix proteins consist of type IV collagen, laminin, fibronectin, entactin, other negatively charged glycoproteins and sulphated glycosaminoglycans such as heparin sulphate.

To form the filtrate, fluid has to pass across both the fenestrated capillary wall and the wall of the nephron prior to entering the Bowman's space.

Clinical box 14.2   Renal failure

Renal failure occurs when glomerular filtration is compromised from a variety of causes, but may also be the consequence of renal tubular function:

- Prerenal – due to depressed renal vascular perfusion so that the hydrostatic filtration forces are reduced (see below). Effective glomerular filtration cannot occur, e.g. from cardiac failure, hypotension from massive blood or fluid loss.
- Renal – due to disease of the nephron; the glomeruli and or microvasculature, or the tubules, e.g. microvascular disease as in diabetes mellitus (see Ch. 3), nephrotoxic drugs, acute tubular necrosis.
- Postrenal – due to obstruction anywhere in the outflow system; the renal pyramid (calyces, pelvis), ureters, down to the bladder neck, or recurrent ascending infections (e.g. pyelonephritis).

Renal failure may be acute or chronic:

- **Acute renal failure** is the sudden deterioration of renal function, which is usually reversible over time. When severe, the consequent fluid and biochemical disturbances may be life-threatening and constitute a medical emergency. Management of acute renal failure is aimed to correct the fluid and biochemical imbalance during the time needed for renal function to recover. Dietary controls of electrolyte, nitrogen and water intake (see Ch. 16); pharmacological interventions (see Ch. 4) and dialysis to remove toxic products of metabolism and excess fluid may be necessary.
- **Chronic renal failure** is a longstanding and progressive impairment of renal excretory function, which may be insidious in onset. The biochemical abnormalities may be undetected for long periods. Causes of chronic renal failure may be congenital (see below), and include glomerular or vascular disease. Treatment is aimed at controlling the biochemical and fluid imbalances (including chronic dialysis), and at the cause, e.g. tight glycaemic control in diabetes mellitus, and to manage complications. Renal transplantation may ultimately be needed.

DEVELOPMENT OF THE KIDNEY

In humans, the embryonic kidneys originate from the intermediate mesoderm (see Ch. 10). The reproductive organs and adrenal cortex also develop from the intermediate mesoderm. The tissues that are destined to become permanent kidneys are preceded by embryonic structures, most of which degenerate and atrophy before birth. There are three stages in the development of these embryonic structures:

- Pronephros
- Mesonephros
- Metanephros.

Pronephros

Cells that develop into the **pronephros** originate in the intermediate mesoderm. Structures known as the cervical nephrostomes, at the level of the fifth cervical to the third thoracic segments, grow as evaginations from the segments to fuse and extend in a caudal direction (downwards) to form a series of ducts, the **pronephric ducts (or nephric ducts)**. Within the ducts, glomeruli develop. The pronephric ducts and glomeruli make up the pronephros. The Wolffian duct forms below the pronephric duct (see Ch. 10). The pronephros is

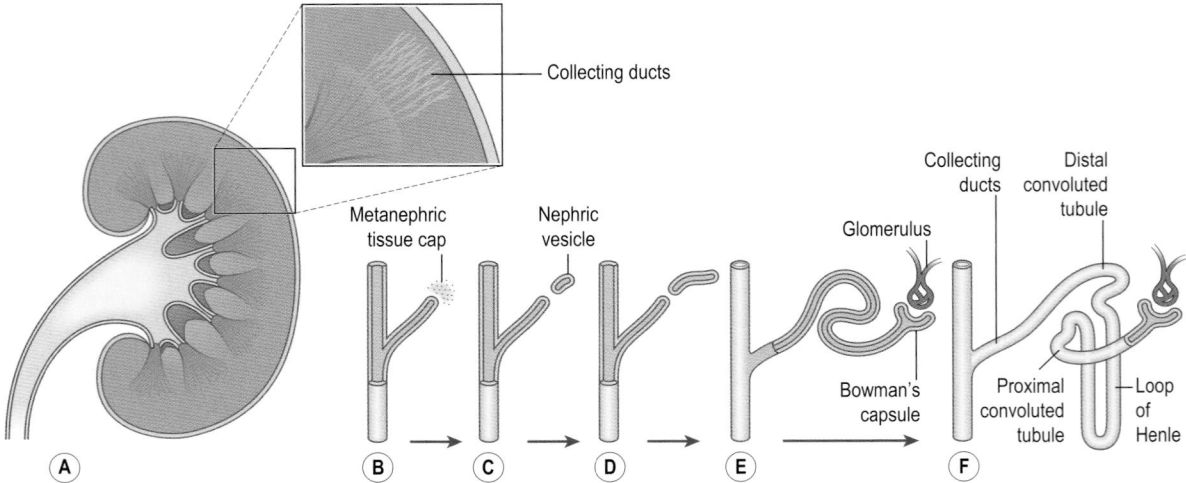

Fig. 14.6 **Development of the renal collecting system and nephrons.** (A) The ureteric buds continue to bifurcate until the 32nd week, producing 1–3 million collecting ducts (B–F). The tip of each collecting duct induces the development of a metanephric tissue cap, which differentiates into a renal vesicle. This vesicle ultimately forms a Bowman's capsule and the proximal and distal convoluted tubules and loop of Henle. Functional nephric units (of the type shown in (E)) first appear in distal regions of the metanephros at 10 weeks. Redrawn with permission from Larsen WJ 1998 Essentials of human embryology. Churchill Livingstone, Edinburgh.

not functional, and rapidly degenerates and disappears at an early stage.

Mesonephros

The **mesonephros** originates in the cell mass on the medial side of the Wolffian duct (from about the sixth thoracic to the third lumbar segment), developing into a series of tubules. One end of the tubules dilates and is invaginated by capillaries to form glomeruli. The mesonephros is functional until the fifth gestational week, but atrophies rapidly from the sixth week onwards.

Metanephros

The **metanephros** is destined to become the permanent kidney. It arises partly from the caudal end of the intermediate mesoderm and partly from the Wolffian duct. At about the fifth or sixth week of gestation, the Wolffian duct develops a diverticulum, the ureteric bud, which eventually becomes the renal pelvis and calyces (proximal and distal convoluted tubules, loop of Henle, collecting tubules), and the ureters. The ureteric bud invades the cell mass of the intermediate mesoderm, when cells from the mesoderm migrate over the ureteric bud and differentiate to eventually form the excretory part of the kidneys, the **nephrons** (the renal cortex, glomeruli). The metanephros migrates upwards to the lumbar region to take up the lumbar position of the adult kidney. The ureters elongate as the metanephros ascends.

PERMANENT KIDNEY

The ureteric buds bifurcate until the 32nd week producing 1–3 million collecting ducts (Fig. 14.6). At the tip of each is a metanephric tissue cap (Fig. 14.6B metanephric blastema, containing cells capable of asexual division and differentiation) which forms the nephric vesicle (Fig. 14.6C). This eventually forms the Bowman's capsule and the rest of the nephron. As the vesicle elongates a capillary complex forms

near one end and invaginates into the tubule to form the Bowman's capsule and glomerulus (Fig. 14.6D–F).

Between the sixth and ninth week the kidneys ascend to a lumbar site just between the adrenal glands (Fig. 14.7). By the tenth week the metanephros has evolved into the cortex and medulla, and each 'tree' of collecting ducts drains into a minor calyx and converges to form the renal papilla. Urine produced by the fetus is excreted into the amniotic fluid but kidney function is not necessary until after birth.

Congenital renal agenesis

Congenital renal agenesis leads to the absence of one (unilateral renal agenesis) or both (bilateral renal agenesis)

Clinical box 14.3   **Congenital malformation of the kidneys and urinary tract**

Congenital malformations of the kidneys and urinary tract are relatively common. Many are asymptomatic and only detected during investigative (e.g. excretion urogram, ultrasound examination) or therapeutic procedures (e.g. laparotomy). Some conditions, however, lead to serious complications such as progressive renal failure, and require surgical interventions or even renal transplantation. The aetiology of the anomalies is generally unknown, but genetic mutation and chromosomal anomalies have been proposed. The congenital defects include:

- Defect in embryonic development owing to abnormal interaction between the ureteric bud and metanephric blastema, which may lead to **agenesis** (failure to develop), **hypo-** or **dysplasia** of the kidneys, **vesicoureteric reflux** (VUR) (see later, Clinical box 14.14) and congenital malformation of the ureters (ectopic or double ureters) among others.
- Hereditary autosomal dominant or autosomal recessive **polycystic kidney disease**.
- Embryological errors with one kidney failing to ascend (ectopic kidney) or the two kidneys fusing to form a horseshoe kidney, which is still functional and is only incidentally detected (Fig. 14.7E).

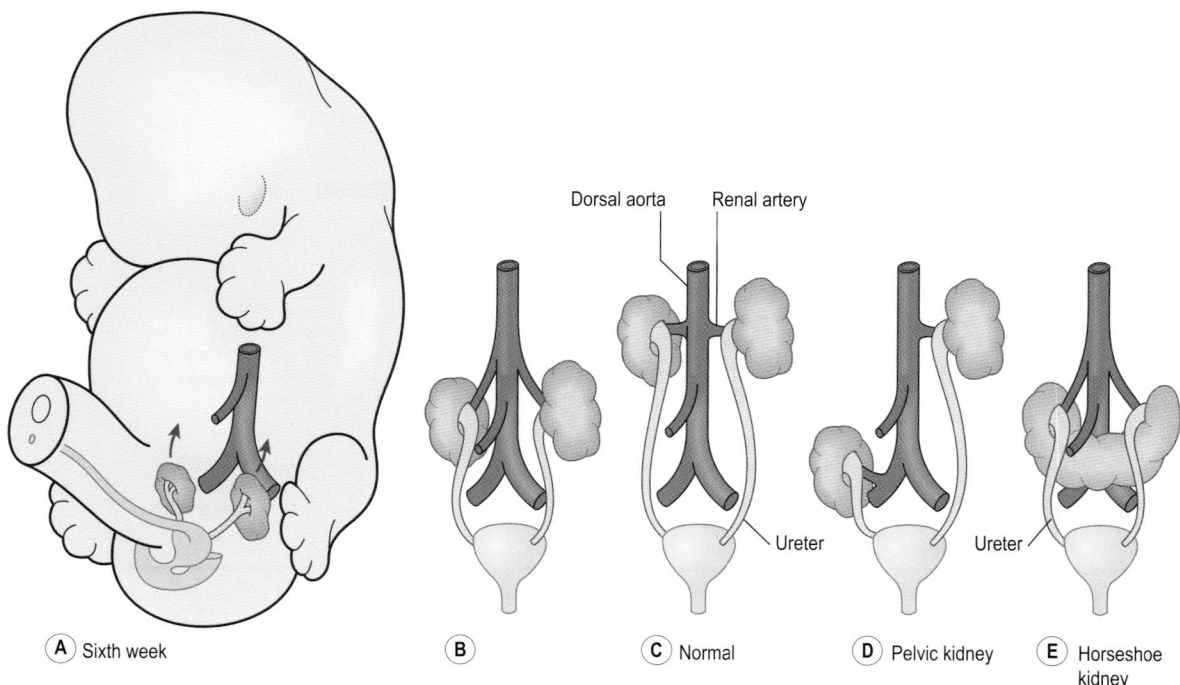

Dorsal aorta   **Renal artery**

Ureter

Ureter

(A) Sixth week   (B)   (C) Normal   (D) Pelvic kidney   (E) Horseshoe kidney

Fig. 14.7 **Normal and abnormal ascent of the kidneys from the pelvis.** (A–C) The metanephroi normally ascend from the sacral region of their definitive lumbar position between the sixth and ninth week. (D) Infrequently, a kidney may fail to ascend, resulting in a pelvic kidney. (E) If the inferior poles of the metanephroi make contact and fuse before ascent, the resulting horseshoe kidney catches under the inferior mesenteric artery. Redrawn with permission after Larsen WJ 1998 Essentials of human embryology. Churchill Livingstone, Edinburgh.

kidneys at birth. Bilateral renal agenesis is rare, but incompatible with life. While in utero, the absence of fetal kidneys leads to a deficiency in amniotic fluid production (**oligohydramnios** or **anhydramnios**). Without amniotic fluid to cushion the fetus, the fetal facial and other features become 'squashed'. The combination of absent kidneys, oligohydramnios and characteristic features is sometimes referred to as **Potter's syndrome** (also called **Potter's sequence, oligohydramnios sequence**). Unilateral renal agenesis is more common, but not life-threatening as long as the single kidney remains healthy.

Polycystic kidney disease

Polycystic kidney disease is characterised by multiple renal cysts. The autosomal dominant form of polycystic kidney disease (ADPKD) is a hereditary disorder presenting in adulthood, with associated other organ abnormalities (e.g. liver cysts). Autosomal recessive polycystic kidney disease (ARPKD) is rare, thought to be due to gene mutation, and fatal in early childhood.

RENAL FUNCTION

In healthy individuals, the kidneys filter 183 L of fluid in 24 hours, excreting 1.5 L to 2 L as urine (see above). They are also involved in the retention of essential nutrients such as protein and glucose; water, acid–base and electrolyte balance; and hormone secretion, as well as the excretion of waste products of metabolism. The complex processes concerned are:

- Filtration
- Reabsorption, which may be passive or selective
- Secretion.

Different parts of the nephron perform different functions. Fig. 14.8 is a simplified diagrammatic representation of how the nephron functions.

GLOMERULAR FILTRATION AND THE PRODUCTION OF PRIMARY URINE

Urine is formed by the capillary hydrostatic pressure forcing the water and salts of plasma through the wall of the glomerular capillaries, most probably through the gaps between the endothelial cells and through the fenestrae (regions of thinning of the wall) in the capillary wall (Fig. 14.5). The fluid then passes between the epithelial podocytes, and between these structures lies the **basement membrane**. This is the filter bed of the kidney and holds back plasma proteins from passing into the nephron (see above).

From measurements of the permeability of molecules of different sizes, all molecules of less than 12 000 molecular weight are filtered into the nephron. This implies that all electrolytes, sugars, amino acids, vitamins, etc., pass easily into the Bowman's capsule and then must be recovered by the rest of the nephron, back into the plasma.

Pore size and macromolecules

If it is assumed that the 'holes' (pores) in the basement membrane are tiny cylinders in the wall of about 1.4 nm in diameter, as the size of the molecule approaches the

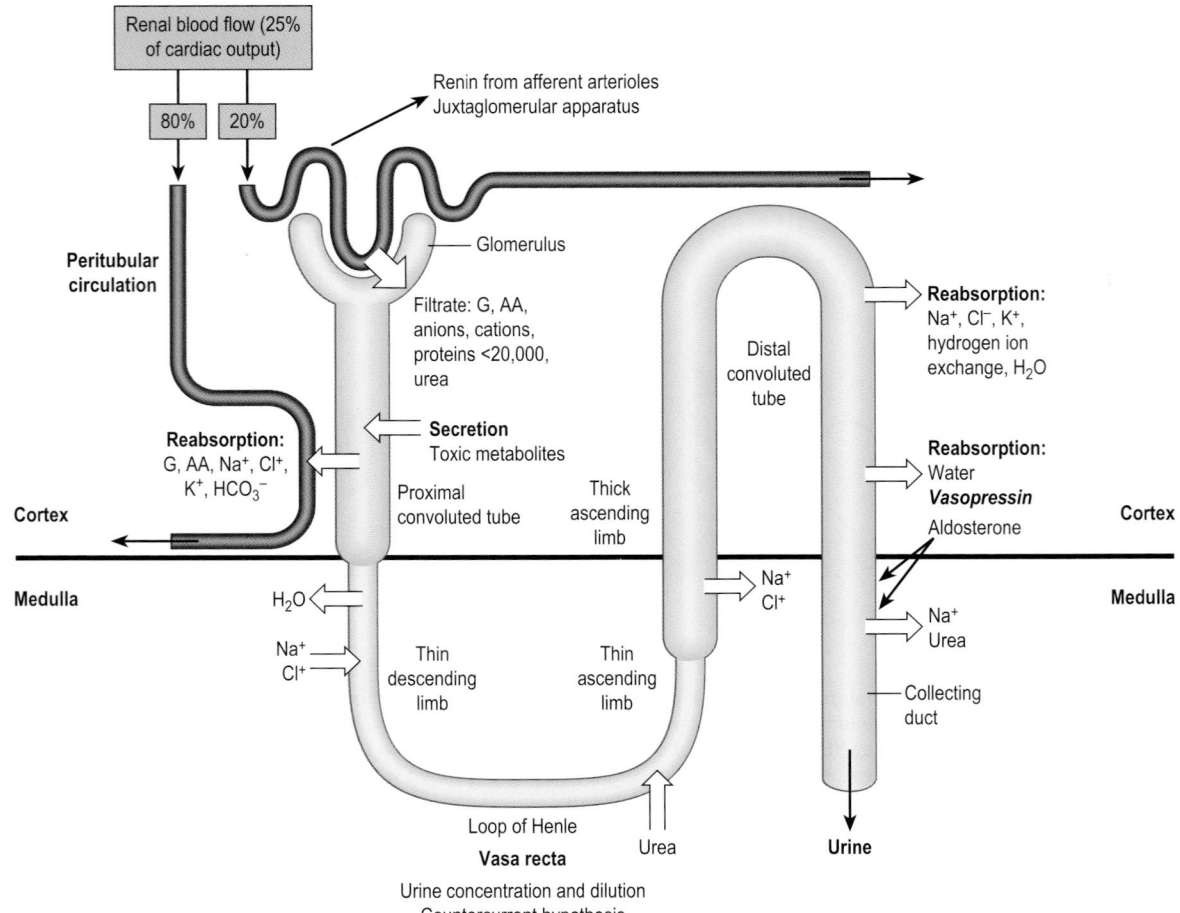

Fig. 14.8 Diagrammatic representation of major transport sites in the nephron. Apart from macromolecules, the glomerular filtrate contains glucose, amino acids, electrolytes such as Na^+, K^+, Cl^-, urea, bicarbonate and water. The PCT is the major site for reabsorption: 99% of the glucose is reabsorbed into the peritubular circulation, also essential nutrients and electrolytes. Bicarbonate reabsorption at the PCT affects renal acid–base homeostasis. Toxic metabolites, cations and anions are also secreted by the PCT. The loop of Henle is the major site for urine concentration according to the countercurrent hypothesis. Further NaCl and water reabsorption takes place in the DCT and CT, controlled by vasopressin and aldosterone. PCT, proximal convoluted tubule; DCT, distal convoluted tubule; CT, collecting tubule; G, glucose; AA, amino acid; G, glucose; HCO_3^-, bicarbonate.

diameter of the pore it will have less and less chance of being filtered. The size of a molecule is usually judged by its molecular weight (MW), but this can be misleading, since some molecules are spherical (globular) whereas others are long and thin. This latter group may get through into filtrate in small amounts by passing 'end on' through the pores, although from their molecular weight it could be assumed that they are far too large; this effect may explain why a small quantity of even the largest proteins do get filtered into the urine, although there may also be a small population of large pores.

However, the most critical factor that affects the filtration of a macromolecule is whether it has a surface charge. Haemoglobin (MW 67 000) escapes into the urine, whereas albumin (MW 62 000) although smaller is not filtered. This is related to the fact that although both molecules are globular proteins, albumin has a negative surface charge, so is held back by the repulsion of the charges on the fibrillar matrix of the basement membrane, whereas haemoglobin is not charged, so it can pass through relatively freely.

In disease states the surface charge on the fibrillar matrix can be disturbed and albumin now appears in the urine (albuminuria), which is a useful warning sign of impending renal failure.

Filtration forces

The hydrostatic pressure (HP) at the afferent arterioles as they enter the glomerulus is about 50 mmHg, which is about 15 mmHg higher than most other systemic capillaries. The capillary hydrostatic pressure only falls by 5 mmHg along the length of the glomerular capillary to 45 mmHg in the efferent arterioles. This large hydrostatic pressure and high permeability of the capillary walls causes a large fraction of fluid and small molecules to be filtered into the Bowman's capsule of the nephron. This 'outward' force is, however, balanced by the opposing pull of the plasma proteins which, being too large to pass through the wall, exert an osmotic force in the opposite direction to the hydrostatic pressure force. This is the colloid osmotic pressure (COP) or oncotic pressure of the plasma proteins and has a value of about 25 mmHg at the start of the glomerular capillaries. The COP gradually rises along the length of the capillary, as water and salts move out of the blood, so increasing the effective concentration of the plasma proteins. By about one third along the length of the glomerular capillary, the COP has risen to about 35 mmHg.

In addition, the movement of fluid into the Bowman's capsule surrounding the capillaries causes a rise in hydrostatic pressure of about 10 mmHg in the tubular pressure within this space, since the exit into the rest of the nephron is narrow. These two pressures balance the hydrostatic pressure so only about 20% of the volume of the blood is filtered into the nephron, as shown in Fig. 14.8. Note that in other systemic capillaries, the pressure in the extracellular fluid (ECF) is usually slightly negative (−0.5 mmHg).

The hydrostatic pressure of the blood draining from the glomerulus is 45 mmHg, as opposed to 12 mmHg in muscle capillaries. This high pressure is needed to drive the blood through the second capillary bed of the peritubular capillaries or through the vasa recta (see Fig. 14.4). The COP of the peritubular blood is also elevated to 30–35 mmHg, which also helps to draw fluid back into the peritubular capillaries.

Proteins

Proteins are mostly held back by the basement membrane. However, a small percentage is filtered and has to be recovered by the cells of the nephron as the filtrate passes down the renal tubule. This recovery is by the process of receptor-mediated endocytosis so the eventual loss of protein into the urine is small, usually about 50–80 mg per 24 hours.

FUNCTIONS OF THE PROXIMAL CONVOLUTED TUBULE (PCT)

The first segment of the tubular portion of the nephron, the PCT, has four main functions.

- It recovers some 70% of glomerular filtrate with respect to the filtered water and electrolytes.
- It reabsorbs most of the filtered sugars, amino acids, nucleosides and other small non-electrolytes.
- It is the prime site for both the recovery of bicarbonate and the generation of new bicarbonate depending on the arterial pCO_2.
- It secretes a number of organic acids and bases, as well as a wide variety of toxic and fat soluble molecules into the urine.

This latter function means that the level of these compounds is higher in the urine than in the blood capillaries (see below). Urinary organic acids and bases, toxic and fat soluble molecules can be in excess of endogenous molecules, from administered drugs or dietary sources. These functions involve a wide range of different types of transport and a large number of different carrier molecules (Fig. 14.9). Most of these processes require energy. The renal metabolic processes are aerobic, and consume large amounts of oxygen, almost equal to cardiac muscle.

Tight junctions

Each epithelial cell of the PCT is joined to those surrounding it by an occluding band of tight junctions close to the apical, or urine, side of the cells (rather like the plastic holding a 'six-pack' of soft drink cans); these junctions can vary in their

'tightness' or permeability. In the PCT they are 'moderately leaky', so although they slow the rate of passage of small molecules between cells, they do not permit steep gradients to be established between the lumen and the blood across the whole epithelium. Any concentration gradients established between the cells on the blood side of the PCT by the transport processes across the cell wall will osmotically draw fluid and some ions through these 'leaky' tight junctions. This process helps to recover water, salts and other small molecules back into the blood by a relatively low energy cost process. This recovery is also aided by **aquaporins** in the PCT cell membrane, which are specific water channels in the cell walls (see below) (Fig. 14.9A). The high permeability of the PCT enables a vast volume of fluid to be recovered at low energy cost. The PCT only uses about 5% of the total energy consumption of the kidney.

The sodium pump

The 'power house' which drives most of the processes in the kidney is the sodium pump (sodium–potassium pump, Na^+/K^+-ATPase pump). All cells in the body have the ability to pump sodium from inside the cell across the cell membrane into the ECF (see Ch. 1). The pump requires energy in the form of ATP, which is generated from oxygen and glucose. The pump must also have K^+ on the outside of the cell, and it usually pumps $3Na^+$ out of the cell for every $2K^+$ transferred in the opposite direction.

The walls of the epithelial cells of the PCT are polarised, which is to say, they have functionally different properties on the luminal (urine) side compared with the blood side of the cell (Fig. 14.9B). The sodium pumps are only found on the blood side of the cell, as tight junctions between the epithelial cells maintain the differential distribution of membrane proteins between apical and basal membranes, and this difference enables the cells to transport ions and non-electrolytes from the urinary filtrate back into the blood.

A rise in intracellular Na^+ concentration increases sodium pump activity, to 'pump' Na^+ ions out of the cell into the ECF. The pumping of sodium out of the cell, and a gradient in the opposite direction for K^+, creates a potential energy gradient across the cell wall that can be used to recover many substances from the glomerular filtrate.

Carrier proteins

In the membranes of all epithelial cells are a number of carrier proteins which can move ions across the cell walls on either the lumen or the blood side of the cell. These carriers use the potential energy of the gradients of Na^+ or K^+ ions set up by the sodium pump to move ions either both in the same direction or one goes 'out' and the other comes 'in'. This arrangement maintains the balance of positive and negative charges across the cell wall, i.e.

- A +ve ion and −ve ion go out together

or

- A +ve ion goes 'out' in exchange for a +ve ion coming 'in'.

The arrangement of these carriers is also different on the two sides of the cell and often certain ions such as K^+ are recirculated; being carried into the cell by one carrier then passing back out again either via an ion selective channel or

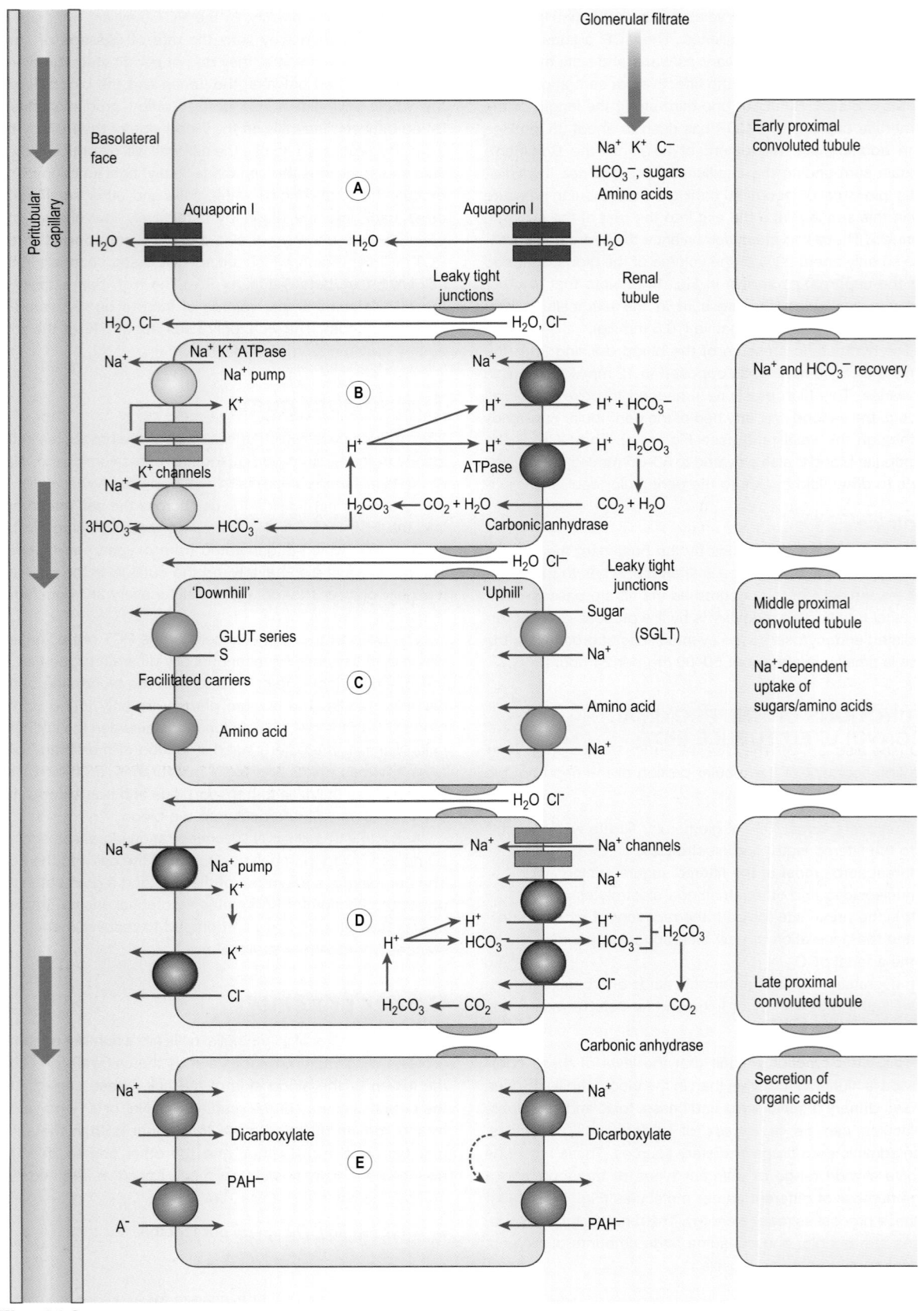

Fig. 14.9 **Functions of the proximal convoluted tubule (PCT).** (A) The glomerular capillaries filter all small ions, sugars and amino acids into the tubule at a rate related to their plasma concentrations and the GFR. (B) Filtered Na^+ is recovered in exchange for H^+ ions and by an ATPase dependent H^+ transport. (C) In the middle PCT sugars and amino acids are recovered by a Na^+ dependent uptake into the cells of the PCT, then moved into the blood by facilitated downhill carriers such as the GLUT series. (D) In the late PCT Na^+ is recovered by Na^+ channels. (E) The transport pathway for organic anion secretion. See text for further details. GLUT, glucose transporter; SGLT, sodium coupled glucose transporter; PAH, para-amino hippuric acid.

on another carrier. The overall effect of these carriers is to recover most of the filtered ions, as well as sugars and amino acids, from the tubular fluid back to the blood (Fig. 14.9B).

Ion channels

There are also membrane-spanning proteins which form ion channels that are selective for a specific ion which will move through a pathway formed by the transmembrane loops of protein. Ions move under the influence of the concentration gradient through these channels across the cell wall. Some ion channels can be in an 'open' state, which permits the ion to pass through, or a 'closed state' when the flow is impeded. These changes in opened or closed state, called 'gating', can be brought about by variation in the membrane potential or by ligands (chemical factors such as acetylcholine (ACh), cyclic nucleotides or G proteins) (see Ch. 4; Fig. 14.9B).

Recovery of bicarbonate by the PCT

Bicarbonate (HCO_3^-) is filtered at the same concentration as the blood, i.e. 24–26 mM, which represents some 4000 mM per 24 hours. The first segment of the PCT has cells which exchange Na^+ for H^+ ions using the Na^+ gradient to 'power' the process. This is an antiport process by which there is a balance in charge and is a major component in the recovery of filtered Na^+ (Fig. 14.9B). There is also an H^+-ATPase dependent process in this section which secretes the H^+ ions into the tubule but it is only a small part of the process and reduces the pH by the end of the PCT to 6.7.

The H^+ produced by these two processes reacts with the filtered HCO_3^- ions to form carbonic acid (H_2CO_3) which immediately dissociates non-enzymatically, to form CO_2 and H_2O (see also Ch. 3). The CO_2, being lipid soluble, crosses the lumen side of the cell membrane where the enzyme **carbonic anhydrase** is present, both bound to the cell wall and in the cytoplasm. In the cell, carbonic anhydrase catalyses the formation of H_2CO_3 from CO_2 and H_2O, speeding up the reaction many-fold, so that H_2CO_3 rapidly forms inside the cell, which again dissociates to form H^+ ions and HCO_3^- ions (Fig. 14.9B).

$$CO_2 + H_2O \rightleftharpoons H_2CO_3 \rightleftharpoons H^+ + HCO_3^-$$

Most of the bicarbonate is thus reabsorbed, and the H^+ ions are excreted in the urine. This is an important process in the renal control of acid–base balance (see below and also Chs 2 and 3).

Some of the H^+ ions are fed into the Na^+/H^+ antiport process so help to recover Na^+ ions. The Na^+ and the HCO_3^- are extruded into the blood on the basolateral side of the cell by the Na^+/K^+-ATPase and by a $Na^+/3HCO_3^-$ carrier (see Fig. 14.9B). These processes recover the filtered HCO_3^- and about 30% of the filtered Na^+; water will osmotically accompany the process, so aiding the fluid and ionic balance. Inhibition of carbonic anhydrase activity thus promotes the excretion of Na^+ and water (see also Ch. 4).

Water

As ions are moved into the ECF on the blood side of the proximal tubular epithelium, both between cells via the 'leaky' tight junctions and into the basal infoldings, osmotic forces are generated which draw water through the cell and across the tight junctions (Fig. 14.9). The passage of water through the lipid bilayer of the cell membranes has been something of a puzzle. The PCT recovers some 67% of 183 L of the glomerular filtrate, which is about 120 L of fluid being recovered over 24 hours. Although the tight junctions between the cells can be classified as moderately 'leaky', the total surface area offered by this paracellular route between the cells would be inadequate to explain this vast movement of water. In addition, since water molecules are partly polar and have a negative charge it is difficult to envisage that this molecule could pass through a lipid bilayer.

Aquaporins

A chance finding from work on the protein content of the red cell membrane identified a special class of proteins – the aquaporins (AqPs). The AqPs are membrane-spanning proteins with the ability to form a specific channel for water through the cell membranes. About 10 classes of aquaporins have been identified with AqP1 being most prevalent on both sides of the cells of the PCT, which explains the unexpected high water permeability of this tissue (Fig. 14.9). These molecules allow the osmotic gradient created by the movement of various electrolytes and non-electrolytes to exert a much greater force than could be predicted, and permit a relatively low expenditure of energy for the vast movement of fluid. The location of other AqPs, especially AqP2, which can be added to the luminal side of the collecting duct cells under the influence of antidiuretic hormone, will be discussed later.

Peritubular capillaries

The PCT and the DCT are enveloped in a dense capillary network, the peritubular capillaries (Fig. 14.4). The recovery of fluid into these capillaries is further aided by the raised COP of 30–35 mmHg of the blood draining from the glomerulus. This also draws water, salts and other molecules into the blood by the Starling mechanism so that by the time this blood passes into the veins it has a normal COP of 25 mmHg.

Sugars, amino acids and other small organic molecules

Sugars, amino acids and other small molecules are recovered from the glomerular filtrate by sodium-dependent carriers found on the luminal side of the PCT cell wall (Fig. 14.9C). Each of these carriers has a special site for the binding of Na^+ and a site for a specific molecular species. There are several carriers for sugars (Na^+-coupled glucose transporter SGLT), five for amino acids, others for ions and many nutrients, each of which are specific for their own molecule. Once Both sites are occupied, the carrier undergoes transformation and the Na^+ and the other molecule on the carrier are now transferred into the cell. This process is termed cotransport and although it does not use energy directly, it does again use the steep gradient for sodium across the cell wall which has been generated by the Na^+ pump on the opposite side of the cell to 'power' the entry of the non-electrolyte 'up' their concentration gradient (Fig. 14.9C). This is secondary active transport (see also Chs 2 and 4).

The Na^+ dependent SGLT cotransport carriers will move their sugar molecules against a concentration gradient. In the first part of the PCT there are SGLT2 carriers, which have a low affinity for glucose, so they will work when there is a high sugar content in the lumen. In the later PCT segment, where the concentration of sugar is low, SGLT1 carriers, which have a high affinity for glucose, will move the sugar against a steep concentration gradient to recover molecules from the filtrate back into the blood.

Since these processes depend upon a finite number of carriers in the cell wall, a sudden large excess of a particular molecule present in the blood will increase the amount filtered into the tubule and cause all the sites to become occupied. When this occurs the process is said to be saturated; the molecules are not fully recovered by the PCT, and will appear in the urine. This condition is seen in diabetes mellitus when glucose appears in the urine (glycosuria), leading to an osmotic diuresis (see also Ch. 3).

Facilitated carriers

Once inside the PCT cell wall, there are other carriers on the blood side for sugars and amino acids called facilitated carriers. This is a type of secondary active transport (see Chs 2 and 3). For sugars these are the GLUT series, with other series for amino acids, ions and other nutrients. These types of carrier move the non-electrolytes only down their concentration gradient into the ECF and then by diffusion into the blood. This type of carrier can also work in the opposite direction and carry sugars, amino acids and other molecules from the blood into the cell when the concentration gradient is reversed (Fig. 14.9C).

Sodium and chloride

The initial recovery of Na^+ is coupled to the Na^+/H^+ antiporter which in turn is dependent on HCO_3^- in the tubule to generate the H^+ ions. The first third of the PCT recovers most of the HCO_3^- ions, so that when its concentration in the tubular fluid falls, the recovery of Na^+ slows. However, to overcome this problem, the next section of the tubule has a Cl^-/HCO_3^- coupled exchange process, so here the HCO_3^- ions are returned to the tubular fluid to help recover Cl^- ions. Now the H^+/Na^+ antiport has more HCO_3^- to react with to help the recovery of more Na^+ ions as well as the Cl^- (Fig. 14.9D).

In this region there are also Na^+ channels which allow Na^+ to enter the cell and be recovered into the blood by the Na^+/K^+-ATPase. This would produce a large potential difference, but Cl^- ions pass through the leaky tight junctions into the intracellular spaces and balance the Na^+ ion charge. Water accompanies these processes so water and salt are recovered (Fig. 14.9).

Secretion of organic anions and cations

Renal tubules can secrete a wide variety of toxic metabolites, both ingested in the diet and produced as byproducts of metabolism, including drugs. These are often organic lipid soluble anions and cations that can cross the cell membrane into the cell. These metabolites could accumulate in the cytoplasm, requiring a specific system of transport to eliminate the molecules from the circulation.

Organic anion transport

Organic anions are mostly weak aromatic and aliphatic organic acids with pKs generally of less than 7. The transporter systems to eliminate organic anions have a wide substrate specificity. At the pH of blood (7.4), these molecules are anions, whereas in the acid pH of the urine, they become undissociated and lipid soluble. The renal tubules are able to secrete these compounds into the lumen so the urinary concentration of these molecules is higher than in the plasma. This is a basis for measuring renal plasma flow by the clearance method described below. Although this secretory mechanism is an advantage for the elimination of unwanted molecules, the broad specificity of the process means that many drug molecules will also be excreted. For example, this was a major problem with penicillin when the bulk of the administered dose was lost into the urine. Probenecid was found to competitively inhibit the secretion of penicillin, so that administration of probenecid together with penicillin maintained the plasma level of the antibiotic (see Ch. 4).

By the use of coloured organic acids the site of secretion was identified as the second S_2 segment of proximal tubules. The mechanism of PCT anion secretion is shown in Fig. 14.9E and some examples of typical compounds are given in Table 14.2. Hippurate is the prime organic anion secreted by the kidney and about 1 g per day is excreted in the urine.

Para-amino hippuric acid (PAH)

There are at least three organic anion transporters, OAT 1–3, which share a 12 transmembrane domain structure related to the sugar transporters. PAH is a model substrate for this process and on the basolateral side of the cell there is a two-stage process (Fig. 14.9E). The first step is the entry of dicarboxylates (α-ketoglutarate and glutarate) cotransported with sodium. The ubiquitous Na^+ pump maintains the low Na^+ in the cell, which enables this cotransport to proceed. Then

Table 14.2 Representative compounds secreted by the renal organic anion and cation transport systems

Anions		Cations	
Endogenous compounds	Drugs	Endogenous compounds	Drugs
Amino acids	Acetazolamide	Acetylcholine	Amiloride
		Adrenaline (Epinephrine)	
Benzoate	Cephalothin	Choline	Amprolium
Bile salts	Chlorothiazide	Creatinine	Atropine
Cyclic AMP	Ethacrynic acid	Dopamine	Cimetidine
Long-chain fatty acids			Hexamethonium
Hippurate	Furosemide	Histamine	Mecamylamine
Hydroxybenzoates	Indometacin	5-Hydroxytryptamine	Morphine
Hydroxyindoleacetic acid	Penicillin G	Noradrenaline (Norepinephrine)	Neostigmine
Oxalate	Probenecid	N-methylnicotinamide	Paraquat
Prostaglandins	Saccharin	Serotonin	Quinine
Urate	Salicylate	Thiamin	Tetraethylammonium

the intracellular dicarboxylate exchanges with an organic anion, in this case PAH, which moves into the cell on the apical (luminal) side of the cell. The PAH is then exported into the lumen on the basolateral side in exchange for another anion such as chloride, urate or hydroxyl ions so the PCT can concentrate PAH to a much higher level than in plasma (200–300 times).

In plasma (pH 7.4), PAH with a pK of 3.8 is 99% ionised whereas in urine with a pH of 4.5, 83% is ionised. The non-ionised fraction can diffuse through the lipid cell membrane, so making the urine more acidic and increasing the secretion of PAH into the urine. This leads to a complete clearance of PAH on a single passage through the kidney.

In contrast, the excretion of some molecules such as probenecid, phenobarbital and salicylic acid can be increased by urinary alkalisation (see Ch. 4). This mechanism is a balance between the pKa, the partition coefficient (Kp) and the pH, so that the excretion of some drugs such as barbital and urate are not increased by urinary alkalisation. PAH has been found to enhance the rate of excretion of water, Na^+, K^+ and HPO_2^- and this is seen in patients receiving massive doses of carbenicillin. This also occurs in starvation where there are increased organic acids derived from fat metabolism (see Ch. 3).

PAH and drug dosage

When the glomerular filtration rate (GFR) falls to 10% or less of normal, hippurate accumulates in the blood and competes for the binding of several drugs such as salicylate, phenytoin, sulfonamides and furosemide. There will be an increased level of the unbound drug in the plasma with a greater therapeutic effect for a given dose. In contrast, when such patients are dialysed, the hippurate is removed so the protein binding now increases and the therapeutic effect of some drugs will be decreased and the dose must be adjusted to allow for this effect.

Efflux transporters and drugs

Efflux transporters are active transport systems that extrude drugs out of cells (see Ch. 4). They require energy to function. These efflux transporters have a broad range of specificity so can handle many molecules. The transport proteins can also be induced or up regulated, so account for the failure of some drugs to continue to act with repeated doses. This effect explains why some anti-cancer agents fail to work after the initial positive response, and may contribute to bacterial multidrug resistance.

Nephrotoxicity

Some drugs can damage the cells of the nephron as they accumulate within the cytoplasm and this nephrotoxicity is related to their uptake in the tubule cells by these processes and the lower ability of the cells to transport these drugs into the urine. Neonates are protected from this damage as their uptake transport system is poorly developed at this stage.

Clinical box 14.4 **Furosemide**

Furosemide is bound to plasma proteins and is not filtered so only passes into the tubule by these secretion processes. Indometacin, aspirin and probenecid compete with this step so reduce the diuretic action of this drug, although they do displace it from the protein binding which increases the entry into the tubule by filtration (see Ch. 4).

Organic cation transport

Many organic cations in the blood are excreted by the kidney where a series of organic cation transporters (OCT) 1–3 are expressed. These are electrogenic organic cation transporters with a broad specificity which suggests they are involved in the first step of secretion of the compounds, moving the molecules across the basolateral membrane. The exit across the brush border is accompanied by an organic cation/H^+ antiporter acting down the lumen/cell H^+ gradient established by the Na^+/H^+ exchange. Table 14.2 gives some examples of these compounds. However, the detailed mechanism of their transport has not been well characterised and work is still in progress, although the structure of the OAT and OCT has been identified.

RENAL FUNCTION TESTS

The symptoms of renal failure can masquerade under an amazing variety of clinical conditions, so it is essential to be able to screen patients using simple low-cost techniques before proceeding to more complex and expensive diagnostic tests.

Blood and urine tests

In routine blood tests a raised level of urea and creatinine are the first signs of possible renal problems, which can be confirmed by testing the urine, where increased levels of protein and tubular debris after centrifugation can often be found. Measurement of the urinary volume over 24 hours and the ability to form concentrated urine, when water intake is restricted, can also be used and will identify both problems within the kidney and of the water control mechanisms.

Osmolarity and specific gravity

Although the osmolarity of urine can be measured directly by the depression of freezing point with an osmometer, a more simple guide is to measure the specific gravity using a hydrometer, which compares the specific gravity of the test fluid with the specific gravity of pure water:

Specific gravity = density of test fluid/density of water

In pure water, the float will sink to a level of 1.000 on the hydrometer. With increasing density of the test solution, the scale on the hydrometer will float to a higher level which is related to the ionic content. Plasma has a specific gravity of 1.010 (285 mOsm). Urine can vary from a specific gravity of 1.035 (1400 mOsm), the most concentrated and dark, down to 1.005 (50 mOsm), the most dilute and pale. Note, however, since the density of fluids varies with temperature and hot fluids are less dense, it is essential to allow the urine to cool to the calibrated temperature of the hydrometer. In hot environments it is necessary to ensure that the hydrometer used is calibrated to the range of climatic temperature.

Although not frequently performed, measurement of the specific gravity of a urine specimen can give an indication of the efficiency of the renal control of fluid balance mechanisms (see below).

Analysing urine

The history of urine analysis can be traced back to ancient Egypt where polyuria and haematuria were mentioned in medical papyri, and by 400 BC, Hippocrates had observed the changes to the colour and odour of urine and its relation

Table 14.3 Urine tests and purpose

Range of tests	Uses
Specific gravity	Athletes to monitor drugs
pH 4.8–7.4	Acid–base disturbances
Leucocytes	Inflammatory disease of the kidney
Nitrite	Presence of bacteria
Protein (albumen)	Renal disease
Glucose	Diabetes mellitus renal threshold 8.3–10 mM
Ketones	Increased fat degradation, gastrointestinal infection in diabetes mellitus
Urobilinogen	Liver disease or increased haemolysis
Bilirubin	Liver damage, hepatitis cirrhosis
Blood	Renal and post-renal bleeding

to disease. Healthy urine should be clear and a straw colour. Other colours can indicate the presence of drugs, blood haemoglobin or bilirubin. The odour of urine can reflect chemical conditions, a fruity odour or acetone in diabetes mellitus and a musty odour indicates hepatic disease, and ingestion of various dietary constituents such as garlic gives other odours. The various penicillins are excreted via the kidney and can impart a strong odour to the urine. By the end of the eighteenth century, the chemistry of urine analysis had progressed to various spot tests and then to test papers, which identify specific constituents present in the urine. Table 14.3 sets out the range of tests commonly in use, and their purpose.

Specialised spectrophotometers can be used to quantify the concentration of various constituents in urine. Microalbuminuria can also be tested for but the test is not quantitative. Alternatively the albumin/creatinine ratio is also useful to give an indication of impending diabetic nephropathy.

Renal handling of molecules

Simple estimates of renal function can be derived from changes in the way that the kidney handles molecules. The kidney can handle molecules in three ways:

- First, a molecule can be simply filtered and then passed unchanged into the urine (Fig.14.10A).
- Second, it can be filtered then reabsorbed as it passes through the PCT, so the final concentration in the urine is less than plasma (Fig.14.10B).
- Finally, a molecule can be filtered and then more can be added to the urine by secretion in the PCT, making the concentration in urine higher than in plasma (Fig.14.10C).

These mechanisms can be studied by the use of a technique called clearance. Water being abstracted from the tubule will alter the concentration in the urine but its effect will depend on the transport of each molecule. Even molecules which are only filtered will be concentrated in the urine by this process.

Renal clearance

The clearance of a molecule is defined as: 'volume of plasma cleared of that molecule per minute'. Since no molecule is fully cleared by the kidney, it is more a concept than a reality. It is a simple way of quantifying the handling by the nephron of various types of molecule. The most useful renal function which can be derived from a clearance measurement is the glomerular filtration rate (GFR).

If the renal excretion, ($U_x \times V$), i.e. the concentration of a molecule in mM in the urine (U_x) multiplied by the volume of urine formed per minute (V), is measured and is divided by the concentration of the molecule in plasma (P_x), we can gain some idea of how the nephron is handling the molecule. This is termed the clearance of a molecule.

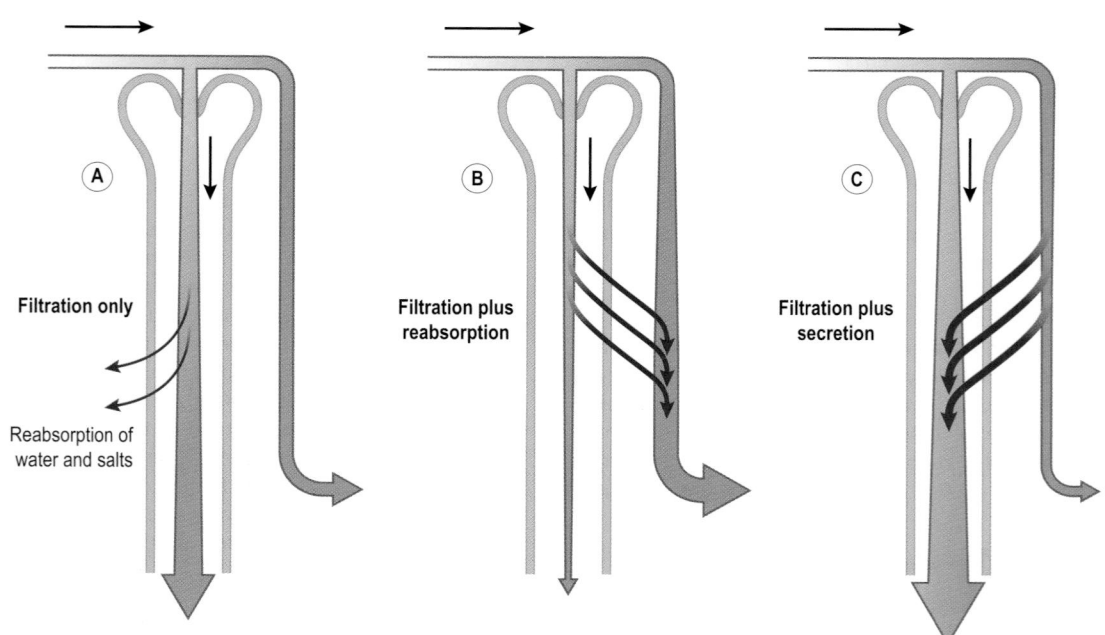

Fig. 14.10 Renal handling of molecules. (A) Molecules can be filtered only and not reabsorbed or secreted, but will still have an increased concentration in the urine due to the fact that fluid is recovered along the nephron. (B) Molecules that are filtered and reabsorbed will have a very low concentration in the urine. (C) Molecules that are filtered and secreted will have an elevated concentration in the urine and very low levels in the blood draining from the nephron.

The clearance of a molecule x is expressed as:

$$C_x = (U_x \times V)/P_x$$

- U_x = the concentration in the urine in mM.
- P_x = the concentration in plasma in mM.
- V = the volume of urine formed per min. i.e. mL/min.

The unit of clearance is mL/min.

Clearance of molecules which are only filtered

If a molecule is filtered and then passes unchanged into the urine, the clearance of such a molecule is an index of the effective glomerular filtration rate of all the nephrons, i.e. the glomerular filtration rate (GFR). The concentration of such a molecule will be raised in the urine, as it will remain trapped in the tubule after filtration, where some 99% of water and other constituents of the filtrate are mostly recovered as they pass along the tubule.

'Inulin' clearance as an index of GFR

In the past, 'inulin' (a plant starch) of molecular weight 5 200, was used for testing renal clearance as a molecule that is filtered then passed unchanged into the urine. 'Inulin' is now no longer available and polyfructans are used instead. Inulin clearance, however, is still a benchmark against which all other methods are judged and the term 'inulin' clearance is still used. To perform a clearance test with 'inulin' (C_{in}), the bladder is first emptied and the 'inulin' injected intravenously as a bolus. Since this molecule is filtered, the level in the blood will rise to a peak value then fall with time, as shown in Fig. 14.11A. The urine is collected for a set period and the concentration of 'inulin' in the urine and the volume formed in mL/min ($U_{in}V$) can be easily determined. The problem, however, remains to find a value of plasma which reflects the average concentration for the period (P_{in}). Various methods have been used to obtain a mean of this value of plasma concentration, including infusing a dilute 'inulin' solution to balance the renal loss as shown by the dotted line in Figure 14.11A, or calculating the area under the curve, but errors in this value have a large effect on the calculation of C_{in}.

Note that whatever level of 'inulin' appears in the blood the same level is filtered into the urine, so the relationship becomes a straight line with a slope of 45 degrees. Fig. 14.11B shows that the clearance C_{in} of this molecule is independent of the blood level.

Values of 'inulin' clearance are in the range of 125 mL/min ± 30 for normal male subjects. This is the value taken as 'normal' GFR. Again, note that the range of C_{in} in normal subjects is quite large, i.e. ± 30 of the population mean value of 125 and depends on body size, age and sex. Females have a lower value than males with a mean of about 90 mL/min being taken as normal. Infants do not achieve adult GFR until they are about 4 years old and cannot fully concentrate their urine until the kidney has matured. With increasing age, renal function begins to decrease above the age of about 65–70.

Creatinine clearance

Creatinine is derived from muscle metabolism and is released from muscles at a constant rate, so has a constant level in the blood. (Note: this is a di-amino acid and must not be confused with creatine.) This molecule makes an ideal marker for GFR since it is endogenous, i.e. occurs naturally in the circulation and the plasma concentration (P_{cr}) is relatively constant. Creatinine clearance, C_{cr}, gives values close to 'inulin', i.e. 125 mL/min, although there is a small component of secretion. However, the error caused by the raised value of urinary creatinine, U_{cr}, is balanced by a plasma chromogen which raises the value of P_{cr} so the errors cancel.

Urea clearance

Urea is also a natural product, but it is reabsorbed and recirculated in the kidney so gives values three-fifths of GFR; urea clearance, C_u, is about 80 mL/min. The ratio of C_{cr} to C_u can be used to reduce variation. C_u does, however, vary with water intake, so if the water intake is low even more is reabsorbed and the value of C_u falls.

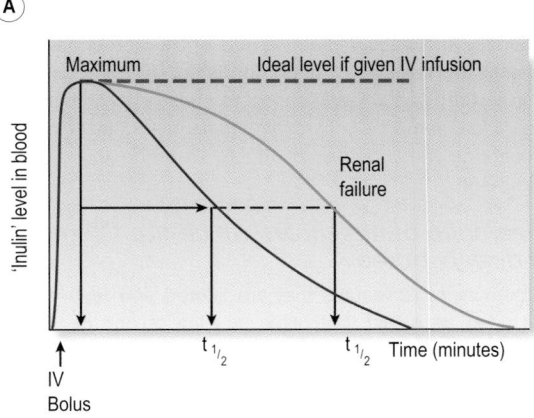

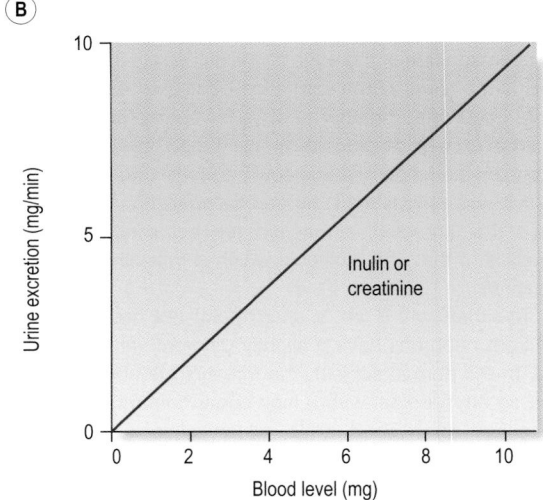

Fig. 14.11 **Inulin clearance.** (A) Molecules that are filtered only, such as 'inulin', can be re-used as an index of GFR. If 'inulin' is given as a bolus into the plasma the level rises rapidly to a maximum then 'falls' off with time as it is filtered. In renal failure the rate of 'fall' is much reduced and by measuring the time to reach a value that was half the maximum, an index of renal function can be derived from the fall off in plasma level. To get a true reading plasma level 'inulin' would have to be infused at a rate to match the filtered loss; since this is not known this is difficult to achieve. (B) Since the urine excretion matches the blood level, it indicates that this molecule is filtered only. IV, intravenous.

Current methods for measuring renal clearance (half life)

Fig. 14.11A shows that the level of 'inulin' in plasma when injected as a bolus decreases with time as it is filtered through the kidney. If the kidney is damaged and GFR is depressed, the rate of 'inulin' filtration with time will be less, and the blood level will fall more slowly (hatched line Fig. 14.11A). This fact can then be used as an indication of renal function. An easily measured molecule, such as ^{51}Cr EDTA (ethylene diamine tetra-acetate, molecular weight 300) is given as a bolus and then the blood level followed for a period of time by taking serial blood samples. EDTA is a molecule which strongly binds to chromium [Cr]. ^{51}Cr is an isotope which emits gamma rays and is easy to count. Initially the counts in plasma samples will rapidly rise to a maximum then decrease over a period. The time can then be taken for the isotope level to fall to half of the maximum, which is the half life ($\frac{1}{2}$) for healthy subjects (Fig. 14.11A). With the progressive deterioration of renal function the $\frac{1}{2}$ gradually increases, indicating loss of filtration capacity, and reflects the number of nephrons which are still functional. This method is quick and cheap and has largely replaced the clearance methods for screening patients for renal failure and monitoring the progress of the GFR during the course of treatment.

Clearance of molecules which are filtered and reabsorbed

Clearance of molecules that are filtered and reabsorbed is not used as a test, but gives an idea of one of the most important functions of the kidney (see Fig. 14.10A). Molecules such as glucose have a very low clearance (0.2 mL/min) since they are actively reabsorbed. The normal plasma level is 4–5 mM and only tiny amounts are found in the urine of normal subjects; however, as the blood level of glucose increases a point is reached – the renal threshold – when glucose appears in the urine at the same rate as 'inulin', etc. This is the result of the saturation of all the carrier sites; i.e. there is a limited number of sites for uptake and, if there is a large excess of glucose in the blood, they all become occupied and now the molecule passes through the PCT, as if it was only filtered. As can be seen from Fig. 14.12A, once the threshold is reached the behaviour of glucose parallels to that of a molecule which is only filtered, such as creatinine.

The threshold is not a sharp point but has a 'splay' as different nephrons have a slightly different value for threshold. In the normal subject, the threshold is about 8–10 mM and so after a meal with a high sugar content, this value is exceeded for a short while, which explains why a small amount of glucose is found in the urine of normal people. The displacement of the glucose response, compared to that of a molecule that is only filtered, is expressed as the tubular maximum, T_m, and represents the total capacity of the kidney to reabsorb glucose. With diabetes mellitus, glucose in the urine is common due to the lack of insulin and high levels of glucose in the plasma, but as the disease progresses, microvascular complications lead to renal damage and a much elevated threshold for glucose. Now little glucose appears in urine, although the plasma levels may be 20 mM or greater (normal 4–5 mM). This is why urine testing for glucose in diabetes mellitus is now no longer used and has been replaced by measuring the glucose level in blood with various reagent strips which give an accurate colour change depend-

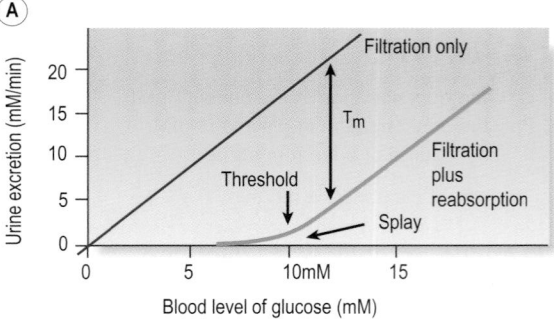

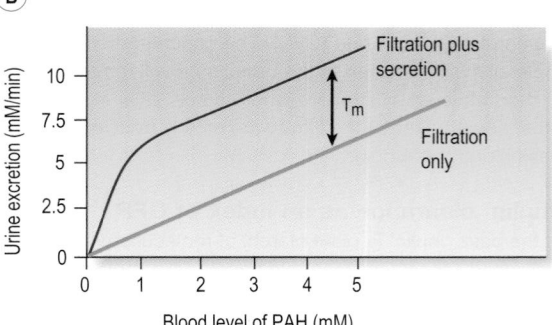

Fig. 14.12 **Clearance of molecules that are filtered and reabsorbed, such as glucose.** (A) Initially no glucose appears in the urine, as it is reabsorbed; however, once the plasma level exceeds the renal threshold glucose is filtered into the urine. This point is related to the availability of carriers to recover the filtered glucose, which eventually becomes saturated. Different nephrons vary in their saturation level so there is a splay in the threshold level. Once the threshold is exceeded, glucose is just filtered and the line is parallel to that of molecules which are only filtered. The displacement of this line gives an index of the tubular maximum, the T_m, for the recovery of glucose. (B) For molecules which are filtered and secreted, the level in the urine is higher than in the plasma. This process will also saturate in most cases. Molecules such as para-amino hippuric acid (PAH) are virtually cleared from the plasma by these processes.

ing on the level of glucose in the blood. This colour is measured by various meters which now can respond in about 10 seconds or less.

Clearance of molecules which are filtered and secreted

Some molecules are both filtered and secreted, such as organic acids and bases, and molecules that are lipid soluble or are toxic and have been converted into glucuronides by the liver (see Ch. 4). With these compounds, more appears in the urine than in the blood as they are secreted into the tubule. As with sugars, this process saturates since there is a finite number of carriers. The process has both a threshold and T_m. The values for clearance of molecules such as PAH (para-amino hippuric acid) are in the region of 650–700 mL/min. Since these compounds are both filtered and secreted, the amount remaining in the blood leaving the nephron is very low and can give an indication of the renal plasma flow (RPF), i.e. the clearance of PAH, C_{PAH} = RPF. Since the PAH is only present in the plasma, the renal blood flow (RBF) can then be calculated by correction with the haematocrit (Hct), i.e.:

$$RBF = C_{PAH}/1 - Hct$$

Use of clearance methods to assess renal function

Renal blood flow (RBF) is about 1.2–1.4 L/min, i.e. one fifth of cardiac output. Thus we can then, by relatively simple methods, obtain the effective GFR and RBF using clearance techniques. The ratio of GFR to RBF is called the filtration fraction (FF) and is about 0.10–0.15; i.e. 20% of the plasma passing through the kidney is filtered into the nephron.

$$FF = GFR/RBF = C_{inulin}/C_{PAH}$$

With the large number of patients with possible renal failure it is essential to take a detailed history and to be able to screen patients using blood tests and simple low cost techniques before proceeding to those which are more complicated and expensive.

Advanced clinical tests

If signs of renal failure are detected on simple testing, a variety of diagnostic tests can then be used to identify the site of the renal dysfunction, e.g. obstruction, by imaging, ultrasound, nuclear medical imaging, computed tomography scans or the gamma camera.

RENAL CONTROL OF FLUID BALANCE

The mechanisms which balance the fluid intake to fluid loss are more precise than those for acid–base and electrolyte balance. The control of these processes reside in an osmoreceptive complex located in the hypothalamus (see Fig. 14.13A) and comprise the subfornical organ (SFO), the organum vasculosum of the lamina terminalis (OVLT) and the median preoptic nucleus (Mn PO), all of which input on to the magnocellular neurons of the supraoptic (SO) and the paraventricular nuclei (PVN) (see Chs 9 and 10). The SO and PVN neurons can act both as osmoreceptors and can also synthesise two peptide hormones – vasopressin and the reproductive hormone oxytocin.

Vasopressin

Vasopressin (or antidiuretic hormone, ADH) is a nonapeptide (nine amino acids, Cys-Tyr-Phe-Gln-Asn-Cys-Pro-Arg-Gly(NH_2)) that has two cysteine residues in positions 1 and 6, linked by a disulphide bridge (see Fig. 14.13B). Antidiuretic hormones evolved very early in evolution and are found in most animal species. In mammals, vasopressin is released from the posterior pituitary in response to a small rise in the osmotic pressure of the plasma usually caused by an increased rate of water loss. There is an inverse relationship between the plasma vasopressin level and the osmolarity of the urine (see Fig. 14.13C). Note, however, that although the volume and concentration of urine vary, the net loss of solute does not, and is maintained constant for a given period. There is thus a mechanism by which the water balance is separated from that of solute.

Normally, the level of vasopressin in the plasma is in the range 2–4 pg/mL and is rapidly increased as the plasma osmolarity changes. This precise matching of the plasma VP level to osmolarity is the central mechanism of water homeostasis (Fig. 14.14A, B). The normal response to a fall in water intake is a rise in plasma osmolarity, and within minutes an increase in the plasma vasopressin level.

Once vasopressin has been synthesised by neurons of the SO and PVN, it is then attached to the transport protein neurophysin as granules, which are then rapidly transported within 30 min to the posterior pituitary, down microtubules in the axons of the neurohypophyseal tract; here it is stored prior to release.

Bursts of action potentials in these axons of the neurohypophyseal tract, in response to a tiny rise in osmotic pressure, cause the release of vasopressin into the bloodstream. However, the slope of this response is steep, and in addition the gradient can be altered by the fluid volume of the extracellular fluid, which will increase or decrease the sensitivity of the response (see Fig. 14.13). Vasopressin can also be released in response to a fall in blood pressure, but the change in blood pressure must be of a much larger magnitude than that of osmolarity.

Vasopressin receptors

Fig. 14.14C shows the cellular action of vasopressin. On reaching the kidney, vasopressin binds to specific V2 receptors located on the basolateral side of the cells of the cortical and medullary collecting ducts. V2 receptors are members of the G protein super family and, when stimulated by vasopressin, cause the activation of an intermediary G protein. This G protein activates a membrane-bound adenylate cyclase that catalyses the conversion of cytoplasmic ATP (adenosine triphosphate) to the second messenger cyclic AMP (cAMP) (see Ch. 4). The cAMP activates protein kinase A, which in turn phosphorylates myofilaments and myofibrils associated with vesicles in the cytoplasm close to the apical side of the tubular wall.

These vesicles contain water permeable channels made up of the preformed AqP2 protein. The vesicles have 'vesicle associated membrane proteins' (VAMP) on their surface which serve to 'dock' with specific sites on the apical membrane of these cells. The AqP2 proteins are then inserted into the membrane by exocytosis, which causes a rapid increase in the water permeability of the apical side of the cells.

On the basolateral side of the collecting duct cells, there are aquaporins 3 and 4 which maintain a high and continuous level of water permeability on this side of the cell. The insertion of AqP2 channels leads to a large increase in the transepithelial water flux within about 9 minutes, so that water is rapidly recovered from the tubule into the blood. The high colloid osmotic pressure of the blood in the peritubular blood vessels also aids the uptake of water in this direction. Once the osmotic pressure of the plasma returns to its normal value as water is reabsorbed, the level of vasopressin falls and the AqP2 channels are returned to the vesicles, and the water permeability of the apical wall rapidly falls within 30 minutes.

When the intake of water is low or there is an increased loss of fluid, such as in hard exercise, the osmolarity of the extracellular fluid rises and the rate of urine production falls with a marked increase in urine concentration. In humans, this can rise to a plasma level of 1400 mOsm (normal plasma is about 285 mOsm). This ability to vary the urine osmolarity from as low as 50 mOsm to 1400 mOsm is independent of solute excretion, which must be kept constant to eliminate toxic metabolites.

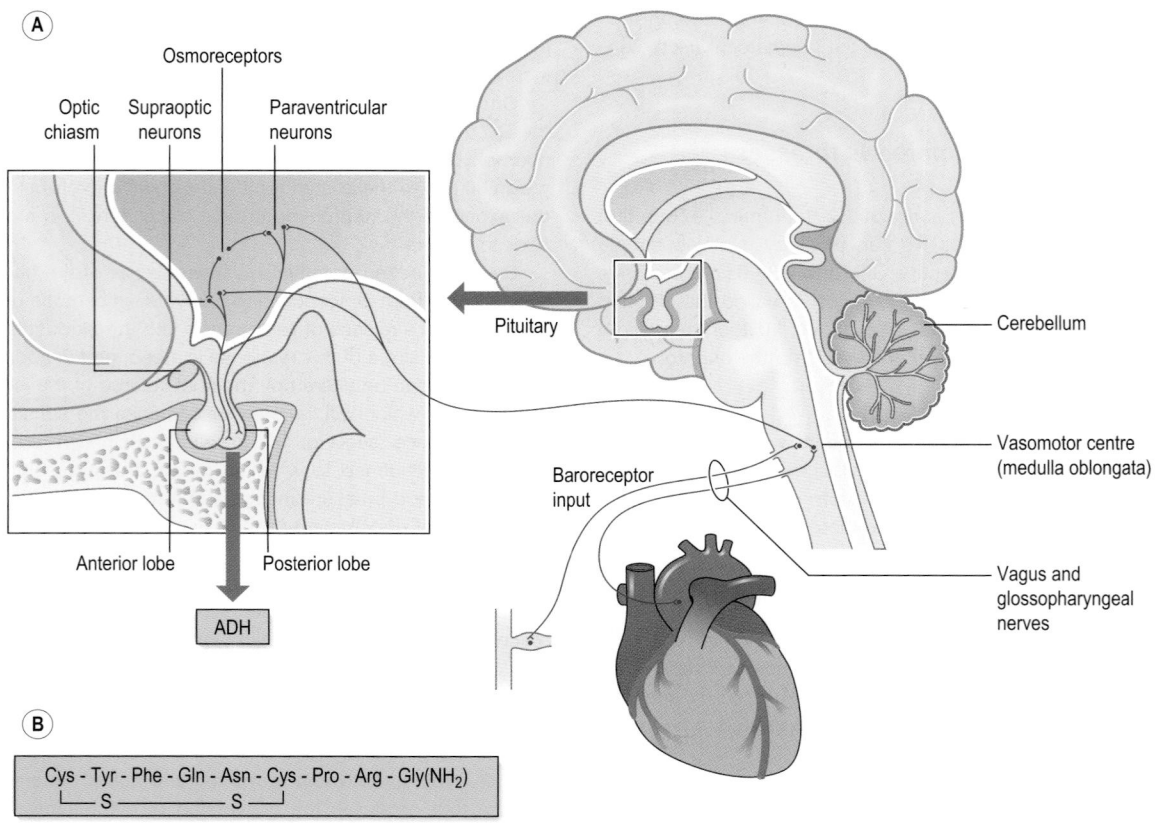

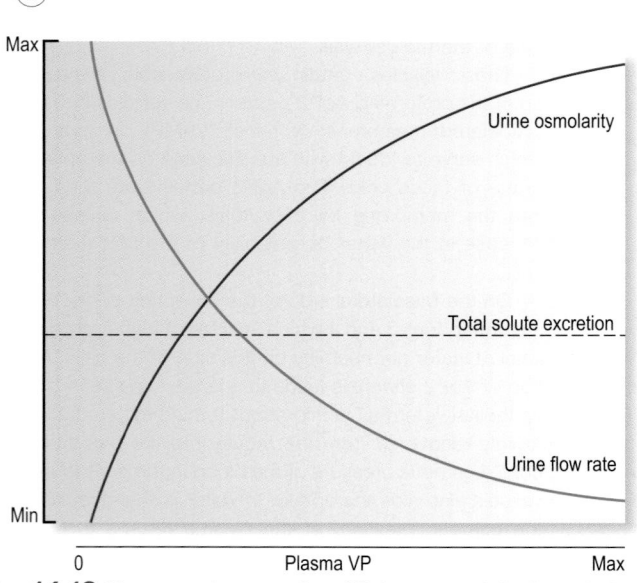

Fig. 14.13 **Vasopressin secretion.** (A) Anatomy of the hypothalamus and pituitary gland (midsagittal section) depicting the pathways of vasopressin (VP) secretion. Also shown are pathways involved in regulating VP secretion. Afferent fibres from the baroreceptors are carried in the vagus and glossopharyngeal nerves. The vasomotor centre includes the solitary tract nucleus. The closed box illustrates an expanded view of the hypothalamus and pituitary gland. (From Koeppen and Stanton 2001, with permission of Mosby, St Louis). (B) The amino acid sequence of vasopressin. (C) Relationship between plasma VP levels and urine osmolarity, urine flow rate, and total solute excretion. (From Koeppen and Stanton 2001, with permission of Mosby, St Louis).

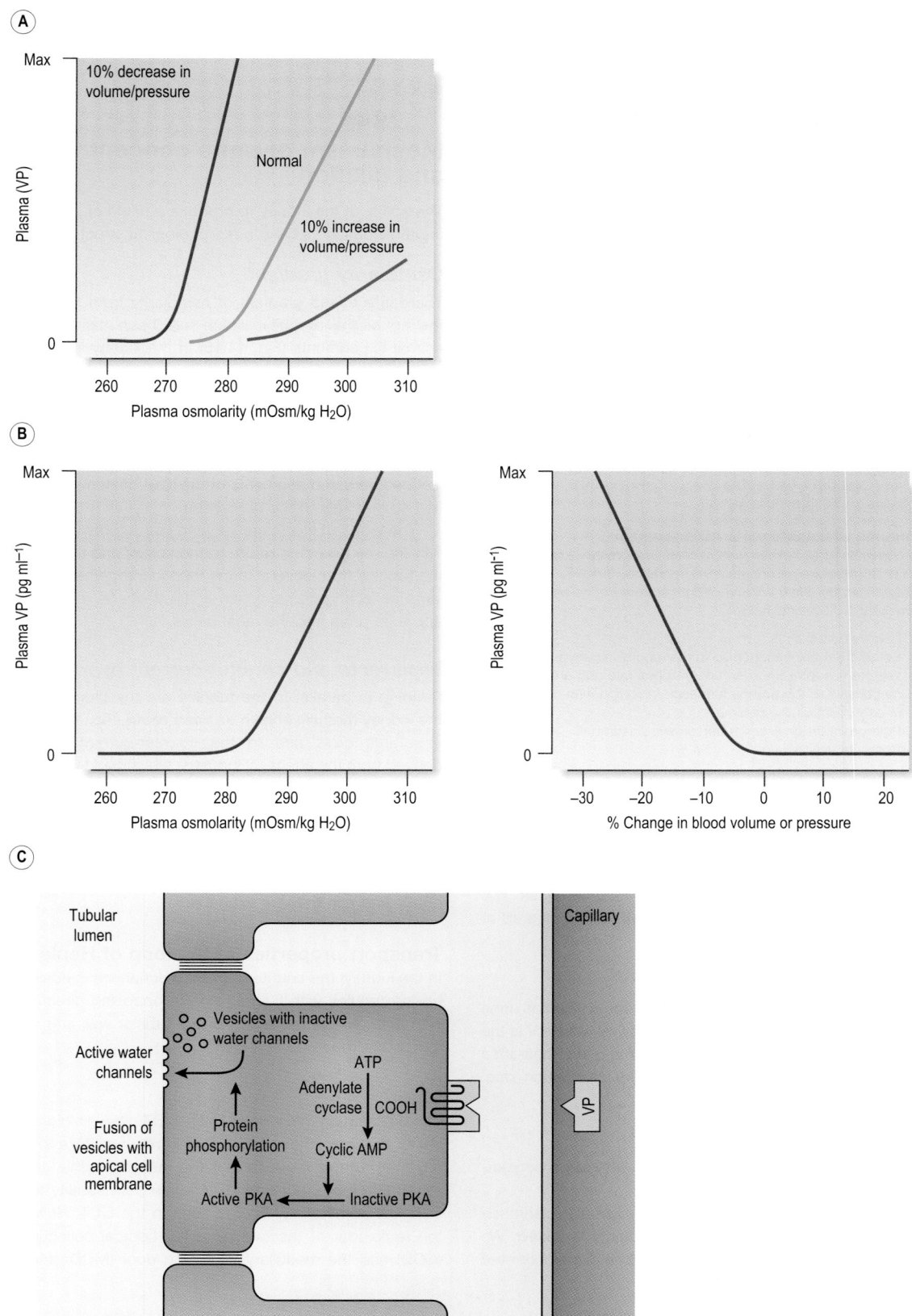

Fig. 14.14 **Action of vasopressin.** Interaction between osmotic and haemodynamic stimuli for vasopressin (VP) secretion. With decreased blood volume and pressure, the osmotic set point is shifted to lower plasma osmolarity values and the slope is increased. An increase in blood volume and pressure has the opposite effect. After Koeppen and Stanton 2001, with permission of Mosby, St Louis. PKA, protein kinase A.

Diabetes insipidus

Diabetes insipidus (DI), 'tasteless urine', is characterised by a high volume of dilute urine with haemoconcentration and polydipsia (excess drinking of water), caused by a lack of vasopressin, either from central hypothalamic damage (permanent DI) or from posterior pituitary damage (temporary DI). Temporary DI recovers because the neurons of the posterior pituitary regenerate. Causes include:

- Iatrogenic post-surgical or post-radiation (cranial)
- Trauma (i.e. head injury)
- Tumours
- Nephrogenic: V2 receptors on the collecting duct become unresponsive to vasopressin, which could be familial or idiopathic
- Psychological: 'hysterical water drinking'.

In normal subjects, water restriction is associated with an increase in the vasopressin level, and this will be paralleled by a rise in the urine osmolarity. DI caused by a hypothalamic lack of vasopressin will not show a rise in vasopressin with water restriction whereas renal insensitivity will show a rise in vasopressin but very little increase in the urine concentration. With the psychological syndrome there will be a normal rise of vasopressin and urine concentration.

Syndrome of inappropriate ADH secretion

The converse of DI is seen with excess vasopressin, known as the syndrome of inappropriate ADH secretion (SIADH), characterised by a low volume of concentrated urine and haemodilution. Causes include:

- Low fluid intake
- Ectopic oat cell carcinomas in the lung or pancreas that secrete vasopressin at an uncontrolled rate and are not responsive to the normal feedback inhibition with changes in osmolarity of the plasma
- Pulmonary lesions, e.g. tuberculosis, pneumonia
- Postoperative anuria.

The production of dilute urine

The kidney can eliminate 'solute free' water to excrete excess water or can conserve water by concentrating the urine. This ability can be measured by using clearance techniques. The osmolar clearance (C_{osm}) is the volume of plasma cleared of solutes each minute.

$$C_{osm} = (U_{osm}/P_{osm}) \times V$$

If the plasma osmolarity (P_{osm}) has the same value as urine osmolarity (U_{osm}), C_{osm} equals the urine flow (V) where V is the rate of urine production in mL/min. The free-water clearance (C_{H_2O}) is the difference between the urine production rate, V and the osmolar clearance.

$$C_{H_2O} = V - C_{osm}$$

A positive value indicates dilute urine whereas a concentrated urine gives a negative value.

In Table 14.4 it can be seen that the osmolar clearance stays constant although the urine osmolarity is varied. We can also calculate the amount of solute 'free' water excreted

(C_{H_2O}) or conserved by subtracting the C_{osm} from the urine flow which is shown in Table 14.4. This again emphasises the ability of the kidney to handle water and solute separately.

Mechanism of urine concentration and dilution

The ability of the kidney to produce a dilute or concentrated urine resides in its unique morphological structure.

Osmolarity gradient

There is a raised gradient of osmolarity from the cortex to the tip of the medulla, which has been demonstrated in animal experiments (Fig. 14.15). If the kidney is sliced horizontally down a renal pyramid, the osmolarity in the cortex is isotonic with the plasma, but as each slice is taken down the pyramid, the osmolarity increases, rising in the desert rodents to some 5000 mOsm at the apex. How this is achieved is still a matter of some debate, but studies using isolated perfused segments of the loop of Henle have identified some clues to the processes.

The loops of Henle are very long structures which plunge into the medulla then return to the cortex and the DCT. Here the tubules from several loops then join together to form the large collecting ducts, which again descend to the medulla and then drain into the renal pelvis.

Vasa recta and counter-current hypothesis

Running in parallel to the tubules are the blood vessels of the kidney medulla known as **vasa recta** (Fig. 14.15). These structures gave rise to the counter-current hypothesis, derived from the chemical industry, which had to concentrate drugs such as penicillin which had been produced in large vats of dilute solution by bacterial fermentation. By having fluids with different solubility for the drug in one arm of a 'U' shaped tube, and using solvents which are immiscible flowing in the opposite direction, the drug is concentrated in one phase and can then be extracted.

Transport properties of the loop of Henle

In the kidney, the counter-current mechanism is achieved by having tubules with fluid flowing in opposing directions but with different permeabilities of the tubular wall and different transport properties.

Water

The descending thin loops of Henle (DTL) have a high permeability to water (Fig. 14.16). This is reduced to a low value after the turn of the loop and the rest of the thin and thick ascending loops of Henle have a low permeability to water. This low permeability is also seen in the DCT. However, in the remainder of the tubule, in the cortical collecting duct (CCD) and the medullary collecting duct (MCD), there is a

Table 14.4	Free water clearance		
Urine state	Concentrated (U_{osm} = 1200)	Dilute (U_{osm} = 150)	Iso-osmotic (U_{osm} = 300)
V (urine excreted)	0.5 mL/min	4 mL/min	2 mL/min
$C_{osm} = (U_{osm}/P_{osm}) \times V$	(1200 × 0.5)/300 = 2 mL/min	(50 × 4)/300 = 2 mL/min	(300 × 2)/300 = 2 mL/min
C_{H_2O}	0.5 − 2 = −1.5 mL/min	4 − 2 = 2 mL/min	2 − 2 = 0 mL/min
Result	Solute free water conserved	Solute free water lost	No loss of free water

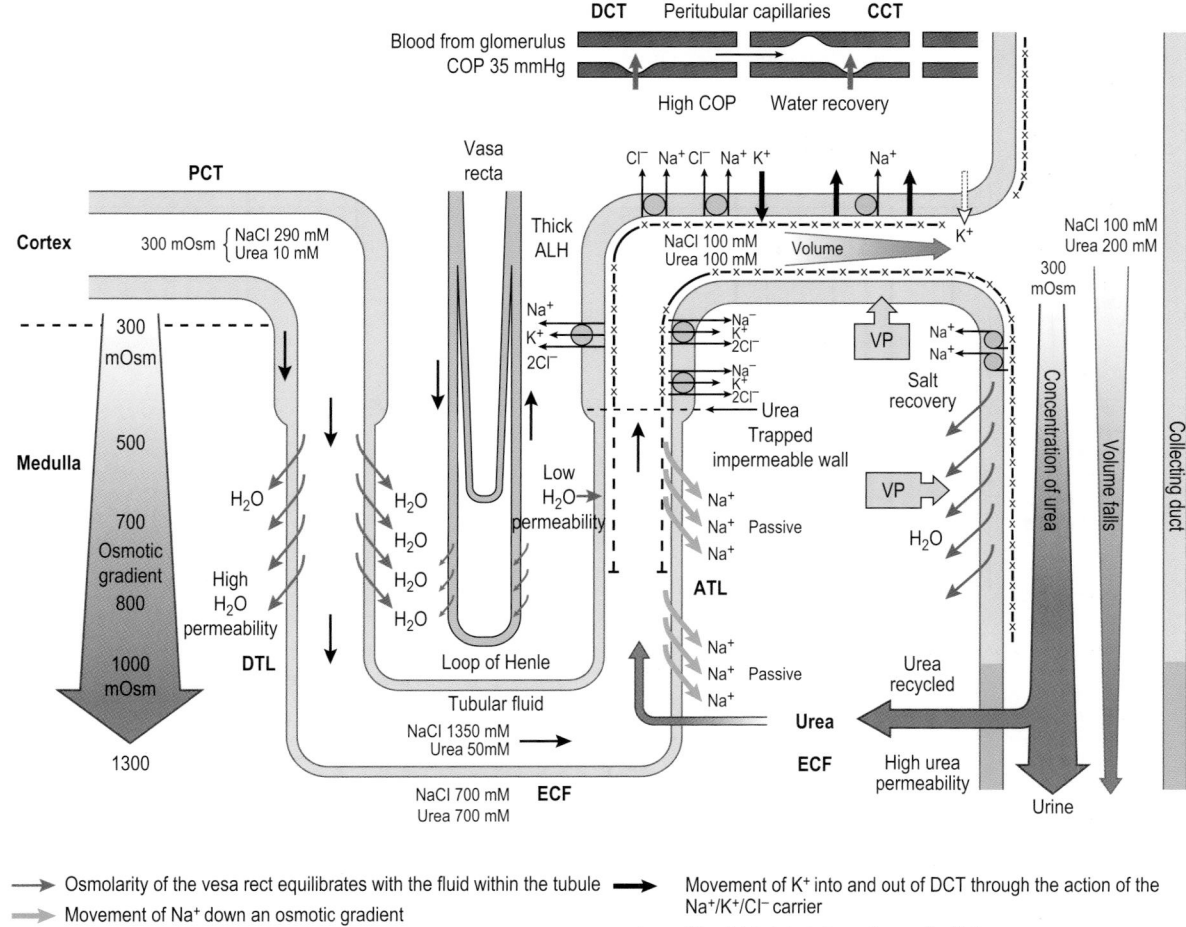

Fig. 14.15 Concentration of urine. On the left side is shown the osmotic gradient from the cortex to the medulla. Fluid passing down the water-permeable descending thin loop will lose fluid drawn out by the osmotic gradient and the tubular fluid becomes concentrated. After the turn in the loop of Henle the wall of the ascending thin loop has a low permeability to water and high salt and urea permeability. On reaching the thick ascending loop the powerful $Na^+/K^+/2Cl^-$ pump recovers ions so the fluid passing into the distal convoluted tubule (DCT) has a low ionic content. In the cortical collecting tube (CCT) water is recovered so the volume of fluid decreases further, but the concentration of urea increases as it is trapped in the tubule by the impermeable wall. As fluid descends the collecting duct, if vasopressin (VP) is present, water is withdrawn and a concentrated urine produced. In the last section of the collecting duct the wall becomes permeable to urea, which is recycled. PCT, proximal convoluted tubule; DTL, descending thin loop of Henle; ATL, ascending thin loop of Henle; ECF, extracellular fluid; ALH, ascending loop of Henle; COP, colloid osmotic pressure.

variable water permeability depending on the presence or absence of vasopressin; with vasopressin present, the permeability to water is high, and it is low when vasopressin is absent (indicated by the solid lines in Fig. 14.16).

The effect of fluid descending the DTLs is that water moves out into the interstitium and the remaining fluid in the tubules becomes concentrated (hypertonic) with a reduction in volume; this volume reduction is under the influence of the osmotic gradient shown in Fig. 14.15. Note: The osmotic gradient is always present to some degree both in diuresis and antidiuresis.

Sodium and chloride

In Fig. 14.17, it can be seen that the passive permeability to sodium also varies along the loop, being high in the outer medulla, but falling in the inner medulla, then rising to a high value in the thin ascending loop of Henle. For the rest of the loop, the passive permeability to Na^+ is low. In contrast, the

active transport for Na^+ is greatly increased in the medullary thick ascending loop of Henle in response to the $Na^+/K^+/2Cl^-$ transport, so that the Na^+ concentration in the fluid rapidly falls and this is the site of action of the loop diuretics (Fig. 14.15) (see Ch. 4).

Counter-current mechanism

The result of the above processes is that Na^+ and Cl^- are pumped out of the ascending loops of Henle into the interstitial fluid, then diffuse back into the descending loops. This is the counter-current mechanism that maintains the high osmolarity in the medulla, which in turn facilitates the recovery of water from the collecting ducts.

Urea

The permeability of the loop to urea is moderately high in the inner medulla, but is very low in the thick ascending loop, in the thin descending loops of Henle and in most of the

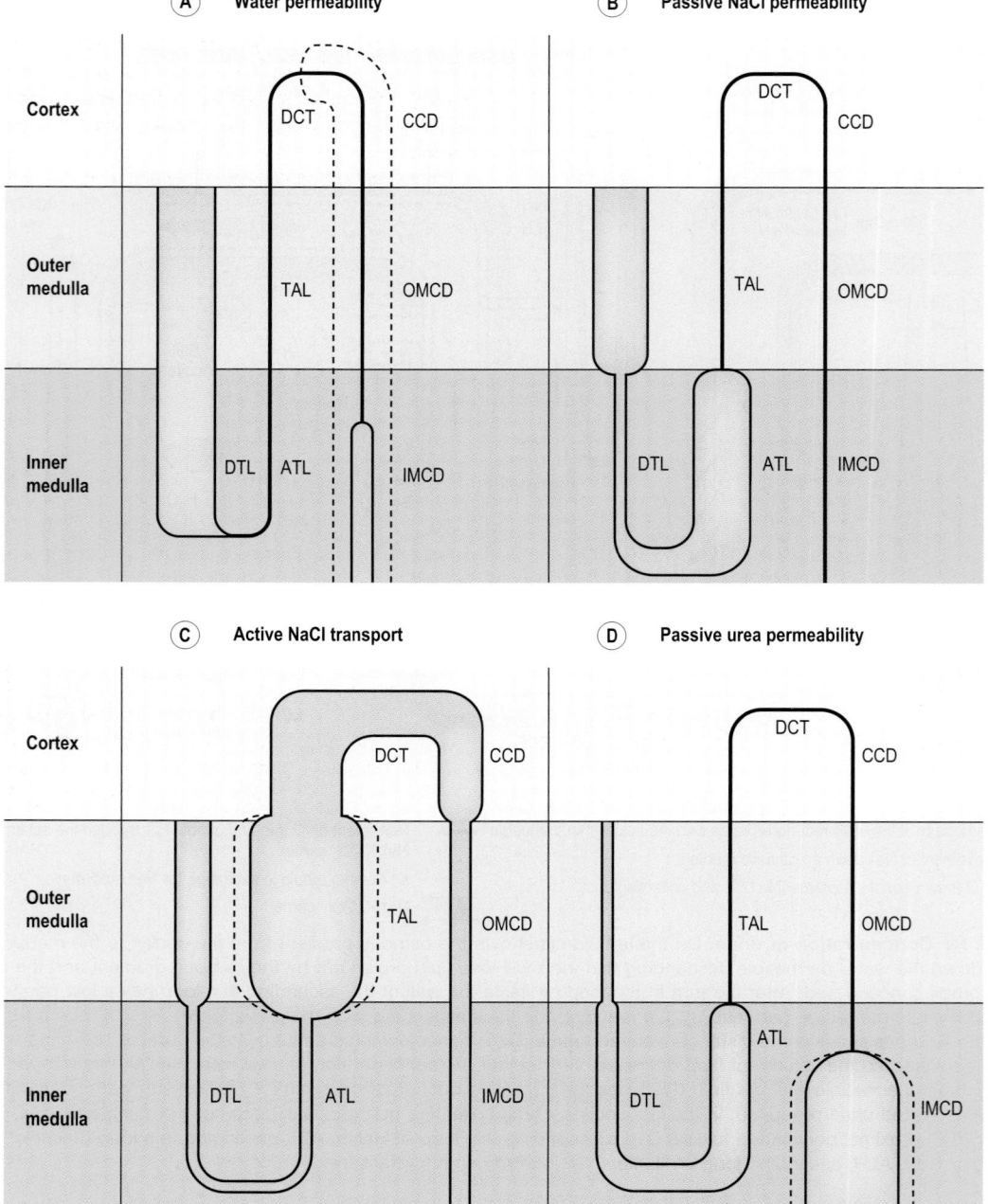

Fig. 14.16 Tubular permeability. Transport and passive permeability properties of the nephron segments involved in the dilution and concentration of urine. The width of the tubular segments is proportional to the magnitude of the parameter. The solid lines depict the situation in the absence of vasopressin. The dashed lines show the effect of vasopressin. DTL, descending thin loop; ATL, ascending thin loop; TAL, thick ascending loop; DCT, distal collecting tubule; CCD, cortical collecting duct; OMCD, outer medullary collecting duct; IMCD, inner medullary collecting duct. After Knepper MA and Rector FC Jr 1991, with permission of WB Saunders.

collecting duct apart from the very last section when its permeability to urea is greatly increased (see Fig. 14.16).

Vasa recta

The vasa recta dips into the medulla and returns to the cortex. The osmolarity of blood in the vasa recta will equilibrate with the fluid within the tubule and supply the cells with oxygen and nutrients without destroying the osmotic gradient. There is a considerable concentration of AqP1 in the

cells of this structure, which allows these processes to proceed rapidly.

Figure 14.15 shows that as fluid moves out of the descending thin loops of Henle into the interstitium, it is carried away by the vasa recta. Within the tubule, the fluid at the bottom of the loop has a high NaCl and urea concentration as water has moved out of the loop. In contrast, the extracellular fluid around the loop has a composition which is very different, with less NaCl and much more urea, than

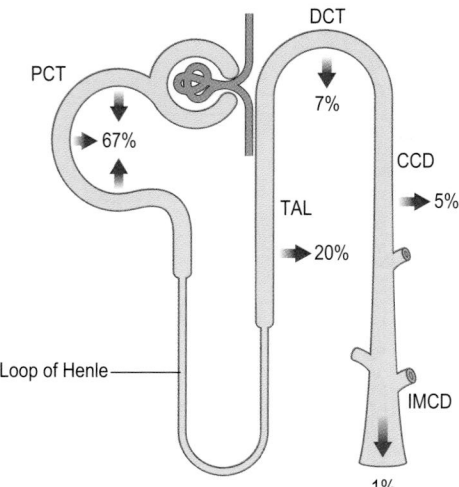

Fig. 14.17 Control of sodium balance. Segmental Na⁺ reabsorption. The percentage of the filtered load of Na⁺ reabsorbed by each nephron segment is indicated. PCT, proximal convoluted tubule; TAL, thick ascending limb; DCT, distal convoluted tubule; CDD, cortical collecting duct; IMCD, inner medullary collecting duct. From Koeppen and Stanton 2001, with permission of Mosby, St Louis.

within the tubule. This difference is achieved by the differences in the wall permeability and the direction of the flow within the loop.

The diluting segment and the DCT

The thick ascending loop of Henle transport processes recover NaCl but leave behind urea; this is the so-called 'diluting segment'. The NaCl passes into the vasa recta and the descending thin loops of Henle, so increasing the concentration in the loop. As the fluid moves up into the DCT, there is a NaCl cotransport process which recovers salt and fluid back into the peritubular vessels. The fluid now entering the collecting duct is hypotonic with a low salt and a high urea concentration recovered in the presence of vasopressin.

Cortical collecting duct

As fluid now enters the CCD and descends into the MCD, more salt and water are recovered, especially in the presence of vasopressin. The urea concentration of the collecting duct fluid rises even higher and now acts as the main 'osmotic' molecule.

Towards the tip of the pyramid there is a sudden increase in permeability (see Fig 14.15) towards urea, and this high permeability allows urea to recirculate from the tubule and reinforces the concentration process. Note that in starvation, when blood urea is low, concentrated urine cannot be formed and fluid is lost, which compounds the problems for the already stressed subject.

If vasopressin is absent, the water permeability of the whole collecting duct is low so dilute urine is formed. However, in this state the gradient between the inside of the tubule and the ECF is very high, so that a considerable fraction of water is recovered by the loop, even though the water permeability is low. Note: The values shown in Figure 14.15 are for illustration only and should not be learnt.

RENAL CONTROL OF SODIUM BALANCE

The control of sodium balance by the kidney depends on the complex interplay between a number of factors, including dietary components, cardiac output and blood pressure, autoregulation within the kidney, and neuroendocrine factors.

For normal body function it is vital that the osmolarity of the plasma and ECF are closely controlled to about 285 mOsm. This control depends on the sodium content of these fluids, which in turn will affect the volume of cells since water can move in and out of the cells depending on the osmotic gradient across the cell membrane. The plasma volume is controlled by a balance between the blood pressure and the colloid osmotic pressure of plasma proteins acting across the capillary walls according to the Starling equilibrium.

On a day-to-day basis, the volume of the ECF depends on sodium content, which is initially kept constant by the addition or excretion of water via the actions of vasopressin. Water can be rapidly lost or gained within 30 min by this mechanism if the osmolarity of plasma changes which, as we have seen, is independent of the control solute. Independent of this fluid homeostasis is the control of sodium balance which is a much slower process, yet over a period of a few days maintains a balance between the sodium intake and sodium loss.

In a diet of natural foods, the content of sodium is relatively low and both humans and animals seek salt (NaCl), both for its value as an essential ion and to improve food flavour. Providing the diet contains 1–2 g of NaCl per day and exercise is moderate (sweat rate low), a human will stay in salt balance with this level of intake. With the added salt in modern processed foods, however, excess salt intake is now a major problem. When we are young, we can consume 100–200 g salt per day and simply excrete the excess salt which is termed **natriuresis** (Information box 14.2). As we age, the ability to excrete excess salt is lost and salt is retained.

Salt balance is mainly controlled via the kidney, but salt can be lost or retained by both the sweat glands and the colon. The hormone aldosterone, released from the adrenal cortex in response to a number of stimuli, can induce these tissues to conserve salt by the upregulation of channels and carriers.

Renal sodium handling

The kidney filters a huge amount of sodium into the renal tubules. Assuming that the GFR is about 180 L/day and the

---

ℹ Information box 14.2   Natriuretic peptides

The atrial natriuretic peptides (ANPs), synthesised mainly in the cardiac atria, promote Na⁺ excretion and lower blood pressure. They are secreted in response to cardiac failure, when the atrial walls are stretched and the ventricles are overloaded. ANP acts on the cells of the renal collecting tubules to prevent Na⁺ entry (see below).

Brain natriuretic peptide (BNP) is secreted by the ventricles. It has similar properties to ANP. Plasma ANP and BNP are increased in heart failure, and is used as a marker for early cardiac failure when there may be no (or few) symptoms.

plasma Na^+ concentration is 145 mM, the renal filtration of Na^+ will be in the region of 26000 mM of Na^+ per 24 hours. Of this vast amount, 99% must be reabsorbed by the nephron to stay in balance. The majority of Na^+ recovery is fixed, and is said to be constitutive with only a small percentage under variable control by the distal tubule, colon and sweat glands. The proportion of Na^+ recovered by the segments of the nephron is shown in Fig. 14.17. Na^+ must first cross from the tubular fluid into the cell across the luminal or apical side of the cell. Since Na^+ ions are polar, they cannot cross a lipid bilayer by simple diffusion and this passage must be carrier mediated.

Sodium recovery

The majority of ion and fluid movement is dependent on the Na^+ gradient generated across the cell by the Na^+/K^+-ATPase pumps located on the blood side of the tubule cells.

The PCT

As previously discussed, from the tubule side of the PCT, non-electrolytes are transported into the cells of the tubule using a sodium dependent cotransporter, which can move these molecules 'uphill' against their concentration gradient using the potential energy of the Na^+ gradient. Non-electrolytes then pass into the blood by facilitated carriers 'downhill', and the sodium which has entered with them is returned to the blood by the Na^+/K^+-ATPase.

The PCT recovers 50–55% of the filtered sodium and water and almost all the glucose, amino acids and nucleosides. A key element of these processes is the Na^+/H^+ antiporter on the apical side of the cell, which recovers Na^+ for H^+ using the Na^+ gradient. The Na^+ then passes to the basolateral side where it is transported back to the blood via the Na^+/K^+-ATPase (Fig. 14.9).

The loop of Henle

The descending thin loop of Henle is water permeable, and as the fluid descends into the medulla the tubule contents are concentrated as the loop is exposed to the increasing concentration gradient in the ECF (see Fig. 14.15). On turning the loop, the wall of the thin ascending loop becomes less permeable to water, but permeable to Na^+ and urea. In all, some 25% of the remaining Na^+ passes from the loop into the ECF and is recovered by the counter-current flow of the vasa recta. The structure of the loop changes again to become the thick ascending loop of Henle, where the powerful $Na^+/K^+/2Cl^-$ carrier removes a further 15% of Na^+ into the cell. This process, which is sensitive to furosemide (see Ch. 4), dilutes the tubule fluid further and this Na^+ is removed from the cell by the usual Na^+/K^+-ATPase. The K^+ is recycled via K^+ channels back into the tubule and the Cl^- exits via Cl^- channels into the blood.

The DCT

In the DCT, which is the connecting segment, the dilute fluid emerging from the loop loses another 5–8% more Na^+ via a thiazide sensitive Na^+/Cl^- cotransport (see Ch. 4).

The collecting ducts

The fluid in the DCT becomes isotonic as salts and water are recovered into the peritubular vessels, aided by the high colloid osmotic pressure of these capillaries, and finally leaves the DCT to enter the collecting ducts. As the fluid descends the collecting ducts, more sodium is recovered by

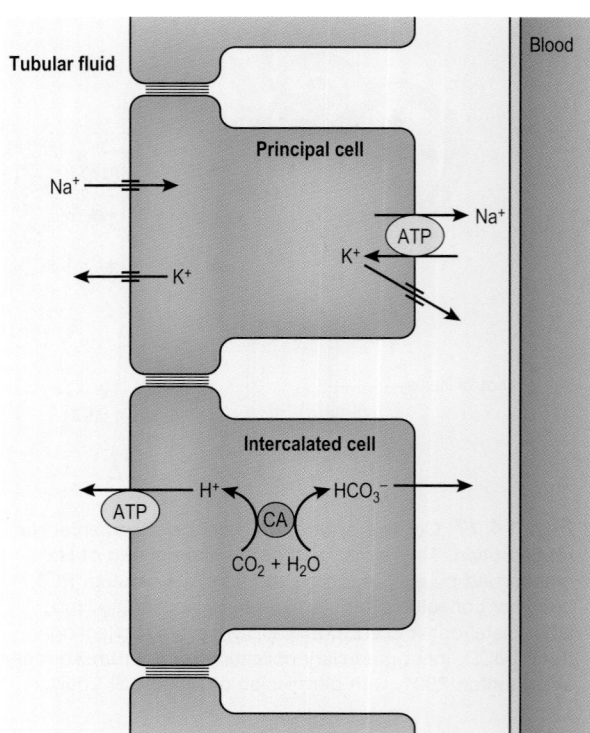

Fig. 14.18 **Autoregulation.** Transport pathways in principal cells and intercalated cells of the distal tubule and collecting duct. ATP, adenosine triphosphate; CA, carbonic anydrase. From Koeppen and Stanton 2001, with permission of Mosby, St Louis.

Na^+/Cl^- cotransport. In this region there are two specific cell types with very different transport properties. The intercalated cells have a H^+-ATPase on the luminal side and can lower the pH of the tubular fluid to pH 4.5, generating in turn new HCO_3^-, which passes back across the basolateral face with Na^+ (Fig. 14.18). In the other cell type, the principal cells, Na^+ passes via Na^+ channels on the apical side into the cells and K^+ exits back into the tubule via K^+ channels in exchange. This K^+ loss into the tubule can cause hypokalaemia (see Ch. 4). Sodium entry into the cells of the collecting ducts occurs through selective Na^+ channels which are opened in response to aldosterone and closed by ANP. With a low level of Na^+ there will be high levels of aldosterone, which will conserve Na^+ so Na^+ loss in urine can be reduced to as low as 1 mM.

Control of GFR by the renal capillaries

Since the amount of sodium entering the renal tubules depends on the GFR it is critical that this filtration process is controlled by a number of mechanisms.

Autoregulation

The first step in sodium balance is to control the hydrostatic pressure driving fluid across the capillary walls; renal glomerular capillaries are unusual in having arterioles at both ends (see Fig. 14.18). These arterioles have sympathetic receptors with different sensitivity to noradrenaline, the efferent arteriole being more sensitive than the afferent, so maintaining the net filtration force when the blood pressure (BP) falls. However, under high levels of sympathetic drive, the renal blood flow can fall and filtration is reduced. Normally, for values of arterial pressures between 70 mmHg and about

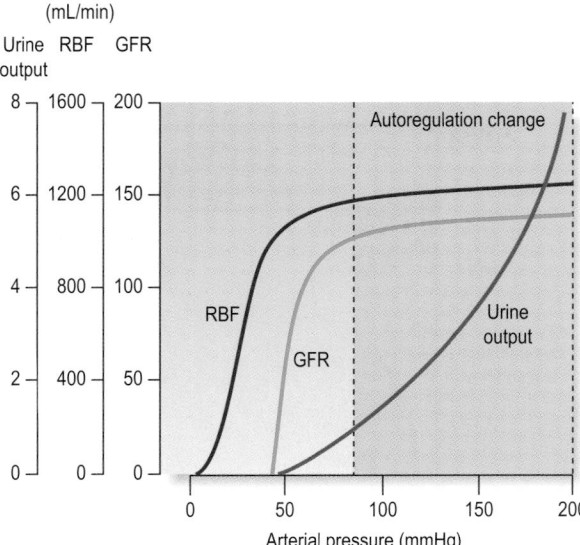

Fig. 14.19 **The independence or autoregulation of renal blood flow (RBF) and glomerular filtration rate (GFR) to changes in blood pressure (BP) above 70 mmHg.** Do note that the lower part of the figure shows that urine flow does increase but only to a small degree as the blood pressure (BP) rises. A further key point is that below a BP of 70 mmHg the RBF and GFR fall with a decrease in BP which can lead to renal failure. From Guyton AC, Hall JE 1996 Textbook of medical physiology, 9th edn. WB Saunders, Toronto, with permission.

180 mmHg the renal blood flow (RBF) and GFR are constant, so that variation in blood pressure does not result in changes in renal haemodynamics and GFR (Fig. 14.19). The rate of urine formation increases with increasing blood pressure, but these changes are small in relation to the large change in blood pressure. Below 70 mmHg the GFR and RBF both fall and such low pressures can cause ischaemia and renal failure.

Glomerular–tubular balance

There is also an intrinsic mechanism in the PCT which increases the reabsorption of fluid and salts in proportion to any changes in the GFR. This may be related to the filtration fraction which would alter the peritubular colloid osmotic pressure, so increasing reabsorption. There may also be a flow dependent factor which increases GFR. These mechanisms ensure that although a single nephron may have a different GFR, the GFRs will match and contribute to the overall balance across the renal bed.

Receptors involved with sodium balance

The Na^+ level in the blood is mainly controlled by the kidney. The 'level' of Na^+ is 'detected' at multiple sites and with a multiple layer sensor system. As has been stated the level of Na^+ reflects the volume of extracellular fluid so there is a need for 'volume' receptors. Since 'volume' cannot be measured directly it can be assessed indirectly by the degree of stretch in the walls of vascular structures containing various low and high pressure baroreceptors.

Baroreceptors

High pressure baroreceptors are located in the walls of carotid arteries and the aorta. These respond to dynamic changes in arterial pressure, being low pressure receptors that can measure an index of 'volume' by the distention of blood vessel walls. These are found in the great veins, atria and ventricles. There are also receptors in the vessels of the liver, the kidneys and the thorax.

The juxtaglomerular apparatus

The juxtaglomerular apparatus (JGA) shown in Fig. 14.20 is a special modified part of the tubule that has three components.

- The first segment of the afferent arteriole, close to the glomerulus, is lined with granular cells which secrete the proteolytic enzyme renin into the blood in response to a fall in Na^+ in the afferent blood supply.
- Second, these cells are also supplied with sympathetic nerves which respond to a fall in arterial pressure.
- Finally, around the afferent and efferent capillaries is a specialised group of mesangial cells through which runs the distal tubule with the specialised macula densa (MD) cells at the interface. The MD cells are especially sensitive to the delivery of chloride ions by the distal tubule. If this delivery is decreased, afferent arteriolar dilation occurs, which may be via prostaglandins and which restores the MD flow; this is termed tubulo-glomerular feedback.

This complex structure; the JGA, responds to:

- The perfusion pressure in the afferent arteriole
- The sympathetic nerve supply to the arterioles
- The 'sodium' concentration in distal tubule as reflected by the chloride delivery.

Renin-angiotension-aldosterone system

The JGA structures are the principal detectors of the renin-angiotensin-aldosterone system. If the ECF volume falls, the pressure distending the afferent arteriole falls, which will cause a sympathetic system discharge onto the afferent arteriolar granular cells. At the same time the supply of sodium '(Cl^-)' ions to the distal tubule falls and these stimuli lead to the release of renin into the blood. Renin is an enzyme which acts on the peptide angiotensinogen, an α-2 globulin in the blood manufactured by the liver. Renin removes a four amino acid fragment to generate angiotensin I (10 amino acids). In various vascular beds, ACE, which is bound to the walls of the blood vessels, mostly in the lung, removes a further two amino acids to form the powerful vasoconstrictor peptide angiotensin II.

Role of angiotensin II and Na^+ control

Angiotensin II has the following actions:

- It is a potent vasoconstrictor of blood vessels, so increases tubular perfusion rate and blood pressure.
- It causes the release of aldosterone from the adrenal cortex.
- It causes the release of vasopressin and stimulates the area postrema, causing thirst.
- It increases the reabsorption of salt by the PCT and activates the sympathetic nervous system centrally.

All these actions cause Na^+ retention, which eventually, by negative feedback, switches off the response.

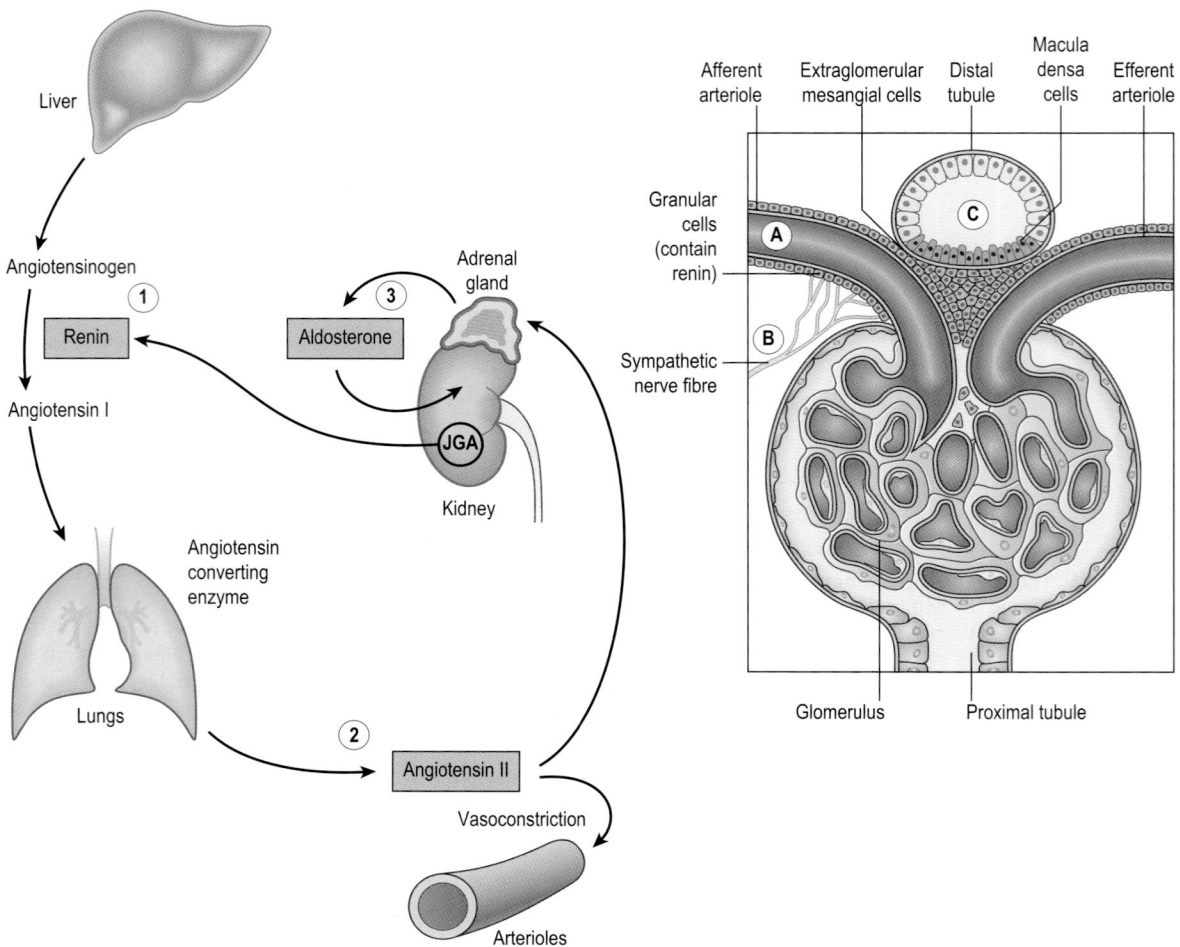

Fig. 14.20 **The renin–angiotensin–aldosterone system.** The numbers 1–3 show the sequence of steps in the activation of the system. The inset shows the juxtaglomerular apparatus (JGA) with major stimuli acting as triggers for renin release. *A* – fall in pressure in afferent arteriole; *B* – release of noradrenaline (norepinephrine) by sympathetic nerve endings on granular cells; *C* – fall in NaCl concentration in distal tubule. Note that angiotensin II has a number of additional actions not shown on this figure. From Field MJ, Pollock CA and Harris DCH 2001 The renal system. Churchill Livingstone, London, with permission.

Aldosterone

Angiotensin II is closely coupled to the release of aldosterone.

- Aldosterone acts on the late part of the DCT and on collecting ducts. It also acts on salivary and sweat glands, and on the colon.
- Aldosterone being lipid soluble crosses the cell wall and binds to a cytoplasmic receptor, and causes the synthesis of Na^+ channel proteins, which increases the uptake of Na^+ by the lumen side of the DCT cells. It also increases the Na^+ transport on the blood side, via Na^+ pump, which raises the cell potential difference (i.e. makes it more negative) and this increases the uptake of Cl^-.
- Aldosterone potentiates the $Na^+/K^+/2Cl^-$ transport in the thick ascending loop of Henle.
- It causes the excretion of H^+ ions by the DCT, therefore if in excess it can cause alkalosis.

Potassium

If the level of K^+ in the plasma is elevated this acts directly on the adrenal cortex to cause the secretion of K^+ into the

lumen by the DCT, which is independent of the renin-angiotensin system.

Clinical box 14.6 **Essential hypertension**

The elevation of blood pressure occurs with age, obesity and genetic factors. However, the role of the kidney and salt is still controversial. While there is no doubt that a high salt intake from processed foods can lead to hypertension, the exact mechanism has not been resolved. In youth, any excess salt is easily excreted but with ageing, this ability is lost. There is, however, no doubt that there is a strong link with the renal handling of salt. Experiments demonstrated that obstructing the renal artery caused hypertension in experimental animals. This response is related to the sodium detection systems within the kidney and the false error signal leads to the release of renin/ angiotensin/aldosterone, thus causing an increase in total peripheral resistance, retention of sodium and expansion of the vascular volume, all of which lead to hypertension. Although a tremendous volume of research has investigated human hypertension, no uniform hypothesis has emerged. Some patients do not have elevated renin or blood volume and do not respond to diuretics so at present this condition is still an enigma. Drugs used in the medical treatment of hypertension are discussed in Chapter 4.

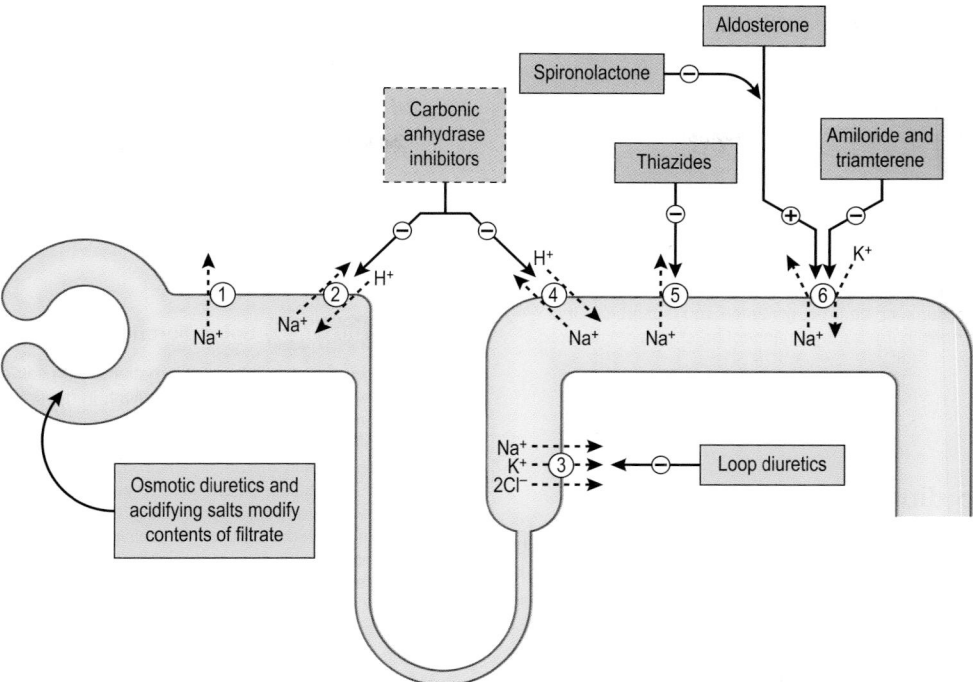

Fig. 14.21 **Main sites of action of diuretics and sodium absorption in the nephron.** (1) Na^+ (passive Cl^- absorption);
(2) Na^+/H^+ exchange; (3) $Na^+/K^+/2Cl^-$ cotransport; (4) Na^+/H^+ exchange; (5) Na^+/Cl^- cotransport; (6) Na^+/K^+ exchange.
Currently used diuretics are shown in *solid boxes*, agents not used for their diuretic action in *boxes with dotted lines*. After
Rang HP, Dale MM and Ritter JM 1999 Pharmacology, 4th edn. Churchill Livingstone, Edinburgh, with permission.

Autoregulation and the DCT

The distal convoluted tubule is limited in its ability to handle
large quantities of salt and water, so the flow of fluid and ions
is also controlled by autoregulation, which is dependent on
the local release of angiotensin II via the MD. Angiotensin
antagonists cause a loss in the ability to autoregulate, so that
as the blood pressure falls, the threshold of the ability to
autoregulate occurs at a 'higher' pressure. Normally, angiotensin II release will increase the efferent arteriolar resistance
as the blood pressure falls, so maintaining GFR.

Tubulo-glomerular feedback

The MD cells not only control the release of renin in response
to a fall in the 'sodium' level but also function in tubulo-
glomerular feedback. A fall in chloride delivery to the distal
nephron will cause afferent arteriolar dilation possibly mediated via prostaglandins. The release of renin via the angiotensin system will cause efferent vasoconstriction. Both of
the above will increase GFR and raise the flow through the
distal tubule towards normal.

Na+ balance summary

Sodium balance within the kidney depends on both physical
factors, such as the cardiac output and blood pressure which
are usually balanced by autoregulation, and on neuroendocrine factors. Autoregulation can be controlled by the 'myogenic mechanism' of the smooth muscles of arterioles which
contract in response to stretch, as is seen in most vascular
beds, but in the kidney, the sympathetic system, acting
through noradrenaline release, can act differentially on the
efferent arterioles to maintain GFR when the blood pressure

falls. The renin-angiotensin-aldosterone system acts to
control not only the GFR, but also the release of renin and
aldosterone, which can upregulate the expression of transporters such as the $Na^+/K^+/2Cl^-$ carrier in the thick ascending
loop of Henle, Na^+/Cl^- cotransport in the DCT and recycling
of urea in the inner medulla. Other neurohormones such as
nitric oxide, ANP, kinin, adenosine, vasopressin and endothelin also play a complex role. This mixture of physical factors
and neuroendocrine influences leads to the mechanism by
which Na^+ balance is achieved.

DIURETICS

When fluid balance is disturbed, if the kidneys are beginning
to function less efficiently or in diabetes, the circulation
becomes overfilled, leading to hypertension. In these states
it is necessary to increase the urine flow with **diuretics** to
reduce the fluid overload in the circulation. The therapeutic
use of diuretics exploits the processes through which renal
resorption of fluid takes place. These drugs have several
sites of action along the nephron, with different mechanisms
of action depending on the processes of water and salt
recovery in the given segment of the nephron.

Most of the 183 L of water filtered into the nephron in 24
hours must be recovered to preserve homeostasis. The bulk
of this fluid (some 70%) is reabsorbed by the PCT, the loops
of Henle recover about 10–20%, leaving the thick ascending
loop, the distal convoluted tubule and the collecting ducts to
recover the final 10%, so only about 1 mL/min passes into
the bladder as urine. The potential sites at which diuretics
can act is shown in Fig. 14.21 (see also Ch. 4).

Osmotic diuresis

Glucose is freely filtered by the capillaries of the nephron, and some 99% is normally recovered by the PCT. If there is an excess of plasma glucose, the recovery process becomes saturated and glucose remains in the tubular lumen; here, since glucose is a small molecule and osmotically active, it retains water in the urine which leads to a brisk osmotic diuresis, salt loss and 'raging thirst', seen in untreated diabetes mellitus. This defect was known from the times of the Ancient Greeks as flies were attracted to the sweet urine (mellitus is Greek for honey). The first test of urine involved tasting a tiny drop of the fluid, which revealed the glucose content of the urine of these patients. The concentration of glucose in both plasma and urine is now measured using 'dipsticks'.

Osmotic diuresis can be used clinically to increase urine flow by using an intravenous infusion of the sugar alcohol, **mannitol**. Mannitol is a small, osmotically active molecule, but is not recovered by the glucose carriers or metabolised, and, being polar, remains trapped in the nephron.

Carbonic anhydrase inhibitors

The recovery of Na^+ by PCT depends on the low intracellular sodium concentration produced by the basolateral sodium pump (see above and Fig. 14.9). On the luminal side of the tubular cell, the exchange of H^+ ions from the cell cytoplasm for Na^+ ions leads to H^+ ions in the tubular fluid. These H^+ ions react with the filtered HCO_3^- ions, which generates CO_2. The CO_2 being lipid soluble passes into the cytoplasm of the PCT cells and is reconverted to H^+ and HCO_3^- ions under the influence of the enzyme **carbonic anhydrase** which is bound to the wall of the PCT cells. The enzyme can be inhibited by a group of **carbonic anhydrase inhibitors** developed from sulphonamides, which were found to cause a mild diuresis. The diuretic effect of carbonic anhydrase inhibition is weak because although it has a major effect on the PCT, the retention of salt and water into the tubule is corrected by the recovery processes further along the nephron.

The thiazide diuretics

Thiazide diuretics block the Na^+/Cl^- cotransport in the distal convoluted tubule (DCT). Examples are chlorothiazide, hydrochlorothiazide and bendrofluazide (see Ch. 4). In this section of the nephron, the cotransport process helps the recovery of Na^+ and Cl^- by the DCT, but although they are well tolerated, the diuresis is relatively mild, since the majority of the salt and water has been removed by the PCT and the thick ascending loop of Henle. They are, however, useful for reducing circulatory volume, especially in the treatment of age-related hypertension. Side effects include potassium loss, increased calcium retention and metabolic alkalosis (see Ch. 4). They also cause vasodilation so are ideal for the treatment of hypertension. They should be avoided in patients with gout as they can cause hyperuricaemia.

Loop diuretics

This relatively newer group of diuretics act on the thick ascending loop of Henle and inhibit the key $Na^+/K^+/2Cl^-$ cotransport process (see Fig. 14.15). This carrier complex recovers large amounts of Na^+ from the lumen of the thick ascending loop so that the fluid entering the DCT has a low osmolarity. Blocking of this process by inhibitors leads to an added load of Na^+ passing into the DCT, which prevents recovery of water by the collecting ducts and cause a brisk dose-related diuresis. Examples include furosemide, bumetanide and ethacrynic acid (see Ch. 4). Loop diuretics act rapidly with a steep dose response curve inducing a profound diuresis. These drugs are rapidly absorbed from the gastrointestinal tract and, being bound to plasma proteins, are not filtered into the nephron but are secreted by the PCT.

Diuretics acting on the late distal tubule and the collecting ducts (K^+ sparing)

Amiloride and triamterene

Amiloride and triamterene are sodium (Na^+) blockers. The principal cells in the late DCT and collecting ducts (see Fig. 14.21) have Na^+ channels in the luminal membrane which leads to the uptake of Na^+ from the tubules; this Na^+ is then returned to the blood via the basolateral sodium pumps. To

Spironolactone is K⁺ 'sparing', so is used in combination with thiazides to prevent K⁺ loss. It is useful in the treatment of primary aldosteronism (adrenal tumours) and in refractory oedema associated with secondary aldosteronism due to cardiac failure, hepatic cirrhosis and nephrotic syndrome. Amiloride is also sometimes used in conjunction with loop or thiazide diuretics. However, both the Na⁺-channel blockers and spironolactone are contraindicated in patients with hyperkalaemia since the K⁺-retention properties of these drugs can be life-threatening.

balance the charge there are K⁺ channels which transfer K⁺ into the tubular lumen. Amiloride and triamterene block these Na⁺ channels, so reduce the recovery of Na⁺ in the late DCT. Although the recovery of Na⁺ by these regions is important it is relatively small and the diuretic effect is limited, but they do prevent excessive K⁺ loss.

Spironolactone

Spironolactone competes with aldosterone, and is a K⁺-sparing diuretic. Aldosterone is the adrenal cortical mineralo-corticoid which is responsible for the control of sodium in the kidney, sweat glands and colon. Aldosterone crosses the basolateral membrane of the late distal tubule and binds to cytosolic membrane receptors which are then translocated to the nucleus. This passage causes the production of multiple gene products which are thought to activate 'silent' Na⁺ channels and Na⁺ pumps and also increase the permeability of the tight junctions. The net effect of these actions is to enhance the NaCl transport back into the blood when Na⁺ is low and cause the excretion of K⁺ and H⁺ ions into the lumen. Spironolactone competitively inhibits the binding of aldosterone to its receptors, leading to a loss of Na⁺ into the urine. The efficiency of this drug does depend on the endogenous level of aldosterone.

RENAL CONTROL OF ACID–BASE BALANCE

The kidney plays a vital role in the control of acid–base balance. The pH of the plasma is held close to 7.4 under normal conditions. This value, which reflects a plasma H⁺ concentration of 40 nM/L, depends on the balance between the concentration of HCO_3^- ions in the plasma, which is mainly controlled by the kidneys, and the arterial pCO_2 which is controlled by the respiratory system (see Chs 3 and 13).

Hydrogen ions

The CO_2 in the circulation is mostly derived from oxidation of glucose and, as the rate of metabolism changes, say in exercise, the increased production of CO_2 is detected by the central and peripheral chemoreceptors, which increase the rate of ventilation so the excess CO_2 is excreted via the lungs and the arterial pCO_2 is kept remarkably constant (see Ch. 13). Since these H⁺ ions can easily be excreted via the lungs, they are termed **volatile**.

The arterial pH therefore depends on the balance between the HCO_3^- concentration and the pCO_2, i.e. kidney/lung. The $[HCO_3^-]$ is the prime buffer in the blood and is therefore affected by the production of **fixed** acids by the biochemical process of the body. These H⁺ ions are defined as 'fixed'

since they can only be excreted via the kidneys. These used to be defined as metabolic H⁺ ions, which can be confusing, so now it is better to use the term non-respiratory H⁺ ions (see below).

Sources of H⁺ ions

Although all H⁺ ions are protons, in biology it is convenient to categorise the H⁺ ions in relation to their sources.

Cell metabolism produces 'volatile' H⁺ ions

The aerobic metabolism of glucose to produce ATP and energy generates some 14 000 mM of H⁺ from bicarbonate (H_2CO_3) which is linked to ventilation and is rapidly adjusted to keep the pH constant. These are primarily 'volatile' H⁺ ions and so can be rapidly 'blown off' or retained by the lungs.

'Fixed' H⁺ ions

'Fixed' H⁺ ions are generated from metabolic processes and the concentration depends largely on the diet. The total amount is relatively small (80–100 mM per 24 h) when compared to the 14 000 mM of 'volatile acid', but the rate of excretion is slow in relation to the acidification process of the renal tubules, which can produce a minimum urinary pH of 4.5. The pH limit of 4.5 is set by the ability of the collecting duct intercalated cell H⁺-ATPase to secrete H⁺ into the tubule, which it can do to about 800 times of the value in the plasma. This value of 4.5 represents a minute concentration of free H⁺ ions equivalent to 0.003 M of H⁺ in the 1–2 L of urine which is produced per day at the rate of about 1 mL/min; it does, however, cause considerable discomfort when passed. The pH of plasma represents 40 nmol/L of H⁺ so 100 mM is still a relatively large concentration.

There are, however, buffers in the urine which allow more H⁺ ions to be secreted into the tubule yet keep the pH above the critical limit of 4.5. The kidneys must excrete H⁺ ions at a rate equal to the rate of extra renal net acid production (0.3–1.0 mM/kg per 24 h).

Sources of non-respiratory H⁺ ions

- Dietary sulphates: Amino acids such as methionine and cysteine, which contain 'S' groups, yield the equivalent of an intake of H_2SO_4 when they are metabolised to urea. In a normal mixed diet this represents an intake of 50–100 mM of 'fixed' H⁺ ions per day. This figure will be much higher for individuals who have a high dietary intake of meat, whereas for a vegetarian diet, the value will be much less.
- Phosphates: A further source of 'fixed' acid is the turnover and breakdown of phospholipids in neurons and DNA which produces the equivalent of some 50 mM of phosphoric acid (H_3PO_4) per day.
- Lactic acid: In health, the arterial pCO_2 only changes in extreme exercise when there is insufficient oxygen to supply the muscles (anaerobiosis) and lactic acidosis occurs (see Chs 3 and 13). The lactic acid, with a pK of 3, dissociates to release ions which act via the peripheral chemoreceptors to drive the ventilation at a rate greater than needed to keep the pCO_2 constant and so disturbs the normal relationship between CO_2 and the rate of ventilation for a given pCO_2. This causes a paradoxical fall in pCO_2 to a small degree. This excess ventilation caused by the raised H⁺ is termed hyperventilation and not the hyperpnoea of normal exercise when the pH is kept constant. Lactic acid is

also produced during surgery when tissues are under perfused and during heart failure when the blood pressure is reduced (see Ch. 3 for lactic acidosis).

Disease states

In disease states excess amounts of fixed acid can be produced, such as the keto acids, α-ketoglutaric and α-hydroxybutyric acids in diabetes mellitus when the supply of glucose is insufficient and fat is metabolised instead (see Ch. 3).

Acid–base balance is vital for life

In comparison to the vast acid load of H_2CO_3, the above figure of 100–150 mM of fixed H^+ ions appears to be small, but it must be remembered that these are strong acids which are not volatile, so can only be eliminated by the kidneys. In renal failure these fixed acids rapidly accumulate leading to acidosis, and if blood pH falls below 6.9, it will result in death (see Ch. 13).

The proteins in the body are used for construction of tissue and for the thousands of enzymes which control all our body functions. These enzymes are complex chains of amino acids folded in a three-dimensional form which brings their active sites to the surface of the molecule in a critical fashion. This folding of a molecule depends on various charged processes (e.g. hydrogen bonds) which are very sensitive to the acidity of their environment. If the body becomes acid, the activities of many of the enzymes change, e.g. conversion of lactate to glucose is decreased by 64% if the pH falls from 7.4 to 7.0.

Renal mechanisms of HCO_3^- control

The kidney can act in three prime ways to maintain the concentration of HCO_3^- ions constant in the plasma (see also Ch. 13).

1. Recovery of filtered HCO_3^-: The rate of filtration of HCO_3^- is directly proportional to the plasma HCO_3^- concentration and the GFR. But since no HCO_3^- is usually found in the urine, the majority of this must be reabsorbed by the nephron. The bulk of HCO_3^- recovery occurs in the PCT (80%), and by the end of the PCT the tubular fluid is acidified to a pH of 6.7 as the concentration of HCO_3^- decreases from 24 mM to 8 mM. There are two processes by which this is achieved.
2. Na^+/H^+ antiporter (see also Fig. 14.9): Na^+ enters the cell down its concentration gradient in exchange for H^+. This antiporter carrier called NHE3 is a one-to-one coupled process of Na^+ for H^+ so is electrically neutral and accounts for 65% of the H^+ secretion. It can be inhibited with amiloride and by lithium which is used in psychiatry and competes with Na^+. In addition, glucocorticoids and thyroid hormones also increase the activity of this antiporter.
3. H^+-ATPase: There is also an H^+-ATPase present which can also transfer H^+ into the tubule lumen of the PCT using ATP which carries the remaining 35% of H^+ secretion (see Fig. 14.9). The H^+ movement into the tubule leads to a reaction with the filtered HCO_3^- to form carbonic acid, which immediately splits into CO_2 and H_2O (see also Fig. 14.9). The CO_2, being lipid soluble, passes into the tubule cells where under the influence of carbonic anhydrase (CA), both bound to the cell walls

and free in the cytoplasm, it rapidly forms carbonic acid, which then splits non-enzymically into H^+ ions and HCO_3^-. The H^+ ions are then used by the antiport carrier again to recover more Na^+ ions. The HCO_3^- ions pass to the basal lateral side of the cell where they are carried across the cell wall to the peritubular capillaries by an electrogenic $Na^+/3HCO_3^-$ carrier. The H^+ formed by the CA-catalysed reaction in the cell is used to recover more filtered HCO_3^- from the PCT (Fig. 14.9).

The Na^+/H^+ antiport can apparently use K^+ instead of H^+, so in alkaline states when the H^+ level falls more K^+ is lost into the tubule, resulting in the condition of hypokalaemic alkalosis. Conversely, in acidosis, less K^+ is lost and hyperkalaemic acidosis can occur as K^+ is retained in the blood. These conditions are observed in vivo, but this explanation may be a little simplistic.

HCO_3^- ions and pCO_2

The recovery of HCO_3^- ions is related to the pCO_2 so if the pCO_2 rises, more HCO_3^- is recovered. Hypercapnia (excess CO_2 in the blood) leads to an increased renal recovery of HCO_3^- and an increase in the HCO_3^-/pCO_2 ratio. This process is relatively slow and takes 2–3 days (see Ch. 13). After haemoglobin, HCO_3^- is the first line key buffer in the plasma. The production of fixed acids such as lactic acid in hard exercise and ketoacidosis in untreated diabetes mellitus leads to a rapid fall in the plasma HCO_3^- concentration by this 'buffering' process. To overcome this acidosis and to return the pH to normal, new HCO_3^- has to be generated and the excess fixed H^+ ion excreted.

Loop of Henle and HCO_3^- ions

The loop of Henle is a key segment for the counter-current hypothesis and the differential permeability of the loops leads to a concentration of tubular fluid at the 'hairpin' turn. The loss of water over electrolytes leads to a rise in the tubular HCO_3^- concentration so the fluid becomes alkaline. This raised HCO_3^- is, however, removed by the thick ascending loop so fluid entering the DCT and the collecting ducts has returned to a low HCO_3^- concentration.

The distal nephron

In the tubular segment from the DCT to the end of the collecting ducts, there are two types of specialised epithelial cell. The principal cells have Na^+ and K^+ channels on their apical side, which lead to K^+ loss when the Na^+ load in the tubule is increased in diuresis. A second cell type, the intercalated cell, has a H^+-ATPase on the apical side and can secrete H^+ ions and can reduce the acidity of the tubule to the minimum pH 4.5, a gradient of $\times 800$. This process leads to the production of more HCO_3^- in the cell, which is then exchanged for Cl^- ions on the basolateral side of the cell. In this case, these are newly generated HCO_3^- ions which can replace the lost HCO_3^- ions in the plasma. The Cl^- is recycled via a Cl^- channel as shown in Fig. 14.9. This H^+-ATPase is induced by mineralocorticoids, such as aldosterone, which accounts for the observed alkalosis seen with excess of this steroid.

Renal buffers

To achieve the excretion of the fixed H^+ ions produced daily yet keep the pH above 4.5, urinary buffers are needed. These

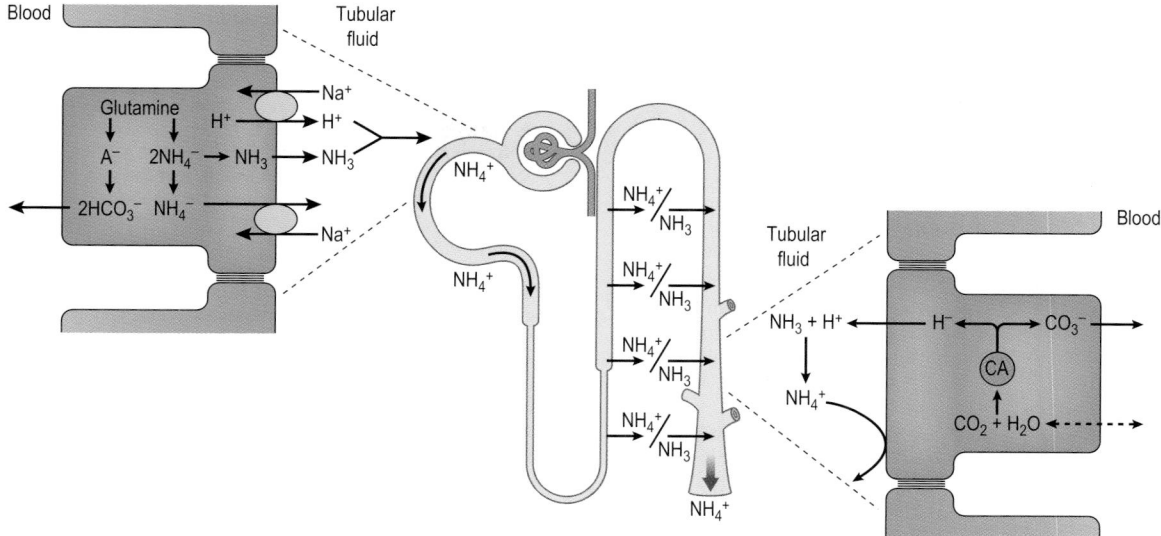

Fig. 14.22 Production, transport and excretion of ammonia by the nephron. Glutamine is metabolised to NH_4^+ and HCO_3^- in the proximal tubule. The NH_4^+ is secreted into the lumen, and the HCO_3^- enters the blood. The secreted NH_4^+ is reabsorbed in the loop of Henle primarily by the thick ascending loop and accumulates in the medullary interstitium, where it exists as both NH_4^+ and NH_3. NH_3 diffuses into the tubular fluid of the collecting duct, and H^+ secretion by the collecting duct leads to accumulation of NH_4^+ in the lumen by the processes of non-ionic diffusion and diffusion trapping. CA, carbonic anhydrase. From Koeppen and Stanton 2001, with permission of Mosby, St Louis.

buffers depend on the urine being acid so although the direct loss of free H^+ is minute, the low pH plays a key role in the excretion of H^+.

Phosphate buffering

In the plasma at pH 7.4 'phosphate' ions depend on the equation:

$$HPO_4^{2-} + H^+ \rightleftharpoons H_2PO_4^-$$

and the equilibrium will lie to the left, since the pK of this reaction is 6.8. In acidic urine at a pH of 4.5, the ratio of HPO_4^{2-} to $H_2PO_4^-$ will switch from 4:1 at pH 7.4 to 1:200 at pH 4.5. This has the advantage of keeping the pH at 4.5 as the added H^+ is 'locked' into the $H_2PO_4^-$. This also saves a cation as there is one less negative charge to balance, usually by a Na^+. Although concentration of HPO_4^{2-} in plasma is low, the molecule is retained in the nephron and with the recovery of water and salts so reaches a concentration of 30–50 mM per 24 h. This can therefore buffer the same amount of H^+ ions, which is about half the daily acid load.

The low urinary pH also has two further effects. First, some molecules with a pK close to 4.5 will become partial buffers so reduce their need for buffering. This is seen with the keto-acids, so their effect on the pH is reduced. Secondly, the synthesis of NH_4^+ from glutamine depends on a low pH.

Ammonium synthesis

Ammonia (NH_3) can exist as ammonium ions (NH_4^+) in the reaction:

$$NH_3 + H^+ \rightleftharpoons NH_4^+$$

which has a pK of 9 and therefore the equilibrium will be far to the right (see also Ch. 3). The proximal tubule is the major site for the synthesis of ammonia mostly from the conversion of glutamine by glutaminase to glutamate. This enzyme is upregulated in acidosis. The reaction yields one ammonia molecule and when the glutamate is further converted to α-ketoglutarate, a further ammonia molecule is produced. The ammonia molecules react with H^+ ions and yield NH_4^+ ions. Since NH_3 is moderately lipid soluble it can cross the apical cell membranes whereas NH_4^+ has a low permeability and becomes trapped in the lumen once this has occurred. NH_4^+ can also travel on the Na^+/H^+ antiporter, which is sensitive to **amiloride**. NH_4^+ ions accumulate in the tubular fluid where the luminal pH is less than in the cell. The PCT H^+ ions are derived from CO_2 and as these are used to produce NH_4^+ this yields an HCO_3^- ion which crosses the basal side of the cell with Na and in this case effectively generates 'new' HCO_3^- ions (Fig. 14.22).

In the loop of Henle, both ionic and non-ionic diffusion occur as the concentration of HCO_3^- is raised by water abstraction. This alkalisation will cause NH_3 to leave the tubule both in the ascending thin loop and the thick ascending loop by non-ionic diffusion and enter the collecting duct with its low pH to again form NH_4^+ ions, which are then trapped in the collecting duct fluid.

The formation of ammonium ions 'absorbs' H^+ ions, so keeping the pH above the critical value of 4.5, and generates new HCO_3^- which replace the base loss by metabolic acidosis. A further advantage is that again the generation of a positive charge as NH_4^+ saves a cation, usually Na^+. In chronic acidosis, the production of NH_3 can be increased six times. Prostaglandins can, however, inhibit ammonia genesis.

In summary, the role of the kidney in excreting fixed H^+ ions is related to the plasma pH, which will induce more ammonia genesis, increase Na/H^+ activity in the PCT and more H^+-ATPase in the collecting ducts. All these factors will help to replace the HCO_3^- lost by non-respiratory acidosis.

Disturbance of acid–base balance occurs when the blood pH deviates from around 7.4, disrupts normal cellular function, and is potentially life-threatening. The types of acid–base disorder are discussed in Chapters 3 and 13. Acid–base disturbance owing to defective renal regulation, otherwise known as metabolic acidosis or alkalosis, is the result of abnormalities in the regulation of 'fixed' H^+ excretion by the kidneys or defective renal buffer systems; bicarbonate, phosphate and ammonium.

Metabolic acidosis

Metabolic acidosis (blood pH <7.4) occurs when there is an increase in acids other than carbonic acid in the blood, with a decrease in plasma bicarbonate concentration, and may arise from:

- Excessive intake of acid
- Excessive fixed H^+ production, as in lactic acidosis and diabetic ketoacidosis (see Ch. 3)
- Decreased renal H^+ excretion, when the distal convoluted tubules fail to excrete H^+ ions, which also features ammonium deficiency and hypokalaemia, and occurs in renal failure.
- Increased renal bicarbonate loss, which may be due to administration of carbonic anhydrase inhibitors (see above), damage to the renal tubules by drugs or heavy metals, or very rarely, a condition known as proximal renal tubular acidosis, associated with low plasma renin and low plasma aldosterone concentrations
- Excessive loss of bicarbonate through the gastrointestinal tract, as in severe diarrhoea, and ileostomy.

Metabolic alkalosis

Metabolic alkalosis (blood pH >7.4) is relatively common, especially in hospital patients, often due to excessive loss of acid gastric contents (vomiting, gastric aspiration) and diuretic use causing chloride or potassium depletion. Severe metabolic alkalosis is life-threatening. Metabolic alkalosis may be due to chloride or potassium depletion, or a mixture of both. The mechanisms for excessive H^+ loss include:

- Loss of sodium, chloride and water in the distal nephron, which promotes potassium and H^+ secretion.
- Potassium depletion, which increases bicarbonate reabsorption in the proximal tubules and stimulates ammonium synthesis.
- Loss of ECF due the action of diuretics, which stimulates renin and aldosterone secretion (autoregulation), but also increases potassium and H^+ excretion.

Ureteric colic, also known as **renal colic** is the symptom of spasmodic, usually severe, pain experienced during the passage of a renal calculus (stone, kidney stone). Renal stones are solid crystals made of a variety of minerals contained in the urine, and are sited either in the kidney or ureters. They vary in size (from <5 mm to >10 cm) and shape, and can occasionally be 'spiky', in the shape of a staghorn; the **staghorn calculus**. Kidney stones are often asymptomatic unless they cause obstruction to the urine outflow, and are only incidentally found on abdominal ultrasound or plain X-ray. They can, however, be passed in the urine, when they cause extreme pain. Pain relief is needed, usually with a non-steroidal anti-inflammatory agent (NSAID), and an antispasmodic is given to relieve ureteric colic (spasm). There are three sites at which the ureters narrow and can act as sites where stones can lodge: just below the renal pelvis, where the ureters pass over the brim of the pelvis, and at the entrance to the bladder (see the dashed lines on Fig. 14.2).

Types of renal stones

Renal stones can be formed from calcium oxalate (the most common form), calcium phosphate, uric acid, magnesium ammonium phosphate or cystine. Although of uncertain aetiology, stones are associated with poor urine output, infection, low pH or a low concentration of factors which inhibit stone formation, such as citrate. Excess dietary intake of protein, sodium and oxalates or overproduction of such compounds has been implicated.

THE URINARY TRACT

Urine from the collecting tubules drains into the renal pelvis after leaving the pyramids. The urine is then carried by the ureters to the bladder, driven by active peristalsis since the pressure in the bladder is greater than in the renal pelvis. Urine stored in the bladder is voided through the urethra. These components constitute the urinary tract (Fig. 14.2).

URETERS

The ureters are composed of two layers of smooth muscle, a circular and a longitudinal layer, but the layers are poorly defined and autonomic ganglia are sparse. Autonomic drugs and their derivatives have little effect on ureteral peristalsis, which is initiated by pacemaker cells in the pelvis. As pressure in the renal pelvis rises to 14 cmH_2O, waves of peristalsis are initiated and the urine is forced towards the bladder at 2–3 cm/s.

The ureteral muscles maintain a tone so the ureters are normally empty unless there is an obstruction, usually a

stone lodged in the lumen. The ureters and bladder are lined with the urothelium, which is a compound epithelium with a specialised structure that is impermeable to CO_2, so can retain high levels of CO_2 in the urine.

The ureters enter the base of the bladder obliquely so are compressed when the bladder muscle contracts at the base of the bladder (Fig. 14.2). In addition the lower section of the ureter is composed of more circular muscle than the initial section and both these properties limit the reflux of the urine into the ureters during normal micturition (passing urine) as the bladder pressure rises when the bladder empties. There is also a reflex which increases ureteric tone as the bladder pressure rises, which also helps to prevent reflux. The kidney can easily be damaged by back pressure and by infection which can enter via this route.

Urinary tract obstruction

The urinary tract can be obstructed by three types of problem:

- Extrinsic – various factors in the abdominal cavity can externally compress the ureters, such as tumours, inflammation, fibrosis, infection, haemorrhage and trauma, which will lead to a decrease in flow of urine into the bladder.
- Intramural – transitional cell cancer, infection, fibrosis and inflammation can all expand the wall and reduce the diameter of the lumen.
- Intraluminal – calculi, bleeding and blood clot formation can also obstruct the ureters.

Congenital problems

A number of congenital problems can interfere with the transfer of urine from the renal pelvis to the bladder such as pelvic/ureteral and ureteral/bladder discontinuity which can

Clinical consequences of urinary tract obstruction

The commonest cause of obstructions of the ureters are stones which are usually radio-opaque. If a stone is of sufficient size it will block the urine flow and cause back pressure on the kidney, which may become a surgical emergency. The obstructed ureter becomes dilated and flaccid (**hydroureter**) as the pressure rises. The lack of urinary flow can lead to the build up of ascending infection, which can in turn lead to renal damage. In the most severe form the whole kidney becomes infected (**pyonephrosis**), which can lead to septicaemia and renal failure. Initially, if the obstruction is relieved, the condition can be reversed and there is post-obstruction diuresis because of retained salts and water. Occasionally, the obstruction causes damage to the AqP2 water channels and a form of nephrogenic DI ensues. If the obstruction is not removed renal scarring occurs and the damage is permanent. Surgical intervention may be required.

Vesicoureteric reflux (VUR)

VUR is the backward flow of urine from the bladder into the ureters or kidneys. Primary VUR is congenital, and thought to be due to an embryonic developmental error leading to defects in the implantation of the ureters into the bladder. Normally, the ureter enters the bladder wall obliquely. Muscular contraction during micturition (voiding urine) compresses the intravesical portion of the ureters, acting as a valve to prevent retrograde urine flow back up the ureters. This mechanism is defective in VUR. Congenital VUR is relatively common, presenting as recurrent urinary tract infections in children, more often in girls than boys. If undetected and untreated, the repeated, ascending infections can lead to pyelonephritis, when the renal pelvis becomes infected, and renal failure may ensue. Medical treatment with long courses of prophylactic antibiotics is used. Surgical intervention to re-implant the ureters in a different site in the bladder may be needed.

cause reflux and the ingress of infection (see Clinical boxes 14.3 and 14.14).

GROSS STRUCTURE OF THE BLADDER

Urine is formed continuously by the kidneys at a rate of at least 1 mL/min so must be stored within the bladder. The bladder consists of three layers of smooth muscle lined with **urothelium**. The outer layer is the longitudinal muscle, the middle is a circular layer and there is an incomplete inner layer; together these form the detrusor urinae. There is also the trigone lying on the floor of the bladder at the back, which is a triangle of muscle between the ureter and the exit from the bladder, the urethra (Fig. 14.2). The ureters enter the bladder through this muscle layer and exit onto the surface of the trigone.

Maintenance of continence

Acting via the pelvic floor, continence is maintained by the sphincters of the bladder and the abdominal pressure compressing the bladder neck (Fig. 14.2). The internal sphincter is an oblique muscle and not well defined. It leads to the urethral sphincter, which is mixed smooth and skeletal muscle, limited by the external sphincter, composed of only striated muscle and under voluntary control. In humans, the urethra is composed of two sets of muscles, the compressor

The cystometrogram

The cystometrogram records the pressure in the bladder as it fills and shows that the pressure rises in three phases. In the initial phase, the pressure rises rapidly to a small degree (Fig. 14.23). The pressure then rises more slowly over phase II. This is receptive relaxation when most of the bladder filling occurs. No contractions occur during this phase until the bladder has filled to 400 mL or so, when the pressure again rises steeply, phase III. This will only occur if the subject has been unable to empty their bladder and will cause a most unpleasant feeling of pain and 'urge to go'. Normal micturition is a complex active process involving both the parasympathetic and sympathetic systems. If the parasympathetic nerves are cut, the tone falls whereas when the sympathetic nerves are cut the tone rises. This process involves the intramural plexuses and is modified by a higher external input. When the bladder is filled externally, a 'blip' is seen as the pressure rises, then it decreases to a mean value. The tone of the bladder is indicated by the slope of phase II; if it is hypotonic it is flat indicating a flaccid bladder and if it is steep, this is a hypertonic over-reactive bladder. Insertion of the catheter into the bladder, and filling it, leads to a guard reflex increasing the tone in the urethra.

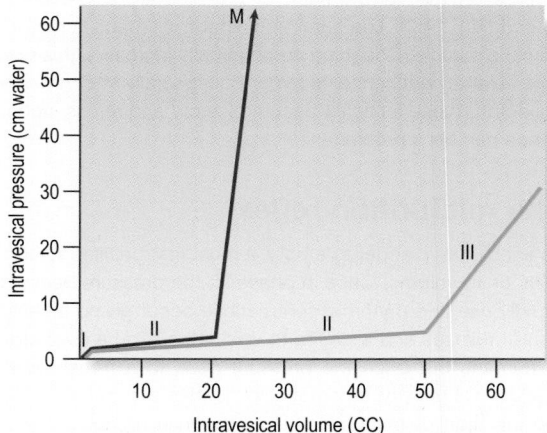

Fig. 14.23 Schematic cystometrogram. M indicates peak pressure during micturition contraction. Segment I, or the initial rise, is segment from zero to first point of inflection. Segment II, or the initial limb, begins at first inflection point and either ends at micturition contraction (*red line*) or, in the absence of micturition reflex, continues into segment III (*green line*). Segment III, or the ascending limb is a sharply rising terminal limb. From Tang PC and Ruch TC 1955 Non-neurogenic basis of bladder tonus. American Journal of Physiology 181(2): 249–257, with permission of American Physiological Society.

urethrae and the bulbocavernosi. These muscles exert a continuous tone which can be measured by a balloon catheter as it is passed into the bladder.

Nerve supply

The motor nerve supply to the bladder is complex, with a parasympathetic supply from the pelvic S2–4 nerves, which has a mixed motor and sensory supply derived from the hypogastric and vesicle plexi. There is a sympathetic supply via the inferior mesenteric ganglia which passes via the hypogastric to the vesical plexus. Finally there is somatic control via S3–S4, the pudic motor control to the external sphincter.

The sensory supply is composed of pain and stretch fibres which receive inputs from a large variety of receptor types within the muscle wall with ascending sensory fibres as well as motor supply. The pelvic sensory fibres carry the desire to void urine.

The sympathetic supply is not vital to micturition, but in males it prevents sperm reflux during ejaculation. The main role of parasympathetic sensory fibres is in relation to the sensation of bladder fullness. Pain is mostly sympathetic.

Bladder filling and tone

Urinary bladder filling and tone can be studied using a double lumen catheter, filling the bladder via one tube and recording the pressure with a transducer connected to the other. Alternatively, a direct recording can be made via a suprapubic needle.

CONTROL OF MICTURITION

The ability of micturition to be controlled is a learned reflex. Both the abdominal pressure and the pelvic floor act to exert a force on the narrow neck of the bladder, so keeping it closed (Fig. 14.2). The outer sphincter in humans is made of somatic muscle. Coughing automatically increases this pressure so aids continence. In females, especially after repeated childbirth, these muscles become flaccid and stress incontinence can be a problem.

The micturition reflex

To enable the bladder to empty, it must first be filled to some 80% of its volume. Once in phase III, the pressure begins to rapidly rise and rhythmic contractions occur giving a sensation of fullness and a desire to void. This can be overridden in humans but once the pressure rises to a threshold the bladder will empty automatically. Under normal conditions the initiation of micturition depends on a graded series of autonomic reflexes, which once started go to completion; however, a normal person can inhibit the process at this stage and interrupt the flow. The micturition reflex depends on ascending signals to the pons and medulla which inhibit the normal descending inhibition and the guard reflex via a spinal route. The detrusor muscle contracts, which mechanically opens the internal sphincter and reflexly inhibits the external sphincter. This process flattens the floor of the bladder so the urethra is now open and fluid flows rapidly out as the detrusor contracts. Fluid flow through the urethra reinforces contraction of the bladder via pelvic plexuses and spinal reflexes. Once the smooth muscle in the bladder wall has maximally shortened, the tension falls and the guard reflex is initiated as the bladder starts to refill.

RENAL DISEASES

The kidney has a large reserve in function so more than 75% can be destroyed before symptoms occur. While this is an advantage in one way in that homeostasis is protected, the onset of renal disease can be insidious and by the time symptoms appear it can be too late to treat the damage. The kidneys protect the organism against acidosis (fixed H^+) and hyperkalaemia (K^+) so, if renal function is lost, it is the consequence of the rise in these factors which could lead to the symptoms of disease and eventual death. Since the large

---

| Clinical box 14.16 | Urinary incontinence |

Failure to control micturition results in **urinary incontinence**, also known as **enuresis**, the involuntary voiding of urine. Until young children learn to control micturition, urine is passed when the bladder is 'full'. **Primary nocturnal enuresis** is the condition in which the child has never been 'dry' at night.

Causes of urinary incontinence
Urinary incontinence may be associated with:

- Bladder defects
- Infection – cystitis, due to incomplete bladder emptying, VUR
- Weakness in bladder musculature – flaccid bladder, detrusor failure.

Bladder outlet defects
- Weakness in pelvic floor muscles leading to incompetence of the urethral sphincter – common in women – usually consequence of parturition, atrophic vaginitis, age.
- Bladder outlet obstruction: prostatic enlargement, bladder calculi.

Neurological bladder defects
- Detrusor overactivity due to defect in central nervous system (CNS) inhibition – conditions include multiple sclerosis, cauda equina lesions, pressure from prolapsed intervertebral disc (S2–4), stroke.
- Intellectual impairment – e.g. **Alzheimer's disease**.

Prostatic enlargement produces problems with micturition
Surgery in the lower abdomen can cause problems with micturition as a high pressure is needed to empty the bladder. In the male, obstruction can occur with benign and malignant growths of the prostate and this hyperplasia presses on the urethra. In this condition, micturition will only occur with a raised pressure. Normally the bladder empties at 30–40 cm of H_2O. However, prostate problems can cause incomplete emptying and chronic retention as the neck cannot be held open. This leads to increased frequency and a small volume is voided on each occasion. Eventually this leads to a flaccid bladder as the urethra is damaged. Removal of the prostate can lead to stress incontinence as the urethra is now too short.

Problems with bladder emptying
Problems in emptying can occur with pain. An infection in the bladder called cystitis causes painful micturition. Spinal shock leads initially to difficulty in filling but with time this ability will return as lower spinal reflexes are still intact. The bladder in these cases can be induced to empty by squeezing the bladder and exceeding the pressure at which the reflex is initiated. Stroking the inner thigh, the Credé manoeuvre, has the same effect.

---

reserve in function 'hides' incipient renal failure, the clinician must always be aware of clues which indicate the onset of renal dysfunction.

Routine blood tests can give early warning in the form of a rise in plasma creatinine and a rise in urea. However, if a patient is elderly with low muscle mass, the plasma creatinine may appear close to normal because of the low level of general metabolism and reduced creatinine production from a limited muscle mass. The same can occur with urea, especially if the intake for protein is reduced for economic reasons, poor dentition with difficulty chewing meat and due to isolation in the elderly.

Falls in the elderly are a major cause of hospital admissions and if bone fractures have occurred, loss of renal function must be considered as an underlying factor leading to calcium deficiency, such as disordered vitamin D production and osteoporosis with loss of calcium. The kidney plays a key role in the production of vitamin D 25-hydroxy-cholecalciferol, which is formed in the liver by a first hydroxylation, undergoes a second hydroxylation in the kidney where it is converted into 1,25-dihydroxycholecalciferol, the active form of vitamin D (see Ch. 3).

GENERAL CLASSIFICATION OF RENAL DISEASE

The kidneys can be damaged by:

- Extrinsic factors such as certain drugs, antibiotics, chemical toxins and bacterial infection such as with *Staphylococcus* in children.
- Intrinsic factors, such as disorders of the immune system, attacking specific tissue in the kidney, such as the basement membrane.
- Secondary intrinsic factors such as a failure of a major organ system where the kidney is under-perfused, such as in heart failure, blockage of a major renal blood vessel leading to a loss in the supply of oxygen and nutrients or liver failure with loss in the production of plasma proteins and upset in colloid osmotic pressure.
- Secondary compensation: the various feedback systems used by the kidney to control sodium balance can be activated. The renin/angiotensin system then leads an inappropriate response, with a fall in renal perfusion as afferent arteriole tone is elevated by angiotensin II and by sympathetic effects as excess noradrenaline is released from the renal nerves. Drugs which inhibit prostaglandin release (e.g. NSAIDs) will have no adverse effects if the kidneys are intact, but may precipitate renal failure in susceptible individuals, because (in renal disease) maintenance of the GFR depends upon the vasodilator effect of prostaglandins.
- Post renal disease. Obstruction of the drainage pathway by blockage of the ureters by stones can lead to back pressure on the nephron which will cause renal damage and, secondary to this, the dilated ureter can be a source of infection which will reflux into the kidneys and lead to septicaemia (see Clinical box 14.13).

ONSET OF RENAL DISEASE

Renal failure can be acute (ARF) with a sudden onset following an upper respiratory tract infection, or chronic with a slow rise in plasma creatinine (CRF), which has an insidious progression with few symptoms at first but eventually increasing problems. A further classification of renal disease can be related to the site of damage, e.g. glomerulonephritis (inflammation of the glomeruli). Tubular disease involves damage to the tubular system that can either be focal and limited in its extent or global and widespread. The site of such changes can be identified by a renal biopsy and careful histological examination, and also by blood chemistry where defects in the immune system can be identified.

ACUTE RENAL FAILURE

Acute renal failure is defined as a sudden fall in renal function. This is accompanied by a fall in GFR and in the ability of the kidney to excrete toxic waste, so the plasma creatinine and urea values rise, which usually takes a week (see Fig. 14.1).

Clinical box 14.17 Nephrotic syndrome and protein loss

The **nephrotic syndrome** is a group of disorders in which the permeability of the glomerular capillaries to protein macromolecules is increased. This leads to heavy proteinuria with values of loss of 3.5 g of protein per day; normally the loss of protein in the urine is 40–80 mg per day. A further consequence is peripheral oedema, which was thought to be due to a fall in colloid osmotic pressure (COP) but now has been identified as the consequence of increased Na$^+$ reabsorption by the collecting ducts leading to overfilling of the vascular space. This excess fluid causes an imbalance between the plasma and interstitial oncotic pressure which can be corrected with corticosteroids.

It is of interest that the rise in Na$^+$ excretion occurs before any changes in the level of albumin so the excess fluid was produced by the inappropriate activation of the renin-angiotensin-aldosterone system.

In nephrotic syndrome the urine sediment is relatively inactive with few cells, which reflects a non-inflammatory injury to the glomerular capillaries. A biopsy usually shows loss of foot processes in the glomerular basement membrane with electron dense deposits but no inflammation. The syndrome appears to reduce the loss of small molecules, which would suggest a loss of the area available for filtration, but an increased number of large pores allowing large protein molecules to be filtered. This loss also includes IgG which is not a charged macromolecule so the effect is not one of a change in surface charge on the fibrillar basement membrane. The site of the increased permeability appears to be the slit diaphragms of the capillary wall.

Clinical box 14.18 Nephritic syndrome

In contrast to the nephrotic syndrome, there may be no proteinuria in the **nephritic syndrome**, although it may be seen in some patients. The urine sediment is active, often containing red cells and white cells with both cellular and granular casts. This syndrome reflects the influx of circulating inflammatory cells such as neutrophils, monocytes, macrophages and lymphocytes into the glomerulus. The severity of the glomerular injury reflects the degree of inflammation. Symptoms range from slight haematuria with no changes in GFR to blockage of blood vessels, a rise in plasma creatinine and a fall in GFR. In this condition there are circulating antibodies against the glomerular basement membrane, immune complex and complement activation and circulating antibodies against neutrophil cytoplasmic antigens.

The urine output falls, and oliguria (less than 400 mL per 24 h) occurs. This may be caused by a decline in renal blood flow, which in turn may be the result of extrarenal factors such as hypotension, dehydration or the oedema of congestive heart failure. In sclerosis of the liver and the nephrotic syndrome, the loss of plasma proteins leads to a decrease in the effective circulating volume and a decline in GFR. This can be diagnosed by careful clinical examination considering skin turgor and hypotension. Urine analysis is normal with a low Na$^+$ and volume in response to the release of vasopressin. The first line of treatment is to restore the fluid balance and the perfusion of the kidney, depending on the underlying cause of the problem.

Acute tubular necrosis

Ischaemia, endogenous and exogenous toxins produce tubular damage which can be very patchy and is a form of

---

acute renal failure. It is the proximal straight tubule which is most sensitive to this damage and leads to intratubular obstruction, then decline of GFR.

Renal ischaemia is the most common cause of acute tubular necrosis (ATN). The effect of the duration of ischaemia is however very variable, some severe damage can occur with a reduction in RBF of only a few minutes whereas little damage is sometimes seen with much larger periods of interrupted flow. Abdominal and cardiac surgery have the highest incidence of ATN, which may relate to damage or stimulation to the neural inputs to the kidney. In the septic patient ATN may be related to the hypotensive effects of endotoxins.

Nephrotoxic agents

The mechanism by which the kidney is able to secrete a variety of toxins and drugs into the urine can malfunction and lead to nephrotoxicity. Antibiotics such as aminoglycosides and amphotericin B, used in the treatment of hospital-acquired infections, result in 10% of the cases of ATN. Occupational exposure to heavy metals also causes ATN and, in the clinical situation, platinum in the form of cisplatin used in cancer chemotherapy can cause renal toxicity. A further problem has been introduced with the increased use of radio-contrast agents in urography and CT scans.

Endogenous toxins such as myoglobin in traumatic muscle crush injury can cause ATN, as do some forms of multiple myeloma associated with a high concentration of immunoglobulin light chains.

Drugs and the elderly

With the elderly and those who have pre-existing renal dysfunction, great care must be taken if drugs with known nephrotoxicity are used. The poor renal function results in the patient being exposed to a higher potentially toxic level as the drug is not cleared from the tubule cells for a longer period of time than in those with normal renal function. Digoxin is a case in point and the failing heart impairs the renal excretion so leading to digoxin toxicity.

Although the values of plasma creatinine and creatinine clearance give early warning of renal impairment in most patients, this can be misleading in the elderly with a low muscle mass, as the creatinine values may be only slightly elevated while renal function is depressed. In addition, if the subject is volume depleted, the conservation of sodium and water can override the normal expected response and may lead to a poor clearance of drugs by tubular secretion. Even if the treatment is terminated, the retention of the drugs in the tubular cells can lead to continued damage. Treatment consists initially of maintenance of fluid and electrolyte balance. The use of diuretics such as **furosemide** and **mannitol** can help but multiple doses should be avoided and

great care taken with fluid balance to avoid pulmonary oedema.

CHRONIC RENAL FAILURE

Chronic renal failure is a clinical syndrome caused by irreversible and progressive renal injury. This condition leads to a rise in plasma creatinine and in blood urea nitrogen (BUN) which is caused by a fall in GFR. In addition, other functions of the kidney are also impaired, such as the failure to secrete hormones such as erythropoietin and calcitriol, which can lead to anaemia and hypocalcaemia. The elevation of plasma urea is referred to as uraemia or azotaemia, and is seen both in chronic and acute renal failure.

Causes of chronic renal failure

Chronic renal failure can be caused by a wide variety of conditions:

- Diabetes mellitus is the commonest, which accounts for some 30–40% of the cases needing dialysis. Type 1 diabetes leads to chronic renal failure after about 10 years, the first signs being microalbuminuria accompanied by diabetic neuropathy and retinopathy. It can also occur in type 2 diabetes, which is also dependent on the duration of the condition and on good glucose control. The mechanisms underlying diabetic nephropathy are discussed in detail in Chapter 3.
- Hypertension is also a major cause of chronic renal failure, which causes thickening of the arterioles and nephrosclerosis, and is limited by reducing the blood pressure.
- The third most common cause of chronic renal failure is glomerulonephritis, which includes conditions such as membranous nephropathy, focal glomerular sclerosis, systemic lupus erythematosus and Goodpasture's syndrome, which reflects immune damage to the glomerular basement membrane.

There are many other causes, such as long-term exposure to lead and other environmental toxins, misuse of analgesics, and various genetic problems such as polycystic kidney disease.

Progression of chronic renal failure

CRF is often a progressive disease but with the appropriate treatment, the damage can be slowed although rarely completely halted. It is thought that the progressive nature of the condition is caused by the remaining healthy nephrons being subject to hyperfiltration and an increased plasma flow with a raised hydrostatic pressure. ACE inhibitors are most useful in the treatment of this progression. The accumulation of uraemic toxins can lead to neurological conditions with seizures and depressed sensory function.

Chronic renal failure and hypertension

The failure in chronic renal failure of the kidneys to excrete adequate water and salt leads to hypertension, which in turn can lead to myocardial infarction and stroke. The disturbance in calcium homeostasis and acidosis leads to bone calcium depletion and osteomalacia. This condition is made worse by the use of aluminium-based antacids taken to bind phosphate.

The progress of chronic renal failure is monitored by plotting the reciprocal of the plasma creatinine against time, and changes in the slope of the line give an indication of whether the rate of renal failure is progressing or slowing.

Erythropoietin

The kidneys secrete the hormone **erythropoietin (EPO)**, which maintains bone marrow production of red cells. A major complication of renal failure has been the loss of red cells owing to the lack of EPO production. Repeated blood transfusions may be necessary to maintain red cell volume. EPO is secreted by the fibroblast-like renal interstitial cells in response to changes in the pO_2 of blood. At high altitude, the pO_2 falls and the EPO is released, which increases red cell mass. This is also seen in chronic obstructive pulmonary disease, where the lung disease results in a low arterial pO_2, leading to polycythaemia (see Ch. 13).

Pharmacological renal damage and chronic renal failure

Table 14.5 lists some of the drugs which can cause acute interstitial nephritis, and renal function must be monitored during their use. The sites of damage vary, with the least

Table 14.5	The nephrotoxicity of some drugs, toxins and endogenous compounds
Aminoglycoside antibiotics	These accumulate in the lysosomes of the PCT cells and can generate reactive species, depending on the number of NH_3^+ groups. Very persistent accumulation for up to 4–6 weeks
Amphotericin	Predominantly produces tubular damage, but acute vasoconstriction may be responsible for rapid reductions in glomerular filtration rate which can return quickly to normal once the drug has been discontinued
Cephalosporins	Acute tubular damage – less frequent with the new generation of compounds
Polymyxin	Tubular damage and also neurotoxic
Rifampicin	Tubular damage and interstitial nephritis
Sulphonamides	Intratubular crystal aggregation may cause obstruction which can be cleared by alkali and fluid administration. Vasculitic damage has also been reported
Tetracyclines	Anti-anabolic and in some cases directly nephrotoxic
Cisplatin	A cytotoxic drug which is also nephrotoxic
Phenacetin	Nephritis
Phenindione	Allergic glomerulonephritis
General anaesthetic agents	Mainly methoxyflurane – produces tubular damage and, as it is metabolised to oxalic acid, crystal deposition within the kidney may cause acute renal failure. This, however, is rare
Radiographic contrast	Strictly not a drug, but mentioned here as reports of nephrotoxicity following intra-arterial injection have been made. Dehydration should be avoided in patients with impaired renal function, and the use of isotonic contrast media may limit renal damage
Endogenous toxins	
■ Myoglobin	Crush injury
■ Haemoglobin	Haemolysis, hypertension
■ Myeloma light chains	Leukaemia
Heavy metals	Environmental toxins
Aluminium	PO_4 = binders and antacids

Clinical box 14.20   Dialysis

Once a patient is oliguric and fails to respond to diuretic treatment, it is better to initiate dialysis at an early stage than wait until hyperkalaemia and uremia develop. Once GFR falls below 10 mL/min renal replacement therapy should be initiated. Although dialysis can maintain most aspects of renal function, phosphate does not exchange easily, so it builds up. Phosphates binders can be given to help correct this problem although, being aluminium based, they can cause toxicity.

Peritoneal dialysis
The patient's peritoneum can act as a dialysis or semi-permeable membrane. Dialysate at body temperature is introduced via a soft catheter into the peritoneal cavity; 1–2 L of fluid can be introduced and left for 1–2 h (Fig. 14.24A). By the use of fluid with an appropriate composition, i.e. lower Na^+ and osmolarity made up with lactate, it is possible to withdraw water, potassium and urea from the patient. The fluid is then drained from the peritoneal cavity and replaced. Using this method it is possible for the patient to carry on a normal life while being dialysed. Much care in the technique is necessary to avoid infection but continuous ambulatory peritoneal dialysis can be continued for many weeks. The total removal of creatinine and urea by this

method may be inadequate but hyperkalaemia and fluid balance can be achieved.

Haemodialysis
A more efficient way of replacing kidney function is to use haemodialysis, with a flat plate or hollow fibre dialyser (Fig. 14.24B). In these the blood flows through the system one way and the dialysate flows in the opposite direction. The membrane is made of various plastics, and permits the rapid removal of waste products in the blood and virtual complete replacement of renal function. A shunt must be constructed between, usually, a peripheral artery and vein so blood can be withdrawn with a roller pump and passed through the dialyser, cleansed and returned to the patient. This process takes 4–6 h and is performed three times per week. With a compliant patient, this can be done at home. This process is also used in haemofiltration which uses a more permeable membrane and can depend on the patient's own blood pressure to drive the blood through the filter. This process is more gentle and can run continuously for several days. Fluid is removed from the patient and a slightly smaller volume returned to balance the electrolytes and fluid volume.

Continued

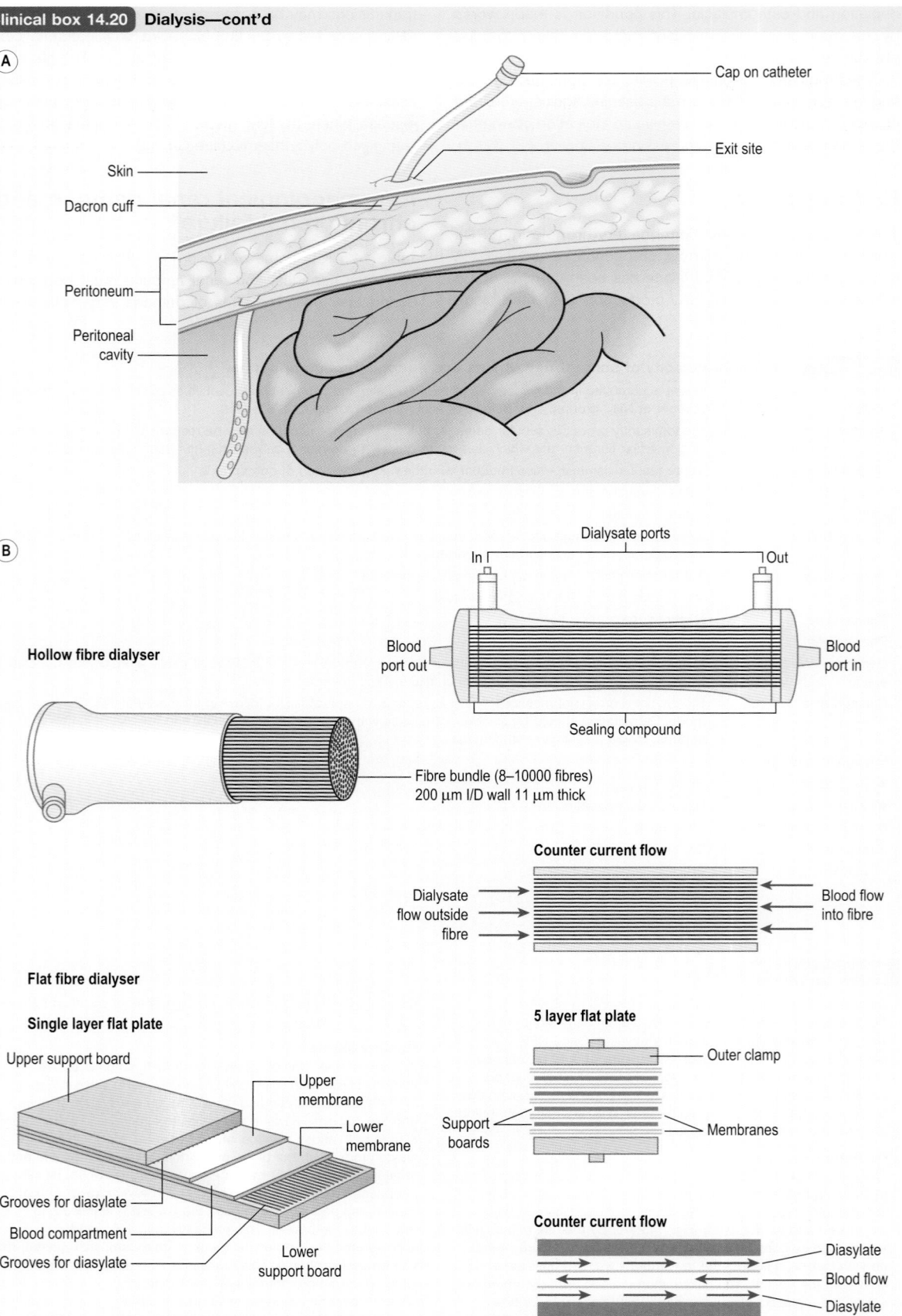

Fig. 14.24 **Haemodialysis.** Diagrams of flat plate and hollow fibre dialysers. Note the arrangements for increasing the surface area of the dialyser membrane. From Thompson FD and Woodhouse CRJ 1987 Disorders of the kidney and urinary tract. Edward Arnold, London, with permission.

common being the glomerulus. However, glomerular damage can be affected by gold and penicillamine used in the treatment of rheumatoid arthritis and to a small extent with NSAIDs. Aminoglycoside antibiotics need particular care as they are secreted by the tubule and can alter glomerular haemodynamics. The nephrotoxicity is related to peak dose rather than the steady state value so a smaller dose given at more frequent intervals is less toxic than a single large dose. Agents such as digoxin and cephalosporin, in contrast, depend on their steady state value and in CRF the dose must be reduced to avoid toxicity. Cephalosporins induce a marked vasoconstriction and a fall in GFR with ischaemic damage in the long term. Note: Absorption of 99% of the water by the nephron can lead to toxic concentration of drugs in the tubule cells.

Analgesic neuropathy is now less common with the withdrawal of combination tablets such as aspirin, phenacetin and caffeine. Chinese herbs such as *Aristolochia frangulin* have been identified as causing interstitial fibrosis and uroepithelial cancer. As with all drugs patients differ in their sensitivity so care must be taken to monitor their effect on renal function.

15

The alimentary system

John Wilkinson

INTRODUCTION

The chemical composition of food is complex and little of it is water soluble, therefore it cannot enter the body fluids unaltered. A series of digestive processes enables food to be broken down and absorbed. These processes take place in the alimentary canal, which consists of the mouth, oesophagus and gastrointestinal tract, and associated exocrine glands producing secretions that act on food.

BASIC FUNCTIONS AND STRUCTURE OF THE ALIMENTARY SYSTEM

The functions of the alimentary canal are concerned with storage, digestion and absorption of food together with the excretion of undigested food and waste products. Digestion is the process of breaking down complex food molecules, by mechanical and chemical methods, into simple ones that can

be absorbed. The digestion products together with salts and water are absorbed into the blood and lymphatic systems. In addition, the alimentary canal serves to protect the body from swallowed noxious agents and bacterial toxins.

Four activities of the alimentary canal can be identified. These are:

- Motility
- Secretion
- Digestion
- Absorption.

Motility is the term used to describe movements of the alimentary canal that are responsible for propelling partly digested food along the canal, and for mixing the food with the digestive secretions in order that digestion and absorption can take place in a regulated manner. These activities are interrelated. In health there is a balance, and we pay little attention to alimentary function. Disruption of one activity in disease leads to an imbalance and we become conscious of gastrointestinal function, e.g. pain and peptic ulceration, diarrhoea, constipation. Coordination of alimentary function depends on the combined action of the nervous, endocrine (circulating hormones) and paracrine (local hormones) systems. The anatomy of the alimentary system and associated glands is shown in Figure.15.1.

- The **mouth** or oral cavity consists of the lips, tongue, gums, teeth, hard and soft palate and the pharynx together with the salivary glands. Food is ingested, mixed with saliva, chewed and swallowed.
- The **oesophagus** is a muscular tube lying in the thorax and abdomen that connects the pharynx to the stomach. It is separated from the pharynx by the upper oesophageal sphincter. Food and drink is propelled to the stomach by the action of the oesophageal muscles.
- The **stomach** lies in the abdomen below the diaphragm. It is separated from the oesophagus and small intestine by the lower oesophageal (cardiac) and pyloric sphincters, respectively.
- The **duodenum** forms the first part of the small intestine. It receives the pancreatic and biliary ducts from the pancreas and liver, respectively.
- The **jejunum** and **ileum** are a continuation of the small intestine. The ileum terminates at the **ileo-caecal junction**.
- The large intestine consists of the **caecum** with the **appendix**, the **colon** (divided into three sections: ascending, transverse and descending) and the **rectum**.
- The **anus** is the opening at the end of the large intestine. An internal and an external anal sphincter control the opening.

BLOOD SUPPLY TO THE GASTROINTESTINAL TRACT

The gastrointestinal tract, liver, gall bladder, pancreas and spleen are supplied with blood from the splanchnic circulation in a number of parallel circuits (Fig. 15.2). Blood is delivered via three major arteries:

- **Coeliac artery** to the liver, gall bladder, pancreas, stomach and spleen
- **Superior mesenteric artery** to the pancreas, small and most of large intestine
- **Inferior mesenteric artery** to the terminal portions of the large intestine and rectum.

The arterial supply divides into a capillary network within the digestive organs that subsequently drains into the hepatic portal vein, which enters the liver. The blood from the hepatic portal vein flows through liver sinusoids before being returned to the heart by the inferior vena cava. The liver also receives about 20–25% of its blood supply from the hepatic branch of the coeliac artery. Blood flow through the splanchnic circulation is enhanced during feeding.

The control of blood flow to the different mucosal and muscle layers (see Fig. 15.7 below) of the gastrointestinal tract is regulated independently. The neural, endocrine and paracrine mechanisms controlling gastrointestinal blood flow are shown in Table 15.1.

Mucosal blood flow is required to:

- Maintain viability of the mucosa
- Provide the precursors for secretory products
- Deliver hormones to their target cells
- Remove absorbed digestion products, toxins and drugs from the mucosa.

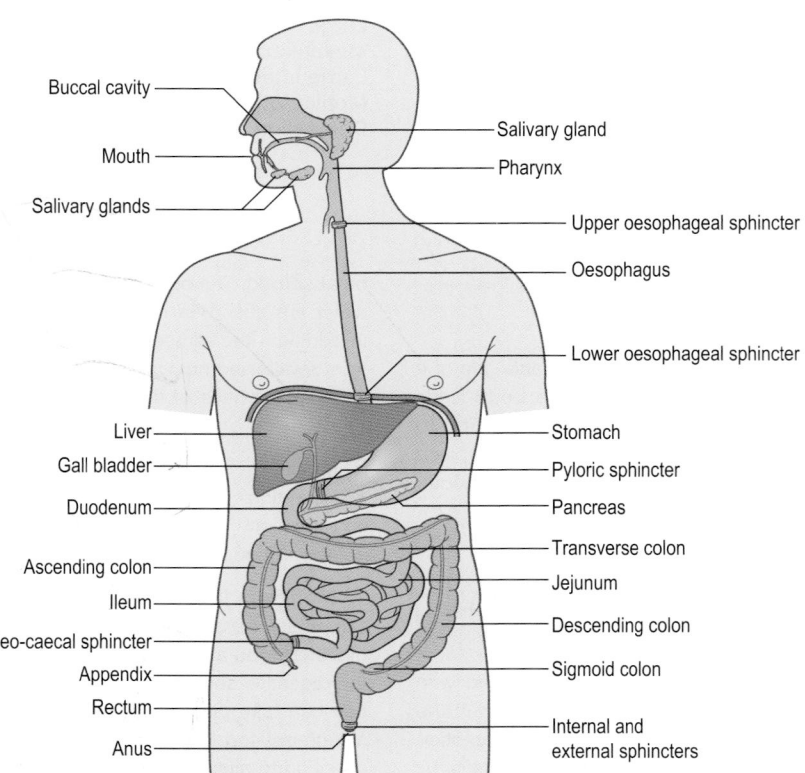

Fig. 15.1 **The alimentary canal and its associated glands.**

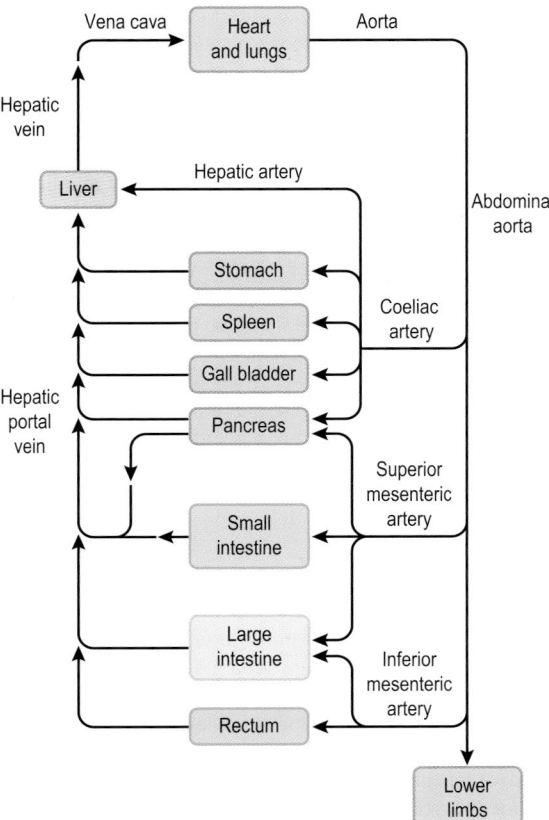

Fig. 15.2 **The splanchnic circulation.**

Table 15.1	Control of gastrointestinal blood flow	
Neural mechanisms	**Vasoconstrictor action (Neurotransmitters)**	**Vasodilator action (Neurotransmitters)**
Parasympathetic nerves		ACh, VIP
Sympathetic nerves	NA via α adrenoceptors	NA via β$_2$ adrenoceptors
Sensory nerves		CGRP, SP, NKA
Enteric nerves		ACh, VIP, NO
Hormonal mechanisms	Catecholamines (mainly adrenaline)	Gastrin
	Angiotensin II	Cholecystokinin
	Vasopressin	Secretin
Local mechanisms	Somatostatin	Adenosine
	Endothelin 1	Low pO_2
		Histamine
		Prostacyclin (PGI$_2$)
		Prostaglandin E$_2$

ACh, acetylcholine; CGRP, calcitonin gene-related peptide; NA, noradrenaline; NKA, neurokinin A; NO, nitric oxide; SP, substance P; VIP, vasoactive intestinal polypeptide.

OVERVIEW OF DIGESTION AND ABSORPTION

Before nutrients can be absorbed, ingested carbohydrates, protein and fat have to be digested. Disruption of the normal mechanisms for either digestion or absorption (malabsorption), or both, leads to disease. Two mechanisms for the digestion of ingested food can be identified. These are:

Clinical box 15.1 Clinical conditions associated with impaired physical digestion

Beginning in the mouth, pain from diseased mucus membranes or dental problems interferes with chewing (mastication), the first step in the process of breaking down large food particles. A number of systemic diseases are associated with oral manifestations. Common conditions include:

- Oral candidiasis (thrush) associated with diabetes mellitus, debilitating illness such as human immunodeficiency virus (HIV)/acquired immune deficiency syndrome (AIDS), cancer and blood dyscrasias, and chemotherapy.
- Mouth ulcers may be due to: infections, e.g. herpes simplex, erythema multiforme (Steven–Johnson syndrome); other ulcerations of the gastrointestinal tract, e.g. coeliac disease, regional ileitis (Crohn's disease), ulcerative colitis, disseminated (or systemic) lupus erythematosus, Behçet's disease; squamous cell carcinoma and other, less common tumours; and trauma including ill-fitting dentures.
- Absence of teeth or neuromuscular defects in old age (e.g. after a stroke) can interfere with mastication.
- Physical digestion in the stomach, i.e. storage of ingested food, mixing the contents to promote fat emulsification, enzyme and acid action, may be impaired through infiltration of gastric musculature by tumour ('leather bottle stomach') affecting motility. Pyloric stenosis from peptic ulceration or tumour delays gastric emptying. Surgical resection (partial gastrectomy) increases the rate of gastric emptying (see later 'dumping syndrome').
- Conditions that affect small intestine motility are usually manifested by increased motility, and may lead to diarrhoea, abdominal pain and discomfort. The irritable bowel syndrome (IBS) is an example. Other causes include infection, food sensitivities, endocrine disease and radiation enteritis.

- Physical digestion
- Chemical digestion.

PHYSICAL DIGESTION

Physical digestion is produced by mechanical activity of the alimentary canal breaking down pieces of food into smaller particles. The food retains its complex chemical structure, but its surface area is increased to expose more sites to enzymic action. Physical digestion takes place in the:

- Mouth
- Antrum and pylorus of the stomach
- Small intestine.

It is dependent upon muscular contractions squeezing and grinding the food, and mixing it with secretions. In addition, bile salts and lecithin act as detergents to emulsify fat globules. These actions are produced by the physical properties of bile salts and lecithin, having fat and water-soluble components in the molecules.

CHEMICAL DIGESTION

Enzymes are responsible for chemical digestion. This involves the hydrolysis of the complex food molecules, that is, being broken up into their simpler constituents, which are capable of being absorbed. Chemical digestion may occur by means of enzyme activity present in the lumen of the alimentary canal or on the luminal-facing membrane of the epithelial cells (enterocytes) in the small intestine.

Carbohydrate digestion

The predominant carbohydrates in the diet are:

- Starch and glycogen (polysaccharides)
- Sucrose and lactose (disaccharides)
- Fructose (monosaccharide).

Starch and glycogen are polymers comprising chains of glucose molecules joined together by α-1,4 glycosidic bonds and at branch points by α-1, 6 glycosidic bonds. Salivary and pancreatic amylases catalyse the hydrolysis of the interior α-1,4 bonds but do not split either the terminal α-1,4 glycosidic bonds or the α-1, 6 glycosidic bonds at the branches of starch and glycogen. The products of amylase action are maltose (a disaccharide), maltotriose (a trisaccharide) and α-limit dextrins (branched oligosaccharides) (Fig. 15.3). However, there are no transport systems for the absorption of these carbohydrates in the intestine. The oligosaccharides derived from starch together with maltose, sucrose, and lactose are further digested by enzymes present on the brush border of enterocytes to their monosaccharides – glucose, galactose and fructose (Table 15.2).

Protein digestion

The various sources of protein for digestion are from food and also desquamated gastrointestinal cells and digestive secretions. Proteins and polypeptides consist of amino acids linked together by a peptide bond formed between the amino terminal of one amino acid and the carboxy terminal of another (see Ch. 2). Protein digestion is accomplished by enzymes (protease or peptidase) hydrolysing peptide bonds either within a polypeptide chain or protein (endopeptidase) or at the free ends (exopeptidase). Thus a protein may be broken down to a mixture of small polypeptides and amino acids.

Protein digestion in the stomach

Peptic cells in the stomach secrete pepsinogens, the precursor of a family of enzymes known as pepsins. The acid contents of the stomach activate pepsinogens to pepsins and denature the structure of proteins. Pepsin is an endopeptidase and specifically hydrolyses peptide bonds containing an aromatic L-amino acid such as phenylalanine or tyrosine. Pepsin is inactivated by the alkaline pH found in the duodenum.

Protein digestion in the small intestine

Protein digestion in the small intestine occurs due to the presence of pancreatic proteases (Table 15.3). The most important are trypsin, chymotrypsin and carboxypeptidase.

These are secreted as precursors into the duodenum and activated by enteropeptidase (enterokinase) secreted by the duodenal and jejunal mucosa. Enteropeptidase activates trypsinogen to trypsin. Once some trypsin is formed it acts autocatalytically to convert more trypsinogen to trypsin and also activates chymotrypsinogen to chymotrypsin. Trypsin, chymotrypsin and elastase are endopeptidases and convert protein into polypeptides. Carboxypeptidases release single amino acids from the carboxyl end of polypeptides. The pancreatic proteases active in the lumen of the intestine produce small peptides and some amino acids before being inactivated by autodigestion. The next stage of protein digestion occurs at the brush border of the enterocytes by the action of peptidases present in the luminal membranes to produce small peptides (di, tri, and tetrapeptides) and single amino acids. Finally, small peptides (usually di- and tri-) are hydrolysed to single amino acids after they have been absorbed into the enterocyte (Fig. 15.3).

Fat digestion

The majority of the fats in the diet are triacylglycerols (triglycerides), consisting of glycerol to which three fatty acids are attached (see Ch. 2). Fats separate from the water phase of the partly digested food in the stomach and empty slowly. The contractile action of the stomach breaks the fat into small droplets and mixes them with the water phase. The nature of fats and their insolubility in the water create difficulties for their digestion by water-soluble lipases. There are three lipases:

- Lingual
- Gastric
- Pancreatic.

The lingual and gastric lipases have acidic pH optima and function in the stomach producing fatty acids and diacylglycerols (diglycerides) by attacking the outer ester linkages between glycerol and the fatty acids.

The major site of fat digestion is in the small intestine. Fat enters the duodenum relatively slowly in order that there is time for the process of emulsification and fat hydrolysis. Fat is emulsified into droplets about 500–1000 nm in diameter by the action of bile salts with their hydrophobic side (fat soluble) dissolving in the fat and their hydrophilic side (water soluble) facing outwards in the water of the intestinal fluid. This process is aided by lecithin and cholesterol, which are also found in bile. The emulsifying agents reduce the surface tension of the fat droplets and keep them apart. These

---

Clinical box 15.2   **Enzyme deficiency**

Deficiencies in enzymes concerned with carbohydrate digestion prevent the breakdown of oligo- and di-saccharides to monosaccharides that can be absorbed, so, instead, these are excreted undigested. This gives rise to diarrhoea after ingesting foods rich in these particular carbohydrates. A common example is milk intolerance due to lactase deficiency, a condition more common in some Asian and Mediterranean countries. It is not a major clinical problem, as most people with lactase deficiency simply avoid milk. A lactose tolerance test is available, but rarely used for adults (see Ch. 3).

Clinical box 15.3   **Enzyme defects in protein digestion**

Deficiency in pancreatic enzyme secretion, notably of trypsinogen and chymotrypsinogen, prevents the conversion of dietary protein into polypeptides for absorption. This can occur in chronic pancreatitis, mainly related to sustained alcohol overuse. Cystic fibrosis sufferers have the same enzyme deficiency. The inability of children with cystic fibrosis to digest protein and fat because of the lack of pancreatic enzymes, trypsin and lipase, leads to nutritional deficiencies in essential amino acids, fatty acids and fat soluble vitamins. High-dose pancreatic enzyme supplements to treat the resulting steatorrhoea, as well as nutritional supplementation, will be necessary.

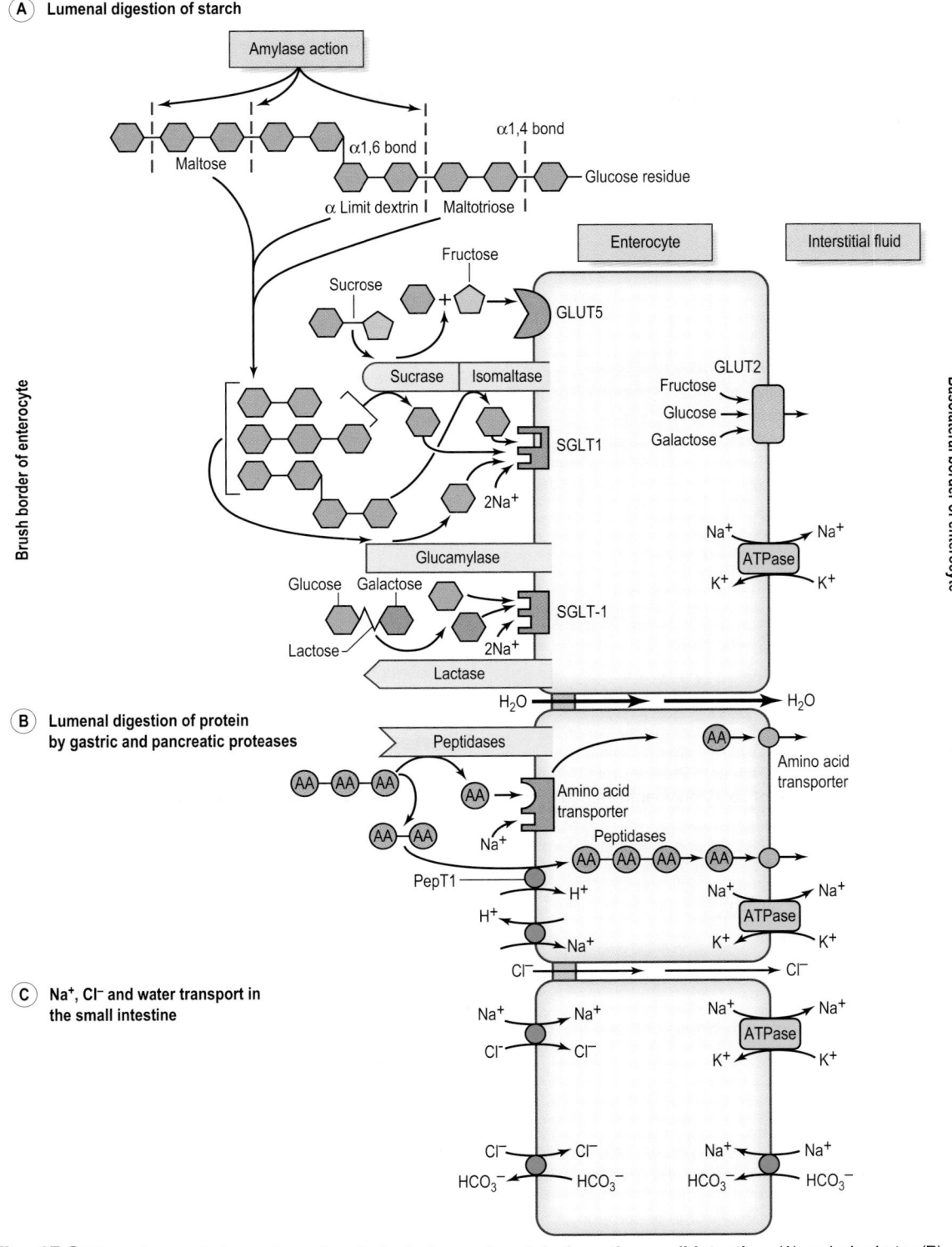

Fig. 15.3 Digestion and absorption of carbohydrates and protein from the small intestine: (A) carbohydrate; (B) protein; (C) electrolytes and water. GLUT2, GLUT5: membrane glucose transporters; SGLT1: sodium glucose-linked transporter; PepT1: peptide membrane transporter.

actions increase the surface area of the ingested fat. This allows an interaction between the water-soluble pancreatic lipase and the ingested fat. Pancreatic lipase (optimum pH 8.0) preferentially hydrolyses the bonds between glycerol and the fatty acid residues at positions 1 and 3 to produce 2-monoacylglycerols (monoglycerides) and free fatty acids.

A small quantity of the 2-monoacylglycerols are hydrolysed to glycerol and a free fatty acid. The presence of fat digestion products, bile salts, cholesterol and phospholipids leads the emulsion to break up into smaller particles, known as mixed micelles, with diameters of up to 5 nm. The bile salts form an outer coat with the fatty digestion products in the centre.

Table 15.2	The action of disaccharidases in the brush border of enterocytes	
Enzyme	**Substrate**	**Products**
Glucoamylase (maltase)	Maltose	Glucose
	Maltotriose	Glucose
	α-Limit dextrins	Glucose
Isomaltase (α-Dextrinase)	α-Limit dextrins	Glucose
Sucrase	Sucrose	Glucose and fructose
	Maltose	Glucose
	Maltotriose	Glucose
Lactase	Lactose	Glucose and galactose

Table 15.3	Gastric and pancreatic proteases	
Precursor	**Activator**	**Protease**
Pepsinogens	Acid	Pepsins
Trypsinogen	Enteropeptidase	Trypsin
Chymotrypsinogen	Trypsin	Chymotrypsin
Procarboxypeptidase	Trypsin	Carboxypeptidase
Proelastase	Trypsin	Elastase

Information box 15.1   Defects in chemical fat digestion

Failure of secretion of pancreatic lipase and deficiency in bile salts affects fat digestion in the small intestine. Pancreatic lipase deficiency occurs in many conditions, including chronic pancreatitis, carcinoma of the pancreas, and cystic fibrosis. Deficiency in bile salts is usually due to obstruction, which may be intra-hepatic, as in cirrhosis of the liver, or extra-hepatic due to gall bladder disease, stones in the biliary tree or tumours. The resulting failure to digest fat leads to the excretion of undigested fat globules in the form of pale, bulky, offensive and sometimes frothy stools that float (steatorrhoea). Steatorrhoea may be confirmed by measuring the fat content of stools. The absorption of fat-soluble vitamins may also be impaired (see below).

The micelles are small enough to diffuse between the microvilli of the enterocytes.

ABSORPTION

Absorption is the term used to describe the transfer of nutrients or their digestion products from the lumen of the alimentary canal to either the blood or lymph. The small intestine possesses efficient mechanisms for the absorption of nutrients and prevents their passage to the large intestine. The presence of nutrients in the large intestine produces diarrhoea resulting from water being drawn into the lumen by osmosis or by bacterial overgrowth. The absorbed molecules have to overcome a barrier (Fig. 15.4) made up of the:

- Unstirred layer of fluid covering the microvilli
- Glycocalyx covering the microvilli
- Luminal plasma membrane
- Cytoplasm
- Basal or lateral border of the cell
- Intercellular space

Clinical box 15.4   Diarrhoea

Disease of the gastrointestinal tract prevents efficient absorption by compromising the transfer of nutrients across the intestinal epithelium. This can be caused by inflammatory processes through infection (gastroenteritis, dysentery, parasitic infestations), immune responses (Crohn's disease, ulcerative colitis, coeliac disease), hereditary digestive enzyme deficiency or through a reduction in surface area after surgical resection.

Clinically, diarrhoea occurs when there is an increase in daily stool weight to more than 300 g, increased fluid content and stool volume, and there is usually an associated increase in frequency of bowel action. Steatorrhoea occurs when there is impaired fat absorption and the stools have a high fat content. Diarrhoea may be:

- Osmotic, when the presence of undigested hypertonic substances draws fluid into the large bowel by osmosis
- Secretory, usually after intestinal resection, in the presence of toxins or laxative use, when fluid and electrolyte absorption is decreased at the same time as an increase in secretion
- Inflammatory, due to damage of the intestinal mucosa through infection or inflammation.

There is increased fluid and electrolyte loss as well as reduced absorption. The fluid and electrolyte loss can lead to severe dehydration and metabolic imbalance. Diarrhoea is one of the leading causes of death among children in developing countries.

- Basement membrane (basal and reticular lamina)
- Plasma membrane of the capillary or lymph vessel.

General principles of absorption

Most carbohydrate, protein and lipid absorption occurs in the small intestine, in the duodenum, jejunum and the early sections of the ileum. These sites, together with the stomach, are also where orally administered drugs are absorbed. Disease of the membranes through which absorption takes place, and defects in the normal mechanisms for absorption, lead to nutritional deficiencies and also adverse or toxic drug effects. Absorption of solutes may occur by either passive or active processes (see Ch. 2).

There are two types of passive diffusion. These are simple diffusion, where small molecules, such as O_2 and CO_2, and fat-soluble molecules diffuse through the lipid bilayer, and facilitated diffusion, where the transported molecule moves through the membrane by means of a protein carrier. In a passive process, the absorbed solute will move from a high to a low concentration. Passive processes do not require the use of energy from cellular metabolism.

Water and some solutes pass through membranes at a faster rate than would be expected from a knowledge of the lipid solubility. This suggests that there are routes through the membrane for water and small hydrophilic solutes. These may be in the spaces between the membrane phospholipids and through specific membrane proteins called aquaporins. Ions can diffuse through specific protein ion channels that span the membrane.

In contrast, an active process involves cellular energy to drive an absorbed solute against either a concentration gradient or an electrical gradient, i.e. an 'uphill' movement from a low to a high concentration or for a charged solute moving to a region of the same charge, e.g. Na^+ ions being transported out of cells. The two types of active transport either

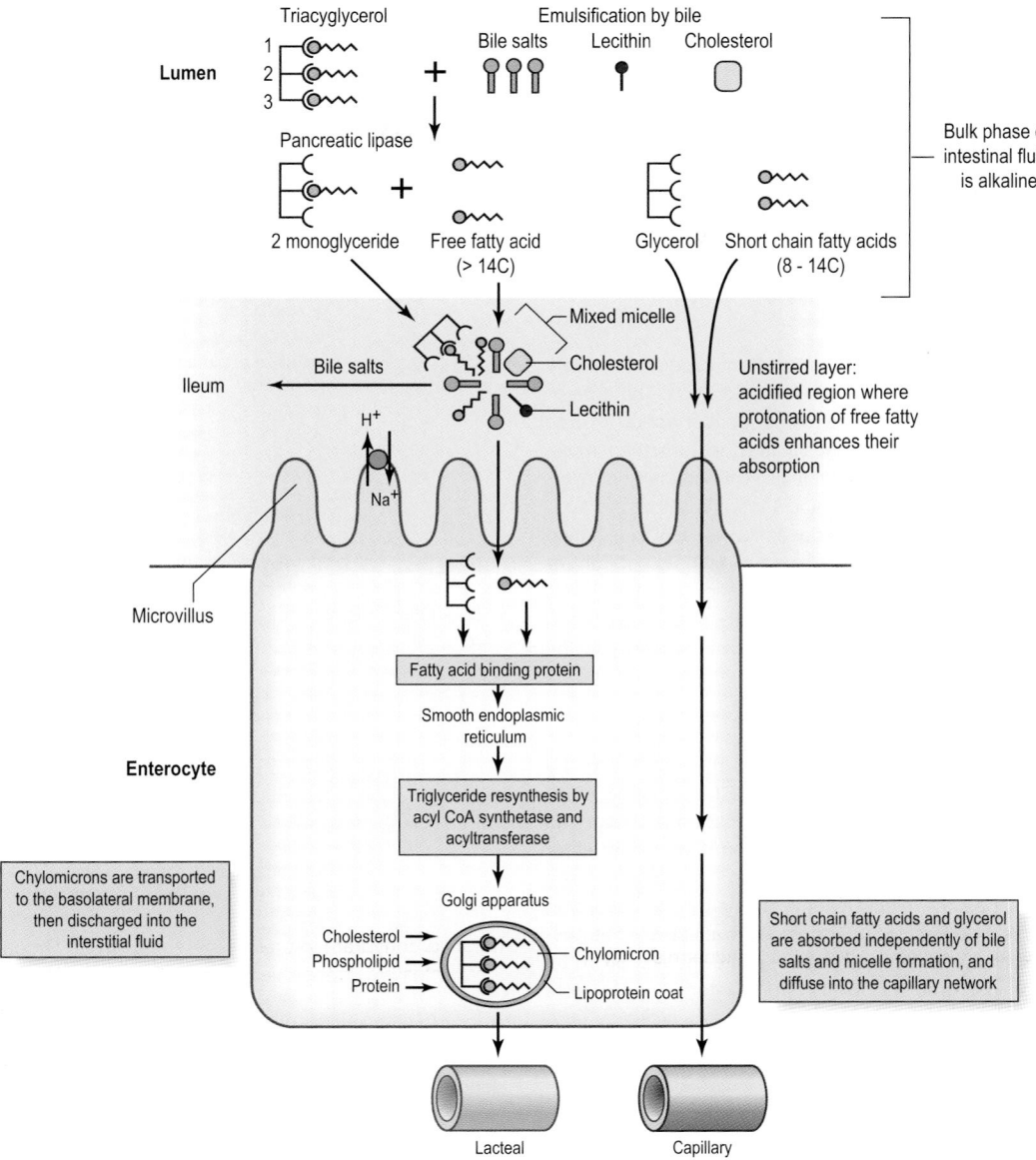

Fig. 15.4 The digestion and absorption of triglycerides.

use ATP directly, as in the Na^+/K^+-ATPase pump, or as a source of energy to power secondary active transport.

For the absorption of many solutes in the alimentary canal there are carrier-mediated mechanisms that use the concentration gradient built up as a result of the primary active transport of Na^+. This process is known as secondary active transport. The carriers have binding sites for the organic molecules and for Na^+. The movement of Na^+ down its concentration gradient can lead to the simultaneous transfer of the organic molecule into the cell against its concentration gradient. Metabolic inhibitors which block the primary active transport system will lead to inhibition of the secondary active transport system once the potential energy stored in the Na^+ concentration gradient across the cell membrane has run down.

Carbohydrate absorption

The carbohydrate digestion products are glucose, galactose and fructose. A small quantity of these sugars is absorbed by passive diffusion through aqueous channels between enterocytes and in the cell membranes. The main transport mechanisms involve carrier proteins in the brush and basolateral borders of enterocytes. All the sugars enter the hepatic portal vein for delivery to the liver.

Glucose and galactose absorption

Glucose and galactose are absorbed by secondary active transport involving a sodium-dependent glucose and galactose transporter (sodium glucose-linked transporter, SGLT1) in the brush border membrane of the enterocyte (see Fig. 15.3). The glucose and galactose compete for the sugar site on the transporter which also binds two Na^+ ions at a different site. Once loaded the transporter moves the Na^+ down its electrochemical gradient into the cell together with either the glucose or galactose. The Na^+ diffuses into the intracellular fluid and is transported out of the cell by the Na^+/K^+-ATPase (sodium pump) on the basolateral membrane. The glucose and galactose accumulate in the cell until they are removed by simple diffusion and facilitated diffusion involving GLUT2, a transporter found in the basolateral borders of the enterocyte.

Fructose absorption

Fructose enters the enterocyte by facilitated diffusion using the specific fructose transporter GLUT5, which does not require the cotransport of Na^+ to function (Fig. 15.3). As with glucose and galactose, GLUT2 transports fructose across the basolateral border of the enterocyte to the tissue fluid.

Protein absorption

The proteases in the gastrointestinal tract produce a variety of peptides and free amino acids for absorption. The enterocytes have a relatively high cytosolic concentration of free amino acids for protein synthesis that, in turn, can make amino acid absorption more difficult. This difficulty is overcome by the absorption of di- and tripeptides that are subsequently hydrolysed by peptidases to release free amino acids within the cell. This hydrolysis maintains a concentration gradient for peptides across the luminal cell membrane. After passing across the basolateral membrane, the absorbed amino acids enter the hepatic portal vein for delivery to the liver.

Di- and tripeptide absorption

Di- and tripeptides are absorbed into the enterocyte by means of a brush border carrier PepT1. The transport of di- and tripeptides is a secondary active transport process. The movement of Na^+ down its concentration gradient, to enter an enterocyte in exchange for a proton moving into the lumen, provides the electrochemical energy for absorbing the peptides (see Fig. 15.3). The PepT1 transporter cotransports H^+ from the lumen and peptides into the cell down an electrochemical gradient for H^+. It is interesting to note the absorption of β-lactam antibiotics (penicillins), and angiotensin-converting enzyme inhibitors (Captopril) is by means of the PepT1 transporter.

Amino acid absorption

There are a number of transport systems (Table 15.4) for L-amino acids in the brush border of enterocytes which require the cotransport of Na^+ to allow the transfer of amino acids against a concentration gradient by means of secondary active transport. Facilitated diffusion of some amino acids also occurs. The presence of carrier systems working in parallel for single amino acids and small peptides in the intestine enhances the overall absorption of amino acids by allowing the uptake of the same amino acid, e.g. glycine in peptide form, as well as free amino acid. Five carrier mechanisms are present in the basolateral borders of enterocytes. Three amino acid carriers not requiring Na^+ to function transport the intracellular amino acids to the extracellular fluid for diffusion into the blood. The Na^+-requiring carriers provide amino acids from the circulation for protein synthesis in crypt cells.

Fat absorption

The process of fat absorption (Fig. 15.4) differs from that of carbohydrate and proteins. Short- and medium-chain-length fatty acids (8–14 C) and glycerol are water soluble and diffuse directly through the luminal and basolateral membranes of

Table 15.4	Amino acid transport systems in enterocytes	
Site and system	**Amino acid transporter**	**Cotransported ion**
Apical membrane		
B	Neutral amino acids, e.g. alanine	Na^+
B°	Neutral and cationic (basic) amino acids, e.g. lysine and also cystine	Na^+
b°ᵗ	Neutral and cationic amino acids	None
X_{AG}^-	Anionic (acidic) amino acids, e.g. glutamate, aspartate	2 Na^+, 1 H^+, inward, 1 K^+ outward
y⁺	Cationic (basic) amino acids, e.g. arginine, lysine	None but will also cotransport small neutral amino acids with Na^+
Imino	Proline and hydroxyproline	Na^+ and Cl^-
β	β amino acids: β-alanine and taurine	Na^+ and Cl^-
Basolateral membrane		
A	Most neutral and imino acids	Na^+
ASC	Neutral amino acids with 3–4 carbons	Na^+
b°ᵗ	Neutral and cationic amino acids	None
L	Neutral amino acids with hydrophobic side chain	None
y⁺	Cationic (basic) amino acids, e.g. arginine, lysine	None but will also cotransport small neutral amino acids with Na^+

the enterocyte to enter the capillaries. The micelles, containing 2-monoacylglycerols and larger free fatty acids (chain length greater than 14 carbon atoms) in their cores, being water soluble, diffuse through the unstirred layer of water at the surface of the enterocyte at a faster rate than can be achieved by fat digestion products alone. The hydrophobic 2-monoglycerides and free fatty acids are delivered by this mechanism to the enterocytes of the jejunum where they are absorbed by diffusion through the lipid portions of the surface of the cell membrane.

The absorbed long-chain fatty acids and 2-monoglyceride bind to a fatty acid binding protein within the enterocyte, thus maintaining the concentration gradient across the cell membrane for these products. The fatty acid binding protein transfers the fatty acids and 2-monoglycerides to the smooth endoplasmic reticulum for the resynthesis of triglyceride by acyl CoA synthetase and acyltransferase. The triglyceride is coated with lipoprotein, derived from cholesterol, phospholipid and apoprotein B in the rough endoplasmic reticulum to form a chylomicron which is transferred to the Golgi apparatus where the protein coat is glycosylated prior to exocytosis across the basolateral membrane. Chylomicrons (diameter 75–600 nm) are too large to enter capillaries but can diffuse through spaces in the walls of lacteals (lymphatic vessels) in the villi. The lacteals drain into larger lymphatic vessels leading to the thoracic lymphatic duct which, in turn, distributes the lymph to the venous system at the junction of the left subclavian vein and left jugular vein.

Bile salt absorption

The bile salts are ionised at intestinal pH and require a carrier mechanism for their absorption. The sodium-dependent carrier is present in the enterocytes of the terminal ileum. Absorption is by means of secondary active transport similar to that described for glucose or amino acid transport. The absorbed bile salts enter the venous system draining the ileum and are transported to the liver in the enterohepatic circulation. The liver extracts the bile salts and secretes them into the bile. The bile salt pool may recirculate two or three times during a large meal.

Vitamins

Vitamins (A, B, C, D, E and K) are organic compounds that the body is unable to synthesise; therefore, they must be absorbed from the small intestine (see Ch. 16).

Water-soluble vitamins

The water-soluble vitamins (B group and C) are absorbed by passive diffusion and in some cases secondary active transport. Specialised sodium-dependent transport systems exist for thiamine (B_1), niacin, folate and vitamin C in the apical membrane of enterocytes. A facilitated transport system is responsible for the exit of niacin, folate and thiamine across the basolateral border.

Vitamin B_{12}

The absorption of vitamin B_{12} (cobalamin) involves a complex series of events. Vitamin B_{12} in food is bound to proteins. The action of pepsins in the stomach releases the vitamin B_{12}. The free vitamin B_{12} binds to glycoproteins, known as R proteins, that are present in the stomach contents derived from saliva and gastric juice. Another glycoprotein capable of binding vitamin B_{12} is intrinsic factor secreted by parietal

---

_i_ Information box 15.2   Vitamin B_{12} malabsorption

Vitamin B_{12} deficiency is caused by the malabsorption of vitamin B_{12}. The commonest cause is **pernicious anaemia**. There is atrophic gastritis leading to a failure in the production of **intrinsic factor**. This is an autoimmune condition, and is associated with other autoimmune diseases, such as thyroid disease and vitiligo. It is sometimes also associated with gastric carcinoma. Intrinsic factor antibodies are present, inhibiting the binding of intrinsic factor to B_{12} in the stomach, and also blocking the vitamin B_{12}–intrinsic factor complex to receptors in the terminal ileum, where B_{12} would normally be absorbed. A 3–6-year store of vitamin B_{12} is present in the liver, so that patients with pernicious anaemia may take years to develop symptoms of anaemia. Treatment is by intramuscular injections of vitamin B_{12}. Other causes of vitamin B_{12} malabsorption include coeliac disease, surgical resection of stomach or ileum, and some drugs.

_i_ Information box 15.3   Vitamin D deficiency

Chronic steatorrhoea could lead to malabsorption of fat-soluble vitamins. Although this could be the cause of vitamin D deficiency (**rickets, osteomalacia**), other factors are anticonvulsant therapy and renal failure, which interfere with vitamin D metabolism.

---

cells. The affinity of intrinsic factor for ingested B_{12} is less than that of R proteins; therefore, most of the vitamin B_{12} in the chyme leaving the stomach and entering the intestine is bound to R protein. Once in the intestine the pancreatic proteases digest the R protein and vitamin B_{12} is free once again. It binds to intrinsic factor, which is resistant to digestion by pancreatic proteases. The vitamin B_{12} intrinsic factor complex passes along the small intestine to the terminal ileum where there are receptors in the brush borders of the enterocytes for the vitamin B_{12} intrinsic factor complex. Binding of the vitamin B_{12} intrinsic factor complex to the membrane receptor triggers endocytosis (receptor-mediated endocytosis) of the complex into the cell. Vitamin B_{12} is released from the complex within the cell and exported across the basolateral border and diffuses into the blood where it binds to transcobalamin II, a transport protein.

Fat-soluble vitamins

The fat-soluble vitamins A, D, E and K entering the small intestine are solubilised by diffusion into micelles containing bile salts and fat digestion products (see Ch. 16). Absorption of these vitamins occurs by diffusion across the brush border of the enterocyte together with fatty acids and monoglycerides. The fat-soluble vitamins are exported to the lymphatic system in chylomicrons.

Absorption of electrolytes and water

Each day about 9 L of fluid enters the alimentary canal. This is derived from the diet (2 L) and the digestive secretions (7 L) (Fig. 15.5). In health about 99% of the water and electrolytes are absorbed into the blood as the fluid passes along the small and large intestine. The major site of fluid absorption is the jejunum and ileum (8.5 L); with a relatively small quantity being absorbed from the colon (0.4 L). The faeces contain about 0.1 L of water. The absorption of water is secondary to the uptake of electrolytes, in particular Na^+ and Cl^-, sugars and amino acids.

Pathways for electrolyte and water absorption

The electrolytes and water may be absorbed by passing between the enterocytes (paracellular route) via aqueous channels, through the tight junctions linking the cells together. The alternative route is by passing through the cells (transcellular route). In the case of electrolytes this may involve both carrier-mediated mechanisms and passage through water-permeable channels (Table 15.5).

Water movement from the lumen of the intestine is secondary to organic and ionic solute movement. The transfer of solutes across the intestinal epithelium creates an osmotic gradient between the lumen and the interstitial fluid and blood. Water is absorbed by osmosis via paracellular and transcellular routes (see Fig. 15.3). Cell membranes contain channels named aquaporins that allow the passage of water. The principle of oral rehydration therapy, used to treat diarrhoea, is based on promoting water absorption by providing an isotonic drink containing glucose and electrolytes, including sodium chloride.

Calcium absorption

Dietary calcium is found in a variety of foods including dairy products. Calcium may exist bound to oxalates, phosphates

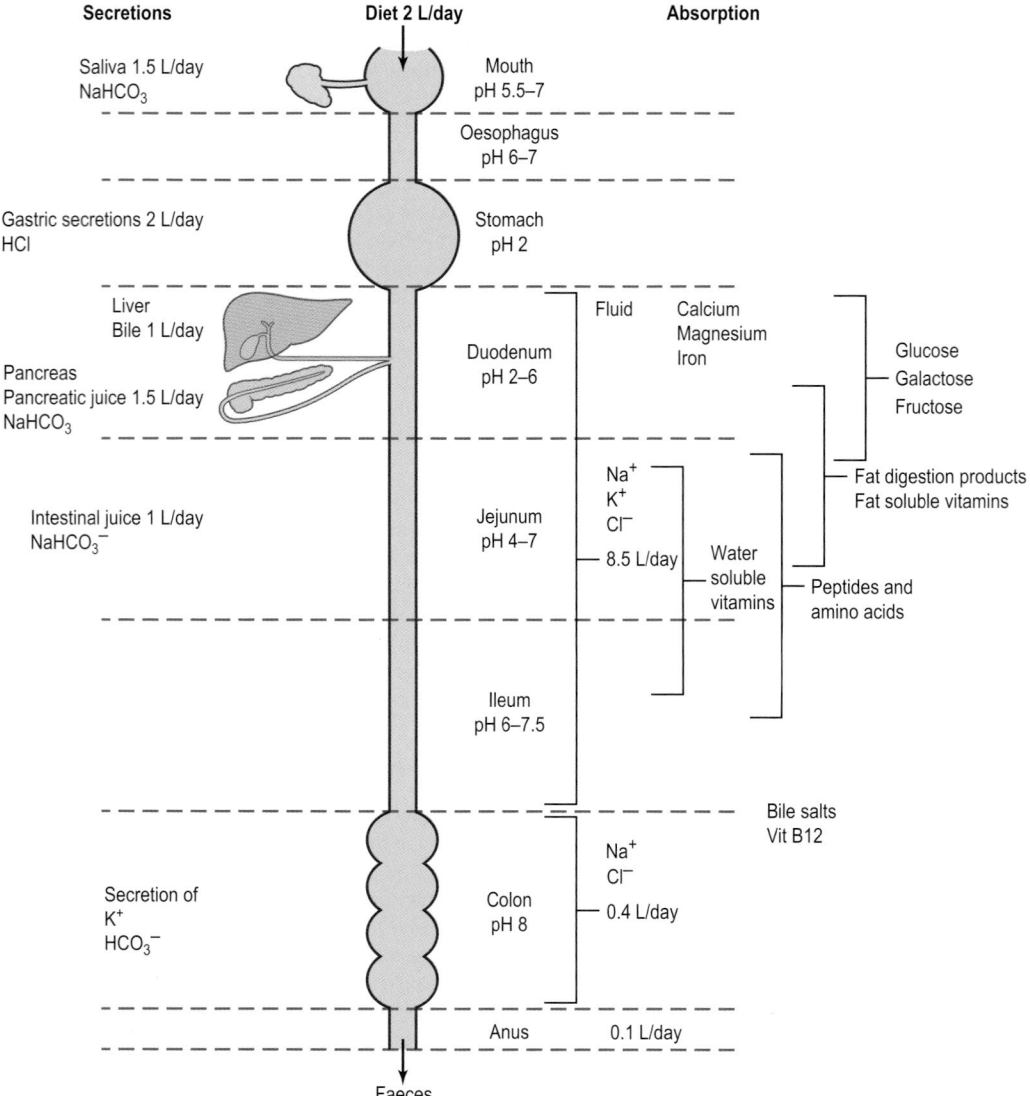

Secretions

Saliva 1.5 L/day
NaHCO$_3$

Gastric secretions 2 L/day
HCl

Liver
Bile 1 L/day

Pancreas
Pancreatic juice 1.5 L/day
NaHCO$_3$

Intestinal juice 1 L/day
NaHCO$_3^-$

Secretion of
K$^+$
HCO$_3^-$

Diet 2 L/day

Mouth
pH 5.5–7

Oesophagus
pH 6–7

Stomach
pH 2

Duodenum
pH 2–6

Jejunum
pH 4–7

Ileum
pH 6–7.5

Colon
pH 8

Anus

Faeces

Absorption

Fluid   Calcium
Magnesium
Iron

Na$^+$
K$^+$
Cl$^-$
8.5 L/day

Water
soluble
vitamins

Glucose
Galactose
Fructose

Fat digestion products
Fat soluble vitamins

Peptides and
amino acids

Bile salts
Vit B12

Na$^+$
Cl$^-$
0.4 L/day

0.1 L/day

Fig. 15.5 **Fluid and electrolyte input into the alimentary canal.**

and phytates or in the ionised form (Ca^{2+}) in the intestine. Ionised calcium is available for absorption by enterocytes in the upper small intestine. The free Ca^{2+} concentration in the cell is low, giving rise to a steep concentration gradient between the lumen and the cytoplasm. Ca^{2+} ions bind to a protein in the brush border and are transported down their concentration gradient into the cell. The free Ca^{2+} concentration in the cytoplasm is kept low by Ca^{2+} binding to calcium-binding proteins that are sequestered in intracellular organelles such as the endoplasmic reticulum. Ca^{2+} ions are exported across the basolateral border of the cell against an electrochemical gradient by active transport. There are two mechanisms:

- Ca^{2+}-ATPase – which uses energy derived from the hydrolysis of ATP to transfer Ca^{2+} out of the cell
- Na$^+$/Ca^{2+} exchanger – in which Na$^+$ moving down its electrochemical gradient into the cell drives Ca^{2+} extrusion.

The Ca^{2+}-ATPase mechanism is the more important one.

Calcium absorption is regulated by 1,25-dihydroxycholecalciferol, (1,25 (OH)$_2$ D$_3$), the active form

of vitamin D which stimulates the synthesis of both calcium-binding proteins and Ca^{2+}-ATPase (see Ch. 10). Note: A high dietary phytate content, as in chapatti flour, may inhibit calcium absorption (see Ch. 16).

Iron absorption

Dietary iron is present in two forms:

- The haem portion of haemoglobin, myoglobin and cytochromes
- An insoluble, non-absorbable state complexed with phytate, tannins and plant fibres. Insoluble iron salts may also form with hydroxide, phosphate and bicarbonate found in digestive secretions.

The acidic conditions of the stomach mobilise the iron compounds by converting the ions from the ferric (Fe^{3+}) to the ferrous (Fe^{2+}) state. Similarly, vitamin C reduces iron to the ferrous state and also forms soluble complexes with it that enhance absorption. Ferric ions are reduced to ferrous ions by duodenal cytochrome b ferric reductase in the brush border of the duodenal enterocyte.

Table 15.5 Electrolyte transport in the small and large intestine

Intestinal region	Na⁺	K⁺	Cl⁻	HCO₃⁻
Duodenum and jejunum	Actively absorbed • Cotransport with glucose, galactose, amino acids • Cotransport with Cl⁻ • Counter transport exchange for H⁺ • Diffusion through aqueous channels	Passively absorbed by diffusion through paracellular pathways as the luminal concentration rises after water absorption	Passively absorbed • Cotransport with Na⁺ • Counter transport exchange for HCO₃⁻ • Diffusion through paracellular channels	Absorbed as CO₂ following neutralisation of secreted H⁺
Ileum	Actively absorbed as above but reduced importance of cotransport with organic solutes	Passively absorbed as above	Passively absorbed • Counter transport exchange for HCO₃⁻ • Diffusion through paracellular channels	Passively absorbed • Counter transport in exchange for Cl⁻ • Diffusion
Colon	Actively absorbed • Via Na⁺ channels • Cotransport with Cl⁻ Stimulated by aldosterone	Secretion Passive leakage from enterocytes through K⁺ channels in their apical membranes when luminal concentration <25 mM Stimulated by aldosterone	Passively absorbed • Cotransport with Na⁺ • Counter transport with HCO₃⁻ • Diffusion through paracellular channels	Secretion Counter transport exchange with Cl⁻

The enterocytes of the duodenum absorb haem and ferrous ions by two separate mechanisms:

1. Haem is absorbed by endocytosis and digested in the enterocyte by haemoxidase to release ferric ions, carbon monoxide and biliverdin. The ferric ions are reduced to ferrous ions that bind to ferroportin 1 in the basolateral membrane for export from the cell.
2. Ferrous ions and a proton bind to a divalent-metal transporter to cross the brush border. The movement of a proton down its concentration gradient into the enterocyte is the driving force for ferrous ion absorption. In the cytosol ferrous ions bind either to a storage protein, apoferritin, to form ferritin or are transferred to ferroportin 1 in the basolateral borders of the cell for export to the tissue fluid.

An additional protein, hephaestin, is considered to have a role in the export of iron from the enterocytes to the plasma. It may be involved in the release of iron from its storage sites and transfer to ferroportin 1 for export to the tissue fluid. Ferrous ions diffuse into the blood and are transported around the body in association with transferrin, a plasma protein.

The absorption of iron needs to be regulated because this metal plays an essential biological role in oxygen transport and redox reactions in cellular respiration. In addition, iron is involved in the formation of reactive oxygen species that may be useful in killing bacteria. However, reactive oxygen species are also toxic to cells when large quantities are produced following excessive iron accumulation (see Ch. 16).

Regulation of iron absorption

Iron transport is stimulated either through erythropoiesis following haemorrhage or moving to high altitude and decreased

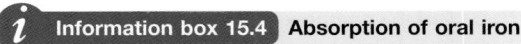

Information box 15.4   Absorption of oral iron

The ferrous state is more readily absorbed than ferric iron, and oral iron supplement formulations are usually in the ferrous state. Iron absorption increases during pregnancy and iron deficiency anaemia. High dietary content of phosphates and phytate (in chapatti flour) can inhibit iron absorption by forming insoluble complexes.

when iron stores are high. The development of the iron absorptive mechanisms in the immature enterocytes of the crypts are controlled by the uptake of transferrin-bound iron from the plasma. In states of iron deficiency the immature enterocyte becomes programmed to increase iron absorption by the upregulation of the divalent metal ion transporter and ferroportin 1 synthesis. An increase in iron accumulation leads to a decrease in the synthesis of the transport systems involved in iron uptake. The accumulation of iron in the enterocyte stimulates apoferritin synthesis and ferritin formation to protect the body from iron overload. The ferritin is released into the intestinal lumen when the enterocytes are shed from the villous tip.

SURFACE ANATOMY OF THE ABDOMEN

The upper abdomen is bound by the lower rib (costal) margins formed by the seventh to tenth costal cartilages, and joined in the middle at the xiphisternum (Fig. 15.6). The lower abdomen extends to the inguinal ligaments and the pubis. The inguinal ligaments appear convex in thin people. To locate the surface positions of abdominal organs, the anterior

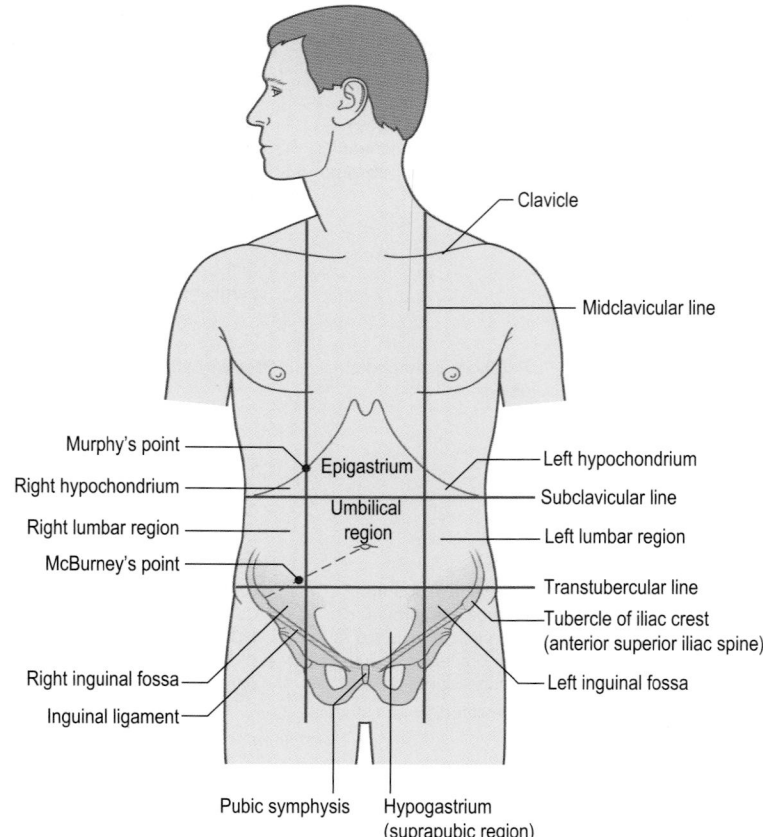

Fig. 15.6 **Surface anatomy of the abdomen.**

surface of the abdomen could roughly be divided into nine regions, or four quadrants. The nine regions are demarcated by two vertical and two horizontal imaginary planes that transect the abdominal cavity.

ABDOMINAL REGIONS

Abdominal regions are demarcated by four imaginary planes into nine regions. The two vertical planes pass through the midclavicular lines. The upper horizontal plane is marked by the lowest edge of the rib cage, the subcostal line, and the lower horizontal plane passes through the line drawn between the tubercles of the iliac crest: the transtubercular line. In practice, the anterior superior iliac spines (ASIS) are easier to feel than the tubercles, which are palpable a little way behind the ASIS. The plane passing through the ASISs is sometimes substituted for the transtubercular plane. From top to bottom in the midline, the regions are epigastric, umbilical and hypogastric (also known as suprapubic). The lateral regions are left and right hypochondrial, lumbar and inguinal (or iliac fossa).

Two important landmarks are McBurney's point, about one third of the way on a line drawn from the right ASIS to the umbilicus, marking the base of the appendix where the point of maximal tenderness is felt in classical acute appendicitis. Murphy's point is roughly below the plane where the midclavicular line crosses the lower margin of the rib cage (costal margin) at about the level of the ninth costal cartilage, and is classically where the fundus of the gall bladder may be found. It is also the point of maximum tenderness in acute cholecystitis.

Epigastric region

Typically, pain and tenderness in the epigastrium are referred from the upper abdominal organs, such as the stomach and duodenum. Palpable masses usually arise from the stomach, and the pulsations of the abdominal aorta can also just be felt in thin people.

Umbilical region

Pain from intestinal obstruction, for example in acute appendicitis, could be referred to the area around the umbilicus. Pain and tenderness from disease of the transverse colon are also located in the umbilical region. The transverse colon is extremely variable in position, sometimes reaching down to the suprapubic region. Tumours of underlying structures and pulsations from the abdominal aorta are palpable here.

Suprapubic (hypogastric) region

Pain and tenderness from the lower bowel, e.g. descending colon and anal canal, bladder and uterus, and sometimes the fallopian tubes, are referred to this region. Enlargement or tumours of the pelvic organs, e.g. bladder and uterus, are palpable here.

Left and right hypochondrium

The spleen is situated behind the left lower ribs. Splenic tenderness and enlargement are felt in the left hypochondrium, although the spleen has to be enlarged to more than three times its normal size to be palpable. The liver and gall bladder are behind the rib cage on the right. An enlarged or tender liver and gall bladder may be palpated in the right hypochondrium.

Left and right lumbar region

The lumbar regions refer to the 'flanks'. Normally, the kidneys lie deep against the posterior abdominal wall and are not palpable. The lower poles of enlarged kidneys may be felt in the lumbar regions. The right kidney is usually lower than the left. Posteriorly, the angles formed by the ribs and the spine are the renal angles where maximal renal tenderness may be felt when the kidneys are dilated or inflamed. The ascending colon may be palpable in the right lumbar region and the descending colon in the left.

Left and right iliac fossa (inguinal region)

Pain and tenderness in the left iliac fossa could be related to problems with the descending or sigmoid colon, whereas signs in the right iliac fossa signify disease of the appendix, caecum or ascending colon. Deep iliac fossa pain may relate to fallopian tube disease. Masses in either iliac fossa are suspicious of underlying tumours, but sometimes a loaded colon or impacted faeces may be palpable.

The pulsations of the femoral artery are easily felt at the midpoint between the anterior superior iliac spine and the pubic symphysis along the inguinal ligament. A weakness in the inguinal canal can cause some abdominal contents to be forced through this potential weakness in the inguinal region when the intra-abdominal pressure is significantly raised, as in coughing and lifting heavy weights. This manifests as palpable 'bulges' medial to the femoral artery when a patient is asked to cough, particularly when standing.

QUADRANTS

For the purposes of description, the surface of the abdomen is also commonly divided into quadrants – the right and left upper and lower quadrants (the gall bladder and liver being palpable in the right upper quadrant, enlarged spleen in the left upper quadrant). The right lower quadrant is where the signs of disease in the appendix and caecum become evident, and the left lower quadrant is where signs of disease of the sigmoid colon become evident.

MICROANATOMY OF THE GASTROINTESTINAL TRACT

The gastrointestinal tract can be considered as a muscular tube 7–10 m in length, consisting of four major layers (Fig. 15.7). From the lumen these are:

- Mucosa
- Submucosa
- Muscle
- Serosa.

There are variations in the general structure related to the functions of the different regions of the gastrointestinal tract.

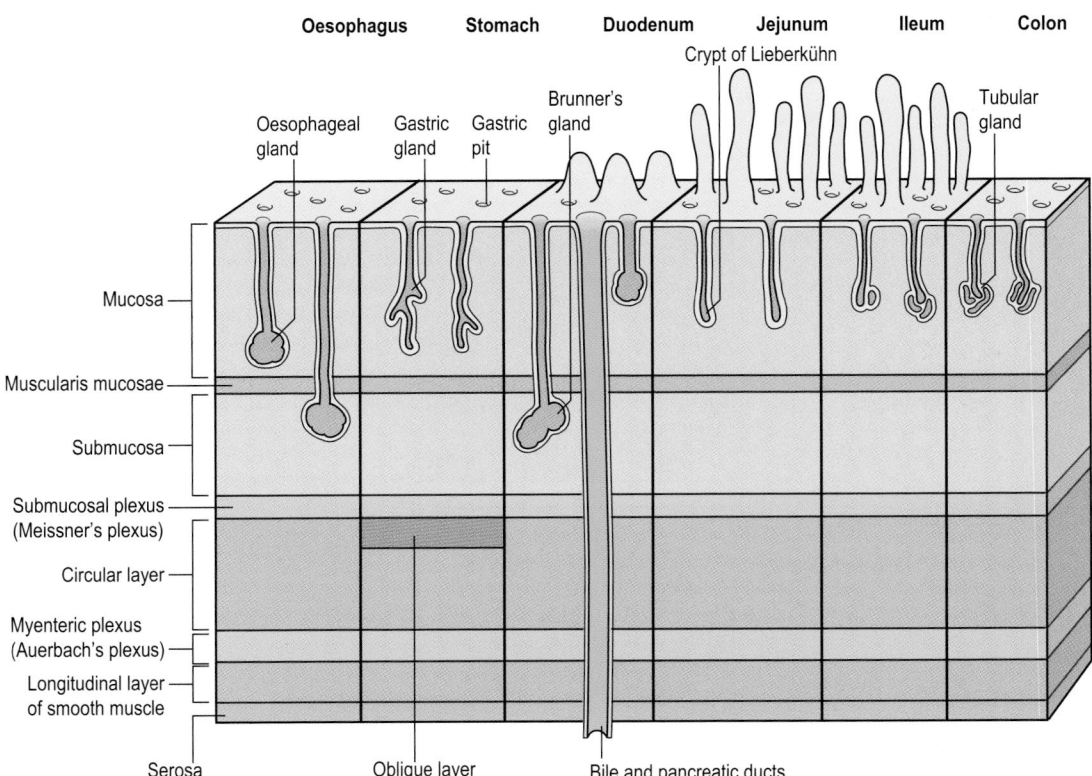

Fig. 15.7 **General organisation of the layers of the alimentary canal together with features of specialised regions.**

The histological structure of the mucosal layers shows the greatest variation (Fig. 15.8). The **mucosa** consists of:

- A lining layer of **epithelial cells** that have secretory and absorptive functions
- The **lamina propria**, a connective tissue support for the mucosa, together with blood vessels and the glandular ducts in some regions
- The **muscularis mucosae**, a thin layer of smooth muscle cells which moves the epithelium, producing mixing activity, and leads to folding of the mucosal layer.

The **submucosa**, which contains connective tissues, blood vessels and lymphatics together with nerves innervating structures within the mucosa.

In most regions of the alimentary canal the external **muscle** consists of two layers of smooth muscle: the inner layer in which the long axis of the muscle fibres is arranged in a circular manner around the canal (**circular muscle**) and an outer layer with the muscle fibres lying along the length of the canal (**longitudinal layer**). Contraction of the circular and longitudinal muscle layers narrows the lumen and shortens the canal, respectively. These muscles are responsible for mixing the food with the digestive secretions and for

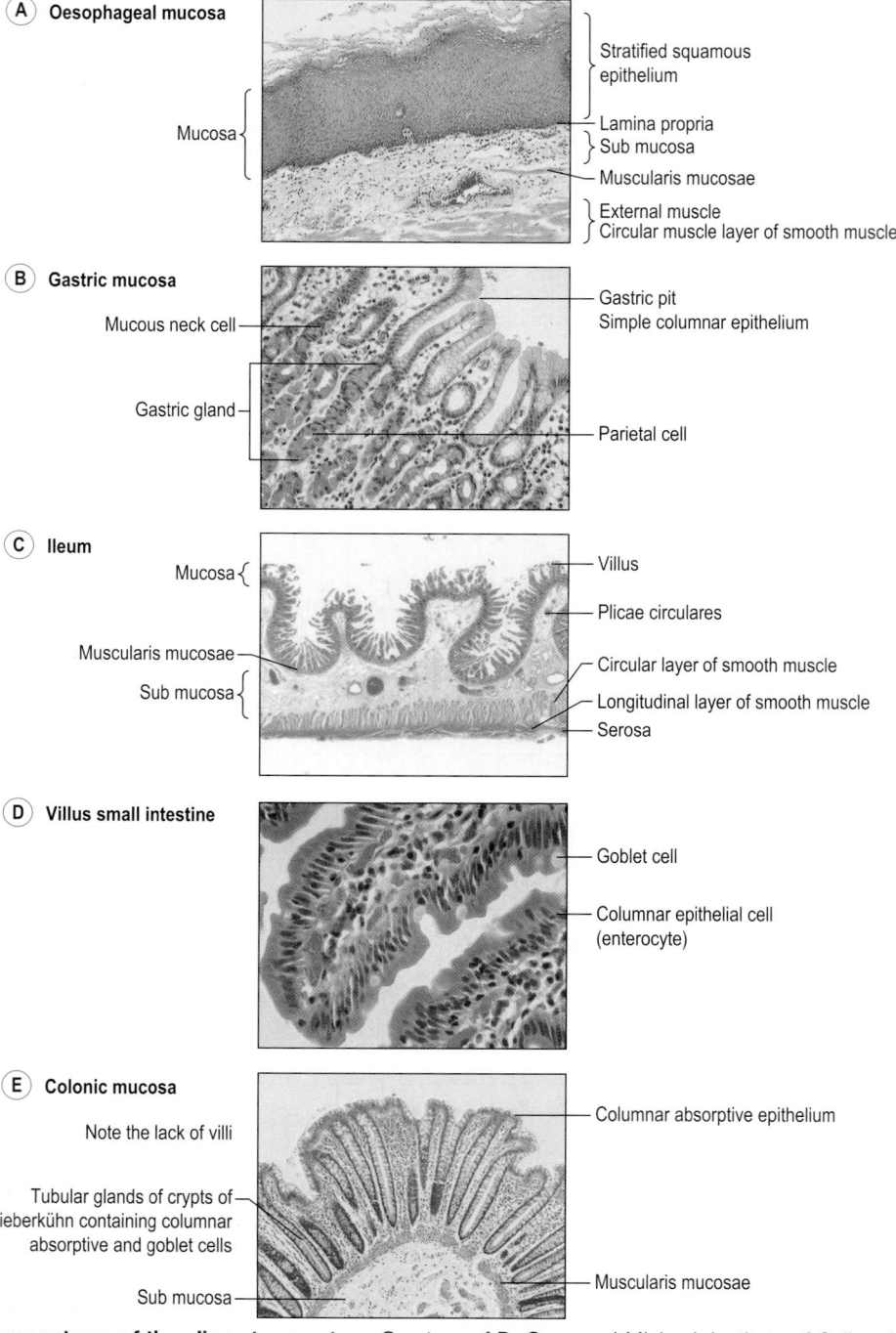

A Oesophageal mucosa

Stratified squamous epithelium

Mucosa
Lamina propria
Sub mucosa
Muscularis mucosae
External muscle
Circular muscle layer of smooth muscle

B Gastric mucosa

Mucous neck cell
Gastric gland

Gastric pit
Simple columnar epithelium
Parietal cell

C Ileum

Mucosa
Muscularis mucosae
Sub mucosa

Villus
Plicae circulares
Circular layer of smooth muscle
Longitudinal layer of smooth muscle
Serosa

D Villus small intestine

Goblet cell
Columnar epithelial cell (enterocyte)

E Colonic mucosa

Note the lack of villi

Tubular glands of crypts of Lieberkühn containing columnar absorptive and goblet cells

Sub mucosa

Columnar absorptive epithelium
Muscularis mucosae

Fig. 15.8 **Microanatomy of the alimentary system.** Courtesy of Dr Gregory J Michael, Institute of Cell and Molecular Science, Barts and The London School of Medicine and Dentistry, Queen Mary University of London.

propelling the contents along the digestive tract. The first third of the oesophagus and the anal sphincter contain skeletal muscle.

The **serosa** is the outermost layer of the alimentary canal and is continuous with the parietal peritoneum lining the inner surface of the body wall. It consists of connective tissues covered with a squamous epithelium.

INNERVATION OF THE ALIMENTARY CANAL

Sensory and motor neurons are found within the wall of the alimentary canal. Major aggregations of neurons are found in:

- **The submucosal plexus** or **Meissner's plexus** on the outer edge of the submucosa adjacent to the circular muscle layer
- **The myenteric plexus** or **Auerbach's plexus** lying between the circular and longitudinal muscle layers.

The plexi are innervated by sensory neurons from the mucosa and muscle layers, and by preganglionic parasympathetic nerves and postganglionic sympathetic nerves from the central nervous system. The nerves, with their cell bodies within the alimentary canal, form the enteric nervous system.

The function of nerves within the alimentary canal is to coordinate muscular, secretory and absorptive activity in order that the digestive tract functions as a coordinated unit. Many functions of the alimentary canal continue to be co-ordinated following the cutting of the parasympathetic and sympathetic nerves innervating the canal. For this reason it may be said that the nerves within the alimentary canal constitute 'a little brain'. The central nervous system (or 'large brain') modifies the action of the enteric nervous system via the parasympathetic and sympathetic branches of the autonomic nervous system.

Table 15.6 shows the hormones and neuropeptides secreted by the alimentary system. Some gastrointestinal hormones and neuropeptides also act centrally on the hypothalamus to control appetite, hunger and satiety (see also Chs 8 and 16).

MOUTH

The mouth or oral cavity consists of the lips, tongue, teeth, gums, and hard and soft palate. Stratified squamous epithelial cells, kept moist by saliva, cover the surface of the oral cavity and tongue. Sensory nerves sensitive to pain, touch and temperature are present in the lining of the mouth together with taste buds in the dorsal surface of the tongue (see Ch. 8). The temperature and taste of ingested food and drink is sampled by the sensory receptors before chewing or drinking begins.

TEETH

In adults there are 32 permanent teeth that have different functions.

- Incisors – chisel shaped teeth for cutting and biting
- Canines – puncture and hold food
- Molars – grind and crush food.

The adult teeth are preceded by 20 deciduous or milk teeth. The deciduous teeth begin to appear at 6 months, the set is complete at 6–8 years and is replaced by permanent teeth at 10–12 years.

TONGUE

The anterior two-thirds of the tongue is composed of skeletal muscle fibres, covered by a layer containing sero-mucous glands and stratified epithelium. The secretions of these glands together with saliva ensures the tongue is moist to facilitate movement during chewing and swallowing food.

MASTICATION

The mastication, or chewing, process physically breaks food into smaller pieces. This voluntary and reflex behaviour serves to:

- Dissolve chemicals in saliva so that they can stimulate the taste buds
- Lubricate the food to ease swallowing
- Mix starch-containing food with salivary α-amylase
- Increase the surface area of food to facilitate digestion in the stomach and duodenum.

The absence of teeth and neuromuscular defects in the elderly after strokes can severely interfere with mastication.

SALIVARY GLANDS

Saliva is an exocrine secretion which enters the mouth from salivary glands by a duct system. There are two types of salivary secretion produced by different cells:

- Serous cells produce a watery secretion
- Mucous cells produce a thick mucus-rich secretion.

In human beings there are three pairs of salivary glands: parotid, submandibular and sublingual (Fig. 15.9). The glands vary in the type of saliva they produce.

The **parotid glands** lie in the cheeks anterior to the ear with their excretory ducts opening into the mouth opposite the second upper molar teeth. They are serous glands producing a watery secretion rich in amylase. These are the largest glands but they produce only 25% of the daily saliva.

The **submandibular glands** lie under the mandible with their excretory ducts entering the mouth under the tip of the tongue behind the central incisor teeth. They secrete 70% of the daily saliva production. These are mixed glands that contain serous and mucous cells, producing a more viscous secretion than the parotid glands.

The **sublingual glands** lie in the floor of the mouth just posterior to the mandible and have many small ducts opening into the mouth, some of them entering the submandibular duct. The cells of the sublingual glands are predominantly mucous cells; therefore, the secretion is thick and viscous due to the presence of mucus. These glands produce 5% of the total daily output. In addition, there are smaller salivary glands scattered over the tongue, buccal cavity and on the inner side of the lips.

Table 15.6	Gastrointestinal hormones and neuropeptides, their source, target organ and action		
Hormone/neuropeptide	**Source**	**Target**	**Action**
Cholecystokinin	I cells in duodenum and jejunum and neurons in ileum and colon	Pancreas Gallbladder	↑ Enzyme secretion ↑ Contraction
Calcitonin gene-related peptide	Enteric neurons Splanchnic afferent nerves	Blood vessels Neurons	↑ Vasodilatation Sensory neurotransmitter
Enkephalins	Enteric neurons	Gastrointestinal smooth muscle Intestinal mucosa	↑ Contraction ↓ Fluid secretion
Enteroglucagon Glucagon-like peptide 1	L cells in the ileum, colon and rectum	Pancreas Stomach	↑ Insulin release ↓ Acid secretion ↓ Gastric emptying
Epidermal growth factors	Salivary and Brunner's glands	Gastrointestinal mucosa	↑ Growth and mucosal protection
Gastric-inhibitory peptide or glucose-dependent insulinotropic peptide	K cells in duodenum and jejunum	Pancreas Stomach	↑ Insulin release ↓ Acid secretion
Gastrin	G cells, antrum of stomach	Parietal cells in body of stomach Enterochromaffin-like cells Gastrointestinal mucosa	↑ Acid secretion ↑ Histamine secretion ↑ Growth
Gastrin-releasing peptide	Enteric neurons	G cells in antrum of stomach	Gastrin release
Ghrelin	Gr or X/A cells in the stomach adjacent to parietal cells	Anterior pituitary Hypothalamus Stomach	↑ Growth hormone release ↑ Feeding ↑ Acid secretion ↑ Motility and gastric emptying
Guanylin	Endocrine cells in ileum and colon	Small and large intestine	↑ Fluid secretion
Motilin	Endocrine cells in upper gastrointestinal tract	Oesophageal sphincter Stomach Duodenum	↑ Smooth muscle contraction migrating myoelectric complex
Neurotensin	N cells, throughout gastrointestinal tract	Gastrointestinal smooth muscle Gastrointestinal mucosa Stomach	Relaxation of LOS ↓ Antral motility ↑ Growth ↓ Acid secretion
Pancreatic polypeptide	Endocrine cells in ileum	Pancreas	↓ Enzyme and fluid secretion
Peptide YY	Endocrine cells in ileum and colon	Stomach Pancreas	↓ Vagally mediated acid secretion ↓ Enzyme and fluid secretion
Pituitary adenylate cyclase-activating peptide (PACAP)	Enteric neurons	Intestinal smooth muscle	Relaxation
Secretin	S cells in small intestine	Pancreas Stomach	↑ HCO$_3^-$ and fluid secretion by pancreatic ducts ↓ Gastric acid secretion
Somatostatin	D cells of stomach and duodenum, δ cells of pancreatic islets	Stomach Intestine Pancreas Liver	↓ Gastrin release ↑ Fluid absorption ↓ Secretion ↑ Smooth muscle contraction ↓ Endocrine/exocrine secretions ↓ Bile flow
Tachykinins: substance P; neurokinin A	Sensorimotor neurons; enteric neurons	Longitudinal and circular layer smooth muscle Enteric nervous system Blood vessels Small and large intestinal mucosa	↑ Contraction Stimulation of inhibitory and excitatory pathways ↑ Vasodilatation ↑ Fluid secretion
Vasoactive intestinal peptide	Enteric neurons Pancreatic neurons	Gastrointestinal smooth muscle Small intestinal mucosa Pancreas	↑Relaxation ↑ Fluid secretion ↑ HCO$_3^-$ and fluid secretion by pancreatic ducts

↑ increase; ↓ decrease; LOS, lower oesophageal sphincter.

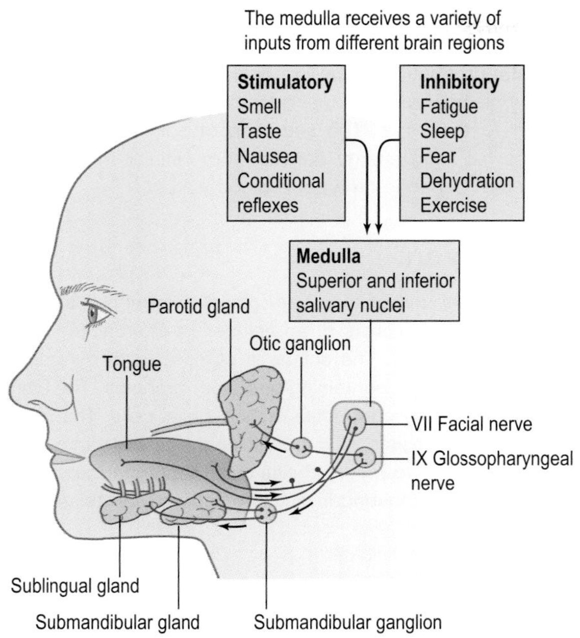

Fig. 15.9 **Position of salivary glands and innervation.**

Clinical box 15.5 Some clinical conditions of the salivary glands

Disease of the salivary glands may lead to impaired secretion of saliva, giving rise to **xerostomia** (dry mouth). This interferes with both chemical and physical digestion of food, and also increases the risk of oral infections and ulceration.

- Mumps is a common childhood infection of the salivary glands, characterised by pain and swelling, which temporarily affects salivation.
- Salivary duct calculi (stones) obstruct the flow of saliva and may cause pain and swelling of the gland.
- Salivary gland tumours are usually benign but may be malignant.
- Some drugs inhibit saliva secretion.
- Sjögren's syndrome is an autoimmune condition in which saliva-secreting cells are destroyed. There may be associated parotid gland enlargement, with ensuing dry mouth. Dry eyes, skin and vagina are also clinical features. This condition can occur in association with other systemic autoimmune diseases (e.g. rheumatoid arthritis, thyroid disease). Difficulty with swallowing because of the lack of lubrication and mouth ulcers and oral infections may be a manifestation of systemic disease (see above).
- 'Water brash' is a symptom in which there is a sudden inflow of saliva into the mouth, but without the stimulation of food. This is sometimes associated with peptic ulceration and inflammatory bowel disease.

FUNCTIONS OF SALIVA

Saliva has three functions. These are:

- Lubrication
- Protection
- Digestion.

Lubrication

The water and mucus in saliva act as lubricants that aid the movement of the tongue to facilitate speech and swallowing of food. You may have noticed that it is difficult to talk when your mouth is dry. Swallowing a number of dry biscuits is also difficult unless they are accompanied by a drink.

Protection

The presence of food debris in the warm and wet environment of the mouth provides ideal conditions for bacterial growth and division. The mouth is protected from metabolic acids produced by bacteria by the buffering action of bicarbonate, phosphate and mucus in saliva. The saliva is saturated with calcium salts at neutral pH, so that the calcium in the teeth does not dissolve. However, calcium from the teeth will dissolve and the formation of dental caries will occur if the pH falls to 5.5, once saliva flow has been reduced after a meal. The presence of protein in saliva forms a protective coat on the teeth surface to reduce the adherence of bacteria and to act as a barrier to acid. In addition, bacterial growth is limited by:

- Lysozyme, an enzyme responsible for breaking down bacterial cell walls
- Lactoferrin, an iron-chelating agent that binds iron to prevent its use by some bacteria requiring iron for growth
- Secretory immunoglobulin A, derived from plasma cells, which provides immunity against bacteria and viruses.

Large volumes of alkaline saliva are produced before vomiting. The alkali neutralises the gastric acid and inactivates the enzyme pepsin when it enters the oesophagus and mouth during vomiting.

Digestion

The digestive function of saliva is to dissolve food so that the chemical constituents can stimulate the taste buds, and to begin chemical digestion of carbohydrate and fat. Saliva contains an α-amylase or ptyalin which starts the digestion of starch by hydrolysing α-1, 4 glycosidic bonds to produce maltose, maltotriose and oligosaccharides known as α-limit dextrans (see Fig. 15.3). Salivary amylase is active over the pH range 4–11 and has an optimum pH 7. Chewing mixes the saliva with food. The amylase present inside a bolus of swallowed food continues its activity in the stomach until the acid in the gastric secretions penetrates the bolus. Up to 75% of starch digestion may occur in the stomach before amylase is destroyed by gastric acid.

Salivary glands present on the tongue secrete a lingual lipase that digests fat. This enzyme is also active in the stomach and intestine.

COMPOSITION OF SALIVA

Saliva consists of water (99%) and dissolved chemicals (1%). In humans, it is less concentrated (hypotonic) than the plasma. The solid materials include organic and inorganic constituents.

Organic constituents

These consist of:

- Amylase (ptyalin)
- Lipase
- Kallikrein

- Lysozyme
- Mucus
- Immunoglobulin A
- Lactoferrin
- Blood group antigens e.g. A and B.

Inorganic constituents

These are electrolytes, mainly Na^+, K^+, Ca^{2+}, Cl^-, I^-, PO_4^{2-} and HCO_3^-. The majority of electrolytes are found in lower concentrations than in the plasma. The exceptions are K^+ and HCO_3^-, which are found in higher contractions. The electrolyte composition and pH of saliva varies with flow rate. The increase in HCO_3^- concentration as flow rate increases accounts for the pH changing from being slightly acidic (pH 5.5–6.1) at resting flow rates to alkaline (pH 7.8) at high flow rates. The K^+ concentration is highest at the lowest flow rate.

SECRETORY MECHANISMS

The total production of saliva per day is 0.75 L to 1 L. The salivary glands produce large quantities of secretion per day relative to their size. The secretion of saliva is an active process requiring energy derived from cellular metabolism that in turn depends on a good blood supply.

The salivon

The functional unit of a salivary gland is termed a **salivon** (Fig. 15.10A). It consists of an acinus, an intercalated duct and a striated duct. The acinus is composed of pyramidal shaped acinar cells containing secretory granules. The acini are surrounded by contractile myoepithelial cells. The intercalated duct consists of cuboidal epithelial cells that may also be attached to myoepithelial cells. Columnar cells containing many mitochondria line the striated ducts. All the

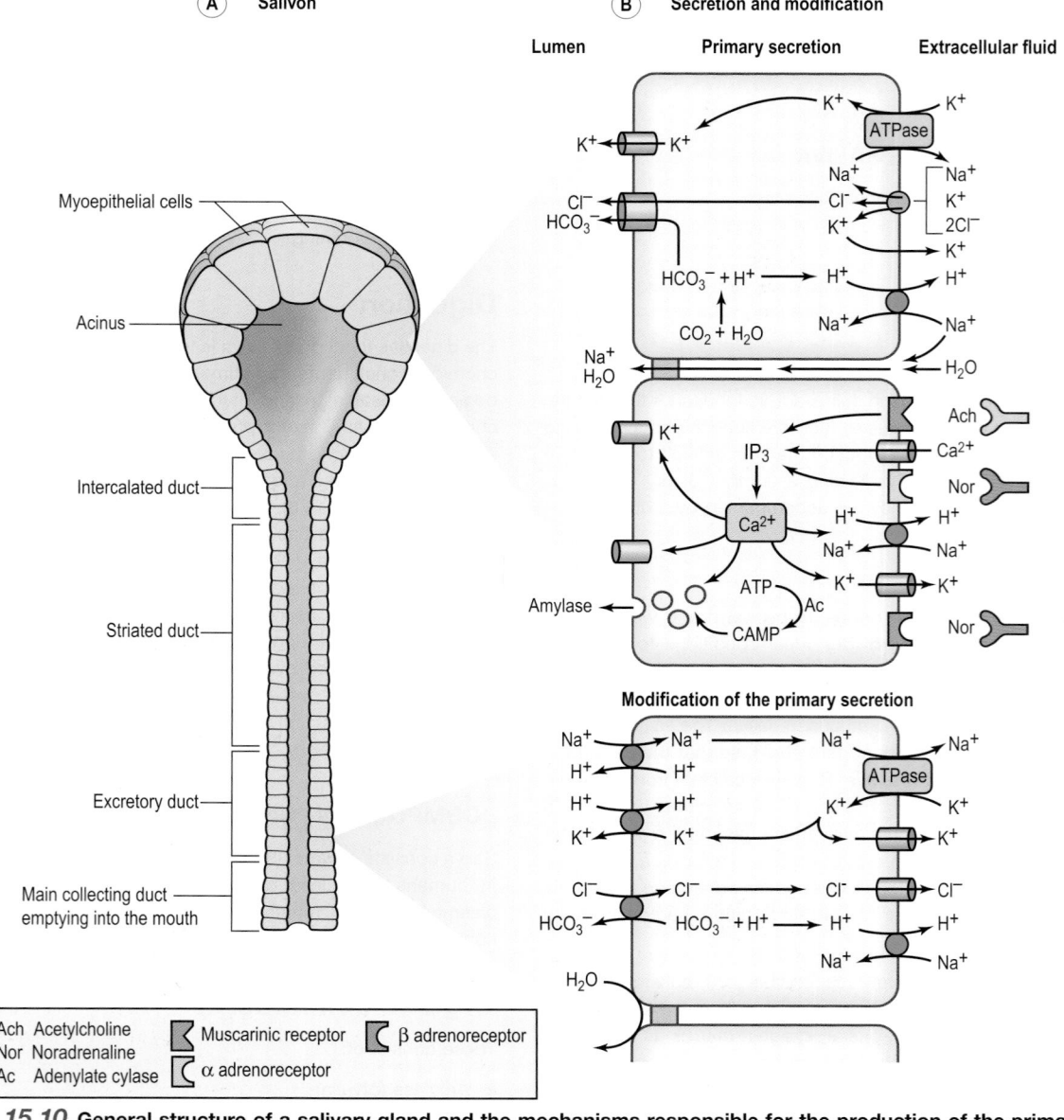

Fig. 15.10 **General structure of a salivary gland and the mechanisms responsible for the production of the primary secretion and its modification.** (A) Salivon. (B) Secretion and modification.

above components lie within a lobule surrounded by connective tissue. Striated ducts from adjacent lobules join together to form interlobular ducts and excretory ducts.

Mechanisms of secretion of saliva

Animal studies have demonstrated that saliva production can take place when the pressure in the duct system is greater than the arterial blood pressure in the arteries supplying the salivary gland. This observation indicates that the process of salivation is not due to the hydrostatic pressure of the blood producing an ultrafiltrate of plasma into the salivary glands and so is different from the production of urine (see Ch. 14). Furthermore, the composition of saliva varies with salivary flow rate. The secretion of saliva is believed to be a two-stage process.

Stage one – the primary secretion

The acinar and intercalated duct cells produce a primary fluid secretion containing amylase and electrolytes. Water moves by osmosis into the lumen of the acini and striated ducts. Experimental evidence indicates that it is either isotonic or slightly hypertonic and has a similar electrolyte composition to plasma.

The production of this primary secretion is an active one that is ultimately dependent upon primary active transport by the Na^+/K^+-ATPase in the basolateral border of the acinar cells (Fig. 15.10B) creating a Na^+ concentration gradient from the extracellular to the intracellular fluid. Na^+, together with Cl^- to maintain electroneutrality, diffuses into the cells. This increases the Cl^- electrochemical potential and creates a diffusion gradient for Cl^- to leave the cell via channels in the apical membrane. The secretion of Cl^- by this mechanism drives the production of saliva. HCO_3^- may also leave the cell via the channel used by Cl^-. The secretion of Cl^- and HCO_3^- is facilitated by the movement of K^+ out of the cell through Ca^{2+}-activated K^+ channels, thus making the interior more electronegative.

K^+ and Na^+ diffuse into the duct system to maintain electroneutrality. K^+ enters the secretion via a channel in the luminal membrane. Na^+ moves through the junctions between the cells to enter the saliva. Water follows the ions and organic constituents of saliva by osmosis.

Stage two – modification of the primary secretion

The striated, intercalated and excretory ducts modify the primary secretion by removing Na^+ and Cl^- and adding K^+ and HCO_3^-. This process is dependent upon the action of Na^+/K^+-ATPase in the basolateral border of the duct cells. As in the acinar cells, this primary active transport mechanism creates the conditions for the secondary transport systems to function. The Na^+/K^+-ATPase lowers the cellular concentration of Na^+ so that an electrochemical gradient exists between the lumen of the duct and the intracellular fluid for the diffusion of Na^+ into the cells. At the apical membrane Na^+ is exchanged for H^+ and Cl^- for HCO_3^- with the result that NaCl is absorbed. The Na^+ is pumped out of the cell across the basolateral border by the Na^+/K^+-ATPase and the Cl^- leaves via a chloride channel. The removal of H^+ by Na^+/H^+ exchange in the basolateral membrane increases the intracellular pH and enhances the exchange of HCO_3^- for Cl^-. Cellular K^+ is secreted into the lumen in exchange for luminal H^+, which is absorbed. In summary, the overall result is that Na^+ and Cl^- are removed and K^+ and HCO_3^- are added to saliva.

The duct cells are relatively impermeable to water. As saliva flows along the duct system more ions are removed than are added and it becomes hypotonic. The final composition of saliva depends upon the flow rate and, as a consequence, on the time that exchanges may take place across the duct cells. At low flow rates there is more time for Na^+, Cl^- re-absorption and K^+ secretion. As the flow rate increases there is less time for ionic exchanges to take place, therefore the Na^+ and Cl^- content of saliva rises and the K^+ content falls. The HCO_3^- concentration of saliva increases with an increase in flow rate due to the action of stimulants of secretion on the acinar cells.

Secretion of organic constituents

Organic constituents of saliva such as amylase and mucus are secreted from zymogen and mucus-filled secretory granules found in the apical border of serous and mucous acini, respectively. Following stimulation of the cells, these granules fuse with the apical membrane, and their contents are secreted by exocytosis.

CONTROL OF SALIVARY SECRETION

The salivary glands are primarily controlled by the autonomic nervous system (see Ch. 4). This is in contrast to the control of gastrointestinal, pancreatic and biliary secretions, which are controlled by gastrointestinal hormones and the autonomic nervous system. Both the parasympathetic and sympathetic divisions of the autonomic nervous system stimulate secretion, but the parasympathetic division is relatively more important.

The smell, taste and chewing of food, in addition to conditioned reflexes associated with the preparation and presentation of food, lead to increased salivary secretion. The sight and thought of food might make you aware of the presence of saliva in the mouth without increasing its flow (as could reading this chapter!). Nausea also stimulates salivation. Sleep, fear, dehydration and exercise inhibit secretion.

Parasympathetic nervous system

The parasympathetic innervation of the salivary acinar cells, ducts and blood vessels arises from the salivary nuclei in the medulla via the facial nerve (cranial nerve VII) to the submandibular and sublingual glands and glossopharyngeal nerve (cranial nerve IX) to the parotid glands, respectively (see Fig. 15.9).

Increased parasympathetic activity stimulates salivary secretion, via the neurotransmitter acetylcholine acting on muscarinic receptors. The synthesis and secretion of amylase and mucus is increased, together with a rise in fluid flow and metabolism of the glands. The myoepithelial cells surrounding the acini and intercalated duct cells contract and expel saliva. Blood flow to the glands is increased by the vasodilator action of vasoactive intestinal polypeptide (VIP) released from the parasympathetic nerves in blood vessels. This action is reinforced by the release of the enzyme kallikrein from duct cells, which release a vasodilator peptide (bradykinin) from α_2-globulins in the plasma. The increased blood supply meets the gland's demand for more oxygen and nutrients to sustain salivary secretion.

Sympathetic nervous system

Sympathetic nerve innervation arises from the thoracic segments 1–3 of the spinal cord and reaches the glands via the superior cervical ganglion. Sympathetic nerve action, via the neurotransmitter noradrenaline (norepinephrine) and the circulating hormone adrenaline (epinephrine), stimulates amylase, K^+ and HCO_3^- secretion via their action on adrenoceptors. Myoepithelial cells are stimulated to contract and expel preformed saliva. Blood vessels are constricted. The vasoconstriction restricts blood flow and salivary secretion.

Intracellular messengers producing salivary secretion

The neurotransmitters acetylcholine and noradrenaline act via their respective receptors to change the concentrations of intracellular second messengers (see Fig. 15.10B), which in turn influence the enzymes and channels involved in the secretory process. Acetylcholine acting via muscarinic receptors increases the free Ca^{2+} concentration within the cells via the production of inositol trisphosphate, which releases Ca^{2+} from intracellular stores, and by the direct influx of Ca^{2+} from the extracellular fluid. Noradrenaline acts via α- and β-adrenoceptors. Stimulation of α-adrenoceptors increases the concentration of free Ca^{2+}. β-Adrenoceptor stimulation activates adenylate cyclase with the formation of cyclic adenosine monophosphate (cAMP). Rises in intracellular Ca^{2+} have a major effect in increasing the fluid secretion, while cAMP influences enzyme and mucus secretion.

PHARYNX AND OESOPHAGUS

The oral cavity gives rise to the pharynx, which continues as the oesophagus and conveys food, drink and saliva to the stomach. The oesophageal mucosa is lined with stratified squamous epithelium. The mucosa and submucosa consists of longitudinal folds, in the absence of a swallowed food bolus. The muscularis mucosae is absent from the upper oesophagus but is developed near the stomach.

The submucosa consists of a network of collagen, and elastic fibres and small blood vessels. A thin layer of mucus produced by mucosal and submucosal glands lubricates the mucosa to aid swallowing. An inner circular layer and an outer longitudinal layer of muscle produce propulsion of a bolus of food to the stomach.

The upper oesophageal sphincter and upper third of the oesophagus in humans consists of skeletal muscle, with the lower third being smooth muscle. The middle third consists of a mixture of skeletal and smooth muscles. Both the skeletal and smooth muscles are arranged in an outer longitudinal and an inner circular layer.

SWALLOWING

The act of swallowing (deglutition) consists of three phases (Fig. 15.11).

Oral or voluntary phase

The process begins with a voluntary action initiated by the closing of the mouth and moving the tip of the tongue to the hard palate in order to separate the bolus of food to be swallowed (Fig. 15.11A). The back of the tongue moves up

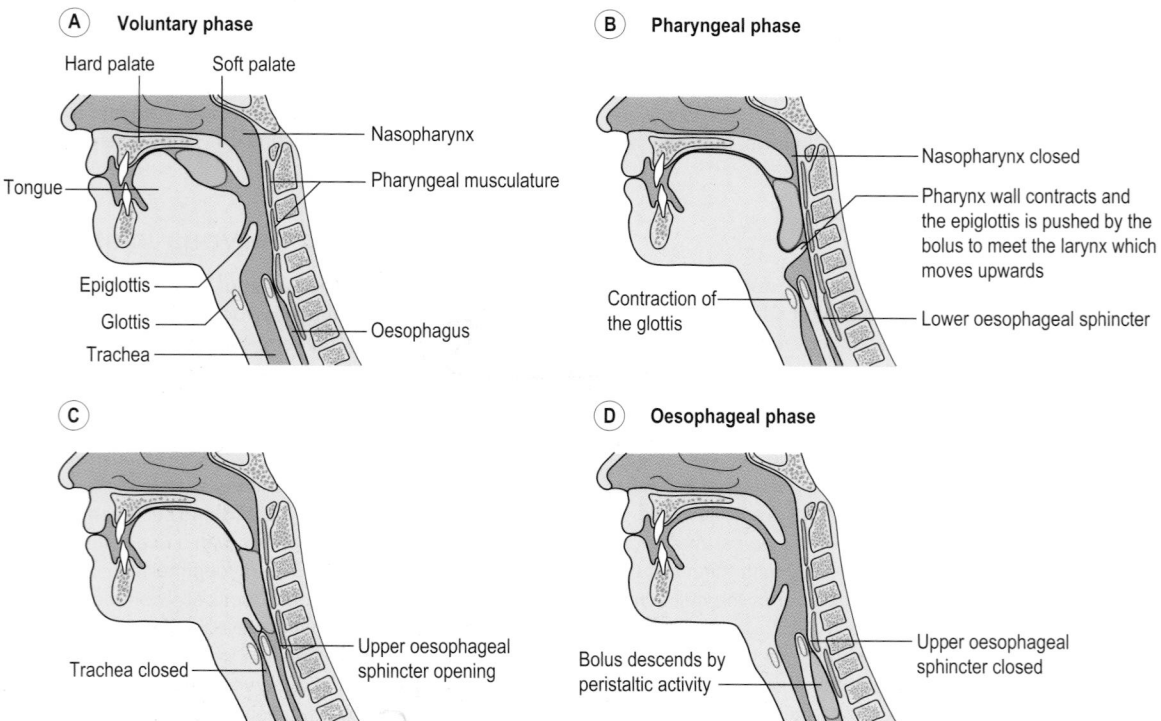

Fig. 15.11 **The major phases of the swallowing reflex.** (A) Voluntary phase. (B, C) Pharyngeal phase. (D) Oesophageal phase.

towards the hard palate and this action pushes the food into the pharynx where mechanoreceptors are stimulated to start the swallowing reflex. Sensory nerve impulses from the mechanoreceptors are propagated in the glossopharyngeal and vagal nerves to groups of neurons lying in the pons and medulla. These coordinate the contractions of skeletal muscles in the pharynx and larynx to deliver the bolus to the oesophagus without it entering the airways. The motor nerve pathways are present in cranial nerves VII, IX, X and XII (see Ch. 8).

Pharyngeal phase

The soft palate moves upwards and constriction of the posterior wall of the pharyngeal wall occurs to separate the oropharynx from the nasopharynx (Fig. 15.11B). In order to prevent food reflux into the nasal passages:

- Ventilation is inhibited
- Contraction of the laryngeal muscles closes the glottis and raises the larynx to create a funnel-like structure to direct the bolus into the oesophagus
- A sequence of peristaltic contractions starting in the upper pharynx propels the bolus of food through the pharynx towards the oesophagus and pushes the epiglottis over the glottis to prevent food entering the trachea
- The bolus passes into the oesophagus through the relaxed upper oesophageal sphincter (Fig. 15.11C).

The mechanisms described above protect against choking during swallowing. Either damage or depression of the neural control mechanism after a stroke or by alcohol or general anaesthetics can lead to the entry of food or vomit into the airways.

Oesophageal phase

The upper oesophageal sphincter contracts once a bolus of food has passed. A peristaltic wave is initiated in the skeletal muscle just below the upper oesophageal sphincter (Fig. 15.11D). This is known as the primary peristaltic wave and its production is coordinated by the 'swallowing centre', a group of neurons distributed in the pons and medulla, via vagal nerve pathways. The circular muscle layer contracts and raises the pressure on the oral side of the bolus and pushes it into an area of low pressure. The longitudinal muscle contraction pulls the oesophagus over the bolus of food. The active muscles relax. This sequence of events is repeated in a distal direction and the wave of contraction travels in the direction of the stomach.

The terminal 1–2 cm of the circular smooth muscle of the oesophagus has a high degree of tension and acts as the lower oesophageal sphincter to prevent gastro-oesophageal reflux. As the bolus of food approaches the lower oesophageal sphincter it relaxes due to action along the vagal nerve pathway, which contains postganglionic neurons utilising vasoactive intestinal polypeptide and/or nitric oxide as a neurotransmitter(s). The peristaltic wave moves down the oesophagus at 2–5 cm/second and takes about 10 seconds to reach the lower oesophageal sphincter. If some of the bolus of food remains in the oesophagus it stimulates sensory nerves that in turn induce another peristaltic wave at the point of distension (see Fig. 15.12). A secondary peristaltic

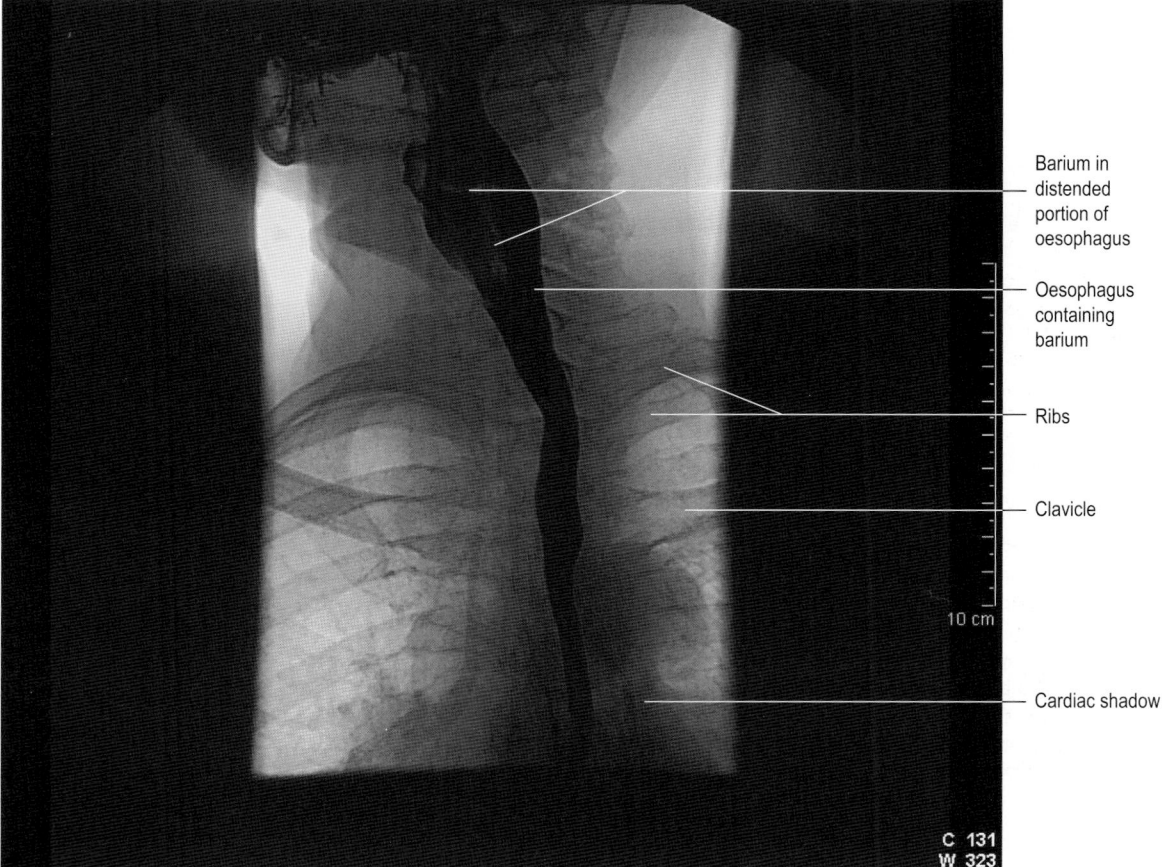

Fig. 15.12 **Barium swallow.** The radio-opaque barium outlines a peristaltic wave in the oesophagus. Courtesy of the Radiology Department, Guys and St Thomas' NHS Foundation Trust.

Disruption of oesophageal motility interferes with normal swallowing. Achalasia is a rare condition in which there is aperistalsis of the oesophagus with a failure of the lower oesophageal sphincter to relax on swallowing. The oesophagus can become dilated, with regurgitation of food. Neurological disorders involving the brain stem, neuromuscular disorders and extreme old age can also be associated with disorders of motility.

Gastro-oesophageal reflux is a normal occurrence, and gastro-oesophageal disease (**GORD**) occurs only when the normal anti-reflux mechanism fails. Persistent reflux of acid gastric contents causes inflammation of the oesophageal mucosa – **reflux oesophagitis** – giving rise to the symptoms of 'heart burn', a burning retrosternal pain after food, hot drinks or alcohol, and made worse by lying down, stooping or bending. Long-standing reflux can result in the replacement of normal oesophageal squamous epithelium by intestinal epithelium (metaplasia or dysplasia), known as **Barretts' oesophagus**. It is more common in middle-aged men, and is premalignant for adenocarcinoma of the oesophagus, requiring careful surveillance with repeated endoscopy and intensive medical therapy. High-grade cases may need mucosal ablation or surgery. **Hiatus hernia** is a condition in which part of the stomach 'herniates' into the chest through a weakness in the diaphragm. Symptoms only appear when there is oesophageal reflux.

Table 15.7	Stomach secretions
Type of secretion	**Constituents**
Exocrine	Hydrochloric acid
	Electrolytes including Na^+ and K^+
	Intrinsic factor
	Pepsinogen
Endocrine	Gastrin
Paracrine	Histamine
	Somatostatin

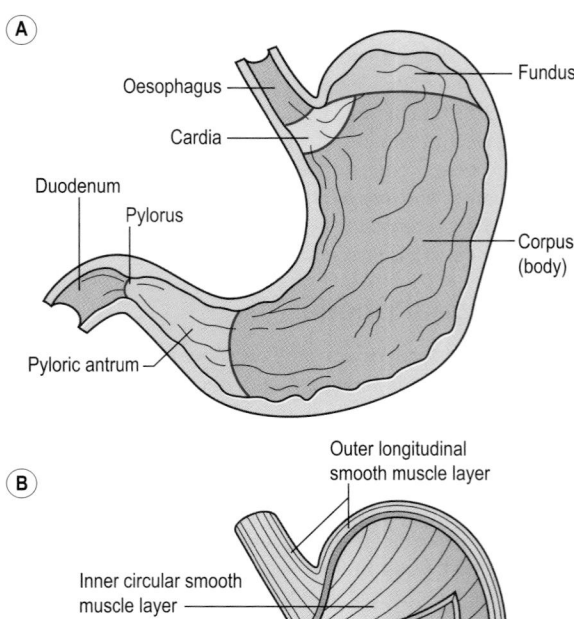

Fig. 15.13 Anatomy of the stomach. (A) Anatomical regions of the stomach. (B) Gastric musculature.

- Cardia
- Fundus
- Corpus (body)
- Pyloric antrum or antrum
- Pylorus.

The cardia lies adjacent to the lower oesophageal sphincter, which guards the entrance to the stomach. The fundus is the upper portion of the stomach, which together with the corpus or body, acts as a reservoir for food and swallowed air. The corpus is the site of secretion of hydrochloric acid, intrinsic factor and pepsinogen by specialised cells in the mucosal lining. The pyloric antrum is the region of the stomach adjacent to the duodenum and is involved in grinding solid food and mixing it with the gastric secretions. Small quantities of liquefied chyme are propelled into the duodenum through the pyloric sphincter.

Gastric musculature

The gastric musculature consists of smooth muscle arranged in distinctive layers. As in other parts of the alimentary canal (see Figs 15.7 and 15.13B), there is an outer longitudinal layer and an inner circular layer which increases in thickness in the antrum and pylorus. Additionally, the fundus and corpus contain a specialised obliquely arranged layer of smooth muscle below the circular layer. The mucosal lining contains a thin layer of muscle, the muscularis mucosae.

The duodenal musculature consists of an outer longitudinal layer, continuous with that of the stomach, and an inner circular layer. A bundle of connective tissue separates the

wave need not be preceded by the oral or pharyngeal phases of swallowing. It may also be induced by the reflux of the gastric contents into the oesophagus. Secondary peristalsis involves neural pathways within the wall of the oesophagus.

STOMACH AND DUODENUM

The stomach is a hollow organ consisting of smooth muscle lined with a secretory mucosa that produces exocrine, endocrine and paracrine secretions (Table 15.7). It receives and stores food temporarily and contributes to digestion by mixing food with gastric secretions to form a semi-liquid material called **chyme**. Chyme is emptied into the duodenum at a controlled rate, in order to allow time for further digestion and absorption of digestion products in the small intestine. In addition, the stomach reduces the entry of bacteria and noxious chemicals into the small intestine.

ANATOMY OF THE STOMACH

Anatomically, the stomach (Fig. 15.13) is divided into five regions:

circular muscle layer of the pylorus from that of the duodenum.

The gastric mucosa

The gastric mucosa is a relatively thick mucous membrane, which is smooth when the stomach is distended but thrown into folds or **rugae** when the stomach is empty. The luminal surface of the mucosa contains gastric pits from which branch tubular shaped glands reaching deeper into the mucosa towards the muscularis mucosae. There are three types of gastric gland:

- Cardiac
- Parietal (or oxyntic)
- Pyloric.

The glandular types, their sites, cell types, their secretion and functions are shown in Table 15.8. The surface layer of all regions of the mucosa contains columnar epithelial cells with nuclei in the basal region. These cells secrete mucus, sodium, potassium and bicarbonate ions. These secretions provide lubrication and act to protect the mucosa from digestion by acid and pepsin. The mucosa of the fundus and body regions contains the oxyntic glands (Fig. 15.14), which are divided into three regions:

- Base
- Neck
- Isthmus.

The base region contains predominantly peptic (or chief) cells. These cuboidal-shaped cells and have well-developed rough endoplasmic reticulum and a Golgi complex typical of cells synthesising protein. These cells are the source of pepsinogen, the precursor of the protease pepsin. This region contains few parietal cells.

The neck region contains parietal (or oxyntic) cells and mucous neck cells. The parietal cells are large rounded cells with a large nucleus and cytoplasm containing many mitochondria and tubulo-vesicles. The presence of many mitochondria are typical of cells needing to provide energy for transport processes, in this case the secretion of hydrochloric acid. The cytoplasm also contains intracellular canaliculi (channels) which open into the lumen of the gland. These canaliculi swell in conditions producing acid secretion. This suggests they are the conduits for the secreted acid to reach the lumen of the gland. The parietal cells also synthesise and secrete a glycoprotein named intrinsic factor, which binds to vitamin B_{12} in the diet to form a vitamin B_{12}–intrinsic factor complex that is absorbed in the terminal ileum.

The mucous neck cells have an irregular shape, with cytoplasm filled with mucous granules along the border adjacent to the lumen of the gland. The isthmus is the region connecting the neck to the gastric pit. It contains a mixture of parietal cells and surface mucous cells. The pyloric gland mucosa consists of chief cells and mucous cells producing pepsinogen and mucus. In addition to exocrine cells, the oxyntic glands and pyloric glands contain endocrine cells.

These hormone-producing cells contain granules near their basal border. The hormones are secreted into the tissue fluid and either act on adjacent cells (a local hormone or paracrine function) or enter capillaries and the hepatic portal circulation before reaching the systemic circulation and being delivered to their target organ via the arterial system (an endocrine function). Some cells such as the G cells of the pyloric antrum possess microvilli that project into the glandular lumen. It is believed that these microvilli contain receptors that are sensitive to the luminal contents and in turn control the secretion of their hormone in response to stimuli. In the case of the G cell, amino acids from the glandular lumen stimulate the release of gastrin. Other

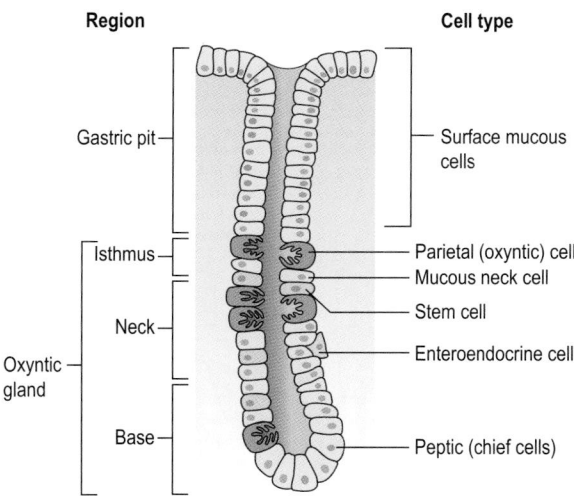

Fig. 15.14 **Structure of an oxyntic gland.**

Table 15.8	Gastric glands, their cell types, exocrine, endocrine and paracrine secretions and functions			
Gland	**Site**	**Cell type**	**Secretion**	**Function**
Cardiac	Adjacent to the lower oesophageal sphincter	Mucous	Mucus	Lubrication
				Protection
Oxyntic	Fundus and corpus	Parietal (or oxyntic)	HCl	Digestion
				Antibacterial
				Activate pepsinogen to pepsin
			Intrinsic factor	Promotes vitamin B_{12} absorption in the ileum
		Peptic (or chief) cell	Pepsinogen	Pepsin – protein digestion
		D cell	Somatostatin	Inhibition of histamine release and acid secretion
Pyloric	Pylorus and antrum	Peptic (or chief) cell	Pepsinogen	Pepsin – protein digestion
		Mucous	Mucus	Lubrication
				Protection
		G cell	Gastrin	Stimulation of gastric acid secretion
		D cell	Somatostatin	Inhibition of gastrin secretion

hormone-containing cells lie adjacent to either the exocrine or endocrine cells and control their function.

For example, enterochromaffin-like cells (ECL cells) containing histamine lie close to parietal cells and stimulate acid secretion. D cells containing somatostatin are also observed to have processes that terminate on parietal cells. Somatostatin is an inhibitor of acid secretion. The position of these cells suggests that they are stimulated by circulating hormones or neurotransmitters to release their products, in order to control adjacent cells in a paracrine manner.

CONTROL OF GASTRIC SECRETIONS

The rate of gastric secretion is determined by stimulatory and inhibitory mechanisms. For convenience, these mechanisms may be considered to occur in three overlapping phases (Fig. 15.15):

1. Cephalic phase
2. Gastric phase
3. Intestinal phase.

STIMULATION OF GASTRIC ACID SECRETION

The basal gastric acid secretion during the inter-digestive period increases when food is anticipated or consumed. The increase in acid secretion occurs by means of mechanisms having their origin in the head (cephalic phase), stomach (gastric phase) and intestine (intestinal phase) (Fig. 15.15).

Cephalic phase

Stimuli such as the thought, sight, smell, taste and chewing of food induce a reflex stimulation of acid secretion via the

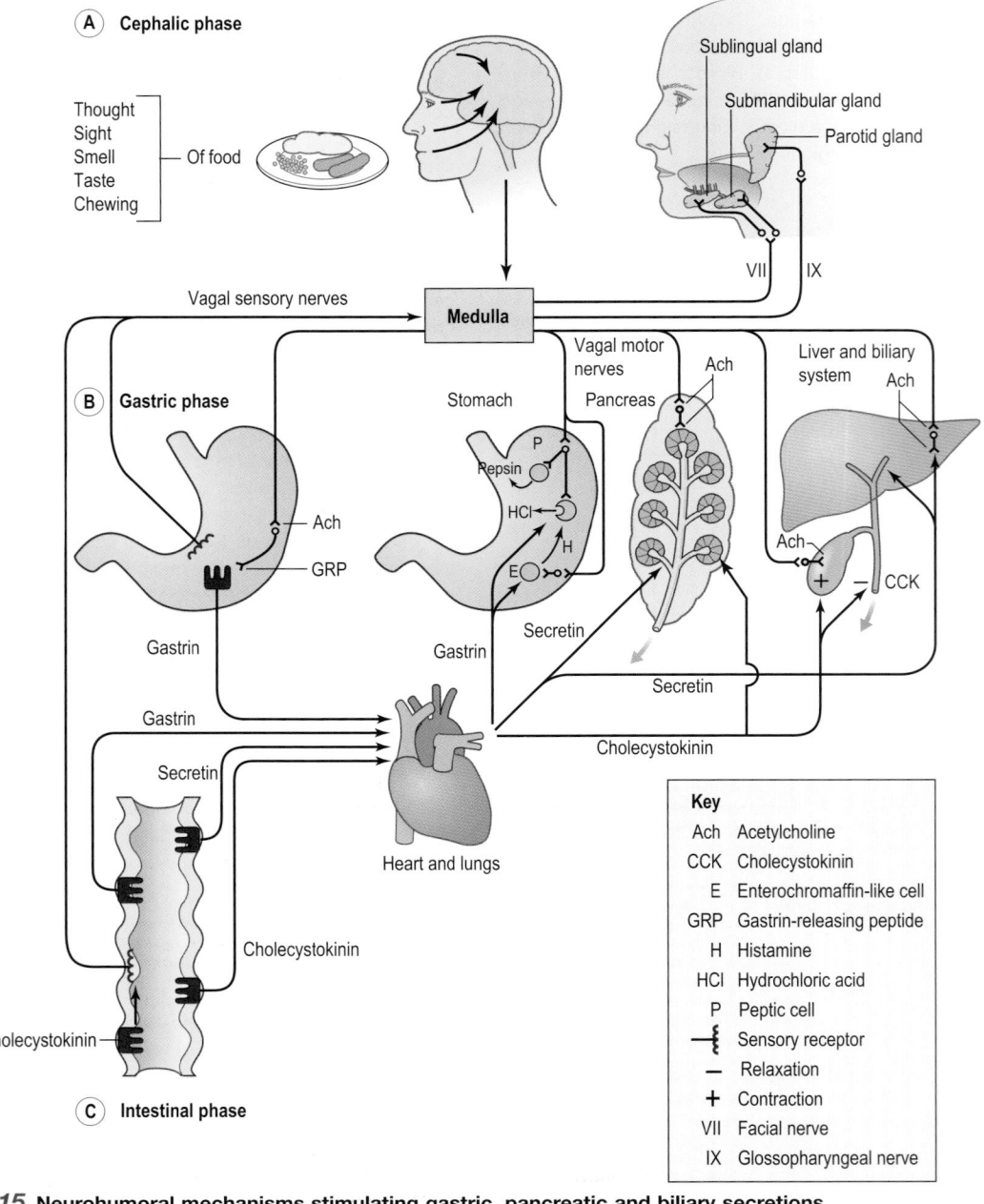

Fig. 15.15 Neurohumoral mechanisms stimulating gastric, pancreatic and biliary secretions.

central nervous system and the vagal nerves. The vagus directly stimulates the parietal cells via the neurotransmitter acetylcholine.

There are two indirect vagal mechanisms of parietal cell stimulation:

- The release of the antral hormone, gastrin, from G cells following vagal stimulation by means of gastrin releasing peptide. The gastrin diffuses into the venous system and is delivered via the heart and arterial system to stimulate the parietal cells of the stomach (an endocrine mechanism)
- The release of histamine from enterochromaffin-like cells as a result of the action of acetylcholine released from postganglionic vagal nerves, and by the action of gastrin. Histamine diffuses from the enterochromaffin-like cells through the tissue fluid to stimulate the parietal cells (a paracrine mechanism).

Gastric phase

This phase is initiated by the presence of food in the stomach and involves physical and chemical mechanisms. Distension of the stomach stimulates stretch receptors that induce vago-vagal and intramural reflexes to induce acid secretion. The chemical composition of food buffers acid secretion and so causes a withdrawal of inhibitory mechanisms preventing gastrin release in addition to releasing gastrin directly. Protein digestion products, particularly the amino acids tryptophan and phenylalanine, are potent stimulants of gastrin secretion. Amino acids are detected by microvilli projecting into the lumen of the pyloric glands from the G cells. Gastrin secreted by the antral G cells consists of 17 amino acids (G17). Other stimulants of acid secretion are Ca^{2+}, caffeine and alcohol.

Intestinal phase

Chyme entering the intestine from the stomach produces a weak stimulation of gastric acid secretion via neural and humoral mechanisms. The upper small intestine contains intestinal gastrin, a peptide consisting of 34 amino acids (G34) that is released by the presence of food. The presence of another stimulant in the intestine, entero-oxyntin, has also been suggested. Entero-oxyntin activity may be due to the action of absorbed amino acids stimulating gastric acid secretion.

INHIBITION OF GASTRIC ACID SECRETION

Cephalic, gastric and intestinal inhibitory phases of acid secretion have been recognised (see Fig. 15.15).

Cephalic phase

1. Withdrawal of vagal nerve activity

   The cephalic phase of stimulation is over once eating is finished and food is removed. This will reduce vagal activity and consequently decrease acid secretion. Emotions, such as fear, sadness and depression, in addition to pain and nausea, act through central nervous mechanisms to inhibit vagal nerve activity from the medulla.

2. Increased splanchnic nerve activity

   Pain and fear lead to increases in splanchnic nerve activity with the release of noradrenaline (norepinephrine), which produces vasoconstriction in the gastric arteries with a reduction in gastric blood flow. The delivery of oxygen, nutrients and gastrin to the stomach is decreased, and gastric acid secretion is inhibited.

Gastric phase

1. Inhibition of gastrin release

   Gastrin release from G cells is controlled by the pH of the antral contents through a negative feedback mechanism. Acid secretion leading to falls in antral pH below 3 inhibits gastrin release, and inhibition is complete when the pH falls to 1.5. This situation will occur towards the end of a meal when the buffering capacity of the gastric contents has been reduced and/or gastric emptying is nearing completion. Two mechanisms may contribute to the inhibition of gastrin release:

   - Changes in pH at the microvilli of the G cells reduce their sensitivity to the stimulatory action of amino acids.
   - Acid stimulates the release of somatostatin from D cell terminals which are directed on to the adjacent G cells. Somatostatin inhibits gastrin release.

2. Inhibition of acid secretion by prostaglandin E_2

   Prostaglandin E_2 (PGE_2), produced in the gastric mucosa, exerts a local regulatory effect to inhibit histamine-stimulated acid secretion. PGE_2 stimulates EP_2 receptors that are negatively coupled to adenylate cyclase, and so inhibit the production of cAMP, the intracellular messenger of histamine. Prostaglandins also reduce the release of histamine and gastrin from ECL and G cells, respectively.

Intestinal phase

The entry of chyme into the small intestine from the stomach induces inhibition of gastric acid secretion. Experimental evidence suggests that a number of neural, hormonal and paracrine mechanisms are involved. These mechanisms, which are responsible for inhibition of acid secretion, need to be clarified.

Acidification of the small intestine inhibits gastric acid secretion. The neural mechanisms include withdrawal of vagal motor nerve activity as a consequence of vagal or splanchnic sensory nerves detecting low intestinal pH, an enterogastric reflex in the splanchnic nerves.

Inhibitory hormonal mechanisms are stimulated by the presence of acid, hypertonic saline, glucose solutions, fats or monoglycerides in the intestine. The hormones involved are described as enterogastrones; that is, chemicals released from the small intestine that inhibit gastric function. There are several candidate enterogastrones:

- Cholecystokinin
- Secretin
- Vasoactive intestinal peptide
- Enteroglucagon/glucagon-like peptide
- Oxyntomodulin
- Gastric inhibitory peptide
- Neurotensin

- Neuropeptide YY
- Somatostatin.

Intravenous infusion of each of the above candidate hormones produces inhibition of acid secretion, but that by itself does not establish a physiological role as an enterogastrone. To do so would require knowledge of the relationship between the delivery of acid, hypertonic and fatty solutions to the small intestine, with the release of the candidate hormones and their delivery to the gastric mucosa during the course of a meal. Inhibition of acid secretion during the intestinal phase may be due to additive or potentiating effects between candidate hormones. Enterogastrones inhibit acid secretion from parietal cells either directly or via the release of somatostatin from D cells adjacent to the parietal cells. An additional mechanism is by the inhibition of gastrin release from the antrum.

The intestinal phase of gastric acid secretion is predominantly inhibitory because removal of part of the small intestine leads to increased acid secretion.

STIMULATION OF PEPSINOGEN SECRETION

Pepsinogen secretion from the zymogen granules in the peptic (chief) cells is controlled in a similar manner to gastric acid secretion. The major mediator stimulating pepsinogen secretion is acetylcholine released from vagal nerves during the cephalic and gastric phases. Acetylcholine acts on muscarinic M_3 receptors on the peptic cell. In addition, acid secretion stimulated by the vagus induces pepsinogen secretion by two mechanisms:

- A local reflex in the intramural cholinergic nerves
- The release of the hormone secretin from the duodenum, which in turn acts on the peptic cells.

Gastrin and cholecystokinin (CCK) are also weak stimulants of pepsin secretion acting via CCK_A receptors. The importance of their role in controlling pepsinogen remains to be determined.

The intracellular messenger for acetylcholine, gastrin and cholecystokinin is Ca^{2+}. Receptor stimulation by these secretagogues leads to the production of inositol trisphosphate to release Ca^{2+} from intracellular stores. Secretin stimulates adenylate cyclase to produce cAMP from ATP. Rises in intracellular Ca^{2+} and cAMP initiate cytoskeletal activity that leads to the movement of zymogen granules containing pepsinogen to the apical surface of the cell, where they fuse with the membrane and discharge their contents by exocytosis.

CELLULAR MECHANISMS OF GASTRIC ACID SECRETION

Morphological changes in parietal cells (Fig. 15.16)

The apical cytoplasm of the parietal cell in the resting state is packed with tubulo-vesicles that contain K^+/H^+-ATPase (proton pump), which secrete H^+ in exchange for K^+. Stimulation of the cell with gastrin, acetylcholine or histamine is accompanied by cytoskeletal movements, causing the migration and incorporation of the tubulo-vesicles into the canalicular membranes. This action produces microvilli on the surface of the canalicular membranes which greatly increases the surface area and the number of proton pumps at the cell surface. Secretion occurs with the opening of K^+ and Cl^- channels in the canalicular membranes. The canaliculi swell when acid secretion begins. The tubulo-vesicles reform at the end of secretion and the microvilli disappear. Parietal cells are rich in mitochondria in order to provide sufficient ATP to power H^+ secretion.

Intracellular messenger for the action of acetylcholine, gastrin and histamine

Acetylcholine and gastrin acting via muscarinic M_3 and CCK_B gastrin receptors, respectively, stimulate phospholipase C which converts phosphoinositol 4,5-bisphosphate (IP_2) to inositol 1,4,5-trisphosphate (IP_3) and diacylglycerol (DAG). IP_3 stimulates Ca^{2+} release from intracellular stores to activate calmodulin-dependent protein kinase. DAG activates protein kinase C. Histamine acting on histamine H2 receptors, activates adenylate cyclase to increase the formation of cAMP from ATP. cAMP-stimulated protein kinase A, Ca^{2+} and protein kinase C are involved in the changes in parietal cell function leading to the onset of acid secretion.

Ion movements during acid secretion

In human beings, it is estimated that during maximal acid secretion, the concentration of H^+ and Cl^- in the parietal cell secretion is 150 mmol/L and 170 mmol/L, respectively. The potential difference across the gastric mucosa with respect to the blood is about −60 mV at rest and falls to −40 mV during stimulation of secretion. Cl^- is secreted against an electrochemical gradient. Protons are moving down an electrical gradient and up a concentration gradient when the pH of the gastric juice is compared with that of the plasma. The secretion of hydrochloric acid requires the expenditure of cellular energy derived from aerobic metabolism. The source of this energy is ATP, produced by the many mitochondria packed into the cell.

Proton pump

The transport processes involved in the production of acid secretion are shown in Figure 15.16. The protons required for acid secretion are derived from water. With the opening of K^+ channels in the canalicular membrane, K^+ diffuses into the canaliculi and stimulates the proton pump from the luminal side to hydrolyse ATP. Protons are pumped into the lumen in exchange for K^+ ions, which are recycled across the canalicular membrane. Cl^- enters the canaliculi from the cytoplasm through Cl^- channels.

The OH^- that remains in the cell is converted to HCO_3^- by reacting with CO_2 in the presence of carbonic anhydrase. Carbon dioxide for this reaction is provided by cellular metabolism and by diffusion from the blood. The HCO_3^- is exchanged for Cl^- across the basal membrane by means of a carrier mechanism. The movement of HCO_3^- down its electrochemical gradient drives the inward transport of Cl^- from the interstitial fluid to the cytoplasm for secretion into the canalicular lumen. The HCO_3^- diffuses into the venous blood leaving the stomach. This produces a rise in the pH of arterial blood and a fall in the acidity of urine after a meal. The phenomenon is referred to as 'the alkaline tide of gastric secretion'.

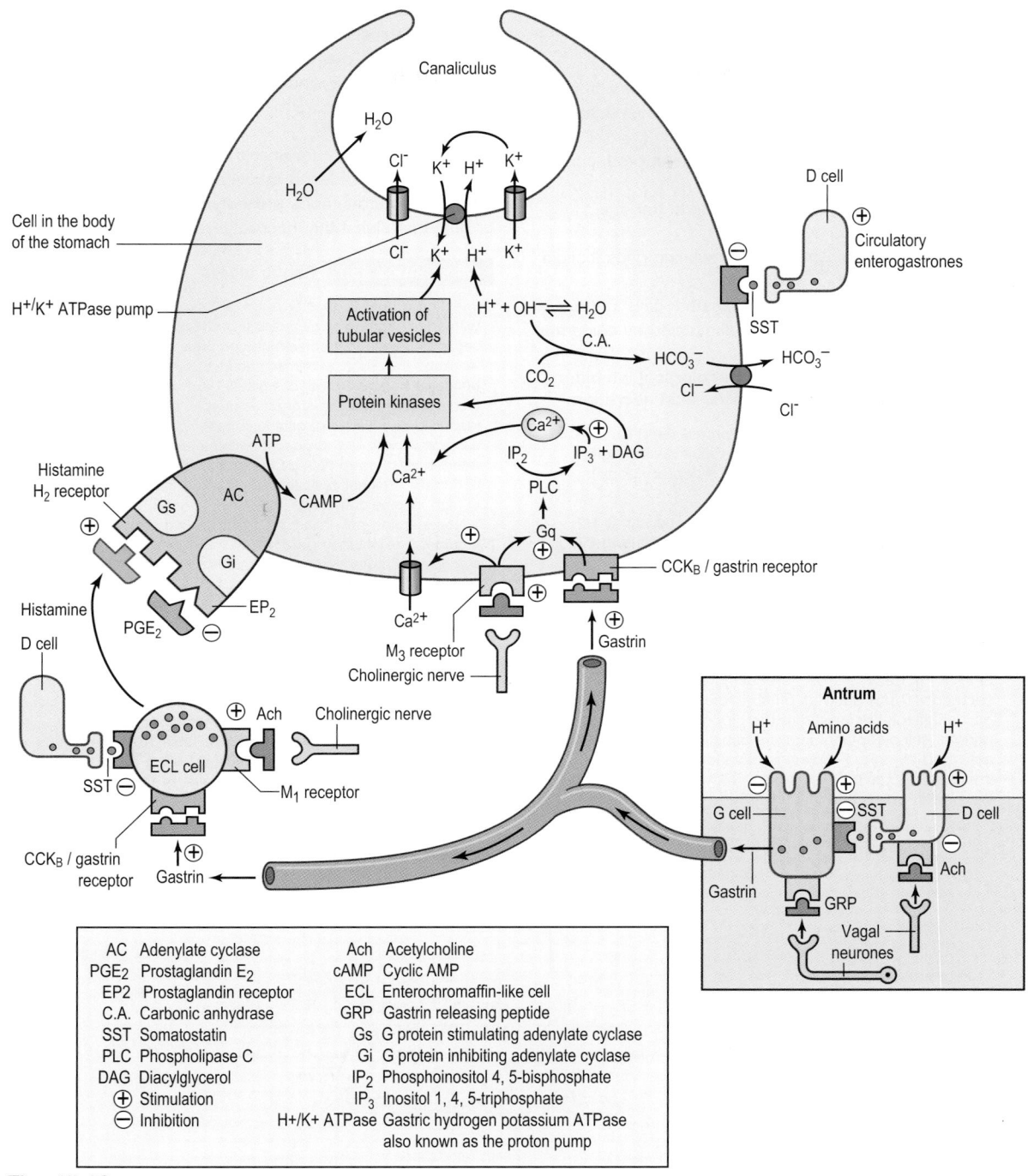

Fig. 15.16 **Physiological mechanisms in the control of gastric acid secretion by the parietal cell.**

Sodium pump

The sodium pump (Na^+/K^+-ATPase) in the basolateral membrane transports K^+ into the cell in exchange for intracellular Na^+. The accumulated K^+ moves down its electrochemical gradient through channels in the basolateral and canalicular membranes, producing a negative intracellular potential.

A Na^+/H^+ exchanger in the basolateral membrane transfers Na^+ into the cell down its electrochemical gradient in exchange for H^+ to provide Na^+ for the sodium pump and subsequent exchange for K^+ to maintain the K^+ content of the cell. Transfer of H^+ out of the cell increases the availability of OH^- to interact with CO_2 to produce HCO_3^-, thereby increasing the drive on Cl^- accumulation in the cell via the Cl^-/HCO_3^- exchanger. The energy for the accumulation of Cl^- within the cell and its diffusion into the canaliculus comes from the action of the sodium and proton pumps. The transfer of HCl into the canaliculus creates an osmotic flow of water to produce the gastric secretion.

GASTRIC MUCOSAL PROTECTION

The ability of the gastroduodenal mucosa to withstand the digestive action of hydrochloric acid, pepsin and bile depends on a number of factors:

- The mucous bicarbonate barrier, where protons are neutralised by bicarbonate ions to produce a neutral pH at the cell surface when the luminal pH is 2
- Phospholipids, covering the epithelial layer producing a protective coat
- Mucus secreted by the epithelial cells to trap the bicarbonate ions
- The action of prostaglandin E_2, stimulating phospholipid and mucus secretion
- The renewal of epithelial cells from stem cells in the neck region of the gastric gland stimulated by epidermal

Information box 15.5 | Pharmacological inhibition of gastric acid secretion

Drugs that inhibit gastric acid secretion are used to promote healing in peptic ulcers and reflux oesophagitis. Commonly used are the histamine H2 receptor agonists and proton pump inhibitors.

- H2 receptor agonists inhibit histamine action at all H2 receptors competitively. The main clinical use is to inhibit gastric acid secretion by inhibiting histamine-, acetylcholine- and gastrin-mediated acid secretion by parietal cells; pepsin secretion is also reduced, with a decrease in gastric juice volume. Familiar preparations include cimetidine and ranitidine.
- Proton pump inhibitors act by the irreversible inhibition of H^+/K^+-ATPase, markedly reducing gastric acid secretion. Drugs such as omeprazole, a substituted benzimidazole, diffuse from the blood through the parietal cell cytoplasm into the canaliculi, where they are activated by acid. Following activation they bind irreversibly to sulphydryl groups in cysteine residues in the proton pump and inactivate it.

growth factor and their migration to cover the luminal surface

- The delivery of bicarbonate ions from the basal border of the parietal cell to the lamina propria by mucosal blood flow, which is maintained by vasodilator neuropeptides, nitric oxide, PGE_2 and PGI_2 (see Table 15.1).

Peptic ulceration

Peptic ulceration occurs when the mucosal protective factors (Fig. 15.17) are reduced or overwhelmed by the action of aggressive factors (**acid**, **proteolytic enzymes** (e.g. pepsin) or **bile**) that digest the mucosal layer.

Clinical box 15.7 | Peptic ulcers

Infection with *Helicobacter pylori*, a Gram-negative organism with spiral morphology, causes ulceration. The bacterium secretes urease that converts blood urea to ammonia, which weakens the mucosal barrier, secretes toxins that destroy epithelial cells and produces platelet-activating factor, a potent ulcerogen and inflammatory mediator. *H. pylori* has also been identified as a cause of gastric cancer. *H. pylori* infection is associated with low socioeconomic status, with a high prevalence of up to 90% of the population in developing countries. A higher prevalence is found in the older population in high-income countries.

Non-steroidal anti-inflammatory drugs (e.g. aspirin or indometacin) inhibit the enzyme cyclooxygenase and reduce the synthesis of protective prostaglandins (PGE_2 and PGI_2) from arachidonic acid, as well as causing irritation. The arachidonic acid is converted to lipoxygenase with the increased production of leukotriene LTB4, which causes neutrophil adhesion to the endothelium of small mucosal blood vessels. This leads to ischaemia, hypoxia, and the release of proteases and reactive oxygen species from neutrophils, all of which damage the mucosa, causing ulceration and mucosal erosions that can bleed.

Ulceration also occurs with vasoconstrictor-mediated reductions in mucosal blood flow (see Table 15.1), caused by trauma and disease. Cigarette smoking, which causes vasoconstriction and mucosal ischaemia, is associated with increased risk of peptic ulceration.

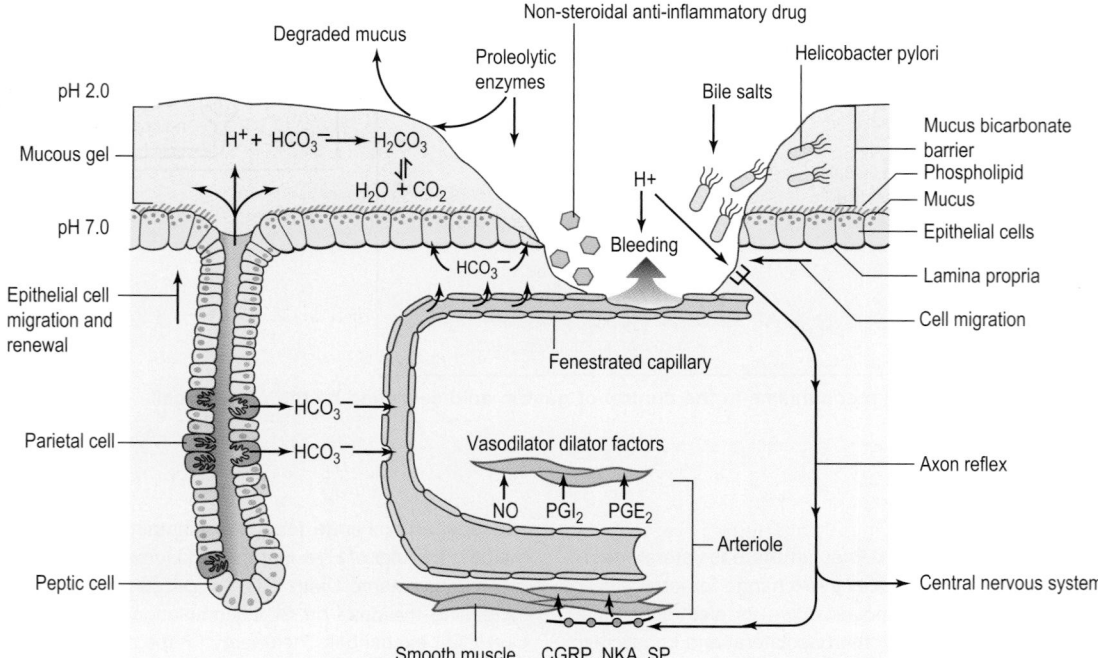

Fig. 15.17 Factors contributing to gastric-mucosal protection and peptid ulceration. Ulcerogenic factors: proteolytic enzymes, bile salts, *Helicobacter pylori*, non-steroidal anti-inflammatory drugs, vasoconstriction. CGRP, calcitonin gene-regulated peptide; NKA, neurokinin A; NO, nitric oxide.

GASTRIC MOTILITY

For the purposes of describing gastric motility, the stomach is divided into two parts (see Fig. 15.13A):

- An upper orad portion containing the fundus and upper two-thirds of the corpus
- A caudad portion containing the lower third of the corpus and the antrum.

GASTRIC MUSCULATURE

The gastric musculature regulates the storage, mixing and emptying of the gastric contents. The smooth muscle cells in the stomach are arranged in four layers (Fig. 15.13B):

1. A longitudinal layer under the serosa and continuous with that of the oesophagus and duodenum
2. A circular layer continuous with that of the circular layers of the oesophagus and duodenum
3. An oblique layer inside the circular layer and found only in the orad region
4. A thin layer, the muscularis mucosae, at the base of the mucosa.

The muscle layers are innervated by intrinsic nerves of the myenteric plexus which receive branches from the submucosal plexus and parasympathetic vagal nerves from the medulla. Postganglionic nerves from the coeliac plexus also innervate the plexus regions.

ELECTRICAL AND CONTRACTILE ACTIVITY OF GASTRIC SMOOTH MUSCLE

The gastric musculature shows rhythmical contractile activity driven by the gastric pacemaker region in the greater curvature of the body of the stomach. This is driven by fluctuations in the membrane potential of the smooth muscles known as the **basic electrical rhythm** (**BER**), **pacesetter potentials** or **slow waves**. The frequency of these slow waves is about three per minute. The slow waves arise from **interstitial cells of Cajal** (**ICCs**). These smooth muscle-like cells occur as a single layer in plexus regions, with overlapping processes extending from the cell bodies of adjacent cells, to form a network providing communication with the smooth muscle layers via gap junctions. Slow wave activity spreads throughout the muscle layers. Some ICCs are found between the enteric nerve terminals and smooth muscles. The smooth muscle membrane potential may reach threshold at the peak of a slow wave potential. At threshold, L-type calcium channels open and an action potential will be generated with an influx of Ca^{2+} into the smooth muscle. The Ca^{2+} initiates contraction of the muscle. The strength of contraction is proportional to the frequency of the action potentials. The electrical activity spreads in a circular direction producing a band of contraction that propagates from the corpus of the stomach towards the antrum. This occurs because the electrical coupling between smooth muscle cells is faster in the circular than the longitudinal direction.

GASTRIC MOTILITY DURING THE INTERDIGESTIVE PERIOD

Contractile activity of the gastric musculature occurs in bursts at 90-minute intervals during the interdigestive period.

These contractions begin in the orad portion of the stomach and sweep towards the antrum, pushing any residues (undigested food, e.g. bones, and other objects that may have been swallowed, desquamated cells, mucus, secretions) into the relaxing duodenum for onward propulsion along the small intestine. These bursts of activity are known as **migrating motor complexes** (**MMCs**). They act to prevent bacterial overgrowth and keep the stomach clean. MMCs depend on the enteric nervous system and are stimulated by the small intestinal hormone **motilin**. The antibiotic **erythromycin** also stimulates MMC production by acting on motilin receptors. Feeding inhibits the MMCs. Vagal nerve activity during the cephalic phase of feeding and gastrointestinal hormones **gastrin** and **cholecystokinin** released during digestion change the pattern of motility to that seen in the fed state.

GASTRIC MOTILITY DURING A MEAL

The pattern of gastric motility during feeding ensures that food is accommodated in the stomach, mechanically broken down, mixed with secretions and emptied into the duodenum at a regulated rate (Fig. 15.18).

Receptive relaxation

Following swallowing, the gastric musculature of the orad portion of the stomach relaxes in order to accommodate food, drink and gastric secretions without an increase in intragastric pressure. This phenomenon is known as receptive relaxation and is produced by the action of VIP and nitric oxide released from enteric nerves (Fig. 15.18A). The enteric nerves respond to such stimuli as:

- Sight, smell, taste of food – cephalic phase
- Oesophageal distension – oesophageal phase
- Gastric distension – gastric phase.

All phases of receptive relaxation include a vagal reflex. Sensory receptors in the oesophagus and stomach, via afferent vagal nerves, activate motor nerve pathways from the medulla to produce receptive relaxation. The reflex is known as a vagovagal reflex. The densest food tends to sink towards the caudad portion of the stomach, leaving the less dense foods such as oils and fat floating on the surface in the fundus. Gradually, the tension in the smooth muscles in the wall of the stomach increases as the gastric contents empty into the duodenum.

Mixing of gastric contents

The presence of food in the stomach stimulates powerful gastric peristaltic activity which begins in the body of the stomach and sweeps towards the antrum at the rate of three contractions per minute (Fig. 15.18A). The lumen of the antrum is narrowed by the contractile activity. Small particles and liquids are pushed towards the pylorus and large particles are forcibly propelled to the corpus of the stomach. This retropulsion of the antral contents into the corpus of the stomach helps to break down the food and mix it with gastric secretions to form chyme.

Gastric emptying

A wave of contraction spreading over the antrum can sweep chyme into the duodenum, where the muscular wall is

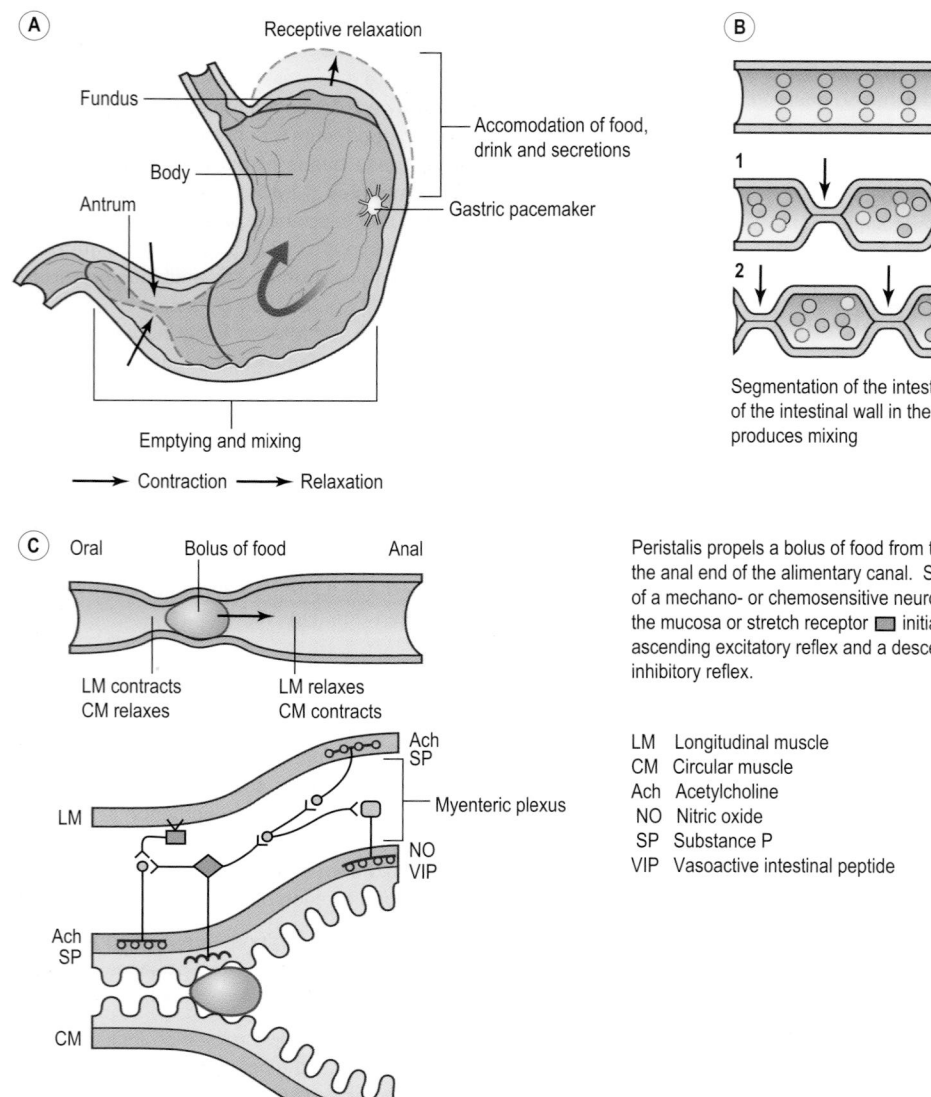

A

Receptive relaxation

Fundus

Body

Antrum

Accomodation of food, drink and secretions

Gastric pacemaker

Emptying and mixing

→ Contraction → Relaxation

B

Segmentation of the intestine. Contraction of the intestinal wall in the sequence 1, 2 produces mixing

C

Oral   Bolus of food   Anal

LM contracts   LM relaxes
CM relaxes   CM contracts

Ach
SP

Myenteric plexus

LM

NO
VIP

Ach
SP

CM

Peristalis propels a bolus of food from the oral to the anal end of the alimentary canal. Stimulation of a mechano- or chemosensitive neuron ◆ in the mucosa or stretch receptor ▭ initiates an ascending excitatory reflex and a descending inhibitory reflex.

LM   Longitudinal muscle
CM   Circular muscle
Ach Acetylcholine
NO   Nitric oxide
SP   Substance P
VIP Vasoactive intestinal peptide

Fig. 15.18 **Gastrointestinal motility.**

relaxed. The powerful peristalsis of the alimentary canal can propel a bolus of food from the oral to the anal end (Fig. 15.15C). Chyme flows from a region of high pressure to one of low. The pyloric sphincter between the antrum and the duodenum acts as a sieve to allow fluid and small particles to enter the duodenum but to retain larger particles in the stomach for further digestion. The motility of the gastroduodenal junction regulates gastric emptying and minimises retropulsion of the duodenal contents into the antrum.

Gastric emptying is regulated in order to match the supply of chyme to the small intestine with the rate at which the chyme can be can digested and absorbed. Overloading the intestine leads to diarrhoea by stimulating peristalsis. The rate of gastric emptying is influenced by:

- the volume and the nature of the gastric contents
- the duodenal contents.

Gastric contents

Liquids empty from the stomach faster than solids, which need to be liquefied. The rate of emptying of liquid meals is approximately proportional to the square root of the volume of fluid remaining in the stomach. Tension in the wall of the stomach is proportional to the square root of the volumes of the gastric contents. Contraction of the gastric musculature may be stimulated either directly by the tension in the smooth muscle cells or by neural activity in either the enteric or vagal nerves.

Oils or liquefied fats will leave the stomach after aqueous solutions, in subjects who are either sitting upright or standing, because they float on the surface of the gastric contents.

Duodenal contents

The composition of the chyme entering the duodenum from the stomach influences the rate of gastric emptying via a number of feedback mechanisms (see Ch. 16). The duodenum is sensitive to the following qualities of the chyme:

- pH
- Osmotic concentration

- Fat
- Amino acids and peptides.

Inhibition of gastric emptying occurs when the duodenal mucosa is exposed to:

- pH <3.5
- Hypertonic solutions
- Fatty acids with a chain length of 12–18 carbon atoms
- Tryptophan.

The neural and hormonal feedback mechanisms initiated by the stimulation of intestinal receptors are not completely understood. Reflex pathways involving both the central nervous system and the coeliac ganglia are present in the vagal and splanchnic nerves. The intestinal hormones, secretin, cholecystokinin and gastric inhibitory polypeptide, probably acting together during a meal, contribute to the inhibition of gastric emptying. The changes in neural and hormonal activity lead to alterations in gastric and duodenal motility. Acidification of the duodenum, for example, reduces gastric contractions and enhances the frequency and size of duodenal contractions. The presence of fats and fatty acids in the duodenum inhibits gastric and duodenal contractions but stimulates pyloric contractile activity.

These changes in gastrointestinal motility reduce the rate of gastric emptying. The inhibitory effects on gastrointestinal motility are known as enterogastrone actions. This name is derived from the hormone postulated to be produced in the intestine (*enteron*, Greek) that inhibits (*chalone*, Greek) the stomach (*gaster*, Greek). A single agent with the properties of enterogastrone has not been identified.

Other factors

Gastric emptying time can be increased by fear, pain and exercise, and reduced by excitement.

NAUSEA, RETCHING AND VOMITING

Vomiting or emesis is a complex series of responses in the gastrointestinal tract, respiratory tract and abdominal musculature leading to the forced expulsion of the gastric and sometimes the duodenal contents. There are three phases:

1. Nausea – a psychological event encompassing the feeling of wanting to vomit and often accompanied by gastric dilatation and upper intestinal contractions propelling the intestinal contents by reverse peristalsis into the stomach. Excessive salivation and pallor of the face may occur.
2. Retching – forceful, involuntary contractions of the diaphragm and abdominal muscles leading to the

cardiac portion of the stomach being forced into the thorax.
3. Vomiting – rapid inspiration followed by reflex closure of the glottis and elevation of the soft palate to prevent vomitus entering the lungs and nasal cavity; contractions of the diaphragm and the abdominal muscles compress the stomach and expel the gastric contents into the oesophagus and mouth through the relaxed lower and upper oesophageal sphincters, respectively.

A variety of stimuli (Table 15.9) induce the complex responses involved in vomiting. The stimuli may be peripheral or central in origin. The hindbrain contains a group of chemoreceptors, known as the **chemoreceptor trigger zone** (CTZ) in the area postrema in the floor of the fourth ventricle that lies outside the blood–brain barrier. Circulating toxic agents stimulate these receptors. Vomiting may result from the summation of signals arising from several sources. Postoperative vomiting in the 24 hours following abdominal surgery may occur as a result of the combined influence of inhalation anaesthetic, the use of opioid analgesics for pain relief and reflexes from irritation to the gastrointestinal tract.

The neural pathways from higher regions of the brain (cortex and limbic system) and from peripheral sensory pathways (gustatory, motion, visual, gastrointestinal, liver) converge in the lateral reticular formation of the medulla

Table 15.9	Causes of vomiting
Central nervous system	Psychogenic factors; certain sights, smells, feelings, nervous dyspepsia, anorexia nervosa and bulimia
	Pain reflexes from injuries and disease, e.g. myocardial infarction
	Motion sickness
	Raised intracranial pressure
	Migraine
Alimentary canal	Pharyngeal irritation
	Distension or obstruction of organs
	Bacterial toxins
	Alcohol
	Therapeutic agents, e.g. non-steroidal anti-inflammatory drugs, antibiotics
	Salts of heavy metals, e.g. copper, mercury, zinc
Metabolic disorders	Diabetes, e.g. ketoacidosis, gastroparesis (delayed gastric emptying)
	Renal failure, e.g. uraemia
Therapeutic agents	Cancer chemotherapy, e.g. cisplatin, doxorubicin
	Radiotherapy
	Dopamine agonists, e.g. levodopa, bromocriptine
	Cardiac glycosides, e.g. digitalis
	Morphine and opioid analgesics
	Selective serotonin reuptake inhibitors, e.g. fluoxetine, paroxetine
Pregnancy	Causes unknown but may involve:
	• Altered function of the alimentary canal – delayed gastric emptying
	• Variation in intra-abdominal pressure
	• Metabolic and hormonal changes
	• Psychogenic factors

Clinical box 15.8   **'Dumping' syndrome**

Dumping describes the symptoms of nausea, vomiting, bloating, sweating, palpitations and feeling faint after a meal in patients after partial gastrectomy or gastro-enterostomy. Decreased gastric emptying time results in the rapid 'dumping' of undigested stomach contents into the jejunum, leading to a rapid fluid influx into the jejunum in order to dilute the hypertonic contents. The pancreas may be stimulated to release excessive insulin, giving rise to hypoglycaemia. The symptoms may also occur in Zollinger–Ellison syndrome, where excessive gastrin secretion leads to over-production of acid, causing peptic ulcer disease. Dumping is also seen sometimes as a complication of cholecystectomy.

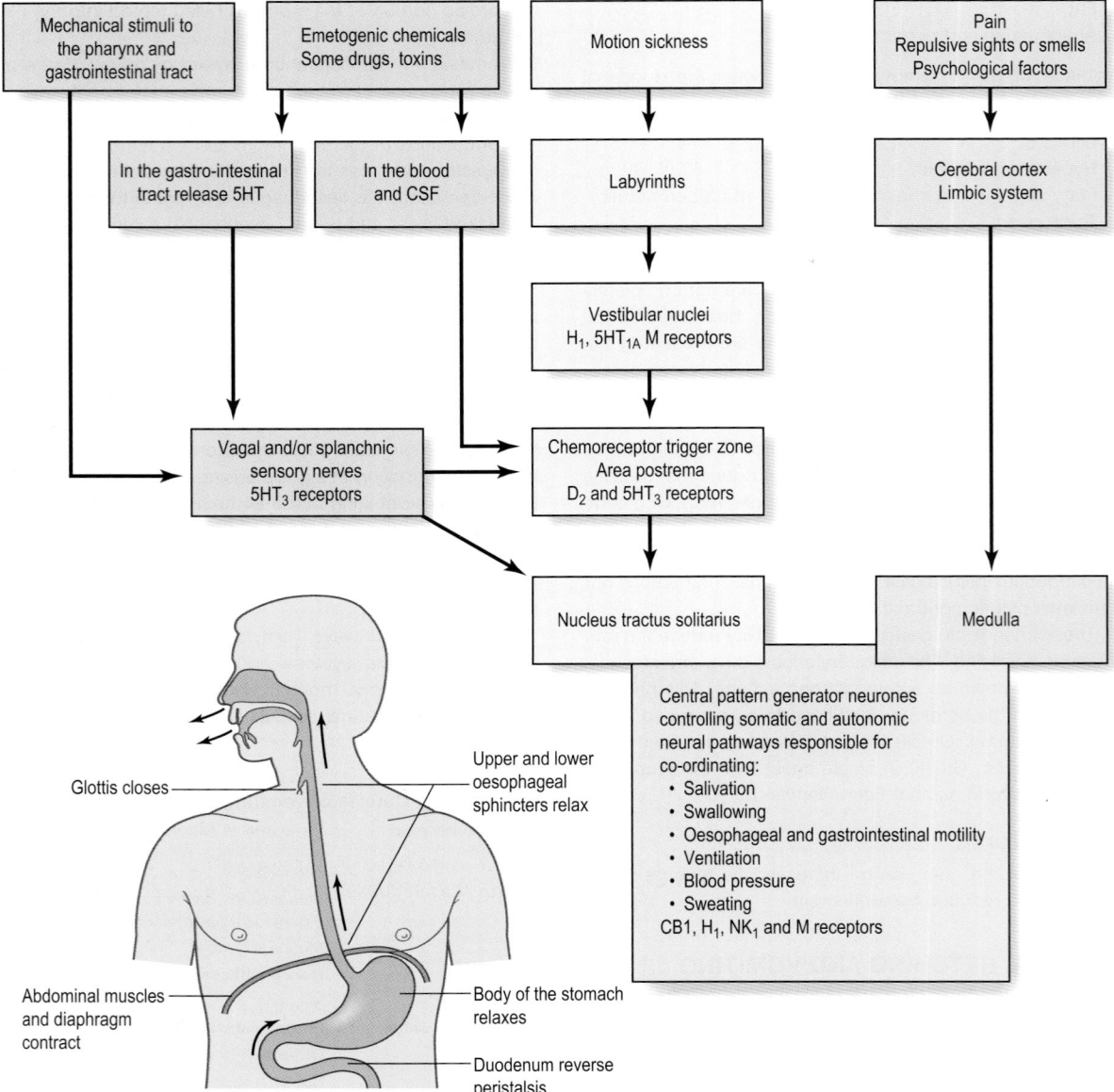

Fig. 15.19 **Stimuli and neural pathways controlling vomiting.** CBI, cannabinoid; D_2, dopamine; $5HT_{1A}$, $5HT_3$, 5-hydroxytryptamine; H_1, histamine; M, muscarinic; NK, neurokinin receptors.

oblongata of the hindbrain to control autonomic and somatic motor nerves involved in the visceral and somatic systems contributing to the vomiting response (Fig. 15.19). The neurons controlling the vomiting response are scattered throughout the medulla oblongata and do not lie in a discrete vomiting centre. The control of vomiting may be better described as being coordinated by a central pattern generator, representing the neuronal circuits involved in regulating the sequence of events in emesis.

EXOCRINE PANCREAS

The exocrine pancreas is responsible for the secretion of enzymes for digesting carbohydrates, proteins and fats. It is composed of a system of ducts and acinar cells grouped into lobules which make up 98% of the pancreatic tissue. The

pancreatic structure resembles that of salivary glands. The remaining 2% of the pancreas is composed of endocrine tissue which produces the hormones insulin and glucagon (see Ch. 10). The exocrine secretion, pancreatic juice, is composed of:

■ enzymes synthesised by acinar cells grouped into lobules
■ an alkaline fluid secreted by the ductular epithelial cells.

The pancreatic juice flows along the main pancreatic duct which empties into the duodenum along with the bile duct (Fig. 15.20).

PANCREATIC ENZYMES

The pancreatic enzymes are synthesized in the rough endoplasmic reticulum of the acinar cells. They are transferred to the Golgi apparatus where they are directed to the condensing vacuoles for packaging into zymogen granules. These

<table>
<tr><td>ⓘ</td><td>**Information box 15.6**</td><td>**Prolonged vomiting can cause acidosis**</td></tr>
</table>

Gastric juice is composed of non-parietal and parietal cell secretions with different electrolyte compositions. Non-parietal cell secretions are produced at a constant flow rate and contain Na^+, K^+, Cl^- and HCO_3^-, while parietal cell secretions are produced at varying flow rates and contain H^+ and Cl^-. The electrolyte composition of gastric juice therefore varies with flow rate. At a low flow rate, the major components are Na^+ and Cl^- with lower concentrations of K^+ and H^+. However, at high flow rates, the major components are H^+ and Cl^- with lower concentrations of Na^+ and K^+.

The HCO_3^- secretion from non-parietal cells is neutralised by H^+ in the parietal cell secretion and can be measured in the absence of H^+ secretion. At all secretory rates the H^+, K^+ and Cl^- concentrations of the gastric juice exceed those in plasma, and the Na^+ concentration is less than that in plasma.

Prolonged vomiting or aspiration of gastric juice can lead to hypokalaemia, metabolic acidosis and death unless intravenous infusions of NaCl, dextrose and K^+ are given. This is particularly important in hyperemesis gravidarum – prolonged vomiting in pregnancy.

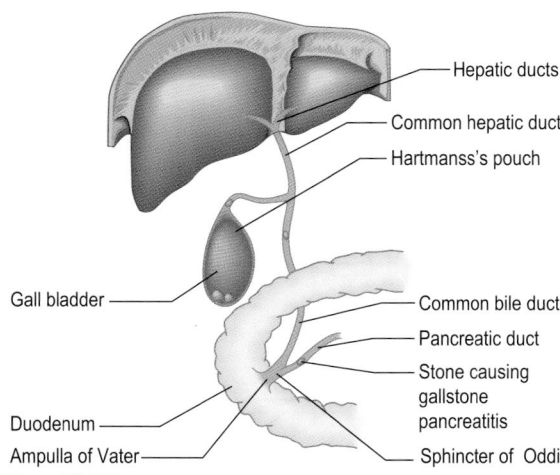

Fig. 15.20 Anatomical relationship between the liver, biliary system, pancreas and the small intestine.
Adapted with permission from Kumar P, Clark M 2005 Clinical medicine, 6th edn. Elsevier Mosby, Edinburgh.

granules are found in abundance at the apical pole of the cell. Each zymogen granule contains several pancreatic enzymes (Table 15.10) whose relative concentration depends on the composition of the diet, e.g. a high carbohydrate diet produces a high amylase component and a reduction in protease.

Mechanisms of enzyme secretion

A rise in the intracellular Ca^{2+} concentration produced by neurohormonal agents (acetylcholine, gastrin and cholecystokinin) acts as a signal to induce exocytosis, in which the zymogen granules fuse with the apical membrane of the acinar cell and the contents are released into the acinar lumen (Fig. 15.21A). In addition to enzyme secretion, the acinar cells secrete a small quantity of isotonic fluid to wash the enzymes into the ducts. The increased intracellular Ca^{2+} concentration, produced by stimulants of enzyme secretion, activates protein kinases which produce an opening of Cl^- channels in the apical membrane. Cl^- diffuses from the cytoplasm to the acinar lumen. The gradient for Cl^- diffusion is maintained by the influx of Cl^- from the interstitial fluid across the basolateral membrane by means of the $Na^+/K^+/2Cl^-$ transporter. This transfer is driven by the Na^+ gradient created by the Na^+/K^+ pump. The electronegative lumen attracts Na^+ to move from the interstitial fluid through cationic channels in the tight junctions between adjacent acinar cells. Water moves from the cells and interstitial spaces to the lumen of the duct system to produce an isotonic secretion.

Alkaline secretion

The pancreas secretes 1–2 L of fluid per day. The pancreatic juice is alkaline (pH ~8) and isotonic to the blood. The major site for the production of the bicarbonate-rich juice is the duct system (Fig. 15.21B). The composition of the secretion varies with flow rate. At low flow rates the major ionic constituents are Na^+ and Cl^-. This contrasts with high flow rates where the predominant ions are Na^+ and HCO_3^-. The concentrations of K^+ and Na^+ at all flow rates are similar to those in

<table>
<tr><td>ⓘ</td><td>**Information box 15.7**</td><td>**Pancreatitis**</td></tr>
</table>

Pancreatic acinar cells are destroyed by acute or chronic inflammation and hereditary factors (e.g. cystic fibrosis), leading to failure to secrete pancreatic enzymes for the digestion of starches, proteins and fats. Nutritional deficiencies then ensue. Causes of pancreatitis include infection, alcohol, gallstones, tumours, heredity, trauma and surgery.

Table 15.10	Pancreatic enzymes		
Enzyme	**Secreted as...**	**Activation**	**Function**
Amylase	Active enzyme		Starch digestion
Trypsinogen	Proenzyme	Activated by enteropeptidase to trypsin which act autocatalytically	Protein digestion
Chymotrypsinogen	Proenzymes	Activated by trypsin	
Procarboxypeptidase			
Proelastase			
Lipase	Active enzymes		Fat digestion
Cholesterol esterase			Cholesterol esters
Phospholipase			Phospholipids
Deoxyribonuclease	Active enzymes		Nucleic acid digestion
Ribonuclease			

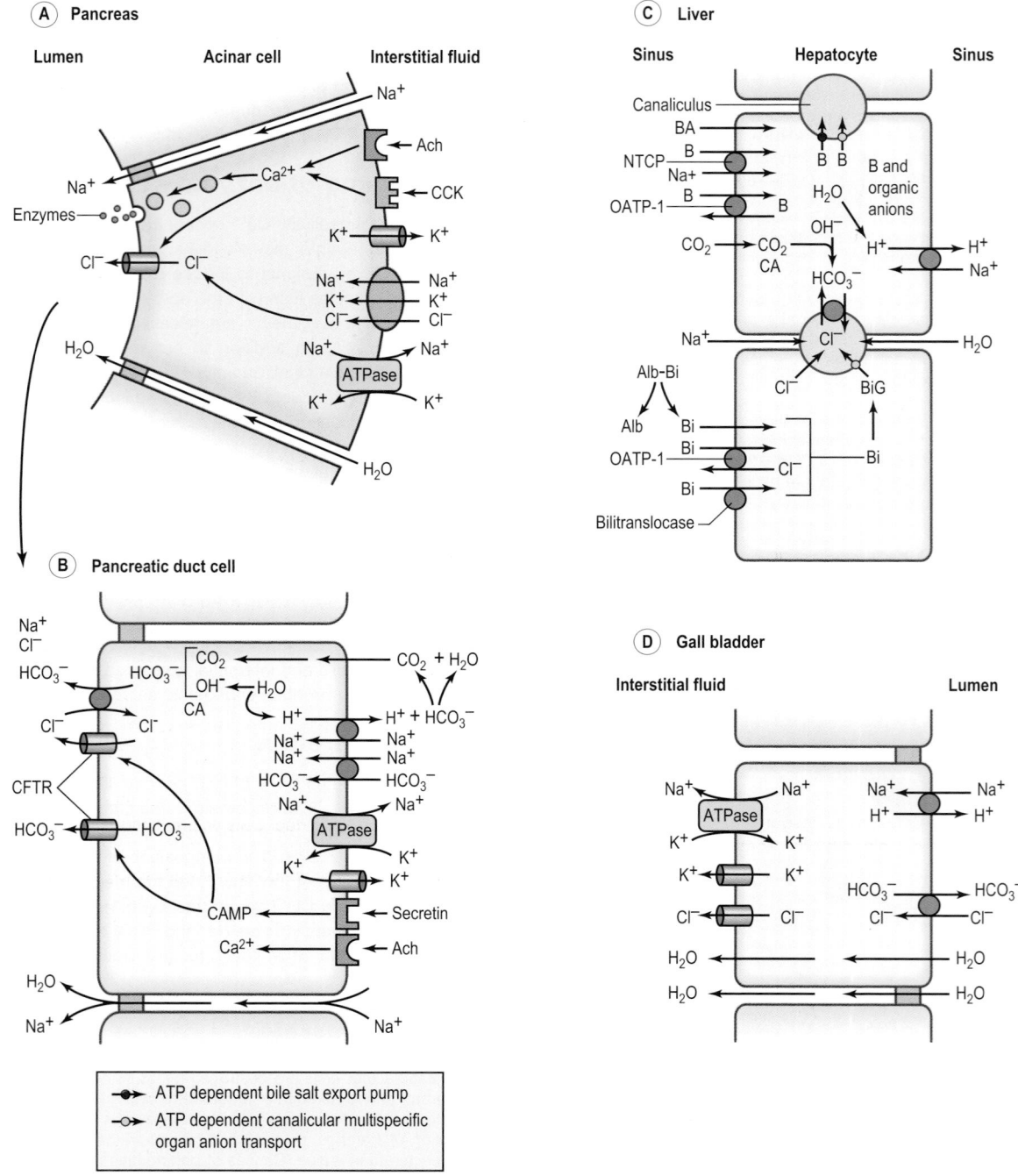

Fig. 15.21 Transport mechanisms involved in the formation of pancreatic juice and bile. ACh, acetylcholine; CCK, cholecystokinin; CA, carbonic anhydrase; CFTR, cystic fibrosis transmembrane regulator; B, bile salts; BA, bile acid; Bi, bilirubin; BiG, bilirubin glucuronide; Alb, albumin; NTCP, sodium taurochlorate cotransporting polypeptide; OATP-1, organic anion transporting protein.

plasma. The concentration of Cl^- falls and that of HCO_3^- rises as flow rate increases.

The reciprocal changes in Cl^- and HCO_3^- concentrations with increases in flow rate may be accounted for by the mixing of two different secretions, one being a NaCl solution produced by the acinar cell, and the second solution being $NaHCO_3$ produced by the duct cells. The NaCl solution predominates at low flow rates. The secretion of $NaHCO_3$ increases with stimulation and dilutes the NaCl solution. At high flow rates, the increased secretion of $NaHCO_3$ leads to a high concentration of HCO_3^- and a low concentration of Cl^- in pancreatic juice.

The pancreatic duct cells can produce HCO_3^- concentrations of 140–150 mM. The HCO_3^- in the duct cells comes from two sources:

- HCO_3^- can be transferred from the interstitial fluid by means of a Na^+-HCO_3^- cotransporter
- CO_2 diffusion from the interstitial fluid.

CO_2, which is lipid soluble, diffuses into the cells where it reacts with water, aided by the action of carbonic anhydrase, to produce carbonic acid. The latter dissociates to produce H^+ and HCO_3^-. The supply of CO_2 is maintained by the duct cells exporting H^+ to the tissue fluid in exchange for Na^+

moving down its concentration gradient into the cells. The H^+ combines with HCO_3^- from the blood to form CO_2 and water.

The basal secretion of HCO_3^- from the duct cell is accounted for by the action of an anion exchanger in the luminal membrane. This mechanism transports HCO_3^- out of the cell into the lumen in exchange for Cl^- uptake. Cl^- is moving down its concentration gradient into the cell. The luminal Cl^- comes from the acinar cells' fluid secretion, and as a result of recycling through channels in the apical membrane of the duct cell.

Stimulation of the duct cells with the hormone secretin leads to enhanced HCO_3^- secretion. The supply of Cl^- is insufficient to account for the concentrations of HCO_3^- achieved. Furthermore, high luminal HCO_3^- concentrations inhibit the Cl^-/HCO_3^- exchange at the apical membrane. The secretion of HCO_3^- under these circumstances is due to a Cl^--independent pathway. The cystic fibrosis transmembrane conductance regulator (CFTR) may serve as the pathway for HCO_3^- secretion to the duct lumen.

The lumen of the duct is electronegative with respect to the interstitial fluid. Na^+ enters the luminal fluid from the interstitial spaces by diffusion down this gradient. The resulting osmotic change draws water into the duct system to produce an isotonic secretion.

CONTROL OF PANCREATIC JUICE SECRETION

The pancreas produces a basal secretion of enzymes and fluid during the interdigestive period. This flow increases in parallel with the intestinal MMC activity. The parasympathetic nervous system is responsible for coordinating this secretory activity, aided by the hormone cholecystokinin.

Pancreatic juice secretion during a meal increases up to 20 times that of the basal secretion. It is determined by stimulatory and inhibitory mechanisms. As with gastric juice this occurs in three overlapping phases: cephalic, gastric and intestinal.

Cephalic phase

The thought, sight, smell, taste and chewing of food produce a reflex vagal nerve stimulation of the pancreatic acinar and duct cells to secrete pancreatic juice. The action of the vagus is mediated by acetylcholine acting on muscarinic M_3 receptors on the acinar and duct cells. Gastrin, released into the circulation by vagal activity to the gastric antrum, also contributes to pancreatic enzyme secretion. Gastrin, which has a similar structure to cholecystokinin (CCK), acts on CCK_A receptors on the acinar cells. Vagal nerve activity produces a pancreatic juice that is rich in enzymes.

Fear acting to increase sympathetic splanchnic nerve activity reduces pancreatic juice secretion. This action is produced by vasoconstriction due to the release of noradrenaline from the splanchnic nerves. Noradrenaline acts via α-adrenoceptors on the vascular smooth muscle, reducing blood flow to the pancreas, which inhibits secretion.

Gastric phase

The gastric phase consists of neural and hormonal components stimulating the pancreas. The gastro-pancreatic reflex is produced by distension of the stomach, leading to the stimulation of stretch receptors with afferent nerves in the vagus conveying information to the medulla. These nerves excite efferent vagal nerves to the pancreas (a vagovagal reflex) by means of the neurotransmitter acetylcholine. Gastrin released by protein digestion products stimulates the pancreatic acinar cells.

Intestinal phase

The intestinal contents play a major role in controlling pancreatic juice secretion. This is achieved by means of the hormones cholecystokinin and secretin, and the enteropancreatic vagovagal reflex.

Cholecystokinin is synthesized by I cells in the duodenal and jejunal mucosa. It is secreted in response to the presence of lipids such as monoglycerides and free fatty acids, amino acids and peptides, but not to carbohydrates or hydrochloric acid in the chyme. In animals, cholecystokinin enters the venous circulation and is delivered to the pancreas to stimulate enzyme secretion via CCK_A receptors situated on the acinar and duct cells. In humans, CCK_A receptors are absent from pancreatic acinar cells. It is suggested that cholecystokinin stimulates CCK_A receptors on vagal sensory nerves to produce a vagovagal reflex secretion of enzymes. The primary role of cholecystokinin is to stimulate enzyme secretion. Cholecystokinin alone has weak effects on fluid secretion but it potentiates the action of secretin.

Secretin is synthesised by S cells in the duodenal mucosa. It is released by hydrochloric acid in the chyme entering the small intestine from the stomach. Bile salts and lipids are much weaker stimulants of secretin secretion than hydrochloric acid. Secretin enters the circulation and is delivered to the pancreatic duct cells where it stimulates bicarbonate and, consequently, fluid secretion.

The **entero-pancreatic reflex** is stimulated by the presence of lipid, peptides and amino acids in the small intestine. The nutrients stimulate vagovagal reflexes with afferent and efferent pathways in the vagal nerves.

Interactions between acetylcholine, cholecystokinin and secretin

Interactions between the neurotransmitter acetylcholine and the hormones cholecystokinin and secretin at the cellular level are important in determining the response of the pancreas to a meal. When the concentration of either cholecystokinin or secretin in the blood during a meal is reproduced, by intravenous infusions of one of the hormones, the response of the pancreas is lower than that observed in a meal. The administration of the drug atropine, to block the action of acetylcholine released from the vagal nerves, or cutting the vagal nerves, reduces the effectiveness of both cholecystokinin and secretin in producing enzyme and bicarbonate secretion, respectively. The results of these observations suggest that when cholecystokinin, secretin and acetylcholine act together, they increase the sensitivity of the pancreas to stimulation. This phenomenon is known as potentiation.

Intracellular messengers for acetylcholine, cholecystokinin and secretin

The actions of acetylcholine, cholecystokinin and secretin depend on the production of intracellular messengers. Acetylcholine and cholecystokinin stimulate muscarinic and cholecystokinin receptors, respectively, in the acinar and duct cells. This results in phospholipase C hydrolysing phosphatidyl inositol to inositol 1,4,5-trisphosphate and diacyl glycerol. Inositol trisphosphate releases Ca^{2+} from stores in the endoplasmic reticulum. The rise in intracellular Ca^{2+} activates calmodulin, which in turn increases the activity of protein kinases and phosphorylation involved in the processes of zymogen granule secretion. DAG activates protein kinase C, which is also involved in enzyme secretion from zymogen granules. The rise in intracellular Ca^{2+} also stimulates fluid secretion by acinar cells, probably leading to the phosphorylation of ion channels involved in the production of the secretion. Secretin stimulates an increase in adenylate cyclase activity to produce cyclic AMP, which in turn activates protein kinase C to promote enzyme and fluid secretion.

Inhibition of pancreatic secretion

Pancreatic function at the end of a meal is returned to the interdigestive state by the lack of stimulatory factors in the alimentary canal. There is an additional inhibitory mechanism that operates from the terminal ileum. The presence of fat in the terminal ileum and colon releases **peptide YY (PYY)**, an inhibitor of pancreatic enzyme secretion.

THE LIVER AND BILIARY SYSTEM

The liver is situated in the right hypochondrium, under the diaphragm, and behind and protected by, the lower ribs. Although embryologically developed from the foregut, the liver performs much more than digestive functions. In health, the liver is not palpable on examination of the abdomen. The lower edge of the liver becomes palpable below the rib cage when the organ is enlarged through disease. The liver participates in a wide variety of processes that are discussed in many chapters in this book. This section is a summary of what the liver does, and what can happen in liver disease.

ANATOMY OF THE LIVER

The liver is a solid, pyramid-shaped organ enclosed by peritoneum. It is the largest internal human organ, weighing between 1.4 kg and 1.6 kg in the healthy adult.

Gross anatomy of the liver

The hepatic portal vein, hepatic artery and common bile duct (see below) enter the liver at the hilum (porta hepatis). The vessels and duct divide into right and left branches. Functionally, the parts of the liver supplied by these branches constitute a larger right and a smaller left lobe. Depending on the blood supply, the liver can be further subdivided into eight segments (Fig. 15.22). This has important clinical implications during surgery, when it is possible to resect individual segments.

Blood supply to the liver

The liver is a highly vascular organ, receiving 25% of the resting cardiac output, and is unique in that it has a dual blood supply of both arterial and venous blood, necessary for the performance of complex liver functions. The hepatic

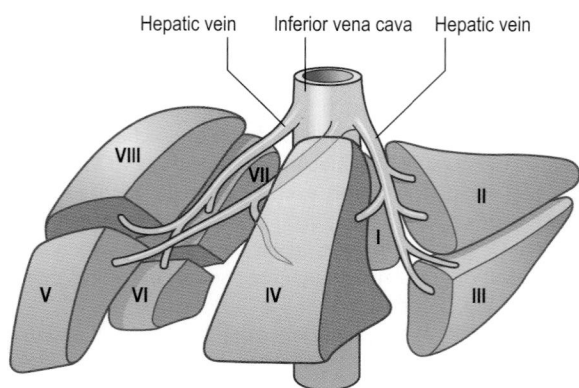

Fig. 15.22 Segmental anatomy of the liver. I, caudate lobe; II-IV, left hemi-liver; V-VIII, right hemi-liver. Adapted with permission from Kumar P, Clark M 2005 Clinical medicine, 6th edn. Elsevier Mosby, Edinburgh.

portal vein and hepatic artery enter the liver through a central area on the ventral surface of the liver, through which the common bile duct also enters. This area is known as the **hilum (porta hepatis)**.

- The portal vein carries blood from the gut, pancreas and spleen. Absorbed nutrients and products of digestion enter the liver directly from the gastrointestinal tract. Senescent (used, spent) red blood cells are delivered from the spleen (see Ch. 12). As much as 75% of the blood supply to the liver is via the portal vein.
- The hepatic artery, arising from the coeliac axis which originates from the abdominal aorta, ensures that the liver cells are well perfused and supplied with oxygen for metabolism.
- The hepatic vein drains into the inferior vena cava.

Microanatomy of the liver

Microscopically, liver cells (hepatocytes) make up the liver parenchyma (substance), forming hepatic plates that are one to two cells thick. The plates are separated from each other by large capillary spaces known as sinusoids. Bile canaliculi run in a network between the hepatocytes, receiving bile secretions, and join to form the intra-hepatic small bile ductules.

The hepatic plates are arranged into a large number of polyhedral liver lobules, which are hexagonal in cross-section (Fig. 15.23). There is a central lobular vein (also known as the terminal hepatic venule) in the middle of each lobule. At the periphery of each polygonal lobule are the portal tracts, which consist of a triad of vessels, also known as the portal triad, consisting of:

- A hepatic arteriole (a branch of the hepatic artery), which supplies oxygenated blood straight from the lungs and heart
- A terminal portal venule, which is a branch of the hepatic portal vein, draining blood from the stomach, intestine, pancreas and spleen
- A bile ductule, which drains into the bile duct, delivering bile (see below).

Arterial blood and portal venous blood mix as the blood flows through the sinusoids from the periphery of the lobule to the central vein. The central lobular veins converge to form

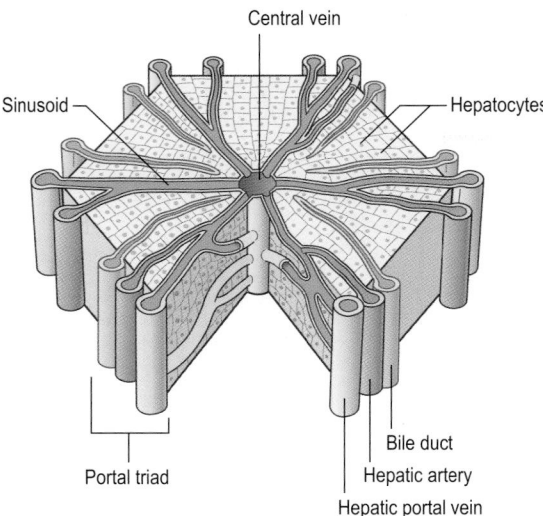

Fig. 15.23 **Microanatomy of a hepatic lobule.** The portal tract consists of a triad of a hepatic arteriole (a branch of the hepatic artery), a terminal portal venule (a branch of the portal vein), and a bile duct, which receives bile from bile ductules. Blood from the portal tract flows through the sinusoids into the central vein.

the hepatic vein, which carries the blood to the inferior vena cava. The sinusoids do not have a basement membrane, and are lined by two cell types:

- Specialised, fenestrated vascular endothelial cells forming a lining with numerous gaps that facilitates transfer of metabolites between the plasma and hepatocytes.
- Mononuclear, phagocytic Kupffer cells that are part of the reticular endothelial system (see also Ch. 12). Kupffer cells, usually situated near the gaps between the endothelial cells, have a role in recycling senescent, non-functioning red blood cells; one of the products is bile.

The hepatocytes are separated from the sinusoids by the space of Disse. The basolateral membranes of the hepatocytes face the space of Disse and are covered with microvilli to create a large surface area to facilitate absorption. The membranes also contain stellate cells that store vitamin A during their quiescent state and produce collagen when activated. The smallest functional unit of the liver is the acinus:

- The liver acinus consists of hepatocytes and sinusoids from two adjacent lobules supplied by one portal tract. Blood flowing through the hepatic sinusoids drains into the central lobular vein, so that there are two to each acinus (Fig. 15.24A).
- The hepatocytes nearest the portal tract, the periportal cells, are well supplied with oxygenated blood from the hepatic arteriole and nutrients from the terminal portal venule (Fig. 15.24B). A difference in oxygen and nutrient concentration arises as the blood flows towards the central lobular vein. Hepatocytes nearest the vein, perivenous cells, are less well oxygenated. This phenomenon is known as metabolic zonation of the liver

where the difference in oxygenation results in differential gene expression and metabolism. For example, periportal cells receive more oxygen than the perivenous cells and have a more oxidative metabolism, whereas the expression of glucokinase is mainly restricted to the perivenous cells (see Ch. 3).

The liver acinus is not to be confused with the basic hepatic lobule. In the acinus, the portal tract is central, with the central lobular veins at the periphery, whereas in the hepatic lobule, the central lobular vein is central with a portal tract at each corner of the hexagon.

FUNCTIONS OF THE LIVER

The liver participates in a wide range of biochemical processes, its functions including metabolism, catabolism, synthesis, elimination of toxic substances and storage. In addition, the liver has an immunological function. Among these functions, the liver has a pivotal role in metabolism, discussed in detail in Chapter 3. The interrelationship of carbohydrate, protein and lipid metabolism to maintain optimum blood glucose concentration is orchestrated in the liver.

The liver and carbohydrate metabolism

The liver has a major role in glucose metabolism to maintain the optimum level of circulating glucose essential to energy metabolism: glucose homeostasis (see Ch. 3).

- Glycogen synthesis and storage: after a carbohydrate-rich meal, glucose is mainly taken up by the perivenous cells, initially to synthesise glycogen. When blood glucose levels are high, e.g. after a meal, the liver stores glycogen.
- Owing to the presence of the enzyme glucose-6-phosphatase (G6Pase), unlike muscle, hepatic glycogenolysis releases glucose directly into the blood stream, thus acting as a reservoir for glucose.
- Gluconeogenesis: the liver is able to synthesise glucose from non-carbohydrate sources (e.g. amino acids and glycerol from fat metabolism), which is an essential source of glucose during starvation when glycogen stores are depleted.

The liver and protein metabolism

As a first step in protein metabolism, the nitrogen component of amino acids delivered to the liver via the portal vein is removed through transamination (catalysed by aminotransferases (also known as transaminases)) and deamination in the liver (see Ch. 3). This function is disrupted in liver disease, and transaminase enzymes are clinical markers of hepatocyte damage (see Clinical box 15.9). One of the products of deamination is ammonia (NH_3), which is toxic and normally removed rapidly via the urea cycle in the liver. The liver thus fulfils its function in protein metabolism by catabolism and detoxification of waste products of metabolism. Protein synthesis is another important liver function.

- Most plasma proteins are synthesised in the liver. Albumin is exclusively produced by the liver, and low plasma concentration, called hypoalbuminaemia, is common in liver disease. The implications for nutritional status, immunity and drug metabolism are discussed in Chapters 4 and 16. (See also Clinical box 15.9).

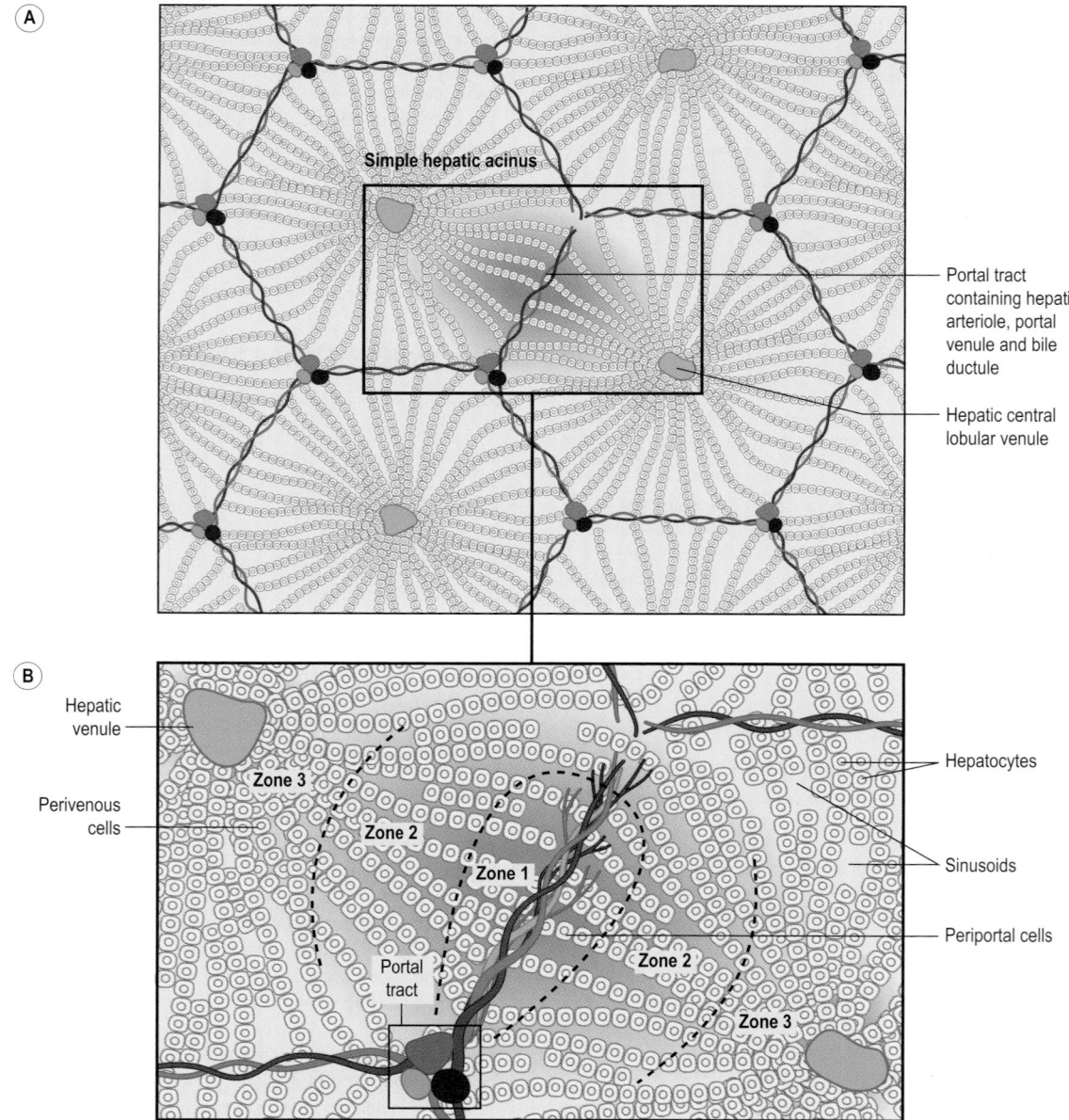

Fig. 15.24 Hepatic acinus and metabolic zonation. Hepatocytes in zone 1, nearest to the portal triad (tract), receive the most oxygen from the hepatic arteriole and nutrients from the portal venule; hepatocytes in the more peripheral zone 3, being more distant, receive less. The difference results in differential oxygenation of the cells, leading to different gene expression and metabolism. Adapted with permission from Young B, Heath JW 2004 Wheater's functional histology, 4th edn. Churchill Livingstone, Edinburgh.

■ The liver also participates in the production of all the coagulation factors: prothrombin, fibrinogen, and factors V, VII, IX, X and XIII. Defective production of one or all of these factors results in coagulation defects, with spontaneous bruising and prolonged bleeding after minor injuries. Laboratory measurement of prothrombin time (PT) assesses the functional concentration of these factors (see Ch. 12).

■ Plasma α- and β-globulins are mostly synthesised by hepatocytes. This function is compromised in liver disease, affecting immunity. (See Clinical box 15.10)

The liver and lipid metabolism

Insoluble dietary lipids are transported to the liver, via the portal vein, as lipoproteins (Ch. 3); the liver has a central role in lipoprotein metabolism. The functions may be summarised to include:

■ Synthesis of triacylglycerol (TAG) and removal of TAG from TAG-rich lipoprotein particles (hepatic triacylglycerol lipase HTGL)

■ Synthesis of very-low-density lipoproteins (VLDL) and high-density lipoproteins (HDL)

■ Synthesis of apolipoproteins that control lipoprotein metabolism

■ Cholesterol: the liver has a major role in both synthesis and catabolism of cholesterol:
  ■ Cholesterol synthesis
  ■ Esterification of free cholesterol to cholesterol ester, catalysed by lecithin-cholesterol acyltransferase (LCAT)

- α_1-Antitrypsin deficiency is a rare genetic disorder associated with about 1% of chronic obstructive pulmonary disease (COPD). Onset of COPD at a young age and a family history are suggestive of α_1-antitrypsin deficiency, and may warrant genotype investigation. When arising in infancy, the condition presents with liver disease.
- Wilson's disease is an autosomal recessive condition in which hepatic caeruloplasmin synthesis is defective. Normally, dietary copper is absorbed from the upper gastrointestinal tract, transported to the liver bound to albumin, and thence incorporated into the copper-containing glycoprotein caeruloplasmin, concerned with plasma copper transport. Caeruloplasmin deficiency leaves the copper free, which is then deposited in the hepatocytes, causing chronic hepatitis, cirrhosis and ultimately liver failure, although the precise mechanism is unclear (see below). Biliary excretion of copper is also compromised. Copper deposits in the central nervous system, kidneys and bone cause further damage. Deposits of copper in the cornea give the characteristic Kayser–Fleischer rings.
- Ferritin, the protein concerned with iron storage, and transferrin, responsible for iron transport, are also synthesised by the liver (see Ch. 12). Although the mechanism of damage is unclear, defective hepatic synthesis of these proteins results in prolonged iron overload in the liver. Hereditary haemochromatosis is a condition in which iron is deposited in the liver (and other tissues), eventually leading to fibrosis (cirrhosis, see below) and liver failure.
- α-Fetoprotein is synthesised by the liver, predominantly in the fetal liver. Elevated maternal plasma α-fetoprotein concentration is used as a screening test for fetal open neural tube defects and as part of the triple test for Down's syndrome. Regenerating hepatocytes synthesise α-fetoprotein, so high concentrations may be associated with carcinoma of the liver.

The acute phase response refers to the body's defence mechanism against infections and inflammation, when the liver synthesises 'acute phase proteins', stimulated by pro-inflammatory cytokines (see Ch. 6). Plasma concentrations rise by 25% or more following the initial challenge, and the magnitude of the response reflects the severity of the infection or inflammatory process. Amino acids are needed as substrate for the increased hepatic protein synthesis. In severe, prolonged inflammatory (including carcinomas) or infective conditions, the amino acids are derived from muscle breakdown, resulting in the muscle wasting of chronic disease (cachexia). Of the acute phase proteins, changes in plasma concentration of C-reactive protein (CRP) are most marked, and values derived from laboratory measurement are used clinically as a marker of infection or inflammation.

- Removal of cholesterol into hepatocytes for excretion as bile salts and sterols
- Steroid and hormone synthesis from cholesterol by the cytochrome P450 system of hepatic microsomal enzymes
- Cytochrome P450 enzymes also participate in the biosynthesis of endogenous substances such as arachidonic acid, a precursor of prostaglandins and thromboxane. Thromboxane induces platelet aggregation and vasoconstriction, which initiates the

normal coagulation mechanisms following injuries (see coagulation cascade, Ch. 12).
- When there is excessive carbohydrate intake, the liver synthesises fatty acids using intermediates from the breakdown of sugars, some amino acids and other fatty acids.

The liver and red blood cells

The red cell membrane, like all cell membranes, is a lipid bilayer containing cholesterol. In severe liver disease, LCAT is decreased so that esterification of free cholesterol to cholesterol ester is reduced, increasing the ratio of circulating cholesterol to cholesterol ester. This changes cell membrane structure. In chronic obstructive liver disease, abnormal liver enzyme activity results in thinning of the red cell membrane, with an increase in membrane surface area, leading to macrocytosis. Microscopically, the abnormal red cells have a central dark area surrounded by a pale ring, giving the appearance of the 'bulls eye' in an archery target; these cells are known as target cells (codocytes).

The respiratory pigments responsible for the transport of oxygen, haemoglobin in red blood cells and myoglobin in muscle, contain haem, a porphyrin with a central iron core (see Ch. 12). Although haem is synthesised in most cells, the liver is the main non-red cell source of haem. The liver is also responsible for the catabolism of haem. Haemoglobin from senescent red blood cells is transported via the portal vein to the liver from the spleen (the graveyard of red blood cells). The spent red cells are phagocytosed by the Kupffer cells, where iron and globin are removed from haem. The iron is released and recycled via transferrin; the globin is also re-used. Haem is then recovered by the Kupffer cells, and the porphyrin ring is broken down to bilirubin for excretion.

Metabolism of bilirubin

Bilirubin, a yellow pigment, is a product of haem catabolism, following the destruction of haem molecules by macrophages. The vast majority of bilirubin (75%) comes from the haemoglobin of senescent red blood cells. Macrophages are part of the reticulo-endothelial system, found in the spleen, bone marrow and the Kupffer cells lining liver sinusoids. After haemoglobin is degraded into haem and globin, the porphyrin ring of haem is cleaved by haem oxygenase, a cytochrome P450 enzyme (see Chs 3 and 4), to biliverdin with the release of iron. Biliverdin, which is water soluble, is enzymically reduced to bilirubin by biliverdin reductase. Bilirubin has low water solubility, therefore it is transported in the blood bound to plasma albumin. On reaching the liver, the bilirubin–albumin complex dissociates and free bilirubin crosses the hepatocyte basolateral membrane by one of three mechanisms: either diffusion or transport by OATP1 or bilitranslocase (see below).

Following uptake by hepatocytes, free bilirubin is transported to the endoplasmic reticulum where it is conjugated with glucuronic acid to form bilirubin glucuronide. The conjugated bilirubin is more soluble and can be excreted by the hepatocyte into the biliary canaliculi via the transporter canalicular multi-specific organic anion transporter (cMOAT), then transported to the gastrointestinal tract via the biliary tree (see below). In the gastrointestinal tract, bacterial flora catabolise conjugated bilirubin to the colourless stercobilinogen (also called faecal urobilinogen), which is oxidised to the coloured stercobilin (also called faecal urobilin) for excretion in faeces.

Bilirubin, being yellow, gives the yellow colouration of bruises and the brown colour of faeces. Excess plasma bilirubin causes jaundice, a yellow discoloration of the skin and sclera (see Clinical box 15.11).

The liver and bile production

Among its many functions, the liver contributes to digestion by secreting bile (Table 15.11). Approximately 0.6–1.2 L is secreted per day in an adult. This exocrine secretion serves not only to aid digestion but also as a route for the excretion of metabolites produced by the liver.

Bile secretion

The components of bile diffuse from the sinusoids through spaces between the endothelium to the space of Disse, from where they are absorbed by the hepatocytes and formed into bile. The apical membranes of adjacent hepatocytes form the walls of the biliary canaliculi into which bile is secreted. The bile then flows through the biliary tree into the duodenum (see Fig. 15.20):

- The biliary canaliculi join together to form bile ductules.
- Bile ductules convey the bile to the bile ducts in the portal tracts at the periphery of the lobule.
- Portal tracts drain into the intra-hepatic bile ducts that join to form hepatic ducts leaving each liver lobe.
- The left and right hepatic ducts join to form the common hepatic duct just outside the liver.
- The common hepatic duct joins the cystic duct from the gall bladder to form the common bile duct.
- Just before its termination in the duodenum, the common bile duct is joined by the pancreatic duct at the ampulla of Vater (hepatopancreatic ampulla).
- The termination of the common bile duct is in the duodenum, marked by an accentuation of its circular smooth muscle layer (Sphincter of Oddi).

Cellular mechanisms of bile secretion

Bile is composed of water, electrolytes, bile salts, cholesterol, phospholipids and bilirubin (Table 15.11). Hepatocytes synthesise the primary bile acids, cholic acid and chenodeoxycholic acid, from cholesterol. These bile acids are metabolised by intestinal bacteria to the secondary bile acids, deoxycholic acid and lithocholic acid. They are absorbed from the intestine and circulate to the liver where they are eventually absorbed by hepatocytes to form bile. The bile acids are conjugated with glycine and taurine to form negatively charged bile salts, which have a greater water solubility than the bile acids at the near neutral pH of the intestinal contents. The enhanced water solubility is important in enabling the bile salts to aid the digestion of fats.

The secretion of bile depends on two separate, active secretory processes:

- Bile-salt-dependent secretion produced by the hepatocytes
- Bile-salt-independent secretion produced by the hepatocytes and duct cells.

Bile-salt-dependent secretion Bile formation begins with the absorption of bile salts and other organic and inorganic ions across the basolateral border of the hepatocyte by a variety of transporters. Bile salt uptake is dependent on two transporters and non-ionic diffusion (Fig. 15.21C).

The Na^+ coupled transporter known as the sodium taurocholate cotransporting polypeptide (**NTCP**) can transfer both conjugated and unconjugated bile salts. The organic anion

---

> **Clinical box 15.11** **Jaundice**
>
> Jaundice (icterus) is characterised by elevated concentrations of bilirubin in the plasma producing a yellow discoloration of the sclera of the eyes, skin and mucous membranes. Jaundice may be characterised as unconjugated hyperbilirubinaemia and obstructive or cholestatic jaundice.
>
> **Unconjugated hyperbilirubinaemia**
> Haemolytic jaundice occurs following excessive haemolysis of erythrocytes in newborn infants, and hereditary, autoimmune and non-immune disorders of erythrocytes. The hepatocytes cannot dispose of the increased amounts of unconjugated bilirubin, which accumulates in the blood (see Ch. 12).
>
> Transient defects in the conjugation of bilirubin may occur in the newborn due to immaturity of the liver in which the glucuronidation pathway is not fully developed, leading to unconjugated bilirubin accumulating in the blood: physiological jaundice. Haemolytic disease of the newborn, due to rhesus incompatibility with maternal blood, results in massive intravascular haemolysis and severe unconjugated hyperbilirubinaemia, which may be complicated by bilirubin deposition in the central nervous system (CNS) – kernicterus – leading to brain damage. Congenital unconjugated hyperbilirubinaemia (e.g. Gilbert's syndrome) may be due to abnormalities in glucuronide conjugation or transport into the biliary canaliculi by cMOAT (see below).
>
> **Obstructive or cholestatic jaundice**
> - Intra-hepatic jaundice: caused by damage to liver cells produced by viruses, drugs, alcohol cirrhosis, or blockage of the intra-hepatic bile ducts leading to a failure of bile secretion.
> - Extra-hepatic jaundice: produced by blockage of the extra-hepatic bile ducts. The obstruction may be due to gall stones in the biliary tree, or due to enlargement of an adjacent organ, such as carcinoma of the head of the pancreas.
>
> Obstructive jaundice, however caused, leads to conjugated bilirubin accumulating in the blood. Some of this water-soluble form of bilirubin is excreted by the kidneys and gives the urine a dark yellow colour. Bile-containing conjugated bilirubin does not enter the intestine, and therefore cannot be transformed by intestinal flora to stercobilin, so that faeces in obstructive jaundice are pale coloured.

Table 15.11	Composition of human hepatic and gall bladder bile	
Component	**Hepatic bile (mmol/L)**	**Gall bladder bile (mmol/L)**
Na^+	150–160	230–240
K^+	4–5	6–14
Ca^{2+}	1.0–2.5	2.5–16
Cl^-	62–112	1–10
HCO_3^-	20–50	8–10
Bile salts	20–40	200–300
Bilirubin	1–3	5–30
Cholesterol	2–4	10–25
Phospholipids	3–7	18–40

transport protein (**OATP1**) also transfers bile acids into hepatocytes in exchange for Cl⁻. In addition, unconjugated bile salts may enter the cell by non-ionic diffusion in their undissociated acid form.

The hepatocytes secrete bile acids and organic anions (e.g. bilirubin, glucuronide, glucuronidated bile acids) across their apical membrane into the canaliculi via two ATP-dependent pumps:

- ATP-dependent bile salt export pump (**BSEP**)
- ATP-dependent canalicular multispecific organic anion transporter (**cMOAT**).

Na⁺ ions accompany the negatively charged bile salts and together they create an osmotic force for water movement into the bile canaliculi. The flow of water from the hepatocytes through the tight junctions between the hepatocytes brings other solutes by solvent drag, producing canalicular bile, which is isosmotic with plasma (~300 mosmol/kg). The bile acids form micelles with cholesterol and phospholipids entering the canaliculi from the hepatocytes. This effectively lowers their concentration and more cholesterol and phospholipid enter the bile.

Bile-salt-independent flow The hepatocytes produce a small bile-salt-independent secretion. The intra-hepatic bile duct cells, called **cholangiocytes**, have a similar function to pancreatic duct cells and produce an isotonic, bicarbonate-rich secretion by the same mechanism as described for pancreatic juice secretion. In summary, the opening of Cl⁻ channels in the apical membranes of the cholangiocytes leads to the diffusion of Cl⁻ into the bile duct, with water movement by osmosis via aquaporin 1 channels. Cl⁻ is exchanged for HCO_3^- produced by cholangiocytes. The bile has a higher concentration of HCO_3^- than the plasma and a lower Cl⁻ concentration. The cholangiocytes have secretin receptors on their basolateral membranes and are stimulated to secrete bicarbonate by the intestinal hormone secretin. This leads to a watery alkaline secretion. Another intestinal hormone, cholecystokinin, potentiates the action of secretin.

The bile ducts also have the ability to reabsorb NaCl and water. This function is observed following removal of the gall bladder.

The liver and drug metabolism

The metabolism of drugs is discussed in detail in Chapter 4. The role of the liver is summarised here as a reminder to the reader. The liver metabolises most drugs, including alcohol. Orally administered drugs are absorbed by the small intestine and transported to the liver via the portal vein, then distributed to the relevant compartments in the body. Outcomes of hepatic drug metabolism include the production of less pharmacologically active metabolites, production of active metabolites that are more potent than the parent drug, conversion of inactive pro-drug to the active drug, production of toxic metabolites and elimination of inactive metabolites.

When in the liver, the drug undergoes:

- First pass metabolism: some drugs, such as glyceryl trinitrate, are completely metabolised and inactivated by the liver so that this class of drugs cannot be administered orally. When a drug is partially inactivated by the liver, producing metabolites with reduced biological activity, a larger dose may be needed. In the elderly or patients with impaired liver function, a drug may not be sufficiently metabolised during first pass metabolism, potentially leading to toxic side effects. In such patients, the usual dose of the drug will need to be reduced.
- Phase I metabolic reactions: these involve microsomal enzymes in the hepatocytes (the mixed function oxidases), of which the cytochrome P450 system is the most important. This mechanism is also known as preconjugation, when the drug undergoes oxidation, reduction and hydrolysis. Oxidation is the most important reaction. Hepatic synthesis of cytochrome P450 enzymes is increased by some classes of drug, a phenomenon known as **enzyme induction**. Enzyme induction increases the rate of phase I reactions. Some drugs cause enzyme inhibition by reducing hepatic enzyme synthesis. These actions lead to reduction or enhancement of the therapeutic effects of drugs, and, particularly when several drugs are administered together, may lead to unwanted side effects. Not all phase I reactions are performed by cytochrome P450 enzymes, some are non-microsomal, located in the hepatic cytoplasm, notably alcohol dehydrogenase and xanthine oxidase (see Ch. 4).
- Phase II metabolic reactions are conjugation reactions where hepatic cytoplasmic enzymes conjugate a phase I metabolite (and sometimes an endogenous substance), most commonly by glucuronidation. The conjugate is nearly always pharmacologically inactive, more water soluble and easily excreted in the urine and/or bile. Conjugation with glutathione is the major pathway for drug detoxification. Unfortunately, some conjugates are more toxic than the parent drug, resulting in hepatotoxicity and potential liver failure. One example is acetaminophen (paracetamol), which taken in overdose is highly toxic (see Information box 4.6, Ch. 4). Some halogenated inhaled general anaesthetics are also hepatotoxic (Ch. 4). Alcohol is toxic to the liver and a major cause of liver disease.

The pharmacokinetics and pharmacodynamics of drugs determine hepatic response. The genes coding for the enzymes, transporters and receptors concerned with drug metabolism vary between individuals, so that each person's response to a drug is variable. Pharmacogenomics, a study of this individual variability, has clinical significance for the future development of medicines.

Immunological functions of the liver

As well as synthesising acute phase proteins necessary for the body's immune mechanisms (see above), immunologically active cells are present in the hepatic reticulo-endothelial system. The body's immune system can be severely impaired when these cells are destroyed in liver disease.

- **Kupffer cells** phagocytise and catalyse bacterial and other antigens absorbed from the gastrointestinal tract, acting as a protective barrier. These antigens are catalysed without the production of antibodies, thus preventing them from reaching and overwhelming other antibody-producing sites.

- The liver also participates in tissue repair. Following challenge from endotoxins, Kupffer cells release cytokines that, in turn, stimulate hepatocytes to release pro-inflammatory cytokines (see Ch. 6).

The liver and hormones

As mentioned previously, steroid hormones are synthesised in the liver. The liver converts inactive hormone to its active form, e.g. cholecalciferol to 25-hydroxycalciferol essential for vitamin D metabolism (see Chs 10 and 16). The liver is also the target for insulin, central for glucose homeostasis (see Ch. 3). The liver inactivates hormones, including insulin, glucagon, glucocorticoids, parathormone, thyroxine, growth and sex hormones. The rate of clearance is variable; for example, insulin is cleared in minutes, steroid hormones take days and thyroxine takes months (see Ch. 10).

Storage function of the liver

The liver is the main storage site for vitamins A, B_{12}, D and K. Iron is stored bound to ferritin in hepatocytes. The liver also functions as a storage site for glycogen.

SOME DISEASES OF THE LIVER

Some clinical conditions resulting from disorders of liver function have already been discussed. In general, liver disease may be the consequence of:

- Hepatocellular damage, when hepatocytes and Kupffer cells are destroyed, and the sinusoids and space of Disse are obliterated. Depending on the cause and severity of the damage, most, if not all, liver functions will be impaired to varying degrees.
- Biliary obstruction, also known as cholestasis, which can occur in small bile ducts intra-hepatically, or in the larger extra-hepatic bile ducts. Jaundice is a clinical manifestation of biliary obstruction and intra-hepatic disease (see Clinical box 15.11).

Hepatocellular disease

Hepatocellular inflammation, known as hepatitis, may be acute or chronic. In acute hepatitis, the portal tracts and lobules are infiltrated by lymphocytes, and the hepatocytes degenerate, become necrotic and are phagocytised. This is followed by fibrosis when the stellate cells are activated to produce collagen (see above). Depending on cause and severity, single or small groups of cells may be affected (focal or spotty necrosis).

More severe damage leads to limited confluent necrosis with collapse of the acinar and lobular architecture (see Fig. 15.25 below). Bridges form between central veins and portal tracts, obstructing portal blood flow, which results in portal hypertension (see below). In the worst case, massive liver necrosis occurs involving numerous hepatic lobules with damage to a substantial part of the hepatic parenchyma. Massive liver necrosis results in fulminant hepatic failure, when encephalopathy develops (see below). Other changes include cholestasis in the acinar metabolic zone 3 and fatty change (steatosis). Steatosis (fatty deposits in hepatocytes) is commonly due to alcoholic hepatitis and drug toxicity.

In chronic hepatitis, lymphoid follicles are present in the portal tracts, which are infiltrated with lymphocytes and plasma cells. Mild to severe inflammation may be present, with further loss of definition in the acinus, changes in the hepatic lobule, confluent necrosis and fibrosis linking (bridging) the portal tracts.

Some causes of hepatitis

Table 15.12 summarises the main causes of hepatitis.

Cirrhosis of the liver

The liver is unusual in having the ability to regenerate. Prometheus, the Titan in Greek mythology, was chained to a rock where an eagle ate his liver every day, but he grew a whole new one every night. Some of the pathological features in liver disease are related to cellular regeneration.

Cirrhosis of the liver is a separate entity from hepatitis, although it may be a consequence of hepatocellular damage caused by hepatitis. Hepatic cirrhosis results from hepatocellular necrosis followed by fibrosis, and nodular regener-

Table 15.12	Causes of hepatitis	
Cause	**Acute hepatitis**	**Chronic hepatitis**
Viral	Hepatitis A–E: commonest cause of acute hepatitis is hepatitis A virus	Hepatitis B, (sometimes plus hepatitis D), hepatitis C
	Epstein–Barr virus (infectious mononucleosis)	
	Cytomegalovirus	
	Yellow fever	
	Herpes simplex	
	Mumps	
	Rubella	
Non-viral, parasitic	Toxoplasmosis	Schistosomiasis
Drugs	Analgesics, e.g. paracetamol	Anti-tuberculosis, e.g. isoniazid
	Halogenated anaesthetics	Antibiotics, e.g. nitrofurantoin, ketoconazole
		Anti-epileptics, e.g. sodium valproate
		Antihypertensives, e.g. methyldopa, amiodarone
		Alcohol (rare)
Autoimmune		Associated with pernicious anaemia, Coomb's +ve haemolytic anaemia, thyroiditis
Genetic		Wilson's disease
		Gilbert's syndrome
		Hereditary haemochromatosis
		Non-alcoholic fatty liver
Other		Chronic hepatitis of unknown cause
		Inflammatory bowel disease (e.g. ulcerative colitis) gives rise to sclerosing cholangitis with subsequent hepatocellular damage, thus strictly a biliary tract disease, and not hepatitis

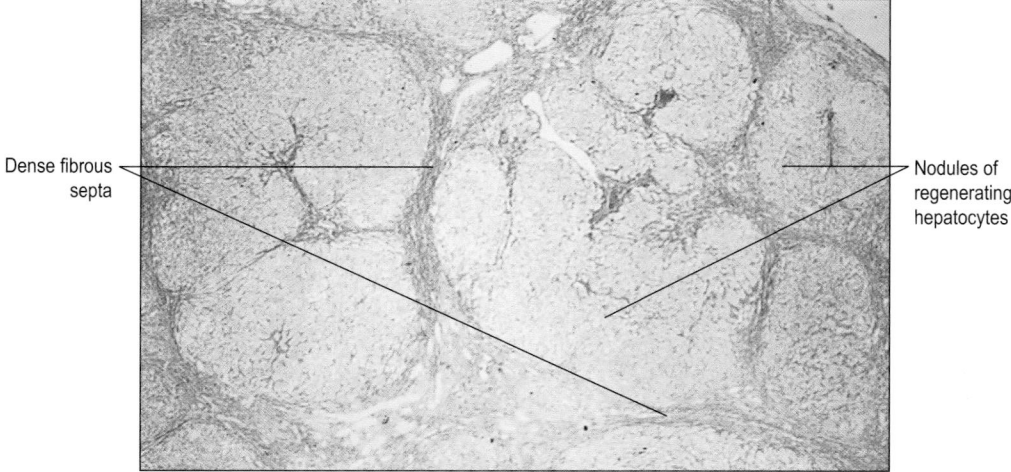

Dense fibrous septa

Nodules of regenerating hepatocytes

Fig. 15.25 **Cirrhosis of the liver.** The specimen is stained with Van Gieson stain so collagen is blue. Note disruption of normal lobular architecture (cf Figs 15.23 and 15.24). Courtesy of Dr Gregory J Michael. Institute of Cell and Molecular Science, Barts and The London School of Medicine and Dentistry, Queen Mary University of London.

ation. The pathology is characterised by dense fibrous septa surrounding variable-sized nodules of regenerating hepatocytes (Fig.15.25). The normal lobular architecture is disrupted, leading to impaired liver function and obstruction to liver blood flow.

World wide, the commonest cause of cirrhosis is viral hepatitis, and the commonest cause of cirrhosis in developed nations is excessive alcohol ingestion. There is no known cure for cirrhosis. Management is aimed at prevention of disease progression and treatment of complications. Occasionally, liver transplantation is the treatment option.

Portal hypertension

Portal hypertension is a serious complication of cirrhosis. The portal vein receives blood from the superior mesenteric and splenic veins, with a normal venous pressure of 5–8 mmHg within it. As a consequence of scarring through fibrosis and distortion of lobular architecture, venous blood flow is obstructed, elevating portal pressure. When the portal venous pressure rises above 10–12 mmHg, portosystemic anastomoses occur in the systemic venous system at sites where the venous system is pliant and collaterals are formed. Dilated collaterals are known as varices. The main sites for portosystemic anastomoses include the gastro-oesophageal junction (oesophageal varices), the rectum (haemorrhoids), and the anterior abdominal wall via the umbilical vein (caput medusae; visible on inspection of the abdomen as snake-like varices radiating from the umbilicus). Oesophageal varices are thin-walled and superficial, thus likely to rupture, causing life-threatening haemorrhage, which may be compounded by coagulation defects.

Ascites

The presence of extracellular fluid in the peritoneal cavity is known as ascites. The mechanisms through which ascites accumulates are uncertain, but possibly include renal water and sodium retention as the consequence of peripheral arterial vasodilatation. Some factors contributing to the formation of ascites include:

Clinical box 15.12 **Clinical features of hepatocellular failure**

The clinical features of hepatic failure are related to the inability of hepatocytes to perform normal physiological functions for enzyme synthesis, protein and coagulation factor synthesis, metabolism and bile production. Measurement of biochemical markers for dysfunction in liver function tests is done when hepatic failure is suspected (see Clinical box 15.13).

Jaundice (see Clinical box 15.11) is not strictly a consequence of hepatocellular failure, but of biliary obstruction from whatever cause. Intra-hepatic biliary obstruction, however, may be a consequence of cirrhosis and hepatitis, when there is distortion of normal hepatic architecture.

Hepatocellular failure may be classified as chronic or acute. Chronic hepatic failure is most commonly seen in cirrhosis, which potentially has many causes, including hepatitis and alcohol misuse. Some patients with chronic hepatitis or in the early stages of cirrhosis may be asymptomatic, but biochemical tests may be abnormal. For example, macrocytosis (abnormal lipid synthesis) and an elevated γ-glutamyl transferase (cholestasis) may be the only clues to alcohol overuse. Other biochemical markers of liver function may be abnormal. Histology ranges from mild to moderate inflammation to cirrhosis, when features of portal hypertension, ascites and porto-systemic encephalopathy may develop progressively.

Primary biliary cirrhosis is a condition in which there is progressive destruction of the bile canaliculi, resulting in cholestasis and eventually hepatocellular necrosis. Over time, this leads to fibrosis, cirrhosis and hepatic failure. The condition predominantly affects women, with onset at over 40 years of age. The aetiology is unknown, but autoimmune mechanisms have been implicated.

Acute hepatic failure occurs when encephalopathy develops over a short period in patients with apparently normal livers. Acute hepatic failure is further classified as subacute when the encephalopathy develops from 2 to 12 weeks of the onset of symptoms (e.g. jaundice), and fulminant when encephalopathy develops in less than 2 weeks. Fulminant hepatic failure occasionally develops in patients with previous liver disease.

Encephalopathy may be indicated by symptoms of altered mental state; such as confusion, disorientation and drowsiness, but may progress to hepatic coma, cerebral oedema and death. A peculiar smell, fetor hepaticus (an offensive odour due to liver disease), may be present on the patient's breath, caused by the presence of volatile, aromatic products of metabolism that accumulate in the blood and are excreted in expired breath.

Clinically, a battery of laboratory biochemical measurements is used as tests of liver function. These tests, however, do not indicate how the liver is functioning at the cellular level, but are markers of cellular dysfunction. Liver function tests are performed on serum or plasma, and include:

- Bilirubin: a marker of haem catabolism. The level of conjugated bilirubin reflects biliary obstruction, while unconjugated bilirubin is a reflection of haemolysis.
- Albumin, prothrombin: markers of protein synthesis
- Transaminases: serum aspartate aminotransferase (AST) and alanine aminotransferase (ALT) are markers of hepatocellular damage.
- Hepatic alkaline phosphatase (ALP) and γ-glutaryl transpeptidase levels reflect cholestasis. Confusingly, ALP could also be raised in bone disease (see Chs 9 and 16).

Other tests that are not specifically liver function tests, but are associated with liver disease include:

- Urea and ammonia: markers of protein catabolism.
- Haemoglobin: anaemia associated with chronic bleeding from oesophageal varices; macrocytosis associated with abnormal lipid synthesis, occurs in alcoholism.
- Cholesterol and triglycerides: reflect abnormal lipid metabolism.
- Immunoglobulins: raised concentrations reflect the reduced phagocytosis of absorbed antigen by Kupffer cells resulting in increased activity at other antibody producing sites.
- α_1-Antitrypsin: deficiency associated with cirrhosis.
- α-Fetoprotein: marker of hepatocellular carcinoma.
- Drug half-life is sometimes measured where drug metabolism is compromised.

- Portal hypertension: this causes a rise in local hydrostatic pressure, which results in increased venous pressure in the capillary beds servicing the intestines and spleen, leading to increased hepatic and splanchnic lymph production and fluid transudation into the peritoneal cavity.
- Increased venous pressure in the splanchnic capillary bed: this reduces water absorption leading to the accumulation of extracellular fluid in the peritoneum. Hypoalbuminaemia due to failure of hepatic albumin synthesis also reduces plasma oncotic pressure, which further reduces water absorption.

Porto-systemic encephalopathy

- Porto-systemic encephalopathy is a neuropsychiatric condition seen in fulminant hepatic failure and advanced cirrhosis, which is potentially reversible, but may lead to coma and death.
- Failure of the liver to metabolise toxic endogenous (e.g. ammonia) and exogenous (e.g. drugs) substances results in an accumulation of these substances in the blood, which circulate to the central nervous system with consequent encephalopathy.
- In portal hypertension, portal blood bypasses the liver through the collaterals, to deliver toxic metabolites directly to the brain, leading to encephalopathy.

GALL BLADDER

The functions of the gall bladder are the storage, concentration and discharge of bile into the intestine. Bile leaving the liver in the hepatic duct between meals is diverted into the gall bladder as a consequence of the closure of the sphincter

Raised concentrations of bile salts, bile pigment (bilirubin from the breakdown of haem) and/or cholesterol may lead to precipitation of these substances in the biliary tree or gall bladder, causing irritation and the formation of gall stones.

- Irritation of the gall bladder wall gives rise to chemical cholecystitis and inflammation.
- Gall stones cause obstruction in the biliary tree with an increased risk of infection – ascending cholangitis and cholecystitis, with further formation of gall stones.
- Obstruction to the common bile duct prevents the secretion of bile into the small intestine so that fat digestion and absorption would be impaired.
- Common bile duct obstruction also prevents the excretion of bilirubin, resulting in clinical jaundice.
- The retention of some drugs and poisons normally excreted in bile could lead to toxicity and other adverse effects.

of Oddi. The gall bladder musculature relaxes to receive the bile. The human gall bladder can accommodate to hold 20–50 mL of bile. Hepatic biliary secretion between meals is about 450 mL.

Bile is concentrated in the gall bladder

In the gall bladder the volume of bile is reduced and concentrated (Fig. 15.21D). The gall bladder concentrates the bile by reabsorbing Na^+, Cl^- and water. Na^+ and Cl^- ions, in the gall bladder lumen, are exchanged for protons and bicarbonate ions, respectively, from the cytoplasm of the epithelial cells. The Na^+ ions are removed from the epithelial cell along the basolateral border by the Na^+ pump. Chloride ions exit the cell via Cl^- channels in these membranes. The observation that the intercellular spaces dilate when fluid is being absorbed suggests that this is the route of fluid absorption. The accumulation of salt in the intercellular space will create an osmotic gradient for the transfer of water from the lumen of the gall bladder. Water passes from the lumen through channels in the membranes and between the cells along this gradient. The resulting solution becomes diluted as it flows towards and through the basement membrane of the epithelium and into capillaries.

The overall result is that the many components of gall bladder bile are more concentrated compared with hepatic bile (see Table 15.11). The bile remains isotonic to plasma because the micelle concentration increases. The aggregates of salts, phospholipids and cholesterol in the micelles have only a small osmotic activity.

The protons secreted by the gall bladder epithelium decrease bile pH and increase the solubility of calcium salts. In turn, this action reduces the possibility of gall stone formation caused by the precipitation of calcium salts. Epithelial cells also secrete mucus to protect their apical membranes from the damaging effects of bile salts. Excessive mucus secretion may contribute to gall stone formation.

Emptying of the gall bladder

Neural and hormonal mechanisms control the emptying of the gall bladder and the expulsion of bile into the intestine

Table 15.13   Structural features of the duodenum, jejunum and ileum

	Brunner's glands	Circular folds	Crypt of Lieberkühn	Villus shape	Paneth cells	Peyer's patches
Duodenum	++	+	+	Broad and short	+	+
Jejunum	−	++	+	Long finger-like	+	+
Ileum	−	+	+	Short finger-like	+	+

+, present; ++, present and distinguishing feature; −, absent.

during a meal. Vagal nerves release acetylcholine to cause gall bladder contraction during the cephalic phase of digestion. Fats in the small intestine stimulate the secretion of **cholecystokinin** that in turn causes smooth muscle contraction in the gall bladder and relaxation of the sphincter of Oddi to allow bile flow along the common bile duct into the intestine. Bile empties into the duodenum during periods in which the musculature is relaxed.

Enterohepatic circulation of bile salts

The liver does not have the capacity to synthesise de novo the quantity of bile salts needed to aid the digestion of fat in each day's meals, so the bile salts have to be recycled from the intestine to meet this need. The enterocytes along the length of most of the intestine are impermeable to conjugated bile salts. This effect maintains a high concentration of bile salts to promote fat digestion and absorption, which is usually complete before the terminal ileum is reached by the chyme.

The enterocytes of the terminal ileum possess transport mechanisms for conjugated and non-conjugated bile salts. A Na^+-dependent bile salt transporter is present in the brush border of the enterocytes that preferentially absorbs the negatively charged conjugated bile salts. The absorbed bile salts probably leave the epithelial cells by an anion exchanger.

Non-conjugated bile salts may be passively absorbed if they become protonated, which removes their negative charges, increasing their lipid solubility. Passive absorption accounts for about 10% of the recycling of the bile salts that can occur along the length of the small intestine and colon. The bile salts are transported in the hepatic portal vein to the liver where they are again extracted and secreted into the bile.

Bile salts that escape absorption from the small intestine are metabolised by colonic bacteria. This can involve deconjugation, which increases their lipid solubility and reabsorption. In addition, bacteria are responsible for the conversion of primary bile acids to secondary bile acids, which may be absorbed. Approximately 5% of the bile salts entering the duodenum are excreted each day. The liver synthesises this quantity each day to make up for the loss. Increases in bile salt excretion are matched by increases in the synthesis in order to maintain the bile salt pool.

SMALL INTESTINE

The small intestine is the major site for the digestion and absorption of food, salts, water and orally administered drugs. The small intestine consists of the:

- Duodenum
- Jejunum
- Ileum.

It serves to:

- Mix digestive secretions with food and propel chyme along the intestine
- Digest and absorb nutrients
- Absorb the constituents of digestive secretions
- Regulate gastric function
- Synthesise and secrete hormones influencing feeding and gastric function
- Defend the body against invasion by microorganisms.

STRUCTURE OF THE SMALL INTESTINE

The generalised structure of the alimentary canal was outlined above. The small intestine is 4–7 m in length. The duodenum is 25–30 cm in length and is recognised externally by an absence of mesentery. There are histological differences between the duodenum, jejunum and ileum (Table 15.13). The surface area of the mucosa is increased by the presence of outgrowths of the submucosa to form circular folds, the plicae circularis or valves of Kerkring, on which are found finger-like projections known as villi. The surface area of the luminal border of the enterocytes is enlarged by the presence of microvilli that create a large surface area for the final stages of digestion and absorption. The total increase in surface area of the intestine produced by the folding the submucosa, mucosa and enterocyte surface is 600 times that of a cylinder with the same internal dimensions as the small intestine.

The villi contain smooth muscle fibres arranged along the length of their core which are attached to the central lacteal, a blind-ended lymph vessel. Contraction and relaxation of the muscle changes the length of the villi and in the process propel lymph along the lacteal vessels. Lymph flows into the lymphatic vessels in the submucosa and onwards through the abdomen to the thoracic lymph duct, which empties its contents into the junction of the left subclavian and internal jugular veins.

The intestinal glands or crypts of Lieberkühn are simple tubular glands lying between the bases of the villi. The crypts contain **stem**, **entero-endocrine** and **Paneth** cells. The stem cells become differentiated into enterocytes and goblet cells as they migrate from the crypts to the tip of the villus. The cells take 3–6 days to reach the tip of the villus where they are extruded and become part of the intestinal juice (succus entericus). The crypts are the source of the intestinal juice, an alkaline fluid similar in composition to extracellular fluid, containing the enzyme enteropeptidase which is responsible for activating trypsinogen. The intestinal juice also contains digestive enzymes derived from extruded enterocytes. The enterocytes begin to synthesise digestive enzymes, develop microvilli and become absorptive cells as they migrate along the villus.

Entero-endocrine cells play a role controlling digestion and local defence mechanisms. They synthesise and secrete intestinal hormones, e.g. cholecystokinin and secretin, and local hormones, e.g. 5-hydroxytryptamine (serotonin). Mechanical stimulation of enterochromaffin cells by the passage of the intestinal contents (chyme, parasites, bacteria) releases 5-hydroxytryptamine and leads to activation of the enteric reflexes, leading to, for example, intestinal fluid secretion and peristalsis. Chemical stimulation of enterochromaffin cells by some anti-cancer drugs produces vomiting via vagal nerve sensory pathways.

The Paneth cells are part of the intestinal defence system against bacteria and parasites. These cells secrete tumour necrosis factor-α (TNF-α), lysozyme and defensins. TNF-α produces inflammation in response to bacteria and parasites. Lysozyme destroys the peptidoglycan bonds in bacterial membranes leading to an influx of water and rupture of the bacteria. Defensins are proteins that produce ion channels in the cell membranes of invading organisms to increase their permeability.

The ileum contains **Peyer's patches** in the submucosa, and they extend into the mucosa where they are covered by an epithelial layer, containing enterocytes, M cells and **dendritic cells**. The M and dendritic cells are capable of taking up antigens and transferring them by exocytosis to the interstitial fluid for processing by macrophages, T and B lymphocytes. Processed antigens produce an immune reaction. The centre of the Peyer's patch contains a germinal centre for proliferating B cells. The Peyer's patches form part of the gut-associated lymphoid tissue (GALT), which includes lymphocytes found between epithelial cells in the intestinal mucosa and in the lamina propria of the mucosa, together with mast cells. The plasma cells secrete IgA antibodies which are transferred by enterocytes to the intestinal lumen, where they react with bacteria and toxins to prevent them becoming attached to epithelial cells. These immunological mechanisms and the non-immunological mechanisms, such as gastric acid secretion, intestinal fluid and mucus secretion, and peristalsis, assist in the defence of the body from luminal pathogens (see Ch. 6).

SMALL INTESTINAL FLUID SECRETION

The enterocytes in the crypts of Lieberkühn are responsible for intestinal fluid secretion. The volume of fluid produced is 1–2 L/day. The production of intestinal fluid secretion is driven by Cl^- secretion from enterocytes. The $Na^+/K^+/Cl^-$ transporter in the basolateral border transfers Cl^- into the cell from the interstitial fluid. The inward movement of the transporter occurs secondary to the action of the Na^+/K^+-ATPase which maintains a low Na^+ concentration in the cell. Cl^- enters the lumen of the intestine by diffusion through Cl^- channels in the apical membrane. These Cl^- channels are a protein known as the cystic fibrosis transmembrane regulator (CFTR). K^+ leaves the cell through K^+ channels in the basolateral border. The intestinal lumen become electronegative and that leads to the flow of Na^+ from the interstitial fluid through paracellular pathways (tight junctions). The movement of NaCl results in an osmotic gradient and the movement of water into the intestine.

In the absence of stimulation there is little fluid secretion. Intestinal fluid secretion is regulated by:

- The enteric nervous system
- Hormones
- Enterotoxins.

Chloride secretion is primarily controlled by the submucosal plexus of the enteric nervous system. Mechanical stimulation of enterochromaffin cells leads to the release of 5-hydroxytryptamine that stimulates sensory neurons to activate secretomotor neurons terminating on enterocytes. The neurotransmitters stimulating the enterocytes are acetylcholine and VIP, via muscarinic M_3 and VIP receptors, respectively. Axon reflexes within the mucosa may also stimulate secretion via substance P acting on neurokinin 1 (NK1) receptors on the enterocytes. Mechanical stimulation of the mucosa also releases prostaglandins, which stimulate the secretomotor neurons. The intracellular messengers for acetylcholine and VIP are Ca^{2+} and cAMP, respectively. The elevation of the intracellular concentration of Ca^{2+} and cAMP leads to stimulation of the enterocytes and fluid secretion.

The intestinal hormone, guanylin, stimulates the guanylin receptor on the apical border of the enterocyte to increase the activity on guanylate cyclase and increase the intracellular concentration of cyclic guanosine monophosphate. This also leads to the opening of the Cl^- channels in the apical membrane. Antigen–antibody reactions at mast cells in the lamina propria and stimulation of these cells by substance P released during axon reflexes lead to histamine release. Histamine stimulates secretion by a direct effect on histamine receptors on the enterocytes and indirectly via cholinergic nerves.

Finally, bacterial toxins (enterotoxins) stimulate enterocytes both directly and by means of enteric reflexes.

SMALL INTESTINAL MOTILITY

In between meals the small intestine undergoes periodic contractile activity at intervals lasting 80–90 minutes. The propulsive waves (known as the migrating motor complexes, MMC) begin in the stomach (see above) and sweep along the small intestine, clearing it of debris and bacteria.

Each MMC consists of four phases:

Phase I a prolonged quiescent period (45–60 minutes) with slow waves.
Phase II a period (30–35 minutes) of action potentials, apparently randomly superimposed on the slow waves, and sporadic contractions. This phase is associated with gastric acid, bile and pancreatic juice secretion.
Phase III a period (2–12 minutes) of activity with action potentials superimposed on each slow wave and regular contractions at the rate of 3 per minute in the stomach and 10–12 per minute in the small intestine.
Phase IV a period in which action potential production and contractile activity reduces and merges into phase I.

The MMC also prevents reflux of bacteria from the large intestine to the terminal ileum. The MMC has been described as the 'housekeeper of the small intestine'. However, within a few minutes of feeding this type of motility ceases.

The small intestine receives chyme from the stomach and digestive secretions from the pancreas, biliary tract and intestinal mucosa. The function of small intestinal motility after eating is to:

- Mix the nutrients in the chyme with the digestive secretions
- Bring the chyme into contact with the epithelial cells to promote the final stages of digestion
- Regulate the rate at which chyme is propelled along the small intestine to the caecum.

Two types of small intestinal motility are needed to fulfil these objectives. Mixing of the chyme with the secretions and bringing the mixture into contact with the mucosa is achieved by the process of **segmentation** (Fig. 15.18B). This is achieved by contractions of the circular muscle layer at short intervals along the intestine. The intestine in between the contracted regions is relaxed. The chyme is propelled a short distance orally and aborally from a point of contraction. The contracted circular muscles relax and are replaced by contractions in the formerly relaxed region. This type of motility will not be very effective in propelling chyme along the intestine to the caecum. It is, however, effective in mixing the chyme with secretions and in breaking up the unstirred layer of fluid adjacent to the epithelial cells to aid nutrient absorption.

Peristalsis propels chyme along the small intestine. This is achieved by contraction of the circular muscle layer on the oral side of the bolus of chyme and relaxation on the aboral side (Fig. 15.18C). The contractile action of the musculature pushes the bolus into the adjacent area of the intestine which is ready to receive it. Peristalsis consists of a repeated pattern of contraction and relaxation of the circular muscle layer of the small intestine. The peristaltic response is controlled by nerves in the enteric nervous system. Distension of the wall of the intestine stimulates mechanoreceptors in the mucosa and muscle layers that synapse with excitatory and inhibitory neural pathways, producing contraction of the circular muscle and relaxation of the longitudinal muscle layers at the point of stimulation. The reflex spreads into the adjoining region ahead of the bolus with the longitudinal muscles being stimulated to contract and the circular muscles to relax to create a dilated region to receive the bolus of chyme. Entry of the bolus stimulates the sensory receptors and the reflex is repeated to propel the bolus along the intestine.

As has been described for the stomach, smooth muscle cells in the small intestine are associated with slow waves of depolarisation to a plateau, followed by repolarisation. Action potentials superimposed on the plateau lead to a contraction. Slow waves are detected in adjacent parts of the intestine and are related in time but do not always give rise to action potentials. A region showing slow waves with action potentials may be separated from another one by a region with slow wave activity alone. This pattern of electrical activity is consistent with segmentation. Interstitial cells of Cajal generate slow wave activity. The frequency of slow waves in the duodenum is about 12 per minute, slowing to 10 per minute in the jejunum and 9 per minute in the ileum. This decline in frequency of pacemaker activity along the intestine is known as the **intestinal gradient**.

Intestino-intestinal inhibitory reflex

If a region of the intestine becomes distended or obstructed, contractile muscle activity in adjacent regions are inhibited. This is a response known as the intestino-intestinal reflex and depends upon the activation of sympathetic nerves via the coeliac ganglion and spinal cord.

Clinical box 15.14 **Causes of small intestine disease**

Diseases of the small intestine disrupt the normal mechanisms of digestion and absorption, giving rise to symptoms of diarrhoea (occasionally steatorrhoea), abdominal pain and discomfort, weight loss and nutritional deficiencies from malabsorption. Causes include:

- Infection – which may be acute or chronic, from gastrointestinal infections and infestations (e.g. *Giardia*), dysentery, cholera, human immunodeficiency virus (HIV) enteropathy, tuberculosis. The diarrhoea may be produced by enterotoxins. For example, the profuse diarrhoea and electrolyte imbalance in cholera is cause by the stimulation of Cl⁻ secretion by the irreversible activation of G proteins by cholera toxin. This leads to fluid loss via increased cAMP in enterocytes.
- Inflammation – which may be autoimmune, associated with connective tissue disorders (e.g. rheumatoid arthritis), ulcerative colitis, regional ileitis (Crohn's disease), gluten sensitive enteropathy (coeliac disease), leads to enterocyte destruction and loss of function.
- Ischaemic – occlusion of arterial or venous blood flow, which occurs more often in the elderly.
- Tumours – either tumours of the small intestine (e.g. adenocarcinoma, carcinoid tumour, polyps – Peutz–Jeghers syndrome), or more distal tumours causing abnormalities in enzyme or other secretions (e.g. Zollinger–Ellison syndrome).
- Radiation – radiation enteritis occurs after pelvic radiation with symptoms of diarrhoea and abdominal pain. This usually resolves after completion of treatment.
- Surgery/trauma – intestinal resection, especially after massive resection.
- Drugs – particularly antibiotics (e.g. amoxicillin), and rarely antibiotic-associated colitis, and drugs that bind to bile salts.

Gastro-ileal reflex

An increase in gastric activity during a meal leads to the gastro-ileal reflex in which propulsive activity of the terminal ileum is increased and its contents are emptied into the caecum via the relaxed ileo-caecal sphincter. This reflex response may be mediated by the extrinsic innervation of the ileum. The gastric antral hormone gastrin and duodenal hormone cholecystokinin have also been implicated in the response. These hormones increase contractile activity in the ileum and relax the ileo-caecal sphincter.

Interruption of the extrinsic innervation of the ileum, as in surgical vagotomy for peptic ulceration, may give rise to chronic diarrhoea.

LARGE INTESTINE

The main function of the large intestine is to absorb water and electrolytes, and to evacuate faeces. The large intestine consists of the:

- Caecum
- Ascending, transverse, descending and sigmoid colon
- Rectum
- Anal canal.

The large intestine serves to:

- Absorb salt and water to produce semi-solid or solid faeces

- Absorb short chain fatty acids produced by colonic bacteria from unabsorbed carbohydrate entering the colon
- Act as a store for faeces
- Expel the faeces.

The mucosa of the colon does not have folds or villi like the small intestine but has numerous tubular glands (crypts of Lieberkühn). These are deeper than in the small intestine (0.4–0.6 mm) and are lined with many goblet cells, enterocytes, stem cells and entero-endocrine cells. The surface enterocytes have microvilli and an absorptive role.

LARGE INTESTINAL FLUID SECRETION

The secretions of the large intestine are similar to those found in the small intestine. However, the volume produced is less and the K^+ and HCO_3^- content is increased together with more mucus. K^+ enters the colonic secretion by both passive and active mechanisms. In the lumen a negative, transepithelial potential difference of up to 25 mV is enough to produce a diffusion of K^+ from the interstitial spaces through the tight junctions to the lumen. Active K^+ secretion occurs as a result of K^+ channels opening in the apical membrane and K^+ diffusion to the intestine. Uptake of K^+ at the basolateral membrane is due to the action of the $Na^+/K^+/Cl^-$ transporter and the Na^+/K^+-ATPase. Aldosterone increases the opening of the K^+ channels in the apical membrane. In addition, aldosterone enhances the absorption of Na^+ from the intestinal lumen leading to a rise in luminal negativity and an increase in passive secretion. It also stimulates the Na^+/K^+-ATPase, subsequently producing a greater active secretion of K^+. VIP and cholera enterotoxin, via an increase in intracellular cAMP, stimulate K^+ secretion. 5-Hydroxytryptamine stimulates a rise in intracellular Ca^{2+}, which also opens apical K^+ channels and promotes secretion. Faecal losses of K^+ by these mechanisms may be significant in secretory diarrhoea.

MUSCULATURE OF THE LARGE INTESTINE

The smooth muscle is arranged in an outer longitudinal and inner circular layers. The longitudinal muscle layer from the caecum to the rectum does not completely cover the large intestine but is arranged in three bands known as the **taeniae coli**. The layer fans out to cover the rectum. The circular muscle layer is continuous from the caecum to the anal canal. The layer becomes thicker to form the internal anal sphincter, which lies adjacent to the external anal sphincter composed of striated muscle.

LARGE INTESTINAL MOTILITY

The large intestine functions as two organs. The proximal part, consisting of the ascending and transverse colon, is the site for the bacterial production of fatty acids and their absorption together with electrolytes and water. Approximately 1.5 L of chyme per day enters the colon from the ileum. The water content of the faeces is 50–150 mL per day. The absorbed water contributes to the maintenance of water balance by the body. Absorption of fluid is aided by the segmental-like activity of the musculature. The colon is divided into segments known as **haustra**. Sequential circular muscle contraction and relaxation cause the position of the haustral folds to change after many minutes. This rate of change of position of the haustra contrasts with the more rapid changes in the position of small intestinal segments, which only last for seconds. This type of motility promotes fluid absorption.

The distal part of the colon (descending and rectosigmoid region) is responsible for the final drying of the faeces and storage before defecation. The contractile movements of sigmoid colon cause retention of the colonic contents in the descending colon. This activity promotes drying of the faeces and a reduction in their volume. The faeces may be retained in the colon for 36 hours or longer in healthy people. In some cases of constipation the contractile activity of the sigmoid colon is enhanced and is absent in diarrhoea. These observations support the view that the contractile activity of the sigmoid colon promotes water absorption from the faeces.

One to three times a day, a propulsive motility described as **a mass movement** drives the faeces in an anal direction. The haustra and segmental activity are abolished for the duration of a mass movement. Mass movements are responsible for propelling faeces into the rectum. Filling of the rectum stimulates sensory receptors that give rise to the desire to defecate. The pattern of colonic motility is similar in both the fed and interdigestive states.

The regulation of colonic motility depends on the interstitial cells of Cajal giving rise to slow wave activity leading to contraction and their modification by the action of the intrinsic and extrinsic nerves. As in other parts of the alimentary canal there are intrinsic nerves with inhibitory and excitatory action on the smooth muscle. These nerves promote mixing and propulsive activity. The excitatory extrinsic innervation is via the vagus and pelvic nerves, with acetylcholine being the major neurotransmitter. The inhibitory extrinsic innervation is provided by the lumbar and sacral branches of the sympathetic nervous system terminating in the intramural plexuses. These nerves tonically inhibit colonic motility via the neurotransmitter noradrenaline. Feeding and distension of the upper regions of the gastrointestinal tract lead to **gastrocolonic reflexes**, in which mass movements are induced via the extrinsic nerve pathways. The afferent pathway is not well defined. The efferent pathway involves the vagus and pelvic nerves to the proximal and distal parts of the colon, respectively. In addition, the hormones gastrin and cholecystokinin are capable of stimulating colonic smooth muscle and may contribute to the response. Distension of the upper colon produces a **colono-colonic reflex** in which activity via the intrinsic nerves and extrinsic sympathetic nerves from the superior and inferior mesenteric ganglia leads to relaxation of the colon.

MOTILITY OF THE RECTUM AND ANAL CANAL

During most of the day the upper portion of the rectum generates segmental activity, which tends to prevent emptying of the colonic contents into the rectum. These movements ensure that the rectum is usually empty. The levator ani muscles making up the pelvic floor are contracted and hold the rectum at an angle of about 90° to the anal canal. This angle helps to maintain continence. The anal canal is tightly closed by the anal sphincters. The rectum fills following a mass movement from the descending and sigmoid colon. Distension of the rectum leads to the urge to defecate. The rectum acts as a storage organ.

DEFECATION

The presence of gas or faeces in the rectum stimulates stretch receptors in its wall and, via the myenteric plexus, stimulates a mass movement in the sigmoid colon and rectum, initiating the **rectosphincteric reflex**. This involves a reflex relaxation of the smooth muscle of the internal anal sphincter and contraction of the striated muscle of the external anal sphincter in order to maintain continence for up to a minute. The rectal contents enter the upper anal canal, producing sensory information that distinguishes between gas, liquid or solid, probably on the basis of the amount of distension produced. Defecation will occur if the circumstances are appropriate and the external anal sphincter relaxes.

Defecation is a reflex activity and is subject to conscious control (Fig. 15.26). The sacral region of the spinal cord (segments S2 to S4) acts to integrate signals from the brain with those from stretch receptors in the rectal wall via afferent fibres in the pelvic nerves. Descending pathways from the cerebral cortex inhibit the somatic motor nerve activity in the pudendal nerves that innervate the external anal sphincter. The tonic flow of nerve impulse to the sphincter producing contraction is interrupted. The external anal sphincter relaxes and peristaltic activity of the rectum expels the faeces. Adopting a squatting position and lowering of the pelvic floor levator ani muscles allows the rectum to come into line with the anal canal. Expulsion of the faeces is aided by the development of high intrathoracic pressure produced by an inspiration followed by expiration against a closed glottis (Valsalva's manoeuvre) with contraction of the abdominal muscles. The intra-abdominal pressure can rise to 200 cm H_2O with the effect of squeezing the wall of rectum and anal canal to aid expulsion of the faeces. In addition, this high intra-abdominal pressure reduces venous return to the heart with possible temporary adverse consequences on blood pressure and the circulation.

If the circumstances are inappropriate the act of defecation is postponed. The internal sphincter contracts and the rectal contents are returned to the colon by retroperistalsis. The sensation to defecate disappears. The faeces are subject to further desiccation and reduction in volume in the colon. Repetition of these events may lead to constipation as the volume of the faeces is reduced and they are less effective at stimulating the stretch receptors in the rectal wall.

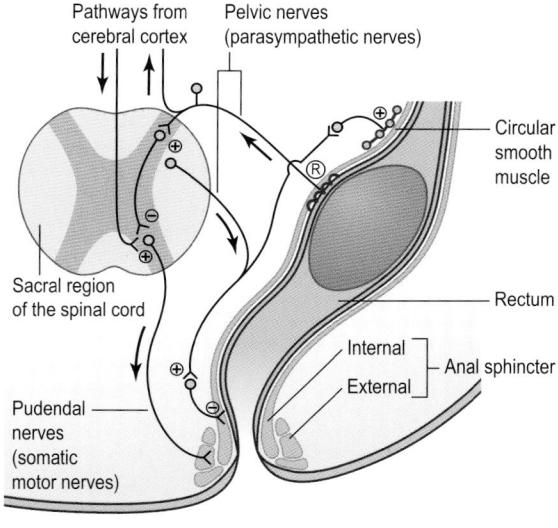

⊕ Stimulation   ⊖ Inhibition   ® Mechanoreceptor

Stimulation of distention sensitive mechanoreceptors produces a reflex contraction on the colonic side of the faeces and a relaxation of the internal and external anal sphincters via the pelvic and pudendal nerves. Pathways from the cerebral cortex can oppose this reflex.

Fig. 15.26 **Postulated neural mechanism for defecation.**

Clinical box 15.15   **Constipation**

Constipation is a complex phenomenon, and is very common. A low dietary fibre intake is a common cause, as are drugs such as diuretics, analgesics and cholinergic drugs. It occurs more often in the elderly. Increasing dietary fibre and fluid intake often relieves constipation. However, it is sometimes associated with serious bowel disease (e.g. intestinal obstruction, colonic cancer, ulcerative colitis), when a change in bowel habit or alternating diarrhoea and constipation are the more significant symptoms. Rarely, a dilated 'megacolon' occurs with chronic constipation. In young patients and children, constipation and megacolon may be due to the presence of a ganglionic rectal segment giving rise to chronic constipation (**Hirschsprung's disease**).

Training small children into a regular bowel habit of defecating at particular times of the day relies on the gastro-colonic reflex, when a natural, large peristalsis is most likely to occur in the colon, inducing defecation.

16

Diet and nutrition

Jeremy Powell-Tuck, Alison Chambers and Jeannette Naish

INTRODUCTION

In 2003, the Director General of the World Health Organization (WHO) unequivocally stated that 'proper nutrition and health are fundamental human rights'. Proper nutrition underpins human health in the sense that it influences growth, physical and intellectual development and the ability to combat disease processes. 'Bad nutrition' or malnutrition whether overnutrition (obesity) or undernutrition, is a major determinant of morbidity and mortality. Knowledge of the principles of nutrition is vital to the understanding of the prevention, diagnosis and treatment of clinical conditions.

DIET

WORLDWIDE DIETARY PATTERNS AND FOOD GUIDES

Human eating habits and dietary patterns change constantly. As average per capita income increases worldwide and the world population is expected to grow by more than 1 billion in the next decade, the combined increase in income and population growth is expected to increase and change the pattern of global food composition.

Eating habits and dietary patterns also vary greatly according to demographic and cultural factors. Historically, most people in the developing world have consumed bulky low-energy diets where half or more of the total energy is supplied by cereals, starchy roots or fruits. Since industrialisation, most people in the developed world have increasingly consumed energy-dense diets, in which less than 25% of the total energy comes from cereals, and consumption of fats, alcohol, meat and dairy products is increased.

Although there is still great disparity between the developed and the developing world's dietary patterns, this distinction has been blurring since the 1970s and 1980s, as the developing world has also become increasingly industrialised. The Food and Agriculture Organization (FAO) of the United Nations was founded in 1945 to collect, analyse, interpret and disseminate information relating to nutrition, food, agriculture, forestry and fisheries. The FAO publishes the world food survey every ten years. Figure 16.1 shows the changes in dietary patterns in different parts of the world over the 20 years from 1981 to 2001. Diets in developing areas have become more energy-dense at the same time as the populations have become less physically active. In contrast, in the developed world, a significant minority of health-conscious people are choosing to consume relatively bulky, low energy-dense diets and may also engage in physically active recreation.

FOOD GUIDES

Many countries have developed their own food guides. These are usually pictorial representations of nutrition recommendations and are usually regularly revised and updated. The food guides are a simple way of summarising the recommended balance of foods in the diet and provide a consistent message regarding dietary advice for the public. Examples can be found on the websites of the various national institutions for nutrition policy.

FOOD LABELLING

In most developed countries, there is public awareness of the healthy eating messages: the connections between diet, health and disease. However, to act on this knowledge, the general population needs nutritional information on specific foods, particularly on processed foods. Therefore, food labelling, quantifying the main nutrients, is important. In the UK (Fig. 16.2), such labelling is compulsory if a nutritional advantage is claimed for the product.

In recent years, manufacturers have started to put more nutritional labels on their products. In the European Union

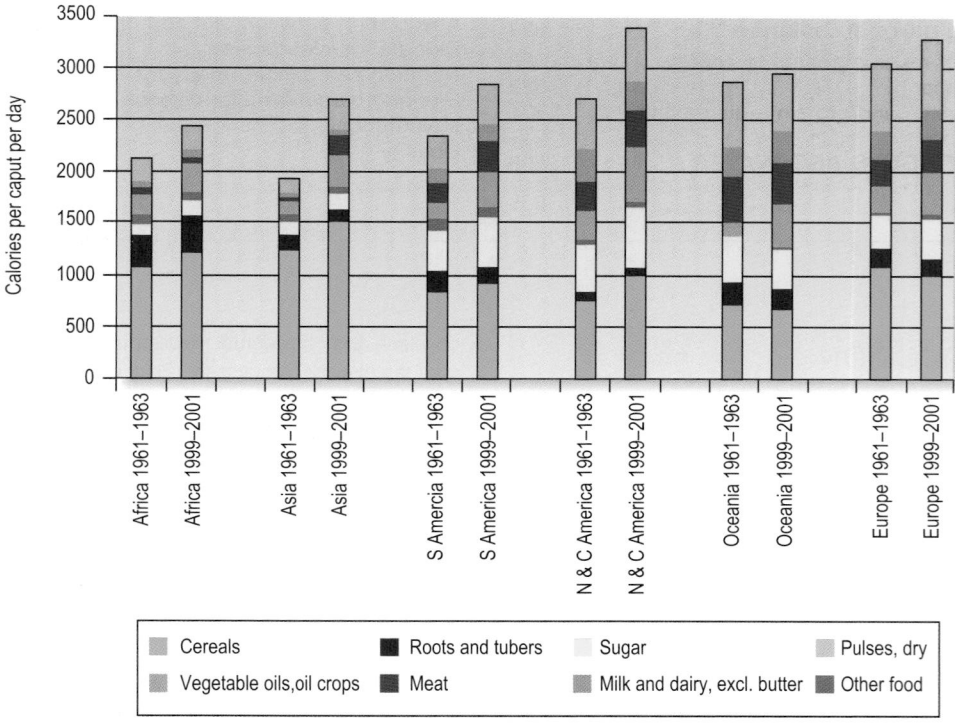

Fig. 16.1 **Dietary patterns in different continents.** *Oceania consists of Australia, New Zealand, Papua New Guinea and Fiji. Reproduced with permission from FAO Statistical Database for Supply Utilisation Accounts and Food Balances domain.

(EU), all food labelling is controlled principally by the Food Labelling Regulation 1996. All packaged food must have a label that states:

- The name of the food
- A list of ingredients in descending order of content, i.e. the first item listed is the largest ingredient
- Storage conditions and durability (best before or use-by date)
- The name and address of the manufacturer, packer or seller established within the EU.

Nutrition claims that the food is a source of a particular nutrient, health claims that the food is in some way beneficial to health, and other claims for particular uses, may be made in relation to certain products. Currently, nutrition and health claims are being reviewed by the EU to ensure that consumers are not being misled.

Food labels are compulsory when nutritional advantages are claimed. Information in the labels is as follows:

- Nutrients – energy (kJ/kcal per kg), protein, fat and carbohydrates are expressed per 100 mL/100 g or per serving.
- More detailed information regarding carbohydrates and fats is sometimes given.
- Vitamins and minerals can only be declared if providing a significant amount (approximately one-sixth of the recommended daily amount).
- Fibre content – this can be analysed by two methods which yield two different results. Currently the UK uses the Englyst method, which measures non-starch polysaccharide. However, the method used by the American Organization of Analytical Chemists (AOAC) is favoured by many UK manufacturers and most other countries and, therefore, may become the European Union standard. The AOAC method provides a higher estimate of fibre content because it measures a much wider range of dietary fibre constituents.
- Salt – this is sometimes expressed as sodium content.

DIETARY REFERENCE VALUES

Dietary reference values (DRVs) provide information on the amount of different nutrients that are needed for maintaining health in different groups of people (Fig. 16.3). Worldwide, there is broad agreement on DRVs based on data from the WHO, FAO and other expert committees of the United Nations. Many countries have produced their own dietary reference standards. For example, from the 1960s onwards, the UK used a single figure for each nutrient: recommended daily intake (RDI) or recommended daily amount (RDA). However, it was found that there was a large potential for misuse and misinterpretation of these single reference points. In response to this a committee was established and in 1991 the dietary reference values (DRVs) guidelines were produced. RDAs were replaced in the UK by three DRVs

Nutritional Information

Typical values	Per serving (1 pie)	Per 100g
Energy	914 kJ	1423 kJ
	218 kcal	339 kcal
Protein	2.3 g	3.6 g
Carbohydrate	31.0 g	48.3 g
of which Sugars	16.6 g	25.8 g
Fat	9.4 g	14.6 g
of which Saturates	1.9 g	3.0 g
Fibre	0.7 g	1.1 g
Sodium	0.1 g	0.1 g

Per serving (1 pie)

218 Calories 9.4 g Fat

Guideline daily amounts

Each Day	Women	Men
Calories	2,000	2,500
Fat	70 g	95 g

Official government figures for average adults

More detailed information regarding carbohydrates and fats is sometimes given

Salt – sometimes given as sodium

Fig. 16.2 **A UK food label.**

EAR Estimated average requirement:
half the population usually needs more than the EAR and half less.

LRNI Lower reference nutient intake:
sufficient for the few people who have low needs, but not meeting the needs of 97.5% of the population (2 standard deviations below the EAR).

RNI reference nutrient intake:
sufficient for about 97.5% of people (2 standard deviations above the EAR). If the average intake of a population is at RNI, the risk of deficiency is very small.

Safe intake:
range for which there is not enough information to estimate RNI, EAR or LRNI. Sufficient for almost everyone but not so large as to cause undesirable effects.

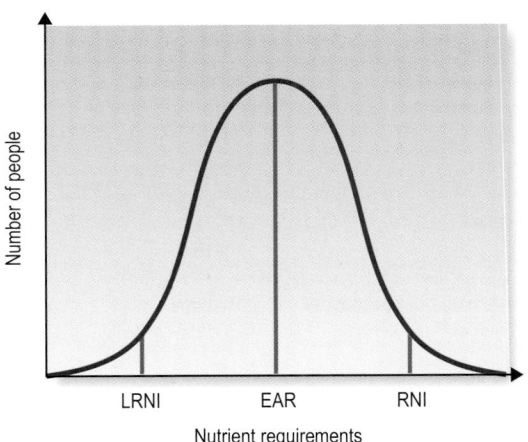

Fig. 16.3 **Dietary reference values for a population.** Reproduced with permission from Department of Health 1991 Dietary reference values for food energy and nutrients for the United Kingdom. HMSO, London (Report on Health and Social Subjects, No. 41).

reference nutrient intake (RNI), estimated average requirement (EAR) and lower reference nutrient intake (LRNI)). The RNI (Fig. 16.3) values are similar to the RDAs, and meet the nutrient needs of the vast majority (97%) of any healthy population. The RNI for different nutrients is set two standard deviations above the EAR, the amount of a nutrient which is needed daily on average in a large population of normal people. The LRNI is set two standard deviations below the EAR and represents a level of usual nutrient intake which is not likely to be sufficient in more than 97% of people. Thus an intake below the RNI does not suggest deficiency, but an intake below LRNI does.

NUTRITIONAL REQUIREMENTS

The major **macronutrients** present in the human diet are proteins, fats and carbohydrates. The present WHO guidelines for a healthy diet for the prevention of chronic diseases were formulated in 2003 (Table 16.1). The recommendations are based on epidemiological and interventional studies that examined the relationship of lifestyle variables, including exercise, smoking, obesity and diet, with:

- Life expectancy
- Incidence of specific diseases, particularly cancer, coronary heart disease and stroke (see later).

VARIATIONS IN NUTRITIONAL REQUIREMENTS

Requirements for most nutrients vary with age and sex, and at times of physiological adaptation, for example during pregnancy, lactation and growth. Appropriate DRVs have thus been produced for these subgroups. In disease states such as infection, trauma, disorders of the gastrointestinal tract or metabolic abnormalities, requirements will vary. The DRVs for one nutrient assume that requirements for energy and all other nutrients are met.

Preconception

Preconceptional nutrition is known to have an impact on ovulation and sperm quality, affecting the fertility of both women and men. It should be remembered that a woman of childbearing age may not be aware of her pregnancy until near the end of the first trimester. Therefore, preconceptual nutritional advice is important and should emphasise a varied and balanced diet and a body weight within a desirable range.

Severe weight loss has an impact on ovulation. Body fat must make up at least 22% of body weight to maintain ovulation. Prolonged undernutrition, as in anorexia nervosa, can result in amenorrhoea. Conversely, obesity can also inhibit ovulation. Weight loss can induce spontaneous ovulation in previously anovulatory obese women. For example, weight reduction in overweight women with polycystic ovarian syndrome (PCOS) leads to ovulation and improves fertility.

Pregnancy

The energy demands of a pregnancy are usually estimated at approximately 323 MJ (77 000 kcal), although variations in activity levels account for major differences in the energy needs of individual women. Over the course of a full-term pregnancy, there should be an approximate weight gain of 12.5 kg, consisting of:

- 2.5 kg body weight
- 3.5 kg infant weight
- 6.5 kg placental weight.

Table 16.1	WHO guidelines for a healthy diet	
Dietary factor	**Goal***	**Important sources**
Fat	15–30	
Saturated fat	10	Meat fat, lard, dripping, butter, cheese and cream
Monounsaturated fat	By difference†	Olive and rape seed oil
Polyunsaturated fat	6–10	Vegetable oils, nuts, eggs, fish and liver
Trans fatty acids	<1	Margarine and other fat spreads
Carbohydrate	50–75‡	
Starches	33	Bread, cereal, rice, potatoes, pasta
Free sugars§	10	Sugar, fruit and cereals
Protein	10–15	Meat and meat products, milk and milk products, eggs, pulses, nuts and seeds
Fibre (non-starch polysaccharide)	18 g/day	Cereals, vegetables, fruit and nuts
Sodium chloride** (sodium)	<5 g/day; 2 g/day	Foods canned in brine, smoked or salted; yeast extract and stock cubes; 'discretionary' (added during cooking or at the table)

*Per cent of daily energy intake unless otherwise stated.
†This is calculated as: total fat − (saturated fatty acids + polyunsaturated acids + *trans* fatty acids).
‡Percentage of total energy including energy from ingested protein and fat, hence the wide range.
§The term 'free sugars' refers to all monosaccharides and disaccharides added to foods by the manufacturer, cook or consumer, plus sugars naturally present in honey, syrups and fruit juices.
 The suggested range should be seen in the light of the joint World Health Organization/Food and Agricultural Organization/United Nations University Expert Consultation on Protein and Amino Acid Requirements in Human Nutrition, Geneva, 9–16 April 2002.
**Salt should be iodised appropriately. The need to adjust salt iodination, depending on observed sodium intake and surveillance of iodine status of the population, should be recognised.

Nutrition during pregnancy

Nutritional requirements increase during pregnancy due to the requirements of the growing fetus, and the mother's body being prepared for parturition and lactation.

- Energy: there are wide variations between individuals. Minimum threshold for maternal weight gain is 6.8 kg. Additional 838 kJ (200 kcals)/day required in the third trimester. Eat according to appetite.
- Protein: an additional 6 g/day to 51 g RNI.
- Vitamins:
  - Folate: poor **folic acid** status is associated with an increased risk of neural tube defects. In most developed countries, all women who are planning a pregnancy are recommended to consider folic acid dietary supplements and to try to include folate-rich foods and foods fortified with folic acid in their diet. Women who become pregnant should supplement their diet immediately (0.4 mg folic acid) until the twelfth week of pregnancy.
  - Vitamin A: an increment of 100 µg/day to 800 µg/day throughout pregnancy. High doses (>1500 µg) are known to be teratogenic.
  - Vitamin D: supplemented to achieve an intake of 10 µg/day.
  - Vitamin C: increase by 10 mg/day to 50 mg/day in the third trimester.
  - Iron: 14.8 g/day, with no recommended increase in pregnancy unless iron stores are inappropriately low at the beginning of pregnancy.

Conditions that affect nutrition during pregnancy are:

- Nausea and vomiting
- Hyperemesis gravidarum
- Cravings, aversions and pica
- Heartburn
- Constipation.

During pregnancy, there are increased requirements for some, but not all nutrients (Clinical box 16.1). The diet must provide sufficient energy and nutrients to:

- Provide extra growth of the breasts, uterus and placenta, and to meet the mother's needs
- Meet the requirements of the growing fetus
- Allow the mother to lay down stores of nutrients for lactation.

Pregnancy is often an ideal opportunity for clinicians to promote healthier eating for the benefit of the baby, immediate family and the wider community, although there has been little research into the effects of this form of intervention.

Lactation

Lactation imposes a heavy nutritional demand on the mother. Requirements for energy, calcium and many other vitamins and minerals are increased. If the nutritional needs of lactation are not met, it is generally the mother who is affected and not the infant. Milk quantity and quality will be maintained at the expense of the maternal stores. Any significant fall in nutritional status, especially calcium, may have long-term consequences for the mother's health, particularly bone health. Lactating women should ingest at least 1200 mg calcium/day. Dehydration can occur if fluids are not replaced – requirement is about 2 L/day.

Aspects of the maternal diet can affect breast milk. High intakes of alcohol and caffeine should be avoided. Strong tasting or highly spiced foods can alter the taste of breast milk, which may cause distress to the infant. Infants who are highly sensitive to allergens such as cow's milk protein can react to, or may be sensitised to, the presence of these antigens in breast milk, although cow's milk exclusion for the mother is rarely justified.

Infancy

Infancy is a period of rapid growth and development. Compared with adults, infants have increased requirements per kilogram of body weight for energy, protein, iron and calcium. Mothers should be encouraged to breastfeed for at least 4 months, because breast milk provides the best form of nourishment. When breastfeeding is not possible, infant formulae, which are based on cow's milk and modified to mimic breast milk, may be used.

NUTRITIONAL STATUS

Assessment of nutritional status identifies individuals who are at risk of under- or over-nutrition. In the hospital setting, **malnutrition** is the major concern as it tends to be under-diagnosed. However, in the general population in the developed world, and increasingly elsewhere too, *obesity* is the major concern because of its associated metabolic syndromes (see below).

There is no single parameter that accurately measures nutritional status. Measures of body composition, functional testing, clinical presentation and laboratory measures all reflect aspects of nutritional status and should be considered together in a nutritional assessment. In children, nutritional status needs to be considered in relation to age, and growth is of major importance.

CHILDREN

The weight and height of children are assessed against standard growth charts to identify whether the weight and height are appropriate for the age of the child. Both are expressed in centiles, which tells us whether a child is above or below the average height or weight for their age, and whether they are growing at the expected rate; that is, whether they are following the same centile over time. Children who become malnourished first lose weight compared with their age and height (**wasting**); with more prolonged undernutrition, their growth becomes affected and height centile diminishes relative to normal or their previous situation (**stunting**). Height centile increase can occur with effective refeeding of malnourished children (**catch up growth**).

MEASURES OF BODY COMPOSITION: ADULTS

Measures of body composition are important in a clinical setting. They allow not only initial assessment but also monitoring of any change in body composition that may be due to disease.

BODY MASS INDEX

To be clinically informative, body weight needs to be expressed as a function of height. The most widely used stature-adjusted weight index is the body mass index (BMI) otherwise known as the Quetelet index (QI). The BMI is a ratio to determine body weight in relation to height; that is, whether a person's body weight is within the expected range for their height.

$$\text{BMI or QI} = \frac{\text{Weight (kg)}}{\text{Height}^2 \text{ (m)}}$$

BMI (QI) is useful for identifying underweight and overweight individuals (Table 16.2). For example, an adult female with a BMI over 30 would have a higher risk for hypertension or type 2 diabetes than one with a BMI of 20, whereas someone with a BMI ≤18.5 would be too thin. BMI, like body weight itself, does not differentiate between fat or lean body mass. Oedema and ascites may result in a higher BMI and an overestimate of muscle mass while heavily muscled individuals, such as body builders or regular attendees at gyms who are over-zealous in their training, may have a BMI that suggests that they are 'overweight'.

ESTIMATING BODY FAT

The percentage of body fat can be estimated by measurements taken at selected anatomical sites where fat is deposited:

- Skinfold thickness
- Arm circumference
- Waist circumference and waist/hip ratio.

Skinfold thickness

Skinfold measurement, also called the 'pinch test', measures the thickness of a fold of skin at selected body sites where adipose tissue is normally deposited, such as over the biceps, triceps, subscapular and suprailiac regions, and thigh and calf muscles. More accurate estimates of adiposity are obtained by measuring skinfold thickness at several sites. In clinical practice, triceps skinfold thickness is most often used as an estimate of body fat reserves.

Arm circumference

The mid upper arm circumference (MUAC) is a useful measure of muscle protein stores (Fig. 16.4). MUAC correlates fairly

Table 16.2	The international classification of underweight, overweight and obese adults according to BMI	
Classification	**BMI (kg/m²)**	
	Principal cut-off points	**Additional cut-off points**
Underweight	<18.50	<18.50
Severe thinness	<16.00	<16.00
Moderate thinness	16.00–16.99	16.00–16.99
Mild thinness	17.00–18.49	17.00–18.49
Normal range	18.50–24.99	18.50–22.99
		23.00–24.99
Overweight	≥25.00	≥25.00
Pre-obese	25.00–29.99	25.00–27.49
		27.50–29.99
Obese	≥30.00	≥30.00
Obese class I	30.00–34.99	30.00–32.49
		32.50–34.99
Obese class II	35.00–39.99	35.00–37.49
		37.50–39.99
Obese class III	≥40.00	≥40.00

Source: Adapted from WHO (1995, 2000, 2004).
BMI values, being ratios, are the same for males and females, and vary with age. Overweight and obesity may impair health, but the degrees of excessive fat accumulation vary between populations. Therefore, the health risk associated with increasing BMI differs for different populations.

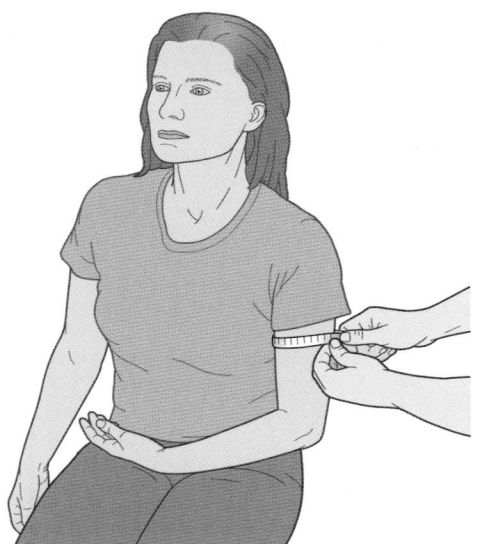

Fig. 16.4 **Measuring arm circumference.** The measurement is taken with a tape measure, midway between the tip of the acromion and olecranon process in the non-dominant arm to the nearest cm, with the dominant arm hanging relaxed.

well with BMI, and has been used as a quick and convenient method of estimating nutritional status of children in field studies and is increasingly being used in adults.

Waist circumference and waist/hip ratio

Strong correlations have been found between subcutaneous and intra-abdominal fat (on computed tomography (CT)), with waist and hip circumferences and waist/hip ratios. Measurement of waist alone may have greater sensitivity for predicting complications of obesity, such as coronary heart disease, than the waist/hip ratio. In Caucasians, a waist measurement of >94 cm in men and >80 cm in women is associated with increased risk. The risk is substantially increased in men with a waist >102 cm and in women >88 cm.

CLINICAL ASSESSMENT OF NUTRITIONAL STATUS

All patients under medical care should be screened for nutritional status; some will need more detailed assessment. The purpose of screening and assessing nutritional status clinically is to identify poor nutrition, and to evaluate the clinical progression of chronic and acute diseases. Usual weight and weight loss or gain are identified and assessed.

'USUAL WEIGHT' AND WEIGHT LOSS/GAIN

'Usual weight' may be constant or variable. If variable, the weight at which the patient feels best should be identified, as well as the weight immediately before illness or when weight loss commenced. Previous records of body weight are helpful. Usual weight allows estimation of **percentage weight loss** once current weight has been measured:

$$\text{Weight loss (\%)} = \frac{\text{Previous weight (kg)} - \text{current weight (kg)}}{\text{Previous weight (kg)}} \times 100$$

Percentage weight gain is calculated by reversing previous and current weights. The timing of the weight change should be noted; whether the weight loss is intentional or unintentional is important:

- In **intentional weight loss** produced by well-designed dieting, the lean body mass component may represent only 25% of the decrease in weight.
- In disease-related **unintentional weight loss**, 60% or more of the loss may be lean.

Weight measurements are distorted by fluid retention or loss. Day-to-day weight measurements are the most accurate clinical guide for assessing changes in hydration.

FOOD INTAKE

Detailed dietary intake is the province of the fully trained dietitian. However, a simple dietary history is often useful to doctors and other clinicians. For example, the number of meals and the quantity, content and variety of snacks consumed can give clues to whether intake is a factor for weight change. Basic enquiries into diet and the timing of meals and snacks can be usefully incorporated into routine questions about lifestyle. The relation of gastrointestinal symptoms with food intake can be of great clinical importance.

Detailed dietary assessment

A full quantitative dietary assessment is time consuming and properly the province of the trained dietitian. Table 16.3 summarises the most commonly used methods of recording intake. Misreporting is common as people can feel guilty or embarrassed about aspects of their diet. In addition, food choices may be influenced when intake is recorded by the patient. All food intake varies by day of the week and season.

Once completed, a dietary record can be analysed into its constituent nutrients by using food composition tables or computer packages based on them. Information on dietary balance, deficiencies and surpluses, specific nutrients and compliance with previously given advice can be obtained from such programs. For example, comparisons can be made with age- and gender-specific DRVs.

MALNUTRITION SCREENING TOOLS

Impressions of nutritional status, such as 'seems to have lost a lot of weight', are often misleading. Malnutrition is common in hospitals, so it is important to screen patients nutritionally. Many hospitals will have their own screening tools that combine features from the history and clinical examination, which are then ranked and combined to produce a score indicating malnutrition risk. In the UK, the Malnutrition Universal Screening Tool (MUST) is a five-step process based on BMI and weight loss designed to identify patients who are at risk of malnutrition or obesity, and includes management guidelines. Another formal assessment tool is the Subjective Global Assessment, used more commonly in the USA and Canada.

Table 16.3	Methods for recording food intake		
Type	**Definition**	**Uses**	**Disadvantages**
Weighed food record	Record with weights of portions served, and plate waste	When a quantified measure of nutrient intake is required, e.g. in specialised research studies	Not all foods fully weighed, as logistically this can be difficult and can lead to poor compliance
Unweighed food record	Estimated record using portions described in household measures (spoon, cups, etc.)	Semiquantitative measure used to identify meal patterns, food choices, e.g. associations between food and symptoms	Can be hard to quantify specific nutrient intakes
24-hour recall	The respondent is asked to recall all food eaten within the past 24 hours	As a quick assessment of food choices/meal patterns	Past 24 hours may not be representative of usual intake
Food frequency questionnaire	A questionnaire consisting of a list of foods. The respondent has to say how often each food is eaten – per day/week/month	For identifying foods eaten less often, which may be of special interest and not included in short-term food records, e.g. when trying to identify certain nutrients consumed over a larger period of time	May not be a good assessment of total diet
Diet history	Respondent is asked detailed questions about usual intake. The aim is to get a comprehensive 7-day estimate of intake	Method used by the majority of dietitians in clinical practice for fast assessment and immediate advice	Information can be difficult to obtain, and often misreported

OTHER MEASUREMENTS OF NUTRITIONAL STATUS

Some laboratory measurements of body composition are set out in Table 16.4. They are not in common clinical use and are used more often in research.

PLASMA PROTEINS

Serum albumin is often incorrectly used as an indicator of nutritional status, because the levels may stay normal in undernutrition uncomplicated by disease. The decrease in serum albumin concentration during infection, cancer, burns and after trauma or surgery is related primarily to increased vascular permeability. While undernutrition may exacerbate disease-related hypoalbuminaemia, albumin concentration primarily reflects a disease process, and it is better considered as an 'index of disease severity' rather than a nutritional indicator. Serum albumin can also be depressed by dilution during refeeding or excessive rehydration. It should be used in combination with some other estimate of the acute-phase response, such as C-reactive protein or the erythrocyte sedimentation rate (ESR).

The same problems apply to other plasma proteins which are used as nutritional indicators, such as pre-albumin, transferrin and retinol-binding protein. However, these may be more sensitive as nutritional indicators because they have a shorter half-life in the circulation and can respond to dietary change more quickly.

VITAMIN STATUS

Vitamin deficiencies can be detected either by biochemical assays or by physical symptoms (see below). The detailed assessment of vitamin status is beyond the scope of this chapter. The relatively common presentation of macrocytic anaemias necessitates vitamin B_{12} and folate assays, but other vitamin deficiencies are unmeasured and often overlooked. Specific deficiency syndromes are outlined below.

MUSCLE STRENGTH

Studies have shown that malnutrition leads to impaired muscle strength, and nutritional support reverses impairment before improvements in weight are seen.

IMMUNOLOGICAL SKIN TESTING

Adequate nutrition is essential for the maintenance of a normal immune system. A total **lymphocyte count** of 800–1200/mm^3 is indicative of moderate protein calorie malnutrition and less than 800/mm^3 indicates severe depletion (normal range 1000–4800/mm^3). Delayed hypersensitivity is particularly affected by undernutrition, and, in the past, skin tests for mumps, tuberculin and *Candida* have been used clinically to monitor nutrition.

ENERGY AND NITROGEN BALANCE

Energy is required for metabolic processes such as active transport of molecules and ions, synthesis of tissue, thermoregulation, and voluntary and involuntary muscle movement. Dietary intake of food provides the body with the macronutrients: carbohydrates, fats and proteins that are converted to energy.

CONVERSION OF MACRONUTRIENTS TO ENERGY

After absorption, food is digested to substrate which is available for energy metabolism. Whatever the macronutrient, most energy ultimately comes from the mitochondrial processing of two carbon fragments linked to a coenzyme, a B vitamin cofactor, in the tricarboxylic acid (TCA or Kreb's) cycle and in oxidative phosphorylation (see also Ch. 3). Figure 16.5 is a simplified representation of the metabolic

Table 16.4   **Investigation/research procedures for measuring body composition**

Measurement	Procedure	Technique	Advantages	Disadvantages
Estimates the fat free mass (bone/ soft tissue) in men and women	DEXA scan	Dual energy X-ray absorptiometry; measures the differential attenuation of X-rays by bones and soft tissue	Good reproducibility	Measurement of % fat in men is less accurate
Lean body mass (LBM)	Total body potassium (TBK)	Whole body monitor detects the natural radioisotope ^{40}K		Interpretation limited if factors that deplete K concentration are present, e.g. diuretic therapy, diabetes and hyperaldosteronism
Elements	Ratio of exchangeable Na^+/K^+	Measured using isotope dilution following administration of $^{22}NaCl$ and H_2O		
Absolute amounts of body fat, protein and minerals	Prompt neutron activation	K, N_2, Na, Cl, Ca and P are measured in a whole body radiation counter after irradiation with fast neutrons. Dose of radiation equivalent to a chest X-ray	Quick procedure (approximately 40 minutes)	The equipment is very expensive
Reflects lean body mass	Total body water – ^2H_2O (D_2O, deuterium oxide)	Estimated by isotope dilution using ^2H_2O or ^3H_2O (T_3O, tritium oxide)	Relatively straightforward and inexpensive technique; is measurable with accuracy in blood, urine or saliva	
Estimates total body water and fat free body mass in healthy adults and children	Bioelectrical impedance analysis (BIA)	Resistance and reactance are measured using an impedance analyser	High reproducibility	Affected by variables such as body position, hydration, consumption of food and drink, ambient skin and air temperature, recent physical activity and conductance of the examination table

pathways that convert carbohydrate, fat and protein to energy.

ENERGY BALANCE

Positive energy balance results in weight gain and the deposition of fat and glycogen, whereas a negative energy balance leads to weight loss and the depletion of glycogen and fat stores. The energy content (calories) of food can be measured by combustion in a bomb calorimeter, a device used to measure the heat produced by combustion of various macronutrients. The word calorimeter is derived from 'calor', the Latin for heat and a calorimeter is a device used for calorimetry, the measurement of heat generated from chemical or physical reactions.

In healthy people, most of the energy in food is absorbed – around 97% of the energy in carbohydrate, 95% in fat and 92% in protein. Less energy is absorbed from protein because nitrogen is metabolised to urea and not fully oxidised, so that some of the energy from protein is not available to the body (see Ch. 3).

Energy consumption

Basal metabolic rate (BMR) is the energy consumption of a normal, post-absorptive (about 12 hours fasting) individual at rest, but not asleep, under thermoneutral conditions. Although BMR varies among people of equal height and weight, owing to ethnic and geographical differences, individual BMRs remain relatively constant over a number of years.

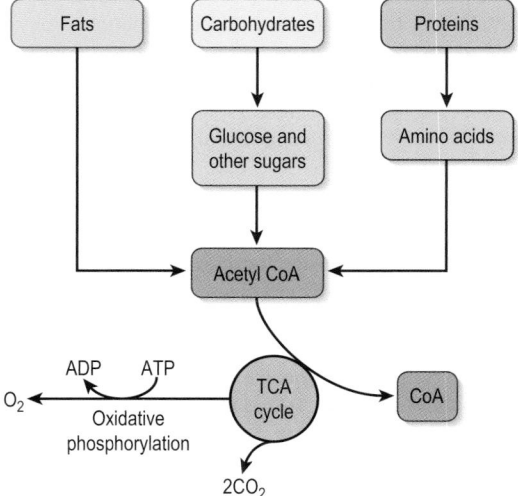

Fig. 16.5 **Metabolic pathways for converting macronutrients to energy.**

Total energy consumption

Total energy consumption is BMR plus increments for:

- Food-induced thermogenesis – approximately 10% energy for a mixed meal.

- Cold-induced thermogenesis – shivering and non-shivering is not usually a big factor in practice in the environment of the developed world.
- Exercise/physical activity.

In practice, BMR plus energy consumption during occupational and non-occupational activity are used for making clinical **estimates** of total energy consumption.

Measuring energy consumption

BMR can be measured at rest by direct calorimetry (direct measurement of heat exchange in a chamber), or indirect calorimetry, which uses a canopy over the head to measure oxygen consumption and carbon dioxide generation from which energy consumption can be calculated. In practice, BMR is estimated from the Schofield (1985) predictive equations, which are based on the analysis of a large number of measurements of BMR and can predict individual BMR reasonably accurately.

Oxygen consumption and carbon dioxide production can also be measured during exercise either by collecting exhaled gases in portable Douglas bags or by studying the subject in a chamber calorimeter. Energy consumption can also be measured by giving the subject a drink of doubly labelled radioactive water and monitoring the relative decay of ^2H and ^{18}O from the body. The difference between the decay of ^2H and ^{18}O allows estimation of CO_2 production and total energy consumption. This method has the advantage that the subject is free to move about.

Total energy expenditure and the effect of physical activity

The total amount of energy used up in a day will depend on the individual's BMR, the nature of their occupation (whether sedentary or labour intensive), and the amount of physical activity undertaken in leisure and the pursuit of sports. The heat derived from food- and cold-induced thermogenesis is not measured separately, but is included in measurements or estimations of energy expenditure.

Energy expenditure during daily living

Daily energy output for the activities of daily living can be estimated from the BMR and the individual's physical activity level (PAL), an index of energy expenditure for physical activity over 24 hours. Energy expenditure during activities of daily living is best measured by the doubly labelled water method, which allows measurements to be made over periods of days or weeks. PAL is expressed as a ratio of total energy expenditure and the resting energy expenditure (BMR). Total daily energy requirement can be calculated from a table of PAL, calibrated for the subject's leisure and work occupation, which provides a multiple by which the estimated BMR can be multiplied. For any one individual, these values are obtained from reference tables (Table 16.5). The most commonly used units are kcal/24 h or kJ/24 h.

An estimated average requirement (EAR) for energy can be calculated by multiplying the BMR by the appropriate PAL (see Table 16.5). The PAL index takes into consideration occupational as well as non-occupational activities because an individual with a sedentary occupation may undertake a lot of non-occupational activity, and vice versa. Physical activity makes a variable contribution to the total energy expenditure, which over average 24-hour periods is nearly always less than the BMR.

An individual at rest would be using energy for maintaining BMR only, i.e. a PAL of 1. Many people in the developed world have sedentary occupations (light activity) and are non-active, or only moderately active, outside work. From the corresponding PAL of 1.4 and 1.5 (Table 16.5), it can be seen that their energy consumption is mainly due to BMR: only about a third of it (0.4–0.5) is due to physical activity. For example, for a woman who has a BMR of 6000 kJ, has a sedentary occupation and is moderately active outside of work, the total daily energy output is:

$$6000 \text{ kJ} \times 1.5 = 9000 \text{ kJ}$$
(4.2 kJ is equivalent to 1 kcal)

Estimates of energy consumption for different types of activity

More accurate estimates of energy consumption during a 24-hour period can be made by keeping a diary of each activity, then calculating the total by adding all the different components. The energy used during each activity is calculated by reference to **physical activity ratios (PAR)** for different activities. PAR is an index of the energy expenditure for the duration of a particular activity compared with a reference activity, such as BMR, expressed as the estimated energy cost **per minute** for the specific activity relative to the measured energy cost **per minute** for the reference activity. This index is used to compare the energy consumption of various activities by different people (Table 16.6).

Energy expenditure during exercise

Energy needs during exercise vary depending on whether it is intense, over a short period (e.g. 100 m sprint), or sustained endurance exercise, such as running a marathon.

Table 16.5	Physical activity levels (PALs)					
Non-occupational activity	Occupational activity					
	Light		Moderate		Moderate/ heavy	
	M	F	M	F	M	F
Non-active	1.4	1.4	1.6	1.5	1.7	1.5
Moderately active	1.5	1.5	1.7	1.6	1.8	1.6
Very active	1.6	1.6	1.8	1.7	1.9	1.7

Source: HMSO 1991 Report of Health and Social Subjects 41.

Clinical box 16.2	Energy needs for sport: advice for sportsmen and sportswomen for optimising performance

The advice on energy intake is aimed at enabling individuals to:

- Compensate for the high energy consumption produced by training and competition to maintain an optimal body weight (water, protein and fat).
- Ensure that the muscles and the liver contain plenty of stored glycogen prior to the event.
- Replace glycogen quickly and optimally after sport or between events.
- Maintain hydration during the sporting activity and salt replacement during prolonged endurance exercise.

Table 16.6	Physical activity ratios for different types of activity	
	PAR	Example activity
PAR 1.2 (range 1.0–1.4)	Lying at rest	Reading
	Sitting at rest	Watching television, reading, eating
	Standing at rest	
PAR 1.6 (range 1.5–1.8)	Sitting	Sewing, playing piano, driving
	Standing	Light kitchen work, ironing, office or laboratory work
PAR 2.1 (range 1.9–2.4)	Standing	Household chores, cooking
PAR 2.8 (range 2.5–3.3)	Standing	Vacuuming, making beds, showering
	Walking	3–4 km/h, cricket
	Industrial	Painting and decorating, machine tool, tailoring
PAR 3.7 (range 3.4–4.4)	Standing	Gardening, sailing,
	Walking	4–6 km/h, golf
	Industrial	Motor vehicle repairs, bricklaying
PAR 4.8 (range 4.4–5.9)	Standing	Chopping wood, heavy gardening, volley ball
	Walking	6–7 km/h
	Exercise	Moderate swimming, gentle cycling, slow jogging
	Occupational	Labouring, digging/ shovelling, felling trees
PAR 6.9 (range 6.0–7.9)	Walking	Uphill with load, cross-country, climbing stairs
	Exercise	Average jogging, cycling
	Sports	Football, tennis, more energetic swimming, skiing

Anaerobic carbohydrate metabolism

During short bursts of intense activity (e.g. sprinting, weight lifting), close to maximum oxygen consumption (VO_2 max) takes place when the exercising muscles depend on their own individual stores of ATP, supported by glucose from the muscle's own store of glycogen. This allows for brief periods when energy consumption is substantially greater than can be supplied by circulating substrates and oxygen. This is called 'anaerobic' metabolism. It builds up lactate and an oxygen debt, which have to be compensated for later. Lactate is recycled to the liver for gluconeogenesis (Cori cycle) (see Ch. 3).

Aerobic carbohydrate metabolism

During more prolonged exercise, 'aerobic' metabolism takes place, in which muscle stores of ATP run out very quickly if they cannot be replenished. Energy during prolonged exercise can be provided by:

Table 16.7	Adult nitrogen balance	
Nitrogen intake (diet)	Nitrogen output (excretion)	
62.5 g protein	Urine	8.50 g (7 g as urea)
	Faeces	0.75 g
	Other	0.75 g
	Total	10.0 g

- The exercising muscle's glycogen stores
- Circulating energy substrate – glucose derived from hepatic glycogenolysis and gluconeogenesis
- Fatty acids derived from adipose tissue.

Training increases the capacity of the muscle mitochondria to oxidise circulating substrate, especially fatty acids, to produce ATP (see below, TCA cycle). This delays the time at which the relevant muscle's glycogen runs out and the athlete becomes especially fatigued ('hits the wall').

NITROGEN BALANCE AND PROTEIN REQUIREMENTS

Nitrogen balance is the difference between the amount of nitrogen that is ingested and the amount lost from the body. It indicates whether the body is **anabolic** or **catabolic** in terms of net protein metabolism; whether the lean tissue is increasing (positive nitrogen balance) or decreasing (negative nitrogen balance). Nitrogen is ingested in the form of dietary proteins, which are metabolised in the liver and excreted, mainly as urea, in the urine.

Dietary nitrogen

Nitrogen makes up about 16% of the weight of most proteins, i.e. 6.25 g protein contains 1 g nitrogen. Table 16.7 shows how a (numerically convenient) intake of 62.5 g protein, which equates with 10 g nitrogen, is balanced quantitatively by nitrogen excretion. Normal adults have a net zero nitrogen balance, with ingestion of food by day balancing losses of nitrogen by day and night. Nitrogen balance is positive during growth, weight regain, pregnancy, and negative during starvation, protein deprivation, nutrient imbalance, trauma and sepsis.

In clinical practice, true nitrogen balance is seldom assessed. Nevertheless, during prolonged artificial nutritional support, it can be helpful to measure urinary losses of nitrogen (if possible), or urea. If a patient is consistently losing more nitrogen than is being provided in a feed over more than a few days, it may become necessary to increase the nitrogen content of the feed to try to achieve closer balance. However, it should be remembered that in the normal individual, a high nitrogen intake results in a high output to balance it: it may not be possible or desirable to achieve balance in a patient who is losing excessive amounts of protein due to sepsis or trauma.

Protein requirements

A positive nitrogen balance is seen during growth (nitrogen intake exceeds excretion), and sufficient nitrogen intake is required for cell renewal and to replace nitrogen excretion in adults. Normal adults in the developed world tend to eat more protein than they need; often more than the RNI of approximately 45 g/day for a non-pregnant woman and 55 g/day for a man.

Protein quality

Twenty amino acids are needed for the manufacture of proteins in humans. Whilst most of them can be synthesised endogenously, eight are essential in the diet because they cannot be endogenously synthesised: isoleucine, leucine, valine, lysine, methionine, phenylalanine, threonine and tryptophan. An additional, ninth, essential amino acid in infants is histidine. The quality of dietary proteins is measured by their essential amino acid content, known as the **amino acid score**. 'High-quality' dietary proteins, formerly known as 'first class proteins', contain similar amounts of essential amino acids as endogenous proteins.

The amino acid score of a dietary protein is measured as the content of individual essential amino acids (mg/g protein) relative to the content present in a hypothetical reference protein which reflects the essential amino acid content of the 'average' endogenous protein. The amino acid content of this reference protein is very similar to milk. Protein quality is quantified as:

$$\text{Amino acid score} = \frac{\text{mg essential amino acid/g (test protein)}}{\text{mg same essential amino acid/g (reference protein)}} \times 100$$

The essential amino acid content of each dietary protein is measured and compared with its content in the standard, or reference protein. The score is expressed as a percentage, the lowest scoring amino acid being the limiting one, and giving the amino acid score for that dietary protein. The closer the essential amino acid content of the dietary protein is to the essential amino acid content of the reference protein, the more *efficient* will be the synthesis of endogenous protein.

Protein quality matters only if protein intake is low and there is not a mixture of proteins in the diet. For example, a vegan diet will only contain plant-derived proteins. Different proteins have different limiting amino acids and so compensate for each other in mixed diets.

Obligatory nitrogen loss

Obligatory nitrogen loss is the amount of nitrogen excreted when protein is excluded from a diet otherwise adequate in energy, electrolytes, minerals, vitamins and trace elements. In this highly artificial situation, the daily excretion of nitrogen in the urine and faeces declines over a few days to a minimum (Fig. 16.6).

Minimum nitrogen requirement

In the absence of growth, nitrogen requirement is estimated by summing the obligatory loss in urine to faecal and other (e.g. skin, sweat) excretions on a protein-free diet (the so-called factorial method). However, an otherwise adequate diet providing only this amount of nitrogen (even as high-quality or first class protein) does not achieve zero balance; the balance remains slightly negative because ureagenesis increases. A better way of finding minimum requirements in adults is by balance studies in which high-quality protein is gradually added to an otherwise complete diet until zero balance is obtained. In children, growth rates must be taken

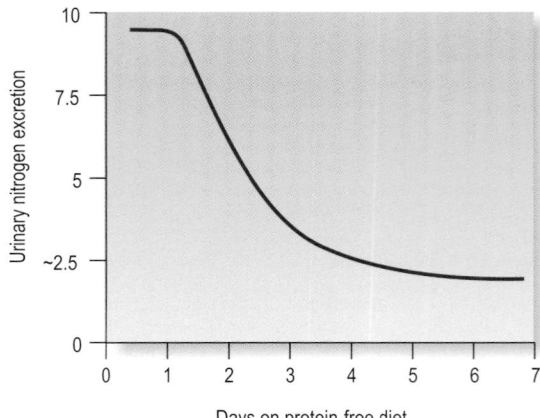

Fig. 16.6 Obligatory nitrogen loss: minimum urinary nitrogen excretion – protein-free diet. Urine nitrogen loss on a protein free, otherwise adequate diet reaches equilibrium of about 2.5 g by about day 5–7. However, if only 2.5 g of nitrogen are supplied in the otherwise protein-free diet, nitrogen losses will increase marginally because of increased ureagenesis, and nitrogen balance is not quite achieved. Slightly more is required for balance.

into account. Adults can maintain nitrogen balance on 96 mg N/kg per day.

Nitrogen excretion

Unlike glucose and fatty acids, amino acids do not have storage depots, so amino acids are stored in structural and functional protein. Most nitrogen is excreted in the urine as urea, with smaller amounts as creatinine and uric acid, for example. The nitrogen containing amino group is removed from the amino acid, and the remaining carbon skeleton is then metabolised for gluconeogenesis and protein synthesis (see Ch. 3). The waste product is ammonia, NH_3, which is highly toxic and rapidly converted to **urea**. Urea is excreted principally through the kidneys. The breakdown of amino acids for use in gluconeogenesis is the main source of urea, and plays a major part in nitrogen balance. When fasting, more amino acids are mobilised for gluconeogenesis, and the metabolic pathways reverse during feeding towards protein synthesis. During feeding, as more protein is eaten, more amino acids are metabolised and more urea nitrogen is excreted so that nitrogen balance is maintained. Losses of nitrogen in the faeces approximate 1 g/day and are relatively constant.

Energy and protein metabolism during fasting and feeding

In healthy people, intracellular metabolism to produce energy is regulated by hormones (Ch. 3). During the fed state, energy stores are laid down for use during periods of fasting (Table 16.8). It is normal to fast overnight or for short periods during the day, but the body adapts if longer periods of fasting occur. The hormones insulin, glucagon, adrenaline, cortisol and growth hormone are involved in the regulation of energy metabolism, exerting short-term effects on the direction of metabolic pathways (Information box 16.1, Fig. 16.7; see also Ch. 3).

Table 16.8	Fuel stores in an average person	
Fuel source	**In weight (g)**	**In energy (kJ)**
Fat		
Plasma free fatty acids	0.4	16
Plasma triacylglycerols	4.0	156
Intramyocellular triacylglycerol	300	11 700
Adipose tissue	12 000	468 000
Carbohydrate		
Plasma glucose	20	360
Liver glycogen	100	1800
Muscle glycogen	350	6300
Whole body protein	10 000	168 000

Source: Adapted from Geissler C, Powers HJ (eds) 2005 Human nutrition 11th edn. Elsevier Science, Oxford.
Note: The principal component of body weight (water) provides no energy. Protein is structural and is therefore not all available for energy production. Glycogen and protein in the body are in the hydrated state and so weigh much more, kilojoule for kilojoule than fat, which is stored in adipose tissue. Adipose tissue contains relatively little water. (4.2 kJ is equivalent to 1 kcal)

ℹ️ Information box 16.1 — Effect of insulin in the fed and fasted states

During the fed state, the active metabolic pathways are for fuel breakdown, storage of excess fuel through glycogen and lipid synthesis, and protein synthesis (anabolism) (see also Ch. 3). These processes are induced by insulin, an anabolic hormone, to:

- Increase glycogen synthesis in the liver and muscle
- Increase hepatic glycolysis
- Increase glucose uptake into muscle
- Increase lipogenesis and decrease lipolysis
- Increase cellular uptake of amino acids and net protein synthesis.

In fasting, which can begin a few hours after the last meal, the direction of the metabolic pathways is reversed to breakdown stored fuels to produce energy. Protein synthesis also slows down. The level of circulating insulin falls. (In the stress of disease or trauma the action of insulin is opposed by increased levels of glucagon, adrenaline, cortisol, and growth hormone). Glycogenolysis, lipolysis, ketogenesis and gluconeogenesis are promoted.

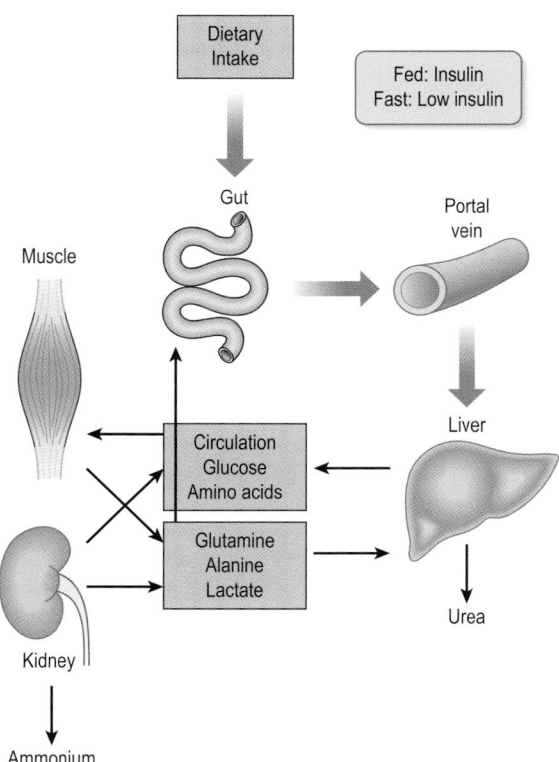

Fig. 16.7 Carbohydrate and amino acid metabolism during fasting and feeding.

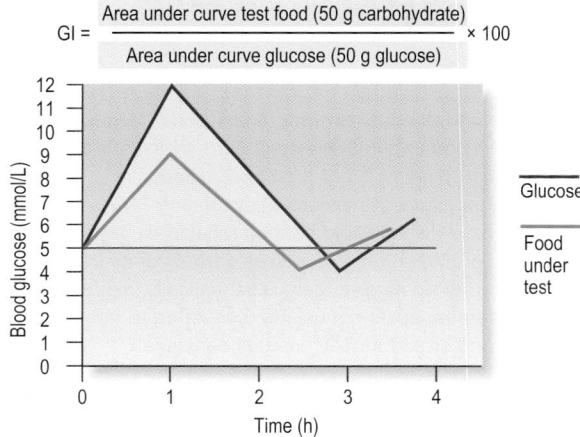

$$GI = \frac{\text{Area under curve test food (50 g carbohydrate)}}{\text{Area under curve glucose (50 g glucose)}} \times 100$$

Fig. 16.8 Glycaemic index (GI).

liver. During brisk exercise, a low insulin state, the exercising muscles take up glucose, which may not be fully oxidised. Lactate is produced and recycled after anaerobic glycolysis back to the liver for gluconeogenesis (Cori cycle) (Ch. 3.)

Fed state

When nutrients are abundant, metabolic processes are geared to the catabolism of macronutrients and anabolism of the excess products for storage against lean times.

Absorbed carbohydrate in the fed state

After a meal, blood glucose rises, as shown in the **blood glucose response curves** in Figure 16.8. Some foods produce a blood glucose response very similar to that of glucose, the reference food; others produce a much flatter curve. Glucose is made available for:

- Metabolism
- Storage as glycogen (principally in muscle and liver)
- In more extreme excess, lipogenesis.

Many physical and chemical characteristics of carbohydrates affect how quickly they are absorbed: reflected in how quickly blood sugar rises and falls after they are eaten. The **glycaemic index** (GI) describes this response in relation to

The anabolic, fed, high-insulin state results in net storage of protein and glycogen. The catabolic, fasted, low insulin state results in mobilisation of, firstly, glycogen for maintenance of blood glucose, and, subsequently, amino acids (especially 3C alanine) as substrate to make 6C glucose (gluconeogenesis–alanine cycle). 5C glutamine is an amino acid which is a major energy substrate for rapidly turning over cells such as enterocytes and lymphocytes. It is partially metabolised there to 3C alanine before this is returned to the glucose (see Fig. 16.8), and foods can be classified as having low, intermediate or high GI (Table 16.9). This is used in the management of diabetes: low GI foods are recommended as an aid to restricting glucose intake. In the UK, low GI foods are recommended to the general population as part of a balanced diet. However, estimating the total GI of a meal is not practical in clinical situations because there are many factors which affect the GI, including:

- Pectin to amylopectin ratio in the food (mainly fruit)
- Degree of ripeness (fruit) and method of preparation (e.g. mashing increases the GI of potatoes)
- Size of the meal
- Addition of fat.

Absorbed fat in the fed state

Dietary fat is about 95% triacylglycerol (TAG) (also known as triglyceride), with cholesterol and phospholipids making up the other main components. Dietary fats in the form of TAG are digested by pancreatic enzymes in the intestine to form free fatty acids and 2-monoacylglycerol (MAG), which are absorbed by the enterocytes (Ch. 15). The enterocytes re-esterify some of the free fatty acids and MAG to synthesise TAGs. Chylomicrons are then assembled from TAGs, cholesterol, apoproteins and phospholipids. Most TAGs enter the systemic circulation as chylomicrons, via the thoracic duct. Medium- and short-chain fatty acids pass directly into the liver via the portal vein. Cholesterol (like bile acids) is absorbed in the last 100 cm or so of the terminal ileum.

In the fed state, the excess of circulating TAG is stored in adipose tissue whose lipid content reflects dietary fatty acid composition. When there is excess carbohydrate intake, it is principally stored as glycogen. Biochemically, dietary carbohydrate can be, but is not usually, converted to fatty acids in the liver and stored as TAG in adipose tissue.

Protein in the fed state

During the fed state, rates of body protein synthesis exceed rates of protein breakdown back to free amino acids, and net protein accumulation (positive nitrogen balance) occurs. The digestion of protein takes place firstly in the stomach by denaturation by stomach acid, then secondly in the small intestine by the action of pancreatic proteases to form a mixture of free amino acids and small peptides, following which a series of carrier systems transport them into the gut cells where they enter the portal blood for transport to the liver. Some amino acids, for example glutamine, are metabolised in preference to glucose in the gut, mainly to alanine (see Ch. 3). Alanine can enter gluconeogenesis, or, together with other amino acids, be used for the synthesis of liver structural or export proteins. Final degradation of amino acids results in the formation of glucose or glycogen from the carbon skeleton, and urea from the amino groups. A relatively small proportion of ingested amino acids, particularly

the branched chain amino acids valine, leucine and isoleucine, say 25%, leave the liver to circulate generally to be available for protein synthesis. The liver therefore acts to protect the rest of the body from sudden potentially toxic surges in free amino acids.

In healthy individuals who have adequate protein consumption, 24-hour dietary intake and excretion of nitrogen should be equal (nitrogen balance). This will include periods of positive nitrogen balance (during feeding), where the rate of protein synthesis is higher than protein catabolism, and periods of negative nitrogen balance (overnight usually), where the rate of synthesis is lower than protein catabolism.

Fasted state

When fasting, metabolic processes tend towards mobilisation of stored energy substrates to meet the energy requirements for maintaining essential biological functions. Metabolic pathways are not independent and in times of substrate deficit the body has the ability to metabolise its stored energy substrates for energy (Fig. 16.9) (Ch. 3).

The need for glucose in the fasted state

During fasting, and after all the glucose from a meal has been metabolised, blood glucose is maintained at a relatively constant 'post-absorptive' level by:

- Drawing on reserves of glycogen in the liver, i.e. glucose is produced via **glycogenolysis** (Ch. 3)
- **Gluconeogenesis**, when glucose is synthesised from lactate or non-carbohydrate (mainly protein) sources in the body (Ch. 3).

The main stores for glycogen are in the liver and muscle. Hepatic glycogenolysis provides an almost immediate source of glucose during short-term fasting (e.g. overnight) for maintaining normal blood glucose concentration. The hormone glucagon activates hepatic glycogenolysis. Skeletal muscle glycogen cannot leave the muscle, so muscle glycogenolysis (activated by adrenaline) does not increase blood glucose and can only meet the energy requirements for muscle contraction during exercise (Ch. 3).

Glucose from hepatic glycogenolysis is sufficient only for between 12 and 24 hours and cannot replace all the glucose needed for essential functions. To meet all the requirements, as hepatic glycogen depletes, gluconeogenesis in the liver and kidneys becomes important. Non-carbohydrate substrates for gluconeogenesis include (Ch. 3):

- Lactate: from anaerobic glycolysis in red blood cells and from active skeletal muscle. Starting with lactate,

Table 16.9	Classification of foods by glycaemic index	
Glycaemic index	**Foods**
High (70–100)	Bread (white or wholemeal), glucose, fruit juices, honey, mashed potatoes
Intermediate (56–69)	Granary bread, rice
Low (<55)	Pulses, beans, peas, legumes, oat and oat-based cereals, pasta, raw fruit

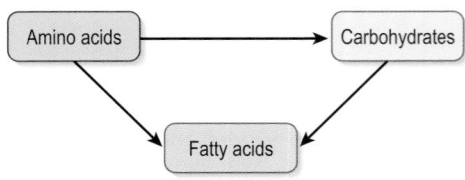

Fig. 16.9 Metabolic pathways of energy substrates in the fasted state. Fatty acids cannot be converted to either carbohydrates or amino acids, but are oxidised via acetyl CoA (if there is plentiful oxaloacetate as a result of glycolysis).

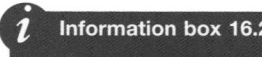

Information box 16.2 — Metabolism of stored energy substrates in the fasted state

During fasting:

- The carbon chains of some (glucogenic) amino acids, particularly alanine, can be converted to glucose
- Fatty acids cannot be converted to glucose or amino acids (only the glycerol component can be a small contributor to glucose)
- Fatty acids can only be oxidised via acetyl CoA entering the TCA cycle if there is plentiful oxaloacetate from glucose or glycogen metabolism.
- Deficiency of oxaloacetate results in acetyl groups forming keto-acids which can be, and are, metabolised during prolonged fasting or starvation. In starvation, as the brain switches from metabolising glucose (derived at first from glycogen and subsequently from protein/amino acids) to keto-acids (derived from fat), it reduces the need for gluconeogenesis from amino acids and therefore 'spares protein'.

gluconeogenesis is conceptually the reverse of anaerobic glycolysis, though there are slight differences in the pathway.

- Glycerol from fat metabolism: TAGs in adipose tissue are broken down to glycerol and free fatty acids by lipolysis (see Ch. 3). These fatty acids cannot be made into glucose. The glycerol component diffuses into the blood-stream to be reconverted to glucose in the liver and kidneys – a minor supply quantitatively.
- Amino acids from protein muscle breakdown: the main amino acids used in gluconeogenesis are alanine and glutamine, from muscle protein hydrolysis.

With prolonged fasting, the body minimises the drain on structural proteins by reducing the need for glucose and therefore gluconeogenesis from protein. This is achieved by muscles using fat for fuel, especially ketones (see below), and the brain adapting to using more ketone bodies.

Decreased insulin – fasting state

The post-absorptive and fasting states are signalled by a low level of circulating insulin associated with raised plasma glucagon concentration (Information box 16.1). This results in glycogenolysis, lipolysis, ketogenesis and net protein breakdown. 5-Carbon (glutamine) and 3-carbon substrates, (alanine, lactate, pyruvate) are cycled back to the liver for gluconeogenesis (see Ch. 3).

Fat in the fasted state

Fatty acids are oxidised, acetyl group by acetyl group, in a process called β-oxidation. Acetyl groups enter the TCA cycle for oxidation by combining with oxaloacetate, derived from glycolysis and regenerated in the cycle (see Ch. 3). During prolonged fasting, gluconeogenesis results in depletion of oxaloacetate, and acetyl groups derived principally from fat are diverted into forming ketoacids, which can be oxidised. The brain, which is normally a major user of glucose, uses glucose less and ketone bodies more. In this way, the body uses ketone bodies derived from fat rather than glucose derived from protein. Water-soluble ketone bodies consist of:

- Acetoacetate
- β-Hydroxybutyrate
- Acetone.

Free fatty acid is mobilised from adipose tissue, and the liver also increases the rate of fatty acid production. Hepatic β-oxidation of fatty acids forms acetyl CoA, which can have one of two metabolic fates:

- React with oxaloacetate to form citrate (and continue to complete oxidation)
- React with acetyl CoA to form acetoacetate and subsequently other ketone bodies.

This is determined by the rate of β-oxidation and the availability of oxaloacetate. If β-oxidation is high and oxaloacetate low, ketone bodies form. Water-soluble ketone bodies from hepatic ketogenesis can be readily transported in aqueous solution in the blood to various tissues (mainly the heart, muscle and the brain). The ketone bodies can cross the blood–brain barrier to become the dominant energy source there.

Prolonged fasting/starvation

During short-term starvation (overnight fast, up to 3 days), glucose from glycogen and, later, ketone bodies, provide fuel for muscle, kidneys and intestine (Table 16.10). With prolonged fasting (more than 3 days), the brain also converts to the use of ketone bodies for more than 50% of its energy metabolism (Table 16.10). This metabolic switch allows glucose to be conserved, reducing the demand to degrade muscle protein for gluconeogenesis (Ch. 3). The concentration of ketone bodies may increase dramatically as starvation continues from days into weeks. The low insulin state of starvation thus has qualitative metabolic parallels with diabetic ketoacidosis.

With prolonged starvation, nitrogen excretion in the form of urea diminishes, reflecting reduction of the drain on protein, but does not go as low as the obligatory minimum loss (the amount of nitrogen lost when dietary protein is excluded, see Fig. 16.6, above) seen in protein deprivation.

Metabolic response to stress: sepsis and trauma

Nutritional support of sick patients requires understanding of the metabolic changes that occur in illness. These occur in

Table 16.10	Fuel used by the brain on days 3 and 40 of a prolonged fast	
Starvation	Day 3	Day 40
Fuel used (g)		
Glucose	100	40
Ketones	50	200
Other glucose	50	40
Endogenous source of fuel used (g)		
Lipolysis	180	180
Muscle protein breakdown	75	20
Hepatic glucose	150	80
Ketones	150	150

Note the increased use of ketones by the brain and the reduced hepatic glucose production by day 40 and the reduction in net muscle protein breakdown.

The clinical effects of starvation reflect the biochemistry. For example, as a result of muscle protein breakdown for gluconeogenesis, there is type II fibre atrophy in skeletal muscle (including respiratory muscle), leaving only the fat burning and posture maintaining (type I) fibres. This results in:

- Wasting and other demonstrable changes in muscle physiology
- Muscle fatigue and decreased ability to do physical work
- Diminished respiratory function (e.g. forced expiratory volume in one second (FEV_1)).

The pulse rate slows and circulating volume and cardiac output decreases.

The ability to produce heat is compromised so that there is increased risk of hypothermia in a cold environment. Respiratory muscle weakness reduces ventilation, increasing the likelihood of respiratory disease (e.g. pneumonia). The patient becomes weak and apathetic.

Information box 16.3   **Cytokines and hormones in illness**

Cytokines are proteins that are produced by a variety of cells in response to exogenous challenge (Ch. 6):

- Pro-inflammatory:
  - Tumour necrosis factor α (TNF-α)
  - Interleukin-1
  - Interleukin-6.
- Classical hormones are secreted by specialised glands mainly in response to stress (Ch. 10):
  - Cortisol
  - Catecholamines
  - Glucagon.

The metabolic responses can be summarised under the following headings:

- Energy metabolism
  - Changes in metabolic rate
  - Increased glucose turnover and insulin resistance
  - Lipid metabolism
- Protein metabolism
  - Changes in whole body protein turnover and nitrogen balance
  - The acute phase response.

response to the secretion of cytokines and classical hormones, and perhaps other unknown factors, considered here separately from the changes that occur simultaneously in the inflammatory response, which are dealt with elsewhere in this book (see Ch. 6).

The BMR rises depending on the severity of the stress and the body temperature of the patient. Burns are notorious for increasing BMR, which may rise to nearly double the normal rate. It should, however, be remembered that it is the *total* energy requirements of the patient that determine how much energy is needed for energy balance. In trauma and sepsis, physical activity almost always reduces dramatically and this reduction in energy need offsets any increase in basal metabolism so the energy requirements of most ill patients are seldom much more than those of active people.

Energy metabolism during illness

Although there is a low level of physical activity during illness, which reduces energy expenditure, other changes use energy and so increase expenditure, for example:

- The inflammatory response (Ch. 6)
- Pyrexia
- Infection
- Sepsis
- Physical trauma (especially burns).

Insulin and the inflammatory response

Blood glucose is raised despite an elevated plasma insulin concentration during stress – 'insulin resistance' (see Chs 3 and 10). This is accompanied by an increase in the levels of pro-inflammatory cytokines and the hormones cortisol, catecholamines and glucagon. The metabolic turnover of glucose is increased.

- There is increased uptake of glucose by immune cells, mediated by non-insulin-dependent systems.
- Glucose metabolism, by both glycolysis and oxidation is increased, with an increase in blood lactate levels so that gluconeogenesis (from lactate) also increases.
- Glycogen synthesis and storage is reduced.

The increase in circulating glucose enables the body to meet the increased energy need during illness.

Protein metabolism in illness

Owing to increased energy needs during trauma and sepsis (see above), amino acids are released from muscle to be made available for gluconeogenesis. Blood glucose level is therefore relatively high and produces a secondary rise in plasma insulin. An elevated blood glucose level in the face of raised plasma insulin is termed **insulin resistance** (see above).

The result of increased amino acid breakdown for gluconeogenesis is an increase in nitrogen excretion, so that unless dietary sources of amino acids increase, there will be a negative nitrogen balance. This effect is enhanced in big and heavily muscled, well-nourished men. It is diminished in a warm environment and in people with a smaller muscle mass. Intake of exogenous amino acids helps to limit protein loss from the body, but urinary nitrogen losses remain high because of sustained protein catabolism. If feeding fails, depletion of tissues becomes a threat to survival.

Protein metabolism and acute phase response in illness

In acute illness, although the rate of protein synthesis increases (in the liver and immune cells), the rate of protein

Information box 16.4   **Energy needs of very sick patients**

In practice, to calculate energy needs for nutritional supplementation of very sick patients:

- Estimate BMR (see above)
- Add a stress factor – usually between 10% and 40% of BMR
- Add a combined factor for activity- and diet-induced thermogenesis
  - Bedbound, immobile: +10%
  - Bedbound, mobile or sitting: +15–50%
  - Mobile on ward: +25 %

Example: The energy requirements for a bed-bound and sitting well-fed man with active inflammatory bowel disease at rest, whose usual BMR is 6000 kJ, will be:

$$6000 \times (10\% \text{ stress} + 15\% \text{ physical activity}) = 7500 \text{ kJ}$$
$$(4.2 \text{ kJ is equivalent to } 1 \text{ kcal})$$

degradation is comparatively higher, resulting in the net loss of body protein from the less essential organs (e.g. muscle). The provision of amino acids in the diet reduces nitrogen losses substantially; however, patients generally do not regain muscle mass until the underlying pathology is resolved.

Protein synthesis provides substrate for the repair of tissue and for host defence mechanisms including the acute phase response. There is a diversion in synthesis away from somatic and circulating proteins, such as albumin, towards acute phase proteins. These include:

- Haptoglobin
- Ceruloplasmin
- α_2-Macroglobulin
- α_1-Antitrypsin
- Fibrinogen
- C-reactive protein
- α_1 Acid glycoprotein.

A prolonged increase in acute phase protein synthesis is accompanied by a reduction in albumin synthesis, one of several causes of clinically observed hypoalbuminaemia, which will not respond to dietary intake until the underlying pathology is successfully treated.

Tracer studies, used more for research, use stable isotopes to determine the rates of amino acid metabolism. These can give a more precise indication of the determinants of nitrogen balance, telling us whether changes in protein synthesis or breakdown to constituent amino acids is dominant. In inflammatory and infective states turnover/breakdown tends to increase if food intake is maintained.

MICRONUTRIENTS AND WATER

Some essential components of the human diet, such as vitamins, electrolytes and trace elements (iodine, zinc, magnesium), are only needed in tiny amounts. Water is another essential part of the diet. Although dietary deficiency of vitamins and minerals is uncommon with a balanced diet in developed countries, supplementation of electrolytes, vitamins and trace metals become important for people on artificial diets or parenteral feeding. The absorption and transport of vitamins and minerals are discussed in Chapter 15.

VITAMINS

Vitamins are organic molecules that are needed in small (microgram to milligram) amounts in the diets of higher animals and man. They are present and serve similar purposes in most forms of life, but humans cannot synthesise them and they have to be ingested in the diet. Although grouped together under 'vitamin', they are not chemically related to each other. They are classified according to their solubility in fat or water. Although only required in small amounts, without them deficiency diseases occur (see below).

Most vitamins function as coenzymes or as antioxidants (see later sections). Except in illness, dietary vitamin deficiencies are relatively rare in developed nations, but seen more often in developing countries, in association with macronutrient malnutrition. Vitamin supplements should not be necessary with otherwise well-balanced diets in people who are not ill or pregnant.

Dietary vitamin supplementation (e.g. ascorbic acid, β-carotene, α-tocopherol) as a means of reducing cardiovascular disease or cancer risk has not been demonstrated to be effective in randomised controlled trials. However, epidemiological studies have shown that a high intake of fruit and vegetables (Mediterranean diet) is associated with reduced cardiovascular morbidity and mortality. The recommendation for an adequate daily intake of fruit and vegetables as sources of micronutrients is uncontroversial.

Vitamins as coenzymes

Some enzymes require the presence of coenzymes or cofactors in order to function (see Ch. 2), of which many are derived from B vitamins. Coenzymes are often involved in oxidation–reduction (redox) reactions, where they act as either electron donors or acceptors. They enable chemical reactions to move in a direction otherwise prevented by an energy gradient.

Vitamins as antioxidants

Protection from damage caused by free radicals may be prevented by the action of a number of antioxidants such as vitamin E, vitamin C, and vitamin A (β-carotene), which form non-reactive, stable radicals.

WATER-SOLUBLE VITAMINS

Water-soluble vitamins are derived from the diet. Apart from vitamin B_{12}, storage is minimal in humans, so that water-soluble vitamin excess or toxicity is unknown. Deficiencies occur either because of poor diet or malabsorption and can lead to disease conditions. It is not generally appreciated how common deficiencies of water-soluble vitamins are among non-alcoholic patients admitted to hospital. For example, subclinical B_1 deficiency can all too easily be converted to clinical deficiency with lactic acidosis if glucose infusions or parenteral nutrition feeds are provided without inclusion of this vitamin.

The B vitamins

The B complex vitamins are coenzymes. In the activated form, they carry electrons and chemical groups in numerous metabolic processes. They are widely distributed in meat, liver, poultry, eggs, dairy products, fish, wholegrain cereals, legumes and grains. Deficiency states often present with multiple B vitamin deficiencies.

Vitamin B_1 (thiamine)

Vitamin B_1 is a coenzyme in carbohydrate metabolism (pentose phosphate, hexose monophosphate pathway) and in pyruvate metabolism. The body stores very little vitamin B_1 so a regular intake is necessary. It is present in the husk of rice, in wheatgerm and in seeds.

Vitamin B_2 (riboflavin)

The coenzymes flavine mononucleotide (FMN) and flavine adenosine dinucleotide (FAD) are derived from vitamin B_2. They are required for carbohydrate and fat metabolism and a wide variety of oxidation and reduction reactions central to all metabolic processes (Ch. 3). Deficiencies lead to angular stomatitis, glossitis, dermatitis, cheilosis and cataracts. Liver, milk, meat, fish and some leafy vegetables are sources of vitamin B_2.

Vitamin B_3 (niacin)

Nicotinic acid and nicotinamide are also known as niacin (vitamin B_3), an essential part of the human diet as it forms the active part of nicotinamide adenine dinucleotide (NAD$^+$) and nicotinamide adenine dinucleotide phosphate (NADP$^+$). Energy for ATP synthesis is derived from oxidation of these nucleotides (see Ch. 3). Both vitamins B_2 and B_3 have a central role in the transduction of energy in the electron transport chain of mitochondria. Niacin can be synthesised from tryptophan in the presence of other B vitamins such as riboflavin, pyridoxine and/or thiamine.

Vitamin B_6 (pyridoxine)

Vitamin B_6 is a cofactor in glycogen and amino acid metabolism. A high dietary protein intake increases pyridoxine requirement.

Biotin

Biotin functions as a coenzyme in lipogenesis, gluconeogenesis and the breakdown of branch chained amino acids (see

Ch. 3). A growth factor for cells, it is synthesised by intestinal flora. Some dietary constituents, such as the raw egg white protein avidin, bind with biotin to prevent its absorption, leading to deficiency. Clinical consequences include dermatitis, depression and muscular pains, but deficiency is very rare outside the context of artificial nutrition.

Pantothenic acid

Pantothenic acid is part of coenzyme A and is widely available in all plant and animal foods. Deficiency in humans is very rare.

Folic acid

The physiologically active, reduced form of folic acid, dihydrofolic acid, acts as a coenzyme in single carbon transfer during nucleic acid (DNA) and amino acid synthesis. Folic acid is therefore most needed by rapidly dividing cells.

Vitamin B$_{12}$ (cobalamin)

Vitamin B$_{12}$, together with folic acid, is involved as a coenzyme in the conversion of homocysteine to methionine (see

above). It also acts as a coenzyme for methylmalonyl CoA mutase. Vitamin B$_{12}$ is synthesised by bacteria and only available in foods of animal origin.

Vitamin C (ascorbic acid)

Vitamin C is essential in the human diet, and abundant in citrus fruits and green vegetables. Ascorbic acid, the physiologically active form, is a reducing agent in hydroxylation reactions. Its role as an antioxidant in preventing cancer and atherosclerosis has attracted much attention but as yet there is no evidence of its effectiveness. It also takes part in the synthesis of adrenaline (epinephrine) and steroids.

Vitamin C deficiency leads to scurvy, a condition in which there is capillary fragility, giving rise to bruising and subcutaneous haemorrhages, bleeding and swollen gums, muscle weakness, anaemia and poor wound healing. Although common in the days of long sea voyages when fresh fruit and vegetables were not available, scurvy is now rare except among the very elderly with poor diets. Vitamin C deficiency is also associated with osteoporosis (see Ch. 9) and immunity is impaired.

FAT-SOLUBLE VITAMINS

Fat soluble vitamins are stored in the liver and adipose tissue. They have to be absorbed with fat and are less easily absorbed from food than water-soluble vitamins. Enthusiastic supplementation, however, can lead to toxicity and overdose. Vitamins A and D function like hormones and are toxic in overdose.

Vitamin A

Vitamin A is a collection of three compounds, retinol, retinal and retinoic acid, collectively known as retinoids. The provitamin is β-carotene, widely distributed in green vegetables; retinol is present in milk, liver, cod liver oil, butter, cheese and margarine. Enough is stored in the liver as retinol palmate to last about a year. Two specialised proteins, serum retinol

---

Clinical box 16.4 Some vitamin B deficiencies

Vitamin B$_1$ deficiency impairs glucose metabolism
The commonest form of thiamine deficiency, beriberi, occurs in populations dependent on rice diets of highly polished rice, which removes the thiamine. Large caloric requirements, as in the catabolic state, can give rise to beriberi. Alcohol inhibits thiamine absorption in the intestines, leading to deficiency. Wernicke–Korsakoff syndrome is the result of thiamine deficiency associated with the combination of chronic alcohol misuse and malnutrition. In thiamine deficiency there are raised levels of pyruvate, which inhibits glycolysis and leads to the accumulation of lactate. The accumulation of both pyruvic acid and lactic acid causes acidosis which, in severe cases, can lead to coma and death.

Vitamin B$_3$ deficiency
Niacin deficiency leads to pellagra, which is rare and is related to some drugs, e.g. isoniazid. Superficial glossitis leads to dermatitis, giving sunburn-like lesions on exposed skin. Pressure sores, diarrhoea, dementia and death ensue. Excessively high doses of niacin are hepatotoxic.

Vitamin B$_6$ deficiency
Pyridoxine is needed for neurotransmitter synthesis (e.g. serotonin, noradrenaline), so deficiency can lead to symptoms of irritability and depression and peripheral neuropathy. Dietary deficiency is rare but peripheral neuropathy associated with administration of the anti-tuberculous drug, isoniazid, is well known. The use of the contraceptive pill can also increase pyridoxine requirement and can theoretically lead to a deficiency state.

Clinical box 16.5 Folic acid deficiency

Deficiency of folic acid is one of the most common vitamin deficiencies. Increased demand, such as during pregnancy and the demand of rapid fetal growth, could precipitate folate deficiency. This feature is also exploited, as antifolate drugs are used against rapidly dividing bacterial cells (antibiotic trimethoprim) and cancer cells (cytotoxic methotrexate).

Folate deficiency causes a macrocytic, megaloblastic anaemia (see Ch 12). The features are similar to vitamin B$_{12}$ deficiency. High intake of folate reduces plasma concentrations of homocysteine.

Clinical box 16.6 Vitamin B$_{12}$ deficiency

Vitamin B$_{12}$ is well stored and deficiency takes months or years to develop. Eventually, deficiency leads to a methionine deficiency in the spinal cord, giving rise to a neurological disorder, subacute combined degeneration of the cord, which can occur without megaloblastic anaemia. The megaloblastic anaemia in vitamin B$_{12}$ deficiency is probably associated with a deficiency of reduced folate (see Ch. 12). For this reason, until the cause is finally established, a macrocytic, megaloblastic anaemia should not be treated with folic acid alone because of the risk of precipitating subacute combined degeneration of the cord.

Vitamin B$_{12}$ is the only water-soluble vitamin stored mainly in the liver. Pernicious anaemia, an autoimmune gastritis which results in lack of gastric intrinsic factor required for the absorption of vitamin B$_{12}$, is one cause of deficiency; gastric resection is a cause of intrinsic factor deficiency. Malabsorption due to chronic pancreatitis can occur as a result of failure to secrete a pancreas-derived activating component of intrinsic factor. Small-intestinal bacterial overgrowth causes deficiency, commonly in the elderly. Extensive (100 cm or more) ileal resection, for example because of Crohn's disease, prevents absorption of vitamin B$_{12}$. Vegans, who eat no animal products, are at risk of dietary vitamin B$_{12}$ deficiency.

Retinol is an intracellular pigment that is bound to rhodopsin in the cells of the retina and acts like a hormone. When exposed to light, it dissociates and initiates the signal to the brain, which is perceived as light. Vitamin A deficiency thus leads to 'night blindness', or visual impairment in poor light. Retinoic acid acts as a typical steroid hormone. It increases the synthesis of proteins controlling epithelial cell differentiation. Deficiency can lead to corneal softening (defective epithelial growth and keratinisation leading to **xerophthalmia**) causing partial and, if severe, permanent blindness. Under famine and starvation conditions, vitamin A deficiency is the commonest cause of blindness. Vitamin A deficiency also occurs in liver failure and in malabsorption as a result of steatorrhoea.

Clinical box 16.8 Vitamin D deficiency

Vitamin D affects Ca^{2+} metabolism and bones (see Ch. 11 for details). Deficiency leads to rickets in children and osteomalacia in adults. This can occur when a lack of sunshine combines with dietary deficiency due to inadequate intake of milk and oily fish, or malabsorption from foodstuffs that bind with dietary vitamin D to prevent absorption.

Clinical box 16.9 Iron deficiency and overload

Iron deficiency anaemia can occur with dietary deficiency, increased demand or excessive blood loss and results in a microcytic hypochromic anaemia:

- Deficiency is seldom due to dietary inadequacy but can be associated with extreme, unbalanced diets such as the vegan diet.
- Increased demand from excessive blood loss in women of childbearing age or from overt or occult gastrointestinal bleeding. Iron deficiency anaemia in men or post-menopausal women should trigger a search for gastrointestinal pathology, particularly colon cancer.
- Malabsorption of iron is rarely a problem but occurs in coeliac disease.
- There is increased demand during both pregnancy and rapid growth in childhood.

Iron overload leads to hepatomegaly and cirrhosis. Excessive iron stores in the liver may be caused by:

- Repeated blood transfusions causing haemosiderosis, for example in β-thalassaemia
- Unusually excessive dietary intake, as in some South African tribes that use iron cooking pots
- Hereditary haemochromatosis.

binding protein (SRBP) and cytosolic binding proteins, are needed to distribute vitamin A from the liver to its active site. High concentrations are toxic, particularly in pregnancy.

Recently, the role of β-carotene as an antioxidant has attracted attention because of the role of retinoids in epithelial cell growth and differentiation. It has been hypothesised that vitamin A is protective against cancers arising from epithelial cells. Although there is some epidemiological evidence of increased cancer risk in populations with very low dietary vitamin A, evidence from randomised controlled trials of effectiveness is not yet available.

Vitamin D (calciferol)

Vitamin D is really a hormone synthesised from cholesterol (produced in the liver) in the skin following exposure to ultra-violet rays in sunlight. Dietary intake is only necessary when exposure to sunlight is inadequate; dietary sources include cod liver oil, eggs, dairy products, fortified milk and margarine. The effect of sunlight leads to the synthesis of ergocalciferol (D_2) and cholecalciferol (D_3), which are further metabolised to hydroxylated derivatives – first in the liver (25 position) and then in the renal tubules (1 position) to 1,25 hydroxyvitamin D_3, the active forms of vitamin D (Ch. 10).

Vitamin E (tocopherols)

Vitamin E is incorporated in the lipid cell membrane structure, lipoproteins and adipose tissues, and is an antioxidant. Although it is associated with fertility in some animals, with a role in spermatogenesis and ovum implantation, there is no proven association in human beings. Widely available in vegetable oils, dietary vitamin E deficiency is rare except in fat malabsorption. In very-low-weight premature infants, vitamin E deficiency causes haemolytic anaemia and thrombocytosis. Dietary sources include seeds, margarines and vegetable oils, especially wheatgerm and sunflower seed oils.

Vitamin K

Vitamin K acts as a coenzyme in activating precursors (clotting factors) produced by the liver in the coagulation cascade (see Ch.12). Dietary deficiency causes haemorrhagic disease. Although dietary deficiency is uncommon, it occurs with fat malabsorption. Coagulation disorders, owing to vitamin K deficiency, can also occur in liver disease (e.g. alcoholic cirrhosis) and in newborn infants. In newborn infants with very immature livers and sterile guts, vitamin K deficiency occurs because it is mostly made by the normal bacterial flora of the jejunum and ileum not present in newborns. Anticoagulants of the dicoumarin group (warfarin or rat poison) act by inhibiting the action of vitamin K. Vitamin K may be used to reverse haemorrhagic conditions from dicoumarin overdose. Dietary sources include green leafy vegetables, vegetable oils and fermented dairy products.

TRACE ELEMENTS: MINERALS

Trace amounts of some minerals are necessary for metabolic processes and are therefore essential in the human diet. All are toxic in high concentrations, and a number of deficiency syndromes have been recognised. Unbound metal ions carry a charge and can lead to the formation of free radicals.

IRON

Iron is essential for many metabolic processes, especially for the oxygen-carrying capacity of haemoglobin (see Ch.12). The average body content of iron is 3–5 g, two-thirds of which is in haemoglobin. Plasma iron is transported as ferric ions (Fe^{3+}) bound to transferrin. It is stored mainly in the liver, spleen or bone marrow as ferritin. Dietary sources include meat, offal, egg yolks, shellfish, some dried pulses and dates, and some green vegetables. Vegans are thus at risk of dietary iron deficiency.

Copper deficiency due to malabsorption occurs in **Menkes'** syndrome, a rare, sex linked, recessive genetic disorder. In children with this condition, there is failure to thrive, mental retardation and bone defects, with characteristic kinky, brittle hair.

Wilson's disease is an inborn error of metabolism and an autosomal recessive disorder. Biliary excretion of copper is severely impaired leading to copper deposits in:

- Liver – resulting in cirrhosis
- Kidneys – with tubular degeneration
- Basal ganglia – causing tremor, involuntary movements and dementia
- Cornea – as Kayser–Fleisher rings.

Clinical box 16.11 **Zinc deficiency**

A very rare hereditary disorder, acrodermatitis enteropathica, is characterised by zinc malabsorption, leading to growth retardation, diarrhoea, hair loss, skin lesions and candida infections. Zinc supplementation reverses all the symptoms. Zinc deficiency can also be caused by increased loss, as in renal disease and major burns. Patients on total parenteral nutrition also need regular assessment of zinc status and supplementation. Zinc depletion prevents wound healing and compromises the immune system so that the patient is more susceptible to infections. Sexual development and spermatogenesis may also be impaired.

COPPER

Copper is incorporated into the oxygenase enzymes, particularly superoxide dismutase, which is a scavenger of superoxide and other reactive oxygen species (see below). It is also necessary for collagen synthesis. Copper deficiency occurs with excessive loss, as in chronic renal dialysis and malabsorption (see Clinical box 16.10).

ZINC

Zinc is involved in many metabolic processes as coenzymes and metalloproteins. Zinc is widely available in all foods. Although of low toxicity, excessive zinc intake interferes with copper absorption and can lead to copper deficiency.

SELENIUM

Selenium is part of the antioxidant glutathione peroxidase and is also found in most cells. Dietary sources include shellfish, offal, Brazil nuts and cereals. Low selenium is thought to impair immune and thyroid function, decrease antioxidant status and increase susceptibility to viral infections. Selenium intake varies worldwide as a result of varying soil composition and therefore the variable selenium content in staple foods such as wheat. Deficiency is rare except for Keshan disease, which is endemic in some areas in China where the soil selenium content is extremely low or absent. Muscle pains and cardiomyopathy may result. Total parenteral nutrition can also lead to selenium deficiency.

MAGNESIUM

Magnesium is an intracellular ion involved in maintaining electropotentials in nerves and skeletal muscle. The amount of magnesium consumed is the main determinant of the amount absorbed, although parathyroid hormone (PTH) and vitamin D probably increase absorption. The main control of plasma magnesium levels is by the kidneys (see Ch. 14).

CALCIUM

Nearly all (99%) the body's calcium in adults is found in the skeleton (about 1 kg). Plasma concentration is about 2.25–2.60 mmol/L. The recommended daily intake of calcium in adults in the UK is:

- Adult (19–50 years) RNI = 700 mg
- Lactation = 700 mg + 550 mg.

Calcium absorption and metabolism are discussed in Chapters 10 and 15. Lack of oestrogen and corticosteroid therapy in particular are implicated in loss of calcium from the skeleton and osteoporosis in later life. Calcium is mainly found in milk and dairy products; vegetables contain a small amount. In some countries (e.g. the UK) flour is fortified with calcium. Calcium requirements increase during pregnancy and lactation. Deficiency is associated with vitamin D deficiency. Adolescent girls frequently do not consume enough calcium. It is estimated that a third of women and a sixth of men will have an osteoporotic fracture at some time in their life.

PHOSPHATE

Phosphate is needed for phosphorylation, an essential process in most metabolic pathways. Daily oral intake for adults is similar to that of calcium. Phosphate is widely available and well absorbed from food, so that dietary deficiency is unknown. Plasma phosphate levels are regulated by PTH (see Ch. 10). Low levels are associated with hyperparathyroidism. High phosphate concentrations are seen in hypoparathyroidism and renal failure.

IODINE

Iodine is a constituent of thyroid hormones. Seafoods and seaweed are rich in iodine. Iodine is also available in milk, which is now the major source of iodine in Western countries. Deficiency causes goitre and brain damage. Endemic goitre occurs in mountainous regions where iodine is absent in the soil. Salt is also iodised to help eradicate iodine deficiency.

FLUORIDE

Epidemiological evidence suggests that dental caries is more prevalent in areas with lower levels of fluoride in drinking water. There are few dietary sources of fluoride apart from shellfish. Fluoridation of drinking water and toothpaste may help. Fluorosis, resulting from fluoride overdose, causes damage to dental enamel with pitting and discoloration.

WATER AND ELECTROLYTES

Water and electrolytes are essential constituents of the human body and are found in three compartments within the body:

- Intracellular fluid (ICF)
- Interstitial fluids
- Plasma.

The typical volumes of fluid distributed in the various compartments are described in Chapters 2 and 4. The intracellular compartment is separated from the extracellular compartment by the lipid cell membrane. In the extracellular compartment, plasma is separated from the interstitial fluids by the capillary membranes. The biochemical composition and volume of body fluids in health are kept constant through homeostatic mechanisms (see Ch. 2). In disease, the control mechanisms are altered, so that there could be disturbance in fluid volume and altered biochemical composition.

WATER

Most of the water in the body is in the lean body mass. The fat-free mass of adults is about 72% water. The amount of water in an adult is therefore dependent on the amount of adipose tissue in their body. Men tend to have a higher percentage of water content than women because women store more fat per unit weight.

Daily water requirements

The water requirement for an average adult varies between 1.5 L and 3 L per day (30–35 mL/kg body weight), of which 0.5 to 1 L is to replace insensible loss; that is, from skin and respiration. The daily output of water is the sum of losses in the urine, faeces and sweat, and will vary according to the environmental temperature, body temperature, amount of physical activity and weight. The amount of water lost in the urine is determined by urine concentration or dilution by the kidneys, which in turn is regulated by vasopressin (also called anti-diuretic hormone (ADH)). The mechanism is discussed in detail in Ch. 14.

The daily water requirement increases substantially during vigorous exercise because of loss through sweating. Children also need more water. To estimate daily fluid balance and fluid requirement in clinical practice, the urine, faecal and other intestinal (e.g. diarrhoea, vomit or gastric aspirate) losses are summed, and then a nominal 500–1000 mL for insensible (sweat) loss are added.

The amount that a person drinks can be in excess of requirement, based on thirst and to some extent habit (Ch. 8). Water is obtained from foods and drinks and from water formed during metabolism. The water formed during metabolism is relatively small at roughly 275 mL/day. For patients who are unable to drink (e.g. postoperatively) or have suffered severe losses, as with burns or haemorrhage, hydration must be maintained by intravenous infusion. Fluid balance can be monitored either by careful input and output charting or by monitoring the changes in body weight from day to day.

ELECTROLYTES

The plasma electrolytes that are clinically important include the sodium and potassium cations (Na^+ and K^+), and the chloride and bicarbonate anions (Cl^- and HCO_3^-). Clinical laboratory measurements of plasma concentration are used for the diagnosis of metabolic disturbances, such as diabetic ketoacidosis, renal failure and so on. Electrolytes are dissolved in water, and as with water, divided into intracellular and extracellular compartments. The molecules dissolved in water contribute to the **osmotic pressure** in their separate compartments (see also Chs 2, 4 and 14). The osmotic gradient created by the different electrolyte concentrations in each compartment enables water to move between the compartments.

Although water is freely diffusible across the barriers between compartments, the movement of water-soluble electrolytes and molecules is restricted by the lipid cell membrane. Water-soluble molecules have to be transported across these membranes via ion pumps, of which the Na^+/K^+-ATPase pump is the most active. The energy-consuming process in which Na^+ is driven out of cells and K^+ is driven into cells is reduced during fasting, so that Na^+ moves into cells and K^+ moves out. The opposite occurs with refeeding (see refeeding syndrome). One of the ion pump's functions is nerve transmission (see Ch. 8). Other ion pumps transport glucose, amino acids and calcium.

WATER AND ELECTROLYTE DEPLETION

Fluid depletion could be due to:

- Severe water deprivation, as in postoperative patients unable to drink, unconscious patients or abnormalities with thirst mechanisms
- Loss of electrolytes and water, as in severe, prolonged vomiting and diarrhoea
- Excess water loss due to pituitary (failure of ADH secretion) or renal (failure to respond to ADH) problems or **diabetes insipidus**
- Excess water loss through osmotic diuresis, e.g. drug induced, hyperglycaemia
- Loss of plasma, as in severe burns
- Haemorrhage, when blood as well as water and electrolytes are lost.

Oral rehydration with water and electrolytes is the method of choice, whenever possible. Intravenous fluid replacement is needed when the fluid loss is severe, the patient is unconscious, or when the patient cannot drink.

Intravenous fluid replacement

A variety of intravenous fluids are available for severely dehydrated patients in whom oral rehydration is contraindicated. Table 16.11 shows the electrolyte content of the principal intravenous fluids used in clinical practice. Note that dextrose saline is a maintenance solution for use when there is no excessive fluid loss or Na^+ depletion, whereas 0.9% ('normal') saline is a replacement solution with a Na^+ content approximating that of plasma. However, compared with plasma values, there is excess Cl^- relative to Na^+, which can result in hyperchloraemic acidosis (i.e. sodium and chloride are equimolar in normal saline whereas there is less chloride than sodium in plasma), so a more physiologically balanced solution such as Hartmann's may be preferable and better tolerated. Both Hartmann's solution and normal saline contain more than a day's requirement of Na^+ per litre. They are therefore fluid replacement and not fluid maintenance solutions and carry the risk of salt and water overload and oedema.

WATER OVERLOAD

Water overload occurs if the intake exceeds renal excretion and is uncommon with normal renal function, except with

Table 16.11	Constitution of solutions for intravenous infusion			
	Na$^+$ (mmol/L)	K$^+$ (mmol/L)	HCO$_3^-$ (mmol/L)	Energy (kJ (kcal)/L)
5% Dextrose	–	–	–	838 (200)
Dextrose saline solution	30	–	–	670 (160)
Normal saline	150	–	–	–
Hartmann's solution	131	5	29 (lactate) +2 mmol Ca	–

very excessive drinking. It does, however, occur if 5% dextrose or a hypo-osmolar solution is infused overenthusiastically. The effect is to dilute sodium content: hyponatraemia (Na$^+$ <135 mmol/L). If uncorrected, hyponatraemic encephalopathy can occur. Hyponatraemia has been reported with excessive intake of sports drinks and water after strenuous exercise, e.g. after running a marathon. It can also occur after excessive dextrose infusions postoperatively, particularly if there is a degree of impaired glomerular filtration. This can be avoided by giving isotonic normal saline.

THE CONTROL OF FOOD INTAKE

The interactions between energy balance and food intake for humans is complex. The increasing prevalence of obesity and its associated disease states has focused attention on the physiological mechanisms that control nutritional intake and energy expenditure. These mechanisms are potential targets for intervention, whether through use of anti-obesity drugs or the use of psychological therapies, in the quest for effective treatment of obesity.

APPETITE AND SATIETY

Appetite refers to a desire to eat, which may be influenced by the sight, taste and smell of food, social and cultural patterns of eating behaviour and psychological factors (e.g. depression). Hunger is the feeling of a pressing need to eat, and satiety is the feeling during, or soon after, a meal that enough has been eaten. Eating as a goal-directed behaviour and motivation for eating (or not) is discussed in Chapter 8. Eating is a basic function to sustain life, which also gives enjoyment. For human beings, satiety does not necessarily terminate eating, and nor is it hunger that always initiates eating.

THE PHYSIOLOGICAL CONTROL OF EATING

A complex system of signals indicating satiety (satiety signals) balances the drive to eat. These include:

- Peripheral signals arising from the gut
- Hormones signalling energy balance and fat stores (Fig.16.10).

These signals are integrated through a network of feedback mechanisms in which the hypothalamus plays the leading role. The brainstem and higher cortical networks also play their part (Fig. 16.11).

PERIPHERAL SATIETY SIGNALS

Satiety signals originating in the gut are carried via afferents in the vagus to the nucleus of the solitary tract (nTS) in the brainstem (Fig.16.11). These signals are initiated by:

- Gastric fullness, a sensation that the stomach is full, and gastric distension, when the stretch receptors in the stomach walls are stimulated by overfilling the stomach, and gastric emptying
- The balance of chemical content in the lumen of the gut
- Peptides and hormones secreted by the stomach and small intestine in response to the presence of food.

Gastric distension and emptying

Filling the stomach leads to distension, which reduces the desire to eat. For example, pyloric ligation (in animal experiments, to prevent gastric contents from entering the duodenum) results in stomach distension that appears to induce

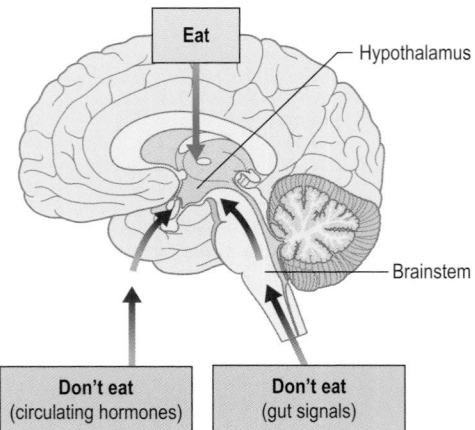

Fig. 16.10 To eat or not to eat. Signal to eat – appetite; signal to stop – satiety. Our innate drive to eat is balanced by competing signals from the body indicating satiety, our fat reserves and overall energy status. Redrawn with permission from Luckman S 2001 Is there such a thing as a healthy appetite? British Society for Neuroendocrinology. Neuro-endocrinology Briefing 14.

satiety. Balloons inflated in the stomach induce satiety in rats. This appears to be true in humans as well: endoscopically placed gastric balloons help obese patients lose weight. Cancer of the stomach is a common pathological cause of early satiety when infiltration of the stomach wall with cancer cells leads to rigidity and limited distension so that smaller than normal feeds make the patient 'feel full'. However, a full stomach does not always stop someone from eating more.

The *rate* of gastric emptying is an important component in determining gastric fullness. It depends upon the physical form of the meal eaten, its volume, energy density, fat content and many other variables, including stress, smoking and whether the food is eaten in a habitual form. In man, for any particular fixed proportions of constituents, the higher the *volume* of a feed, the *slower* the gastric emptying. Animal studies indicate that slower gastric emptying gives rise to a greater sense of satiety.

Balance of chemical contents in the gut

The presence of food in the duodenum, jejunum and ileum delays gastric emptying, probably mediated by intestinal receptors for acidity, osmolality, fat, glucose and amino acids. A jejunal infusion of a mixture of casein hydrolysate, oleic acid and maltose, designed to simulate the composition of normal chyme in the jejunum, inhibits gastric acid secretion and delays gastric emptying. The results of altering the proportions of the constituents in the infusion suggest that carbohydrate and fat have the principal inhibiting effect on acid secretion, whereas carbohydrate, fat and protein delay stomach emptying.

Peptides and hormones

A variety of peptides and hormones are secreted by the stomach and small intestine in response to the presence of

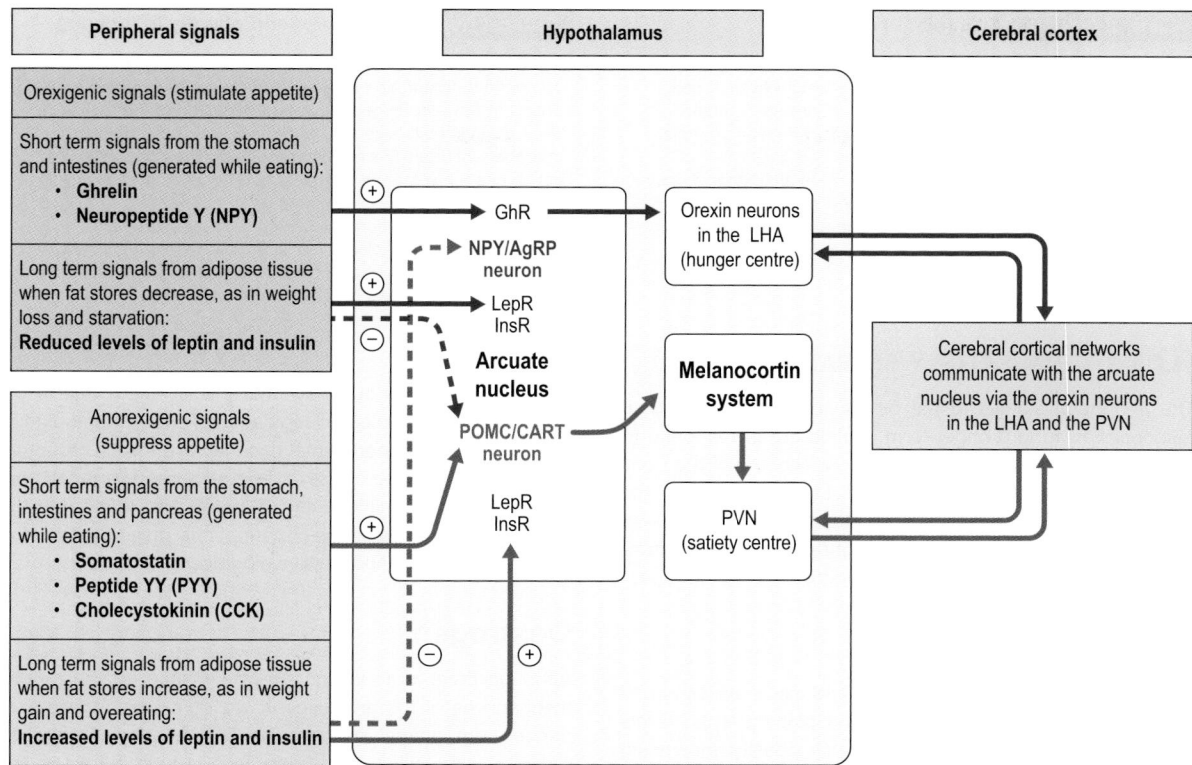

Fig. 16.11 Diagram of postulated pathways for the regulation of appetite and energy balance. Hunger (during starvation and weight loss) increases appetite and reduces energy expenditure. Satiety should reduce eating and increase energy expenditure. Increased secretion of leptin and insulin from fat stores after weight gain inhibits the NPY/AgRpP neuron, resulting in reduced appetite, whereas reduced leptin and insulin levels during starvation inhibit the POM/CART neuron so that appetite is stimulated. Corticotropin releasing hormone (CRH) stimulates the anorexigenic pathway. Plasma levels are raised in response to stress and in anorexia nervosa. Thyrotropin releasing hormone (TRH) increases thermogenesis and thus energy expenditure. AgRP, agouti-related peptide; NPY, neuropeptide Y; POMC pro-opiomelanocortin; CART, cocaine and amphetamine regulated transcript; PVN, paraventricular nucleus; LHA, lateral hypothalamic area; LepR, leptic receptor; InsR, insulin receptor; GhR, ghrelin receptor.

food, stimulating the pancreas to secrete digestive enzymes and hormones, the gall bladder to contract and empty bile into the duodenum, promote or inhibit stomach and gut motility, and act as short-term chemical signals to inhibit excessive eating (see also Ch. 15). Among these, the best characterised include:

- **Cholecystokinin** (CCK) – a hormone secreted in the duodenum, jejunum and terminal ileum in response to the presence of food. CCK reduces appetite and inhibits eating. It also acts as a neurotransmitter in the hypothalamus to inhibit eating (see below).
- **Glucagon-like peptide-1** (GLP-1) – the ileal brake is a signal which reduces gastric emptying and inhibits upper intestinal motility when food reaches the ileum. It is mediated by GLP-1, which is cleaved from proglucagon and expressed in the gut, pancreas and brain.
- **Oxyntomodulin** – also proglucagon-derived and secreted by ileal cells in proportion to ingested calories, this peptide lessens hunger and food intake.
- **Peptide YY** (PYY) – secreted in the ileum and colon and also part of the 'ileal brake'. It is related to neuropeptide-Y (NPY, see below), inhibits pancreatic exocrine secretion and slows down gastric and small bowel transit of food. Intestinal PYY reduces appetite

(whereas hypothalamic NPY increases food intake) but the effect may be independent of central pathways.

PERIPHERAL HUNGER SIGNALS

Peripheral hunger signals arise from the intestine, mediated by the hormone ghrelin. Hunger is not usually experienced until after near-complete gastric emptying (about 1.5–3 hours after eating) and peaks about 2–4 hours after onset. Hunger ratings in experimental subjects continue to increase after complete gastric emptying, indicating that while an empty stomach may give rise to hunger, it cannot be the whole cause.

Ghrelin

Ghrelin is a unique gut-mediated, orexigenic gut peptide hormone secreted by gastric epithelium (also kidneys). It is a natural ligand for the growth hormone secretogogue (GHS; activates the secretion of growth hormone) receptor (GHS-R). It increases hunger (orexigenic effect), growth hormone secretion and fat stores, and is also found in the hypothalamus. Ongoing research may elucidate its role in energy homeostasis and obesity (see below).

Clinical box 16.12   Ghrelin in disease

Plasma concentrations of ghrelin in patients with anorexia nervosa are higher than normal. As body weight rises to near normal levels, ghrelin concentration falls. Conversely, ghrelin levels are lower in obese people compared with lean controls. The relationships between the conditions and ghrelin concentration are not yet clear. Ghrelin levels are extremely high in the plasma of patients with Prader–Willi syndrome, characterised by extreme obesity and an almost insatiable appetite.

Clinical box 16.13   Leptin and obesity in humans

Recently, cousins with severe early-onset obesity were found to be leptin deficient, and a family with obese adult members were found to have leptin gene mutation. Mutation of the leptin receptor gene has also been reported, where the affected members of a family were grossly obese. The conclusion that leptin has a pivotal role in appetite and obesity control is very tempting.

Administration of recombinant leptin to subjects with congenital leptin deficiency led to dramatic weight loss and appetite reduction, but giving leptin to obese subjects without congenital defects has not shown the same effects.

LONG-TERM SATIETY SIGNALS

The peripheral signals to eat or not to eat are short-term responses to food. Longer-term signals are in response to the overall energy requirements and expenditure of the body – energy homeostasis (see Fig. 16.11). Discovery of the hormone **leptin** in 1994 led to the understanding of how endocrine and metabolic signals might orchestrate the integration of food intake, energy expenditure and fat storage.

Leptin

Leptin is a hormone synthesised and secreted by white adipose tissues (see Fig. 16.11), and plasma leptin levels reflect the size of fat stores, rising with obesity. Increasing plasma leptin concentration has the effect of a satiety signal on the hypothalamus to increase satiety and suppress appetite (anorexigenic). It also increases basal metabolic rate (BMR) and energy expenditure when the hypothalamus activates the peripheral nervous system to increase fat breakdown for gluconeogenesis. Leptin may be regarded not only a satiety signal but also as an adipostatic signal. In this sense, adipose tissue acts as an endocrine organ. During starvation, plasma leptin concentration falls. The effect is to increase appetite and eating (orexigenic) and to decrease BMR in order to conserve energy. It has been shown that in animals, low circulating leptin also inhibits growth and reproduction.

Leptin resistance

The discovery of leptin led to a massive increase of research into the control of appetite and obesity to find more effective medical treatments for overeating and obesity. Initially tested on mice with an obese gene (*ob/ob*) and deficient in leptin, intravenous or intraventricular injection of recombinant leptin resulted in reduced feeding and weight loss. It also abolished hyperglycaemia, hyperinsulinaemia and diabetes. Increasing doses produced larger effects. Further experimental evidence suggests that *ob/ob* mice with a diabetes gene are unresponsive to leptin, despite high plasma concentrations. These findings suggest that **leptin resistance**, either due to leptin deficiency or unresponsive leptin receptors, may contribute to a voracious appetite and obesity.

Leptin resistance has similarities with insulin resistance, which may be due to defective transport into the hypothalamus (specifically the arcuate nucleus) or blockade of leptin action. The cellular mechanisms are as yet poorly understood.

Insulin

Before leptin was discovered, research was focused on the role of insulin on human energy homeostasis. Evidence from animal experiments suggests that insulin has a role in the central (brain) physiological regulation of energy homeostasis (see Fig. 16.11). Experimental mice lacking insulin receptors in the brain became obese. It has also been reported that intraventricular administration of insulin and leptin into the brain potentiates the action of peripherally given CCK to stop feeding, leading to sustained weight loss.

Oestrogen

Although there is as yet no direct evidence for the cellular mechanisms of the anorexigenic action of oestrogens, evidence from animal experiments is emerging. Oestrogen receptor expression has been localised in parts of the hypothalamus, namely the arcuate nucleus. Oestrogen appears to target the anorexic pro-opiomelanocortin (POMC) neuron (see below).

CENTRAL NEUROENDOCRINE REGULATION OF EATING

The feedback networks and neurobiology concerned with the regulation of nutrient intake in human beings is extremely complicated, and the subject of much recent research. The hypothalamus is the major site where the diverse signals are integrated. To simplify matters, both **orexigenic** (increase eating) and **anorexigenic** (inhibit eating) pathways are considered here (see Fig. 16.11).

Biotechnical experiments (cloning and brain imaging techniques) have found leptin receptors in the arcuate nucleus of the hypothalamus. When melanocortin, also found in the arcuate nucleus, was shown to be anorexigenic, the anatomical proximity of the leptin receptors to the melanocortin system led to the conclusion that leptin affected the melanocortin metabolism pathway. This is currently thought to be the most important component in the regulation of eating and energy balance.

Melanocortin system

Melanocortin peptides include adrenocorticotropin and melanocyte-stimulating hormones (α-MSH), which determine skin and hair colour. Activation of the melanocortin pathway is essentially anorexigenic (see Fig. 16.11) – it inhibits eating and increases BMR. The melanocortin system, found in the arcuate nucleus of the hypothalamus, integrates the long-term energy homeostatic signals to the hypothalamus with the short-term peripheral satiety and hunger signals received via the nTS in the brain stem. It is also thought that the arcuate nucleus acts as a 'sensor' of changes in blood glucose levels.

Although research into the relationship of the melanocortin system and obesity is in its early stages, with fascinating new information yet to emerge, a melanocortin–obesity syndrome has been postulated. Two families have been found to have this rare syndrome, which is characterised by red hair, gross obesity and adrenocorticotropic hormone (ACTH) deficiency.

The complex neural networks in the arcuate nucleus contain neurons that both activate and inhibit melanocortin receptors (see Fig. 16.11):

- Pro-opiomelanocortin (POMC) and cocaine-amphetamine regulated transcript (CART) neurons activate the melanocortin pathway (anorexigenic).
- NPY and agouti-related peptide (AgRP) neurons inhibit the melanocortin pathway (orexigenic).

The arcuate melanocortin system is central to the action of leptin on energy homeostasis, and would appear to be a promising target for therapeutic intervention in medical conditions such as morbid obesity, type 2 diabetes and eating disorders leading to cachexia. In theory, pharmacological or genetic manipulation of either the POMC/CART or NPY/AgRP circuits could correct these defects.

POMC/CART neuron

Leptin (and insulin) signalling in the arcuate nucleus stimulates the production of POMC and CART, increasing activity in the melanocortin pathway. This has been shown to suppress appetite and eating behaviour in animals.

Melanocortin and β-endorphins are produced by the gene encoding POMC. With respect to appetite and obesity regulation, POMC activates the anorexigenic melanocortin pathway in the arcuate nucleus, and also has expression in the nTS in the medulla (see below). It has been demonstrated that POMC neurons in the arcuate nucleus contain CART.

CART also activates the anorexigenic melanocortin pathway. It was originally identified in animal experiments as a transcript induced by cocaine and amphetamine. This was later refuted, so that CART may be a misnomer, despite human cocaine and amphetamine addicts being anorexic. CART neurons are also found in the lateral hypothalamus.

NPY/AgRP neuron

AgRP and NPY are neurotransmitters in the hypothalamus. CCK and somastatin from the gut also act as neurotransmitters in the brain. Leptin suppresses the synthesis of the orexigenic peptides NPY and AgRP. Abnormal NPY expression may be one part of the cause of obesity. AgRP is a recently discovered neuropeptide found in the arcuate nucleus. A growing body of evidence indicates it has a major role in the regulation of mammalian feeding behaviour. AgRP has been shown to antagonise the action of melanocortin peptides. The exact mechanism of AgRP and agouti protein action has been difficult to study.

AgRP inhibits the melanocortin pathway, but there is no feedback mechanism, so that although there is a mechanism to increase eating via AgRP expression, there is apparently no reverse mechanism to the POMC neuron to inhibit eating. This could explain why the central control mechanism for eating is more directed towards feeding than fasting, a point

Research into the effect of melanocortin on the cardiovascular system and sexual function is in its infancy. The actions are complex and involve diverse cellular mechanisms. Early evidence indicates that melanocortin has an effect on heart rate and blood pressure which, if chronic, might explain the long-term complications of medical conditions such as obesity and diabetes. It also has an effect on how the body eliminates excess sodium (natriuresis). Administration of melanocortin in animal experiments induces inflammation, and brain melanocortin receptors are thought to control sexual behaviour.

Upper gastrointestinal tract peptides and neurotransmitters released in response to the presence of food (see above) are carried via vagal afferents to the nTS.

- **CCK:** there is early evidence from animal experiments that brainstem POMC neurons may transmit CCK satiety signals to the hypothalamus. Further clues may come from the link between the intraventricular injection of leptin and insulin with the enhanced effect of peripherally administered CCK.
- **Ghrelin:** most of the evidence for the mechanisms of the action of ghrelin has been derived from animal experiments. It appears that vagal afferents carry ghrelin signals to inhibit POMC neurons in the nTS. The inhibited nTS neurons then send further signals to the arcuate nucleus to synapse with the NPY neuron. Ghrelin signalling on the brain is thereby mediated by NPY/AgRP in the arcuate nucleus to increase appetite and feeding. There is also evidence indicating that there may be anatomical links between ghrelin and NPY, and that ghrelin may activate NPY directly.

in favour of survival for wild animals, but not necessarily for humans.

Orexins

Orexin neurons (A and B) are found in the lateral hypothalamus. Activation of these neurons in animal experiments increases feeding. Early evidence suggests that low plasma leptin concentrations during fasting have an excitatory effect on orexin neurons, and that the effects of excitatory signals greatly outweigh the effects of inhibitory signals.

Peripheral satiety signals

Identification of POMC expression in the brainstem, close to the nTS, suggests that there is neuroendocrine coordination between the melanocortin system in the hypothalamus and the brainstem, integrating the long-term, adipostatic control of appetite and body weight with the more short-term, acute signals from the gut.

Endocannabinoid system

Cannabis has been known to increase the appetite, and has been used as a medicine for nausea and vomiting for centuries. More recently, a synthetic analogue has been prescribed for nausea, vomiting and weight loss in patients with terminal cancer and acquired immune deficiency syndrome (AIDS). In the 1990s, first the cannabinoid receptors (CB), then the human endogenous ligands for cannabinoid receptors, now known as **endocannabinoids**, were discovered. The endocannabinoid system consists of the endogenous ligand, the receptors and the enzymes that synthesise and degrade them. Animal experiments indicate that the endocannabinoid system is active in central and peripheral sites. The brain endocannabinoid system may have two effects:

- Increases the motivation to eat palatable (high fat) food via cortical reward mechanisms, and thus reinforces eating behaviour
- Regulates short-term levels of orexigenic/anorexigenic mediators in the hypothalamus.

The endocannabinoid system is activated after transient fasting, which increases appetite, reduces satiety and eventually increases body fat accumulation and reduces BMR. Endocannabinoid levels are high in fasting and low during feeding. Changes in endocannabinoid levels appear inversely related to plasma leptin concentration.

Overactivity of the endocannabinoid system

It has been postulated that chronic, sustained overactivity of the central endocannabinoid system may contribute to obesity and metabolic syndromes. The 'hyperactivity' may occur in response to high fat diets, and leptin resistance associated with obesity. Stress may also have a part to play, which may explain the weight gain that sometimes accompanies depression.

DIET AND DISEASE

Diet is strongly implicated in the aetiology of some of the most prevalent diseases: obesity and its complications including coronary heart disease, hypertension and therefore heart failure and stroke, and many cancers. Nonetheless it has proven difficult to demonstrate causality between diet and disease because of the huge size and economic cost of the clinical trials needed to do so.

Much depends on epidemiological association of disease with diet and then animal studies to test hypothetical mechanisms. Other approaches are case–control and cohort studies, which have validity only if they follow a large enough sample of the general population over a sufficiently long period (see Ch. 7). Most studies create a highly artificial situation in which changes are made in the amount of a single nutrient. This is confounded by diet being made up of a large number of foods, each containing many macro- and micronutrients, and that a change in one type of food with the intention of changing one nutrient in the diet will also change other nutrients. Furthermore, the difficulties are compounded by the fact that there is a variable latent effect between (repeated) exposure to nutrient intake and pathological response.

ASSOCIATION BETWEEN DIET AND DISEASE

Given the difficulties involved in research, it is remarkable how much progress has in fact been made in defining the effects of diet and dietary change. Diet is estimated to explain around 30% of cancers in the Western world, rather less, perhaps 20%, in the developing countries. Theories regarding ageing, formation of atheroma and cancer are based on the effects of cellular damage by free radicals.

Reactive oxygen species or free radicals

Oxygen atoms bind together by sharing electrons (paired) in their outer shells to form O_2 molecules (see Ch. 2). When the outer shells are full, the molecule is stable and inert (or unreactive). During chemical reactions, the bond between electrons sometimes splits to give a free, unpaired electron. The molecule is know as a 'free radical'. Reactive oxygen species are oxygen molecules that have gained an extra, unpaired electron, and are known as **superoxide** when a single electron is added.

The molecule containing the oxygen radical becomes highly unstable and reactive, because it tries to 'steal' an electron from another molecule to stabilise itself. Within cells, the free oxygen radical captures an electron from the nearest molecule, which loses an electron and becomes a free radical. This sets off a chain reaction that ends by disrupting the cell. Thus reactive oxygen species are toxic, causing tissue damage. However, they have a positive role in immunological defence systems where they enter cancer or bacterial molecules and disrupt them.

At human body temperatures, O_2 is stable. The vast majority of O_2 in the body is used in producing energy (90%) and in redox reactions (9%). Less than 1% is converted to free radicals (reactive oxygen species). Free radicals are alleged to play a role in more than 60 different health conditions, including ageing, cancer and atherosclerosis.

Formation of reactive oxygen species

Free radicals are highly reactive compounds that are formed in the body during normal metabolic processes or introduced from the environment. Oxygen, although essential to life, is the source of the potentially damaging free radicals. Environmental sources of free radicals include exposure to ionising radiation (from industry, sun exposure, cosmic rays, and medical X-rays), ozone and nitrous oxide (primarily from automobile exhaust), heavy metals (such as mercury, cadmium and lead), cigarette smoke (both active and passive), alcohol, unsaturated fat and other chemicals and compounds from food, water and air.

Metal ions are normally bound to transport or storage proteins (e.g. iron on haemoglobin, myoglobin or methaemoglobin). In cells, metal ions that are not bound to protein donate electrons to O_2 to form reactive oxygen species.

Body defence against cancer or invading bacteria

Phagocytic action of white blood cells involves enzymic action that adds an electron to the O_2 molecules around the bacteria to form **superoxide**, which reacts with itself to give another reactive oxygen species, hydrogen peroxide. Hydrogen peroxide destroys the bacteria by generating free radicals that eventually disrupt the cells.

ⓘ Information box 16.6 **Redox reactions**

- **Oxidation** occurs when a molecule loses an electron – an oxidising agent therefore is a molecule that gains an electron. Oxygen is a common oxidising agent.
- **Reduction** occurs when a molecule gains an electron – a reducing agent is therefore a molecule that loses an electron.

Oxidative stress

Oxidative stress occurs when the production of reactive oxygen species exceeds the body's defences against them.

Defence against reactive oxygen species – antioxidants

The antioxidant defences are both endogenously produced and dietary and can be summarised to be:

- Enzymatic: superoxide to hydrogen peroxide, hydrogen peroxide to water (catalase and glutathione peroxidase)
- Non-enzymatic: glutathione, urate, ubiquinones, albumin, bilirubin, vitamins A, E, C, β-carotene.

There are normal metabolic processes that 'mop up' the tiny amount of free radicals produced:

- Proteins that bind metals such as iron and copper (transport and carrier protein) trap metal ions that activate redox reactions.
- Detoxifying enzymes that mop up metal ions – **superoxide dismutase**, **catalase**, **glutathione peroxidase**.
- Anti-oxidant vitamins A, C and E are reducing agents that donate H atoms to free radicals caused by action of reactive oxygen species in proteins, lipids, and DNA (see later); for example, vitamin A protects against damage by sunlight.

DIET AND CARCINOGENESIS

Diet can influence carcinogenesis through general mechanisms, which apply to most or all cancers, or through specific toxicities which increase the risk of a particular cancer. Epidemiological studies suggest that certain dietary components increase the risk of cancer, whereas others appear to be protective (Table 16.12). The evidence that cancer is preventable by consuming a balanced diet comes from:

- Differences in incidence between communities
- Changes in incidence in migrant people
- Changes in incidence over time
- Identification of causes in animal research
- Intervention trials (randomised controlled trials).

Dietary constituents can be directly mutagenic, usually by forming mutagen-DNA adducts (Table 16.13). Mutagens can be diluted. It may be their dilution effect in the colon that gives dietary non-starch polysaccharides, such as fibre and resistant starch, their protective effect against colon cancer.

Antioxidants

One general protective component that emerges repeatedly in population studies is a generous intake of fruit and vegetables. A possible mechanism is that the presence of antioxidants, such as vitamin C, carotenoids (e.g. lycopene from tomatoes), fat-soluble vitamin E and the trace element selenium, inhibit oxidation and therefore DNA damage and tumour initiation. Lycopene, a carotenoid pigment found in red fruits, which concentrates in prostate tissue, has been particularly implicated as protective in prostate cancer. Evidence from clinical trials, however, has not convincingly demonstrated the effectiveness of supplementation with these substances in prevention of cancer. Folic acid is alleged to be protective through its effect on DNA methyla-

Information box 16.7 Factors associated with oxidative stress

- Cells of the immune system produce excessive amounts of reactive oxygen species in response to overwhelming infections and cancers, and to 'challenges' that may be local, as in arthritis and atherosclerosis, or systemic, as in systemic lupus erythematosus.
- Deficiencies in antioxidant enzymes and/or vitamins.
- Excessive products of certain types of enzyme reactions e.g. fatty acid oxidation (see Ch. 3).
- Metal overload, as the result of repeated blood transfusions in thalassaemia major.
- Drugs, such as antibiotics and cytotoxic agents, and alcohol and nicotine from tobacco smoking.
- Environmental factors (including diet).
- Hyperbaric oxygen.

Table 16.13 Mutagenic dietary constituents

Food	Mutagen	Cancer produced
Red/processed meat, especially char-grilled	Polycyclic hydrocarbons, heterocyclic amines, N-nitroso compounds	Colon
Fatty foods	Saturated fat	Breast, colon,
Salt fish	Salt and nitrosamines	Oral cavity, nasopharynx, oesophagus and stomach
Alcohol	Alcohol + smoking combined especially	Oropharynx and oesophagus; breast
Mouldy/rancid foods	Aflatoxin	Hepatocellular

Table 16.12 Dietary components associated with increased cancer risk

Dietary factor	Proposed reason for increased risk	Type of cancer
Excessive food intake: obesity	A result of its effects on oestrogen production.	Breast; colorectal; endometrial
High intake of meat and meat products	Increased exposure to carcinogens such as heterocyclic amines or N-nitroso compounds	Colorectal; breast; prostatic; pancreatic
Lack of fruit and vegetables	Fruit and vegetables have a protective effect due to a wide range of antioxidants, vitamins and anticarcinogens	Colorectal; lung; prostatic; cervical; breast; pancreatic; gastric; oesophageal
Lack of dietary fibre	Low-fibre diets pass along the gastrointestinal tract slower, thus the mucosa is exposed to potential carcinogens for longer.	Colorectal; pancreatic

Source: COMA 1998 (this report discusses the evidence of associations as being not, moderately, or strongly consistent).

The Committee on Medical Aspects of Food Policy (COMA) working party has produced guidelines on dietary practices intended to reduce the risk of the most common types of cancer:

- Maintain a healthy body weight.
- Consume a variety of fruits and vegetables (at least five portions/day).
- Eat plenty of cereal food – whole wheat or wholemeal.
- Limit consumption of red meat to no more than 90 g/day (or 8–10 portions/week).
- Moderate alcohol consumption (3–4 or 2–3 units per day for men and women, respectively).
- Avoid high dose supplements as a means of cancer protection.

tion. Hypermethylation can lead to the inactivation of genes that suppress tumour formation.

Obesity

Obesity is another main general nutritional risk factor for cancer. This is particularly true for those cancers that may be influenced by hormones (e.g. post-menopausal breast, prostate, endometrium, testis), because excess adipose tissue results in the increased production of oestradiol. Obesity also increases the risk for cancers of the pancreas, oesophagus, kidney and colon. Bile salt excretion and oesophageal reflux are also increased in obese individuals.

NUTRITION AND CANCER TREATMENT

From diagnosis onwards there are many aspects of cancer that can affect nutritional status:

- Reduced appetite (depression and anxiety)
- Physical symptoms such as dysphagia, early satiety and food-induced abdominal pain can impair intake; malabsorption and increased losses can also be caused by cancer
- Abdominal symptoms, taste changes, nausea, vomiting, pain, diarrhoea due to anti-cancer treatment
- Dry mouth (xerostomia), sore mouth or oesophagitis due to mucositis
- Increased metabolic rate (due to tumour load and cytokine production).

Treatment for cancer, whether curative or palliative, can involve surgery, radiotherapy, chemotherapy, or a combination of all three. However, nutrition is also important. The main aims of nutritional therapy are to:

- Restore or maintain good nutritional status, to enable patients to better metabolically handle the stress of treatment(s) and to recover, especially from surgery
- Overcome complications of treatment by providing nutritional support, e.g. advising on a soft diet or enteral nutrition in those who have problems swallowing, and providing artificial nutrition to those who cannot eat enough
- Improve outcome – the prevention of weight loss and protein energy malnutrition can enhance immune responses and improve quality of life. Bone marrow

Hyperlipidaemia and hypercholesterolaemia
Hyperlipidaemia refers to elevated plasma levels of total lipids, whereas cholesterol is a component of plasma lipids. Plasma cholesterol is widely accepted to be correlated with CHD risk. This is challenged by some authorities on the grounds that the correlation is weak, and, within populations, is probably biased by familial hyperlipidaemias. Efforts have been made to influence the incidence of CHD, or to slow its development (secondary prevention after an index clinical presentation such as a heart attack), by changes in plasma cholesterol. Modest reductions can be achieved by reducing saturated fat intake and increasing dietary polyunsaturated fats. However, such interventions have not been as successful in reducing CHD as drug intervention with statins.

Control of cholesterol
Dietary saturated fat is a more important determinant of plasma cholesterol level than dietary cholesterol. This is because cholesterol is synthesised from acetyl CoA by all tissues (see Ch. 3). In contrast, dietary cholesterol is delivered to cells as low-density lipoprotein (LDL), which binds to a membrane receptor and is transported into the cell. This process inhibits endogenous cholesterol production, but in certain severe forms of hypercholesterolaemia the inhibition fails and overproduction ensues; this failure is genetically determined. Some lesser forms of hypercholesterolaemia may be related to less severe genetic polymorphisms, which might mimic this process in a milder form. Such individuals may gain most benefit from a diet low in saturated fat.

Correction of hyperlipidaemia (see also Ch. 3) has a major impact: a 1% reduction in population blood cholesterol is associated with a 3% reduction in the risk of coronary heart disease.

- **If no lipid profile is available**: the dietary approach is to advise low total fat (especially saturated fatty acids), high soluble fibre, and reduced alcohol, with replacement of refined carbohydrates by complex carbohydrates.
- **If a lipid profile is available**: the dietary approach depends on the specific picture of dyslipidaemia, advice being matched to the desired effects (Information box 16.9).

The emphasis of advice differs slightly according to the specific picture of dyslipidaemia.

suppression, for example, is prolonged in the presence of poor nutrition.

At all stages of the disease, the dietitian has an important role. Early referral will result in better nutritional therapy.

DIET AND CARDIOVASCULAR DISEASE

Epidemiological studies have shown an association between diet, coronary heart disease (CHD), peripheral vascular disease (PVD) and stroke. The main disease process underlying cardiovascular disease is atherosclerosis (see Chs 3 and 11). Age, sex and family history are unmodifiable risk factors for cardiovascular disease, but there are many modifiable risk factors that are diet related. A poor diet can indirectly influ-

Lipid profile	Dietary advice
Raised total and LDL cholesterol; normal HDL cholesterol and TAGs	Reduce SFA intake, partially substitute with MUFA Encourage sources of soluble fibre Moderate sources of dietary cholesterol if excessive
Raised TAG; normal total LDL and HDL cholesterol	If obese, encourage weight loss by reduction of SFA Replace high intakes of refined CHO with more complex sources Reduce or avoid alcohol intake
Raised total and LDL cholesterol and TAG	If obese, encourage weight loss by reduction of total and SFA Partial substitution with MUFA Replace high intakes of refined CHO with more complex sources Reduce or avoid alcohol intake Moderate sources of dietary cholesterol if excessive
Low HDL cholesterol	Encourage regular exercise Modest alcohol intake (1–2 units per day) can be encouraged Moderate sources of dietary cholesterol if excessive

CHO, carbohydrates; MUA, monounsaturated fatty acid; SFA, saturated fatty acid; LDL, low-density lipoprotein; HDL, high-density lipoprotein; TAG, triacylglycerol.

ence the development of cardiovascular disease by increasing obesity and associated risk factors such as hypertension, hypertriglyceridaemia and type 2 diabetes.

Dietary prevention of atherosclerosis

Dietary prevention of atherosclerosis focuses on:

- Preventing the accumulation of lipid and its composition
- Changing the composition of circulating and stored lipid
- Reduction of the process of oxidation or glycation
- Prevention of hypertension, which increases the risk of infarction.

Atherogenesis

Excess LDL (due to smoking, hypercholesterolaemia, hypertension or diabetes) leaks from plasma into the extracellular space, where it becomes oxidised. Oxidised LDL is cytotoxic to endothelial cells, promotes inflammation, and is immunogenic. Its products are mitogenic and attract macrophages. The abnormality in the arterial wall that starts as oxidised LDL is taken up there by macrophages. Lesions progress from fatty streaks to atherosclerotic plaques as a result of lipid deposition, connective tissue proliferation and fibrin and thrombus accumulation. Atherogenesis is similar to a process of chronic inflammation within the arteries. The artery becomes narrowed. A tear in the plaque is often the precipitating cause for the formation of a large thrombus, which may occlude the artery and cause infarction, whether myocardial, cerebral or peripheral.

Prevention focuses on the accumulation of the lipid and its composition, on the reduction of the process of oxidation or glycation, and the prevention of hypertension, which increases the risk of infarction. As LDL per se is not toxic, the oxidation process is important in the accumulation of modified lipid in the vessel wall. Oxidised LDL also inhibits the production of nitric oxide (a vasodilator) in the endothelium. Oxidation is inhibited by vitamin E. Oxidation processes *may* be modified by dietary and endogenous antioxidants.

Vitamins C and carotenoids are present in vegetables and fruits, while vitamin E comes especially from seed and vegetable oils. Dietary intake of these nutrients is inversely proportional to the incidence of coronary heart disease.

Homocysteine

Hyperhomocysteinaemia is associated with an increased risk of coronary heart disease. Homocysteine is a sulphur-containing amino acid that is derived from, and can be reconverted to, methionine. Folic acid and vitamin B_{12} are needed for the conversion of homocysteine to methionine. Homocysteine can also be converted to cysteine in a process that requires vitamin B_6. Folic acid and vitamin B_{12} and B_6 supplements, particularly combined, reduce plasma homocysteine, but it is not known whether such supplementation reduces coronary heart disease morbidity and mortality.

Diet and hypertension

In patients with hypertension, diet is an important element in the prevention of cardiovascular disease. This is particularly important for patients with metabolic syndrome (or syndrome X), consisting of:

- Hypertriglyceridaemia with low HDL cholesterol
- Insulin resistance (fasting glucose 6.1 mmol/L or more)
- Central obesity (waist circumference >102 cm men and >88 cm women)
- Hypertension (blood pressure 130/85 mmHg or more).

This syndrome arises from interplay between genetic propensity (e.g. defective insulin receptor genes), sedentary lifestyle and poor diet. Patients are at risk of diabetes, coronary artery disease, left ventricular failure and stroke. Treatment involves preventive diet, weight loss, exercise and medication.

Dietary approach to hypertension

Excessive alcohol is associated with hypertriglyceridaemia, hypertension and stroke. High vegetable intake is preventive.

> **Information box 16.10** **Recommendations for a cardioprotective diet**
>
> - Maintain an ideal weight.
> - Increase consumption of fish – especially oily fish.
> - Increase consumption of fruit and vegetables (at least five servings a day).
> - Replace saturated fats with monounsaturated fats.
> - Divide fat intake between at least three regular meals per day.
> - Reduce total fat intake and replace with foods containing complex starches.
> - Avoid excessive alcohol intake.
> - Limit salt intake.

An appropriate diet includes fruits, vegetables, low-fat dairy foods, grains, poultry, fish and nuts and with a reduction in fats, red meat, sweets and sugar-containing drinks.

Large-scale population studies, such as the Intersalt Study, have established the relationship of sodium intake with raised blood pressure. Sodium restriction is well recognised as being effective in hypertension; the Mediterranean diet (see below) enhances the effect of sodium restriction in reducing blood pressure.

Cardioprotective diets

Epidemiological evidence has highlighted the lower risk of cardiovascular disease in the Mediterranean population. Randomised controlled trials support a Mediterranean diet as cardioprotective in high-risk populations (Information box 16.10). Nevertheless, these guidelines should be viewed in the context of a general healthy diet, and lifestyle factors should also be considered, including smoking cessation, increased physical activity and stress management.

Some therapeutic diets

In some diseases, a specific therapeutic diet is an integral part of treatment, and the importance of adherence to such diets should not be underestimated. The following sections aim to describe briefly the general dietary principles and the significance of dietary therapy in some relatively common disease states.

Dietary treatment of coeliac disease

Coeliac disease is an inflammatory disorder of the gut with a strong genetic susceptibility. It is caused by an immune reaction to gluten, resulting in an inflammatory infiltrate in the lamina propria of the proximal small intestine with flattening of the villi, an increased proportion of intra-epithelial lymphocytes to enterocytes and increased crypt cell proliferation (see Ch. 15). This leads to malabsorption of all macro- and micronutrients, particularly fat-soluble vitamins and calcium. The condition is commonest in Caucasians, with a prevalence of around 1:300 in Europe and North America.

Diet is the single most important factor in the treatment of coeliac disease. Symptoms usually improve within a few weeks of following a gluten-free, well-balanced diet, and the intestinal mucosa recovers within a few months. Gluten-containing foods, however, are a source of other essential nutrients, such as trace minerals and vitamins. A totally gluten-free diet may lead to deficiency states. For this reason, in the UK, in 1996 the British Society of Gastroenterology recommended all treatment and follow-up should be supervised by a dietitian.

Dietary restrictions in renal disease

The main aims of dietary management in renal disease are to limit the consequences of deteriorating renal function by maintaining nutritional status and minimising complications. Diet is modified only in severe or end-stage disease, when appetite is often severely suppressed and weight loss common. Dietary management of the renal patient has to be closely linked to clinical management and renal replacement therapy. Blood biochemistry should be regularly monitored and treatment adjusted accordingly.

Protein

Protein intake has to be adequate to avoid malnutrition. Low-protein diets cause problems with compliance and may negatively impact on nutritional status, putting the patient at a higher risk of morbidity at the onset of haemodialysis. Current daily recommendations suggest a protein intake of 0.8–1.0 g/kg body weight for conservative management of chronic renal failure. This is increased slightly to 1.2 g/kg ideal body weight in haemodialysis and continuous ambulatory peritoneal dialysis (see Ch. 14).

Energy

There must be sufficient energy provided to prevent weight loss. In haemodialysis and continuous ambulatory peritoneal dialysis, energy requirements are often taken to be greater than or equal to 147 kJ/kg of ideal body weight (IBW). Malnutrition, which is linked to a poor outcome, is prevalent in 40–50% of patients on haemodialysis and continuous ambulatory peritoneal dialysis.

Potassium

Potassium restriction is often necessary because the ability to excrete potassium is impaired in chronic renal failure. This can lead to hyperkalaemia, causing cardiac arrhythmias or cardiac arrest. Blood biochemistry monitoring will indicate whether a low potassium diet is required. Potassium is abundant in a normal diet, and rich sources are found in pure fruit juices, bananas and any fruit or vegetable which has not been boiled in water. The intake of these foods should be restricted. The intake of meat, cheese, milk and fish should also be reduced if necessary.

Phosphate

Hyperphosphataemia is common in chronic renal impairment. High-protein foods tend to be high in phosphate, so limiting phosphate without limiting protein can be difficult. Phosphate binders are commonly prescribed, such as calcium carbonate or calcium acetate, which have the added advantage of providing extra calcium.

Sodium and fluid

In renal failure, sodium and fluid retention lead to oedema and hypertension. A no-added salt (<100 mmoL/day) diet is advised if the patient has oedema or hypertension. Fluid restriction is usually required only during end-stage renal failure when urine output has diminished: fluid intake is often restricted to 500 mL plus the previous day's urine output.

Information box 16.11   General dietary advice for people with diabetes

When assessing the diet of an individual with diabetes it is important to ensure:

- Three regular meals per day. Snacks are not essential but may be needed if the patient is treated with insulin to prevent hypoglycaemia or 'hypos' between meals.
- Complex carbohydrate or starchy foods are included at each main meal, e.g. bread, potatoes, rice, pasta or breakfast cereals. Ideally these should be high fibre or wholemeal varieties for general health purposes.
- Avoidance of sugar and sugary foods. Complete exclusion is not necessary but moderate consumption encouraged as far as possible.
- A diet low in fat, especially if the patient is overweight. Saturated fats should make up no more than 10% of energy intake in the light of cardiovascular risk and hyperlipidaemia.
- A high fibre diet rich in fruit and vegetables.

Dietary control in diabetes mellitus

Dietary principles for type 1 and type 2 diabetes are very similar, the main emphasis being on improving glycaemic control, thus:

- Alleviating acute and chronic symptoms of hyperglycaemia
- Reducing the risk of cardiovascular disease and other diabetic complications
- Achieving, or maintaining ideal body weight.

Many patients presenting with type 2 diabetes are initially treated with diet alone. The doctor, dietitian and diabetes nurse specialist should work closely to ensure the delivery of nutritional advice tailored to the patient's needs and medication, with monitoring and evaluation of progress.

Exercise in diabetes

Being overweight is a risk factor for type 2 diabetes, and weight reduction to a desirable range improves glucose tolerance. Daily exercise benefits the diabetic patient by lowering blood glucose and free fatty acids and reducing insulin resistance. Exercise also helps weight control, and reduces the risks of cardiovascular disease.

Lipid lowering

A lipid-lowering diet is incorporated into the diabetic diet because most people with diabetes have hyperlipidaemia. Disturbance of lipid metabolism in relation to poor glycaemic control means that those with diabetes have a greater risk of cardiovascular disease. Cigarette smoking must be discouraged. Lipid-lowering drugs are also highly effective.

Artificial nutrition

The term nutritional support is used to describe the provision of artificial feeds to maintain or improve nutritional status during illness. Nutrition should be supplied by the simplest, safest, most cost-effective approach. Supplementation of the patient's diet using ordinary nutrient-dense foods is the first step. If this is unsuccessful, liquid sip feeds may be introduced to provide some or all of the food needed. If this line of approach fails then artificial nutrition may be required:

Clinical box 16.18   Indications and methods for enteral feeding

Enteral feeding is used if the patient is unable to:

- Eat or drink (unconscious, etc.)
- Eat *enough* (poor appetite, abdominal pain, etc.)
- Swallow (oropharyngeal dysfunction after a cerebrovascular accident, oesophageal benign or malignant stricture, etc.)
- Empty their stomach normally (trauma – especially to head or abdomen, postoperative ileus, cerebral palsy, gastric outflow obstruction, diabetic autonomic neuropathy, etc.)
- In addition, it is sometimes used as primary treatment of inflammatory bowel disease or intestinal fistula.

Nasogastric tubes can be placed through oesophageal strictures, and nasoduodenal or nasojejunal tubes can be placed endoscopically, radiologically or surgically if the patient is vomiting due to poor gastric emptying (e.g. paralytic ileus, diabetes or head injury) or has partial gastric outflow obstruction (e.g. peptic ulcer or gastric or pancreatic neoplasm). A clear feeding regimen should be planned to encompass breaks. A rest period of 4 hours is usually advised to allow gastric pH levels to normalise, reducing infection. Three methods of infusion are used:

- Bolus feeding – the delivery of 100–300 mL of feed over a 10–30-minute period.
- Gravity feeding – continuous drip feeding by adjusting the roller clamp on a giving set.
- Continuous feeding – which requires a pump. Feed is infused at a specified rate. Some patients encounter abdominal discomfort, bloating or diarrhoea at higher rates.

Enteral feeds may be used in the hospital, usually in the short- to medium-term where per nasal tubes are the norm, or long term in the community when feeds are usually infused through a gastrostomy or, in the context of delayed gastric emptying, a jejunostomy placed endoscopically, radiologically or surgically.

- **Enteral nutrition** – consists of feeding liquid, artificial food via a nasogastric or nasojejunal tube directly into the stomach or small intestine, respectively.
- **Parenteral nutrition** – this is intravenous feeding.

Nutritional assessment, discussed earlier in this chapter should be performed to estimate nutritional needs before starting artificial feeding, whether or not standard 'off the shelf' feeds are to be used. Calculation of fluid and electrolyte needs is part of this process. For enteral feeding, standard proprietary 'polymeric' adult and paediatric formulae are available. 'Predigested' (elemental or peptide-containing 'oligomeric') feeds are also used in severe maldigestion, for example in chronic pancreatitis.

Enteral nutrition

Enteral feeding is preferred to parenteral nutrition because it helps maintains gut mucosal integrity, and is physiologically more normal. It also costs less. The route of delivery will depend on the patient's condition.

Complications of enteral feeding

The most common complications of enteral feeding are:

- Tube blockage
- Oesophageal reflux or aspiration into the lungs
- Refeeding syndrome is a risk in malnourished and fasted patients (see below).

The risks of these are increased if the tube becomes displaced. Gut infections, constipation, nausea, distension,

Clinical box 16.19   Complications of parenteral nutrition

The disadvantages of parenteral feeding are the complications it can cause. These can be divided into:

- **Metabolic** – fluid overload, hyper- or hypoglycaemia, electrolyte imbalance.
- **Refeeding syndrome** – this can occur with oral, enteral and parenteral feeding. Glucose load in an undernourished patient can produce salt and water retention and heart failure, hypokalaemia, hypophosphataemia, hypomagnesaemia and acidosis.
- **Physiological** – disturbed liver function (fatty liver, cholestasis, biliary sludge and stasis).
- **Catheter related** – infection, thrombosis, peripheral thrombophlebitis, catheter blockage/splitting, extravasation.
- **Technical** – pump malfunction.

Complications related to central venous catheter insertion include air embolism, pneumothorax, chylothorax, cardiac arrhythmias and brachial plexus injury. Patients are monitored to detect catheter related complications, especially early sepsis and electrolyte imbalance.

When parenteral feeding is discontinued, oral or enteral feeding should be slowly introduced with reduction in parenteral nutrition. The speed at which this occurs will depend on the speed of returning intestinal function and the duration of parenteral feeding.

dumping syndrome and diarrhoea may also occur. Gastrostomies and jejunostomies may be complicated by peritonitis or abdominal wall sepsis.

Parenteral nutrition

Parenteral feeding is a method of delivering nutrition intravenously when the gastrointestinal tract is not functioning or is inaccessible. The term **total parenteral nutrition** implies that no other food is being taken intestinally, although it is often loosely used as a synonym for parenteral nutrition. Based on the patient's calculated requirements, parenteral feeds have to be nutritionally complete and contain a full complement of vitamins, trace elements and minerals, and prepared under sterile conditions. Excess feeding could be lethal.

Parenteral feeding is indicated only when enteral intake is impossible, insufficient or undesirable. It is most often used during ileus in the context of critical illness. It can be used in the long term at home for patients with chronic intestinal failure due to short bowel or to intestinal pseudo-obstruction. Parenteral nutrition is delivered through peripheral or central veins. The choice is dictated by the state of the arm veins, the osmolarity of the feed, and the proposed duration.

MALNUTRITION

Here, malnutrition is taken to mean undernutrition, as in common usage. This could be from insufficient daily intake of protein and energy, inadequate micronutrient intake or an unbalanced intake of macronutrients (see later).

- Macronutrient malnutrition: related to severe, prolonged deficiency in protein and energy intake, known as **protein–energy malnutrition (PEM)**. This will usually also be associated with deficiencies in micronutrient intake. Sustained PEM leads to loss of muscle mass and fat. Starvation, an extreme form of PEM could be

Clinical box 16.20   Consequences of malnutrition

PEM causes numerous conditions that may lead to further disease:

- Reduction in BMR
- Potassium loss and relative sodium retention
- Increased intracellular sodium
- Lean body mass reduction (reduction in total body and intracellular potassium)
- Decreased plasma volume
- Muscle wasting, especially of type 2 fibres
- Loss of adipose tissue
- Increased muscle fatigue, reduced ability to do physical work
- Reduced cardiac output
- Reduced diaphragmatic function
- Decreased delayed hypersensitivity
- Susceptibility to infection
- Decreased cold-induced thermogenesis
- Mental apathy.

fatal if continuous for 2–3 months, depending upon initial body stores of fat and protein, and micronutrient status.
- Micronutrient deficiency: inadequate intake of vitamins and trace minerals in the diet (see later).
- Unbalanced macronutrient intake: 'over'-nutrition leads to obesity (see later). Unbalanced diets may be deficient in micronutrients.

In developing nations, whole populations may suffer from sustained, long-term malnutrition due to:

- Failure of crops, famine
- Failure of agricultural, economic and transport policies
- Conflict (war)
- Poverty
- Natural disasters such as earthquakes, tsunamis.

Although malnutrition in developed nations could also arise from poverty, the pattern is more of an unbalanced intake of macronutrients, which can lead to undernourishment, or 'overnourishment' (obesity).

Malnutrition and disease states

Malnutrition is commonly caused by or associated with disease:

- Anorexia: psychological – depression, eating disorder, e.g. anorexia nervosa, reduced central control of appetite in cancer
- Inability to eat or swallow, persistent vomiting
- Increased energy expenditure and net protein breakdown (catabolic state): cancer, burns, wounds, sepsis, postoperative state (see below).
- Side effect of drugs
- Immobility, e.g. old age.

Diagnosis of malnutrition

Malnutrition may not be easily recognised, particularly in hospital, and is associated with many medical conditions. Formal screening or assessment processes should be followed to document weight loss and weight for height quantitatively (see above).

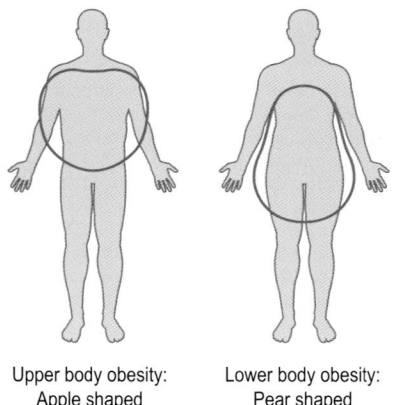

Upper body obesity:
Apple shaped

Lower body obesity:
Pear shaped

***Fig. 16.12* Obesity classified according to body fat distribution**: health risks are higher with upper body obesity.

<table>
<tr><td>Clinical box 16.21</td><td>Increased risk of disease associated with obesity</td></tr>
</table>

Obesity, defined as BMI >30, carries an increased risk for:

- Diabetes (especially type 2)
- Coronary heart disease
- Hyperlipidaemia
- Hypertension
- Stroke
- Gall stones
- Some cancers (breast and colon for example)
- Infertility
- Sleep apnoea/respiratory problems
- Arthritis
- Joint and back pain
- Poor self-esteem.

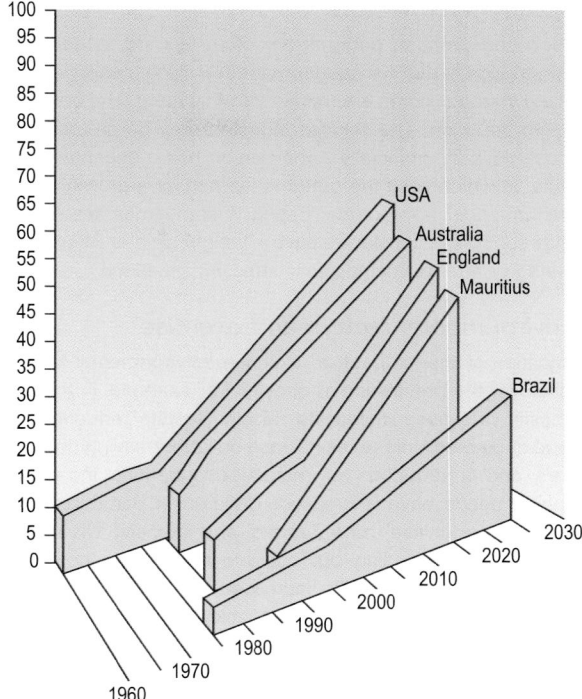

***Fig. 16.13* Worldwide prevalence of obesity.** Redrawn with permission from The Global Challenge of Obesity and the International Obesity Task Force. IOTF 2002. Figure 3. www.iuns.org/features/obesity/obesity.htm (The International Association for the Study of Obesity (IASO) is an umbrella organisation for national obesity associations which comprises 52 member associations, representing 56 countries. IOTF is the policy arm of IASO.)

OBESITY

Obesity is the result of excess fat deposition in adipose tissue. In clinical practice, obesity is defined as Quetelet Index or BMI of 30+ (see above). It is only in relatively recent times that the impact of obesity on general health has been recognised (Clinical box 16.21). Risks to health rise with increasing BMI, especially as it increases above 30, and also depends on body fat distribution (Fig 16.12).

Obesity can be seen as a condition of affluence; its prevalence is increasing in developed countries, but it is also becoming common in the developing world. Over two-thirds of adults in the developed world have a BMI over 30 (Fig. 16.13). Of even more concern is the rise in childhood obesity, predisposing the next generation to the associated health risks. Obesity is now considered as one of the most important public health concerns of our time.

Aetiology of obesity

The cause of obesity is the prolonged excess of energy input over output (energy imbalance), causing the body to store the unused energy as fat deposits in adipose tissue. Each kilogram of adipose tissue represents the storage of about 29 330 kJ (7000 kcal). Just 838 kJ (200 kcal) per day excess might therefore be expected to result in an increase in weight of about 11 kg in a year if there was no compensatory increase in energy expenditure. Basal metabolic rate is closely related to lean body mass, which rises only a little as people become obese (adipose tissue is about 75% fat, 25% lean). It is thus remarkable how well the body balances energy intake to expenditure day by day.

It might be imagined that there would be teleological advantage in storing some energy at least in times of plenty, to guard against times of food shortage; it is precisely this safety mechanism which promotes obesity during prolonged periods in which shortage is never experienced. Once a person has become obese and the fat stores have been established, s/he will remain obese if energy input and output remain equal. An increase in energy intake above expenditure depends on the following:

- Appetite and the mechanisms involved in control (see above)
- Psychogenic and social aspects of eating (see later and Ch. 8)
- Exercise and environmental factors
- Genetic factors.

Obesity tends to run in families but this is not necessarily entirely genetic; nonetheless genetic factors may play a part through appetite regulation. BMR correlates with lean body mass, and obese people do not have a lower BMR than non-obese people, because their lean body mass is modestly elevated compared with non-obese people.

Psychogenic factors

Food consumption patterns are often learned. A common assumption is that we need to eat three filling meals per day. Many young children are trained into this habit, and continue it into adult life. The calories ingested may be greater than those utilised, especially if the person has a sedentary lifestyle, in which case the patterns learned as a growing child are no longer appropriate. Eating is sometimes associated with comfort or tension release – weight gain is often seen during or after psychologically stressful situations.

Environmental factors and exercise

Because of their impact on exercise, environmental factors influence the prevalence of obesity. For example, in the UK, obesity has been increasing rapidly despite reductions in food and energy intake. As reliance on labour-saving devices, cars and a reduction of manual occupations increases, energy needs have decreased. Children in particular have fewer opportunities to run around, and intensive UK school curricula are crowding out sporting and leisure activities. Coinciding with this is the increased consumption of high-energy convenience meals and snacks.

As a race, humans have evolved to guard against energy deficit more efficiently than energy excess (see above), hence the resulting prevalence of obesity in times of plenty. This becomes particularly important when previously rural/agrarian populations change to a more Westernised and urban mode of living; a classic example of this is the Pima Indians in southern USA. The traditional diet of the Sierra Madre (Mexico) Pima Indians is a low-fat diet (15% of energy as fat). They are physically active as farmers and sawmill workers. But in the past 50 years lifestyle changes in the Pimas of Arizona, who now consume a high-fat diet (50% of energy as fat) and lead a more sedentary lifestyle, have resulted in an epidemic of obesity and diabetes. The Pimas of Mexico have a much lower incidence of obesity and diabetes than their genetic kindred in Arizona.

Treatment of obesity

There are three categories of treatment for obesity:

- Dietary
- Pharmacological
- Surgical.

The latter two categories should not be viewed as an alternative to diet, but complementary.

Dietary management

The long-term goal of any dietary management programme is to change eating habits, behaviours and attitudes for life. Ideally, a multidisciplinary team approach is taken with attention given to any psychological factors influencing behavioural patterns. Weight-reducing diets should be attainable and flexible. It is important that they encourage a general healthy eating pattern that can be continued after the desirable amount of weight has been lost (see Information box 16.12 for example).

A slow but steady rate of weight loss is likely to be more effective than extremely restrictive diets that not only can reduce metabolic rate, but also are impractical and can result in difficulties with compliance. Diets that reduce overall intake will inevitably mean a reduction not only of energy but

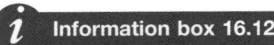

Information box 16.12 | **Example of a weight-reducing diet**

The diet must provide a deficit in energy balance, reducing intake to below energy requirements. The easiest way of doing this is to reduce total fat intake because fat is the highest energy-containing food (38 kJ/g). For example, a reduction of 2100–4200 kJ per day should result in a weight loss of 0.5–1 kg per week, allowing for an energy value of about 29 330 kJ per kg adipose tissue which is made up of about 75% fat and 25% lean tissue. This is considered a healthy rate of weight loss that minimises loss of lean body mass, and maximises energy liberated from adipose stores.

also of other nutrients; thus some patients may benefit from vitamin or mineral supplements.

A psychological model for dietary modification

Advice for weight reduction from changing eating behaviour may be complied with better if it fits in with the psychological model for dietary modification. When dietary modification is needed to achieve a healthier state, the objective is to modify aberrant eating behaviour to achieve appropriate change. This is, however, a one-dimensional view of the patient–practitioner relationship. It is necessary to consider how the patient feels about changing habits – they may not want, or feel they need, to make any changes.

Since it was first developed in the early 1980s, the cycle of change model (Fig. 16.14) has been influential in our understanding of behaviour, especially of addictive behaviours (see also Ch. 8 for details of addiction). Change can be understood as a six-step repeating process with central features of resistance and resilience. Knowledge of where a patient is in the cycle of change makes it easier to begin the process of achieving change. A person can enter or leave the cycle at any point. It is usual for people to travel through the cycle a few times before reaching a stable change. For example, if an obese patient is in the pre-contemplative stage; that is, they are unaware, unwilling or too discouraged to change, then giving weight-reducing advice at this time will be a waste of time. In this situation, discussion of the risks associated with obesity and the advantages of losing weight will be of greater benefit, with the idea of moving the patient into the contemplative or decision stage.

Pharmacological management

Various drugs for decreasing the degree of hunger or the absorption of fats are now being clinically prescribed to help combat obesity.

Appetite suppression

Sibutramine is a centrally acting appetite suppressant which blocks the re-uptake of serotonin (known to suppress appetite) and noradrenaline (which can effect metabolic rate). The increase in serotonin concentration in the synaptic cleft thus decreases food intake. Adverse reactions include an increase in heart rate and a smaller reduction in blood pressure. The effectiveness of appetite suppressants is limited because people do not eat purely in response to hunger.

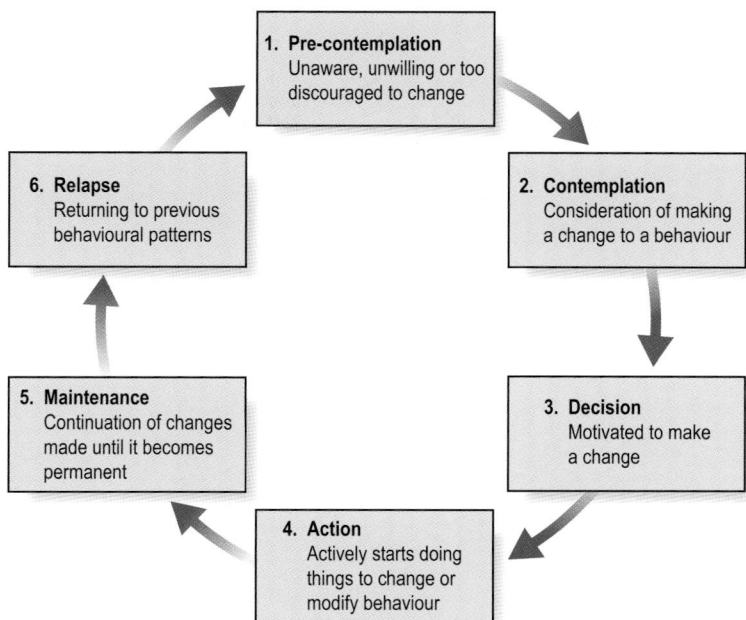

Fig. 16.14 **Six stages in the cycle of change.**

The figure shows a circular diagram with six boxes connected by arrows:

1. **Pre-contemplation** Unaware, unwilling or too discouraged to change

2. **Contemplation** Consideration of making a change to a behaviour

3. **Decision** Motivated to make a change

4. **Action** Actively starts doing things to change or modify behaviour

5. **Maintenance** Continuation of changes made until it becomes permanent

6. **Relapse** Returning to previous behavioural patterns

Inhibition of fat absorption

Orlistat is a pancreatic lipase inhibitor, which binds to dietary fat and so blocks its digestion and absorption. To minimise the risk of adverse gastrointestinal effects caused by the unabsorbed fat in the bowel, patients have to reduce their habitual fat intake to less than 30% of total energy. Consequences of failure to comply with fat restriction include fatty loose stools and faecal incontinence. Trials of orlistat suggest increased weight loss and prolonged maintenance of weight reduction. However, this may be due to reduced intake rather than decreased absorption.

Surgical management

Surgical procedures are an effective but last resort for treatment, performed only in individuals classified as morbidly obese or severely obese with significant disease (e.g. high blood pressure or diabetes). Long-term complications include nausea, vomiting, diarrhoea, heartburn, malabsorption and vitamin deficiency. There are two main types of bariatric surgery:

■ Malabsorptive surgery: the length of the digestive tract (gut) is shortened, thus reducing the amount of food absorbed by the body. This type of surgery involves creating a bypass by joining one part of the intestine to another.
■ Restrictive surgery: consists of sewing parts of the stomach together or fitting a tight band around the body of the stomach to make a small pouch for food to enter, thus restricting the capacity of the stomach. This restriction of the size of the stomach makes the patient feel full after eating a small amount of food.

Increasing physical activity

Unfortunately, as obesity develops, there is a tendency for physical activity to decline. Physical exercise improves glucose tolerance and diminishes insulin resistance. Regular exercise can increase energy expenditure and metabolic rate – its most important role in maintenance of weight loss. Any increase in physical activity will be of some benefit, including walking up stairs instead of taking the lift, or walking instead of using a car. This is important for severely obese people who are limited in the kind of activity they can undertake.

Prevention of obesity

The best treatment for obesity is prevention:

■ Prevention of weight gain in lean subjects
■ Prevention of any further weight gain in already obese adults
■ Adequate nutritional education about a balanced diet for school children. Fatness at the age of 13 is a strong predictor of adult obesity, and the earlier in life obesity develops the greater the risk of mortality.

Index

Note: Page numbers in *italics* refer to figures and page numbers in **bold** refer to tables.

Thiamine see Vitamin B₁